All Life is Yoga

Sri Aurobindo

Textbook of Medical Physiology

Fourth Edition

All Life is Yoga

Sri Aurobindo

Textbook of Medical Physiology

Fourth Edition

Gopal Krushna Pal

MBBS, MD (Physiology), **PhD, DSc, BNYT, MD** (AM), **MD** (Yoga), **MABMS, FABMS, FABAP, FSAB, FRSB** (UK)

Professor (Senior Scale), Department of Physiology,
Program Director and Faculty In-Charge, Advance Center for Yoga,
Jawaharlal Institute of Postgraduate Medical Education and Research (JIPMER)
Dean (Faculty of Medicine), Pondicherry University,
Honorary Professor, Sri Aurobindo International Center of Education, Puducherry.
Former Dean, JIPMER, Karaikal, Puducherry, India.

Co-Authors:

Pravati Pal

MBBS, MD, MABMS, BNYT, MD (AM)

Professor, Department of Physiology, JIPMER, Puducherry, India

Nivedita Nanda

MSc, PhD (Medical Biochemistry), **BNYT**

Additional Professor, Department of Biochemistry, JIPMER, Puducherry, India.

AHUJA'S
AHUJA PUBLISHING HOUSE
KNOWLEDGE YOU NEED. CAUSE YOU DESERVE

AHUJA PUBLISHING HOUSE

ELSEVIER

RELX India Pvt. Ltd.
Registered Office: 818, Indraprakash Building,
8th Floor, 21, Barakhamba Road, New Delhi-110001
Corporate Office: 14th Floor, Building No. 10B, DLF Cyber City,
Phase II, Gurgaon-122002, Haryana, India

AHUJA'S
Ahuja Publishing House.
Knowledge You Need. Calibre You Deserve

Ahuja Publishing House
Registered Office: C-8/124 B
Lawrence road, Delhi-110035, India

Textbook of Medical Physiology, 4th edition, GK Pal

First Edition, 2007; Second Edition, 2011; Third Edition, 2019; Third Updated Edition, 2020

ISBN: 978-81-312-6599-4
e-Book ISBN: 978-81-312-6600-7

This 4th edition of Textbook of Medical Physiology, by GK Pal is co-published by arrangement with RELX India Pvt. Ltd. and Ahuja Publishing House.

Notice

This co-pub edition has been undertaken by Ahuja Publishing House having address at C-8/124 B Lawrence road, Delhi-110035, India, at its sole responsibility. Practitioners and researchers must always rely on their own experience and knowledge in evaluating and using any information, methods, compounds or experiments described herein. Because of rapid advances in the medical sciences, in particular, independent verification of diagnoses and drug dosages should be made. To the fullest extent of the law, no responsibility is assumed by Elsevier, Ahuja Publishing House, authors, editors or contributors in relation to this co-pub edition or for any injury and/or damage to persons or property as a matter of products liability, negligence or otherwise, or from any use or operation of any methods, products, instructions, or ideas contained in the material herein.

Printed in India by S. K. Printer's

Dedicated at the lotus feet of

Srima, the Divine Mother

and

Sri Aurobindo, the Divine Master

All can be done if God-touch is there.

Sri Aurobindo

The Authors

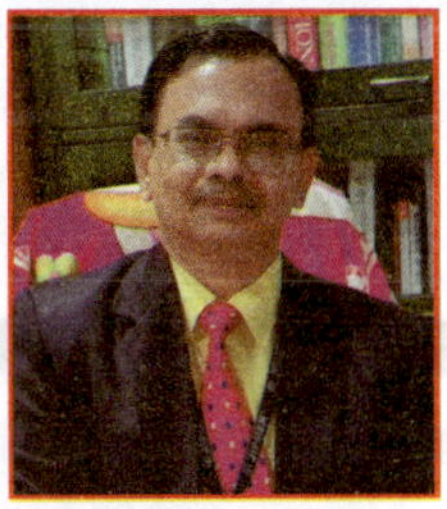

Dr. Gopal Krushna Pal, MD, PhD, DSc, is Professor (Senior Scale) of Physiology, at Jawaharlal Institute of Postgraduate Medical Education and Research (JIPMER), Pondicherry. He completed his medical graduation at V. S. S. Medical College, Burla, (Sambalpur University), Odisha, in 1986. Then he practiced medicine under residency scheme for a brief tenure at Ram Monohar Lohia Hospital, New Delhi, and All India Institute of Medical Sciences, New Delhi. He did his MD and PhD in Physiology from JIPMER, Pondicherry. Dr. Pal has been teaching physiology for more than three decades. Dr. Pal, an internationally acclaimed physiologist joined Physiology by choice and predilection and for his deep devotion for the subject.

Dr. Pal joined as a permanent faculty member at JIPMER, Pondicherry, following his selection through UPSC in 1996. His performance at the UPSC interview for the post of Assistant Professor was outstanding for which Dr. Pal was awarded **Five Advance Increments in Salary by UPSC** at the time of joining the post at JIPMER, which is an exceptional achievement, rarely awarded by UPSC for such recognition of merit. G. K. Pal was awarded **University Gold Medal** for securing the highest mark in the subject Medicine in final MBBS examination, and the **Shyamabati Dubey Award** for his outstanding performance in the same. He has received many awards and medals for securing highest positions in various debate and essay-writing competitions during his premedical and medical studies.

Dr. Pal is a medical researcher par excellence. His special research experience is in neurophysiology of food and water intake, regulation of body weight, obesity, diabetes, gestational diabetes, hypertension, gestational hypertension, HRV, BRS, experimental physiology and Yoga. He has published more than **220 research papers** in reputed national and international journals. He has **5480 research citations** in Google Scholar and **2560 citations** in Research Gate (RG) , a remarkable and unique research achievement by an academician in Physiology. He has **RG Score of 38.90**.

Dr. Pal is the recipient of **Dr. N Padmanabhan Memorial Award** of the Indian Association of Biomedical Scientists (IABMS) for *best research work in physiology*, for the year 1991. He was awarded **A V Tilak Parvathy Devi Prize** by the Indian Association of Physiologists and Pharmacologists (APPI), for *best research work in Neuroendocrinology*, twice, first-time for the year 1998, and second-time for the year 2007. Dr. Pal is the recipient of coveted **ICMR Scientist Award for Biomedical Research** from Indian Council of Medical Research for his *outstanding contribution in the field of Neurophysiology of Ingestive Behaviours* for the year 1998. He has received **Dr. D. S. Munagekar Award** from Indian Medical Association for the *best research publication by a medical scientist* for the year 2002. Dr. Pal was awarded **SIRI Research Award** by IABMS for *best research work in Neurophysiology of Stress* for the year 2003. He is also the recipient of **Dr. Sushila Thakur Prakriti Mandir Prize** for the year 2004 from APPI for the *best research publication in the field of Yoga, Natural Health and Naturopathy*. Association of Physiologists of Odisha bestowed **Dr. R. N. Sen Memorial Oration Award** on Dr. Pal in the year 2005, in recognition of his *outstanding contribution in the field of Neurophysiology*. Dr. Pal has received **Prof. R. C. Shukla Oration Award** from APPI for best research publication in cardiovascular physiology for the year 2008. Dr. Pal has received **Professor J. N. Maitra Memorial Oration Award** from Physiological Society of India (PSI) for his outstanding contribution in the field of academics and research in Physiology for the year 2009. He also received **Dr. M. L. Gupta Prize** from APPI for the year 2010 for best contribution in medical education in Physiology. Dr. Pal is the recipient of **Dr. B. K. Anand Research Prize** of APPI for the year 2011 for best research publication in Physiology. He has received **Bharat Jyothi Award** from India International Friendship Society for the year 2015 for his best contribution in Medical Education and Research. Dr. Pal is the recipient of Professor **K. P. Puthuraya Best Teacher Award** from APPI for the year 2017. He has received **Professor S. Subramaniam Memorial Oration Award** of IABMS for the year 2018 for his best research contribution in the field of Biomedicine. Recently, Dr. Pal has been awarded the most prestigious **JIPMER Scientific Society Faculty Oration Award** for the year 2020 and **M.K.Nambiar Memorial Oration Award** of IABMS for the yerar 2021 for his notable contributions in clinical research and biomedical research, respectively.

Many postgraduate and undergraduate medical students who have performed research projects of ICMR, KVPY and DST under the guidance of Dr. Pal have received various awards like Dr. Leela Krishnamurthy Award, Dr. N. Padmanabhan Memorial Award, ICMR Studentship Award, and so on. Under the guidance of Dr. Pal, four MBBS students of JIPMER have received Kishore Vaigyanik Protshahan Yojna Award (**KVPY Award**) in medicine stream from DST, New Delhi.

In recognition of his immense contribution in biomedical research, Dr. Pal was conferred with the **Fellowship Title (FRSB)** of Royal Society of Biology, UK (London) in the year 2020. He is also the recipient of **Fellowship Title** of IABMS, Society of Applied Biotechnology, and Federation of Biotechnology. For his contribution in the field of biomedical research, the **New York Academy of Sciences** has nominated him as an honorary member of the academy.

Dr. Pal is an astute organizer. As convener and organizing secretary, he had organized Golden Jubilee Celebration of Utkal Divas at VSS Medical College, Burla, in the year 1985. He was the General Secretary of Sri Aurobindo Youth Organization of Odisha from 1983 to 1987. He has organized many annual conferences, and various symposia and seminars, CME and workshops of IABMS, APPI, ASSOPI and of the institute and ACYTER, JIPMER. Currently, Dr. Pal is the **President of IABMS, Vice-President of FIPS and General Secretary of ASSOPI**.

Dr. Pal has been appointed as examiner for medical universities in Tamil Nadu, Kerala, Karnataka, Andhra Pradesh, Odisha, Maharastra, Gujarat, Rajasthan, Jammu and Kashmir, Delhi and Pondicherry. He is a subject expert for National Board of Examinations (DNB), UPSC, INIs and other apex selecting bodies of the nation. He is also a member of board of studies of many medical universities. Dr. Pal has been nominated as member of Governing Body of ICMR for three years (2021-2024).

Dr. Pal is an expert reviewer and editor for many national and international journals. He was Editor-in-Chief (2006– 2009) of the journal 'Biomedicine', the official publication of IABMS, and Editor (Physiology) of IJPP (2009-2012), the official publication of APPI. Currently, Dr. Pal is **Editor-in-Chief** of International Journal of Clinical and Experimental Physiology (IJCEP).

Dr. Pal has already **authored four other medical textbooks** such as Comprehensive Textbook of Medical Physiology, Textbook of Practical Physiology, Textbook of Practical Physiology for Dental Students and Textbook Medical Physiology for Dental Students. For his keen interest in practice of yoga and as an ardent follower of The Mother and Sri Aurobindo, Dr. Pal with his family has settled in the divine land of Pondicherry for the spiritual progress and fulfilment through practice of integral yoga. He is closely associated with Sri Aurobindo Ashram at Pondicherry. Dr. Pal is an Honorary Professor at Sri Aurobindo International Center of Education (SAICE), Puducherry.

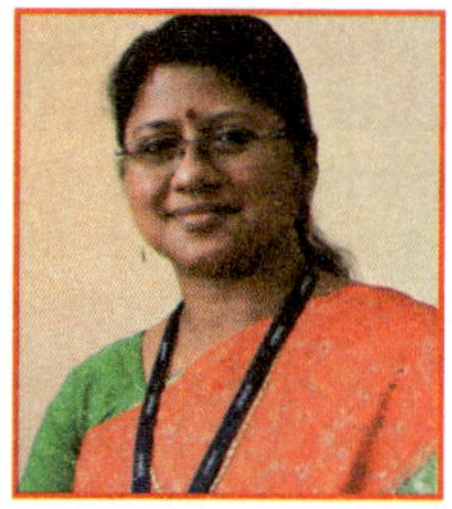

Dr. Pravati Pal, MBBS, MD, MABMS, is Professor of Physiology, in JIPMER, Pondicherry. She obtained her MBBS degree from VSS Medical College, Sambalpur University, Odisha, in 1993 and MD in physiology from JIPMER, Pondicherry in 1998. She has been actively involved in teaching and research in physiology. Her fields of interest are electrophysiology, physiology of nerve and muscle, endocrinology and neurophysiology.

Dr. Pal has had an outstanding academic and research career. She was the **third rank holder** in Odisha in HSC Examination and ***topper among the girls*** in the state of Odisha, for which she was awarded the most coveted **Gauri Shankar Memorial Award**. For her exceptional performance at the MD examination, she was awarded **Distinction and Gold Medal in the subject**. She was also awarded the **Vaithilingam Venkatasubba Reddiar Medal** by Pondicherry University for her best performance in the PG examination. For best research work in physiology, she received the **Dr. N Padmanabhan Memorial Award** from the IABMS, for the year 1998. She has received **Niranjan Bishnupriya Award** for the best research paper presented at Annul Conference of Association of Physiologists of Orissa in the year 2005. She has published many research papers in national and international journals. Dr. Pal has received **Sikshsa Ratan Puraskar** from India International Friendship Society (IIFS), New Delhi for the year 2010, for her outstanding contribution in the field of medical education and research. She is the recipient of the coveted **Prof. K. P. Puthraya Award** for best teacher in Physiology for the year 2013, and **A. V. Tilak Parvathy Devi Prize** of APPI for best research publication in Endocrinology, for the year 2016. She has 125 research publication and **1673 citations** in Google Scholar. Her **h index is 24** and i-10 index is 46.

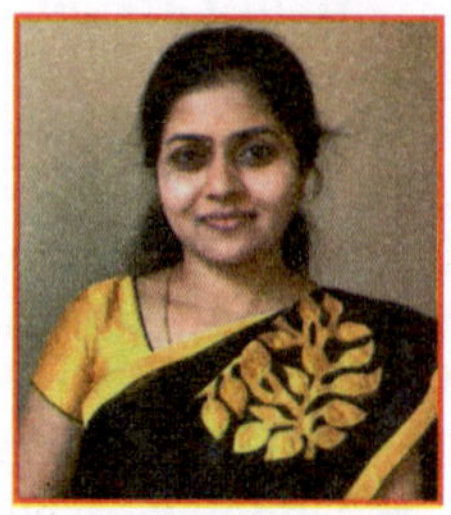

Dr. Nivedita Nanda is presently working as an Additional Professor in the Department of Biochemistry, JIPMER, Puducherry. She has obtained her postgraduation in M. Sc. (Medical Biochemistry) and PhD from JIPMER. Her fields of research interest are oxidative stress, thyroid dysfunctions, neurochemistry of immunity and ingestive behaviours, and metabolomics and proteomics of cardiovascular risks. Dr. Nivedita has an excellent academic and research career. She was **among the best-tenth rank holder** in HSC Examination in the state of Odisha. For the research work during her post-graduation, she was awarded **Dr. N Padmanabhan Memorial Award** from the Indian association of biomedical scientists, for the year 2002. She has received **ABAP Young Scientist Award 2011** of Association of Biotechnology and Pharmacy, for the year 2011, **Prof. G. K. Pal Award** of APPI for best research publication in IJPP for the year 2012, and **Sri BM Patil Memorial Award** of ASSOPI for the best research work by a scientist below the age of 45 years, for the year 2018. She is the recipient of most coveted the **Thangam Vasudevan Award** of IABMS for the best research work in the Field of Biomedicine for the year 2021. She has published 86 research papers in national and international journals. Dr. Nanda has **1088 citations** in Google Scholar. Her h index is 19 and i-10 index is 26.

You must do the work as an offering to the Divine and take it as part of your sadhana.

The Mother (of Sri Aurobindo Ashram)

Acknowledgements

At the outset, we would like to acknowledge the contribution of two medical institutes that have given us the base and the pillars for acquiring medical knowledge; first, the VSS Medical College, Burla, Sambalpur, Odisha, and the second, Jawaharlal Institute of Postgraduate Medical Education and Research (JIPMER), Puducherry, the premier and apex institute in medical education in India. Also, we would like to acknowledge the contribution of great medical teachers who have guided us to reach this level in our life.

For preparing the manuscript of the present edition of the book we are especially thankful to Ahuja Publishing House, New Delhi and Elsevier Publications, New Delhi, for providing us all the resources required for updating the recent advancement in medicine and constantly encouraging us to complete the task of writing. In this regard, we rightly acknowledge the timely help extended to us by Mr. Umesh Ahuja and Mr. Tarun Ahuja, Directors, Ahuja Book Company Pvt Ltd., New Delhi, and Ms. Nimisha Goswami, Director Content Strategy, Elsevier India. We sincerely acknowledge the contribution of Mr. S. Janarthanan, Graphic-designer, Auroville, for preparing the manuscript of the entire book in a short time including the preparation of pictures of many complex drawings, flowcharts and graphs. Authors are sincerely thankful to M. Renugasundari, PhD Scholar, Physiology Department, JIPMER, for her technical support in preparation of competency chart and proof-reading of some portion of the manuscript. We sincerely thank our all department colleagues and residents, well-wishers inside and outside JIPMER for always showering their love and affection on us. We are very much thankful to the undergraduate and postgraduate students of JIPMER and other institutes who have been constantly requesting us to write this book in a new structured format, suitable to their learnings.

Our children Dr. Auroprajna Pal, JR in Forensic Medicine, AIIMS, Bhubaneswar, and Auroprakash Pal, final MBBS student, JIPMER, Puducherry, have been the constant source of our inspiration in all our endeavours. We shall fail in our duty if we do not appreciate the contribution of our sister Ms. Sabita Nanda, who has helped in typing manuscripts of many chapters of the book. We always owe our achievements to our parents late Mrs. Anupama Nanda, late Dr. Artatran Nanda, late Sri Mrutyunjay Pal and Srimati Malati Mani Pal for showering on us their love and blessing to come to the greater heights in our life. We take this opportunity to express our heart-felt thanks to our friend and mentor late Ms. Kumud Ben of Sri Aurobindo Ashram, who had constantly been supportive to us during all our difficult times.

G. K. Pal
Pravati Pal
Nivedita Nanda

A drop of practice is better than an ocean of theories, advices and good resolutions.

The Mother (of Sri Aurobindo Ashram)

Preface to Fourth Editon

Physiology is the key subject in medical science. With new revised curriculum of Medical Council of India (now, NMC), 2019, which is more objective-oriented, clinically-focussed and skill-based integrated programme, physiology is the most suitable subject for implementation of such a new syllabus in medical profession in India. As Physiology provides the knowledge and basis of medical practice, it is the subject for effective integration with clinical and paraclinical subject. Thus, in the new curriculum, Physiology will be the major link for integration among all the subjects. The present edition of the book is thoroughly revised in the light of new National Medical Commission (NMC) guidelines for undergraduate medical curriculum.

Competency map in the tabular format with reference to chapter and page number and citation of of competency code inside the relevant places in text, have been provided. The 'learning objectives' of each chapter have been totally revised to make them more structured as 'must know' and 'desirable to know' categories that are suitable for the new objectivised NMC syllabus. Clinical application and applied aspects have been made more updated and revised. More numbers of 'Clinical Notes' and 'Important Notes' have been added to this edition, to make the student understand and remember the physiological basis of clinical applications in medicine. New chapters on Aviation and Space Physiology, Physiology of Stress, Physiology of Yoga and Meditation, Brain Death, Free Radical Generation and Oxidative Stress, Glucose Homeostasis and Pathophysiology of Diabetes, Physiology of Thymus Gland, Pathophysiology of Cyanosis, Pathophysiology of Renal Failure, and Body Fluid Volume Homeostasis have been added to this edition.

All major concepts and advances in physiology have been thoroughly incorporated in the text. The presentation of the texts, especially to explain key concepts have been made more structured with more point-wise (bulleted) description. Multiple choice questions that are part of all assessments have been given at the end of each chapter. All feedbacks from the students and faculty on the previous editions of the book have been incorporated in the new edition. We wish that this totally revised fourth edition of 'Textbook of Medical Physiology' will fulfil all the requirements and aspiration of our readers. We request our readers to provide us the feedback and inputs through mail (email ID given below)

G. K. Pal
Pravati Pal
Nivedita Nanda
Email: gkpalphysiology@gmail.com

Preface to the First Edition

Physiology as a subject has a central place in medical science. It plays a critical role in learning the principles of medicine. Without sound knowledge of body functions, it is practically impossible to study and understand the bodily abnormalities. From functions to dysfunctions, drug-preparation to medicine-prescription, disease-treatment to diseaseprevention, all have physiological basis and approach; and therefore, require the help of knowledge in Physiology. Physiology as a medical subject has changed over years from its non-clinical and pre-clinical format to the pro-clinical subject as Applied and Clinical Physiology. Starting from clinical investigations like ECG, EEG, EMG, nerve conduction studies, evoked potentials, autonomic-function tests, pulmonary-function tests and so on to bed-side management of patients require knowledge and proficiency in Physiology. In fact, Physiology department in a good medical institute provides all such facilities and opportunities. It is not far for superspeciality courses to start in subjects of Applied and Clinical Physiology. However, the growth of Physiology as a medical topic depends a lot on us, who practice physiology as a teacher, clinician and researcher. The glory of physiology depends on the image of the physiologists.

In India, Physiology as a subject in medical curriculum has changed immensely since 1997, especially after introduction of new Medical Council of India (MCI) syllabus. The duration of first MBBS course was reduced by one-third, from its original one-and-half years to one year. Moreover, students practically get about eight months to study the fi rst MBBS subjects, as enough time is spent in initial adjustment to new environment, language and profession. This has increased the responsibilities on teachers in physiology to complete the course within the stipulated period and make the students learn the subject within a short span of time. Therefore, there is a need for reshaping the subject, integrating it with other subjects of medicine and amalgamating the basic knowledge of physiology for its application in medicine.

The present book has made a sincere effort in all these directions. Emphasis has been made on providing the concepts of all aspects of physiology including the basic knowledge, regulation and integration of body functions, application of knowledge in medicine, pathophysiological basis of occurrence of common dysfunctions, and their physiological basis of management (investigations and treatment). All systems and topics start with introduction, which emphasizes the importance of learning that section in clinical medicine. Hence, the readers should not miss the introductory part before studying the topic proper. All complex and important physiological processes are highlighted by simplified step-wise descriptions, especially with the help of flow charts. Most of the data pertaining to their relevance in physiology and medicine have been summarized in tabular form. All important concepts are highlighted in the form of golden boxes.

Understanding will be incomplete without learning the content of these boxes. The clinical aspects have been noted as Applied Physiology at the end of each topic. After the publication of our Physiology Practical Book, students and teachers in Physiology have been consistently requesting me to write a Text Book of Physiology. With all their wishes and blessings, fi nally the book has been made available to them. This is a project in evolution, which needs feedback from our readers for its further growth and development. The year 2006 is particularly important for two golden events. First, JIPMER completed its Golden Jubilee year; and the institute is further aspiring to progress to the pinnacle ofmmedical education and training through greater autonomy in its academics and administration. The Mother of Sri Aurobindo Ashram in early nineteen-thirties had a vision of a great medical education center to come up at the place where JIPMER stands now. Therefore, it is imperative to remember the second, and the foremost golden event of the year; that is, the Golden Jubilee year of Supramental Descent. The Supramental Light-Force-Consciousness was made available by the Mother to the subtle physical environment of the earth atmosphere on 29th of February, 1956, which aims at progressive evolution of human consciousness to its greater heights. Thus, in these two golden moments of our time, we pray that with the Grace of the Divine Mother we all become the effective media for transmitting the medical wisdom for the advancement of our profession in particular and the society in general.

Dr. G. K. Pal

Each nation is a Shakti or power of the evolving spirit in humanity and lives by the principle which it embodies. India is the Bharata Shakti, the living energy of a great spiritual conception, and fidelity to it is the very principle of her existence.

For by its virtue alone has been the secret of her amazing persistence and perpetual force of survival and revival.

Sri Aurobindo

Contents

Part B : Heart

Part C : Circulation

Part D : Applied and Clinical Aspects of CVS

SECTION VI: RESPIRATORY SYSTEM 363 – 446

SECTION VII: GASTROINTESTINAL (GI) SYSTEM 447 – 521

Part I: Introduction and Functional Organization

Part II: GI Secretions

Part III: GI Motility

Part C : Motor System

Part D : Hypothalamus, EEG & Sleep; Limbic & Higher Functions; CSF

SECTION XII: SPECIAL SENSES 937 – 1000

Part A : Vision

Part B : Hearing

Part C : Smell and Taste

SECTION XIII: INTEGRATIVE PHYSIOLOGY 1001 – 1065

Competency Map in Physiology

Competency Code	Competency	Core (Y/N)	Chapter Nos.	Page Nos.
	PHYSIOLOGY			
Topic: General Physiology				
PY1.1	Describe the structure and functions of a mammalian cell.	Y	3	12–20
PY1.2	Describe and discuss the principles of homeostasis.	Y	2	7–11
PY1.3	Describe intercellular communication.	Y	3	20–23
PY1.4	Describe apoptosis – programmed cell death.	Y	3	26–28
PY1.5	Describe and discuss transport mechanisms across cell membranes.	Y	4	33–42
PY1.6	Describe the fluid compartments of the body, its ionic composition & measurements.	Y	6	47–52
PY1.7	Describe the concept of pH & Buffer systems in the body.	Y	135	1036,1037
PY1.8	Describe and discuss the molecular basis of resting membrane	Y	5,18	45,46,
	potential and action potential in excitable tissue.			151–153
PY1.9	Demonstrate the ability to describe and discuss the methods used to demonstrate the functions of the cells and its products, its communications and their applications in Clinical care and research.	Y	2	3–26
Topic: Haematology				
PY2.1	Describe the composition and functions of blood components.	Y	7	55–58
PY2.2	Discuss the origin, forms, variations and functions of plasma proteins.	Y	7	57, 58
PY2.3	Describe and discuss the synthesis and functions of Haemoglobin and			
	explain its breakdown. Describe variants of haemoglobin.	Y	10	75–77
PY2.4	Describe RBC formation (erythropoiesis & its regulation) and its functions.	Y	9	67–71
PY2.5	Describe different types of anaemias & Jaundice.	Y	11,12	80–83, 85,86
PY2.6	Describe WBC formation (granulopoiesis) and its regulation.	Y	14	96–98
PY2.7	Describe the formation of platelets, functions and variations.	Y	16	126–129
PY2.8	Describe the physiological basis of hemostasis and, anticoagulants. Describe bleeding & clotting disorders (Hemophilia, purpura).	Y	16,17	125, 138–142
PY2.9	Describe different blood groups and discuss the clinical importance of blood grouping, blood banking and transfusion.	Y	13	87–95
PY2.10	Define and classify different types of immunity. Describe the development of immunity and its regulation.	Y	15	110–120
PY2.11	Estimate Hb, RBC, TLC, RBC indices, DLC, Blood groups, BT/CT.	Y	9,10, 13, 14	65,78, 79,90, 96,99, 103,104, 105,107 Practical skills
PY2.12	Describe test for ESR, Osmotic fragility, Hematocrit. Note the findings and interpret the test results etc.	Y	9	66, 67
PY2.13	Describe steps for reticulocyte and platelet count.	Y	9, 16	72,131 Practical skills

Competency Code	Competency	Core (Y/N)	Chapter Nos.	Page Nos.
Topic: Nerve and Muscle Physiology				
PY3.1	Describe the structure and functions of a neuron and neuroglia; Discuss Nerve Growth Factor & other growth factors/ cytokines.	Y	15,18, 19,94	122, 145–148, 161,771
PY3.2	Describe the types, functions & properties of nerve fibers.	Y	19	158,159
PY3.3	Describe the degeneration and regeneration in peripheral nerves.	Y	19	160,161
PY3.4	Describe the structure of neuro-muscular junction and transmission of impulses.	Y	20	163–166
PY3.5	Discuss the action of neuro-muscular blocking agents.	Y	20	166,167
PY3.6	Describe the pathophysiology of Myasthenia gravis.	Y	20	167,168
PY3.7	Describe the different types of muscle fibres and their structure.	Y	21,22, 23	171–176, 188,192, 193
PY3.8	Describe action potential and its properties in different muscle types (skeletal & smooth).	Y	21,22, 23	180,181, 183–186, 193-196
PY3.9	Describe the molecular basis of muscle contraction in skeletal and in smooth muscles.	Y	21,23	176–179, 194,195
PY3.10	Describe the mode of muscle contraction (isometric and isotonic).	Y	21	181
PY3.11	Explain energy source and muscle metabolism.	Y	22	186–188
PY3.12	Explain the gradation of muscular activity .	Y	NA	Practical
PY3.13	Describe muscular dystrophy: myopathies.	Y	22	189,190
PY3.14	Perform Ergography. Y NA Practical	Y	NA	Practical
PY3.15	Demonstrate effect of mild, moderate and severe exercise and record changes in cardiorespiratory parameters.	Y	133	1019
PY3.16	Demonstrate Harvard Step test and describe the impact on induced physiologic parameters in a simulated environment.	Y	NA	Practical
PY3.17	Describe Strength-duration curve.	Y	18	150
PY3.18	Observe with Computer assisted learning (i) amphibian nerve - muscle experiments (ii) amphibian cardiac experiments.	Y	NA	Practical
Topic: Gastro-Intestinal Physiology				
PY4.1	Describe the structure and functions of digestive system.	Y	56	449–453
PY4.2	Describe the composition, mechanism of secretion, functions, and regulation of saliva, gastric, pancreatic, intestinal juices and bile secretion.	Y	58,59, 60,61, 62	462–464, 467–469, 470–472, 478–482, 486–488, 491–494
PY4.3	Describe GIT movements, regulation and functions. Describe defecation reflex. Explain role of dietary fibre.	Y	63,65, 66, 138	498,499, 506–508, 512–515, 516,517, 1050
PY4.4	Describe the physiology of digestion and absorption of nutrients.	Y	67	518–521
PY4.5	Describe the source of GIT hormones, their regulation and functions.	Y	57	454–458
PY4.6	Describe the Gut-Brain Axis.	Y	62	492
PY4.7	Describe & discuss the structure and functions of liver and gall bladder.	Y	61	484–487
PY4.8	Describe & discuss gastric function tests, pancreatic exocrine function tests & liver function tests.	Y	59,60, 61	472–474, 482,483, 485,486

Competency Code	Competency	Core (Y/N)	Chapter Nos.	Page Nos.
PY4.9	Discuss the physiology aspects of: peptic ulcer, gastrooesophageal oesophageal reflux disease,v omiting, diarrhoea, constipation, Adynamic ileus, Hirschsprung's disease.	Y	59,64, 65,66	474,475, 503,509, 510,514, 517
PY4.10	Demonstrate the correct clinical examination of the abdomen in a normal volunteer or simulated environment.	Y	NA	Practical skills
Topic: Cardiovascular Physiology (CVS)				
PY5.1	Describe the functional anatomy of heart including chambers, sounds; and Pacemaker tissue and conducting system.	Y	27,29, 31	231–233, 245–248, 274,275
PY5.2	Describe the properties of cardiac muscle including its morphology, electrical, mechanical and metabolic functions	Y	28, 29	238–242, 244,245
PY5.3	Discuss the events occurring during the cardiac cycle.	Y	31	268–272
PY5.4	Describe generation, conduction of cardiac impulse.	Y	29	248–250
PY5.5	Describe the physiology of electrocardiogram (E.C.G), its applications and the cardiac axis.	Y	30	254–257, 259,260
PY5.6	Describe abnormal ECG, arrythmias, heart block and myocardial Infarction.	Y	30	260–266
PY5.7	Describe and discuss haemodynamics of circulatory system.	Y 3	4	293–295
PY5.8	Describe and discuss local and systemic cardiovascular regulatory mechanisms.	Y	38	326–328
PY5.9	Describe the factors affecting heart rate, regulation of cardiac output & blood pressure.	Y	32,37	285,286, 311–324
PY5.10	Describe & discuss regional circulation including microcirculation, lymphatic circulation, coronary, cerebral, capillary, skin, foetal, pulmonary and splanchnic circulation.	Y	36, 39,40, 47	303–308, 329–341, 344,345, 395–399
PY5.11	Describe the patho-physiology of shock, syncope, and heart failure.	Y	39,42, 43	332, 351–355, 356–359
PY5.12	Record blood pressure & pulse at rest and in different grades of exercise and postures in a volunteer or simulated environment.	Y	NA	Practical skill
PY5.13	Record and interpret normal ECG in a volunteer or simulated environment.	Y	NA	Practical skill
PY5.14	Observe cardiovascular autonomic function tests in a volunteer or simulated environment.	Y	NA	Practical skill
PY5.15	Demonstrate the correct clinical examination of the cardiovascular system in a normal volunteer or simulated	Y	NA	Practical skill
PY5.16	Record Arterial pulse tracing using finger plethysmography in a volunteer or simulated environment.	Y	NA	Practical skill
Topic: Respiratory Physiology				
PY6.1	Describe the functional anatomy of respiratory tract.	Y	44	363–368
PY6.2	Describe the mechanics of normal respiration, pressure changes during ventilation, lung volume and capacities,	Y	45,46, 47	371–387, 389–394,

Competency Code	Competency	Core (Y/N)	Chapter Nos.	Page Nos.
	alveolar surface tension, compliance, airway resistance, ventilation, V/P ratio, diffusion capacity of lungs.			399,400
PY6.3	Describe and discuss the transport of respiratory gases: Oxygen and Carbon dioxide.	Y	48	402–410
PY6.4	Describe and discuss the physiology of high altitude and deep sea diving.	Y	50,52	425–427, 434,435
PY6.5	Describe and discuss the principles ofa rtificial respiration, oxygen therapy, acclimatization and decompression sickness.	Y	51,52, 54	431,432, 435,440
PY6.6	Describe and discuss the pathophysiology of dyspnoea, hypoxia, cyanosis, asphyxia; drowning, periodic breathing.	Y	47,51, 53	399, 428–431, 436–438
PY6.7	Describe and discuss lung function tests & their clinical significance.	Y	55	443–446
PY6.8	Demonstrate the correct technique to perform & interpret Spirometry.	Y	NA	Practical skill
PY6.9	Demonstrate the correct clinical examination of the respiratory system in a normal volunteer or simulated environment.	Y	NA	Practical skill
PY6.10	Demonstrate the correct technique to perform measurement of peak expiratory flow rate in a normal volunteer or simulated environment.	Y	NA	Practical skill
Topic: Renal Physiology				
PY7.1	Describe structure and function of kidney.	Y	86	709–714
PY7.2	Describe the structure and functions of juxta glomerular apparatus and role of renin-angiotensin system.	Y	86	715–718
PY7.3	Describe the mechanism of urine formation involving processes of filtration, tubular reabsorption & secretion; concentration and diluting mechanism.	Y	87, 88, 89	722–727, 731–740, 744–748
PY7.4	Describe & discuss the significance & implication of Renal clearance.	Y	87	725
PY7.5	Describe the renal regulation of fluid and electrolytes & acidbase balance.	Y	88,91, 135	740–742, 752–756, 1035-1038
PY7.6	Describe the innervations of urinary bladder, physiology of micturition and its abnormalities.	Y	93	762–765
PY7.7	Describe artificial kidney, dialysis and renal transplantation.	Y	92	760,761
PY7.8	Describe & discuss Renal Function Tests.	Y	92	757–760
PY7.9	Describe cystometry and discuss the normal cystometrogram.	Y	93	763
Topic: Endocrine Physiology				
PY8.1	Describe the physiology of bone and calcium metabolism.	Y	77	624–631
PY8.2	Describe the synthesis, secretion, transport, physiological actions, regulation and effect of altered (hypo and hyper) secretion of pituitary gland, thyroid gland, parathyroid gland, adrenal gland, pancreas and hypothalamus.	Y	70,71, 72,73, 74,75, 76,77	542–544, 546–557, 559–564, 566–577, 580–598, 600–605, 606–623, 631–635
PY8.3	Describe the physiology of Thymus & Pineal Gland.	Y	78	638–640
PY8.4	Describe function tests: Thyroid gland; Adrenal cortex, Adrenal medulla and pancreas.	Y	73,74, 75,76	577,578, 593,604, 621,622
PY8.5	Describe the metabolic and endocrine consequences of obesity & metabolic syndrome, Stress response. Outline the psychiatry component pertaining to metabolic syndrome.	Y	111, 137, 138	888, 1044-1046, 1051
PY8.6	Describe & differentiate the mechanism of action of steroid, protein and amine hormones.	Y	68,69	526, 536–541

Competency Code	Competency	Core (Y/N)	Chapter Nos.	Page Nos.
PY10.8	Describe and discuss behavioural and EEG characteristics during sleep and mechanism responsible for its production.	Y	112	894–897
PY10.9	Describe and discuss the physiological basis of memory, learning and speech.	Y 1	14,115	911–917, 919,920
PY10.10	Describe and discuss chemical transmission in the nervous system. (Outline the psychiatry element).	Y	95	776–778, 783–787
PY10.11	Demonstrate the correct clinical examination of the nervous system: Higher functions, sensory system, motor system, reflexes, cranial nerves in a normal volunteer or simulated environment.	Y	NA	Practical skills
PY10.12	Identify normal EEG forms. Y 112 893,894	Y	129,130	993,994,
PY10.13	Describe and discuss perception of smell and taste sensation.			996–999
PY10.14	Describe and discuss patho-physiology of altered smell and taste sensation.	Y	129,130	994,999, 1000
PY10.15	Describe and discuss functional anatomy of ear and auditory pathways & physiology of hearing.	Y	125,126, 127	973–978, 979–981, 982–986
PY10.16	Describe and discuss pathophysiology of deafness. Describe hearing tests.	Y	128	988–990
PY10.17	Describe and discuss functional anatomy of eye, physiology of image formation, physiology of vision including colour vision, refractive errors, colour blindness, physiology of pupil and light reflex.	Y	118,119, 120,122, 123,	939–945, 946–950, 951–954, 964,965, 967–969
PY10.18	Describe and discuss the physiological basis of lesion in visual	Y	121	956,962, 963
PY10.19	Describe and discuss auditory & visual evoke potentials.	Y	124,128	972,990
PY10.20	Demonstrate (i) Testing of visual acuity, colour and field of vision and (ii) hearing (iii) Testing for smell and (iv) taste sensation in volunteer/ simulated environment.	Y	122,123, 128,129, 130	961,962, 969,989, 990,994, 1000
PY11.1	Describe and discuss mechanism of temperature regulation.	Y	132	1006-1015
PY11.2	Describe and discuss adaptation to altered temperature (heat and cold).	Y	132	1015,1016
PY11.3	Describe and discuss mechanism of fever, cold injuries and heat stroke.	Y	132	1016,1017
PY11.4	Describe and discuss cardio-respiratory and metabolic adjustments during exercise; physical training effects.	Y	133	1022-1031
PY11.5	Describe and discuss physiological consequences of sedentary lifestyle.	Y	133	1030
PY11.6	Describe physiology of Infancy. N 137 1042, 1043			
PY11.7	Describe and discuss physiology of aging; free radicals and antioxidants.	N	137	1046-1048
PY11.8	Discuss & compare cardio-respiratory changes in exercise (isometric and isotonic) with that in the resting state and under different environmental conditions (heat and cold).	Y	132	1011
PY11.9	Interpret growth charts. Y 137 1042			
PY11.10	Interpret anthropometric assessment of infants.	Y	137	1042
PY11.11	Discuss the concept, criteria for diagnosis of Brain death and its implications.	Y	112	901
PY11.12	Discuss the physiological effects of meditation.	Y	139	1063,1064
PY11.13	Obtain history and perform general examination in the volunteer / simulated environment.	Y	NA	Practical
PY11.14	Demonstrate Basic Life Support in a simulated environment.	Y	54	441,442

Section I

General Physiology

Oh India, land of light and spiritual knowledge!
Wake up to your true mission in the world,
Show the way to union and harmony.

The Mother
(of Sri Aurobindo Ashram)

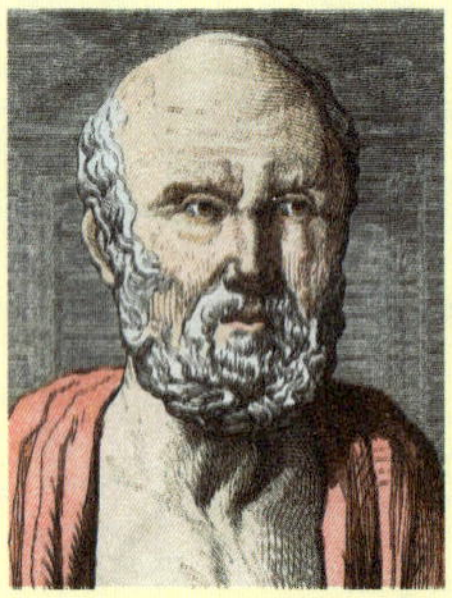

Hippocrates was a teacher at the School in the Health Temple at Cos. Writings of the group are distinguished by a high ethical tone, keen observation, logical application of existing ideas and cautious judgment. Hippocrates established the popular ethics of medical practice for physicians, which is commonly known as **'Hippocratic Oath'** that all physicians solemnly pledge at the time of obtaining their degrees to start medical practice

Reference: Jones WHS and Withington ET. *The works of Hippocrates.* 4 volumes. London, Heinemann Publication: 1923.

'Hippocratic Oath' with modification is as follows.....

I solemnly pledge to consecrate my life to the service of humanity; I will give to my teachers the respect and gratitude that is their due;
I will practice my profession with conscience and dignity;
The health of my patient will be my first consideration;
I will respect the secrets that are confided in me, even after the patient has died;
I will maintain by all the means in my power, the honor and the noble traditions of the medical profession;
My colleagues will be my sisters and brothers;
I will not permit considerations of age, disease or disability, creed, ethnic origin, gender, nationality, political affiliation, race, sexual orientation, social standing or any other factor to intervene between my duty and my patient;
I will maintain the utmost respect for human life;
I will not use my medical knowledge to violate human rights and civil liberties, even under threat;
I make these promises solemnly, freely and upon my honor.

Chapter 1

Importance of Physiology in Medicine

Learning Objectives

<u>On completion of study of this chapter:</u>

The student will be able to (must know):

1. Understand the importance of physiology in learning principles of pharmacology, pathology and medicine.
2. Appreciate the role of physiology in medical practice.
3. Realize the value of physiology knowledge for conducting medical research.

The student may also be able to (desirable to know):

1. Know that physiology helps in integral progress in human life.

Physiology is the study of body functions, their mechanisms, and regulations in all living organisms. Human physiology is study of the functions of various cells, organs and organ systems of human body. Medical Physiology is the application of human physiology for understanding the pathophysiology of diseases and the physiological basis of management of diseases.

PHYSIOLOGY FOR LEARNING MEDICINE

Physiology: the Mother of Medicine

Medical physiology provides the knowledge to understand that homeostasis (internal balance of body systems) is that basis of normal health and disharmony between systems results in bodily dysfunctions. The knowledge in physiology helps to understand, diagnose and treat the diseases. For an example, for diagnosis and management of acute myocardial infarction (AMI), the physician should know the physiology of coronary circulation to understand how change in coronary hemodynamics produces AMI. He understands the mechanism and spread of pain of AMI to appreciate the radiation of myocardial ischemic pain and learns the electrophysiology of cardiac muscle to appreciate the ECG abnormalities in AMI. The knowledge of physiological basis of drug actions helps him provide the treatment of AMI. Similarly, treatment of other diseases requires adequate knowledge in physiology to understand, diagnose and manage.

Physiology for Learning all Subjects

A medical student with ample knowledge in physiology learns Pharmacology. Pharmacology in principle is an extension of physiology. For an example, learning pharmacotherapy for bronchial asthma the student understands the use of catecholaminergics especially β receptor agonists that cause immediate bronchodilation and provide relief. In physiology, he has learned that sympathetic stimulation causes relaxation of bronchial smooth muscle by releasing norepinephrine acting through β receptors. Similarly, mechanisms of action of all of drugs has physiological basis. Thus, knowledge in physiology is important for learning pharmacology.

Physiology is **useful for learning Pathology**. For an example, a student learns in physiology that neutrophil is the first line of defence against acute infection and monocyte is the defence for chronic infection. Therefore, when he examines a histology slide and finds abundant neutrophils in the microscopic field, immediately he comprehends the infection or inflammation is of acute nature, and when he observes plenty of monocytes or macrophages in the slide, he understands the tissue has chronic inflammation. Likewise, understanding pathological basis of diseases requires the basic knowledge in physiology. Genesis of all diseases has a *pathophysiological basis*.

Knowledge in physiology is essential **for learning Medicine**. Etiopathogenesis, clinical manifestation, diagnosis and management of all diseases have the physiological basis. Application of physiology in medicine is **clinical physiology**. Physiology has application in all branches of medicine such as surgery (surgical physiology), gynecology, ophthalmology, otorhinolaryngology, pediatric medicine, endocrinology, oncology, gastroenterology, pulmonology, neurology, cardiology and so on.

PHYSIOLOGY FOR MEDICAL PRACTICE

Physiology for Becoming a Good Physician

The knowledge in physiology guides a physician not only to understand the pathophysiology and diagnosis of diseases, but also to adhere to rational treatment for the disease. Presently, in medical practice, there is tendency to provide prompt symptomatic relief by prescribing a list of analgesics and antibiotics as modern men want immediate improvement. There is no time, interest and knowledge for an assisted-natural remission of the disease. However, this type of management does not help the patient in the long-term basis. Nevertheless, some diseases require immediate and judicious treatment by modern antibiotics and therapeutics.

The mankind is presently inflicted by chronic ailments such as hypertension, heart disease and diabetes mellitus. For treatment of such diseases especially in the early stage, lifestyle modifications like dietary alteration, reduction in stress level, practice of mental relaxation, regular physical exercises and yoga are very useful. Usually, these non-pharmacological practices are known to improve health. Medicines should be prescribed only when these natural means fail to check the disease.

Physiology educates that effective treatment of many diseases requires **improvement of body immunity**. For, example, fever due to acute inflammation is a natural manifestation of the disease and part of the defense mechanisms of the body. Therefore, instead of immediately prescribing antibiotics, physician can reassure the patient that the body heals itself. Administration of higher antibiotics and analgesics suppresses the immunity of the patient that exposes him to various infections. For example, a simple boil (cellulitis), which heals by itself, does not warrant prescription of antibiotics. A doctor should assure the patient about the natural course of the boil and may advise him for warm fomentation on the part that improves blood flow to the region and facilitates the process of healing. Conversely, treatment by antibiotic may halt the healing process of the boil and in some cases produces antibioma (tumor due to antibiotics). A doctor should know that **frequent use of antibiotics suppresses the immune system** of the body. A physician with ample knowledge in physiology helps patient in facilitating the natural remission and recovery without prescribing higher medicines. This is the physiological basis of treatment. Thus **"A good physician is a physiologist, and a good physiologist is a physician".**

Physiology for Prevention of Diseases

Knowledge of pathophysiology of a disease process helps physician to adopt the measures that prevent the diseases. For example, a physician who understands that regular physical exercises with healthy diet retard the process of atherosclerosis and oxidative stress and prevent cardiovascular, cerebrovascular and many metabolic diseases, he himself practices healthy lifestyle and encourages his patients to do so. Thus, a good physiologist-physician plays a bigger role in the prevention of diseases and improvement health in the community.

PHYSIOLOGY FOR MEDICAL RESEARCH

Physiology is the mother of medical research. The inventions and discoveries in medical science and advances in medicine are mainly due to research contributions from physiology. Therefore, from its inception in 1901, Nobel Prize in the field of medical sciences has been designated as Nobel Prize in 'Physiology or Medicine'. Many Nobel Prize winners in medicine starting from Emil Adolph Von Behring (1901), Sir Ronal Ross (1902), Prof. Finsen NR (1903), Prof. Ivan Petrovich Pavlov (1904) to Harvey J. Alter, Michael Houghton and Charles M. Rice (2020) are scientists or physicians who have worked in the medical fields related to physiology. Etiopathogenesis of the diseases and physiological basis of management are explained mainly due to research-discoveries in physiology.

Significant contribution of Scientist

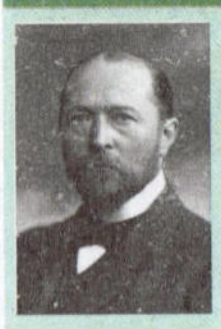

Emil A. Von Behring (1854-1917) Prof. Behring was awarded first Nobel Prize in Physiology or Medicine, 1901, for his work on physiology of immunity and serum therapy, especially its application against diphtheria. This opened the path in the domain of medical therapy, a victorious weapon against illness and deaths. He developed quantitative methods for the bioassay of antisera and antitoxins.

Basic and Clinical Research

Research in basic and clinical physiology has advanced knowledge in clinical medicine. Basic research reveals the mechanism and pathophysiology of diseases, whereas clinical research unravels the management and prevention of diseases. Usually, clinicians will not have time for research. However, collaborative research with clinical departments creates more research interest in clinicians, improves their outlook for research, yields clinical output of research, and promotes interactive coordination between the departments. Physiologists should invite participation of physicians in the research to ensure application-based outcome in clinical research.

Significant contribution of Scientist

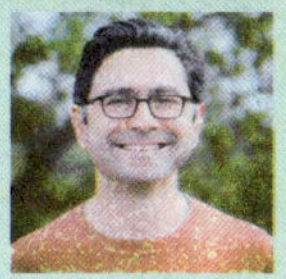

Ardem Patapoutian

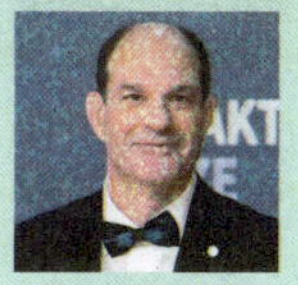

David Julius

Nobel Prize in Physiology or Medicine for the year 2021 was awarded jointly to **David Julius and Ardem Patapoutian** for their discoveries of **receptors for temperature and touch.**

To be noted here that ***Joseph Erlanger and Herbert Gasser*** received the Nobel Prize in Physiology or Medicine in 1944 for their discovery of different *types of sensory nerve fibers* that react to distinct stimuli, for example, in the responses to painful and non-painful touch, temperature etc.

PHYSIOLOGY FOR INTEGRAL PROGRESS

Physiology for Integral Knowledge

Physiology provides the knowledge for keeping good health. In addition, physiology provides the knowledge for integral health. Physiology makes us learn the importance of harmonious working of body systems. Derangement of any of the system of body leads ultimately to dysfunction of other systems, as the systems works as an integrated unit. Thus, integral health depends on the growth of all systems of the body, which happens by exercise, yoga, good nutrition and sleep.

Physiology for Spiritual Progress

The fundamental aim of our terrestrial existence is to attain perfection: perfection in physical growth, beauty, mind and intelligence and perfection in inner progress. A progressive evolution of consciousness is spirituality. Spiritual progress can easily be enhanced with improvement of body physiology. For example, practice of pranayama not only improves breathing capacity and oxygenation of the body, but also causes purification of mind and vital and enhances the cognitive faculties. In yoga, subtle physical bodies and centers such as heart center, spinal-cord center, pineal center, etc. have been described. It has been said that concentration on these specific centers releases the spiritual energy from the center that helps in enriching the mind and body. Knowledge in anatomy and physiology help concentrate and release energy from the centers. A physiologist with sincere aspiration is privileged for acquiring higher knowledge, force, and consciousness. Even, teaching physiology to students is among the best methods of calming the body and mind, and getting connected with the higher forces.

To study human physiology is an opportunity, to become a physiologist is a privilege, to enlighten others the physiological basis of health-promotion is a joy, and to practice physiology for integral progress is the golden prospect in life. Thus, the **Physiology is for Progress and Prosperity** (PPP).

Exam Questions

1. Briefly describe the importance of physiology in the study of medicine.
2. Briefly explain with example how knowledge in physiology helps to understand, pharmacology, pathology and medicine.

Multiple Choice Questions

1. **Who is the first scientist to receive Nobel prize in Physiology or Medicine?**
   A. Ronald Ross
   B. Patrovich Pavlov
   C. Von Behring
   D. Charles Sherrington

2. **What was the area of research for Nobel prize in Physiology or Medicine for the year 2020?**
   A. Molecular mechanism of circadian rhythm
   B. Adaptation of cell to oxygen availability
   C. Cancer therapy by immunomodulation
   D. Discovery of Hepatitis C Virus

Answers

1. C **2. D**

Chapter 2

Functional Organization of Human Body and Principles of Homeostasis

Learning Objectives

On completion of study of this chapter:

The student will be able to (must know):

1. Name various systems of the body and understand the physiological organization of these systems.
2. Define homeostasis.
2. Name scientists who gave the concept of milieu interior, and who coined the term homeostasis.
3. Explain the feedback mechanisms of homeostatic regulation.
4. Give the examples of homeostatic regulations.

The student may also be able to (desirable to know):

1. Describe the mechanisms of negative and positive feedback regulations.
2. Understand that dysfunctions are mainly due to failure of homeostatic regulations.

FUNCTIONAL ORGANIZATION OF HUMAN BODY

Physiologically, the human body is made up of different systems. Each body system is made up of organs and tissues, and each tissue is composed of cells. Cells are the functional and anatomical units of the body.

Cell as the Unit of the Body

The fundamental unit of a living organism is the cell. The body is made up of cells that specialize into tissues in various organs for carrying out specific functions. There are about 100 trillion cells in a human body. While about 75 trillion cells are present in organ systems, about 25 trillion cells are present as red cells in the blood. Thus, red cells are most abundant of any particular type of cells in the body.

Unicellular vs Multicellular Organisms

Unicellular Organisms

In unicellular organisms such as ameba, the processes that sustain life are carried out by a single cell. They have following characteristics:

1. O_2 and soluble nutrients enter the cell by simple diffusion, and macromolecules of nutrients are ingested by phagocytosis.
2. Metabolic waste products, including CO_2 diffuse out of the cell and undigested materials are removed by exocytosis.
3. Presence of contractile proteins in the cell enables it to move by pseudopodia away from noxious stimuli or towards food.
4. Reproduction is achieved by simple cell division and asexual reproduction.

Multicellular Organisms

In multicellular organisms such as animal and man, the cells are organized into tissues (nerves, muscles, connective tissue, lymphoid tissue, epithelial tissue, blood etc.); and the tissues are organized into larger units known as organs (e.g. kidney, liver etc.). The tissues and organs are further organized into functional systems meant for performing various body functions. They have following characteristics:

1. Developed systems meant for carrying out specific functions. Examples are, cardiovascular system for circulation of blood, respiratory system for oxygenation of tissues, etc.
2. Ingestion of nutrients, digestion and absorption of nutrients and the process of cellular metabolism are elaborate.

3. Highly developed systems of regulation of body functions.
4. Controlled system of locomotion.
5. Reproduction is usually sexual.

Major Physiological Systems

Functionally, the body systems can be broadly divided into:

1. The *system for supplying nutrition to the body*, which is achieved by the gastrointestinal (GI) system.
2. The ***systems to support the body for locomotion and external works***. The movements are performed by the muscles and bones (the musculoskeletal system), and the nerves supplying the skeletal muscles.
3. The ***systems for internal communication, integration and regulation***: The communication between the cells and organs and control of organ systems is achieved by the circulating blood, gaseous exchange at tissue level through respiration, the hormones secreted from endocrine glands, and the neurons innervating the tissues. The **regulations of body functions** are carried out primarily by the nervous system and the endocrine system. Hence, regulation of any particular body function is usually discussed under two major categories: the *neural regulation* and the *hormonal regulation*.
4. The ***systems for reproduction***: Reproduction is accomplished by the reproductive organs.
5. The ***systems for excretion***: Though kidney is the major organ of excretion, lower parts of GI tract (colon, rectum, and anal canal) and skin also contribute to excretion of wastes from the body.
6. The ***system for protection***: Protection of the body is carried out by two major systems: the Immunity System and the Integumentary System. **Immunity system** mainly consists of leucocytes and lymphoid tissues. Neutrophils, monocytes and lymphocytes are the major defence of the body. Neutrophils and monocytes kill invaders by phagocytosis, whereas lymphocytes take part in specific immunity. **Integumentary system** consists mainly of skin and its appendages. The skin covers the body and provides mechanical protection, in addition to chemicals secreted from sweat glands and specialized cells provide protection.

The major body systems are:

Musculoskeletal or Locomotor System: This system enables the body adopt posture against gravity and move about in the environment. This is mainly for execution of works.

Blood: The blood serves as transport medium for conveying nutrients and oxygen to all the cells, and for delivering waste products from tissues to the organs that excrete them (the lungs and kidneys). Blood contains cells that take part in body defence mechanisms and provide immunity.

Cardiovascular or Circulatory System: The heart is the central pump that generates pressure for flow of blood in the blood vessels that serve as vehicular system for blood to flow.

Respiratory system: The respiration is responsible for delivering atmospheric oxygen to the blood, and excreting CO_2 produced by the cells of the body.

Gastrointestinal or Alimentary System: The GI system serves to ingest, digest, and absorb nutrients, water and electrolytes, and excrete undigested or unabsorbed waste matter.

Urinary or Excretory System: The urinary system consists of kidneys, ureter and urinary bladder. It excretes waste products from the body and plays a major role in maintaining *composition of body fluids*.

Endocrine System: Hormones secreted by various endocrine glands serve mainly regulatory functions. They control metabolism, growth, development and reproductive functions.

Reproductive System: Reproductive organs and genital structures ensure maintenance of progeny and the species.

Nervous System: The nervous system is mainly for co-ordination, communication and regulation of body functions.

Integumentary System: It consists mainly of skin and its appendages. The skin by covering the body provides mechanical protection to the body. Skin plays important role in temperature regulation.

PY1.2

PRINCIPLES OF HOMEOSTASIS

Homeostasis: Definition & Concept

Homeostasis is defined as the *maintenance of the constancy of the internal environment of the body*.

In 19th century, ***Claude Bernard***, a French physiologist, was first to introduce the concept of **milieu interiéur**, which means the internal environment of the body.

Significant contribution of Scientist

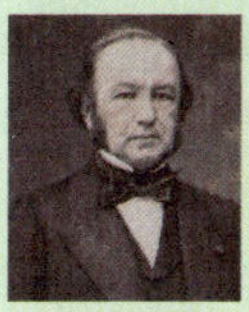

Claude Bernard C. Bernard (1813 – 1878), was a great French physiologist and genius of all time. He introduced the concept of **milieu interiéur**, preservation of the internal stability despite changes in the external environment, which was later utilized to understand the mechanism of '*homeostasis*'. He was the first to provide satisfactory explanation for the *mechanism of action of any drug*.

Extracellular Fluid as the Internal Environment

About 60% of the total body weight is water, which means a man weighing 70 kg has a total water content of about 42 liters, of which 28 L is present inside the cells and 14 L is present outside the cell.

- The electrolyte composition of the extracellular fluid roughly resembles that of seawater, which is rich in sodium and chloride, and poor in potassium.
- The intracellular fluid contains more potassium and less sodium-chloride.

In 1929, an American physiologist **Walter Bradford Cannon** coined the term ***'homeostasis'*** (*homoios* means 'like' and *stasis* means 'standing still') to describe the phenomenon of the constancy of the internal environment. He described that the capacity of self-regulation is the cause for maintenance of steady states in the body, which occurs due to coordinated integration of various physiological mechanisms.

Control Systems of the Body

There are multiple control systems in the body that operate within the organ systems to control functions of the body as whole or the function of a system. They control many vital parameters such as electrolytes, pH, body temperature etc., within the normal range, which is essential for survival of the being (Table 2.1).

Table 2.1 | Normal range and approximate short-term nonlethal range of some important parameters of the body.

Parameters (Unit)	Normal Range	Approximate short-term nonlethal limit
Plasma pH	7.35 – 7.45	6.9 – 8.0
Plasma K^+ (mmol/L)	3.5 – 5.0	1.5 – 9.0
Body Temperature (°F)	97 – 98.8	65 – 110
CO_2 (Venous blood) (mmHg)	35 – 45	5.0 – 80
Plasma Na^+ (mmol/L)	135 – 146	115 – 175
Plasma HCO_3^- (mmol/L)	24 – 32	8.0 – 45
Blood Glucose (mg/dL)	60 – 99	25 – 1500

Control systems work through **feedback mechanisms** (see below). The major control systems of the body are as follows:

1. **Neural Control:** Neural control of body functions is the instantaneous and most effective control mechanism.
2. **Hormonal Control:** Hormones secreted from endocrine organs are important for regulation of metabolic functions, growth and development. Hormones also influence functions of many organs such as heart, brain, kidney, stomach, intestine, and so on.

Significant contribution of Scientist

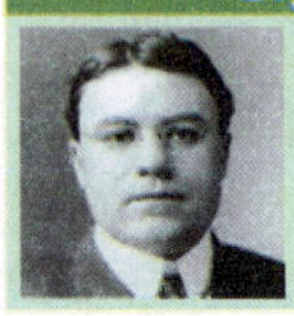

W. B. CANON

W. B. Canon (1871 – 1945) was first to coin the term homeostasis and describe its mechanism. He analyzed the mechanisms of internal regulations of body activity. He described the relation of endocrines to emotions and studied neuro-endocrine functions.

3. **Renal Control:** Kidneys play an important role in homeostasis. Regulation of body fluid volume and composition is vital for normal body functions.
4. **Chemical Control:** Various chemicals such as pH, PCO_2, PO_2 of body fluids, and concentration of electrolytes, ADP, adenosine etc. in plasma influence functions of organs or organ systems. Hormonal and chemical controls are combinely known as **humoral control**.
5. **Thermogenic Control:** Body temperature directly controls enzymatic and metabolic activities. Alteration in body temperature affects cardiovascular, respiratory and neuronal functions.
6. **Circadian Control:** Day-night variation in body functions is due to the circadian control. The center of circadian regulation is the suprachiasmatic nucleus located in the hypothalamus.

Homeostatic Mechanisms

Homeostasis is the stability of the internal environment. Homeostasis of composition of internal environment and various body parameters is the vital requirement for functioning of the body, which is achieved by operation of feedback mechanisms.

Feedback Systems of Homeostatic Regulations

Homeostatic regulation is mainly achieved through the feedback mechanisms that operate to safeguard a set point already set for the physiological variable. The stimulus for feedback control is a change in the level of the variable, which is detected by the sensor (the receptors) that activate the feedback system which in turn triggers a response to bring the variable back to the normal range of the set point and restores homeostasis.

Negative Feedback

The negative feedback mechanism is the usual mechanism of homeostatic regulation.

- When a **variable is raised above the set point**, the negative feedback mechanism triggers processes that *inhibit the formation of the variable* (Flowchart 2.1).
- When the **variable is lowered below the set point**, negative feedback system *withdraws the inhibition* to allow production of the variable.

Components of Negative Feedback System

Negative feedback control system requires a sensor that detects the change in variable, a control center that receives input from the sensor and initiates command signal, and an effector that evokes responses according to the command signal directed from the control center (Flowchart 2.2). There are priorities in homeostatic control system (Application Box 2.1)

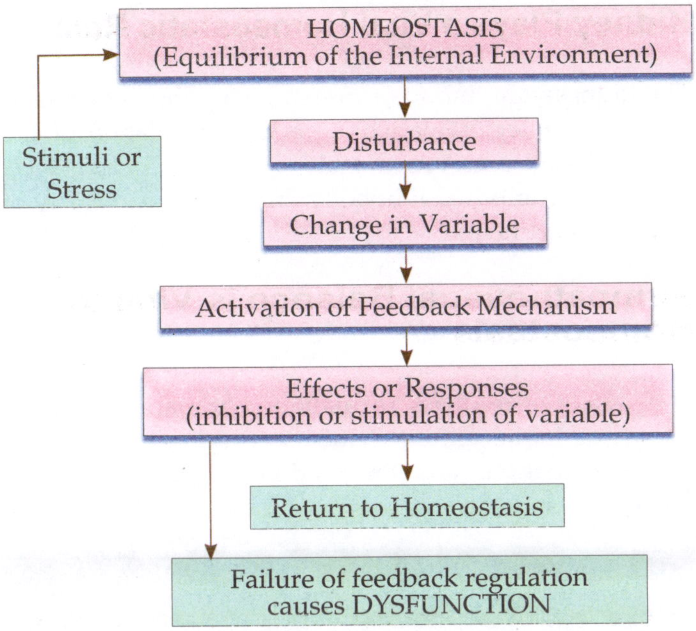

Flowchart 2.1: Feedback mechanism of homeostatic regulation. Note, failure of feedback control leads to the dysfunctions or diseases.

The Sensor: The sensor contains receptors that monitor the change of the variable and provide sensory signals to the control center of the changes detected. The examples are carotid sinus and aortic arch that contain baroreceptors in their wall and detect change in pressure in their lumen.

The Control Center: Usually, control centers are located in the central nervous system, especially in the brain. For example, centers for blood pressure regulation are located in medulla and the hypothalamus.

The Effector: The effector is the target organ that produces the response. For example, blood vessels and heart are the effector organs for blood pressure regulation.

- Depending on the rate of sympathetic and vagal discharges, the effector organs change their activities to achieve the target effect.

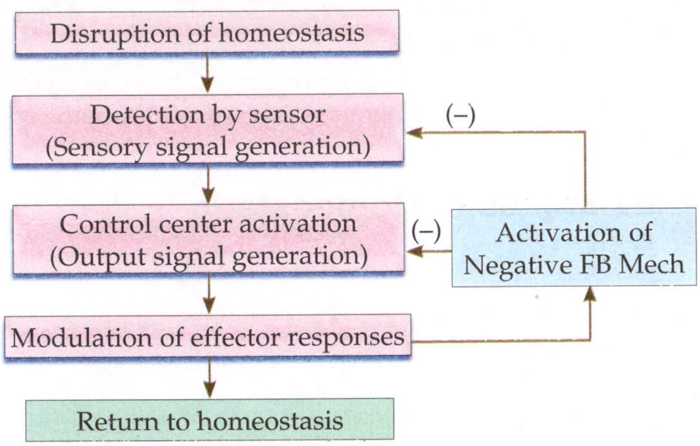

Flowchart 2.2: Components of negative feedback control system. Minus sign depicts inhibition. FB Mech: Feedback Mechanism.

- When the deviation is the increase in the variable above the set point, the effector will be inhibited, and inhibition continues until the variable is reduced to the normal set point.
- Reverse process is initiated when the variable is reduced below the set point.

IMPORTANT NOTE

Gain in Homeostatic Control: The magnitude of efficiency with which homeostatic control system maintains a balanced condition is determined by the gain in the negative feedback regulation. This can be calculated by noting the difference in the system with the intact feedback and without the feedback. Gain is calculated as correction divided by error (Gain=Correction/Error). Gain in baroreceptor control of BP could be 2 [40 (correction)/20 (error)). That means, the disturbance that increases BP does so only one-third as much as would occur if the control system were not present. The gain in control system for other homeostatic processes such as temperature regulation is very high, as high as 30.

Positive Feedback

In a positive feedback system, increase in the variable triggers processes that further increase the variable. Therefore, this control mechanism does not operate to provide homeostasis. The variable stimulated the production of another variable or subsequent variables, which in turn stimulates the production of the primary variable (Flowchart 2.3). Thus, positive feedback mechanism is a vicious cycle that terminates only when the stimulus applied to trigger is withdrawn or the process itself is self-terminated. Hence, positive feedback can sometimes be harmful (Application Box 2.2).

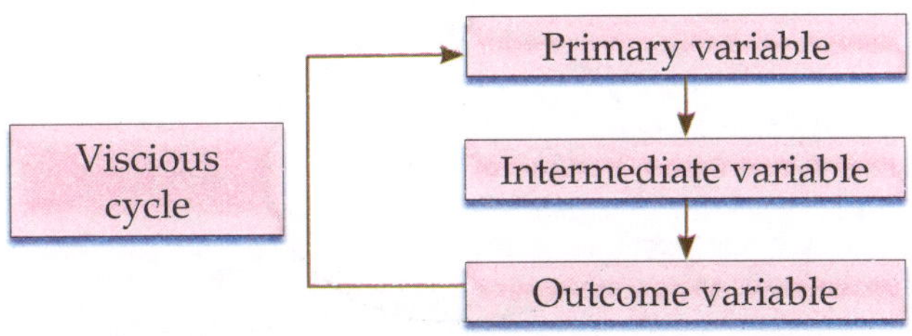

Flowchart 2.3: Schema of positive feedback system. Note that outcomes variable in this system stimulates the primary variable, which in turn further stimulates the production or activity of outcome variable. Plus sign indicates stimulation.

Application Box 2.1

Priorities in homeostatic controls: Life-saving regulatory mechanisms normally take precedence over those that are activated routinely. For example, regulation of body temperature on exposure to extreme weather gets priority over the control of gastric emptying in similar conditions. Similarly, activation of withdrawal reflex in response to a noxious stimulus, which protects the body from injury, takes precedence over other somatic reflex and visceral reflexes.

Examples: Typical example of positive feedback regulation is the parturition reflex initiated by oxytocin.

- Towards term, when the head of the matured fetus presses on the uterine cervix, the cervical distension sends signal to posterior pituitary to release oxytocin.

- Oxytocin increases the excitability of myometrium and causes uterine contraction.
- Contraction of uterus further pushes the fetus onto the cervix, and cervical distension further increases oxytocin release that promotes uterine contraction, and the vicious cycle continues till the baby is delivered.

Other examples of positive feedback mechanisms:

1. **LH Surge:** This is increased luteinizing hormone (LH) secretion leading to ovulation. Normally, estrogen inhibits LH secretion. But, before ovulation, estrogen provides positive feedback to LH secretion that results in LH surge.
2. **The Hodgkin's Cycle:** Sodium influx that causes upstroke (depolarization) of nerve or muscle action potential (Fig. 2.1). Opening of few sets of sodium channel provides positive feedback for opening of other sodium channels that results in massive sodium influx causing depolarization.
3. **Activation of Digestive Enzymes:** The activation of digestive enzymes pepsinogen and trypsinogen by pepsin and trypsin respectively.
4. **Enzyme Cascade Hypothesis of Coagulation:** Activation of one clotting factor, which acts as an enzyme to activate the next clotting factor in the coagulation cascade.

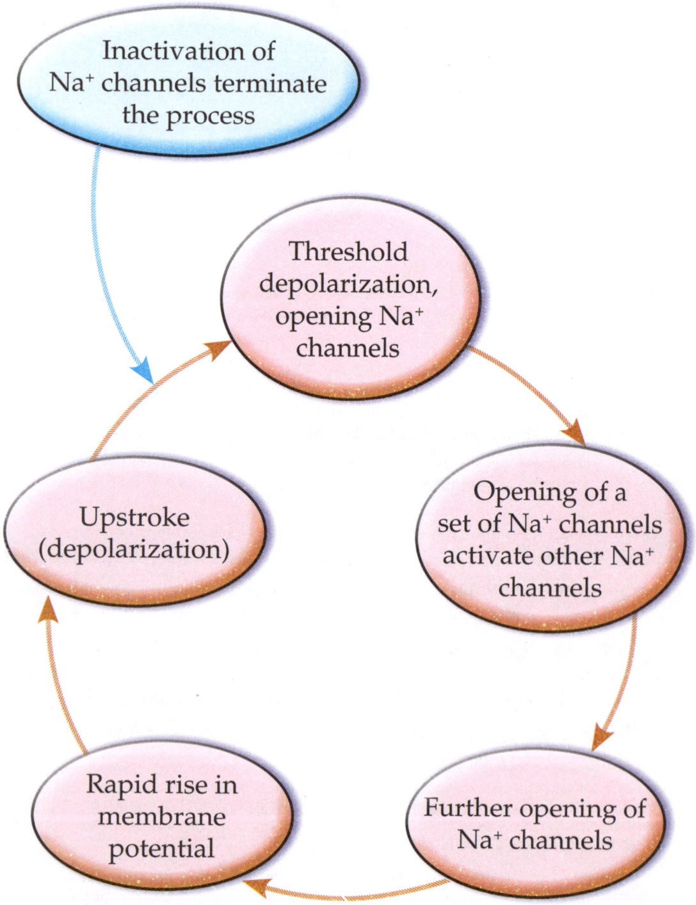

Fig. 2.1: Hodgkin's cycle as an example of positive feedback mechanism. In this, opening of a set of Na^+ channels activates opening of subsequent sets of Na^+ channels (+ve feedback) that leads to depolarization of the cell.

Kidney Plays a Vital Homeostatic Role

The kidneys are important organ for the homeostasis of many physiological variables such as regulation of the arterial blood pressure and blood volume, pH balance, electrolyte composition of body fluids, and osmolarity of fluid compartments.

Sympathovagal Balance is Vital to Homeostasis

The system of feedback regulation is primarily based on the neural inputs and mechanisms, which is called as the neural regulation. Neural regulation has the advantage of immediate and effective control of the parameters.

Application Box 2.2

Positive feedback can sometimes be detrimental and cause death: Positive feedback mechanism sets a vicious cycle that continues to increase the level of the variable until the stimulus that has triggered the response is withdrawn. Increase in the variable beyond a physiological limit could be detrimental. For example, intravascular coagulation triggered by release of tissue factor from damaged tissue, if not stopped after formation of clot at the site of injury can lead to formation of clots beyond the site and in other blood vessel and lead to disseminated intravascular coagulation (DIC). In fact, one of the mechanisms of DIC is release some coagulants from damaged tissue that triggers a vicious cycle for formation clots and dissemination of intravascular clots. Therefore, homeostatic mechanisms are usually operated by negative feedback systems.

- The autonomic regulation of visceral functions dominates all other regulatory mechanisms.
- As sympathetic and vagal stimulation to the organs have opposite influences, a balance between them, which is known as **sympathovagal balance** is essential for smooth conduct of cardio-respiratory, endocrinal and other visceral and metabolic functions.
- Chronic autonomic dysregulation (sympathovagal imbalance) that leads to dyshomeostasis and dysfunction has been reported to be the major contributor to degeneration, decay and premature death.

Examples of Homeostatic Regulations

There are many examples of homeostatic regulations; few are given below.

Body Temperature Regulation: The temperature of the body is maintained within a narrow range of 96°F to 98.4°F. Increased temperature above normal is called as fever and below is called as hypothermia. During fever, the body activates controlling mechanisms to increase heat loss through cutaneous vasodilation and sweating. When hypothermia develops, the body responds by decreasing heat loss through vasoconstriction and by increasing heat production through shivering.

Blood Pressure Regulation: The normal systolic and diastolic pressures in adults range between 100 to 120 mmHg and 60 to 80 mmHg respectively. Sudden rise or fall in pressure initiates many neural and humoral mechanisms to restore blood pressure within the normal range (for details, refer 'Regulation of blood pressure').

Regulation of Hormone Secretion: Secretion of many hormones such as thyroxine, cortisol etc. from their respective endocrine tissues is regulated mainly by negative feedback mechanisms. Increase in hormone concentration in plasma inhibits their production and decrease in concentration facilitates their secretion mainly by altering the synthesis of their regulating trophic hormones. This forms the physiological basis of diagnosis of these hormonal disorders.

Intracellular Homeostasis

Though, traditionally homeostasis (constancy of internal environment) refers to the stability of extracellular fluid volume and composition, it is also applicable to intracellular fluid and intracellular conditions. Rather, the primary objective of homeostasis is to maintain intracellular homeostasis that promotes cell or tissue or organ functions.

- Homeostasis is greatly affected by intracellular activities. For example, pH homeostasis, temperature homeostasis, Na^+ homeostasis, K^+ homeostasis etc. depend mainly on intracellular enzyme activities and cell metabolism.
- Similarly, intracellular milieu is largely influenced by changes in the ECF volume and composition.

Hence, homeostasis is achieved primarily by the coordinated and balanced interaction between intracellular and extracellular environments of the body.

Exam Questions

1. Describe the feedback mechanisms of homeostatic regulations and give examples for each.
2. With help of an example, explain the positive feedback mechanism.

Multiple Choice Questions

1. **Which of the following is NOT true about the painting "The Great Lady Anatomy"?**
   A. The painting is more than 600 years old
   B. It is considered the first scientific picture of human stucture
   C. It is the picture of a lady named Anatomy
   D. Was painted by Leonardo da Vinci

2. **The number of cells present in human body are about**
   A. 100 trillion
   B. 100 billion
   C. 10 billion
   D. 10 trillion

3. **The biggest organ of the human body is**
   A. Interstitium
   B. Stomach
   C. Mesentery
   D. Liver

4. **Temperature regulation is the most important function of**
   A. Cardiovascular system
   B. Excretory system
   C. Endocrine system
   D. Intgumental system

5. **Which of the following scientists coined the term 'Homeostasis'?**
   A. E H Starling
   B. Claude Bernard
   C. W. B. Canon
   D. William Harvey

6. **All of the following are examples of positive feedback control system EXCEPT**
   A. LH surge during menstrual cycle
   B. Na^+ entry through leaky sodium channels
   C. Activation of clotting factors
   D. Uterine contraction by oxytocin during parturition

Answers

1. C **2. A** **3. A** **4. D** **5. C** **6. B**

Chapter 3

Cell and its Functions, Intercellular Connections, Physiology of Genetics, and Apoptosis

Learning Objectives

On completion of study of this chapter:

The student will be able to (must know):

1. Illustrate the structure of cell membrane and list the functions of cell membrane.
2. Briefly describe the structure and functions of various cell organelles and the nucleus.
3. Name various cytoskeletons and molecular motors & give their functions.
4. Classify intercellular junctions and give their functions.
5. Briefly explain the importance of gap junction in health and disease.
6. Classify cell adhesion molecules and give their functions.
7. Appreciate the application of genetics in physiology.
8. Understand the physiology and importance of apoptosis.

The student may also be able to (desirable to know):

1. Explain the basic principles of genetics, chromosomal disorders, and functions of DNA & RNA.
2. Understand the basic principles of recombinant DNA technology, polymerase chain reaction and blotting techniques.
3. Learn the genetic basis of cancer and principle of gene therapy.
4. Explain the mechanism of apoptosis.

PY1.1

CELL AND ITS FUNCTIONS

The cell is the structural and functional unit of tissues. A cell consists of three fundamental structures: cell membrane, cytoplasm containing organelles, and the nucleus (Fig. 3.1).

1. The *cell membrane* or the plasma membrane is the boundary in all animal cells that surrounds the cytoplasm.
2. The *cytoplasm* contains organelles. The **organelles** in animal cells are mitochondria, ribosome, peroxisome, lysosomes, centrioles, endoplasmic reticulum and Golgi apparatus. Cytoplasm also contains **filamentous cytoskeletal structures** such as microfilaments, intermediate filaments and microtubules.
3. The *nucleus* is present at the center of the cell.

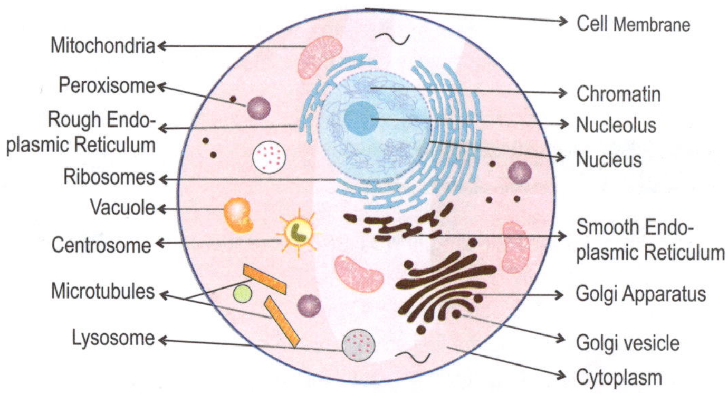

Fig. 3.1: Structure of a cell

Cell Membrane

Structure of Cell Membrane

The cell membrane is basically a double layer of lipid molecules having thickness of 7–10 nm, into which are inserted or attached various protein molecules (Fig. 3.2). Lipids constitute about 42% of the dry weight of the membrane, protein constitutes 55% and carbohydrate constitutes 3%.

Fluid-Mosaic Model of Membrane

The widely accepted membrane model is the *Fluid-Mosaic Model* described by **Singer and Nicolson in 1972**. According to this model:

1. Cell membrane consists of a double layer of phospholipid that contains protein molecules.
2. The model is called fluid mosaic model as the membrane **lipids are present in the fluid form** that allows the

flexibility of the membrane without disturbing the structural integrity.

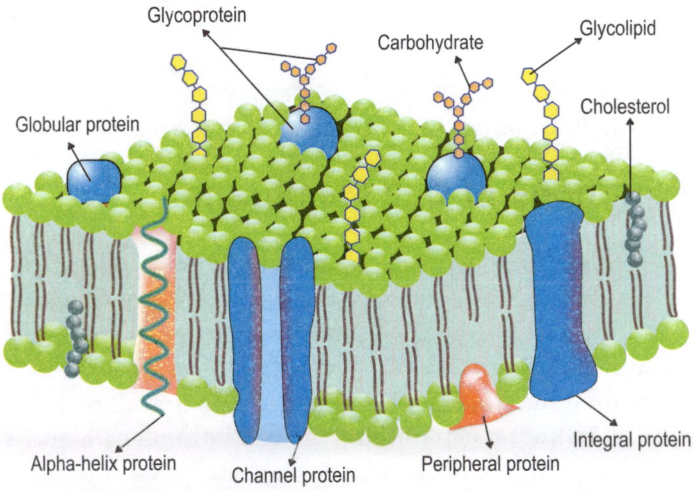

Fig. 3.2: Structure of cell membrane.

3. The membrane proteins are loosely attached and float in the fluid phospholipid bilayer.
4. Translational diffusion: This is the rapid and random redistribution (diffusion) of protein and phospholipid molecules that occurs within the plane of the membrane.
   - This occurs rapidly for phospholipids, which can move several micrometers per second.
   - The fluidity of the membrane is mainly dependent on the lipid composition of the membrane.

Lipid Bilayer

The major lipids in the cell membrane are phospholipids, glycolipids and cholesterol.

1. The **phospholipids** are phosphatidylcholine, sphingomyelin, phosphatidylserine and phosphatidyl-ethanolamine.
2. **Glycolipids** are generally found in the outer layer.
3. **Cholesterol** is incorporated into the hydrophobic regions of the membrane, and serves to reinforce the lipid permeability barrier.

IMPORTANT NOTE

The fluidity of cell membrane depends on its cholesterol-phospholipid ratio.

- In eukaryotes, this ratio is about 1:1.
- Higher cholesterol content reduces the fluidity of the membrane.
- Phospholipid molecules can move freely within the specific layer, but not from one layer to another..

Amphipathic nature of lipids: Lipids are *amphipathic* ('amphi' means both) molecules as their head or polar region is hydrophilic and tail or nonpolar region is hydrophobic. Hydrophobic tail ends are directed towards the center and the hydrophilic head is located to periphery of the membrane. Thus, hydrophilic head of lipid molecules faces the aqueous phase from both inside and outside the cell.

Functions of the Lipid Bilayer

The main function of the lipid bilayer of a cell membrane is to create a **permeability barrier** between the interstitial fluid and the cytoplasm.

- The permeability of a substance depends on whether it is lipid-soluble or water-soluble.
- Lipid soluble substances like oxygen and alcohol can pass easily through the cell membrane, whereas water soluble substances like urea and glucose can not pass easily.
- Thus, lipid bilayer makes the membrane semipermeable.

Membrane Proteins

The protein content of membrane is 50–60% of the membrane mass.

IMPORTANT NOTE

The protein content of biological membrane depends on the function of the membrane.

- In the Schwann cell, the cell membrane is concerned with insulating the nerve axon, which is mainly the function of lipids. Therefore, protein constitutes less than 25 per cent of the membrane.
- In membrane of mitochondria, which is involved in cell metabolism, 75 per cent of the membrane is protein..

Membrane proteins are of two types: integral proteins and peripheral proteins (Fig. 3.3).

Integral Proteins

Membrane proteins that span the entire thickness of the membrane are known as integral proteins or **transmembrane proteins**. The functions are as follows:

1. Channel proteins: **Channels or pores** are integral proteins through which water-soluble substances like glucose and electrolytes can diffuse across the cell membrane.
2. Carriers: Carrier proteins transport substances through cell membrane by **facilitated diffusion**; for example transport of glucose through glucose transporter.
3. Ion pumps: Membrane proteins serve as pumps for active transport of ions across the membrane; for example **Na^+–K^+ ATPase** that pumps K^+ into the cell and Na^+ out of the cell against their concentration gradient.
4. Receptor and enzyme proteins: Integral proteins that are present towards the outer half of the membrane usually serve as receptors and usually those on

the inner half serve as enzymes. G protein coupled receptors belong to this category of proteins.

5. **Antigenic functions:** Complex membrane proteins such as *glycoproteins* act as antigens on the surface of the cell; for example **blood group antigens** in the membrane of red cells.

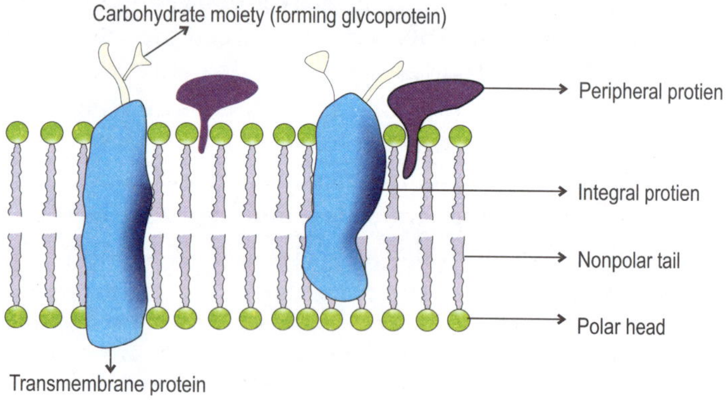

Fig. 3.3: Arrangement of proteins in the membrane.

Peripheral Proteins

Protein molecules are inserted lightly in the outer or inner border of the membrane or just bound to the surface of the membrane, are called peripheral proteins.

They are of **two types**: intrinsic and extrinsic proteins.

Intrinsic Proteins: They are present on *inner surface of the membrane*. They usually serve as **enzymes or anchor proteins** for cytoskeleton and other microfilaments that maintain cell shape.

Extrinsic Proteins: They are present on the *outer surface of the membrane*.

- They serve as **cell adhesion molecules** for anchoring cells with basal lamina and with neighboring cells.
- They can be removed without disrupting the membrane.

Membrane Carbohydrates

On the external surface of the cell membrane is loosely covered by a carbohydrate layer known as the cell coat or **glycocalyx**.

- These carbohydrates are usually ***oligosaccharides*** that are covalently linked to membrane proteins forming **glycoproteins** or lipids forming **glycolipids**.
- Some are also polysaccharide chains of proteoglycans, the integral membrane protein.

Thus, the outer surface of the lipid bilayer is covered by a layer of glycoproteins and glycolipids.

Functions of the Glycocalyx

1. Glycocalyx serves as a protective coat. Carbohydrate is negatively charged and therefore prevents negative particles like protein molecules to interact between cells.
2. Some of the transmembrane glycoproteins like selectins recognize and bind with specific oligosaccharides on other cell membranes, and therefore, permit temporary cell-to-cell adhesion. Such temporary adhesion occurs between neutrophils and endothelial cells at the site of inflammation. Stronger adhesion between cells is formed by integral membrane proteins such as integrins.
3. Some carbohydrate molecules serve as receptors.

Functions of Cell Membrane

1. Cell membrane maintains a constant and distinctive **intracellular environment**, which is essential for functioning of the organelles. For example, the intracellular fluid has lower concentration of sodium and chloride, low pH, but higher concentration of potassium, organic phosphates and magnesium.
2. Cell membrane **maintains the cell volume** by actively transferring ions across it, especially by pumping sodium ions out of the cell.
3. In neurons and muscle cells, it **maintains a potential difference** between intracellular and extracellular surfaces, which enables cells to respond to various stimuli.
4. Cell membrane helps in **recognizing foreign cells or antigens** so that they can be destroyed by phagocytes.

Cell Organelles

Mitochondria

Mitochondria are the 'power house' of the cell. They are abundant in cells that have high rate of metabolism such as in liver, cardiac muscle etc.

Structure

Mitochondria consist of two important components: **membranes and matrix.**

Mitochondrial Membranes: Mitochondrion has two layers of membranes: the outer and inner membranes.

- The inner membrane is folded into multiple incomplete septa like structures called **cristae** (Fig. 3.4). Cristae are rich in many enzymes like cytochromes b, C_1, C, a and a_3, NADH dehydrogenase, succinate dehydrogenase, electron transferring flavoproteins, carnitine-palmitoyl transferase etc.
- **Number of cristae** is more in resting state of mitochondrion, but ***decreases with activity***, hence less in the respiring state.

Mitochondrial Matrix: The region enclosed by the inner membrane is called matrix.

- An amorphous material fills the matrix, which contains enzymes involved in the Kreb's citric acid cycle and fatty acid oxidation (Table 3.1).
- Matrix also contains several strands of DNA, ribosomes and enzymes for synthesis of proteins coded by the mitochondrial genome.

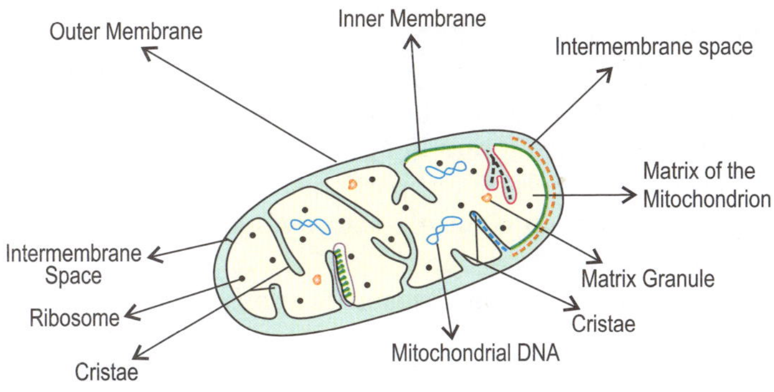

Fig. 3.4: Structure of mitochondria

Table 3.1 | Important mitochondrial enzymes.

A. Membrane enzymes
I. Enzymes of outer membrane
1. Cytochrome b_5 and b_5 reductase
2. Fatty acyl coA synthase
3. Phospholipase A
II. Enzymes of inner membrane
1. Cytochrome b, C1, C, a and a3
2. NADH & succinate dehydrogenases
3. β-OH-butyrate dehydrogenase
4. Carnitine-palmitoyl transferase
B. Enzymes in inter-membrane space
1. Adenylate kinase
2. Nucleoside diphosphokinase
3. Sulfite oxidase
C. Enzymes in the matrix
1. Pyruvate dehydrogenase complex
2. Citrate synthase
3. Isocitrate & malte dehydrogenases
4 Fatty acid oxidation system
5. Ornithine transcarbamoylase
6. α-oxoglutarate dehydrogenase

Functions

1. The inner membrane contains the **cytochromes** of the electron transport system and the associated **enzymes for oxidative phosphorylation**.
2. The **TCA cycle** takes place in the matrix.

- The initial breakdown of proteins, carbohydrates and fats occurs in the cytoplasm of the cell, and the end products that enter mitochondria as acetyl-CoA combines with oxaloacetate to from **citric acid**.
- The end products of the citric acid cycle (**Kreb's cycle**) are CO_2, H_2O and ATP.
- Thus, formation of ATP is the main function of mitochondria.

Clinical Aspects

The disease that affects mitochondrial energy transduction is called ***Luft's Disease***. Mitochondria are also damaged by free radicals (oxidative aging) and age-related other degenerations.

IMPORTANT NOTE

Mitochondria have a short lifespan and are constantly renewed. As they have strands of DNA they are capable of self-replication as well as protein synthesis.

Endoplasmic Reticulum

The endoplasmic reticulum (ER) consists of a network of anastomosing membranous **tubules**, **vesicles**, and flattened **cisternae** (Fig. 3.5).

- The membranes of ER are continuous with the outer membrane of nucleus and are also connected with Golgi apparatus.
- ER is the site of the **synthesis of proteins and lipids** for the membrane of the cell and organelles, and **secretory vesicles** of the cytoplasm.
  They are of **two types**: rough ER and the smooth ER.

Rough Endoplasmic Reticulum

When surface of ER is studded with ribosome, the organelle is called rough ER (RER) or **granular ER** as it gives a 'rough' or 'granular' appearance to it.

- RER are present in more number in cells that are *actively involved in protein synthesis* like acinar cells of pancreas and neurons.
- In neurons, **Nissl garanules** are modified RER.

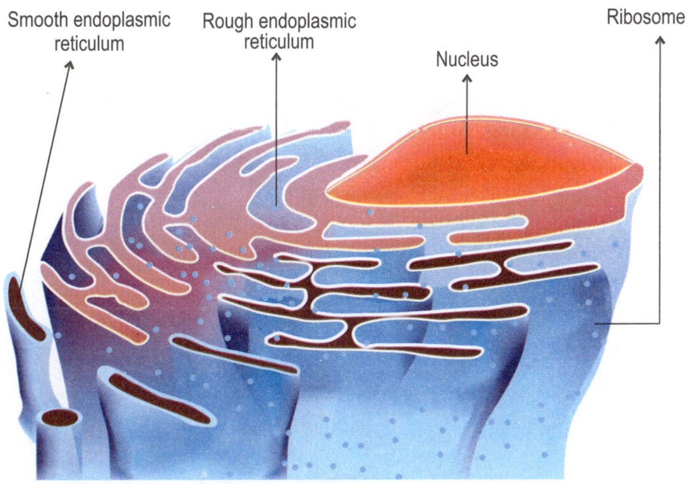

Fig. 3.5: Endoplasmic reticulum. Note the presence of ribosome on the surface of rough ER.

Functions of RER:

1. It is concerned with **protein synthesis**. Therefore, it is abundant in cells of endocrine glands and cells secreting digestive enzymes.
2. It also plays some role in **glycosylation**, i.e., conjugation of carbohydrates with proteins to form glycoproteins, a function which it shares with the Golgi apparatus.

Smooth Endoplasmic Reticulum

When ribosomes are not attached to the surface of ER, the organelle is called smooth ER (SER) or **agranular ER** as its surface has 'smooth' or 'agranular' appearance.

Functions of SER:

1. It is concerned with the **synthesis of lipids**. Hence it is abundant in cells that synthesize cholesterol, steroid hormones and phospholipids.
2. In muscles, it is called **sarcoplasmic reticulum**, which is specialized for the ***storage of calcium ions*** that is released during excitation-contraction coupling.
3. SER is part of **intracellular transport system** as it is continuous with the RER and Golgi apparatus.
4. It is also the site for the **detoxification or neutralization** of hormones and toxic substances.

Golgi Apparatus

The Golgi apparatus (GA) is also known as **dyctyosome**. It is present in all cells and generally located close to the nucleus.

It appears as flat vesicles that are dilated peripherally and stacked together in a bunch as **stacks of cisternae**.

Anatomically and functionally it is closely associated with endoplasmic reticulum.

Functionally GA has two main regions: *cis* and *trans*. The region nearer to the nucleus is the cis face (***cis Golgi***) and the region close to the membrane is the trans face (***trans Golgi***) (Fig. 3.6).

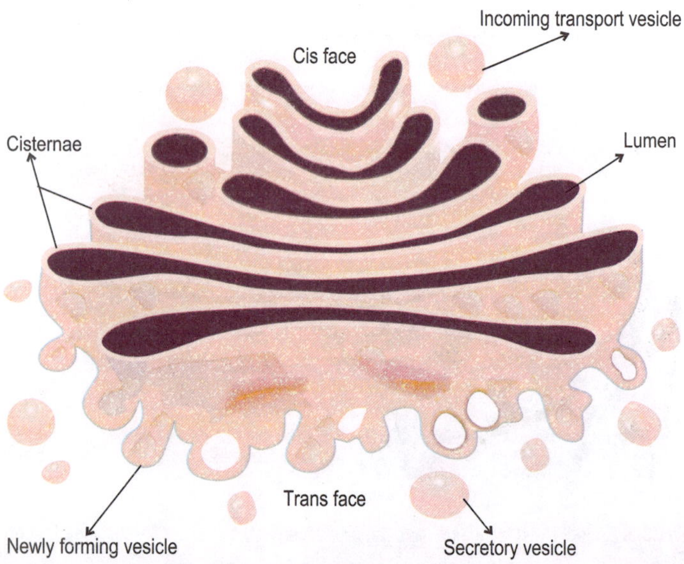

Fig. 3.6: Golgi apparatus. Note the cis-face and trans-face.

Major functions of GA:

1. It is the **site for packaging** of secretory products into the ***secretory granules***.
2. It is the site for the **incorporation of carbohydrates** into the newly synthesized proteins to form ***glycoproteins***.
3. **Primary lysosomes are formed** in GA.
4. **Transports material** to other organelles and cell surface.

Lysosomes

Lysosomes are membrane-bound spherical organelles that contain a variety of **hydrolytic enzymes** meant for intracytoplasmic digestion. More than 40 different lysosomal enzymes (lysozymes) have been isolated. Some important lysozymes are listed in Table 3.2.

- Lysosomes are found in almost all animal cells except erythrocytes. They are particularly abundant in **cells having high phagocytic activity** such as neutrophils and monocytes.
- In granulocytes, the lysosomes appear as **cytoplasmic granules**.
- During phagocytosis, the phagosome containing bacteria, viruses etc. fuse with the lysosomes and lysosomal enzymes digest these foreign organisms. Therefore, lysosomes are known as ***autophagosomes***.

Lysosomal enzymes function best in acidic pH: The pH interior of lysosome is about 5, compared to outside pH 7.2 of cell cytoplasm. This is due to **H^+-ATPase**, the proton pump present on the lysosomal membrane that pumps protons (H^+) from cytosol into the lysosomal interior against its electrochemical gradient. The lysosomal enzymes are **acid hydolases** as they function best in acidic pH.

IMPORTANT NOTE

Acid phosphatase is used as a marker for lysosomal activity.

Table 3.2 | Important lysosomal enzymes.

A. Proteolytic enzymes
1. Cathepsins (proteinases)
2. Collagenases
3. Elastase
B. Lipolytic enzymes
1. Lipases & phospholipases
2. Fatty acyl esterases
C. Carbohydrate splitting enzymes
1. α-glycosidase
2. β-galactosidase
3. Hyaluronidase
4. Aryl sulphatase
D. Nucleic acid hydrolyzing enzymes
1. Ribonuclease & deoxyribonuclease
E. Other enzymes
1. Acid phosphatases
2. Catalase

Types of Lysosomes

There are **three forms of lysosomes**: primary lysosomes, secondary lysosomes and residual bodies.

Primary Lysosomes: They are formed with hydrolytic enzymes synthesized by rough endoplasmic reticulum and packaged in the Golgi apparatus. They are generally referred to as **storage vacuoles**.

Secondary Lysosomes: They are formed by fusion of lysosomes with endosomes, hence called **endolysosomes**.

Tertiary Lysosomes: They are formed by fusion of **autophagic vacuoles** with primary lysosomes, hence called **phagolysosomes**.

IMPORTANT NOTE

Residual Bodies: The undigested remnants in the lysosomes are called as residual bodies. They are excreted by exocytosis.

Functions of Lysosome

1. **Digestive organelle:** Lysosomes contain many enzymes essential for **intracellular digestions**.
2. **Bactericidal:** Lysosomes **kill and remove infective organisms** and foreign bodies.
3. **Fertilization of ovum:** **Acrosome,** located on the head of spermatozoa is a specialized lysosome that contains many hydrolytic enzymes. Acrosome plays an important role in **penetration of ovum by sperm**.
4. **Autolysis:** When a cell is damaged or ruptured, the enzymes liberated within the cytoplasm digest the cytoplasmic contents, a process known as *autolysis*. The autolytic enzymes are mainly lysosomal enzymes.
5. **Housekeeping:** Lysosomes remove intracellular products of metabolism from the cell (Clinical Note 3.1.)

Clinical Note 3.1

Lysosomal storage diseases: Congenital absence of lysosomal enzymes leads to accumulation of materials in the lysosome causing lysosomal storage diseases (Table 3.3).

Table 3.3 | Common lysosomal storage diseases.

Disease	Enzyme deficiency	Unique features
Fabry disease	α-galactosidase A	Cutaneous angiokeratomas and hypohydrosis.
Gaucher disease	Acid β-glucosidase	Hepatosplenomegaly, and skeletal dysplasia.
Niemann-Pick disease	Sphingomyelinase	Mental retardation, seizures, lung failure.
Tay-Sachs disease	β-hexaminidase A	Mental retardation, macrocephaly and hypercusis in infants.
Hurler disease	α-L-iduronidase	Mental retardation, coarse facies, CVS involvement.
Pompe disease	Acid α-glucosidase	Myocardiopathy

Ribosomes

Though ribosomes are usually present on the **surface of endoplasmic reticulum**, they are also present as free organelles in the cytoplasm.

- They contain about 85% of RNA of the cell.
- They are the major site of protein synthesis.

RNA is also present in nucleus, mitochondria and cytoplasm, and consequently protein synthesis occurs in these structures too.

Peroxisomes

Peroxisomes are small spherical organelles having diameter of about 0.5μ, and therefore denoted as **microbodies**. They are formed by budding or by division of smooth endoplasmic reticulum.

- They are referred to as **subcellular respiratory organelles**. But they do not have energy-coupled electron transport system.
- They contain **oxidases** that promote ***oxidation of lipids*** (especially omega-oxidation of long chain fatty acids) forming acetyl coA and hydrogen peroxide (H_2O_2), and **catalases** that liberate oxygen from H_2O_2.
- With the help of **peroxins**, the protein chaperons, various proteins with specific signal sequence are directed to peroxisome.
- The membrane of peroxisome contains a number of **specific proteins that transport substances** between peroxisome matrix and cytosol.
- Peroxisome matrix contains **more than 50 enzymes** that are involved in many metabolic reactions of lipids (long chain fatty acids, plasmalogen, cholesterol, bile acids) purines, amino acids and H_2O_2 (Application Box 3.1).

PPA Receptors: Proliferation of peroxisome is caused by many synthetic products that act on receptors in the nuclei of cells, known as **peroxisome proliferation activated receptors** (PPARs).

Application Box 3.1

Peroxisomes protect from oxidative stress (OS): H_2O_2, a potent oxidant produced during metabolic reactions is one of the agents for oxidative stress. H_2O_2 is destroyed by catalase, a peroxisomal enzyme, which is designated as an antioxidant for combating OS. Thus, peroxisomes protect cells from the toxic effects H2O2. Hence, Increased catalase activity is one of the markers of OS.

- PPARs are members of nuclear receptor superfamily. On activation they bind to DNA and produce changes in mRNA production.
- PPARs have extensive physiologic effects and affect many tissues and organs.

Diseases of Peroxisomes

Zellweger syndrome: Peroxisomes may be abnormal or absent, which occurs due to mutations in the gene encoding peroxins or peroxisomal enzymes. It is characterized by profound **neurologic impairment**, accumulation of very-long chain fatty acids, abnormalities in synthesis of bile acids and **marked reduction of plasmalogens**. The child usually dies within a year.

Infantile Refsum disease: Another similar genetic disorder is **infantile Refsum disease**, which is less severe and only few proteins are affected.

Centrosomes

Centrosome is located close to the nucleus in eukaryotic animal cells. It is formed by two **centrioles** placed at right angle to each other that are present within the amorphous pericentriolar material.

Centrioles: Centrioles are short cylindrical structures made up of **microtubules placed in group of three** (triplets) that run longitudinally in the wall of centrioles.

- There are **nine sets of triplets** arranged at regular intervals in the wall of each centriole.
- The subunits of microtubules in centrosome are **γ-tubulins**.
- Centrosomes are *microtubule-organizing center* (MTOCs).

Functions

Centrosomes regulate chromosome movement during cell division. They duplicate themselves and move apart from each other to the poles of mitotic spindle to monitor the process of cell division.

Cytoskeleton

Cytoskeleton is an intracellular system of fibers that not only maintains the structural integrity of the cell, but also allows appropriate change in cell shape for cell mobility and participation of cell in various physiological activities. It consists of **microfilaments, microtubules and intermediate filaments**.

These cytoskeletal elements are made up of different cell proteins (Table 3.4).

Table 3.4 | Protein subunit and diameter of cytoskeletal elements of cell.

	Microfilament	Intermediate filament	Microtubule
1. Shape	Double stranded helical arrangement	Tubular hollow	Long, non-branching
2. Diameter	7 nm	10 nm	25 nm
3. Basic protein units	Actin	Various proteins	Tubulin
4. Location in cell	Forms a network adjacent to cell Core of microvilli Contractile elements of muscle	Extend across cytoplasm connecting desmosome and hemidesmosome The nuclear lamina In skin epithelium as keratin	Mitotic spindle Core of cilia
5. Major functions	Essential element of contractile element of muscles	Provide mechanical strength and link cells together	Provides network for movement of organelles, Movement of cilia

Microfilaments

Microfilaments are long solid filaments (Fig. 3.7A) having diameter of about 7 nm. They are made up of **actin**.

- Actin is the **most common cell protein** that accounts for about 15% of total protein in the cells.
- Actin in the globular form is called **G actin**, which is the unpolymerized actin subunit.
- G actin subunits polymerize to form the filamentous actin, referred to as **F actin**.
- In vivo, actin filaments polymerize and depolymerize.

In **cells with microvilli** on their epithelial surface, microfilaments extend into the microvilli.

Functions

1. Microfilaments are the major **contractile fibers** of the cell that help in **change of cell shape and cell movement**.
2. As microfilaments exhibit **contractile phenomena** within the cytoplasm, they help in ***phagocytosis, transport and secretion*** of cellular materials, cell contraction, **cell discharge**, movement of secretory granules etc. For example, in platelets they facilitate release reaction (**platelet release**).
3. Filamentous actin helps in **movement of chromosome and cell division**.
4. Through *anchoring proteins*, F actin fibers attach to various cytoskeletal structures and interact with membrane bound proteins.
5. Microfilaments project into the microvilli present on the epithelial surface such as on the intestinal mucosa, and extend up to the tip of microvilli. They help in **microvilli movement**.
6. Microfilaments in the **lamellopodia** (lamellar extensions from cell that occur at the time of cell crawling) help in *cell movement on a surface*.
7. Actin filament interacts with **integrin receptors** to form ***focal adhesion complexes (FAC)***. FAC serve as **points of traction** with the surface over which cell pulls itself.
8. Microfilaments are also used by some molecular motors as tracks.

Microtubules

Microtubules are **long hollow tubular structures** (Fig. 3.7B) having diameter of about 25 nm, including the wall thickness. The inner cavity diameter of microtubules is about 15 nm. They are made up of subunits of globular proteins called **tubulins** that are arranged in a closely packed helical manner.

- Tubulins in microtubules are of two types: **α-tubulin** and **β-tubulin**, except the tubulins in centrioles that are γ-tubulins.
- The α and β-tubulin subunits form heterodimers that aggregate to make tubular structures of stacked rings.
- Each ring in microtubule usually contains **13 subunits**.

Disassembly and Assembly: A unique property of tubulin subunits is their property of *disaggregating (disassembly)* and *re-aggregating (assembly)*. Therefore, microtubules form a dynamic cytoskeletal framework of the cell. The process of assembly and disassembly may occur simultaneously.

- Interaction with GTP facilitates microtubule formation.
- Microtubule growth is **temperature sensitive** with cold conditions favoring disassembly.

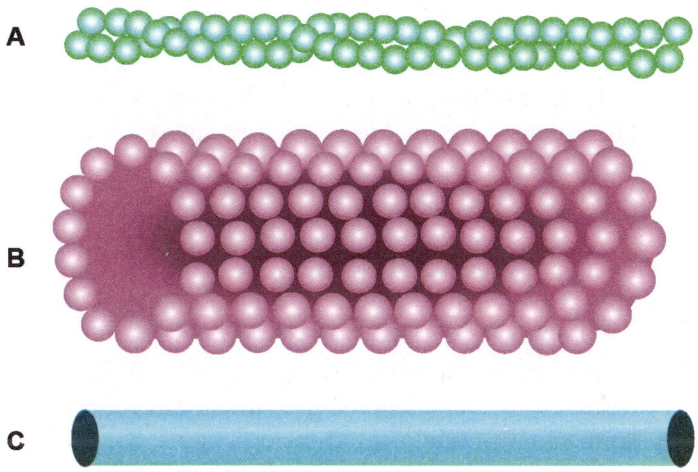

Fig. 3.7: Microfilament (A), Microtubule (B), and Intermediate filament (C).

- Many drugs act by inhibiting microtubule assembly (Clinical Note 3.2).

Clinical Note 3.2

Cytotoxic drugs act by inhibiting microtubular functions: Cancer chemotherapeutic agents such as vincristine and vinblastine promote disassembly of microtubules. Paclitaxel, another anticancer drug binds with microtubules and stabilize them against depolymerization, prevent formation of mitotic spindles and cells die. Colchicine inhibits microtubule assembly.

In cells with cilia and flagella, microtubules extend into these structures. Kinesin and dynein are microtubule-based molecular motors.

Functions

1. Microtubules serve as **cytosolic guide rails** for transport of substances within the cytoplasm or transport of secretory granules to the cell membrane. They help in transport of vesicles and organelles from one part of the cell to another.
2. They contribute to the maintenance of **cell strength and cell shape**.
3. They help in the **formation of spindles** that move chromosomes during mitotic cell division.
4. They are the pillars for structure and **function of cilia**.
5. They contribute to **cell motility**.

Cilia: Cilia beat in a synchronous whip-like fashion and allow a directional flow. Each cilium is an outgrowth of a basal body situated beneath the cell membrane, which has the property of reproducing itself.

- In each cilium, there is an **axoneme** that typically consists of ***nine doublets of microtubules*** that run circumferentially from base to the tip while a single pair of microtubules runs centrally (9+2 arrangement).
- All microtubules in cilia are linked together by protein cross-linkages that form the axoneme.
- In cilia, dyneins are present close to axoneme, called ***axonemal dyneins***.

The coordinated interaction between tubulins of axoneme and axonemal dyneins promotes ciliary movement.

Basal body is present at the base of axoneme, which has arrangement of microtubules in nine sets of triplets similar to that of arrangement in centriole.

Intermediate Filaments

These are filamentous structures made up of various subunits (Fig. 3.7C). The average diameter of these filaments varies from 8 to 14 nm.

Functions

1. They connect the nuclear membrane to the cell membrane and also membranes of cell organelles. Therefore, the major function of these filaments is to **integrate the organelles within the cytoplasm.**
2. They form supple skeletal network for the cell and **resist rupture of cell** from external pressure.
3. Intermediate filament proteins are cell markers (Clinical Note 3.3).

Clinical Note 3.3

Intermediate filament proteins are cell markers: Proteins of intermediate filaments are cell specific. Therefore, they are frequently used as cellular markers. For example, cytokreatin is the marker of epithelial cells, whereas vimentin is the marker of fibroblast.

IMPORTANT NOTE

In the absence of microfilaments, cells easily rupture. Blister formation in skin is common in humans when these filaments are absent or abnormal.

Molecular Motors

Molecular motors help in the movement of various cell parts, proteins and organelles within the cell cytoplasm. They are **100-kDa ATPases**.

- They have **two domains**: the domain that attaches with cargo (the cell part to be moved) and the other domain attaches with microtubules or actin filaments.
- The domain attaching with microtubules or actin is the head part that **contains ATPase**, which causes hydrolysis of ATP to provide *energy for movement of molecules*.

Types: Molecular motors can be broadly divided into **two categories**: microtubule-based and actin-based.

Microtubule-based Molecular Motors

Microtubule-based molecular motors make movement of molecules along the microtubules. They are mainly kinesin and dynein.

Kinesin

The conventional kinesin is a *double-headed molecule* that transports its cargo towards the negative terminal of microtubules. One head attaches with microtubule and the other head with the cargo.

- Some kinesins **move cargo** towards the positive terminal of microtubules.
- Other kinesins are involved in **cell divisions** such as mitosis and meiosis.

Dynein

Dynein is also a *double-headed molecule*. There are **two types** of dynein: cytoplasmic form and axonemal form.

Cytoplasmic Dynein: It functions like that of conventional kinesin that **moves cargo** towards the negative terminals of microtubules.

Axonemal Dynein: **Cilia and flagella** contain dynein-based molecular motors that are axonemal type. Thus, these dynein molecules are responsible for **beating of cilia and flagella**.

Actin-based Molecular Motors

Actin based molecular motors make **movement of molecules along the actin filaments**. These are mainly **myosin I – V**. However, there are 18 types of myosins.

- **In myosin II,** the head binds with actin and pulls actin by bending the neck region.
- **In myosin V,** the heads of myosin molecules walk on the microfilaments one after another.

Functions: Myosin molecules perform various functions like muscle contraction, contraction of intestinal villi, cell migration etc.

The Nucleus

Structure of Nucleus

All living cells in humans **except red blood cells** contain nuclei. Platelets are cellular fragments. Nucleus is bound by a **bilayer nuclear membrane** that surrounds the **nucleoplasm**. The nucleus contains nucleoplasm and **nucleolus**.

Nuclear Membrane

The nuclear membrane is a double-layered membrane. The space between the two membranes is called **perinuclear cisterns**. In some cells, nuclear membrane is in continuity with the membrane of endoplasmic reticulum.

- There are circular openings in the nuclear membrane known as **nuclear pores** that serve as passages for the exchange of materials between the cytoplasm and the nucleoplasm, especially for the *transport of mRNA and proteins*.
- There are two **special transport proteins** in the nuclear membrane, known as ***importins*** and ***exportins*** that regulate transport of molecules across nuclear membrane.
- Another nuclear membrane protein known as **Ran**, plays organizing role in these transport mechanisms.

Nucleoplasm

The nucleoplasm is the nuclear matrix, which is a gel like ground substance that contains genetic material in the form of DNA.

- When cell is not dividing, the genetic material is present in the form of tangled mass called **nuclear chromatin** and when cell division begins, the tangled mass unwinds and appears as distinct strands known as **chromosomes**.
- The nuclear chromatin is made up of **coiled strands of DNA**, bound to large quantities of basic proteins (histones).

Nucleolus

The nucleus contains nucleolus, a patchwork of granules **rich in RNA**. There may be multiple nucleoli in a nucleus, especially in developing cells. Nucleoli **synthesize ribosomes**.

Functions of Nucleus

Nucleus regulates cell functions.

1. It contains DNA that is responsible for transmission of hereditary traits.
2. It also contains RNA that is essential for protein synthesis.
3. Nucleus is the main regulator of cell division.

PY1.3

INTERCELLULAR JUNCTIONS

In tissues, junctions formed between the cells are called intercellular junctions or **intercellular connections**. In epithelial tissues that line the free surfaces such as skin, and basement membrane of tubular structures and cavities of the body such as alimentary tract, kidney tubules and urinary bladder, the cells are bound tightly together by specialized **intercellular junctions** (Fig. 3.8).

Types

Functionally, **intercellular junctions** or connections are of **two types**: junctions that tie cells together and Junctions that allow transfer of ions and small molecules (Table 3.5).

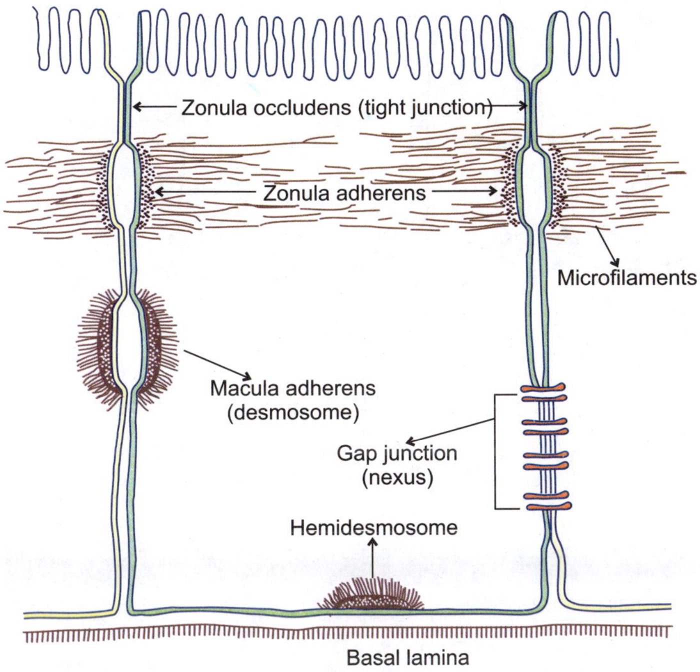

Fig. 3.8: Intercellular junctions

Table 3.5 | Intercellular junctions
A. Junctions that tie cells together
1. Tight junctions
2. Anchoring junctions
a. Cell to cell anchoring junctions
- Desmosome
- Zona adherens
b. Cell to basal lamina anchoring junctions
- Hemidesmosome
- Focal adhesion
B. Junctions that allow transfer of ions and small molecules
1. Gap junctions

Tight Junctions

Tight junctions are commonly found in the epithelium of the GI tract, nephrons, urinary tract, hepatobiliary tract, and choroid plexus. They are also called **zonula occludens**. Tight junctions are typically located towards the *apical region of the cells* (Fig. 3.8).

- At tight junctions, the outer layer of the cell membrane of neighboring cells fuses with each other that **obliterates the intercellular space** close to their apical margin.
- They are **made up of ridges**, half of which is contributed by both neighboring cells and each half is bound tightly to each other. Therefore, they practically form the **barrier for transport** of solutes and solvents from the lumen into the interstitial space and between cells.
- However, they contain ion and water channels that make them **selectively leaky**, though the degree of leakiness varies in different epithelia.

The proteins: The membrane proteins that contribute to formation of tight junctions belong to **three main families**: **occludin, claudins** and **junctional adhesion molecules** (JAMs). Many other membrane proteins from cytosolic side interact with tight junctions.

Functions of Tight Junctions

1. In general, they form **selective permeability barrier** that prevent transport of macromolecules from the luminal fluid into the interstitial space. Thus, macromolecules pass only through the epithelial cell as vesicles (vesicular transport).
2. Due to the presence of **leaky channels**, small size water-soluble particles are permitted through tight junctions. However, the degree of permeability varies.
   - For example, **in the gut**, Na^+ ions pass fairly freely, while **in the urinary bladder**, the passage for sodium is almost nil.
   - Also, the permeability of a substance through tight junctions can be increased, depending on the *osmolality gradient* across the epithelium. This forms the **paracellular transport** of solutes and solvents.
3. **In the brain**, tight junctions between endothelial cells of cerebral blood vessels contribute to the effectiveness of ***blood-brain barrier***.
4. **In the ciliary bodies**, they form ***blood-aqueous barrier*** between the cells of inner non-pigmented epithelium.

Anchoring Junctions

Anchoring junctions are of **two types**: cell to cell anchoring junctions and cell to basal lamina anchoring junctions.

Cell to Cell Anchoring Junctions

Cell to cell anchoring junctions are desmosome and zonula adherens.

Desmosomes: Desmosomes are the junctions characterized by focal thickening of two adjacent cell membranes (Fig. 3.8).

- **Intermediary filaments** from cytosol are attached to the thickened areas.
- The intercellular space between the two membrane thickenings also contains filamentous materials such as **cadherins**.
- Extracellular portions of many membrane proteins are also present in this space.

Zonula Adherens: Zonula adherens is located below the base of tight junctions (Fig. 3.8).

- It is the *major site of attachment for intracellular microfilaments*.
- Cadherins are present in the intercellular space at this junction.

Cell to Basal Lamina Anchoring Junctions

Cell to basal lamina anchoring junctions are hemidesmosome and focal adhesion.

Hemidesmosomes: In appearance, they look like *half of desmosomes*, and therefore are called hemidesmosome (Fig. 3.8).

- Microfilaments are attached to it intracellularly.
- In contrast to presence of cadherins in desmosome, hemidesmosomes contain integrins.

Focal Adhesions: Focal adhesions connect cell to the basal lamina. Intracellularly, they are associated with actin filaments. Therefore, they assist in cell movement.

Gap Junctions

Structure

Gap junctions are called **nexus** between the cells at which the intercellular space is narrowed from its 25 nm diameter to 3 nm. They are made up of special transmembrane proteins known as **connexons**. The connexons from the membrane of two adjacent cells are lined up with one another (Fig. 3.9).

- Each connexon is formed by six identical protein subunits called **connexins**.
- Connexin surrounds an aqueous channel and when connexon of adjacent cells are aligned, the aqueous channels of both cell membranes become a continuous one. This allows substances of adjacent two cells to pass though the channel without passing through the ECF.
- The diameter of the channel is about 2 nm.
- As connexons connect the cytoplasm of adjacent cells through their aqueous channels. Water, ions, amino acids, sugars and hormones can pass from cell to cell through them.

As connexons keep the adjacent cell membranes at a fixed gap, the junction is named as 'gap junctions'. Mutation occurs in the connexin genes (Clinical Note 3.4).

Clinical Note 3.4

Mutation of connexon genes: In humans, there are about 20 different genes that code for connexin proteins. Mutation of these genes results in diseases that are specific for tissues. For example, mutation of a specific connexin gene that produces Charcot-Marie-Tooth disease, exclusively affects peripheral neurons. Therefore, peripheral neuropathy is the outstanding feature of this disease.

Functions

1. **Electrical synapse:** As the pores of gap junction are larger than ligand-gated or voltage-gated channels, passage of substances is easier through them. Gap junctions easily allow ions to pass through and serve as *electrical synapses*. They permit rapid propagation of electrical activity from cell to cell. Therefore, tissues with gap junctions between cells behave as **physiological syncytium** (Application Box 3.2).
2. Gap junctions also permit **passage of organic solutes** such as sugars and amino acids with molecular weight upto 1000 from cell to cell.
3. **Chemical messengers and hormones** are also exchanged between cells through gap junctions.

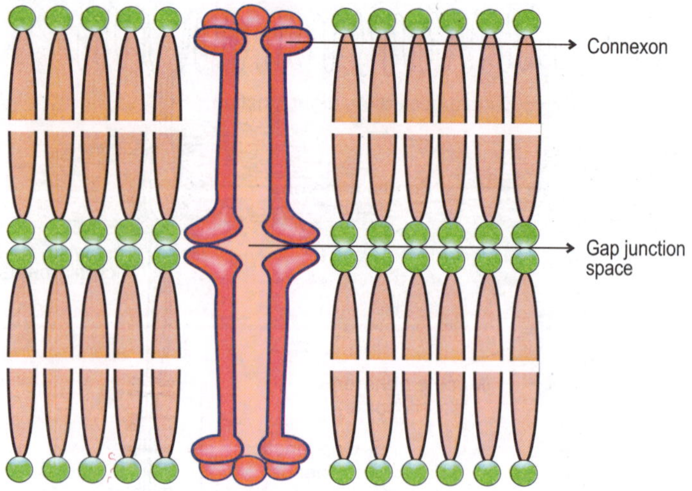

Fig. 3.9: Structure of gap junction. Note, gap junction is formed by connexons apposing on each other from adjacent cells. Each connexon is formed by six subunits of connexin that surrounds the channel.

Regulation of Gap Junction Functions

Though transports of ions through gap junctions is not an active process, their activities are regulated by **intracellular calcium** concentration and **cytosolic pH**. Increase in any of these parameters can prevent transport through gap junctions by closing their channels.

Functional syncytium: Gap junctions are present abundantly in heart muscle. As they serve as electrical synapses, electrical impulses pass easily from cell to cell in cardiac muscle. Thus, stimulation of one muscle cell in heart results in activation of all muscle cells. This makes **cardiac muscle a functional syncytium.**

- **Ventricular and atrial muscles** are *two separate syncytia* as they are separated by non-conducting septa.
- Gap junctions are also present in **visceral smooth muscles** that conduct electrical impulses from cell to cell. Hence, visceral smooth muscles also have syncytial behaviour.

Cell Adhesion Molecules

Cells are attached to each other and to the basal lamina by cell adhesion molecules (CAMs) that are present *abundantly at intercellular connections* or junctions. By their property of adhesions between the cells, they **provide stability to the tissue**.

Application Box 3.2

abundantly in heart muscle. As they serve as electrical synapses, electrical impulses pass easily from cell to cell in cardiac muscle. Thus, stimulation of one muscle cell in heart results in activation of all muscle cells. This makes cardiac muscle a functional syncytium.

Systems of Binding

They have both extracellular and intracellular bindings.

Extracellular Binding: Many of CAMs bind to membrane proteins called **laminins**.

- Laminins are cross-shaped large membrane molecules that have *multiple receptor domains* on the extracellular matrix.
- CAMs bind to these extracellular receptor domains.

Intracellular Binding: CAMs pass through the cell membrane to expose into the interior of the cell and *attach with the cytoskeleton* inside the cell. This intracellular binding of CAMs with cytoskeletal structures **enhances strength** of cell adhesions.

Nature of Binding

CAMs exhibit both homophilic and heterophilic bindings.

Homophilic Bindings: In homophilic bindings, CAMs attach with **similar molecules** present on the other cells.

Heterophilic Bindings: In heterophilic bindings, CAMs attach with **different molecules** of other cells.

Types of CAMs

Though there are confusions on classifying CAMs, they can be broadly categorized into **four varieties**: Integrins, IgG superfamily proteins, cadherins and selectins.

Integrins: Integrins are heterodimeric proteins that bind to various receptors.

IgG Superfamily Proteins: CAMs belonging to IgG superfamily are immunoglobulins.

Cadherins: These are calcium dependent molecules that mediate homophilic binding.

Selectins: They have carbohydrate binding domains that resemble lectin-like structure.

Functions of CAMs

1. They **zip cell to cell**. Cell adherence is strengthened by CAMs.
2. For their attachment with cytoskeleton, they play role in **cell movement**.
3. **Cellular signals** are transmitted out of the cell or extracellular signals are transmitted into the cell via CAMs.
4. They play significant role in **inflammation and wound healing**.
5. CAMs **prevent apoptosis**.

PY1.9

PHYSIOLOGY OF GENETICS

Mendel's work in 1886 that hereditary characteristics are transmitted to offsprings by separate units laid the foundation of genetics. Later, Johannied, the Danish botanist in 1909 termed these units as genes and, Morgan the American geneticist established that the hereditary characteristics are transmitted on chromosomes.

IMPORTANT NOTE

Loss of cellular contact from extracellular matrix due to defects in CAMs **hastens the process of apoptosis.**

Significant contribution of Scientist

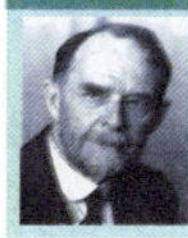

Thomas Hunt Morgan (Nobel Prize in Physiology' 1933)
The Nobel Prize was awarded to T. H. Morgan for his discoveries concerning the role played by the chromosome in heredity.

Chromosomes

The term chromosome was coined by Waldeyer in 1888. Chromosomes transmit the genetic information from parents to offspring.

- There are **46 chromosomes** in cells of all tissues *except gametes* that contain 23 chromosomes. Autosomes are present in somatic cells and sex chromosomes in gametes.
- Each chromosome consists of **two chromatids** that are connected at the **centromeres**. Each chromatid is composed of **two chromonemes.**
- Though chromosomes are formed mainly by DNA, they also contain RNA, the basic protein histones, complex proteins, organic phosphorous compounds and inorganic salts.

The DNA

Deoxyribonucleic acid (DNA) is found in bacteria, and mitochondria and nuclei of all eukaryotic cells. DNA is the component of chromosome.

- **Chromosomes** are made up of a *mammoth molecule of DNA*, which is about 2 m in length. However, DNA is accommodated in the nucleus as most part of it at intervals is *wrapped around histone proteins* to form **nucleosomes.**
- About **25 millions of nucleosomes** are present in a nucleus.
- The complex of DNA and the histone protein is called **chromatin.**
- As cell division begins, acetylation of histone loosens the coiling and pairs of chromosomes become visible.

Functions of DNA

1. DNA as part of chromosome **transmits genetic characteristics** (hereditary features) from generations to generations.
2. It possesses information required for the **synthesis of RNA and cell proteins** (including enzymes).
3. It controls **cell division.**

The Genome

Each chromosome contains only one type of long-chain DNA molecule. DNA is the component of chromosome that carries the *genetic message* (blueprint of heritable characteristics) of the cell. The total genetic information stored in chromosomes of a cell is known as **the genome.**

- The human genome contains about **3 billion nucleotide pairs**, and in diploid cells they are organized into 23 pairs of chromosomes (all cells of the body except the gametes).

- In each pair, one is derived from the mother and the other from the father. However, in males, the *X* chromosome is inherited from the mother, and the *Y* chromosome from the father.
- The *X* and *Y* chromosome are concerned with the determination of sex, and therefore they are called **sex chromosomes**.
- The *XX* are necessary for development of the female and *XY* pair is necessary for development of the male.
- Gametes (sperm and ovum) have half this number of chromosomes, and therefore are said to be haploid cells. During fertilization of an ovum by a sperm, the diploid number is restored, so that each cell carries 23 chromosomes from each parent.

The Genes

The gene is the functional unit of DNA. A gene is defined as the portion of DNA responsible for the **production of a single RNA molecule**.

- Each chromosome contains myriad of genes. The genes do not exercise their powers all the time. The inherent control mechanisms are such that only selected genes are switched on at any given time.
- Though, the DNA of each cell in a multicellular organism has same DNA sequence and same genetic capabilities, the difference between different cell types lies in the differences in genetic expression.

Gene Expression

The genetic expression of each cell type is selective, and therefore, the protein synthesis is different in different tissues. Genetic expression occurs in **two broad steps**: transcription and translation (Flowchart. 3.1).

Transcription

Transcription is the process in which **RNA is synthesized from DNA**. In this process, the genetic information stored in DNA is transferred to the RNA.

- During the process of formation of RNA, the relevant part of the DNA double helix unwinds and exposes the gene unit, which is then copied.
- The DNA strand that directs the synthesis of mRNA through complementary base pairing is called **template strand** (also called, coding strand or sense strand) and the other DNA strand is called **noncoding strand** or antisense strand.
- The enzyme *RNA polymerase* carries out transcription by binding to a site on DNA called **promoter site**.

Translation

This is the process by which genetic message transferred to mRNA from DNA is **converted into polypeptide chain** containing *specific sequence of amino acids*.

- The mRNA is processed from the primary RNA transcript; the process known as maturation in which introns (non coding sequences) are cut and released while joining the two adjacent exons (coding sequences).
- Each gene unit is organized into **three components**: regulatory DNA sequences (named repressor, promoter and operator), exons and introns. Only the exons and introns contain the *genetic code*.

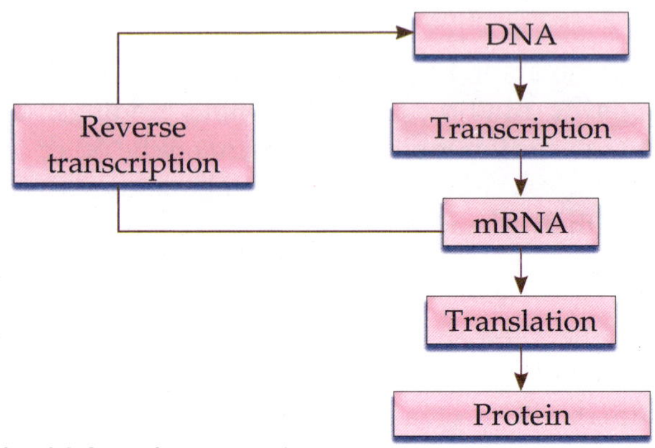

Flowchart 3.1: Steps of gene expression

Steps of Protein Synthesis

Protein synthesis occurs in **three major steps**.

1. **Amino acid activation:** In the presence of enzyme aminoacyl tRNA synthase, amino acids react with ATP, get activated and get attached to specific tRNA.
2. **Translation:** Translation occurs in three steps such as *initiation* (translation of mRNA with formation of initiation complex), *elongation* (elongation of polypeptide chain by sequential addition of amino acids to the growing end) and *termination* (termination of polypeptide synthesis evoked by nonsense codon).
3. **Post-translational modification:** Post-translational modifications such as proteolytic degradation, hydroxylation, glycosylation etc. make the protein more functional.

Regulation of Gene Expression

Gene expression is regulated by following mechanisms.

1. **Gene amplification:** Enhancement of gene expression can cause drug resistance. For example, amplification of the gene coding for dihydrofolate reductase causes development of drug resistance by cancer cells to chronic administration of methotrexate.
2. **Gene rearrangement:** This enhances the generation of antigen specific immunoglobulins.
3. **Regulation through transcription factors:** Transcription factors regulate interaction of protein with specific segments of DNA.
4. **Regulation through mRNA:** Modification of mRNA activity is the major mechanism of regulation of gene expression.

The RNA

Ribonucleic acid is a single chain made of several polynucleotides (polymer of ribonucleotides). Unlike DNA, which is double stranded, the RNA is a **single strand**. RNA is present in the nucleus, cytoplasm, ribosomes and to some extent in mitochondria.

RNA **differs from a DNA** strand in many aspects such as:

1. RNA chain is much shorter in length than the DNA chains.
2. The sugar-phosphate backbone contains ribose instead of deoxyribose.
3. The base thymine is replaced by uracil.

Types of RNA

There are three types of RNA, and they have different functions.

1. **Messenger RNA:** Messenger RNA (mRNA) is formed in the nucleus and enters cytoplasm for protein synthesis. It forms the **template that directs the synthesis of protein** molecules within ribosomes.
2. **Transfer RNA:** Transfer RNA (tRNA) **conveys specific amino acids** to the site of protein synthesis.
3. **Ribosomal RNA:** Nucleolus is the site of synthesis of ribosomal RNA (rRNA), which is **associated with many proteins** to form ribosomes, the protein-synthesizing machine.

Application of Genetics In Medicine

Recombinant DNA Technology

Recombinant DNA technology in genetic engineering refers to the process in which a **DNA fragment of interest is transferred** from one organism to a self-replicating genetic element such as a **bacterial plasmid**, which involves cutting, modifying and joining DNA molecules using enzymes such as DNA ligase and others. It is performed in **four stages**.

Stage 1: This is the **stage of creation of a copy of gene** essential for the purpose. This can be done by making a copy of the gene from its mRNA, by synthesizing the gene artificially or by chopping a part of DNA with restriction enzymes and searching for the part with the required gene.

Stage 2: This is the **stage of joining the gene to a vector molecule,** in which the generated gene is attached to the vector DNA for cloning. The usual vectors are *plasmids, cosmids and bacteriophages*.

Stage 3: This is the **stage of introduction of vector DNA into the host cell** to produce *chimeric DNA* or recombinant DNA.

Stage 4: This is the **stage of cloning of the chimeric DNA**. The chimeric DNA contained in a vector is introduced into bacterial cells by the process called *transfection*.

- The host cell allows multiplication of the chimeric DNA of the vector that leads to production of large number of identical target **cloned DNA molecules.**
- The cloned DNA is released form the vector by cleavage, which is isolated, characterized and used for different purposes.

Uses of Recombinant DNA Technology

1. **Synthesis of hormones:** By recombinant DNA technology, hormones like insulin, growth hormone, erythropoietin etc, can be produced in large amount for therapeutic purposes.
2. **Laboratory diagnosis:** Diagnosis of diseases like AIDS has become simple by using recombinant DNA technology.
3. **Gene therapy:** It is useful in therapy for certain genetic defects.
4. **Use in forensic medicine:** DNA fingerprinting technique is useful in solving medicolegal cases.
5. **Use in agricultural purposes:** Recombinant DNA technology is used in generating genetically engineered plants to enhance the yield of crops.

PCR & Blotting Techniques

Polymerase Chain Reaction (PCR)

PCR is a specific and very rapid method of **amplifying a target DNA sequence**.

- This involves **denaturation of DNA** (separation of double stranded target DNA into single strands by heating), **cooling the single DNA** strand followed by **DNA amplification**.
- The DNA amplification is achieved by formation of **new DNA strand** in the presence of enzyme DNA polymerase and the substrate deoxyribonucleotide triphosphate.
- PCR causes million-fold amplification of target DNA in a very short span of time.

Uses: PCR is **highly sensitive** and can detect the presence of even a single molecule of DNA. It is used for **quick diagnosis of diseases, DNA fingerprinting and sex identification**.

Blotting Techniques

Blotting techniques are methodical techniques used for the **identification of a particular DNA, RNA or a protein**. There are southern blotting (for DNA), northern blotting (for RNA) and western blotting (for protein).

Southern Blotting: In southern blotting, DNA is extracted from the cells like leucocytes and cleaved into fragments by ***restriction endonucleases***.

- These DNA fragments are separated and denatured.
- Then they are transferred onto a sheet of nitrocellulose paper from the agarose gel, a process called blotting.

- Then DNA fragments are fixed to the membrane usually by ultraviolet cross-linking. Then the DNA is labeled (tagged) to form hybrid complexes.
- Following the hybridization reaction, the membrane is washed and regions of hybridization are identified by autoradiography.

Southern blotting is used for techniques like ***DNA fingerprinting*** and for ***detection of mutant gene*** that causes diseases like cystic fibrosis.

Northern Blotting: This is similar to southern blotting except that the **RNA is identified** instead of DNA. Northern blotting is used for ***analysis of gene expression*** in a particular tissue.

Western Blotting: It is used for identification of specific proteins.

- First, the SDS polyacrylamide gel electrophoresis is performed for the separation of various proteins in a protein mixture.
- Then the electrophoresed protein bands are transferred from SDS polyacryl amide gel to a nitrocellulose membrane.
- Afterward, identification of protein is done by using a labeled antibody probe.

Western blotting along with ELISA is a **confirmatory test for HIV**.

Cloning

Cloning means production of many **identical copies of a molecule**. There are four types of cloning: Gene cloning, reproductive cloning, embryo cloning, tissue cloning.

Gene Cloning

Gene cloning is also referred to as ***DNA cloning*** or ***recombinant DNA technology***.

- This is the process of transfer of a specific DNA fragment of one organism to a self-replicating genetic component of the cloning vector such as bacterial plasmid.
- Following transfer of the DNA fragment, the molecule is propagated in the host organism.

Uses: Gene cloning is used widely in genetic engineering for **sequencing of genomes** and in **gene therapy**.

Genetic Screening

Genetic screening is the detection of the *genetic variations in a human being*. It is used for diagnosing diseases at various stages such as prenatal diagnosis, diagnosis of carrier states and for prognostic diagnosis.

Prenatal Diagnosis

Prenatal diagnosis aims at identifying the **health problems in the fetal stage** and therefore has preventive applications. This is performed by **chorionic villus sampling, amniocentesis** and pre-implantation diagnosis.

Diagnosis of Carrier States

A group of people carry and transmit the disease without suffering from it. The **identification of such carrier people** is important in preventing the spread of disease in the community. The examples of carrier states include sickle cell anemia, cystic fibrosis and phenylketonuria etc.

Prognostic Diagnosis

Some diseases like diabetes mellitus or Huntington's chorea that are present in childhood are likely to occur in genetically susceptible individuals when they become adult or middle aged. Genetic screening of such people can help identify the **susceptibility of the disease** and helps in preventing the disease to occur at a later stage.

Gene Therapy

Hereditary disorders occur due to transmission of defective genes. Gene therapy aims at providing the correct copy of the gene concerned. This is achieved by **gene replacement** (replacement of a mutant gene with a normal gene), **gene correction** (correction of the specific bases of DNA) and **gene augmentation** (insertion of a foreign DNA into the genome of a cell to rectify the genetic defect).

Somatic Cell Therapy: In humans, somatic (nongametic) cells are used in the gene therapy as changes in these cells cannot be inherited.

- Cells are isolated with the defective gene from the patient and grown in culture. Then they are **transfected** with a remedial gene construct.
- Transfected cells are then **transfused back** into the patients.
- It is successfully tried in **cystic fibrosis** of the lung and severe combined immuno-deficiency syndrome (**SCID**).
- **In cancer**, gene therapy is very useful, in which oncogenic gene is inactivated by introducing a gene such as tumor suppressor gene. This selectively kills the cancer cells.

PY1.4

APOPTOSIS

Apoptosis (Greek word meaning *'falling off'* or *'dropping off'*) is the **programmed cell death**. It is a distinct process from necrosis (cell death due to injury). Apoptosis has genetic control. **Genes of the own cells** play important role in this programmed cell death. Examples of apoptosis are:

IMPORTANT NOTE

Decreased apoptosis a cause of malignancy: Apoptosis plays an important role in removal of unwanted cells, degenerated cells, **potentially harmful cells and self-reactive cells** from the body. Therefore, decreased apoptosis has been implicated in the genesis of ***malignancy and autoimmune diseases***.

1. Death of neurons in central nervous system during brain development and synapse formation.
2. During fetal development, degeneration of many tissues like web in the fingers.
3. Many blood cells like eosinophils undergo apoptosis.

Mechanisms of Apoptosis

Stimuli

Activation of cysteine proteases in the cell called **caspases** triggers apoptosis. Normally, caspases are present in the inactive form in the cell, and stimulated by external and internal stimuli.

Molecular Mechanisms

Initiation of Apoptosis

Stimuli signaling programmed cell death act either on the cell membrane or intracellularly.

- Usually, it is triggered by absence of stimuli that are normally required for normal cell survival such as absence of certain hormones, growth factors, cytokines, etc.
- Activation of receptors like receptors of TNF initiates programmed cell death.
- Intracellular stimuli may include heat, radiation, hypoxia, etc.
- Genetically programmed events.

Regulation of Apoptosis

Once apoptosis is initiated, certain intracellular proteins provide signal for the final programmed cell death, which actually determine the outcome. Apoptosis depends on the **balance between proapoptotic and anti-apoptotic proteins**.

Proapoptotic proteins: BAX and BAC

Anti-apoptotic proteins: BCL-2, BCL-XL, MCL-1

Proteins that regulate between proapoptotic and anti-apoptotic proteins: BAD, BIM, BID, Puma and Noxa

BCL-2: BCL2 is a protein which is equivalent to CED9, the cell death gene found in nematodes. BCL2 is located in the outer mitochondrial membrane and control apoptotic process by binding to various cytosolic proteins.

- Usually it binds to **BAX and BAD** proteins that are known to *promote apoptosis*.
- It may also bind with **BCLXL** protein that *inhibits apoptosis*.

Significant contribution of Scientist

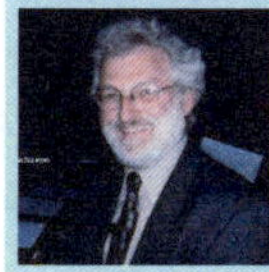

John E Sulston

The 2002, Nobel Prize in Physiology and Medicine was awarded to Sydney Brenner, Horvitz and John E Sulston for their work identifying genes that control apoptosis. The genes were identified by studies in the nematode C Elegans and these same genes function in humans for apoptosis.

- Another binding protein present in the cytosol is the **proapoptotic protease activating factor** (apzaf1), which is a mammalian counterpart of gene CED4 of nematode.

Thus, apoptosis depends on binding of BCL2 with pro-apoptotic and antiapoptotic proteins.

Other apoptotic regulator proteins: Other regulator proteins of apoptosis are TP53 (p53) protein, caspases, BAX and certain viruses such as adenovirus, papilloma virus, hepatitis B virus, etc.

Steps of Apoptosis

Stimuli (external/internal)
↓
FAS receptor activation (cytotoxic T cell)
↓
Ceramide generation and activation of caspase
↓
Mitochondrial injury
↓
DNA damage
↓
Formation of nuclear protein TP53 (induction fo cell death protein BAX)
↓
Cytoplasmic and chromatin condensation
↓
Formation of apoptotic bodies
↓
Apoptosis
↓
Phagocytosis (removal of apoptotic bodies)

Flowchart 3.2: Major steps of apoptosis

Apoptosis occurs in following major steps (Flowchart 3.2).

1. **FAS receptor activation:** CD 95 or FAS, the surface receptor present on cytotoxic T cells when comes in contact with the target cell, is activated. This leads to ***activation of caspases*** and subsequent proteolysis.
2. **Ceramide generation:** Hydrolysis of sphingomyelin on the cell membrane generates ceramide. Ceramide causes mitochondrial injury.
3. **DNA damage:** Damage by various agents and activated oxygen species like free oxygen radicals leads to

apoptosis. DNA injury influences nuclear protein TP53 that induces the synthesis of cell death promoting protein BAX.

4. **Cell shrinkage:** Cell reduces in size and cytoplasmic condensation occurs.
5. **Formation of apoptotic bodies:** Apoptotic bodies are formed as described below.
6. **Phagocytosis:** The dead apoptotic cells and their fragments are identified and engulfed by phagocytes.

Changes in Apoptosis

Pathophysiologic Changes

Changes in apoptosis confuses with the changes in necrosis.

Necrosis: In necrosis, cytoplasm is *homogenously eosinophilic*, and nuclear changes are **pyknosis** (condensation and clumping of nucleus), **karyolysis** (disintegration of the nucleus) and **karyorrhexis** (nucleus fragments into small bits and disperses into cytoplasm).

Apoptosis: In apoptosis, there is *condensation of nuclear chromatin and cell fragments* into **apoptotic bodies** that are phagocytosed by macrophages (Fig. 3.10).

The characteristic changes in apoptosis include the following:

1. May involve single cells or a cluster of cells. The apoptotic cells become round or oval and reduce in size. The cytoplasm becomes **intensely eosinophilic** containing condensed or fragmented nuclear chromatin material. Typically, *inflammatory response around apoptosis is absent*.
2. Though cytoplasm is reduced, organelles remain almost normal.
3. Cell membrane convolutes with formation of membranebound spherical structures called **apoptotic bodies** that contain compacted organelles.
4. **Chromatic condensation** occurs around the periphery of nucleus.
5. **Phagocytosis** of apoptotic bodies occurs by macro phages.

Biochemical Changes

Biochemical changes include:

1. **Proteolysis** of cytoskeletal proteins.
2. Crosslinking of protein molecules.
3. **Fragmentation of nuclear chromatin** by *activation of nuclease*.
4. A glycoprotein molecule called **thrombospondin** and a phosphoprotein called **phosphatidylserine** appear on the outer surface of apoptotic bodies, which facilitate recognition by macrophages for phagocytosis.

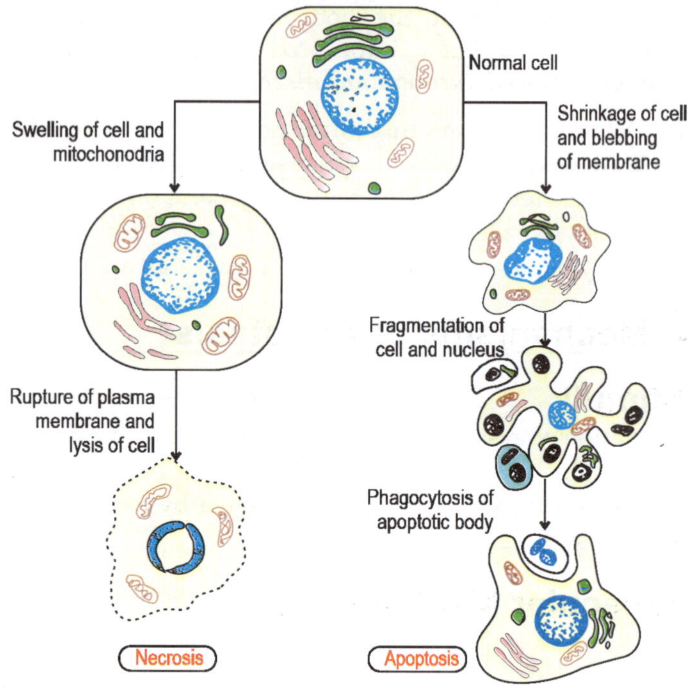

Fig. 3.10: Morphological changes between apoptosis and necrosis.

Detection of Apoptosis

Apoptosis cane be identified by:

1. DNA fragmentation assay by electrophoresis
2. TUNEL Staining
3. Demonstration of chromatic condensation by H&E/Feulgen/Acridine-orange staining
4. Estimation of cytosolic cytochrome-c, activated caspase, and annexin-V.

Applied Aspect

Apoptosis is linked to pathophysiology of diseases.

A. Disorders with reduced apoptosis (survival of abnormal cells)

1. Cancer
2. Autoimmune diseases

B. Disorders with increased apoptosis (excessive loss of cells)

1. Neurodegenerative diseases: Alzheimer's disease, Parkinson's disease, Huntigton's disease
2. Ischemic injury such as myocardial infarction and stroke may be associated with increased apoptosis.

Exam Questions

1. Describe the structure and functions of cell membrane.
2. Describe the structure, functions and dysfunctions of mitochondria.

3. Describe the structure, functions and dysfunctions of lysosomes and peroxisomes.
4. Describe the structure and functions of various cytoskeletal proteins.
5. Describe the structure and functions of molecular motors.
6. Describe the structure and functions of gap junctions.
7. Describe the structure and functions of cell adhesion molecules.
8. Describe the basic principle and application of genetics in physiology.
9. Describe the mechanism, regulation and applied aspects of apoptosis.

Multiple Choice Questions

1. **The contribution of lipids to dry weight of the cell membrane is about**
   A. 15% B. 22% C. 55% D. 42%
2. **All of the following are functions of cell membrane, EXCEPT:**
   A. Regulation of acid base balance
   B. Maintenance of cell volume
   C. Recognition of antigens
   D. Transportation of ions
3. **Which of the following proteins is NOT present in RBC membrane?**
   A. Band-3 protein
   B. Spectrin
   C. GLUT-2
   D. Glycophorin
4. **The H+ concentration in lysosome is**
   A. Less than H+ concentration in cytoplasm
   B. Same as H+ concentration in microtubules
   C. Same as H+ concentration in cytoplasm
   D. More than H+ concentration in cytoplasm
5. **All of the following are cell adhesion molecules, EXCEPT:**
   A. Ankyrin
   B. Integrin
   C. Cadherin
   D. Selectin
6. **The cytoskeletal structure includes all of the following, EXCEPT:**
   A. Intermediate filaments
   B. Golgi apparatus
   C. Microfilaments
   D. Microtubules
7. **Which of the following are known as 'Power houses' of the cell?**
   A. Lysosomes
   B. Peroxisomes
   C. Mitochondria
   D. Nucleus
8. **Which of the following statements is true for mitochondria?**
   A. Major site of cellular oxidation of nutrients
   B. Membrane contains cytochrome
   C. Number of cristae is less in resting state
   D. Luft's disease is a mitochondrial dysfunction
9. **All of the following are intercellular junctions, EXCEPT:**
   A. Zonula adherens
   B. Focal adhesion
   C. Hemidesmosome
   D. Hemicholinium
10. **All of the following are molecular motors, EXCEPT:**
    A. Myomesin
    B. Myosin II
    C. Dynein
    D. Kinesin
11. **The lipid bilayer of the cell membrane allows passage of all EXCEPT:**
    A. Oxygen
    B. Urea
    C. Alcohol
    D. Carbon dioxide
12. **The enzyme having a vital role in the regulation of apoptosis is:**
    A. Citrate synthase
    B. Cathepsin
    C. Caspase
    D. Catalase
13. **All of the following help in the detection of apoptosis, EXCEPT:**
    A. TUNEL staining
    B. Estimation of cytochrome-c
    C. DNA fragmentation assay
    D. Estimation of arylsulfatase
14. **Which of the following enzyme is used in PCR technique?**
    A. RNA polymerase
    B. DNA polymerase
    C. Acid phosphatase
    D. Reverse transcriptase
15. **The short and long arms of chromosome are respectively termed as:**
    A. q and r arms
    B. p and q arms
    C. c and d arms
    D. q and p arms
16. **The identification and mapping out of the chromosome is known as:**
    A. Karyotyping
    B. Crystallography
    C. Western blotting
    D. Tissue cloning

Answers

1. D	**2. A**	**3. C**	**4. D**	**5. A**	**6. B**	**7. C**
8. C	**9. D**	**10. A**	**11. B**	**12. C**	**13. D**	**14. B**
15. D	**16.A**					

Chapter 4

Transport Across the Cell Membrane

Learning Objectives

On completion of study of this chapter:

The student will be able to (must know):

1. Name common ion channels in the membrane; and name different types of carrier proteins with examples.
2. Classify transport processes and list the differences between passive and active transport mechanisms.
3. Define, list the factors affecting and give the mechanism of diffusion, facilitated diffusion and osmosis.
4. Illustrate competitive inhibition in carrier-mediated transport.
5. Define filtration, bulk flow, solvent drag and Donnan effect, and give example for each.
6. Describe the primary and secondary active transport processes.
7. Describe the structure, mechanism of action and functions of Na^+-K^+ ATPase.
8. Elucidate the mechanism of endocytosis, exocytosis and transcytosis

The student may also be able to (desirable to know):

1. Describe the gating of ion channels.
2. Define the concept of osmole and application of osmosis in clinical conditions.
3. Describe other types of ATPases..

Passage of substances through cell membrane occurs by the following **three processes**: diffusion, passage through channels or carrier proteins, and endocytosis and exocytosis.

MEMBRANE CHANNELS

Membrane proteins that constitute channels are integral proteins that span entire width of the membrane. Normally, they are formed by several polypeptide subunits. Along the length of the integral protein, an aqueous pore is present around which the polypeptide subunits are arranged.

- Ions pass through the aqueous pore from one side of the membrane to the other without entering through the lipid bilayer.
- Channels are often selective due to presence of a **selectivity filter** that permits specific ions to pass through the channel (Fig. 4.1).

Types of Channels

Protein channels are broadly divided into two types: ion channels and water channels

Ion Channels

Sodium and potassium channels are extensively studied membrane channels. Usually, a polypeptide subunit forms **a gate** at one end of the channel that opens in response to a specific stimulus (Fig. 4.1).

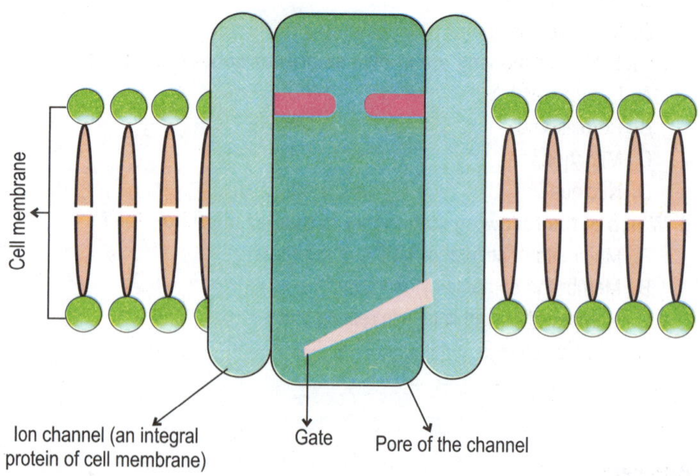

Fig. 4.1: A typical ion channel. An ion channel is a pore in the integral protein of the membrane. Note, there is selectivity filter at one end that allows the selective passage of ions through the channel, and there is gate at other end that on activation opens the channel.

- Opening of the gate opens the channel and allows the ions to rapidly move (108 ions per sec) through the channel.
- However, the **selectivity filter** permits specific ions to pass through and makes *ion channels are often selective*.

Sodium Channels

Sodium channels have been studied in detail among all the ion channels.

- It has subunits surrounding an aqueous pore of about 0.5 nm in diameter. The inner surface of the pore is negatively charged.
- It is selective for passage of sodium.
- Sodium channel is blocked by **tetrodotoxin**.

Potassium Channels

There are many types of potassium channels.

- They are about 0.3 nm in diameter.
- Potassium channels are blocked by *tetraethyl ammonium* or **4-aminopyridine**.

Calcium and Chloride Channels

There are various channels for Ca^{++} and for Cl^-.

- **Ca^{++} channels** can be voltage-gated, ligand-gated and stretch sensitive.
- **Cl^- channels** are dimeric and pentameric (e. g. $GABA_A$ & glycine receptors). Cystic fibrosis transmembrane conductance regulator (CFTR) proteins located on apical membrane of pancreatic duct epithelial cells are Cl^- channels.

Water Channels

Water channels in the cell membrane are **aquaporins**. There are 13 types of aquaporins in mammals. Aquaporins 1 to 4 are located in kidney tubular epithelial cells that are involved in water reabsorption.

Gating of Ion Channels

Some of the ion channels remain always open, and therefore they are referred to as **non-gated channels**. However, many ion channels open and close by gates. There are **three general mechanisms of gating**: voltage-gating, ligand-gating and mechanical-gating.

Voltage Gating

Change in the membrane potential beyond a certain threshold value opens or closes the gate of the ion channels. Therefore, they are called voltage-gated channels. Ion channels in excitable tissues such as nerve and muscle are mainly voltage-gated channels like Na^+, K^+ and Ca^{++} channels.

Mechanism of Gating

The exact mechanism of voltage-gating is not known. It is believed that alteration in membrane potential induces movement of some charged amino acids in helical segment of the channel protein that causes a **conformational change** of the channel protein, which in turn opens or closes the gate and allows the ions to pass through the channel rapidly.

Gating for Na^+ channels: For Na^+ channels, the gate is located on the outer end of the channel (Fig. 4.2A).

- The **gate closes** the outer opening of the channel ***when the cell is at RMP*** (–70 mV in nerve, –90 mV in muscle and –50 mV in pacemaker tissue).
- When *inside becomes less negative*, the **gate opens** and Na^+ influx occurs that leads to first, formation of local response and later, the genesis of action potential.

Gating for K^+ channels: For K^+ channels, the gate is located on the inner end of the channel (Fig. 4.2B).

- The **gate closes** the cytoplasmic opening of the channel when the ***cell is at RMP***.
- When interior becomes less negative and *approaches towards positivity*, more and **more gates open** and K^+ efflux occurs that leads to first, reversal of depolarization potential and later, the repolarization of action potential.
- **Opening of K^+ channels is slower** than the opening of Na^+ channels. Therefore, the *phase of repolarization is less steep* than the phase of depolarization.

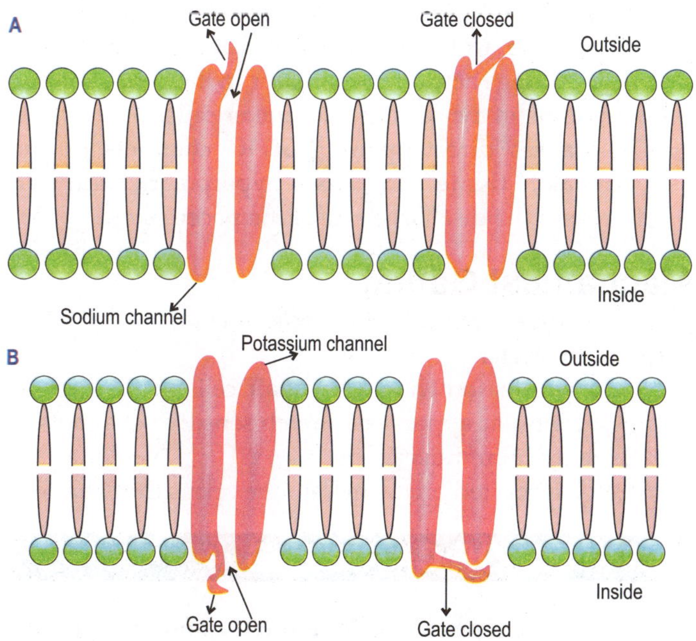

Fig. 4.2: Gating mechanisms of ion channels. Arrow indicates passage of ion through the channel when the gate is open. Note, the gate is present towards the outer side of the membrane in sodium channel (A) and towards inner side of membrane in potassium channel (B).

Ligand Gating

Interaction of the channel with a **ligand** (hormone or neurotransmitter) causes opening or closure of the channel. Hence, the channels are called **ligand-gated channels**. As the ligand is a chemical agent, the gating is also called **chemical gating**.

Mechanism of Gating

The chemical agent **binds with the specific receptor** protein on the membrane and brings about **conformational change** in the protein that in turn directly or indirectly opens the channel. Nicotinic and muscarinic cholinergic receptors are examples.

Nicotinic Cholinergic Receptor: Nicotinic cholinergic receptor channel in postsynaptic neuromuscular junction is a ligand-gated ion channel. Acetylcholine released at the nerve ending binds with these receptors and opens the ion channels that generate post-synaptic potential.

Muscarinic Cholinergic Receptors: Acetylcholine at the parasympathetic endings binds with muscarinic cholinergic receptors on the membrane of GI smooth muscle cells and activates G protein, which in turn activates the enzyme that causes production of second messengers such as cyclic AMP or Ca^{++}. The second messengers activate enzymes like kinase that act on the ion channel by phosphorylation.

Other examples: Other examples are the action of noradrenaline on β-adrenergic receptors on the smooth muscle cell.

Direct opening of channels: The receptor for the hormone or neurotransmitter may also be the channel itself, so that the action by the ligand is direct on the channel.

- For example, acetylcholine released at parasympathetic nerve endings acts on the receptor in the post-synaptic membrane in the cardiac pacemaker cells.
- This causes direct **opening of K^+ channels in the pacemaker tissue** and causes hyperpolarization that decreases the discharge rate of the pacemaker.

Mechanical Gating

Some of the channels are *mechanosensitive* and they **respond to stretch**.

- For example, ion channels in hair cells in the cochlea and vestibular apparatus, stretch sensitive channels in the ventricular muscles etc.
- Stretch imparted on the membrane opens the channels.

TYPES OF CARRIERS

There are **three types of carrier proteins**: uniport, symport and antiport (Fig. 4.3).

Uniport

Uniport is the carrier protein that **transports only one substance**. For example, Na^+ channels transport Na^+ and K^+ channels transport K^+.

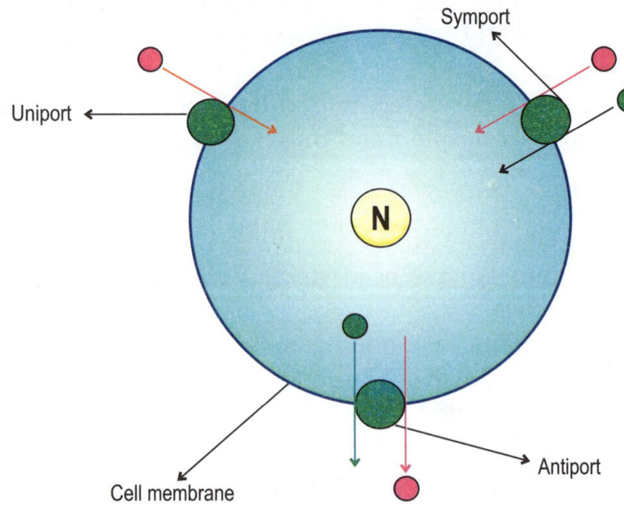

Fig. 4.3: Types of carrier proteins in the cell membrane. Note, uniport transports only one substance, symport transports two different substances in the same direction and antiport transports substances in opposite direction.

Symport

Symport carriers transport **two or more substances** from one side of the membrane to the other **in the same direction.**

- Transport of Na^+ and glucose from the lumen of the intestine or kidney tubule into the epithelial cells through the same carrier protein is an example of symport mechanism.
- Such substances are said to be **co-transported**.

Antiport

Antiport carriers transport substances **in opposite directions** in which one substance is transported to the inside of the cell and other substance from inside the cell to the outside.

- Substances transported in opposite directions by one carrier are said to be **counter-transported**.
- A typical antiport carrier is the **sodium-potassium pump**, which is operated by Na^+-K^+ ATPase. It actively transports 3 Na^+ out of the cell, and 2 K^+ into the cell for each molecule of ATP hydrolyzed.
- Another example is **Na^+–H^+ exchanger** found in the proximal tubular cells of the nephron in which the inward facilitated diffusion of Na^+ is coupled with the outward diffusion of H^+.

Characteristics of Carrier-Mediated Transport

Carrier-mediated transport systems exhibit **two important properties**: Competition for the carrier protein and the saturation of the transport process.

Competitive Inhibition: Presence of **different molecules with similar structure** generates competition for the same carrier protein for their transport, which results in competitive inhibition of the process. For instance, the presence of *ketoses in intestinal content decreases the reabsorption of aldoses* by the gut .

Saturation Kinetics: The number of carrier proteins in a membrane is limited. Therefore, the rate of carrier-mediated transport reaches a maximum which is known as **transport maximum or Tm**.

- The Tm cannot be exceeded by increasing the concentration of the substance.
- Thus, the carrier-mediated transport exhibits saturation kinetics.

PY1.5

TRANSPORT PROCESSES

Classification

Table 4.1 | Types of transport processes

A. Passive transports
1. Simple diffusion
2. Facilitated diffusion
3. Osmosis
4. Filtration
5. Bulk flow
6. Solvent drag
B. Active transports
1. Primary active transport
2. Secondary active transport
C. Vesicular transports
1. Exocytosis
2. Endocytosis
D. Transport across epithelia
1. Transcellular transport
2. Paracellular transport

Transport mechanisms through cell membrane can be broadly divided into **three types**: passive transport, active transport and vesicular transport (Table 4.1). There is another mechanism of transport called as transport across epithelia.

Special Features

Passive Transports

There are two common features of passive transport processes (Table 4.2). These are:

(a) **Transport is downhill:** In passive transports, the substances pass through the membrane from both sides, however, net movement occurs **down the electrochemical gradient**.

(b) **Transport does not require metabolic energy:** Passive transport does not require utilization of ATP. Examples are simple diffusion, facilitated diffusion, osmosis, filtration, bulk flow and solvent drag.

Active Transport

Active transport differs from passive transport by its **utilization of energy**. The common features of active transport are (Table 4.2):

1. **Uphill transport:** Transport occurs against the electrochemical gradient of the substance.
2. **Requires energy:** Energy utilized for transport is derived from the breakdown of ATP. Hence, they are susceptible to metabolic poisons.
3. **Exhibits saturation kinetics:** This is because of limitation in the rate of availability of carriers or supply of energy.

The active transport mechanisms are:

1. Primary active transport
2. Secondary active transport

Vesicular Transport

This transport has no relation with the concentration gradient. However, it may utilize metabolic energy.

Vesicular transport mechanisms are:

1. Exocytosis
2. Endocytosis

Table 4.2 | Differences between active and passive transport processes.

	Active transport	Passive transport
1. Nature of transport	Against electrochemical gradient	Along the gradient
2. Utilization of energy	By hydrolysis of ATP	Not needed
3. Saturation Kinetics	Is a feature	May not be present

SIMPLE DIFFUSION

Definition: Diffusion is the process of passive transport in which molecules move from the area of higher concentration to the area of lower concentration.

- Examples are transport of O_2, CO_2, urea, ammonia and ions.
- In simple diffusion, **random movement of molecules** occurs.
- The net movement of molecule ceases when the concentration of molecule on both sides becomes equal and a **diffusional equilibrium** is achieved.

Factors Affecting Rate of Diffusion

Factors determining the rate of diffusion across the cell membrane can be broadly divided into **two categories**: (a) properties of the substance and (b) the properties of the membrane.

Properties of the Substance

Properties of the substance that determine diffusion through membrane are mainly of **two types**: (a) concentration and electrical gradients of the substance, and (b) permeability of the substance through the membrane.

Effect of Concentration & Electrical Gradients

The concentration or **the chemical gradient** of the substance is primarily responsible for the direction of transport of the substance (Fig. 4.4). The electrical potential difference (**electrical gradient**) also influences. Usually, substances move along both the electrical and chemical gradients (transfer along the **electro-chemical gradients**).

- Electrochemical gradient is mainly used for the ions.
- For gases, concentration gradient is expressed as partial pressure, and for water as hydraulic pressure.

Role of Thermal Energy: In a liquid or gas, all particles are in constant and random motion due to **thermal energy**.

- The **motion varies directly with temperature**.
- The motion is absent at absolute zero temperature.
- This random movement of particle provides the physical basis for diffusion of solutes and gas molecules in body fluids and across the cell membranes.

Unidirectional Flux: When two liquids are separated by a semi-permeable membrane, the number of particles in the liquid striking a unit area from each side of the membrane at any given time is **proportional to the concentration of the substance** on that side. These particles succeed in passing through the membrane along the gradient, which is called as *unidirectional flux*.

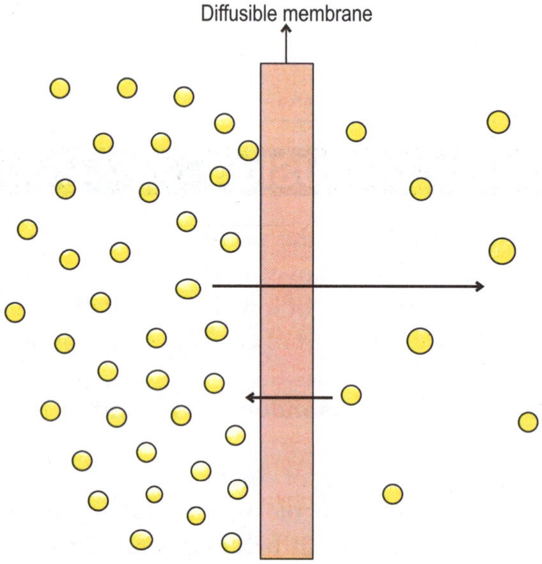

Fig. 4.4: Diffusion across the cell membrane. The molecules move in both directions, but the movement is more from higher to lower concentration of solutes. The length of arrow indicates the magnitude of movement.

Unidirectional flux is thus proportional to the **concentration of the substance** in the liquid.

Similarly, the unidirectional flux of the particles in the *opposite side* of the membrane is proportional to the concentration of the substance on that side of the liquid.

Hence, **net diffusion** is the *difference between the opposing unidirectional fluxes*.

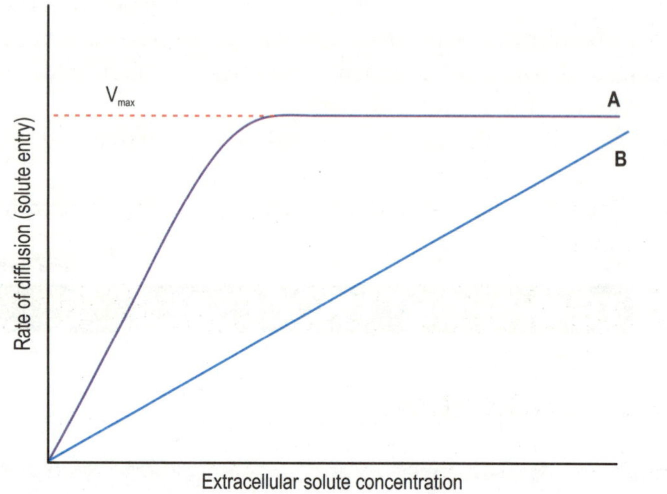

Fig. 4.5: Rate of diffusion (solute entry into the cell) by carrier mediated or facilitated diffusion (A) and simple diffusion (B). In simple diffusion, though a linear relationship exists between the rate of diffusion and concentration of solute throughout the process, total quantity of solutes transported is less due to slower rate of diffusion. In facilitated diffusion, though diffusion does not increase further after reaching V_{max} (maximum rate), the total amount of solutes transferred is more due to higher rate of diffusion.

Diffusion across the membrane ceases when the balance between the fluxes from both sides becomes zero.

A distinguishing feature of simple diffusion is the linear relationship between solute concentration and rate of diffusion (Fig. 4.5).

Permeability of the Substance

Permeability refers to the **ease at which substances pass through** the membrane.

The **factors that determine** the permeability are:

1. **Lipid-solubility:** As the membrane is a lipid bilayer, the permeability is **proportional to their lipid solubility** of the substance.
2. **Molecular size:** For water-soluble substances like ions that pass through aqueous channels, permeability is **inversely proportional to their molecular size**.
   - For example, a cation like Na^+ attracts more water in its hydration shell than K^+. The atomic weight of Na^+ is 23, whereas that of K^+ is 39.
   - However, the effective molecular size of the hydrated Na^+ is larger than K^+.
   - Therefore, K^+ permeability at rest is much more than the permeability of Na^+.
3. **Charge on the molecule:** Since membrane is polarized with its **negative interior**, cations easily enter from outside into the cell and anions in the opposite direction.

4. **Temperature:** Rate of diffusion is **high at higher body temperature** as temperature facilitates motion of molecules in the solution.
5. **Distribution of channels in the membrane:** The **number of protein channels** for the substance in the membrane determines the permeability of the substance through the membrane.
6. **Pressure gradient:** In addition to the electrochemical gradients of the substance, the **fluid pressure gradient** also contributes to the diffusion of the membrane. Diffusion is *more from high pressure to low pressure*, as the pressure causes greater number of molecules to hit the membrane.

Properties of the Membrane

In addition to the concentration gradient of the substance across the membrane, two membrane properties influence diffusion: i) the **cross-sectional area** and, ii) **thickness of the membrane**. These factors are governed by **Fick's law of diffusion**.

Fick's Law: The rate of diffusion of a molecule through a membrane is proportional to the surface area (A) available for diffusion, and inversely proportional to the thickness of the membrane (T).

According to Fick's law, for a substance whose inside and outside concentrations are respectively C_i and C_0 mmol/l:

Net Rate of Diffusion (J) = $\frac{-DA}{T} \times (C_i - C_0)$, where D is the diffusion coefficient.

The minus sign indicates that the direction is down the concentration gradient.

As thickness of biological membranes is fairly constant at 10^{-6} cm, D/T simplifies to the permeability coefficient 'P' of the membrane, and:

$$\text{Flux} = -P \times A\,(C_i - C_0)$$

FACILITATED DIFFUSION

This is also called **carrier-mediated diffusion**, as the process of diffusion is facilitated by a carrier protein in the membrane. Like simple diffusion, facilitated diffusion is also a **downhill transport** that *does not require energy*.

Features of Facilitated Diffusion

It differs from simple diffusion by four features: faster rate of transport, saturation kinetics, competitive inhibition and specificity (Table 4.3).

1. **Faster Rate of Transport:** Carrier-mediated (facilitated) diffusion allows the transport of polar or hydrophilic molecules at a **much faster rate** than the simple diffusion.

2. **Saturation Kinetics:** In facilitated diffusion, the *number of carrier proteins available determines the rate of diffusion*.

- When all the available binding sites on the carrier proteins are occupied, the system operates at the maximum capacity. This is called **saturation point**.
- However, the rate of diffusion is faster in facilitated diffusion than the simple diffusion, which occurs at a much slower rate due to no involvement of carrier protein.
- Thus, the net diffusion in facilitated type is more than in simple type (Fig. 4.5).

3. **Competitive Inhibition:** Many substances ***share same carrier protein*** for their transport. When more than one such substance is present on the same side of the membrane, they compete to bind with the carrier protein.

- Thus, one substance ***decreases the transport of the other***.
- For example, transport of D-glucose across the epithelial membrane slows down once D-galactose is present along with it as they share same glucose transporter.

4. **Specificity:** The carrier proteins are **often specific** for different molecules. For example, the carrier protein for protein does not transport cholesterol or fatty acid.

Factors Affecting Facilitated Diffusion

Factors that influence simple diffusion also affect facilitated diffusion as described above. However, the major factor is the **number of carrier proteins available** for the transport.

- Sometimes, facilitated diffusion is also operated by other factors like **hormones**.
- For example, transport of glucose by GLUT-4 into muscles and adipose tissue is insulin-dependent.

Table 4.3 | Differences between simple diffusion and facilitated diffusion.

	Simple diffusion	Facilitated diffusion
1. Mode of diffusion	No carrier molecule Involved	Carrier molecule involved
2. Saturation kinetics	No saturation kinetics, diffusion is linear.	Has saturation kinetics. No increase in diffusion once saturation is reached.
3. Competitive inhibition	Absent	Substances that share the same carrier protein compete for transport
4. Rate of diffusion	May be slow	Faster
5. Specificity	No specificity	Carrier protein may be specific

OSMOSIS

Definition: Osmosis is defined as the process of movement of solvent from the solution with the lower concentration of solutes to the solution with higher concentration of solutes, when both the solutions are separated by a semipermeable membrane.

- A solution with lower solute concentration contains proportionately more water molecules than a solution with higher concentration of solutes.
- A semipermeable membrane allows the passage of solvent, not the solute.
- Therefore, net flux of water (solvent) through a semipermeable membrane occurs from a solution of lower solute concentration to that of higher solute concentration (Fig. 4.6).

Osmotic Effectiveness of a Substance

A substance to be osmotically effective should not be transferred to another compartment and should not be metabolized.

- Protein is ***osmotically most effective*** as it is neither transferred from nor metabolized in the compartment.
- Other examples are various complex polysaccharides such as dextran. Sodium chloride is also osmotically effective even though Na^+ and Cl^- ions can diffuse through the cell membrane.

Osmotic Pressure

Osmotic pressure is the minimum pressure applied to the solution with higher solute concentration to prevent osmosis.

- It depends on the number of molecules or the ions dissolved in a solution rather than the nature of chemical composition.

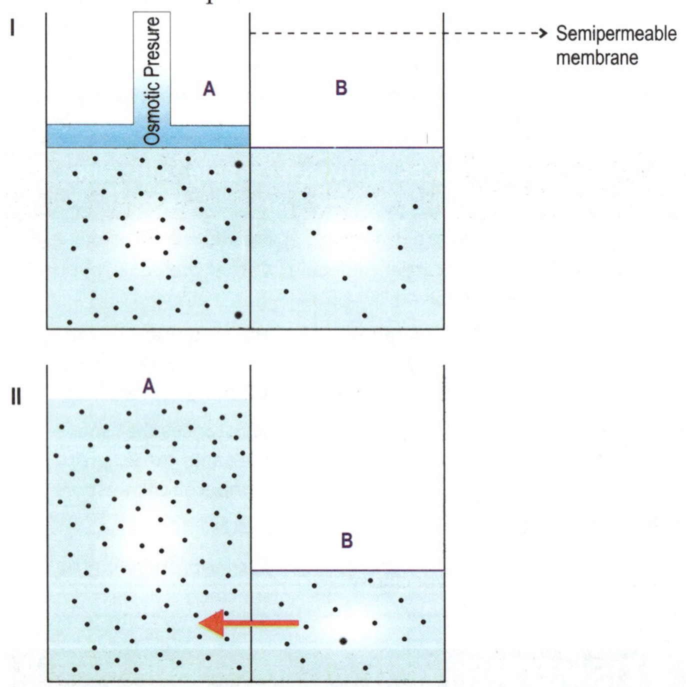

Fig. 4.6: The process of osmosis. **I:** Compartment A containing more osmotically active solutes is separated by a semipermeable membrane from compartment B containing less solutes. Solvent movement from B to A is prevented by application of osmotic pressure on A. **II:** Solvent (not the solute) moves from B to A (indicated by arrow mark) till osmotic equilibrium is reached, which results in increase in volume of A.

- Osmotic pressure in body fluid is mainly exerted by osmotically active solutes dissolved in the fluid such as colloidal substances.
- Hence, the osmotic pressure is called **colloidal osmotic pressure.** Oncotic pressure prevents edema formation (Application Box 4.1).

Application Box 4.1

Oncotic pressure determines rate of capillary filtration: In the plasma, the colloidal particles are proteins. The osmotic pressure due to presence of plasma proteins is called oncotic pressure, which is 25 mm Hg. **Oncotic pressure** opposes filtration across the capillary membrane. Therefore, edema occurs in hypoproteinemia.

OTHER TRANSPORT PHENOMENA

Filtration, Bulk Flow, Solvent Drag

Filtration: Filtration is the process by which fluid is forced through a membrane mainly because of the difference in hydrostatic and oncotic pressures on two sides.

- Water moves out of capillaries when the net hydrostatic pressure exceeds net osmotic pressure and from interstitial space into the capillaries when the net osmotic pressure exceeds the net hydrostatic pressure. This is filtration.

Bulk Flow: When filtration results in movement of greater quantity of water, the process is called **bulk flow**.

Solvent Drag: During bulk flow of water, it carries with it, dissolved particles (solutes), a phenomenon known as **solvent drag**.

Donnan Effect

Presence of nondiffusible ion on one side of the membrane affects the distribution of other ions to which membrane is permeable. This results in asymmetrical distribution of ions across the cell membrane.

Gibbs-Donnan effect

The asymmetrical distribution of ions across the cell membrane at equilibrium has the following effects:

i) There will be an electrical difference across the cell membrane whose magnitude can be determined by **Nernst equation** (details given in next chapter).
ii) Because of presence of protein anions ($prot^-$) in the cells, there are more osmotically active particles in the cells than the interstitial fluid.

- This can lead to osmotic swelling and rupture, which is prevented by Na^+–K^+ pump that produces net movement of positive charge out of the cell and keeps the inside and outside of the cell in osmotic equilibrium.

- Thus, normal cell volume and pressure depend on Na^+ - K^+ pump.

Nonionic Diffusion

Ions are present either in undissociated (non-ionic) or dissociated (ionic) form. In ionic form they can not be easily transported across the cell membrane as membrane is charged. However, in their undissociated (nonionic) form they diffuse through the membrane easily. This is called nonionic diffusion.

- Many ions in the body pass the membrane in undissociated form and then, they dissociate to their ionic form once they reach the other side of the membrane.
- Nonionic diffusion occurs regularly along the epithelial membrane of kidney and GI tract.

ACTIVE TRANSPORT

In active transport processes, substances are transported against their electrical and chemical gradients. There are **three common characteristics** of active transport mechanisms:

1. **Uphill Transport:** The transport occurs **against the electrochemical gradient** of the substance transported.
2. **Utilizes Metabolic Energy:** Energy utilized for the active transport is derived from the **breakdown of ATP**. Therefore, mechanisms that prevent the supply of ATP hinder the active transport process.
3. **Exhibits Saturation Kinetics:** Like any carrier-mediated transport, this has also a **saturation point** for limitation in the rate of availability of carriers and the supply of energy.

Types: There are **two types** of active transports:

1. Primary active transport
2. Secondary active transport

Primary Active Transport

Primary active transport is the transport mechanism that **directly utilizes metabolic energy** for the transport process. The mechanism is operated by **ion pumps.**

- In this process, the solute is transported *against its electrochemical gradients* with the help of energy. The **energy is derived from ATP**.
- The ion pumps hydrolyze ATP to ADP and use energy in the third phosphate bond for the transport process. As the ion pumps hydrolyze ATP, these are also called **ATPases**.

Types of ATPases: The commonly occurring ATPase is **Na^+–K^+ ATPase** or **Na^+–K^+ pump**.

Other ATPases are: Calcium ATPases, H^+–K^+ ATPase and H^+–ATPase (Table 4.4).

- They are also classified into **P-type** (phosphorylation type), **V-type** (vacuolar type), **F-type** (energy coupling factor type) and **ABC transporters**.

MDR-1 protein: Multidrug resistance 1 protein that pumps anticancer drug out of cancer cell that causes drug resistance in treatment of cancer.

Table 4.4 | Types of ATPases, their location and functions.

Types	Example	Location in cell
P-type	Na^+–K^+ ATPase Ca^{++} ATPase H^+–K^+ ATPase	Plasma membrane Sarcoplasmic reticulum Plasma membrane
V-type	H^+ ATPase	Lysosomal membrane
F-type	Mitochondrial ATP synthase	Inner mitochondrial membrane
ABC transporters	CFTR protein MDR-1 protein	Plasma membrane Plasma membrane

CFTR protein: cystic fibrosis transmembrane regulator protein involved in genesis of cystic fibrosis; MDR-1 protein: multidrug resistance 1 protein.

Na^+-K^+ ATPase

Na^+–K^+ ATPase is primarily responsible for maintaining the high K^+ and low Na^+ concentration inside the cells.

Structure

The Na^+–K^+ ATPase is made up of an **α and a β subunit.**

- At the cytoplasmic side, the α subunit has ATPase activity and binding sites for 3 Na^+, ATP and phosphate (Fig. 4.7).
- At the extracellular side, it has binding sites for 2 K^+ and ouabain.
- The phosphate group is bound to an aspartic acid residue of the α subunit.

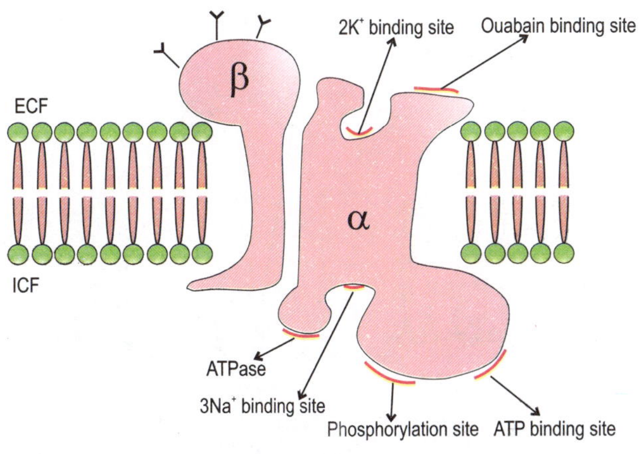

Fig. 4.7: Structure of Na^+-K^+ ATPase. It has a small β subunit and large α subunit. The extracellular surface of α subunit contains binding sites for two K^+ and ouabain, and intracellular surface has binding sites for three Na^+ and one ATP, a phosphorylation site and an ATPase site.

Significant contribution of Scientist

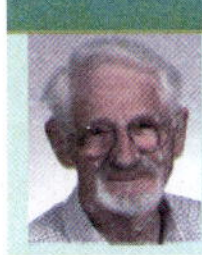

Jens Christian Skou The Na^+-K^+ pump was discovered in 1957 by Danish physiologist Prof. Jens Christian Skou of Aarhus University, He received the **Nobel Prize in Chemistry** together with **Paul D. Boyer** and John E. Walker for his discovery of Na^+-K^+ ATPase.

Functions

The Na^+–K^+ ATPase pumps **three Na^+ ions out of the cell** and **two K^+ into the cell**. This is called a *P-type ATPase*, as the carrier protein is phosphorylated during the process.

It serves many important cellular functions:

1. **Cytosolic ion concentration:** Na^+-K^+ pump opposes Na^+ to accumulate in the cell and K^+ to exit from the cell along their concentration gradient. Thus, it maintains **high K^+ and low Na^+** in the cell.
2. **Cell volume:** By maintaining ion concentration on both sides of the cell, Na^+-K^+ pump **regulates water movement** across the cell membrane.
   - This maintains **intracellular water content** and therefore, the cell volume.
   - Failure of Na^+-K^+ pump activity can lead to cell swelling and rupture.
3. **Protein synthesis:** The primary function of Na^+-K^+ pump is to maintain a high intracellular concentration of K^+, which is essential for protein synthesis.
4. **Resting membrane potential (RMP):** Na^+-K^+ pump also maintains RMP by maintaining ion gradients across the cell membrane.
5. **Hormone actions:** Na^+-K^+ pump mediates action of many hormones on the cell. Some important examples are **thyroxine, aldosterone and insulin**.

Mechanism of Action

1. First, binding of three Na^+ and one ATP molecule to their respective sites on α subunit activates the enzyme ATPase that *catalyses the hydrolysis of ATP to ADP* liberating high energy phosphate bond (**phosphorylation**).
   - This phosphorylation of α subunit by ATP causes conformational change in the carrier protein that **transfers three Na^+** from inside to the outside of the cell (Fig. 4.8).

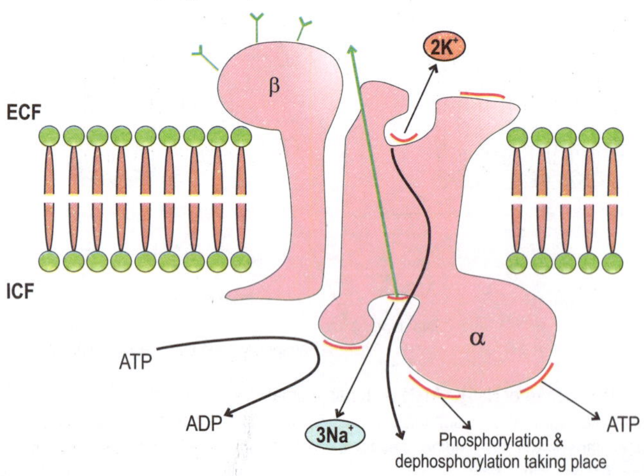

Fig. 4.8: Mechanism of action of Na^+-K^+ ATPase. Binding of three Na^+ and one ATP on α subunit activates ATPases that converts ATP to ADP. This causes phosphorylation of α subunit that changes its configuration and transfers 3 Na^+ to ECF. K^+ binds to K^+ binding site on the extracellular surface that causes dephosphorylation of α subunit and transfers 2 K^+ from ECF into the cell. Thus, three Na^+ are pumped out for entry of two K^+ into the cell.

2. In the next step, two K^+ bind to the outer side of the α subunit, and this leads to the *hydrolysis of the aspartic acid-phosphate bond* (**dephosphorylation**).
   - This in turn causes ***re-conformational change*** in the α subunit that **transfers two K^+** from outside to the inside of the cell.
   - Re-conformational change of the carrier protein also returns to its original conformation.

Thus, during one cycle of *conformational* (phosphorylation) and *re-conformational* (dephosphorylation) change in the α subunit of Na^+-K^+ ATPase, **three Na^+ ions are pumped out** of the cell and **two K^+ into the cell**, and one ATP is hydrolyzed.

Regulation of Na^+-K^+ Pump

Activation: Many hormones, chemicals and drugs act by increasing Na^+-K^+ pump activity such as **thyroxine, insulin, aldosterone**, G-actin etc.

Inhibition: Many hormones and chemicals act by decreasing Na^+-K^+ pump activity such as **dopamine, digitalis** metabolic poisons like DNP (2,4 dinitrophenol) etc. (Clinical Note 4.1). Hypoxia and hypothermia inhibit Na^+-K^+ pump activity.

Clinical Note 4.1

Digitalis inhibits Na^+-K^+ pump: Cardiac glycosides like ouabain or digitalis used in the management of heart failure inhibit Na^+-K^+ pump. This accumulates Na^+ inside the cell that decreases Na^+ gradient from outside to inside. Calcium efflux through sodium-calcium exchanger in the membrane utilizes sodium gradient. Hence, decreased sodium gradient decreases calcium efflux causing increase in cytosolic calcium concentration that promotes myocardial contractility.

Other Common ATPases

Ca^{++} ATPase: Ca^{++} ATPase is present in all cell membranes, membrane of endoplasmic reticulum and sarcoplasmic reticulum in muscle cell.

- The Ca^{++} pump actively transports calcium out of the cell.
- Maintains a higher concentration of calcium in the ECF (10^{-3} molar) compared to the ICF (10^{-7} molar).

H^+–K^+ ATPase: The H^+–K^+ pump is present on the luminal membrane of **parietal cells of stomach** and the **intercalated cells of the distal nephrons**. In stomach, it mediates HCl secretion and in kidney it secretes H^+ into the tubular fluid.

H^+ ATPase: There are 2 types: V-type and F-type.

1. *V-type ATPase:* The H^+ pump or **the proton pump** located on the membrane of *lysosome and endoplasmic reticulum* is a V-type ATPase. It ***pumps H^+ (proton)*** from cytosol into these organelles.
2. *F-type ATPase:* The proton pump in the *inner mitochondrial membrane* is an F-type ATPase. It ***synthesizes ATP*** by utilizing energy stored in the proton gradient created by respiratory chain.

ABC Transporters: ATP-binding cassette (ABC) transporter proteins use energy derived from ATP for transporting a variety of compound out of the cells, those include ions, steroids, peptides, bile acids, drugs and xenobiotics.

- As drugs are transported out of the cells, they are known as **MDR 1 protein** (multidrug resistance 1 protein).
- Cells in the organs that usually express MDR proteins are liver, kidney and GI tract.
- **CFTR protein** (cystic fibrosis transmembrane regulator protein), belongs to this superfamily of ABC transporters (Application Box 4.2).

Secondary Active Transport

Many cells have several carrier mechanisms that transfer one solute against its concentration gradient by using the energy generated by gradient of another solute. Usually, **Na^+ is the driver solute** for most of these mechanisms.

Application Box 4.2

ABC transporters produce drug resistance in cancer cells: ABC transporters cause expulsion of cytotoxic drugs from cancer cells. This decreases effective concentration of drugs in the cells needed for killing cancer cells. Hence, cancer cells become resistant to anticancer chemotherapy. Examples are **MDR 1** protein (multi-drug resistance-associated protein 1) and **BRCP** (breast cancer resistance protein).

- Energy created by **Na^+ gradient** is utilized for transport of other solutes.
- The Na^+ gradient is generated and maintained by Na^+-K^+ pump.
- Though the transport system by itself does not directly utilize energy, it depends on the function of Na^+-K^+ pump.
- Therefore, when the pump is inhibited by a blocking agent, transport process stops.

In Kidney and GIT

Typical example of secondary active transport is the **reabsorption of glucose from the kidney tubule or intestine.**

- The **primary active transport of Na^+** out of the basal and basolateral membranes of the proximal tubules of the nephron and the small intestine ***by Na^+-K^+ pump*** leads to **decreased concentration of Na^+** in the cytosol of the epithelial cells.
- This causes **facilitated diffusion of Na^+** from the lumen into the cells.
- The **carrier protein** that transfers Na^+ from the luminal fluid into the cell ***also transports glucose*** in the *same direction* (Fig. 4.9).
- Thus, the carrier protein is a **symport** that transports glucose simultaneously with sodium. The symport also *transports amino acids and other solutes*.

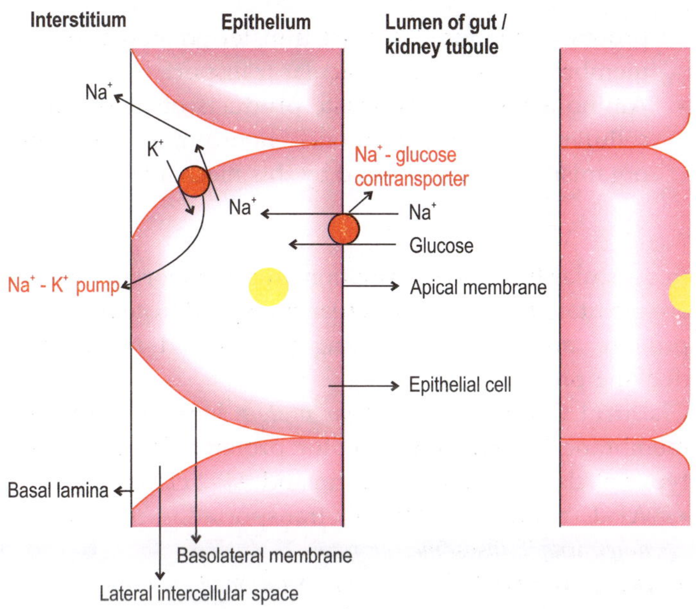

Fig. 4.9: Mechanism of secondary active transport (in kidney or intestine). Na^+-K^+ pump located on basolateral membrane actively pumps sodium out of the cell that decreases cytosolic sodium and creates gradient for transport of sodium from lumen into the cell. The carrier protein (symport) that transports sodium also transports glucose into the cell. Thus, transport of glucose is the secondary active transport.

- The carrier protein may also be an **antiport** counter-transporting hydrogen ion (in the nephron) out of the cell for bringing in sodium (Application Box 4.3).
- Since the transport depends on primary active transport of sodium by the Na^+-K^+ pump, it is known as a secondary active transport.

Application Box 4.3

The carrier protein may also be an antiport: The example of carrier protein being an antiport in secondary active transport is the counter-transporting hydrogen ion in the nephron out of the cell for bringing in sodium (Na^+-H^+ exchanger). Another example is Na^+-Ca^{++} exchanger in cardiac cell.

Characteristic Features: As the carrier protein for secondary active transport system is an integral membrane protein it exhibits **competitive inhibition and saturation kinetics.** However, it differs from the usual carrier transport for its exclusive **dependence on primary transport mechanism** (the pump) and for transporting **against its own electrochemical gradient**.

VESICULAR TRANSPORT

The transport process that occurs by either **fusion of vesicle** or **formation of vesicle** is called as vesicular transport.

- Fusion of vesicle with the cell membrane occurs in **exocytosis** and formation of vesicle from the cell membrane occurs in **endocytosis**.
- **Macromolecules** such as large protein molecules can not be transported by diffusion or active transport

process. Therefore, they are transferred across the cell membrane mainly by vesicular transport.

- Amino acids, sugars, waste products of metabolism, cellular secretions, hormones, neurotransmitters and organisms are transported by this mechanism.

Role of Vesicular Transport Proteins

In vesicular transport, formation and transport of vesicles are facilitated by some vesicular transport proteins. These proteins are: clathrin, coating proteins, dynamin and docking proteins.

Clathrin: Clathrin is a *fibrillar protein* located in the cell membrane beneath the receptor protein. There are **two types** of clathrins: AP-1 clathrin and AP-2 clathrin.

- **AP-1 clathrin** helps in transportation *from Golgi apparatus to lysosome*.
- **AP-2 clathrin** helps in *transportation of endosomes*.

Coating Proteins (COP): There are **two types** coating proteins: COP I and COP II. Coating proteins help in transportation of vesicles *between endoplasmic apparatus and Golgi apparatus*.

Dynamin: Dynamin helps in **formation of vesicles from cell membrane**, especially in clathrin-mediated endocytosis.

Caveolin: Cell membrane contains **caveoli** that are membrane indentations coated with ***caveolin***, the protein that facilitates *endocytosis of various proteins*.

Docking Proteins: Before exocytosis of vesicles, **docking of vesicles** occurs.

Docking proteins facilitate *attachment of vesicle with membrane*.

Examples of docking proteins are **V snare protein and T snare protein** (for details, refer "Synaptic Transmission")

Types Vesicular Transports

Vesicular transports are of **three types**: endocytosis, exocytosis and transcytosis.

Endocytosis

Endocytosis is the process of transport in which a substance is **taken into the cell by means of vesicle formation**.

- A region of plasma membrane is pinched off to form an endocytic vesicle that causes internalization of the substance to the cell.
- The vesicle may contain fluid and dissolved solutes or particulate material.
- The size of the vesicle varies from 0.1 μm to 2 μm.

Mechanisms of Endocytosis

Endocytosis occurs by **two mechanisms**: constitutive and clathrin-mediated.

Constitutive Endocytosis: Endocytosis by *constitutive pathway* occurs in almost all cells. It is called 'constitutive'

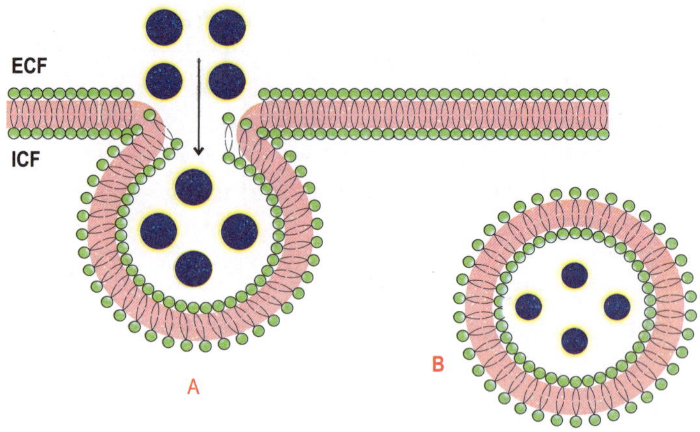

Fig. 4.10: Constitutive Endocytosis. **A:** Formation of vesicle; **B:** Separation of vesicle from the membrane.

as the process occurs continually and does not require any specific stimulus.

- The molecule or the substance makes contact with the cell membrane that invaginates to form an endocytic vesicle.
- The non-cytoplasmic side of the membrane then fuses and the vesicle is pinched-off into the cytosol.

Thus, it occurs in **two major steps**: formation of vesicle and separation of vesicle from the membrane (Fig. 4.10).

Clathrin-mediated Endocytosis: Endocytosis occurs in three steps:

1. Receptors are concentrated in small pits called **coated pits**, beneath which clathrins are present. The attachment of the macromolecules to the receptors stimulates invagination of the coated-pit, enclosing the molecule and a small portion of the ECF, forming a vesicle.
    - Clathrin molecule forms a geometrical array that surrounds the vesicle (Fig. 4.11).
    - Once the vesicle formation is complete, clathrin molecules detach from the vesicle and recycle to the membrane.
2. The endocytic vesicle detaches from the cell membrane.
3. Fusion of the endocytic vesicle with lysosomes that empty their **acid hydrolases** into the vesicle leading to the digestion of the substances in the vesicle.

Types of Endocytosis

Endocytosis is of **three types**: phagocytosis, receptor-mediated endocytosis and pinocytosis.

Phagocytosis: Phagocytosis, otherwise called '**cell-eating**', is the process of ingestion of large particles or microorganisms by specialized cells called phagocytes.

- In this process, the phagocytic cells such as macrophages and neutrophils engulf bacteria, foreign particles and tissue debris and digest them with the help of lysosomal enzymes.
- For details, refer 'Lysosomes' in the previous chapter)

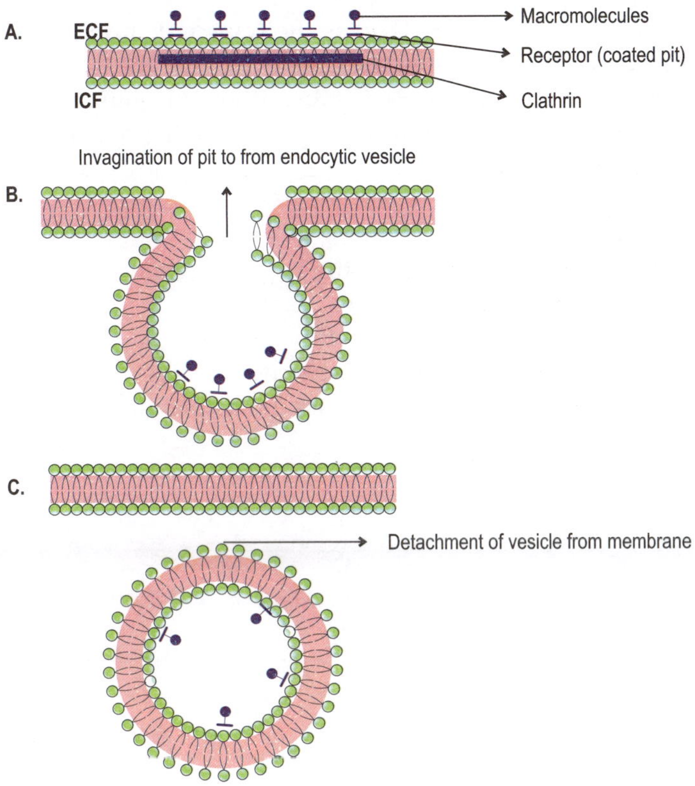

Fig. 4.11: Mechanism of clathrin-mediated endocytosis. **A:** Location of clathrin molecules and receptors for macromolecules. **B:** Attachment of macromolecules with receptors causes invagination of coated pit forming endocytic vesicle. **C:** Detachment of vesicle from the membrane into the cell.

Receptor-mediated Endocytosis: In this process, extracellular molecule binds with the specific receptor on the cell membrane. Receptors are concentrated at a depression on membrane called **coated-pits**.

- Once the external molecule attaches with receptor, the coated-pit pinches off from the membrane in the form of an **endocytic vesicle** causing rapid internalization of the molecule.
- Hormones, growth factors, transport-proteins, viruses etc. enter cells by receptor-mediated endocytosis.

Pinocytosis: Pinocytosis is the **fluid-phase endocytosis** or '**cell drinking**' by which substances in solution in extracellular fluid are internalized to the cell.

- It is a continuous process that occurs in most cells of the body.
- The stages in pinocytosis are same as endocytosis except that the endocytic vesicle contains fluid instead of solid particles.

Exocytosis

Exocytosis is the export from the cell, which is reverse of endocytosis. By exocytosis, hormones, neurotransmitters, digestive enzymes and undigested foreign particles are released form cells.

- Before exocytosis, the molecules are synthesized in endoplasmic reticulum and packaged in Golgi apparatus to form the **transport vesicles**.
- The vesicles then move to the cell surface, fuse with the cell membrane and release their content by exocytosis (Fig. 4.12), which requires ATP and Ca^{2+}.

Emiocytosis: Emiocytosis is the term refers to exocytosis of specific hormones and granules.

Mechanism of Exocytosis

Exocytosis occurs in **two pathways**: constitutive and regulated.

Constitutive Exocytosis: This type of exocytosis is seen in almost all cells.

- By this mechanism, some proteins are continuously secreted by the cells.
- For example, secretion of mucus by goblet cells of small intestine.

Regulated Exocytosis: In regulatory exocytosis, macromolecules that are stored in the vesicles fuse with cell membrane and release their content in response to specific extracellular stimulus.

- This is the major mechanism of rapid secretion of hormones, neurotransmitters and digestive enzymes in response to specific stimuli.
- This is also called **non-constitutive exocytosis.**

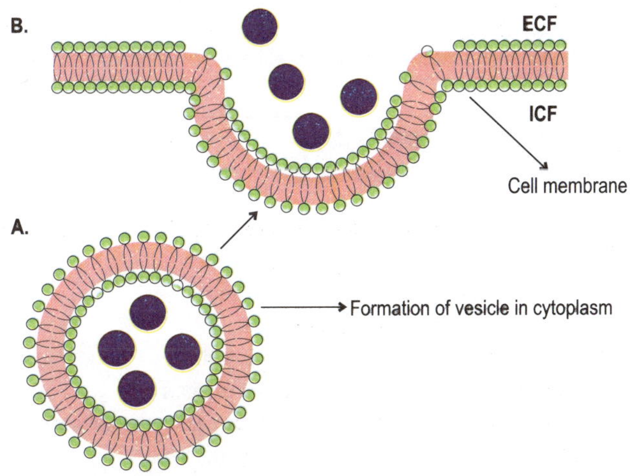

Fig. 4.12: Constitutive exocytosis, which occurs in two major steps. (A) Formation of exocytic vesicles; (B) Fusion of vesicles with the membrane and discharge of its content into ECF.

Transcytosis

When vesicular transport is limited within the cell, the process is called transcytosis or **cytopemisis**. Vesicles are formed within the cell and transported in the cytoplasm.

TRANSPORT ACROSS THE EPITHELIA

There are **two mechanisms** for transport across the epithelia: transcellular transport and paracellular transport.

Transcellular transport: This is the **transport through the cell** i. e. from lumen through apical surface into the cytosol and from there through basolateral space or through basal membrane into the interstitial fluid.

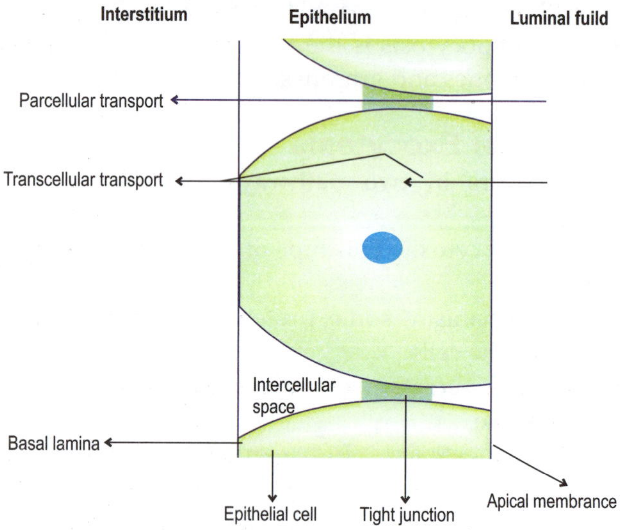

Fig. 4.13: Paracellular and transcellular transports. Paracellular transport occurs through the junction between the cells and transcellular transport occurs through the cell.

Paracellular transport: This is the transport **through the tight junctions between the cells** bypassing the transport through cells (Fig. 4.13). Reabsorption of sodium and glucose in kidney tubule and intestine is the example of transport across the epithelia.

Ultrafiltration

Ultrafiltration through the glomerular capillary endothelium and Bowman's capsule epithelium is a **special transport mechanism** through epithelia. However, in ultrafiltration, transfer of substances occurs mainly due the difference in pressures across the epithelium.

Exam Questions

1. Describe the mechanism of diffusion and osmosis. List the differences between diffusion and facilitated diffusion.
2. Describe the structure, mechanism of action and functions of Na^+-K^+ pump. List the differences between primary and secondary active transport.
3. Describe the mechanism of different types of gating of ion channels. Add a note on carrier proteins.

Multiple Choice Questions

1. Transport of ions across a semipermeable membrane is known as:
A. Endocytosis B. Osmosis
C. Exocytosis D. Transcytosis

2. The process of cell drinking is termed as
A. Transcytosis B. Exocytosis
C. Phgocytosis D. Pinocytosis

3. Which of the following can NOT be true for calcium channels?
A. Utilise energy B. Ligand-gated
C. Stretch-sensitive D. Voltage-gated

4. All of the following are true for active transport, EXCEPT?
A. ATP hydrolysis occurs B. Along the electrical gradient
C. Against the concentration gradient
D. Exhibits saturation kinetics

5. Which of the following statement is true for osmolality of a solution?
A. It is the number of moles per liter of water
B. It is the number of osmoles per kg of water
C. It is affected by temperature
D. It is not linked to osmotic pressure

6. The coupling ratio of Na^+-K^+ ATPase is:
A. 2:1 B. 1:2
C. 2:3 D. 3:2

7. The rate of diffusion of a molecule through a membrane is inversely proportional to:
A. Concentration gradient B. Thickness of the membrane
C. Diffusion coefficient D. Surface area for diffusion

8. All of the following have extracellular sites on Na^+-K^+ ATPase, EXCEPT:
A. ATP B. Sodium
C. Potassium D. Phosphorylation

9. Compared to facilitated diffusion, simple diffusion:
A. Exhibits saturation kinetics B. Shows competitive inhibition
C. Shows specificity D. Has slower rate

10. All of the following are functions of Na^+-K^+ ATPase, EXCEPT:
A. Inhibits protein synthesis B. Maintains cell volume
C. Maintains RMP D. Mediates action of thyroxine

11. Which of the following has slowest transport rate across cell membrane?
A. Urea B. Oxygen
C. Carbon dioxide D. Vitamin A

12. Receptor-mediates endocytosis involves:
A. Cathepsin B. Clathrin
C. Syntaxin D. Synaptvinobrevin

13. Caveolin is used in:
A. Constitutive exocytosis B. Regulated exocytosis
C. Receptor-mediated endocytosis D. Facilitated diffusion

Answers

1. B	2. D	3. A	4. B	5. C	6. D	7. B
8. C	9. D	10. A	11. A	12. B	13. C	

Chapter 5

Membrane Potential

Learning Objectives

On completion of study of this chapter:

The student will be able to (must know):

1. List the factors that contribute to the membrane potential.
2. Give the normal values of RMP of different excitable tissues and equilibrium potential of important ions.
3. Understand the concept of Donnan effect and Nernst equation
4. Give the values of concentration of ions in ECF and ICF and the equilibrium potential for each ion.
5. Briefly explain the mechanism of genesis and maintenance of RMP.

The student may also be able to (desirable to know):

1. Explain the concept of Gibbs-Donnan Equilibrium.
2. Explain the concept of Nernst Equation
3. Explain the concept of Goldmann-Hodgkin-Katz Equation.

BASIC PRINCIPLES

The cell membrane separates intracellular fluid from extracellular fluid. An electrical potential difference exists across the membrane of all living cells with the inside being negative in relation to the outside. This **potential difference** is called membrane potential.

- At resting state of the cell, the membrane potential is called **resting membrane potential** (RMP). The RMP is different in different tissues (Table 5.1).
- **In a nerve cell, the RMP is –70 mV**. When the *neuron is stimulated*, membrane potential changes and inside of the cell becomes positive due to depolarization. The membrane potential during this state of activation is called ***action potential***.
- RMP plays an important role in ***deciding the degree and duration of action potential***, as the RMP is the level from where the phase of depolarization starts.
- In some tissues like visceral smooth muscles, RMP fluctuates.

Table 5.1 | RMP of important excitable cells.

Cell	RMP (mV)
Neuron	−70
Skeletal muscle	−90
Cardiac muscle	−90

Factors Contributing to Membrane Potential

Membrane potential is mainly due to *distribution of ions across the cell membrane*, which results mainly from the **selective permeability** of the cell membrane to various ions at rest.

However, membrane potential is influenced by **various forces** affecting the ion distribution.

1. Selective permeability of the cell membrane to various ions
2. Gibbs–Donnan equilibrium
3. Nernst equation
4. Goldmann-Hodgkin equation

Selective Permeability of Membrane to Various Ions

The cell membrane is selectively permeable. Some ions are highly permeable, some are less permeable and others impermeable. The permeability mainly depends on the **molecular weight and the radius of ions** in their hydrated form (Table 5.2).

- Though the ions like Na^+, K^+, Cl^- and HCO_3^- are diffusible through the membrane, the **permeability is more for K^+**.
- Though the particle size of K^+ is large (atomic weight 39) as compared to Na^+ (atomic weight 23), the

permeability for K^+ is 500 to 1000 times greater than that for Na^+ for its **effective radius**.

- The membrane is practically *impermeable to intracellular proteins and organic phosphates*.

Table 5.2 | Molecular weight and radius of hydrated ions and other substances.

Ions/substances	Mol Wt	Radius
K^+	39	0.12
K^+	39	0.12
Cl^-	35.5	0.12
H2O	18	0.12
Ca^{++}	40	0.15
Na^+	23	0.18
Urea	60	0.23
Glucose	180	0.38
Albumin	69,000	7.50

Gibbs-Donnan Membrane Equilibrium

When two solutions containing ions are separated by a semipermeable membrane, at equilibrium, each solution will be *electrically neutral*.

- That means, the **total quantity of cations** will be *equal to total quantity of anions*.
- Also, the **product of diffusible ions** on one side of the membrane *will be equal* to product of diffusible ions on the other side of the membrane.

This is called Gibbs-Donnan membrane equilibrium.

For example, two solutions A and B containing sodium and chloride ions are separated by a semipermeable membrane. Then, according to Gibbs-Donnan equilibrium, **each solution should be electrically neutral** (Fig. 5.1), which means, $(\text{cations})_A = (\text{anions})_A$, and $(\text{cations})_B = (\text{anions})_B$ or,

$(Na^+)_A = (Cl^-)_A$ and, $(Na^+)_B = (Cl^-)_B$

The product of **diffusible ions on both sides will also be equal**, which means, $(\text{diffusible cations})_A \times (\text{diffusible anions})_A = (\text{diffusible cations})_B \times (\text{diffusible anions})_B$ Or, $[(Na^+)_A \times (Cl^-)_A] = [(Na^+)_B \times (Cl^-)_B]$

Thus, the ratio of diffusible ions will be:

$$\frac{(\text{Diffusible cations})_A}{(\text{Diffusible cations})_B} = \frac{(\text{Diffusible anions})_B}{(\text{Diffusible anions})_A}$$

$$\text{Or, } \frac{[Na^+]_A}{[Na^+]_B} = \frac{[Cl^-]_B}{[Cl^-]_A}$$

Thus, there will be **equal and balanced distribution** of ions at equilibrium.

However, when a non-diffusible ions 'X' is added on one side (let us say, side A), then as per Gibbs'-Donnan equilibrium principle, the **distribution of diffusible ions will change** to maintain electroneutrality of both sides (Fig. 5.2).

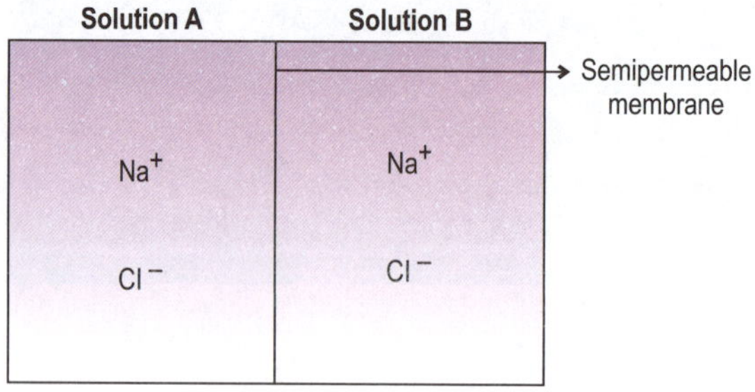

Fig. 5.1: Gibbs Donnan equilibrium. Na^+ and Cl– are equally distributed on both side of semipermeable membrane, in solution A and B.

For both solutions to be electrically neutral:

$(Na^+)_A = (Cl^-)_A + (X^-)_A$ and, $(Na^+)_B = (Cl^-)_B$

Therefore, $(Na^+)_A + (Cl^-)_A + (X^-)_A > (Na^+)_B + (Cl^-)_B$

Also, for the product of diffusible ions on two sides to be equal,

$(Na^+)_A \times (Cl^-)_A = (Na^+)_B \times (Cl^-)_B$

Thus, $(Na^+)_A > (Na^+)_B$, and $(Cl^-)_A < (Cl^-)_B$

Consequently, there is **unequal distribution of diffusible ions** on both sides. Therefore, at equilibrium, Na^+ is more on the side which contains non-diffusible anions 'X' (side A) and Cl^- is more on the other side i.e., B. However, their *concentration ratios are equal*.

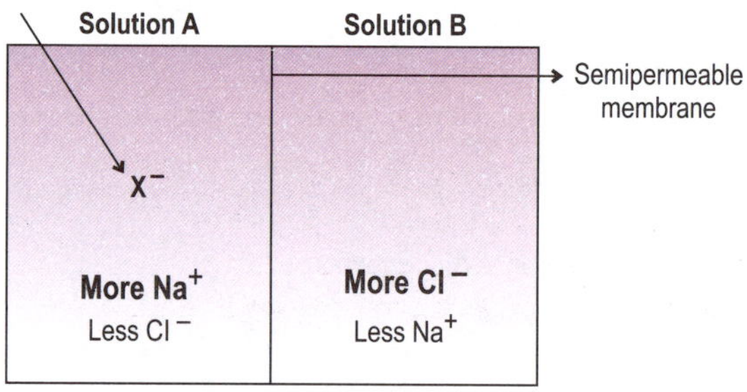

Fig. 5.2: When nondiffusible anion (X^-) was added to the solution A, more Cl^- is transferred to B to maintain balance of anion on both sides. Consequently, more Na^+ is transferred to solution A to maintain electroneutrality of both sides.

Same analogy is applicable to intracellular fluid (ICF) and extracellular fluid (ECF). **ICF contains non-diffusible anions** like proteins and organic phosphate. Therefore, asymmetrical distribution of diffusible ions occurs across the cell membrane with **cations being more inside than the outside**. Therefore, at rest, **interior of the cell is negative** to the exterior (discussed below in genesis of RMP).

Nernst Equation

As described above, in accordance with Gibbs'-Donnan equilibrium, *asymmetrical distribution* of diffusible ions occurs across the cell membrane with **more cation (K^+) present inside.**

- Therefore, K^+ will try to diffuse into the ECF from ICF, which is **opposed by the electrical gradient**, created by *presence of non-diffusible anions* inside the cell.

- Thus, finally equilibrium is reached between the concentration gradient and the electrical gradient resulting in *diffusion potential* (**equilibrium potential**) across the cell membrane.

The magnitude of this equilibrium potential is determined by Nernst equation:

$$E_{(m)} = -\frac{RT}{ZF} \ln \frac{(Conc)_i}{(Conc)_o}$$

Where,

$E_{(m)}$: Equilibrium potential (in millivolts) of the ions at which efflux and influx of the ions are equal
R : The natural gas constant (8.316 joules/degree).
T : The absolute temperature
F : The faraday constant (Number of coulomb/mole of charge = 96,500 coulomb/mole)
Z : The valency of the ion
ln : Natural logarithm
$(Conc)_i$: The concentration of the ions in the intracellular fluid
$(Conc)_o$: The concentration of the ions in the extracellular fluid

At normal body temperature (37°C), converting from the natural log to the base 10 log and replacing some of the constants with numerical values, the equation can be simplified to:

$$E_{(m)} = \pm 61 \log \frac{(Conc)_i}{(Conc)_o}$$

Thus, Nernst equation helps in calculating the equilibrium potential for each ion individually (Table 5.3).

Table 5.3 | Concentrations (mmol/L) of important ions in ECF & ICF and their equilibrium potential (EP) in a mammalian spinal motor neuron.

Ions	ECF	ICF	EP (mV)
Na^+	150	15	+ 60
K^+	5.5	150	–90
Cl^-	125	9	–70
HCO_3^-	21	5	–25
Calcium	2.5	10^{-4}	+130

Goldmann-Hodgkin-Katz Equation

The magnitude of the membrane potential at any given time depends on the **distribution of Na^+, K^+ and Cl^-** and on the **permeability of each of these ions**.

- The role of different ions in the generation of membrane potential is accurately described by Goldmann-Hodgkin-Katz (GHK) equation or also called **Goldmann's constant field equation**.

$$V = \frac{RT}{F} \ln \frac{P_{K+}[K^+]_o + P_{Na+}[Na^+]_o + P_{Cl-}[Cl^-]_i}{P_{K+}[K^+]_i + P_{Na+}[Na^+]_i + P_{Cl-}[Cl^-]_o}$$

Where,
V : membrane potential,
R : gas constant,
T : absolute temperature,
F : Faraday constant,
ln : natural logarithm
P_{K+}, P_{Na+} and P_{Cl^-} : permeabilities of the membrane to K^+, Na^+ and Cl^-, and $_i$ and $_o$ refer to inside and outside of the cell respectively.

Effects of Goldmann constant field equation:

1. Important ions that generate membrane potentials in nerve and muscle fibers are sodium, potassium and chloride.
   - The voltage of membrane potential is determined by the **concentration gradient** of each of these ions.
2. The relativity of importance of each ion in determination of the voltage depends upon **the membrane permeability of individual ion.**
3. *Cation concentration* from inside the membrane to outside is responsible for electronegativity inside the membrane.
   - Due to concentration gradient, **cations diffuse to outside of the cell** leaving the non-diffusible anions inside the cell.

PY1.8

GENESIS OF RMP

Resting membrane potential (RMP) is the membrane potential at rest. In neurons, the RMP is –70 mV. The RMP is created due to following reasons.

1. **Permeability of the membrane to K^+:** Normally, K^+ is more inside and less outside the cell (Table 5.3). Therefore, a concentration gradient exists for K^+ from inside to outside that facilitates K^+ to diffuse out of the cell.
   - At rest, **permeability of the membrane to K^+ is higher** than any other ion. Therefore, K^+ easily diffuses out of the cell (Fig. 5.3), though this is opposed by the electrical gradient.
   - As, K^+ is the major intracellular cation, its diffusion creates negativity inside the cell.
   - The **permeability of the membrane to K^+** is the *major cause of RMP*.
2. **Permeability of the membrane to Na^+:** At rest, ECF Na^+ is more than the ICF Na^+. Therefore, there is a concentration gradient for Na^+ from outside to inside, for which Na^+ diffuses into the cell.
   - However, at rest membrane is **less permeable to Na^+** (Fig. 5.3) than to K^+.

- Therefore, K^+ exit is not balanced by Na^+ entry (more K^+ goes out).
- Hence, interior of the cell remains relatively negative.

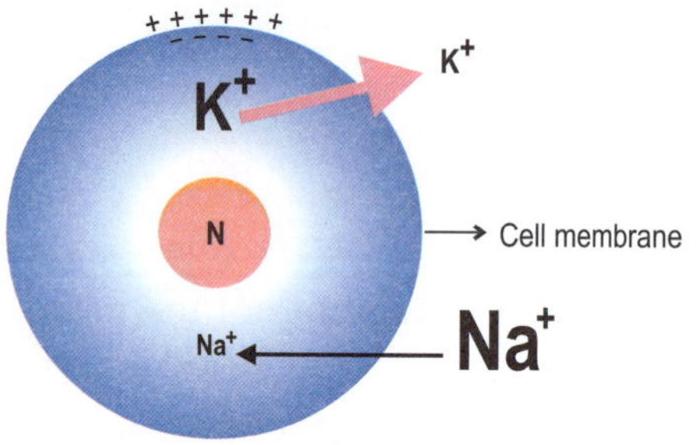

Fig. 5.3: Genesis of resting membrane potential (RMP). At rest, cell membrane is more permeable to K^+ than to Na^+. Hence, K^+ efflux is more than the Na^+ influx resulting in exit of more cations from the cell that creates relative negativity inside. This is the major cause of genesis of RMP. Direction and thickness of arrow indicate direction and magnitude of movement of ions. Size of letters for ions indicates their relative concentration in ECF and ICF. N: Nucleus.

3. **Permeability to anions:** Exit of more cations from the cell should be accompanied by proportionate exit of anion to maintain electroneutrality.
   - However, exit of K^+ (the cation) is not accompanied by exit of same number of anions as **permeability of anions at rest is also not same** as that of K^+.
   - Therefore, more negative ion remains inside.
4. **Role of Na^+-K^+ pump:** The role of Na^+-K^+ pump is to **maintain RMP** rather than to generate it. However, Na^+-K^+ pump also contributes to the genesis of RMP, as it is an **electrogenic pump**.
   - It pumps out three Na^+ for two K^+ to come in.
   - Therefore, it pumps more cations out of the cell and less into the cell.
   - Thus, **less cations are taken inside**, which in other words, a *relative negativity is created inside* (Application Box 5.1).

Application Box 5.1

Negativity is only along the membrane: It should be noted that the number of ions that are responsible for membrane potential is a very small fraction of the total number of ions actually present inside the cell. In the cell, the cations and anions are present in equal proportion except along the membrane. Therefore, negativity is created and maintained only close to the membrane.

Maintenance of RMP

K^+ diffusing out of the cell and Na^+ diffusing into the cell will come to halt once the concentration gradient ceases to exist for both the ions. However, that does not happen, as **Na^+-K^+ ATPase helps in building the concentration gradient**.

- It serves to pump back the Na^+ that diffuses into the cell and K^+ that diffuses out of the cell.
- Thus, Na^+-K^+ pump plays an **important role in maintaining RMP**.

Exam Questions

1. What is Donnan effect and how does it contribute to the membrane potential?
2. Briefly explain the mechanisms of genesis and maintenance of resting membrane potential.

Multiple Choice Questions

1. **Most diffusible ion in an excitable tissue is:**
   A. Sodium
   B. Phosphate
   C. Chloride
   D. Potassium
2. **If intracellular conc. of K^+ is 10 mM and extracellular conc. is 100 mM, calculate equilibrium potential of K^+ based on Nernst equation.**
   A. 10 mM
   B. 100 mM
   C. 60 mM
   D. – 90 mM
3. **Nernst potential of K^+ is :**
   A. – 90 mV
   B. – 70 mV
   C. +70 mV
   D. + 90 mV
4. **Equilibrium potential of an ion is calculated by:**
   A. Gibbs-Donnan equilibrium
   B. Nernst equation
   C. Goldman equation
   D. Katz equation
5. **What is the effect on membrane, if extracellular concentration of K^+ is decreased.**
   A. Decreased magnitude of RMP
   B. Increased negativity of membrane
   C. Increased magnitude of RMP
   D. Decreased negativity of membrane
6. **RMP is mainly due to the permeability of the membrane to:**
   A. Sodium
   B. Potassium
   C. Chloride
   D. Magnessium

Answers

1. D 2. C 3. A 4. B 5. B 6. B

Chapter 6

Body Fluids

Learning Objectives

On completion of study of this chapter:

The student will be able to (must know):

1. Give the normal values of total body water (TBW) as % of body weight in different age groups in males and females.
2. Name different body fluid compartments, total fluid present in the compartment and composition ions in each compartment.
3. Give the % distribution of body water in different body fluid compartments.
4. Give the characteristics of an ideal indicator used for measuring body fluid volumes.
5. Name the indicator used and understand the basic principle and method of measurement of body fluid volume of different compartments.
6. Define osmolarity and osmolality and give their normal values in plasma.
7. Explain why dehydration is common and often severe in children.
8. Define pH and give normal values of pH of blood.

The student may also be able to (desirable to know):

1. Describe the methods of measurement of fluid volumes of different body fluid compartments.

Cell functions depend on fluids present both outside and inside of the cell. Body fluid is compartmentalized into intracellular and extracellular fluid compartments.

Body Fluid Content: The body composition of a **normal adult male** on average consists of 15% fat, 18% proteins, 7% minerals and 60% water.

- The **total body water** (TBW) as percentage of body weight on average is **about 60%** in adult males, which is about *10% more than adult females* (Table 6.1).
- **In infants** and children, though TBW as percentage of body weight is more than in adults, their absolute water content is *significantly less*.
- **In elderly people** in both the sexes, TBW is about **10% less** than their adult counterparts.
- **In females**, TBW is *less than in males* due to relatively ***greater amount of adipose tissue*** (subcutaneous fat) in them.

Table 6.1 | TBW as % of body weight.

Age	Males	Females
Infants	65 – 70	65 – 70
Children (upto 9 yrs)	60 – 65	59 – 62
10 – 17 yrs	58 – 60	55 – 58
18 – 39 yrs	58 – 64	48 – 55
40 – 59 yrs	52 – 58	45 – 50
60 yrs and above	50 – 55	42 – 48

Of total body water, about two-third is present in intracellular compartment and one-third in extracellular compartment (Table 6.2).

Table 6.2 | Distribution of total body water (TBW) in ECF and ICF compartments in a 70 kg adult male.

Compartment	% of body weight	% of body water	Volume
TBW	60	100	42L
ECF	20	33	14L
ICF`	40	67	28L

PY1.6

BODY FLUID COMPARTMENTS

Extracellular Fluid Compartment

Fluid present in the spaces outside the cell constitutes extracellular fluid (ECF) compartment. This includes plasma, interstitial fluid and transcellular fluid (Fig. 6.1).

Plasma

Plasma is the fluid part of the blood. It constitutes about 25% of the ECF, which is about 5% of the total body weight (Table 6.3).

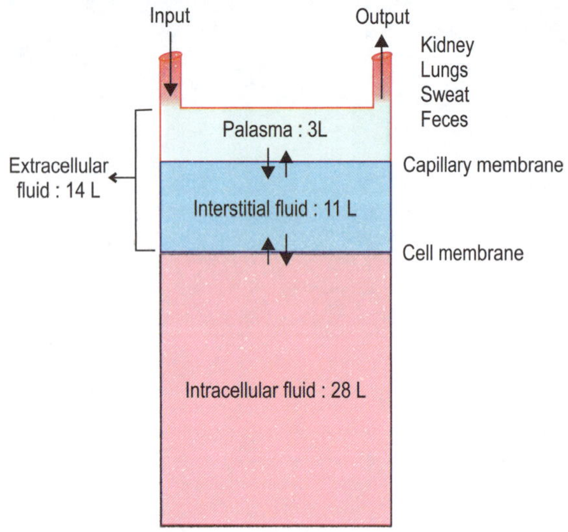

Fig. 6.1: Distribution of body fluids in body fluid compartments. Arrows indicate exchange of fluid between the compartments.

Table 6.3 | Distribution of extracellular fluid (ECF) in a 70 kg adult male.

Compartment	% of ECF	% of body weight	Volume	% of body water
Plasma	25	4 – 5	3.5L	8
Interstitial and transcellular fluid	10.5	15	10.5L	25

Volume of plasma can be calculated from blood volume and PCV (packed cell volume) as:

$$\text{Plasma volume} = \text{Blood volume} \times \frac{100 - \text{Hematocrit}}{100}$$

Blood Volume & Red Cell Volume: Blood volume is the plasma volume and blood cell volume.

- Blood volume is about 80 ml/kg of body weight or 8% of the total body weight.
- **Red cell volume** is the volume occupied by the circulating red cells.
  - It is determined by subtracting plasma volume from total blood volume.
  - However, it is also calculated by injecting **red cells tagged with radioactive isotopes** such as ^{51}Cr, ^{59}Fe or ^{32}P. Fraction of red cell tagged is measured after proper mixing has occurred.
- Total blood volume is **less in children** (Application Box 6.1).

Application Box 6.1

Dehydration is common and rapid in children: Ratio of ECF volume to ICF volume is larger in infants and children than in adults. However, as the total volume of ECF is much smaller in children than in adults. In addition, the regulatory mechanisms for maintaining ECF volume are not well developed in infants and children. Therefore, dehydration is more common and occurs rapidly in these age groups.

Interstitial Fluid

It is the ECF volume present in the **space between the cells** (ECF outside the vascular system).

- Interstitial fluid surrounds all cells except blood cells and includes lymph (lymph constitutes 2–3% of the total body weight).
- It is in constant motion throughout the body and is exchanged rapidly with the circulating blood.
- Interstitial fluid volume is about **15% of body weight**.
- It *can not be measured directly* as substances used for it rapidly equilibrate with plasma.
- It is calculated by subtracting plasma volume from ECF volume.

Transcellular Fluid

Transcellular fluid represents fluid **in the lumen of structures** lined by epithelium.

- It includes fluid in the secretion of exocrine digestive glands, cerebrospinal fluid (CSF), pleural, peritoneal, synovial and pericardial fluids, intraocular (aqueous and vitreous humors) fluids, bile, luminal fluids of the gut and fluid in the cochlea and kidney tubules.
- The total transcellular fluid volume is **1.5% of body weight**, which is about 1L.

Intracellular Fluid Compartment

Intracellular fluid (ICF) is the fluid contained **within the cells of the body**.

- It constitutes about **two-thirds of total fluid** of the body.
- It can not be measured directly.
- It is measured by subtracting ECF volume from total fluid volume.

MEASUREMENT OF BODY FLUID VOLUMES

General Concept

The volume of fluid compartment is usually measured by the **indicator dilution principle**, which is based on the following relationship:

$$C = \frac{A}{V} \quad \text{i.e., } V = \frac{A}{C}$$

where, A is the amount of a substance injected intravenously, V is the volume in which the substance is distributed and C is the final concentration attained.

Characteristics of an Indicator

1. Should be relatively easy to measure.
2. Should remain in the compartment being measured.

3. Should not change the fluid distribution in the compartment being measured.
4. Should be non-toxic.
5. Must mix evenly throughout the compartment being measured.
6. Should remain unchanged by the body during the mixing period or the amount changed must be known.

Principle of Measurement

Size of fluid compartment is measured by injecting a substance and then calculating the volume of fluid in which the test substance is distributed. This is called the **volume distribution.**

- Volume distribution of the injected substance is equal to the **amount injected divided by concentration of the substance** in the sample.
- If indicator *leaves the compartment* by excretion or metabolism during the time allowed for mixing, then calculation is done as follows:

$$\text{Volume distribution} = \frac{\text{Amount injected} - \text{Amount removed}}{\text{Final concentration of the substance}}$$

Measurement of ECF Volume

The ECF volume is difficult to measure, as the limit of this space is ill-defined, and few substances mix rapidly in all parts of the space while remaining exclusively extra-cellular.

Principle of Measurement

Volume Distribution Principle

ECF volume is measured by **volume distribution principle.**

Using Inulin: Inulin, a polysaccharide having mol wt of 5200.

- **Radioactive inulin** is prepared by substituting ^{14}C for one of the carbon atoms of the molecule.
- Radioactive inulin levels are easily determined by counting the samples with suitable radiation detectors.

Other substances used: Also, **Cl^-** ($^{36}Cl^-$ and $^{38}Cl^-$), **^{82}Br, mannitol and sucrose** are used for measurement of ECF volume.

- Cl^- is largely extracellular. Therefore, radioactive isotopes of **Cl^- ($^{36}Cl^-$ and $^{38}Cl^-$)** are used for the purpose. However, ECF volume determined by using Cl^- is greater than actual volume as some Cl^- is also present in intracellular fluid.
- **^{82}Br, sulphate, thiosulphate, thiocyanate and ferrocyanide** are also used for measuring ECF volume. As these ions interchange with Cl^- in the body, they *determine greater values* for ECF.
- **Mannitol and sucrose** have also been used to measure ECF volume.

Methods of Measurement

Measurement of Plasma Volume

Plasma volume is measured by **two dilution methods.**

First Method: In the first method, the substance used **neither leaves the vascular system nor penetrates red cells.** Examples are:

i) **Evans Blue Dye** (T-1824) that remains bound to plasma proteins.
ii) **Radio-iodinated human serum albumin** (RISA) i.e. serum albumin labeled with radioactive iodine.
   - It slowly escapes from circulation into the interstitial fluid.
   - Suitable sample of injected solution and plasma samples obtained after injection are counted in a scintillation counter.
iii) **Radio-iodinated gamma globulin and fibrinogen.** These substances generally do not leak out of the blood stream.

Second Method: In this method, radioisotopes of phosphorus (^{32}P), iron ($^{55,59}Fe$) and chromium (^{51}Cr) are used that **penetrate and bind to red cells.** Therefore, the red cells volume i.e. volume occupied by all the circulating RBCs in the body can be measured by injecting tagged red cells intravenously.

- After thorough mixing has occurred, fraction of the RBCs that is tagged is measured.
- Commonly used tag is ^{51}Cr, which is attached to the red cells by incubating in a suitable 'Cr' solution.

Then, plasma volume is calculated by using the formula:

$$\text{Plasma volume} = \frac{100 - \text{PCV}}{100} \times \text{Blood volume}$$

(PCV is packed cell volume, which is practically the red cell volume)

Measurement of Interstitial Fluid Volume

Interstitial fluid volume cannot be measured directly as it is difficult to sample and no substance penetrates exclusively in this compartment.

- Substance that equilibrates in interstitial fluid also equilibrates in plasma.
- Therefore, the interstitial fluid volume is estimated as the difference between ECF volume and plasma volume.

Measurement of ICF Volume

Intracellular fluid (ICF) volume cannot be measured directly by dilution principle as no substance remains confined only to this compartment. It is *determined indirectly* by subtracting ECF volume from total body water (TBW). Thus, **first TBW is measured**.

Measurement of TBW: Measurement of TBW is performed by **indicator dilution principle**.

- **Deuterium oxide** (D_2O, heavy water) is usually used as it has properties that are slightly different from H_2O. However, in *equilibration experiments* for measuring TBW, it gives accurate results.
- **Tritium oxide** and **aminopyrine** can also be used for measuring TBW.

Note: Measurement of red cell volume, plasma volume, effective blood volume is described in next chapter.

IMPORTANT NOTE

Volume of different body compartments can be approximately calculated by following formulae.
Total body water = 0.6 × Body weight
Intracellular fluid volume = 0.4 ×Body weight
Extracellular fluid volume = 0.2 × Body weight
Interstitial fluid volume = 0.75 × ECF
Plasma volume = 0.25 × ECF

IONIC COMPOSITION OF BODY FLUIDS

Basic Features

1. The distribution of electrolytes varies in body compartments.
2. **Sum of the concentrations** of the cations equals the sum of the concentrations of the anions in respective compartments. This makes the fluid in each compartment **electrically neutral**.
3. Na^+, Ca^{++}, Cl^- and HCO_3^- are largely extra cellular (Table 6.4) and K^+, Mg^{++}, organic phosphates (PO_4^{3-}) and proteins ($prot^-$) are mainly intracellular.
4. Essentially, almost all the **K^+ in the body is in exchangeable pool**, whereas only **65% – 70% of Na^+ is exchangeable**.
5. Solutes that are exchangeable are **osmotically active**.
6. Almost all of the body **Ca^{++}** (in bone) and most of the body **Mg^{++}** (in bone and cells) are **non-exchangeable** (Fig. 6.2).

Table 6.4 | Concentration (mmol/L of H2O) of major ions in ECF (plasma) and ICF.

Ions	ECF	ICF
Na^+	145	12
K^+	5	140
Ca^{++}(ionized)	1.2	0.1 µmol/L
Mg^{++}	1.5	20

Table 6.4: Contd....

Cl^-	110	5
HCO^{3-}	27	10
$PO4^{3-}$	2	60

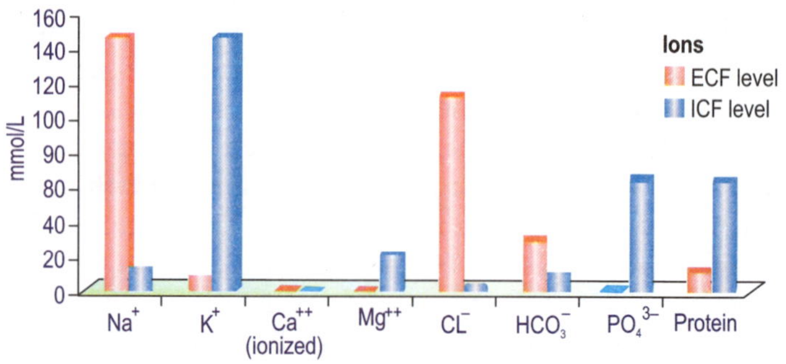

Fig. 6.2: Comparison of electrolytes and protein in ECF (orange bars) and ICF (blue bars) expressed as millimole per liter (mmol/L). (ECF: extracellular fluid; ICF: intracellular fluid)

Units for Measuring Solutes

Moles

The mole is the standard unit for expressing the amount of substances in the SI unit system. A mole is the **gram-molecular weight of a substance**, i.e. the molecular weight of a substance, in grams.

- Each mole (mol) consists of approx. 6×10^{23} molecules.
- Thus, 1 mole of KCl = 39 + 35.5gm = 74.5 gm (i.e. sum of atomic masses of all the atoms in the molecule).

Millimole: The **millimole** (mmol) is 1/1000 of a mole. Thus, 1 mmol of KCl = 74.5 mg.

Principles

1. The concentrations of two different substances on the basis of number of grams per liter of solution do not indicate how many molecules of each compound are present. Therefore, concentrations **in units of grams per liter** are often used when the chemical *structure of the solute is unknown*.
2. When the *structure of a molecule is known*, concentrations are expressed as **moles per liter**.
   - This provides a unit of concentration based upon the number of molecules of the solute in solution.
   - Thus a solution containing 74.5 gm of KCl in 1 liter of solution is said to be one-molar (1M or 1 mol/L) solution of KCl.
3. Since 1 mole of any molecule will have the same number of molecules (6×10^{23}), 1M solution of KCl contains the same number of solute molecules per liter as 1 M solution of glucose or any other substance.

Osmole and Milliosmole: The concentration of osmotically active particles is usually expressed in osmoles (osm).

- One **osmole** equals the gram molecular weight (i.e. one mole) of the substance divided by the number of freely moving particles each molecule liberates in solution.

- The **milliosmole** (mosm) is 1/1000 of 1 osm.

i) If a solute is a **non-ionizing compound** like glucose, one osmole is equal to 1 mole of solute particle. Thus, 1 molar solution of glucose has a concentration of 1 osm (1 osmole per liter).

ii) If the solute is an **ionizing compound** like NaCl, each ion is an osmotically active particle.
  - Therefore, in 1 molar solution of NaCl, NaCl would dissociate into Na^+ and Cl^- ions, so that each mole in solution would supply two osmoles of solute per liter of solution.
  - Similarly, one mole of $CaCl_2$ would dissociate into Ca^{++}, Cl^- and Cl^-, and thus, supplying 3 osmoles.

Equivalents

The equivalent is the standard unit for expressing the solutes in the body which are in the form of **charged particles**.

- One equivalent (Eq) is 1 mole of an ionized substance divided by its valency. One mole of KCl dissociates into 1 Eq of K^+ and 1 Eq of Cl^-.
- One Eq of K^+ = 39 gm/1 = 39 gm; whereas 1 Eq Ca^{++} = 40gm/2 = 20gm. The milliequivalent (mEq) is 1/1000 of 1 Eq.

Normality: The normality (N) of a solution is the number of gram equivalents in 1 liter. Therefore, 1 N solution of hydrochloric acid (HCl) contains 1 + 35.5 gm/L = 36.5gm/L.

Osmolarity and Osmolality

Definitions: Osmolality of a solution refers to the number of osmoles (number of osmotically active particles) dissolved in a kilogram of solvent. Osmolarity refers to the number of osmoles in one liter of plasma.

Unlike osmolality, the value in osmolarity is affected by the volume of *other solutes* in the solution.

Osmolarity is also *affected by temperature*.

Though osmotic pressure is determined by osmolality, the difference between osmolality and osmolarity is negligible.

Osmolarity is frequently used in physiology for its easy measurement.

IMPORTANT NOTE

Osmole is important:
Note that the important factor determining the osmotic pressure of a solution is the **concentration of the particles released in solution** (i.e. the osmoles), not the size, shape or charge of the particles.

- Osmotically active substances in the body are dissolved in water.
- As the density of water is 1, osmolal concentration is expressed in osmoles per liter (osm/L) of water.

Plasma Osmolality

The total **sum of all the particles** in plasma determine its osmolality, and *over 90 per cent* of the osmolality of plasma is **due to NaCl**.

- The plasma proteins contribute very little, even though their molecules are large in size.
- The normal **plasma osmolality is 290 mOsm per kg**, out of which *270 mOsm is due to the effect of NaCl*.

Tonicity

Tonicity refers to the **osmolality of a solution in relation to plasma** (same osmotic pressure or freezing-point depression as plasma).

- Solutions, which have osmolality same as that of plasma, like 0.9 % NaCl, are said to be **isotonic**, and those with lower osmolality are said to be **hypotonic**.
- Solutions with higher osmolality than that of plasma are said to be **hypertonic**.

Osmotic lysis of red cells in hypotonic solution: The solution of 0.9 % NaCl is isotonic, and therefore, red cells do not change their shape and size in this solution. In hypotonic solutions, red cells undergo osmotic lysis due to endosmosis and in hypertonic solutions they shrink due to exosmosis (Clinical Note 6.1)

Clinical Note 6.1

Hyperosmolal coma: In diabetes, increased plasma osmolality due to very high plasma glucose concentration causes shrinkage of cells. Especially, dehydration of brain cells leads to coma, which is an acute medical emergency. In chronic renal failure, very high urea and creatinine can cause encephalopathy.

Effects of metabolism and shifting of solutes: A solution may be isotonic initially, but **later it becomes hypotonic** if the osmotically active particles are transferred into the cell or metabolized.

- For example, 5% glucose solution is isotonic and remains so temporarily when infused intravenously.
- However, as glucose is rapidly metabolized, the net effect of infusion is like the infusion of a hypotonic solution.
- Therefore, **infusion of normal saline** (0.9% NaCl) is preferred **in volume depletion**, as described above.

Note: Details of control of water balance and osmolality of body fluid compartments are described in the Chapter 136, "Body Fluid Volume Homeostasis".

H^+ Concentration of Body Fluids and Concept of pH

The hydrogen ion concentration of body fluids is expressed as H^+ or pH (negative logarithm of H^+).

$pH = -\log_{10}[H^+]$

The pK: When pK (K is the ionization or dissociation constant) of a buffer system is known, it is possible to determine the effective pH range of the buffer. Hence, pK = negative log of K (–log K) and is equal to the pH at which half of the acid molecules are dissociated and half are undissociated.

Blood pH: Blood pH is 7.35 – 7.45, at the range of H^+ conc. 20 – 126 mEq/L. Acidosis refers to blood < 7.35 and alkalosis refers to pH of blood > 7.45.

Note: Details of pH-buffer system and acid-base balance are described in the chapter "Principles of acid-base homeostasis", Chapter 134.

Exam Questions

1. Give the normal values of distribution of total body water in different compartments in a normal adult male. Describe the method of measurement of plasma volume.
2. In a tabular format, give the concentration of three important cations and three important anions in ECF and ICF. Describe the method of measurement of ECF volume.

Multiple Choice Questions

1. In a person weighing 60kg, the total body water is:
A. 15 L B. 25 L
C. 35 L D. 45 L

2. In a person weighing 70kg, the ICF is:
A. 14 L B. 28 L
C. 35 L D. 42 L

3. All the following statement are true about total body water (TBW), EXCEPT:
A. In elderly, the TBW is 24% less than their adult counterparts
B. In females, TBW is less than males
C. In infants, TBW to total body weight ratio is greater
D. It can be measured by Tritium oxide

4. Which the following is measured by using Deuterium oxide?
A. Intracellular fluid B. Extracellular fluid
C. Total body water D. Red cell volume

5. All the following statements are true, EXCPT:
A. Intracellular fluid is 67% of total body water
B. Extracellular fluid is 33% of total body water
C. Plasma is 8% of total body water
D. Interstitial fluid is 15% of total body water

6. Next to Na+, which the following ion has maximum concentration in plasma?
A. K+ B. Cl-
C. HCO3- D. PO43-

7. Next to K+, which the following ion has maximum concentration in ICF?
A. Mg++ B. Cl-
C. HCO3- D. PO43-

8. Radio-isotope of chromium (51Cr) is used for measurement of:
A. Red cell volume B. Intracellular fluid
C. Extracellular fluid D. Total body water

9. After injection of 30mg of a substance into a compartment, 2mg was excreted and final concentration was 2mg/L. The volume of compartment is:
A. 15 L B. 28 L
C. 14 L D. 2 L

10. All the following statements are true for interstitial fluid, EXCPT:
A. It's volume is 15% of total body weight
B. It is about 10.5 L
C. It is measured by 82Br
D. Lymph is included under Interstitial fluid

Answers

1. C	2. B	3. A	4. C	5. D	6. B
7. D	8. A	9. C	10. C		

Section II

Blood

"An illness of the body is always the outer expression and translation of a disorder, a disharmony in the inner being; unless this inner disorder is healed, the outer cure cannot be total and permanent.

Sri Aurobindo"

Chapter 7

Introduction to Blood, and Plasma Proteins

Learning Objectives

On completion of study of this chapter:

The student will be able to (must know):

1. Define blood and give the composition and functions of blood.
2. Say wat is buffy coat and give uses of buffy coat preparation
3. Give the normal value of blood volume in adults and children.
4. Give the composition and functions of plasma.
5. Name the plasma proteins give their normal values, and list the functions of plasma proteins.
6. Give the uses of fresh frozen plasma.

The student may also be able to (desirable to know):

1. Describe the methods of blood volume measurement
2. Describe the functions of plasma proteins

THE BLOOD

Blood is defined as *liquid connective tissue that fills the heart and blood vessels*. The normal blood volume in an average adult is **5–6 liters**, which accounts for about **8% of the body weight**.

Composition of Blood

PY2.1

Blood consists of two components: cells and fluid.

1. The **cellular component** comprises of different formed elements, and the **fluid component** is the plasma. The **formed elements** are red blood cells (erythrocytes), white blood cells (leucocytes), and platelets (thrombocytes).
2. The **plasma** consists of about 55% of the total blood volume which is made up of water and solid particles. When blood is collected in an anticoagulated tube and allowed to settle by centrifugation, three layers are distinctly visible.

Buffy Coat: The upper plasma layer is separated from lower red cell mass by a thin **buffy coat** (Fig. 7.1).

- The buffy coat contains **leucocytes and platelets**.
- In diseases, abnormal cells are found in the buffy coat like **LE cells** in systemic lupus erythematosus and atypical or *primitive blood cells* (atypical mononuclear cells, promyelocytes, metamyelocytes, blast cells, megakaryocytes etc.) in malignant or premalignant conditions.
- Also, ***buffy coat preparation*** may be useful for the detection of bacteria, fungi or parasites within neutrophils, monocytes or circulating macrophages.

IMPORTANT NOTE

Buffy Coat Smear: Blood films prepared from buffy coat is useful in the detection of these abnormal in blood such as LE Cells and atypical cells.

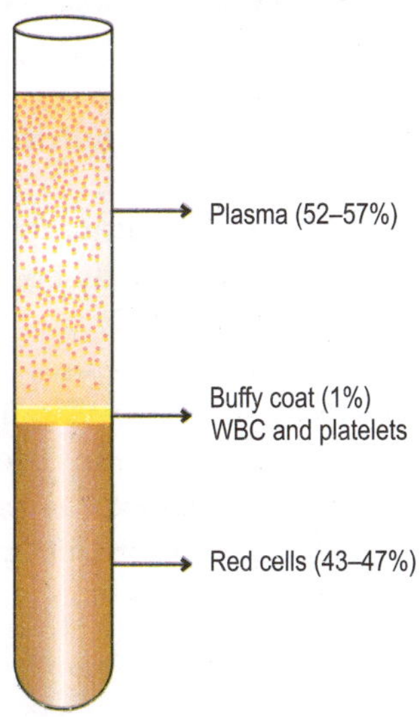

Fig. 7.1: Appearance of centrifuged blood. Note, about 1% of blood forms the buffy coat (present between plasma and red cell mass) that mainly contains WBC and platelets.

Functions of Blood

1. **Respiratory functions:** Blood transports oxygen from lungs to tissues, and carbon dioxide from tissues to the lungs.
2. **Transport medium:** Blood acts as the medium for transport of various substances such as hormones, chemicals, nutrients, vitamins, etc between different parts of the body.
3. **Temperature regulation:** Blood plays an important role in temperature regulation.
   - Blood circulation conducts heat from the interior of body to the surface through blood vessels.
   - Vasoconstriction preserves body temperature and vasodilation facilitates heat dissipation from the body.
4. **Excretory function:** Blood helps in excretion of waste materials by transporting them from different parts of the body to the kidney.
5. **Water homeostasis:** 55% of blood is plasma and 92% of plasma is water.
   - In conditions of hypovolemia such as diarrhea and vomiting, mechanisms are activated to increase the water content of blood.
   - Thus, by maintaining blood volume, water homeostasis (*volume homeostasis*) of the body is maintained.
6. **Acid-base balance:** Blood contains plasma proteins and hemoglobins.
   - **Protein and Hb buffers** play important role in maintaining acid base balance of the body.
   - Also, **bicarbonate** in blood buffers the acids.
7. **Immunity:** Blood contains **lymphocytes** that mediate *cellular immunity* and **antibodies** that mediate *humoral immunity*.
   - Blood also contains cells and chemicals such as **compliment proteins** that take part in *nonspecific defenses* of the body.
8. **Storage function:** Blood serves as **temporary reservoir** for electrolytes, nutrients, chemicals, hormones, etc.
9. **Body color:** Blood provides natural color to the body. In anemia and hypovolemia, body becomes pale.
10. **Nutritive functions:** Blood delivers all nutrients such as glucose, lipids, proteins, vitamins, minerals, etc. to the tissues of the body for their utilization and storage.
11. **Oncotic pressure:** The albumin present in blood exerts osmotic pressure, known as oncotic pressure that controls capillary filtration and **prevents edema formation**.

Blood Volume

The total blood volume can be roughly calculated as **70–80 ml/kg of body weight**.

- **In adult males**, the total volume of blood is about 5–6 liters and **in females** about 4.5–5.5 liters.
- **In children**, though the absolute volume of blood present is significantly less than adults, the volume expressed per kg of body weight is more (80–90 ml/kg-BW).

Blood volume is also expressed *per square meter of body surface area*, which is normally **2.8 lit/m²** of the body.

Effective Blood Volume: Effective blood volume = the total blood volume – the volume that is sequestrated.

- This means the volume which is present actually in the circulation that helps in perfusion of tissue.
- However, it is difficult to estimate the sequestered volume of blood in the visceral organs.

The Plasma

Plasma is the **fluid component** of blood which constitutes about **55% of the total blood volume**. The remaining 45% are cells (formed elements).

Composition of Plasma

Plasma constitutes water and solids (Table 7.1). Water content of plasma is about 92% of the total plasma (Fig. 7.2). The major solute (solid) content is the plasma proteins, which constitutes about 7% of the plasma and other solutes make up the rest 1%.

Table 7.1 | Composition of plasma.

1. **Water :** 92%
2. **Solids or Solutes :** 8% (plasma proteins constitute 90% of solids)
a. **Inorganic**
i. Anions: Chloride, bicarbonate, phosphates, sulphates, etc.
ii. Cations: Na^+, K^+, Ca^{++}, Mg^{++} etc.
b. **Organic**
i. Colloids: Plasma proteins
ii. Crystalloids: Glucose, lipid, urea, uric acid, etc.

Clinical Box 7.1

Fresh Frozen Plasma: In some conditions, plasma needs to be stored for years for future analysis, for which plasma is stored frozen below –20°C. This is called fresh frozen plasma (FFP), which can be stored upto 7 years in a blood bank. However, to preserve clotting factors plasma should be frozen within 6 hours after collection. FFP is used for plasmapheresis (therapeutic plasma exchange).

If the **whole plasma** is to be used for investigations, blood is collected with anticoagulants (*anticoagulated blood*). Fresh frozen plasma can be stored for years (Clinical Box 7.1).

Serum

During blood coagulation, a soluble plasma protein called **fibrinogen is removed** from plasma as it is utilized in the formation of fibrin (the blood clot). Plasma without clotting factors is called **serum** (Application Box 7.1).

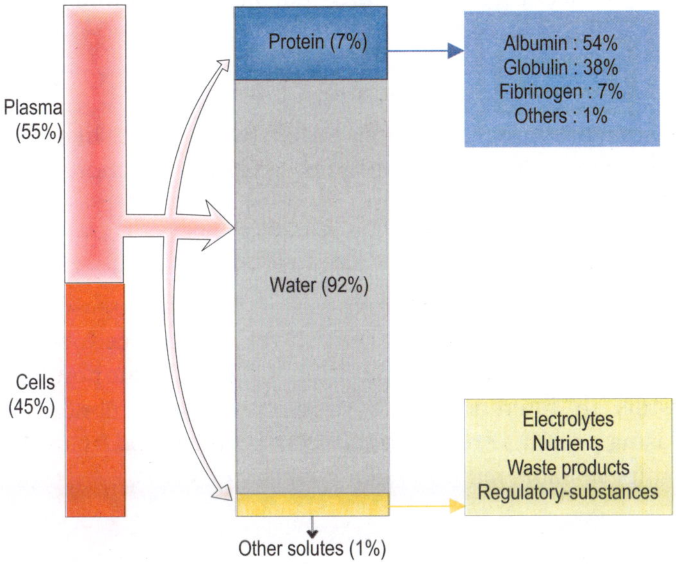

Fig. 7.2: Constituents of plasma

Application Box 7.1

Separating plasma and serum: Plasma is separated by centrifuging anticoagulated blood. The serum is separated from blood by allowing the blood to coagulate (serum = blood – fibrinogen and other clotting factors)..

Uses of Serum:

1. Many **biochemical tests** are performed by separating serum from blood by allowing the blood to clot (*coagulated blood*). Serotonin content of serum is high as platelets release serotonin during clotting.
2. Serum is also used as a supplement to **cell culture media**.
   - Serum ensures a better environment for growth of cells *in vitro* as it contains all nutrients, sugar, proteins, hormones and other factors.
   - **Fetal calf serum** is used often for *growth of human cells*.

PY2.2

PLASMA PROTEINS

Plasma proteins are the major solute constituents of plasma. The normal plasma protein concentration is 6–8 g/100 ml of plasma.

Types of Plasma Proteins

Plasma proteins are of 3 types: albumin (4–5.5 g%), globulin (1.5–3 g%), and fibrinogen (0.3 g%). Plasma proteins are formed mainly in the liver.

Albumin: It is formed in the liver. It has half-life of about 20 days and its molecular weight is 66000.

- Being smallest in diameter among the plasma proteins, in kidney diseases with glomerular injury it appears early in urine (**albuminuria**).
- Albumin determines colloidal osmotic pressure (oncotic pressure) of plasma.

Globulin: This is formed in the liver, cells of reticuloendothelial system and plasma cells.

Globulins are divided into three categories: α (α_1, α_2), β (β_1, β_2) and γ.

- The molecular weight of globulins is 90000–156000.
- Globulins include different *transport proteins* like transferrin, ceruloplasmin, hemopexin, etc. They form different *lipoproteins* in combination with lipids in plasma.
- **Antibodies** (immunoglobulins) are ***γ-globulins*** that are formed by plasma cells.

IMPORTANT NOTE

Albumin-Globulin ratio (AGR) is important: The AGR is 1.7:1 (1.2 to 2.2:1).

- In many diseases, AGR is altered.
- Detection of AGR helps in diagnosing and assessing the prognosis of some diseases.

Fibrinogen: The molecular weight is 340000. It is produced in the liver.

- It plays an important role in **blood coagulation**.
- It also contributes to the viscosity of plasma and determination of ESR.

Functions of Plasma Proteins

1. **Osmotic pressure (OP):** The osmotic pressure of plasma due to plasma proteins is called oncotic pressure, which is normally **25 mmHg**.
   - OP retains fluid in the vascular compartment and therefore, ***prevents loss of fluid from capillaries into the interstitial tissue space***.
   - **Decrease in OP** due to hypoproteinemia as occurs in liver and kidney diseases leads to **edema formation** due to escape of water into the interstitial tissue space.
2. **Viscosity:** Plasma protein contributes to about 50% of the viscosity of blood (red cells account for remaining 50%).
   - The viscosity depends on the *molecular shape of the plasma protein*.
   - Therefore, the fibrinogen molecules that are elongated and fibrillar in shape contribute more to blood viscosity than albumin molecules that are ellipsoid in structure.
3. **Immunity**: Antibodies are plasma proteins (**gamma globulins**).
   - Antibodies mediate humoral immunity that protects the body from infections, especially extracellular pathogens and from the effect of toxic substances.
4. **Coagulation**: Blood clotting depends on **concentration of fibrinogen** that forms fibrin thread, the final step

in blood coagulation. Also, other clotting factors like prothrombin are plasma protein.

5. **Transport:** Plasma proteins serve as **carrier molecule for transport** of various substances like hormones, drugs, metals, etc.
6. **Buffering:** Plasma proteins form an important buffering system of the body called **protein buffers**. This helps in **acid-base balance** of the body.
7. **Protein store:** Plasma proteins serve as **mobile protein reserve** of the body, which can be utilized for tissue growth, especially in situations of protein depletion.
8. **Synthetic function:** Plasma proteins provide substrate for the **synthesis of protein hormones** like erythropoietin, etc. and various enzymes
9. **Determination of ESR:** ESR mostly depends on the concentration of fibrinogen in the plasma.
   - **Fibrinogen facilitates rouleux formation**, which in turn increases the rate of sedimentation of red cells.
   - Therefore, conditions in which fibrinogen concentration is more like acute inflammations, ESR is more.

Separation of Plasma Proteins

Plasma proteins can be separated by methods like salt separation, paper electrophoresis, Cohn's fractionation, ultracentrifugation, immunochemical analysis etc.

- Determination of concentration of various fractions is useful for estimation of albumin-globulin ration (AGR) and for diagnosis & prognosis of different diseases.

Plasmapheresis: These are broad range of procedures in which **extracorporeal separation of blood components** results in filtered plasma product. Usually, abnormal plasma proteins are separated from whole blood by using semipermeable membranes.

Exam Questions

1. Give the composition of blood and the functions of each component.
2. What is buffy coat, and how is it prepared? List the uses of buffy coat.
3. Name the plasma proteins, and briefly describe the functions of plasma proteins.
4. What is normal albumin-globulin ratio, and what is its clinical significance?

Multiple Choice Questions

1. Which of the following contributes to oncotic pressure of plasma?
A. Fibrinogen
B. Prothombin
C. Globulin
D. Albumin

2. All of the following are true for the plasma concentration, EXCEPT:
A. Fibrinogen: 3 g/dL
B. Albumin: 4 to 5.5 g/dL
C. Total protein: 6 to 8 g/dL
D. Globulin: 1.5 to 3 g/dL

3. All of the following are functions of the plasma proteins, EXCEPT:
A. Are important buffering system
B. Help to decrease the blood pressure
C. Contribute to immunity
D. Serve as carriers for some hormones

4. Which of the following is NOT synthesized in liver?
A. Prothrombin
B. Albumin
C. Gamma-globulin
D. Fibrinogen

5. The contribution of plasma proteins to the body's total buffering capacity is
A. 5%
B. 15%
C. 25%
D. 35%

6. All of the following are true for buffy coat layer, EXCEPT:
A. Blast cells are found in malignant condition
B. Separates plasma and WBCs
C. Contains platelets
D. Useful for detection of LE cells in systemic lupus erythematosus

Answers

1. D 2. A 3. B 4. C 5. B 6. B

Chapter 8

Bone Marrow and Hemopoiesis

Learning Objectives

On completion of study of this chapter:

The student will be able to (must know):

1. Name the types of bone marrow and give their functions.
2. Appreciate the importance of myeloid-erythroid ratio in bone marrow.
3. Define hemopoiesis and name the sites of hemopoiesis in different stages.
4. Differentiate medullary and extramedullary hemopoiesis.
5. Name the sites of hemopoiesis in different age groups.
6. Name the types of stem cells in bone marrow.
7. Briefly describe regulation of hemopoiesis.

The student may also be able to (desirable to know):

1. Describe the functional organization of bone marrow.
2. Describe the regulation of hemopoiesis.

BONE MARROW

Bone marrow is the site of hemopoiesis. There are **three types of bone marrow**: red marrow, yellow marrow and white marrow.

Red Marrow

The red marrow is the active marrow and is red in colour. It consists of many blood vessels that contain sinusoidal capillaries.

Marrow Stroma: It principally consists of a network of sinuses that originate at the endosteum from cortical capillaries and terminate in the collecting vessels that enter the systemic circulation.

- Hematopoiesis takes place in the **intersinus spaces**. Red cells are formed in the **erythroid nests**.
- Endothelium and reticular cells are the sources of cytokines that profoundly influence hemopoiesis.

Effect of Age: Red bone marrow is present in almost **all bones of the body at birth**.

- However, with advancement of age red marrow is replaced by fatty tissue and slowly becomes inactive.
- At the **age of 20–30 years**, red marrow of long bones ceases to produce cells, and active marrow is *limited to the membranous bones* like skull bones, vertebrae, ribs, sternum and pelvic and pectoral girdles (Fig. 8.1).

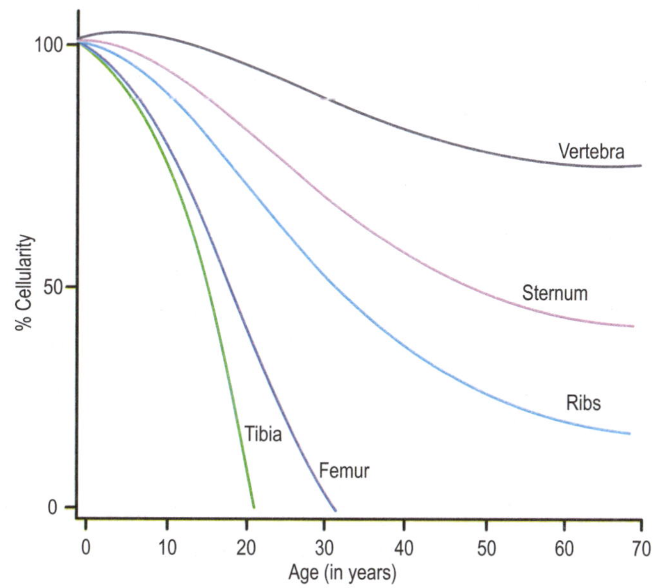

Fig. 8.1: Hemopoietic activity after birth. Note, though hemopoiesis ceases in tibia and femur by third decade of life, it continues throughout life in vertebra, sternum and ribs.

Yellow Marrow

The yellow marrow contains less blood vessels and more **fat cells and fibro-fatty tissue.** Differences between red and yellow marrow are listed in Table 8.1.

- The yellow marrow **does not participate in hemopoiesis**.
- Fat cells replace hematopoietic cells in the bones of hands, feet, legs and arm at about age of 20 years.

White Marrow

In very old individuals, a gelatinous transformation of fat to a **mucoid material** occurs in bone marrow. This type of marrow in *elderly persons* is called white marrow.

Table 8.1 | **Differences between red and yellow bone marrow.**

	Red Marrow	Yellow Marrow
1. Activity	Red in color, and contain active hemopoietic tissue	Yellow in colour, and inactive
2. Cellularity	Highly cellular; contains all types of hemopoietic cells	Very less cellular; contains more fat cells
3. Sites	In adults, it is restricted to vertebrae, sternum, ribs, clavicles, pelvic bones, skull and ends of humerus and femurs.	In all other bones except ends of long bones, and axial skeletons

Bone Marrow Examination

Usual **indications** for bone marrow examination are:
1. Anemias: Aplastic anemia & refractory anemias
2. Aleukemic leukemia & differentiation of leukemias
3. Myelofibrosis and myelosclerosis
4. Multiple myeloma
5. Agranulocytosis
6. Megaloblastic anemia
7. Thrombocytopenic purpura

Procedure: Bone marrow examination is usually done by **needle aspiration** and **bone marrow biopsy**. The usual sites of aspirations are sternum (sternal puncture), ileac crest and spinous process of vertebra.

Purpose: Examination of stained marrow smear is performed for assessing **cellularity of the marrow**, **effectiveness of hemopoiesis** (erythropoiesis, leucopoiesis and thrombopoiesis), **myeloid-erythroid ratio**, and presence of **tumor cells**, plasma cells, LD bodies (Leishman Donovan bodies as seen in Leishmaniasis), and malaria parasites.

Myeloid-Erythroid Ratio: In red bone marrow, cells are mostly of myeloid series, which constitute about 70–75% of the cell mass. The erythroid series constitutes about 25% of the marrow cell mass.
- Thus, the *myeloid-erythroid ratio* (MER) in the bone marrow is 3:1 (Application Box 8.1).
- But in the peripheral blood, red cells are much more than the white cells, ***leucocyte-erythrocyte ratio*** being 1:700.

HEMOPOIESIS

Hemopoiesis is the process of formation (development, maturation and release) of blood cells.

This is also called **hematopoiesis**.

Application Box 8.1

MER in bone marrow preserves leucocyte population in peripheral blood: The average life span of red cell is 120 days, whereas white cells stay in peripheral blood for few hours to few days. Therefore, to preserve white cell population in peripheral blood nature has provided more white cell precursors in bone marrow. This (more myeloid cells in the marrow) helps to replace adequate leucocytes in the blood as leucocytes have shorter life span than erythrocytes in circulating blood.

Sites and Stages of Hemopoiesis

Sites of hematopoiesis depends on the ***stage of hematopoiesis***.
- During **intrauterine life**, hematopoiesis occurs first in the **yolk sac**, and later in the **liver and spleen**.
- **After birth**, hematopoiesis is confined to **bone marrow**.

Hematopoietic Microenvironment: The environment in these organs (yolk sac, liver, spleen and bone marrow) where hematopoiesis takes place is called hematopoietic microenvironment.

Stages of Hematopoiesis

Hematopoiesis occurs in **three stages**: mesoblastic, hepatic and medullary.

Mesoblastic Stage

Mesoblastic stage is the stage of development of blood cells **in the yolk sac and non-yolk sac** regions during ***embryonic stage of intrauterine life***.
1. **Yolk sac:** Yolk sac contains cells with multilineage differentiating capabilities that start functioning as early as **second week** of gestation.
2. **Non-yolk sac regions:** The few non-yolk sac regions that participate in hematopoiesis are **paraaortic splanchnopleura** (PSP) and **aorta-gonad mesonephros** (AGM) regions.
   - PSP region gives rise to B-cell progenitors.
   - AGM region contains pluripotent stem cells.

Early lymphoid precursors have also been identified in the **day-8 yolk sac**. Also, lymphohematopoietic stem cells have been detected in vivo in the **9th day yolk sac**.

Hepatic Stage

During **second trimester** of pregnancy, hemopoiesis takes place in the **liver and spleen**. This is called hepatic stage.
1. **In liver:** In liver, hematopoiesis starts as early as **5th week of gestation**, which reaches its peak in 5th month and **ceases at birth** (Fig. 8.2).
2. **In spleen:** In spleen, hematopoiesis occurs mainly in the ***second trimester*** and the degree of hematopoiesis is *quite less* than that in the liver.

Medullary Stage

Formation of blood cells in the bone marrow is called **medullary hemopoiesis**.

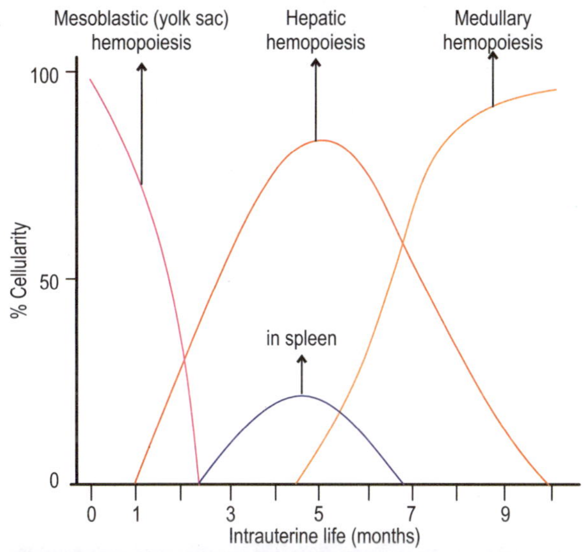

Fig. 8.2: Hemopoietic activity during intrauterine life.

- Marrow cavities in the bone appear as early as **5th month of fetal life**, and soon they become hemopoietic. *In initial phase*, bone marrow is the exclusive site for granulocytic and megakaryocytic proliferation, during which erythropoietic activity is confined to liver.
- Erythropoiesis in bone marrow occurs effectively **towards the end of third trimester** of pregnancy and then **continues throughout life**.

Extramedullary Hemopoiesis: **After birth**, hemopoiesis stops in liver and spleen and gets **confined only to the bone marrow**. When hemopoiesis occurs *in liver and spleen in postnatal life*, is called **extramedullary hemopoiesis**.

IMPORTANT NOTE

Extramedullary hemopoiesis after birth is abnormal: Hematopoiesis does not occur in liver and spleen during post-natal life (after birth). However, when the demand for blood cells is more than the rate of production, hematopoiesis occurs in liver and spleen. Such **extramedullary hemopoiesis** after birth is considered **abnormal.**

Rate of Medullary Hemopoiesis

Bone marrow is one of the largest organs in the human body.

- It produces about **6 billion cells** (2.5 billion red cells, 2.5 billion platelets and 1 billion granulocytes) *per kg of body weight per day* in adolescents and adults.
- However, the rate of production is adjusted to the needs of day-to-day life.

Sites of Medullary Hemopoiesis

Bone marrow is the sole site of erythropoiesis in human beings.

In long bones: In long bones, active marrow ***regresses rapidly*** after first decade of life and **ceases to produce cells** between ***20–30 years*** of life (refer Fig. 8.1).

In membranous bones: Hemopoiesis continues to occur in active marrow of **vertebrae, pectoral and pelvic girdles, ribs, sternum and skull**. However, with age the degree of hemopoiesis also decreases in these bones.

Steps of Hemopoiesis

Hematopoiesis occurs in the bone marrow from **hematopoietic stem cells**. The mother hematopoietic stem cell is the **pluripotent stem cells** (PPSC), also called as **hemocytoblast**. Stem cells develop into progenitor cells that further develop into precursor cells and matured cells (Flowchart 8.1).

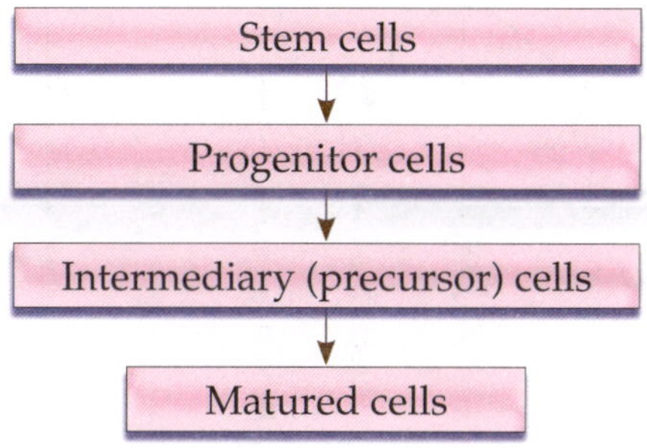

Flowchart 8.1: General steps of hemopoiesis.

Stem Cells

Stem cells in the bone marrow have **two important properties**: self-renewal and differentiation.

Self-Renewal: This is the property of **duplicating themselves**. Due to self-renewal, the bone marrow never goes out of stock for stem cells and ***stem cell reserve*** is maintained.

Differentiation: This is the property of **developing into specific lineage of cells**. Due to differentiation, stem cells develop into **progenitor cells** of various cell lines.

Types of Stem Cells

pluripotent stem cells produce **two groups of stem cells**: myeloid stem cells and lymphoid cells. Fig. 8.3).

Myeloid Stem Cells: Myeloid stem cells are **pluripotent (tri-lineage)** in nature that give rise to **three types of progenitor cells.** These are:

1. **Erythroid progenitors** that form erythroid series for red cells.
2. **Granulocytic-monocytic progenitors** that form granulocytes (neutrophil, eosinophil, and basophil), and monocytes.
3. **Megakaryocytic progenitors** that form platelets.

Lymphoid Stem Cells: Lymphoid stem cells are **unipotent stem cells** (UPSC) that produce only ***cells of lymphocyte series***.

Progenitor Cells

Progenitor cells develop from stem cells.

- Progenitor cells form **colony forming units** (CFUs) that give rise to different types of blast cells.

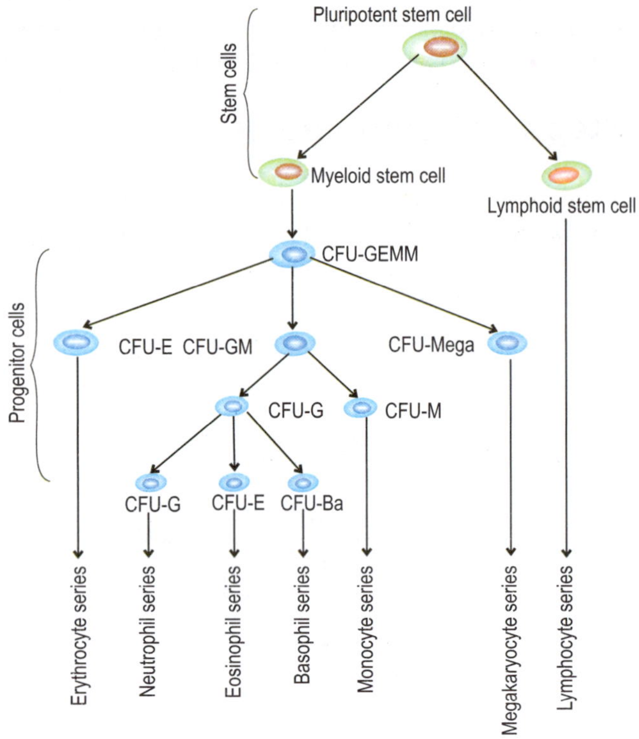

Fig. 8.3: General outlines of hemopoiesis in bone marrow.

- ***Myeloid stem cells*** differentiate into **CFU-GEMM**, i. e. CFU for granulocyte, erythrocyte, megakaryocyte and monocyte.

CFU-GEMM develops into ***three major CFUs*** (Fig. 8.3).

1. **CFU-E:** CFU-E is the CFU for erythroid series that form ***proerythroblast***, which in turn develops into **precursor cells of erythroid series**.
2. **CFU-GM:** CFU-GM is the multilineage CFU that in turn forms CFU for granulocytes ***(CFU-G)*** and CFU for monocytes ***(CFU-M)***.
   - CFU-G develops into **myeloblast** that differentiates into ***three lineages*** of granulocytes (neutrophil, eosinophil, and basophil).
   - CFU-M develops into **monoblast** that differentiates into monocyte.
3. **CFU-Mega:** CFU-Mega differentiates into **megakaryoblast** that in turn forms platelets.

Types of Hemopoiesis

Hemopoiesis is broadly divided into **three types**: erythropoiesis, leucopoiesis and thrombopoiesis.

- **Erythropoiesis** is the development of red cells.
- **Leucopoiesis** is the development of leucocytes.
- **Thrombopoiesis** is the development of platelets.

The pluripotent stem cell (hemocytoblast) differentiates into myeloid and lymphoid stem cells, which forms precursor cells that further develop into five **major blast cells** of five different cell lines (Fig. 8.4).

- **Proerythroblast** forms erythroid series for development of red cells.
- **Myeloblast** differentiates into three lineages of **granulocytes series** (neutrophil, eosinophil, and basophil).
- **Monoblast** differentiates into monocytes.
- **Lymphoblast** develops into lymphocytes.
- **Megakaryoblast** forms platelets.

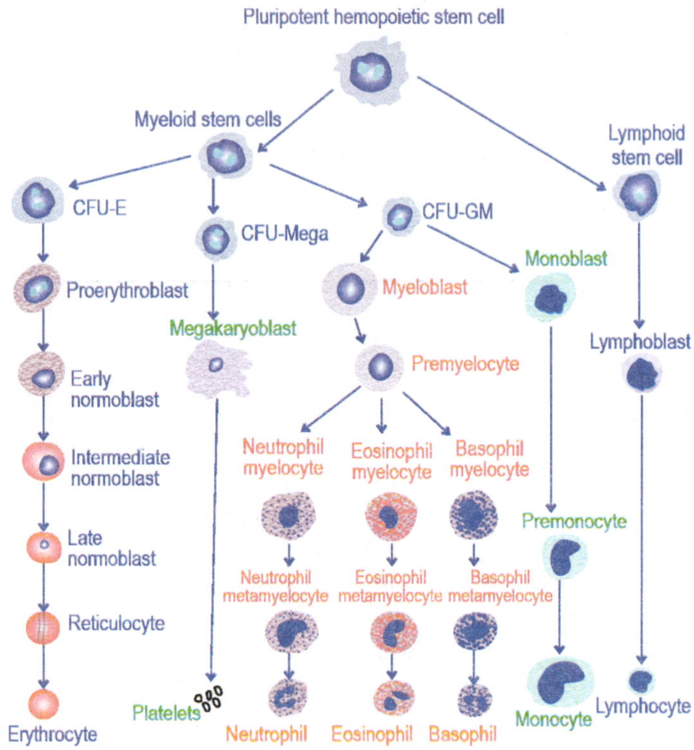

Fig. 8.4: Hemopoietic activities in bone marrow. Note, stem cells through precursor cells gives rise to blast cells of different series: proerythroblast for erythropoietic series, myeloblast for granulocytic series (neutrophilic, eosinophilic and basophilic), monoblast for monocytic series, megakaryoblast for megakaryocytic (platelet) series, and lymphoblast for lymphocytic series.

Regulation of Hemopoiesis

Hemopoiesis is regulated by various **cytokines**. Cytokines that influence development of blood cells are called **hemopoietic growth factors** (HGFs).

- As many of them stimulate development of CFU, they are also called **colony stimulating factors** (CSFs).
- Many of them are nonspecific, influencing more than one cell line, whereas few of them are specific in their actions.

Hemopoietic Growth Factors

The major HGFs are listed in Table 8.2.

1. **Erythropoietin:** It is secreted from kidney and stimulates **development of erythrocyte precursors**.
2. **Interleukins (IL):** There are many interleukins, IL_1 to IL_{11}.
   - IL_5 controls eosinophil development.
   - IL_2 and IL_4 control lymphocyte development.
   - IL_1 and IL_2 control monocyte-macrophage development, etc.

3. **Colony stimulating factors:** There are three major groups of CSFs: M-CSF, G-CSF and GM-CSF.
   - **M-CSF** controls development of monocyte precursors.
   - **G-CSF** controls growth of granulocyte precursors.
   - **GM-CSF** promotes proliferation of both granulocytes and monocytes.
4. **Other growth factors:** Colony stimulating factor 1 (*CSF 1*) that influences macrophage development, leukemia inhibitory factor (*LIF*) that controls growth of megakaryocyte and stroma cell derived cytokine (*SCDC*) that influences B cell differentiation.

Table 8.2 | Target cells of hemopoietic growth factors (HGFs).

Cell lineage	Cytokines (HGFs)
1. Erythroid-BFU	Erythropoietin, IL_3, IL_4 and GM-CSF.
2. Erythroid-CFU	Erythropoietin
3. Neutrophil-Macrophage	GM-CSF
4. Macrophage	CSF-1, IL1 and IL_8
5. Neutrophil	G-CSF
6. Eosinophil	IL_5 and IL_3
7. Megakaryocyte	IL_3, IL_1, IL_6, IL_4, GM-CSF and LIF.
8. Basophil- Mast cell	IL_3, and GM-CSF
9. B lymphocytes	IL_7, IL_4, IL_5 and SCDC
10. T lymphocyte	IL_2, erythropoietin and GM-CSF

Exam Questions

1. Name the types of bone marrow and list the differences between them.
2. List the indications of bone marrow examinations.
3. Briefly describe the stages of hemopoiesis.
4. With the help of a schematic diagram, briefly describe the steps of medullary hematopoiesis.
5. Give a short note on hemopoietic growth factors.

Multiple Choice Questions

1. Which of the following is true for red marrow?
A. In adults, present in radius and ulna
B. Contains only hemopoietic cells of erythroid series
C. Yellow in colour
D. Highly cellular

2. The hepatic stage of hemopoiesis starts in:
A. 5th month of gestation
B. 3rd month of gestation
C. 5th week of gestation
D. 3rd week of gestation

3. Which of the following is NOT a property of stem cell?
A. Proliferation
B. Stains brightly with Rhodamine
C. Differentiation
D. Self-renewal

4. The medullary stage of hemopoiesis starts in:
A. 5th month of fetal life
B. 7th month of fetal life
C. 9th week of fetal life
D. After birth

5. Which of the following is NOT a bone marrow?
A. White marrow
B. Yellow marrow
C. Red marrow
D. Orange marrow

6. Which of the following is NOT an important growth factors for RBC?
A. SCDC
B. GM-CSF
C. IL-4
D. Erythropoietin

7. Which of the following is an important growth factor for eosinophil?
A. IL-1
B. IL-2
C. IL-3
D. IL-4

8. Red marrow of long bones ceases to produce cells after the age of ?
A. 10-20 years
B. 20-30 years
C. 40-50 years
D. 60-70 years

Answers

1. D 2. C 3. B 4. A 5. D 6. A 7. C 8. B

Chapter 9

Red Blood Cells: Structure, Functions, Development (Erythropoiesis), and Destruction

Learning Objectives

On completion of study of this chapter:

The student will be able to (must know):

1. Give the dimensions of red cell and normal values of red cell count in males and females.
2. List the functions of red cells.
3. Appreciate the importance of learning red cell fragility.
4. List the common variations in hematocrit.
5. List the factors affecting ESR, give normal values of ESR and list the variations in ESR.
6. Give the stages & sites of erythropoiesis, describe the steps of erythropoiesis & regulation of erythropoiesis.
7. Give the source and functions of erythropoietin.
8. Give the normal count of reticulocyte and alteration in reticulocyte count in different conditions.
9. Understand reticulocyte response & reticulocyte index.
10. Give the sites and process of red cell destruction.

The student may also be able to (desirable to know):

1. Describe the regulation of erythropoietin production
2. Describe the fate of destroyed red cells.

RED BLOOD CELLS

The red blood cells or erythrocytes ('erythros' means red) are the major cellular elements of blood.

Structure and Functions

Red Cell Dimensions

Human red cell is a circular, non-nucleated and biconcave disc (Fig. 9.1).

Shape : Biconcave
Size : 7.5 (7 to 8) μm in diameter
Thickness : 2 μm at the periphery and 1 μm at the center
Surface area : 140 μm^2
Volume : 87 μm^3 (78 to 94 μm^3)

The advantages of biconcavity of red cells:

1. When exposed to hypotonic environment, red cells **withstand lysis** to a greater degree as they swell to a larger extent to attain spherical shape before bursting.
   - They **do not lyse easily** when blood is hypotonic.
2. The surface area of the red cell is much greater than that of a sphere of the same size, which **increases the area for exchange of gases** (oxygen and carbon dioxide).
3. It helps in **easy folding of red cells** and therefore, *facilitates their movement* through the narrow capillaries.

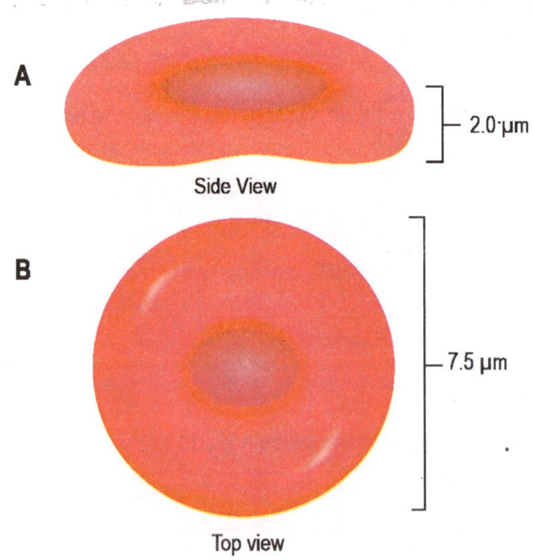

Fig. 9.1: Shape of red cells. **A.** the side view when the cell is kept vertical (Note, the thickness is 2 μm at the periphery and 1 μm at the center). **B.** the surface view (Note, the diameter of the cell is 7.5 μm).

Red Cell Composition: Red cells are composed of water 62.5%, hemoglobin 35%, and other substances 2.5%.

Abnormal red cells: Abnormal red cells (Fig. 9.2) such as microcytes (small cells), macrocytes (big cells), poikilocytes

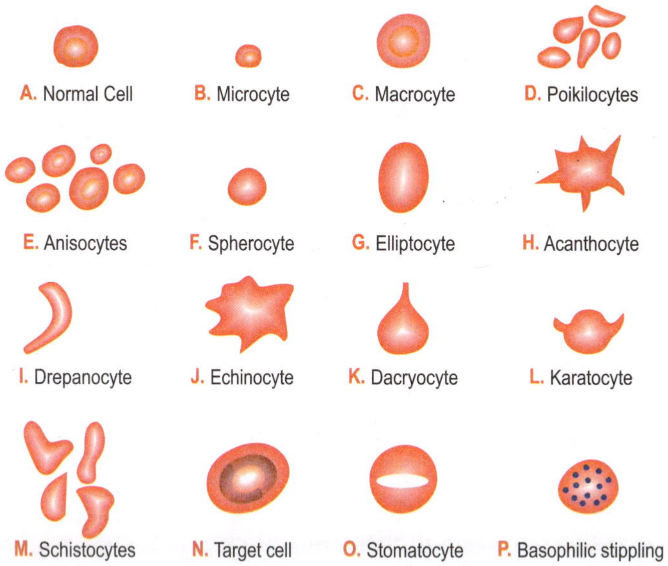

Fig. 9.2: Normal and abnormal red cells. (A) Normal red cell; (B) Microcyte; (C) Macrocyte; (D) Poikilocyte; (E) Anisocyte; (F) Spherocyte; (G) Elliptocyte; (H) Acanthocyte; (I) Drepanocyte (sickle cell); (J) Echinocyte (burr cell or crenated cell); (K) Dacryocyte; (L) Keratocyte; (M) Schistocytes, (fragmented red cells); (N) Target cell; (O) Stomatocyte; (P) Basophilic stippling.

(different shapes), spherocytes (spherical), elliptocytes (elliptical), acanthocytes (irregular shape), drepanocyte (sickle cell), echinocyte (burr cell), dacrocytes (tear drop), keratocyte (with a pair of spicules), schistocyte (fragments of cell), target cells (central deep stain area), stomatocyte (slit-like area in center), and basophilic stippling are seen in different pathological conditions.

IMPORTANT NOTE

Punctate basophilia: When coarse basophilic ***dark blue granules*** are seen in red cells, it is called punctate basophilia. It is seen ***in chronic lead poisoning***.

- It is also seen in other heavy metal poisoning, thalassemia, megaloblastic anemia, infections and liver disease.
- Sometimes in lead poisoning, Cabot's ring (ring shape or figure of 8) at the periphery of red cells or Howell Jolly bodies (small nuclear fragments appear in cytoplasm) are found in erythrocytes.

Red Cell Count

PY2.12

In adult males : 4.5 – 6 (average 5.2) millions per cu mm of blood

In adult females : 4 – 5.5 (average 4.7) millions per cu mm of blood

In newborns : 6 – 8 millions per cu mm of blood

In children : 3 – 5 millions per cu mm of blood

The count is more in infants mainly due to hemoconcentration.

- The count rapidly decreases to its lowest level at about 2–4 months.
- Then, count slowly increases from one year of life to reach about 5 millions/mm^3 at about 10 years.

Life Span of Red Cells: Red cells usually live for 120 days. Aged red cells are destroyed by tissue macrophage system.

Specialities of RBC Membrane

In addition to the general features of a membrane, red cell membrane contains two special proteins: integral and peripheral proteins.

Integral Proteins: Two special types of integral proteins are found in red cell membrane. These are glycophorins and band-3 proteins.

1. **Glycophorins** are glycoproteins that contain 60% carbohydrate and 40% protein.
   - There are **five types** of glycophorins: A, B, C, D and E.
   - ***Glycophorin-C*** provides stability and shape to the red cell membrane, and its deficiency leads to elliptocytosis.
2. **Band-3 protein** (***anion exchanger-1***) is a dimeric protein, which acts as 'pore' or transport protein that exchanges bicarbonate and chloride ions in the capillaries of lungs.

Peripheral Proteins: The inner surface of red cell membrane contains two special proteins that are linked to the cytoskeleton and are essential for ***stabilization of membrane and biconcave shape*** of the cell. These are spectrin and ankyrin.

- Spectrin is a fibrous protein attached to cytoskeletal proteins and ***maintains cell shape***.
- Ankyrin has has two domains: one binds with spectrin and other with N-terminal region of band-3 protein that extends into cytoskeleton.
  - Ankyrin maintains red cell membrane integrity.
  - Hereditary spherocytosis and elliptocytosis occur due to defects in these membrane proteins (Application Box 9.1).

Deformability of red cells: An important determinant of red cell survival is its deformability (membrane plasticity).

- When red **cells become rigid** (less deformable), the viscosity of blood increases and cells are lysed while passing through the splenic pulp.
- The *primary cause* of decreased deformability is **due to spherocytosis** of the cell rather than stiffening of their membrane.

Application Box 9.1

Common membrane defects: Deficiency of ankyrin and spectrin results in membrane defects like **spherocytosis, elliptocytosis and poikilocytosis** etc. These defects also make the cells rigid so that the cells are destroyed prematurely.

Metabolism of Red Cells

Red cells have no nuclei, mitochondria and ribosomes. Therefore, adequate synthesis of proteins and lipids does not occur in red cells.

- Red cells depend mostly on **glucose metabolism** for their energy supply.
- 90% of glucose is oxidized by EM pathway and 10% by HMP shunt.

- **Glucose-6-phosphate dehydrogenase** (G-6-PD) is the main enzyme for HMP shunt that generates NADPH, keeps glutathione in reduced state, which is a strong reducing agent and prevents damage to the red cell.
- Therefore, G-6-PD deficiency interferes with red cell functions (Application Box 9.2).

Application Box 9.2

G-6-PD deficiency causes hemolysis: In the absence of G-6-PD, an *inborn error of metabolism*, red cells are susceptible to the damages due to oxidation. Therefore, **hemolytic anemia** is common in G-6-PD deficiency. Especially, hemolysis is facilitated on exposure to anti-malarial drugs, though these individuals are generally malaria resistant.

Functions of Red Cells

1. The most important function of red cell is to **transport oxygen** from lungs to the tissue. This is due to the presence of hemoglobin in the red cell which has high affinity for oxygen.
2. Hemoglobins also participate in **carbon dioxide transport** from tissues to lungs and maintenance of **acid base balance**.
3. Red cells contribute to 50% of **viscosity of blood**.
4. Absence or presence of antigen on red cell membrane confers **blood group** of the individual, which is essential for blood donation or transfusion.

Physiological Aspects

Fragility of Red Cells

The ***tendency of the cells to hemolyze*** is called fragility of the cells. Usually, red cell fragility is of **two types**: mechanical and osmotic.

Mechanical Fragility

Lysis of red cells due to **mechanical stress** and strain is called ***mechanical fragility***. When red cells pass through capillaries and splenic pulp, their membrane undergoes mechanical stress.

- A red cell passes about **three lakh times though capillaries** during its life span, which makes the cell more fragile due to mechanical stress.
- Membrane of **older red cells** becomes stiff that increased mechanical stress and makes them vulnerable to rupture.
- Red cell **membrane defects** increase mechanical fragility.

Osmotic Fragility **PY2.11**

Osmotic fragility is defined as the ease with which the red cells are ruptured when they are exposed to hypotonic solutions.

- It assesses the integrity of red cell membrane.
- The **osmotic fragility test** helps in the diagnosis of anemia in which the physical properties of the red cells are altered.

In isotonic solutions: In an **isotonic solution**, the solution of equal concentration as that of red cell content, the red cells remain intact. Such a solution has same tonicity with that of plasma. Examples are 0.9% NaCl, 5% glucose, 10% mannitol and 20% urea.

In hypertonic solutions: When suspended in **hypertonic solution**, a solution with more tonicity (> 0.9% NaCl), red cells shrink due to loss of water from them by *exosmosis*.

In hypotonic solutions: Red cells absorb water by *endosmosis*, when kept in **hypotonic solutions**, a solution with less tonicity (< 0.9% NaCl). Endosmosis results in hemolysis due to swelling and rupture of the cells.

Alteration in Osmotic Fragility

When the rate of hemolysis of red cells is increased, the **osmotic fragility is said to be increased**, and when the rate of hemolysis is decreased, the **osmotic fragility is said to be decreased**.

- Increased osmotic fragility denotes **decreased resistance of cells to rupture**.
- As the resistance of the red cell membrane to rupture is related to its geometric configuration, **red cells that are spherical** demonstrate *increased hemolysis*, whereas **red cells that are flat like** sickle cells demonstrate *decreased hemolysis*.

Normal Value & Variations

Normally, osmotic fragility begins at 0.45 to 0.50 and completes at 0.30 to 0.33.

A. Conditions of Diminished Fragility:

1. Iron deficiency anemia
2. Thalassemia
4. Sickle cell anemia
3. Obstructive jaundice
4. Post-splenectomy

B. Conditions of Increased Fragility:

1. Hereditary spherocytosis
2. Congenital hemolytic anemia

Packed Cell Volume or Hematocrit

Hematocrit is the fractional volume of blood that erythrocytes occupy. Hematocrit or packed cell volume (PCV) is the volume of packed red cells following centrifugation.

- The hematocrit is a **reliable index of the red cell population**, as it provides useful information about the red cell mass.

Normal Value & Variations

Adult male : 46% (40–50%)
Adult female : 42% (37–47%)

Hematocrit **decreases** in conditions of decreased red cell count and **increases** in conditions of increased red cell count.

- When cells are deformed as occurs in *spherocytosis or sickle cell disease*, more plasma is trapped between the packed cells, which gives a **false high result**.

Erythrocyte Sedimentation Rate

Red cells have the property of **rouleaux** (piling one on the other) formation (Fig. 9.3).

- The piled red cells are heavier. Therefore, when whole blood is allowed to settle, sedimentation of erythrocytes is facilitated due to the presence of rouleaux.
- The rate, at which the red cells fall (sediment), is known as the erythrocyte sedimentation rate (ESR).

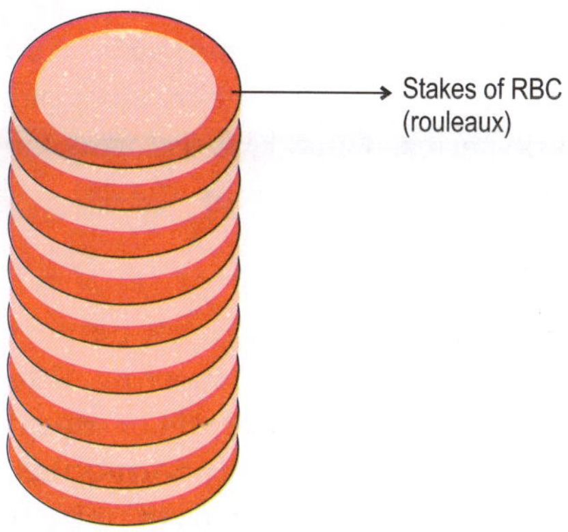

Fig. 9.3: Rouleaux formation

Factors Affecting ESR

ESR depends on **3 major factors**: shape and number of red cells, size of rouleaux, and the plasma factors. Other factors also contribute.

Shape and Number of Red Cells: The **biconcave shape favors** rouleaux formation. Therefore, ESR is less in hereditary spherocytosis and sickle cell anemia.

- Increase in red cell mass increases viscosity of blood and decreases ESR.
- ESR is less in polycythemia and more in anemia (except in sickle cell anemia).

Size of Rouleaux: ESR depends on the mass of the falling particles, i.e. the size of rouleaux (the red cell aggregates).

- The *larger the size of rouleaux, the faster is the fall.* Therefore, the factors that increase the size of rouleaux facilitate ESR.
- Increase in red cell size without change in their shape increases the size of rouleaux.

Plasma Factors: The size and number of rouleaux mainly depends on the **fibrinogen** concentration of plasma. **Globulin** content of plasma also contributes.

- **In normal blood**, red cells remain separate as they have negatively charged surface and tend to repel one another.
    - **In pathological conditions**, when **fibrinogen concentration increases** in plasma, fibrinogen neutralizes the charges on red cells and removes the repelling forces. This facilitates rouleaux formation.
- **In some conditions**, in addition to fibrinogen, other plasma factors called as **acute phase-reactants** (APRs) increase in the blood.
    - APRs neutralize the charges on the red cell surface and facilitate rouleaux formation. Therefore, ESR increases in **acute infections and noninfective inflammations**.
    - Rise in **C reactive protein** in the plasma in acute rheumatic fever is an example of such APRs.
    - In **malignancies and collagen diseases**, ESR increases due to rise in plasma level of **globulin**.

Other Factors: Body **temperature** and **plasma viscosity** affect ESR. Increased temperature increases ESR by decreasing viscosity. When, the medium for sedimentation (the plasma) becomes thicker, rate of sedimentation decreases.

IMPORTANT NOTE

ESR is high in acute inflammation: Increased level of acute phase reactants increases ESR in inflammation and infection.

Normal Values & Variations

In Wintrobe method:

Males : 0 – 9 mm/hr
Females : 0 – 20 mm/hr

In Westergren method:

Males : 3 – 5 mm/hr
Females : 5 – 12 mm/hr

Physiological Variations

1. Pregnancy: During pregnancy ESR increases due to increase in plasma fibrinogen content.
2. ESR is more during menstrual bleeding, & parturition
3. ESR is more in female

Pathological Variations

Increase in ESR:

1. Tuberculosis
2. Acute inflammation like cellulitis
3. Chronic inflammation like arthritis
4. Malignancy
5. All types of anemias except membrane defects like hereditary spherocytosis and sickle cell disease
6. Collagen diseases like rheumatoid arthritis, SLE
7. Chronic infections like chronic tonsillitis

Decrease in ESR:

1. Polycythemia
2. Sickle cell anemia, hereditary spherocytosis
3. Hypofibrinogenemia
4. Hyperviscosity syndromes

PY2.4

ERYTHROPOIESIS

Definition

Erythropoiesis is the process of formation or production of red cells.

Sites of Erythropoiesis

During intrauterine life: In intrauterine life, erythropoiesis takes place in yolk sac, spleen and liver, and in bone marrow sequentially.

1. **Mesoblastic stage**: First takes place in the mesoderm of yolk sac and mesoderm of the body. During this stage, erythropoiesis is intravascular.
2. **Hepatic stage**: From the 5th week of gestation, erythropoiesis takes place in the liver and spleen
3. **Medullary stage**: From the 5th month of intrauterine life, the bone marrow starts forming red cells (***intrauterine medullary erythropoiesis***).
   - Erythropoiesis in bone marrow is very slow in second trimester.
   - Medullary erythropoiesis becomes *more effective towards end of third trimester*.

After birth: After birth, **bone marrow** becomes the sole site of erythropoiesis ***(medullary erythropoiesis)***.

- **Till adolescent period**, marrow cavity of all bones is involved in erythropoiesis, after which erythropoiesis regresses in the limb bones.
- **After the age of 20–30 years,** erythropoiesis is mostly limited to sternum, ribs, vertebrae, skull, pelvic and pectoral girdles (refer Fig. 8.1; Chapter 8).
- **Extramedullary erythropoiesis** in postnatal life is always considered **abnormal**.

Stages or Steps of Erythropoiesis

There are four major stages or **steps of erythropoiesis**: stem cells, progenitor cells, precursor cells and mature cells (Fig. 9.4). Each stage has sub-stages.

During erythropoiesis, following cellular changes take place in general:

1. Cell size progressively reduces.
2. Size of nucleus and number of nucleoli decreases, chromatin material condenses and finally nucleus disappears.
3. Staining reaction of cytoplasm changes from deep basophilic to polychromatophillic (acidophilic plus basophilic) and finally to acidophilic type. This occurs mainly due to gradual reduction in quantity of RNA material.

Stem Cells

Pluripotent Stem Cells

Pluripotent stem cells have two unique properties: 1) self renewal, and 2) differentiation. As they renew themselves, at no time bone marrow is depleted of stem cells. They also develop (differentiate) into the subsequent progenitor cells.

Committed Stem Cell

There are of two types: stem cells for myeloid series and for lymphoid series.

1. **Myeloid stem cells** form erythroid series, megakaryoid series, monocytic series and granulocytic series (refer Fig. 8.3 and 8.4; Chapter 8).
2. **Erythroid stem cells** give rise to progenitor cells for erythroid cell lines. There are two progenitor cells: BFU-E and CFU-E.

Progenitor Cells

There are **two types** of progenitor cells: 1) BFU-E and 2) CFU-E.

- **BFUs-E** are burst forming units-erythroid progenitor cells that give rise to large number of CFU-erythroid cells.
- **CFUs-E** are colony forming units-erythroid progenitor cells that give rise to moderate number of blast cells of erythrocytic series. Thus, BFU-E forms CFU-E, which in turn forms blast cells (erythroblasts).

Precursor Cells

Precursor cells are **blast cells**, the first to be morphologically identifiable cells in the bone marrow. Precursors for erythrocytes are called **erythroblasts** or **normoblasts**.

- Normoblasts develop from **pronormoblasts**.
- There are three successive forms of normoblasts: early, intermediate and late (Fig. 9.4).

Pronormoblast

Pronormoblasts (**proerythroblast**) are the first blast cells to appear in bone marrow and the **first identifiable cells of erythrocyte series**.

Following are the characteristics of pronormoblast.

1. This is a large cell, having diameter of about 20–25 µm. Cell is irregularly rounded or slightly oval.
2. The cytoplasm is less in amount, occupies about 20% of the cell.
   - Presence of ***high concentration of polyribosomes*** makes the cytoplasm intensely basophilic.
   - Cytoplasm has *high content of RNA*, which indicates vigorous protein synthesis in the cell.
3. The nucleus is large and occupies 80% of the cell. It contains multiple nucleoli.
4. Mitosis is present.
5. Hemoglobin is not yet formed in the cell.

Early Normoblast (Basophilic Erythroblast)

Early normoblast or **early erythroblast** is the first erythroblast to appear in bone marrow. The features are:

1. Diameter of these cells is 15–18 µm.
2. Cells exhibit active mitosis.
3. Cytoplasm is scanty, deep blue and basophilic.
   - The basophilic cytoplasm is due to continuation of many polyribosomes in it.
   - Therefore, early normoblast is also called **basophilic erythroblast**.

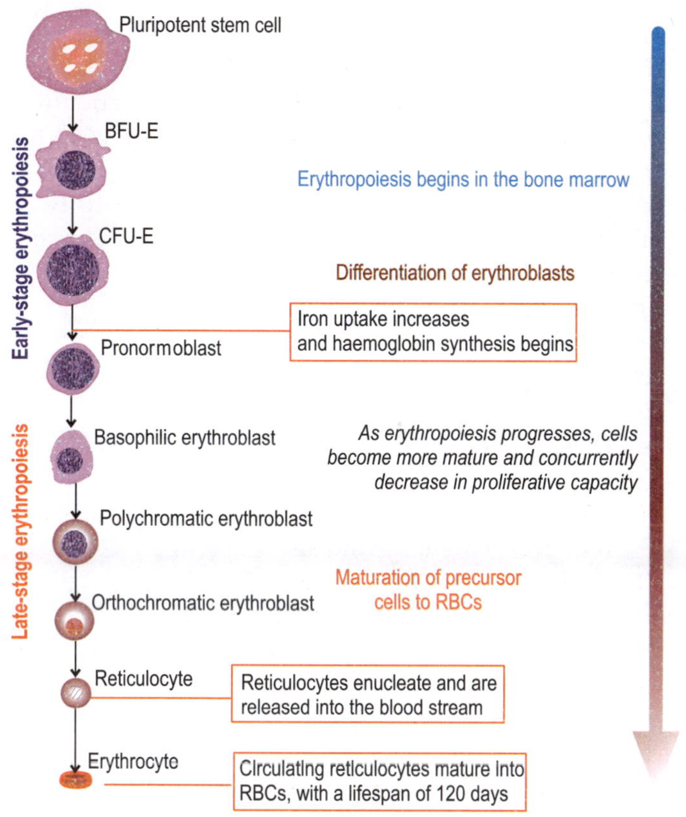

Fig. 9.4: Stages of erythropoiesis. Note that cell size decreases in each stage. Nuclear size also decreases and finally nucleus disappears in reticulocyte stage.

4. Nucleus is large and occupies three-fourth of the cell area.
   - Nucleus is composed of dark violet **heterochromatin clumps** interspersed with pink clumps of euchromatin.
   - The chromatins are connected by linear strands. This often gives nucleus the ***appearance of wheel spokes.***
5. **Hemoglobin appears first time** in these cells in erythropoiesis.

Intermediate Normoblast (Polychromatic Erythroblast)

This is also called **intermediate erythroblast**. Following are features:

1. The cell is smaller than the early normoblast, having the diameter of 12–15 µm.
2. The cytoplasm changes from blue to pink as hemoglobin dilutes the polyribosome content.
3. Nucleus is small and occupies about half of the cell area.
   - The distribution of heterochromatin clumps in nucleus gives the appearance of **checkerboard pattern**.
   - There are no nucleoli.
4. Hemoglobin synthesis increases, which makes the cell acidophilic.
   - The presence of RNA material makes the cytoplasm eosinophilic.
   - Thus, mixture of acidophilic hemoglobin and eosinophilic RNA in cytoplasm makes it **polychromatic**. Therefore, intermediate normoblast is also called ***polychromatic erythroblast***.
5. Mitosis is sluggish in intermediate normoblast.

Late Normoblast (Orthochromatic Erythroblast)

This is also called late erythroblast. This is produced by final mitosis in the erythropoietic series.

The features are:

1. This is smallest in the erythroblastic series (7–12 µm in diameter) and mitosis is absent.
2. Cytoplasm is ***deeply eosinophilic*** giving the appearance of an orthochromatic cell. Hence, this is also called **orthochromatic erythroblast.**
3. Nucleus is small and pyknotic at the beginning.
   - Sometimes, dark nuclear chromatin materials are arranged in a typical pattern to give the appearance of a *cart-wheel*.
   - Finally, the pyknotic nucleus disintegrates.
4. Hemoglobin synthesis increases and almost completes in this stage.

Mature Cells

Reticulocytes

Reticulocytes are also called as *juvenile red cells.*

- They have full complement of hemoglobin.
- They are slightly larger than red cells.
- They have a network of reticular nuclear material. The reticular network is nothing but the remnants of disintegrated organelles, and especially of the nuclear fragments.
- Due to the presence of reticular network, the cells are called reticulocytes. The reticulum is stained by **supravital stains.**
- Hemoglobin synthesis continues to some extent in some reticulocytes.
- The reticulocyte count is 0–1 per cent of red cells in adults (details of reticulocyte are given below).

Erythrocytes

Erythrocytes are the final cells in erythropoiesis. They are biconcave discs, having diameter of about 7.5 µm.

Duration of Erythropoiesis

The total period for erythropoiesis is about 7 – 9 days. It takes 5 to 7 days for progenitor cells to become reticulocyte and another 2 days for reticulocytes to become red cells.

Regulation of Erythropoiesis

Feedback mechanisms controlling erythropoiesis are of **two types**: functional feedback and end-product feedback.

Functional Feedback: Red cells supply oxygen to the

tissues, and therefore oxygen requirement of the tissue is the major functional feedback for red cell production. **Erythropoietin** is the chief mediator of this functional feedback.

End-Product Feedback: The end-product feedback is due to the **products of red cell destruction**. Though the precise mediator of this feedback is not clearly identified, stimulatory effects of **hemin** on erythropoiesis.

Factors Controlling Erythropoiesis

Various factors effectively control erythropoiesis. They are broadly be divided into **three categories**: hormonal, dietary and others (Table 9.1).

Table 9.1 | Factors controlling erythropoiesis
A. Hormonal factors
1. Erythropoietin
2. Androgens
3. Estrogen
4. Thyroxine
5. Anterior pituitary hormones
- Growth hormone
- TSH, ACTH, LH, FSH, Prolactin
6. Corticosteroid
7. Interleukins.
B. Dietary factors
1. Vitamins (vitamin B_{12}, folic acid, vitamin C)
2. Proteins
3. Minerals (iron, copper, cobalt and nickel)
C. Other factors
1. Intrinsic factor
2. Chemical factors
3. Environmental factor (hypoxia)
4. Drugs

Hormonal Factors

Erythropoietin

Source: Erythropoietin is produced mainly by the **interstitial cells in peritubular capillary bed of kidney**.

- To some extent, it is also produced by juxtaglomerular cells and extraglomerular mesangial cells of kidney.
- Kidney secretes about 85% of erythropoietin (Clinical Note 9.1).

The rest **15% comes from liver**. The nonparenchymal cells (Kupffer cells) of liver and perivenous hepatocytes produce erythropoietin.

Structure: Erythropoietin is a *glycoprotein* containing 165 amino acids.

- There are four oligosaccharide chains attached with polypeptide chain.
- These oligosaccharide chains are necessary for the physiological activity of erythropoietin.

Mechanism of Action: Erythropoietin acts on erythropoietin receptors that belong to ***cytokine receptor superfamily***.

- The receptor has **tyrosine kinase activity**.
- Binding of erythropoietin with its receptor initiates activation of a cascade of **serine and threonine kinases** that finally leads to **activation of JAK-2 protein**.
- Formation of **JAK and other signaling proteins** bring about changes in cell functions in a similar way like that of growth hormone.

Functions: Erythropoietin stimulates erythropoiesis in several ways.

1. It acts mainly on the **progenitor cells and early precursors**.
   - It especially stimulates BFU-E and CFU-E to form pronormoblasts.
   - It decreases cell cycle length of precursor cells, and therefore, enhances mitosis.
2. It facilitates **maturation of normoblasts**.
3. It increases hemoglobin synthesis in normoblasts.
4. It acts on the stem cells to promote their transformation towards erythroid series.
5. It stimulates early release of reticulocytes into circulation.

Regulation of Erythropoietin (EPO) Production: Factors regulating Ep production can be divided into factors increasing and factors decreasing the production.

Factors Increasing EPO Production: Hypoxia, low blood volume, anemia, lung diseases and hormones like epinephrine, nor-epinephrine, androgen, thyroxine, prolactin, ACTH etc. facilitate Ep production.

- Hypoxia stimulates erythropoiesis by increasing erythropoietin production.
- This is the mechanism of polycythemia that occurs at high altitude.

Factors Decreasing EPO Production: Estrogen inhibits erythropoiesis. Adenosine antagonist such as theophylline decreases erythropoietin secretion.

Metabolism: Ep is inactivated mainly in liver. The half-life of Ep in circulation is about 5 hours.

> **Clinical Note 9.1**
>
> **Renal disease causes anemia:** As kidney is the major source of erythropoietin, chronic renal diseases that reduce renal mass significantly, produce anemia. Anemia is also produced following nephrectomy.

Interleukins and GM-CSF

1. **Interleukin 1, 3 and 5** that are produced mostly from T-cells *stimulate erythropoiesis* mainly acting on stem cells to convert them to the progenitor cells.
2. **GM-CSF** (granulocyte-macrophage colony stimulating factor), which is produced from T-cells, endothelial cells, and fibroblasts *stimulates production of committed stem cells.*

Androgens

Androgens **stimulate erythropoiesis**. Thus, red cell count is more in males after puberty.

- Androgen stimulates erythropoietin production.
- Also, it directly stimulates erythropoiesis.

Estrogens

Estrogens **inhibit erythropoiesis**.

- Estrogen inhibits erythropoiesis by **inhibiting erythropoietin production** and also by decreasing the response of stem cells to erythropoietin.
- Estrogen inhibition of red cell production is more **prominent in hypoxic conditions**. Therefore, Monge's disease (erythrocytosis in chronic mountain sickness) is less common in females.

Thyroxine, Cortisol & Growth Hormone

1. **Thyroxine stimulates erythropoiesis**, by stimulating erythropoietin production.
2. **Growth hormone stimulates erythropoiesis** by increasing the mitosis and maturation of erythroid precursors.
3. **Cortisol** produces *mild erythrocytosis*.

Dietary Factors

Iron

Iron is the raw material for synthesis of heme component of hemoglobin. Therefore, iron deficiency results in hypochromic microcytic anemia.

Vitamin B_{12} and Folic Acid

These two vitamins are necessary for **maturation of red cell precursors** as they promote DNA synthesis.

Folic Acid: For synthesis of DNA, thymine is required, and **tetrahydrofolate** is necessary for thymine synthesis, which is formed from folic acid.

- **Tetrahydrofolate** *promotes formation of deoxythymidilate from deoxyuridylate*, which is required for synthesis of DNA.
- Thus, folate deficiency leads to arrest of mitosis and chromosome division in the absence of DNA synthesis.

Vitamin B_{12}: It promotes **conversion of methyltetrahydrofolate to tetrahydrofolate**. Therefore, vitamin B_{12} deficiency also causes arrest of chromosomal division.

IMPORTANT NOTE

Megaloblastic anemia in deficiency of folic acid and vitamin B_{12}: In deficiency of these two vitamins, megaloblasts are produced in the bone marrow, causing megaloblastic anemia. Megaloblasts produce macrocytes, that manifests as **macrocytic anemia**.

Protein

Protein is essential for **synthesis of globin** component of hemoglobin. Therefore, **protein deficiency** is invariably associated with *hypochromic anemia*.

Other Nutritional Factors

- **Vitamin C** helps in absorption of iron. Therefore, vitamin C deficiency causes anemia.
- Other minerals like **copper and cobalt** influence hemoglobin formation. Thus, deficiency of these minerals leads to anemia.

Other Factors

Intrinsic Factor

Intrinsic factor is secreted from **oxyntic cells of stomach** along with hydrochloric acid.

- It helps in absorption of vitamin B_{12} ***(extrinsic factor of Castle)*** from terminal part of ileum.
- Therefore, intrinsic factor deficiency produces megaloblastic anemia (**pernicious anemia**).

Environmental Factors

Hypoxia due to any cause increases erythropoiesis by increasing erythropoietin production. Hypoxia occurs at **high altitude**, and commonly seen in **cardiac and respiratory diseases**.

Drugs and Chemicals

Vasoconstrictor agents like catecholamines, nucleotides like cAMP, NAD, NADP, products of red cell destruction (hemolysates), cobalt salts and thyroxine **stimulate erythropoiesis**.

Effective & Ineffective Erythropoiesis

Under normal conditions, most of the red cells produced in the marrow are actively alive or have the potential to live a normal life span. This is called **effective erythropoiesis**. However, a fraction of red cell production is ineffective with destruction of **nonviable red cells** either within the marrow or shortly after they are released into circulation.

- When percentage of production of these nonviable red cells is increased, the erythropoiesis is called **ineffective erythropoiesis**.
- Ineffective erythropoiesis is suspected when **reticulocyte count is normal** *despite erythroid hyperplasia of marrow*.

Reticulocytes

Reticulocytes are **juvenile red cells** in the bone marrow. They develop into mature red cells and few of them pass into circulation along with red cells.

Structure: Reticulocytes are slightly bigger than red cells (Table 9.2). Reticulocytes do not possess nuclei but contain a network of reticulum in the cytoplasm that represents the *remnants of basophilic cytoplasm* (the RNA material) of the precursor cells.

IMPORTANT NOTE

The basophilic stippling represents precipitation of RNA materials in the cytoplasm. Such stippling is seen in red cells in toxic conditions such as heavy metal poisoning, especially in **lead poisoning**.

- On **vital staining** with cresyl blue, the reticular network appears in the form of heavy wreath, or clumps of small dots, or as a faint thread connecting two small nodes (Fig. 9.5).
- The ribosomal and cytoplasmic remnants of reticulocytes pick up **supravital stain** when the stain is allowed to penetrate cells while in the living condition.
- In diseased conditions, the stained basophilic RNA materials present in the form of clumps in the cytoplasm appear as discrete blue particles (**punctate basophilia**).

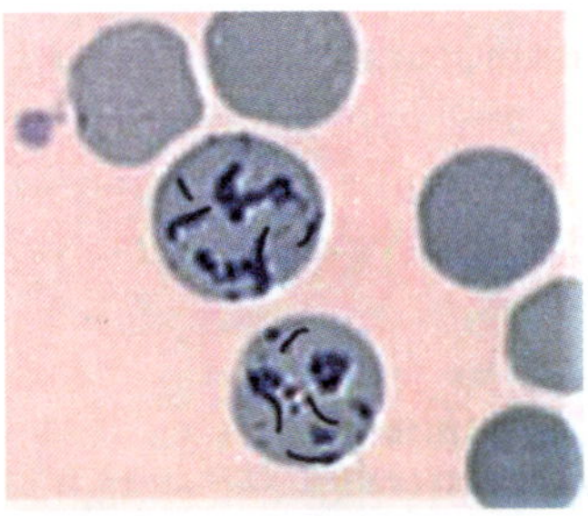

Fig. 9.5: Reticulocytes, as appear after supravital staining.

Table 9.2 | Differences between reticulocytes and red cells.

	Reticulocytes	Red cells
Size	8	7.5 μm
Nuclear material	Present	Absent
Count	Very few (<1% of red cells)	Plenty (5 milliond/mm^3)
MCHC*	Less	More

* MCH is same in both the cells

Development: Reticulocytes are produced in the bone marrow from late normoblast.

- The **nucleus is removed** from the late normoblast to become reticulocyte.
- With the release of young red cells into the circulation, a few reticulocytes are also released.
- When the bone marrow releases red cells at an increased rate, more reticulocytes are released. Thus, the number of reticulocytes in the peripheral blood **is an index of erythropoiesis** (Application Box 9.3).

Normal Count: Normal reticulocyte count **in adult is 0–1%** of the red cells.

- In newborns, the count is 2–6 %.
- The number falls during the first year of life to less than 1% and then the level is maintained throughout life.

Application Box 9.3

Reticulocyte count indicates bone marrow activity: Reticulocytes are the immediate precursors of red cells. Therefore, when the demand for red cells in the body is increased, reticulocyte formation and release are also increased. Thus, reticulocyte count increases along with red cell count.

Reticulocyte Response

The reticulocyte count is performed to assess the **therapeutic response of anemias to treatment**. With initiation of therapy, new red cells are formed and released rapidly into the circulation, and many reticulocytes are also released. This increases reticulocytes in blood, which is called *reticulocyte response*.

- Reticulocyte response indicates a **favorable response to treatment**.
- This is typically observed at the beginning of treatment for **pernicious anemia and iron deficiency anemia**.

1. When **vitamin B_{12} is administered** for treatment of pernicious anemia, the number of reticulocytes increases in the blood, which indicates that the patient is responding well to treatment.
2. Similarly, when **iron is administered** in the treatment of iron deficiency anemia, reticulocyte number increases.

IMPORTANT NOTE

Reticulocyte count is carried out to assess the response of patient to the treatment in pernicious anemia and iron deficiency anemia.

Alteration in Reticulocyte Count

Reticulocytosis: Increase in reticulocyte count is called as reticulocytosis. This is seen in various physiological and pathological conditions.

Physiological: **Newborns and infants** have higher count than adults. Count is more at **high altitude**.

Pathological: Hemolytic anemia, acute hemorrhage, during treatment for deficiency anemias (reticulocyte response), and any condition that stimulates bone marrow to produce red cells.

Reticulocytopenia: There is no physiological reticulocmytopenia. It is seen in aplastic anemia, myxedema, hypopituitarism and leuco-erythroblastic anemia.

Reticulocyte Count in Ineffective Erythropoiesis: Reticulocyte count **remains almost normal** in ineffective erythropoiesis (described above). In fact, ineffective erythropoiesis is suspected when *reticulocyte count is normal despite erythroid hyperplasia of marrow.*

Leuco-erythroblastic Reaction: This term is used to describe the presence of immature myeloid and nucleated red cells in the peripheral blood, which occurs as a consequence of disturbance of the bone marrow architecture by abnormal tissues. This is seen in secondary carcinoma of bone, myelofibrosis, postsplenectomy states, thalassemia major, multiple myeloma, and COVID-19 infection.

Reticulocyte Index

Effective erythropoiesis is estimated by reticulocyte count, which is normally expressed as the % of red cells. However, it can also be expressed as the **total number of circulating reticulocytes per unit of blood**. i.e.,

Absolute reticulocytes = reticulocyte percentage × red cell count

To use reticulocyte % as a measure of the rate of red cell production, the **% may be corrected for the hematocrit**. This is called as **reticulocyte index**.

$$\text{Reticulocyte index} = \text{Reticulocyte \%} \times \frac{\text{Actual Hct}}{\text{Normal Hct}}$$

DESTRUCTION OF RED CELLS

The average lifespan of normal red cell is 120 days. After red cells live their normal life, they become less deformable and more rigid, and get ruptured while passing through capillaries.

Mechanisms of Destruction

There are two mechanisms of red cell destruction: intravascular and extravascular.

Intravascular Destruction

Red cells destruction in the circulation (intravascular demise) is less frequent. If there is a defect in the membrane, hemolysis in circulation is facilitated.

- For example, in *paroxysmal nocturnal hemoglobinuria*, complement complexes create holes in the red cell membrane that promotes intravascular hemolysis.
- Intravascular destruction is also common in *cardiac valve hemolysis* and *microangiopathic hemolytic anemia*.

Extravascular Destruction

Macrophages in liver and spleen trap and senescent red cells. **Two important changes** in senescent red cells that make them vulnerable to mechanical destruction or phagocytosis by macrophages: decreased deformability and alteration in surface properties.

Decreased Deformability: Deformability of red cells helps them to easily pass through the narrow capillaries and splenic pulps.

- The **biconcave shape** and to some extent the **viscosity of hemoglobin solution** in the cell *facilitate the ability of red cells to deform.*
- Decreased deformability due to **change in shape** as occurs in spherocytosis or elliptocytosis, and **increased internal viscosity** as occurs in sickle cell or Hb-C disease, make the red cells vulnerable to lysis while passing through the splenic pulp.

Alteration in Surface Properties: Binding of **antibodies or complement** components to the surface of red cells, changes the chemical composition of the membrane.

- Especially, **binding of IgG or C_3** causes *oxidation of membrane components.*
- This is detected by macrophages that ingest red cells.

Fate of Destroyed Red Cells

Fate of destroyed red cells depends on whether the cells were destroyed intravascularly or extravascularly.

Intravascular Destruction

Destruction of red cells in circulation (**hemolysis**) releases hemoglobin (Hb) into plasma, which is then converted to **heme and globin** (Flowchart 9.1).

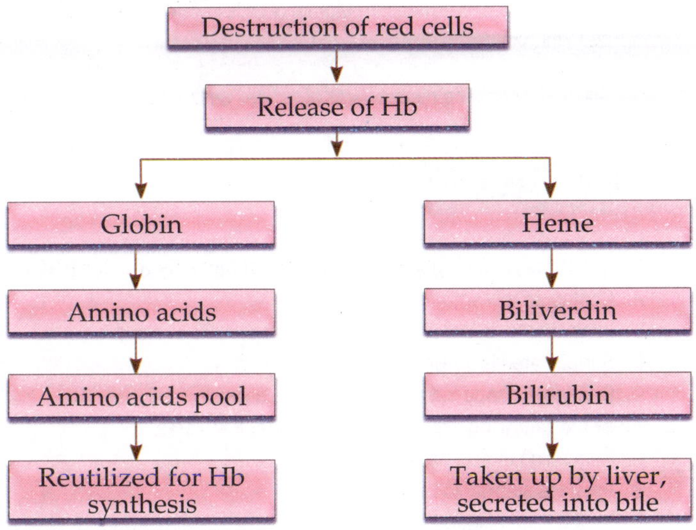

Flowchart 9.1: Fate of destroyed red cells.

- In plasma, Hb binds with **haptoglobin** (Application Box 9.4).
- The **Hb-haptoglobin complex** is transported to liver, where the heme of Hb is converted to iron and **biliverdin** by *heme oxygenase.*
- Biliverdin is further degraded to **bilirubin**. Increased hemolysis causes *hyperbilirubinemia* or **hemolytic jaundice** (described in Chapter 12)
- **Heme in the plasma** binds with **haemopexin**, a plasma glycoprotein.
- When the capacity of haemopexin to bind with heme is saturated, heme binds with albumin to form **methemalbumin**.

Application Box 9.4

Plasma haptoglobin level indicates hemolysis: In intravascular hemolysis, Hb-haptoglobin complex clears haptoglobin from plasma. Therefore, haptoglobin content of the plasma is **decreased in hemolysis** and the degree of decrease is apparently proportionate to the rate of hemolysis. Therefore, estimation of plasma haptoglobin level is an **index of hemolysis.**

Extravascular Destruction

In the phagocytic cells (macrophages), red cells are degraded by lysosomes into lipids, protein and heme.

- Heme is catabolized to bilirubin.
- Globin (protein) is reprocessed in their catabolic pathways.

IMPORTANT NOTE

Fecal and urinary urobilinogen indicate rate of hemolysis: Bilirubin formed from destruction of red cells regardless of their site of destruction is finally excreted through bile into the GI tract.

In the intestine, bilirubin is converted to urobilinogen by bacterial reduction.

A small fraction of ***urobilinogen*** is absorbed from intestine and excreted through urine.

Thus, **fecal and urinary urobilinogen contents** *are indices of the rate of hemolysis.*

Exam Questions

1. Briefly describe how different factors influence ESR. List 4 common causes each of increased and decreased ESR.
2. With the help of a schematic diagram of cells in different steps of erythropoiesis, describe the process of erythropoiesis. Briefly describe the regulation of erythropoiesis.
3. What is reticulocyte response. Briefly explain its physiological and clinical significance.
4. Briefly describe the mechanisms of red cell destruction. Give a note on fate of destroyed red cells.

Multiple Choice Questions

1. Which of the following statement is NOT completely true for RBCs?
A. Contribute to viscosity of blood
B. In newborns, the count is 6 – 8 millions per mm3 of blood
C. Surface area is 14 µm2
D. Biconcave shape increases the surface area

2. All of the following are functions of RBCs, EXCEPT:
A. Regulation of acid base balance
B. Provides stability to blood
C. Recognition of blood group antigens
D. Transportation of gases

3. Which of the following factors does not affect ESR?
A. Iron content of blood
B. Temperature
C. Shape of red cells
D. Fibrionogen content of blood

4. Biconcave shape and flexibility of RBC is maintained by:
A. Actomysin
B. Glutathion
C. G6PD
D. Ankyrin

5. The RBCs:
A. Shrink in a solution of 0.7% NaCl
B. Depend on mitochondria for ATP production
C. Remain intact in 20% urea solution
D. Are 4 - 5 µm in diameter

6. The erythropoiesis process to be completed, takes:
A. 3 days
B. 7 days
C. 28 days
D. 120 days

7. Erythropoietin increases RBC count by all of the following, EXCEPT:
A. Early differentiation of stem cells in the bone marrow
B. Increased synthesis of erythropoietinogen from liver
C. Increased synthesis of Hb in precursor cells
D. Increased release of reticulocytes from bone marrow

8. All of the following help in the maturation of RBCs, EXCEPT:
A. Iron
B. Folic acid
C. Intrinsic factor of Castle
D. Vitamin B12

9. Senescent RBCs are removed from blood by:
A. Monocytes in blood
B. Macrophages in spleen
C. Neutrophils in blood
D. Histiocytes in tissues

10. Ineffective erythropoiesis is characterized by:
A. Normal reticulocyte count and erythroid hyperplasia of marrow
B. Increased reticulocyte count and normal marrow
C. Decreased reticulocyte count and normal marrow
D. Increased reticulocyte count and erythroid hyperplasia of marrow

Answers

1. C 2. B 3. A 4. D 5. C 6. B 7. B 8. A 9. B 10. A

Chapter 10

Hemoglobins and Blood Indices

Learning Objectives

On completion of study of this chapter:

The student will be able to (must know):

1. Name the types of Hb and give the major steps of Hb synthesis.
2. Give the normal values of Hb in males and females and list the functions of Hb.
3. List the physiological and pathological variations in Hb concentration.
4. Name the various Hb complexes and common conditions in which they are found.
5. Give the values of blood indices and name common conditions of their alteration.

The student may also be able to (desirable to know):

1. Describe the physiological aspects of hemoglobin complexes.
2. Describe the clinical significance of blood indices.

PY2.3

HEMOGLOBINS

Hemoglobin (Hb) is a conjugated protein pigment present in red cells and constitutes more than 90% of dry weight of these cells.

Structure of Hb

Hb is made up of heme and globin.

Heme: Heme is a complex molecule, made up of a series of **tetrapyrrole rings**, terminating in *protoporphyrin*, with a ***central iron atom***.

Globin: This is a protein substance that consists of **two pairs of polypeptide chains**. Each amino acid chain is attached to a heme moiety to form a single Hb molecule.

Synthesis of Hb

Formation of Hb requires heme and globin. Heme is formed in mitochondria and globin in ribosomes (Flowchart 10.1).

- **Succinyl-CoA**, an intermediary product of TCA cycle combines with glycine to form **α-amino-β-ketoadipic acid** with the help of pyridoxal phosphate, which in turn forms **α-amino-δ-levulinic acid** (ALA) in the presence of ALA synthase.
- ALA is converted to **porphobilinogen**, which forms **protoporphyrin-IX**.
- Ferrous iron is introduced into protoporphyrin-IX and in the presence of heme synthase, **heme is formed.**
- **Globin**, the protein component formed by ribosome combines with heme to form Hb.

As iron and amino acids are raw materials for synthesis of heme and globin, iron and protein deficiencies lead to Hb deficiency.

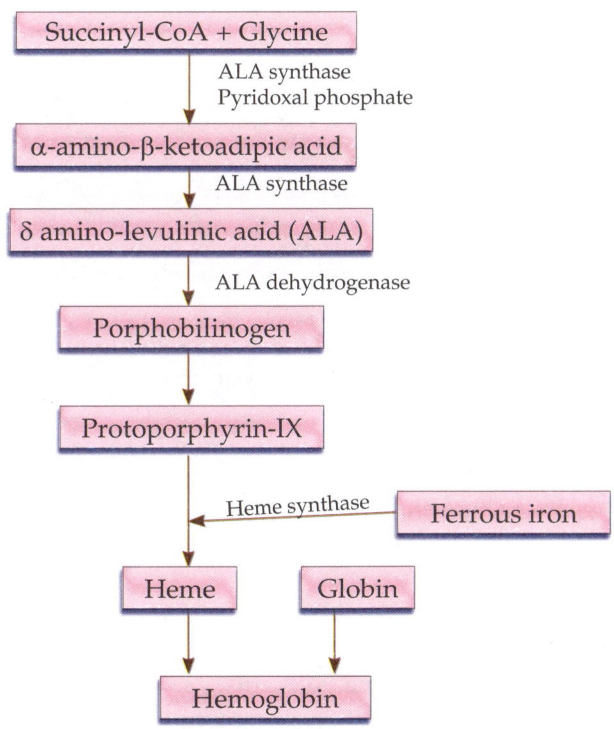

Flowchart 10.1: Steps of hemoglobin synthesis.

Types of Hemoglobin

Hemoglobins can be broadly divided into normal and abnormal types (Table 1). **Normal hemoglobins** are adult Hb, fetal Hb and embryonic Hb, and **abnormal hemoglobins** are Hb S, Hb C, Hb D, Hb E and unstable Hb.

Normal Hemoglobins

Adult Hemoglobins

Adult Hb are of two types: Hb A and Hb A_2.

Hemoglobin A (Hb A): Hb A is the major Hb and comprises about **97 % of hemoglobin** of adult red cells.

- It consists of **two α and two β chains** with the structural formula $\alpha_2\beta_2$.
- Hb A is detected in small amount in the fetus as early as the eighth week of intrauterine life.
- During the first few months of post-natal life, Hb A replaces Hb F and the adult pattern is fully established in 6 months.

Hemoglobin A_2 (Hb A_2): This is the minor hemoglobin in the adult red cells. It has the structural formula of $\alpha_2\delta_2$.

- Hb A_2 is present in very small amounts at birth and reaches the **adult level of 3 %** during the first year of life.
- Its concentration increases in some anemias.

Table 10.1 | Types of Hb

A. Normal Hb
Adult Hb
Fetal Hb
Embryonic Hb
B. Abnormal Hb
Hb S
Hb C
Hb D
Hb E
Unstable Hb

Fetal hemoglobin (Hb F)

Hb F is the **major hemoglobin in intrauterine life**. It has the structural formula of $\alpha_2\gamma_2$.

- Hb F accounts for 70 to 90 % of hemoglobin at term.
- It then **falls rapidly to 25 % in one month**, and 5 % in six months.
- The **adult level of 1 %** is not reached in some children until puberty.
- Hb F concentration in adults increases in some types of anemia, hemoglobinopathies, and sometimes in leukemia.

Hemoglobin Bart's (Hb Bart's): This is the minor hemoglobin present in fetal life.

- It consists **of 4 gamma (γ) chains,** γ_4.
- Hb Bart's concentration **increases in fetal life in thalassemia**.

Embryonic Hemoglobins

These hemoglobins are confined to the very early stages (embryonic stage) of development. There are 3 embryonic hemoglobins:

1. **Gower Hb 1:** It consists of 2 zeta and 2 epsilon chains ($\zeta_2\varepsilon_2$).
2. **Hb Gower 2:** It consists of 2 alpha and 2 epsilon chains ($\alpha_2\varepsilon_2$)
3. **Hb Portland:** It consists of 2 zeta and 2 gamma chains ($\zeta_2\gamma_2$).

Abnormal Hemoglobins

There are **four clinically important abnormal hemoglobins**: Hb S, Hb C, Hb D, and Hb E. These are present in different hereditary hemoglobinopathies. The most commonly encountered hemoglobin is **Hb S** which consists of $\alpha_2\beta_2$, but in the beta chain, **valine is substituted for glutamic acid at the sixth position.** Hb S is present in sickle cell anemia.

Unstable hemoglobins are hemoglobin variants that undergo denaturation, and precipitate in the red cells as ***Heinz bodies***. Unstable hemoglobins are present in some form of congenital non-spherocytic hemolytic anemia.

Physiological Aspects

Normal Values

Adult males: 14 to 18 (16 ± 2) g/dL of blood
Adult females: 12 to 16 (14 ± 2) g/dL of blood

In newborns, hemoglobin concentration is normally **16 to 22 g/dL,** which occurs mainly due to hemoconcentration.

- Hb decreases to 9 to 14 g/dL at about two to four months of age.
- By ten years of age, the normal hemoglobin concentration will be 12 to 14 g/dL.
- There may be a slight decrease in hemoglobin level after 50 years of age.

Functions of Hb

Hemoglobin serves **four important functions.**

1. **Gas Transport:** It transports **oxygen from lungs to the tissues** by forming ***oxyhemoglobin*** and **carbon dioxide** from tissues to lungs by forming ***carbaminohemoglobin***.
   - When fully saturated, 1g of hemoglobin carries **1.34 ml of oxygen**.
   - Thus, **oxygen carrying capacity** of blood can be calculated easily if the value of blood hemoglobin concentration is known. For example, if Hb is 15 g %, 100 ml of blood will carry 15 × 1.34 = 20.7 ml ofo xygen.
   - The oxygen molecules combine with hemoglobin to form **oxyhemoglobin.**

- Hemoglobin returning with carbon dioxide from tissues is called **reduced hemoglobin.**

2. **Hb as Buffer:** Hemoglobin **acts as a buffer** in maintaining blood pH.
3. Hb serves to destroy physiologically important nitric oxide molecule.
4. It imparts red color to the blood. Erythrocytes look red due to the presence of hemoglobin in them, which is a red pigment.

Variations in Hb Concentration

Conditions that Decrease Hb Concentration

Physiological: **Children** have values lower than that in adults and **women** have values lower than that in males. **Hb is less during pregnancy** due to hemodilution.

Pathological: Hb is less in different types of **anemia** (details are given in next chapter). However, **relative decrease** in Hb concentration occurs in different pathological conditions that produce hemodilution like excess ADH secretion as occurs in pituitary tumors.

Conditions that Increase Hb Concentration

Physiological: Hb level is high at **high altitude** that occurs due to **hypoxia**.

- Hb is more in newborns.
- In excessive sweating, relative increase in Hb occurs due to hemoconcentration.

Pathological: Hb concentration increases in conditions that **produce hemoconcentration** like severe diarrhea, vomiting etc; and **conditions that produce hypoxia** like congenital heart disease, emphysema etc. It may also be due to **polycythemia vera** (for details, see next chapter).

Hemoglobin Ligands (Complexes)

Besides its binding with oxygen to form **oxyhemoglobin,** Hb combines with other chemicals and gases to form **Hb-complexes.** The common Hb complexes are given below.

Nitrosohemoglobin: Nitric oxide (NO) is a physiologic ligand of Hb. Binding of Hb with NO destroys NO and forms nitrosohemoglobin by formation of **nitrosyl heme.**

Carbaminohemoglobin: Carbon dioxide (CO_2) is a physiologic ligand of Hb.

- Binding of CO_2 with Hb leads to formation of carbaminohemoglobin.
- CO_2 combines with globin, not with heme.
- It helps in transport of CO_2 from tissues to lungs.

Carboxyhemoglobin: Carboxyhemoglobin, also called **carbomonoxyhemoglobin** is formed when heme of Hb combines with **carbon monoxide** (CO).

- Hb binds with CO about **200 times** than that of oxygen. Therefore, it readily combines with CO even when CO is present in low concentration.
- However, formation of carboxy-Hb is reversible.
- Concentration of Carboxy-Hb is very low in normal persons.
- **In smokers** its concentration is high, ranging from **1 to 10g/dL.**

Methemoglobin: Methemoglobin is Hb in which iron has been oxidized from ferrous to **ferric state.**

- Methemoglobin is not capable of reversibly binding with oxygen.
- Therefore, in methemoglobinemia oxygen carrying capacity is grossly reduced.

Cyanmethemoglobin: Cyanmethemoglobin or **hemiglobincyanide** is formed by the action of cyanide anion (CN^-), for example potassium cyanide (KCN^-) with Hb. This combination is reversible.

- **Hemiglobin** is the hemoglobin in which the *iron has been oxidized by cyanide* to the ferric state.
- Hemiglobincyanide is the methemoglobin bound to cyanide ions.

Sulfhemoglobin: Sulfhemoglobin is formed on exposure to some toxic agents, usually sulfur containing drugs and chemicals.

- In sulfhemoglobin, the iron is in ferrous state, but oxygen affinity is about 100 times lower than the normal Hb.
- Once sulfhemoglobin is formed, it is irreversible and remains throughout the life of the carrier RBC.

Glycosylated or Glycated Hemoglobin: Binding of glucose with protein (globin) of Hb results in glycosylated or glycated hemoglobin.

In one fraction of Hb A, known as **Hb A1$_C$** glucose is attached to terminal valine in β chain.

In normal individuals, **glycated Hb is 4 to 5.6%** of total Hb. Its concentration increases in hyperglycemia.

Applied Physiology

Hb Destruction

Hb destruction occurs with destruction of red cells (hemolysis) releasing heme and globin.

- Globin returns to the body's metabolic pool where its amino acids are subsequently reutilized.
- The porphyrin ring of heme is cleaved by the microsomal enzyme, *heme oxidase*, yielding **biliverdin.**
- The biliverdin is further reduced to form **bilirubin** by *biliverdin reductase* (Refer, Flowchart 9.1, Chapter 9).

In acute hemolysis, Hb casts block renal tubules and cause tubular necrosis (Application Box 10.1).

Application Box 10.1

ARF and Tissue Hypoxia: In hemolysis, hemoglobin is released into blood (hemoglobinemia) and gets filtered in the renal tubules to appear in the urine (hemoglobinuria). In tubules, hemoglobin forms casts and blocks lumen of tubules causing **acute tubular necrosis** or acute renal failure (ARF). Hemoglobinemia also increases blood viscosity that affects cardiac output and hemodynamics. Hb deficiency causes tissue hypoxia.

Hemoglobin Estimation

PY2.11

Hemoglobin estimation is the most frequently ordered laboratory test in clinical practice. As it is more convenient, estimation of hemoglobin is preferred to the total RBC count to detect anemia.

Estimation of Glycated Hb

Glycated-Hb (HbA1c) is measured in the conditions of prolonged hyperglycemia that indirectly reflects the **glycemic control in diabetes**. It is used in detecting **severity of diabetes**.

- As per WHO criteria, if HbA1c is more than 6.5%, it is considered abnormal (Table 10.2).
- Its concentration increases in conditions in which blood glucose is chronically elevated like diabetes mellitus, Cushing syndrome, hyperthyroidism etc.
- As per ADA (American Diabetic Association) criteria:

HbA1c: 4% - 5.6%: **Normal**
HbA1c: 5.7% - 6.5%: **Prediabetes**
HbA1c: > 6.5%: **Diabetes**

Table 10.2 | The average blood glucose at various levels HbA1c.

HbA1c	Blood Sugar level
HbA1c 4%	68 mg/dL
HbA1c 5%	90 mg/dL
HbA1c 6%	120 mg/dL
HbA1c 7%	152 mg/dL
HbA1c 8%	183 mg/dL
HbA1c 9%	212 mg/dL
HbA1c 10%	240 mg/dL

IMPORTANT NOTE

Glycated Hb (HbA1c) reflects glycemic control in diabetics: When blood glucose is chronically elevated for **more than three months**, glycated Hb is formed in more quantity. Therefore, instead of fasting blood glucose, emphasis is given more on estimation of glycated Hb for assessing glycemic control in diabetic patients on therapy. Thus, glycated Hb is *an index of chronic hyperglycemia* in diabetic subjects.

PY2.11

BLOOD INDICES

The values of hemoglobin, PCV and total RBC count are used to calculate red cell volume and red cell hemoglobin content and concentration. These are called **red blood cell indices**. Determination of these indices is of considerable clinical importance and is widely used in the **classification of anemia**.

Mean Corpuscular Volume

Definition: Mean corpuscular volume (MCV) is the **average volume of an RBC expressed in femtoliters** (1 fL = 10^{-15} L).

Esimation: If the PCV and the number of red cells per liter are known, MCV is calculated by dividing the volume of red cells per liter by the number of red cells per liter.

$$\text{MCV (fL)} = \frac{\text{Hematocrit (\%)} \times 10}{\text{RBC count in millions/mm}^3}$$

Where, the factor 10 is introduced to convert the hematocrit reading (in %) from volume of packed red cells per 100 ml to volume per liter.

For example, if the hematocrit reading is 40%, and the red cell count is 5 millions, then MCV is calculated as:

$$\text{MCV} = \frac{40 \times 10}{5} = 80 \text{ fL.}$$

Normal Value: The MCV in normal adults is between **78 and 96 fL**.

Interpretation: The MCV is the **index of the size of red cells.**

- It depicts whether the red cells are microcytic, normocytic or macrocytic.
- If the **MCV is less than 80 fL**, the red cells are considered ***microcytic***.
- If **MCV is greater than 96 fL**, they are considered *macrocytic*.

Mean Corpuscular Hemoglobin

Definition: The mean corpuscular hemoglobin (MCH) is the **average weight of hemoglobin content in an RBC expressed in picograms** (1 pg = 10^{-12} g).

Estimation: It is calculated by dividing the hemoglobin content of 1 liter of blood (in g/L) by the number of RBCs in 1 liter.

$$\text{MCH (pg)} = \frac{\text{Hb (g/dL)} \times 10}{\text{RBC count in millions/mm}^3}$$

For example, if the hemoglobin content is 14 g/dL, and the RBC count is 5 millions:

$$\text{MCH} = \frac{14 \times 10}{5} = 28 \text{ pg.}$$

Normal Value: The normal range for MCH is **27 to 33 pg**.

Interpretation: It may be as high as 50 pg in macrocytic anemia, or as low as 20 pg or less in hypochromic microcytic anemia.

Mean Corpuscular Hb Concentration

Definition: The mean corpuscular hemoglobin concentration (MCHC) is the **average hemoglobin concentration per unit volume of packed red cells**.

Estimation: It is expressed as g/dL, or percent.

$$\text{MCHC (\%)} = \frac{\text{Hb (g/100 ml)}}{\text{PCV/100 ml}} \times 100$$

For example, if the hemoglobin concentration is 15 g/dL and hematocrit is 40 %:

$$MCHC = \frac{15}{45} \times 100 = 33.3\ \%.$$

Normal Value: The normal range of MCHC is between 33 and 37 g/dL (or %).

Interpretation: MCHC above 40 % indicates malfunctioning of the instrument or error in the calculation of the manual measurements used, as an MCHC of 37% is near the upper limits for hemoglobin solubility, thus limiting the physiologic upper limit of the MCHC. **In hypochromic anemias**, the hemoglobin concentration is reduced and values as low as 20 to 25 % are not uncommon.

Color Index (CI)

Definition & Estimation: This is the **ratio of hemoglobin percent and RBC percent.**

$$CI = \frac{\text{Hb percent}}{\text{RBC percent}}$$

100 % of Hb = 14.8 g/100 ml.

100 % of RBC = 5 millions/mm^3

Normal value: The normal range of CI is between 0.85 and 1.10.

Interpretation: CI less than 0.85 indicates hypochromic anemia.

Exam Questions

1. Classify hemoglobins and give examples for each. Give the structure and significance of each type of Hb.
2. Name the hemoglobin complexes and briefly describe their functions.
3. What is glycated Hb, and what is its normal value. Briefly explain the clinical utility of estimation of HbA1c.
4. Name the blood indices, give their definitions and normal values.

Multiple Choice Questions

1. All of the following are physiological (nomal) Hb, EXCEPT:
- A. Hb F
- B. Hb S
- C. Hb A
- D. Hb A2

2. HbA1c level in a normal healthy adult is:
- A. 7 - 8.5%
- B. 6 - 7.6%
- C. 4 - 5.6%
- D. 1 - 2.6%

3. The number of oxygen molecules carried by each Hb molecule is:
- A. 8
- B. 6
- C. 4
- D. 2

4. All of the following are Hb-complexes, EXCEPT:
- A. Embryonic Hemoglobin
- B. Carboxyhemoglobin
- C. Nitrosohemoglobin
- D. Carbaminohemoglobin

5. All of the following are true, EXCEPT:
- A. Affinity of Hb for CO is more than for oxygen
- B. Binding of Hb to sulphur is irreversible
- C. In methemoglobin, iron is in ferric state
- D. Binding of Hb to cynide anion is irreversible

6. Normal value of MCHC is:
- A. 38 - 45%
- B. 33 - 37%
- C. 27 - 32%
- D. 22 - 26%

7. Normal value of MCH is:
- A. 40 – 45 pg
- B. 34 – 39 pg
- C. 27 – 33 pg
- D. 22 – 26 pg

8. When Hb level is 10 gm%, 100 mL of blood will carry approximately:
- A. 20.7 mL of oxygen
- B. 13 mL of oxygen
- C. 10 mL of oxygen
- D. 7.4 mL of oxygen

9. Which of the following statement is true?
- A. Hemoglobinemia causes vasoconstriction
- B. Protoporphyrin from Hb gets recycled
- C. Binding of carbondioxide to Hb is called carboxyhemoglobin
- D. Increased temperature increases the affinity of Hb to oxygen

10. Binding of oxygen to hemoglobin takes place in about:
- A. 1.3 second
- B. 1 second
- C. 0.1 second
- D. 0.01 second

Answers

1\. B 2. C 3. C 4. A 5. D 6. B 7. C 8. B 9. A 10. D

Chapter 11

Pathophysiology of Anemia and Polycythemia

Learning Objectives

On completion of study of this chapter:

The student will be able to (must know):

1. Define and classify anemia and give the common causes of each category of anemia.
2. Give the salient blood picture of common types of anemia.
3. List the types and causes of polycythemia.

The student may also be able to (desirable to know):

1. Explain the etiopathogenesis and blood picture of common anemias.
2. Briefly describe the blood picture and bone marrow picture of polycythemia vera.

PY2.5

ANEMIA

Anemia is defined as **decreased red cell count or hemoglobin** content of blood.

- Detection of anemia is usually performed by **estimating Hb content** of blood.
- Clinically, anemia is detected by assessing the **degree of paleness** usually by looking at the ***lower palpebral conjunctiva*** or nail beds.
- Detection of *morphological types* of anemia depends on **blood indices**.

Causes and Classification

Anemias can be classified either morphologically or etiologically.

Common causes of anemia are:

1. Inadequate supply of nutrients resulting in **deficiency anemias** (deficiency of iron, vitamins and proteins)
2. Aplasia of bone marrow.
3. Anemia associated with chronic diseases
4. Anemia associated with renal failure
5. Anemia due to inherited diseases (e.g. thalassemia)
6. Anemia due to blood loss

However, anemia is **classified etiologically into two types**: decreased red cell production and increased red cell destruction (Table 11.1)

Table 11.1 | Classification of anemia

Classification of anemia
A. Decreased red cell production
1. Stem cell failure
– Aplastic anemia
– Anemia of leukemia
2. Progenitor cell failure
– Pure red cell aplasia
– Chronic renal failure
– Chronic diseases
3. Precursor cell failure
– Megaloblastic anemia
– Iron deficiency anemia
– Thalassemia
– Hemoglobinopathies
B. Increased red cell destruction or loss
1. Acquired causes
– Acute blood loss
– Hypersplenism
– Micro- and macroangiopathic
– Antibody mediated
2. Hereditary causes
– Membrane defects
– Enzyme defects
– Globin defects

Morphological Classification

Hypochromic Microcytic Anemia: MCV, MCH, and MCHC are below normal.

- Such subnormal red cell indices correspond to **microcytosis and hypochromia** of red cells in the blood film.
- This occurs due to the result of a defect in red cell formation in which **hemoglobin synthesis is impaired** to a greater extent.

- The common examples are **iron deficiency anemia** and **thalassemia**.

Normochromic Normocytic Anemia: MCV, MCH, and MCHC are within the normal range.

- Size and hemoglobin concentration of the red cells are normal in the blood film.
- It is usually seen in **blood loss anemia, hemolytic anemia** and **aplastic anemia**.

Macrocytic Anemia: The MCV is above the upper limit of the normal.

- It corresponds to **macrocytosis of red cells** in the blood film.
- The red cells are usually **normochromic**.
- The typical example of is **megaloblastic anemia** that occurs due to deficiency of vitamin B_{12} or folic acid.

Etiological Classification

Blood Loss Anemia

Acute Hemorrhage: Anemia in acute hemorrhage depends on the **extent of blood loss**. Activation of ***compensatory mechanisms*** to expand the blood volume *causes hemodilution* and aids to decrease in hemoglobin content.

Chronic Hemorrhage: Chronic hemorrhage commonly occurs in following conditions.

1. **Gastrointestinal blood loss:** Peptic ulcer, hemorrhoids, carcinoma of the stomach and colon, esophageal varices, chronic gastritis, ulcerative colitis, hookworm infestation etc.
2. **Respiratory diseases:** Respiratory diseases that produce epistaxis, hemoptysis as occurs in pulmonary tuberculosis or bronchogenic carcinoma produce anemia.
3. **Genitourinary disease:** Diseases that cause hematuria and hemoglobinuria produce anemia.
3. **Diseases of genital tract:** In females, loss of blood from genital tract like menstrual disorders (menorrhagia, metrorrhagia) and uterine pathologies produce anemia.

Aplastic Anemia

Aplastic anemia is the anemia due to **impaired red cell production**.

- Marrow examination shows a near **absence of hematopoietic precursor cells**.
- Aplastic anemia is commonly produced by **cytotoxic and cancer chemotherapeutic drugs** and **irradiation** of bone marrow.

Hemolytic Anemia

Hemolytic anemia results from increase in the rate of **red cell destruction**. Defects causing premature red cell destruction may be divided into **two broad categories**: intracorpuscular and extracorpuscular.

- Common **intracorpuscular defects** are hereditary spherocytosis and thalassemia.
- Common **extracorpuscular defects** are hemolytic diseases of newborn, incompatible blood transfusion, drug-induced anemia, and burns.

Common Anemias

Iron Deficiency Anemia (IDA)

This is the **commonest form of anemia** in the developing countries.

- It usually occurs due to **deficiency of iron in the diet**.
- Anemia is **microcytic hypochromic** type (microcytic and hypochromic cells in blood smear) (Fig. 11.1).
- **Micronomoblasts** are seen in bone marrow with ***decreased marrow iron store***.

Etiopathogenesis: Three major factors are involved in the pathogenesis of IDA.

1. **Increased demand** for iron as occurs in ***pregnancy, lactation and growing children***. IDA is common in these groups.
2. **Inadequate intake** due to ***nutritional deficiency***.
3. **Chronic blood loss** like bleeding peptic ulcer, piles, worm infestations, epistaxis, hemoptysis etc.

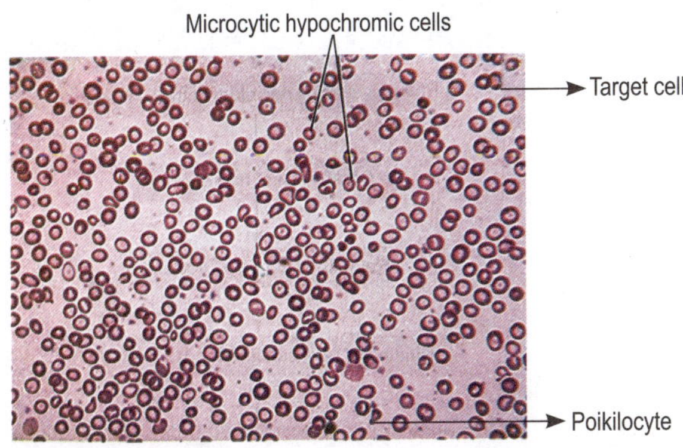

Fig. 11.1: Peripheral blood smear of a patient of iron deficiency anemia. Note red cells are mostly microcytes with severe hypochromia, anisocytosis, poikilocytosis and target cells: *Courtesy*: Fig. 12.3, Page 248, Concise Pathology by Geetika Khanna Bhattacharya, Elsevier, 2021.

Hereditary Spherocytosis

This is a form of *hereditary hemolytic anemia* in which the fundamental abnormality is the **deficiency of spectrin** in red cell membrane.

- Spherocytes are less deformable and susceptible to hemolysis.
- The **usual features are** anemia, jaundice, enlarged spleen, and may present with gall stone.
- The **blood picture** typically shows ***anemia with spherocytosis*** (presence of many spherocytes in blood smear) (Fig. 11.2), increased osmotic fragility, hyperbilirubinemia, and reticulocytosis.
- Usually, anemia is **normocytic and normochromic**.
- **Splenectomy** helps in improving the condition.

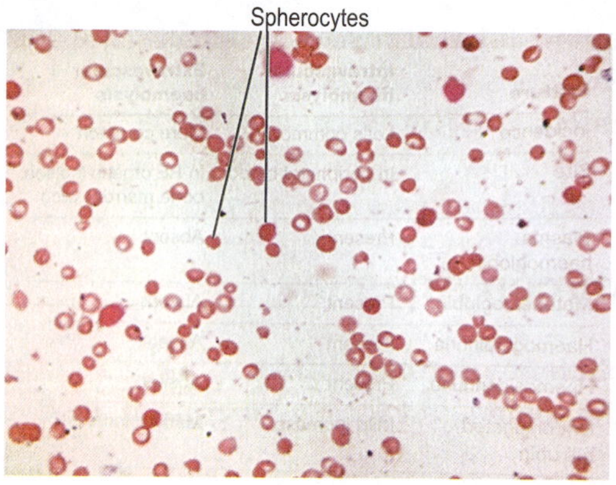

Fig. 11.2: Peripheral blood smear of a patient of hereditary spherocytosis. Note red cells are mostly spherocytes: *Courtesy*: Fig. 12.6, Page 258, Concise Pathology by Geetika Khanna Bhattacharya, Elsevier, 2021.

Sickle Cell Anemia

This is a hereditary disorder in which red cells contain an abnormal hemoglobin called **Hb S**.

- In Hb S, **glutamic acid is replaced by valine** *at sixth position of beta chain.*
- In the *deoxygenated state*, red cells take the shape of a sickle and undergo **intravascular hemolysis**.
- Diagnosis is usually made by **sickling test** (sickling of red cells when the blood sample is mixed with a reducing agent like sodium metabisulphite), **hemoglobin solubility test** (relative insolubility of reduced Hb S in phosphate buffer), and **hemoglobin electrophoresis**.
- **Hypersplenism** is usually associated.
- The anemia is usually **normochromic and normocytic,** with presence of sickle cells (Fig. 11.3).

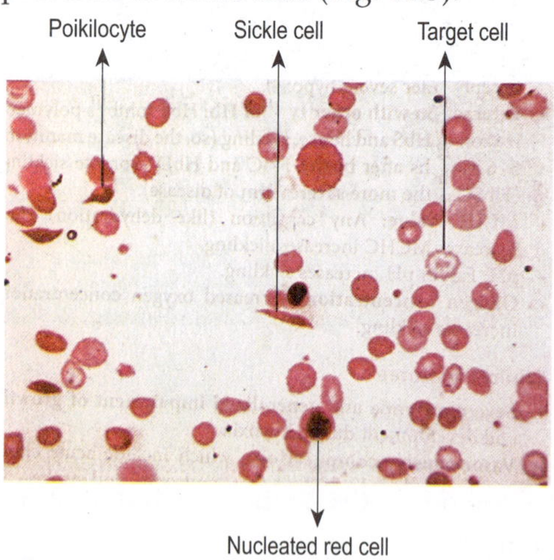

Fig. 11.3: Peripheral blood smear of a patient of sickle cell disease. Note few red cells are sickle cells, poikilocytes and target cells: *Courtesy*: Fig. 12.7, Page 260, Concise Pathology by Geetika Khanna Bhattacharya, Elsevier, 2021.

Thalassemia

Thalassemia is a genetic defect in which the rate of ***synthesis of*** one or more types of ***hemoglobin polypeptide chain is decreased.***

- There are **two major classes** of thalassemia: **α thalassemia** and **β thalassemia,** in which α and β globin genes are involved respectively.
- This causes decrease in the respective polypeptide chain of Hb.
- There are many homozygous and heterozygous, and major and minor forms of the disease.

β Thalassemia Major: In β thalassemia major, anemia develops in **first few months of life** and becomes progressively severe.

- **Splenomegaly**, hepatomegaly and skeletal deformities are common.
- Though anemia is usually **microcytic and hypochromic** (Fig. 11.4), all forms and combinations are not uncommon.

α Thalassemia: Anemia of α thalassemia (failure to synthesize α chain) is ***more hemolytic*** than dyserythropoietic.

- Thalassemias are diagnosed by ***hemoglobin electrophoresis***, demonstration of **Hb-H inclusions** (in the absence of sufficient alpha chains, excess of beta or gamma chains aggregate to form Hb-H), assessment of rate of globin chain synthesis, alkali denaturation test, and acid elution test.

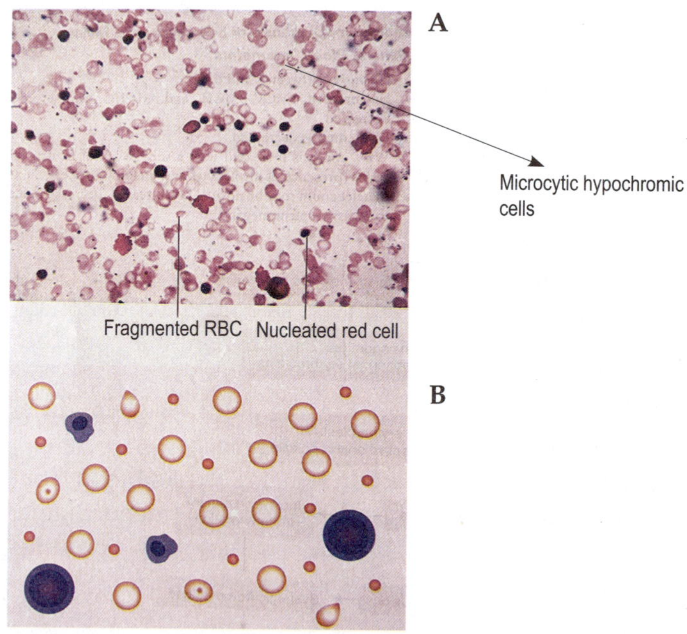

Fig. 11.4: Peripheral blood smear of a patient of β thalassemia major (A), and a schematic picture (B). Note red cells are mostly microcytic hypochromic with anisocytosis, poikilocytosis. There are tear drop cells and nucleated red cells: *Courtesy*: Fig. 12.8, Page 262, Concise Pathology by Geetika Khanna Bhattacharya, Elsevier, 2021.

Pernicious Anemia

This is a **megaloblastic anemia** that occurs due to **deficiency of intrinsic factor** (IF) secreted from oxyntic cells of stomach leading to **vitamin B_{12} deficiency**.

- **Common causes** are chronic gastritis, gastric atrophy and partial gastrectomy.
- The blood picture depicts **macrocytic** normochromic anemia (Fig. 11.5).
- **Hypersegmented neutrophils** are also seen.

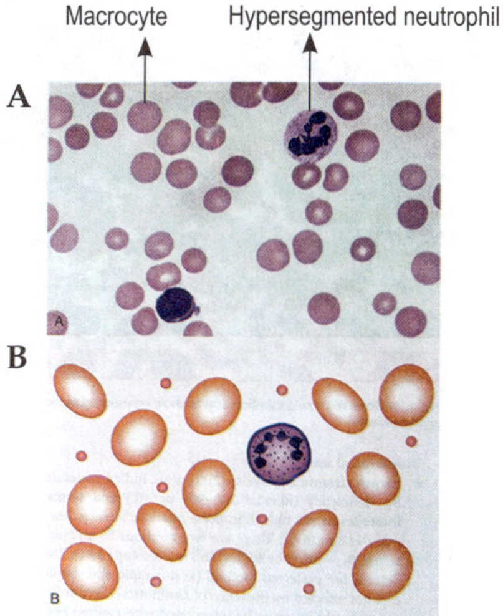

Fig. 11.5: Peripheral blood smear of a patient of pernicious anemia (A), and a schematic picture (B). Note the anemia is megaloblastic with red cells mostly macrocytic, but normochromic. Hypersgmented neutrophil is seen. *Courtesy*: Fig. 12.4, Page 253, Concise Pathology by Geetika Khanna Bhattacharya, Elsevier, 2021.

POLYCYTHEMIA

Though, polycythemia strictly denotes increase in all cell types of blood, traditionally it refers to **increase in number of red cells**.

Types

Polycythemia is broadly divided into **three forms** (Table 11.2).

- The **primary form** is the *polycythemia vera*.
- The **secondary forms** are secondary to other conditions or diseases.
- The ***relative or apparent polycythemia*** is not true polycythemia, but a spurious increase in red cells due to dehydration.

Table 11.2 | Types of polycythemia.

Types of polycythemia
A. Primary polycythemia - Polycythemia vera
B. Secondary polycythemia (secondary erythrocytosis) 1. Appropriate increase in erythropoietin secretion - High altitude - Congenital heart disease with right to left shunt. - Chronic pulmonary diseases - Chronic smokers 2. Inappropriate increase in erythropoietin secretion - Renal tumors, renal cyst, hydronephrosis - Liver tumors (mainly hepatocarcinoma) - Brain tumors (cerebellar hemangioma) - Endocrine disorders (pheochromocytoma, virilizing ovarian tumors, Batter syndrome)
C. Apparent (relative) polycythemia - Dehydration; Redistribution of body fluid

Polycythemia Vera

Polycythemia vera is an **abnormality of hematopoietic stem** cell in which a single stem cell is transformed into a cell having selective growth advantage that gradually becomes the major source of marrow precursors.

- Disease commonly starts in **6th decade of life**, and usually presents with headache, **plethora** (a ruddy complexion), pruritus, thrombosis and GI bleeding.
- For plethoric appearance of patients, the disease is also called **polycythemia rubra vera**.
- **Bone marrow** is characteristically **hypercellular.**
- *Erythrocyte count* is **very high**.
- Leucocytosis with absolute **neutrophilia and thrombocytosis** are common.
- The disease is treated by **phlebotomy** (removal of about 500 ml of blood in 2 to 4 days time).
- **Myelosuppresive drugs** like hydroxyurea and busulfan are also prescribed to inhibit marrow activity.

Multiple Choice Questions

1. Iron deficiency anemia is:

A. Macrocytic hypochromic
B. Microcytic hypochromic
C. Normocytic hypochromic
D. Normocytic normochromic

2. In moderate to severe anemia, all of the following are reduced, EXCEPT:

A. 2,3-diphosphoglycerate levels in RBC
B. Exercise capacity
C. Cardiac output
D. Arterial PO2

3. All of the following are features of macrocytic anemia, EXCEPT:

A. Increased MCHC
B. Hypersegmentation of neutrophils
C. Howell-Jolly bodies
D. Basophilic stippling

4. Which of the following statement is NOT true?

A. Hemolytic anemia is normocytic normochromic
B. Nutritional deficiency is commonest cause of anemia in developing countries
C. In sickle cell anemia, glutamic acid is replaced by valine in ▯ chain
D. In hereditary sphereocytosis, osmotic fragility is decreased

5. All of the following are true, EXCEPT

A. Increased intravascular hemolysis in sickle cell anemia
B. Increased hematopoietic precursor cells in aplastic anemia
C. Hereditary sphreocytosis is an autosomal dominant disorder
D. Pernicious anemia occurs in gastric mucosal atrophy

6. All of the following can cause polycythemia, EXCEPT:

A. High altitude
B. Chronic smokers
C. Chronic alcoholism
D. Congenital heart disease

Answers

1. B 2. C 3. A 4. D 5. B 6. C

Chapter 12

Pathophysiology of Jaundice

Learning Objectives

On completion of study of this chapter:

The student will be able to (must know):

1. Define jaundice and give normal value of serum bilirubin.
2. Outline the steps of bilirubin metabolism.
3. Classify jaundice and list causes of each.
4. Give the physiological basis of causation of jaundice.
5. List the differences in laboratory findings of different types of jaundice.

The student may also be able to (desirable to know):

1. Describe the physiology of bilirubin metabolism
2. Explain the pathophysiology of jaundice

PY2.5

Jaundice is **defined as** the yellowish discoloration of sclera, skin and mucous membrane due to the deposition of bilirubin. This happens due to **hyperbilirubinemia**.

- The **normal plasma bilirubin** level is ***0.2–0.8 mg/dL***.
- Jaundice is detected clinically only when the bilirubin level exceeds 2 mg/dL.
- Bilirubin level between 0.8–2 mg/dL is called **latent** or **subclinical jaundice**.
- Jaundice first appears in sclera because bilirubin has high affinity for scleral protein called **elastin**.

BILIRUBIN METABOLISM

After the average lifespan of 120 days, aged red cells are trapped and destroyed by the macrophages of mononuclear phagocytic system (MPS) that are present in spleen, liver, etc.

- **Macrophages** split hemoglobin into heme and globin (Fig. 12.1).
- **Heme** is catabolized to **biliverdin,** which is further reduced to **bilirubin**.

Steps of Bilirubin Metabolism

In Blood: Bilirubin enters the blood stream and forms a complex with albumin (Fig. 12.1). **Albumin-bilirubin complex**. This complex is *split in the liver* and bilirubin enters liver cells, whereas albumin stays back in the blood.

In liver cells: In liver cells, bilirubin undergoes **three-step metabolism**: uptake, conjugation and excretion.

1. ***Uptake:*** Bilirubin in the hepatocyte binds with **ligandin**, a cytoplasmic protein. Bilirubin-ligandin complex prevents bilirubin to return back to the blood.
2. ***Conjugation:*** Hepatocytes conjugate bilirubin with **glucuronic acid**, which takes place in the endoplasmic reticulum and involves *UDP-glucuronic acid* and *glucuronyl transferase*. This forms **bilirubin glucuronide** (Fig. 12.1).
3. ***Excretion:*** Bilirubin glucuronide is excreted from hepatocytes into the biliary canaliculi. This is an active process and is the *rate-limiting step* in the hepatic bilirubin metabolism.

In Intestine: Bilirubin glucuronide is excreted in bile to be discharged into the small intestine.

- In large intestine, bilirubin is acted upon by the bacterial flora, where glucuronic acid is split, and bilirubin undergoes a series of reduction reactions to from **stercobilinogen.**
- About 80% of stercobilinogen is oxidized to **stercobilin**, which is excreted in stool. Stercobilin is a brownish compound that *imparts brown color to the stool.*
- Remaining 20% stercobilinogen is absorbed to **enter the enterohepatic circulation**.

A part of the absorbed stercobilinogen enters the general circulation and is **filtered and excreted by the kidneys**. In urine, the stercobilinogen is called **urobilinogen**.

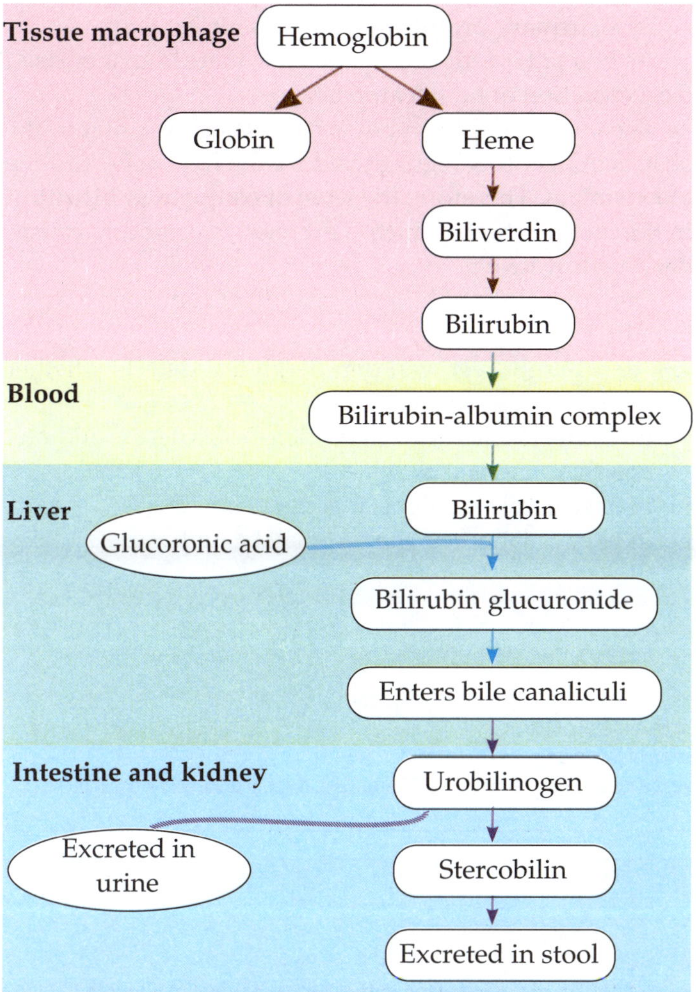

Fig. 12.1: Bilirubin metabolism and excretion: GT: Glucuronyl transferase.

TYPES OF JAUNDICE

Though traditionally jaundice is divided into **three types** such as hemolytic, hepatic and obstructive; physiologically, the **causes of jaundice** are divided broadly into **two categories**: increased production of bilirubin and decreased excretion of bilirubin.

Increased Production of Bilirubin: This occurs due to **increased hemolysis**. Therefore, the jaundice is called **hemolytic jaundice**.

Decreased Excretion of Bilirubin: Bilirubin excretion is impaired when liver cannot conjugate bilirubin efficiently, which is called **hepatic jaundice**, or when conjugated bilirubin cannot be excreted in bile due to biliary obstruction, which is called **obstructive jaundice**.

- Hepatic jaundice commonly occurs in **viral hepatitis**.
- Obstructive jaundice is commonly seen in **gall stones** (stone in the common bile duct) or **stricture of bile duct**.

Hemolytic Jaundice

This occurs due to increased hemolysis (Table 12.1). Excessive production of bilirubin leads to more conjugation of bilirubin in liver.

Table 12.1 | Causes of hemolytic jaundice.

A. Inherited disorders
1. Spherocytosis, elliptocytosis
2. Glucose 6-PD deficiency
3. Pyruvate kinase deficiency
4. Sickle cell anemia
B. Acquired disorders
1. Microangiopathic hemolytic anemia
2. Paroxysmal nocturnal hemoglobinuria
3. Spur cell anemia
4. Immune hemolysis
- Warm and cold antibodies
- Hemolytic diseases of newborn
- Incompatible blood transfusion
5. Drug-induced (rifampicin, probenacid)
6. Burn

- Thus, more quantity of **bilirubin glucuronide** is delivered to the intestine.
- Consequently, the amount of **stercobilinogen** formed in the intestine is increased.
- This leads to increased excretion of **fecal stercobilinogen and urinary urobilinogen.**
- Bilirubin in plasma forms a complex with albumin, the **albumin-bilirubin complex,** which can't be excreted in the urine. Therefore, hemolytic jaundice is **acholuric jaundice** (absence of bilirubin in urine).
- Liver function tests are usually normal.

IMPORTANT NOTE

Stool is dark-brown colored in hemolytic jaundice: As bilirubin is bound to protein, there is no excretion of bilirubin in urine. Hence, hemolytic jaundice is called **acholuric jaundice**. But, increased fecal stercobilinogen causes **dark-brown colored stool**.

Hepatic Jaundice

In hepatic jaundice, not only the conjugation of bilirubin is impaired, but also some amount of conjugated bilirubin is not excreted in bile.

- The conjugated bilirubin diffuses back into the bloodstream. Consequently, conjugated bilirubin **(bilirubin glucuronide)** is excreted in the urine.
- This makes **urine yellow** due to the presence of urinary bilirubin.
- Bilirubin excreted in bile is reduced. Hence, **fecal stercobilinogen and urinary urobilinogen are reduced** (Table 12.2).
- Plasma albumin-globulin ratio is altered.
- **Neonatal jaundice** could be due to defective conjugation of bilirubin (Clinical Note 12.1)

Clinical Note 12.1

Physiological jaundice: This is seen in some newborns and therefore this is also known as **neonatal jaundice**. It is common in premature babies and neonates having low birth weight. The jaundice usually appears on the second or third day of life and disappears within a week. It occurs due to subnormal activity of glucuronyl transferase that impairs conjugation of bilirubin in hepatocyte. It is unlikely to be due to hemolysis.

Table 12.2 | Differences in laboratory tests between three types of jaundice

	Hemolytic	Hepatic	Obstructive
Hyperbilirubinemia	Mild	Moderate	Severe
Fecal stercobilinogen	Increased	Decreased	Absent
Urinary urobilinogen	Increased	Decreased	Absent
Urinary bilirubin	Absent	Present	Present
Van den Bergh test	Indirect	Biphasic	Direct
Liver function	Normal	Impaired	May be impaired

Obstructive Jaundice

In obstructive jaundice, no bile reaches the intestine. Hence, neither bilirubin nor bile salts is present in the intestine.

Therefore, **no fecal stercobilinogen is formed**, and stool becomes **clay colored**.

Also, **urinary urobilinogen is absent**.

As bile salt is reduced in intestine, there is an increased fecal excretion of fat (**steatorrhea**).

The conjugated bilirubin accumulates proximal to the obstruction, and is regurgitated by the liver cells into the bloodstream. Therefore, the level of **conjugated bilirubin in the blood is high,** which is excreted in urine and causes **deep yellow urine**.

Due to prolonged biliary stasis, liver functions may be impaired.

van den Bergh Test: van den Bergh test detects whether bilirubin is conjugated or not.

- In hemolytic jaundice, van den Bergh test is indirect positive.
- In obstructive jaundice, it is direct positive.
- In hepatic jaundice, the test may be biphasic.

Exam Questions

1. With the help of a schematic diagram, briefly describe the major steps of bilirubin metabolism.
2. Classify jaundice and briefly explain the pathophysiology of different categories of jaundice.
3. List the differences in laboratory findings in hemolytic, hepatic and obstructive jaundice. Briefly explain the difference in color of urine and stool in three types of jaundice.

Multiple Choice Questions

1. Which of the following statement is NOT true?
   A. Normal serum bilirubin level is 0.2-0.8mg/dL
   B. Stercobilinogen is a brown-colored compound
   C. Hepatocytes form bilirubin glucoronide
   D. Bilirubin-albumin complex is split in the liver

2. The excretion of conjugated bilirubin by hepatic cells into bile canaliculi is:
   A. A carrier-mediated process
   B. By diifusion
   C. An active process
   D. Facilitated by increased viscosity

3. The severity of intravascular hemolysis is indicated by decrease in level of:
   A. Urobilin
   B. Billiverdin
   C. Hemopexin
   D. Haptoglobin

4. Which of the following is true for unconjugated bilirubin?
   A. Do not bind to brain tissue
   B. Excreted in urine
   C. Forms covalent complex with albumin
   D. Soluble in alcohol

5. Compared to unconjugated bilirubin, conjugated bilirubin:
   A. Has lower level in serum
   B. Serum albumin binding is high
   C. Shows indirect van den Bergh reaction
   D. Not soluble in water

6. Neonatal jaundice
   A. Always due to hemolysis
   B. Common in low birth-weight babies
   C. Persists for many weeks
   D. Always pathological

Answers

1. B 2. C 3. D 4. D 5. A 6. B

Chapter 13

Blood Groups and Physiological Basis of Blood Transfusion

Learning Objectives

On completion of study of this chapter:

The student will be able to (must know):

1. Understand the physiological basis of blood grouping.
2. Learn the concept of agglutinogens and agglutinins.
3. Define Landsteiner's law & give its physiological basis.
4. Learn the basis of Rh system & the mechanism of Rh incompatibility.
5. Give the features and treatment of erythroblastosis fetalis.
6. List the indications of blood transfusion.
7. Appreciate the concept of universal donor, universal recipient, and major & minor cross matching.
8. List the changes in red cells following storage of blood.
9. List the hazards of blood transfusion.

The student may also be able to (desirable to know):

1. Explain the mechanism of inheritance of blood groups.
2. Describe the procedure of transfusion.
3. Explain the role of H antigen in ABO typing.
4. Give the importance of Bombay blood group.
5. Explain the basis of hazards of blood transfusion.

Human red cells contain numerous surface proteins called **blood group antigens**. Depending on the antigens present on red cell membrane, the corresponding **antibodies are usually absent** in the plasma of that individual. This forms the physiological basis of blood groups and principle of blood transfusion.

- The blood group antigens are called **agglutinogens** and the antibodies against them are called **agglutinins**.
- There are more than **30 blood group systems** and **400 antigens** in human beings.
- Many of them have *cold antibodies* that do not react at body temperature. Therefore, only few of them are immunologically active.
- The blood group systems important for blood transfusion are **ABO and Rh systems**.

Uses of Blood Groups

1. Characterization of red cell antigen and antibodies forms the basis of **compatibility testing for blood transfusion**. ABO and Rh blood groups are usually displayed in the identity cards of individuals.
2. The blood group antigens have provided the scientific basis for understanding ***hemolytic diseases*** of the newborn and ***autoimmune hemolytic anemias***.
3. Blood group antigens play some important role in **susceptibility to infections** by malaria parasites, bacteria and viruses. Also, few blood groups provide resistance to some diseases (details given below).
4. Red cell antigens are also **associated with clinical disorders**. Absence of certain red cell antigens is associated with specific dysfunctions, and certain inherited and acquired diseases are associated with alteration of red cell antigen expression. These associations have led to understanding of pathophysiology of these pathologic processes.
5. Medicolegal experts take the help of characterization of red cell antigen and antibodies in establishing the **identity of the father** in cases of *disputed paternities* (also, the identity of the mother in cases of disputed maternity).
6. Recent research reports indicate that specific blood groups are associated with **human traits, personalities, and behaviors**. Therefore, blood groups could be associated with behavioral ailments.

PY2.9

ABO SYSTEM

ABO system is the most important for blood transfusion as ABO agglutinogens are highly antigenic.

- Physiologically, it is most significant due to natural occurrence of A and B antibodies in the plasma of individuals who lack corresponding antigen on their red cells.

- In addition, transfusion of incompatible ABO blood groups instantly leads to serious consequences.

ABO Agglutinogens

Types

In ABO system, there are **two antigens:** antigen A and antigen B.

- A antigen has two sub-types: A and A_1.
- The genes for antigens for ABO system are ***ABO genes located on chromosome 9***.

Occurrence

These antigens are present on the **membrane of red cells**.

- They are also found in **other tissues** like salivary gland, testes, lungs, kidney and pancreas.
- Therefore, they are secreted in minute quantity in saliva, pancreatic secretion and seminal fluid.
- Some individuals, especially blood group O, secrete blood **group H antigens in saliva** and other body fluids; they are called **H secretors**.

Time of Appearance

ABO antigens are present since fetal life. They **first appear at sixth week** of intrauterine life.

- At birth, the concentration is about one-fifth of concentration in adults.
- Concentration rises slowly to reach a significant level at puberty and reaches **maximum at 15–17 years of life.**
- Therefore, for collection of blood for blood transfusion, the **age of the donor** *should be minimum of 15 years.*

Chemical Nature

Blood group antigen A and B are complex *oligosaccharides.*

There is **difference in their terminal sugars**.

For agglutinogen A, terminal sugar is N-acetyl galactosamine, and for agglutinogen B, terminal sugar is galactose.

Blood Groups Based on Antigens

Based on the presence or absence of A and B antigens on the red cell membrane individually or in group, four blood groups have been described.

Group A : Antigen A is present
Group B : Antigen B is present
Group AB : Both A and B antigens are present
Group O : Neither A nor B antigen is present

Subtypes: A antigen has two sub-types, A and A_1.

- Group A is subdivided into two groups: the **group A_1** containing A and A_1 antigens, and **group A_2** containing A antigen alone.
- Similarly, the AB blood group is subdivided into A_1B and A_2B blood groups.

Distribution

In the Indian population, the distribution of the ABO blood group is as follows:

A : 27 %
B : 31 %
AB : 8 %
O : 34 %

In the A blood groups, A_1 is 75 % and A_2 is 25 %.

Role of H Gene and H Antigens

The expression of A and B antigens are dependent on the **presence of H genes**. Most of the individuals are homozygous for the H gene.

- A and B red cell antigens are glycoproteins, and their formation starts with basic precursor substances, which is first converted to H substance (by transferase) under the influence of H gene.
- H substance is partially converted under the influence of A and B genes (and specific transferase) into A and B antigens. Some of the H substance remains unconverted.
- Since O group individuals do not have A and B genes, neither A nor B antigen is formed, and these have only H substance (H remain unchanged).
- A, B and H antigens may be detected in the saliva and other body fluids also. Such individuals are called ***secretors***, while the remaining without it are ***non-secretors***.

IMPORTANT NOTE

Secretors and Non-secretors: The individuals who secrete A, B and H antigen substances in the saliva and other body fluids are called **secretors** and those who do not are called **non-secretors**.

Bombay Blood Group

In 1952, Bhende, Bhatia and Deshpande discovered a new blood group called as Bombay blood group (Phenotype Oh).

- These individuals lack the H gene, and therefore the *basic precursor substance can't be converted into H substance*. This in turn results in failure to form A or B antigen.
- When their blood sample is tested for routine AB grouping, they will be labeled as blood group O. However, their serum contains anti A and anti B and anti H antibodies.
- These individuals, therefore whenever needed should be transfused with only Bombay blood group.

ABO Agglutinins

Types

In ABO system, agglutinins are of **two types:** anti-A (α) and anti-B (β). The α agglutinin has **two subtypes**, α proper and α_1.

Occurrence

These antibodies are found in plasma. Generally, an antibody is formed against a particular antigen when there is exposure to that antigen. But blood group antibodies are **naturally occurring antibodies.**

- Blood group antibodies are formed without prior exposure to the antigens, and they are present in the blood of individuals in whom the respective antigens are absent.
- The mechanism of development of blood group antibodies (as naturally occurring) is not known.

Time and Mechanism of Appearance

Anti–A and anti-B agglutinins are **not formed during fetal life** and are *absent at birth.*

- They appear in the **second week of neonatal life** and increase very slowly in concentration to attain the **peak level at about 10 years** of life.
- The exact **mechanism of formation** of agglutinins in the absence of their corresponding agglutinogen is not clearly known.
  - It has been proposed that **intestinal bacteria and food contain antigens** similar to that of blood group agglutinogens.
  - Therefore, when the baby starts eating and food gets absorbed from intestine, antigens are absorbed into the blood.
  - As these antigens are recognized as **non-self antigens** by the body's immune system, they stimulate antibody production.
  - However, these antigens are present in **very low concentration** and antibodies against them are **produced very slowly**; therefore, antigen-antibody reaction does not occur (Application Box 13.1).
  - Moreover, antigens are removed by phagocytic cells.

Application Box 13.1

ABO incompatibility does not cause hemolytic diseases of newborns: ABO antigens are also expressed in other tissues, and therefore, ABO compatibility is of significant consideration in organ transplantations. However, in newborns, ABO incompatibility rarely causes clinical hemolytic disease because antibodies against A and B antigens are predominantly IgM that do not cross the placenta during fetal life, and antigens A and B are not well developed at birth.

Chemical Nature

The α and β agglutinins are **globulins** and belong to **Ig M category**. Therefore, they **do not cross the placenta**.

- They function efficiently at low temperature, i. e. between 5° to 20° C.
- Therefore, they are called **cold antibodies**.

Agglutinins against Blood Groups

As antibodies are directed against the antigens, the **individuals with blood group A antigen** on the red cell membrane do not have anti-A antibody, rather ***possess anti-B antibody*** in their plasma, and **persons with blood group B** do not contain anti-B, rather have ***anti-A antibody*** in their plasma (Table 13.1).

- Similarly, individuals with blood group AB do not have any antibody and individuals with blood group O have both the antibodies in their plasma.
- These facts were first noted and described by **Karl Landsteiner** in 1900, and his theory is popularly known as **Landsteiner's law**.

Significant contribution of Scientist

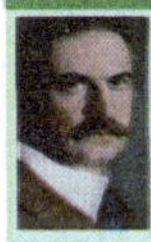

KARL LANDSTEINER (1868-1943):

Karl Landsteiner discovered isoagglutinin in human blood in 1900, leading to recognition of human blood groups and success of blood transfusion. For his work on blood groups, He received Nobel Prize in Physiology 1930.

Landsteiner's Law

This law states that **if a particular agglutinogen is present** on the red cell membrane of an individual, the **corresponding agglutinin must be absent** in his plasma. Conversely, if the agglutinogen is absent in the red cells, the corresponding agglutinin must be present in the plasma.

- This law holds good for ABO system.
- However, the second part of the law does not apply for Rh and many other blood group systems as there are no naturally occurring agglutinins in these systems.

Antigen and Antibodies for ABO Blood Groups: Thus, in ABO system (Table 13.1):

1. **Blood group A** has antigen A on the red cell membrane and anti-B antibody in the plasma.
2. **Blood group B** has antigen B on the red cell membrane and anti-A antibody in the plasma.
3. **Blood group AB** has both antigens A and B on the red cell membrane and no antibodies in the plasma.
4. **Blood group O** has no antigens on the red cell membrane and possesses both agglutinins anti-A and anti-B in the plasma (Fig. 13.1).

Table 13.1 | Occurrence of antigens and antibodies in ABO system.

Blood group	Antigen (on RBC)	Antibody (in plasma)
A	A	Anti-B
B	B	Anti-A
AB	A and B	Nil
O	Nil	Anti-A and anti-B

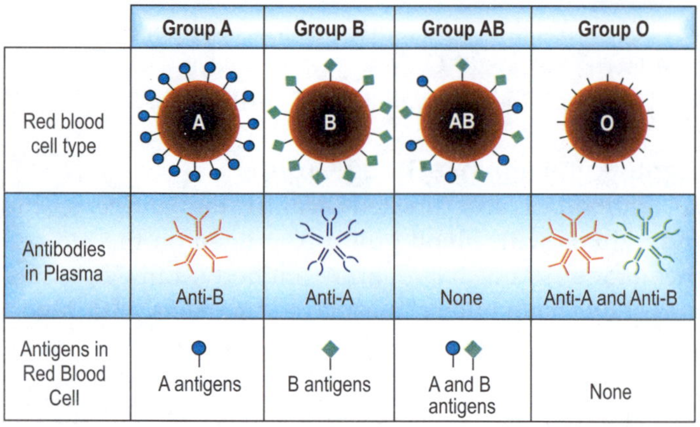

Fig. 13.1: Distribution of antigen on red cell membrane and antibodies in plasma in ABO system of blood group.

PY2.11

Blood Grouping: Blood grouping is performed by suspending the red cells of the person's blood group to be checked in the anti-A and anti-B antisera that are commercially available. If the agglutination (**clumping of red cells**, as checked under the microscope) is present, red cells contain that particular antigen (Fig. 13.2).

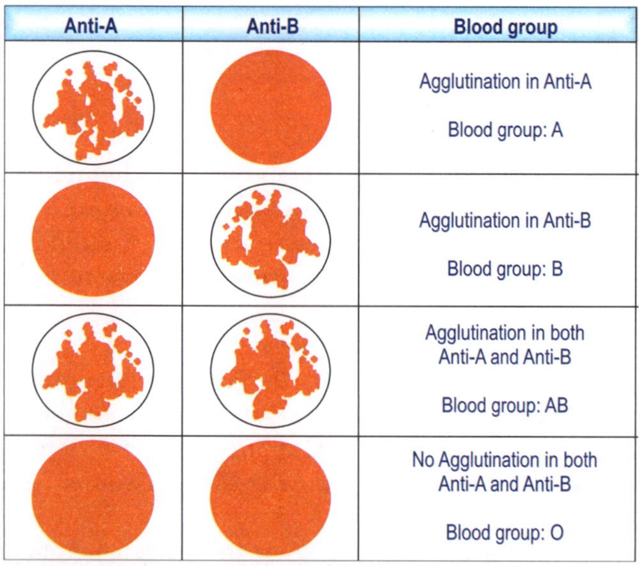

Fig. 13.2: Method of blood grouping.

Inheritance of ABO Blood Groups

Blood groups are genetically determined. Normally, presence of a blood group antigen is a **dominant characteristic**. Therefore, the antigen is present in the phenotype irrespective of the genotype (Table 13.2).

There are **three types of genes**: O, A and B. Therefore, a person can have any of the six possible genotypes: OO, OA, OB, AA, BB, and AB.

Table 13.2 | ABO phenotypes and their possible genotypes.

Phenotype (blood group)	Genotype
A	AA, AO
B	BB, BO
AB	AB
O	OO

Gene O is genetically not important. Therefore, the respective phenotype may be A or B or AB or O (Application Box 13.2).

For example, if blood group of one parent is A and other parent is B, then there is possibility of child having any of the four blood group of ABO system (Fig. 13.3).

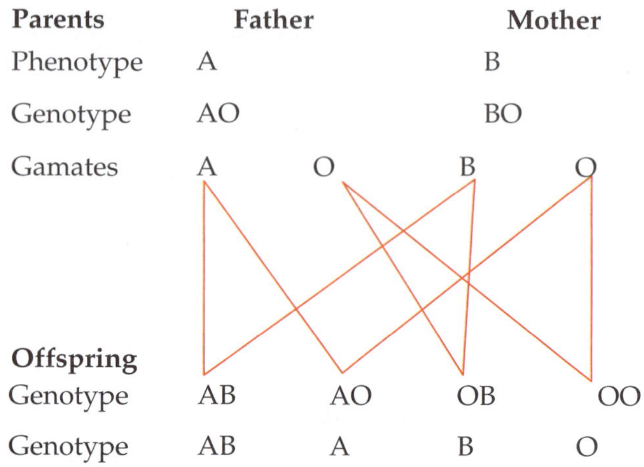

Fig. 13.3: Inheritance of ABO antigen.

Application Box 13.2

Disputed paternity: When the blood group of a child and the mother is known, it can be told whether the man in suspicion could have been the father of the child or not. However, blood group can never prove that a particular man is the father of a particular child. This is because the blood group of the man can be one out of several other possible men. Therefore, determination of blood group gene only helps to identify, not confirms the identity. MNS system is more useful in this regard.

Rh SYSTEM

The Rh (Rhesus) system is the second most important blood group system in transfusion medicine. This was first described in Rhesus monkeys in 1940 by Landsteiner and Weiner; hence it is called Rh system.

Rh Antigens

In Rh system, there are **six antigens**, but there are ***no naturally occurring antibodies***.

- The antigens are C, D, E, c, d and e.
- Out of these six antigens, immunologically most active is the **D antigen**.
- Thus, in Rh system, there are two blood groups: **Rh positive** (D antigen present) and **Rh negative** (D antigen absent).
- The *gene for Rh antigen* is the RHD and RHCE genes that are located on **chromosome 1**.

The antigens of Rh system participate in **cation transport and membrane integrity** of red cells. Rh antigens are membrane proteins *found in red cell membrane*, not in any other tissues.

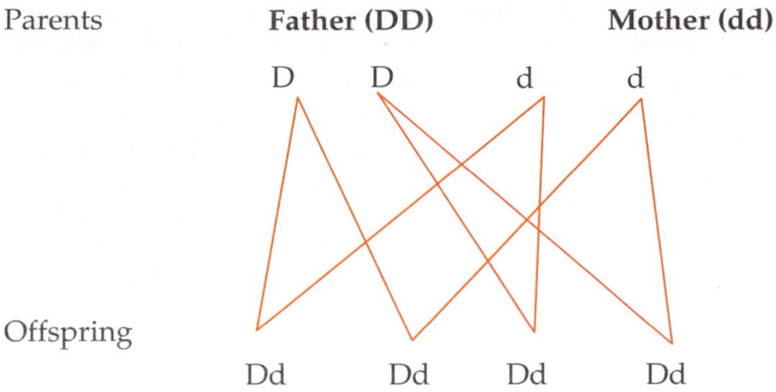

Fig. 13.4: Inheritance of Rh antigen.

Inheritance: Rh antigen is inherited as dominant gene.

- In Indian population, **95 to 98% are Rh +ve** and 2 to 5% are Rh –ve.
- Rh +ve individual may have **homozygous (DD)** or **heterozygous (Dd)** genotypes.
  - Usually, 60% of Rh +ve individuals have Dd genotype and 40% have DD genotype.
  - The genotype of Rh –ve person is dd.
- If one of the parents is homozygous positive and the other is homozygous negative, all offsprings will be heterozygous positives (Fig. 13.4).
  - Similarly, if the father and mother are homozygous negatives, all offspring will be homozygous negatives, and
  - when one of the parents is heterozygous positive and the other homozygous negative, 50% of offspring will be heterozygous positive and 50% will be homozygous negatives.

Rh Antibody

The antibody in the system is called **anti-D antibody**, which is produced only when an Rh negative individual receives the Rh positive blood.

- These antibodies develop very slowly in the first encounter; but form rapidly following subsequent encounters.
- Rh antibody is of **Ig G type,** which can cross placental barrier.
- Hence, if antibodies are present in mother's blood, can be **transferred to the fetus**.
- Rh antibody is ***best reactive at body temperature***, and therefore, designated as **warm antibody**.

Rh Incompatibility

Rh incompatibility occurs when an **Rh negative individual receives Rh positive blood**.

- Normally, when an Rh-negative person receives Rh-positive blood, there will be **no immediate reactions** as Rh negative individual does not normally has anti-Rh antibody.
- However, the donor's red cells induce an immune response in the recipient to synthesize anti-Rh antibodies, which takes about **two to four months to reach a significant titer**.
  - But by that time the donor's red cells die their natural death within 120 days.
  - The anti-Rh antibody cannot produce any harm to the recipient's red cells because the Rh-negative recipient's red cells contain no Rh antigens.
- But, if the same Rh-negative person who has already received a **Rh-positive blood before**, receives a second Rh positive transfusion later, the anti-Rh antibodies are synthesized in large amount immediately by the memory cells.
  - This antibody reacts against the donor cells and causes reactions of mismatch transfusion.
  - Thus, the Rh negative individual can safely receive Rh positive blood once in life time.

In Pregnancy: The similar Rh incompatibility occurs in pregnancies when ***Rh negative mother bears Rh positive fetus***, which leads to **erythroblastosis fetalis**.

Erythroblastosis Fetalis

Etiopathogenesis

This is a **hemolytic disease of the newborn** which occurs due to **Rh incompatibility** when an Rh-negative mother carries Rh positive fetus during pregnancy.

- Usually, no reaction occurs in the first pregnancy.
- However, at the time of delivery **during placental separation**, a small amount of ***fetal blood leaks*** into the maternal circulation. This induces formation of **anti-Rh agglutinins** in the mother.
- Therefore, **in subsequent pregnancies**, the anti-Rh agglutinin from mother, which is predominantly IgG type ***crosses placenta*** to enter fetal circulation and causes hemolysis.
- In third and subsequent pregnancies, the degree of hemolysis becomes severe.

Clinical Features

The features are mainly **due to hemolysis**. Hemolysis leads to **anemia**, extramedullary hemopoiesis and neonatal **hyperbilirubinemia**. If the hemolysis is severe, the fetus may die *in utero* or if the fetus is born alive, he may have the following features.

1. **Anemia:** Anemia is proportionate to the degree of hemolysis.
2. **Hemolytic jaundice:** Occurs due to hemolysis. **Serum bilirubin** level may be ***more than 25mg%*** in severe cases.
3. **Generalized edema:** Edema occurs in the whole body ***due to anemia and hypoproteinemia***. This is called **hydrops fetalis**.

4. **Kernicterus:** This is a neurologic syndrome with major **motor deficits** that occurs due to the ***deposition of bilirubin in the basal ganglia.***
   - **Hyperbilirubinemia** occurs due to hemolysis.
     - Basal ganglia have more affinity for bilirubin.
     - However, bile pigments *cannot cross the blood-brain barrier* (BBB) in adults.
     - Therefore, hemolysis ***in adults does not produce kernicterus.***
   - *BBB is not fully developed* in fetuses, infants, and children. In them, bilirubin enters brain and gets deposited in the basal ganglia.
   - Therefore, hemolysis ***in infancy and early childhood causes kernicterus.***
   - The dysfunction mainly manifests in the form of **motor dysfunctions**.
5. **Extramedullary hemopoiesis:** Due to severe anemia, extramedullary hemopoiesis occurs, for which **erythroblasts** (nucleated red cells) are released into the blood.
   - Erythroblasts are seen in plenty in peripheral smear.
   - Hence, the disease is called erythroblastosis fetalis.

Treatment

About 50% of the fetuses and newborns with erythroblastosis fetalis have mild hemolysis and do not require treatment.

In severe cases, the major modalities of treatment are: intrauterine fetal transfusion, exchange transfusion and phototherapy.

1. **Intrauterine fetal transfusion:** If the disease is diagnosed in fetus and found to be severe, the treatment is intrauterine fetal transfusion. Presently, the fetal transfusion is carried out by **intraperitoneal route**, which has replaced the direct intravascular fetal transfusion.
2. **Exchange transfusion:** The treatment of newborns with severe anemia, jaundice and hydrops is exchange transfusion soon after birth.
   - Exchange transfusion removes sensitized red cells, bilirubin and maternal antibody from the plasma.
   - A **double-volume exchange transfusion** (2 x 80 ml/kg) replaces 90% of the infant's blood volume with antigen negative red cells.
   - Blood chosen for exchange should be **ABO negative, Rh negative** and cross-matched against mother's blood.
3. **Phototherapy:** Intensive phototherapy is very effective in **reducing serum bilirubin level** (Clinical Note 13.1).

Prevention

Erythroblastosis fetalis is prevented by administering a **single dose of anti-Rh antibodies** in the form of **Rh immunoglobulin** during the post-partum period following the first delivery. The disease can also be prevented by **passive immunization** of the mother with a small dose of Rh immunoglobulins during pregnancy.

> **Clinical Note 13.1**
>
> **Phototherapy for neonatal jaundice:** Bilirubin in excess is toxic to the body, especially it produces neurotoxicity. However, bilirubin, on exposure to light undergoes structural and configurational isomerization and photo-oxidation. These changes in bilirubin make it less toxic and less lipophilic products that are excreted efficiently without hepatic conjugation. Therefore, phototherapy is the primary ***treatment for unconjugated hyperbilirubinemia*** in newborns. *Neonatal jaundice* is mainly hemolytic and unconjugated.

OTHER BLOOD GROUP SYSTEM

The other blood groups of clinical importance are MNS system, H system, Lewis system, Ii system, PI system, Duffy system, Kidd system, Lutheran system, etc. The MNS system is used mainly for medicolegal issues in physical identification, and the other systems are mostly used for assessing the susceptibility to diseases. Blood group associated diseases are listed in Table 13.3.

Table 13.3 | Blood group associated diseases.

A. Diseases due to occurrence blood groups.		
Group A	:	Carcinoma of salivary glands, stomach colon, rectum, uterus and ovary; ITP; coronary thrombosis, pernicious anemia
B	:	E coli UTI, gonorrhea
O	:	Peptic ulcer, rheumatoid arthritis, typhoid fever, von Willebrand disease
Le	:	Sjögren syndrome
Fya/b	:	Vivax malaria
K	:	Chronic granulomatous diseases
Rh –ve	:	Autoimmune hemolytic anemia
Ii	:	Hemoglobinopathies
B. Blood group associated with disease resistance		
Pl/Pk	:	E coli pyelonephritis
Fyab	:	Plasmodium vivax malaria
C. Absence of antigen associated with diseases		
Rhnull	:	Hereditary stomatocytosis, hemolytic anemia
Kx	:	Hereditary Acanthocytosis
D. Diseases associated with alteration of antigens		
Weak AB	:	Leukemia, Hodgkin disease, aplastic anemia
Weak Rh, K	:	Autoimmune hemolytic anemia
Weak MN	:	Bacterial infection, preleukemia, leukemia
Acquired A	:	Myelogenous leukemia
Acquired B	:	Bacterial infections, GI lesions
Acquired K	:	Enterococcus faecium infection
Acquired Jkb	:	E. faecium and micrococcus infections

PHYSIOLOGICAL BASIS OF BLOOD TRANSFUSION

Indications for Transfusion

1. Acute blood loss (whole blood is preferred).
2. Chronic anemia (thalassemia and sickle cell disease)
3. Bone marrow failure.
   - Leukemia
   - Aplastic anemia
   - Bone marrow infiltration by neoplastic cells
4. Purpura (platelet transfusion is preferred)
5. Clotting factor deficiencies (fresh frozen plasma is preferred). In hemophilia, cryoprecipitate of factor VIII is given.
6. Preparation for surgery and during surgery
7. Burns

Procedure of Blood Transfusion

Safety transfusion should always include:

i) Selection of appropriate donor
ii) ABO and Rh typing
iii) Cross matching
iv) Antibody screening of the patient (to detect the presence of clinically significant antibodies).

Selection of Appropriate Donor

Healthy donors free from transfusion-transmissible diseases should be identified for blood transfusion.

- Ideally, the **age of the donor** should be ***18 years or above*** and preferably should not be above 60 years.
- Donor should be voluntarily willing to donate blood.
- The **hemoglobin status** of the donor should be estimated. There should be minimum of 12 g% Hb in female, and 13 g% Hb in male donors.
- Donor must be **screened for** AIDS, hepatitis, lymphomas, and protozoal organisms like malaria, filaria etc.

ABO and Rh Typing

ABO incompatibility causes immediate reactions and may even kill the persons. The Rh incompatibility causes delayed reactions.

- Therefore, ABO and Rh compatibility must be ensured before any transfusion.
- The concept of **universal donor and recipient** helps in this process.

Universal Donor

The blood group O negative (O group and Rh –Ve) persons are considered to be the universal donor because their **red cells contain no antigens**.

- Therefore, their blood cells on transfusion to any individual do not cause agglutination reaction.
- Hence, blood group O –Ve can be given to any individual.

Universal Recipient

The **blood group AB positive** (AB group and Rh +Ve) individuals are considered to be the universal recipient because their plasma contains no antibodies.

- Therefore, they can safely receive blood from any one as they do not cause agglutination reaction against any blood cells.

Cross-Matching

In addition to ABO and Rh systems, there are many other minor blood group systems. Hence, ***cross-matching should always be done*** to eliminate the possibilities of any form of mismatching.

Major Cross-Matching

In major cross-matching, the **cells of the donor are directly matched against the plasma of the recipient**. As it is important to ensure that antibodies present in the recipient's plasma do not harm the donor's red cells, this cross-matching is called major cross-matching.

- The **ABO agglutinogens** are ***highly antigenic*** and produce agglutination even in low concentration.
- Therefore, though donor's red cells are less in quantity than the recipient, they produce agglutination reactions.
- **ABO agglutinins** do ***not react highly***, as they are **cold antibodies**.
- Moreover, donor's agglutinin is ***diluted in large volume of recipient's plasma***, hence not capable of inducing agglutination reaction.

Therefore, it is important to match donor's agglutinogen (red cells) against recipient's agglutinin (plasma).

Minor Cross-Matching

In minor cross-matching, the **donor's plasma is checked against the red cells of the recipient**. It is called minor cross-matching, because it is not very important to assess the reactivity of donor's agglutinin against recipient's cells.

- This is because; small volume of the donor's plasma is diluted in a large volume of the recipient's plasma.
- Therefore, the agglutinin titer of donor's plasma falls to such a low level after transfusion that they are unlikely to damage the red cells of the recipient.
- However, for full compatibility, minor cross-matching should also be performed.

Antibody Screening of the Patient

The patient who receives transfusion, his serum should be screened for various antibodies like autoantibodies that may react against the donor's cells and cause hemolysis.

Blood Collection and Storage

Collection of Blood

Usually, 350 ml of blood is collected from a single donor at a time. The blood mixes with 50 to 70 ml of **anticoagulant consisting of citrate, phosphate and dextrose (CPD).**

- **Disodium hydrogen citrate** is used instead of trisodium citrate as anticoagulant, because this favors *fall of pH which* is required for survival of red cells.
- Donors are advised not to donate blood for at least next three months.

Autologous Donor Blood: When the donor is the recipient himself, the blood collected is called autologous donor blood and the transfusion is called autologous transfusion.

- This can be done prior to a planned surgery.
- The Hb of the person should be more than 12.5 g%.
- Blood is collected every 72 hours upto 72 hours prior to surgery or till the Hb level has not gone below 11g%.
- Usually 2 to 4 units of blood of 250 ml each can be collected.
- The same blood (recipient's own blood) is used during surgery.

Storage of Blood

Blood is stored in the blood bank **at 4°C.**

- Stored blood for transfusion should ideally be **used within 2 weeks** of storage.
- However, blood should not be used if it is stored for more than 3 weeks, because gross hemolysis occurs after this period.

Red Cell Changes During Storage

Red cells undergo rapid changes during storage in simple citrate solutions even at 4° C. During cold storage, the changes that occur are mainly due to **reduction of metabolism** of cells.

The changes are:

1. **Increase in sodium and decrease in potassium** concentration in the red cells.
   - This occurs due to decreased active transport of ions across the cell membrane.
   - At low temperature, **Na^+-K^+ pump activity is grossly decreased.**
   - This results in net increase in the total base and water of the cell.
   - The inhibition of Na^+-K^+ pump increases intracellular sodium concentration that causes water to enter the cell by endosmosis.
2. **Cells swell and become more spherocytic.**
   - This results in *spontaneous hemolysis.*
   - Leucocytes and platelets almost totally disappear within 24 to 48 hrs of storage.
3. The **ATP content in the cell decreases** and inorganic phosphate concentration increases.
   - This is due to imbalance between phosphorylation and dephosphorylation processes in the cell.

Changes in Stored Blood after Transfusion

Within 24 hours of transfusion, the cell metabolism greatly increases.

- Consequently, the **sodium is extruded** from the cells and the **potassium is drawn back** into the cells.
- The ***volume, shape, and fragility*** of the red cells come back to normal **within 24 to 48 hours.**
- Red cells show **80% of survival 24 hours after transfusion** if the transfusion is given ***within 14 days*** of storage of the blood.
- But the survival rate greatly decreases if the blood is stored for more than 2 weeks.
- Blood should never be used after 30 days of storage.

Hazards of Blood Transfusion

Blood transfusion, even in ideal condition carries risks of adverse reactions. Mostly, transfusion reactions occur due to human error.

I. **Due to Mismatched Transfusion:** When an incompatible blood is transfused, the mismatched transfusion reaction occurs immediately.
   - The reaction is primarily due to agglutination of donor's red cells followed by their hemolysis.
   - This is called **acute hemolytic transfusion reactions.**
   - Usually, it occurs due to ABO incompatibility.
   - The severity of the reaction depends on the degree of hemolysis.

The **complications of mismatched transfusion** are:

1. Shivering and fever (febrile reactions)
2. Hemoglobinemia and hemoglobinuria
3. Jaundice
4. Acute renal failure

Renal failure occurs due to:

i) **hemoglobin casts** blocking the renal tubules and damaging the tubules,
ii) release of toxic substances from the lysed red cells causes renal vasoconstriction, and
iii) circulatory shock.

5. **Hyperkalemia** (due to release of potassium ions from red cells). This may cause ***cardiac arrest in diastole.***

II. **Due to Faulty Techniques of Giving Blood:** Due to wrong method of transfusion, following complications may arise.

1. **Thrombophlebitis:** This is a common complication in those who receive repeated transfusions.
2. **Air Embolism:** Air enters the venous circulation and

gets lodged at the outlet of the right ventricle and blocks the flow of blood to the lungs.

- Death may occur in severe cases.
- Use of plastic bags has reduced this complication.

III. **Due to Massive Transfusion**: This occurs when **more than 10 units of blood** are given within 24 hours or when the total blood volume is exchanged within 24 hours.

- This leads to **circulatory overload**.
- Cardiac arrhythmias and even sometimes cardiac arrest occur due to high potassium level in the stored blood.

IV. **Febrile Reaction:** The patient feels cold and may get rigor due to rise in body temperature. This occurs mainly due to **presence of pyrogens** in the transfusion apparatus.

IV. **Allergic Reactions:** This is less frequent and is characterized by itching, erythema, nausea, vomiting, and in severe cases may cause anaphylactic reactions.

VI. **Transmission of Diseases**

1. Hepatitis
2. Malaria
3. AIDS
4. Syphilis

Exam Questions

1. Describe the physiological basis of blood grouping in ABO system, with reference to agglutinogens and agglutinins.
2. Define Landsteiner's law and explain its application in blood transfusion.
3. Give the physiological basis of Rh incompatibility. List the features of erythroblastosis fetalis and explain how it can be treated and prevented.
4. What is cross matching. Describe the basis of universal donor and universal recipient.
5. Describe the changes in red cells following storage, and list hazards of blood transfusion.

Multiple Choice Questions

1. ABO agglutinogens are present in all, EXCEPT:
A. Sweat B. Saliva
C. Seminal fluid D. Pancreatic secretion

2. In "ABO" blood groups, agglutinogen first appears at:
A. 6th day of fetal life B. 6th week of fetal life
C. 6th month of fetal life D. Birth

3. The blood groups A, B, AB and O with aggutiniogens (A, B) and agglutinins (α, β) can be depicted as:
A. A, B, AB, $\alpha\beta$ B. Aα, Bβ, AB$\alpha\beta$, $\alpha\beta$
C. Aβ, Bα, AB$\alpha\beta$, $\alpha\beta$ D. Aβ, Bα, AB, $\alpha\beta$

4. The maximum titre of blood group agglutinins is reached at
A. 10 weeks of fetal life B. Birth
C. 10 months of age D. 10 years of age

5. ABO blood group agglutinins belong to the following globulin type:
A. Ig E B. Ig M
C. Ig A D. Ig G

6. What is the minimum amount of Rh+ve blood required to induce Rh antibodies in an Rh-ve individual?
A. 50 mL B. 25 mL
C. 10 mL D. 0.5 mL

7. All of the following changes would occur in blood after 10 days of storage, EXCEPT:
A. Increased prothrombin time
B. Increased plasma potassium concentration
C. Decreased dextrose level
D. Decreased lactic acid level

8. A man with blood group B cannot be biological father of a child with AB blood group, if the mother is:
A. Having blood group AB B. Having blood group A
C. Having blood group B D. Rh negative

9. Earliest sign of transfusion reaction is:
A. Oliguria B. Chill and rigor
C. Jaundice D. Hemoglobinuria

10. Glucose is added to stored blood to:
A. Provide nutrition B. Increase haemoglobin content
C. Decrease lactic acid level D. Prevent hemolysis

11. All of the following statements are true for cold antibodies, EXCEPT:
A. Antibodies of ABO blood group
B. IgG type
C. Active between 5°C and 20°C
D. Do not cross the placenta

12. The ideal anticoagulant for storage of blood in the blood bank is:
A. EDTA B. Double oxalate
C. Disodium hydrogen citrate D. Trisodium citrate

13. Fresh blood refers to blood which is transfused:
A. Within 1 hour B. Within 6 hours
C. Within 24 hours D. Immediately

14. Erythroblastosos fetalis in the first pregnancy is prevented by:
A. Immunization of the mother by Rh immunoglobulins during pregnancy
B. Fresh blood transfusion to the baby immediately after birth
C. Immunization of the mother by Rh immunoglobulins soon after birth
D. Destruction of Rh-positive cells in the fetus by Anti-Rh antibodies

15. A person with absence of anti - B and anti- Rh agglutinin in plasma can NOT have the blood group:
A. B-positive B. B-negative
C. AB-positive D. O-negative

16. Before blood transfusion, it is necessary to have:
A. Recipient's cells matched with donor's cells
B. Recipient's plasma matched with donor's cells
C. Recipient's plasma matched with donor's plasma
D. Recipient's cells matched with donor's plasma

Answers : 1. A 2. B 3. D 4. D 5. B 6. D 7. D 8. C 9. B 10. A 11. B 12. C 13. C 14. A 15. D 16. B

Chapter 14

White Blood Cells

Learning Objectives

On completion of study of this chapter:

The student will be able to (must know):

1. Classify leucocytes & give % distribution of leucocytes in blood.
2. Give the steps of leucopoiesis.
3. Elucidate the structure and functions of each leucocyte, & list the causes of increase and decrease of each leucocyte.
5. Explain the mechanism of phagocytosis & killing by neutrophil.
6. Describe the role of eosinophil in allergy.
7. List the components of mononuclear-phagocyte system.
9. Appreciate the role of leucocytes in body defence mechanisms.
10. Define and classify leukemia.

The student may also be able to (desirable to know):

1. Describe the steps and regulation of leucopoiesis.
2. Understand the life history of leucocytes.
3. Describe the different neutrophilic granules and their functions.
4. Describe the content of eosinophil granules and their functions.
5. Describe the functions of monocytes and macrophages.
6. Briefly describe different leukemias

Leucocytes or white blood cells perform mainly the defence functions of the body. Leucocytes are of **two types**: granulocytes, containing granules in the cytoplasm, and agranulocytes, without cytoplasmic granules.

PY2.11

Table 14.1 | Types of leucocytes and their distribution in peripheral blood as differential leucocyte count (DLC) and absolute count.

Leucocytes	Percentage (DLC)	Absolute count (per cu mm)
A. Granulocytes		
1. Neutrophils	50 – 70	2000 – 2750
2. Eosinophils	1 – 4	40 – 440
3. Basophils	0 – 1	20 – 80
B. Agranulocytes		
1. Monocytes	2 – 8	1500 – 4000
2. Lymphocytes	20 – 40	500 – 800

- The **granulocytes** are neutrophils, eosinophils and basophils and **agranulocytes** are lymphocytes and monocytes (Table 14.1).
- After their short life in circulation, leucocytes enter tissues of the body.
- In the tissue, monocytes become macrophages, a component of mononuclear phagocyte system.

PY2.6

LEUCOPOIESIS

Leucopoiesis is the development of leucocytes.

Stages of Leucopoiesis

The **pluripotent stem cells** in the bone marrow give rise to **committed stem cells**.

The committed stem cells in the bone marrow are broadly of two types: **myeloid stem cells** and **lymphoid stem cells**.

- The stem cells for **lymphoid series** form lymphocytes.
- The stem cells for **myeloid series** are ***trilineage stem cells*** that form stem cells for three kinds of precursor cells (refer, Fig. 8.4, Chapter 8):
  1. Erythroid series for red cells
  2. Megakaryoid series for platelets
  3. Stem cells for granulocyte-monocyte series

Stem Cells of Granulocyte-Monocyte Series: The stem cells for granulocyte-monocyte of myeloid series give rise to **progenitor cells** (**colony forming units** or CFUs) named as CFU-GM (Fig. 14.1).

- **CFU-GM** is the phagocytic series progenitor cell that on further differentiation from **CFU-G** (for neutrophils, eosinophils and basophils) and **CFU-M** (for monocytes).
- **CFU-G** further subdivides into **three CFUs**: CFU-G for neutrophil, CFU-Eo for eosinophil, and CFU-Bas for basophil.

- The CFUs form **blast cells**.
- Thus, CFU-G forms respective **myeloblasts** (neutrophil-myeloblast, eosinophil-myeloblast and basophil-myeloblast) for neutrophil, eosinophil and basophil, and CFU-M forms **monoblast** that develops into monocytes.

In general, myeloblasts form **promyelocytes**, promyelocytes form **myelocytes**, myelocytes form **metamyelocytes** that develop into **mature leucocytes**.

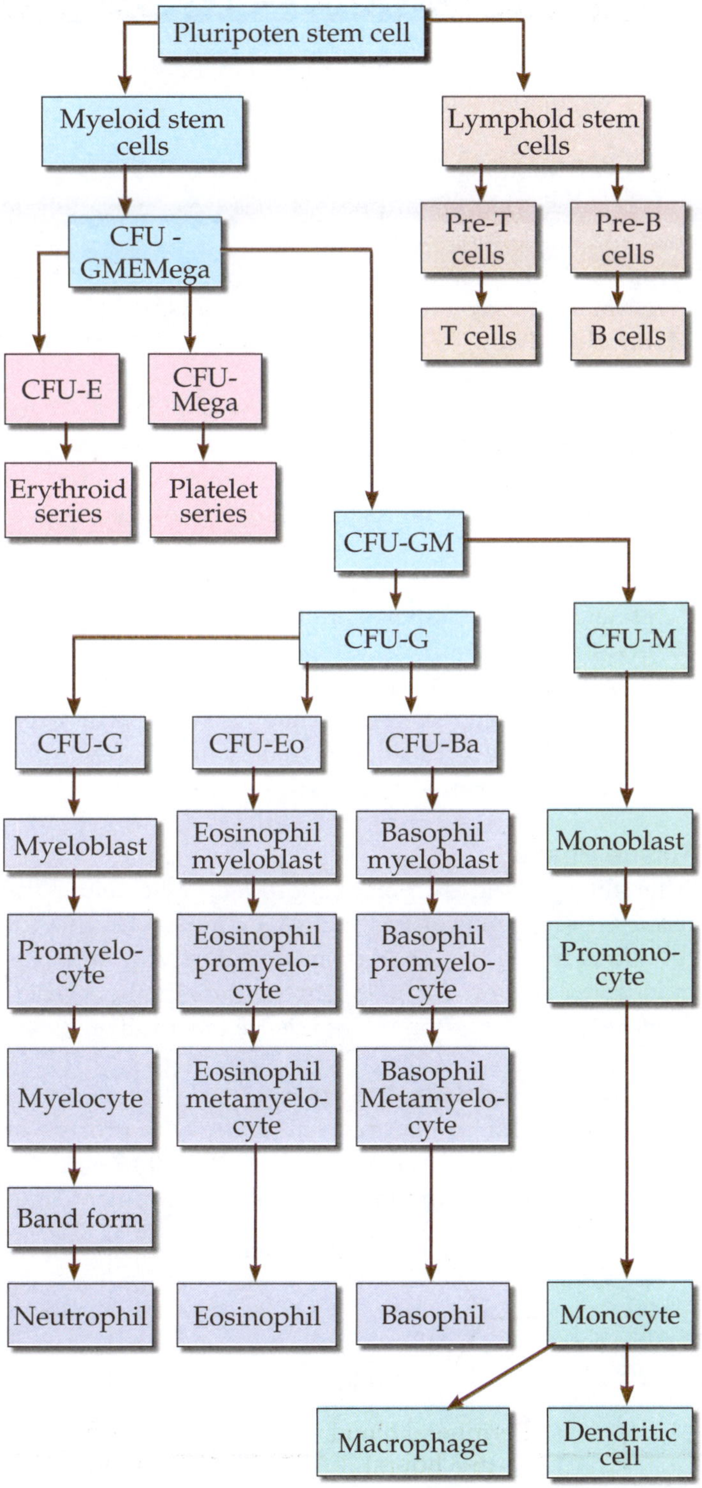

Fig. 14.1: Stages of leucopoiesis.

Colony-Forming Units

Colony forming units (CFUs) are **progenitor cells** that develop from committed stem cells.

- There are different CFUs for different cell lines.
- They possess the properties of stem cells and can not be distinguished morphologically.
- However, **CFU-GM** (as described before) forms respective blast cells for different leucocytes.

Blast Cells

These are *earliest precursor cells* of leucocyte development that are ***morphologically distinguishable***.

- The blast cells for neutrophils are **myeloblasts**, for eosinophil are **eosinophil-myeloblasts**, and basophils are **basophil-myeloblasts**, for monocytes are **monoblasts** and for lymphocytes are **lymphoblasts**.
- The blast cells are ***large cells*** (16–20 µm) with ***large nucleus*** containing *multiple nucleoli*.
- The **nucleoli are prominent features** of blast cells and are the sites of assembly of ribosomal proteins and r-RNA.
- The cytoplasm is scanty.
- Cells are **actively mitotic**.

Myeloblasts: The earliest precursor cells **for neutrophils** are myeloblasts.

- They have scanty blue cytoplasm with 5–10 nucleoli in a large nucleus.
- There are separate myeloblasts for eosinophils (**eosinophil-myeloblasts**) and basophils (**basophil-myeloblasts).**

Monoblasts: These are the blast cells for monocytes. As they resemble myeloblasts morphologically, they are also called myelo-monoblasts.

Lymphoblasts: These are blast cells for lymphocytes.

- They have fewer nucleoli.
- Nuclear chromatins are clumped.

Promyelocytes and Promonocytes

The promyelocytes and promonocytes develop from myeloblasts and monoblasts respectively.

- The cells are large, and cytoplasm is granular.
- Nucleus is round and condensed and contains **less nucleoli**.
- Cells are mitotic.
- **Promonocytes are larger cells** (larger than myeloblasts) that on further development form monocytes.
- The promyelocytes are also larger cells and contain large population of **peroxidase-positive granules**.

Myelocytes

Myelocytes have diameter of about **12–20 µm**.

- They contain round concentric nucleus. **Nucleoli are absent**.

- Cells show some degree of mitosis. About *three cell divisions* occur in this stage of maturation.
- The characteristic feature of this stage is appearance of **peroxidase negative specific granules**.

Metamyelocytes

The diameter of metamyelocyte is **12–18 µm**. The cells are non-dividing (**no mitosis**) and have mixed granule populations.

Matured Cells

Neutrophils developed from metamyelocytes are **juvenile neutrophils** (band forms) that further grow into **matured neutrophils** (segmented neutrophils). **Eosinophils and basophils** develop from their respective metamyelocytes.

Regulation of Leucopoiesis

Leucopoiesis is mainly regulated by various **cytokines**, especially, colony stimulating factors (CSFs), interleukins and tumor necrosis factors (TNFs).

Interleukins

IL-1, IL-6 and IL-3 promote maturation of **stem cells.**

- **IL-5** helps in development of **eosinophil,** and therefore, IL-5 is also called **eosinophilic growth factor.**
- **IL-3 and IL-4** facilitate development of **basophils**.
- **IL-2 inhibits** myelopoiesis.

Colony Stimulating Factors

Important colony stimulating factors (CSFs) that influence leucopoiesis are GM-CSF, G-CSF and M-CSF.

GM-CSF: This is the **granulocyte-monocyte colony stimulating factor** (GM-CSF) secreted by fibroblasts, vascular endothelial cells, monocytes and T lymphocytes.

- GM-CSF stimulates differentiation and proliferation of **pleuripotent stem cells into committed cells.**
- GM-CSF also helps in differentiation of **CFU into granulocyte and monocyte precursors** and their further development **into mature cells.**

G-CSF: This is the **granulocyte colony stimulating factor.**

- It is produced by monocytes, endothelial cells and fibroblast.
- It helps in development and functions of granulocytes.

M-CSF: This is the **monocyte colony stimulating factor.** This is also called CSF-1.

- It is produced by fibroblasts, endothelial cells and macrophages.
- It promotes proliferation of monocytes and macrophages, and also stimulates functions of monocytes.

Tumor Necrosis Factor

Tumor necrosis factors (TNFs) help in proliferation and differentiation **of stem cells.**

LIFE HISTORY OF LEUCOCYTES

Leucocytes have mainly **three phases** in their life: marrow phase, circulation phase and tissue phase.

Marrow Phase

This is the **development phase**. It has two pools: mitotic pool and maturation pool.

Mitotic Pool: The cells during development from **myeloblasts to myelocytes** undergo mitosis.

Maturation Pool: This is the phase of maturation of **metamyelocytes into mature cells.**

Circulation Phase

The matured cells are released into circulation and remain in circulation **for few hours** (**circulation pool**) before they enter the tissues.

- At rest, many leucocytes especially neutrophils, adhere to the endothelial lining of blood vessels (called **margination pool)** in addition to circulating in the blood (**active circulation pool**).
- In conditions of increased hemodynamics such as exercise, the **leucocytosis** occurs mainly due to ***disruption of margination*** of leucocytes.

Tissue Phase

After their activities in circulation, leucocytes enter the tissues (**tissue pool** of leucocytes). Granulocytes live for **few days** in the tissues (Application Box 14.1), whereas monocytes remain for a longer period. In the tissues, monocytes are transformed into **tissue macrophages**.

Duration of Leucopoiesis

From myeloblast to matured leucocytes, the process of development usually **takes 10 days** (Fig. 14.2). About 5 days are spent in the mitotic pool (development upto

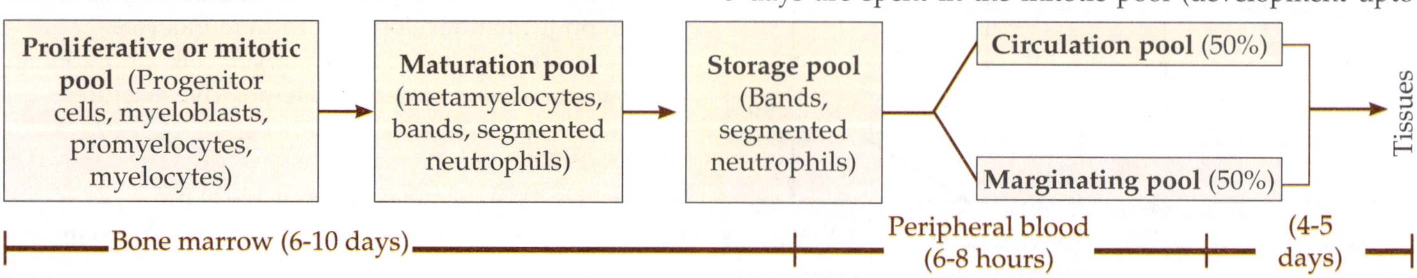

Fig. 14.2: Life history of leucocytes.

myelocytes) and another five days are utilized in the maturation pool (development from metamyelocyte to the mature cells).

Application Box 14.1

Apoptosis of leucocytes: Apoptosis is the programmed cell death. This is a physiologic phenomenon of elimination of mature cells from the body. Biochemically, apoptosis occurs due to internucleosomal DNA fragmentation, and morphologically, by nuclear and cytoplasmic condensation. The apoptotic cells are phagocytosed by macrophages. Senescent neutrophils and eosinophils undergo apoptosis.

NEUTROPHILS

Neutrophils constitute 50 to 70% of leucocytes in blood. They are **highly phagocytic,** and they form the major defense **against acute bacterial (pyogenic) infections**.

Structure

The major identifying features are:
1. Size of neutrophils varies between 10–14 µm.
2. Cytoplasm contains **fine pink colored granules** (Fig. 14.3A and 14.3B)
3. Nucleus is **multilobed** and the lobes are connected by thin strand.
4. Nucleus may contain **Barr body** (Application Box 14.2).
5. The nucleus of **juvenile neutrophil** is single lobed (*band form*).
6. The **oldest neutrophils** may have 6 or 7 lobes in their nucleus (Fig. 14.4).

Application Box 14.2

Sex determination: In females, sex chromatin is present in 2 – 5% of neutrophils as a drumstick appendage attached to the nuclear lobe (Barr body). Drumstick appendage of chromatin is about 1 µm in length attached to the nucleus by a thin chromatin strand. Presence of Barr body indicates 2X chromosomes. Thus, it helps in determination of gender as female.

A. Neutrophil in blood smear (Leishman stain)

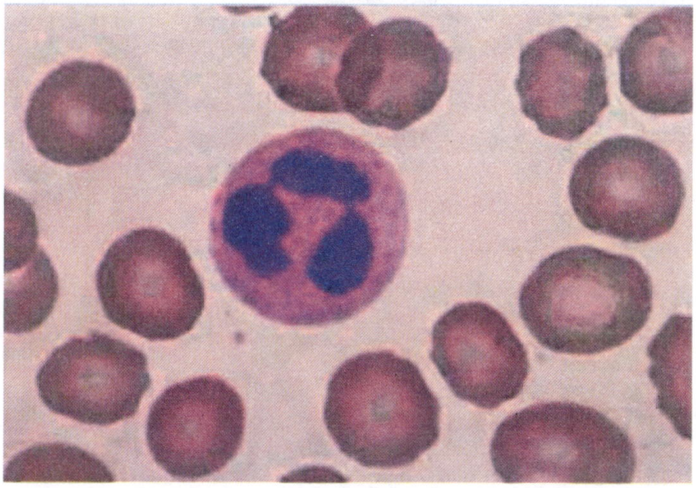

B. Schematic diagram of neutrophil

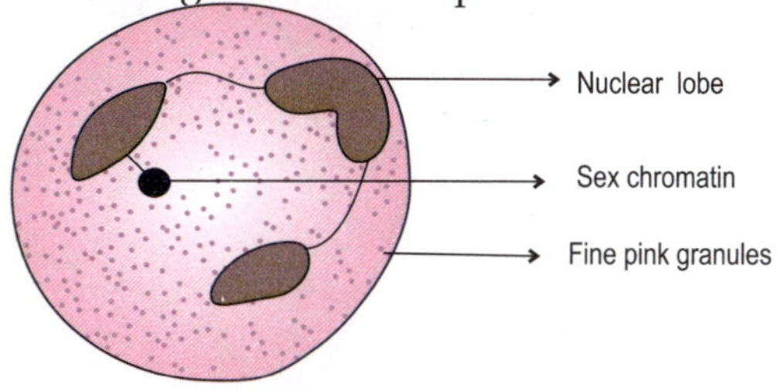

Fig. 14.3: Structure of neutrophil, as appears in a stained smear **(A)**, and drawn schematically **(B).** Note the presence fine pink granules in cytoplasm, and the sex chromatin (Barr body) attached to the lobe of the nucleus.

Arneth Count

Based on the nuclear lobes, neutrophils are classified as N_1 to N_6/N_7 (Fig. 14.4). This is called **Arneth count.**
- Normally, N_2 and N_3 constitute most of the neutrophils in peripheral blood.
- Presence of **younger neutrophils** (mostly N_1 and N_2) indicates stimulation of bone marrow, which is called ***shift to left*** (Fig. 14.5).
- Presence of **older cells** (mostly N_4 and N_5) indicates suppression of bone marrow (***shift to right***).
- **Hypersegmented nucleus** of neutrophils is typically seen in ***megaloblastic anemia*** that occurs due to folate and vitamin B_{12} deficiency (refer, Fig. 11.5, Chapter 11).

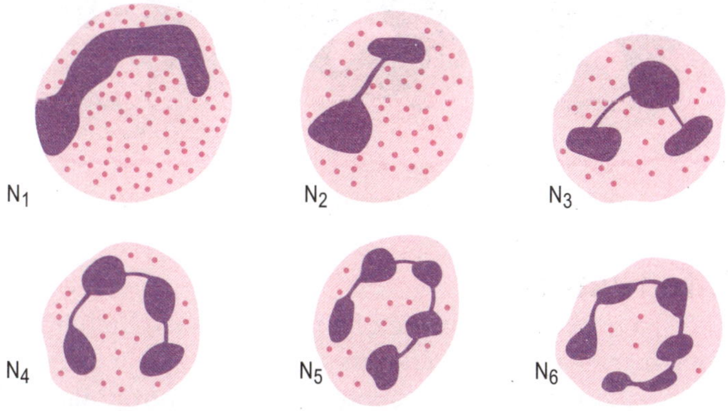

Fig. 14.4: Stages of neutrophil as described in Arneth count. Note, N1 is the youngest (band form) and N_6 or N_7 is the oldest cell.

Granules of Neutrophils

Neutrophils have **four types of granules**: primary or azurophilic granules, secondary or specific granules, tertiary granules and secretory granules.

Primary granules: These **azurophilic granules** that contain myeloperoxidase, lysosomal enzymes, elastase, proteinase, α_1-antitrypsin and perforins (bactericidal-permeability increasing proteins). Contents of azurophil granules kill bacteria and cause tissue destruction during inflammation.
- The primary granules become abnormal to form **Auer bodies** in acute myeloid leukemia.
- Abnormalities of granules are seen in **Chediac-Higashi syndrome** as large blue granules (Fig. 14.6A) (Clinical Note 14.1).

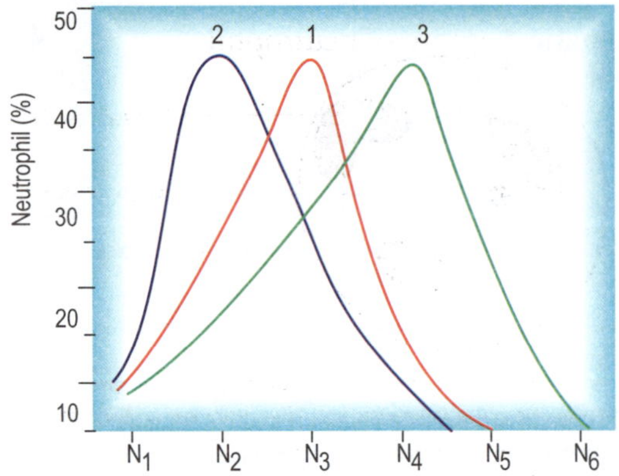

Fig. 14.5: Arneth count. 1. Normal Count; 2. Shift to left (younger neutrophils); 3. Shift to right (Older neutrophils).

Secondary granules: These are **specific granules** and contain lactoferrin, gelatinase and lysozyme.

- Lysozyme is microbicidal and lactoferrin is antibacterial.
- Abnormalities of specific granules are **Alder-Reilly anomaly** showing large lilac inclusions (Fig. 14.6 B) and **May-Hegglin anomaly** showing numerous basophilic inclusions (Fig. 14.6 C).

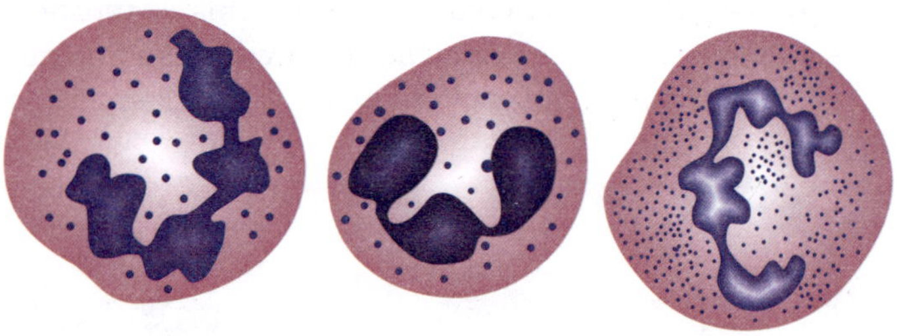

A B C

Fig. 14.6: Neutrophil granular abnormalities in: **A:** Chediac Higashi Syndrome; **B:** Alder-Reilly anomaly; **C:** May-Hegglin anomaly.

Life History

They have four stages in their life: marrow pool, circulation pool, margination pool and tissue pool.

- In peripheral blood, about 50% of neutrophils are present in circulation pool and remaining 50% remains in the margination pool (Fig. 14.2).
- After their usual *life in circulation* for about **6 to 8 hours**, neutrophils ***enter tissues*** where they live for **about 4 days**.

Clinical Note 14.1

Chediac-Higashi syndrome: This is an autosomal recessive disease of abnormality of neutrophil azurophilic granules, characterized by occulocutaneous albinism and increased susceptibility to infection. The garanules fuse to form megagranules. There is absence of elastase, cathepsin-G and defensins that leads to severe infections.

Neutrophil Count PY2.11

Normally, neutrophils constitute 50–70% of the total leucocytes in the peripheral blood. Neutrophil count alters in various conditions (Table 14.2).

Table 14.2 | Conditions that alter neutrophil count.

A. Neutrophilia
1. Physical stimuli: Exercise, pain, labor, surgery
2. Emotional stimuli: Panic, stress
3. Infections: **Acute bacterial infections**
4. Inflammation, burn, infarction, trauma
5. Drugs: Epinephrine, glucocorticoids
7. Endocrine disorders: ACTH excess, Cushing's syndrome
8. Meyloproliferative diseases
B. Neutropenia
1. Congenital: Kostmann syndrome
2. Infections: **Typhoid** and paratyphoid fevers
3. Drugs: Chloromphenicol, phenylbutazone, phenytoin
4. Aplastic anemia
5. Viral infections: Measles, influenza
6. Hypersplenism
7. Autoimmune diseases: SLE, Felty syndrome

Functions

Neutrophil is **actively phagocytic** and contain antimicrobial and bactericidal chemicals in their granules. Neutrophils are the **first line of defense against acute bacterial infections**.

Neutrophil Phagocytosis

Phagocytosis is the process of ingestion and killing of microbes or a foreign substance by a phagocyte.

- Actively **phagocytic cells** are neutrophils, monocytes and macrophages.
- **Steps of phagocytosis** by neutrophil include chemotaxis, diapedesis and adherence, ingestion and illing (Fig. 14 .7).

Chemotaxis

Chemotaxis is the process of migration of neutrophils to the site of infection.

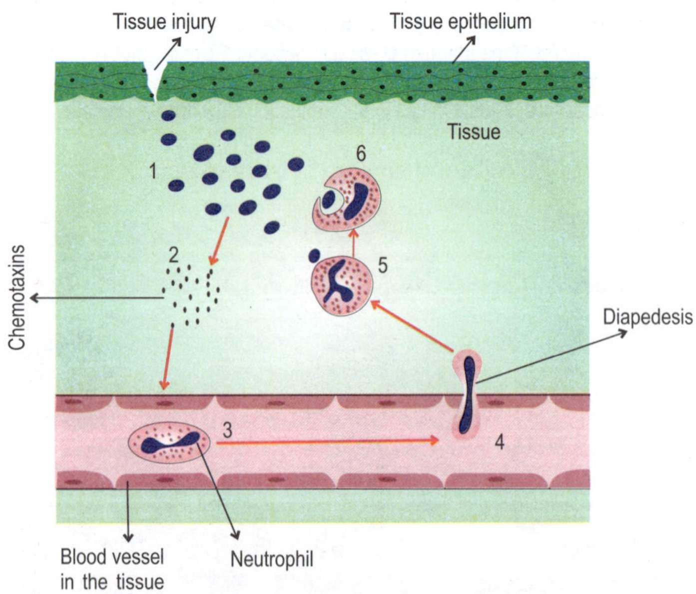

Fig. 14.7: Mechanism of phagocytosis by neutrophil. 1: Invasion of organism into the tissue; 2: Release of chemotaxins from organism and injured tissue; 3: Chemotaxis; 4: Diapedesis; 5: Opsonization and adherence; 6: Ingestion and killing.

- The chemical substances released from the site of infection attract neutrophils to the site. They are called **chemotaxins** (*taxin* means movement) or ***chemoattractants.***
- Chemotaxins are microbial products or chemicals secreted from leucocytes or damaged tissue.
- Complement proteins, especially **C5a and C3** act as chemotaxins.
- During chemotaxis, neutrophils change their shape and become **highly ameboid**.
- Chemotaxins ***stimulate bone marrow*** to produce more neutrophils.

Diapedesis

Neutrophils pass through the capillary endothelial cells to the site of infection, by the process called diapedesis.

Neutrophils **adhere tightly** to endothelial lining with the help of **L-selectins**.

By **ameboid movement**, neutrophils squeeze through the space between endothelial cells.

Opsonization and Adherence

The process by which the bacteria are made tasty to the phagocyte is called **opsonization**.

- The chemicals that facilitate the process of opsonization are called **opsonins**.
- **IgG antibody, C5a and C3b** are known opsonins.
- Bacteria coated by opsonins bind to the receptor on the neutrophil membrane.
- The attachment of membrane of phagocyte to the membrane of microbe is called **adherence**.
- Opsonization facilitates the process of adherence.

Ingestion (Endocytosis)

Adherence facilitates **motor activity** of neutrophils.

- The membrane of phagocyte extends projections from both the sides to encroach on to the microbe.
- These extensions are called **pseudopodia**.
- Pseudopodia finally surround the microbe and form phagocytic vesicle (***phagosome***).

Killing

The bactericidal (killing of bacteria) mechanisms can broadly be divided into **two types**: nonoxidative and oxidative.

Nonoxidative Mechanisms: Neutrophil granules contain a wide variety of ***antibacterial chemicals*** such as degradative enzymes, proteases, defensins and cationic proteins.

- **Lysozyme** that hydrolyzes the cell wall of bacteria and **lactoferrin** that sequesters iron (iron is required for bacterial growth) are nonoxidative components of bacterial killing.
- **Defensins** (α and β defensins) released from azurophil granules have unusual cyclic structure and kill bacteria by disrupting their outer membrane and breaking single-strand DNA structure.

Oxidative Mechanisms: Activated neutrophils produce a number of **oxygen metabolites** that are antimicrobial.

- The metabolites are **superoxide anion** (O_2^-), H_2O_2, **free hydroxyl radicals** (OH·), **hypochlorous acid** (HOCl) and **singlet oxygen** ($'O_2$).
- These reactive metabolites are generated by a nicotinamide adenine dinucleotide phosphate **(NADPH)-dependent oxidase** that reduces molecular oxygen to O_2^-.
- The oxidase is quiescent in resting neutrophils and is stimulated following neutrophil activation and promotes **O_2^- formation.**
- ***O_2^- is the most effective*** oxidant metabolite.
- **Myeloperoxidase**, the enzyme of primary granules facilitate **conversion of Cl^- to HOCl**, which is also a potent oxidant.

Respiratory Burst: Activation of ***NADPH oxidase*** is associated with increased oxygen intake of neutrophil (Application Box 14.3). This is called **respiratory burst.**

Interaction of two mechanisms: Nonoxidative mechanism facilitates the oxidative mechanism of killing. The protease enzymes of neutrophil granules produce a **killing zone** around the activated neutrophil by damaging the tissue, which helps the oxidant metabolites to promote their bactericidal properties.

Application Box 14.3

CGD occurs due to defective NADPH-oxidase: In chronic granulomatous disease (CGD), a genetic disorder, neutrophils fail to generate O2– and related metabolites. Neutrophils and monocytes ingest catalase positive microorganisms but can not kill them due to lack of adequate active oxidants that result from decreased NADPH-oxidase activity. This leads to formation of chronic granulomas, the abnormal inflammatory tissue reactions.

IMPORTANT NOTE

Phagocytic Dysfunction: When neutrophil is activated, its cytosolic calcium concentration increases that facilitates contraction of microfilaments, microtubules and myosin-1 filaments. This promotes diapedesis and phagocytosis.

- **Neutrophil hypomotility**, a primary phagocytic dysfunction of neutrophil, decreases phagocytic activity.
- There are about 15 primary disorders of neutrophil function.

EOSINOPHILS

Eosinophils are known for their protective function **against allergy**. Like neutrophils, eosinophils produce proinflammatory mediators.

- Eosinophils have short life span in circulation but **live longer in tissue**. There are 100 eosinophils in tissue to 1 eosinophil in peripheral blood.

- Eosinophils are present in the epithelia of respiratory, gastrointestinal and genitourinary tract.
- Their production and function are mainly influenced by IL-5.

Morphology

Eosinophils have size same as that of neutrophils.

- Eosinophil **granules are coarse and brick red** in color in blood smear stained by Leishman stain (Fig. 14.8).
- **Nucleus is usually bilobed** and the lobes are separated by a thick strand. This gives eosinophil nucleus an appearance of a pair of ***spectacles***.
- The granules are plenty, and sometimes encroach onto the nucleus.

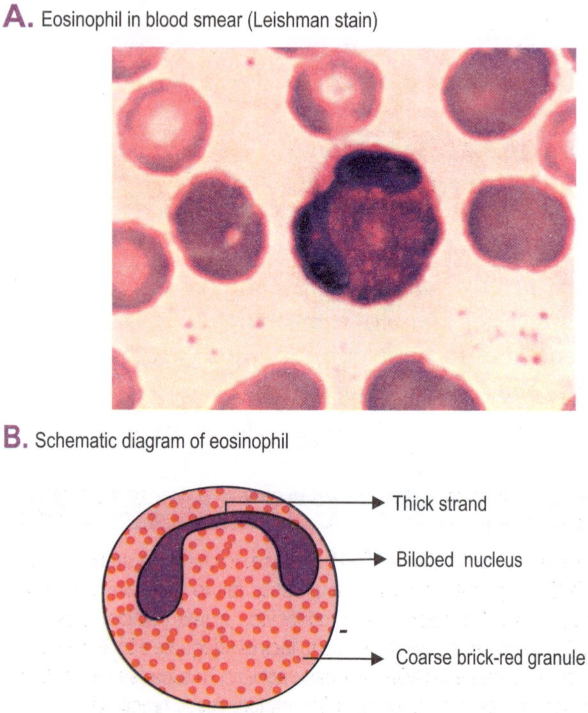

Fig. 14.8: Structure of eosinophil, as appears in a stained smear (A), and drawn schematically (B). Note the presence of many large-sized brick-red granules in cytoplasm.

Table 14.3 | Eosinophil-derived chemicals.
A. Granule derived chemicals
- Major basic protein
- Eosinophil cationic protein
- Eosinophil peroxidase
- Eosinophil-derived neurotoxin
- Lysophospholipase, Phospholipase D
- Arylsulphatase, Acid phosphatase
- Catalase, Histaminase, Hexoseaminidase
B. Cytokines (may or may not be secreted from granules)
- GM-CSF, TNF-α, TGF-α and TGF-β
- Macrophage inhibition factor (MIF)
- $IL_{1\ to\ 6}$, IL_8 and IL_{12}
C. Lipid-derived chemicals
- Leukotriene C, Thromboxane B_2
- Platelet activating factor (PAF)
- PGE_1 and PGE_2

Chemicals Secreted by Eosinophils

Chemicals secreted from eosinophil are divided into **three categories**: chemicals from granules, cytokines, and lipid-derived chemicals (Table 14.3).

Eosinophil Granular Contents

The granules of eosinophil contain following major chemicals.

1. Major basic protein
2. Eosinophil cationic protein
3. Eosinophil-derived peroxidase
4. Eosinophil-derived neurotoxin
5. Cytokines
6. Other chemicals

Major Basic Protein (MBP): MBP is toxic against many intestinal parasites and their larvae.

- Eosinophil **adheres with the IgG coated larva** and secretes MBP into the integument of the larva that causes damage to the larval tissue.
- MBP is also **toxic to pneumocytes and epithelial cells** of respiratory tract and makes the bronchial tree ***hyper-responsive to bronchoconstrictors***.
- Therefore, worm infestations are usually associated with respiratory symptoms.

Eosinophil Cationic Protein (ECP): ECP is rich in arginine and **toxic to helminthic parasites and tracheal epithelium**.

- ECP along with eosinophil-derived neurotoxin produces **neurotoxicity**.

Eosinophil Peroxidase (EP): EP is a heme containing protein.

- It is **toxic to the adult parasites and pulmonary tissue**.
- When combined with H_2O_2, its toxicity increases.

Eosinophil-Derived Neurotoxin (EDN): EDN is a glycosylated protein having striking **ribonuclease activity**. It is **toxic to the neural tissues** of parasites.

Cytokines: The important eosinophil cytokines are $IL_{1\text{-}6}$, IL_8 and IL_{12}, GM-CSF, macrophage inhibition factor (MIF), TGF α and β and TNF-α.

- **TGF-α** mediates in wound healing.
- **Interleukins** such as IL_5, IL_3 and GM-CSF act in autocrine fashion as eosinophil growth factor.
- **MIF** plays a role in the genesis of adult respiratory distress syndrome.

Other Chemicals: Lysophospholipase constitutes 10% of eosinophil proteins.

- The **other enzymes** secreted from eosinophils like phospholipase D, arylsulphatase-B, acid phosphatase, catalase and histaminase take part in ***eosinophil-mediated inflammatory reactions*** and ***killing of parasites***.

Functions

Like neutrophils, eosinophils migrate to the tissues.

- The chemoattractant for eosinophils is **eosinophil chemotactic factor of anaphylaxis** (ECF-A).
- ECF-A facilitates tissue accumulation of eosinophils.

Eosinophils participate in **two important defense mechanisms** of the body:
1. Against helminthic infections
2. Against allergy.

In Helminthic Infections

Eosinophils attack intestinal parasites especially the larva of S. mansoni, Trichinella spiralis, Toxocara canis, N. brasilensis, Fasciola hepatica, roundworms and hook worms. They attack the larva **opsonized by IgG, IgE and complements**.
- First, eosinophils attach themselves to the larva, which activates the eosinophils.
- Within about 3 hours, activated eosinophils **secrete their granular content** onto surface of the larva.
- Once, the tegument is breached, eosinophils **crawl under it** and **secrete toxic mediators** that destroy the tissues of larva and **phagocytose the larva**.
- In this process, **degranulation** of eosinophils occurs.

In Allergy

In allergic condition like **bronchial asthma**, eosinophils play a major role in pathogenesis.
- *Bronchial hyper-reactivity* is correlated with **eosinophilia and airway eosinophil content**.
- Inhibition of airway eosinophilia **by glucocorticoid** causes improvement in bronchial hyper-responsiveness and asthmatic symptoms.
- Though, glucocorticoid causes eosinopenia by eosinophil apoptosis, the main mechanism is the **inhibition of production of IL_5 and IL_3** from type 2 helper cells.
- It is suggested that asthma is an **eosinophil-mediated disease** driven by type-2 helper lymphocytes that secrete IL_5 and IL_3.

Table 14.4 | Causes of eosinophilia and eosinopenia.

Causes
A. Eosinophilia
1. Helminthic infections: Ascariasis (roundworm), filariasis, toxocariasis, ancylostomiasis (hookworm), echinococcosis etc.
2. Allergic diseases: Bronchial asthma, allergic rhinitis, atopic dermatitis, urticaria, food allergy, hay fever
3. Drugs (drug allergy)
4. Tropical pulmonary eosinophilia
5. Addison's disease
B. Eosinopenia
1. Glucocorticoid therapy
2. Cushing's syndrome
3. Aplastic anemia
4. Drug-induced agranulocytosis

Alterations in Eosinophil Count PY2.11

The normal eosinophil count is 2–4%, or **40–440 per µl of blood** (absolute count). When the count is more, is called **eosinophilia**, and when less is called **eosinopenia** (Table 14.4).

BASOPHILS

Basophils are least frequent blood cells. They account for **0 to 1% of leucocytes** in blood. Though they recruit into tissues, unlike eosinophils they ordinarily do not reside in the tissue. Structurally, they resemble mast cells.

Morphology

Basophils

Identifying features of basophils are (Fig. 14.9):
1. The size is same as of neutrophils (10 – 14 µm).
2. The nucleus is usually **'S' shaped**.
3. Nuclear chromatin shows marked condensation.
4. The **granules are bluish and large in size** and more in number. As cell is **heavily studded with granules**, nucleus is often not visible.
   - Granules are surrounded by membranes and contain dense particles called *Chracot-Lyeden crystals*.
   - **Basophil granules** secrete histamine, chondroitin sulphate, tryptase, carboxypeptidase A, cathepsin G, leukotrienes, eosinophil chemotactic factor of anaphylaxis (ECF-A), neural protease and MBP.

Functions

Basophils and mast cells are mainly involved in **allergic reactions**.
1. **Role in acute allergic reactions:** Basophils and mast cells have receptors for Fc region of IgE.

A. Basophil in blood smear (Leishman stain)

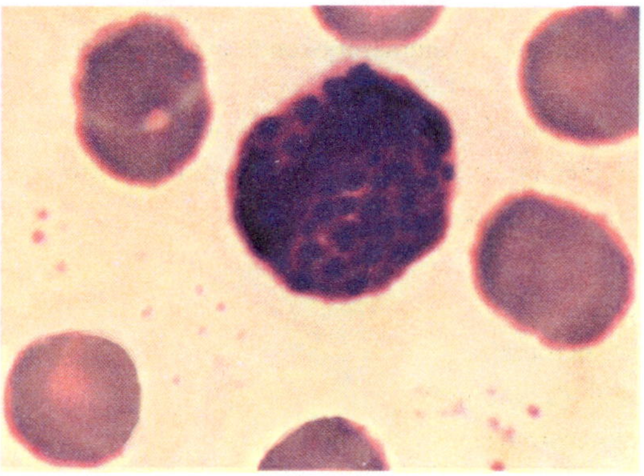

B. Schematic diagram of basophil

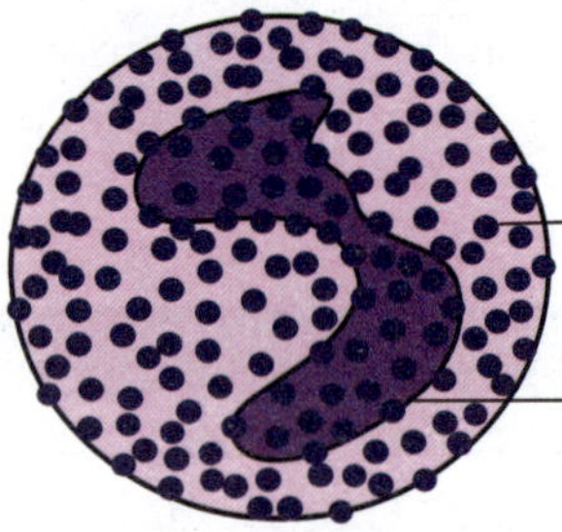

Fig. 14.9: Structure of basophil, as appears in a stained smear (A), and drawn schematically (B). Note the cell is studded with large bluish granules.

- Binding of IgE to these cells initiates degranulation that leads to release of histamine.
- Acute allergies such as acute rhinitis, urticaria, food allergy etc. are mediated by this mechanism.
- Massive release of histamine occurs in **anaphylaxis,** the acute systemic allergy that causes vasodilation and inhibition of cardiac output resulting in acute hypotension.

2. **Role in chronic allergic reactions:** Basophils and mast cells also contribute to **late-phase reactions**.
   - In chronic allergic conditions such as bronchial asthma, basophils and mast cells are **recruited to the site of allergy**.
   - Especially, mast cells **secrete cytokines** that attract leucocytes, eosinophils and basophils, which in turn mediate chronic allergy.
   - This mechanism of pathogenesis of *late-phase reaction* is termed as **mast cell-leucocyte cascade**.
3. **Role in T-cell dependent responses:** Activation of mast cells in the affected tissues along with infiltration of basophils occurs in a variety of T cell dependent immunological responses.
4. **Role in host defense:** Basophils and mast cells play critical role in host resistance to some **viral, bacterial and parasitic infections.** These cells increase in conditions like chicken pox, small pox and tuberculosis.

Table 14.5 | Alteration in basophil count

A. Basophilia
1. Allergic and inflammatory conditions: Ulcerative colitis, urticaria, drug and food allergy
2. Infections: Chicken pox, small pox, influenza
3. Endocrinal disorder: myxedema (hypothyroidism)
4. Basophilic leukemia
5. Polycythemia
B. Basopenia
1. Cortisol therapy
2. Cushing's syndrome
3. Hyperthyroidism

Normal Count

PY2.11

Normal basophil count is **0–1%,** and absolute count is **20–80 per µl of blood**. Mast cells are normally not found in blood. Increase in basophil count is called **basophilia** and decrease in count is called **basopenia** (Table 14.6).

Mast Cells

Basophils resemble mast cells, but mast cells are different cells. Mast cells **reside in the tissues**. They are round or elongated cells with **nonsegmented nucleus.**

- **Granules** are numerous, but smaller in size.
- **Granules** secrete histamine, heparin, cathepsin, ECF-A and neural protease.
- **Two types** of mast cells: ***mucosal mast cells*** (present in the mucosa) and ***connective tissue mast cell.***

Differences between basophils & mast cells are given in Table 14.6.

Table 14.6 | Differences between basophils and mast cells.

	Basophils	Mast cells
Origin	Bone marrow	Bone marrow
Reside in	Blood	Tissue
Life span	Few days	Few months
Growth factor	IL-3	SCF
Major secretion	Histamine, IL-4	Histamine, heparin
Receptors for	IgE, IgG	IgE

Mastocytosis: Secondary increase in mast cell count occurs in allergic conditions like asthma, and connective tissue disorders like rheumatoid arthritis.

Primary increase in mast cell count occurs in systemic disorders such as urticaria pigmentosa, mast cell leukemia etc, and are called as ***systemic mastocytosis.***

MONOCYTES

Monocyte is the **second line of defense against** microbial infections.

- After spending life in blood, monocytes enter the tissues and get transformed into **macrophages**.
- Monocytes and macrophages are important components of ***mononuclear phagocyte system***.

Morphology

Monocytes are the **largest blood cells**. The identifying features are:

1. Diameter varies between **12–25 µm**.
2. The nucleus occupies half of the cell and remains eccentrically. **Cytoplasmic-nuclear ratio** is 50:50.
3. Often the **nucleus is reniform** (kidney shaped), but may be horse-shoe shaped, round or irregular (Fig. 14.10).

4. There are nuclear chromatin clumps that give the nucleus a **nonhomogenous** or **stringy appearance**.
5. Cytoplasm is abundant and **ground glass** in appearance.
6. Though monocyte is traditionally classified as agranular leucocytes, fine pink-purple granules are present in about 30% of cells. The *monocyte granules* contain hydrolytic enzymes such as acid phosphatase and lysozymes.

Surface Receptors: Monocytes have a number of receptors on its surface such as Fc receptors for IgG, IgA and IgE, receptors for complements, cytokines, insulin, glucocorticoid and angiotensin.

- Monocytes and macrophages express **HLA class II and their receptors** on their surface that ***help in antigen presentation***.

A. Monocyte in blood smear (Leishman stain)

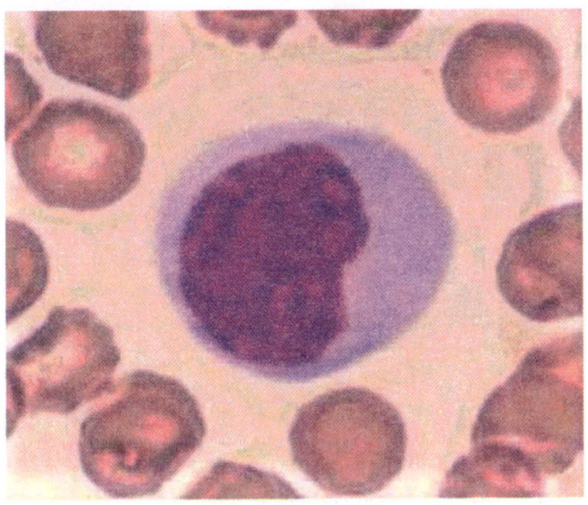

B. Schematic diagram of monocyte.

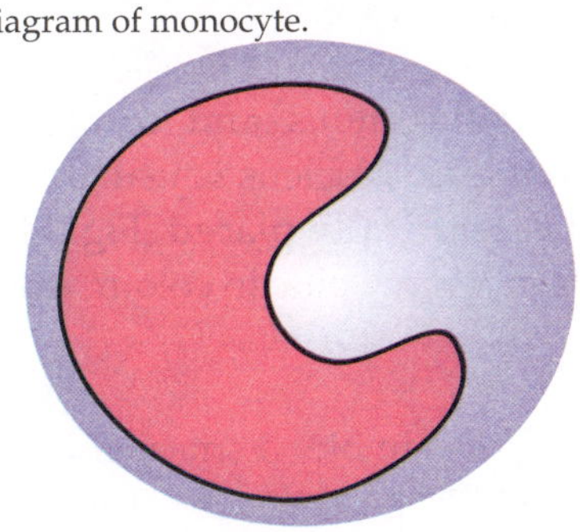

Fig. 14.10: Structure of monocyte, as appears in a stained smear (A), and drawn schematically (B). Note the ground-glass or turbid cytoplasm. Nucleus is spongy in appearance and cytoplasmic-nuclear ratio is about 50:50.

Functions

1. **Phagocytosis and microbial killing:** Monocyte is an **active phagocyte**.
    - The presence of various **surface receptors** facilitates recognition of various organisms to be phagocytosed.
    - Organisms are **killed by oxidants** produced by NADPH oxidase and nitric oxide synthase, and intracellular **hydrolytic enzymes**.
    - Monocyte is the **second line of defense** against infections.
2. **Antigen presentation:** Monocyte is an important antigen presenting cell (APC).
    - Partially digested product of the antigen (Ag) attaches with the MHC II molecules (**MHC+Ag**) on the surface of monocyte.
    - **T cells are activated** when they encounter MHC+Ag present on the APC membrane.
    - This is the **first step** in the activation of ***cellular immunity***.
3. **Release of cytokines and enzymes:** Monocyte secretes various chemokines such as **IL-1 and IL-6** that are essential for ***coactivation of immunological responses***.
    - **TNF-α and interferons** that facilitate killing of viruses and other microbial organisms.
    - **Growth factors** like GM-CSF, M-CSF, TGF and PDGF promote leucopoiesis and erythropoiesis.
    - Monocytes by secreting **complement factors** augment the local tissue defense responses.
    - Monocyte releases **various enzymes** like collagenase, elastase, plasminogen activator etc. that participate in wound healing and tissue remodeling.

Life Span

Monocytes ***in circulation*** have a wide range of half-life between **10–72 hours**.

- From circulation they ***enter tissues*** and live **few weeks to months**. The average life in tissues is three months.
- However, in tissue, they are transformed into **tissue macrophages** and live for years.

IMPORTANT NOTE

Monocytes are more in chronic inflammation: If there is tissue infection or inflammation, initially the monocyte numbers are less than neutrophils. But, if inflammation persists for more than 12 hours, monocytes predominate over neutrophils.

Normal Count

PY2.11

Normal monocyte count is **2–8%,** and the average absolute count is **400/μl of blood**. Increase in count is called **monocytosis** and decrease in count is called **monocytopenia** (Table 14.7).

Table 14.7 | Causes of alteration in monocyte count.

A. Monocytosis
1. Acute and chronic monocytic leukemia
2. Hodgkin's disease
3. Glucocorticoid therapy
4. Polycythemia vera
5. Postsplenectomy state
7. Cytomegalovirus infection
8. Collagen diseases
9. Malaria, Kala azar
B. Monocytopenia
1. Aplastic anemia
2. Septicemia

- The monocyte count is more in neonates and infants, which is about 1000/µl of blood.
- Men tend to have slightly higher monocyte count than women. However, in adults count more than 800/µl of blood is considered as monocytosis.

Macrophages

Monocytes are transformed into macrophages in the tissues. Macrophages in different tissues form **mononuclear phagocyte system** (Table 14.8).

- On becoming macrophage, there is increase in **cell size, number of cytoplasmic granules** and increase in heterogeneity of the cell shape.
- The average diameter of macrophages varies from **25 to 50 µm**.
- Cytoplasm contains **multiple large azurophil granules**.
- They contain all the surface receptors that are present in monocytes.
- In chronic tissue inflammations, macrophages are converted into **multinucleated giant cells** that are highly phagocytic and microbicidal.

Table 14.8 | Distribution of cells of mononuclear phagocyte system.

A. In blood
- Monocytes
B. In bone marrow
- Monoblasts, Promonocytes
C. In tissues
- Kupffer cell in liver
- Osteoclasts in bone marrow
- Alveolar macrophages in lungs
- Histiocytes in connective tissue
- Microglia in brain
- Red pulp macrophages in spleen
- Macrophages in lymph nodes and thymus
- Mesangial cells in kidney
- Dendritic cells/histiocytes in skin
- Type A cells in synovium
D. In body cavities
- Pleural macrophages, peritoneal macrophages
E. In inflammatory tissues
- Epitheloid cells, multinucleate giant cells

LYMPHOCYTES

Lymphocytes are morphologically divided into **small and large lymphocytes**, and functionally divided into T cells, B cells and NK cells.

Morphology

Small Lymphocytes

Small lymphocytes are same in size to that of red cells. They **constitute 35%** (20–50%) of total lymphocytes. The identifying features are:

1. Size: 6–9 µm in diameter.
2. Ovoid or kidney shaped nucleus with **densely packed nuclear chromatin**.
3. Nucleus is usually eccentrically placed and occupies about **90% of the cell** area (Fig. 14.11).
4. There is a thin rim of bluish cytoplasm that **does not contain granules**.

A. Small lymphocyte in blood smear (Leishman stain)

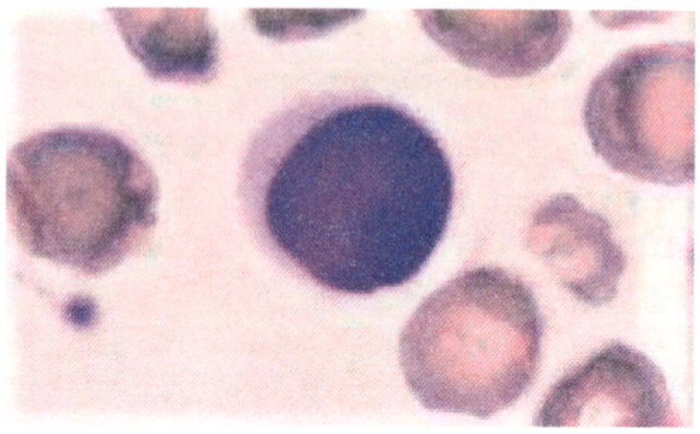

B. Schematic diagram of small lymphocyte

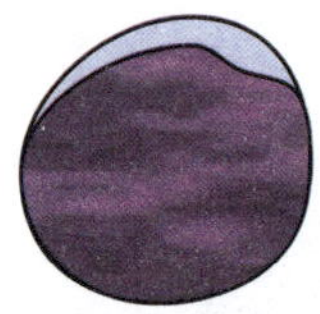

Fig. 14.11: Structure of small lymphocyte, as appears in a stained smear (A), and drawn schematically (B). Note, nucleus occupies 90% of cytoplasm.

Large Lymphocytes

Large lymphocytes constitute **65% of total lymphocytes**. The identifying features are:

1. **Size:** 10–15 µm in diameter (Fig. 14.12 A).
2. **Nucleus is homogenous and compact** with dense nuclear chromatins. Nucleus is usually oval or kidney shaped and **eccentrically placed** (Fig. 14.12 B).
3. The **cytoplasm** is navy blue in colour, **does not contain granules**.

A. Large lymphocytes in blood smear (Leishman stain)

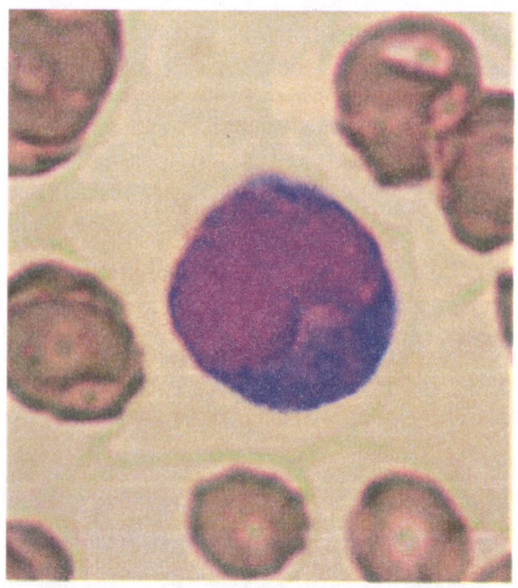

B. Schematic diagram of large lymphocyte

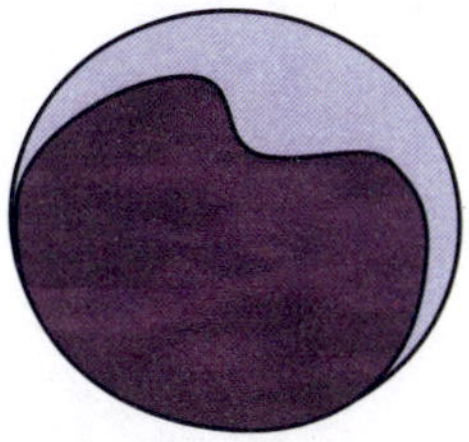

Fig. 14.12: Structure of large lymphocyte, as appears in a stained smear (A), and drawn schematically (B). Note, eccentrically placed nucleus.

Normal Count & Functions PY2.11

Normal lymphocyte count is 20–40% of total leucocytes. The absolute count is 500 – 8000 per cu mm of blood. Increase in count is called lymphocytosis and decrease in count is called lymphocytopenia (Table 14.9).

Table 14.9 | Causes of lymphocytosis and lymphocytopenia.

A. Lymphocytosis
- Infectious mononucleosis
- Whooping cough (Bordetella pertusis)
- Tuberculosis
- Postsplenectomy
- Acute and chronic lymphocytic leukemia
- Monoclonal B-cell lymphocytosis
B. Lymphocytopenia
- Aplastic anemia
- Glucocorticoid therapy
- Severe combined immunodeficiency states

Functionally, lymphocytes are divided into three categories: B cells, T cells and NK cells.

- **B cells** on stimulation are transformed into **plasma cells** that secrete antibodies. B cells mediate ***humoral immunity***.
- **T cells** mediate ***cellular immunity***.
- **NK cells** mediate ***natural and nonspecific*** immunity.

Summary of Blood ells

- To summarize, blood cells are formed elements of blood (Table 14.10).

Erythrocytes are anuclear cells having diameter of 7 to 8 µm that are primarily meant for ***transport of oxygen*** from lungs to the tissues.

Leucocytes are of various sizes and they mainly play role in ***defence mechanisms***.

Platelets are anuclear and smaller cells (cellular fragments) that principally participate in ***homeostasis***.

LEUKEMIA

Definition

Leukemia is defined as a **malignant neoplasia of hemopoietic cells** in which there is **abnormal proliferation of leucocytes and their precursors** resulting in appearance of ***abnormal and immature leucocytes*** in the peripheral blood associated with *very high leucocytosis*, and *infiltration of tissues* by leukemic cells. The total leucocyte count is usually very high, except in aleukemic leukemia.

Table 14.10 | Summary of the formed elements in blood.

Cells	Count	Features	Functions
Red blood cells (erythrocytes)	5.4 million/mm³ in males; 4.8 million/mm³ in females	7-8 µm diameter, biconcave discs, without a nucleus, life span about 120 days.	Transports oxygen and carbon dioxide
White blood cells (leukocytes)	4000-11,000/mm³	Live for a few hours to few days	Kill pathogens (body defence)
1. Neutrophils	50 - 70% of all WBCs	10-14 µm diameter; nucleus is multilobed, connected by thin strands of chromatin; cytoplasm has fine, pink granules.	Phagocytosis of organisms (first line of defence)
2. Eosinophils	1 - 4% of all WBCs	10-14 µm diameter; nucleus is bilobed; coarse brick-red	Combat the effects of histamine in allergic reactions, kill parasitic worms.
3. Basophils	0 - 1% of all WBCs	10-14 µm diameter; nucleus is bilobed or irregular in shape; large cytoplasmic granules are deep blue-purple	Release heparin, histamine, and serotonin in allergic reactions that promote overall inflammatory response
4. Lymphocytes	20 - 40% of all WBCs	Small lymphocytes are 6-9 µm in diameter; Large lymphocytes are 10-14 µm in diameter; nucleus is round or slightly indented; cytoplasm forms a clear rim around the nucleus	Mediate immune responses
5. Monocytes	2 - 8% of all WBCs	12 - 25 µm diameter; nucleus is oval or kidney-shaped or horseshoe-shaped; cytoplasm turbid in appearance.	Phagocytosis (after transforming into tissue macrophages).
Platelets (thrombocytes)	150,000-400,000/mm³	2 - 4 µm diameter, cell fragments, no nucleus.	Form platelet plug in hemostasis (temporary hemostatic plug)

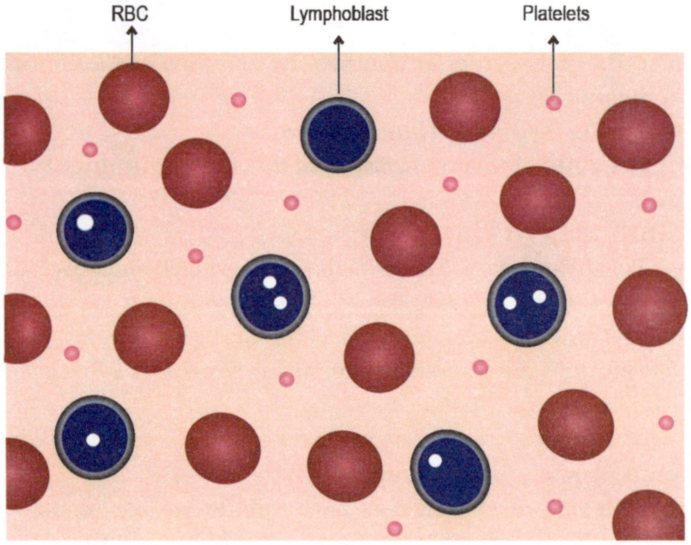

Fig. 14.13: Blood picture (schematic) of acute lymphoblastic leukemia. Note the presence of many lymphoblasts.

Types

Leukemia is classified into **two main categories**: myeloid (myelocytic) and lymphocytic leukemia. These two varieties are sub-classified into **acute and chronic types**.

Acute Lymphoblastic Leukemia

Acute lymphoblastic leukemia (ALL) is primarily a disease of children and young adults.

- This constitutes **80% of childhood acute leukemias**.
- The **usual presentations** are anemia or hemorrhage, infective lesions of the mouth and pharynx, fever, prostration, headache and malaise.
- Generalized ***lymphadenopathy, splenomegaly*** and ***hepatomegaly*** are common.
- The typical **blood picture** is of *anemia and thrombocytopenia*, with a moderate or marked increase in white cells, the majority of which are blast cells '**lymphoblasts**' (Fig. 14.13).

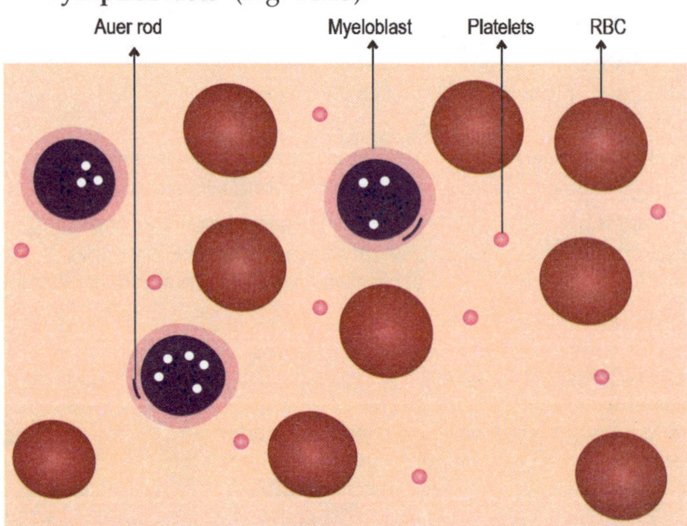

Fig. 14.14: Blood picture (schematic) of acute myeloblastic leukemia. Note the presence of many meyloblasts, and Auer rods in myeloblast.

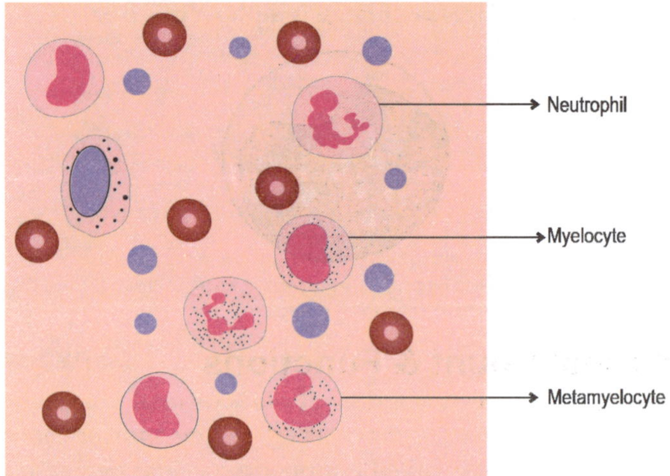

Fig. 14.15: Blood picture (schematic) of chronic myeloid leukemia. Note ethe presence of many myelocyte, metamyelocyte and neutrophils.

Acute Myeloblastic Leukemia

Acute myeloblastic leukemia (AML) primarily affects **adults between the ages of 15 and 40 years**.

- It constitutes only **20% of childhood leukemias**.
- The presentation is like that of ALL, but lymphadenopathy and hepatosplenomegaly is not common.
- Blood picture presents anemia, thrombocytopenia, and moderate to high leucocytosis.
- More ***than 60% of leucocytes*** in the peripheral blood are blast cells (**myeloblasts**) (Fig. 14.14).

Chronic Myeloid Leukemia

Chronic myeloid leukemia (CML) accounts for about **20% of all cases of leukemia**.

- It is primarily a disease of **adults between 30 to 60 years** of age with the peak incidence in the 4th and 5th decades of life.
- Onset is usually slow with **nonspecific features** like anemia, weight loss, weakness, and easy fatigability.
- **Splenomegaly is the outstanding physical sign.**
- Hepatomegaly may be present, but lymph node enlargement is rare.

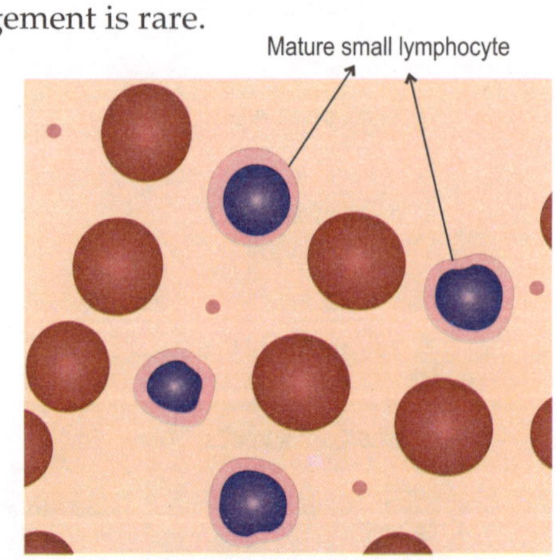

Fig. 14.16: Blood picture (schematic) of chronic lymphocytic leukemia. Note the presence of many lymphocytes (mature small lymphocytes).

- Markedly elevated total leucocyte count usually **more than one lakh cells** per cubic mm of blood is seen commonly.
- **Neutrophils and metamyelocytes** constitute most of the circulating cells (Fig. 14.15).
- Blasts cells are present rarely except in the blastic crisis.

Chronic Lymphocytic Leukemia

Chronic lymphocytic leukemia (CLL) is the most indolent of all leukemias.

- It occurs typically in **persons over 50 years of age**.
- Males are affected twice as frequently as females.
- Patients present with nonspecific symptoms.
- **Lymphadenopathy** *is the outstanding physical sign.*
- Hepatosplenomegaly may be present.
- Mild to severe increase in leucocyte count is seen. More than 90% of leucocytes are mature lymphocytes (Fig. 14.16).

Multiple Choice Questions

1. **All of the following are phases in the life history of a leucocyte, EXCEPT**
   A. Circulation phase
   B. Tissue phase
   C. Hepatic phase
   D. Marrow phase
2. **All of the following have phagocytic function, EXCEPT:**
   A. Macrophage
   B. Mast cells
   C. Monocytes
   D. Neutrophils
3. **Which of the following is NOT present in eosinophil granules?**
   A. Histamin
   B. Acid phosphatase
   C. Lysophospholipase
   D. Catalase
4. **The granules of neutrophil are considered as lysosomes, because:**
   A. They take both acidic and basic stains
   B. They release peroxidise enzyme
   C. Their enzymes can hydrolyse any substrate
   D. They are morphologically identical to lysosomes
5. **During chemotaxis, neutrophils**
   A. Become highly ameboid
   B. Release lysozymes
   C. Leukopoiesis is inhibited
   D. Engulf the bacteria
6. **Which of the following is NOT a product of myeloid stem cell?**
   A. Basophils
   B. Platelets
   C. T cell
   D. RBC
7. **Life span of leukocyte in blood is about**
   A. 4-6 hours
   B. 6-10 days
   C. 6-8 weeks
   D. 120 days
8. **During exercise, the major mechanism of increased leukocyte count is:**
   A. Increased release of neutrophils from bone marrow
   B. Disruption of margination by leucocytes
   C. Stimulation of myeloblastic activity
   D. Stimulation of granulopoiesis
9. **Neutrophil count decreases in all, EXCEPT:**
   A. Typhoid fever
   B. Malaria
   C. Chloramphenicol administration
   D. Acute bacterial infection
10. **All of the following are true about leukemia, EXCEPT:**
    A. Immature cells in the peripheral smear
    B. Infiltration of bone marrow by leukemic cells
    C. Total leukocyte count is always very high
    D. Infiltration of tissues by leukemic cells
11. **Which of the following is NOT true about monocyte?**
    A. Second line of defence
    B. Phagocytic
    C. Count decreases in malaria
    D. Releases cytokines IL-1
12. **Which of the following is NOT true about neutrophil?**
    A. The primary granules are peroxidise positive
    B. Acts as an antigen presenting cell
    C. Count increases in burn and infarction
    D. Hypersegmented nucleus is seen in megaloblastic anemia
13. **Which of the following is NOT true about relative lymphocytosis?**
    A. Lymphocyte percentage is more than 40%
    B. Absolute lymphocyte count is normal
    C. Seen in Cushing's syndrome
    D. Seen in children below 2 years
14. **In which of the following condition, neutrophils fail to generate O2- ?**
    A. Acute myeloblastic leukemia
    B. Chronic granulomatosus disease of childhood
    C. Chronic myeloid leukemia
    D. Amyotrophic lateral sclerosis
15. **All of the following are components of mononuclear phagocyte system, EXCEPT:**
    A. Mesangial cells in kidney
    B. Promonocyte
    C. Osteocyte
    D. Monoblast
16. **Immediate hypersensitivity reaction is mediated by granules of?**
    A. Eosinophil
    B. Basophil
    C. Neutrophil
    D. Dendritic cell

Answers

1. C	2. B	3. A	4. C	5. A	6. C
7. A	8. B	9. D	10. C	11. C	12.B
13. C	14. B	15. C	16. B		

Chapter 15

Immunity

Learning Objectives

On completion of study of this chapter:

The student will be able to (must know):

1. Classify immunity.
2. Classify lymphocytes and give their functions.
3. List the nonspecific defence mechanisms of the body.
4. Name primary & secondary lymphatic organs and give their functions.
5. Describe the mechanism of cellular immunity.
6. Describe the mechanism of humoral immunity
7. Name the antibodies and give their functions.
8. Understand physiology of immune responses.
9. Appreciate the role of complement system in immunity.
10. Explain the mechanism of immunological tolerance.
11. Understand the basis of transplant rejection and its prevention.
12. Name immunological disorders & give one example for each.

The student may also be able to (desirable to know):

1. Describe the mechanism of innate immunity.
2. Describe the development of immune mechanisms.
3. Describe the process of presentation of antigen and the role of MHC antigen in it.
4. Describe the mechanism of immunity by the complement system
5. Describe various immunological disorders.

Mammalians are endowed with various defense mechanisms that can broadly be divided into **specific and non-specific defenses**. The specific defense mechanisms of the body are collectively known as immunity.

Types of Immunity PY2.10

The ability of the body to defend against invading agents is called immunity. The invader may be a living organism or a nonliving substance.

- Immune responses broadly involve *two steps*: **First,** the recognition of pathogen or the foreign material, and, **Second,** the reaction to eliminate it.
- Largely, **immune responses** are of *two types*: innate or non-adaptive and acquired or adaptive (Table 15.1).
- *Innate immunity* is mostly **nonspecific** that include phagocytosis, inflammation, release of cytokine and antibacterial peptides from phagocytes and inflammatory cells, activation of complement system etc.
- *Acquired immunity* is **specific** in which a distinct set of lymphocytes are activated by specific antigens and eliminate them by specific mechanisms.

Table 15.1 | Types of immunity.

A. Innate (non-adaptive) immunity
1. Nonspecific defenses
2. Relatively specific defense by NK cells
B. Acquired (adaptive) immunity
1. *Naturally acquired*
a) Active immunity (usually through infections)
- Cellular immunity
- Humoral immunity
b) Passive immunity (transfer of antibody from mother)
- Ig G via placenta
- Ig A via breast feeding
2. *Artificially acquired*
a) Active immunity
- vaccination
b) Passive immunity
- i.v. injection of antibodies such as anti-D immunization of Rh –ve mother.

NONSPECIFIC DEFENSE

Nonspecific defense (**innate immunity**) mechanisms include mechanical defense, chemical derense and defense by natural killer cells, phagocytosis, inflammation and fever.

Mechanical Defense

Skin and Epidermis: Skin and epidermis are **physical barriers** of the body to check the entry of organisms into the body.

- **Severe infection** occurs ***in burns*** due to loss of skin.

Mucous Membranes: Mucous membrane mechanically traps the organisms and secretes chemicals that inhibit the organisms.

Mucus: Mucus secreted by mucosal epithelium traps microorganisms, especially in the respiratory, gastrointestinal and genitourinary tracts.

Hairs: Almost all openings (entry points) of the body such as nostrils, ears, eyes, anus, urethra and vagina (in females) are guarded by hairs.

- They **filter microorganisms** and **prevent their entry** into the body.

Cilia: Cilia present in mucous membranes filter microorganisms.

Tear: Tear secreted from lacrimal apparatus washes the microbes and dilutes the chemical substances produced by microbes.

Saliva: Saliva washes microbes from the oral cavity and keeps the mouth and teeth clean. Saliva contains **antimicrobial chemicals**.

Urine: Urine flow during micturition washes microbes from urinary tract.

Chemical Defense

Acidic pH of Skin: Acidic pH of skin inhibits growth of micro-organisms.

Bactericidal Substance of Sebum: Sebum is the secretion of the glands in the skin.

- It contains ***bactericidal substances*** like **unsaturated fatty acids** that kill microbes.

Chemicals in Body Secretions: Antimicrobial substances like **lysozyme** secreted in saliva, tears, sweat and other body secretions inhibit growth of micro-organisms.

Acidic pH of Stomach and Vagina: Strongly **acidic pH of gastric secretion** kills many micro-organisms and also destroys toxins in the stomach.

- **Low pH of vaginal secretion** also prevents entry of microbes into the body.

Complement Proteins: The complement proteins activated in response to entry of microorganisms into the body kill organisms by **facilitating opsonization, phagocytosis** and **osmotic lysis**.

Interferons: These are secreted from activated lymphocytes and **kill viruses**.

Defense by NK Cells

NK cells or **natural killer cells** are third category of lymphocytes that are **neither B nor T cells**.

- They have the ability to kill a **wide variety of microorganisms** and **tumor cells**.
- They do not mature in thymus.
- Unlike B and T cells, they **lack surface antigen receptors**.
- They are **large granular cells** (Fig. 15.1)
- They constitute about **15% of total lymphocytes** in the body.
- They are present in the spleen, lymph nodes, bone marrow and blood.

Mechanism of Killing: They kill microbes by following mechanisms.

1. **Osmotic lysis** by incorporating ***perforins*** into the surface of the microbes.
2. They release interferons that **activate phagocytosis** and immunity.
3. They possess **Fc receptors** that allow them to ***kill antibody coated viruses***.

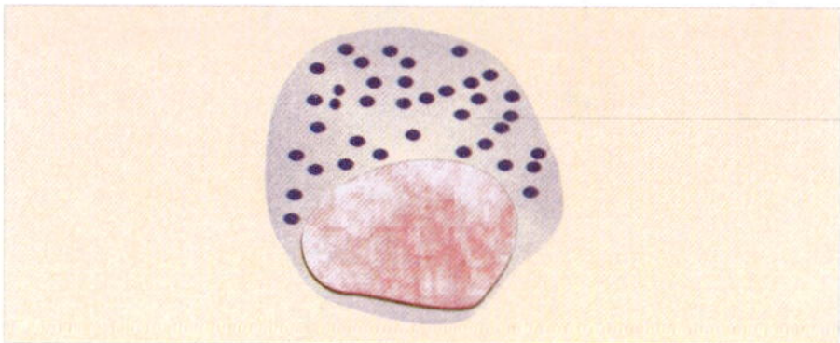

Fig. 15.1: Natural Killer cell. Large cells with granular cytoplasm.

Defense by Phagocytic Cells

Granulocytes (neutrophils, eosinophils and basophils), **monocytes and macrophages** kill micro-organisms by phagocytosis. Details of phagocytosis by neutrophils are described in previous chapter.

- Monocytes transform themselves into **macrophages** in the tissue.
- The macrophages that are mobile in the tissues are called **wandering macrophages**.
- The **fixed macrophages** are present in specific tissues of the body.
- These macrophages are mononuclear cells and are important component of **mononuclear phagocyte system** (MPS).

MPS include the following (Fig 15.2):

1. Kupffer cells of the liver
2. Alveolar macrophages in the lungs
3. Microglia of brain
4. Tissue macrophages in the spleen and lymph nodes
5. Osteoclasts in bone
6. Mesangial cells in kidney
7. Histiocytes in connective tissues
8. Langerhans cells in the skin

Defense by Inflammation and Fever

Inflammation

The response of the tissue to injury is known as inflammation. It is characterized by appearance of **four**

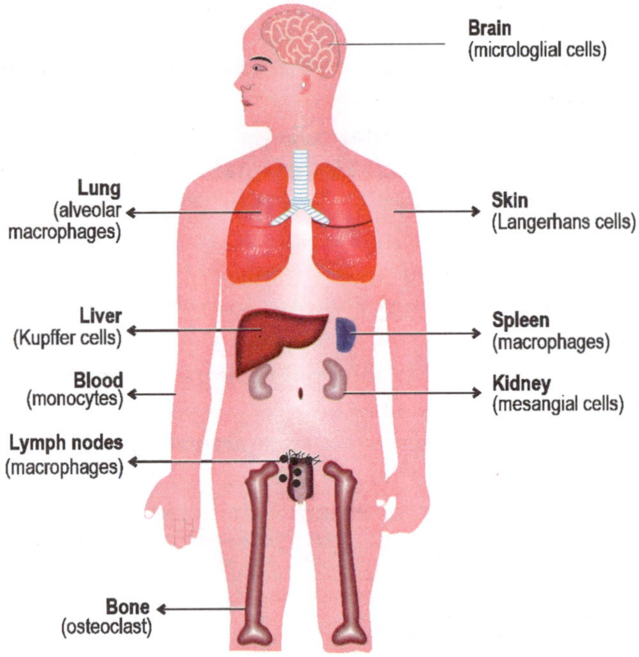

Fig. 15.2: Cells of mononuclear phagocyte system.

features in sequence: rubor (redness), dolor (pain), calor (increased temperature) and tumor (swelling).

Stages of Inflammation: There are **three stages of inflammation**: vasodilation and increased permeability, phagocyte migration and phagocytosis, and tissue repair (Fig. 15.3).

1. **Vasodilation** allows more blood to flow and **increased permeability** allows fluid to escape into the tissue. This happens by **histamine and bradykinin** released from the inflammatory cells.
2. **Phagocytes migrate** to the site of injury by diapedesis and chemotaxis, engulf the organisms by **phagocytosis** and kill them.
3. **Tissue repair** is the healing stage in inflammation, which is facilitated by migration of **fibroblasts and macrophage** to the site that repair the epithelium by secreting **growth factors**.

Role of NF-κB: Recent evidence suggests that a transcription factor, called **nuclear factor-kappa B** (NF-κB), plays an important role in inflammation.

- Normally, NF-κB is bound to another cytoplasmic protein called **IκBα**, and this ***binding keeps NF-κB in an inactive state.***
- Viruses and cytokines that induce inflammation **separate NF-κB from IκBα**.
- NF-κB then migrates to nucleus and attaches with the DNA.
- This induces the **transcription of genes** for formation of various chemicals that participate in inflammation.
- Thus, NF-κB stimulates synthesis and secretion of **mediators of inflammation**.
- **Acute phase reactants** (APRs) produced during inflammation induce systemic responses (Application Box 15.1).

IMPORTANT NOTE

Cortisol increases the production of IκBα: Anti-inflammatory drugs like cortisol increase the production of IκBα in the cell, and therefore, prevent the activation of NF-κB, that inhibits inflammation.

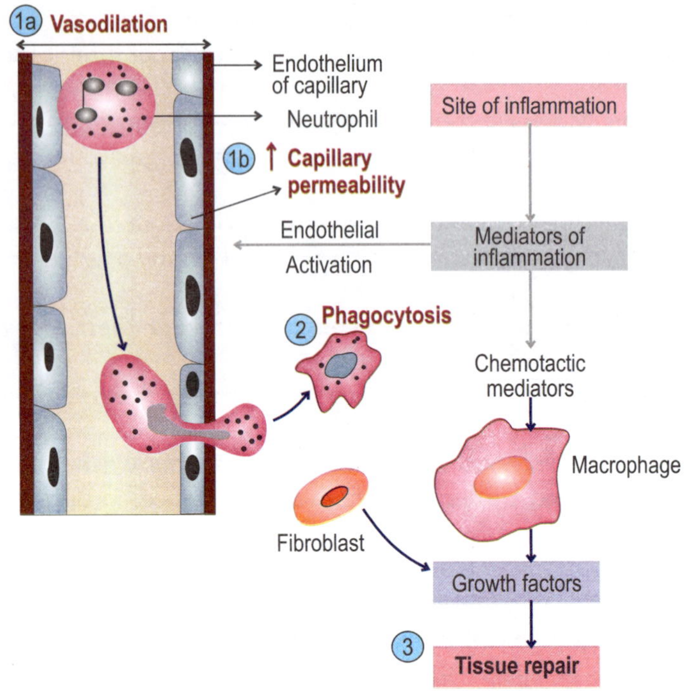

Fig. 15.3: Steps of inflammation. **1a**: Vasodilation that increases blood flow to the area; **1b**: Increased capillary permeability; **2**: Phagocytosis by neutrophil; **3**: Tissue repair (after few days) by macrophage and fibroblast that secrete growth factors.

Application Box 15.1

APRs are markers of inflammation: Acute phase reactants (APRs) are **C-reactive protein** (CRP), orosomucoid protein, fibrinogen, haptoglobin, serum amyloid protein A and C3 complement protein. The first to appear in acute inflammation is CRP. The ***plasma level of CRP*** is an important marker of inflammation.

Fever

Fever is one of the protective phenomena of the body against infections.

- Increased body temperature **prevents growth of micro-organisms**.
- Fever also **facilitates the actions of interferon** and different body enzymes that ***inhibit the growth*** of many microorganisms.

SPECIFIC DEFENCE MECHANISMS (Acquired Immunity)

Acquired immunity is broadly divided into **two categories**: the cellular (cell mediated) immunity and humoral (antibody mediated) immunity. Cellular immunity is mediated by **cytotoxic T cells** (killer cells) and humoral immunity is mediated by **antibodies** formed by **plasma cells**.

Development of Immunity

Development of immunity is the development of lymphocytes. Immunity develops in response to an antigen, which is generally an infective organism or a nonliving substance.

- A specific antigen stimulates the development of a specific set of lymphocytes. Functionally, lymphocytes are of *two types*: **T and B cells.**
- The major sites of lymphocyte development are the **primary lymphoid organs.**
  - For T cell, primary lymphoid organ is thymus.
  - For B cell, primary lymphoid organ is **bursa equivalent** (bone marrow).
- In these organs, lymphocytes differentiate from their precursors that originate from the bone marrow and proliferate and mature into functionally potent cells.
- In mammals, ***T cells mature in thymus***, and ***B cells mature in bone marrow*** *and fetal liver* (Flowchart 15.1).

After their maturity, they circulate in blood and migrate to **secondary lymphoid organ** where they reside (Table 15.2).

- Secondary lymphoid organs **are lymph nodes, spleen and gut associated lymphoid organs.**
- Enlargement of lymph nodes and spleen indicates infection (Clinical Note 15.1).

Table 15.2 | Distribution of T and B cells in various lymphatic tissues of the body.

Lymphoid tissue	T cell %	B cell %
Origin	Bone marrow	Bone marrow
Thymus	100	0
Bone marrow	10	90
Spleen	45	55
Lymph node	60	40
Blood	80	20

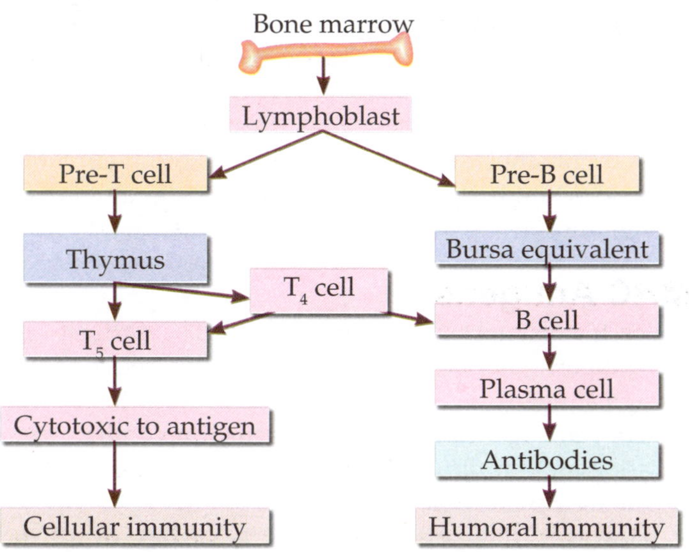

Flowchart 15.1: Development of immunity. Note, helper cell (T4 cell) induces both cellular and humoral immunity.

Clinical Note 15.1

Lymphadenopathy & splenomegaly indicates infections or pathology: Lymph nodes draining a particular area get enlarged (lymphadenopathy) in response to infection or inflammation in that area. For example, axillary lymphadenopathy indicates infection, tumor or malignancy in the mammary gland. Thus, it helps in detecting the site of pathology. Splenomegaly is a common feature of lymphomas, leukemias and chronic parasitic infections like malaria and kala azar.

Development of T cells

Mechanism of Development

T cells develop in the thymus. Therefore, they are called **thymus-dependent cell** or T cell.

- The **Pre-T cells** or precursor cells migrate to thymus in response to chemotactic signals that are periodically emitted from the thymus.
- **β_2-microglobulin** is a putative chemoattractant for pre-T cells.
- The **epithelial cells, macrophages and interdigitating cells** in thymus are rich in MHC class II antigens. They help in the differentiation of pre-T cells into T cells.
- Especially, epithelial cells in the peripheral areas of cortex called **thymic nurse cells** secrete IL-7, which supports proliferation of pre-T cells and their differentiation into **T cells.**
- As T cells mature they migrate to the medulla, and mature T cells migrate **into the lymph nodes, spleen, bone marrow**, other tissues and blood.

Changes during Development

During their processing (differentiation and proliferation) in the thymus, they undergo **two major changes** that confer on them the ability to recognize and kill the antigens.

1. **Formation of specific receptors on T cells:** The receptors to recognize the antigen are formed on T cell surface (Fig. 15.4A). These are called **T cell receptors** (TCR).
   - There are **four types** of polypeptides for TCR: α, **β, γ and** δ.
   - However, only two sets are present in TCR.
   - The combinations are either ***αβ* or** γδ**.**
   - Accordingly, TCR are either ***αβ* TCR** or γδ **TCR.**
   - The T cells with αβ TCR are called ***αβ* T cells,** and T cells with γδ TCR are called **γδ T cells.**
   - About 95% of circulating T cells are αβ T cells and 5% are γδ T cells.
2. **Synthesis of chemokines to kill antigens:** The cells acquire capacities to from various chemokines that are capable of killing invading organisms.
   - Important chemokines are **lymphotoxin and interferons.**

Types of T cells

There are **three types of T cells**: the helper T cells (T_4 cells), cytotoxic T cells (T_8 cells), and memory T cells.

Helper T cells (T_4 cells): The helper T cells are called T_4 cells as they contain CD4 protein on their cell surface.

- They are known as helper or **inducer cells** as they assist in induction of both cellular and humoral immunity.
- There are two sets of helper T cells:
  - **Type 1 helper cells** (T_H1 cells) that assist in *cellular immunity*.
  - **Type 2 helper cells** (T_H2 cells) that assist in *humoral immunity*.

Cytotoxic T cells: These are called T_8 cells as they contain **CD8 protein** on their cell membrane.

- They are called cytotoxic or **killer cells** as they kill invading organisms by inducing cytotoxicity.

Memory T cells: A small subset of T cells remains in the tissue as memory T cells.

- On subsequent exposure to similar challenges, they are activated immediately and proliferate to millions of T cells.
- Memory T cells **live a long life**, may be the entire life of the individual.
- They induce **prompt and focused** cell-mediated immune response.

Development of B Cells

The lymphocyte precursors that enter the **bursa equivalents** like fetal liver and bone marrow in mammals form B cells. They are called B cells as they develop in the bursa equivalent tissues (hence, bursa-dependent cells or B cells).

In the birds, a lymphoid tissue is present near the cloaca (the bursa of Fabricius) where pre-B cells develop into B cells.

However, in mammals there is no such bursa, but they have **bursa equivalents**.

Changes during Development

During their development in bursa equivalents, B cells acquire **receptors to recognize** antigen and **receptors for various cytokines**, and most importantly the ***genes for immunoglobulin synthesis***.

- Each clone of B cell lineage is committed for making only one specific antibody against a specific antigen.
- This is the central principle of ***clonal selection theory*** of antibody production.

Cells Formed: B lymphocytes once mature in bursa equivalents migrate to lymph nodes, bone marrow, blood and other tissues.

1. **Plasma Cells:** On specific immunologic stimulation, B cells undergo transformation to form plasma cells that produce **large quantities of antibodies**.
   - Plasma cells are not normally found in blood.
   - Antibodies formed by plasma cells kill or neutralize antigens.
2. **Memory B cells:** A small set of B cells form memory B cells.
   - The memory B cells persist for many years.
   - Induce prompt and heightened humoral immunological responses.

Antigens

Definition: Antigens are living organisms or substances that on entry into the body induce specific immunological reactions.

Properties: Antigens have **two important properties**: immunogenicity and reactivity.

1. **Immunogenicity** is the ability to provoke an immune response i. e., to stimulate the production of specific antibody or proliferation of specific T cells or both.
2. **Reactivity** is the ability of the antigen to react specifically with an antibody or a cell or both.

An antigen that possesses both the properties is defined as a **complete antigen**. An antigen that has the reactivity but lack immunogenicity is called **partial antigen** or a **hapten**.

Types: Antigens may be the entire **micro-organisms** like a bacterium or a virus, or a part of the organism like capsule of the virus, flagella of bacteria or the cell wall of the organism.

- The antigen may also be a **non-microbial substance,** such as pollen, egg white, transplanted tissue or incompatible blood cells.

Chemical Nature: Antigens are large complex molecules.

- Usually, they are **protein in nature**.
- However, nucleoproteins, glycoproteins, or large polysaccharides also behave as antigens.
- Usually, T cells respond to protein antigens, whereas B cells respond to proteins and non-protein antigens.

Antigenic Determinant: Specific portion of an antigen that triggers the immunological reaction is called antigenic determinant or **epitope**.

- Usually, an antigen possesses many antigenic determinants, each of which induces production of a specific antibody or proliferation of a specific set of T lymphocytes.

MHC Antigens

Major histocompatibility complex or MHC antigens are self-antigens that help in identifying and rejecting the foreign antigens.

- They are also called **HLA antigens** (human leucocyte associated antigens), as they were first identified on the membrane of leucocytes.
- However, they are present on the **surface of all the body cells** *except in red cells* (remember, red cells contain blood group antigens).

- Though MHC antigens are responsible for rejection of transplanted tissues, their normal function is to ***identify the foreign antigens and present them to the T cell*** for induction of cellular immunity.
- The ***recognition of an antigen*** is the first step in activation of immunological responses.

Types of MHC Antigens

There are **two types** of MHC antigens: type 1 or MHC I, and type 2 or MHC II antigens.

- **MHC I antigens** are present on the cell membranes of all body cells except red cells.
- **MHC II antigens** are present on the surface of antigen presenting cells (APCs), thymus cells and activated T cells (Fig. 15. 4B).

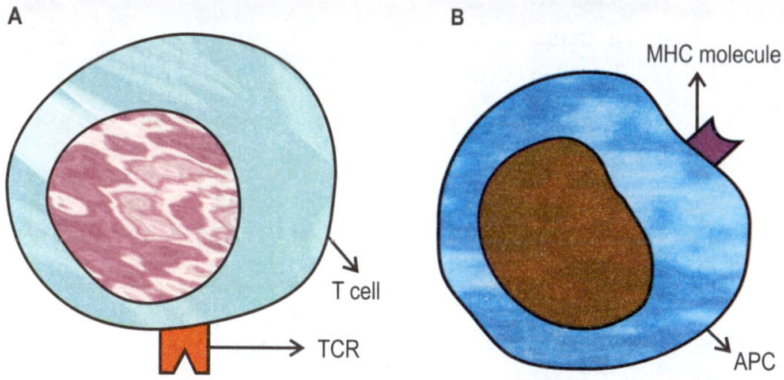

Fig. 15.4: **A:** T cell Receptors (TCR); **B:** Major histocompatibility complex (MHC) molecule expressed on the surface of antigen presenting cell (APC).

Mechanism of Action of MHC Antigens

When a peptide fragment of a self-cell protein is picked up by the MHC antigen and expressed on the surface of the APC along with MHC proteins, T cells ignore it.

- However, when the peptide fragment is of a foreign protein (antigen), **T cells recognize it** and get activated that induces immunological responses.

MECHANISM OF CELLULAR IMMUNITY

Antigen on entry into the body directly does not induce cellular immunity unless presented to the T cells by the antigen presenting cells (APCs). T cells are then activated and proliferated to destroy or eliminate the antigen. Thus, cellular immunity has **three major steps**:

1. Antigen recognition, processing, and presentation
2. Activation and proliferation of T cells
3. Elimination of the invader

Antigen Recognition, Processing & Presentation

The cells that process and present antigens to the T cells are called **antigen presenting cells** (APCs). APCs include **macrophages, dendritic cells** and **B cells**.

Steps of Antigen Presentation

There are **five major steps** in antigen presentation (Fig.15.5).

1. **Ingestion of the antigen:** Antigens are ingested by APCs by endocytosis.
2. **Digestion of the antigen and formation of vesicles:** Following phagocytosis, antigen is digested partially by the lysosomal enzymes and form phagosome within the cytoplasm of APCs.
   - The *phagosomal vesicles* contain peptide fragments of antigens.
   - Simultaneously, MHC II molecules are formed in the cell (*MHC vesicles*).
3. **Fusion of vesicles:** The phagosomal vesicles containing peptide fragments of antigen combine with the vesicles containing MHC II molecules.
   - These two vesicles merge to **form single vesicle**.
4. **Binding of peptide fragments with MHC II molecules:** Following fusion of vesicles, antigen fragments bind with MHC II molecules.
   - The fused vesicles containing MHC II and antigen fragments (Ag -MHC complex) **undergo exocytosis**.
5. **Expression of MHC-Ag complex on the membrane of APC:** During the process of exocytosis, the MHC-Ag complex is **incorporated into the cell membrane** of APC.
   - When APC containing this MHC-Ag complex comes in contact with a particular T cell, the complex **attaches with T-cell receptor** (Fig.15.6).
   - Consequently, the T cell gets activated that triggers cellular immunity.

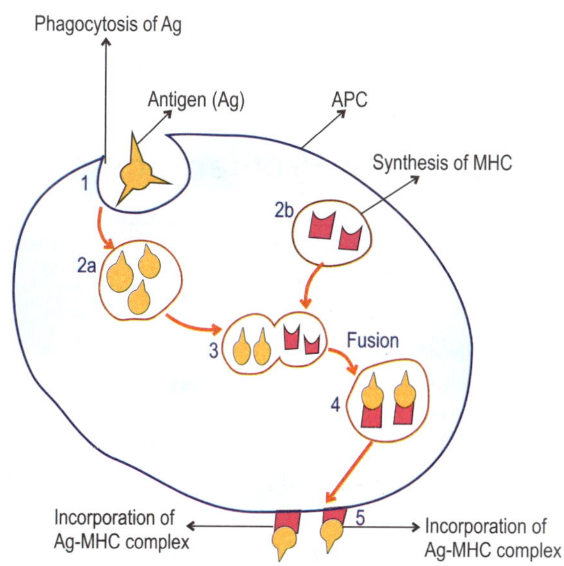

Fig. 15.5: Steps of antigen processing and presentation by antigen presenting cell (APC). **1:** Phagocytosis of antigen (Ag); **2a:** Partial digestion of Ag into its peptide fragments in the vesicle; **2b:** Synthesis of MHC-II molecule; **3:** Fusion of vesicles containing Ag fragments and MHC molecules; **4:** Single vesicle containing antigen fragments attached to MHC molecules; **5:** Incorporation of MHC-Ag complex on the membrane of APC during exocytosis.

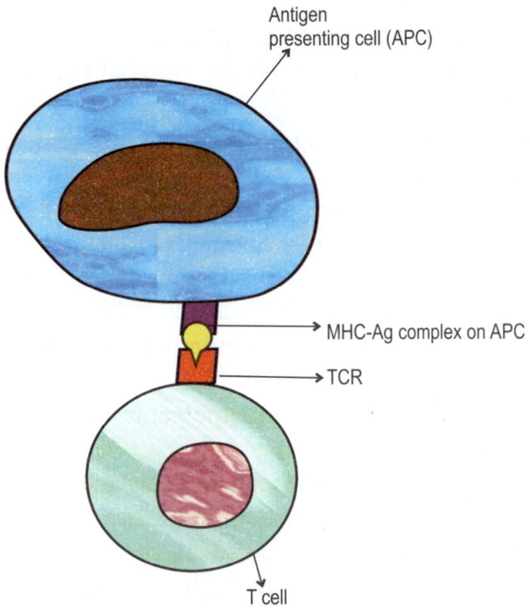

Fig. 15.6: Recognition of antigen by T cell. Note, MHC-Antigen complex attaches with T cell receptor for recognition of the antigen and induction of immunity.

Immunologic Synapse: Antigen presenting cell (APC) contacts T cell. T cell receptors are surrounded by **adhesion molecules**. These protein molecules on surface of T cells bind to APC when the two cells transiently join. The junction, i.e., the space between the T cell and APC is called immunologic synapse.

- The activity at this synapse **permits the T cell activation** to occur.
- It is now generally accepted that **two signals** are necessary to produce activation.

1. One is produced by the ***binding of the digested antigen to the T cell receptor***.
2. The other is produced by the ***joining of the surrounding proteins in the synapse***.
   - If the first signal occurs but the second does not, the T cell is inactivated and becomes unresponsive.

Activation and Proliferation of T cells

Activated T cell undergoes differentiation and proliferation into the **effector T cells** (Fig. 15.7).

Activation of T cells: When TCRs come in contact with MHC-Ag complex located on the surface of the APCs, T cells are activated. This is the first step in induction of cellular immunity.

Proliferation and differentiation of T cells: The activated T cells with proper **co-stimulation by IL_2** released from T_H1 cells undergo proliferation and differentiation into **two sets of T cells**: cytotoxic T cells, and memory T cells.

- The **cytotoxic T cells** are also called T_8 cells or killer T cells as they kill and eliminate the microbes.
- The **memory T cells** are programmed to recognize the original invading antigen in future, when the body is re-exposed to the similar antigens.

Elimination of the Invader

The cytotoxic T cells kill the invading microbes by following **three major mechanisms**.

1. **Cytolysis:** Killer cells synthesize and secrete perforins and incorporate them into the membranes of the invading organisms.
   - **Perforins** are water channels that freely allow water to enter the microorganism along the osmotic gradient.
   - The invading cell swells and finally undergoes **osmotic lysis**.
2. **Release of lymphotoxin:** Activated T cells secrete lymphotoxins that kill the microbes.
   - **Tumor necrosis factor** (TNF-β) is a known lymphotoxin.
3. **By interferons:** Killer cells secrete **gamma-interferon** (γ-IFN) that is mainly antiviral. γ-IFN promotes phagocytic activity of neutrophils and macrophages by opsonization.

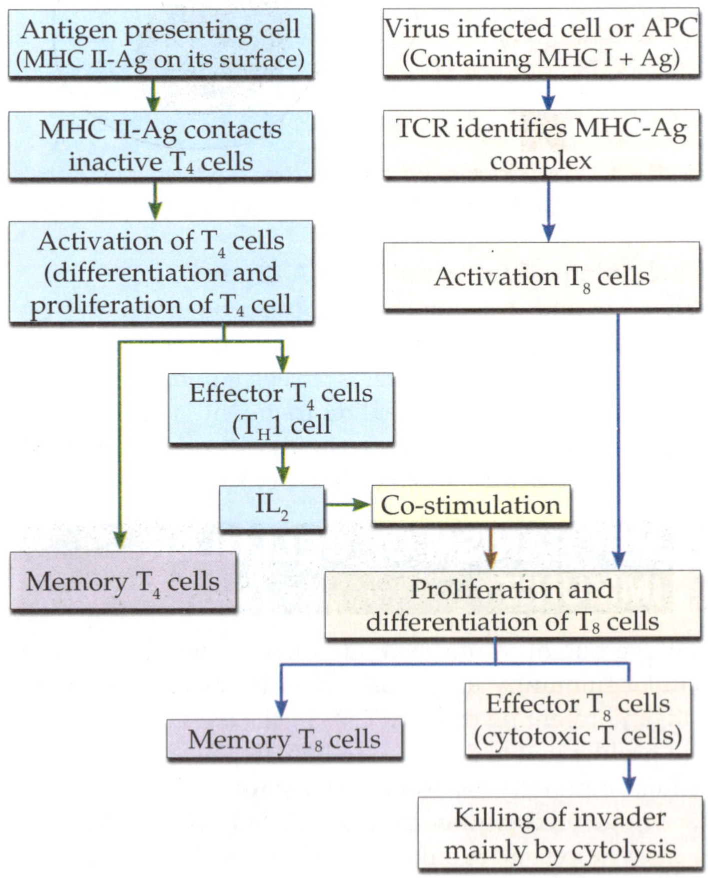

Fig. 15.7: Mechanism of cellular immunity.

Cellular immunity is activated mainly against **intracellular pathogens and tumor cells**, as in:

1. Viral infections
2. Fungal infections
3. Tumor cells, especially cancer cells
4. Transplanted cells

5. Chronic bacterial infections like tuberculosis, brucellosis, etc.
6. Parasitic infections

MECHANISM OF HUMORAL IMMUNITY

Humoral immunity is mediated by **antibodies that are produced by plasma cells.** Plasma cells are normally not present in the blood. In response to an antigen, B cells are activated and differentiated into plasma cells.

Steps of Humoral Immunity

Activation of humoral immunity involves six steps (Fig. 15.8):

1. Presentation of antigen
2. Activation of B cells
3. Differentiation of B cells into plasma cells
4. Proliferation of plasma cells and antibody production
5. Killing of the invaders by antibodies that include activation of complement system
6. Formation of memory B cells and subsequent immunological responses

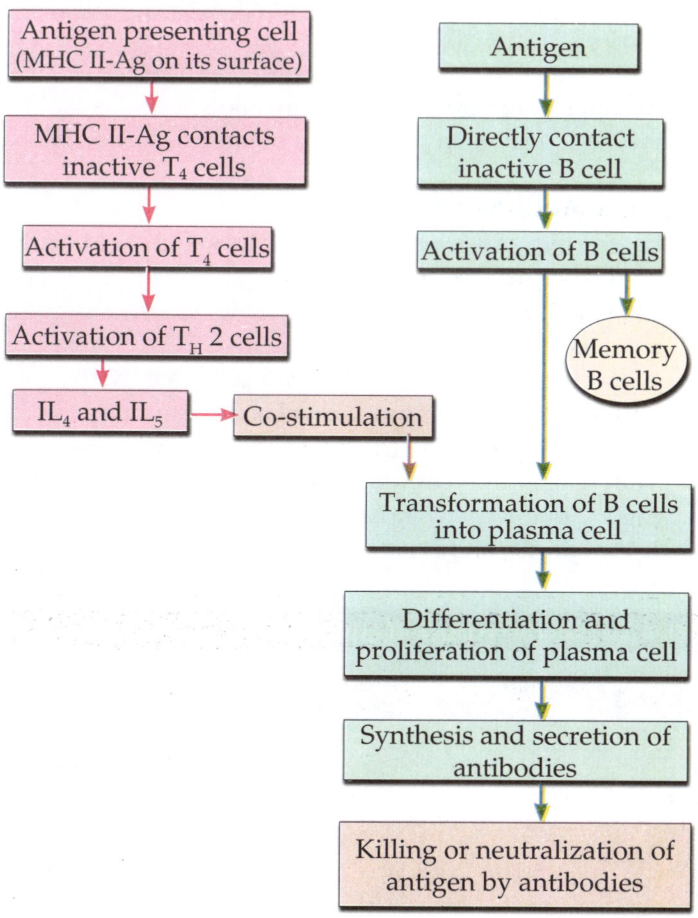

Fig. 15.8: Mechanism of humoral immunity.

Presentation of Antigen

As **B cells themselves are APCs**, antigen presentation through other APCs is not a must for induction of humoral immunity. However, MHC-Ag complex on an APC can activate B cells.

Activation of B Cells

When an antigen binds directly to the receptors present on the surface of the B cells, the B cells are activated.

- B cells are also activated when they come in contact with MHC-Ag complex presented by other APCs.
- This process is accentuated by the **co-stimulation by IL-4 and IL-5** secreted from T_H2 cells.

Differentiation of B cells into Plasma Cells

The activated B cell **enlarges in size** and undergoes complete transformation to become **plasma cell.**

- Plasma cell has more cytoplasm containing numerous rough endoplasmic reticulums.
- The enlarged B cell appears almost like a lymphoblast. Therefore, this differentiation is also called as **blast transformation.**
- **Co-stimulation by T_H2 cells** facilitates the process of transformation.

Proliferation of Plasma Cells and Antibody Production

Plasma cells then undergo proliferation to form millions of plasma cells.

- They **secrete large quantity of antibodies.**
- A specific antigen stimulates activation of specific B cells that undergo proliferation of a **selective clone** of plasma cell. This is called **clonal selection** of plasma cell.
- Specific clone of plasma cells produces specific antibodies.

Killing of the Invaders

Antibodies attack antigens and destroy them by following mechanisms.

1. **Neutralizing antigen:** Antibodies neutralize the antigens. For example, antigens detoxify the bacterial toxins and prevent them to induce immunological reactions.
2. **Immobilization of microbes:** Antibodies prevent the motility of bacteria thereby inhibit their spread to the surrounding tissue.
3. **Activation of complement system:** Antibodies (antigen-antibody complex) activate the **classical pathway of complement system** by activating C1 and complements kill organisms.
4. **Precipitation of antigens:** Antibodies cause agglutination and precipitation of antigens.
   - By this mechanism, soluble antigens become insoluble.

- Insoluble antigens are easily phagocytosed by phagocytic cells.

5. **Facilitation of phagocytosis:** Antibodies enhance phagocytosis by opsonizing the antigen.
   - Opsonization is the process by which microbes or antigens are made tasty to phagocytes for ingestion by coating antigen with **opsonins like antibody, complement proteins** etc.
6. **Provide immunity to newborns:** IgG antibody can easily cross placenta and enter fetal circulation from the maternal blood. Thus, it provides immunity to newborns. IgA antibody from the maternal milk also provides immunity to the newborn.

Formation of Memory B cells and Subsequent Immunological Responses

A small subset of activated B cells differentiates into **memory B cells**.

- Memory B cells respond quickly and vigorously to the same antigens on subsequent exposures.
- The immunological responses on second and subsequent exposures to antigen are more in intensity and duration than on first exposure.
- This is called **secondary immunological response**.
- These memory B cells live a longer life, may be the life of the individual.

Types of Humoral Immune Responses

There are **two types** of immune responses: the primary response and the secondary response.

Primary Response

When antigen enters the body first time, the immune response induced is called primary response.

- The **antibodies are formed slowly** with a latent period of about *four days to four weeks*.
- The concentration of antibodies rises gradually and attains a **smaller peak** (Fig. 15.9).
- Though IgM and IgG antibodies contribute to the primary response, the response is **mainly due to IgM**.
- Also, antibody titer in primary response returns back to normal level within few days to weeks.

Secondary Response

When the same antigen enters the body for the second time, the immune response triggered is the secondary response.

- It occurs **rapidly and intensely**, which is due to the **immunological memory**. Antibodies are formed rapidly.
- Therefore, concentration of antibody rises fast (**fast rising slope**), reaches a **greater peak**, **falls very slowly** and usually **never returns back to normal**.
- The antibodies in the secondary response are primarily of **IgG type**.

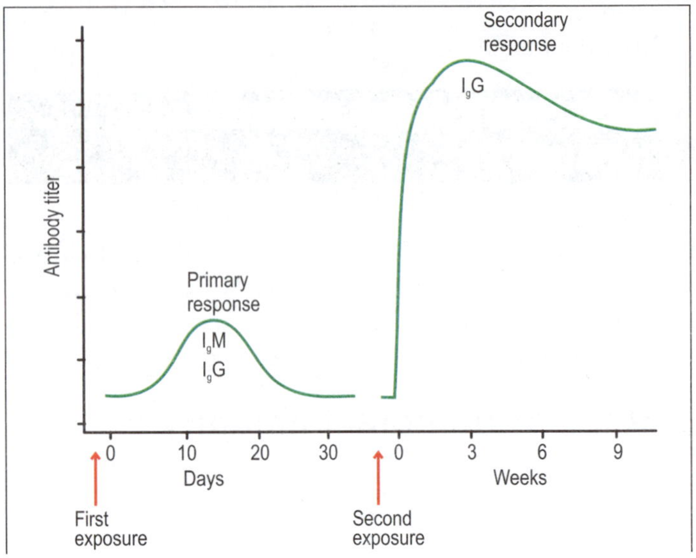

Fig. 15.9: Primary and secondary immunological responses.

Antibodies

Antibodies are **immunoglobulins** (Ig).

- Ig binds specifically with the **antigenic determinant** of the antigen. This binding triggers the production of further antibodies.
- Binding of antigen with Ig is like the key fitting into the lock.
- There are specific antigen receptors on B cells.
- Binding of specific antigen with the specific receptor on B cell, results in **production of specific antibody**.

Types of Antibodies

There are **five types of antibodies**: IgG, IgA, IgM, IgD, and IgE (summarized in Table 15.3).

- They are produced in response to specific stimuli (specific antigens).
- A specific clone of B cells that are activated by specific antigenic stimulus produce specific antibody, i. e. monoclonal antibody (details, given below).
- The concentration of **IgG in plasma is maximum** (1000 mg%), followed by IgA (200 mg%), IgM (120 mg%), IgD (3 mg%), and IgE (0.05 mg%).

Table 15.3 | Characteristics of antibodies.

Characteristics	IgG	IgA	IgM	IgD	IgE
1. Structure	Monomer	Monomer	Pentamer with	Monomer	Monomer
2. Heavy chain	$\gamma_1, \gamma_2, \gamma_3, \gamma_4$	α_1, α_2	μ	δ	ε
3. Additional chain	Nil	J, SC	J	Nil	Nil
4. Molecular weight	150	160 – 385	900	180	190

Table 15.33: Contd...					
5. Plasma level (mg%)	1000	200	120	03	02
6. Half-life (days)	21	06	05	03	02
7. Complement activation	Yes	Yes	Yes	No	No
8. Transfer through placenta	Yes	No	No	No	No

Functions of Antibodies

Different antibodies play different role in immunological responses.

IgG: **Complement fixation** by classical pathway
IgA: Localized **protection in body secretions** like tear, salivary and intestinal secretions, etc.; complement fixation by alternate pathway
IgM: Complement fixation by classical pathway
IgD: **Antigen recognition** by B cells
IgE: **Histamine release** from mast cells and basophils; also has reagin activity

COMPLEMENT SYSTEM

There is a **group of plasma proteins** designated as complement proteins as they **complement the effects of antibodies** in destroying antigen. These proteins constitute the complement system.

- Though there are more than 30 complement proteins, eleven are categorized in this system and are designated as **C1–C9**.
- C1 is further divided into **C1q, C1r, and C1s** (thus, total is 11).
- Complement proteins are normally present in the *inactive form*. Once activated, they exert their immunological and inflammatory actions and boost the humoral immune mechanism.

Mechanisms of Activation

There are **three mechanisms** of complement activation: classical pathway, alternative pathway and mannose-binding lectin pathway.

Classical Pathway

In this process, **C1 binds with immunoglobulin** attached to an antigen. This binding triggers a sequence of events that **activates other complement proteins**.

- This is similar enzyme cascade pathway of blood coagulation in which one activated protein activates the other protein (Fig. 15.10).
- Once, antigen-antibody complex activates C1, activated C1 (C1a) activates C2 and C4.
- Activated C2 and C4 (C4b, and C2a) activates C5, which (C5a) in turn activates C6, C7, C8, and C9.
- These activated complement proteins kill microorganisms and facilitate inflammation by following mechanisms:

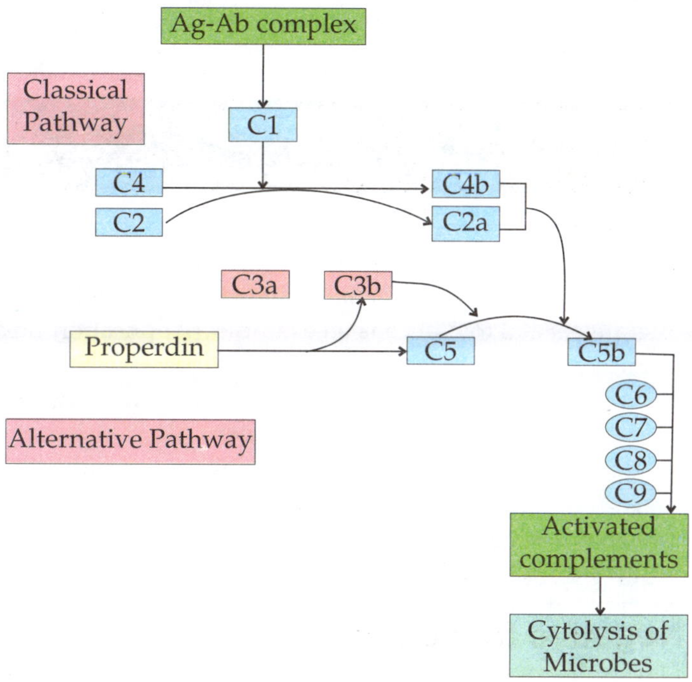

Fig. 15.10: Activation of complement system.

1. **C3a, C4a, and C5a: Promote phagocytosis** by facilitating chemotaxis, releasing histamine from mast cells, and causing arteriolar dilation.
2. **C3b: Promote opsonization** (makes the bacteria tasty to the phagocytes).
3. **C5b, C6, C7, C8, and C9:** Cause **cytolysis** of the microbes.
   - The activated complements incorporate **perforins** (pore-forming molecules) into the membranes of microbes.
   - This results in transport of ions and water into the microbes through the pores, which finally result in **osmotic lysis** of microbes.

Alternative Pathway

This is also called **properdin pathway** as the key protein in the plasma for this pathway is the **properdin**.

- In this system, a circulating protein called **factor-1**, recognizes the polysaccharide unit present on the surface of microorganisms (but not in the normal mammalian cells).
- The interaction of factor-1 with the polysaccharide on microbes triggers a reaction that activates C3 and C5.
- Once C3 is activated, it activates other complement proteins (Fig. 15.10).

Mannose-Binding Lectin Pathway

The plasma protein lectin binds with **mannose group on the surface** of bacteria, which activates complement proteins.

The complement system activates B cell, and thus serves as the link between innate and acquired immunity. Following apoptosis, complement proteins help in disposing the debris.

MECHNISMS OF SELF-RECOGNITION (Immunological Tolerance)

Self-recognition is the process by which own MHC proteins **do not recognize self-antigens** (identify only foreign antigens). This is due to the mechanism of **immunological tolerance.** Fetal tolerance is an example. (Application Box 15.2).

- Immunological tolerance is defined as **unresponsiveness of the individual to an antigen**.
- Immunological tolerance to self-antigen provides the physiological basis for self-recognition.
- Development of immunological tolerance is based on the process of negative and positive selections.

Negative Selection

During the process of development of T cells in thymus, cells with TCR that recognize peptide fragments of self proteins are eliminated while cells with TCR that do not recognize peptide fragments of self proteins are retained.

- This occurs either due to **deletion** (the self-reactive T cells undergo apoptosis) or **anergy** (the self-reactive T cells remain unresponsive to immunologic stimulation).

Application Box 15.2

Fetal tolerance: Though fetus that grows in the mother's uterus is **genetically a different** organ (fetal graft) and foreign tissue immunologically, is not rejected during pregnancy like rejection of a transplanted organ. This is an example of **immunological tolerance**, which is due to four mechanisms:

1. During the formation of placenta, trophoblast cells that separate the mother and fetus **do not express MHC I and II antigens**, and therefore, loose their immunogenicity. Instead, placenta expresses, HLA-G a nonpolymorphic antigen. Therefore, antibodies against fetal tissue do not develop.
2. Placenta has **Fas ligand** on its surface which attaches to the T cells. This attachment causes apoptosis of T cells destined to react against fetal tissue.
3. **Alpha fetoprotein** (AFP) that is formed during fetal development causes suppression of T and B cells that react against fetal graft.
4. High level of progesterone during pregnancy is believed to suppress immunity against fetal tissue.
5. Maternal tissue fails to recognize HLA antigen of trophoblastic cells as the entire trophoblastic mass is covered by a coat of fibrinoid material, known as ***Nitabuch's layer***. The fibrinoid material of this layer, probably due to its negatively charges, repels the lymphocytes.

Clonal Deletion: During embryonic life, the clone of T cell and B cells containing receptors that **react against self-antigens are selectively removed** from the body during their thymic and bursal development, so that they are ***not available in postnatal life*** to react against self antigens.

- These self reactive lymphocytes undergo apoptosis.

Clonal Anergy: The self-reactive clone of T and B cells those remain alive during post-natal life lose the capacity to be activated in response to self-antigens.

- This is because they **lose the activity of their receptors and lymphokine systems** to react against self antigens, which may be due to the **immune suppression** of these cells by body's self regulating systems.
- This state of idleness is called clonal anergy.

Positive Selection

Immunological tolerance is also achieved by positive selection in which the T cells that are **capable of recognizing self-MHC molecules** during their thymic development **survive** and those that do not recognize undergo apoptosis.

- The T cells recognize MHC- self antigen complex as the self antigens and do not react against them.

APPLIED PHYSIOLOGY

Organ Transplantation

Tissue or organ transplantation involves replacement of an injured or diseased tissue or organ by a new tissue or organ. Commonly transplanted organs are skin, kidney, bone and liver.

- The transplanted tissue is rejected as the recipient develops an immune response against the transplanted organ, which is a foreign tissue to him.
- **Transplant rejection** is due to the **activation of cellular immunity** against the transplanted tissue.
- The rapidity at which the organ is rejected depends on degree of matching of MHC antigen (HLA antigen) of donor with the HLA antigen of the recipients.

Types of Transplants

1. **Autograft:** Transplantation of a tissue from **one part of the body to another part** of the same individual is called autograft.
    - The best example is the skin graft.
    - Autograft is **never rejected**.
2. **Isograft:** Transplantation of organs between the **genetically identical individuals**.
    - The best example is the transplantation of *tissues from the identical twin*.
    - Isograft is also **not rejected**.
3. **Allograft:** This is the transplantation of organs between **individuals of the same species**, but with different

genetic background.
- The example is transplantation from an individual other than identical twin.
- Allograft is **rejected**.

4. **Xenograft:** This is a transplant from or **between different species**.
   - For example, transplantation of organ between animal and man.
   - Commonly used xenograft is the physiological dressing using animal skin over severe burn surfaces.
   - Xenograft is rejected fast.

Prevention of Transplant Rejection

A number of treatments are available to prevent rejection of a transplanted organ. These are:

1. **Immunosuppressive drugs:** The commonly used drug is **azathioprine**.
   - This is a purine antimetabolite that kills T lymphocytes.
   - Individual on azathioprine is ***susceptible to severe infection*** because of immunosuppression.
2. **Glucocorticoid therapy:** Glucocorticoids have strong immunosuppressive activity.
   - They inhibit proliferation of cytotoxic T cells by **inhibiting the production of interleukin 2** (IL-2) from T_4 cells.
3. **Antilymphocyte globulins:** These are monoclonal antibodies produced against T lymphocytes. They **inhibit T cell activity**.
4. **Antibiotics:** Antibiotics usually used for the prevention of transplant rejection are **cyclosporine, tacrolimus and rapamycin.**
   - ***Cyclosporine*** is a fungal extract and ***tacrolimus*** is an antibiotic of fungal origin.
   - They **prevent T cells** from *transcribing the IL-2 gene* by preventing dephosphorylation of NF-AT, a transcription factor.
   - ***Rapamycin*** prevents activation of IL-2 receptor from producing T cell differentiation and proliferation.
5. **Monoclonal antibodies:** They prevent activation and proliferation of T cells.

Monoclonal Antibodies

Monoclonal antibodies are antibodies prepared from a **single clone of B or plasma cells**. They are obtained by **fusing a B cell with a tumor cell** that produces antibodies in large quantity.

Method of Production

An animal is immunized by injecting a particular antigen.

- The animal is then sacrificed and the **antibody producing cells** are extracted from the spleen of the animal.
- The antibody producing cells are fused to the **myeloma cells** that are obtained from B lymphocyte tumor in a patient suffering from multiple myeloma.
- Fusion of myeloma cell with antibody producing cell results in formation of a **hybridoma** which grows to become an antibody producing tumor.
- The fused cells (hybridoma cells) are separated, and **every single cell is allowed to form a clone** of cells.
- The single clone of hybridoma cells **produce specific antibody** consisting of heavy or light chains of spleen cell or of myeloma cells. These are called monoclonal antibodies.

Uses of Monoclonal Antibody

Monoclonal antibodies are used in a wide variety clinical spectrum.

1. For measurement of drug level in patient's blood.
2. Diagnosis of allergic diseases, hepatitis, sexually transmitted diseases etc.
3. Detection of cancer in the early stage.
4. Preparation of vaccines.
5. Prevention of transplant rejection.
6. Treatment of autoimmune diseases.

Immunological Disorders

Allergy

This is a **hyper-reactive response** of the body to an antigen which is usually tolerated by others. There are **two types** of allergies: the ***local allergy*** such as urticaria and the ***systemic allergy*** (anaphylaxis).

Hypersensitivity Reactions

There are **four types** of hypersensitivity reactions:

Type I Reaction or Anaphylaxis: In this reaction, the individual **over-reacts to a sensitized allergen**.

- The antigen-antibody complexes release **histamine and slow-releasing substance A** from mast cells and basophils.
- Histamine produces bradycardia, decreased cardiac output and rapid vasodilation leading to acute hypotension, often called as **anaphylactic shock**.
- It is an *acute medical emergency* that requires prompt treatment.

Type II Reaction or Cytotoxic Reaction: This reaction is caused by IgG or IgM antibody, which is directed ***against antigen present on person's red cells***.

- Incompatible blood transfusions, hemolytic diseases of newborn and autoimmune hemolytic anemias are examples.

Type III Reaction or Immune Complex Disease: In this reaction, the antigen and antibodies form complexes that escape phagocytosis.

- These **immune complexes** *are deposited on the basement membrane* of the blood vessels and induce inflammation.
- Examples are glomerulonephritis, systemic lupus erythematosus (SLE) and rheumatoid arthritis.

Type IV Reaction or Delayed Hypersensitivity Reactions: These reactions are **mediated by macrophages** that are activated by T cells.

- Allergens (antigens) are taken up by APCs and presented to T cell.
- This causes proliferation of T cells, some of which migrate to the location of allergen entry into the body.
- There, they secrete cytokines and induce inflammatory reactions.
- The best example is the **skin test for tuberculosis**.

Autoimmune Diseases

Normally, the immune system does not react against self-proteins. In some conditions, immune system **fails to neglect self-antigens** and triggers immune reaction against body's own antigens. This results in autoimmune diseases.

- This may be due to the **persistence of T cells or B cells** *that are active against self-antigens*.
- Especially, *failure of the process* that removes antibodies against self-antigens leads to formation of **autoantibodies**.
- Autoantibodies may **eliminate the receptors** or **activate the receptors**.
  - Example of destruction of receptors is **myasthenia gravis**, in which antibodies formed against nicotinic cholinergic receptors destroy the receptors.
  - Example of activation of receptors is **Grave's disease**, in which antibodies formed against TSH receptors stimulate receptors.

Immunodeficiency States

Immunodeficiency diseases are classified into **two categories**: congenital or primary and acquired or secondary.

Congenital Immunodeficiency Syndromes: There are list of diseases in which severe combined immunodeficiency (SCID) occurs due to defects in development in either cellular or humoral immunity.

Acquired Immunodeficiency Syndrome (AIDS): AIDS occurs due to infection by **human immunodeficiency virus** (HIV).

- HIV is a **retrovirus** that binds to CD4 protein on the surface of helper cells and **decreases number of circulating T_4 cells**.
- Helper cells are required for induction of both cellular and humoral immunities. Thus, HIV infection causes **severe immunodeficiency** state that predisposes the individual to **all type of serious infections and malignancies.**
- The disease is **transmitted by** blood, semen, or vaginal secretions or through breast feeding. The usual mode of transmission is **sexual contact.**
- The usual **clinical features** are fever, lymphadenopathy, sore throat, diarrhea and weight loss.
- Oral candidiasis, anogenital herpes simplex infection, *Pneumocystiis carinii* pneumonia, cryptococcus meningitis and cytomegalovirus infections are common.
- Finally, the patient dies due to **secondary infection or cancer**. The commonest malignancy is ***Kaposi's sarcoma***.

Cytokines PY3.1

Cytokines or **immunokines** are a group of hormone-like substances that usually act in a **paracrine fashion** to control immunological responses.

- They are secreted from activated lymphocytes, macrophages, endothelial cells, glial cells, etc.
- They are **classified into**: interleukins, tumor necrosis factors (TNF), interferons, transforming growth factors (TGF) and GM-CSF.

Interleukins

Important interleukins are **IL-1 to IL-13**.

- They are produced by macrophages, activated T cells, APCs, NK cells, mast cells and other somatic cells.
- Their functions are summarized in Table 15.4.
- IL-1 is called **endogenous pyrogen** as it produces fever and induces anorexia.

Tumor Necrosis Factors (TNF)

There are **two types** of TNFs: TNF-α and TNF-β.

- **TNF-α** is produced by activated macrophages. It acts like interleukin-1.
- **TNF-β** is produced by activated type 1 helper cells. The physiological effects are same as TNF-α.

Interferons (IFN)

There are **three types** of IFNs: IFN-α, IFN- β, and IFN-γ.

IFN-α: This is produced by macrophages, neutrophils, and other somatic cells.

- It prevents growth of viruses (antiviral).
- It also activates macrophages and NK cells, and induces the expression of type I MHC on all somatic cells.

IFN- β: Same as IFN-α.

IFN-γ: Secreted by activated type 1 helper cells and NK cells.

- It induces expression of MHC I on all somatic cells and MHC II on APCs.
- It activates macrophages, neutrophils and NK cells.
- It stimulates cellular immunity. It is also antiviral.

GM-CSF

Functions of GM-CSF have been discussed in 'leucopoiesis'.

Table 15.4 | Source and important functions of common cytokines.

Cytokines	Source	Functions
IL1	Macrophage & monocyte	Activation of cellular immunity, activation of 1 inflammation, and hemopoiesis.
IL2	T_H1 cells	Stimulates cellular immunity, NK cells and macrophages.
IL3	T cell	Activates hemopoiesis
IL4	T_H2 cells, mast cells, basophils &	Stimulates humoral immunity, activates monocytes, eosinophils, IgE class switching
IL5	T_H2 cells, mast cells & eosinophils	Stimulates eosinophil development
IL6	T_H2 cells, fibroblast & macrophages	B cell differentiation, production of acute phase proteins (ARP), activation of lymphocytes
IL 8	T cells and macrophages	Chemotaxix of neutrophils and basophils
IL11	Osteoblasts, fibroblasts	Stimulates hemopoiesis and production of ARP
IL 12	Macrophage and B cell	Stimulates synthesis of IFNγ, activates T_H1 cell
TNFα	T cell, B cells, NK cell & Macrophage	Promotes inflammation
TNFβ	B cells & T_H1 cells	Promotes inflammation
IFNα and β	Virally infected cells	Kill viruses
IFNγ	T_H1 cells, NK cells	Activation of macrophage, inhibition of T_H2 cells
TGFβ	T cell, B cells, & Mast cells	Suppresses immunity
GM-CSF	T cell, B cells, NK cell & Macrophages	Stimulates granulopoiesis & monocyte production

T_H1 cells: Type 1 helper cell; T_H2 cells: Type 2 helper cell; TNF: tumor necrosis factor; IFN: interferon; TGF: Transforming growth factor

Exam Questions

1. Describe the nonspecific defense mechanisms (innate immunity) of the body.
2. List the functions of NK cells and briefly describe the mechanism of killing by NK cell.
3. Describe the steps of inflammation as a defence mechanism of the body.
4. Describe the process of development of T cells and B cells.
5. Name antigen presenting cells (APCs). Describe the steps of antigen presentation by APCs.
6. Describe the mechanism of cellular immunity.
7. Describe the mechanism of humoral immunity.
8. Name the complement proteins. Describe the role of complement system in immunity.
9. What are the immunological responses? List the differences between them.
10. What is immunological tolerance. Describe the mechanisms of immunological tolerance.
11. Describe how transplant rejection can be prevented.
12. Describe the steps of monoclonal antibody production in the laboratory. List the uses of monoclonal antibody.

Multiple Choice Questions

1. If thymus is removed in childhood:
- A. Cellular immunity is lost, but humoral immunity will remain intact
- B. Humoral immunity is lost, butcellular immunitywill remain intact
- C. Bothcellular andhumoral immunity will remain intact
- D. Bothcellular and humoral immunity will be lost

2. Which of the following is a secondary lymphoid organ?
- A. Bone marrow
- B. Spleen
- C. Thymus
- D. Fetal liver

3. All of the following are true about plasma cell, EXCEPT:
- A. Formed from B cells
- B. T helper cell co-stimulates to form plasma cell
- C. A specific antigen stimulates a selective clone of plasma cell
- D. The specific clone of plasma cell secrets IgG, IgA, IgM, IgD, IgE

4. Autoimmune diseases are usually due to
- A. Decreased suppressor T cells
- B. Decreased memory T cells
- C. Stimulation of suppressor T cells
- D. Stimulation of memoryT cells

5. Which of the following antibodies can easily cross the placenta?
- A. IgA
- B. IgD
- C. IgG
- D. IgM

6. Which of the following transplant is least tolerated?
- A. Iso graft
- B. Allograft
- C. Autograft
- D. Xenograft

7. **All of the following complements cause cytolysis of microbes, EXCEPT:**
   A. C4a
   B. C5b
   C. C6
   D. C9
8. **Which of the following complement promote opsonisation of bacteria?**
   A. C3a
   B. C3b
   C. C7
   D. C8
9. **All of the following complements promote chemotaxis, EXCEPT:**
   A. C3a
   B. C4a
   C. C5a
   D. C5b
10. **All of the following are true for secondary response of humoral immunity, EXCEPT:**
   A. The antibodies are primarily of IgM type
   B. Occurs speedily and intensely
   C. Antibodies attain a greater concentration
   D. Antibody titre falls very slowly
11. **Which of the following statement is NOT true?**
   A. Drug allergy is caused by cytotoxic T cell
   B. Immunity is suppressed in patients on ACTH therapy
   C. Immunoglobulin A is a reagin antibody
   D. C-reactive protein level is increased in acute inflammation
12. **Which of the following statement is NOT true?**
   A. Natural immunity is non-specific to a particular micro-organism
   B. Memory T cells survive for 4 - 6 days
   C. Acquired humoral immunity is a major defence against bacterial infection
   D. Antigen –antibody complex activates complement system by classical pathway
13. **Which of the following statement is true?**
   A. Erythromycin is an immune-suppressant drug
   B. Endemic goitre is an autoimmune disorder
   C. Rejection of transplant is due to activation of complement system
   D. Glucocorticoid inhibits immunity by inhibiting production of IL2
14. **Perforins are?**
   A. Pinocytosed molecules
   B. One type of interleukins
   C. Pore forming molecules
   D. Phagocytosed molecules
15. **Which of the following is NOT an autoimmune disease?**
   A. Hashimoto's thyroiditis
   B. Insulin dependent diabetes mellitus
   C. Non-insulin dependent diabetes mellitus
   D. Mysthenia gravis
16. **Anaphylaxis reaction results from liberation of all, EXCEPT:**
   A. Bradykinin
   B. Interleukin
   C. Histamin
   D. Eosinophil chemotactic factor -A
17. **Which of the following is NOT true for NK cells?**
   A. Kill microbes by osmotic lysis
   B. The killing process is facilitated by MHC antigen
   C. Constitute 15% of total lymphocytes
   D. Kill antibody-coated viruses
18. **Which of the following cell can become antigen presenting cell in humoral immunity?**
   A. Monocyte
   B. Neutrophil
   C. T cell
   D. B cell
19. **Which of the following is NOT an antigen presenting cell?**
   A. T cell
   B. B cell
   C. Dendritic cell
   D. Macrophage
20. **Which of the following is the major T-cell population?**
   A. Memory T cell
   B. Helper T cell
   C. Suppressor T cell
   D. Cytotoxic T cell

Answers

1. D	2. B	3. D	4. A	5. C	6. D	7. A	8. B	9. D	10. A	11. C
12. B	13. D	14. C	15. C	16. B	17. B	18. D	19. A	20. B		

Chapter 16

Platelets

Learning Objectives

On completion of study of this chapter:

The student will be able to (must know):

1. Define hemostasis and list the major steps in hemostasis.
2. Name the steps of thrombopoiesis.
3. Correlate the structural modifications in platelet with their functions.
4. List the properties of platelet and give their significance.
5. Explain the role of platelet in Hemostasis.
6. List the causes of thrombocytosis and thrombocytopenia.
7. List the platelet function tests.
8. Understand common platelet dysfunctions.

The student may also be able to (desirable to know):

1. Describe the steps and the regulation of thrombopoiesis.
2. Describe the properties of platelets in relation to platelet functions.
3. Describe platelet function tests.

PY2.8

Hemostasis is defined as the process of **arrest of bleeding** while maintaining blood in a fluid state within the vascular system. The vascular injury initiates a series of events in sequence that finally forms clot at the site of injury and prevents loss of blood from the body.

Steps of Hemostasis

Hemostasis occurs in **three stages**: vasoconstriction, temporary hemostatic plug formation and blood coagulation (Fig. 16.1).

Vasoconstriction: Immediate response of blood vessel to injury is vasoconstriction.

- Contraction of vascular smooth muscle to injury is **initially a mechanical response** (stretch-induced contraction).
- Later, vasoconstriction is maintained and potentiated by **secretion of vasoconstrictor** substances from the activated platelets.

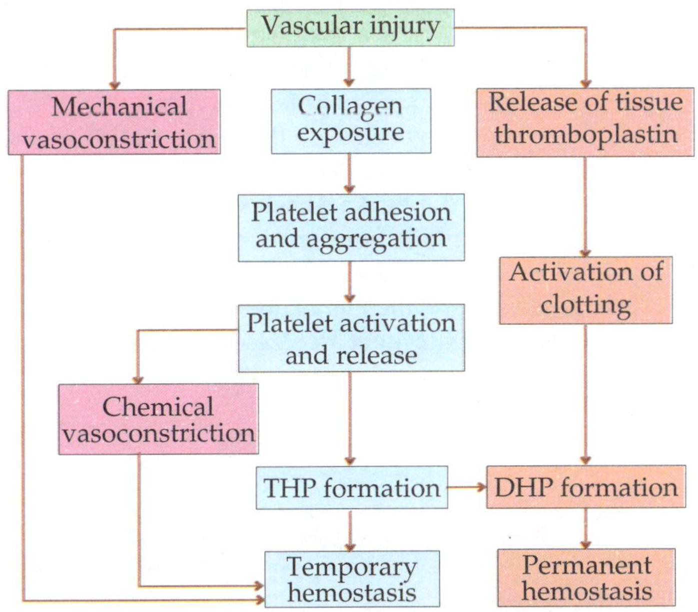

Fig. 16.1: Mechanisms of hemostasis. THP: temporary hemostatic plug; DHP: definitive hemostatic plug.

Temporary Hemostatic Plug Formation: Formation of **platelet plug** at the site of injury is called *temporary hemostatic plug*.

- This occurs due to three properties of platelets: **adhesion, aggregation, and release reaction**.
- Platelets **adhere to the injured surface** and **aggregate to each other** at the site.
- Activated platelets ***release several chemicals*** (**platelet release**) that further facilitate vasoconstriction, adhesion and aggregation.

Blood Coagulation: Immediately following injury, the **clotting mechanisms** of blood is initiated.

- This results in formation of blood clot (**definitive hemostatic plug)** at the site of injury that stops bleeding.

PY2.7

DEVELOPMENT OF PLATELETS

The development of platelets is called **thrombopoiesis** or ***thrombocytopoiesis.***

- They are anuclear fragments of **megakaryocytes**.
- Megakaryocytes are the giant cells in the bone marrow.

Stages of Development

The stages of platelet development are as follows (Flowchart 16.1):

1. Stem cells (Pluripotent stem cells, Committed stem cells and CFU-Mega)
2. Megakaryoblast
3. Megakaryocytes (Basophil megakaryocyte, granular megakaryocyte and mature megakaryocyte)
4. Platelets

Megakaryocytes: Platelets develop from myeloid stem cells that from CFU-Mega, which in turn develop into megakaryoblast (refer Fig. 8.4, Chapter 8).

- Megakaryoblast forms megakaryocytes that grow in three stages: basophil megakaryocyte, granular megakaryocyte and mature megakaryocyte.
- Matured megakaryocytes are the largest cells in bone marrow.

Features of matured megakaryocytes are:

1. These are **polyploid bone marrow cells** (polyploidy means increased amount of DNA in the nucleus). They have horse-shoe shaped large nucleus.
2. The cells are still **bigger in size** (more than 25 to 50 μm).

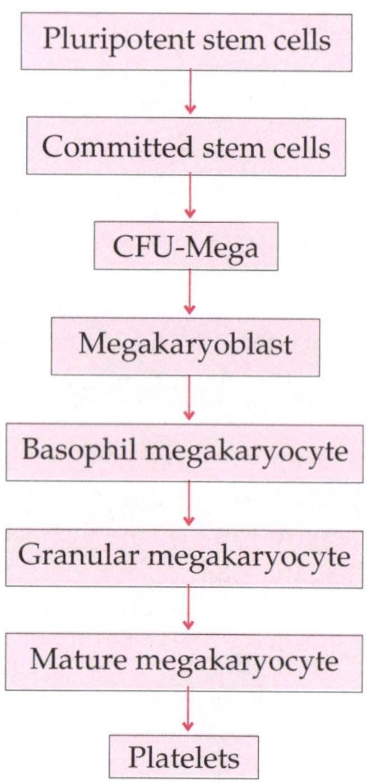

Flowchart 16.1: Stages of thrombopoiesis. CFU-Mega: colony forming unit of megakaryocyte.

3. Cytoplasm contains numerous **granules of different kinds**. ***Four types of granules*** have been described in megakaryocyte: α-granules, dense granules, lysosomal granules and myeloperoxidase granules.

Platelet formation: Megakaryocytes form platelets by pinching off bits of cytoplasm and extruding them into the circulation.

- On average, each megakaryocyte produces about 1000 to 3000 platelets.
- Normally, platelet production per day is about 35,000 to 45,000 per microliter of blood.

Regulation of Thrombopoiesis

The production and release of platelets from bone marrow remains normally constant.

- The production of platelets is **enhanced by** removal of platelets from blood (*thrombocytopheresis*) and **decreased by** transfusion of platelets.
- This indicates that a **feedback regulatory mechanism** exists for platelet production.

Thrombopoietin, interleukins and GM-CSF control thrombopoiesis.

Thrombopoietin: Thrombopoietin is produced mainly from **liver parenchymal cells**. To some extent, it is also formed in kidney.

- Though the naturally occurring thrombopoietin for medical uses is not very effective, ***commercial thrombopoietin*** have been synthesized by recombinant technology and used in thrombocytopenia.
- Thrombopoietin **stimulates differentiation and proliferation of megakaryocytes.**

Interleukin: IL-1, IL-3, IL-6 and IL-11 stimulate platelet production.

GM-CSF: GM-CSF produced by monocytes, T cells, fibroblasts and endothelial cells simulates erythropoiesis, granulopoiesis and thrombopoiesis.

Life History

Platelets have the half-life of about **4 days**.

- They survive in circulation for about 8–12 days.
- The aged platelets are removed from circulation by **reticuloendothelial cells in spleen.**
- Therefore, **platelet count increases after splenectomy** and decreases in splenomegaly.

STRUCTURE AND FUNCTIONS

Platelet Morphology

Though platelets are subcellular elements, their membrane and cytoplasmic modifications help them to effectively participate in hemostasis. They have **highly developed cytoskeletal and canalicular system** suited for their functions.

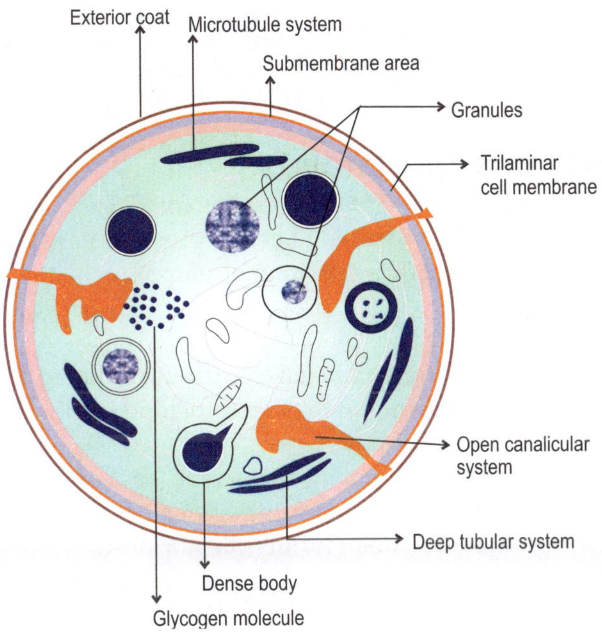

Fig. 16.2: Structure of a platelet. Note the extensively developed cytoskeletal systems, canalicular system and granules in platelet.

Dimensions

Platelets are small, anucleated, granular and spherical or oval bodies.

- Their diameter ranging from **1.5 to 3.0 μm**.
- Frequently they **change their shape** with very long and thin processes extending out from their body called as **filopodia**.

Cell Membrane

Cell membrane is covered by an **exterior glycocalyx coat** (Fig. 16.2) that contains glycoprotein receptors, glycolipids.

- The cell membrane is a **trilaminar unit** consisting of a bilayer of phospholipids in which cholesterol, glycolipids and glycoproteins are embedded.
- **Glycoproteins** aid to ***prevent adherence*** of platelets to the normal vascular endothelium.
- **Glycoprotein receptors** (GPIIb/IIIa) help in *adhesion and aggregation of platelets*.
- Platelets have receptors on their cell membrane for collagen, ADP, von Willebrand factor and fibrinogen.

Cytoskeletal Systems

Cytoskeletal systems in platelets are membrane and cytoplasmic cytoskeletal systems.

Membrane Cytoskeleton

A network of **spectrin molecules** is present in the cell membrane, which connects to the actin filaments that and membrane of open canalicular system.

- **Filamin 1** (actin binding protein) interacts with membrane glycoprotein and actin present below the membrane and connects them to the transmembrane spectrin network.
- Thus, **filamin 1 provides stability** to the membrane and ***discoid shape*** of the platelets.
- Other membrane proteins include **talin, vinculin and vimentin**.
- Membrane cytoskeleton plays important role in **platelet spreading** following their adhesion to the vascular endothelium.

Cytoplasmic Cytoskeleton

Cytoplasm contains a well-developed contractile system, which consists of an **extensive network of microtubules** and **microfilaments**.

Microtubules: There is a sub-membrane microtubular system consisting of many microtubules. Microtubules are made up of α and β tubulins. Cytosolic motors like *dynein and kinesin filaments* are also associated with microtubules. Microtubules ***provide membrane stability and support the discoid shape*** of the cell.

Microfilaments: Platelet microfilaments consist mainly of **actin molecules** that polymerize into microfilamentous bundles. Few myosin filaments are attached to actin filaments. Actin and myosin filaments constitute **contractile system** in platelets that helps to **change the shape of platelets** and discharge their granular content to the exterior through canaliculi (**cell release**).

Cellular Systems

There are two cellular systems: open canalicular system and dense tubular systems.

Open Canalicular System: There are many canaliculi in the platelets that open to the exterior.

- They form the **conduits for discharge** of contents of granules.
- This extensive open canalicular system **enhances the degree and rate of platelet release**.

Dense Tubular System: This is a **closed system of channels** formed by residual endoplasmic reticulum present close to the open canalicular system.

- This **sequesters the ionized calcium**.
- The membrane of tubular system contains ***peroxidase activity***, and the interior contains **calreticulin**, a calcium binding protein that ***helps in calcium accumulation***.
- Release of calcium from dense tubular system **facilitates platelet release**.

Cytoplasmic Organelles

Platelet contains numerous peroxisomes, mitochondria, lysosomes and granules.

Platelet Granules

Platelet granules are of two types: the alpha granules and dense granules.

Alpha Granules: There are about 50–80 alpha granules per platelet.

- They are 200 nm in diameter.
- They contain various chemicals (Table 16.1).

Dense Granules: There are about 3–8 dense granules per platelet.

- They are also called **dense bodies**.
- They have diameter of about 20–30 nm.
- They contain chemicals like serotonin, ADP, calcium, ATP etc.

Table 16.1 | Contents of platelet granules.

A. Contents of alpha granules
1. von Willebrand factor
2. Thrombospondin, β-Thromboglobulin
3. PDGF (platelet derived growth factor)
4. PAF (platelet activating factor)
5. Platelet factor 4 (platelet phospholipid)
6. Fibronectin, plasminogen, platelet fibrinogen
7. α_2-Plasmin inhibitor, α_1-Protease inhibitor
8. Proaccelerin, coagulation factors V and XI
9. Tissue plasminogen activator (tPA)
B. Contents of dense granules
1. Serotonin
2. ADP, Calcium, ATP
3. Pyrophosphate

Properties of Platelets

Platelets have **three unique properties**: adhesion, aggregation, and activation & release.

Adhesion

Platelets easily adhere to the **damaged vascular endothelium**. This is called **platelet adhesion**.

- Platelets have the tendency to stick to the **exposed collagen** of the injured vessel wall (Fig. 16.3A).
- Adhesion is facilitated by **von Willebrand factor**.
- However, platelets **do not adhere** to the *normal vessel wall*.

Aggregation

Platelets not only stick to the injured vessel wall but also to each other.

- The property of platelets to **stick to each other** is called platelet aggregation (Fig. 16.3B).
- **Fibrinogen, thrombin, GPIIb/IIIa and PAF** promote platelet aggregation.

Activation and Release

Platelets are activated when they bind to collagen or to each other.

- The activation is **facilitated by thrombin and ADP.**
- The activated platelets **change their shape** and discharge their granular contents.
- The ***discharge of the granular content*** to the exterior through open canalicular system is called **platelet release** (or secretion).
- This is also called **release reaction**, which is facilitated by chemicals released from platelet granules.

Functions of Platelets

Important functions of platelets are as follows:

1. **Temporary hemostasis:** Platelets prevent bleeding by forming plugs at the site of injury (temporary hemostatic plug). Platelets also promote vasoconstriction by producing serotonin that helps in hemostasis.
2. **Blood coagulation:** Platelets contribute to blood coagulation by releasing platelet factor 4, and synthesizing clotting factor V and XI.
3. **Clot retraction:** Platelets promote clot retraction, which is essential for stabilization of clot.
4. **Thrombolysis:** Platelet influences fibrinolysis.
5. **Phagocytosis:** Platelets phagocyte smaller molecules like immune complexes and viruses.
6. **Storage and transport:** Platelets synthesize, secrete and transport many chemical substances as listed in Table 13.1.

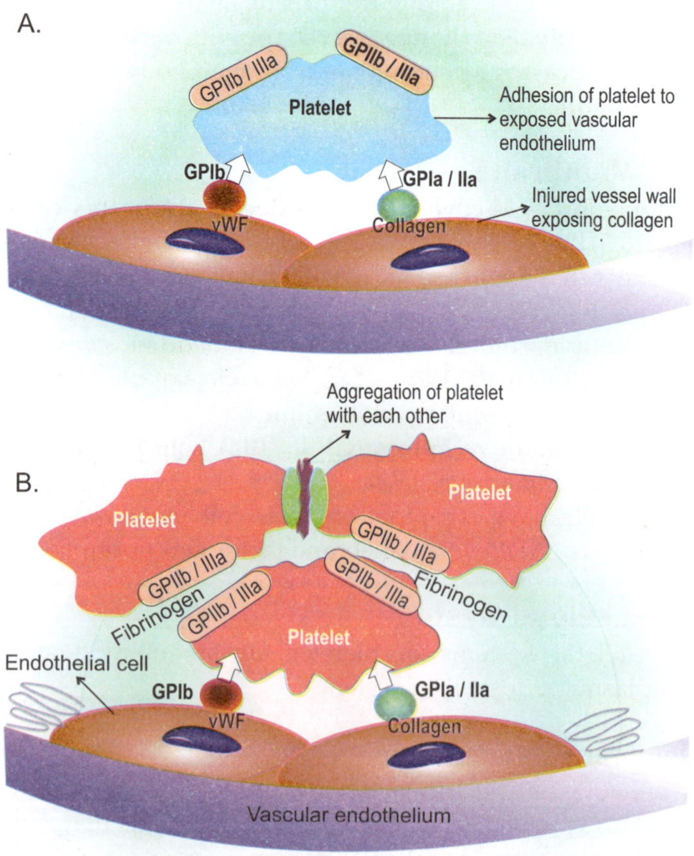

Fig. 16.3: Platelet adhesion to injured vascular endothelium **(A)**; and aggregation of platelet to each other **(B)**. Note exposed collagen and von Willebrand factor (vWF) facilitate adhesion, and Fibrinogen, GPIIb/IIIa facilitate aggregation.

7. **Vascular growth:** Platelets help in growth of vascular endothelium by secreting platelet–derived growth factor (**PDGF**). PDGF is also produced by macrophages and endothelial cells. PDGF is synthesized in three forms: PDGF-AA, PDGF-BB and PDGF-AB (containing either of the two polypeptide chains A or B).

Normal Count & Variations PY2.13

Normal count of platelet is **1.5–4 lakhs/mm³** of blood.

Thrombocytopenia: Thrombocytopenia is defined as the platelet count **less than 1.5 lakhs/mm³** of blood.

- But, bleeding occurs when platelet count decreases below 40,000/mm³ of blood. Therefore, platelet count below 40,000/mm³ of blood is called **critical count**.
- However, **severe internal bleeding** occurs when count is **below 10,000/mm³ of blood.**
- Thrombocytopenia commonly occurs in ITP, aplastic anemia, hypersplenism, acute leukemia, cytotoxic chemotherapy and radiation (Table 16.2).
- About 70% of platelets released from bone marrow are present in circulation and 30% are **sequestered in spleen**.
- Therefore, **splenectomy** usually causes ***thrombocytosis*** and **hypersplenism** invariably causes ***thrombocytopenia***.

Thrombocytosis: Thrombocytosis commonly occurs in polycythemia vera, chronic myeloid leukemia, iron deficiency anemia, splenectomy, chronic infection, surgery and following acute hemorrhage.

Table 16.2 | Variations in platelet count.

A. Thrombocytosis
1. Essential thrombocythemia
2. Other **meyloproliferative diseases** like polycythemia rubra vera, CML etc.
3. Familial thrombocytosis
4. Acute blood loss
5. **Iron deficiency**
6. **After splenectomy**
7. Malignancies
8. **Drugs:** vincrisitine, epinephrine
9. After surgery
10. Chronic infection
B. Thrombocytopenia
1. Hereditary thrombocytopenias like Fanconi anemia, Alport syndrome, May-Hegglin anomaly etc.
2. Hypersplenism
3. Idiopathic thrombocytopenic purpura (ITP)
4. HIV infection
5. Aplastic anemia
6. Massive transfusion of stored blood
7. Drugs: Heparin, quinidine, quinine, rifampicin etc.
8. Acute leukemia
9. Cytotoxic chemotherapy
10. Irradiation of bone marrow

ROLE OF PLATELET IN HEMOSTASIS

Hemostasis is the **arrest of bleeding**. Hemostasis occurs in **two major steps**: temporary hemostasis and the definitive hemostasis.

- Following injury to blood vessels, platelets aggregate at the site of injury and seal the opening in the vascular tree. This is the first and important step in prevention of bleeding, which is called **temporary hemostasis**.
- Simultaneously, mechanisms of blood coagulation are also activated that forms blood clot, the processes combinely known as **definitive hemostasis**.
- Though platelet is essential for temporary hemostasis, it also contributes to **blood coagulation and clot retraction**.
- Platelet also controls **thrombolysis**.

Role in Temporary Hemostasis

Immediate hemostasis following vascular injury is achieved by formation of **platelet plug** (also called, **platelet thrombus**) at the site of injury.

- As platelet thrombus can be washed away, unless supported by a clot, this is called **temporary hemostatic plug**.
- Temporary hemostatic plug formation depends on **adhesion, platelet aggregation, and release reaction.**

Platelet Adhesion

Platelets adhere to the exposed vascular wall, which is called platelet adhesion (Fig. 16.4A). Especially, exposed **collagen** and **von Willebrand factor** in the injured vessel wall attract platelets as platelets have receptors for them on their cell membrane.

Platelet adhesion is also controlled by following factors:

1. **The depth and degree of injury:** Deeper and extensive injuries have more platelet aggregation due to release of **more quantity of PAF** from the tissue.
2. **Site of injury:** Platelet aggregation is more in mucocutaneous tissue than muscluloskeletal tissues.
3. **Age of the individual:** In elderly individuals, the aggregation is less.
4. **The hematocrit:** Increased number of red cells increases platelet aggregation by **forcing the platelets to the periphery** of the blood stream.
    - Therefore, in anemia efficiency of platelet plug formation is less.
5. **Speed of blood flow:** When blood **flow is faster**, platelets *do not get adequate time* for ***adhesion.***
    - Sluggishness of blood flow facilitates platelet adhesion.
6. **Size of blood vessel:** Adhesion is more in smaller vessels.

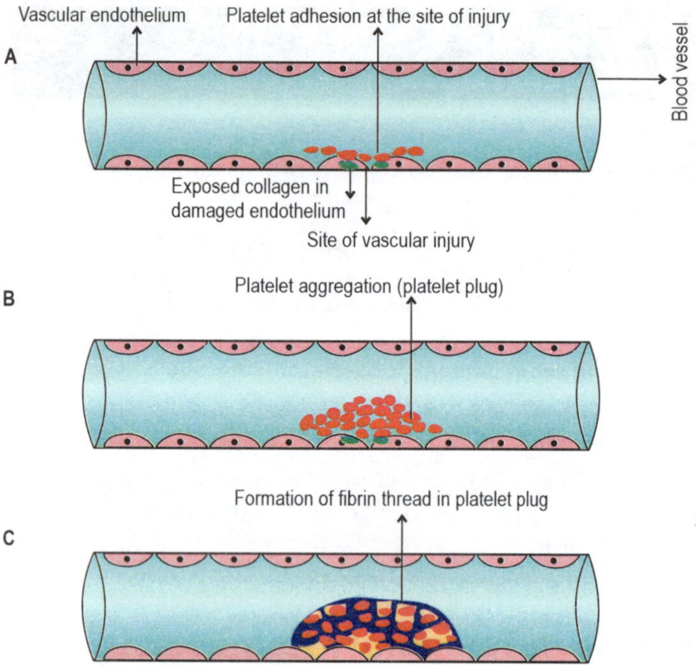

Fig. 16.4: Role of platelet in hemostasis. **A:** Platelet adhesion at the site of vascular injury. Note, exposed collagen of damaged vascular endothelium promote adhesion; **B:** Platelet aggregation; **C:** Formation of fibrin threads in and around the aggregated platelets (definitive plug formation).

Platelet Aggregation

Platelet adhesion is immediately followed by platelet aggregation at the site of injury (Fig. 16.4B).

- **Fibrinogen** and **thrombin** promote platelet aggregation.
- Simultaneously, platelets are activated, and activated platelets release chemicals from their granules.
- These chemicals, especially **ADP** and **platelet activating factor** (PAF) further facilitate platelet aggregation (Application Box 16.1).
- Thus, accumulation of more platelets at the site of vascular injury facilitates the process of temporary hemostatic plug (platelet thrombus) formation.

Application Box 16.1

Use of ADP inhibitors: ADP facilitates platelet thrombus formation. There are ADP receptors on the surface of platelets. Three types of ADP receptors have been identified on platelet membrane: P2Y1, P2Y2 and P2X1.

- ADP released from dense granules during platelet activation binds with ADP receptors on platelet membrane and facilitates platelet aggregation that promotes platelet thrombus formation.
- Therefore, inhibitors of ADP (ADP receptor antagonists that prevent platelet aggregation) have been clinically tried in the prevention of myocardial infarction and stroke.

Platelet Activation and Release

Adhesion of platelets to damaged vascular endothelium activates the platelets.

- Polymerization of microfibrillar actin occurs in activated platelets that results in **pseudopodia or spicules formation**.
- Platelets are also activated by **tissue factors and chemicals** released from granules of the platelets, especially PAF. Thrombin and ADP also promote activation.
- The activated platelets release various chemicals from their granules to the exterior via canalicular system; the process is called **release reaction** or **platelet release**.

Following are the **mechanisms of platelet release**:

1. **Through platelet activating factor (PAF): Platelet adhesion** activates platelets. Activation of platelet is **facilitated by PAF**, a cytokine secreted from neutrophils, monocytes and platelets.
   - PAF acts via G-proteins and activates **phospholipase-C and diacylglycerol** (DAG).
   - DAG increases cytoplasmic calcium by **promoting calcium release** from dense tubular systems that are present close to open canaliculi.
   - Calcium causes **contraction of microfilaments** that helps in movement of granules to the open canalicular system.
   - Membranes of granules fuse with the membranes of canaliculi and the contents of granules are **released into the canaliculi by exocytosis**.
   - From canaliculi, chemicals are transferred to the exterior of the cell.
   - During this process, platelets **change their shape** and exhibit movement.
2. **Through thromboxane and serotonin:** Formation of DAG activates the enzyme **phospholipase A_2**, which converts membrane phospholipid into **arachidonic acid**.
   - Arachidonic acid is converted to **endoperoxides** by cyclooxygenase.
   - Endoperoxides in turn form **thromboxane A_2** (TX-A_2).

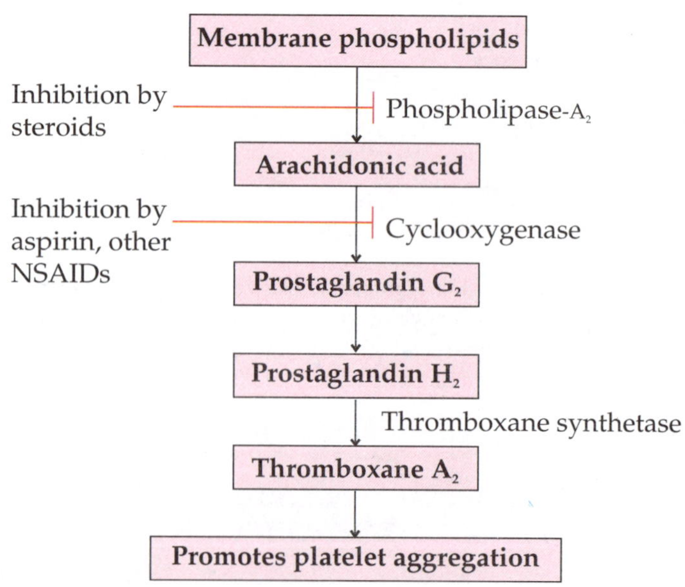

Flowchart 16.2: Synthesis of thromboxane A_2 that promotes platelet aggregation.

- $TX-A_2$ is a potent vasoconstrictor and **promotes platelet aggregation** (Flowchart 16.2).
- **Serotonin** released from platelet produces vasoconstriction and promotes hemostasis.

3. **Through thrombospondin and thrombonectin:** Thrombospondin and thrombonectin released from platelet granules facilitate the activity of contractile system and further **promote exocytosis** of granules and release of their content to the exterior.

Role in Temporary Hemostasis

Role in Blood Coagulation

Platelet factor 4 (PF4) acts as a cofactor for blood coagulation (for details, refer next chapter).

- Activation of platelet leads to increased platelet coagulant activity.
- Platelets **accelerate thrombin formation**.
- Platelet synthesizes **coagulation factor V and XI**.
- Platelet phospholipids accelerate the formation of **Va, VIIIa and XIa.**
- Va is essential for conversion of **prothrombin to thrombin**.

Role in Clot Retraction

If platelets are present in the clot in a test tube, within minutes to hours, the **clot contracts**, extruding a very large fraction of serum. This is called clot retraction.

- The **platelet filopodia** extends into fibrin clot and **fibrin strands tug** with filopodia.
- Thus, shrinkage of platelet with contraction of filopodia causes **internalization of fibrin** that causes clot retraction.
- In vivo, the phenomenon akin to clot retraction is the **consolidation of the thrombus**, which not only firmly **seals the opening in the injured vessel**, but also **facilitates wound healing**.
- Clot retraction also ***prevents the process of thrombolysis***.
- Platelet deficiency prolongs the clot retraction time.

Role in Thrombolysis

Role of platelet in fibrinolysis is complex. Both profibrinolytic and antifibrinolytic actions of platelets have been demonstrated.

- **Profibrinolytics** like thrombospondin, tPA and plasmin are synthesized by platelets.
- However, **antifibrinolytics** like plasminogen activator inhibitor-1 and α_2-antiplasmin are also secreted from platelets.
- It appears that **antifibrinolytic effects** of platelets predominate over their profibrinolytic effects in vivo as platelet rich thrombus is known to resist thrombolysis.

IMPORTANT NOTE

Use of aspirin: Aspirin inhibits platelet aggregation by inhibiting the membrane enzyme cyclo-oxygenase. Cyclo-oxygenase facilitates thromboxane A_2 formation that facilitates platelet aggregation and causes vasoconstriction. Therefore, **disprin** (soluble aspirin) is used in treatment and prevention of myocardial infarction and stroke.

Platelet Function Tests

1. **Platelet count**
   Decreased platelet count is associated with prolongation of bleeding time. Clinically, bleeding occurs when platelet count is less than 40,000/mm^3 of blood (**critical count**).
2. **Bleeding time (BT)**
   BT assesses integrity of platelets.
   - BT is prolonged in thrombocytopenia and thrombasthenia.
   - In **thrombasthenia** platelet count is normal but functionally platelets are abnormal.
3. **Platelet aggregation tests**
   Ability of platelets to aggregate is assessed with the help of **aggregometer**.
4. **Platelet adhesiveness test**
   Platelet's ability to adhere is tested by allowing anticoagulated blood to pass through a plastic tube containing glass beads, during which platelets stick to the beads.
   - Platelet adherence is measured by estimating the platelet retention in the tube.
5. **Clot retraction time**
   When blood is collected without anticoagulant, clotted blood retracts and 50% retraction occurs by the end of one hour.
   - Clot retraction completes at the end of 18 to 24 hours.
   - When retraction is less than 50% in one hour, thrombocytopenia or platelet malfunction is reported.

PLATELET DYSFUNCTIONS

Idiopathic Thrombocytopenic Purpura (ITP)

ITP is a **primary autoimmune purpura** characterized by thrombocytopenia which usually occurs due to formation of **antibody against platelets**. It occurs in **two forms**: childhood ITP and adult ITP.

- **Childhood ITP** is common but less severe and occurs equally in both genders that usually resolves spontaneously in six months.
- **Adult ITP** is less common and occurs predominantly in females.

The **common feature** of the disease is bleeding that usually occurs spontaneously.

- Skin is the commonest site of hemorrhage, exhibiting petechiae or ecchymoses.
- Bleeding occurs from mucus membranes in the form of epistaxis (bleeding from the nose), or bleeding-gums.

Diagnosis is made by demonstrating thrombocytopenia, anemia, and anti-platelet antibodies in the patient.

The **treatment** consists of administration of corticosteroids, and splenectomy.

Thrombocytopenia in Pregnancy

Thrombocytopenia is common during pregnancy and usually asymptomatic.

- A form, called **gestational thrombocytopenia** causes excessive bleeding during parturition.
- Another form is associated with **pre-eclampsia**.

Neonatal Autoimmune Thrombocytopenia (NATP)

NATP occurs in newborns and platelet count is less than 50,000/cumm of blood.

- It may be associated with autoimmune hemolytic anemia.
- **Antibodies** are demonstrated *against platelet specific alloantigens*.
- NATP is **treated by** platelet transfusion, steroid and immunoglobulins.

Exam Questions

1. Give the steps of hemostasis. Describe the process and importance of temporary hemostatic plug formation.
2. List the steps of thrombopoiesis. Briefly describe the regulation of thrombopoiesis.
3. List the properties of platelets. Describe how structural modifications in platelet facilitate its functions.
4. Describe the role of platelet in hemostasis.
5. Name platelet function tests and give their normal values.

Multiple Choice Questions

1. Thrombocytosis occurs in:
A. Hypersplenism B. After surgery
C. Acute leukemia D. Massive transfusion of stored blood

2. Thrombocytopenia occurs in:
A. Acute blood loss B. Iron deficiency
C. Polycythemiarubravera D. Dengue fever

3. Platelet membrane contains receptors for all of the following, EXCEPT:
A. ADP B. Platelet activating factor
C. Blood group antigens D. Fibronectin

4. All of the following are released from dense granules of platelets, EXCEPT:
A. Pyrophosphate B. Proaccelerin
C. Calcium D. ATP

5. All of the following can be features of purpura, EXCEPT:
A. Prolonged BT
B. Decreased platelet count
C. Decreased vitamin K level
D. Increased capillary fragility

6. Asprin inhibits the enzyme:
A. Alpha-1-protease B. Thromboxane synthatase
C. Phospholipase D. Cyclooxygenase

7. The percentage of clot retraction that occurs at the end of one hour is:
A. 10% B. 30% C. 50% D. 80%

8. Which of the following statements is NOT true?
A. Thrombocytopenia decreases the clot retraction time
B. Clot retraction time is a reliable screening test for platelet function
C. The clot contracts down to 40% of its original volume
D. The contractile proteinthrombosthenin promotes clot retraction process

9. Platelets survive in the circulation for about:
A. 2-3 days B. 5-6 days
C. 8-12 days D. 20-25 days

10. Which of the following is not well developed in platelets?
A. Cytoplasmic cytoskeletal system
B. Dense tubular system
C. Actomyosin filament system
D. Open canalicular system

11. Which of the following statement is NOT true about platelets?
A. Adhesion is facilitated by von Willebrand factor
B. Aggregation is inhibited by thromboxane A2
C. Activation is facilitated by glycoprotein IIb-IIIa
D. Aggregation is inhibited by prostacyclin

12. Which of the following is NOT a function of platelets?
A. Serotonin production
B. Vascular growth
C. Phagocytosis of immune complexes
D. Thrombolysis

13. Idiopathic thrombocytopenic purpura:
A. Is a genetically transmitted disease
B. Is due to decreased formation of platelets
C. Is predominant in adult females
D. Corticosteroids worsens the condition

Answers

1. B	2. D	3. C	4. B	5. C	6. D
7. C	8. A	9. C	10. C	11. B	12. A
13. C					

Chapter 17

Blood Coagulation

Learning Objectives

On completion of study of this chapter:

The student will be able to (must know):

1. Name the clotting factors.
2. Describe the mechanisms (intrinsic and extrinsic) of blood coagulation.
3. Understand the importance of clot retraction.
4. Explain the mechanism of fibrinolysis.
5. List the functions of plasmin and appreciate the role of plasmin activators
6. List the anticoagulants, and give their mechanism of action and uses.
7. List the investigations for bleeding disorders.
8. Enumerate the common abnormalities of coagulation.

The student may also be able to (desirable to know):

1. Describe regulation of blood coagulation.
2. Describe anticlotting mechanisms.
3. Describe the tests to assess integrity of intrinsic and extrinsic pathways of blood coagulation.

The **definitive hemostasis** is the coagulation of blood, the process which is simultaneously activated along with the activation of platelets. Coagulation of blood occurs due to **activation of clotting factors** (coagulation proteins) that are normally present in their inactive form in plasma.

Clotting Factors

There are known 12 clotting factors (Table 17.1) depicted as factor I to XIII (factor VI absent). Later, few more were added to the list.

MECHANISM OF BLOOD COAGULATION

Blood coagulation occurs in **three major stages**:

1. Activation of Stuart Prower factor (formation of prothrombin activator)
2. Formation of thrombin from prothrombin
3. Formation of fibrin from fibrinogen

Table 17.1 | Clotting factors

Factor I	: Fibrinogen
Factor II	: Prothrombin (α_2 - globulin)
Factor III	: Tissue thromboplastin
Factor IV	: Calcium ion
Factor V	: Proaccelerin
	: Factor VI does not exist
Factor VII	: Proconvertin
Factor VIII	: Antihemophilic factor [antihemophilic globulin (AHG) or antihemophilic factor A].
Factor IX	: Christmas factor (antihemophilic factor B)
Factor X	: Stuart Prower factor,
Factor XI	: Plasma thromboplastin antecedent (antihemophilic factor C)
Factor XII	: Hageman factor, contact factor
Factor XIII	: Fibrin stabilizing factor (Laki-Lorand factor)
HMW-K	: High-molecular weight kininogen (Fitzgerald factor)
Pre-K	: Prekallikrein (Fletcher factor)
Ka	: Kallikrein
PL	: Platelet phospholipid
Inhibitors	
	: Protein C
	: Protein Z
	: Thrombomodulin
	: Antithrombin III
	: Tissue factor pathway inhibitor
	: Protein Z-dependent protease inhibitor

Activation of Stuart Prower Factor (Factor X)

Activation of **Stuart Prower factor** or factor X is the key to blood coagulation.

- Factor Xa is called **prothrombin activator** as it activates prothrombin to form thrombin.
- Therefore, this is also called stage of prothrombin activation.

This is achieved by two pathways: the intrinsic pathway and the extrinsic pathway (Fig. 17.1).

Intrinsic Pathway

Intrinsic mechanism of prothrombin activation occurs in **four steps**.

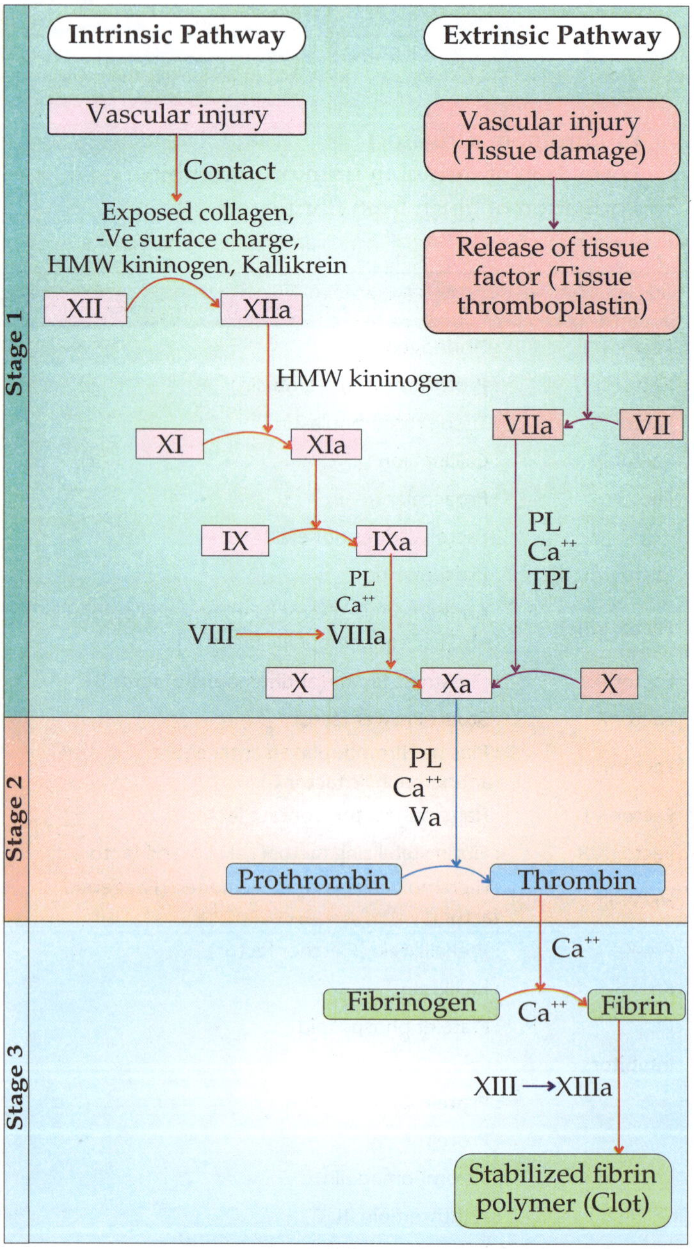

Fig. 17.1: Mechanism of blood coagulation. TPL: tissue thromboplastin; PL: platelet phospholipids.

Step 1 (Activation of XII)

Activation of intrinsic pathway starts with **contact of Hageman factor** (factor XII) with a ***negatively charged surface*** *or* ***exposed collagen*** of the injured vessel wall.

- High molecular weight kininogen **(HMW kininogen) and Kallikrein** act as *cofactors to facilitate* the activation of factor XII.
- Exposed collagen stimulates platelet adhesion and aggregation before initiating blood coagulation.

Step 2 (Activation of XI)

Activated XII (XIIa) converts **XI to its active form (XIa)**.

- This step is accelerated in the presence of **HMW kininogen**.

Step 3 (Activation of IX)

XIa then converts **IX to IXa**, which is accentuated by VIIa.

- **Calcium** accelerates this process.

Step 4 (Activation of X)

Final step in activation of prothrombin activator is activation of X.

- IXa causes activation of **X to Xa**, the activated Stuart Prower factor.
- The membrane **phospholipid, calcium and activated factor VIII** act as cofactors for the activation of Stuart Prower factor.

Formation of VIIIa is the key: Formation of VIIIa is crucial to the process of activation of X.

- Factor VIII circulates as a complex with vWF.
- Separation of VIII from vWF activates VIII.
- Activation of VIII is facilitated by Xa and thrombin, the factors that are the consequences of formation of VIIIa.
- Thus, activation of factor VIII and further activation of clotting mechanism become a vicious cycle.

IMPORTANT NOTE

Enzyme Cascade Hypothesis: In the intrinsic system of blood coagulation, activation of one clotting factor acts as an enzyme for the activation of next factor that leads to sequential activation of subsequent factors in a series of steps. Therefore, the intrinsic process of blood coagulation is called **enzyme cascade hypothesis**.

Extrinsic Pathway

Extrinsic pathway of blood coagulation occurs in **three steps**.

Step I (Release of TPL)

Key to the clotting mechanism is the release of tissue thromboplastin (TPL) from the injured tissue.

- As TPL is the **tissue factor** which is viewed as extrinsic to circulating blood, this system of blood coagulation is called extrinsic system of clotting.

Step II (Activation of VII)

TPL converts factor VII to its active form (VIIa).

- This is the **key step in extrinsic mechanism**.
- VIIa directly activates not only X (Stuart Prower factor), but also IX (Christmas factor).
- Thus, it also influences intrinsic mechanism of activation of factor X.

Step III (Activation of X)

VIIa converts X to Xa. This process is accelerated in the presence of **calcium, platelet phospholipid and TPL**.

Though there are intrinsic and extrinsic systems of blood coagulation, these two systems do not operate independently; they are activated simultaneously and they complement each other.

Formation of Thrombin from Prothrombin

This is the second stage of blood coagulation in which activated Stuart Prower factor (Xa) converts prothrombin to thrombin, in the presence of platelet phospholipid, calcium and **activated factor V (Va)**.

- Factor Va acts as cofactor for acceleration of this process.
- Therefore, it is also called as proaccelerin or accelerator globulin.

Factor II: Factor II is **prothrombin**, a vitamin K-dependant protein formed in liver.

- Prothrombin forms **thrombin**, which is basically a ***proteolytic enzyme*** having molecular weight of 34,000 dalton.
- Thrombin is formed rapidly and in large amount as both intrinsic and extrinsic mechanisms stimulate its formation.

Functions of Thrombin in Blood Coagulation

1. It converts **fibrinogen to fibrin monomers** by removing fibrinopeptides A and B from fibrinogen.
   - Fibrin monomers then form fibrin polymers (clot).
2. It **activates formation of prothrombin activator** by stimulating the **activation of VIII, V, and XIII**.
   - Thus, it provides *positive feed-back* to the coagulation process.
3. It is a potent **activator of platelets**.
4. It **activates procarboxypeptidase B** that inhibits plasmin-mediated fibrinolysis.
5. It has also **anticlotting activity**.
   - It binds to cofactor thrombomodulin on endothelial cells that allows protein C to be activated (see below).
   - Thus, thrombin balances the coagulation and anticoagulation processes in the body.
6. It helps in **repair of vessel wall**.
   - It has growth factor and cytokine like activities that play role in inflammation, wound healing and atherosclerosis.

Inhibitors of Thrombin: The primary inhibitor of thrombin in plasma is **antithrombin III. Heparin cofactor II** also inhibits thrombin.

Formation of Fibrin from Fibrinogen

This is the final stage of blood coagulation in which **thrombin acts as an enzyme to convert fibrinogen to fibrin**. In this process, first, the fibrin monomers are formed and afterward, they are polymerized to fibrin thread (blood clot). This occurs in **three steps**:

1. Proteolysis of soluble fibrinogen
2. Polymerization of fibrin monomers
3. Stabilization of fibrin polymer

Proteolysis of Soluble Fibrinogen

Fibrinogen has **three domains**: two peripheral (D) domains and one central (E) domain.

- Thrombin binds with central domain and proteolytically releases two fibrinopeptides A and B from amino terminals of Aα and Bβ chains of each fibrinogen molecules.
- Release of fibrinopeptides leads to the formation of fibrin monomer (Flowchart 17.1).

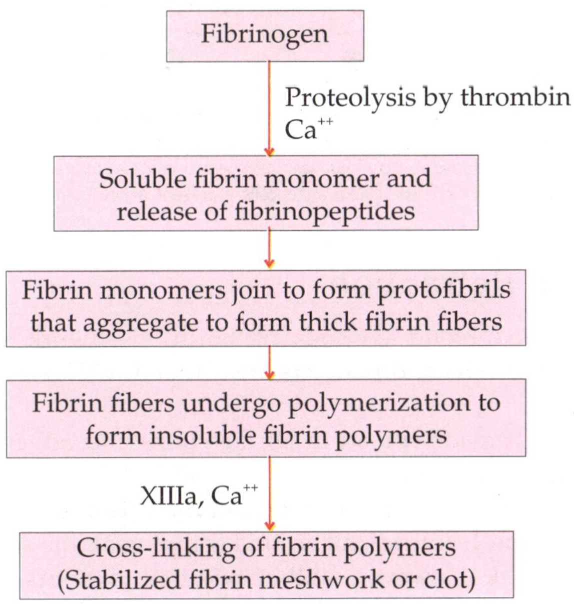

Flowchart 17.1: Mechanism of fibrin stabilization

Polymerization of Fibrin Monomers

Fibrin monomers join to form **protofibrils**.

- About **15 to 20 protofibrils aggregate** to from thick fibers of fibrin.
- Protofibrils also branch out to form into a **meshwork of interconnected thick fibrin fibers**. This is called *polymerization of fibrin monomers*.

- **Thrombin** initiates the process of polymerization and simultaneously **activates XIII**.
- XIIIa completes the process of polymerization.

Stabilization of Fibrin Polymer

Fibrin stabilizing factor (XIIIa) stabilizes the fibrin polymers by cross-linking them.

- XIII is converted to XIIIa **by thrombin**.
- Calcium acts as a cofactor for this conversion.
- **Covalent cross-linking** of fibrin polymers provides adequate strength to the fibrin thread and to the fibrin meshwork.
- The **stabilized fibrin meshwork** is the blood clot.
- **Red cells and platelets are trapped** inside the fibrin meshwork to give the volume to the clot (Fig. 17.2A).

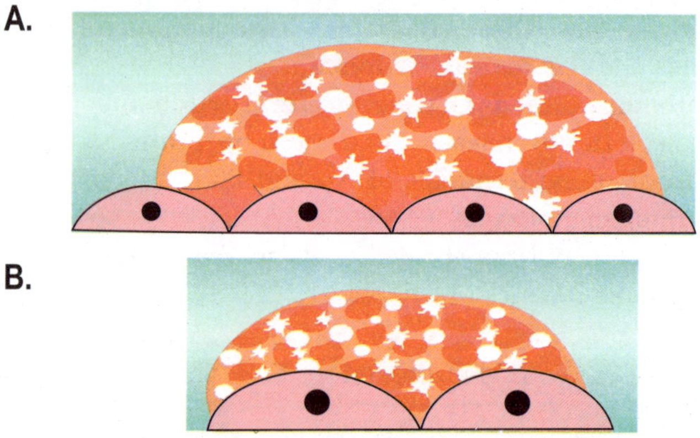

Fig. 17.2: **A:** Clot at the site of injury. Note, red cells (red colored spherical structures) and platelets (white colored spherical and spiculated structures) are trapped within the meshwork of fibrin thread (yellow materials interspersed between the red and white cells). **B:** Retracted clot. Spiculated white cells represent activated platelets with pseudopodia.

Clot Retraction

The clotted blood consists of fibrin meshwork containing red cells and platelets are trapped within it (Fig. 17.2A).

Fibrin threads spread in all directions and adhere to the endothelial wall.

- When blood is allowed to **clot in a test tube**, the fibrin mesh spreads all around trapping all the serum within it. However, within minutes to hours, **clot shrinks expressing serum** out of it (Fig. 17.2B). This phenomenon is called ***clot retraction***.
- The process of clot retraction is believed to occur in vivo that causes **consolidation of thrombus** (intravascular clot).
- **Clot retraction is the function of platelets**. For effective clot retraction to occur, normally functioning platelets must be present in adequate number.
- Retracted clot **decreases the efficiency of thrombolysis** (fibrinolysis). Therefore, a thrombus rich in platelets is **resistant to fibrinolytic agents**.

Mechanism of Clot Retraction

The platelets form spicules (**filopodia**) that extend along the fibrin threads.

- Fibrin strands **tug with the filopodia**.
- Also, **protofibrils** of thick fibrin strand get **embedded within the filopodia** by the action of membrane cytoskeleton.
- Later, **platelets shrink** with contraction of their filopodia (Fig. 17.2B).
- This causes **internalization of fibrin within the contracted platelets**. Thus, *retraction of clot* occurs.
- **Thrombin and calcium** accelerate clot retraction.
- ***Glycoprotein IIb/IIIa receptors*** on platelets facilitate clot retraction.

Functions of Clot Retraction

A retracted clot is a **consolidated and stable thrombus**, which not only firmly seals the opening in the injured vessel, but also has other functions.

The functions of retracted clot are as follows.

1. Retracted clot strongly **seals injured vessel**.
2. It facilitates **wound healing**.
3. It **prevents thrombolysis**.

Prolongation of Clot Retraction Time

Normally, clot retraction begins within thirty seconds after clot formation. However, the process of retraction is **very slow**.

- About 50% retraction occurs at the end of one hour and **completes in 18 to 24 hours**.
- Clot retraction time is said to be prolonged when **retraction is less than 50%** at the end of one hour.
- In **Glanzmann thrombasthenia**, deficiency of IIb/IIIa receptors results in inhibition of clot retraction that causes prolongation of clot retraction time.
- **Platelet deficiency** also prolongs the clot retraction time.

ANTICLOTTING MECHANISM (Fibrinolysis)

The process of coagulation automatically initiates the anticlotting mechanisms so that intravascular clot does not spread beyond the site of injury.

Mechanism of Fibrinolysis

Fibrinolysis occurs in three steps:

1. Activation of protein C
2. Activation of plasmin
3. Fibrinolysis

Activation of Protein C

- **Thrombin** which is produced by clotting mechanism

acts as an enzyme to **activate protein C** to its active form.

- The anticlotting mechanism activated by thrombin can also be initiated by **thrombomodulin**, a hormone secreted from endothelial cells of blood vessel.
- **Thrombomodulin** activates protein C (Fig. 17.3).

Activation of Plasmin

Activated protein C **inactivates the inhibitors of plasmin activator**.

- This in turn ***activates plasminogen activator***, which promotes formation of **plasmin** from plasminogen.
- Activated protein C along with its cofactor protein S also **inactivates Va and VIIIa** into their respective inactive forms.
- This aids in prevention of coagulation.

Fibrinolysis

Plasmin acts as an enzyme to cause fibrinolysis (lysis of clot).

This process is ***facilitated by cofactors*** thrombin, tissue-type plasminogen activator and urokinase-type plasminogen activator.

Fibrin is degraded by plasmin to **fibrin degradation products** (FDP) (Clinical Note 17.1). The details of fibrinolysis by plasmin are given below.

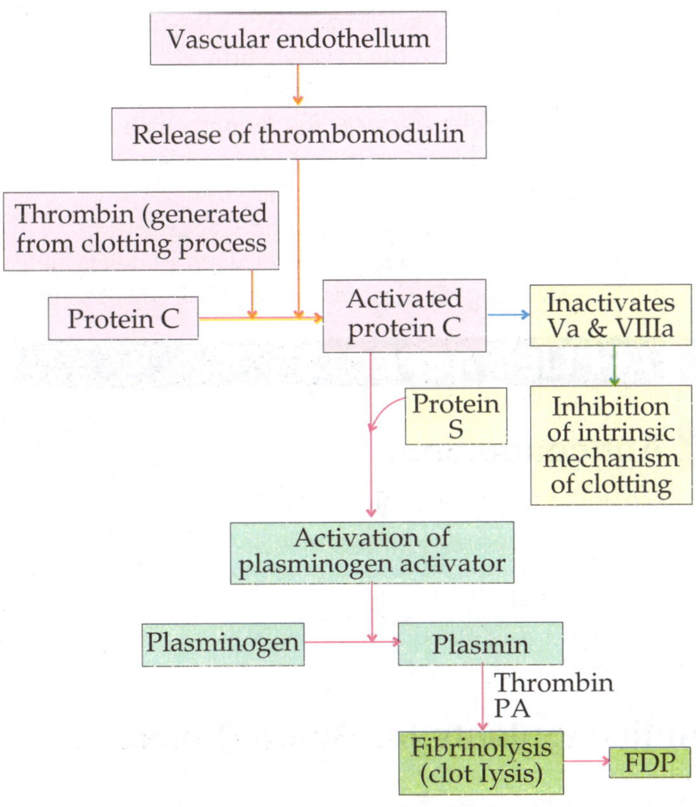

Fig. 17.3: Anticlotting (fibrinolysis) mechanism. PA: plasminogen activators (t-PA, u-PA); FDP: fibrin degradation product. Note, fibrinolysis occurs in three major steps: activation of protein C, activation of plasmin and fibrinolysis.

Clinical Note 17.1

FDP level indicates the rate of fibrinolysis: Activation of clotting process as occurs in DIC (see below) activates the anticlotting mechanism (fibrinolysis). Fibrinolysis causes accumulation of FDP in plasma which is subsequently excreted in urine. Hence, measurement of FDP in urine is an index of rate of fibrinolysis as well as intravascular coagulation.

Plasmin

Plasmin is formed from plasminogen by the action of plasminogen activator.

Functions of Plasmin

Functions of plasmin can be broadly divided into two categories: Fibrinolytic actions and nonfibrinolytic actions.

Fibrinolytic Actions

Plasmin cleaves both fibrinogen and fibrin.

- Plasmin **cleaves α and β chains** within the D domain of fibrinogen that releases Aα and Bβ fragments.
- Degradation of fibrin by plasmin results in production of **fibrin degradation products** (FDP), such as **D-dimers**.

Nonfibrinolytic Actions

Plasmin has many functions other than fibrinolysis.

1. Plasmin is involved in **tissue remodeling**.
2. Plays a role in **inflammation** and tumor cell invasion.
3. Controls **ovulation** and embryogenesis.
4. Regulates development of neurons.
5. Plasmin plays a role in **activation of growth factors**.
6. Helps in **proliferative response** of blood vessels to injury.

Plasminogen Activators

There are two plasminogen activators: the tissue plasminogen activator and urokinase.

Tissue plasminogen activator (t-PA): t-PA is a polypeptide having 527 amino acids.

- Fibrin facilitates t-PA activity by increasing affinity of t-PA for plasminogen.

Urokinase: Urokinase plasminogen activator (u-PA) is a glycoprotein consisting of 411 amino acids.

- Physiologically, u-PA is a more effective activator of plasminogen than t-PA even in the presence of fibrin (Clinical Note 17.2).
- **Streptokinase** is a variant of urokinase.

Clinical Note 17.2

t-PA and urokinase for treatment of AMI: t-PA and urokinase for their fibrinolytic activity are used for lysis of intra-coronary clot in acute myocardial infarction (AMI). t-PA is very effective for this purpose as it causes lysis of clot at the site of thrombosis.

Applied Aspects

Inhibitors of Fibrinolysis

Inhibitors of fibrinolysis are divided into two categories: plasmin inhibitors and plasminogen-activator inhibitor (PAI). Plasmin is inhibited α_2**-antiplasmin** and α_2-**macroglbulin**. PAI are secreted by placenta, monocytes and tumor cells.

Fibrinolytic Deficiency

Fibrinolytic deficiency is usually due to **plasminogen deficiency**. Usually this is congenital. Hypofibrinolysis is seen in pregnancy (Clinical Note 17.3).

Enhanced Fibrinolysis

This usually occurs due to congenital or acquired *loss of fibrinolytic inhibitor activity*.

- ***Deficiency of*** α_2**-antiplasmin** is a common cause.
- **Acquired** α_2**-antiplasmin deficiency** may be seen in liver disease, DIC, nephritic syndrome and thrombolytic therapy.

Clinical Note 17.3

Pregnancy is a hypofibrinolytic state: In pregnancy, overall fibrinolytic activity is reduced. This leads to increased fibrin deposition, as suggested by increased D-dimer levels. The PAI levels also increase in pregnancy. The hemostatic and fibrinolytic imbalance is increased in preeclampsia and eclampsia. This predisposes to intravascular thrombosis.

REGULATION OF BLOOD COAGULATION

Blood coagulation at the site of injury is a life-saving process as it prevents loss of blood volume. Fluidity of blood and absence of thrombosis (intravascular clot) are important physiological states that are essential for normal circulation and blood supply to tissues of the body.

The balance between coagulation and anticoagulation is due to play of various regulatory mechanisms.

1. **Dynamism of blood flow:** When the rate of blood flow decreases, as occurs in vascular stasis, intravascular coagulation is facilitated. Thus, a dynamic flow prevents intravascular coagulation.
2. **Role of vascular endothelium:** Damage to vascular endothelium initiates the clotting mechanism by exposing its collagen and negatively charged particles.
    - Once adequate hemostasis is achieved, **thrombomodulin**, a hormone secreted by endothelial cells of blood vessel prevents further blood coagulation by ***activating protein C-protein S complex***.
    - Also, **protease inhibitors AT-III** and tissue factor pathway inhibitor are expressed on the surface of the endothelial cells.
    - Endothelial cells also **inhibit platelet activation** by releasing prostacyclin and EDRF that inhibit platelets.
3. **Heparin-Antithrombin-III system: Heparin** is a naturally occurring anti-coagulant, secreted from mast cells and basophils.
    - Heparin acts by **activating antithrombin III** activity.
    - Heparin-antithrombin III complex **prevents activation of clotting factor IX, X, XI and XII.**
4. **Negative feedback by thrombin:** Thrombin, which is a major mediator of blood coagulation, initiates the process of **anticlotting mechanism** (fibrinolysis).
    - Thus, coagulation is an autoregulatory process.
5. **Role of Liver:** Many **coagulation factors** are plasma proteins, **produced mainly in the liver**.
    - Therefore, in liver diseases, clotting time is prolonged.
    - Also, liver plays an important role in **preventing intravascular coagulation** by ***removing activated clotting factors*** from blood.
6. **Role of platelets:** In addition to its role in primary hemostasis, platelets contribute to coagulation in various ways.
    - Following platelet activation, **platelet phospholipids** (platelet factor 3 and 4) released to their surface act as cofactors to accelerate the formation of **Va, VIIIa and XIa**.
    - Also, factor IXa formed by VIIa–tissue factor complex binds to the platelet surface.
    - This leads to the formation of IXa-VIIa complex on the platelet surface, following which factor X is recruited from the plasma to the platelets and is **activated to Xa** on platelet membrane.
    - As platelets adhesion and aggregation are localized at the injured vessel wall, platelets help in **restricting clotting reactions** to the site of injury.

APPLIED ASPECTS

Anticoagulants

PY2.8

Anticoagulants prevent blood from clotting. They are mainly used:

1. For collection of blood sample for laboratory investigations
2. For preserving blood for transfusion
3. For anticoagulation therapy

Anticoagulants for Blood Collection

Anticoagulants commonly used are EDTA, trisodium citrate, double oxalate, sodium fluoride, and heparin.

EDTA (ethylenediamine tetra-acetic acid): The **sodium and potassium salts of EDTA** are the commonly used and most powerful anticoagulants.

- It acts by its **chelating effect on the blood calcium**.
- It **inactivates calcium** by forming insoluble complex with it.

Sodium Citrate: Trisodium citrate is the commonly used anticoagulant in coagulation studies.

- It **prevents coagulation by inactivating calcium ions**.
- It is usually used for determination of prothrombin time, partial thromboplastin time and estimation of ESR by Westergren method.

Double Oxalate: It contains **ammonium and potassium oxalates**.

- Potassium oxalate alone causes shrinkage of red cells whereas ammonium oxalate increases their volume.
- Hence, double oxalate is also called as **balanced oxalate**.
- The oxalates form an insoluble complex with the calcium in the blood, and thereby prevent coagulation.

Sodium Fluoride: Sodium fluoride is used mainly for collecting blood specimen *for plasma glucose estimation*.

- Fluoride is an **inhibitor of glycolytic enzymes** and thus prevents loss of glucose.
- However, as fluoride is *not a strong anticoagulant*, it is mixed with the oxalate.

Oxalates: Oxalates of sodium, potassium, ammonium or lithium act as anticoagulant.

- They form **insoluble complexes with calcium**.

Heparin: Heparin is a natural constituent of blood.

- It prevents coagulation for approximately 24 hours by neutralizing thrombin.
- It **facilitates action of antithrombin III**. Thus, it *prevents formation of fibrin from fibrinogen*.
- Usually, it is used at a concentration of **10–20 IU per ml of blood**.
- It is *commonly used* for osmotic fragility test, blood gas determination and pH assays.
- It is also used in **anticoagulation therapy** and in preventing blood coagulation during animal experiments.

Anticoagulants for Anticoagulation Therapy

Anticoagulants are used for **treatment or prevention of thrombosis** (intravascular clots).

They are usually required for:

1. Management of thrombotic diseases like venous thromboembolism
2. Placement of mechanical heart valves as heart valve prosthesis is associated with risk of thromboembolism
3. Prevention of thromboembolism in chronic nonrheumatic atrial fibrillation
4. Prophylaxis after attacks of cerebral ischemia
5. Management of ischemic heart disease
6. Peripheral vascular diseases
7. Placement of central venous catheters.

Types: Anticoagulants used in anticoagulation therapy are of **two types**: oral and intravenous.

Oral Anticoagulants

Routinely used oral anticoagulants are vitamin K antagonists, glycosaminoglycans, inhibitors of factor Xa and inhibitors of thrombin.

Vitamin K Antagonists

The four ***vitamin K-dependent coagulation factors*** are II, VII, IX and X.

- They undergo **post-translational γ-carboxylation** of approximately 10 glutamic acid residues, which is necessary to enable them **to bind calcium** and to localize enzymatic processes to a phospholipid surface like membrane of activated platelet.
- When **γ-carboxylation is reduced** by 1 to 6 glutamic acid residues, coagulation activity of factors II, VII, IX and X is ***impaired significantly***.

Warfarin: The commonly used vitamin K antagonist is **warfarin**. This is a coumarin derivative.

Warfarin **inhibits γ-carboxylation** of about 3 to 10 glutamic acid residues, especially of **factor II** (prothrombin).

- Warfarin achieves this by ***inhibiting the reductase enzymes*** that cause formation of *vitamin* KH_2 (Fig. 17.4).
- **Vitamin** KH_2 is required for γ-carboxylation of vitamin K-dependent coagulation factors.

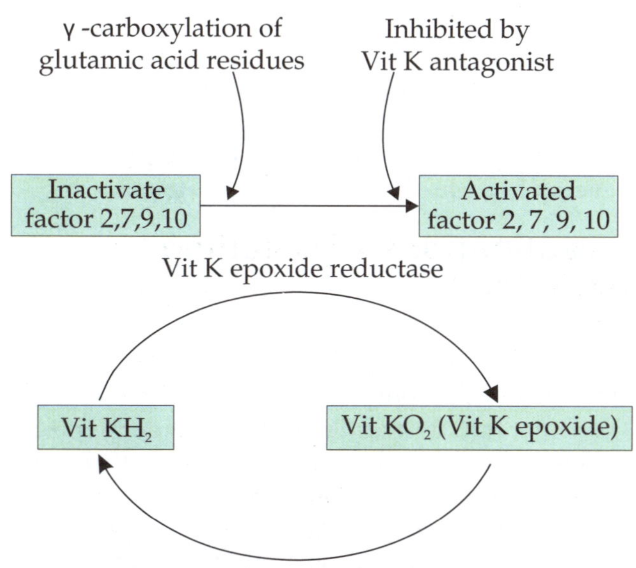

Fig. 17.4: Mechanism of action of vitamin K antagonist in the prevention of blood coagulation. Factors 2, 7, 9 and 10 are vit. K dependent clotting factors. Vitamin K antagonists inhibit both Vit K epoxide reductase and Vit K reductase that are essential for Vit KO_2 and Vit KH_2 formations. Vit. KH_2 is required for γ-carboxylation of these clotting factors that activate them.

- During the process of γ-carboxylation, vitamin KH_2 is converted to **vitamin K-epoxide** by *vitamin K epoxide reductase*, and vitamin K-epoxide is converted back to vitamin KH_2 by *vitamin K reductase*.

- **Both these enzymes are inhibited** by coumarin derivatives such as warfarin.

Dicoumarol: Dicoumarol is another commonly used vitamin K antagonist.

Glycosaminoglycans

Oral heparin sulfate and iduronyl-glycosaminoglycan are used as anticoagulants.

Inhibitors of Thrombin

Many **low-molecular weight selective inhibitors** of thrombin have been recently identified and are under clinical trials.

Intravenous or Subcutaneous Anticoagulants

Most commonly used intravenous anticoagulants are **heparin and hirudin.**

Heparin

Anticoagulant activity of heparin is due to its **facilitation of the effects of antithrombin III** (AT-III).

- AT-III inactivates thrombin, Xa and IXa.

Hirudin

Hirudin is a naturally occurring most **specific inhibitor of thrombin**.

- It is also produced by recombinant DNA technology.
- It **directly inactivates thrombin** by binding to the active site and main fibrinopeptide binding region of thrombin.
- It has been tried in the treatment of acute coronary syndrome, patients undergoing coronary angioplasty and deep vein thrombosis.
- It is mainly used as anticoagulant **in patients who develop heparin-induced thrombocytopenia**.

Investigations of Bleeding Disorders

Bleeding disorders are primarily due to the defects in formation of either in temporary hemostatic plug or in definitive hemostatic plug.

Therefore, **initial investigations** aim at differentiating these two primary defects.

If it is a **coagulation disorder**, tests are performed to ***detect the deficiency of clotting factor*** that has caused the disease and also to assess whether the **defect is in intrinsic or extrinsic system**.

A. Tests that Detect Defects in Temporary Hemostatic Plug

1. Bleeding time
2. Capillary fragility test
3. Platelet aggregation test
4. Platelet adhesiveness test

B. Tests that Detect Defect in Definitive Hemostatic Plug

1. Clotting time
2. Prothrombin time
3. Prothrombin consumption test
4. Partial thromboplastin time
5. Activated partial thromboplastin time
6. Thrombin time
7. Plasma recalcification time
8. Clot retraction time

Common Abnormalities of Coagulation

Hemophilia A

Etiology: Hemophilia A, also known as **classical hemophilia**, is a bleeding disorder that occurs due to **deficiency of factor VIII**.

- **Women are carriers** and generally do not suffer from the disease as they are protected by the second X-chromosome which is usually normal.

Clinical Features: The disease manifests with the ***bleeding tendency*** which appears in infancy, but in mild cases may appear in adult life.

- **Soft tissue hematomas** and **hemarthroses** (bleeding into joints) leading to severe *crippling hemarthropathy* are highly characteristic of the disease.
- **In severe cases, *spontaneous hemarthropathy*** from infancy is the common feature.
- **In mild to moderate cases**, continuation of hemorrhage secondary to trauma or surgery is the feature.
- Bleeding usually persists from days to weeks inspite of formation of clots.
- Bleeding may also occur spontaneously into tissues, and cavities of the body.

Diagnosis: Patients have **prolonged activated partial thromboplastin time** (APTT).

- Prothrombin time (PT) and BT are normal.
- Assay of factor VIII in plasma is diagnostic.

Treatment: The treatment consists of **transfusion of fresh blood** (as on storage factor VIII is rapidly lost), or transfusion of **factor VIII-concentrate**.

- Fresh-frozen plasma and cryoprecipitate both contain factor VIII.

Christmas Disease (Hemophilia B)

Etiology: Christmas disease or hemophilia-B occurs due to **deficiency of factor-IX** (antihemophilic factor-B or Christmas factor).

- This is a **sex-linked recessive** hemorrhagic disease.

Features: The disease is clinically indistinguishable from hemophilia A.

- Bleeding episodes are clinically identical to those in hemophilia A.

- Therefore, this is also called hemophilia-B.
- Hematoma, hemarthroses and crippling hemarthropathy occur.

Diagnosis: In most cases, PT is normal and **partial thromboplastin time (PTT) is prolonged.**

- Specific assay of factor IX coagulant activity confirms diagnosis.

Treatment: The specific treatment of hemophilia B is the **replacement of factor IX**.

von Willebrand Disease

Etiology: von Willebrand disease (vWD) is the most common inherited bleeding disorder in humans that occurs due to **deficiency of von Willebrand factor** (vWF).

- vWF plays a central role in hemostasis as it serves as a **carrier for factor VIII** and is essential for **adhesion of platelets** to the injured vessel wall.
- Therefore, deficiency of vWF leads to **defects in the formation of both temporary and definitive hemostatic plugs**.

Clinical Features: Mucocutaneous bleeding epistaxis, easy bruising, hematoma, menorrhagia and GI bleeding are common.

- Hemarthroses and muscle hematoma may occur.

Diagnosis: As vWF is primarily responsible for platelet adhesion, **prolongation of bleeding time** is a standard screening test for vWD.

- However, *clotting time is prolonged or normal* depending on the degree of deficiency of factor VIII.
- Quantitative and functional **assays of plasma vWF** are diagnostic.

Treatment: Desmopressin (DDAVP), an analogue of ADH increases factor VIII activity, vWF-Ag concentration and ristocetin cofactor activity.

Disseminated Intravascular Coagulation (DIC)

Definition and Etiology: DIC is a clinicopathological syndrome in which there is **widespread intravascular coagulation** that occurs due to **procoagulants** that are introduced into or produced by blood circulation.

- The procoagulant activity overcomes the natural anticoagulant mechanisms.
- This is a hemorrhagic disorder in which **diffused intravascular coagulation** results in defects of hemostasis.
- In this disease, coagulation factors and platelets are overutilized.
- The commonest procoagulant stimulus is the **tissue factor exposure** to the blood.

This is **usually seen in:**

1. Septic abortions
2. Amniotic fluid embolism
3. Gram-negative septicemia
4. Fungemia
5. Severe trauma
6. Burns (burn sepsis)
7. Snake bite
8. Sometimes in hemolytic transfusion reactions.

Features: The clinical manifestations of DIC include two important features: i) **multiorgan dysfunctions** caused by widespread microembolism, and ii) **bleeding** caused by consumption of platelets, fibrinogen, factor V and factor VIII.

- Therefore, this is also called **consumption coagulopathy**.
- There is also activation of secondary fibrinolysis (hence, also called **defibrination syndrome**).

Diagnosis: Laboratory features include thrombocytopenia, hypofibrinogenemia, **increased D-dimer** and **fibrin degradation product** (FDP) and prolonged PTT, PT and thrombin time (TT).

Diagnosis is usually done by demonstrating **FDP in urine** and decreased concentration of coagulation factors and fibrin monomers in blood.

Treatment: Treatment is based on early diagnosis, elimination of the precipitating factors, and replacing coagulation factors and platelets.

- Blood component therapy is needed for those who bleed excessively.

Thrombosis

Thrombus is an **intravascular clot.**

- Normally, a balance is maintained between the processes of coagulation and anticoagulation.
- Three factors (**Virchow's triad**) predispose to the formation of thrombosis.

The **3 factors** are:

1. **Endothelial injury:** Injury to vascular endothelium occurs in chronic and sustained hypertension, ulcerated atherosclerosis, arterial diseases etc.
    - Injured site becomes the **site for platelet adhesion and aggregation** and **intravascular clot formation**.
2. **Sluggishness of blood flow:** Stasis of blood promotes thrombosis.
3. **Hypercoagulability of blood:** Increased **activity of procoagulants** such as fibrinogen, prothrombin and other coagulants leads to thrombosis.

Platelet aggregation at the site of injury initiates the process of thrombosis. *Venous thrombosis* is more common than arterial thrombosis.

Example: One common example is thrombosis of **lower limb veins in varicosities**.

- **Deep vein thrombosis** is not uncommon.
- Thrombosis also occurs in **cardiac chambers and valve leaflets**.

Thromboembolism

The major complication of thrombosis is **thromboembolism.**

Emboli are dislodged from thrombus and circulate to be lodged in microcirculation in visceral organs such as brain (**cerebral embolism**), lungs (**pulmonary embolism**), heart (**coronary embolism**) and intestine (**intestinal embolism**).

Coronary and cerebral thrombosis leads to *ischemic tissue death **(infarction)**,* which causes heart attack and stroke respectively.

Treatment: Prophylactic anticoagulation and **antiplatelet therapy** is the mainstay of prevention of complications of thrombosis.

Exam Questions

1. Describe the mechanism of blood coagulation.
2. Describe the intrinsic / extrinsic mechanism of blood coagulation
3. Describe the mechanism of fibrinolysis.
4. List the functions of plasmin. Briefly describe the plasminogen activators and inhbitors of fibrinolysis.
5. Classify anticoagulants. Briefly describe the mechanism of action of vitamin K antagonists.
6. Classify the tests performed to investigate bleeding disorders. Briefly describe the pathophysiology of DIC.

Multiple Choice Questions

1. The first and immediate event in hemostasis is:
A. Platelet adhesion B. Activation of factor XII
C. Vasoconstriction D. Platelet aggregation

2. Normally, blood does not clot inside a blood vessel, because:
A. Collagen is not exposed in vascular endothelium
B. Heparin from mast cells lyses the clot
C. Vitamin K abntagonists are present in blood
D. Thrmbomodulin–protein C complex causes fibrinolysis

3. All of the following are true for Intrinsic pathway of coagulation, EXCEPT:
A. Does not require factor VII
B. Activated factor VIII is crucial for activation of factor X
C. Triggered by injury to body tissues
D. Proceed slowly than extrinsic pathway

4. Heparin acts by facilitating action of:
A. Vitamin K B. Prothrombin activator
C. Plasmin inhibitor D. Antithrombin III

5. All of the following are features of enzyme cascade system, EXCEPT:
A. Activated enzymes in turn activate other inactive enzymes
B. Negative feedback regulation
C. Gradual amplification
D. Facilitated by several cofactors

6. Lack of Vitamin K does not cause deficiency of:
A. Proaccelerin B. Proconvertin
C. Christmas factor D. Stuart-Prower factor

7. Hemophilia is:
A. Autosomal recessive B. X-linked recessive
C. Females suffer more than males
D. Replacement with prothrombin improves the condition

8. All of the following detect defects in coagulation pathway, EXCEPT?
A. Prothrombin time B. Clotting time
C. Clot retraction time D. Activated partial thromboplastin time

9. Streptokinase, used in acute myocardial infarction for the lysis of intracoronary clot:
A. Inactivates activated clotting factors
B. Inhibits thrombin
C. Facilitates release of heparin
D. Activates plasminogen

10. Administration of aspirin in low dose prevents myocardial infarction by:
A. Not allowing the clots to stabilize
B. Inhibiting platelet aggregation
C. Activating the fibrinolytic mechanism
D. Decreasing the clotting factors

11. Which of the following is the glass or contact factor?
A. Factor XIII B. Factor XII
C. Factor XI D. Factor IX

12. All of the following are functions of thrombin, EXCEPT:
A. Facilitates repair of injured vessel wall
B. Activates factor XIII
C. Activates formation of prothrombin activator
D. Inhibits the platelets

13. Which of the following does NOT activate fibrinolytic system?
A. Trypsin inhibitor B. Protein C
C. Stress D. Glucocorticoids

14. Which of the following is a cofactor in stabilization of fibrin polymer?
A. Magnesium B. Phospholipid
C. Calcium D. Tissue thromboplastin

15. Which of the following is NOT true about von Willebrand disease?
A. Most common inherited bleeding disorder
B. Desmopressin is useful in less severe cases
C. Factor VIII level is increased
D. Mucocutaneous bleeding is the commonest presentation

16. Which of the following is NOT true about temporary hemostatic plug?
A. Can be dissolved by anticoagulants
B. Gets converted to definitive hemostatic plug by fibrin
C. Seen following injury to vessel wall
D. It is a plug formed by aggregation of platelets

Answers

1. C 2. A 3. C 4. D 5. B 6. A 7. B 8. C 9. D 10. B 11. C
12. D 13. A 14. C 15. C 16. A

Section III

Nerve and Muscle

"*Never forget that you are not alone.*
The Divine is with you, helping and guiding you.
He is the companion who never fails,
the friend whose love comforts and strengthens.
Have faith and He will do everything for you.

The Mother
(of Sri Aurobindo Ashram)"

Chapter 18

Structure and Functions of Neuron, Nerve Potentials and Propagation of Nerve Impulse

Learning Objectives

On completion of study of this chapter:

The student will be able to (must know):

1. Name the different parts of a neuron and give their functions.
2. Know the mechanism of genesis of electrotonic potentials.
3. Define rheobase, chronaxie & utilization time and draw the strength-duration curve.
4. Draw a labeled schematic diagram of nerve action potential (AP) and describe the ionic basis of each phase of AP.
5. Define refractory periods (ARP & RRP) of nerve AP and explain their importance.
6. Explain the mechanism of propagation of AP and appreciate the importance of saltatory conduction.
7. List the differences between graded potential and action potential.

The student may also be able to (desirable to know):

1. Describe the process of axoplasmic transport.
2. Describe the details of ionic basis of nerve potentials.

The neuron is the structural and functional unit of the nervous system. The neuron is an excitable cell which transmits messages in the form of **action potentials**. There are about **86 billion neurons** present in the human brain and **69 million neurons** in spinal cord.

STRUCTURE OF A NEURON

Though neuron occurs in diverse shapes and sizes, basically it has **three parts**: a cell body, dendrites, and an axon that ends at axon terminal (Fig. 18.1).

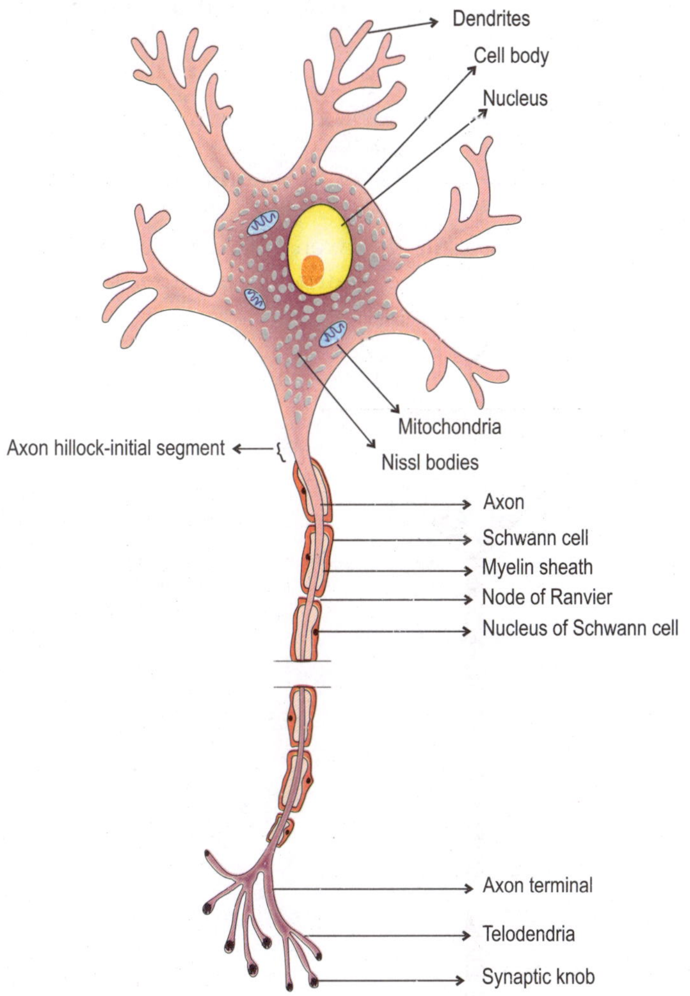

Fig. 18.1: Parts of a neuron.

Cell Body

Cell body, also known as soma or **perikaryon** is the center of the neuron. It contains the nucleus and cytoplasm containing cell organelles.

- **Cell organelles** are mainly numerous Nissl granules, many mitochondria, Golgi apparatus and lysosomes.
- **Nissl granules** (also called as Nissl bodies) are rough endoplasmic reticulum.
- **The nucleus** usually contains one nucleolus.

- Though the neuron is an active cell, it has ***lost the capacity to regenerate*** as indicated by the absence of centriole.
- The soma at one end gives rise to small branching processes called **dendrites** and at the other end a long process called **axon**.

Dendrites

The numerous short extensions from the cell body are called dendrites.

- They **increase the cell surface area** of the neuron many folds.
- In neurons of cerebral and cerebellar cortex, small knobby projections called **dendritic spines** further increase the surface area.
- Dendrites **receive the incoming signals** from other cells and ***transmit them to the cell body***.
- On an average, there are about **10,000 dendrites per neuron** present in the CNS.

Axon

Axon or the axis cylinder of the neuron forms the nerve fiber.

- The cytoplasm in the axon is known as **axoplasm** that contains mitochondria, Golgi apparatus, and cytoskeletal proteins.

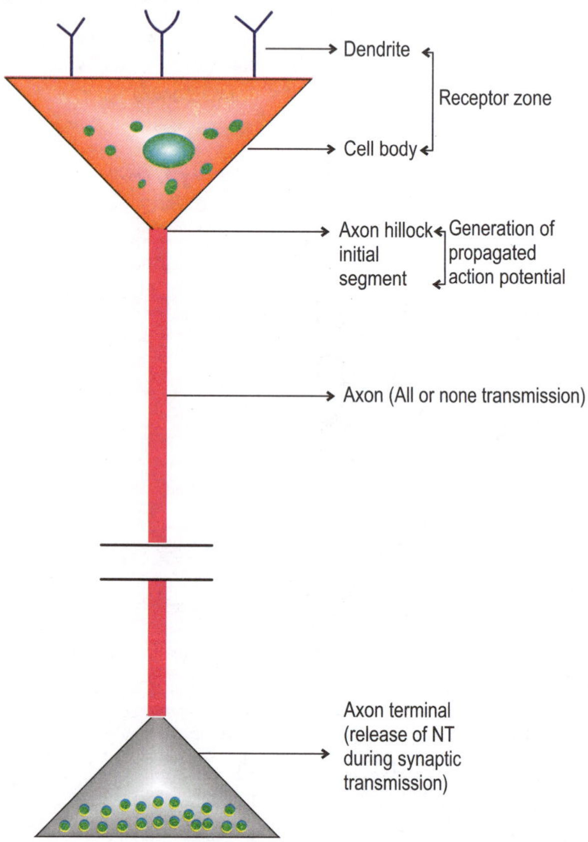

Fig. 18.2: Major functions of different parts of a neuron. NT: neurotransmitter.

Axon Hillock–Initial Segment: The axon arises from a thickened, tapered area of the cell body called the **axon hillock.**

- The initial portion of the axon is known as the **initial segment**.
- The axon hillock continues as initial segment, and this part is known as **axon hillock–initial segment** portion of the neuron.
- The **action potential is generated at the initial segment** in motor neurons and at the first node of Ranvier in sensory neurons (Fig. 18.2).

Axon Terminal: The terminal part of axon **loses myelin** and divides into several branches.

- The endings form bulb like enlargements called **terminal buttons** or synaptic knobs.
- The buttons contain neurotransmitter vesicles.

Axonal Growth: During development of a neuron, axonal growth depends on the interaction between the growing axon and the surrounding tissue environment.

- At the growing end is present a **growth cone**, which is motile and contains actin.
- The **direction of axonal growth** is determined by ***cell adhesion molecules***, influenced by trophic factors secreted from target cells and guided by glial cells.

Types of Axons

Axons are of **2 types**: myelinated & unmyelinated.

Myelinated Axons

In the peripheral nervous system (PNS), myelinated axons have a sheath around them formed by the **Schwann cells.**

- The large diameter somatic nerve fibers and preganglionic fibers of the autonomic nervous system are myelinated.
- In CNS, myelination is carried out by **oligodendrocytes**.

Role of Schwann Cell in Myelination

The double layers of the membrane of a single Schwann cell **wrap several times** (about 100 times) over **1 mm length** of the axon forming a covering of **8–10 µm thickness**.

- The adjacent layers stick to each other tightly with the help of a protein called **protein zero** (P_0) present in the Schwann cell membrane.
  - **Mutation of P_0** causes ***defective myelination*** and decreased conduction as occurs in various peripheral neuropathies.
- The **nucleus of the Schwann cell** lies beneath the plasma membrane ***in the outermost layer***.
- Thus, the myelin sheath extending along the length of an axon is **formed by many Schwann cells**, which are ***present at regular intervals*** along the course of the axon.
- The gaps between the Schwann cells are called the **nodes of Ranvier**.

- The membrane at the node is exposed to the ECF.
- Each node is **0.5–1.0 μm in length** and the internodal distance is 1–2 mm.

Objectives of Myelination: Myelination has following three main objectives:

1. Increases the speed of conduction
2. Reduces energy expenditure by the cell
3. Provides a protective covering to the axon.

Timing of Myelination During Development: Myelination of different types of nerve fibers takes place at different times.

- The **sensory fibers of the dorsal column system** first get myelinated, which occurs at **4th–5th month** of intrauterine life.
- The **corticospinal tract fibers** start myelinating at **two months of age** and the process gets ***completed at about 2nd year of life***, when the child has learned to walk.

Significant contribution of Scientist

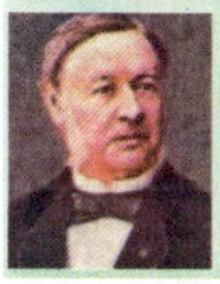

Theodor Schwann (1810 – 1882)

T. Schwann advanced the concept of cellular organization of living beings and described the structure of neurilemma (covering of the nerve). He is popularly remembered for his discovery of myelin sheath of axons; hence these cells are known as **Schwann cells**.

Unmyelinated Axons

Unmyelinated axons *do not have myelin sheath* (Table 18.1).

- Somatic nerve fibers of **very small diameter**, **postganglionic sympathetic neurons** of the autonomic nervous system, **dorsal root fibers** and most of the fibers in invertebrates are unmyelinated.
- The **speed of conduction** of impulse is **slower** in unmyelinated nerve fibers.

Table 18.1 | Difference between myelinated and unmyelinated nerves

Myelinated nerves	Unmyelinated nerves
1.Have axons of large diameter.	Have axons of small diameter.
2. Axons surrounded by concentric layers of Schwann cell plasma membrane.	Axons surrounded by cytoplasm of Schwann cells.
3. Nerve impulse jumps from one node to the other node, which is called saltatory conduction	Nerve impulse travels uniformly along the axolemma.
4. Density of voltage gated Na^+ channels are more (about 350 to 500/μm² at initial segment, and 2000 to 12,000 /μm² in node of Ranvier).	Na^+ channels are less in axons (about 110 /μm²).
5. Saltatory conduction seen in myelinated nerves is fast and consumes less energy.	Conduction seen in unmyelinated nerves is slow and consumes more energy.
6. Examples: All preganglionic fibers in ANS. In PNS, fibers more than 1μm in diameter.	All post-ganglionic fibers in ANS. In PNS, fibers less than 1μm in diameter.

Axoplasmic Transport

Transfer of substances between cell body and axon terminal is called axoplasmic transport.

- Axoplasmic transport can be **abolished by** application of colchicine, dinitrophenol, azide, cyanide and prolonged anoxia.

Types: There are **2 types** of axoplasmic transport: anterograde and retrograde.

Anterograde Transport

The transport of materials from the cell body **towards the axon terminals** is known as anterograde transport.

- Various **neurotransmitter vesicles** from the cell body are transported to nerve endings through axoplasmic transport.

Axoplasmic transport may be **fast or slow.**

1. **Fast axoplasmic transport** occurs at a speed of about 400 mm/day, which is accomplished by kinesin. a microtubule associated protein that transports many organelles, vesicles and membrane glycoproteins.
2. **Slow axoplasmic transport** occurs at the rate of about 0.5–2 mm/day. Various structural proteins like actin, neurofilaments and microtubules are transported by slow transport.

Retrograde Transport

Transport **from the axon terminals to the cell body** is known as retrograde transport.

- It occurs at a speed of about **200 mm/day**, brought about by ***dynein***, another microtubule associated protein.

The examples of retrograde transport are:

i) **Transport of chickenpox virus**, known as varicella zoster from nerve terminal to cell body that causes herpes simplex.

ii) **Transport of** tetanus toxin from motor neuron ending to the cell body.

iii) **Transfer of nerve growth factor** from presynaptic terminal to the soma.

iv) **Reuptake of synaptic transmitters:** Neurotransmitters like norepinephrine (NE) released at the nerve terminals are rapidly removed from the synaptic cleft by reuptake into the presynaptic neuron.

In the presynaptic terminal, NE is repackaged into vesicles or deaminated by mitochondrial monoamine oxidase.

- Some of the vesicles may be transported back to the cell body and this may provide a **feedback signal** to the cell body for further synthesis of transmitters.

Neuronal Ion Channels

Like any other cell membrane, neuronal membrane possesses numerous ion channels like Na^+, K^+, Ca^{++}, Cl^- etc. They are broadly categorized into **three types**:

i) Nongated or leaky channels
ii) Gated (voltage -gated, ligand- gated and mechanical- gated)
iii) ATP-driven pumps.

Resting State: In the resting state, the membrane is permeable to many ions like Na^+, K^+, Cl^- etc. through **leaky channels.**

- Permeability is **more to K^+** that mainly contributes to the genesis of resting membrane potential (RMP) of –70 mV.
- The RMP is maintained by Na^+-K^+ ATPase.

Active State: In the active state, the **depolarization and repolarization** phase of action potential occurs due to sequential activation of voltage-gated **Na^+ and K^+ channels.**

- These channels are present throughout the axon, where they participate in the initiation and propagation of action potentials.
  i) The **voltage-gated Na^+ channels** are concentrated at the ***nodes of Ranvier.***
  ii) The **voltage-gated Ca^{++} channels** are mainly present at the ***axon terminals,*** where they play important role in the secretion of neurotransmitters.
  iii) The **mechanical-gated Na^+ channels** are involved in the genesis of receptor potential in the *somatic sensory nerve endings.*
  iv) **Ligand-gated ion channels** are present predominantly on *dendritic spines, dendrites and cell body* of the neuron.

Distribution of Na^+ channels: In myelinated neurons, the number of Na^+ channels **per square micrometer of membrane** in different segments of the neuron is as follows:

1. At cell body: 50–75
2. At initial segment: 350–500
3. On the surface of the myelin: 25
4. At the nodes of Ranvier: 2000–12,000
5. At the axon terminals: 20–75

- Thus, the channels are concentrated in areas where the action potential is **first initiated** (initial segment) and in regions where it is **regenerated** (nodes of Ranvier) during its propagation.

In unmyelinated neurons, about **110 Na^+ channels** are present ***per square micrometer*** of the axonal membrane.

- Abnormalities of channels are called **channelopathies** (Clinical Note 18.1).

Clinical Note 18.1

Channelopathies: The diseases caused due to the structural or functional changes in the various ion channels are known as channelopathies, which include episodic and spinocerebellar ataxias, some forms of epilepsy and familial hemiplegic migraine.

Terms often used for Membrane Potentials

Certain terms are used to explain the change in membrane potentials.

Excitability: The ability of the cells to **generate action potential** in their membrane is known as excitability.

Polarized: When there is a **voltage difference** between the inside and outside of the membrane, the membrane is said to be polarized.

- At rest, the interior of the cell is –70 mV in comparison to outside.

Depolarizing Stimulus: When a stimulus allows influx of positive charges or efflux of negative charges, it **decreases the membrane potential** (i.e. the membrane potential approaches towards zero) and the stimulus is called a depolarizing stimulus.

Depolarized: A membrane is said to be depolarized when the membrane potential becomes **positive or less negative** in relation to RMP.

Repolarization: After the depolarization phase, return of the potential towards the resting value is known as repolarization.

Hyperpolarized: Similarly, as the interior of the cell **becomes more negative** in relation to RMP, due to influx of negative charges or removal of positive charges, the membrane is said to be hyperpolarized.

- In this state, the membrane potential is more negative in relation to RMP.

GENESIS OF NERVE POTENTIALS

When a stimulus is applied to a neuron, it induces ions to flow across the membrane and alters the ionic balance on both sides of the membrane, producing a **voltage change.** The voltage changes lead to ***generation and propagation of the electrical signals*** in the axon from one end to the other. These generated signals are of **two types:**

i) **Electrotonic or graded potentials** that spread the signal over short distances, and
ii) **Action potentials** that transmit message throughout the length of the plasma membrane. Another type of response seen in neuronal membrane is called **local response.**

Electrotonic Potentials

Definition

Electrotonic or graded potentials are **local, non-propagated potentials** of small magnitude, in response to a depolarizing or hyperpolarizing stimulus of lesser strength.

Types

Electrotonic potentials are **two types:** catelectrotonic and anelectrotonic.

Catelectrotonic Potential: When a membrane is electrically stimulated, the ***cathodal end*** of the stimulator evokes a **depolarizing response** called catelectrotonic potential.

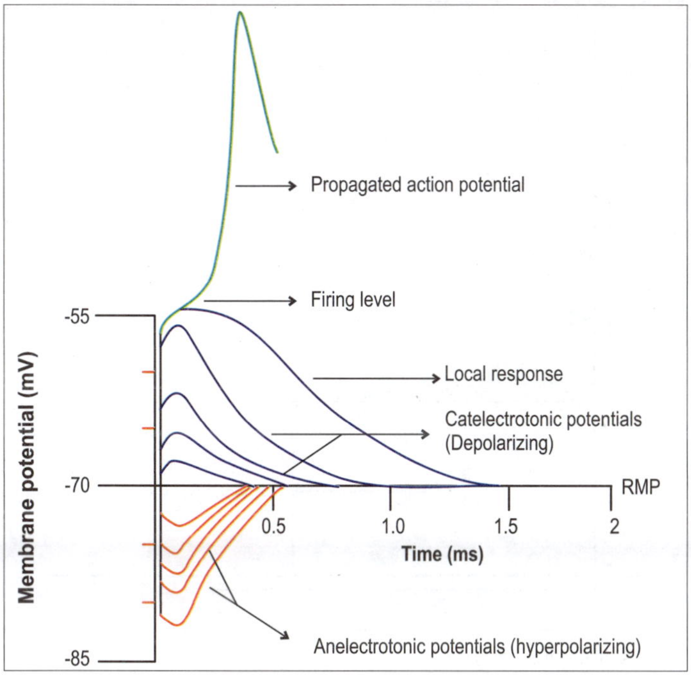

Fig. 18.3: Electrotonic potentials and local response. RMP: resting membrane potential.

- The graph displays *upward waveform*.

Anelectrotonic Potential: The **hyperpolarizing potential** produced due to stimulation at the ***anodal end*** is known as anelectrotonic potential (Fig. 18.3).

- The graph displays *downward waveform*.

Mechanism

In the resting state, anions are lined along the interior of the membrane and cations along the exterior of the membrane.

Stimulus of Smaller Strength: With the application of a cathodal stimulus of smaller strength across a small area of the plasma membrane, **few Na^+ ions enter** through the sodium channels into the cell.

- At that instant, **at the site of stimulus**, the inside of the ***membrane becomes positive*** compared to the previous resting state due to accumulation of cations.
- The magnitude of the change in membrane potential depends on the **quantity of positive charges** entering the cell.

Stimulus of Greater Strength: With application of **greater strength of stimulus**, more positive charges enter into the cell and the **voltage change is larger**.

Graded Potential: The term graded potential comes from the fact that the potential change **increases in a stepwise manner** with application of increasing strength.

- Graded potentials are recorded from the membranes of **dendrites and cell body**.

After Effects

Following the graded potential, the **repolarizing forces try to neutralize** the disturbance in RMP, created by the Na^+ entry.

- As a result, **K^+ tends to come out** of the cell and Cl^- **enters** through the leaky channels to maintain the electrical neutrality.
- Also, **Na^+ moves away** by diffusion from the site of stimulus that decreases amplitude of the graded potential with time.
- Moreover, the **ionic disturbance** produced (more sodium and less potassium inside) due to the application of the stimulus ***is eliminated by*** increased activity of the **Na^+-K^+ ATPase** that pumps $3Na^+$ out and $2K^+$ in.
- All these lead to the gradual return of the membrane potential towards the resting value.

Decremental Conduction

When recorded near the site of stimulus, the amplitude of the potential is larger and **recorded at a farther place, *it is smaller.***

- The potentials die out within 3 mm from the site of stimulus.
- If recorded immediately after the application of the stimulus, the amplitude is larger and **with delay in recording**, the ***amplitude is smaller***.
- Thus, it **decays progressively with time and distance**, which is called *decremental conduction*.

Properties of Graded Potential

1. **Graded in nature:** The potential change **increases in a stepwise manner** with application of increasing strength of stimulus i.e. the ***magnitude of potential change is proportionate to the stimulus strength.***
2. **Decremental conduction:** Graded potentials decay progressively with time and distance.
3. **Depolarizing or hyperpolarizing nature:** If the change in potential primarily depends on the type and strength of the stimuli (Fig. 18.3).
   i) With application of increasing strength of stimulus, more positive charges enter the cell and the amplitude of the wave ***rises proportionately***.
   ii) When the membrane is stimulated with anodal end, due to entry of negative charges or removal of positive charges, the membrane potential becomes more negative; the graph displays a ***downward waveform***.

Thus, graded potentials can occur in either a depolarizing or a hyperpolarizing direction.

3. **Summation:** Graded potentials also exhibit the ***property of summation***; i.e. if a second stimulus is applied before the potential produced by the first stimulus has disappeared, **both the potential changes are added together** producing a ***larger or prolonged wave*** in the recording.
   - This happens due to the arrival of more Na^+ ions at the site of stimulus before neutralization of all

the positive charges accumulated by the first stimulus.

- Similarly, the anelectrotonic potentials exhibit the property of summation.

Forms of Graded Potentials

According to the site of genesis, they are described differently. For example:

End-plate potential: recorded from skeletal muscle membrane at neuromuscular junctions.

Receptor potential: recorded from sensory nerve endings.

Synaptic potential: recorded from membrane of post-synaptic neurons at neuro-neuronal junctions.

Pacemaker potential: recorded from pacemaker cells in the heart, intestine.

Local Response

As the axon is stimulated with slowly increasing strength of stimuli, the amplitude of the electrotonic potential gradually rises.

- When the membrane potential is **decreased by 7 mV**, the pattern of graded potential is altered.
- The **response becomes greater** than what is expected for that strength of stimulus. This ***enhanced response*** is known as local response.
- Similar to the graded potential, the local response gradually **dies out with increasing distance**.
- Local response is seen **only with a depolarizing stimulus** of lower strength, and not with a hyperpolarizing one.

Ionic Basis of Local Response

As the applied cathodal stimulus is progressively raised from zero, the **influx of Na^+ ions** through the leaky sodium channels ***proportionately increases***.

- Consequently, the membrane potential gradually **decreases from –70 to –63 mV**.
- At that point of time, the **voltage-gated sodium channels start opening**, which allows entry of some more Na^+ ions.
- The **extra Na^+ ions** entering into the cytoplasm are added to the existing Na^+ influx, resulting in local response.

Strength and Type of Stimuli

With a gradual increase in stimulus strength, as the membrane potential approaches a value of –55 mV, the neuron starts generating action potentials.

- The process is often termed as ***firing* or *discharge*** of the neuron and the membrane potential at –55 mV is known as the **firing level** or **threshold**.
- The stimulus that brings the membrane potential to –55 mV is known as threshold stimulus.

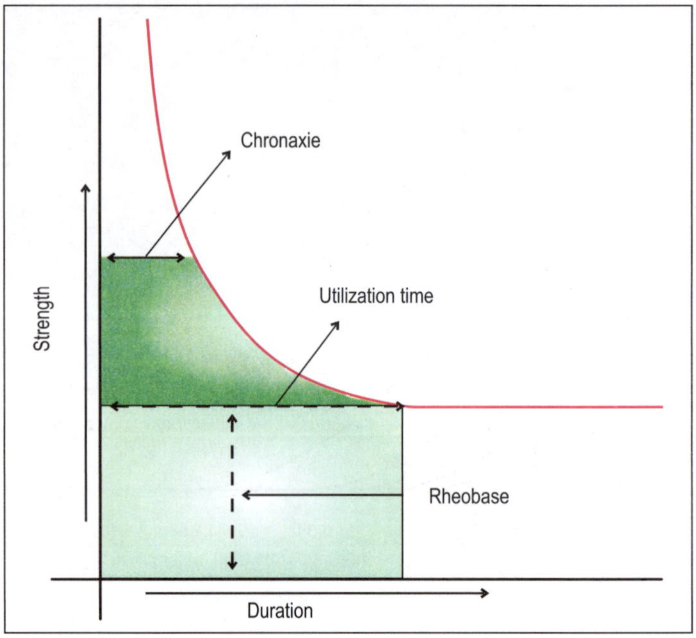

Fig. 18.4: Strength-duration curve.

Threshold Stimulus: It is defined as the **lowest strength of stimulus** that ***elicits an action potential***.

Subthreshold Stimulus: The stimulus less in strength than the threshold is known as subthreshold stimuli.

Suprathreshold Stimulus: The stimulus higher in strength than the threshold is known as suprathreshold stimulus.

Strength-Duration Relationship

Strength and duration of a stimulus have a complimentary role in determining the excitability of a tissue. These two parameters are **inversely related** to each other.

The relationship between the strength and duration of stimuli depicted in graph form is known as **strength-duration curve** (Fig. 18.4).

Rheobase: To excite a tissue, the **lowest amplitude of current** required is termed as rheobase.

Utilization Time: The minimum time for which the rheobase must be applied to elicit an action potential is known as utilization time.

- A stimulus weaker than rheobase does not excite the tissue and a stimulus stronger than rheobase requires less time (less than utilization time) to elicit a response.

Chronaxie: It is the **time required** for a stimulus of ***double the rheobase strength*** to produce an action potential.

- Usually, chronaxie gives us a better idea about the excitability of a tissue.
- Lesser the chronaxie, greater is the excitability.
- Nerves have a shorter chronaxie compared to muscles.

Accommodation

If the **intensity of a stimulus is raised slowly** to the threshold value, the tissue ***fails to produce an action potential*** because it adapts to the stimulus. This phenomenon is known as accommodation.

- During the slow depolarization, some of the voltage-gated Na^+ channels start opening at a membrane potential of –63 mV.
- But they soon get inactivated before another set of channel opens as the membrane takes longer time to arrive at the next level of potential.
- Thus, the sufficient number of activated sodium channels that are required to fire an action potential is never accomplished.

Action Potential

Definition

Action potential is defined as a **transient change in membrane potential** of about 100 mV, which is *conducted along the axon* in an ***all-or-none fashion***.

- It is characterized by a **gradual depolarization to threshold**, and a **rapid ascent** in the membrane potential followed by a **rapid descent**.
- It travels along the axon with the **same shape and amplitude** being regenerated at regular intervals.

The action potential is also known as an **impulse** or **spike potential**.

Duration and Amplitude

The duration of a single nerve action potential is about **1 msec**, during which the membrane potential sharply rises from –70 to +35 mV, and then returns to its resting value.

Latent Period

Latent period is the interval between the application of the stimulus and the onset of action potential.

- **Duration** of latent period depends on the distance between stimulating and recording electrodes and the type and diameter of nerve fiber.

Phases of an Action Potential

A typical action potential has a phase of **depolarization** and a phase of **repolarization**.

Phase of Depolarization

Depolarization is recorded as an **upstroke** during which the membrane potential approaches zero and then becomes positive.

- It consists of **slow depolarization** to threshold (***local response***), **rapid rising phase**, **overshoot** and **peak**.
- During the overshoot, membrane potential crosses the zero or isopotential level and at the peak, it reaches +35 mV.

Phase of Repolarization

Repolarization is recorded as **down-stroke** during which the membrane potential returns to the resting level.

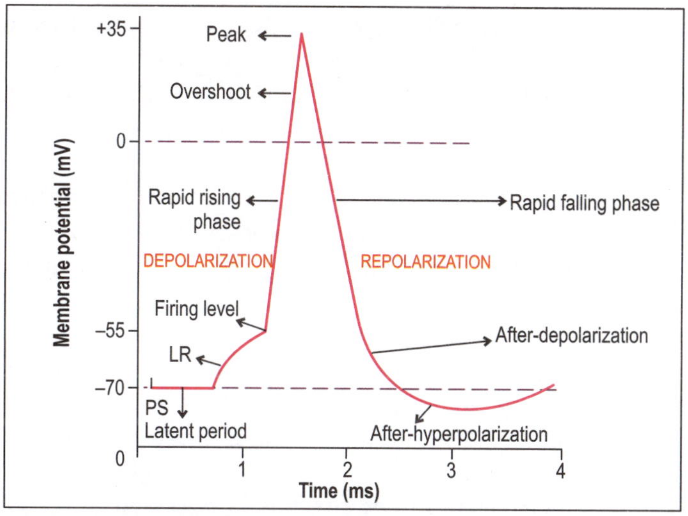

Fig. 18.5: Phases of action potential recorded from a neuron. Note, depolarization phase consists of local response, rapid rising phase, overshoot and peak; and repolarization phase consists of rapid falling phase and after-depolarization. LR: local response; PS: point of stimulation.

- It includes a **rapid falling phase** and slower terminal part called **after-depolarization**.

After-Hyperpolarization

The phase of repolarization is followed by an **after-hyperpolarization phase** during which the membrane potential undershoots (becomes more negative) and then returns back to the resting level (Fig. 18.5).

Ionic Basis of Action Potential

Depolarization

Depolarization is due to **opening of voltage-gated Na^+ channels,** causing massive *influx of sodium ions.*

- The **early part of local response** is due to entry of sodium ions through the leaky channels.
- When the membrane potential **is about –63 mV**, few of the ***voltage-gated Na^+ channels*** begin to open.
- The influx of Na^+ through leaky channels and later through opening of few voltage-gated Na^+ channels decreases the membrane potential **from –70 mV to –55 mV**.
- At this **threshold potential,** there is simultaneous opening of ***large number of the voltage-gated Na^+ channels,*** increasing the membrane permeability to sodium ions **several hundredfold.**
- This leads to **massive influx of sodium** ions producing a swift, large and **steep depolarization,** raising the membrane potential **to +35 mV.**
- Thus, a change in membrane potential occurs by 105 mV, from the resting value of –70mV to +35mV.

At threshold level, the number of Na^+ channels that have already opened, cause concomitant opening of almost all the Na^+ channels in the stimulated part of the membrane. This is an example of **positive feedback control** (Application Box 18.1). This leads to simultaneous **autoactivation** of huge number of Na^+ channels.

Membrane potential remains below Na^+ equilibrium potential: Though depolarization is due to opening of voltage-gated Na^+ channels, membrane potential does not reach equilibrium potential for Na^+, which is +60 mV, due to **three following factors**:

1. At the peak of the action potential, **sodium influx abruptly ceases** due to the abrupt closure of Na^+ channels, as opening of Na^+ channels is a ***transient phenomenon***.
   - Na^+ channels open very fast and also close very fast.
   - The speedy closure is due to rapid **autodeactivation**.
2. The voltage-gated potassium channels being fully open, this **allows the exit of positively charged K^+ ions**.
3. The **electrical gradient for Na^+ is reversed** after the overshoot that slows further sodium entry.

> **Application Box 18.1**
>
> **Hodgkin's cycle:** At threshold level of action potential, prior opening of few Na+ channels leading to further opening of many other Na+ channels is called Hodgkin's cycle. This is an example of **positive feedback** control in which a stimulus triggering an event further facilitates the process. During an action potential, approximately 20,000 **Na+ ions** enter into the cell.

Repolarization

Repolarization is due to ***opening of voltage-gated K^+ channels*** causing **efflux of K^+.**

- The **K^+ channels** are sensitive to the same depolarization that opens the voltage-gated Na^+ channels, but they **open more slowly**.
- **At the peak** of the action potential, the voltage-gated Na^+ channels enter a closed state whereas the voltage-gated ***K^+ channels are fully open***.
- The **membrane permeability** to potassium ions ***increases several times*** causing increased **potassium efflux**.
- The K^+ concentration is **much higher inside** the cell and at the peak of the action potential, ***outside of the membrane is negative relative to inside***, which is positive at +35 mV.
  - These **two factors** favour the electrochemical gradient for potassium efflux.
- Repolarization is contributed by ***decline in sodium influx***.
- The termination of action potential due to activation of voltage-gated potassium channels is a **negative feedback process**.

Following rapid repolarization, when the membrane potential drops close to RMP, the inside of the membrane becomes negative that limits the efflux of potassium.

- Thus, **after-depolarization phase** is due to the ***slower exit of potassium ions*** that considerably decreases the rate of repolarization and makes the repolarization curve oblique (less steep).

After-hyperpolarization

At the RMP level, though most of the voltage-gated K^+ channels are closed, some of them still remain open allowing **continued efflux of K^+ ions**.

- Consequently, the membrane potential **continued to become more negative** resulting in ***prolonged and slow undershoot***, which is called the phase of after-hyperpolarization.
- Finally, the K^+ channels completely close, restoring the membrane potential to the RMP level.

Ionic Conductance during Action Potential

Conductance of an ion means the ease with which the ion passes through the membrane.

- It indicates the **permeability of the membrane to the ion**.
- Conductance is **reciprocal of resistance** offered by the membrane and the potential gradient across the membrane hindering the passage of the ion.

Na^+ Conductance: The Na^+ conductance **rises gradually from the RMP to the firing level**.

- Then **increases very rapidly to reach a peak**, just before the peak of the action potential.
- After that it **declines rapidly** and returns to the base line.

K^+ Conductance: The K^+ conductance rises after the rise in Na^+ conductance.

- Initially, K^+ conductance increases at a *slower rate*.
- Then the rate rises, attains a **peak much after the peak of Na^+ conductance.**
- And then **decreases very slowly** to reach the base line.

Thus, compared to Na^+ conductance, **K^+ conductance has slower rise, lesser magnitude** and much ***slower and prolonged return*** to the baseline (Fig. 18.6).

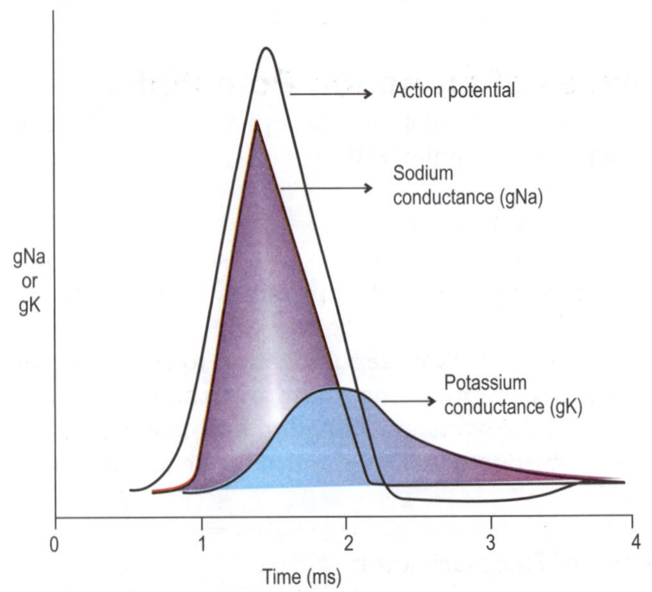

Fig. 18.6: Conductance of sodium and potassium across the membrane during action potential.

Ionic Activity after the Action Potential

At the end of an action potential, there is more sodium and less potassium inside the cell. The ionic composition is restored by **increased activity of the Na^+-K^+ ATPase**.

- The number of ions taking part in generation of a single action potential is very little compared to the total number of ions present in the cell.
- About 1 of every one million Na^+ ions enters the cell and same number of K^+ ions comes out of the cell during an action potential.
- This produces a negligible change in the intracellular ionic concentration.

IMPORTANT NOTE

Ionic balance after A.P. is a must: If this small ionic imbalance that happens following each action potential is not restored, then following repeated generation of action potentials, it would be difficult to generate action potentials further. This is because slowly the concentration gradients of sodium and potassium across the membrane will cease to exist.

Effects of Extracellular Ionic Changes

1. When **extracellular Na^+ concentration is decreased**, the amplitude of the action potentials becomes smaller than usual because the concentration gradient for Na^+ that drives sodium into the cell is reduced.
2. When **extracellular Na^+ concentration is increased**, the amplitude of the action potentials may increase.
3. When **extracellular K^+ concentration is decreased**, the membrane potential becomes ***more negative*** as the resting K^+ efflux is favoured by the increased concentration gradient across the membrane.
4. When **extracellular K^+ concentration is increased**, the membrane potential come closer to the firing level and the membrane becomes ***more excitable***.
5. When **extracellular Ca^{2+} concentration is decreased**, the electrical potential difference across the membrane is decreased, as the inside becomes less negative compared to outside.
   - The RMP come closer to the firing level, so that, the magnitude of depolarization needed to reach the firing level is less.
   - Hence, decrease in extracellular Ca^{++} concentration increases the excitability of the tissue, as observed in hypocalcemic tetany, occurring in hypoparathyroidism.
6. If **extracellular Ca^{2+} concentration is increased**, the RMP goes away from the firing level due to increased potential difference across the membrane. Consequently, the magnitude of depolarization needed to reach the firing level is more, decreasing the tissue excitability.

Ion Channel Blockers

Na^+ Channel Blockers

The drugs like lidocaine, procaine etc. and neurotoxins like tetrodotoxin, saxitoxin etc. **block the voltage-gated Na^+ channels** and hinder the generation of action potentials.

Local Anesthetics: Lidocaine and procaine are used as local anesthetics.

- When injected into the tissue, the ionizable hydrophobic drug molecules diffuse readily through the plasma membrane and **block transmission** of somatic sensations.
- **Axons with smaller diameter are more sensitive** to the local anesthetics than the large diameter fibers.

Membrane Toxins: The neurotoxins like **tetrodotoxin** (TTX) and **saxitoxin** (STX) cause paralysis. Ingestion of tissues containing small quantity of these toxins can lead to death.

K^+ Channel Blockers

The voltage-gated K^+ channel blockers are **tetraethylammonium** (TEA) and **4-aminopyridine** (4-AP).

Na^+-K^+ ATPase Blocker

Drugs like digitalis and dinitrophenol **block the Na^+–K^+ ATPase pump**.

All-or-None Law

Definition

All or none law states that the action potential occurs **with a constant amplitude and shape** irrespective of magnitude of the stimulus.

- A **subthreshold stimulus** fails to excite the tissue.
- Only a stimulus of **threshold magnitude** elicits an action potential.
- If **suprathreshold stimuli** are applied, the action potentials resulting from them have the same amplitude, duration and form as those produced by threshold stimuli, provided the experimental conditions remain same (Fig. 18.7).

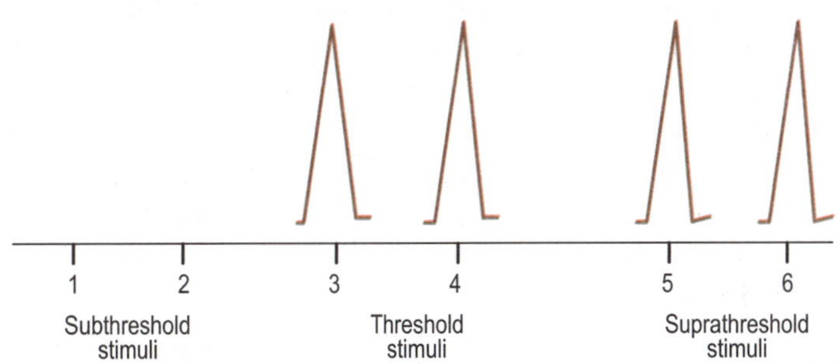

Fig. 18.7: All or none law for action potential. Note, subthreshold stimuli (1 & 2) do not evoke formation of action potential, whereas, threshold (3 & 4) and suprathreshold (5 & 6) stimuli evoke similar action potentials.

Mechanism

The voltage-gated Na^+ channels open instantaneously as soon as 15 mV of depolarization (firing level) is achieved following the application of threshold stimulus, and thereafter the membrane automatically attains another +90 mV of depolarization (–55 to +35 mV).

- Thus, once the threshold level is reached, the **magnitude of sodium influx becomes independent of the stimulus factor.**
- Therefore, a **stimulus with extra strength** (higher threshold stimulus) that produces greater degree of initial depolarization (>15mV) practically **does not add more** to the formation of action potential.
- Thus, as a rule, once the action potential is formed, it **appears with its maximum size and shape**, otherwise it does not form at all.
- This is called all-or-none law of action potential.

Refractory Periods

During the action potential, the stimulated area of the membrane remains unresponsive to a second stimulus, and later it requires a greater degree of depolarization to get excited again.

- The **length of time during which the membrane is unresponsive** *to a second stimulus no matter how strong is the stimulus*, is known as refractory period.
- The periods of total and relative refractoriness are known as absolute and relative refractory periods respectively.

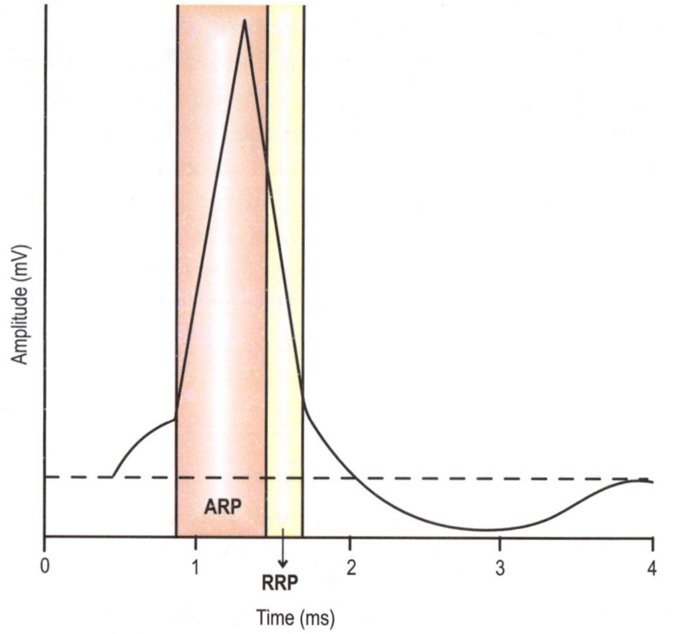

Fig. 18.8: Refractory periods of nerve action potential. ARP: absolute refractory period; RRP: relative refractory period.

Absolute Refractory Period (ARP)

Definition & Duration

ARP is defined as the period in the action potential during which, application of a **second stimulus of any strength and duration does not produce another action potential.**

- The ARP corresponds to the period from the time the firing level is reached *until repolarization is about one-third complete* (Fig. 18.8).
- Thus, it is the time **from the firing level to one-third of repolarization**.

Mechanism

At the peak of the action potential, the **voltage-gated sodium channels close** and they remain in that inactivated state for some time before returning to the resting state.

- These sodium channels can reopen in response to a second stimulus, only after attaining the resting state.
- Hence, even a stronger stimulus will not produce a second action potential, and the membrane is said to be in its ARP.

Physiological Importance

ARP limits the number of action potentials that the nerve can fire in a given period of time.

ARP serves **two important functions**:

1. ARP determines the **rate of discharge of nerve fiber.**
   - Generally, **large diameter nerve fibers** have an ARP of about 0.4 msec, with a firing rate of 2500 impulses per second,
   - **Small diameter fibers** have an ARP of about 4 msec, with a firing rate of 250 impulses per second.
2. ARP is also responsible for the **one-way conduction of action potentials**.

Relative Refractory Period (RRP)

Definition & Duration

RRP is defined as the period following ARP during which, application of a suprathreshold stimulus can elicit a second action potential.

- The RRP starts from the **end of ARP to the beginning of after-depolarization** (that means from one-third of repolarization to end of repolarization).

Mechanism

The following **two factors** contribute to RRP:

1. All the sodium channels present at the site of stimulus **do not attain the open state or resting state exactly at the same time.**
   - For example, few of them open when the membrane potential is –63 mV, causing local response.
   - Similarly, at RRP level, some of them have returned to their initial resting and can allow the influx of Na^+.
2. A suprathreshold stimulus can **spread to larger area** over the membrane and **open extra voltage-gated sodium channels** that can contribute to take the membrane potential to firing level.

Thus, only a suprathreshold stimulus and not any threshold stimulus can open up sufficient number of sodium channels to elicit an action potential during the RRP.

Excitability of the Membrane: The excitability of the membrane depends on the phases of the action potential.

- Close to the firing level, the membrane is most excitable.
- Excitability decreases, as the potential moves away from the firing level.
- During the ARP, it is least excitable.

INITIATION AND PROPAGATION OF ACTION POTENTIAL

Initiation of Action Potential

The genesis of action potentials requires presence of large number of voltage-gated ion channels that are present mostly on the axons.

- The action potential is first initiated in the specialized areas in the axon called the **first node of Ranvier** in sensory neurons and **initial segment-axon hillock area** in motor neurons.
- These areas are known as **trigger zones** that have a very high concentration of voltage-gated sodium and potassium channels.
- The synaptic potentials generated at dendrites or cell body are **integrated and transmitted to the axon hillock**.
- If the integrated potential **is sufficient to depolarize** the membrane of the axon hillock to firing level, action potential is generated.

Propagation of Action Potential

Once formed, the action potential is regenerated at regular intervals to be transmitted from the initial segment of the axon to the axon terminal. This is known as the propagation of action potential.

- The speed and mode of propagation of action potential is different in myelinated and unmyelinated axons.

The **speed of conduction** of the impulse depends on **two factors**:

1. **Myelination:** Conduction velocity is **more in myelinated axon** and is proportionate to the degree of myelination.
2. **Diameter of the axon:** Conduction velocity is proportionate to the diameter of the fiber.
   - As large diameter fibers have less cytoplasmic resistance, flow of ions across the membrane is easier.
   - Hence, fibers with larger diameter have faster rate of conduction.

In Unmyelinated Axon

At the site of genesis of action potential, large influx of positive charges into the membrane occurs, which is known as **current sink**.

1. The **positive charges diffuse away** from the site of accumulation.
   - The adjacent membrane, which is in its resting state, has a potential of –70 mV.
   - This potential difference allows the positive charges to flow toward the adjacent negative area.
   - Consequently, ***the potential of the adjacent membrane decreases*** and **reaches the threshold value**, as the fraction of Na^+ ions that move to the nearby negative area are sufficient enough to bring the **adjacent membrane to the firing level**.
   - This results in ***opening of the voltage gated Na^+ channels*** present in that area, firing an action potential.
2. Similarly, from the site of second action potential, **positive charges flow to the adjacent resting membrane** and decrease its potential to the threshold level.
   - This ***activates the voltage gated Na^+ channels*** present in that part of the membrane resulting *in another action potential*.
3. In this manner, **each point of the membrane gets depolarized** to the firing level and produces an action potential.
   - As the depolarization and repolarization phases of the ensuing action potentials are repeated, there is **a sequential opening and closing** of sodium and potassium channels along the axonal membrane (Fig. 18.9).
4. The action potential does not move by itself but helps to **generate a new action potential** in the membrane ahead of it.
   - As the number of voltage gated Na^+ and K^+ channels are distributed uniformly along the axon, the action potential arriving at the end of the axon is almost identical in appearance to the initial one.
   - Thus, due to the **local current flow** produced following an action potential, there is **serial depolarization** of the adjacent membrane to the firing level and action potential travels, being successively regenerated along the membrane in an all-or-none manner.

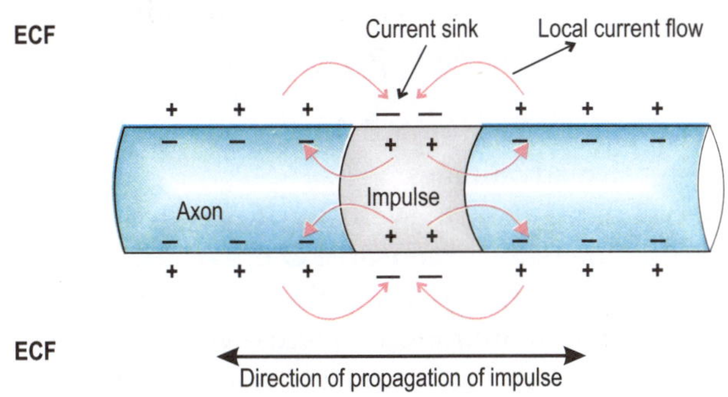

Fig. 18.9: Propagation of action potential in unmyelinated axon.

5. At the same time, in the exterior of the membrane, the negative area (generated by the stimulus due to withdrawal of positive charges) attracts flow of positive charges from the adjacent regions toward the site of stimulus.
   - Thus, on both sides of the site of action potential, a **circular pattern of current flow** occurs across the membrane; i.e. inside the membrane, positive charges flow away from the site of action potential, whereas outside the membrane, positive charges flow towards the site of action potential.
   - This circular pattern of current flow tries to restore the resting potential of the membrane where the action potential was previously generated.

In Myelinated Axon (Saltatory Conduction)

Myelin acts as an insulator and does not allow free flow of ions across the membrane.

1. Therefore, massive Na^+ influx does not occur in the myelinated portion of the membrane and **positive charges flow to the adjacent area**.
   - Also, in the myelin sheath, the concentration of positive charges does not decrease fast because of less 'leakage'.
   - This helps the charges to spread farther along the axon.
2. The local current (the positive charges) **travels like a graded potential** and dies away 37% of its maximal strength over a distance of about 3 mm.
   - As the internodal distance is 1–2 um, the local current **arrives at the adjacent node of Ranvier** and decreases its membrane potential.
3. Most importantly, the **voltage gated Na^+ channels are present in large numbers** at the nodes of Ranvier.
   - Therefore, as soon as the nodal membrane gets depolarized to threshold level, an action potential is quickly fired.
   - Thus, in the myelinated axon, the **action potential is generated at each node of Ranvier** (Fig. 18.10).
4. The action potential rapidly proceeds from one node to the other and pause at each node to get regenerated.

Therefore, the mode of propagation of action potential in myelinated axon is known as **saltatory conduction** (Latin word *'saltare'* means to jump).

Advantages in Myelinated Axon

There are **two advantages**:

1. In myelinated axon, the **velocity of conduction is faster**.
2. Myelination helps to **conserve energy**.
   - As the ionic flux occurs only at the nodes of Ranvier, the **total membrane area** across which ionic balance to be restored **is much less** in myelinated axon.
   - Moreover, in unmyelinated axons, voltage-gated channels open throughout the axonal length causing activation of larger number of Na^+-K^+ ATPase and higher expenditure of energy.

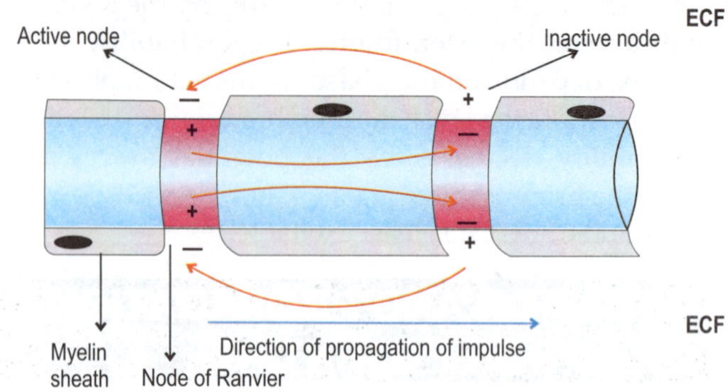

Fig. 18.10: Propagation of action potential in myelinated axon.

Direction of Propagation of Action Potential

In the motor neuron, the action potential is conducted from axon hillock toward axon terminal. In the sensory neuron, it propagates from the first node of Ranvier toward CNS. This is called **anterograde conduction** of impulse.

- The axon contains a large number of voltage gated Na^+ channels that promotes **quick generation of an action potential** in the axonal membrane next to the trigger zone.
- Following depolarization, the area on the membrane where action potential was produced becomes refractory. Therefore, **action potential does not travel back** towards the trigger zone.
- Though local currents from the site of next action potential tend to bring the membrane toward threshold value, the area of the **membrane of previous action potential does not fire** an action potential, as the *sodium channels in that portion remain inactivated*.
- Hence, the action potential **can be conducted only in the direction** away from the site of previous action potential.

Differences between Graded Potential & Action Potential

The major differences are listed in Table 18.1.

Table 18.1 | Differences between graded potentials and action potentials.

	Graded potential	Action potential
1. Amplitude	Amplitude is proportional to the strength of the stimulus	Once threshold potential is reached, amplitude remains same irrespective of the strength of the stimulus
2. Conduction	Travels in a decremental fashion; amplitude gradually decreases with time and along distance	Conducted in an all-or-none manner; appears with the same amplitude and shape all along the axon

Table 18.2: Contd...

3. Summation	Can be summated	Cannot be summated
4. Nature	Can be a depolarizing or hyperpolarizing potential	Always a large depolarizing potential
5. Mechanism	Due to opening of ligand-gated or leaky ion channels	Due to opening of voltage-gated ion channels
6. Properties	Does not have a threshold or refractory period	Have a threshold and refractory period

Exam Questions

1. Draw a suitable diagram of electrotonic potentials. Describe the ionic basis and physiological significance of these potentials.
2. With the help of a suitable diagram, describe strength-duration relationship of stimuli.
3. Draw a schematic diagram of an action potential recorded from a neuron. Describe the ionic basis of each phase of action potential.
4. Define all or none law and refractory periods. Give the ionic basis of these phenomena.
5. With the help of a suitable diagram, describe the initiation and propagation of action potential in myelinated and unmyelinated neurons.
6. List the differences between graded potential and action potential. Explain why action potential can not be summated.

Multiple Choice Questions

1. The maximum density of sodium channels on a neuron are present at:

A. Axon terminal B. Axon hillock
C. Dendrites D. Cell body

2. All of the following are true for dendrites, EXCEPT:

A. Receptive short processes emerging from cell body
B. Highly branched
C. Nissle granules are never present
D. The potentials generated do not obey all-or-none law

3. Development of myelin sheath in central nervous system depends on:

A. Astrocytes B. Oligodendrocytes
C. Schwann cells D. Ependymal cells

4. The maximum rate of axonal transport is:

A. 10 mm per day B. 40 mm per day
C. 100 mm per day D. 400 mm per day

5. Example of unipolar neurons is:

A. Brush cells of cerebellum B. Spinal motor neuron
C. Olfactory receptor neuron D. Dorsal root ganglion cell neurons

6. The potential at axo-dendritic synapse corded by:

A. EEG electrodes
B. ECG electrodes
C. Nerve conduction study electrodes
D. Microelectrodes

7. Rheobase denotes:

A. Firing rate of neuron
B. Specificity of impulse transmission
C. Duration of action potential
D. Strength of current

8. Which of the following statements is true for neuronal metabolism?

A. To maintain RMP, the Na+-K+ pump uses 7% of total energy
B. In the absence of oxygen, the conduction in neuron stops immediately
C. Neurons are rich in vitamin B1
D. Resting neuron does not use phospholipids for energy

9. All of the following are factors for nerve growth, EXCEPT:

A. Leukemia inhibitory factor
B. Neurotrophin-3
C. Neurotensin
D. Platelet-derived growth factor

10. All of the following are true about myelination, EXCEPT:

A. Motor fibers complete myelination later than sensory fibers
B. Schwann cell sheath is called neurilemma
C. Increases energy expenditure as the impulse jumps from node to node
D. Patchy destruction of myelin occurs in multiple sclerosis

11. In the neuron, the site of generation of graded potential is:

A. Initial segment B. Axon terminal
C. Node of Ranvier D. Dendrites

12. Which of the following is a sodium channel blocker?

A. Lidocaine B. Nitroglycerinel
C. Nifedipine D. Tetraethylammonium

13. All of the following are true for absolute refractory period (ARP) in neuron, EXCEPT:

A. Responsible for one-way conduction
B. Large diameter axons have longer ARP than small diameter axons
C. Determines the rate of action potential
D. Due to sodium channels remaining in the inactivated state

14. Which of the following is a potassium channel blocker?

A. Procaine B. 4-aminopyridine
C. Tetrodotoxin D. Saxitoxin

15. All of the following are true for action potential, EXCEPT:

A. Can be summated
B. Requires threshold stimulus
C. Does not show decremental response
D. Generated at first node of Ranvier in first order sensory neuron

16. In the neuron, chronaxie denotes:

A. Conduction velocity B. Rate of firing
C. Strength of stimulus D. Excitability

Answers

1. B	2. C	3. B	4. D	5. A	6. D
7. D	8. C	9. C	10. C	11. D	12. A
13. B	14. B	15. A	16. D		

Chapter 19

Classification and Properties of Nerve Fibers, Nerve Injury and Other Applied Aspects

Learning Objectives

On completion of study of this chapter:

The student will be able to (must know):

1. List the properties of nerve fibers.
2. Know what is orthodromic and antidromic conduction and give example for each.
3. Classify nerve fibers and give their functions.
4. Describe the degenerative (Wallerian degeneration) following nerve injury.
5. List the regenerative changes in nerve after nerve injury.
6. Name common diseases affecting nerve fibers and their causes.

The student may also be able to (desirable to know):

1. Describe the properties of nerve fibers.
2. Describe the factors affecting nerve regeneration.

PY3.2

PROPERTIES OF NERVE FIBERS

Important properties of the nerve fibers are as follows.

1. Excitability
2. Conductivity
3. Unfatigability
4. Refractory period
5. All or none law
6. Summation
7. Accommodation

Excitability

Excitability is the property by virtue of which cells or tissues respond to changes in the external or internal environments.

- The production of a wave of depolarization demonstrates that a nerve has been excited.
- Strength and duration of the stimulus, and extracellular Ca^{2+} influence excitability.

Conductivity

Action potential is generated in the nerve fiber on stimulation, a, is propagated along its entire length to the axon terminal. If the action potential is initiated in the middle part of axon, it can travel in both directions.

Summation

Application of a subthreshold stimulus does not evoke an action potential. However, if subthreshold stimuli are applied in rapid succession, they are summated and they produce an action potential. This property is called summation.

Accommodation

Application of continuous stimuli may decrease the excitability of the nerve fiber, a phenomenon called accommodation. More than nerve fiber, it is nerve endings that adapts. This decreases the transmission of impulse across the neurons.

Unfatigability

Nerve fibers cannot be fatigued, even when they are stimulated continuously. This is because the nerve fibers primarily conduct impulses (propagation of action potential) that do not involve expenditure of energy.

Refractory period and 'All or none law 'of nerve fibers have already been described in the previous chapter.

Compound Nerve Action Potential

Compound nerve action potential is the **property of a mixed nerve**. When an action potential is recorded from a nerve as part of nerve conduction study or muscle function, a compound action potential is recorded.

- As a mixed nerve is made up of a group of nerve fibers with varying diameter and properties (sensory and motor fibers), the action potential has **different peaks in descending order** representing in general from thicker fiber to thinner fibers from left to right of the action potential.

CLASSIFICATION OF NERVE FIBERS

Based on function, nerves are classified as motor, sensory and secretomotor, and based on myelination they are classified as myelinated and unmyelinated. Most widely appreciated classification is of **Erlanger and Gasser**, which is based mainly on their diameter and conduction velocity.

Erlanger and Gasser Classification

This is based on their **diameter and conduction velocities**. Broadly fibers are classified into **three categories**: A, B and C.

Type A Nerve Fibers

These are **fastest conducting fibers** with conduction velocity ranging from **70 to 120 m/sec**. The fiber diameter varies from **12–20 μm**. Type A fibers are further subdivided into α, β, γ and δ fibers (Table 19.1).

1. **Aα fibers** supply extrafusal fibers in skeletal muscles and also carry proprioception.
2. **Aβ fibers** carry touch pressure sensation and act as motor fibers.
3. **Aγ fibers** supply intrafusal fibers in muscle spindles.
4. **Aδ fibers** are mainly fast conducting nociceptive fibers.

Type B Nerve Fibers

These are **preganglionic autonomic afferent and efferent fibers**.

- They have a **diameter of less than 3 μm** and conduction velocity ranging from **3 to 15 m/sec**.

Type C Nerve Fibers

These are unmyelinated fibers. They are subdivided into **two broad categories**:

1. Dorsal root fibers that carry various sensations and have **diameter of 0.4–1.2 μm** and their conduction velocity varies from **0.5 to 2 m/sec**.
2. Postganglionic sympathetic fibers with diameter 0.3–1.3 μm and conduction velocity of 0.7 to 2.3 m/s (Table 19.1).

Table 19.1 | Classification of nerve fibers

Fiber types	Fiber diameter	Conduction velocity (m/s)	Function
Aα	12–20	70 –120	Somatic motor and proprioception
Aβ	5 – 12	30 – 70	Touch-pressure
Aϒ	3 – 6	15 – 30	Motor to muscle spindle
Aδ	2 – 5	12 – 30	Pain, cold and touch
B	< 3	3 – 15	Autonomic preganglionic fibers
C-dorsal root fiber	0.4 – 1.2	0.5 – 2	Somatic sensations
C-sympathetic fiber	0.3 – 1.3	0.7 – 2.3	Postganglionic sympathetic fibers

Numerical Classification

Sensory nerve fibers are typed into Ia, Ib, II, III and IV. A comparison of the numerical classification and the later classification is shown in Table 19.2.

Table 19.2 | Numerical classification of sensory fibers.

Types	Origin	Fiber types
Ia	Primary spindle afferent from annulospiral ending	A α
Ib	From Golgi tendon organ	A α
II	Secondary spindle afferent from flower spray endings. Also from touch and pressure receptors	A β
III	Mainly from pain and cold receptors,	A δ
IV	Mainly from pain and temperature	C fibers in dorsal root

Classification by Susceptibility to Various Agents

(Hypoxia, Pressure and Local Anesthetics)

Hypoxia: Type **B fibers** are most susceptible to hypoxia. Type C is the least susceptible.

Pressure: Type **A fibers** are most susceptible to pressure and type C is the least. This is because of fiber diameters.

Local anesthetics: Type **C fibers** are most susceptible to local anesthetics and type A is least susceptible.

NERVE INJURY

When a nerve is sectioned, the distal part of the nerve separated from the cell body degenerates. This is called **Wallerian degeneration**.

- The proximal portion of the axon still attached to the cell body then develops a **growth cone** and grows distally toward the distal portion; the changes associated are known as **regenerative changes**.
- The soma gets informed about the injury by absence of substances transported retrogradely from the axon terminals.

Significant contribution of Scientist

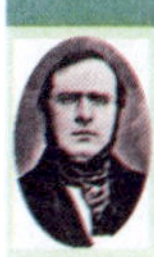

Augustus Volney Waller (1816 – 1870): described peripheral degeneration of nerve fibers after sectioning the main trunk of the nerve, the central stump remaining alive. He is widely known for changes in neurons following injury, which is popularly known as Wallerian degeneration.

Grading of Nerve Injury

Based on severity, nerve injury is typed into **five degrees**:

1. **First-degree injury** is transient loss of function that occurs due to a mild pressure on the nerve.
   - The temporary loss of function is mainly caused by local ischemia following obstruction to the blood flow.
   - Nerve fibers completely recover within few hours to few weeks.
2. **Second degree injury** includes severe nerve damage with intact endoneural tube.
   - This occurs due to severe and prolonged pressure on the nerve.
   - The regeneration is delayed but complete as endoneural tube is intact.
3. **Third degree injury** is the severe damage to the nerve fiber that interrupts endoneural tube.
4. **Fourth degree injury** refers to a severe damage to the nerve associated with disorganization of nerve fasciculi.
5. **Fifth degree injury** is the complete transection of nerve. The degenerative changes occur early.

Degenerative Changes (Wallerian Degeneration) PY3.3

The degenerative changes occurring in the distal segment of the axon are called **Wallerian degeneration.**
The changes are as follows (Fig. 19.1 A to D):

1. **Transmission of impulse:** Shortly after the injury, synaptic transmission occurring at the axon terminal stops within hours.
2. **Axonal changes:** The axon swells and the ***terminals retract from the postsynaptic target***.
   - Gradually over a period of several weeks, the **axon and all its terminals degenerate**.
   - If the axon is myelinated, **round fatty enlargements** form all over the myelin sheath that looks like a series of beads (Fig. 19.1B).
   - The myelin sheath breaks down but the ***myelinating cells remain viable*** (Schwann cell in the PNS and oligodendrocyte in the CNS).
   - The debris created by the disintegration of the axon and its myelin is devoured by macrophages and Schwann cells in the PNS and microglia in the CNS. The phagocytic process is **rapid in the PNS** than in the CNS.
3. **Effect of stimulation:** On stimulation, the distal axon can conduct an action potential upto 3 days; this ability is impaired from 3rd to 5th day, and action potential cannot be initiated after the 5th day.
4. **Changes in soma and the stump:** Following injury, degenerative changes are seen in the soma and to some extent in the proximal stump.

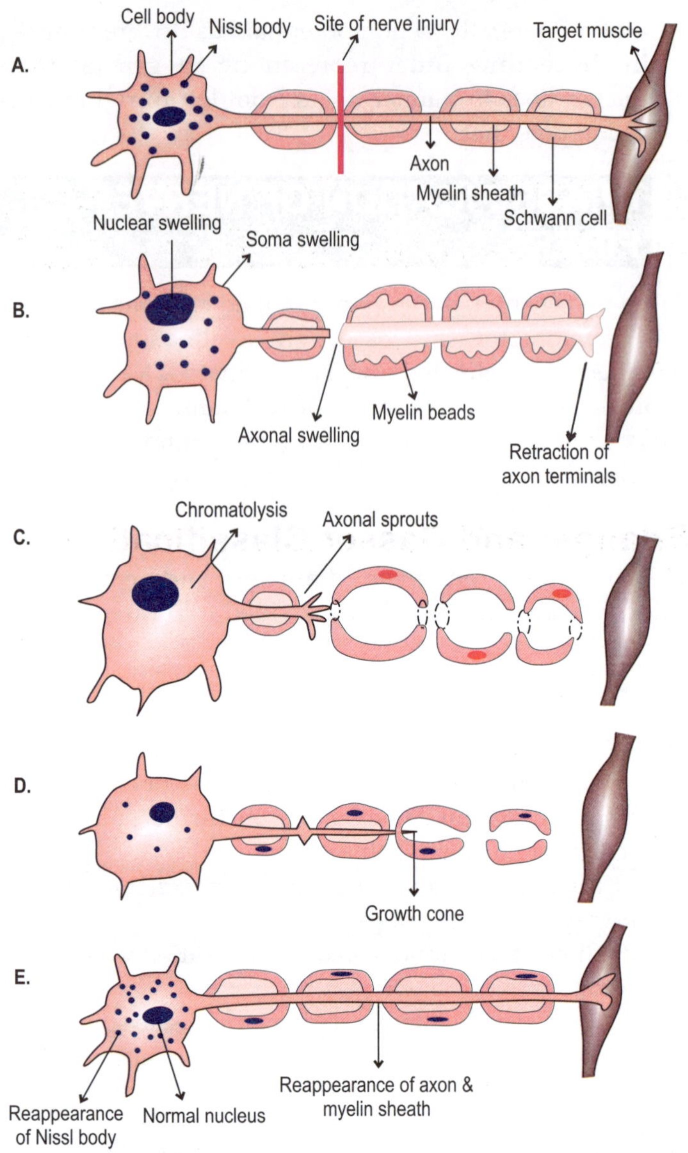

Fig. 19.1: Changes in neuron following nerve injury. **A:** Normal neuron with indication for site of section; **B:** Immediate change depicting swelling of soma, swelling of nucleus which is eccentrically placed, swelling of axon distal to the section, beading of myelin sheath and retraction of axon terminal from target tissue; **C:** Continuation of degenerative changes depicting chromatolysis, disappearance organelles in soma cytoplasm, disintegration of axon and degeneration of myelin sheath, and beginning of regeneration in the form of sprouting from proximal stump of axon; **D:** Regenerative changes with reduction in soma swelling, appearance of few Nissl bodies, development of growth cone and initiation of myelination; **E:** Normalization of the soma and axon with reestablishment of axon contact with the target muscle.

These changes are known as **retrograde degeneration**. The changes are:

i) **Cell body swells** and become rounded.
ii) The **nucleus also swells** and moves to an eccentric position (Fig. 19.1B).
iii) Endoplasmic reticulum instead of being closer to the nucleus reassembles around the periphery of the cell body.
iv) The ribosomes appear disorganized.
v) The *Nissl granules gradually disintegrate* and are stained weakly with basic dyes; this is known as **chromatolysis** (Fig. 19.1C).

Regenerative Changes

The soma tries to repair the axon by synthesizing new structural proteins that fills up and distends the cisterns of the rough endoplasmic reticulum.

- This is known as **axonal reaction**.
- Chromatolysis is **reversible**, if the neuron survives and reestablishes its contact with the appropriate target.

Axonal Changes

The proximal end of the axon develops **many sprouts** (Fig. 19.1C).

1. The sprouts elongate by formation of a **growth cone** at their growing ends (Fig. 19.1D).
2. The Schwann cells that had survived the degeneration ***multiply and form rows*** along the pathway previously taken by the disintegrated distal axon.
3. Out of the many sprouting branches, one branch finds the way through the Schwann cells and finally *reinnervates the original target structure*.
4. The regeneration rate of the growing axon is about 1–4 mm/day.
5. The Schwann cells then lay down their bilayered membrane to ***form the myelin sheath*** around the newly formed axon.

Somatic Changes

The soma regains its size.

- Number of Nissl granules slowly reappears.
- Other organelles also reappear.
- The cell loses excess fluid and regains its normal size. The nucleus occupies the central position (Fig. 19.1E).

Changes in Target Structure

Following degeneration of the nerve, the neurotransmitter release at axonal terminal decreases.

1. Decreased neurochemical at the synaptic cleft leads to **up-regulation of the receptors** in the target structure.
2. Therefore, when neurotransmitter is released following regeneration, the response of the target tissue to the neurotransmitter is increased.
   - This is called **denervation hypersensitivity** (for details, refer to next chapter).

Transneuronal Degeneration

It is the degeneration of a neuron **due to loss of input from or loss of output to the adjacent neuron**, a phenomenon usually seen in central nervous system.

1. When a neuron is over stimulated by a neurotransmitter such as glutamate (excitotoxic) and dies, it leads to damage to the neighboring neurons.
   - It is called **anterograde transneuronal degeneration** (dying forward) or trans-synaptic degeneration when the damage to a neuron results in degeneration of its postsynaptic neuron.
   - It is seen in late stage of ***brain injury***.
2. When a neuron loses its trophic support from its target neurons and dies, it is called **retrograde transneuronal degeneration** (dying backward).
   - It is seen in ***amyotrophic lateral sclerosis***.

Factors Influencing Regeneration

Successful axonal and somatic regeneration depends mainly on four factors: severity of the injury, degree of damage to the cell body, site of injury and secretion of neurotrophins.

Severity of Injury

If the gap between the proximal and distal parts is more than 3 mm, the multiple outgrowths intermesh and form a tumor like swelling called **neuroma**.

1. If neuroma is formed, successful regeneration can never occur.
2. If the neuroma involves sensory fibers, pain is felt at the site when touched.

Condition of Soma

If the axonal damage is close to the cell body, a larger part of the neuronal membrane and cytoplasm is lost. In such situations, the neuron often dies instead of regenerating.

Location of Injury

In the CNS, a single oligodendroglia sends out many processes to myelinate several (around 15) axons. Therefore, even though the axonal sprouting occurs, the ***oligodendroglia cannot form a path*** along which the sprouts can grow.

- Besides, ***glial scars*** formed by astrocytes pose obstruction in the pathway of the growth cone.
- Hence, axons in the CNS regenerate less successfully than axons in the PNS.

Neurotrophins

When specific neurotrophins are administered to the site of injury, the growth of the regenerating sprout is enhanced and enmeshing of the branches does not occur.

OTHER APPLIED ASPECTS

Demyelinating Diseases

Multiple Sclerosis

In multiple sclerosis, **patchy loss of axonal myelin** occurs at several areas in the nervous system, resulting in decreased conduction velocity along the fiber.

1. The pathways commonly affected are ***pyramidal tracts, cerebellar tracts, medial longitudinal fasciculus, optic***

nerve and posterior columns.

2. The symptoms vary depending on the site of affection. The usual symptoms are **sensory abnormalities** (decreased or abnormal sensations or pain), **muscle weakness**, fatigue, spasticity, optic neuritis, diplopia and ataxia (poor coordination).

Demyelinating Form of GBS

In demyelinating form of *Guillain-Barre syndrome,* loss of myelin causes abnormal conductions.

Exam Questions

1. Briefly describe the properties of nerve fibers.
2. Describe the physiological basis of Erlanger-Gasser classification of nerve fiber.
3. Describe the Wallerian degenerative changes and regenerative changes that occur following nerve injury. Give short note on factors that promote neuronal growth

Multiple Choice Questions

1. The type of nerve fiber most susceptible to pressure is:
A. C fiber B. B fiber
C. Aβ fiber D. Aδ fiber

2. Group B nerve fibers:
A. Are autonomic preganglionic
B. Are autonomic postganglionic
C. Carry crude touch
D. Carry temperature

3. Which of the following type nerve fiber carries proprioceptive sensation?
A. B fiber B. Aα fiber
C. Aγ fiber D. Aδ fiber

4. Primary spindle afferents from annulospiral endings are of type:
A. Ia fiber B. Ib fiber
C. II fiber D. IV fiber

5. Antidromic conduction can be seen at:
A. Axon
B. Dendrites
C. Axon terminal of motor neuron
D. Chemical Synapse

6. Which of the following statement is true for excitability of neuron?
A. Not affected by strength of current
B. Not affected by duration current
C. Muscles are more excitable than neuron
D. Decrease in ECF Ca^{2+} increases the excitability

7. Compound nerve action potential is:
A. Affected by length of axon
B. Elicited only from motor neurons
C. Affected by strength of stimulus
D. Does not depend on types of fibers in the nerve

8. The type of nerve fiber most susceptible to hypoxia is:
A. Aα B. Aβ
C. B D. C

9. Neuropraxia is a type of:
A. Physiological conduction block
B. Damage to endoneurium
C. Complete damage to axon
D. Complete demyelination of axon

10. The percentage of sensory fibers in a motor nerve is:
A. 40% B. 10%
C. 5% D. 0%

11. Which of the following statement is NOT true for neuronal regeneration?
A. Injury close to cell body leads to less successful regeneration
B. Gap between proximal and distal end of axon when less than 3 mm, produces a neuroma
C. Less successful in CNS than in peripheral nerve injury
D. Neurotrophins play an important role

12. All of the following are regenerative changes following nerve injury, EXCEPT:
A. Schwann cells form rows
B. Soma swells
C. Nissl granules reappear
D. The rate of growing axon is 1-4mm/day

13. All of the following are true for compound nerve action potential, EXCEPT:
A. Shows multiple peaks
B. Is property of a mixed nerve
C. Obtained by extracellular recording
D. Peaks at left are from thinner fibers and at right from thicker fibers

14. Which of the following is NOT a feature of Wallerian degeneration?
A. Terminals retract from postsynaptic target
B. Axonal end develops many sprouts
C. Schwann cells remain viable
D. Conduction stops shortly after injury

15. The neurons may get irreversible damage if exposed to hypoxia for:
A. 24 minutes B. 8 minutes
C. 1 minute D. 30 seconds

16. Which of the following is NOT true for multiple sclerosis?
A. Abnormal pain sensation
B. Weakness of muscles
C. Incordination of movement
D. Increased thickness of myelin sheath

Answers

1. C	2. A	3. B	4. A	5. A	6. D
7. C	8. C	9. A	10. A	11. B	12. B
13. D	14. B	15. B	16. D		

Chapter 20

Neuromuscular Transmission

Learning Objectives

On completion of study of this chapter:

The student will be able to (must know):

1. Draw the schematic diagram of neuromuscular junction (NMJ).
2. Describe the events of neuromuscular transmission at presynaptic, synaptic and postsynaptic parts of NMJ.
3. Define end plate potential and outline its mechanism.
4. Classify neuromuscular blockers and give their mechanism of action.
5. Learn the physiological basis of causation of myasthenia gravis & the basis of its treatment.
6. Understand the phenomenon of denervation hypersensitivity and it application.

The student may also be able to (desirable to know):

1. Discuss the detailed process of neuromuscular transmission.
2. Explain the pathophysiology of Lambert-Eaton syndrome.

The junction between a motor neuron and a muscle fiber is known as the neuromuscular junction (NMJ). This is also called **myoneural junction** or **motor end plate.**

PY3.4

STRUCTURE OF NEUROMUSCULAR JUNCTION

The anatomy of neuromuscular junction may be broadly divided into **three parts**: Presynaptic, synaptic and postsynaptic portions.

Presynaptic Portion (Axon Terminal)

The neurons innervating skeletal muscle fibers are known **as motor neurons.**

- They have their cell bodies in anterior horn of the spinal cord or in the brainstem.
- Their axons are myelinated and are the **largest-diameter axons** *in the body*.

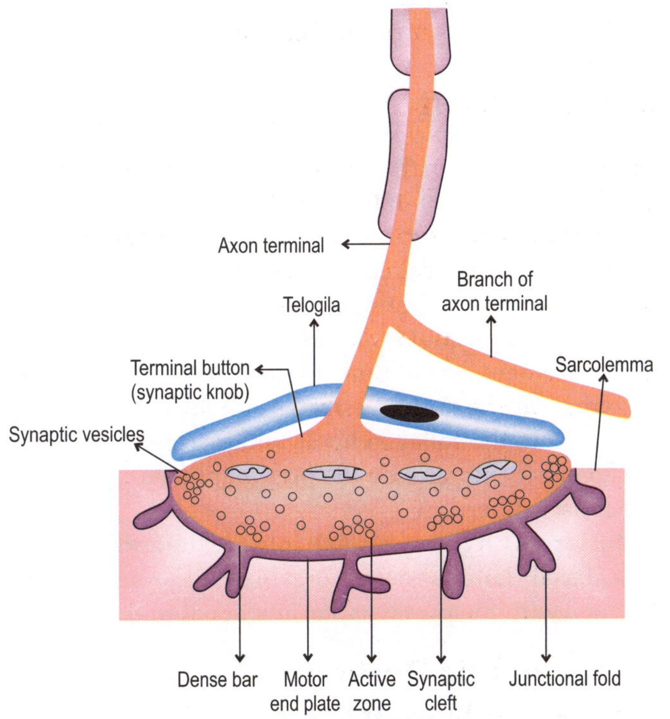

Fig. 20.1: Structure of neuromuscular junction. Note that acetylcholine vesicles are clear vesicles that are clustered at active zones in the terminal buttons opposite to junctional folds. Junctional folds are invagination of motor end plate into the muscle cell that contains more acetylcholine receptors and increase surface area for generation of electrical activities.

The **features of presynaptic portion** of NMJ are:

1. As the axon of motor neuron approaches the muscle fiber, it **loses its myelin sheath** and divides extensively into ***several fine branches*** of about 2μm in diameter, called **axon terminals**.
2. The terminals are covered by Schwann cells, known as **teloglia** (glial cells at terminals).
3. Each terminal forms a junction with a single skeletal muscle fiber, midway along its length.

- Thus, each muscle fiber is supplied by one motor neuron terminal.
- The motor neuron, including its axon and axon terminals and the muscle fibers supplied by it are called a **motor unit**.

4. Each terminal is expanded at its end to form a knobby structure, called **synaptic knob *(terminal button)*,** which contains neurotransmitter vesicles and plenty of mitochondria (Fig 20.1).
   - The terminal button lies in the groove (**synaptic trough**) on the surface of the muscle fiber, but outside the muscle cell membrane.
   - Presence of large number of mitochondria indicates higher metabolic activity at terminal region.
5. The vesicles are clustered around specific points called **active zones.**
   - The membrane at the active zones is modified to form **dense bar** that contains numerous **voltage-gated Ca^{2+} channels.**
   - These channels mediate Ach release.

Synaptic Cleft

This is the gap between the terminal button and the muscle fiber, which is about **40–100 nm wide.**

- The muscle fiber is covered by a layer of amorphous connective tissue called the ***basement membrane*** or ***basal lamina***, consisting of collagen, glycoproteins and other extracellular matrix proteins.
- The basement membrane in the cleft contains the enzyme ***acetylcholine-esterase*** (AchE), which is anchored to the collagen fibrils and is secreted into the basement membrane by the presynaptic terminal and the muscle fiber.
- AchE **rapidly hydrolyzes Ach into acetate and choline.** The basal lamina helps organize the presynaptic buttons with the postsynaptic junctional folds.

Postsynaptic Portion (End Plate Membrane)

The postsynaptic portion of the neuromuscular junction is known as the ***end-plate membrane*** (**motor end-plate**). This is the part of the sarcolemma that lies directly under the terminal button (Fig 20.1).

- The area of the endplate membrane increases many times as it is thrown into several folds called **junctional folds.**
- The endplate membrane contains numerous **ACh receptors** (AchR), which are concentrated at the crests of the junctional folds. It also contains voltage-gated Na^+ channels.

ACh receptors at NMJ: Ach receptors (AChR) at NMJ are **nicotinic type**.

- An average end plate contains about **15–40 million AchR**, which accounts for about ***10,000 AchR per square micrometer*** of end-plate membrane.
- The AchR protein is a **chemically gated ion channel** that undergoes a configurational change and opens when two molecules of Ach bind to it.
- The channel is **blocked by α-bungarotoxin.**
- Because of its larger pore diameter (0.8 nm), AChR is **permeable to both $Na^+$and K^+.**
- But, as the electrochemical gradient is favorable for Na^+entry, *more sodium moves in* than potassium coming out resulting in **net Na^+influx.**
- AchR allows the **passage of only cations** because the anions are repelled by the fixed negative charges present in it.

MECHANISMS OF NEUROMUSCULAR TRANSMISSION

Neuromuscular transmission (NMT) is the transmission of impulse from the motor neuron to the skeletal muscle fibers supplied by the neuron.

Mechanisms involved in NMT are broadly divided into **three parts**: presynaptic events, synaptic-cleft events and postsynaptic events.

Presynaptic Events

The purpose of presynaptic mechanism is to release acetylcholine into the synaptic cleft.

This occurs in **following steps:**

1. Arrival of an action potential at the axon terminal **depolarizes the membrane** of the terminal buttons.
2. This causes activation and **opening of the voltage-gated calcium channels**, which leads to **calcium influx.**
3. Increased cytoplasmic calcium concentration increases movement of microtubules and microfilaments that leads to **migration of neurotransmitter vesicles** to the inner surface of the presynaptic membrane.
4. The vesicles **fuse with the membrane** and discharge their contents into the synaptic cleft by **exocytosis.**
   - Various **membrane proteins** present in the vesicular membrane as well as in the neuronal membrane are involved in the fusion process.
   - Effective interaction between **synaptobrevin,** a vesicular membrane protein with **syntaxin,** a neuronal membrane protein occurs in the presence of **SNAP-25,** α/γ **SNAP, NSF** and many other associated proteins.

Quantal Release

Depolarization of the terminal button causes synchronous releases of about **60–200 vesicles** from different parts of the presynaptic membrane.

- All the vesicles are roughly of the same size.

- Each vesicle contains around **4000–10,000 Ach molecules.**
- The vesicle or the multimolecular ***packet of ACh*** is known as **quanta**, and the process of release is known as **quantal release** of neurotransmitter.
- With each action potential, the presynaptic terminal discharges about the same amount of neurotransmitter, collectively known as a '**quantum** of neurotransmitter' or ***'quantal content'***, which is synonymous with "number of vesicles released".

Events at the Synaptic Cleft

The released Ach molecules diffuse across thesynaptic cleft and **bind to the receptors present at the postsynaptic membrane**.

1. On their way to the end plate membrane, some Ach molecules are **hydrolyzed by AChE**, and some *diffuse out of the synaptic cleft.*
2. However, the amounts that arrive at the end-plate region and get bound to AchR, is sufficient enough to produce an action potential in the muscle fiber.

Events at the End Plate

The major purpose of postsynaptic mechanism is to **generate action potential in sarcolemma** adjacent to end plate. This occurs in **following steps** (Flowchart 20.1):

1. The binding of ACh to AChR in the end-plate membrane allows Na^+ influx, producing a graded potential known as **end plate potential (EPP).**
2. EPP decreases the membrane potential to the firing level and opens the voltage-gated Na^+ channels resulting in an **action potential** at the membrane adjacent to the end plate region.
   - The voltage-gated Na^+ channels are present all over the sarcolemma.
3. The action potential propagates along the sarcolemma and T-tubule network, activating the contractile machinery.
   - As the motor end-plate is present at the middle of a muscle fiber, action potential ***propagates in both directions***.
4. The binding of ACh to AChR is **loose and reversible**.
   - Soon ACh diffuses away and gets **rapidly hydrolyzed by AChE *to acetate and choline*.**
   - The action of ACh is terminated.
5. This leads to ***closure of ion channels, cessation of end plate potential*** and consequently action potential.
6. The acetate diffuses away into the extracellular fluid and choline is taken up by the presynaptic terminal to be reused for the synthesis of new ACh.

All these events at the neuromuscular junction occur in a **few milliseconds** and can be ***repeated several times*** per second without fatigue.

Arrival of an action potential at the axon terminal

↓

Depolarization of the membrane of the terminal buttons.

↓

Activation and opening of the voltage-gated calcium channels

↓

Calcium influx into terminal button

↓

Calcium-mediated exocytosis of acetylcholine vesicle and Ach release

↓

Binding of Ach to Ach receptors in the end-plate membrane

↓

Na^+ influx resulting in local depolarization & formation of end plate potential (EPP)

↓

EPP brings membrane potential to firing level & generates action potential

↓

Spread of action potential to the T-tubule

Flowchart 20.1: Steps of neuromuscular transmission.

End Plate Potential (EPP)

The EPP is like a **graded potential**, the amplitude of which is proportionate to the amount of neurotransmitters released.

- The EPP is always a **depolarizing potential.**
- EPP decays slowly with time and distance from the end plate region, which is known as **decremental conduction**.
- Stimulation of a single motor neuron produces an EPP of about 70 mV.
- EPP of this magnitude is much bigger than that required (15 mV) to bring the membrane potential to firing level (Application Box 20.1).
- Therefore, stimulation of a motor nerve always produces **action potential in all the muscle fiber** supplied by it; i.e. all the muscle fibers in a motor unit contract in response to discharge of its motor neuron.
- Due to this 10-fold safety factor, stimulation of a motor neuron never fails to excite an action potential in the muscle fibers of its motor unit.
- This reserve helps to elicit muscle contraction even in different pathological situations like:

Application Box 20.1

Safety factor of EPP: A stimulated motor neuron produces an EPP of about 70 mV. Under normal circumstances, the amount of neurotransmitters released is enough to activate about 10 times the number of receptors required to produce an EPP that can bring the membrane potential to firing level.

i) decrease in number or function of AchR receptors,
ii) decline in the quantity of Ach released, and
iii) abnormal voltage-gated Na^+ channels in the end plate region.

Miniature End Plate Potential

When the motor nerve is at rest, spontaneously occurring potentials of minute amplitude (0.1 to 4 mV) are recorded from the endplate membrane. These potentials are known as **miniature end plate potential** (MEPP).

1. They occur **several times a second** and have all the properties of an EPP.
2. MEPP occurs due to *release of the contents of a single Ach vesicle* by exocytosis (**a quantal event**) that opens around **2000 Ach channels** in a very small area of the end plate membrane.

PY3.5

BLOCKADE OF NEUROMUSCULAR TRANSMISSION

The neuromuscular transmission is disrupted at different steps by **drugs, chemicals, toxins and trauma**. The blockade can occur at presynaptic or postsynaptic level.

Presynaptic Blockade

Interruption of events taking place at the presynaptic axon terminal leads to **impaired calcium influx** causing ***decreased vesicle release***.

Botulinum Toxins

The bacterium *Clostridium botulinum* releases a toxin that causes a paralytic disease called **botulism.**

1. The botulinum toxin is one of the most potent natural toxins, a minute amount of which causes serious illness.
2. The **lethal dose** for an adult human is around 2 to 3 µg.
3. Botulinum toxin B, D, F and G **inactivate synaptobrevin**, a vesicle membrane protein that is required for the binding and fusion of ACh vesicles with the plasma membrane of the axon terminal.
4. Botulinum toxin A and B **act on SNAP-25** and toxin C **breaks down syntaxin**.
5. Thus, the botulinum toxin **inhibits the release of acetylcholine** from the axon terminals resulting in cessation of muscle contraction (***flaccid paralysis***) (Clinical Note 20.1).

Clinical Note 20.1

Clinical Uses of Botulinum Toxin: The paralytic effect of botulinum toxin is utilized for ***therapeutic and cosmetic purposes***. Local injections of highly diluted toxin ***(botox treatment)*** produce muscle relaxation at the desired site.

- It is injected into the lower esophageal sphincter to treat achalasia cardia;
- into extra-ocular muscles to decrease their overactivity, which is used in the management of strabismus and blepharospasm;
- into facial muscles to reduce aging-related skin wrinkle, and
- is used in cases of cervical dystonia.

However, it can also be a lethal bioterrorism agent by dispersing it as an aerosol or by contaminating the food supply.

Hemicholinium

The drug inhibits choline uptake by the presynaptic terminal resulting in depletion of Ach.

- Consequently, the EPP decreases and action potential cannot be formed.

Postsynaptic Blockade

A variety of agents can act on the postsynaptic membrane interfering with generation of EPP by different mechanisms. They may be classified into **competitive blockers and depolarizing blockers**.

Competitive Blockers

Competitive blockers are agents that compete with Ach to bind to AChR on endplate membrane. Examples: **Curare and Gallamine.**

- Attachment of the competitive blocker to AChR does not lead to opening of ion channels, as it does not have the biological activity of ACh.
- Moreover, it does not get hydrolyzed by AChE.
- So, the Ach binding sites in the receptors **remain occupied permanently**.
- In these conditions, motor nerve releases ACh, but **ACh fails to bind to its receptor** resulting in absence of EPP and lack of muscle contraction.

Curare

Curare is a plant product used as a South American arrowhead poison for hunting.

- The animal hit by such arrow suffers from **paralysis in all skeletal muscles** including the respiratory muscles.
- Consequently, the animal dies of asphyxiation.

Gallamine

Gallamine is given before surgery to **relax the skeletal muscles**.

- It reduces the required dose of general anesthetic as well as bleeding and other complications.
- As the respiratory muscles are also relaxed, patients are supported with artificial ventilation.

Depolarizing Blockers

Drugs like **succinylcholine** and **carbamylcholine** have the biological activity of ACh, but they are ***not hydrolyzed by AChE***. Therefore, their action is **long lasting**.

- When they bind to AChR, the **ion channels remain open** in the end plate.
- The maintained depolarization keeps the ***voltage-gated Na^+ channels in an inactivated state*** and ***blocks subsequent action potentials***.

There are other drugs that produce the blockade by inactivating AChE reversibly or irreversibly.

Reversible AchE inhibitors

These agents **compete with ACh to bind to AChE**, thereby, prevent the hydrolysis of ACh by AChE.

- The accumulated ACh at the synaptic cleft binds to AchR, leading to a **depolarizing block**.
- This is of use in diseases like **myasthenia gravis**, where excess ACh is a requirement in the face of decreased AChR.
- **Neostigmine** and **physostigmine** (eserine) are examples of reversible AChE inhibitors.
- Their attachment with AchE decreases, when the concentration of the drug falls and so the block is removed after some time.
- This block can be **overcome by application of curare** that attaches to AChR and reduces the effect of excess ACh on the end plate membrane.

Irreversible AchE inhibitors

The **organophosphorous compounds** (pesticides like parathion, malathion and baygon) and **nerve gases** used in chemical warfare like disopropylfluro-phosphate (DFP) and sarin, **bind to AChE very tightly**.

- This binding is irreversible.
- Lack of hydrolysis of ACh produces **sustained depolarization** of the end plate resulting in no further contractions in response to subsequent nerve stimulation.
- Poisoning with these agents lead to **skeletal muscle paralysis** and death from asphyxiation.
- Nerve gases also cause accumulation of ACh at the cardiac pacemaker cells.
- Therefore, in cases of nerve gas exposure, **atropine** (a muscarinic receptor antagonist) **is given as antidote**.

NEUROMUSCULAR DYSFUNCTIONS

Myasthenia Gravis — PY3.6

It is a neuromuscular disorder of **autoimmune nature**, characterized by weakness and fatigability of skeletal muscles that gradually worsens as the muscles are used.

Etiology

Myasthenia gravis results from a **decrease in the number of AChR** present on the motor end plate due to production of **circulating autoantibodies** against these receptors.

- Moreover, the ***postsynaptic folds are flattened***, or simplified.
- Due to these changes, though **ACh is released normally**, the magnitude of the ***end plate potential falls below the threshold*** for initiating a muscle action potential.

The **anti-AChR antibodies** have following *three major functions*:

i) They compete with Ach to bind to AChR, producing receptor blockade.
ii) They induce endocytosis of AChR.
iii) They damage the postsynaptic membrane.

Features

1. **Fatigue:** Normally, on repeated stimulation of the motor nerve, the amount of ACh released per action potential gradually decreases (**presynaptic rundown**). But the amount is enough to generate an EPP well above the threshold level.
   - In myasthenic patients, due to the postsynaptic changes along with the presynaptic rundown, after a few motor nerve impulses, the successive contractile responses become feebler, causing **fatigue**.
   - So there is **decremental response to repetitive nerve stimulation** on EMG recording from the affected muscle.
2. **Women** ***are affected more*** than men in a ratio of 3:2.
3. **Muscle Weakness**: The weakness increases during prolonged use of the muscle and improves after rest or sleep.
   - Thus, the patient feels better in the morning, but **symptoms aggravate towards evening** or after exertion.
3. **Ptosis:** The **extraocular muscles and eyelids** are often involved early in the course of the diseases.
   - Therefore, **diplopia and ptosis** (drooping of eyelids) are early symptoms.
4. **Proximal limb muscles** are commonly affected.
5. In severe cases, respiratory muscle paralysis leads to death.

Physiological Basis of Treatment

Current modalities of treatment are as follows.

1. **Administration of AChE inhibitors:** Drugs such as **pyridostigmine and neostigmine** increase the concentration of ACh at the neuromuscular junction.
2. **Thymectomy:** Thymectomy is helpful, as the immune responses mediated by **T cells** are part of the pathophysiologic mechanisms.

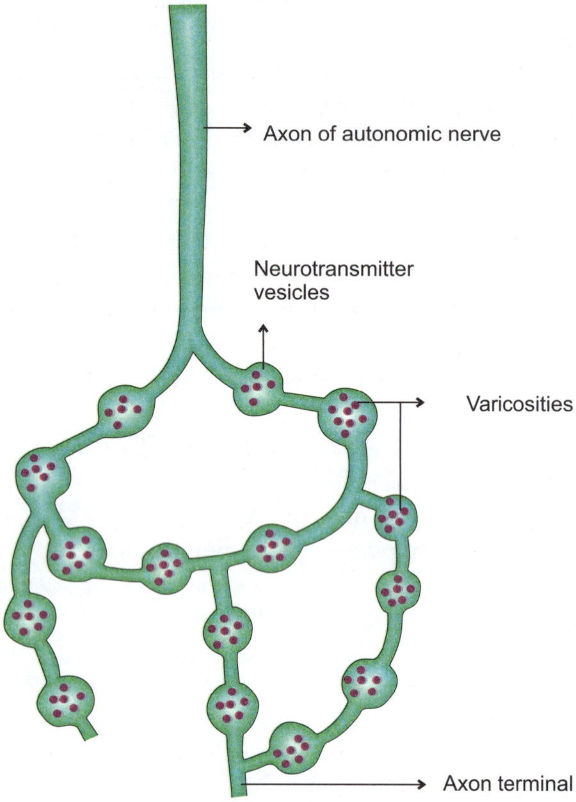

Fig. 20.2: Termination of autonomic neurons on smooth muscle. Note, axon does not end with typical neuromuscular junction. Rather, axon has numerous dilations (varicosities) on its course that contain neurotransmitter vesicles.

- It blunts down the immune response and improves the condition.

3. **Immunosuppression:** Immunosuppressive drugs **glucocorticoids and azathioprine** are useful. They inhibit the immunological mechanisms.
4. **Plasmapheresis:** Plasmapheresis removes AChR antibodies from plasma.

Lambert-Eaton Myasthenic Syndrome

It is a presynaptic disorder of the neuromuscular junction due to production of **autoantibodies against voltage-gated Ca^{2+} channels**.

- The decreased Ca^{2+} influx in the presynaptic axon terminals results in impaired ACh release from the nerve endings.
- The muscular weakness is primarily seen in the limb muscles. Patients show **incremental response to repetitive nerve stimulation** as Ca^{+2} level raises with each action potential.
- Thus, with prolonged contractions, muscle strength increases.

NERVE ENDINGS IN SMOOTH & CARDIAC MUSCLES

The smooth and cardiac muscle cells are innervated by autonomic nervous system. There are **no well-defined end plate** regions or precise synaptic terminals.

1. Especially **in smooth muscles**, the neurotransmitter vesicles are present **in dilated areas of the axon** all along its length.
   - These dilated portions (swellings) are known as **varicosities** (Fig. 20.2).
2. On stimulation of the neuron, the neurotransmitters are released and then diffused to the adjacent muscle fibers, initiating action potentials in many fibers simultaneously.
3. In a noradrenergic nerve, there can be as many as 20,000 varicosities per neuron. This type of synaptic arrangement is called **synapse en passant**.
4. The depolarizing potentials produced in the smooth muscle cells are known as **excitatory junction potentials** (EJPs).
5. EJPs are like **graded potentials** and can be summated.
6. The hyperpolarizing potentials produced in the smooth muscle cells are known as **inhibitory junction potentials** (IJPs).

DENERVATION HYPERSENSITIVITY

When a neuron is cut and the distal axon degenerates, the target tissue innervated by its synaptic terminals becomes more reactive to the neurotransmitter secreted at the nerve endings. This ***phenomenon of increased responsiveness*** is known as **denervation hypersensitivity**.

- This is seen in **both skeletal and smooth muscles.**
- Due to degeneration of the nerve endings, the chemical is no more released from the terminals.

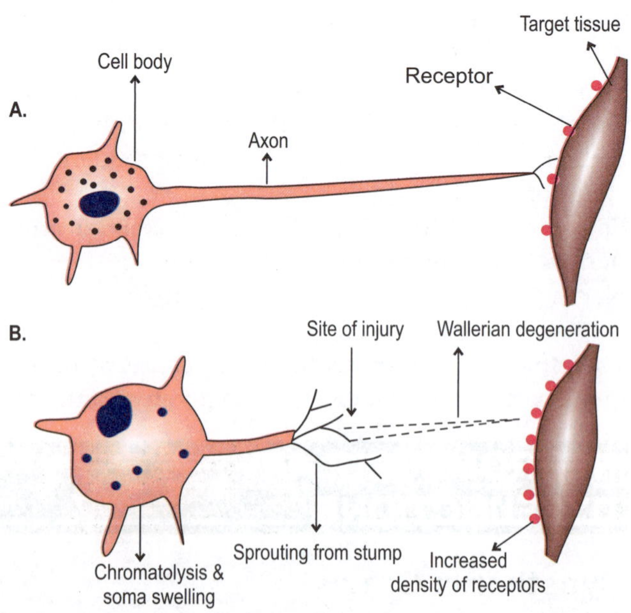

Fig. 20.3: Denervation hypersensitivity following erve injury. Note the increased density of receptors in the target tissue (B) compared to the normal one (A) that increases responsiveness of the tissue to the neurotransmitter.

- The tissue reacts to the neurotransmitter present in the circulation, where concentration of the chemical is lower than at the synaptic endings.

The hypersensitivity occurs due to **three reasons**:

1. **Increased number of receptors** at the postsynaptic membrane (**up-regulation**).
   - Both number and distribution of receptors increase.
   - For example, after degeneration of the motor nerve, the AChRs appear all over the sarcolemma (Fig. 20.3B), whereas normally they are confined to the end plate region only (Fig. 20.3A).
2. **Increased responsiveness** (sensitivity) of receptors to the chemical.
3. In case of noradrenergic neurons, the reuptake of neurotransmitter molecules by the presynaptic terminals is decreased resulting in **higher plasma noradrenaline concentration**.

Exam Questions

1. With the help of a schematic diagram of neuromuscular junction, describe the mechanism of neuromuscular transmission.
2. Describe the mechanisms of end-plate potential.
3. Classify neuromuscular blockers and give their physiological mechanisms.
4. Explain the phenomenon of denervation hypersensitivity.

Multiple Choice Questions

1. The number of motor endplate (s) innervated by one motor neuron is:
A. 10 B. 6 C. 2 D. 1

2. The myoneural junction is:
A. Present in CNS B. Present in uterine myometrium
C. Present in the myocardium D. Motor endplate

3. The glial cells covering the presynaptic terminal at motor endplate are called:
A. Teloglia B. Microglia
C. Astrocyte D. Ependymal cells

4. All of the following are present in high concentration in the neuromuscular junction, EXCEPT:
A. Acetylcholinesterase B. Glycoprotein
C. Glycine D. Collagen

5. The neurotransmitter released at neuromuscular junction is:
A. Adrenaline B. Acetylcholine
C. Serotonin D. Neurotrophin

6. The width of synaptic cleft is about:
A. 2-5μm B. 6-15nm C. 20-30μm D. 40-100nm

7. All of the following statements are true for presynaptic terminal, EXCEPT:
A. Contains plenty of mitochondria
B. Contains plenty of voltage-gated K+ channels
C. The vesicles are clustered around the active zones
D. The synaptic knob lies in the synaptic trough

8. Which of the following statement is NOT true for end plate membrane?
A. It is the postsynaptic portion of the neuromuscular junction
B. Contains numerous voltage-gated Na+ channels
C. Junctional folds decreases its area
D. Contains numerous Ach receptors

9. Which of the following statement is NOT true for Ach receptors (AchR) at neuromuscular junction?
A. Muscarinic type
B. Blocked by bungarotoxin
C. Density is 10000 AchRs per square micrometer
D. Allows passage of only cations

10. Which of the following statement is true for end plate potential?
A. Can be summated
B. Produced by opening of voltage-gated Na+ channels
C. Can be depolarizing or hyperpolarizing
D. Decreases the membrane potential to firing level

11. The depolarization of presynaptic membrane
A. Is due to Ach binding to Ach receptor
B. Occurs after exocytosis of vesicles
C. Is produced by end-plate potential
D. Leads to opening of voltage-gated Ca++ channels

12. In denervation hypersensitivity:
A. Plasma epinephrine level decreases due to sympathetic denervation
B. Seen in smooth muscles
C. Ach receptors disappear from sarcolemma
D. Decreased responsiveness of the receptors to the neurotransmitter

13. Which of the following is a presynaptic blocker?
A. Botulinum toxin B. Physostigmine
C. Gallamine D. Carbamylcholine

14. Which of the following is a depolarizing blocker?
A. Hemicholinium B. Succinylcholine
C. Curare D. Sarin

15. Which of the following statement is true?
A. Synapse en passant arrangement is seen in cholinergic neuron
B. Discharge from a single presynaptic neuron in a smooth muscle can active only a single muscle fibre
C. Neurotransmitter vesicles are present in varicosities in smooth muscle
D. Excitatory Junctional potentials are produced in skeletal muscle

16. Which of the following statement is true for myasthenia gravis?
A. Decremental response to repetitive nerve stimulation is absent
B. Symptoms improve towards evening
C. The endplate membrane folds are flattened
D. Increase in Ach receptors at motor endplate

Answers

1. D	2. D	3. A	4. C	5. B	6. D
7. B	8. C	9. A	10. D	11. D	12. B
13. A	14. B	15. C	16. C		

Chapter 21

Muscle: Structure, Functional Organization, Excitation-Contraction Coupling and Molecular Basis of Skeletal Muscle Contraction

Learning Objectives

On completion of study of this chapter:

The student will be able to (must know):

1. Understand the arrangement of muscle fibers and fibrils in skeletal muscle.
2. Name the contractile proteins in the skeletal muscle and give their functions.
3. Outline the structure and functions of myosin and actin filaments and mention their functions.
4. Draw the labeled diagram of sarcomere.
5. Draw the picture of sarcotubular system (STS) and explain the role of STS in in muscle contraction and relaxation.
6. Describe the process of excitation-contraction coupling in skeletal muscle.
7. Understand the cross-bridge cycle and the molecular mechanism of.
8. List the types of muscle contraction and the differences between them.

The student may also be able to (desirable to know):

1. Describe the structure and functions of muscle proteins.
2. Describe the role of STS in muscle contraction and relaxation.
3. Explain the mechanism and objectives of cross-bridge cycle.

Muscles are classified into **three types**:

1. Skeletal muscle
2. Smooth muscle
3. Cardiac muscle.

Skeletal muscle, as the name implies, is attached to the skeleton (bones).

- The contraction in skeletal muscle is initiated by **discharge of the motor neuron supplying it**.
- Skeletal muscle is capable of **rapid force development and shortening**.
- It can **maintain contractile force** for relatively *longer periods*.

STRUCTURE OF SKELETAL MUSCLE

A typical skeletal muscle contains many **muscle bundles or fascicles**. Each fascicle consists of large number of muscle fibers arranged parallel to each other. Connective tissue layers in the muscle bundles are epimysium, perimysium and endomysium (Fig. 21.1).

1. The connective tissue layer around the muscle is called **epimysium**.
2. The layer covering each fascicle is known as **perimysium.**
4. The layer surrounding each muscle fiber is termed as **endomysium**.

The blood vessels and nerves supplying the muscle fibers are present within the perimysium. All the three layers are made up of **collagen and elastin** that helps to transmit the force from the muscles to the bones. Muscles are usually attached to bones by collagen fibers known as tendons.

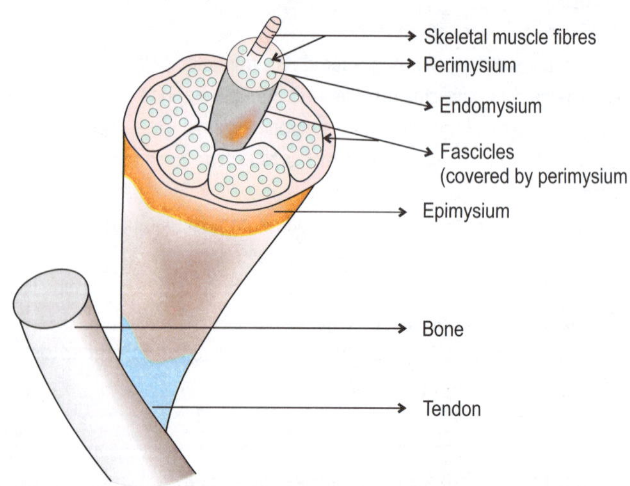

Fig. 21.1: The muscle bundle. Note the arrangement of epimysium, perimysium, and endomysium.

Myocyte

The structural unit of muscle is muscle fiber that is a single skeletal muscle cell (myocyte).

- The cell membrane of myocyte is known as ***sarcolemma*** and the cytoplasm as ***sarcoplasm***.
- The muscle fibers are long, cylindrical, ***multinucleated cells***, extending the entire length of the muscle, and attach to tendons at both ends.
- They are **10–100 µm in diameter** and may extend up to 20 cm in length.
- In embryonic fibers, the nuclei are centrally placed; but following differentiation after birth, they lie beneath the sarcolemma, hence peripherally placed (Fig. 21.2A).

The **important functions of sarcolemma** are:

1. It **transmits the wave of depolarization** originating at the motor end plate over the entire cell surface to initiate contraction.
2. Besides **shielding the muscle fiber**, the sarcolemma contributes to the parallel **elastic resistance** i.e. the resistance to stretch offered by all the connective tissue layers.
3. It has ***no gap junctions***, thereby promotes **electrical separation** between fibers.

Myofibrils and Organelles PY3.7

Characteristically, the sarcoplasm is filled with myofibrils that extend along the axis of the cell and are connected to the tendons at both ends of the muscle fiber.

1. Each myofibril is 1 µm in diameter and consists of cylindrical bundles of two types of **myofilaments** that are referred to as thick and thin filaments.
2. The sarcoplasm contains the usual cytoplasmic organelles including mitochondria (sarcosomes), sarcoplasmic reticulum, and Golgi apparatus.

Striations: The most striking feature of skeletal muscle is the **presence of striations** due to alternate light and dark bands throughout the length of the fiber as seen through a light microscope (Fig. 21.2B).

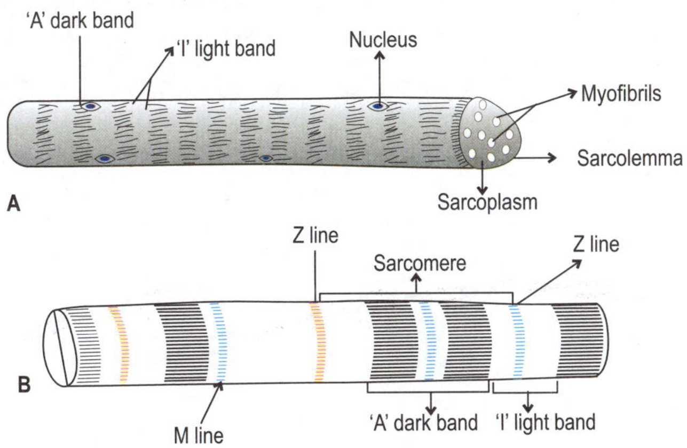

Fig. 21.2: A: Structure of a myocyte (muscle cell). Note the presence of nuclei peripherally, and alternate light and dark bands. B: Striations in myocyte, which is due to presence alternate dark (A) and light (I) bands.

1. The dark band is also called **A band** because it is *anisotropic to polarized light*.
2. The light band is known as **I band** because it is *isotropic to polarized light*.

Each myofibril is made up of units called **sarcomere** that contains different muscle proteins (see below).

Muscle Proteins

There are **three types of proteins** in skeletal muscle:

1. **Contractile proteins:** myosin and actin
2. **Regulatory proteins:** troponin and tropomyosin
3. **Attachment proteins:** titin, nebulin, alpha actinin, desmin, myomesin and dystrophin

Contractile Proteins

There are two contractile proteins in skeletal muscle: **myosin and actin**.

Myosin

These are thick filaments in muscle.

- The thick filaments are **polymers of myosin II** (MW 480,000).
- Myosin filament is a **bundle of myosin molecules**.
- The **heads of myosin molecules** (cross bridges) project from the filaments that are arranged in a helical manner (Fig. 21.3).

The filament is composed of following units:

1. Two intertwined heavy chains,
2. Two regulatory light chains, and
3. Two alkali (essential) light chains.

The myosin II has *three regions*: **two globular heads, neck** (hinge region) and a **long tail** (Fig. 21.3).

Myosin Head

Each head is made up of amino terminal portions of one heavy chain forming a complex with two light chains, one regulatory and one alkali.

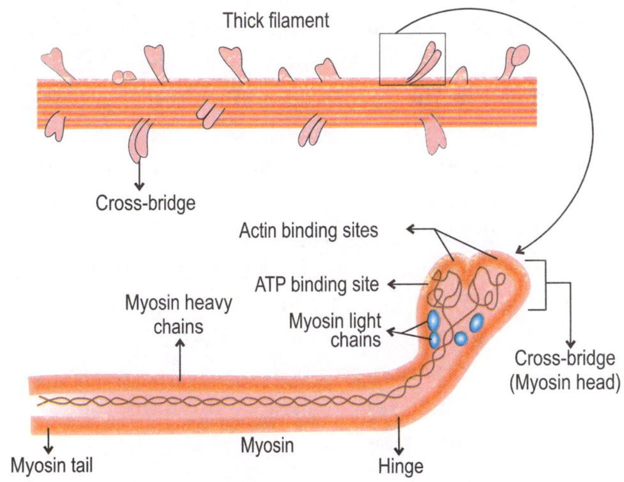

Fig. 21.3: Structure of myosin molecule.

- The myosin head contains **two binding sites**, one for actin and one for ATP (Fig. 21.3).
- The **ATP binding site** functions as an ATPase (hydrolyzes ATP).
- The carboxy terminals of the heavy chains coil around each other in an alpha-helical configuration forming a long rod-like tail.
- The **alkali light chain** stabilizes the myosin head and the **regulatory light chain** regulates its ATPase activity.

Myosin Tail

The tail of each myosin molecule **lies along the axis** of the thick filament, and the two globular heads extend out to the sides, forming the *cross-bridges*.

Myosin Hinge

In the hinge region, the tail joins the globular head.

Arrangement of Myosin Molecules: The myosin molecules aggregate with a definite directional arrangement, such that their **tail-ends are directed towards the center** of the thick filaments creating a bare region in the middle consisting of myosin tails only, while the **globular heads point away from both sides** of the tail.

- The site of the reversal of polarity of myosin molecules is the **M line** where slender cross connections preserve the organization and alignment of the thick filaments in the sarcomere.
- Besides titin, proteins like myomesin and C- protein contribute to the bipolar organization and packing of the thick filaments.

Actin

These are **thin filaments,** and they are made up of actin molecules.

The actin filament (**F-actin**) is made up of globular molecules of **G-actin** (Fig. 21.4).

- **G-actin** is a globular protein with a diameter of 4–5nm and MW 42,000.
- G-actin molecules (monomers) are joined from front to back into long chains that wind about each other forming a double stranded alpha helical filament known as **F-actin** (or filamentous actin) that forms the backbone of the thin filament.
- The cytoskeletal protein **nebulin** extends along the length of the F-actin and plays a role in the regulation of the length of the thin filament.
- Each actin monomer contains **binding sites** for myosin, tropomyosin, troponin I, and other actin monomers.
- As the F-actin undergoes a half–turn every seven G-actin monomers, a groove is formed down the length of the helix which is occupied by the long, filamentous protein **tropomyosin**.
- Each thin filament contains **300–400 actin molecules** and **40–60 tropomyosin molecules**.

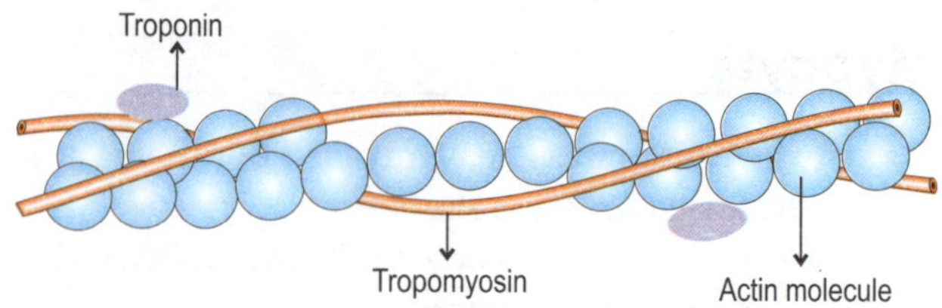

Fig. 21.4: Structure of actin filament. Note, actin (thin) filament is made up of actine molecules.

Regulatory Proteins

Regulatory proteins are **tropomyosin and troponin.**

Tropomyosin

Tropomyosin is a rod-shaped molecule (MW 70,000) composed of **two strands of polypeptides** intertwined in an alpha helical configuration with a ***length approximately equal to seven actin monomers***.

- It is located in the groove between two chains of actin (Fig. 21.5).
- The tropomyosin molecules are connected to one another serially that extends over the entire actin filament covering myosin-binding sites on the actin monomers.
- The **function** of tropomyosin is to ***interfere with*** the *binding of myosin head to actin.*

Troponin

Troponin is a complex of **three proteins**: Troponin T, Troponin I and Troponin C (Fig.21.5)

Troponin T: Troponin T has molecular weight 30,000.

- It **binds the troponin complex to tropomyosin**.

Troponin I: Troponin I (MW 22,000) binds the troponin complex to actin.

- It is called I, because it **inhibits the binding of actin** to myosin by blocking the myosin binding site on actin.

Troponin C: Troponin C (MW 18,000) **binds to calcium**.

IMPORTANT NOTE

Interaction of troponin with tropomyosin: Each troponin complex interacts with one tropomyosin molecule, which in turn interacts with seven actin monomers.

- The troponin complex also interacts directly with the actin filaments.
- Troponin is known as the regulatory protein in the contraction of skeletal muscle.

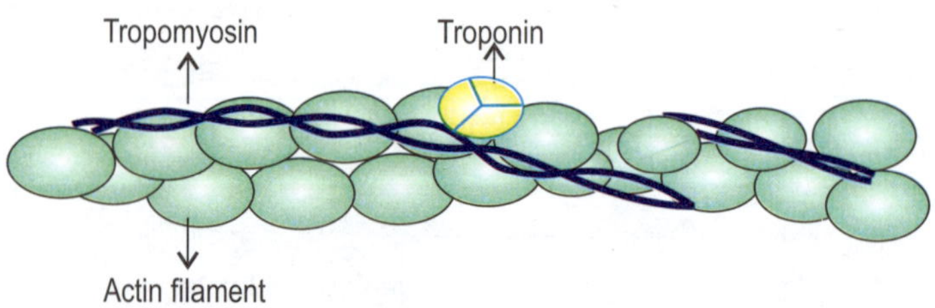

Fig. 21.5: Structure of tropomyosin and troponin. Note the double helical structure of tropomyosin and the three components (I, T and C) of troponin.

Attachment Proteins

Titin

It is a large, elastic, filamentous, cytoskeletal protein, which extends from the Z line to the M line.

- It provides framework for the thick filaments by **connecting the Z line to the M line.**
- It *prevents overextension of the thick filaments* and maintains the central location of the A band.

Nebulin

This is a large, filamentous protein that extends along the length of the thin filaments.

- It is reported to play a role in *stabilizing the length of the actin filaments* during muscle development.

Alpha Actinin

Alpha actinin **anchors** the thin filaments to the Z line.

Desmin

Desmin is present in the intermediate filament of cytoskeleton of myocyte.

- It **connects the Z line to the sarcolemma**.
- It also connects myofibrils to each other.

Dystrophin

It is a large rod like protein that anchors the thin filaments to the membrane spanning protein **beta-dystroglycan**, which in turn is connected to the extracellular matrix protein **laminin** through alpha-dystroglycan.

- Dystrophin helps in **transfer of force** *from the contractile system to extracellular regions* through the transmembrane proteins.
- These proteins are disrupted in the group of genetic diseases called **muscular dystrophy**.
- Absence of these proteins or their mutations leads to muscle degeneration, weakness and even death.

Myomesin

It is present in the region of M disc.

- It **binds the tail end of myosin** filament to the disc.

Sarcomere

Sarcomere (In Greek; *sarco* means muscle, and *mer* means part) is the structural and functional unit of myofibril. A single myofibril may be composed of hundreds or thousands of sarcomeres that are joined end-to-end.

- In each myofibril, thick and thin filaments are **arranged in a repeating pattern** in the form of sarcomere (Fig. 21.2B).
- Sarcomere is **defined** *as the portion of the muscle fibril between two successive Z lines.*
- The *average length* of a sarcomere is **2 µm**.

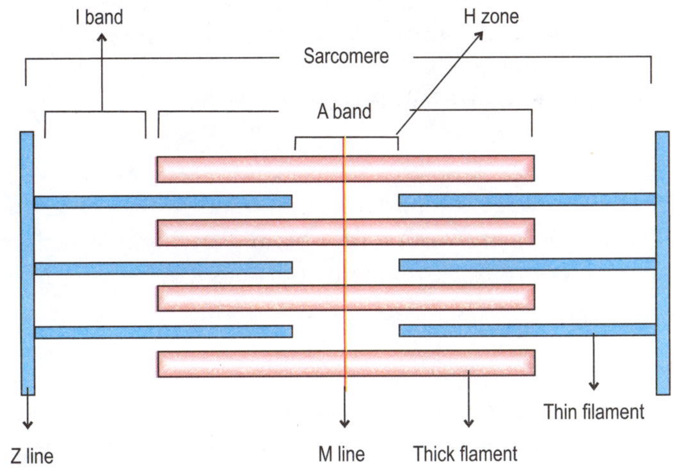

Fig. 21.6: Structure of a sarcomere.

Structure

Electron micrographic studies reveal the detailed structure of sarcomere (Fig. 21.6).

Z line

The Z line or **Z disc** is a network of interconnecting proteins.

- It is oriented perpendicular to the axis of the muscle fiber.
- The thin filaments are anchored to the two sides of each Z line by **alpha actinin**.

Thin Filament

Each thin filament is **1 µm long and 7 nm in diameter**.

- It is composed of the contractile proteins: actin, tropomyosin and troponin in a **ratio of 7: 1: 1.**
- From the Z line, the thin filaments project in parallel arrays towards the center of the sarcomere where they **overlap a portion of the thick filaments.**
- Thus, each sarcomere contains **two sets of thin filaments**, one at each end.
- The Z disc not only binds the thin filaments of a single myofibril together, but connections between the Z discs also anchor each myofibril to its neighbors.

Thick Filament and A band

The parallel array of thick filaments located in the middle of each sarcomere produces **A band**.

- The thick filament is **1.6 µm long and 10 nm in diameter.**
- It consists of the protein **myosin** (see above).

I Band

I band lies between the ends of A bands of two adjacent sarcomeres and includes those portions of the thin filaments that **do not overlap** the thick filaments. The Z line bisects I band.

- **During muscle contraction**, the length of the sarcomere (the distance between two Z lines) decreases. This results in ***shortening of I band*** but, length of A band remains unchanged.

- Thus, **sarcomeric length** *is decided by the length of I band.*

H Band

H band (H zone) is a narrow, light band in the center of A band. This is the portion of A band showing no overlap (represented by thick filaments only) as can be seen in a relaxed muscle.

M Line

A transverse M line runs through the middle of H band. The M line contains proteins that bind the parallel array of thick filaments.

1. Besides, the cytoskeletal protein, titin binds the thick filaments to the Z lines.
2. In fact, **titin filaments** extend from Z line to M line and thus, are linked to M-line proteins, thick filaments and Z line proteins.
3. Therefore, it plays a key role in ***organizing & maintaining regular array of thick filaments*** in the middle of each sarcomere.

Hexagonal & Triangular Arrangement

A cross section through the overlap region of A band shows that each thick filament is surrounded by a **hexagonal array of six thin filaments**, and each thin filament is surrounded by a triangular arrangement of three thick filaments (Fig. 21.7).

Cross-Bridges

The globular heads of myosin II project from the surface of the thick filaments toward the thin filaments and bridge the gap between them.

1. These projections are known as **cross-bridges** (Fig. 21.8).

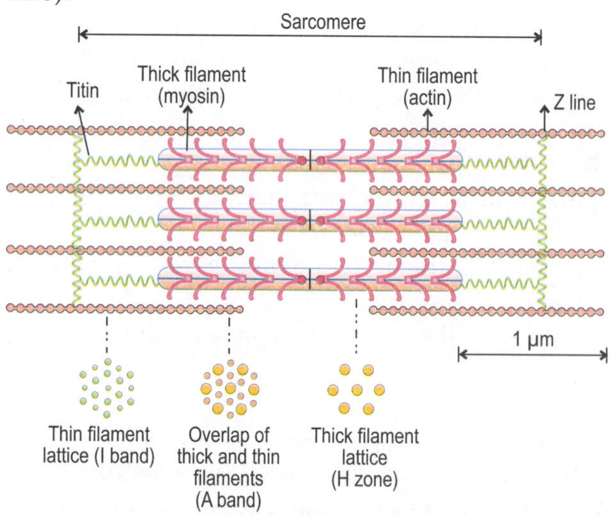

Fig. 21.7: Hexagonal and triangular arrangement of thin and thick filaments. A cross section through the overlap region of A band shows that each thick filament is surrounded by a hexagonal array of six thin filaments, and each thin filament is surrounded by a triangular arrangement of three thick filaments.

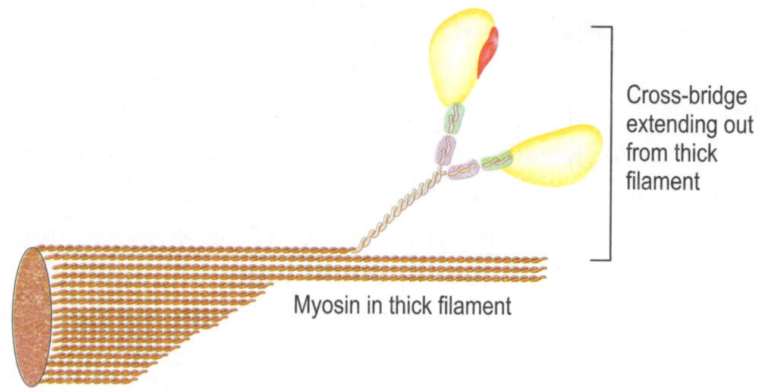

Fig. 21.8: The structure and position of cross-bridge.

2. During muscle contraction, they attach to the thin filaments and pull them.

Sarcotubular System

Inside a muscle fiber, fibrils are surrounded by **membranous structures** known as sarcotubular system. The relationship of sarcotubular system with the I and A bands of sarcomere in a myofibril is shown in Fig. 21.9.

Structure

It consists of sarcoplasmic reticulum and T (transverse) tubules.

T-tubules

The T-tubules, also called **sarcotubules** are tubular extensions of the sarcolemma, about **0.03 μm in diameter**.

- They penetrate to the center of the muscle fiber and surround the individual myofibrils at the junctions of A and I band (Fig 21.9).
- The lumen of the T tubule **contains extracellular fluid**, which is a continuation of the ECF surrounding the muscle fibers.
- Once initiated, an **action potential is rapidly conducted** along the sarcolemma over the surface of the muscle fiber as well as **into the interior** of the muscle cell by the ***way of the T-tubules*** so that deep lying myofibrils are fast activated.

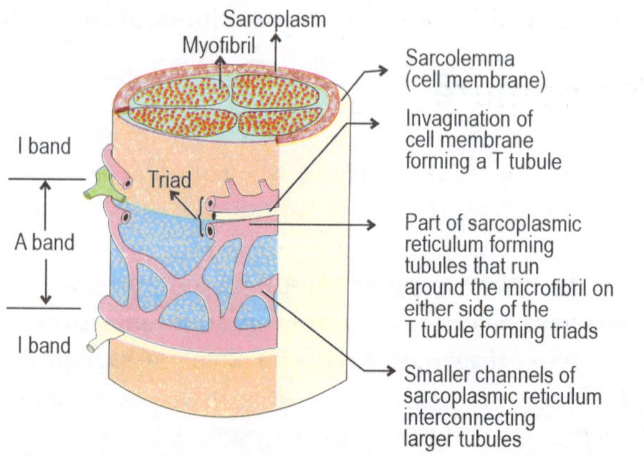

Fig. 21.9: Arrangement of sarcotubular system in the myofibril. Note the relationship of sarcoplasmic reticulum and T-tubules with I and A bands of sarcomere, in a myocyte.

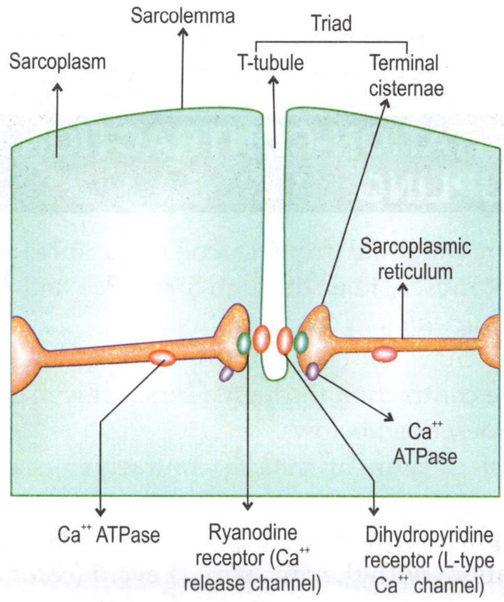

Fig. 21.10: Structure of sarcotubular system. Note the arrangement of triad (central T tubule and two adjoining cisternae)

Sarcoplasmic Reticulum

The sarcoplasmic reticulum (SR) in skeletal muscle corresponds to the endoplasmic reticulum found in other cells.

1. It forms an elaborate **membranous network** having extensive anastomosis around each myofibril and runs parallel to the myofilaments.
2. The slender tubules, about **0.04 µm in diameter**, have an elongated portion in the middle and dilated region at both ends known as lateral sacs or **terminal cisternae**.
3. The cisternae lie in close contact with the T-tubules **at the A-I junction**.
4. The combination of the T-tubule membrane and its two neighboring cisternae is called a **triad** (Fig 21.10), which plays a vital role in linking membrane action potentials to muscle contraction (details see below). In cardiac muscle, it forms a diad due to the presence of one cistern.

Receptors & Channel Proteins in STS

The T-tubules are separated from the terminal cisternae by a narrow space of about 12–14 nm that contains areas of densities known as *'feet'*. The junctional feet involve two integral membrane proteins, one in the T-tubule membrane, and the other in the membrane of the terminal cistern.

1. The T-tubule protein is a modified ***voltage-sensitive calcium channel*** known as the **dihydropyridine (DHP) receptor**. It is so named because it is blocked by the drug dihydropyridine.
2. The DHP receptors are **L-type calcium channels** and they are clustered in groups of four called *'tetrads'*.
3. Primarily the receptor acts as a ***voltage sensor*** *rather than a calcium channel*.
4. The portion of the terminal cisternae membrane that faces the T-tubules contains proteins known as the **ryanodine receptors**. They are so called because they bind to the plant alkaloid ryanodine. They mainly act ***as calcium release channels***.
5. There is also **calcium ATPases** present on the membrane of SR that pumps calcium back into the SR.

Functions

Role of STS in Muscle Contraction & Relaxation

Sarcotubular system (STS) plays a vital role in muscle contraction as it links T-tubular action potentials (excitation) with calcium release from the SR that activates the contractile machinery (**contraction**).

- When calcium is pumped back into the SR, decline in cytoplasmic calcium level leads to muscle **relaxation**.
- Thus, STS is crucial in both contraction and relaxation process by mediating ***calcium release*** and ***calcium uptake.***

Mechanism of Calcium Release

Following depolarization at the motor end plate, action potentials propagate along the sarcolemma and down the T-tubule membrane.

- Depolarization of the triad region of the T-tubules induces *conformational changes* in each of the four DHP receptor proteins, which leads to a ***conformational change in the ryanodine receptor*** resulting in **opening of the ryanodine receptor channel**.
- Calcium is thus released from the terminal cisternae of the SR into the cytoplasm, **activating cross-bridge cycling**.
- The entire process, starting from depolarization of the T-tubule membrane to the initiation of the cross-bridge cycling is termed *excitation-contraction coupling*.
- Further, conformational change in DHP receptor allows calcium entry from the ECF into the cytoplasm through the DHP receptor channel and this ***increase in calcium level*** inside the cell can as well ***activate the ryanodine receptors*** resulting in calcium release.
    - This mechanism is known as **calcium-induced calcium release** (CICR).
    - However, this pathway has a much lesser role in contraction of skeletal muscle.
- CICR plays an important role in cardiac muscle contraction.
- Increase in Ca^{2+} concentration near the sarcoplasmic reticulum is known as ***calcium spark***.

Mechanism of Calcium Uptake

The membrane of the SR contains a **protein called SERCA** (Sarcoplasmic Endoplasmic Reticulum Calcium ATPase).

This is so named as it is present in all cells in connection with the endoplasmic reticulum.

- The protein is a **Ca^{2+} ATPase** that **pumps free calcium ions** from the sarcoplasm to the SR, from where the calcium ions are moved to their storage sites in the terminal cisternae.
- The pump **relocates two molecules of Ca^{2+}** into the SR for each molecule of ATP hydrolyzed.
- It becomes active **as soon as the Ca^{2+} concentration** in cytoplasm ***becomes high***.
- In the terminal cisternae, a Ca^{2+} binding protein called **calsequestrin**, favors ***storage of calcium at high concentration***.
- With decrease in cytoplasmic calcium concentration, contractile activity ceases and **relaxation process begins** (Flowchart 21.1).

Normally, Ca^{2+}-Mg^{2+} ATPase pumps Ca^{2+} into longitudinal part of SR; from there Ca^{2+} is transferred into cisternae and get stored

↓

Action potential arrives at T tubule and gets transmitted deep into the T tubule.

↓

Opens voltage-gated Ca^{2+} channels deep in the T tubules, located in dihydropyridine receptor.

↓

Conformational change in ryanodine receptor, resulting in calcium release into sarcoplasm.

↓

Calcium diffuses in sarcoplasm to bind with troponin C to cause muscle contraction.

↓

Autoactivation of Ca^{2+}-ATPase that pumps Ca^{2+} from sarcoplasm into the SR.

↓

Ca^{2+} binds with calsequestrin in fluid of cisternae and remains stored there.

↓

Decrease in sarcoplasmic Ca^{2+} concentration that causes muscle relaxation.

Flowchart 21.1: Role of sarcotubular system in muscle contraction and relaxation.

Functions of STS:

1. It transfers action potential from the surface of the muscle fiber to the interior, closer to the myofibrils.
2. It raises cytoplasmic calcium concentration by calcium release from SR.
3. It ensures muscle relaxation by calcium reuptake by SR
4. The cisternae of SR act as storage sites for calcium.

EXCITATION-CONTRACTION COUPLING

The **action potential** from sarcolemma **spreads to the interior** of muscle fiber through T tubules and ***increases sarcoplasmic calcium*** concentration.

- The calcium diffuses to **troponin C and induces muscle contraction** through a series of well controlled steps (described below).
- Role of calcium in muscle contraction is discussed below.
- This phenomenon of **pairing of electrical event** (excitation) **with the mechanical event** (contraction) is called **excitation-contraction coupling**.

Mechanism of Contraction

The term contraction means attachment of myosin heads to actin and **activation of the cross bridge cycles** so that force is generated with shortening of muscle fibers.

Sliding-Filament Theory

In 1957, **A.F. Huxley** proposed 'Sliding-Filament Theory' of muscle contraction.

- Shortening of a muscle fiber occurs due to **sliding of thin filaments over thick filaments** toward the center of the sarcomere (described below in 'molecular mechanisms of muscle contraction').
- It was observed that the **length of A band does not change** during contraction, but **the H zone and I band decrease in width** and the Z lines move closer together.

Significant contribution of Scientist

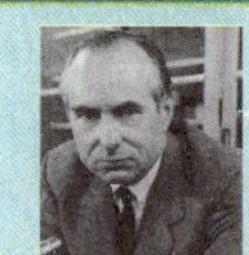

Sir Andrew Fielding Huxley (1917–2012) an English physiologist discovered the basis for propagation of nerve impulses (action potential) earned him Nobel Prize in Physiology or Medicine in 1963 for the "Sliding filament theory" of muscle mechanics. He was conferred a Knight Bachelor by Queen Elizabeth II in 1974, and was appointed to the Order of Merit in 1983. .

Molecular Basis of Muscle Contraction PY3.9

The **sliding motion of the filaments** occurs as a result of a *cyclic interaction* between the ***myosin cross bridges and the actin filaments***, in the presence of calcium and ATP.

- This is known as the **cross-bridge theory** or the **ratchet theory** as the strokes are similar to the action of a ratchet.
- The force generation and shortening are produced at the cross-bridge sites where the chemical energy stored in the muscle is converted into mechanical energy.

Role of Troponin, Tropomyosin & Calcium

Calcium ions provide the most important chemical link in the regulation of muscle protein interactions during the course of excitation-contraction coupling.

- **In resting skeletal muscle**, cytoplasmic calcium ion concentration is low, which is about 10^{-7}M in the region of the myofilaments.
  - Troponin I is attached to myosin binding site on actin and partially covers the myosin binding site.
  - Rest of myosin binding site is covered by tropomyosin filament.
- Thus, in normal condition, **troponin I and tropomyosin inhibit myosin-actin interaction**.
- Troponin T is attached to tropomyosin.
- Each tropomyosin molecule is **held in this blocking position** by troponin that is bound to both tropomyosin and actin.
- Thus, the **troponin-tropomyosin complex** behaves as a ***relaxing protein*** that prevents undesirable contraction.

Troponin-Tropomyosin Interaction

Following **propagation of action potential** along the sarcolemma and down the T tubules, **calcium is released** from the SR and **calcium concentration rises to 10^{-4} M** in the sarcoplasm, which accounts for about ***1000-fold rise*** of the ion.

- Calcium **binds to troponin C** and induces a conformational change in the troponin molecule.
- This result in **shifting of troponin I from the actin filament** (Fig. 21.11 A), allowing tropomyosin to move deeper into the actin groove, **unmasking the myosin binding sites** (Fig. 21.11 B).
- The conformational change alters the position of troponin T that **drags tropomyosin away** from the myosin-binding sites.
- The exposure of the binding sites allows **myosin heads to interact** with actin and engage in **cross-bridge cycling**.
- Thus, the troponin-tropomyosin complex **regulates the contraction of skeletal muscle**.

As the regulation of the contractile process by calcium is implemented through the actin filaments, it is also called **actin-linked regulation**.

Role of Calcium

An **increase in cytoplasmic Ca^{2+}** concentration triggers the contractile process by **removing the inhibition** on cross bridge cycling. On the contrary, **decrease in cytoplasmic Ca^{2+} concentration** leads to ***detachment of calcium from troponin*** that reverses the process and turns off contractile activity.

ok

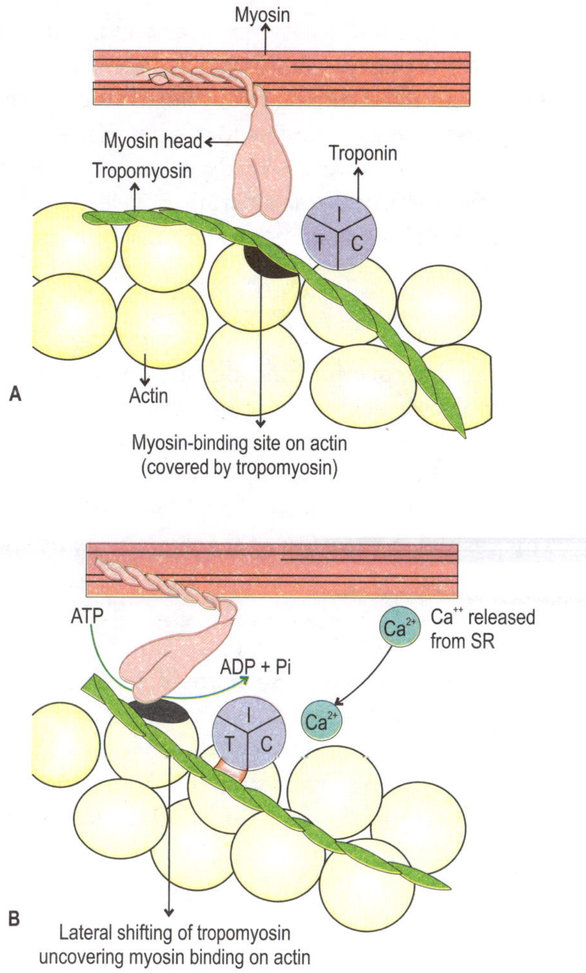

Fig. 21.11: A: Role of troponin-tropomyosin interaction in muscle contraction. Binding of calcium with troponin C induces conformational change in the troponin molecule, which shifts troponin I from the actin filament. **B:** Simultaneously troponin T that drags tropomyosin away from the myosin-binding site on actin. Exposure of this binding site allows myosin heads to interact with actin and engage in cross-bridge cycling. Note, ATP is converted to ADP during this interaction.

1. **In skeletal muscle**, increase in cytosolic calcium in response to a single action potential is usually sufficient to saturate all troponin-binding sites on actin filaments.
   - At a calcium **concentration of 10^{-4}M**, there is ***full force development***, and the *contractile system is fully saturated*.
   - With further increase in concentration, there is only small increase in the force.
2. **In cardiac and smooth muscle**, the amount of calcium regulates the degree of actin-myosin interaction as the contractile system is **only partially saturated** under normal conditions.

Cross Bridge Cycle

The sequence of events that occur during the interaction between the myosin cross-bridges and the actin molecules is termed as a cross-bridge cycle.

- During each cycle, **cross bridge** (myosin head) ***attaches to thin filament*** causing displacement of thick filament over thin filament followed by **detachment of myosin head in a repetitive fashion.**

- **ATP is required** during the cycle; for the movement of the cross bridge as well as for its detachment.
- However, all the cross-bridges *do not go through the same phase* at any instant during a cycle. This helps in a smooth and sustained contraction.

Events in the Resting Muscle

When the muscle is at rest, the cytoplasmic ATP gets attached to its specific binding site in the head of the myosin molecule and the globular head is not attached to actin.

- The intrinsic ATPase activity of the myosin head **breaks down ATP to ADP and Pi** (Fig. 21.12A).
- This results in ***rotation of the myosin head*** around the hinge in such a way that the globular head is positioned at 90° angle in relation to the thick filament, pointing towards, but not attached to the thin filament.
- This rotation **moves the myosin head about 10 nm along the thin filament**, so that, the head is positioned against a new actin molecule.
    - This resting conformation is known as the **energized state** or the ***'cocked position of the myosin head'*** in which, energy is stored in the form of Pi, similar to the potential energy stored in a coiled spring.

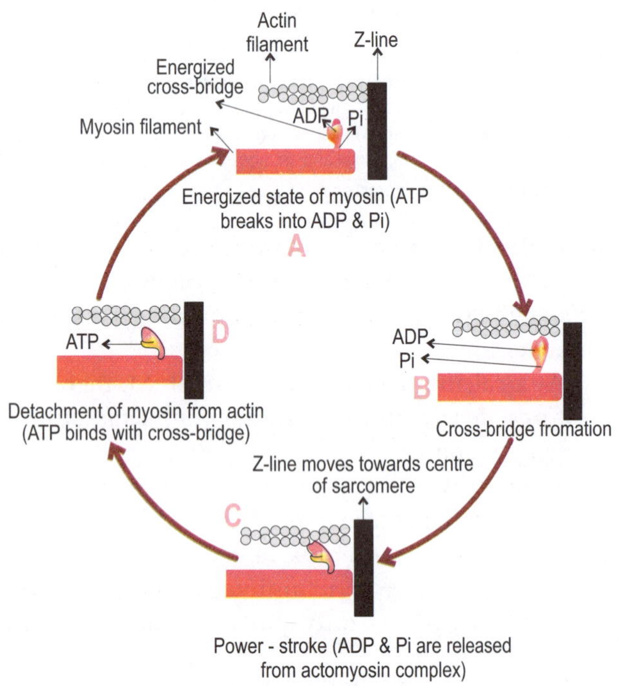

Fig. 21.12: Cross-bridge cycle. **A:** Resting state (cross-bridge is energized by braking down of ATP to ADP and Pi that provides energy; **B:** Myosin head-ADP-Pi complex develops more affinity for actin and bind with actin to form actomyosin complex; **C:** Myosin Head pulls actin filament that moves Z line towards center of sarcomere (power-stroke), and actomyosin complex is free of ADP and Pi; **D:** ATP binds with myosin head and detaches it from actin filament (detached state).

- When most of the cross-bridges in a muscle are in this energized state, it keeps the muscle in a **relaxed state.**
    - ATP hydrolysis in the resting muscle keeps the muscle prepared for future contraction.

Events in the Stimulated Muscle

When action potential arrives at the T-tubules, calcium is released from the SR and the myosin-binding sites on actin are exposed.

1. The ***myosin-ADP-Pi complex has higher affinity for actin***. The charged or energized myosin head binds to actin, forming *the actomyosin complex*, also called **cross-bridge formation** (Fig. 21.12B).
2. The binding of myosin head to actin has **two effects:**
    i) First, Pi is released from myosin head producing the **power stroke** i.e. a conformational change in which the myosin head bends on the hinge at an angle of about 45 degrees pulling the actin filament about 11 nm toward the center of the sarcomere (Fig. 21.12C).
    ii) Secondly, the binding causes the **dissociation of ADP** from the myosin head leaving the actomyosin complex in a **rigid state.**
    - That means the myosin head stay attached to the actin molecule in the same position and at a 45° angle with respect to the thick and thin filaments.
3. For detachment to occur, a **new molecule of ATP must bind to the myosin head** and initiate next cycle.
    - Usually, the sarcoplasmic ATP concentration in normal physiological conditions is always adequate to produce the necessary detachment of cross-bridges.
    - So, the ADP-free actomyosin complex *(**attached state**)* quickly binds to ATP.
4. Binding to ATP **decreases the affinity of myosin for actin** resulting in detachment of cross-bridges from the thin filaments, called as **detached state** (Fig. 21.12D).
5. Soon after, **ATP hydrolysis** occurs and the myosin head attains the **energized state.**

If Stimulation Continues: If the stimulus for contraction persists, i.e. the **sarcoplasmic Ca^{2+} remains elevated**, then myosin-binding sites on actin get exposed and the next cross bridge cycle ensues.

- The **cycle can go on** as long as the sarcoplasmic Ca^{2+} remains high, ATP is available, and the ***physiological limit to shortening*** has **not been** reached.

Effects of Cross-Bridge Formation

During contraction, being attached to an actin molecule, each myosin cross-bridge pivots around its hinge.

- Each thick filament has **500–600 myosin heads**, and each one can pivot about ***five times per second*** during a rapid contraction.
- One stroke of a cross-bridge produces **11 nm displacement of the thin filament** over the thick filament.

- As long as the muscle is stimulated, these swiveling motions of many cross-bridges with each cross-bridge repeating its cycle many times, **drag the thin filaments** attached to successive Z lines towards the center of the sarcomere, producing **large displacements of the thin filaments**.
- This leads to **decrease in the sarcomeric length** and ultimately muscle shortening.
- **When shortening does not occur** as in isometric contraction, the repetitive binding and pull on the actin generate tension.

Role of ATP in Cross-Bridge Formation

ATP is required for the **detachment of myosin head from the thin filaments**.

1. If most of the cross-bridges in a muscle **remain in the detached state**, it would produce **relaxation** in the muscle.
2. ***Not all the cross bridges*** *remain in the detached state* even in a completely relaxed muscle; some of them bind to actin and generate tension that **contributes to the tone of the muscle**.
3. If cellular ATP stores are depleted, as happens after death, the cross-bridges cannot detach and it is called a **rigor cross bridge**, the cycle stops there and the filaments remain in the attached state. This produces stiffening in the muscle, known as ***rigor mortis*** (Clinical Note 21.1).

Clinical Note 21.1

Rigor mortis: Stiffening of the muscle after death is called rigor mortis. Within 3 to 6 h of death, the depletion of ATP fails to detach the cross-bridge. Therefore, muscle remains in a state of contraction or rigidity. The rigidity of rigor mortis completes in about 12 h and disappears about 40 to 60 h after death due to disintegration and putrefaction of muscle fibers.

Cross-Bridge Cycle is a Four-Step Process

The process of cross-bridge cycle occur **in four main steps** (Fig. 21.12A to D, as depicted above):

1. ATP hydrolysis in the myosin head leading to energized state of the myosin.
2. Cross-bridge formation in the presence of increased calcium.
3. Release of Pi and ADP from myosin head producing power stroke.
4. Binding of ATP to myosin head causing detachment of myosin from actin.

During muscle contraction, Z lines move towards M line that decreases sarcomeric length (muscle shortening), and **during muscle relaxation,** Z lines remain wide apart (Fig. 21.13).

- In this process of contraction and relaxation, **A band remains constant** and **changes occur in I band and H zone**.

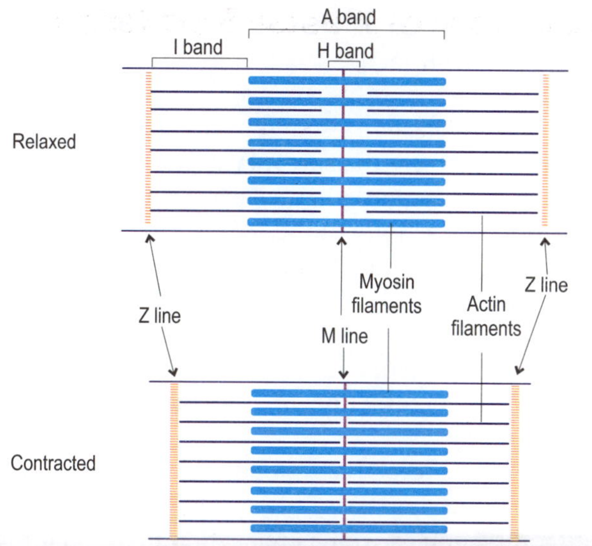

Fig. 21.13: Length of sarcomere and width of A, I and H bands in relaxed and contracted muscles. Note, in contract state, I and H bands almost obliterate, whereas A band remains same in both contracted and relaxed states.

- In extreme contracted state, I band and H zone almost obliterate.

In Summary: Molecular basis of skeletal muscle contraction is summarized in Flowchart 21.2.

Propagation of action potential in the motor axon

↓

Release of acetylcholine that generates action potential in the sarcolemma

↓

Inward spread of depolarization along T tubules into the muscle

↓

Release of calcium from the terminal cisternae increasing sarcoplasmic Ca^{2+} concentration

↓

Binding of Ca^{2+} to troponin C that uncovers the myosin binding sites on actin

↓

Attachment of myosin head to actin initiating cross-bridge cycle

↓

Sliding of thin filaments over thick filaments towards the center of the sarcomere

↓

Decrease in sarcomeric length producing muscle shortening

Flowchart 21.2: Major steps of molecular basis of skeletal muscle contraction.

Mechanism of Muscle Relaxation

Like muscle contraction, relaxation is also **an active process**.

- The **Ca^{2+}ATPase** present on the membrane of SR **pumps Ca^{2+} from the sarcoplasm** into the SR.
- If no further action potential arrives at the myoneural junction, the activity of Ca^{2+}ATPase **decreases calcium concentration** in the vicinity of the myofilaments to a very low level.
- Consequently, **very few calcium ions are available** to bind with troponin.
- This leads to **cessation of interaction** between actin and myosin.
- The contractile activity stops and relaxation process begins (Flowchart 21.3).

Thus, contraction as well as relaxation in skeletal muscle requires energy in the form of ATP.

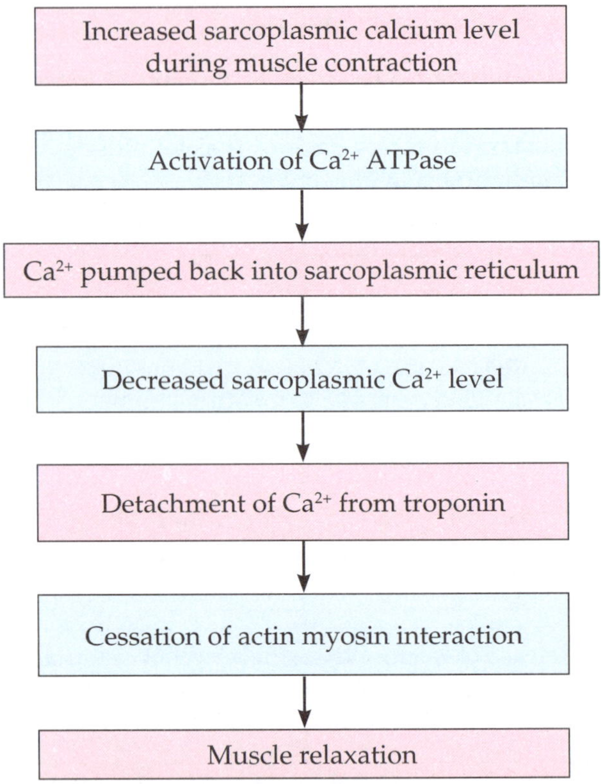

Flowchart 21.3: Major events in skeletal muscle relaxation.

Action Potential & Contractile Response PY3.8

Action Potential

The **resting membrane potential** of skeletal muscle is **–90 mV**.

- The **duration** of the action potential is **2–4 ms** and **absolute refractory period is 1–3 ms** (Fig. 21.14A).
- The **depolarization phase** of the action potential is due to ***sodium influx*** and **repolarization** is a manifestation of ***potassium efflux***.

The action potential produces a state of increased cytosolic calcium concentration, which activates the contractile apparatus long after the electrical activity in the membrane has ceased.

Contractile Response

The action potential spreads at a speed of 5 m/sec along the sarcolemma and down the T tubules to activate the myofilaments.

1. A **twitch** is defined as the mechanical response of single muscle fiber to an action potential consisting of a phase of contraction followed by a relaxation phase.
2. When the action potential and the twitch contraction are plotted on the same time scale, the contractile response begins about 2 ms after the onset of the action potential (Fig. 21.14B). This delay is known as the **latent period**, during which the **Excitation-Contraction Coupling** takes place.

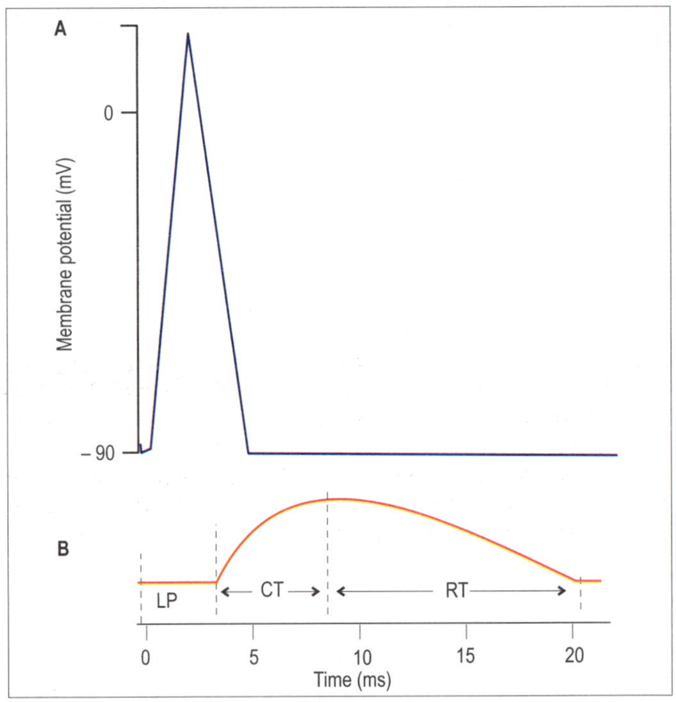

Fig. 21.14: Comparison of electrical and mechanical responses of skeletal muscle. **A:** Action potential recorded from skeletal muscle fiber; **B:** Simultaneous recoding of contractile response on same time scale. LP: latent period; CT: contraction time; RT: relaxation time.

Contraction & Relaxation Time

Calcium released during a twitch can fully activate the contractile machinery, but the relaxation process starts soon after; so, the magnitude of peak tension developed is relatively low.

- The duration from the start of the contractile response to the attainment of peak tension is the **contraction time** and from the point of peak tension to the end of contractile response is the **relaxation time**.
  - The **duration of the twitch is about 7.5 ms** in the fast muscle fiber and **about 100 ms** in slow muscle

fiber. Normally, twitches occur occasionally in a healthy person.
- In the clinics, twitches are usually elicited while testing the tendon jerks (myotatic reflexes).
- In **lower motor neuron diseases**, presence of twitches that occur spontaneously helps to establish the diagnosis.

PY3.10

TYPES OF CONTRACTION

Tension is the force of the contracting muscle acting on an object. **Load** is the force exerted on the muscle by an object, i.e. weight of the object against which muscle tension acts.
- Thus, muscle tension and load act against each other.
- When an object is to be lifted, muscle tension has to be more than the opposing load.

Contractions are of two types:
1. Isometric contraction
2. Isotonic contraction

Isometric Contraction

When muscle contraction is associated with **no apparent change in muscle length**, the phenomenon is called isometric contraction. The muscle develops tension but does not shorten or lengthen; for example, when somebody is trying to lift a heavy object.
1. During this type of contraction, the cross bridges bind with the actin molecules and attempt to pull them but cannot drag the thin filaments because the load is greater than the tension exerted by the muscle fiber. This exerts a force on the thin filament, the **isometric tension**.
2. If isometric contraction is continued, cycling cross bridges again and again bind to the same actin molecules.
3. According to the law of physics, if displacement is zero (position of the object does not change), the work done (force × displacement) is also nil, though force is generated and energy is spent. Thus, in isometric contraction **no external work is done**.
4. Isometric tension can be recorded with the help of an isometric lever when the muscle is stimulated to contract with its two ends held at fixed points.

Isotonic Contraction

When muscle contraction is associated with **no apparent change in muscle tone**, the phenomenon is called isotonic contraction.
- The shortening of the muscle fiber occurs due to sliding of thin over thick filaments. Examples of such muscle contractions are walking, running, lifting an object etc.
- Isotonic contraction is also known as ***concentric contraction***.

The major difference from isometric contraction is that in isotonic contraction, ***the external work is done*** (Table 21.1).

Table 21.1 | Differences between isometric and isotonic contractions.

	Isometric	Isotonic
1. Length of muscle	Remains same	Shortening occurs
2. Tension	Tension increases	No change
3. External work	No work done	Work is done

Processes in Isometric and Isotonic Contractions

When an object is **to be lifted**, initially tension increases in the muscle till it becomes equal to the downward pulling force (due to the weight of the object) without any change in muscle length i.e. the ***fibers undergo isometric contraction.***
1. Once the tension in the muscle is greater than the opposing load, shortening contraction of the muscle lifts the object and brings it to the new position; here the fibers undergo isotonic contraction.
2. Now, if the object is to be held in space in the new position, the fibers undergo isometric contraction, the tension generated being just equal and opposite to the load of the object.
3. Pushing against a wall is an example of isometric contraction if the elbow does not bend during the act i.e. the distance between shoulder and hand remains unchanged.

Exam Questions

1. Name the muscle proteins and give their functions.
2. Draw a labelled diagram of a sarcomere in relaxed and contracted state of the muscle.
3. Describe the role of sarcotubular system in muscle contraction. What is excitation-contraction coupling? Describe the molecular basis of muscle contraction.
4. What is cross bridge cycle? Describe the changes in electromechanical processes during different phases of cross bridge cycle
5. Briefly describe the relationship between electrical and mechanical response in skeletal muscle.

Multiple Choice Questions

1. **All of the following are components of thin filament, EXCEPT:**
   A. Actin B. Titin C. Troponin D. Tropomyosin
2. **All of the following occur during skeletal muscle contraction, EXCEPT:**
   A. A band does not change B. H zone reduces
   C. Two Z lines come closer D. I Band becomes wider
3. **The length of myosin filament in skeletal muscle is:**
   A. 1.6 mm B. 16 μm
   C. 1.6 μm D. 1.6 nm
4. **In the extreme contracted state of skeletal muscle, the width of**
   A. I band disappears B. I band increases
   C. H band increases D. A band decreases
5. **Which of the following is a regulatory protein in skeletal muscle contraction?**
   A. Myosin B. Actin
   C. Tropomyosin D. Nebulin
6. **Which of the following is NOT a sarcolemmal protein?**
   A. Sarcoglycan B. Dystroglycan
   C. Dystrophin D. Calmodulin
7. **In the sarcomere, the A band is so called because:**
   A. It is the constant length band
   B. It is the central important band
   C. It is anisotropic in its refractive index
   D. It is the first band to be discovered
8. **All of the following are present in skeletal muscle sarcotubular system, EXCEPT:**
   A. Calmodulin B. Rynodine receptor
   C. Calsequestrin D. Dihydropyridine receptor
9. **Which of the following favors storage of calcium in skeletal muscle sarcoplasmic reticulum?**
   A. Calsequestrin B. Calbindin
   C. Calcineurin D. Troponin
10. **In the extreme stretched state of skeletal muscle, the width of :**
    A. A band decreases
    B. H band increases
    C. I band decreases
    D. A band increases
11. **The function of Troponin-tropomyosin complex is:**
    A. To cover myosin binding sites on actin
    B. To facilitates myosin head to deliver its power stoke
    C. To regulate dihydropyridine-rynodine interaction
    D. To provide maximum elastic resistance during contraction
12. **All of the following favors the skeletal muscle contraction to continue, EXCEPT**
    A. High level of sarcoplasmic ATP
    B. Thin filaments touch the H zone
    C. Thin filaments touch the M line
    D. Increased level of sarcoplasmic calcium
13. **The latent period in nerve muscle preparation is due to time taken for all of the following, EXCEPT:**
    A. Activation of the contractile mechanism
    B. Overcoming the viscous resistance of the muscle
    C. Pumping back of calcium to sarcoplasmic reticulum
    D. Conduction of impulse along the axon from the point of stimulus
14. **The termination of skeletal muscle contraction occurs when**
    A. Reduction in sarcoplasmic calcium concentration
    B. Reduction in cytoplasmic calcium concentration
    C. Ach is hydrolyzed by acetylcholinesterase
    D. Closure of Rynodine channels occur
15. **During isometric contraction of skeletal muscle, there is:**
    A. External work is done
    B. Decrease in muscle length
    C. Increase in muscle length
    D. Increase in muscle tension
16. **Which of the following muscle mainly undergoes isometric contraction?**
    A. Interossei of hand
    B. Extraocular muscles
    C. Lumbricals of hand
    D. Quadriceps femoris
17. **In skeletal muscle fiber:**
    A. During relaxation, calcium diffuses back to sarcoplasmic reticulum
    B. The function of calcium is to expose the myosin binding sites on actin
    C. A single motor neuron discharge is not sufficient to activate contractile machinery
    D. Depolarization of the T-tubule follows binding of Troponin C to calcium
18. **Which is NOT true for excitation contraction coupling in skeletal muscle?**
    A. It links cross bridge formation with sliding of actin over myosin
    B. It links depolarization in T tubules with sliding of actin over myosin
    C. It links electrical and mechanical event
    D. It couples action potential and cross bridge cycling
19. **Which of the following do not favor rigor mortis?**
    A. Extremely cold environment
    B. Decrease in sarcoplasmic ATP level
    C. Decrease in sarcoplasmic calcium level
    D. Myosin head remaining attached to actin
20. **During skeletal muscle contraction, the cytoplasmic calcium concentration rises**
    A. 1,000 times
    B. 100 times
    C. 50 times
    D. 4 times

Answers

1. B	2. D	3. C	4. A	5. C	6. D
7. C	8. D	9. A	10. B	11. A	12. C
13. C	14. B	15. D	16. D	17. B	18. A
19. C	20. A				

Chapter 22

Properties of Skeletal Muscle and Applied Aspects

Learning Objectives

On completion of study of this chapter:

The student will be able to (must know):

1. List the properties of skeletal muscle and understand their functional importance.
2. Name the energy sources in skeletal muscle and explain the mechanism of oxygen debt.
3. Define the motor unit and give the concept of size principle.
4. Outline the physiological mechanisms of muscle fatigue.
5. Elucidate the mechanism of rigor mortis.
6. Name muscle fiber types and list differences between them.

The student may also be able to (desirable to know):

1. Describe the properties of skeletal muscle.
2. Explain the mechanism of muscle fatigue and rigor mortis.

PY3.8

PROPERTIES OF SKELETAL MUSCLE

Important properties of skeletal muscles (in addition to the properties like contractility, excitability, fatigability etc.) are:

1. Summation of contraction
2. Staircase Phenomenon
3. Tetanization
4. Post-tetanic potentiation
5. Length-tension relationship
6. Load-velocity relationship

Summation of Contraction

When stimuli are **applied in quick succession**, the contractile responses are added to produce a higher response. The action potential of the skeletal muscle is brief (1–4ms) compared to its twitch duration.

- When a stimulus is applied, the absolute refractory period of the action potential is over by the time contraction starts.

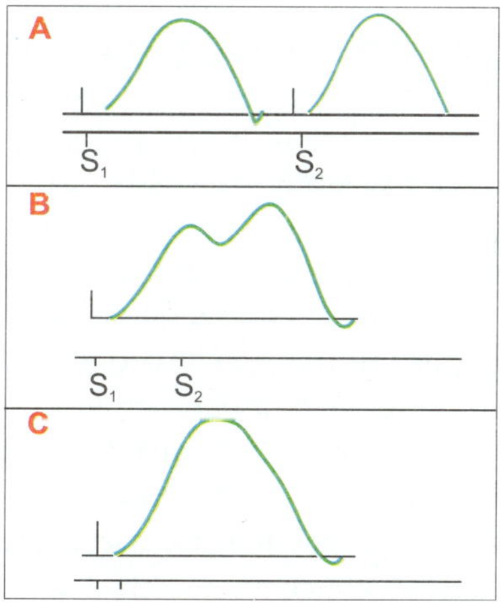

Fig. 22.1: Summation of contraction. **A:** Second stimulus (S2) was applied after the contractile response of first stimulus (S1) was over; **B:** S2 was applied in the contraction phase of S1; **C:** S2 was applied close to the latent period of S1. Note, second stimulus applied before relaxation period of first response, leads to summation of contraction and increases in magnitude of contraction.

- If the next stimulus is applied quickly, the second twitch is produced when the contraction phase of the first twitch is still continuing, and therefore the phase of contraction of the second twitch is added to the phase of contraction of the first twitch, resulting in a **summated contractile response,** which is higher in amplitude than a single twitch (Fig. 22.1 A to C).
- The **Ca^{2+} released due to the second stimulus is added** to the Ca^{2+} released by the first stimulus, producing a higher sarcoplasmic Ca^{2+} concentration that results in a ***bigger contractile response***.
- Thus, repeated stimulation of the muscle before the relaxation produces a phenomenon known as **summation of contractions**.

The **contractile elements have no refractory period**, they do not follow all or none law and contraction can continue till Ca^{2+} and ATP are available.

Staircase Phenomenon

If a skeletal muscle is **stimulated rapidly** (but below the tetanizing frequency) with suprathreshold stimuli, there is **progressive increase** in the force of contraction for the first few contractions, until a maximum uniform tension per contraction is reached. This is the staircase phenomenon or **treppe** (in German). Treppe is also seen in cardiac muscle. In 1871, **Henry Pickering Bowditch** first described Treppe in the frog's heart.

- During repeated and rapid stimulation, if a second contraction occurs during the relaxation phase of the first one, the **amplitude of the second twitch will be higher** than the first one (Fig. 22.2A).
- This is because when the muscle has not completely relaxed, the **cytoplasmic calcium concentration remains elevated** as all the calcium released due to the first stimulus have not been pumped back into the sarcoplasmic reticulum.
- This leftover calcium is added to the calcium released during the second contraction and results in greater amplitude.
- Also, the heat produced during preceding contraction **decreases sarcoplasmic viscosity** and *facilitates the enzymatic activity* that increases the height of succeeding contractions.
- Thus, if subsequent contractions occur before the relaxation phase of the previous one is over, first few twitches gradually increase in amplitude.
- This is called staircase phenomenon as the graph is in an ascending order, like a staircase.
- The amplitude does not increase after a few contractions as the calcium level becomes saturated.

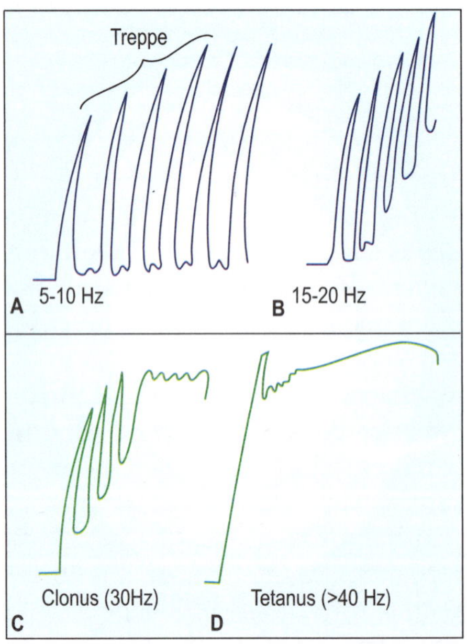

Fig. 22.2: Effect of frequency on muscle contraction and tension. **A:** at frequency of 5–10 Hz, treppe (staircase phenomenon) occurs; **B & C:** at frequency of 15–30 Hz, clonus (partial tetanus) occurs; **D:** at frequency of 40 Hz or above, tetanus occurs.

Tetanization

If the muscle is stimulated repeatedly at a **very high frequency**, continuous activation of the contractile mechanism occurs without any relaxation, resulting in a sustained contraction known as **tetanus** (tetanic contraction).

1. In **Clonus** *(incomplete or unfused tetanus)*, there are periods of incomplete relaxation between the maintained contractions (Fig. 22.2 B and C).
2. While the frequency of the action potentials progressively increases to tetanizing frequency, the tension generated in the muscle gradually rises and summated until a maximal **tetanic tension** is reached in **complete tetanus** *(fused tetanus)*, there is no relaxation between the contraction phases (Fig. 22.2D..

Beyond this, tension does not increase further with increase in frequency of the action potentials.

Critical Frequency: The critical frequency (CF) at which summation of contractions occurs differs from muscle to muscle since it depends on the twitch duration of a fiber.

$$CF = \frac{1}{\text{Twitch duration (in sec)}}$$

For example, a fiber has twitch duration of 10 ms or 0.01s. The CF for this fiber will be 1/0.01s = 100/s.

When a muscle is stimulated with a frequency more than CF, summation of contractions occurs. Stimulation of the muscle with less than CF produces distinct contractions with intermittent relaxations.

Mechanism: Following a single action potential, **enough Ca^{2+} is released** to expose all the myosin binding sites on actin molecules.

- But, the attachment of activated myosin heads to these sites takes time.
- Also, the **Ca^{2+} concentration starts decreasing** as the pumping back of Ca^{2+} into the sarcoplasmic reticulum commences immediately.
- Therefore, all the cross-bridges are not engaged and the **tension generating mechanism is not saturated**.
- In a ***tetanic contraction***, more and more Ca^{2+} is released with each successive action potential, exhausting the pumping-back mechanism.
- Thus, the cytosolic calcium remains at a constantly high level so that all the myosin-binding sites on the thin filaments are available.
- Therefore, the **tension generated during tetanic contraction is very high.**

IMPORTANT NOTE

1. A fast muscle needs a larger CF and a slow muscle needs a smaller CF to summate the contractions.
2. The tension generated during a complete tetanus is usually about four times that of a single twitch.

Such contraction occurs in a disease called ***tetanus*** caused by the organism clostridium tetani.

Post-Tetanic Potentiation

When a single stimulus is applied to a muscle **immediately after the tetanic contraction** is over, the amplitude of contraction is higher than that of a single twitch. This phenomenon is known as *post-tetanic potentiation*.

1. Following tetanic contraction, the **released Ca^{2+} takes some time to be pumped back** into the sarcoplasmic reticulum.
2. This left over Ca^{2+} is **added to the Ca^{2+} released by the next single stimulus** resulting in a higher cytosolic Ca^{2+} level and therefore, a bigger contraction.

Length-Tension Relationship

Isometric tension developed in a muscle depends on the initial length of the muscle.

1. When the muscle fiber is stretched, the tension registered by it is known as the **passive tension**, which is due to the ***elongation of the elastic titin filaments***, not due to activation of the contractile elements.
2. If this **stretched muscle is stimulated**, the tension developed by it is known as the **total tension**.
3. At any length, the amount of tension actually generated by the cross-bridge movements is known as the **active tension**, which is the total tension minus passive tension.

The length-tension relationship graph (Fig. 22.3) shows that within physiological limit, the tension is directly proportional to length i.e. tension in the muscle increases, as the length is gradually increased.

- The length of the muscle prior to contraction is called the **initial length**.
- The length of the muscle at which it develops ***maximal isometric active tension*** is known as the **optimal length** or **resting length**, beyond which the tension generated on stimulation decreases until the muscle fibers are injured by the stretch.
- In a relaxed state, if the **tendon is cut** from its bony attachment, the muscle ***shortens about 20 per cent***.

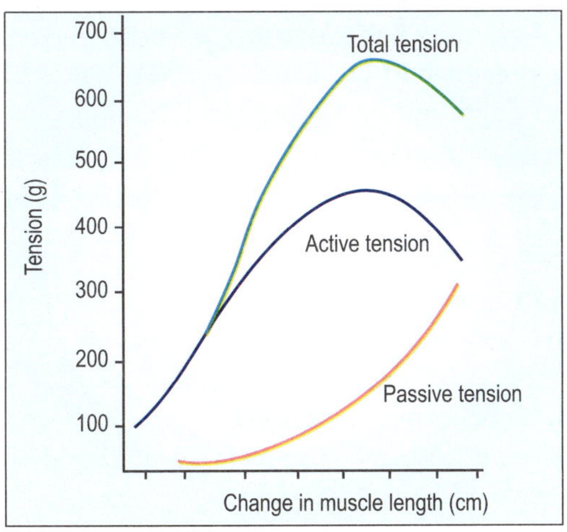

Fig. 22.3: Length-tension relationship in skeletal muscle.

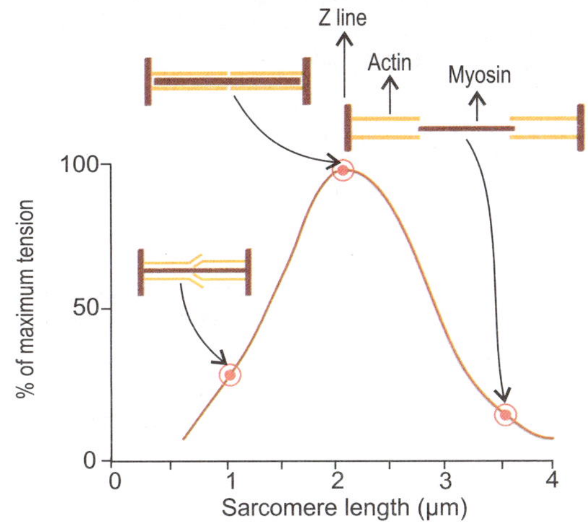

Fig. 22.4: Active tension developed at different sarcomere length. Note, interaction between actin and myosin is maximum at the peak of active tension, which corresponds to resting muscle length.

- That means muscles are under some stretch in the resting state.
- This stretch of resting muscles generates maximum tension on stimulation.
- Therefore, **resting length** is the muscle length at which maximum response is produced when it is stimulated.

Length-Tension Relationship in a Sarcomere: Based on sliding filament mechanism, the amount of tension generated depends on the total number of cross-linkages formed by actin-myosin interactions.

1. **At resting length**, there is maximum overlap between actin and myosin filaments that causes maximum tension development.
2. As the **muscle is stretched** beyond this length, *overlap of thick and thin filaments decreases progressively* and the ***active tension developed declines*** proportionately, - and when there is no overlap, the tension generated becomes nil (Fig. 22.4).
3. On the contrary, when the **length becomes less** than the resting length, *overlap decreases* and the ***tension declines***.
4. With **further reduction in length**, the *thin filaments overlap each other* at the center of the sarcomere so that the binding sites on actin are in the bare area of the thick filaments, producing **minimal tension**.
   - The **optimal sarcomeric length** in frog muscle is **2.0–2.2 μm.**

Load-Velocity Relationship

When a muscle contracts against a load (isotonic contraction), the **velocity of fiber shortening is inversely proportional to the degree of load.**

1. When there is **no load**, the muscle contracts with ***maximum velocity*** and the *velocity decreases with increasing load on the muscle* (Fig. 22.5).
2. When the **load becomes equal to the maximal isometric tension**, the ***shortening velocity is zero***.

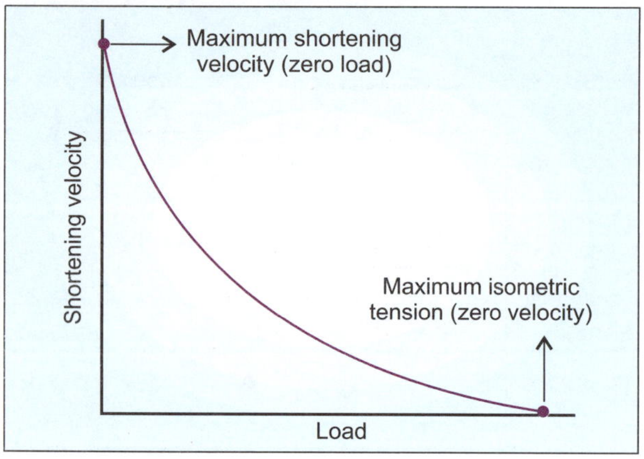

Fig. 22.5: Load-velocity relationship.

3. If the **load increases further**, the muscle lengthens (**lengthening contraction**).

Mechanism: The **rate of cross bridge cycling** in a muscle, which depends on its ***ATPase activity***, *determines the shortening velocity of that muscle.*

- In general, **a light load offers less resistance** to the sliding of the filaments so that thin filaments move quickly over thick filaments allowing few cross bridges to form at a time, producing ***less tension and faster contraction.***
- **Increasing the load** on a cross-bridge slows its forward movement during a power stroke and reduces the ATP hydrolysis,
    - the slower contraction allows more time for actomyosin interaction and ***greater tension development***.

Thus, for any given load, the shortening velocity is maximal when the muscle is at its resting length.

1. When a muscle is stretched by a load prior to start of contraction, the condition is known as **free-loaded** (**pre-loaded**).
2. When the load is applied to the muscle after it starts contracting, the condition is called **after-loaded**.

PY3.11

Energy Sources in Skeletal Muscle

Adenosine Tri-Phosphate

Adenosine Tri-Phosphate (ATP) is the immediate source of energy for contraction in skeletal muscles.

- During ATP hydrolysis, the **terminal high-energy phosphate bond** of ATP ***splits to form ADP and Pi***, with release of **7.3 kcal for each mole of ATP hydrolyzed.**
- ATP → ADP + Pi + 7.3 kcal

The functions of ATP in muscle are as follows:

1) It supplies the **energy required for cross-bridge movement** during muscle contraction.
2) ATP binding to myosin **breaks the actin-myosin interaction** and allows the cross-bridge cycle to continue.
3) It provides **energy to the Ca^{2+}-Mg^{+} ATPase pump** that transports Ca^{2+} back into the SR and initiates relaxation.
4) The **Na^{+}-K^{+} pump in the sarcolemma utilizes the energy** derived from ATP hydrolysis to maintain the membrane excitability (RMP).

In resting muscle, less ATP molecules are present in the sarcoplasm.

- Once contraction is initiated, ATP store can sustain contraction for fraction of a second.
- For contractions to continue, muscle requires an enormous supply of ATP, which has to be generated immediately.

ATP is regenerated by ***three other pathways***:

1. Phosphorylation of ADP by **creatine phosphate**
2. Oxidative phosphorylation of ADP in the mitochondria
3. Phosphorylation of ADP by the break-down of glucose to CO_2 and H_2O.

Creatine Phosphate

Creatine phosphate (CP) is also called **phosphorylcreatine**.

Phosphorylation of ADP by creatine phosphate is a very rapid, non-oxidative process, which provides ATP by **transfer of a phosphate group from CP to ADP**, catalyzed by the enzyme ***creatine kinase*** (CK).

$$CP + ADP \xrightarrow{CK} C + ATP$$

The concentration of CP is about five times that of ATP in the resting muscle.

- The ATP supplied by this mechanism sustains contractions for a few seconds.
- During recovery period, the concentration of CP is restored back to the normal level by addition of ATP formed by glycolysis to creatine (C).
- Also, some mitochondrial ATP transfers its phosphate group to creatine.

$$C + ATP \xrightarrow{CK} CP + ADP$$

At rest and during light exercise, muscle utilizes ***free fatty acids*** as its energy source.

During moderate to heavy exercise, *metabolism of glucose and glycogen* has the primary role to generate ATP.

- **In the presence of O_2**, *aerobic glycolysis* takes place, the end products being CO_2, H_2O and 38 molecules of ATP.
- **If the O_2 supply is inadequate**, *anaerobic glycolysis* delivers lactic acid and 2 ATP per molecule of glucose.

Oxygen Debt

During rapid strenuous activity, even with the high respiratory rate and maximum possible dilation of the blood vessels, *ATP generated by aerobic glycolysis is not rapid* to meet with body's energy need.

- In that case, **anaerobic glycolysis** occurs to fulfill the ATP demand.
- For example, when a person ***runs for an hour***, around **95% of the energy** spent comes from **aerobic glycolysis**

and only 5% from anaerobic glycolysis whereas in a ***100-meter dash*** completed in 10 seconds, 85% of the energy is derived from anaerobic glycolysis.

After the exercise is over, body has to accomplish the following functions:

1. Convert the surplus lactate into pyruvate
2. Replenish the ATP and CP stores in the muscle
3. To replace the O_2 that came from myoglobin.

For all the above functions, O_2 is required.

- Therefore, even after the termination of the exercise, the ***respiratory rate remains high for some time*** according to the severity of the exercise.
- The **amount of extra oxygen taken up by the body above the basal O_2 consumption** following exercise is known as ***oxygen debt*** (Application Box 22.1).

Muscle Fatigue

When a skeletal muscle is repeatedly stimulated, the tension developed by the muscle decreases gradually. The **decrease in muscle tension** *because of previous contractile activity* is known as muscle fatigue.

Application Box 22.1

Effects of training: Trained athletes can increase muscle oxygen consumption greatly than the nonathletes. They can also effectively utilize free-fatty acids.

- Thus, they sustain exercise without loss of glycogen and accumulation of lactate.
- Hence, oxygen debt in them is much smaller even for severe exercise.
- They also practice more carbohydrate meal several days before the final competition to increase their muscle glycogen store.

- There is decline in the amplitude of contraction as well as the shortening velocity, and the relaxation period is prolonged.
- Fatigue can be of **early or late onset** and the rate of its progress can be **fast or slow**.

In general, the **factors affecting skeletal muscle fatigue** are:

1. The types of fibers present in the muscle
2. The intensity and duration of the exercise
3. Availability of nutrients like oxygen and glucose
4. Accumulation of metabolites like lactic acid, H^+, K^+ and substance P
5. Previous regular training of the similar type of activity
6. CNS factor

CNS Factor: Out of all the factors, the CNS factor plays an important role in delaying the muscle fatigue. **Motivation and encouragement** significantly prolong the duration of exercise.

- Secretion of certain **neurotransmitters** by sensory inputs from the exercising muscle influences fatigue.
  - One probable mechanism they activate is the **endorphin system**.
  - The degree and source of encouragement also affect fatigue significantly.
- A muscle that fatigues early, also **recovers early** and the one that takes longer time, also recovers late.

Rigor Mortis

During the cross-bridge cycle, binding of ATP to the myosin head breaks the actin-myosin interaction and brings in relaxation of the muscle.

- **If cellular energy stores are depleted**, as happens after death, the **cross-bridge detachment cannot** occur due to lack of ATP.
- Therefore, the *myosin heads remain in the attached state.*
- Following death, the **cytoplasmic calcium concentration remains elevated** because of following reasons:

1. Calcium is not pumped back into the sarcoplasmic reticulum in the absence of ATP.
2. Ca^{2+} diffuses from ECF into the cytoplasm.
3. The inactive membrane of the SR cannot hold back Ca^{2+}, which diffuses out of SR to the sarcoplasm.

- The raised cytoplasmic calcium concentration initiates contraction by exposing the myosin heads on actin and permitting **formation of cross-bridges that do not detach** due to lack of ATP.
- This leads to stiffness in the muscle, which is known as **rigor mortis**.
  - It starts about 3 to 4 h after death and gets ***completed in about 12 h*** after death.
  - The stiffness ***disappears 48 to 60 h after death*** due to disintegration of muscle proteins.

Heat Production in Muscles

During muscle contraction, most of the energy is spent in the form of heat, part of the energy is used to do the work and a small portion is used to build up the ATP stores.

- The amount of heat generated can be measured accurately with the help of sensitive thermocouples.

The heat generated is of the **following types**:

a) **Resting heat:** When the muscle is at rest, the heat generated **due to basal metabolism** is known as resting heat.

b) **Initial heat:** Initial heat is the heat liberated during muscle contraction **in excess of resting heat**. It can be further divided into two parts.

   i) **Activation heat:** It is produced after the muscle is stimulated and before the contraction starts.

   ii) **Shortening heat:** It is released during isotonic contraction and is proportionate to the degree of shortening.

c) **Relaxation heat:** When a previously shortened muscle **returns to its original length**, the heat generated is known as relaxation heat.

d) **Recovery heat:** This is the heat produced by the **metabolic processes to restore the muscle to its resting state**, in excess of resting heat.

- The recovery heat is liberated for a prolonged period and is equal in magnitude to the initial heat.

PY3.7

Fiber Types in Skeletal Muscle

Skeletal muscle fibers are classified into two categories: type I and type II (Table 22.1).

Type I Muscles Fibers

Muscles consisting mainly of type I fibers are red muscles.

1. Have **many capillaries and high myoglobin.**
   - This ensures an increased blood flow to supply more oxygen.
2. Have plenty of mitochondria and myoglobin,
   - Synthesize ATP by oxidative phosphorylation; hence named as **oxidative fibers.**
3. Have **low myosin ATPase activity**, they break down ATP slowly;
   - Thus, rate of cross-bridge cycling is less, causing a **decreased contraction velocity.**
   - Hence, known as the **slow fibers.**
5. More **resistant to fatigue**; remain contracted for longer time, thereby help maintain posture.
   - Therefore, type I fibers in back and proximal limb muscles are known as ***postural muscles.***

Type II Muscles Fibers

Type II fibers are mainly **white muscles.**

- Have a greater contraction velocity.
- Carry out **fine, precise movements.**
- Examples are intrinsic muscles of the hand and extra ocular muscles of the eye.

Table 22.1 | Differences between type I and II muscle fibers

	Type I	Type II
1. Other names	Slow; red; oxidative	Fast; white; glycolytic
2. Contraction velocity	Slow	Fast
3. Myosin ATPase	Low	High
4. Ca^{2+}-pumping capacity of SR	Low	High
5. Rate of fatigue	Slow	Fast
6. Fiber diameter	Moderate	Large
7. Size of motor unit	Small	Large
8. Glycogen content	Low	High
9. Glycolytic capacity	Low	High
10. Oxidative capacity	High	Low
11. Mitochondria	Numerous	Less
12. Myoglobin content	High	Low
13. Capillaries	Many	Few
14. Primary source of ATP production	Oxidative phosphorylation	Glycolysis

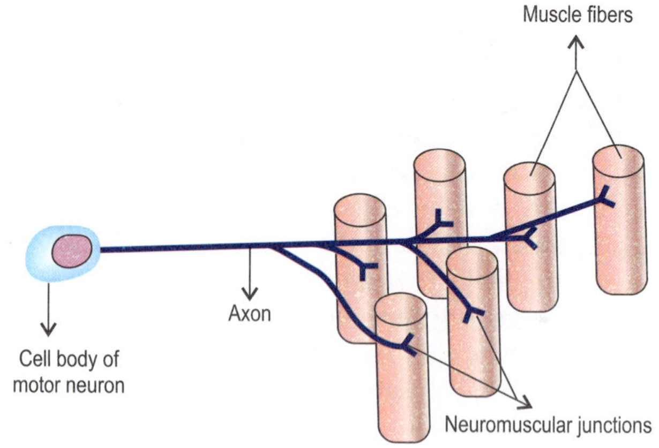

Fig. 22.6: Structure of a motor unit.

Motor Units

Definition

A motor unit consists of a **single motor neuron, its axonal branches and all the muscle fibers** supplied by them (Fig. 22.6).

Size of a Motor Unit

When a motor neuron discharges, contraction is produced in all the muscle fibers supplied by it. The size of a motor unit can be **large or small** depending on the number of muscle fibers innervated by it.

1. **In the intrinsic muscles of the hand**, one motor neuron innervates **less than ten muscle fibers.**
   - So, stimulation of a motor unit produces a small rise in tension.
2. **The back muscles** have **hundreds or a thousand muscle fibers** per motor unit.

- Activation of a single motor unit causes a large increase in tension.

Recruitment of Motor Units

When a single motor neuron discharges, there is some rise in muscle tension. If additional motor neurons fire, there is further increase in tension, as there is **increase in the number of active motor units.**

- The **process of activating a greater number of motor units** is called *recruitment of motor units.*

Hand Muscles: In hand muscles, gradual activation of motor units produces a stepwise increase in muscle tension because, with activation of each new unit, a small amount of tension is added.

- As the tension goes up in a graded manner, it can precisely be regulated.
- Therefore, **muscles for skilled movements have smaller motor units**, for which ***finer regulation of muscle tension*** is of primary importance.

Trunk & Proximal Limb Muscles: In back muscles, with recruitment of additional motor units, each time a huge amount of tension is added.

- Therefore, the back muscles are useful in **maintenance of posture**.
- In these muscles, there is need to develop **a greater tension** to resist the downward pull of the gravity (Application Box 22.2).

Application Box 22.2

Asynchronous discharge of motor units prevents fatigue: The motor units discharge asynchronously. When some of the motor units are active, other units are silent. Afterward, the active units go to rest and the silent units become active.
- At any instant of time, the inputs from different units are summated and this results in a smooth contraction of the muscle.
- This also helps the muscle to work for longer time without being fatigued.

Size Principle

Usually the large diameter, fast conducting motor neurons innervate the muscle fibers of the fast motor units and the small diameter, slow conducting motor neurons innervate muscle fibers of the slow motor units. This is called the *size principle*.
- As the strength of contraction gradually increases, the **small motor units are recruited initially**, followed by the recruitment of large motor units.
- Thus, during the activity of mild to moderate intensity, the **less fatigable, oxidative fibers mostly take part** in the contractile activity, whereas the ***glycolytic fibers are recruited during more intense contraction***.
- In general, a muscle has **both types of motor units** (Application Box 22.3).

Application Box 22.3

Nature of exercise determines type of muscle fibers: Proportion of fast & slow motor units determines the overall strength, fatigability or contraction velocity of a muscle. There are both types of motor units in a muscle.
- Regular practice of isometric exercise increases the number of slow fibers.
- Practice of isotonic exercise increases the percentage of fast fibers.

Whole-Muscle Contraction

A **whole muscle** (for e.g. biceps or triceps) consists of **many muscle fibers** that are organized into **several motor units**. For contraction of a whole muscle, CNS regulates the **recruitment of more motor units** and by increasing the **frequency of discharge** of the motor units.
- The motor units discharge **asynchronously** that results in a *smooth and sustained contraction* **preventing early fatigue** of the muscle.
- The **total tension** developed in a muscle depends on the **number of active fibers** at any instant during contraction, which is decided by following factors:
  i). The total number of active motor units
  ii). The number of fibers present in each motor unit
  iii). The type of fibers present in each motor unit (based on the initial length of the fiber, its diameter and fatigability)

Muscle Strength

The strength of a muscle is measured by the **maximum load it is capable of lifting**.
- The strength of human skeletal muscles is about **3–4 kg/cm²**, a value typical of all mammals.
- In the same age group, **males have a higher value** than females, the ratio being **1: 0.65.**
- The male hormone ***testosterone*** contributes to better development and growth of skeletal muscles.
- **Genetic make-up** plays a role.
- **Regular training** enhances muscle power.

APPLIED ASPECTS

Muscular Dystrophy PY3.13

Muscular dystrophy (MD) occurs due to **mutations in the genes** coding for dystrophin-glycoprotein complex.

Duchenne Muscular Dystrophy

This commonest MD, also called **pseudohypertrophic MD,** an *X-linked recessive disease.*
- Affects mostly male children.
- Characterized by **progressive muscular weakness** by age 4, and **hypertrophy** of affected muscles (mainly calf muscles, and pelvi-femoral muscles.
- Cardiomegaly is common
- Typically, the child uses his hands to climb up, while getting up from the floor.
- By age 12 they are no longer ambulatory, and death occurs by age 30.
- Disease occurs due to **absence of dystrophin** in the muscles, caused by mutations of the dystrophin gene.
- **Dystrophin gene** is a large gene, located in the **p21 region of the X chromosome**.

Baker's Muscular Dystrophy

Baker's muscular dystrophy (BMD) is a less severe and rare form MD.
- It is similar in presentation to Duchenne MD, but patients often survive into adulthood.
- In BMD patients, **dystrophin is reduced in amount or present in an abnormal form**.

Laminin 2 Mutation: In several forms of MD, **laminin 2,** a protein for connections between the exterior of muscle cells and the extracellular matrix, **is absent along with dystrophin**.

Myopathies

Mutations in the gene coding for the protein **desmin**, causes skeletal and cardiac myopathies.

Metabolic Myopathies: Metabolic myopathies occur due to **mutations in the genes coding for various enzymes**

involved in the metabolism of carbohydrates, proteins and fats.

- In these patients, muscle breakdown occurs due to accumulation of toxic metabolites.

Inflammatory Myopathy: Poliomyelitis is an inflammatory myopathy in which, *weakness of proximal limb muscles* is an early feature.

- It is due to **destruction of motor neurons** present in the anterior horn of spinal cord by the poliovirus resulting in paralysis of skeletal muscles.
- Death may occur due to respiratory failure.

Other Muscle Diseases

Myotonia

These are conditions where muscle relaxation is prolonged after voluntary contraction. They are due to **abnormal genes on chromosomes 7, 17 or 19** that lead to ***malfunction of Na^+ or Cl^- channels.***

Focal Dystonias

Dystonia means **faulty contraction**. When it is limited to a small and specific region of muscles, so it is called focal dystonia.

- These are **neuromuscular disorders** characterized by **involuntary and repetitive or sustained skeletal muscle contractions** that cause ***twisting, turning or squeezing movements*** in a body part.
- The common dystonias are: **spasmodic torticollis and cervical dystonia** that usually affect neck and shoulder muscles, **blepharospasm** that affects eyelid muscles, **strabismus and nystagmus** that affect extraocular muscles, **writer's cramp** that affect finger muscles.
- **Injection of botulinum toxin** into the affected muscles is a treatment of these disorders.

Muscle Sprain

Muscle sprain often occurs during sports activity or physical labor due to overstretching or forced extension of an active muscle.

- Very often the **myotendinous junction is injured** or at times there is separation of the fibers.
- **Treatment** includes ice packs, rest, immobility and analgesics.

Muscle Cramp

This is a painful condition due to **involuntary tetanic contraction of skeletal muscle**.

- It is caused by generation of **nerve action potentials at a very high rate.**
- Usually occurs in **electrolyte imbalances** in ECF surrounding both the muscle and nerve fibers due to **over-exercise or persistent dehydration.**

Exam Questions

1. Describe the properties of skeletal muscle. Add a note on rigor mortis.
2. Explain the property of length-tension relationship and load-velocity relationship in skeletal muscle and give their physiological significance.
3. Define oxygen debt and describe the mechanism and importance of oxygen debt. Add a note on energy sources in muscle.
4. What are the types of muscle fibers and list the differences between them?
5. Define motor unit. Explain the phenomenon of motor unit recruitment and size principle.

Multiple Choice Questions

1. **Compared to type II muscle fibers, type I muscle fibers have:**
   A. Low Ca++ -pumping capacity of sarcoplasmic reticulum
   B. Less mitochondria C. High glycogen content
   D. High myosin ATPase
2. **Which of the following leads to staircase phenomenon?**
   A. Increased Troponin level in the thin filaments
   B. Summation of contractions
   C. More calcium available in the sarcoplasm in subsequent contractions
   D. Subsequent depolarization opens greater number of rynodine receptos
3. **The muscle length at which it develops maximal isometric active tension is called:**
   A. Resting length B. Active length
   C. Maximum length D. Initial length
4. **The amount of tension actually generated by the cross-bridge movement of muscle is called:**
   A. Central Tension B. Passive tension
   C. Total tension D. Active tension
5. **Twitch of a single motor unit is called:**
   A. Tremor B. Myoclonic jerk C. Fasciculation D. Chorea
6. **The heat produced after the muscle is stimulated and before the contraction starts is known as:**
   A. Shortening heat B. Activation heat
   C. Resting heat D. Recovery heat
7. **All of the following factors can delay fatigue, EXCEPT:**
   A. Release of dopamine
   B. Elevated plasma K+ level
   C. Moderate rise in plasma glucose level
   D. Previous regular training of similar type of activity
8. **Which of the following statement is NOT true about muscle tetanus?**
   A. Critical frequency is more if twitch duration is less
   B. Summation of contractions occur at critical frequency and above
   C. Periods of incomplete relaxation produces clonus
   D. Tension developed is two times that of a single contraction

Answers

1. A 2. C 3. A 4. D 5. C 6. B
7. B 8. D

Chapter 23

Smooth Muscle

Learning Objectives

On completion of study of this chapter:

The student will be able to (must know):

1. Name the types of smooth muscle and give their structural specialities.
2. Describe the mechanism of smooth muscle contraction.
3. Appreciate the difference in smooth and skeletal muscle contraction.
4. List the properties of smooth muscle.
5. List the differences between skeletal, smooth and cardiac muscle.

The student may also be able to (desirable to know):

1. Describe the properties of smooth muscle and cardiac muscle.
2. Explain functional differences between skeletal, cardiac & smooth muscles.

Smooth muscles are mainly present in the visceral organs and blood vessels. The **distinctive features** in smooth muscles are:

1. **Absence of regular pattern of cross-striations** as found in skeletal and cardiac muscles, hence the name *smooth muscles*.
2. The **nerve supply** to smooth muscles is through the branches of **autonomic nervous system**.
3. The **length-tension relationship** is not linear as in skeletal and cardiac muscle.
4. Smooth muscles can **remain contracted for relatively longer periods** without expenditure of much energy, a property that endows them with a ***better metabolic economy***.

TYPES OF SMOOTH MUSCLES

In some organs, groups of smooth muscle fibers behave as ***syncytium***, like that of cardiac muscles and in few other organs they follow the functional properties of skeletal muscles. Based on this, they are classified into two types: **single-unit** smooth muscles, and **multiunit** smooth muscles.

Single-Unit Smooth Muscle

The muscle fibers in single-unit smooth muscles are connected to each other by **gap junctions**.

- The action potential spreads rapidly to all the fibers of the unit.
  - Therefore, contraction occurs simultaneously in all the fibers.
- Due to this **synchronous electrical and mechanical activity**, the fibers behave as a **syncytium** or a single unit.
- They form the **walls of hollow viscera** such as the gastrointestinal tract, ducts of digestive glands, the ureters and urinary bladder, the uterus and small diameter blood vessels.
- As they are present in many visceral organs, they are also called **visceral smooth muscles**.

Multiunit Smooth Muscle

Multiunit smooth muscles **do not have gap junctions**; therefore, they do not act as a syncytium.

- They resemble *skeletal muscles functionally* as they are largely under neural control, though not under voluntary control.
- They are abundantly innervated by the fibers of the autonomic nervous system.
- Examples are intrinsic muscles of the eye (ciliary body and iris), muscle in the large airways to the lungs, precapillary sphincters, and piloerector muscles.

Functional Organization

Types of arrangement of smooth muscle fibers are of **three types**:

1. **Circular:** Circular pattern of arrangement is seen in the **blood vessels, airways and sphincters**.

- **In vessels and airways,** contraction of the muscles ***narrows the diameter of the passage*** and reduces the flow.
- **In sphincters,** the contraction can *totally block the passage* and stop the flow.

2. **Circular and Longitudinal:** Circular and longitudinal organization is found in **GI tract**.
   - **Inner circular** muscle layer and **outer longitudinal** muscle layer regulate movements of intestine and promote the ***mixing and forward movement of the digested food***.
3. **Circular, Longitudinal and Oblique:** Circular, longitudinal and oblique arrangement is typically found in the **uterus and urinary bladder**.
   - When the increased contents of these viscera stretch these muscles, they contract and ***decrease the volume*** by expelling the contents.

PY3.7

STRUCTURE

The **special features** of smooth muscles are as follows:

1. The cells are quite **small in size** compared to the whole tissue.
   - The small size of cells is an advantage for smooth muscle for precisely controlling visceral functions.
2. Each smooth muscle fiber is a spindle-shaped cell, **100–300 µm long and 5–10 µm in diameter** at the middle (Fig. 23.1).
3. Smooth muscle cells contain a **single elongated nucleus** at the center and few mitochondria.
4. The cell ***derives energy*** mainly from **glycolytic pathway**.
5. The **sarcoplasmic reticulum is well developed** only in some types of smooth muscles; in others it is rudimentary.
6. Myofilaments are organized differently.
   - There are **no sarcomeres** and **striations are not visible** (Fig. 23.2).
6. There is **lack of an organized T tubular system**.
7. The cell membrane shows invaginations called **caveolae** that increase the surface area.

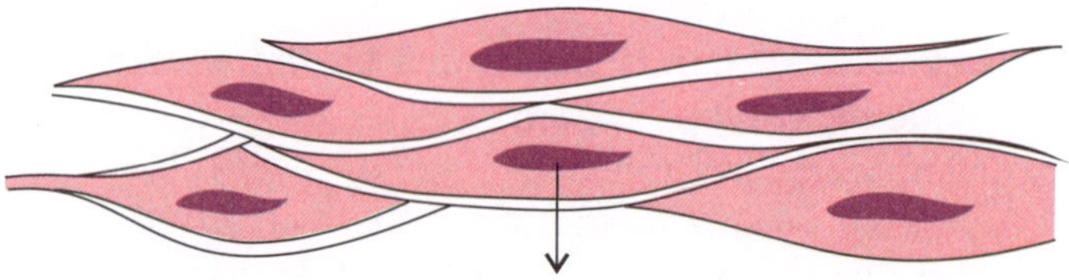

Fig. 23.1: Structure of smooth muscles. Note the spindle shaped nature of cells with single elongated centrally placed nucleus.

Myofilaments

The cytoplasm contains three types of myofilaments: **thick, thin, and intermediate**.

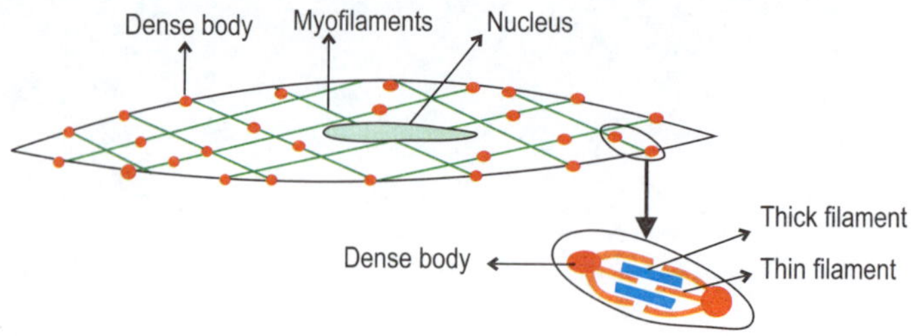

Fig. 23.2: Structure of smooth muscle cell.

In addition, the cytoplasm contains a calcium-binding protein called **calmodulin**, which is structurally related to troponin.

Thick Filaments

The thick filaments are about 2.2 µm long and composed of myosin molecules that are not arranged in a regular pattern around the axis of the filament as in the skeletal muscle.

- They are interspersed among the thin filaments (Fig. 23.2) and are much fewer than in skeletal or cardiac muscle.

Intermediate Filaments & Dense Bodies

The diameter of intermediate filaments is about 10 nm, which is present between that of the thick and thin filaments.

- Intermediate filaments **provide cytoskeletal support** and have negligible roles in contractile activity.

Dense Bodies: Small, electron-dense, dark areas called dense bodies are present throughout the cytoplasm, as well as attached to the cell membrane.

- Those associated with the cell membrane are often called membrane-associated dense bodies or patches, or **focal adhesions**.
- Dense bodies are functionally ***analogous to the Z lines*** in skeletal muscle fibers.

Thin Filaments

In smooth muscles, thin filaments are composed of **actin and tropomyosin** molecules, but *troponin protein complex is absent*.

Functional Organization of Filaments

The relationship between the thick and thin filaments is poor and they are less well organized.

1. Due to absence of an organized arrangement of contractile apparatus, the ***length tension relationship*** in the smooth muscles is **very much flexible**.
2. The **thick and thin filaments** are ***obliquely oriented*** to the long axis of the cell.
3. The **actin filaments anchor to the dense bodies** by means of the protein ***α-actinin***.
4. During the sliding-filament mechanism, the gap between the actin filaments reduces and the shortening force is transmitted through the dense bodies to the

plasma membrane producing contraction of the muscle fiber.

Organization of Muscle Fibers

The smooth muscle fibers are **organized in sheets** and the cells are connected to adjacent cells by short strands of connective tissue.

1. Most importantly, the cells are linked to each other by **gap junctions**, by which many cells are ***activated at a time by single action potential***.
2. With the help of the stroma and the gap junctions, the **mechanical as well as electrical activities of the cells are coupled**, so that contraction occurs in an integrated and coordinated fashion.

Innervations of Smooth Muscles

Smooth muscles exhibit a **spontaneous, slow wave rhythm**. Neural stimulation only modulates (increases or decreases) this basic pattern.

- Branches of the autonomic nervous system innervate the smooth muscles, most of which are supplied by **sympathetic** as well as **parasympathetic fibers**.
  1. In response to a nerve action potential, neurotransmitters are secreted from the **numerous varicosities** present along the axon, and then *diffuse to the adjacent tissues* (refer, Fig. 20. 3, Chapter 20).
  2. Since the release of neurotransmitters is not confined to the axon terminals, **specialized neuromuscular junctions are absent** in smooth muscles.
  3. Unlike the skeletal muscle, the **receptors for neurotransmitters are not gathered** at the neuromuscular junctions, they are scattered along the postsynaptic membrane.

ELECTRICAL PROPERTIES

Unlike the skeletal muscle where the stimulus arrives in the form of an all-or-none action potential, in smooth muscles the contraction may or may not be preceded by an action potential.

Characteristic Electrical Activities

When the stimulus is excitatory, the membrane potential decreases and it increases in response to an inhibitory stimulus.

- The **membrane potential** of visceral smooth muscles is variable (no fixed resting potential), ranging from **–30 mV to –70 mV** with an average of –50 mV.
- The visceral smooth muscle shows **spontaneous oscillations in a wave like pattern**.
  - Some of the oscillations lead to **action potentials** that may occur in the *rising or falling phase* of the wave.
- The **multiunit smooth muscles** *do not discharge spontaneously*; they also do not respond to stretch.
- Most of the visceral smooth muscles **generate action potentials inherently.**
  - Any stimulus acting on it only alters the rate and pattern of action potentials formed.
- The **shapes of action potentials** vary widely, which may be a **spike, or action potential** with a ***prolonged plateau, or multiple spikes***, superimposed on the membrane potential (Fig. 23.3). Other forms of spikes or action potentials of smooth muscle have been described in GI system.
- In some cells, in response to stimuli like hormones or mechanical stretch, the membrane potential shows a graded change that may culminate into an action potential.

Action Potential

PY3.8

The action potentials are generally of **low amplitude**, which is about 60 mV, and the duration is around 100 ms.

- ***The depolarization phase*** is caused by influx of calcium from ECF due to the opening of voltage-gated Ca^{2+} channels.
- Compared to the striated muscles, the **upstroke of actions potential is prolonged** in smooth muscles, because the ***Ca^{2+} channels take more time to open*** than the Na^{+} channels.
- The **repolarization phase** occurs ***due to closure of Ca^{2+} channels***, which occurs slowly.
  - Opening of voltage-gated K^{+} channels contributes towards the later part of repolarization.
- Action potentials are generally observed in visceral smooth muscles.
- Some smooth muscle cells contract without any change in membrane potential.

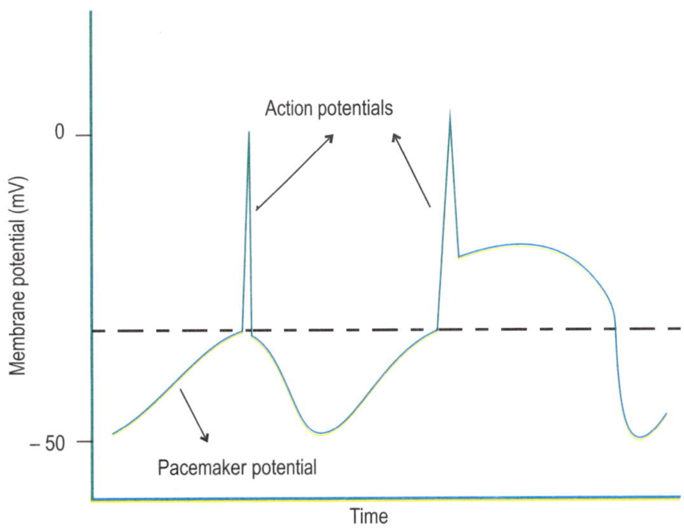

Fig. 23.3: Electrical activities (pacemaker potential and action potential) in smooth muscle.

Junctional Potential

Generally, action potentials are not observed in multiunit smooth muscles.

- Instead, in response to neurotransmitters like Ach, ***local depolarization*** called **junctional potential** is recorded.
- This **spreads electrotonically** along the muscle fiber and decreases the membrane potential **causing calcium influx** through the opening of **voltage-gated Ca^{2+} channels**, leading to contraction.

Pacemaker Potential

In addition to action potentials, pacemaker potentials are recorded in visceral smooth muscle.

- Unlike cardiac muscle, the pacemaker activity *is not generated at a fixed location*; rather it **shifts from place to place**.
- In visceral smooth muscles like intestine, pacemaker activities occur **at several sites** at the same time and then they **travel for a short distance** in the muscle.

MECHANISM OF CONTRACTION

Role of Calcium

PY3.9

As in other muscle types, changes in **sarcoplasmic calcium ion concentration** plays a major role in smooth muscle contraction.

- The cytosolic calcium concentration is increased mainly by **entry of calcium from the interstitial fluid** (**calcium influx**) or to some extent by its *release from cytoplasmic calcium stores* (**calcium release**).
- The cytosolic calcium concentration **decreases due to:** i) **binding of calcium to calmodulin**, ii) **pumping back** of calcium to the SR and, iii) **calcium efflux**.

Calcium Influx

Calcium influx occurs through voltage-gated Ca^{2+} channels, ligand-gated Ca^{2+} channels and a few leaky channels.

- The ECF calcium concentration is about 12000 times than that of the cytoplasm (1,200,000 nmol/L in ECF versus 100 nmol/L in cytoplasm).
- This high ***inwardly directed gradient*** favours calcium entry into the smooth muscle as soon as calcium channels open.

Calcium Release

Calcium release from the SR takes place by **two mechanisms**.

1. **IP_3-mediated pathway** activated by second messengers.
2. **Calcium-induced calcium release** (CICR) mechanism in which, some amount of calcium influx stimulates further calcium release from the SR.

Binding of Calcium to Calmodulin

Binding of calcium to calmodulin starts when cytoplasmic calcium concentration **is above 10^{-7} M** and is **completed at 10^{-4} M.**

Pumping Back of Calcium to the SR

Pumping back of calcium to SR is mediated via a **Ca^{2+} ATPase** present on the membrane of SR.

Calcium Efflux

Calcium effluxto the ECF occurs by **Na^{+}-Ca^{2+} antiport**, a process of secondary active transport and by **Ca^{2+}-ATPase**, both the mechanisms being present on the cell membrane.

Molecular Basis of Contraction

The following **step-wise processes** take place sequentially to culminate in muscle contraction.

1. Rise in cytosolic calcium mainly due to **calcium influx from ECF**.
2. Calcium **binds to calmodulin** and activates **myosin light-chain kinase** (MLCK).
   - **Calmodulin** is a small protein associated with MLCK, which is a *Ca^{2+}-calmodulin dependent protein kinase*.
   - When calmodulin binds with four calcium ions, *MLCK is activated.*
3. **Activated MLCK** utilizes one molecule of ATP and causes **phosphorylation of the myosin head** (*regulatory light chains* of myosin, on serine at position 19).
   - The phosphorylation process **activates myosin ATPase** enzyme present in the myosin head.
4. The activated myosin ATPase **hydrolyses one ATP molecule**.
   - As a result, the energized myosin head *(Myosin-ADP-Pi complex)* **binds with actin** producing the power stroke and pulls the thin filament towards the center of the thick filament.
   - **ADP and Pi are released** during this process.
   - Thus, **increased myosin ATPase** activity ***initiates the cross-bridge cycle*** and results in shortening due to the **sliding-filament mechanism**.
5. The **cross-bridge detaches** from actin when another ATP molecule attaches to myosin head *reducing its affinity for actin*.
   - Then, the myosin ATPase enzyme hydrolyses the ATP resulting in the attachment of myosin head with actin and the **next cross-bridge cycle** ensues.
6. Thus, the **cross-bridge cycle continues**, provided that the *myosin head remains phosphorylated*.
7. The cross-bridge cycle continues as long as the required cytoplasmic calcium concentration is maintained, because ***phosphorylation depends on cytosolic calcium level*** (Flowchart 23.1).

IMPORTANT NOTE

In skeletal muscles, contraction proceeds with activation of thin filament proteins **(actin-linked regulation)**, whereas in smooth muscles, the process of contraction is myosin based **(myosin-linked regulation)**.

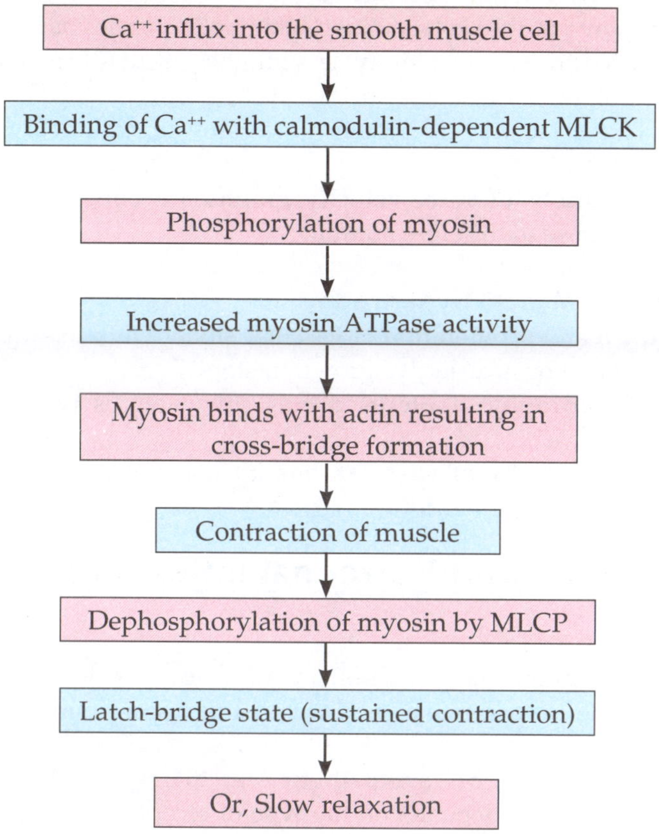

Flowchart 23.1: Major events of smooth muscle contraction and relaxation. MLCK: Myosin light-chain kinase; MLCP: Myosin light-chain phosphatase.

Mechanism of Relaxation

Relaxation is brought about by **dephosphorylation of myosin** light-chain by the enzyme **myosin light-chain phosphatase** (MLCP). This enzyme is constantly active during the periods of relaxation or contraction.

- During contraction, the rate of **MLCK-induced phosphorylation exceeds** the rate of MLCP-induced dephosphorylation and therefore, amount of **phosphorylated myosin increases in the cell**, which allows the contraction to proceed.
- When the cytoplasmic **calcium concentration decreases**, *calcium is detached from calmodulin* resulting in **decline in MLCK activity**.
- Consequently, the activity of MLCP predominates causing **dephosphorylation of myosin**;
  - the myosin ATPase enzyme ***remains inactive***, and **relaxation ensues**.

Thus, **phosphorylation and dephosphorylation** of the myosin light-chain is regulated by ***respective rise and fall of cytosolic calcium concentration***.

Types of Contraction

Unlike the skeletal muscles that demonstrate either twitch or tetanic contraction waves on stimulation, the smooth muscles exhibit phasic or tonic type of contraction.

Phasic Contraction: In phasic type, the degree of phosphorylation, the rate of cross-bridge cycle and the cytoplasmic calcium concentration **return to the resting value** following the phase of contraction.

Tonic Contraction: During tonic contraction, the above-mentioned parameters **do not return to the resting value**, rather they remain elevated above the baseline.

- However, their activity remains less than their peak activity, producing a **sustained tension** in the muscle at a lower level of MLCK phosphorylation that occurs with less expenditure of energy.
- This is possible due to the operation of **latch-bridge mechanism**.

Latch-Bridge Mechanism

Muscle in this state of sustained tension is known as the **latch-state**, in which dephosphorylation of attached cross-bridges occurs in an environment of elevated cytosolic calcium level.

- When MLCP-induced dephosphorylation of myosin light-chain takes place, it **does not bring about dissociation** of myosin from actin *until the cytoplasmic calcium concentration falls* below a critical level.
- This **attached cross-bridges** following dephosphorylation are known as the **latch-bridges** (Flowchart 23.1).
- In this process, the rate of cross-bridge cycle is decreased due to slower rate of detachment of cross-bridges.
  - That means the cross-bridges **spend more time in an attached state**.
- Therefore, the **ATP utilization is less**, which enables the visceral smooth muscles to have sustained contractions with less expenditure of energy.
- The force of this sustained contraction **can be graded** over a wide range because the cytosolic calcium concentration can be finely regulated over a wide range.

From the latch-state, the **relaxation of the muscle** occurs when the cytoplasmic **calcium concentration falls below 10^{-7} M.**

PROPERTIES OF SMOOTH MUSCLE

The properties of visceral smooth muscles may be divided into **3 categories** (Table 23.1):

Many electrical properties of smooth muscles are described above. Other important properties are discussed below.

Contractile Response

In response to a stimulus, the visceral smooth muscles show a **prolonged contraction** that has a slow initiation and the relaxation also takes longer time.

- The **latent period is 100–200 msec**; the **contraction period can be 200–500 msec** or even more.
- The relaxation period extends into few hundred milliseconds.

Table 23.1 | Properties of smooth muscle.

Properties
A. Morphological properties
1. Lack of striations
2. Absence of Troponin
3. Absence of T-tubules
4. Absence of well-developed neuromuscular junctions
B. Electrical properties
5. Presence of gap junctions (syncytial property)
6. Excitability
7. Variable RMP and shifting pacemakers
8. Variable action potentials
C. Mechanical properties
9. Tonus
10. Plasticity
11. Slow and prolonged contractile response
12. Length-tension relationship
13. Force-velocity relationship
14. Muscle hypertrophy

Muscle Tone

Visceral smooth muscles are continuously in a state of spontaneous irregular contraction known as **tonus**, which occurs due to generation of ***basic slow wave rhythm***.

- In blood vessels, especially the arterioles, this muscle tone helps to maintain the blood pressure without much expenditure of energy.
- The *multiunit smooth muscles* **do not exhibit** the inherent muscle tone.

Length-Tension Relationship

The length-tension relationship is variable in smooth muscles.

- When a smooth muscle is stretched, it **initially shortens** and exerts tension.
- If the stretch is maintained, gradually the tension decreases.
- If the stretch is increased, the tension may not rise proportionately or at a particular length, the tension may increase considerably.
- Thus the relationship is **highly inconsistent**.
- The ***adaptability*** of the smooth muscle *to the new length with less increase in tension* is known as **plasticity**, which is based on the latch-bridge phenomenon.

Stress Relaxation: In blood vessels, this feature is also known as stress relaxation that helps to maintain BP within the normal range in-spite of sudden rise in pressure.

Receptive Relaxation: In hollow viscera like stomach, large volume of food and fluid can be accommodated without an undue increase in internal pressure, called receptive relaxation.

Force-Velocity Relationship

Compared to the skeletal muscles, smooth muscles have a low myosin ATPase activity, less number of cross-bridges and a slower rate of cross-bridge cycling.

- These factors contribute to a **slower contraction velocity**.
- A **variety of force-velocity graphs** are obtained in response to different stimuli.

Smooth Muscle Hypertrophy

Growth and proliferation of vascular smooth muscles are stimulated by a variety of growth factors.

- **Hypertrophy of uterus** during pregnancy is typical example.
- **Hypertrophy of vascular smooth macules** occurs in chronic hypertension.

Neural and Hormonal Influences

Autonomic Control

The autonomic nervous system influences the intrinsic rhythmic or pacemaker activity of the visceral smooth muscles.

- The effect of **sympathetic or parasympathetic** stimulation depends on the type of receptor involved and the second messenger(s) released subsequently.
- For example, in GI system parasympathetic stimulation is excitatory and sympathetic is inhibitory, whereas the effects are opposite in blood vessel.

Hormonal Control

Nitric Oxide (NO): NO is released from the endothelial cells binds to the receptors present on the sarcolemma of vascular myocyte.

- The NO-receptor complex stimulates *guanylyl cyclase* and **forms cGMP**, which activates **cGMP-dependent protein kinase**.
- This protein kinase produces **relaxation of vascular smooth muscle** by: i) increasing calcium reuptake by SR, ii) opening of Ca^{2+}activated- K^+ channels and, iii) decreasing IP_3-induced Ca^{2+}release by inhibiting phospholipases C.

Other Hormones: **Angiotensin II** acting via AT II receptors, **vasopressin** and **endothelin** stimulate contraction of smooth muscles by releasing IP3. **Adenosine** causes relaxation by increasing the level of cAMP.

Cardiac Muscle

Muscles present in heart are **cardiac muscles**. Though they are structurally close to skeletal muscle they **demonstrate many properties of smooth muscles**. The details of cardiac muscles are described in Chapter 27,28, in CVS.

General features of cardiac muscles are:

1. Cardiac muscle is an **involuntary**, but **striated** muscle.
2. The fibres are branched and attached with each other closely.
3. **Intercalated discs** are present at the point of contact of two muscle fibres.
4. Numerous **gap junctions** are present in the intercalated disc that make cardiac tissue **functional syncytium**.
5. They show **well developed sarcoplasmic reticulum** with plenty of cytoplasm, **mitochondria** and rich in glycogen.

Salient features are depicted to differentiate it from skeletal muscles and smooth muscles (Table 23.2)

Differences Between Three Muscle Groups

Differences between skeletal, cardiac and smooth muscles are summarized (Table 23.2).

Table 23.2 | Differences between skeletal, cardiac and smooth muscles

	Skeletal muscle	Cardiac muscle	Smooth muscle
	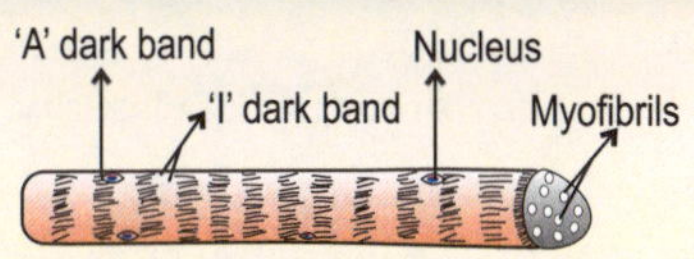	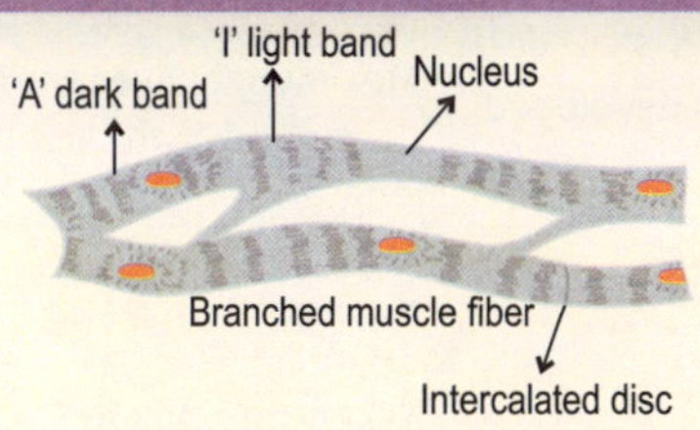	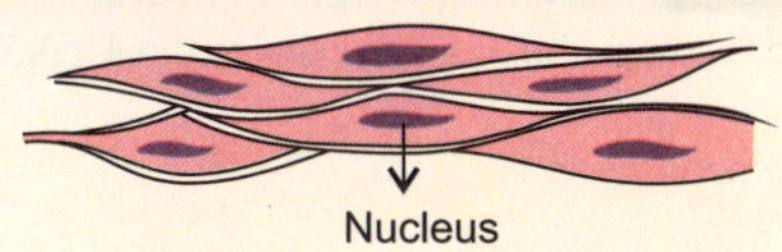
A. Morphological properties 1. Distribution	Fixed to bones, Form body muscle	Heart only, not attached to bone	(A) Single (visceral) unit smooth muscle in hollowed viscera eg: Intestine, Bronchi, Uterus, Ureters. (B) Multi unit smooth muscle in capillary muscle. Iris in eye, pilo-meter muscle of skin; muscle in blood vessels.
2. Striations	It has well developed striations, therefore, also called striated muscle	Also show cross striations	Lack cross striations, therefore also called 'plain' muscles.
3. Size and shape	Cylindrical, 1-40 mm Long, 50-100μm Diameter; multi--nucleated cells	Short, cylindrical, 100 μm long and 15 μm diameter; single nucleus; forms a branching network	Spindle (Elongated), single nucleus, variable sizes
4. Sarcoplasmic reticulum	Well developed	Well developed more than in the skeletal muscle.	Poorly developed
5. Syncytial structure	Non-syncytial	It is functionally syncytial in character.	Functionally syncytial in character
6. Sarcotubular system	Present;T system at A-I junction; terminal cistern prominent.	Present;T system at A-I junction; terminal cistern prominent.	Present, but not so characteristic
7. Nerve supply	By somatic nerves and by special nerve endings	Via two branches of ANS with ganglia and free nerve terminals.	Via two branches of ANS with ganglia and free nerve terminals.
8. Control and rhythmicity	Voluntary control, no rhythmicity	It contracts rhythmically and spontaneously in the absence of external innervation, by pacemaker drive	Rhythmicity: two types (i) regular and (ii) irregularly discharging pacemaker
9. Blood supply and oxygen consumption	840mL/min (3-4 mL 100 gm/min) with moderate oxygen consumption	Abundant, 250mL/min (80mL/100 gm/min) with high O_2 consumption	350mL/min (1.4 mL per 100 gm/min) with less O_2 consumption
B. Electrical Properties 10. RMP	-90mV	-90mV	-50mV (Range between -30mV to - 70mV), Fluctuating

11. Action potential (AP)	Rapid depolarization Spike duration is 2-4ms Total amplitude120mV, Conduction velocity 5mts/sec	rapid depolarization, 15 to 20mV produces, AP duration 250ms, Amplitude 100Mv, variable speed of conduction	Variable (rapid rise and fall in action potential). Total duration 50msec. Total amplitude upto 60 mV, variable speed of conduction.
C. Mechanical Properties 12. Mechanical events	Contraction starts 2 msec after the start of depolarization, before repolarization ends. Can summate the contractile response, Tetanization occurs	More than half of mechanical contraction is over during absolute refractory period. Tetanization does not occur.	Muscle starts to contract approximately 200 msec after the start of the spike (150msec after the spike is over). Peak contraction is reached approximately 500msec after the spike. Tetanus is seen.
13. Duration of muscle twitch	Varies with types of muscle fibres; 7.5 msec in fast muscles, 100msec in slow muscles.	One & half times the total duration of action potential.	Approximately 1,000msec
14. Excitation contraction coupling	Rapid process, time from initial depolarization to initiation of contraction is 10 msec.	More rapid process time (< 10msec)	Very slow process
15. All or none law	Applicable, true for single muscle fibre.	Applicable, true for whole of the atria or ventricles.	Applicable, true for single muscle fibre.
16.Length tension relationship	Maximum active tension is developed at the optimal length	Maximum active tension is developed at the optimal length	Shows property of plasticity.
17. Phenomenon of fatigue	Occurs	Not seen	Possible but difficult to demonstrate.
D. Metabolic Properties 18. Energy utilization	Under basal state 20% by fats. >60% from carbohydrates; 20% by proteins.	65% by fats, 25% by carbohydrates; and 10% by ketones bodies & amino acids.	Low, mainly provided by the carbohydrates & fats.

Exam Questions

1. Describe the mechanism of smooth muscle contraction.
2. Describe the properties of smooth muscle.
3. Explain the role of calcium in smooth muscle contraction and give a note on latch bridge mechanism.
4. List the differences between skeletal muscle, cardiac muscle and smooth muscle.

Multiple Choice Questions

1. **Which of the following is true in smooth muscle?**
   A. Cytoplasmic Ca^{++} concentration increases by entry of Ca++ from interstitial fluid
   B. The stimulus follows all-or-none law
   C. Depolarization is due to opening of voltage-gated Na+ channels
   D. Repolarization is mainly due to opening of voltage-gated K+ channels
2. **Smooth muscle contraction is regulated by:**
   A. Actin B. Myosin
   C. Troponin D. Tropomyosin
3. **Increase in cytoplasmic calcium during smooth muscle contraction is due to**
   A. Serine kinase B. cGMP
   C. cAMP D. IP3-DAG
4. **Compared to multiunit smooth muscles, the single unit smooth muscles:**
   A. Are less abundant B. Are absent in the walls of hollow viscera
   C. Have gap junctions D. Do not behave as a syncytium
5. **In smooth muscle contraction, calmodulin activates:**
   A. Myosin light-chain kinase B. Magnesium ATPase
   C. cGMP dependent kinase D. cAMP dependent kinase
6. **All of the following are present in smooth muscle, EXCEPT:**
   A. Calcium B. Actin C. Troponin D. Myosin
7. **The contraction in smooth muscle**
   A. Depends on cellular calcium stores
   B. Is initiated when myosin binding sites are uncovered by tropomyosin
   C. Is sustained with low cytoplasmic calcium concentration
   D. Is inhibited with dephosphorylation of myosin
8. **All of the following are true for visceral smooth muscles, EXCEPT:**
   A. Sarcoplasmic reticulum is poorly developed
   B. Show the property of plasticity
   C. Have twitch duration of 50 ms
   D. Have resting membrane potential of -50mV
9. **All of the following is absent in smooth muscles, EXCEPT:**
   A. Cross striations B. T-tubules
   C. Well-developed neuromuscular junctions D. Gap junctions
10. **In latch state of smooth muscles:**
    A. Phosphorylation of myosin light chain takes place
    B. Cross-bridges spend more time in an attached state
    C. ATP utilization is more
    D. Contraction cannot be graded

Answers

1. A 2. B 3. D 4. C 5. A 6. C
7. D 8. C 9. D 10. B

Section IV

Autonomic Nervous System

*Let us work as we pray.
For indeed work is the body's
best prayer to the Divine..*

The Mother
(of Sri Aurobindo Ashram)

Chapter 24

Functional Organization and Functions of Sympathetic and Parasympathetic Systems

Learning Objectives

On completion of study of this chapter:

The student will be able to (must know):

1. Comprehend the importance of autonomic neural regulation of body functions.
2. Understand the functional organization of ANS.
3. Identify the arrangement of pre- and post-ganglionic fibers of both divisions of ANS.
4. Name the sympathetic ganglia & appreciate segmental distribution of sympathetic fibers to visceral organs.
5. Understand the importance of basal sympathetic and parasympathetic tone.
6. Mention effects of sympathetic & parasympathetic stimulation to various organs & the receptors mediating the effects.
7. Describe the physiology of fight-or-flight response.

The student may also be able to (desirable to know):

1. Explain the differences between sympathetic & parasympathetic systems.
2. Appreciate the role of sympathovagal balance in achieving good health.

Autonomic nervous system (ANS) can be broadly categorized into five parts:

1. Maintenance of homeostatic conditions of the body.
2. Regulation of visceral functions.
3. Control body's responses to environmental changes.
4. Coordination of responses to exercise and stress.
5. Assisting the endocrine system to regulate systemic, metabolic and reproductive functions.

FUNCTIONAL ORGANIZATION

ANS is traditionally divided into two subdivisions: **sympathetic** and **parasympathetic**, based on their anatomic, functional and neurochemical properties. **Enteric nervous system** is considered to be the *third division* of ANS.

Sympathetic System

The cell bodies of sympathetic system are located in the thoracic and abdominal segments of the spinal cord and sympathetic ganglia are present as a chain close to the vertebral column.

This system is called the **thoracolumbar division of the ANS** (Fig. 24.1).

Parasympathetic System

1. The cell bodies of parasympathetic system are found in the brainstem cranial nerve nuclei (**cranial**

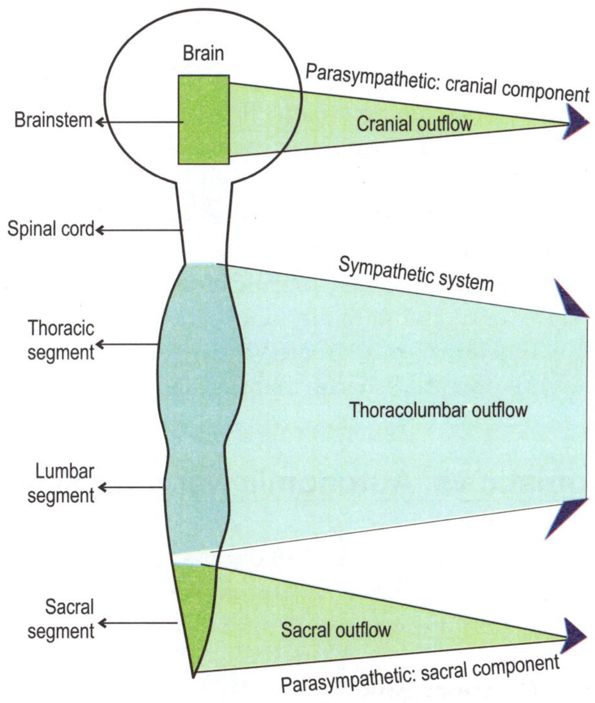

Fig. 24.1: General view of sympathetic (thoracolumbar) and parasympathetic (craniosacral) outflow of autonomic nervous system.

component), and in the most caudal part of the spinal cord (spinal or **sacral component**).

2. Hence, it is also termed as **craniosacral division of ANS.**

Enteric Nervous System

The enteric nervous system (ENS) is the local neural network in GI system which has strong anatomical and physiological link with ANS. Therefore, ENS is considered as the **third division of ANS**. It is concerned with the regulation of gastrointestinal functions.

Functional Characteristics

The sympathetic system is described as the *adrenergic system* for its adrenaline (or noradrenaline) like actions and parasympathetic system as the *cholinergic system* for its acetylcholine like actions. The important functional characteristics of these two systems are as follows:

1. The sympathetic division is primarily meant for **utilization of metabolic resources** and execution of **emergency responses** of the body, whereas the parasympathetic division helps in **restoration and build-up of the body's energy reserve**. Therefore, sympathetic system is **system of utilization** of energy and parasympathetic system is the system of storage of energy.
2. Almost all the organs are supplied by both sympathetic and parasympathetic nerves and usually they are **activated in a reciprocal fashion**. Therefore, when the discharge rate in one division is increased, the rate in the other division is decreased.
3. In some organs, sympathetic and parasympathetic systems work ***synergistically***. For example, to enhance gastrointestinal secretions, when parasympathetic stimulation increases volume and enzyme content, sympathetic activation contributes to increased mucus content of the secretory product.
4. Few structures such as systemic blood vessels and skin receive only sympathetic innervation and therefore, their functions are regulated by alteration in the rate of sympathetic discharge to these structures.

Somatic vs. Autonomic Nervous System

The nervous system contacts all organs and tissues of the body via the sensory system **(afferent innervation)**, motor system **(efferent innervation)** and the ANS.

Central Connections

1. The **efferent axons (lower motor neurons) of somatic system** originate from ventral horn of the spinal cord and innervate the skeletal muscle.
2. **In ANS**, efferent pathway consists of two or three-neuron tract with one or two synapses interposed between the center and the effector cells.
   - The cell bodies of autonomic motor neurons are located in the *intermediolateral horn of spinal cord* or in the specific *brainstem cranial nerve nuclei.*
   - The efferent fiber emerges from CNS as the **preganglionic axon** and then synapses with the cell bodies of neurons located in a peripheral ganglion.
   - The neuron from the ganglion then projects as **postganglionic axon** to the effector cells (usually a visceral organ).

Reflex Arc

The somatic nervous system collects information from the external environment, whereas the ANS collects information usually from inside the body, i. e. the changes in visceral structures.

Receptors

- Receptors are located in the body surface or in the musculoskeletal system in somatic system.
- In ANS, the receptors are present in the visceral structures.

Afferent Pathway

- The **afferent neurons of somatic system** enter spinal cord via dorsal root and terminate on interneurons in of dorsal horn or on motor neurons in the ventral horn.
- The **afferent neurons of ANS** enter spinal cord in a similar fashion, but they terminate on autonomic efferent neurons having their cell bodies in *intermediolateral horn* (ILH) of spinal cord.

Central Neurons

- **In somatic system,** cell body of a motor neuron is located in the ventral horn of the spinal cord. The afferent neuron may contact motor neuron directly or through interneurons.
- **In ANS,** the cell bodies of central neurons are located in ILH of spinal cord on which the afferent neuron directly terminates.

Efferent Neurons

- **In somatic system,** motor neurons originate from ventral horn and terminate directly on effector organ, which is usually a skeletal muscle.
- **In ANS,** there are two neurons between the CNS and the effector organ.
   - *The first efferent neuron* is the **pre-ganglionic neuron** that has cell body in the intermediolateral horn of spinal cord or in the cranial nerve nuclei in brain stem.
   - *The second efferent neuron* is the **post-ganglionic neuron** that has cell body in the ganglia outside the spinal cord (Fig. 24.2) or in the effector organ.

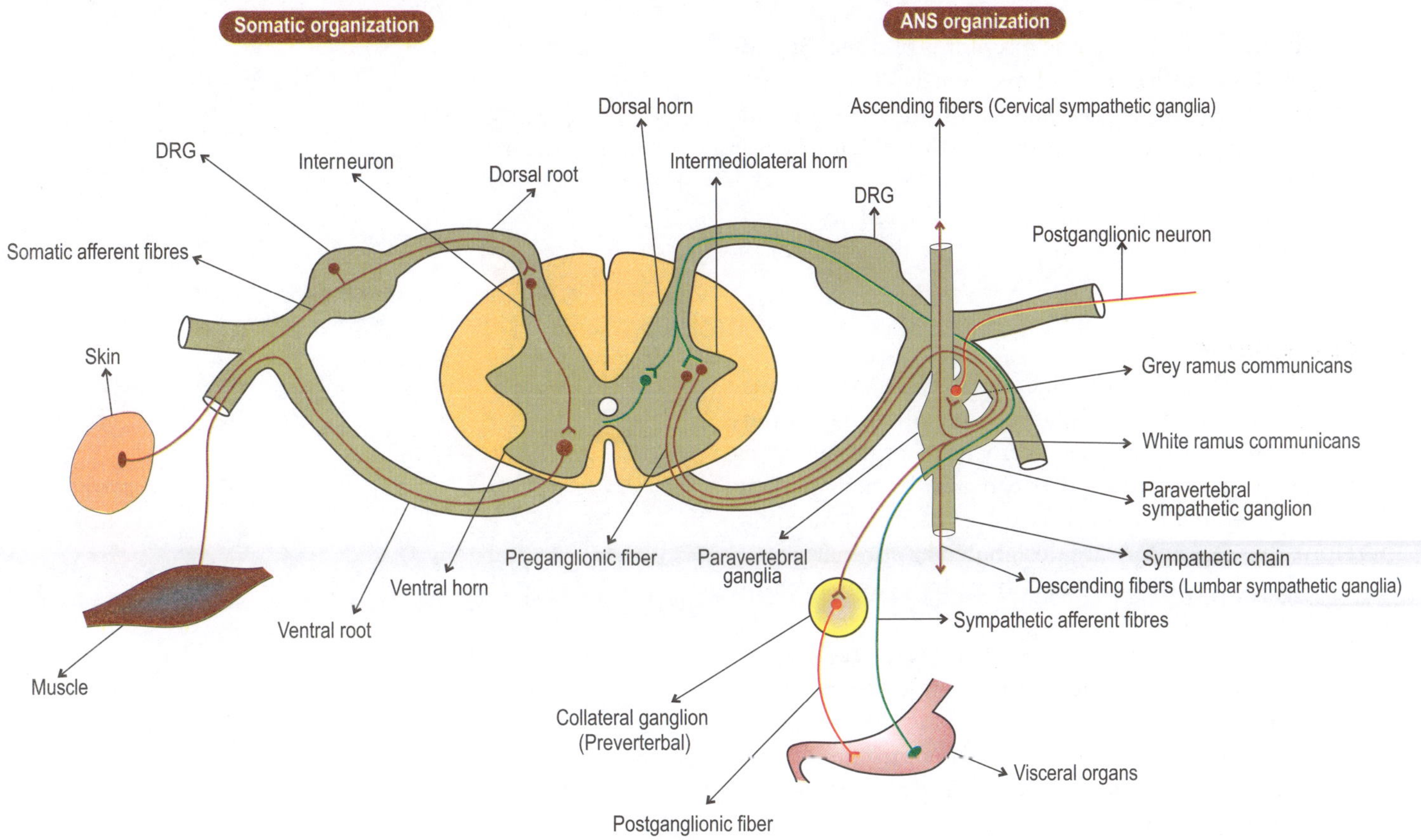

Fig. 24.2: Differences between segmental organization of somatic nervous system and ANS (mainly sympathetic component). DRG: dorsal root ganglion.

Effector Organs

Somatic motor nerves innervate skeletal muscles. The efferents ANS innervate are visceral organs.

NEUROTRANSMITTERS OF ANS

In ANS, postganglionic axons terminate in **varicosities**, the swellings enriched in synaptic vesicles that release the transmitter into the extracellular space surrounding the effector cells (refer Fig. 20.3, Chapter 20). The neurotransmitters in ANS are acetylcholine, noradrenaline and others. (Fig. 24.3)

Acetylcholine

Acetylcholine is the neurotransmitter at the following nerve terminals (**cholinergic fibers**) in ANS:

1. Preganglionic nerve terminals of both the sympathetic and the parasympathetic divisions.
2. All parasympathetic postganglionic neurons.
3. Postganglionic sympathetic neurons to sweat glands and blood vessels in skeletal muscle.

Cholinergic Receptors: The synapse at preganglionic nerve terminals utilizes **nicotinic receptors** similar to that found at neuromuscular junction. The synapse between the postganglionic neuron and the target tissues utilizes **muscarinic receptors** (Fig. 24.4).

1. The receptor classification is based on the response of the synapses to the alkaloids nicotine and muscarine at respective type of synapse.

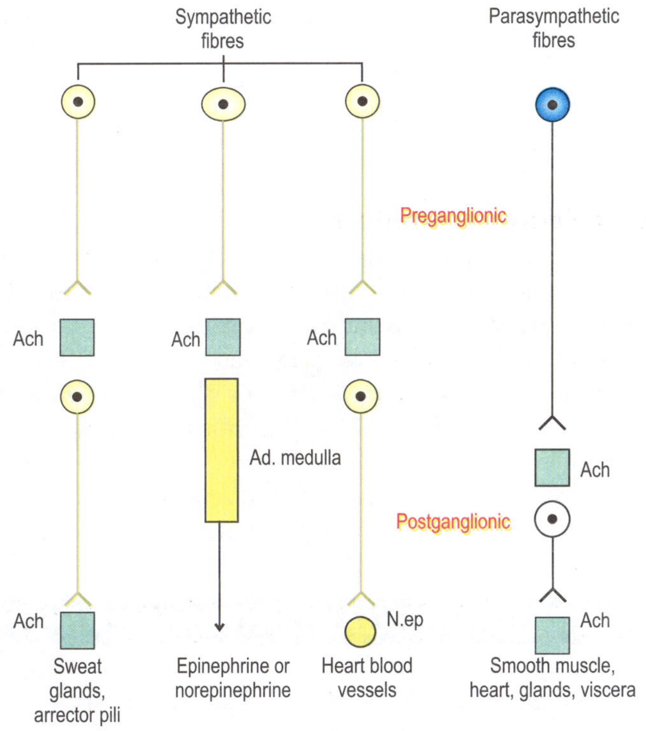

Fig. 24.3: The autonomic efferent fibers and neurotransmitters released by their terminals.

- The nicotinic receptor is blocked by *hexamethonium* in autonomic ganglion, in contrast to blockade by *curare* at neuromuscular junction.
- The muscarinic receptor is blocked by *atropine*.

- The nicotinic cholinergic receptor is of **direct ligand-gated type** as it contains ion channel in it.
- The muscarinic receptor is of **indirect ligand-gated type** as it uses a G protein to mediate effector functions.

2. The action of acetylcholine is terminated by *acetylcholinesterase*, the enzyme present at the cholinergic synapses.

Norepinephrine

Noradrenaline (NA) or norepinephrine is the neurotransmitter at postganglionic sympathetic nerve terminals (**adrenergic fibers**). NA released from adrenergic synapses utilize adrenergic receptors that can also be activated by adrenaline or epinephrine released from adrenal medulla. Therefore, these receptors are designated as adrenergic.

Adrenergic Receptors: These receptors are broadly classified into two types: α and β (Fig. 24.3).

1. **The α receptors** respond more to NA and less to epinephrine, and least to isoproterenol, the synthetic catecholamine.
2. **The β receptors** respond best to isoproterenol and epinephrine and less to NA. Propranolol is the antagonist for β receptors.

Subclassification: Each class of receptors is further classified as α_1 or α_2, and β_1, β_2 or β_3.

- The adrenergic receptors are of the **indirect ligand-gated type** as they utilize G protein for their effects.
- The α_1 **receptors** activate phospholipase C.
- The α_2 **receptors** inhibit adenylyl cyclase, whereas β ***receptors*** stimulate it.

Other Neurotransmitters

In ANS, especially in the intrinsic plexuses of the gut many amines, amino acids and active peptides are widely distributed as **co-neurotransmitters**. For example, ***neuropeptide Y*** is co-released by vasoconstrictor nerve, ***vasoactive intestinal polypeptide*** (VIP) and ***calcitonin-gene-related peptide*** (CGRP) are released along with cholinergic nerve terminals. ***Nitric oxide*** is another neurotransmitter produced by autonomic fibers. The term **non-adrenergic non-cholinergic** fibers apply to such nerves.

GENERAL ORGANIZATION OF ANS

Organization of ANS occurs at five different levels: cortical organization, hypothalamic organization, brain-stem organization, spinal organization and peripheral organization.

Cortical Organization

Cortical areas controlling functions of ANS are mainly **limbic areas and prefrontal cortex**.

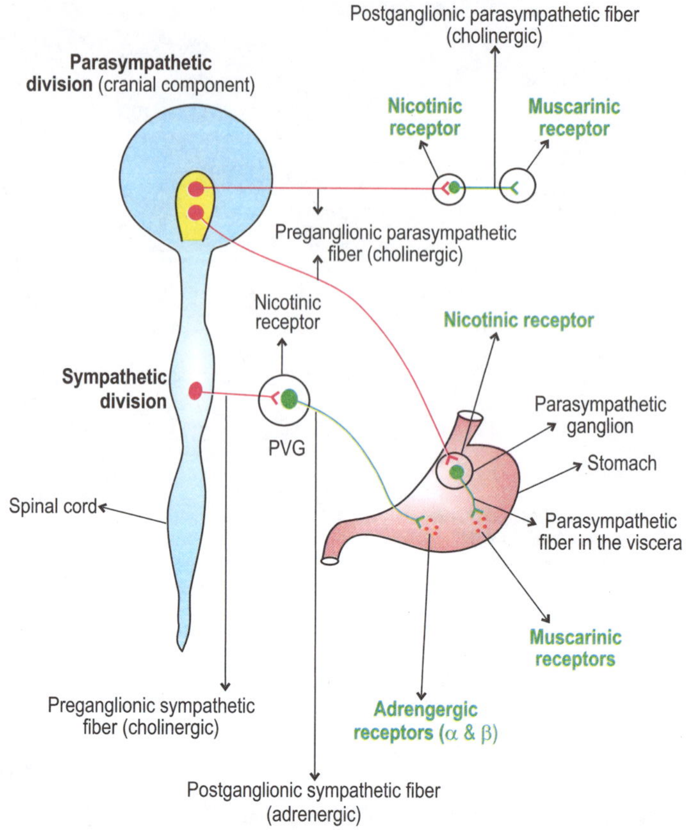

Fig. 24.4: Distribution of fibers (cholinergic and adrenergic) and receptors (nicotinic, muscarinic and adrenergic) in sympathetic and parasympathetic divisions of autonomic nervous system. PPG: pterygopalatine ganglion; LG: lacrimal gland; PVG: paravertebral ganglion of sympathetic trunk.

- The sympathetic responses to emotion originate in the limbic and prefrontal cortical areas.
- These areas *activate sympathetic system* by stimulating hypothalamic and brain-stem areas that have influence on the system.

Hypothalamic Organization

Hypothalamus considerably influences autonomic functions. Hypothalamus via hypothalamo-pituitary axis controls secretions of major endocrine glands.

- For its profound influence on autonomic responses, Sherrington had correctly pointed out that hypothalamus is the **head-ganglion** of sympathetic nervous system.

Brain stem Organization

Brain-stem areas contain major nuclei of ANS. These are broadly classified into two categories: parasympathetic nuclei and sympathetic nuclei.

Parasympathetic Nuclei: The **cranial outflow** of parasympathetic system originates from **cranial nerve nuclei** that are located in the brain-stem. The cranial nerves that carry parasympathetic fibers are oculomotor (III cranial nerve), facial (VII cranial nerve), glossopharyngeal (IX cranial nerve) and vagus (X cranial nerve).

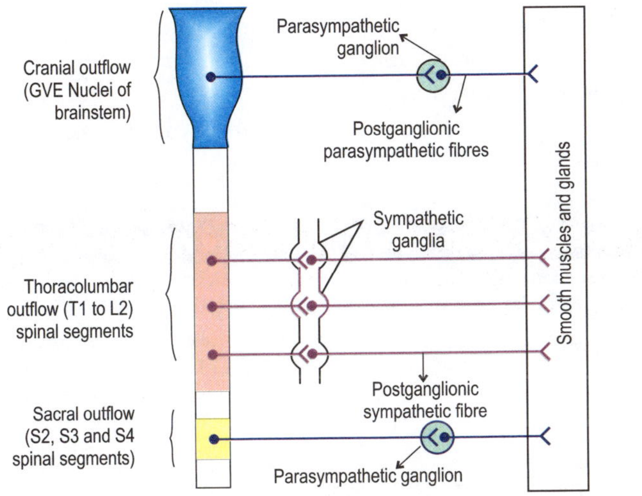

Fig. 24.5: Spinal and peripheral organization of parasympathetic (craniosacral outflow) and sympathetic (thoracolumbar outflow) systems. Note that the preganglionic fibers are smaller in sympathetic compared to parasympathetic system. GVE: General visceral efferent.

1. ***Nucleus tractus solitarius*** (NTS) in the medulla receives general visceral sensation via IX and X cranial nerves.
   - It is also closely connected with reticular formation containing cardio-respiratory centers. Therefore, NTS mediates respiratory and cardiovascular responses to autonomic activation.
   - Special visceral sensations in VII, IX and X cranial nerves reach NTS.
2. ***Edinger-Westphal nucleus*** in the midbrain is the nucleus of III cranial nerve.
3. ***Salivary nucleus*** is located in pons and ***dorsal motor nucleus of vagus*** in medulla.

Sympathetic Nuclei: Sympathetic fibers originate from ***vasomotor center*** in the medulla and project to the intermediolateral horn of spinal cord via bulbospinal pathway.
- Nucleus gigantocellularis and parvocellularis in the reticular formation on stimulation depress activity of vasomotor center.
- Stimulation of NTS inhibits sympathetic outflow and stimulates vagal activity.

Spinal and Peripheral Organization

Cell bodies of autonomic efferent neurons are located in the intermediolateral column of the spinal cord. Sympathetic (**thoracolumbar outflow**) and parasympathetic (**craniosacral outflow**) outputs of ANS and their ganglia are described below (Fig. 24.5).

SYMPATHETIC SYSTEM

Functional Anatomy

Preganglionic Neurons

Cell bodies of preganglionic neurons of the sympathetic division are located in the intermediolateral horn of the thoracic (T_1 to T_{12}) and upper lumbar (L_1 to L_3) segments of spinal cord. Hence, sympathetic division is known as **thoracolumbar outflow** of ANS.

- The preganglionic neurons come out of the spinal cord via ventral roots.
- After the merger of dorsal and ventral roots, spinal nerve emerges.
- Sympathetic preganglionic axons leave the spinal nerve via the white rami communicantes and enter the paravertebral sympathetic ganglia, which is an interconnected chain located on both sides of the vertebral column.

Preganglionic fibers have any of the following destinations (Fig. 24.2):

1. Preganglionic fibers emerging from spinal cord **synapse with cell bodies of postganglionic neuron located in the paravertebral sympathetic ganglion** at the same spinal cord level. The postganglionic sympathetic axons then travel in the cervical and lumbosacral spinal nerves. However, few fibers of sympathetic ganglion chain extend above and below the spinal level.
2. The chain of sympathetic ganglia **extends above and below** the thoracolumbar spinal levels, in which branches of preganglionic fibers ascend to the cervical levels or descend to the sacral level. Thus, preganglionic axons may synapse with postganglionic neurons in the paravertebral ganglion at the same level, or ascend up or descend down to the several spinal segments and then synapse with the postganglionic neuron.
   - **Preganglionic axons that ascend to cervical level** arise from T_1 to T_5 and form three major ganglia: superior, middle and inferior cervical ganglia.
   - **Preganglionic axons descend below L_3**, form two additional lumbar and at least four sacral ganglia. Preganglionic fibers ***synapse with postganglionic neurons in these sympathetic ganglia*** **that are present beyond the thoracolumbar segments** of spinal cord.
3. The preganglionic axons may pass through the paravertebral ganglia *en route* without synapsing there to terminate in a **pre-vertebral ganglion (collateral ganglion)**, which is located close to the organ (Fig. 24.2).

Postganglionic Neurons

1. Postganglionic neurons **for somatic structures** such as sweat glands, piloerector muscles, cutaneous blood vessels and blood vessels of skeletal muscles leave the paravertebral ganglion in the gray rami communicantes and reenter the spinal nerve to supply the target tissues.
2. Postganglionic neurons **to head, heart and lungs** originate in the cervical or upper thoracic paravertebral

ganglia and proceed to the organs as *separate nerves*, for example the cardiac nerve to the heart, or as *perivascular plexuses* of axons that accompany arteries.

In general, **in sympathetic system**, the preganglionic fibers are smaller than the postganglionic fibers (Application Box 24.1), whereas **in parasympathetic system**, the preganglionic fibers are much longer than the postganglionic fibers (Fig. 24.3 and Fig 24.4).

Sympathetic Ganglia

Sympathetic ganglia are of **three types**: paravertebral, prevertebral and terminal.

Paravertebral Ganglia

There are two paravertebral chains of ganglia on either side of the spinal cord. Each chain has 22 or 23 ganglia.

Cervical Ganglia: There are **three cervical ganglia**: superior, middle and inferior.

1. The **superior cervical ganglion** provides sympathetic fibers that innervate the structures in the head. These sympathetic fibers travel in the perivascular plexus along the carotid arteries and innervate radial muscle of the iris that causes dilation of the pupil, supply Muller's muscle that assists in elevating the eyelid, and innervate lacrimal and salivary glands. Therefore, diseases involving this pathway produce prominent ophthalmic signs.
2. The **middle and inferior cervical ganglia** innervate structures in the chest, including the trachea, esophagus, heart and lungs. Often, inferior cervical ganglion and first cervical ganglion fuse to form **stellate ganglion**.

> **Application Box 24.1**
>
> **Intrinsic cardiac adrenergic cells:** Evidences indicate that few postganglionic sympathetic neurons are embedded in the cardiac tissue like that of postganglionic neurons of parasympathetic systems that are usually located in the visceral organs. These neurons form intrinsic cardiac adrenergic cells (ICAC). Secretion from ICAC accounts for about 15% of adrenaline and noradrenaline content of the heart. It is believed that during fetal and early childhood, catecholamine content of ICAC plays an essential role in development of the heart.

Thoracic Ganglia: There are about 12 thoracic ganglia. Fibers from these ganglia supply mainly thoracic structures.

- Preganglionic fibers from T_1 and T_2 supply structures in head and neck,
- from T_3 and T_4 supply thoracic viscera,
- from T_5 to T_9 supply structures in upper limb, and
- from T_6 to T_{12} supply upper abdominal viscera (Table 24.1).

Lumbar and Sacral Ganglia: There are **three lumbar ganglia** for three lumbar segments. However, there are **two additional lumbar** and at least **four sacral ganglia** that are present below the lumbar segments.

- Preganglionic fibers from T_{10} to L_2 supply structures in lower limbs, and
- from L_1 and L_2 supply lower abdominal viscera (Table 24.1).

Table 24.1 | Segmental distribution of sympathetic fibers.

Preganglionic neurons from spinal segments	Structures innervated by postganglionic fibers
T_1 and T_2	Dilator pupillae, Muller's muscle, blood vessels and sweat glands of head & neck.
T_3 and T_4	Heart, esophagus, trachea, bronchi and lungs.
T_5 to T_9	Blood vessels and sweat glands of upper limbs.
T_6 to T_{12}	GI tract, liver, urinary tract, adrenal medulla & spleen.
T_{10} to L_2	Blood vessels and sweat glands of lower limbs.
L_1 and L_3	Bladder, uterus, fallopian tube, testes, vas deferens, seminal vesicle and prostate.

Prevertebral Ganglia

Postsynaptic neurons for the abdominal and pelvic visceral organs arise from the pre-vertebral ganglia. They are also called **collateral ganglia**. There are *three major prevertebral ganglia*: celiac, superior mesenteric and inferior mesenteric.

1. **Celiac ganglion:** The preganglionic axons for celiac ganglion originate in the T_5 to T_{12} spinal levels and provide innervation to the stomach, small intestine, liver, pancreas, gallbladder, spleen and kidneys.
2. **Superior mesenteric ganglion:** The preganglionic fibers for superior mesenteric ganglion originate primarily in T_{10} to T_{12} and innervate the small and large intestines (Fig. 24.6).
3. **Inferior mesenteric ganglion:** The preganglionic fibers for inferior mesenteric ganglion originate from L_1 to L_3 and innervate the lower part of colon, rectum, urinary bladder and reproductive organs.

Terminal Ganglia

These are located in the organ innervated by sympathetic fibers. Examples are adrenal medulla, heart, pancreas and urinary bladder.

Adrenal Medulla: Adrenal medulla is a neuroendocrine structure, innervated by *preganglionic sympathetic fibers* originating in the lower thoracic spinal segments that travel in lesser splanchnic nerve.

- It is considered as a **modified sympathetic ganglion,** as it contains postganglionic cells.
- Preganglionic fibers terminate on the **chromaffin cells** (modified ganglion cells), that synthesize epinephrine and norepinephrine.

Other Terminal Ganglia: Some of the cells in heart, pancreas and urinary bladder are modified postganglionic

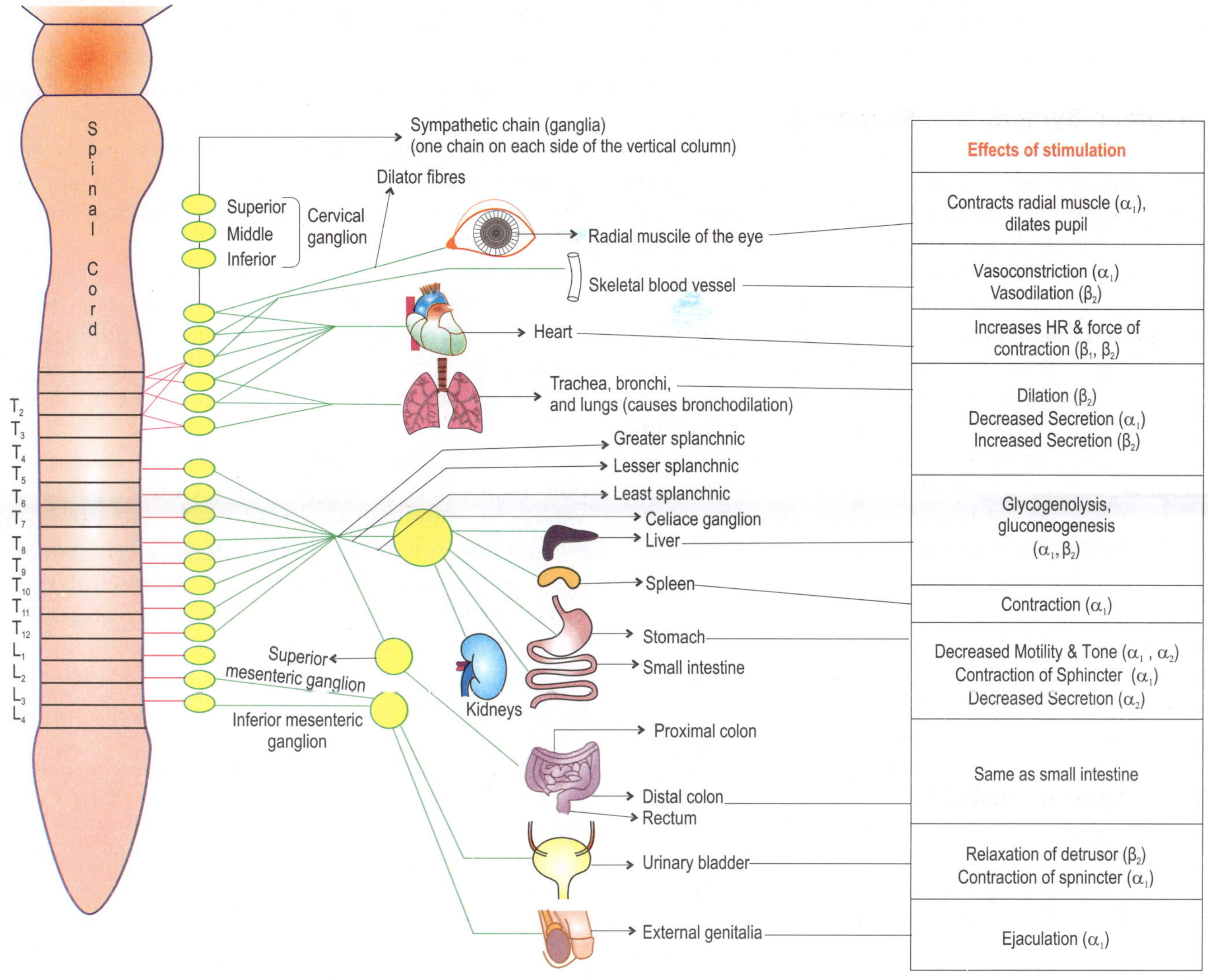

Fig. 24.6: Innervation of organs by sympathetic division of ANS. Note that preganglionic fibers are small and postganglionic fibers are long in sympathetic system.system.

cells. The postganglionic cells in heart (**intrinsic cardiac adrenergic cells**) influence development of heart during fetal life.

Neurotransmitters

All preganglionic fibers are cholinergic and sympathetic postganglionic fibers are **adrenergic** that secrete either **noradrenaline or adrenaline** (described above). However, there are few sets of **postganglionic sympathetic cholinergic fibers**.

- These are postganglionic sympathetic fibers *supplying sweat glands and blood vessels of skeletal muscles*.
- Evidences suggest that blood vessels of heart, lungs, kidney and uterus also receive some cholinergic innervation.

Sympathetic Responses

Sympathetic activities are broadly of **two types**: basal level activity at rest and widespread responses following activation.

Basal Sympathetic Activity

The sympathetic fibers have a basal rate of discharge at rest, called **basal sympathetic tone**.

1. The resting sympathetic tone influences many visceral functions. For example, normal blood pressure at rest is due to the basal rate of discharge in sympathetic fibers supplying blood vessels, which is also known as *vasoconstrictor tone*. Alteration in BP occurs mainly by changes in this sympathetic vasoconstrictor tone (Application Box 24.2). For example, to achieve a target increase in BP during exercise, sympathetic stimulation increases heart rate and myocardial contractility and intensifies vasoconstriction.
2. Profound decrease in BP following spinal cord transaction is due to decrease in vasoconstrictor tone.

Sympathetic Reactivity: Increase in sympathetic discharge in response to challenges imposed on the body such as orthostatic stress, hand-grip, immersion of hand in cold water etc. represent the reactivity of sympathetic system to various stimuli. This forms the basis of sympathetic function tests (described in next chapter).

Widespread Sympathetic Response

Another characteristic feature of sympathetic stimulation is that it produces **widespread organ responses**. Example of a widespread response is *fight or flight reaction* (see below). The widespread response to sympathetic activation is due to **two fundamental properties**: divergence of sympathetic outflow and activation of adrenal medulla.

Sympathetic Divergence: The number of postganglionic axons emerging from the paravertebral chain of ganglia is greater than the number of preganglionic neurons originating from the spinal cord, the **ratio of postganglionic to preganglionic neurons being 100:1**. Therefore, effector tissues innervated by sympathetic fibers are more.

- This basic *principle of divergence* enables the sympathetic system to produce widespread responses by simultaneously modulating functions of many effector organs.
- The divergence is due to branching of the preganglionic sympathetic axons in the paravertebral chain of ganglia that makes synaptic connections with multiple postganglionic neurons both above and below their original level of emergence from the spinal cord.

Role of Adrenal Medulla: The adrenal medulla, a *neuroendocrine gland*, is a **modified sympathetic ganglion**.

- The **chromaffin cells** of the adrenal medulla secrete epinephrine and norepinephrine directly into the bloodstream in response to activation by sympathetic preganglionic fibers and modulate many organ functions.
- Thus, adrenomedullary secretion by sympathetic activation forms the **physiological basis of divergence** for widespread sympathetic responses.
- Circulating epinephrine plays a bigger role in mediating widespread responses as its secretion is considerably more than that of norepinephrine.

Application Box 24.2

Sympathetic tone represents the stress level: The sympathetic tone primarily depends on the influence of vasomotor center (VMC) on ILH of spinal cord. VMC receives input from many areas of the brain including limbic system and hypothalamus. Hence, in stress vasomotor tone increases that in turn increases sympathetic tone. Therefore, relaxation of the mind ensures decrease in stress level and sympathetic tone of the individual.

Effects of Sympathetic Stimulation

Effects of sympathetic stimulation are summarized in Table 24.2. Effects are mediated by release of noradrenaline from sympathetic nerve endings and adrenaline and noradrenaline from adrenal medulla. Catecholamines elicit their effects by acting on **adrenergic receptors**.

Adrenergic receptors are broadly divided into **two types**: α and β.

- The α receptor has two subtypes: α_1 and α_2; and β receptor has three subtypes: β_1, β_2 and β_3.
- Generally, β receptors are more sensitive to adrenaline and α receptors to noradrenaline.

Effects of α_1 Stimulation: α_1 receptors are present in vascular smooth muscles of cutaneous and splanchnic circulation, sphincters of bladder and GI tract and radial muscles of iris.

- Stimulation of these receptors causes contraction or constriction of the structures in which they are present. They are equally sensitive to adrenaline and noradrenaline.
- The effects are mediated by formation of **intracellular IP_3**.

Effects of α_2 Stimulation: α_2 receptors are present in presynaptic nerve endings, wall of GI tract, platelets and adipocytes. Stimulation of these receptors often causes relaxation or inhibition of the structure. The effects are mediated by **decreased formation of intracellular cAMP**.

Effects of β_1 Stimulation: β_1 receptors are present in SA node, AV node and ventricular muscle.

- Stimulation of these receptors causes excitation of these structures. They are more sensitive to adrenaline than noradrenaline.
- The effects are mediated by increased formation of **intracellular cAMP**.

Effects of β_2 Stimulation: β_2 receptors are present in blood vessels of skeletal muscles, bronchial smooth muscles and wall of GI tract.

- Stimulation of these receptors causes relaxation of these structures. They are more sensitive to adrenaline than noradrenaline.
- The effects are mediated by change in the level of **intracellular cAMP**.

Effects of β_3 Stimulation: β_3 receptors are present in adipose tissues. Stimulation of these receptors causes lipolysis. The effect is mediated by increase in the level of **intracellular cAMP**.

Table 24.2 | Effects of sympathetic and parasympathetic stimulation

Effector organ	Sympathetic	Parasympathetic
Eye		
Dilator papillae	Contraction (α_1) (dilation of pupil)	–
Sphincter pupillae	–	Contraction (constriction of pupil)
Ciliary muscle	Relaxation (β_2)	Contraction
Muller's muscle	Contraction (α_1)	-
Glands		
Lacrimal gland	–	↑ secretion
Nasal glands	↓ secretion (α_1)	↑ secretion

Table 24.2: Contd....		
Salivary glands		
Secretion	Amylase secretion	↑ secretion
Blood vessel	Constriction (α_1, α_2)	Dilation
Heart		
SA node	↑ heart rate (β_1, β_2)	↓ heart rate
AV node	↑ conductivity (β_1, β_2)	↓ conductivity
Conduction paths	↑ conductivity (β_1, β_2)	↓ conductivity
Atria	↑ contractility (β_1, β_2)	↓ contractility
Ventricles	↑ contractility (β_1, β_2)	↓ contractility
Blood vessels		
Cutaneous	Constriction (α_1)	No supply
Skeletal muscle	Dilation (β_2) Constriction (α)	No supply
Visceral	Constriction (α_1)	No supply
Coronary	Dilation (β_2) Constriction (α_1, α_2)	Dilation
Cerebral	Constriction (α_1)	Dilation
Pulmonary	Constriction (α_1) Dilation (β_2)	Dilation
Renal	Constriction (α_1, α_2) Dilation (β_1, β_2)	No supply
Systemic veins	Constriction (α_1, α_2) Dilation (β_2)	No supply
Lungs		
Bronchioles	Dilation (β_2)	Constriction
Glands	↑ secretion (β_2) ↓ secretion (α_1)	
Skin		
Sweat glands	Less secretion	↑ secretion
Pilomotor muscle	Contraction (α_1)	No supply
GI tract		
Motility and tone	Decrease (α_1, β_1, β_2)	Increase
Sphincter	Contraction (α_1)	Relaxation
Secretion	Inhibition (α_2)	Stimulation
Gall bladder	Relaxation (β_2)	Contraction
Liver	Glycogenolysis and gluconeogenesis (α_1, β_2)	–
Pancreas		
Islets	↓ secretion (α_2) ↑ secretion (β_2)	↑ secretion
Acini	↓ secretion	↑ secretion
Adrenal medulla		
Secretion	↑ secretion of Epinephrine & NE	–
Urinary system		
Detrusor muscle	Relaxation (β_2)	Contraction
Trigone-Sphincter	Contraction (α_1)	Relaxation
Ureter	Contraction (α_1)	Relaxation
Other structures		
Male sex organ	Ejaculation (α_1)	Erection
Uterus	Contraction (α_1) Relaxation (β_2)	Variable
Adipose tissue	Lipolysis (α_1, β_1, β_2)	None
Pineal gland	↑ melatonin secretion (β)	None
JG cells	↑ renin secretion (β_1)	None

Fight-or-Flight Response

The fight-or-flight response is a typical widespread response of sympathetic activation. This occurs in critical situations of life when one has to either fight the situation or flee from the situation. Though many components of the responses are due to direct effects of sympathetic stimulation, secretion of catecholamine from adrenal medulla contributes considerably. The effects are as follows:

1. **Sympathetic stimulation of CVS** *increases blood pressure* due to increased cardiac output and vasoconstriction. Also, *redistribution of the blood flow* occurs to skeletal muscles and heart from splanchnic and cutaneous territories so that ***performance enhances***.
2. In lungs**, increased exchange of blood gases** occurs due to *stimulation of the respiratory rate and dilation of bronchiolar tree*. This **increases supply of oxygen** to the tissues.
3. Sympathetic stimulation to salivary gland **decreases salivary secretion**. However, *secretion of mucus increases proportionately*, permitting lubrication of the mouth despite increased ventilation and reduced salivation.
4. **Supply of metabolic substrates increases**, which is an essential component of effective stress reaction. The demand for increased supply of substrates like glucose and fatty acids is met by the actions of circulating epinephrine on hepatocytes and adipocytes. **Glycogenolysis** increases plasma glucose concentration and **lipolysis** promotes plasma free fatty acid level.
5. **Sympathetic stimulation to sweat glands** causes *secretion of a watery fluid*, and *evaporation of body heat*. **Cutaneous vasoconstriction** with concurrent sweat gland activation causes *cold, clammy skin* of a frightened individual.
6. **Activation of piloerector muscles** of hair follicles causes hair-standing-on the skin. The hair erection

helps in *preservation of body temperature* or gives a *ferocious appearance* to threaten the enemy.
7. **Pupillary dilation** *enhances visual acuity* and perception to make the individual environmentally maximal alert.
8. **Stimulation of brainstem reticular system** makes the individual maximally alert and mentally conscious to take appropriate decisions in quick successions.
9. Activity of **bowel and bladder** *temporarily ceases* due to constriction of sphincters.

PARASYMPATHETIC SYSTEM

The parasympathetic system is the **craniosacral outflow** of ANS.

1. In contrast to the stimulation of sympathetic system that causes widespread responses, parasympathetic activation causes **localized responses** and the divergence is minimal (Table 24.3).
2. This is because the **divergence ratio** of the presynaptic output to postsynaptic output is about 1:15, in contrast to 1:100 in sympathetic system.
3. Also, there is no circulating hormonal mechanism to aid to the divergence of parasympathetic activation.

Table 24.3 | Differences between functional organization of sympathetic and parasympathetic systems

Feature	Sympathetic system	Parasympathetic system
Origin	Thoracolumbar outflow (cell bodies of of preganglionic fibers are located in IML horn of thoracic and lumbar segments of spinal cord).	Craniosacral outflow (cell bodies preganglionic fibers are located in brainstem cranial nerve nuclei and sacral segments of spinal cord).
Preganglionic fibers	Short and cholinergic	Long and cholinergic
Ganglia	Located close to spinal cord, forms chain of paravertebral ganglia.	Located close to the target organ or in the organ
Postganglionic fibers	Long, unmyelinated and adrenergic	Short, myelinated and cholinergic
Ratio of pre to postganglionic fibers	1:100	1:1 to 1:15
Organs innervated	Almost all organs of the body	Mainly visceral organs
Responses	Widespread	Localized
Impact on body energy	Utilizes energy	Restores energy

Functional Anatomy

Parasympathetic ganglia are located either close to the organ or embedded in the organ. Therefore, preganglionic neurons are much longer than postganglionic neurons.

Cranial Component

Cell bodies of preganglionic neurons are located in the brainstem. Hence, this component is also called **brainstem parasympathetic division.**

- Brainstem parasympathetic neurons innervate structures in the head, neck, thorax and abdomen.
- Parasympathetic axons from brainstem travel in III, VII, IX, and X cranial nerves.
- Nuclei of these cranial nerves are present in the tectum in midbrain, pons and medulla.

Cranial Nerve III: The **oculomotor nerve** originates from tectum of the midbrain.

1. The cell bodies are located in the **Edinger-Westphal nucleus**. The preganglionic axons terminate on the cell bodies of postganglionic neuron in **ciliary ganglion** (Fig. 24.7).
2. The postganglionic axons enter eyeball near the optic nerve and innervate *sphincter pupillae* that control the diameter of the pupil, the *ciliary muscle* that focuses the lens for accommodation for near vision and the *choroidal blood vessels*.
3. Optic nerve projects to tectum and provides input for ocular reflexes.

Cranial Nerve VII: The preganglionic fibers in facial nerve emerge from the **superior salivary nuclei** in the rostral medulla and then pass from the facial nerve into the greater superficial petrosal nerve to synapse in the **pterygopalatine ganglion** (Fig. 24.7).

1. The postganglionic fibers innervate the *lacrimal gland and the glands of nasal and palatal mucosa*.
2. Another set of preganglionic fibers in the facial nerve travel via the chorda tympani nerve to synapse in the **submandibular ganglion**.
3. These postganglionic fibers from submandibular ganglion innervate *submandibular and sublingual glands*. Stimulation of this nerve **increases saliva production**.

Cranial Nerve IX: The glossopharyngeal nerve originates form the **inferior salivary nuclei** in the medulla. The preganglionic fibers terminate in **otic ganglion.**

1. The postganglionic axons join the auriculotemporal branch of 5th cranial nerve to innervate parotid gland, where they *facilitate secretion of saliva.*
2. **Chemosensory information** of blood gasses from carotid bodies and **baroreceptor information** of blood pressure from carotid sinus are transmitted to the medullary cardiovascular centers via glossopharyngeal afferents.

Cranial Nerve X: Vagus nerve arises from the **nucleus ambiguous** and **dorsal motor nucleus of vagus** in the medulla. Vagus nerve comprises up to *75% of total parasympathetic activity*.

1. **Preganglionic fibers** travel in the vagus nerve to ganglia located in the organ, i. e., in the heart and lungs and in the intrinsic plexuses of the GI tract.
2. Sympathetic **postganglionic fibers** intermingle and travel in the same nerve trunk with the parasympathetic preganglionic fibers to the target tissues. This forms the **vagosympathetic trunk**.
3. The **right vagus nerve** has more influence on SA node and left vagus on AV node. Thus, vagal stimulation **slows the heart rate**.
4. The vagal efferents to lungs cause **bronchoconstriction** and increase bronchial secretion.
5. Vagal fibers innervate esophagus, stomach, small intestine and large intestine upto two-third of transverse colon. On GI tract, vagus nerve **stimulates motility and secretory functions**. Acetylcholine and VIP are the transmitters of the postganglionic neurons.
6. There are vagal innervations of kidneys, liver, spleen and pancreas.

Sacral Component

Sacral parasympathetic neurons innervate structures in the pelvis.

1. **Preganglionic fibers** originate in the intermediolateral gray column of the sacral segments S_2, S_3, and S_4 of spinal cord.
2. The preganglionic fibers terminate in ganglia in or near the viscera that include descending colon, sigmoid colon, rectum, internal anal sphincter, urinary bladder and the reproductive organs (Fig. 24.7).

Parasympathetic Functions

Parasympathetic system **restores body's energy reserve.** Favourable conditions in both external and internal environments herald parasympathetic activation.

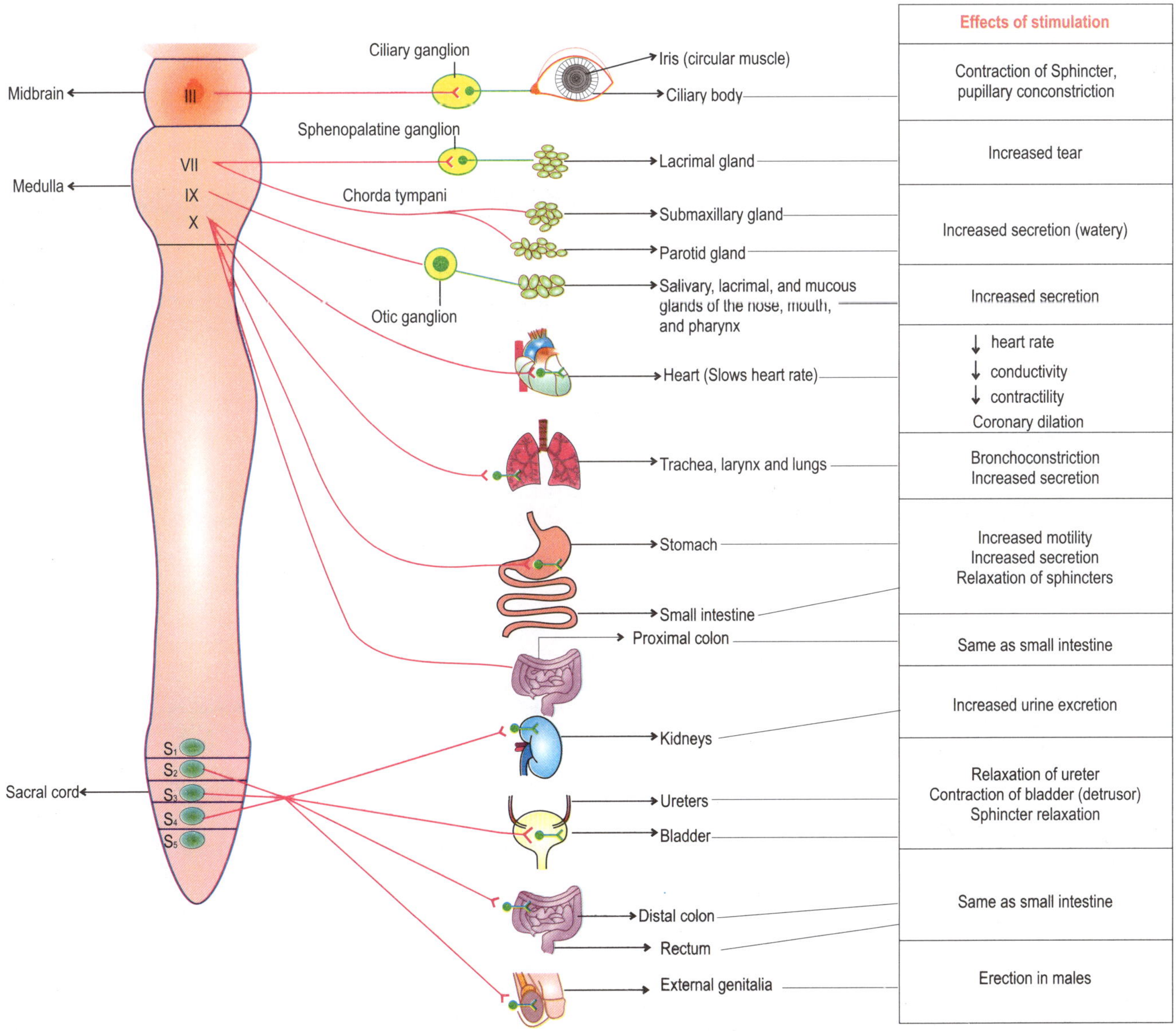

Fig. 24.7: Innervation of organs by parasympathetic division of ANS. Note that preganglionic fibers are longer in parasympathetic system. The post ganglionic fibers are much smaller, either close to the organ or located in the organ.

1. Except on cardiovascular system, most parasympathetic effects are stimulatory, especially for the processes that facilitate energy storage and physical growth (Clinical Box 24.1).
2. They stimulate intestinal motility, secretion, digestion and absorption.
3. They promote reproductive functions.

Neurotransmitters and Receptors

Most of the **parasympathetic fibers are cholinergic.** Acetylcholine is the neurotransmitter in both pre- and postganglionic fibers. The cholinergic receptors are muscarinic and nicotinic.

Muscarinic Receptors: Cholinergic muscarinic receptors are present in **heart, smooth muscles and glands**. These receptors are activated by acetylcholine and muscarine.

1. Activation of these receptors produce *inhibitory effects on heart*, for example, decreased heart rate, and *excitatory effects on smooth muscle and glands*, for example, increased GI motility and secretion etc.
2. Effects are mediated by **decreased cAMP formation** in the cytosol of cardiac cells and **direct opening of K^+ channels** in nodal tissues of heart.
3. In smooth muscles and glandular tissues, effects are mediated by **intracellular IP_3 and Ca^{++}**.
4. Muscarinic receptors are **blocked by atropine**.

Nicotinic Receptors: Cholinergic nicotinic receptors are present in **autonomic ganglia** (both sympathetic and parasympathetic), **neuromuscular junctions** and **adrenal medulla**. These receptors are activated by acetylcholine and nicotine.

1. Activation of these receptors produces *excitatory effects* on target tissue.
2. Effects are mediated by **direct binding of acetylcholine to α subunits** of the receptors.
3. Receptors also contain Na^+ and K^+ channels.
4. Nicotinic effects are **blocked by ganglion blockers** such as hexamethonium that prevent action of acetylcholine in the ganglia and at neuromuscular junction by curare drugs.

SYMPATHOVAGAL BALANCE

As discussed before, sympathetic activation causes energy expenditure and parasympathetic activation restores energy. Therefore, people with hyper-sympathetic behavior are mostly anxious, restless, do not deposit fat and are more sensitive to stress. Individuals with hyper-parasympathetic temperament are mostly lazy, sluggish and develop obesity. Therefore, a balanced sympathetic and parasympathetic state i.e., a **stable sympathovagal balance** is required to attain energy homeostasis and to preserve good health (Clinical Box 24.2).

Clinical Box 24.2

Sympathovagal imbalance (SVI) is the major cause of metabolic syndrome: Energy dyshomeostasis resulting from SVI is the major cause of obesity, diabetes, hypertension and heart diseases. Stress is the common contributor to SVI. Therefore, regular practice of yoga is advised to attain sympathovagal homeostasis.

Exam Questions

1. With the help of schematic diagram, depict the innervation of organs by sympathetic nervous system and briefly describe sympathetic functions.
2. With the help of schematic diagram, depict the innervation of organs by parasympathetic nervous system and briefly describe parasympathetic functions.
3. List the major differences between sympathetic and parasympathetic functions of cardiovascular, gastrointestinal, endocrine and reproductive systems.
4. Describe the fight and flight response.
5. Briefly explain the importance of sympathovagal balance and imbalance

Multiple Choice Questions

1. **Which of the following is true about ANS?**
   A. Higher center of integration is medulla oblongata
   B. Preganglionic fibers of parasympathetic system is loner than postganglionic fibers
   C. Ratio of preganglionic to postganglionic fiber id 20:1
   D. Conduction velocity in autonomic fibers is same as somatic fibers.
2. **Which of the following is true about parasympathetic system?**
   A. Postganglionic fibers are close to the viscera
   B. Parasympathetic ganglia are located close the organ or in the organ
   C. Intrinsic cardiac adrenergic cells in the heart are postganglionic cells.
   D. Nuclei of cranial part of parasympathetic system reside in vasomotor center in medulla.
3. **Which of the following is not a parasympathetic nucleus?**
   A. Edinger Westphal nucleus
   B. Nucleus Tractus Solitarius
   C. Nucleus gigantocellularis in vasomotor center
   D. Nucleus ambiguous
4. **Which of the following is NOT a co-transmitter in ANS?**
   A. VIP
   B. CGRP
   C. GABA
   D. Neuropeptide-Y
5. **Sympathetic outflow from spinal cord is from:**
   A. T1 – L3 B. C3 – L1
   C. T5 – L1 D. C5 – L1

6. Which of the following is not a ganglion of sympathetic system?
   A. Stellate ganglion
   B. Ciliary ganglion
   C. Celiac ganglion
   D. Superior mesenteric ganglion
7. Which of the following is not true about sympathetic system?
   A. Preganglionic fibers are longer than postganglionic fibers
   B. Preganglionic to postganglionic fiber ratio is about 1: 100
   C. Preganglionic fibers can ascend or descend down several spinal segments to synapse with postganglionic neurons
   D. Preganglionic fiber can pass through paravertebral ganglia without synapsing there to terminate in a prevertebral ganglion (collateral ganglion) located close to the organ.
8. Sympathetic fibers to heart, lungs, esophagus, trachea and bronchi originate from spinal cord segments:
   A. T1 and T2
   B. T 3 and T4
   C. T5 and T9
   D. T6 to T12
9. Which of the following is not true of adrenal medulla?
   A. It is a modified sympathetic ganglion
   B. Preganglionic sympathetic fibers terminate on chromaffin cells
   C. Preganglionic fibers to adrenal medulla originate in lower thoracic spinal segments that travel in lesser splanchnic nerve
   D. Chromaffin cells secrete more norepinephrine than epinephrine
10. Which of the following is the cause of widespread response in sympathetic stimulation?
   A. Ratio of sympathetic postganglionic to preganglionic fibers is 100:1
   B. Secretion of catecholamines from adrenal medulla
   C. Both A and B
   D. Basal sympathetic tone is more than parasympathetic tone
11. Postganglionic fibers are longer in:
   A. Sympathetic system
   B. Parasympathetic system
   C. It is of same length in both sympathetic and parasympathetic systems
   D. Enteric nervous system
12. All are effects of sympathetic stimulation EXCEPT:
   A. Increased conduction velocity
   B. Increased heart rate
   C. Increased refractory period of cardiac muscle action potential
   D. Increased contractility of cardiac muscle
13. During fight or fight response, which of the following is responsible for increase in local muscle blood flow?
   A. Sympathetic mediated cholinergic vasodilation
   B. Release of local vasodilators in muscle
   C. Release of vasodilators such as histamine from endocrine glands
   D. Activation of parasympathetic fibers that have cholinergic vasodilation effects
14. Sympathetic stimulation increases blood flow to all EXCEPT:
   A. Cutaneous circulation B. Coronary circulation
   C. Cerebral circulation D. Renal circulation
15. Stimulation of postganglionic sympathetic neurons leads to all EXCEPT:
   A. Fast EPSP
   B. Slow EPSP
   C. Fast IPSP
   D. Slow IPSP
16. Sympathetic nerve fibers innervating sweat gland release:
   A. Noradrenaline
   B. Adrenaline
   C. Acetylcholine
   D. Dopamine
17. Which of the following is NOT part of fight or flight response?
   A. Decreased bowel and bladder functions
   B. Decreased salivary secretion
   C. Stimulation of brainstem reticular activating system
   D. Cutaneous vasodilation
18. Parasympathetic outflow is from which segments of spinal cord?
   A. C2-4
   B. T2-4
   C. L2-4
   D. S2-4
19. Preganglionic fibers are longer in:
   A. Parasympathetic system
   B. Sympathetic system
   C. Same length in both sympathetic and parasympathetic
   D. Variable in both
20. Which of the following is not a direct effect of acetylcholine?
   A. Decrease in BP
   B. Increase contraction of heart
   C. Decrease in HR
   D. Decrease in conduction
21. Which of the following is not a nucleus of parasympathetic (cranial) nerve?
   A. Edinger-Westphal nucleus
   B. Superior salivary nucleus
   C. Inferior salivary nucleus
   D. Dorsal respiratory nucleus
22. Stimulation of vagus nerve results in all EXCEPT:
   A. Bronchoconstriction
   B. Increased motility of GI Tract
   C. Increased gastric secretion
   D. Increased blood pressure
23. Which of the following is NOT true regarding receptors of parasympathetic system?
   A. Muscarinic receptors are present in organs such as heart, endocrine glands, smooth muscles.
   B. Nicotinic receptors are present in autonomic ganglia
   C. Muscarinic receptors are blocked by curare drugs
   D. Nicotinic receptors are blocked by ganglion blockers such as hexamethonium

Answers

1. B	2. D	3. C	4. C	5. A	6. B	7. A
8. B	9. D	10. C	11. A	12. C	13. A	14. A
15. C	16. C	17. D	18. D	19. A	20. B	21. D
22. D	23. C					

Chapter 25

Autonomic Dysfunctions, Autonomic Function Tests and Spectral Analysis of Heart Rate Variability

Learning Objectives

On completion of study of this chapter:

The student will be able to (must know):

1. Name common autonomic disorders.
2. Understand the pathophysiology of Horner's Syndrome.
3. Classify autonomic function tests (AFTs) and understand their basic principle.
4. Learn application of sympathetic and parasympathetic function tests.
5. Understand the principle and application of heart rate variability.

The student may also be able to (desirable to know):

1. Describe the AFTs and their clinical interpretation
2. Describe the use of HRV in clinical physiology.

AUTONOMIC DYSFUNCTIONS

Autonomic disorders are broadly termed as **autonomic failures**.

Types of Autonomic Failures

Autonomic failures are of two types: primary and secondary.

Primary Autonomic Failure

Primary autonomic failure is **idiopathic autonomic dysfunction** that invariably manifests as *orthostatic hypotension*.

Secondary Autonomic Failure

Secondary autonomic failure occurs in various diseases.

- Commonly seen in **diabetes**, amyloidosis, beriberi, syringomyelia, tabes dorsalis and subacute combined degeneration of spinal cord.
- It also occurs in patients receiving **sympatholytic drugs** of those who have undergone **surgical sympathectomy**.
- Autonomic imbalance also occurs in patients with **prolonged bed rest**.

Features of Autonomic Dysfunctions

Autonomic dysfunctions manifest as multiple organ dysfunctions as autonomic nerves innervate many visceral organs.

Cardiovascular Features: Usual manifestation is **orthostatic hypotension**. **Tachycardia** may also be seen.

Gastrointestinal Features: Either *constipation or diarrhea* can occur. Dysphagia is not uncommon. Dryness of mouth occurs frequently.

Renal Features: Increased **frequency of micturition** is the usual feature. Nocturia and incontinence may occur.

Reproductive Features: In males, **erectile dysfunction** is common. **Premature ejaculation** is also common in males. In females, **decreased vaginal lubrication** during sexual act is common.

Sudomotor Features: **Anhidrosis or hypohidrosis** is common. Heat intolerance and hyperhidrosis may occur.

Neurological Symptoms: Weakness, lethargy and giddiness.

Treatment

Treatment should start immediately for the cause of the disease, if it is of secondary variety of autonomic failure. Treatment otherwise is mostly symptomatic depending on the nature of the failure.

Diseases Affecting Sympathetic System

Horner's Syndrome

This is a syndrome (described by Johan Horner) of autonomic dysfunction, characterized mainly by:

1. Presence of **ptosis** (drooping of the upper eyelid)
2. **Miosis** (constriction of pupil)
3. **Facial anhidrosis** (*lack of sweating* on the affected side of face and neck).

Etiology: Horner's syndrome is a condition of **oculo-sympathetic paralysis**. Horner's syndrome commonly occurs in ***malignancy of cervical lymph nodes*** that presses on cervical sympathetic chain, and ***Pancost tumor of lungs***.

Pathophysiology: Clinical manifestations of this syndrome occur due to **interruption of sympathetic nerve supply to the head and neck**.

1. Center (**connector neurons**) for the sympathetic outflow to head and neck lies in lateral horn cells of first thoracic segment of spinal grey matter. Proximally it gets supraspinal control through reticulospinal tract descending from brainstem reticular formation.
2. **Preganglionic sympathetic fibres** for head and neck arising from 1st thoracic segment ascend through cervical part of sympathetic chain.
3. After relay in cervical sympathetic ganglia, **postganglionic fibres** are distributed to head and neck through ***following branches***.
   - **Lateral branches:** Gray rami to join cervical spinal nerve to arterial wall and sweat gland.
   - **Medial splanchnic branches.**
   - **Internal carotid branch:** It runs along internal carotid artery to enter inside the cranium. Apart from vascular branches, fibres along ophthalmic artery, entering the orbit supply dilator pupillae and part of levator palpebrae superioris.

A patient may suffer from Horner syndrome **due to lesion of anyone of following three levels** of sympathetic pathway for head and neck.

1. **First neuron lesion:** Affecting reticulospinal tract.
2. **Second neuron lesion:** Affecting first thoracic segment of spinal gray matter.
3. **Third neuron lesion:** Affecting cervicothoracic (stellate) ganglion.

Physiological basis of Clinical Features: **Ptosis** occurs due to paralysis of Muller's muscle, and **miosis** occurs due to paralysis of dilator pupillae. **Anhydrosis** is due to decreased sympathetic activity.

i. **Miosis:** Constriction of pupil due to unopposed action of sphincter pupillae for non-functioning dilator pupillae.
ii. **Ptosis:** Partial dropping of upper eyelid due to paralysis of levator palpebrae superioris.
iii. **Anhidrosis:** dryness of one half of the face with head and neck due to impaired secretion of sweat gland.
iv. **Flushing or blanching of same half of face** due to loss of vasoconstrictor effect on skin.

Raynaud disease

It is a vasospastic disease due to **hyperactivity of vasoconstrictor sympathetic fibres** affecting digital arteries of fingers.

- It is a bilateral disorder which is precipitated by exposure to cold and smoking. In smokers, **nicotine aggravates** vasospasm.
- Clinical manifestations are **pain, pallor and cyanosis** due to impaired vascular supply.
- Fingertips show black discoloration with formation of **dry gangrene**.

Buerger Disease

It is **arterial occlusive disease** of lower limb.

- Ischemia of muscle of leg causes pain due to muscular cramps intermittently.
- Therefore, the disorder is named as **intermittent claudication**.

Diseases Affecting Parasympathetic System

Argyll Robertson Pupil

It is a disorder in a patient of neurosyphilis due to **lesion of pretectal nucleus** of midbrain which is one of the cell stations in light reflex pathway.

- The disease is characterized by **narrow pupil with no reaction to light** due to interruption of light reflex pathway.
- In case of Argyll Robertson pupil, accommodation reflex is not disrupted as it does not pass through pretectal nucleus.

A simple formula to remember manifestation of Argyll Robertson pupil.

Argyll Robertson pupil is ARP (Accommodation reflex preserved), PRA (Pupillary reflex absent)

Adie tonic pupil

This is a syndrome characterized by flowing clinical presentations.

i. Diminished or **absent light reflex** due to disorder of function sphincter pupillae.
ii. Slow or **delayed dilation of pupil** in the dark.
iii. Slow or **delayed accommodation** to near vision because of ciliary muscle which is responsible for increase of curvature of lens.

All the above features are supposed to be due to suppression of parasympathetic ocular function.

3. Frey syndrome

It is a clinical condition that is found to occur following **healing of a penetrating wound** of face over parotid gland.

- During healing process, injured nerves of this area of face communicate with one another, as done by

auriculotemporal nerve supplying parasympathetic postganglionic *secretomotor fibres to parotid gland* with **great auricular nerve** supplying sweat glands of this area of face.

- So, stimulation of salivary secretion during mastication of food causes **sweating of area of face** supplied by great auricular nerve.

AUTONOMIC FUNCTION TESTS

Autonomic function tests (AFTs) are performed to confirm the clinical diagnosis of autonomic dysfunctions and to assess the degree of sympathetic and parasympathetic involvement in the process of dysfunction.

AFTs are classified as:

A. Tests for cardiovascular autonomic functions

1. Heart rate and Blood pressure (BP) response to standing
2. Heart rate and BP response to passive tilting
3. Heart rate response to deep breathing
4. Valsalva ratio
5. BP response to handgrip
8. Cold pressure test
9. Norepinephrine spillage technique
10. Standing to lying ratio
11. Spectral analysis of heart rate variability (HRV)
12. Analysis of blood pressure variability including baroreflex sensitivity

B. Tests for sudomotor functions

1. Sympathetic skin response
2. Thermo-regulatory sweat test (TST)
3. Quantitative sudomotor axon reflex test (QSART)

C. Vasomotor test

1. Laser Doppler Velocimetry for skin blood flow measurement
2. Cold pressor test

D. Tests for pupillary functions

1. Cocaine test
2. Adrenaline test

E. Tests for bladder functions

1. Test for sphincter-detrusor dysynergia
2. Cystometrogram

F. Other methods

1. Muscle sympathetic nerve activity (MSNA)

Tests for Cardiovascular Autonomic Functions

Heart Rate Response to Standing

Changing the posture from supine to standing, heart rate increases immediately by about 10 to 20 beats per minute.

- On standing, the heart rate increases until it reaches a maximum at about the 15th beat, after which it slows down to a stable state at about 30th beat.
- The ratio of R-R intervals corresponding to the 30th and 15th heart beat is called **the 30:15 ratio.**
- The 30:15 ratio is a ***measure of parasympathetic function***.
- However, relative **bradycardia at 30th beat** depends also on the **sympathetic reactivity**.
- The normal 30:15 ratio is 1.15 – 1.12 at 21 to 30 yrs and 1.12 to 1.10 at 31 to 40 years of age.
- This ratio decreases with age. Ratio less than 1.04 is considered abnormal.

Blood Pressure Response to Standing

The changes in blood pressure on standing are studied to assess the **integrity of the sympathetic system.**

- Immediately on standing, blood pressure falls, which activates baroreceptor reflex and blood pressure **returns to normal within 15 seconds.**
- When there is **sustained fall** in systolic pressure more than 20 mm of Hg or diastolic fall more than 10 mm of Hg within three minutes of standing, ***orthostatic hypotension*** is said to be present.

Norepinephrine (NE) Spillage Technique

NE level in plasma is measured in supine position and after 5 minutes of standing. The difference in level of NE represents alteration in **sympathetic-hormonal reactivity.**

Heart Rate Response to Tilting

Heart rate response to **head up tilt** (HUT) is a useful tool in the diagnosis of autonomic dysfunctions. It is more accurate because the active change of position is avoided by passively tilting the subject on a tilt-table. Moreover, variation in time taken by individuals to stand and the manner in which they stand from supine position is avoided in this method.

- On changing from recumbent to operate position on a tilt table to 60 to 80-degree HUT, **pooling of venous blood** of about 30% occurs in the peripheral vascular compartment, especially in lower limbs.
- This decreases cardiac filling pressure and stroke volume by about 40%.
- **Heart rate rises** immediately due to **withdrawal of parasympathetic activity** and afterward due to **increased sympathetic activity**.

Standing to Lying Ratio (SLR)

Heart rate (RR interval) response to lying down from standing posture is assessed by continuous recoding of ECG.

- Following lying from standing position, **increase in venous** return produces **reflex bradycardia.**
- Ratio of **longest RR interval in standing** to **shortest RR interval in lying** down is calculated as SLR.
- Value of SLR **below 1** is considered as abnormal.

Heart Rate Response to Deep Breathing

The variation of heart rate with respiration is known as **sinus arrhythmia**. Inspiration increases and expiration decreases heart rate.

- This is primarily mediated via **parasympathetic control** of heart.
- Pulmonary stretch receptor, and cardiac mechanoreceptors and baroreceptors contribute to sinus arrhythmia.
- The difference between the **maximum and minimum heart rate** during a deep breathing is called **deep breathing difference** (DBD).
- DBD is more than 15 beats per minute in normal individual. It **assesses the parasympathetic activity**.
- DBD decreases with age.
- It is one of the ***best parasympathetic reactivity tests***.

Normal values of DBD at different age group are:

10 to 40 years : > 18 beats per minute
41 to 50 years : > 16 beats per minute
51 to 60 years : > 12 beats per minute
61 to 70 years : > 8 beats per minute

E:I Ratio: Usually, subject is asked to inhale deeply for five seconds and then exhale for five seconds for six cycles. The ratio of ***shortest RR interval in inspiration to longest RR interval in expiration*** is calculated for each, which is called expiration-inspiration ratio (E/I ratio). The average E/I ratio of six cycles in a normal young individual is about 1:20. The E/I ratio decreases with age (Table 25.1).

Table 25.1 | Normal values of E:I ratio.

Age (years)	E:I ratio
16 to 20	: > 1.23
21 to 25	: > 1.20
26 to 30	: > 1.18
31 to 35	: > 1.16
36 to 40	: > 1.14
41 to 45	: > 1.12
46 to 50	: > 1.11
51 to 55	: > 1.09
56 to 60	: > 1.08
61 to 65	: > 1.07
66 to 70	: > 1.06

Normally, instead of DBD expressed in terms of beats per minute, **E:I ratio** is usually considered for assessing parasympathetic reactivity to deep breathing.

DBD is abnormal in **multisystem atrophy, progressive autonomic failure, diabetes mellitus, autonomic neuropathy and CNS depression**.

Valsalva Ratio

The Valsalva ratio is a measure of parasympathetic and sympathetic function.

- The test is performed by closing both nostrils and then blowing into a tube connected to sphygmomanometer. By putting strain, blowing pressure is maintained at 40 mmHg for 15 seconds.

Valsalva Maneuver

Valsalva maneuver has **four phases** (Fig. 25.1). The changes in heart rate are due to alterations in BP.

Phase I: Phase I consists of the ***onset of strain***. In this phase, there is transient increase in blood pressure that lasts for a few seconds. This occurs due to increased intrathoracic pressure and mechanical compression of the great vessels. However, ***heart rate does not change*** much.

Phase II: This is the ***phase of straining***. In the early part of this phase, venous return decreases, which in tun decreases cardiac output and blood pressure. This change persists for 4 seconds. In the later part of this phase blood pressure returns towards normal, which occurs due to increased peripheral resistance as a result of sympathetic vasoconstriction. However, ***heart rate increases steadily*** throughout this phase due to ***vagal withdrawal*** (in the early phase) and ***sympathetic activation*** (in the later phase).

Phase III: This phase occurs following the ***release of strain*** during which there is transient decrease in blood pressure lasting for a few seconds. This is caused by mechanical displacement of blood to pulmonary vascular bed, which was under increased intrathoracic pressure. There is **little change in heart rate.**

Phase IV: This is the phase that occurs with ***further release of strain***. The blood pressure slowly increases and ***heart rate proportionately decreases***. It occurs following 15 to 20 seconds after release of strain and lasts for about 1 minute or more.

The cardiovascular changes occur due to increase in venous return, stroke volume and cardiac output.

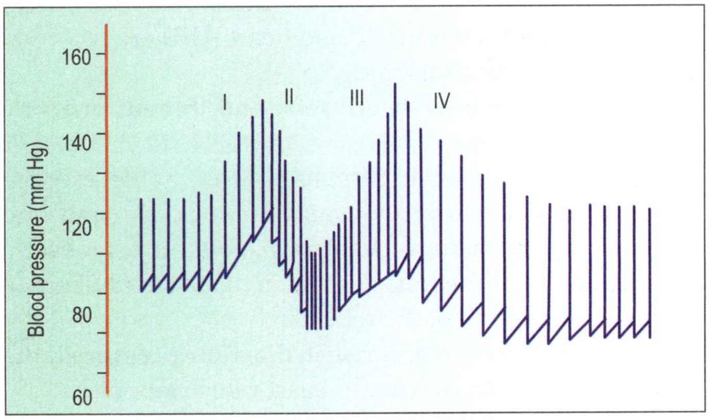

Fig. 25.1: Blood pressure changes during different phases (I, II, III, IV) of the Valsalva maneuver.

Valsalva ratio is the ratio of minimal heart rate in phase IV to maximum heart rate in phase II as depicted in terms of RR interval.

$$\text{Valsalva ratio} = \frac{\text{Longest R-R interval during phase IV}}{\text{Shortest R-R interval during phase II}}$$

Clinical Correlation: Valsalva ratio **more than 1.45 is considered to be normal**.

- Ratio 1.2–1.45 it considered borderline, and ratio less than 1.2 is regarded abnormal.
- The normal ratio is different at different age group (Table 25.2).
- Valsalva ratio is also affected by gender, posture of subject in which recording is done, expiratory pressure, duration of strain and level of yoga practice of the subject.

Table 25.2 | Normal values of Valsalva ratio at different age.

Age (years)	Valsalva ratio
10 to 40	: > 1.5
41 to 50	: > 1.45
51 to 60	: > 1.40
61 to 70	: > 1.35

Changes in Valsalva ratio occur due to **changes in cardiac vagal efferent** and ***sympathetic vasomotor activity***, which are stimulated by carotid sinus and aortic arch baroreceptors and other intrathoracic stretch receptors.

- *Failure of heart rate to increase during strain suggests a* ***sympathetic dysfunction*** *and failure of heart rate to slow down after the strain suggests* ***parasympathetic dysfunction***.

BP Response to Sustained Hand Grip

Hand-grip test is an isometric exercise in which the subject is asked to maintain handgrip against resistance.

- Resistance usually offered by using a handgrip dynamometer at a **30% of maximum voluntary contraction for 5 min.** BP and heart (HR) are recorded before and after the handgrip.
- In hand-grip test, **heart rate and blood pressure increase**.
- These cardiovascular responses to isometric exercise are mediated partly by central motor command and partly by mechanical changes or both, in response to contraction of the muscles that activate small fibers in the afferent limb of the reflex arch.
- The normal response is **rise in diastolic pressure more than 15 mm Hg** and rise in heart rate by about 30%.
- The blood pressure rise is due to *increased sympathetic activity* and heart rate rise is due to *decreased parasympathetic activity*.
- The responses to handgrip test are usually not dependent on age.
- Isometric handgrip test is one of the **best sympathetic reactivity tests**.

Cold Pressure Test

This test is performed by submerging the upper limb of the subject in ice cold water at 4°C for 30 to 60 sec. and BP is recorded before and after the procedure. The submersion of hand in cold water increases systolic pressure by about 20 mm Hg and diastolic pressure by 10 mm Hg.

- The afferent limb of the reflex pathway is somatic fibers whereas the efferent pathway is the sympathetic fibers.
- Thus, it assesses sympathetic activity.
- Cold pressor test is one of the ***best sympathetic reactivity tests***.

Analysis of BPV and BRS

Blood pressure variability (BPV) including baroreflex sensitivity (BRS) is a newer method of assessing autonomic reactivity to various stimuli, such as orthostatic challenge and injection of chemicals and drugs that changes the blood pressure.

- This is assessed by **continuous blood pressor variability** (BPV) measurement.
- Sensitivity of baroreceptors to change in dynamic component (fluctuations) of blood pressure is an important marker of **sympathetic and parasympathetic** systems. Thus, it is a reflection of integration of both the components.
- BRS is expressed as ms/mmHg. BRS **20 ms/mmHg or more** indicates good autonomic tone and improved CV health.
- BRS less than 20 ms/mmHg reflects poor cardiovascular (CV) health, and BRS less than 15 ms/mmHg is an indicator of increased CV risk.

Spectral Analysis of HRV

Recently, spectral analysis of heart rate variability (HRV) has evolved as a sensitive tool for assessing integrity of sympathetic and parasympathetic functions and for determining the **sympathovagal balance**. (Details given below)

Tests for Sudomotor Functions

Sympathetic Skin Response

Sympathetic skin response (SSR) helps in studying the functions of **peripheral sympathetic cholinergic (sudomotor) fibers** by evaluating the changes in resistance of skin in response to electrical stimuli.

- SSR is age dependent and is present in both hands and feet till the age of 60.
- Composition of surface electrodes, stimulus frequency,

skin temperature, and mental state of the subject affect the parameters of SSR.

- The latency and amplitude of SSR are measured.
- The amplitude of SSR in hand is 1.6 mV and in feet is 2.1 mV.
- SSR is helpful in diagnosing multisystem atrophy, progressive autonomic failure, diabetes, uremic patients and alcoholic neuropathy.

Thermoregulatory Sweat Test (TST)

Assessment of **sweating response to heat** also assesses sudomotor functions.

- The subject's body temperature is raised by 1°C by exposing to heat of the electric heater.
- Sweating response is studied by demarcating the area of sweating with the help of iodide starch or quinizarin powder that changes the color of the moist skin.
- Absence of sweating in TST indicates sympathetic pre- and post-ganglionic lesions.

Quantitative Sudomotor axon Reflex Test

Quantitative sudomotor axon reflex test (**QSART**) is a measure of regional autonomic function by Ach-induced sweating.

- In this test, Ach is injected intradermally and the sweat production rate is assessed.
- Reduced or absence of sweating indicates post-ganglionic lesion of sudomotor fibers (sympathetic fibers concerned with sweating)

Tests for Pupillary Functions

Pupillary function tests assess the function of sympathetic nerve supplying iris. Two tests usually performed are: cocaine test and adrenaline test.

Cocaine Test

Dilation of pupil is observed following instillation of 4% cocaine on both eyes. Cocaine prevents reuptake of norepinephrine at adrenergic nerve endings. Therefore, pupils dilate in response to cocaine, but, Horner's pupils do not.

Adrenaline Test

Instillation of 1:100 or 1% noradrenaline on eyes dilate Horner's pupil more than normal pupil. This is due to the mechanism of denervation hypersensitivity of Horner's pupil.

AFTs Sympathetic & Parasympathetic Functions

AFTs to assess Sympathetic & Parasympathetic Functions are listed Table 25.3.

Table 25.3 | Specific tests to assess sympathetic & parasympathetic functions.

A. AFTs for assessment of sympathetic functions:
1. BP response to standing/tilt
2. Cold pressor test
3. Isometric hand-grip
4. Galvanic/sympathetic skin response
5. Thermoregulatory sweat test
6. Tachycardia ratio
7. Valsalva ratio
8. NE spillage test
9. LF and LFnu of HRV
B. AFTs for assessment of parasympathetic functions:
1. Resting heart rate: Basal heart rate is a good index of parasympathetic functions as heart rate in resting conditions is a measure of vagal tone. Resting HR more 75 indicates poor vagal tone and is considered as a CV risk.
2. 30:15 ratio
3. E:I ratio
4. Valsalva ratio
5. Bradycardia ratio
6. Baroreceptor sensitivity
7. Standing to lying ratio
8. HF and HFnu of HRV

SPECTRAL ANALYSIS OF HEART RATE VARIABILITY

Heart rate variability (HRV) is the **cardiac beat-to-beat variation** (variation in cardiac cycle length), a physiological phenomenon that occurs mainly due to variation in cardiac activity during the respiratory cycle (***respiratory sinus arrhythmia***) at rest, though the circadian rhythm, environmental factors and exercise also contribute to it.

- As SA nodal discharge is largely controlled by **parasympathetic (vagal) influence**, and ***sinus arrhythmia is primarily due to alteration in vagal tone*** in inspiration and expiration, **HRV is mainly influenced by vagal activity**, though both the divisions of ANS influence it.
- HRV has been considered as a ***sensitive indicator of autonomic function***, especially for the assessment of **sympathovagal balance**.

Basic Principle

The basic principle is that beat to beat variation in SA nodal discharge as recorded by ECG is computed and analyzed by the software for determination of spectral indices of HRV.

- There are **two types** of HRV recordings: the **short-term HRV recording** done for 5 min, and day-night **long-term HRV recording**.
- Though long-term HRV recording is the ideal one for robust HRV analysis, the **short-term HRV recording** is usually performed in research and clinical investigations.

- The brief procedure of **short-term recording** as depicted in the *Task Force Report on HRV*

HRV Components

The power spectrum of HRV in humans usually reveals **three spectral components**: HF, LF and VLF (Fig. 25.2).

HF component: High-frequency (HF) component is caused by **vagal tone** during the respiratory cycle.

LF component: Low-frequency (LF) component of HRV is usually characterized by an oscillatory pattern with a period of 10 seconds. LF component mainly represents **sympathetic power**. However, ***parasympathetic drive*** also contributes to it.

VLF component: Very low frequency (VLF) component accounts for all other heart rate changes, including those associated with thermoregulation and humoral (especially, **rennin-angiotensin mechanism**) and local factors.

Calculation of Time Domain Indices

In a continuous ECG record, each QRS complex is detected, and the so called normal to normal (NN) intervals (i. e. all intervals between adjacent QRS complexes resulting from sinus node depolarization) or instantaneous heart rate is determined. Simple time domain variables that are calculated include (Table 25.4):

1. **The mean RR**
2. **SDNN:** Standard deviation of normal to normal interval.
3. **RMSSD:** Square root of the mean squared differences of successive normal to normal intervals.
4. NN50: Number of pairs of adjacent NN interval differing by more than 50 ms in the entire recording.
5. pNN50: NN50 count divided by the total number of all NN intervals.

Table 25.4 | Selected time domain indices.

Variable	Physiological significance
SDNN	Overall vagal modulation of cardiac functions from beat to beat
RMSSD	Vagal modulation of cardiac functions on short-term basis
SDNN index	Same as SDNN

Calculation of Frequency Domain Indices

Frequency domain variables that are usually calculated include **total power** (TP), **low frequency** (LF) component, LF component expressed as ***normalized unit*** (LFnu), **high frequency** (HF) component, HF component expressed as ***normalized unit*** (HFnu) and **LF/HF ratio** (Table 25.5).

Normalizing spectral powers are calculated by the formula as follows:

1. LF nu = LF x 100 (TP – VLF)
2. HF nu = HF x 100 (TP – VLF)
3. LF/ HF ratio = Ratio of LF to HF spectral powers

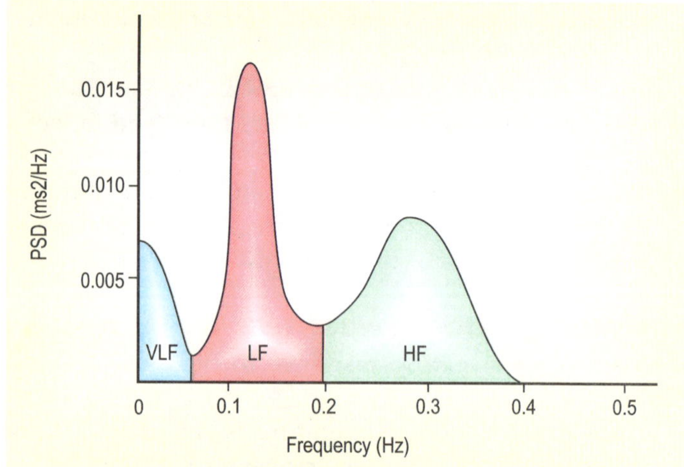

Fig. 25.2: Distribution of very low frequency (VLF), low frequency (LF) and high frequency in HRV power spectrum. Note, in this picture, the total power (TP) was 920 ms^2, of which VLF was 70 ms^2, LF was 420 ms^2 and HF was 430 ms^2.

Table 25.5 | Selected frequency domain measures of HRV.

Variable	Frequency Range	Physiological significance
TP (ms^2)	Approximately <0.4 Hz	Overall vagal potency of cardiac modulation, i.e., the heart rate variability
VLF (ms^2)	0 – 0.04 Hz	Integrity of renin-angiotensin system
LF (ms^2)	0.04 – 0.15 Hz	Mainly, cardiac sympathetic drive
LF-normalized (LFnu)		Cardiac sympathetic modulation, independent of other powers of modulation
HF (ms^2)	0.15-0.4 Hz	Cardiac parasympathetic drive
HF-normalized (HFnu)		Cardiac parasympathetic modulation, independent of other powers of HRV
LF/HF		Sympathovagal balance

TP: total power; nu: normalized unit

Importance of HRV Analysis

Physiological Significance

HRV analysis is used to precisely assess the **efficiency of cardiac vagal drive** of the individual, as it reflects the heart rate variability that occurs mainly due to **sinus arrhythmia**.

Thus, physiologically HRV is the function of the **cardiac vagal drive**.

- The **HF component** of HRV *indicates the cardiac vagal drive* of the individual:
- The **LF component** of HRV *mainly indicates the cardiac sympathetic drive.*
- **Increased LF-HF ratio** reflects *increased sympathetic activity* (Fig. 25.3) that is invariably associated with **decreased TP**, and **decreased LF-HF** ratio indicates *increased parasympathetic and decreased sympathetic activity* that is invariably associated with **increased TP** (Fig. 25.4).

Frequency Domain Results

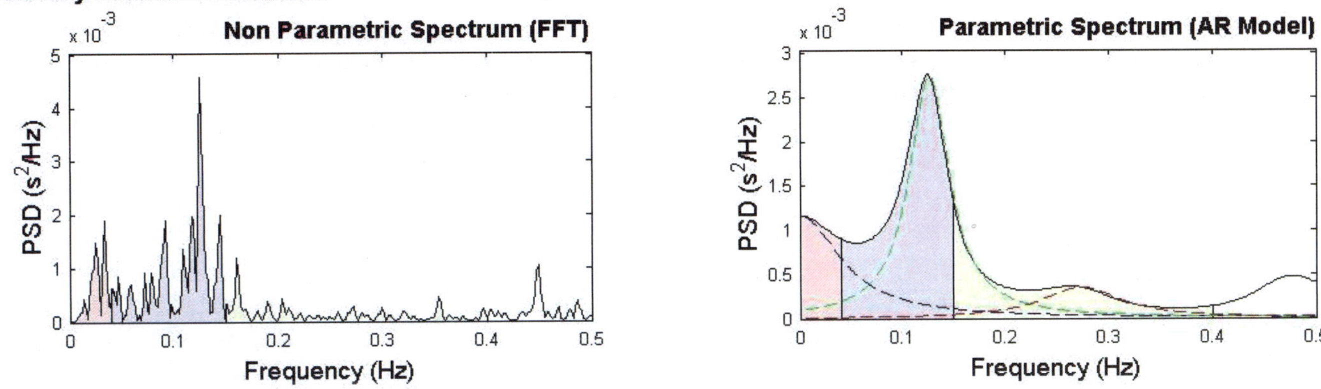

Frequency Band	Peak (Hz)	Power (ms^2)	Power (%)	Power (n.u.)
VLF	0.0332	22	15.4	
LF	0.1250	89	62.7	74.0
HF	0.1602	31	22.0	26.0
LF/HF			2.852	

Frequency Band	Peak (Hz)	Power (ms^2)	Power (%)	Power (n.u.)
VLF	0.0000	61	21.1	
LF	0.1270	189	65.9	64.6
HF	0.2734	37	13.0	12.7
LF/HF			5.077	

Fig. 25.3: Frequency domain indices of HRV analysis of a subject having increased sympathetic activity. Refer Fig. 25.2 for PSD of VLF, LF and HF of HRV. Note, as depicted in parametric spectrum, LF Power (ms^2) is significantly increased (189 ms^2) compared to HF Power, which is grossly reduced (37 ms^2) and LF-HF ratio is increased to 5.077. Also, TP is only 287 (VLF 61+LF 189+HF 37).

Frequency Domain Results

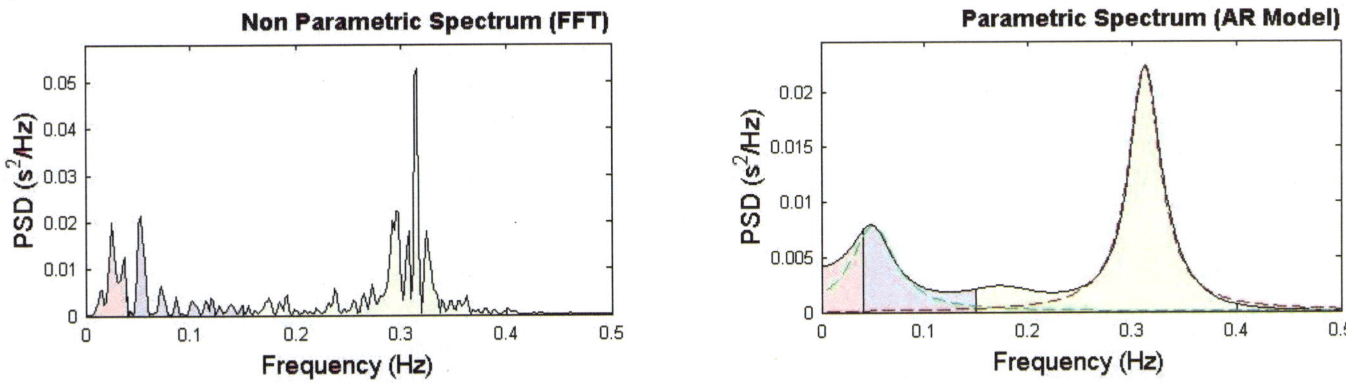

Frequency Band	Peak (Hz)	Power (ms^2)	Power (%)	Power (n.u.)
VLF	0.0254	247	15.2	
LF	0.0527	312	19.2	22.7
HF	0.3145	1063	65.5	77.3
LF/HF			0.293	

Frequency Band	Peak (Hz)	Power (ms^2)	Power (%)	Power (n.u.)
VLF	0.0000	0	0.0	
LF	0.0508	557	30.0	28.4
HF	0.3105	1301	70.0	66.3
LF/HF			0.428	

Fig. 25.4: Frequency domain indices of HRV analysis of a subject having more parasympathetic activity. Refer Fig. 25.1 for PSD of VLF, LF and HF of HRV. Note, as depicted in parametric spectrum, HF Power (ms^2) is significantly increased (1301 ms^2) compared to LF Power, which is much less (557 ms^2) and LF-HF ratio is increased to 0.428. Also, TP is 1858 (VLF 0+LF 557+HF 1305), which is quite high and reflects increased HRV, the indicator of good CV health.

- The **sympathovagal balance** is assessed by the **LF-HF ratio**:

1. **Total power** (TP) of HRV indicates the **magnitude of heart rate variability**. TP is the single most HRV parameter to assess the strength of vagal modulation of the heart.
2. **Decreased TP** (decreased overall cardiac vagal modulation) has been implicated with future adverse **cardiovascular (CV) morbidities** and mortalities

Clinical Note 25.1

Decreased TP is the marker of CV Risk: TP power reflects the total power of vagal modulation. Decreased TP indicates poor vagal tone and decreased strength of HRV. Less TP alone is a good predictor of adverse CV event. TP less than 100 is associated with sudden cardiac death. More TP is protective to the heart.

3. HRV could be used as a **sensitive tool in the prediction of CV risks.**

4. Presently, HRV is used as a **prognostic tool in conditions like post-myocardial infarction** and cardiac transplantation.
5. The most important application of HRV analysis is the surveillance of post-infarction and diabetic patients.
6. HRV gives information about the sympathetic–parasympathetic autonomic drives, and used as tool for assessment of **autonomic imbalance**.
7. Decreased HRV is well correlated with the **risk of sudden cardiac death** in patients with heart disease.
8. **Improvement in HRV** and CV health are observed in interventions like **exercise and yoga.**

Exam Questions

1. Classify autonomic disorders. Briefly describe the physiological basis of clinical features of Horner's syndrome.
2. Classify autonomic function tests. Briefly describe one important test each to assess sympathetic and parasympathetic function.
3. List the frequency domain and time domain indices of HRV and give their physiological significance. Briefly describe the clinical application of HRV.

Multiple Choice Questions

1. Which of the following neural structure in NOT involved in autonomic control?
A. Premotor cortex
B. Prefrontal cortex
C. Amygdala
D. Hypothalamus

2. In Argyll-Roberson pupil:
A. Direct light reflex is preserved
B. Accommodation reflex present
C. Indirect light reflex is preserved
D. Pupillary reflex present

3. Which of the following is NOT a feature of Horner syndrome?
A. Ptosis
B. Flushing of same half of face
C. Mydriasis
D. Facial anhidrosis

4. In Adie pupil, all are true EXCEPT:
A. Diminished light reflex
B. Delayed accommodation to near vision
C. Delayed dilation of pupil in darkness
D. Tonically constricted pupil

5. Which of the following is a parasympathetic function test?
A. Galvanic skin response
B. Deep breathing difference
C. Cold pressor test
D. Isometric handgrip test

6. Orthostatic hypotension is said to be present, when sustained fall in:
A. SBP > 40mmHg, DBP >20mmHg
B. SBP > 50mmHg, DBP >25mmHg
C. SBP > 10mmHg, DBP >5mmHg
D. SBP > 20mmHg, DBP >10mmHg

7. A more accurate sympathetic reactivity test will be:
A. Isometric handgrip test
B. HRV Analysis
C. Norepinephrine spillage technique
D. Tachycardia ratio

8. A more accurate parasympathetic reactivity test will be:
A. 30:15 ratio
B. HFnu and TP of HRV analysis
C. Heart rate response to deep breathing
D. Bradycardia ratio

9. Which of the following pressure indicates increased sympathetic activity in isometric handgrip test?
A. Increase in SBP > 10 mmHg
B. Increase in DBP > 15 mmHg
C. Increase in DBP > 25 mmHg
D. Increase in DBP > 8 mmHg

10. HRV mainly denotes:
A. Coronary sympathetic activity
B. Cardiac sympathetic drive
C. Cardiac vagal drive
D. Renal sympathetic activity

11. Which of the following HRV index is a sympathetic marker?
A. HFnu
B. LFnu
C. RMSSD
D. TP

12. Which of the following is NOT true about HRV?
A. The parameters are highly variable
B. It can be used more as a prognostic marker than a diagnostic tool
C. Long-term HRV recording is ideal for cardiovascular risk assessment
D. HRV is a precise AFT for cardiovascular ailments

Answers

1. A	2. B	3. C	4. D	5. B	6. D	7. A	8. C
9. B	10. C	11. B	12. D				

Section V

Cardiovascular System

"*People with small and narrow minds are in love with their narrowness and attached to their own limited ideas, feelings, opinions, preferences, and get disturbed, angry or full of doubt if anyone tries to make them think more widely.*

Sri Aurobindo"

Chapter 26

Functional Organization of Cardiovascular System

Learning Objectives

On completion of study of this chapter:

The student will be able to (must know):

1. Understand the functions of heart as a central pump.
2. Name the types of blood vessels and give their functions.
3. Name the divisions of vascular system and give their functions.
4. List the differences between systemic and pulmonary circulations.
5. Learn the importance of central and peripheral blood volumes.

The student may also be able to (desirable to know):

1. Describe types of blood vessels based on their histological specializations.
2. Explain the differences between systemic and pulmonary circulations.

Cardiovascular system consists of a central pump, **the heart** that propels blood into circulation, and an extensive **network of blood vessels** that circulates blood throughout the body.

HEART

The **primary function** of the heart is **to pump blood** into circulation.

- The forceful ejection of blood creates energy for the blood to circulate in the blood vessels.
- The heart consists of a dual pump (the right and left pumps) that ejects blood into two serial circuits: the systemic and pulmonary circulations (Fig. 26.1).
- The right pump is the right ventricle that propels blood into the pulmonary circulation for exchange of gases in the lungs.
- The left pump is the left ventricle that propels blood into the systemic circulation to supply oxygen and nutrients to the tissues.
- The output of each pump at rest is about 5 lit/min.
- This accounts for about 400 million liters of blood pumped by the heart during the lifetime of a person who lives about 70 years, which is enough to fill a lake of 1 km long, 40 m wide and 10 m deep.
- Pumping of blood is increased many-fold in daily routine works, exercise, emotion etc.

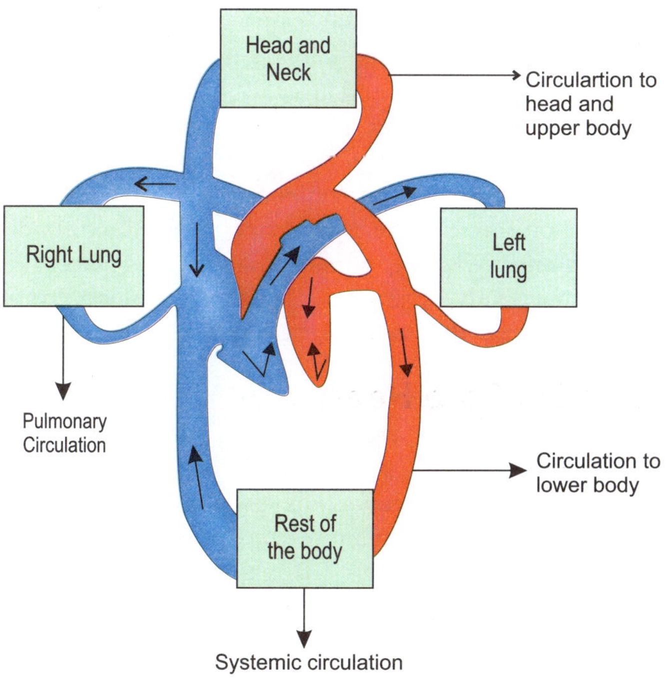

Fig. 26.1: Arrangement of systemic and pulmonary circulations. Note that the right pump (right ventricle) propels blood into pulmonary circulation and the left pump (left ventricle) pumps blood into systemic circulation.

Chambers of the Heart: Heart has **four chambers**: two atria and two ventricles.

- The right atrium and right ventricle constitute right side of the heart (sometimes, called as right heart, especially by clinicians).
- The left atrium and left ventricle constitute the left side of the heart (or the left heart).

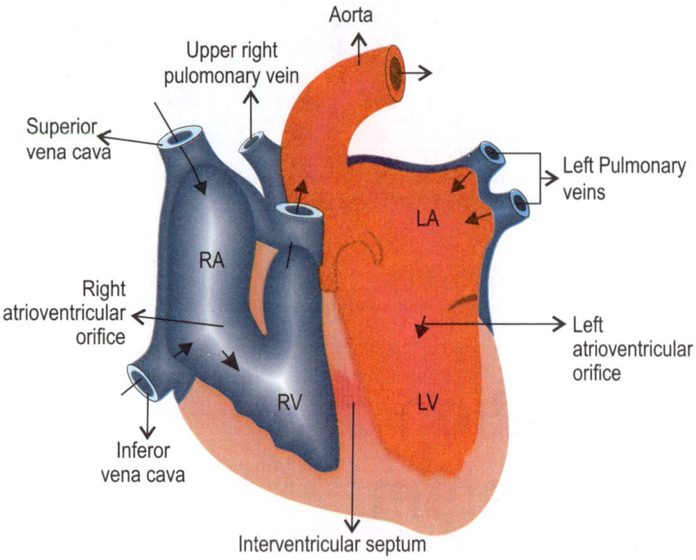

Fig. 26.2: Chambers of the heart and the direction of flow of blood (indicated by arrow) through the chambers. RV: Right ventricle; LV: Left ventricle; RA: Right atrium; LA: Left ventricle.

Right side of the Heart

Right side of the heart consists of right atrium and right ventricle (Fig. 26.2).

- The right atrium receives blood from different parts of the body through superior and inferior vena cava and empties blood into the right ventricle.
- The right atrioventricular valve or the tricuspid valve guards the flow of blood from right atrium to right ventricle and prevents flow of blood in backward direction.
- The right ventricle pumps blood into the pulmonary circulation through the pulmonary trunk (the pulmonary arteries) where gaseous exchange takes place.
- Pulmonary valve prevents back flow of blood from pulmonary trunk into the right ventricle.

Left side of the Heart

Left side of the heart consists of left atrium and left ventricle (Fig. 26.2).

- The left atrium receives oxygenated blood from the pulmonary circulation via pulmonary veins and empties blood into left ventricle through left atrioventricular valve or mitral valve.
- The mitral valve ensures unidirectional flow of blood from the left atrium to the left ventricle.
- Left ventricle pumps blood into the systemic circulation through the aorta.
- The aortic or the semilunar valve, which is present at the base of aorta prevents back flow of blood into left ventricle from the aorta.

BLOOD VESSELS

The blood vessels form a **close system** of tubes (*the vascular system*) that transport blood from the heart to the tissues and return blood from the tissues to the heart (Fig. 26.3).

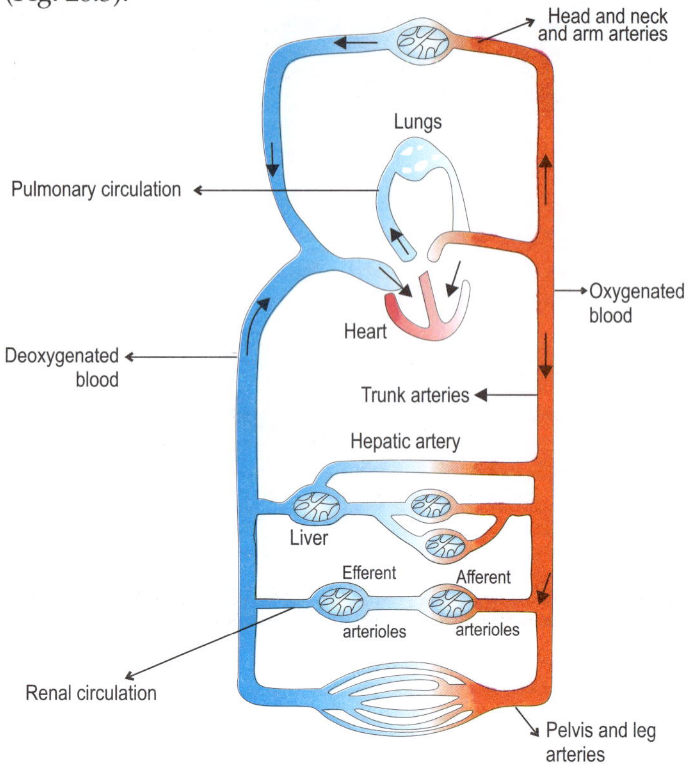

Fig. 26.3: Overview of cardiovascular system (CVS). Note CVS is a closed system that transports oxygenated blood from heart to tissues and returns deoxygenated blood from tissues to the heart. Pulmonary circulation is much smaller in comparison to systemic circulation.

Functional Histology of Blood Vessels

Generally, the blood vessels have **three layers**: the tunica externa (adventitia) or the outer coat; tunica media (the muscle layer) or the middle coat; and the tunica interna (intima) or the inner layer (Fig. 26.4).

1. **Tunica externa** consists of ***elastic tissues and collagen fibers***.
2. **Tunica media** consists of ***smooth muscles and elastic tissues***.
   - In tunica media, the smooth muscles are arranged circularly around the lumen of the blood vessels.
   - Therefore, contraction of the smooth muscles as occurs in sympathetic stimulation leads to vasoconstriction, and relaxation of the smooth muscles as occurs in sympathetic inhibition leads to vasodilation.
3. **Tunica intima** is composed of an ***endothelial cell lining***, which is a simple squamous epithelium. This is called the **vascular endothelium**.

Components of Vessel Wall

In accordance with three layers of blood vessels, ***four important components*** form the vascular wall: the **endothelial cells, elastic tissue, smooth muscles and fibrous tissue** (collagen fibers).

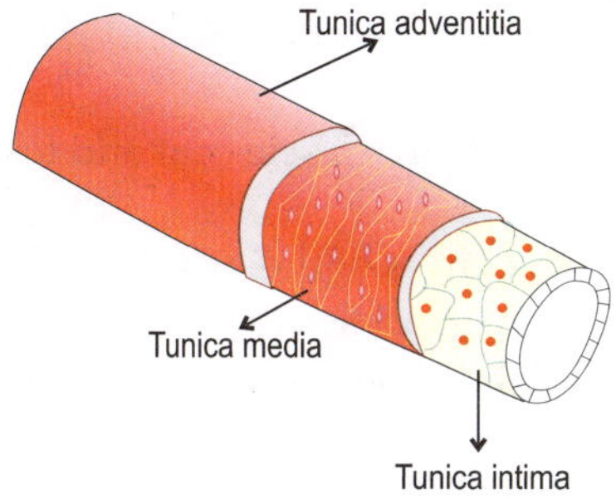

Fig. 26.4: Layers of the wall of a blood vessel (an artery). Note three layers (adventitia, media and intima) from outside to inside.

- Distribution of these components in various blood vessels determines their functional significance (Fig. 26.5).
- They also influence the ratio of wall thickness to the internal diameter that significantly contributes to their role in hemodynamics.

Endothelial Cells

Endothelial cells form the inner lining of all blood vessels, known as **vascular endothelium**.

- Endothelial cells are present as a single continuous layer.
- Tight junctions and other intercellular connections keep the endothelial cells adhered to each other.
- In capillaries, the vessel wall is formed only by a layer of endothelial cells present on the basal lamina.
- This makes them suitable for exchange of substances between blood and tissues.
- However, the transport of substances across the capillary wall depends on how tightly the cells in the endothelium are adhered together.
- For example, tight junctions of endothelial cells of capillaries in brain are very tight, which contributes to the effectiveness of blood brain barrier, whereas in liver they are not so tight, which allows easy capillary filtration.
- Endothelial cells also secrete many chemicals and hormones that control cardiovascular functions.

Elastic Tissue

The amount of elastic tissue present in the vessel wall determines the **ability of the vessel to stretch**.

- The percentage of elastic fibers in aorta and large arteries is more in comparison to their other components.
- Therefore, these vessels have more compliance.
- Elastic fibers are made of elastins and microfibrils.
- Elastins are protein molecules formed by nonpolar amino acids such as glycine, alanine, valine and proline.
- Microfibrils are minute fibril strands made up of glycoproteins.
- Elastin molecules assemble along with microfibrils to form a network of fibers that is highly capable of stretching.

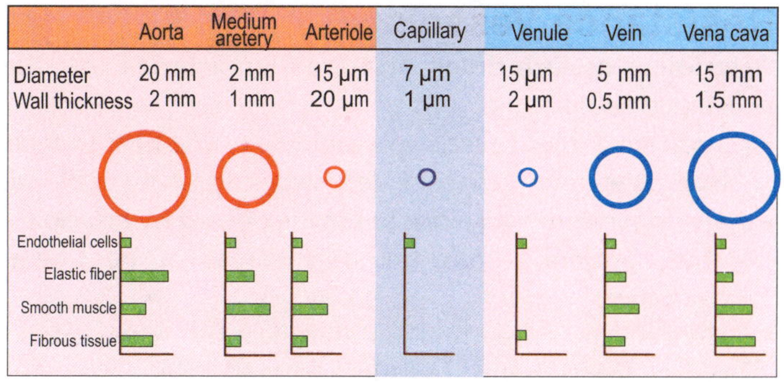

Fig. 26.5: Comparison of distribution of different components of vessel wall in aorta and large arteries, arteries, arterioles, capillary, venules, veins and vena cava. Also note the difference in diameter of vessel to wall thickness.

- Elastic fibers are abundant in arteries and veins, less in arterioles, and absent in capillaries and venules.

Smooth Muscle

Smooth muscle is **present in all vessels except capillaries and venules**.

- The quantity of smooth muscles is more than elastic fibers in arterioles, metarterioles and small arteries. Therefore, these vessels serve as resistance vessels.

Fibrous Tissue

In blood vessels, fibrous tissue is primarily made up of **collagen fiber**s, which are mainly type **I and III collagens**.

- Fibrous tissue is present in all parts of vascular tree except capillaries.
- It prevents distention of vessels and increases wall tension.

Physiological Classification of Blood Vessels

Functionally, blood vessels are classified into **four categories**: Windkessel vessels, resistance vessels, exchange vessels and capacitance vessels.

Windkessel Vessels

The **aorta and large arteries** are Windkessel vessels. Windkessel, a German word, means an **elastic reservoir.**

- The aorta and large arteries have more elastic elements in their wall (Fig. 26.5).
- Therefore, these vessels have higher compliance.
- During systole, their wall stretches to accommodate the blood ejected by ventricles, and during diastole, their wall recoils back to presystolic position.
- This recoiling effect is called Windkessel effect.
- The Windkessel or the recoiling effect pushes blood in forward direction during diastole.
- Blood in blood vessels is pushed forward during systole by the force created by ventricular ejection and during diastole by the force created by arterial recoiling.
- Thus, blood flow is continuous during both the phases of cardiac cycle.

Resistance Vessels

Arterioles, metarterioles and smaller arteries are the resistance vessels.

- They have thick muscle coat and less elastic fiber in their wall. Therefore, they provide resistance to flow of blood.
- The maximum resistance to flow is offered by arterioles. Thus, arterioles form the major seat of peripheral resistance.
- Hence, the pressure falls significantly when blood passes through the arterioles.

Exchange Vessels

Capillaries are thin vessels as their wall is formed only by a **single layer of endothelial cells**.

- The blood flow is sluggish in capillaries due to more total cross-sectional area of these vessels.
- These two factors (thin wall and sluggish flow) favor exchange of gases and nutrients along the capillary wall.
- Therefore, capillaries are called exchange vessels.

Capacitance Vessels

Normally, more than **60% of the total blood** is present in the venous compartment.

- Veins can accommodate still larger amount of blood without increasing much pressure in them.
- Therefore, large and small veins are called capacitance vessels.

Divisions of Vascular System

The vascular tree consists of **three systems**: the arterial system, the system of capillary networks and the venous system.

Arterial System

The arterial system consists of the aorta, large arteries, smaller arteries, arterioles and metarterioles.

Arteries

Arteries have **thick tunica media**.

- The smooth muscles of arteries are extensively innervated by sympathetic fibers of the autonomic nervous system.
- Therefore, sympathetic stimulation results in vasoconstriction and sympathetic inhibition leads to vasodilation.
- The arteries are specifically susceptible to atherosclerosis.

Arterioles

Arteries branch out to form the arterioles.

- Arterioles regulate the resistance to flow through the various organs of the body.
- Thus, they control distribution and rate of blood flow to the organs.
- Arterioles have thick muscle coat and few elastic fibers in their wall.
- The ratio of thickness of the wall to the diameter of the vessel is high in arterioles.
- Therefore, contraction or relaxation of the smooth muscles in arteriolar wall allows them to readily control the vessel caliber.
- Hence, arterioles are the main resistance vessels.

IMPORTANT NOTE

Arterioles are 'stopcock' of the circulation: Due to thick muscle coat in arterioles, they are the resistance vessels and control blood flow to the organs. Arterioles serve as the **'stopcock' of the circulation.**

Metarterioles

Arterioles terminate in metarterioles.

- Metarterioles are histologically same as that of arterioles except that the muscle coat is thin, and the lumen is smaller.
- A flap of smooth muscle called precapillary sphincter is present at the end of the metarterioles or arterioles.
- This sphincter regulates blood flow to the capillaries.

System of Capillary Network

The system of capillary network originates from arterioles and metarterioles.

- It consists of extensively branched, small and thin-walled vessels.
- They are made up of only the tunica interna, a single layer of endothelial cells.
- This makes them suitable for exchanging materials between the blood and the tissues.
- Capillaries are therefore called the exchange vessels.
- The circulation of blood through the capillaries is called the microcirculation.

IMPORTANT NOTE

Slow blood flow in capillaries due to large CSA: Due to their extensive branching networks, the total cross-sectional area (CSA) of capillaries is quite large (Table 26.1).

- Hence, blood flow is very slow in this segment of circulation.
- This facilitates the process of transcapillary exchange.

Table 26.1 | Total cross-sectional area (CSA) of different parts of circulatory system.

Parts	Total CSA (Cm^2)
Aorta	2.5
Small arteries	20
Arterioles	40
Capillaries	2500

Table 26.1: Contde....	
Venules	250
Small veins	80
Vena cavae	8

Venous System

The venous system starts from capillaries. It consists of **collecting venules, venules, and small and large veins**.

Venules

Venules is to collect blood from the capillaries and drain into the veins.

- These small vessels have thinner muscular wall that form the low-pressure collecting system.
- Like arterioles, venules are innervated by sympathetic fibers.
- Contraction or relaxation of the venules contributes to the overall size of the venous compartment.

Veins

Venules unite to form veins that join together to form larger veins.

- Veins have thin muscle coat.
- About two-thirds of blood volume in the systemic circulation is present in the veins (Fig. 26.6).
- Therefore, veins serve as the blood reservoir.
- The veins in the limbs, especially in the lower limbs contain valves within.
- Venous valves facilitate venous return.

SYSTEMIC Vs PULMONARY CIRCULATION

The circulatory system consists of **two important parts**: the systemic circulation and the pulmonary circulation.

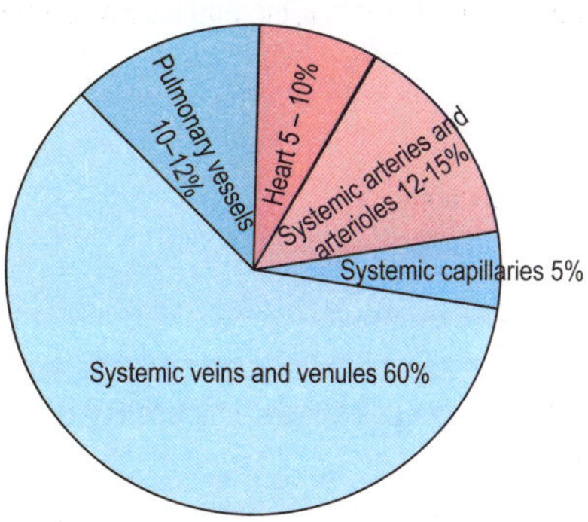

Fig. 26.6: Percentage distribution of blood volume in different vascular compartments.

Systemic Circulation

The circulation of blood through the systemic vascular bed is called systemic circulation. This is also called the peripheral circulation or the greater circulation.

- This is the major circulation as it contains 80–85% of the total volume of blood.
- It provides oxygenated blood to different parts of the body and drains venous blood back to the heart.
- The pressure in the arterial compartment in systemic circulation is high.
- The systolic pressure is 100 to 140 mmHg.
- Pressure drops progressively as the blood flows from the arteries to the veins.
- The arteries and arterioles have thicker walls and narrower lumen and are richly innervated by the sympathetic fibers (Table 26.2).
- They have high resting vasoconstrictor tone.
- Thus, they provide higher resistance to blood flow.
- The capillaries are longer and narrower.
- Therefore, systemic capillaries also provide resistance to blood flow.

Table 26.2 | The major differences between systemic and the pulmonary circulations.

	Systemic Circulation	Pulmonary Circulation
1. Synonyms	Peripheral or greater circulation	Central or lesser circulation
2. Pressures	High pressure	Low pressure
- Systolic press	100–140 mm Hg	20–30 mm Hg
- Diastolic press	60–90 mm Hg	5–15 mm Hg
- Mean pressure	100 mm Hg	15 mm Hg
- Pulse pressure	20–50 mm Hg	10–15 mm Hg
3. Arteries	Thick wall and narrow lumen	Thin wall and large lumen
4. Arterioles	Thick wall and narrow lumen	Thin wall and large lumen
5. Capillaries	Long and narrow	Short and wide
6. Resting sympathetic tone	High vasoconstrictor tone at rest)	Absent (lack vasoconstrictor tone)
7. Peripheral resistance	High	Low
8. Capillary blood flow	Continuous	Pulsatile

Pulmonary Circulation

The circulation of blood through the pulmonary vascular bed is called pulmonary circulation. This is also called the **central circulation** or the **lesser circulation**.

1. It is the minor circulation as it contains **only 10 to 12% of the total blood volume**.
2. It provides a **low resistance pathway** for the entire output of the right ventricle to traverse through the lungs.

Significant contribution of Scientist

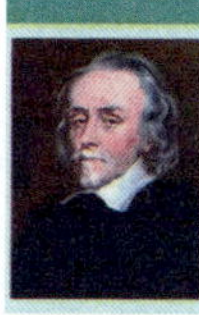

William Harvey (1578 – 1657) was first to study extensively the details of blood circulation through arteries, described the functions of venous valves and clarified circulation of blood through lungs. As a distinguished teacher and physician, his lecture notes on circulation in 1616 are monuments forever.

3. The **arteries have thin wall** and **large lumen**.
   - Arteries have rich sympathetic innervations.
   - But unlike that of systemic arteries they lack resting vasoconstrictor tone.
4. The **arterioles have thin wall and larger lumen**.
   - Therefore, pulmonary arterioles provide low resistance to flow.
5. The **capillaries are shorter and wider**.
   - Consequently, resistance is also less in capillaries.

Thus, the vessels in the pulmonary circulation are primarily designed to provide **a low resistance circulation** for the entire output of the right ventricle to pass through them.

IMPORTANT NOTE

Pulmonary Circulation is a low resistance circuit: The output of the right ventricle is same as the output of the left ventricle.
- Same equal amount of blood is ejected by right ventricle into a much smaller pulmonary circulation.
- Therefore, the nature has provided a low resistance circuit for the pulmonary vascular bed to accommodate and quickly transfer the right ventricular output to left side of the heart.

VOLUME DISTRIBUTION IN VASCULAR COMPARTMENTS

Five to six liters of blood is present in an adult weighing 70 kg.
- 10–12% of blood volume is present in pulmonary circulation, 5–10% in heart and 80–85% in systemic vessels (Fig. 26.6).
- In pulmonary circulation, the blood is almost equally distributed amongst arteries, capillaries and veins.
- In systemic circulation, about three fourth of blood (75% of systemic circulation, or 60% of the total) is present in venous compartments.
- Though, only 5% of the blood volume is present in capillaries, capillary blood is important for tissue oxygenation and nutrition.

Central vs. Peripheral Blood Volume

Blood volume is divided into central or thoracic and peripheral or extra-thoracic blood volume.

Central Blood Volume

The central blood volume is the volume of blood present in pulmonary circulation, heart, superior vena cava, intrathoracic portion of inferior vena cava and aorta.
1. It constitutes about **25% of the total blood volume**.
3. Central blood volume is important as it **determines the atrial filling and cardiac output**.
3. **Central venous pressure** is a good indicator of central blood volume, as the compliance of intrathoracic vessels apparently remains same.

Peripheral Blood Volume

The peripheral blood volume is the volume of blood that is mainly present in veins of the extremities, abdominal cavities and head and neck.
1. It constitutes about **75% of the total blood volume**.
2. Contribution of volume of blood in head and neck to the peripheral pool is less, as it is less in quantity.
   - Therefore, mainly it is blood in limb and abdominal veins that constitute the peripheral blood volume.
3. **Shift of blood from peripheral pool to central pool** is physiologically important, as it finally determines the cardiac output (Clinical Note 26.1).

Clinical Note 21.1

Both central & peripheral blood volumes are important: Alteration in total blood volume due to any cause affects both central and peripheral blood volumes. For example, in acute hemorrhage fall in central blood volume, which is detrimental to life, is quickly compensated by shift of blood from the peripheral compartment. Failure of the compensatory mechanisms decreases ventricular end-diastolic filling and cardiac output.

Exam Questions

1. Name the types of blood vessels. Describe how their functional histology is correlated with their functions.
2. List the differences between systemic and pulmonary circulation and give physiological basis of four important differences.
3. What is central blood volume. Briefly explain the importance of central venous pressure.

Multiple Choice Questions

1. **Which of the following is NOT true?**
   A. Fibrous pericardium prevents over-distension of heart
   B. Normally, the amount of pericardial fluid is 35mL
   C. Pericardial fluid reduces friction between the two layers
   D. Excess accumulation of pericardial fluid is called pericardial effusion
2. **Left ventricle has more muscle mass compared to right ventricle because:**
   A. By the nature of evolution
   B. LV consists of four groups of fibers whereas RV consists of only two groups of fibers
   C. Left coronary artery supplying the left ventricle has greater flow
   D. LV does more work to propel the blood compared to the RV
3. **Windkessel vessels are:**
   A. Medium sized arteries B. Arteries in upper and lower limbs
   C. Aorta and large arteries D. Large arteries and small arteries

Answers

1. B 2. D 3. C

Chapter 27

Functional Anatomy of Heart, Cardiac Muscle and Cardiac Innervation

Learning Objectives

On completion of study of this chapter:

The student will be able to (must know):

1. Give a note on functional anatomy of heart.
2. Have a concept of pericardial layers of heart and of pericardial effusion.
3. Understand the specialty of histology of cardiac muscles.
4. Appreciate cardiac muscle as functional syncytium.
5. Learn the myocardial contractile system and arrangement of sarcotubular system.
6. Explain the length-tension relationship of cardiac muscle.
7. Define Frank-Starling law of the heart and explain its physiological mechanisms.
8. List the effects of vagal and sympathetic stimulations of heart.

The student may also be able to (desirable to know):

1. Describe the myocardial contractile system.
2. Describe the properties of cardiac muscle.
3. Describe the innervation of the heart.

PY5.1

FUNCTIONAL ANATOMY

The size of the heart of an individual is approximately the size of his or her closed fist.

- The average weight of the heart is about 300 g in adults.
- The heart is covered and protected by pericardium.
- The heart consists of **four chambers**: two atria (right and left) and two ventricles (right and left).

Pericardium

The covering of heart is called **pericardium**. It is **a double-layered sac** that covers and protects the heart (Fig. 27.1).

Fibrous Pericardium

The outer layer is the fibrous pericardium, which is made up of dense irregular connective tissue.

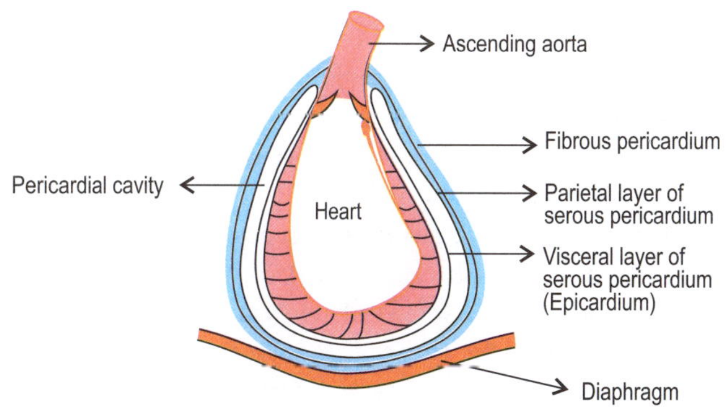

Fig. 27.1: Layers of the pericardium. Note the reflections of fibrous and serous pericardium.

- For its toughness and inelasticity, the fibrous pericardium prevents overdistension of the heart.

Serous Pericardium

The inner layer is the serous pericardium, which is further made up of **two layers**.

Parietal Pericardium: The outer layer of the serous pericardium is the **parietal pericardium**, which is in close contact with the fibrous pericardium.

Visceral Pericardium: The inner layer of the serous pericardium is the **visceral pericardium,** which is in close contact with the surface of the heart.

Pericardial Cavity

The space between the two layers of the serous pericardium is called the pericardial cavity.

- The serous fluid present in the pericardial cavity is the pericardial fluid.
- Normally, the amount of pericardial fluid is about 15 ml.
- The function of pericardial fluid is to reduce friction between the layers of the pericardium when heart expands or contracts.

- When fluid accumulates in excess in the pericardial cavity as occurs in pericarditis, the condition is called pericardial effusion (Clinical Note 27.1).

Clinical Note 27.1

Cardiac tamponade: When very large amount of fluid accumulates in pericardial cavity, the condition is called *cardiac tamponade*.

- Cardiac tamponade may occur due to bleeding into the pericardium (hemopericardium) as occurs in heart injury or in severe acute pericarditis
- In such a condition, the expansion of heart is severely restricted due to compression on ventricles from pericardial sac.
- In extreme cases, it may be life threatening due to gross reduction in cardiac output.

Cardiac Chambers

Heart is made up of four chambers: **two atria** (right and left) and **two ventricles** (right and left).

Right Atrium: Right atrium receives blood from different parts of the body via inferior and superior vena cava. This is called **venous return**.

- It empties blood into the right ventricle through tricuspid valve, which is largely passive.
- Only about 20% of the blood is transferred by atrial contraction (atrial systole).

Left Atrium: Left atrium receives blood from the pulmonary circulation via four pulmonary veins and empties blood into the left ventricle via the **mitral valve**.

Right Ventricle: The right ventricle pumps blood into pulmonary circulation through the **pulmonary semilunar valves**.

- The peak pressure generated by the right ventricular contraction is about 25 mmHg.

Left Ventricle: The left ventricle pumps blood into the systemic circulation through the **aortic semilunar valves**.

- The peak pressure generated by the left ventricular contraction is about 120 mmHg.

Cardiac Valves

The cardiac valves are present at the junction between the chambers and at the output orifices of the ventricles. There are **two atrioventricular valves** and **two semilunar valves**.

- They are made up of thin flaps (leaflets) of fibrous tissue covered with endothelium, which are firmly attached to the valve rings (Fig. 27.2).
- The orientation of the valves allows unidirectional flow of blood through the heart and the movement of the valve leaflets opens or closes the valves.

Atrioventricular Valves

They are located between the atria and ventricles. The left atrioventricular valve is the **mitral valve**, which has two cusps (bicuspid valve). The right atrioventricular valve is the **tricuspid valve**.

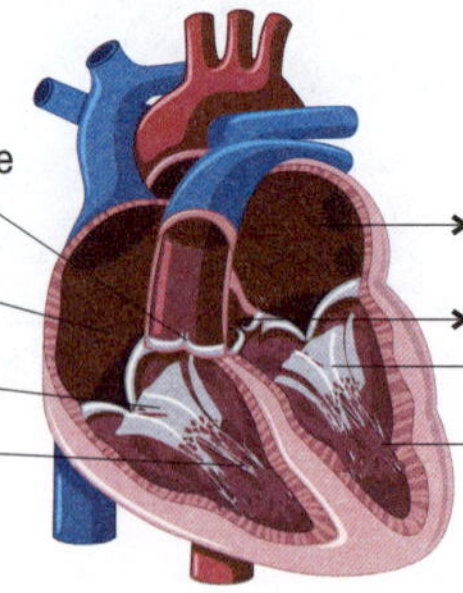

Fig. 27.2: Cardiac chambers and cardiac valves. Note the structure of semilunar (pulmonary and aortic) valves and atrioventricular (tricuspid and mitral) valves.

- The size of the cusps of the atrioventricular valves is more than the size of atrioventricular orifice (Fig. 27.2).
- Therefore, when valves are closed there is adequate overlapping of the valve leaflets, which totally prevents leakage of blood back into the atrium.
- The chordae tendineae (strong ligaments arising from the papillary muscles) are attached to the free edges of the valves, which prevents eversion of the valves during systole (Fig. 27.3).

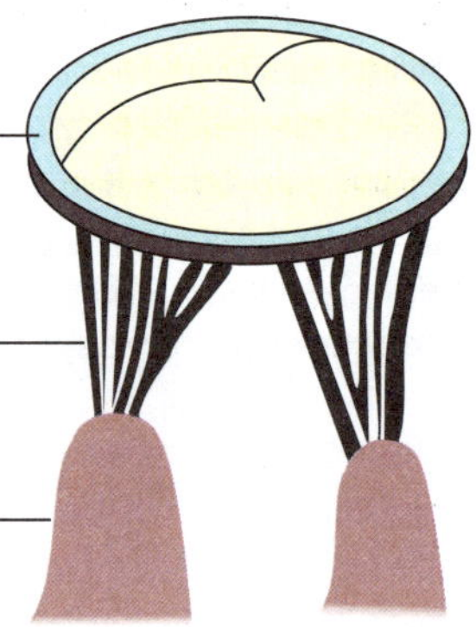

Fig. 27.3: Attachment of chordae tendineae with a cardiac valve. Chordae tendineae are attached with free edges of valve leaflets that prevent their eversion during systole.

Semilunar Valves

These are located at the outlet orifice of the ventricles: **pulmonary valve** at the orifice of right ventricle and **aortic valve** at the orifice of left ventricle (Fig. 27.2).

- These valves consist of three cusps that are attached to the valve rings.
- At the beginning of ventricular systole, the cusps open and blood is propelled from ventricles.
- Towards the end of systole when the blood flow reverses (from aorta towards the ventricle), the cusps snap and prevent regurgitation of blood into the ventricles.

Wall of Heart Chambers

The wall of heart chambers has **three layers**: epicardium, myocardium, and endocardium (Fig. 27.4).

Epicardium

This is the outermost layer.

- In fact, it is the visceral layer of the serous pericardium.

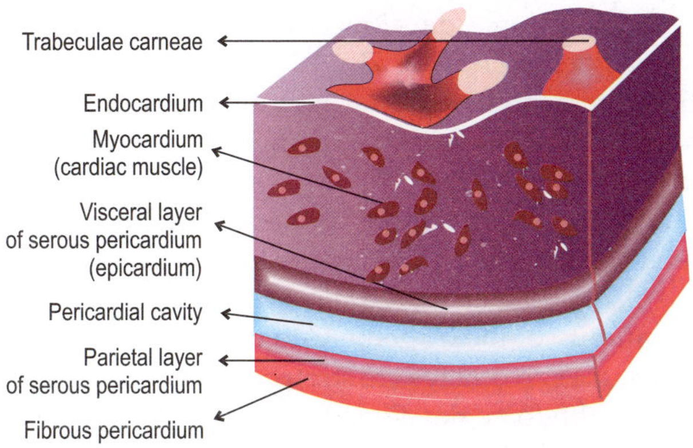

Fig. 27.4: Layers of the heart wall.

- It is made up of mesothelium and connective tissue.

Myocardium

The middle layer is the myocardium that consists of the cardiac muscle.

- Myocardium forms the bulk of the ventricles, which is primarily responsible for ventricular pump activity.
- Wall of atria is thinner than the wall of ventricles.
- The wall thickness is proportionate to the pressure generated by the chambers to propel blood.
- Atrial wall is thinnest (2 mm thick) as the blood from atria enters ventricles mostly passively.
- The left ventricular wall thickness is 10 mm as left ventricle generates maximum pressure to pump blood into the systemic circulation, and right ventricular wall thickness is 5 mm as right ventricle generates less pressure to pump blood into the pulmonary circulation (Fig. 27.2).
- The muscles of the ventricles are arranged mostly spirally around the lumen of the chambers.

Endocardium

This is the inner wall of the heart.

- It consists of a layer of endothelium overlying a thin layer of connective tissue.
- It is continuous with the endothelial lining of large vessels that originate from the heart.

CARDIAC MUSCLE

Heart muscle is classified as striated muscle. The myocardial fibers are separated from each other by sarcolemma.

- The nucleus of the muscle cell is centrally placed.
- The muscle fibers are branched.
- At the junctions of branching of fibers, there are specialized areas known as intercalated discs (Fig. 27.5).
- Intercalated discs contain many gap junctions.
- Gap junctions are electrical synapses through which the wave of depolarization can easily pass through from cell to cell.
- Therefore, when a cardiac muscle cell is stimulated, the electrical impulse spreads rapidly to the other muscle cells and heart contracts as a single unit. Thus, cardiac muscles act as a functional syncytium.

Heart as a Functional Syncytium

A syncytium is defined as a **tissue containing cells with no boundaries** (the *nuclei are free in the protoplasm*).

- Thus, syncytial tissue acts as a single unit. The example of a structural syncytium is the muscles in the body-wall of the earthworm.
- In heart, the myocardial fibers are indeed separated from each other. Therefore, myocardial tissues are not anatomical syncytium.
- However, they are physiological syncytium as functionally they behave like a single unit due to presence of numerous gap junctions.
- In fact, there are two syncytia in the heart: the atrial syncytium, and the ventricular syncytium.
- This is because the atria are completely separated from the ventricles by a fibrous band of tissue known as atrioventricular ring.
- Therefore, atria and ventricles are functionally two separate units.

Myocardial Contractile System

Though myocardial cells differ from skeletal muscle cells in few aspects, the **contractile mechanisms in both the tissues are almost similar**.

- The myocardial contractile unit consists of sarcomeres that contain thick and thin filaments.
- Thick filaments are myosin filaments and thin filaments are actin filaments.
- As in the skeletal muscle, shortening of cardiac muscle occurs by the sliding filament mechanism.
- An important difference is that skeletal muscle cells contain few mitochondria whereas the cardiac muscle cells are rich in mitochondria, which allows them for rapid oxidation of substrates to produce ATP.

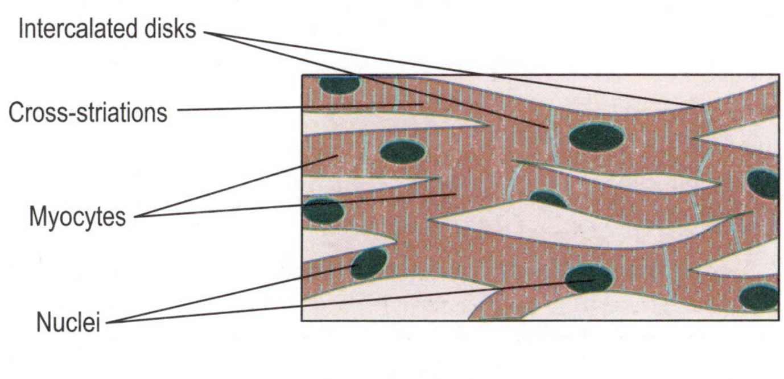

Fig. 27.5: Structure of cardiac muscle. Note the branching of fibers and presence of intercalated disks.

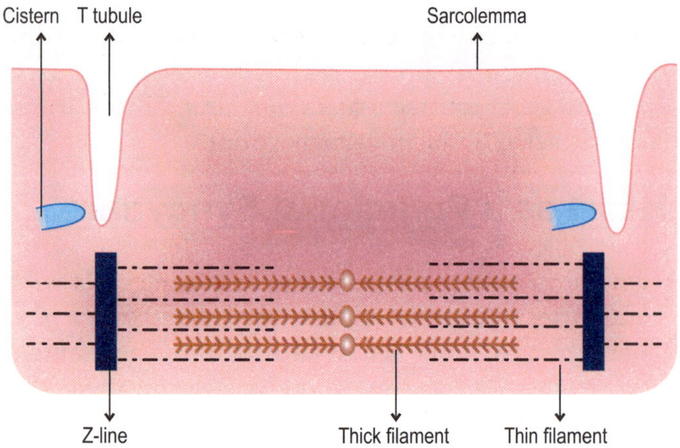

Fig. 27.6: Location of sarcotubular system (T tubule and cistern) in cardiac muscle. Note that it is in the form of a diad (one T tubule and one narrow tubular cistern) and located at Z line instead of at A-I junction as in skeletal muscle.

Sarcotubular System

The sarcotubular system is **well developed** in the myocardial cells.

- It consists of transverse tubules (T tubules) and sarcoplasmic reticulum (cisterns).
- The T tubules are present as deep invagination of the sarcolemma into the muscle fibers at the Z line (Fig. 27.6), which is present at A-I junction in the skeletal muscle (Table 27.1).
- T tubules are almost continuous with the interstitial fluid for which they play important role in muscle contraction.
- T tubules are more developed in ventricular myocytes than the atrial myocytes, and the diameter of T tubule in ventricular muscle cell is more than double the diameter of T tubules in skeletal muscle cell.
- Sarcoplasmic reticulum is present in close association with T tubular system forming a diad that contains one T tubule and one cistern (Fig. 27.7), which is triad (one T tubule and two cisterns) in the skeletal muscle.

Table 27.1 | Difference between the sarco-tubular system of cardiac and skeletal muscle.

	Cardiac muscle	Skeletal muscle
1. Sarcomeric organization	Less regular	Quite regular
2. Location of T tubules	At Z line	At A-I junction
3. Diameter of T tubules	More	Less
4. L tubules (tubular part of cistern)	Narrow tubular cistern	Large dilated cistern
5. Association of T tubule and cistern)	Diad (one T tubule and one cisterns)	Triad (one T tubule and two cisterns)

Length-Tension Relationship

The length-tension relationship of cardiac muscle is similar to that of skeletal muscle.

- The active force developed is maximum within the optimal length (Fig. 27.7).
- The interaction of thick and thin filaments and the number of cross-bridge formation are maximal within this optimal length.
- The increase in length of sarcomere increases the sensitivity of the myofilaments to calcium.
- It is also explained that stretch of myocardium increases the affinity of the troponin C to calcium.
- When the sarcomeres are stretched beyond the optimal length, the force developed decreases due to decrease in the overlap and interaction between the thick and thin filaments.
- This decreases cross-bridge formation.
- The length-tension relationship is implicated to explain the physiological activities of the heart.

Frank-Starling Law of the Heart

This law states that the **force of contraction is directly proportional to the initial length** of the muscle fiber, ***within the physiological limit.***

- This is also known as Starling's Law of the heart.
- This explains how the increase in preload or end-diastolic volume increases cardiac output.

Mechanisms: There are **four mechanisms** to explain Frank-Starling Law:

1. With increased end-diastolic volume, the initial length of the muscle fiber increases due to increase in chamber size that stretches the muscle fibers.
   - With increased stretch of muscle fibers, the interaction between thick and thin filament increases, which increases the force of contraction.
2. The stretch of muscle fibers ***opens the stretch-sensitive calcium channel*** on the muscle cell membrane.

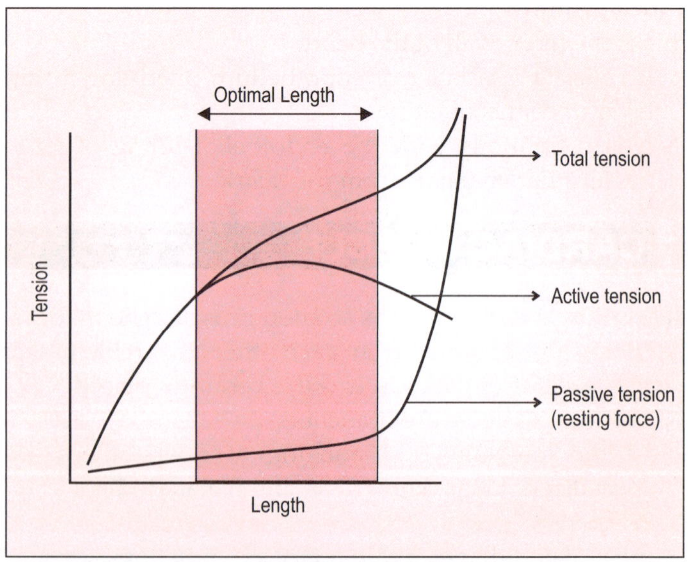

Fig. 27.7: Length-tension curve of cardiac muscle. Note that over a range of length (that represent ventricular volume), the total force (tension) increases with length. The resting force increases steeply immediately after the optimal length, which is physiologically protective to the heart as it prevents overdistension due to overfilling of ventricle.

- This increases the calcium influx into the myocardial cell. Thus, force of contraction increases.

3. Increase in intracellular calcium ions due to calcium influx from ECF induced by stretch, increases the further ***release of calcium from sarcoplasmic reticulum*** by activating the ***calcium-induced calcium channels*** present on the membrane of this cell organelle.
   - Increased intracellular calcium increases the force of contraction.
4. Stretch of myocardium ***enhances the affinity of troponin C for calcium.***
   - This increases the binding of calcium to troponin C, which enhances the force of contraction.

Significant contribution of Scientist

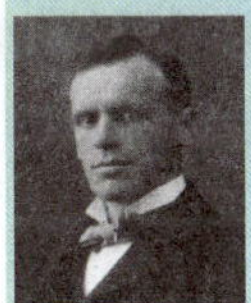

Ernest Henry Starling (1866 – 1927), was a great teacher and researcher in physiology. He studied the osmotic effects of serum proteins on fluid movements along the capillaries, for which the mechanism of capillary filtration is popularly known as Starling hypothesis, and the factors are called Starling forces. He described length-tension relationship of cardiac muscle, which is popularly known as Starling's law or Frank-Starling law of the heart.

Excitation-Contraction Coupling

The mechanism of excitation-contraction coupling in cardiac muscle is similar to that of skeletal muscle.

- However, the appropriate concentration of sodium and potassium in addition to the concentration of calcium is essential for excitation and contraction of cardiac muscle.
- These ions are needed for the generation of the resting membrane potential (RMP), the action potential and the pacemaker potential of cardiac tissues.
  i) K^+ is mainly required for the RMP and therefore determines the excitability.
  ii) Na^+ and Ca^{++} are mainly required for action potential
  iii) K^+ and Ca^{++} are mainly required for pacemaker potential
  iv) Concentration of Ca^{++} is required for the muscle contractility.

Effects of alterations in these ions:

Decreased Extracellular Na^+: Na^+ is required for ***action potential*** of cardiac muscle. Therefore, decreased extracellular Na^+ concentration ***decreases excitability*** of the heart.

Decreased Extracellular K^+: Decreased extracellular K^+ does not affect excitability significantly.

Increased Extracellular K^+: An increase in K^+ concentration in the ECF causes *depolarization and loss of excitation* that finally results in ***cardiac arrest in diastole.***

Increased Extracellular Ca^{++}: An increase in extracellular Ca^{++} *increases the force of contraction*, and if the concentration is very high it causes ***cardiac arrest in systole*** (calcium rigor).

Decreased Extracellular Ca^{++}: The decreased extracellular Ca^{++} concentration decreases the force of contraction and eventually ***cardiac arrest occurs in diastole.***

Mechanism of E-C Coupling

When excitation (the wave of depolarization) of the cardiac muscle spreads into the muscle cells through the T tubules, ***Ca^{++} is released*** from the sarcoplasmic reticulum. Calcium also enters the cytosol from the interstitial fluid.

- In fact, the Ca^{++} that enters the cell from the interstitial fluid triggers Ca^{++} release from the sarcoplasmic reticulum.
- The Ca^{++} then binds with the troponin C and the calcium-troponin complex interacts with the tropomyosin that uncovers the active site between the thick and thin filament.
- This allows the cross-bridge cycling, which causes muscle contraction.

Influence of Cytosolic Ca^{++}: Alteration in cytosolic Ca^{++} alters the force of contraction. Therefore, mechanisms that increase the cytosolic Ca^{++} increase the force of contraction, and the mechanisms that decrease the cytosolic Ca^{++} decrease the force of contraction.

For example, epinephrine enhances myocardial contractility by increasing the cytosolic Ca^{++}.

Cytosolic Ca^{++} can be increased by **two mechanisms**:

i) By increasing the Ca^{++} in the ECF.

ii) By decreasing the Na^+ gradient across the sarcolemma.

Influence of Cytosolic Na^+: The Na^+ gradient can be decreased either by increasing the intracellular Na^+ or by decreasing the extracellular Na^+.

- The increase in cytosolic Na^+ retards the sodium-calcium exchange, which decreases the Ca^{++} removal from the cell so that concentration of Ca^{++} in the cell increases.
- The decreased ECF Na^+ causes less Na^+ to enter the cell, so that less Ca^{++} is exchanged for Na^+, which results in accumulation of Ca^{++} in the cell.
- The cardiac glycosides like digoxin increase the force of contraction by inhibiting Na^+-K^+ ATPase that results in accumulation of intracellular Na^+.
- This decreases the sodium-calcium exchange and allows Ca^{++} to accumulate in the cell.

Contractility

This is defined as the **change in peak isovolumetric force at a given initial fiber length** (at a particular end-diastolic volume).

- It represents the performance of ventricle at a given preload or afterload.
- The increased contractility represents increase in developed force and velocity of contraction.

Capillary Density

Myocardium is **highly rich in capillaries.**

- There is almost one capillary for one muscle fiber in cardiac muscle in comparison to one capillary for 100-500 muscle fibers in skeletal muscles.
- Due to anatomical closeness between the capillary and the muscle fiber, the diffusion distance (the distance between the capillary membrane and the sarcolemma) is very less, which facilitates delivery of oxygen and nutrients and removal of carbon dioxide and waste products.

CARDIAC INNERVATION

Both the **sympathetic and parasympathetic divisions** of the autonomic nervous system innervate the heart (Fig. 27.8). In general, stimulation of parasympathetic decreases and stimulation of sympathetic increases activities of the heart.

The cardiac pacemaker (SA node) activity is tonically influenced by both parasympathetic and sympathetic systems.

In basal conditions, **parasympathetic or vagal tone is more than the sympathetic tone**.

- Therefore, normally the resting heart rate is the function of the vagal tone.

The **ventricular muscle** is predominantly **supplied by the sympathetic fibers** and the parasympathetic innervation of ventricle is sparse.

- Therefore, myocardial contractility is greatly influenced by sympathetic discharge.
- Hence, stroke volume is the function of sympathetic tone.

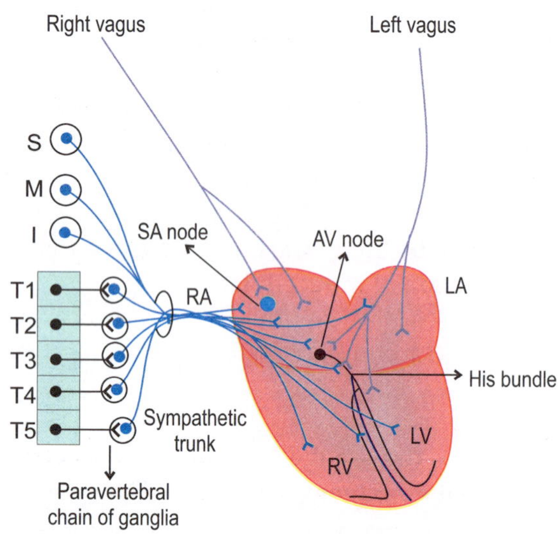

Fig. 27.8: Innervation of the heart. Note that right vagus predominantly supplies SA node and right atrium, and left vagus predominantly supplies AV node, bundle of His, and left atrium. There is sparse vagal innervation of ventricles. Sympathetic fibers heavily innervate both atria and ventricles. S, M, and I are superior, inferior, and middle cervical ganglia, respectively. T1–T5 are 1st to 5th thoracic vertebrae, respectively. RA, LA, RV, and LV are right and left atria and ventricles.

Parasympathetic Innervation

The cardiac parasympathetic (vagal) fibers originate from the **three vagal nuclei** present in the medulla oblongata: **nucleus tractus solitarius, dorsal motor nucleus of vagus** and **nucleus ambiguous**.

- The preganglionic parasympathetic fibers traverse in the vagus nerve on both the sides.
- The ganglion cells are mostly located in the cardiac tissues and the postganglionic fibers are present in the heart itself.

Difference in Right & Left Vagi: There are differences in cardiac innervation by the right and left vagi (Fig. 27.8).

- The right vagus mainly innervates right atrium and SA node.
- Therefore, stimulation of right vagus strongly inhibits heart rate.
- The left vagus predominantly innervates the left atrium, AV node and the bundle of His.
- Therefore, stimulation of left vagus slows or blocks AV nodal conduction.
- However, stimulation of either of the nerves can inhibit functions of both the nodes, as there is sufficient overlap in nodal innervation by both the vagi.
- The innervation of ventricles by the vagi is sparse.
- Therefore, parasympathetic stimulation does not significantly affect the force of contraction.

Effects of Parasympathetic Stimulation: Vagal stimulation to heart results in:

1. **Negative chronotropic** effect (decreased heart rate)
2. **Negative dromotropic** effect (decreased rate of conduction)
3. **Negative bathmotropic** effect (decreased excitability of the heart)
4. **Negative inotropic** effect (decreased myocardial contractility)

Basal Heart Rate Vs. Intrinsic Heart Rate

Basal Heart Rate

Basal heart rate is the heart rate in resting condition. This is also called **resting heart rate**.

- SA nodal activity is primarily under the control of vagus nerve.
- Therefore, the basal heart rate depends on the vagal tone (Application Box 27.1).

Intrinsic Heart Rate

Intrinsic heart rate is the SA nodal discharge without autonomic influence. Following **denervation of heart** i. e., abolition of influence of sympathetic and parasympathetic influence by blocking noradrenergic and cholinergic transmissions, **heart rate increases** from basal rate of about 70 per minute to about post-denervation rate of 120 per minute.

The increase in heart rate following denervation (intrinsic heart rate) indicates that normally vagal tone dominates over sympathetic tone for the control of heart rate.

Application Box 27.1

Basal heart rate is the function of vagal tone: Resting heart rate is an index of parasympathetic activity. As vagus nerve inhibits SA nodal discharge, the individual with high vagal tone has lower basal heart rate. Resting heart rate is an important marker of parasympathetic functions.

Sympathetic Innervation

The cardiac sympathetic fibers originate in the intermediolateral gray column of the spinal cord starting from **lower two cervical segments** to the **upper five thoracic segments** (Fig. 27.9).

- The preganglionic fibers, after emerging from the spinal cord enter the paravertebral chain of ganglia.
- The cell bodies of the postganglionic fibers are located in the superior, middle and inferior cervical ganglia.
- The fibers traverse along the adventitial surface of the blood vessels to reach the heart.
- The sympathetic fibers innervate the atria, nodal tissues and conducting pathways, and pierce ventricles to extensively supply the myocardium (Fig. 27.8).

Difference in Left & Right Sympathetic Fibers: There is some difference in distribution of left and right sympathetic fibers supplying the heart.

1. **The right side of the sympathetic division** mainly supplies SA node, right atrium and right ventricle, whereas the **left sympathetic fibers** mainly supply the AV node, left atrium and the left ventricle.
2. Thus, stimulation of **right sympathetic nerve predominantly affects the heart rate** whereas stimulation of **left sympathetic nerve mainly affects the myocardial contractility**.
3. However, there is adequate overlap in innervation of heart by both sides of the sympathetic fibers.
   - Therefore, stimulation of either side of sympathetic nerve can affect both rate as well as force of contraction.

Cardiac sympathetic tone: At rest, there is adequate tonic discharge in the sympathetic nerve supplying the heart. This is called the **sympathetic tone**.

- However, as stated above, normally the influence of vagal tone on SA node predominates over the sympathetic tone.
- Therefore, the basal heart rate is an index of vagal tone rather than sympathetic tone.

Effect of Sympathetic Stimulation: Cardiac sympathetic stimulation results in:

1. **Positive chronotropic** effect (increased heart rate)
2. **Positive inotropic** effect (increased myocardial contractility)
3. **Positive dromotropic** effect (increased rate of conduction)
4. **Positive bathmotropic** effect (increased excitability of the heart).

Exam Questions

1. Describe the special histological modifications in cardiac muscle and give their physiological significance.
2. Describe the myocardial contractile systems. List the differences in sarcotubular systems in cardiac and skeletal muscles.
3. With the help of a suitable diagram, describe the length-tension relationship in cardiac muscle.
4. Define Frank-Starling law of the heart, and briefly explain the mechanisms of this law.
5. With the help of a suitable diagram, depict the cardiac vagal and sympathetic innervations. Briefly explain the differences between the effects of vagal and sympathetic stimulation of the heart.

Multiple Choice Questions

1. **Fibers of internodal pathways are :**
   A. Modified nerve fibers
   B. Modified atrial muscle fibers
   C. Conduct impulses rapidly at a speed of 5mts/sec
   D. Have large number of noradrenergic receptors
2. **Which of the following has the highest conduction velocity?**
   A. HIS bundle B. Purkinje fibers
   C. Internodal pathways D. Ventricular muscles
3. **Which of the following is true about myocardial contractile system?**
   A. T tubule is located at A-I junction
   B. Diameter of T tubule is less than that of T tubules in skeletal muscle
   C. Sarcomeric organization is less regular than that of skeletal muscle
   D. Association of T tubule with cisterns form a triad
4. **SA node is the primary pacemaker of the heart, as it:**
   A. Is capable of generating the impulse
   B. Decides speed of conduction of impulse
   C. Allows immediate transmission of cardiac impulse throughout the heart
   D. Determines the rate at which the heart beats
5. **Which of the following is true about intercalated discs?**
   A. Present exclusively at the middle part of sarcolemma
   B. Permit neurotransmitters to easily pass through them
   C. They contain numerous gap junctions
   D. Provide high resistance bridges for the spread of excitation from one cardiac muscle fiber to another
6. **Which of the following is true about vagal innervations of heart?**
   A. There is sufficient overlap in nodal innervations
   B. Right ventricle is richly innervated by right vagus
   C. Vagal influence on SA Node is less than the sympathetic influence at rest.
   D. Left vagus sparsely innervates AV node.

Answers : 1. B 2. B 3. C 4. D 5. C 6. A

Chapter 28

Properties of Cardiac Muscle

Learning Objectives

On completion of study of this chapter:

The student will be able to (must know):

1. List the properties of cardiac muscle.
2. Appreciate the hierarchy of pacemaking activity in cardiac pacemakers.
3. Explain why cardiac muscle can't be tetanized.
4. Understand the application of all-or-none law, compensatory pause and staircase phenomenon.
5. Elucidate the length-tension relationship, frequency-force relationship and load-velocity relationship of cardiac muscle.

The student may also be able to (desirable to know):

1. Describe properties of cardiac muscle.

Cardiac muscles are endowed with **special properties** to ensure **unfatigable work of heart as a pump** throughout life.

The **properties** of cardiac muscles are: **PY5.2**

1. Automaticity
2. Rhythmicity
3. Conductivity
4. Contractility
5. Excitability
6. Distensibility
7. Long refractory period, for which cardiac muscle can't be tetanized.
8. Functional syncytium
9. Extrasystole and compensatory pause
10. All or none Law
11. Staircase phenomenon
12. Length-tension relationship
13. Frequency-force relationship
14. Load-velocity relationship

In experimental conditions, the properties from number **1 to 6 can be studied in a beating heart** and number **7 to 12 can be studied in a quiescent heart** (which is performed by placing Stannius ligatures).

SPECIAL PROPERTIES

Automaticity

Automaticity is the property of automatic beating of the heart.

- Heart continues to beat even when it is completely denervated or isolated (but artificially perfused) from the body.
- The ability of the cardiac muscle to continue to **contract regularly** even in the ***absence of its nerve supply*** is referred to as **automaticity**.
  - This occurs due to the ***spontaneous generation of impulses*** by the SA node, the **primary pacemaker of the heart** that displays pacemaker potential.
- Automaticity is also the property of **other potential pacemakers** of the heart like AV node, His-Purkinje system, ventricular muscle etc.

Rhythmicity

Heart not only beats automatically, but also rhythmically at regular intervals.

- Rhythmicity refers to the rhythmic excitation of the heart.
  - This is called **autorhythmicity**.
- This occurs due to **rhythmic discharge** of the pacemaker, the SA node.
  - Thus, heart rate is the function of cardiac pacemaker.
  - SA node is the **primary pacemaker**.
- The rate of discharge of SA node is 60–100 per minute, the highest among all the pacemakers.
  - Therefore, the **normal heart rate is 60–100 per minute**.

Pacemaking Tissues in the Heart

Normal heart has three intrinsic pacemaking tissues: SA

node, AV node and His-Purkinje fibers. When the intrinsic pacemakers fail to discharge, ventricular muscle generates the pacemaking potential.

- The term 'pacemaking-activity' refers to the spontaneous time-dependent depolarization that leads to action potential in an otherwise quiescent cell or tissue.
- Any of the pacemakers can initiate the heartbeat.
  - However, the pacemaker with highest frequency triggers the action potential that propagates throughout the heart.
  - The SA node being the fastest pacemaker, override the activity of all other pacemakers.
  - Therefore, SA node is the primary pacemaker.
- Thus, till SA node is functioning normally, heart beats according to SA nodal rhythm. Cardiac pacemakers have a hierarchy among themselves (Table: 28.1).

IMPORTANT NOTE

Secondary Pacemakers: When SA node is defunct, the failure of SA nodal rhythm results in activation of AV node, the next in the hierarchy to take over the pacemaker activity. Thus, AV node and other cardiac pacemakers are called secondary pacemakers.

Table 28.1 | The rate of discharge of potential pacemakers of heart.

Pacemaker tissue	Rate/min
SA node	60 – 100
AV node	40 – 60
His bundle	25 – 40
Purkinje fiber	25 – 40
Ventricular muscle	15 – 30

Demonstration of Hierarchy of Pacemakers: The hierarchy of pacemakers can be demonstrated experimentally, usually in frogs by placing **Stannius ligatures**. In this experiment, the normal cardiogram is recorded, which denotes rate of sinus venosus, the natural pacemaker in frog's heart.

- The **first Stannius ligature** is placed between the sinus venosus and atria, i.e. on the white cresentic line, and the cardiogram is recorded.
  - This reflects the ***atrial rhythm***, which is slower than the normal sinus rhythm as the impulses are generated in the atria (Fig 28. 1).
- The cardiogram is then recorded after placing **second Stannius ligature**, which is placed between the atria and the ventricles.
  - This records ***ventricular rhythm*** as the impulses are generated in the ventricle, which is slower than the atrial rhythm.

Conductivity

The cardiac tissues conduct impulses generated in the heart.

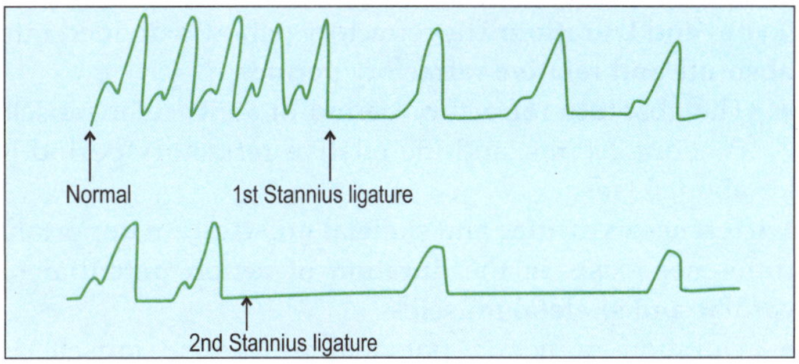

Fig. 28.1: Effects of Stannius ligatures on frog heart's activities. The first ligature decreases heart rate and the second ligature further decreases it.

- Impulse produced in SA node is conducted by **specialized conducting pathway** to the ventricular muscle.
- The impulse then **spreads rapidly in cardiac muscle** to the different parts of the heart.

Contractility

Cardiac muscle contracts in response to a stimulus.

- Ventricular contraction enables heart **to pump blood** into the circulation.
- The **increased contractility increases cardiac output** and decreased contractility decreases cardiac output.

Excitability

Cardiac muscle is an excitable tissue like nerve and other muscles.

- Excitability is the **ability of the cardiac muscle to respond** to different stimuli.
- Cardiac excitability can be **altered by various factors** like concentrations of ***ions and hormones***, and most importantly the ***state of autonomic activity*** i. e., the sympathetic and parasympathetic tones.
- **Sympathetic stimulation has positive bathmotropic** (increased excitability) effects and ***vagal stimulation has negative bathmotropic*** (decreased excitability) effects.

Distensibility

This is the ability to stretch. This occurs due to the property of **compliance (stretchability)** of the cardiac muscle.

- This property helps in **adequate filling** of atrial and ventricular chambers during their respective diastole.
- Ventricular distensibility decreases due to increased stiffness of cardiac muscles as occurs in cardiomyopathy and infiltrative diseases.
  - This **decreases end-diastolic volume**, which in turn decreases stoke volume.

Long Refractory Period

The **action potential of ventricular muscle** has a long refractory period.

Definition of Refractory Period: This is the period during which muscle ***does not evoke a response no matter how strong is the stimulus***.

Types and Duration: The refractory period is divided into **absolute and relative refractory periods.**

- The **absolute refractory period** of ventricular muscle is about 200 ms, and the **relative refractory period** is about 50 ms.

Difference in cardiac and skeletal muscles: An important difference exists in the **duration of action potential of cardiac and skeletal muscles.**

- Duration of action potential of **cardiac muscle is 250 ms,** which is almost same as the duration of the mechanical response.
- In **skeletal muscle,** the duration of action potential is maximum **about 5 ms,** which is much less than the duration of mechanical response.

In Ventricular Muscle

In ventricular muscle, as the duration of action potential is almost same as the duration of its mechanical response, the **refractory period extends to the most part of the mechanical response** (Fig 28.2B).

- Therefore, in cardiac tissues, always a ***new action potential generates a fresh mechanical response.***
- Consequently, a *fresh contraction cannot occur* before the completion of the previous mechanical response.
- Thus, ***mechanical responses of ventricular muscle cannot be merged,*** and therefore **cardiac muscle cannot be tetanized** (Application Box 28.1).

In Skeletal Muscle: In skeletal muscle, **mechanical responses can be merged,** and muscle can be tetanized, as the duration of action potential is much shorter than the duration of mechanical contraction (Fig 28.2A).

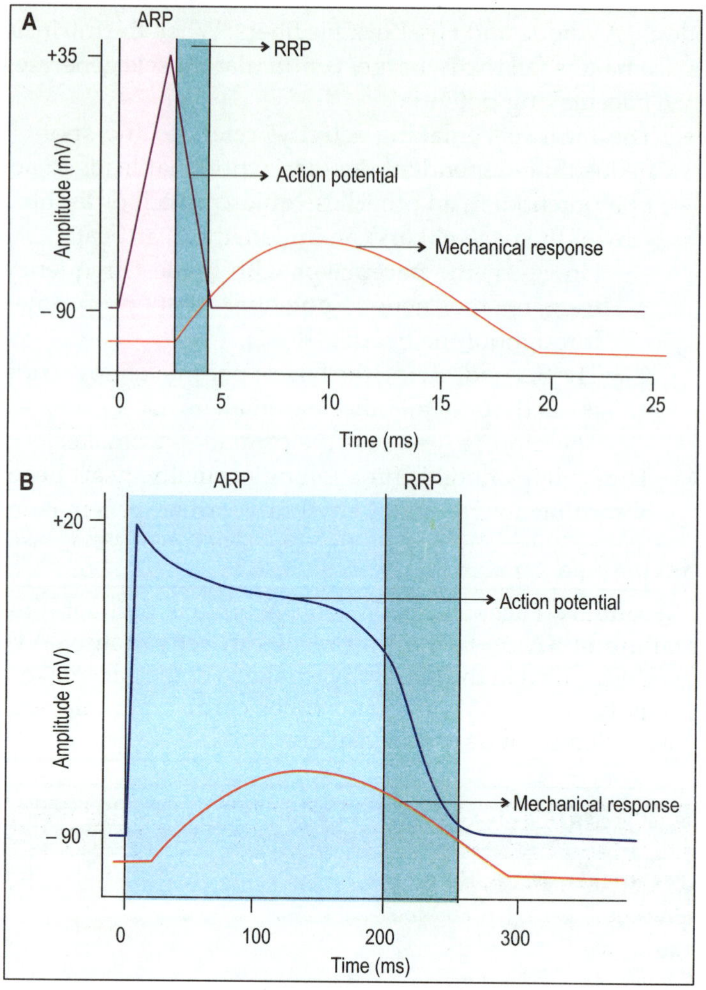

Fig. 28.2: Relationship between electrical and mechanical responses in cardiac **(B)** and skeletal **(A)** muscles. Note, in cardiac muscle, due to long refractory period, a greater part of the mechanical response falls in the absolute refractory period (ARP) of the action potential, whereas in skeletal muscle, the mechanical response starts almost after the ARP. Therefore, skeletal muscle can be tetanized, but not the cardiac muscle. RRP: relative refractory period.

Application Box 28.1

Long refractory period is very useful: Long refractory period is a unique property of the cardiac muscle that provides safety to the heart as it prevents tetanization of heart muscle.

Functional Syncytium

Cardiac muscle is a functional syncytium due to the presence of **numerous gap junctions.**

- Therefore, all muscle fibers contract almost simultaneously.
- There are two syncytia in heart: **atrial and ventricular syncytia** (details are given in previous chapter).

Extrasystole & Compensatory Pause

Extrasystole

When a sufficiently **stronger stimulus is applied in the relative refractory period** in an experimental recording of normal cardiogram, an ***extra contractile response*** occurs. This is called *extrasystole*. This ***contraction occurs earlier*** than the normally expected one (Fig. 28.3).

- **Extrasystole** is not uncommon in real life, and it may not be always pathological.
- Usually, the extra-stimulus arises from an ectopic focus in the ventricle.

Compensatory Pause

The natural stimulus (impulse arising from the SA node) **falls in the refractory period of the extrasystole** and does not evoke a response.

- Therefore, the natural contraction is missed.
- Hence, **a long pause** is recorded following the extrasystole, which is called **compensatory pause** (Fig. 28.3).
- Post-Extrasystolic Potentiation: The **magnitude of contraction** following the compensatory pause is **usually a higher one** as the ventricle gets more time for filling during the pause.
- The ***increased end-diastolic volume*** increases the force of contraction by Frank-Starling mechanism.
    - This is called **post-extrasystolic potentiation** (PEP).
- PEP can also occur ***independent of ventricular filling.***

- PEP may be an intrinsic mechanism of the heart that occurs due to **accumulation of more amount of calcium ions** in the myocardial cell during the compensatory pause.

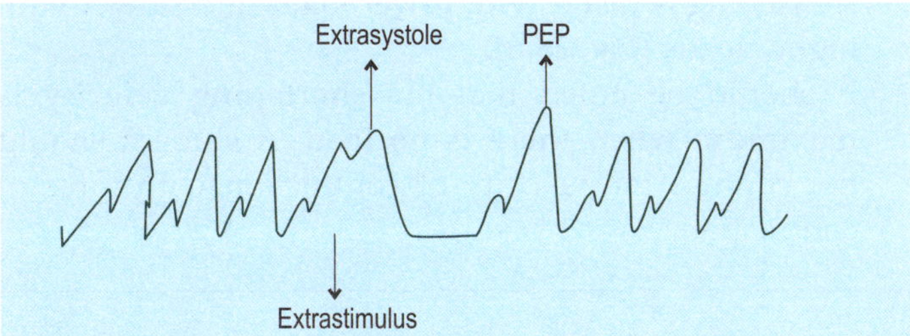

Fig. 28.3: Demonstration of extrasystole in a normal cardiogram of frog. CP: compensatory pause; PEP: post-extrasystolic potentiation.

All or None Law

Heart muscle follows all or none law.

Definition: All or none law states that the **magnitude of response of a tissue to stimuli remains same irrespective of the strength of stimuli.** That means, if the tissue responds, it responds optimally or it does not respond at all.

- When the stimulus is of **subthreshold strength**, the muscle does not respond to it at all, and if the stimulus is of **threshold intensity**, the muscle exhibits the optimum response.
- The **height of contraction does not increase** following the application of **suprathreshold stimulus** (Fig. 28.4). This is called all or none law.

Mechanisms: All or none law occurs due to **two reasons**:

i) All or none nature of the **action potential**

ii) **Syncytial nature** of the heart muscle, which behaves as a single functional unit.

Environment should not change: All or none law is applicable only when the conditions (**both internal and external environment) remain same.**

- The response will change if the condition is changed.
  - For example, if heart is stimulated following the sympathetic activation, the magnitude of contraction increases.
  - In this case, the ***excitability and contractility of the heart is changed*** by sympathetic stimulation and therefore the change in magnitude of contraction.

Staircase Phenomenon

Concept: If a quiescent heart (following application of second Stannius ligature) is stimulated repeatedly keeping the interval between the stimuli just less than 10 s, the **magnitude of first 3–4 contractions progressively increases** (Fig. 28.5). This is called staircase phenomenon.

- It appears that the staircase phenomenon violates the principle of all or none law, but in fact it is not so, because each stimulus alters the condition for the next stimulus.

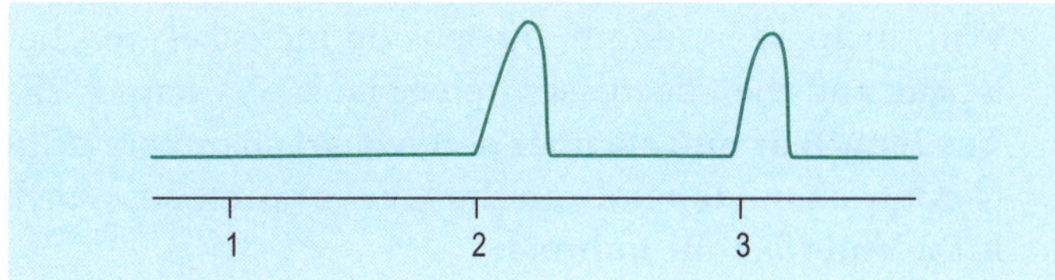

Fig. 28.4: Demonstration of all or none law in heart muscle of frog. 1: subthreshold stimulus; 2: threshold stimulus; 3: suprathreshold stimulus. Note, subthreshold stimulus does not evoke a response and suprathreshold stimulus does not change the height of contraction.

Mechanisms: There are **three mechanisms** of staircase phenomenon:

1. The amount of **calcium ion released** during each contraction is **not completely pumped back** into the sarcoplasmic reticulum as the second stimulus is applied within 10 s.
   - Therefore, some ***residual amount of calcium is left*** prior to the next stimulus.
   - This **increases the quantity of calcium available** to the contractile machinery in the next stimulus (the calcium left in the previous contraction plus the calcium released by the present stimulus).
   - Therefore, the second stimulus evokes a bigger response. Similarly, subsequent 2 to 3 stimuli progressively increase the magnitude of contraction.
2. During the first contraction, the **temperature in the myocardial cells increases** which ***enhances the enzymatic activity*** for the muscle contraction.
   - Therefore, the second stimulus acts under the **beneficial effect of increased enzymatic activity** of the first one.
   - Similarly, few subsequent stimuli progressively increase the height of contraction.
3. The first contraction **decreases the viscosity** of the sarcoplasm due to increased temperature.
   - Thus, the resistance provided by the sarcoplasm for the second and subsequent contractions is significantly lower than the first one.
   - This increases the magnitude of few subsequent contractions.

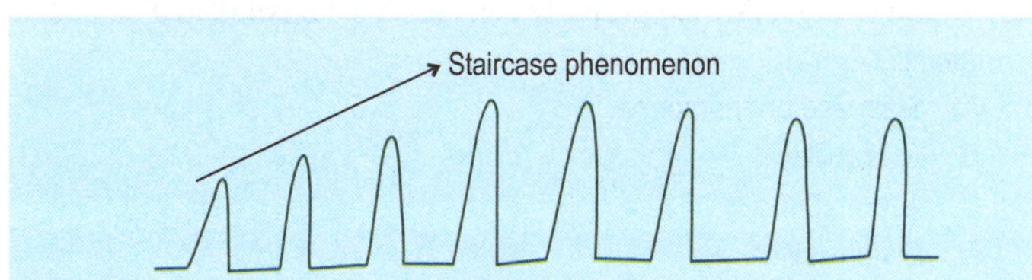

Fig. 28.5: Demonstration of staircase phenomenon in heart muscle of frog. Note, gradual increase in the height of tracings for first four contractions, which then remains same for subsequent contractions.

Length -Tension Relationship

The force of contraction is **directly proportional to the initial length** (the length of the muscle fiber prior to the contraction) of the muscle fiber, within the physiological limit, which is known as the **Frank-Starlings Law of the heart.**

- With increase in length, the tension increases, reaches a peak and then decreases (refer Fig. 27.7, Chapter 27).
- The **length of muscle fiber** of the heart chambers prior to contraction **depends on the level of preload**, which is the **enddiastolic volume**.
  - Thus, as the ventricular filling increases (the increase in end-diastolic volume), the stroke volume increases.
- This is called **heterometric autoregulation** of cardiac output.

Frequency-Force Relationship

Increase in force of contraction due to increase in heart rate (frequency) is known as frequency-force relationship.

- This is known as Bowditch phenomenon as described by H. P. Bowditch (1840-1991).
- However, increase in myocardial performance is restricted to a limited increase in frequency.

Load-Velocity Relationship

The relationship of **velocity of shortening to the load imparted on muscle** with which the muscle contracts, is called the load-velocity relationship.

1. The velocity of contraction is **inversely proportional** with the load that acts against it.
2. The velocity of muscle shortening, or contraction decreases with increasing afterload. That means, shortening is **faster with lower loads** and slower with higher loads (Fig. 28.6).
3. It should be noted that the **shortening velocity is maximum when there is no load**. A student should not confuse the velocity of contraction with force of contraction.

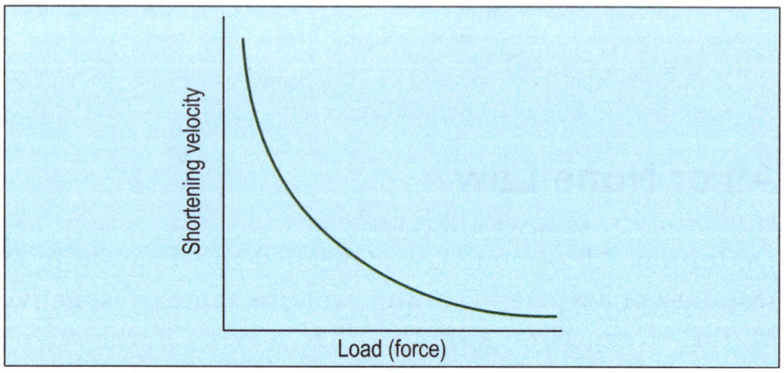

Fig. 28.6: Relationship of load with velocity of contraction. As afterload increases the velocity of shortening of cardiac muscle fiber decreases. A similar relationship exists in skeletal muscle.

Exam Questions

1. Describe the properties of cardiac muscle.
2. Name the six important properties of cardiac muscle. Explain why cardiac muscle cannot be tetanized.
3. What is the rate of discharge of cardiac pacemakers? How can the hierarchy of pacemakers be demonstrated in the cardiac tissue?
4. How do the cardiac muscle act as functional syncytium? Briefly explain the physiological significance of it.
5. Define extrasystole. What is the cause of compensatory pause? What is the physiologic significance of post-extrasystolic potentiation?
6. Explain the length-tension relationship, frequency-force relationship, and load-velocity relationship in cardiac muscle.

Multiple Choice Questions

1. **Cardiac muscle cannot be tetanized because:**
   A. Cardiac muscle has a rich blood supply
   B. Heart has abundantly supplied by sympathetic and vagal fibers
   C. Its absolute refractory period is longer
   D. It has high myoglobin content
2. **Which of the following property can ideally be studied in a quiescent heart?**
   A. Staircase phenomenon
   B. Excitability
   C. Autorhythmicity
   D. Distensibility
3. **Afterload causes:**
   A. Partial contraction of contractile element (CE) of the muscle with stretching of series- elastic elements (SEE)
   B. Partial contraction of CE of the muscle without stretching of SEE
   C. Complete contraction of CE of the muscle without stretching of SEE
   D. Complete contraction of CE of the muscle with stretching of SEE
4. **For cardiac muscle, velocity of shortening of the muscle (Vmax) can be used as a measure of:**
   A. Conductivity
   B. Rhythmicity
   C. Excitability
   D. Contractility
5. **Under basal conditions, caloric need of heart is largely met by:**
   A. Protein
   B. Fatty acids
   C. Ketone bodies
   D. Carbohydrates
6. **All of the following are true of extrasystole, EXCEPT;**
   A. It is an extra contraction of the ventricle due to sympathetic overdrive
   B. The long pause following the extrasystole is known as compensatory pause
   C. Following compensatory pause, ampliitude of contraction is greater
   D. It is elicited by a stronger stimulus applied in relative refractory period

Answers

1. C 2. A 3. D 4. D 5. B 6. A

Chapter 29

Electrophysiology of the Heart, and Origin and Propagation of Cardiac Impulse

Learning Objectives

On completion of study of this chapter:

The student will be able to (must know):

1. Draw the labeled diagrams of fast and slow response action potentials and give their ionic basis.
2. Draw a levelled diagram of pacemaker potential and give the ionic basis of it.
3. Explain the effects of sympathetic and vagal stimulation on pacemaker potential.
4. Appreciate the spread of impulse in conducting system of the heart.

The student may also be able to (desirable to know):

1. Describe the electrical properties of the cardiac muscle.
2. Describe the fast and slow response action potentials of cardiac tissues.

The **resting membrane potential** (RMP) of the **cardiac muscle fiber is –90 mV** and of Purkinje fibers is –95 mV. The RMP of pacemaker tissues is about –60 mV.

- There are **many ionic currents** in different cardiac tissues.
- The ionic currents are due to the ***presence of various ion channels*** in the cell membrane.
- Many ionic currents interact and combine uniquely to produce action potentials in cardiac tissues.

IONIC CURRENTS IN CARDIAC TISSUES

There are **four major types** of ionic currents in cardiac tissues: the sodium current, calcium current, potassium currents and pacemaker current. Functions of these currents are summarized in Table 29.1.

Pacemaker Current (I_f)

The pacemaker current (I_f) is found in SA and AV nodal cells.

- The channel underlying this current is a **nonspecific cation channel** called **HCN** (Hyperpolarization-activated Cyclic Nucleotide-gated) channel.
- **HCN channels** conduct **both Na^+ and K^+**.
    - Therefore, the reversal potential of I_f is about –20 mV, between the Nernst potentials for K^+ (about –90 mV) and Na^+ (about +60 mV).
- The HCN channels have the **funny property** (hence called **'f' channel**) such that they do not conduct at positive potentials, but their activation is slow (100 ms), and the current does not inactivate.
    - Thus, I_f produces an **inward, depolarizing current** as it is slowly activated at the end of phase 3.
- These channels are also known as **'h' channels** (I_h) as they are activated following hyperpolarization.
- I_f contributes to **pacemaker potential**.

Table 29.1 | Major membrane currents in cardiac tissues.

Current	Type of channels involved	Functions
I_{Na}	Voltage-gated Na^+ channel	Produces Phase 0 of fast response action potential (FRAP)
I_{CaL}	L-type Ca^{2+} channel	Produces Phase 2 of FRAP Produces Phase 0 of slow response action potential (SRAP)
I_{CaT}	T-type Ca^{2+} channel	Contributes to later part of pacemaker potential
I_{Kr}	Inward rectifying K^+ channels	Maintains RMP (phase 4) of cardiac muscle cells
I_{TO}	Outward transient rectifying K^+ channels	Contributes partially to phase 1 of FRAP
I_{Ks}	Outward delayed rectifying K^+ channels	Produces Phase 3 of FRAP Produces Phase 3 of SRAP Contributes to early part of prepotential by its closure
I_{KG}	G protein activated K^+ channels	Hyperpolarization of membrane in phase 4 of FRAP & SRAP

Table 29.1: Contd...		
I_{KATP}	ATP sensitive K^+ channels	Play role in electrically regulated contracting behaviour
I_f	Mixed cation channel for both Na^+ & K^+	Contributes to pacemaker potential

Note: FRAP occurs in atrial and ventricular muscles and Purkinje fibers, and SRAP occurs in SA and AV nodes. However, in SA and AV nodal cells, I_K and I_{CaT} contribute significantly **to the phase 4 depolarization** i. e., the prepotential or pacemaker potential.

PY5.2

ACTION POTENTIALS IN CARDIAC TISSUES

Normally, two types of action potentials are seen in the heart: the slow response action potential and the fast response action potential. Action potentials recorded from different tissues are depicted in Fig. 29.1.

Fast Response Action Potential

Fast response type of action potential is recorded from **atrial and ventricular muscles and Purkinje fibers**.

Phases and Ionic Basis

Typically, **five phases** (phases 0-4) are observed in a fast response action potential as recorded from ventricular muscle fibers (Fig. 29.2).

Phase 0

This is the **phase of rapid depolarization and overshoot**.

- As soon as the membrane potential reaches threshold, rapid depolarization (a **steep rise in the spike**) occurs.
- This is due to **sudden increase in the permeability** of the membrane **to sodium ions**, which occurs due to hundredfold **opening of voltage-gated sodium channels.**
- The sodium ions **enter rapidly** into the myocardial cells.

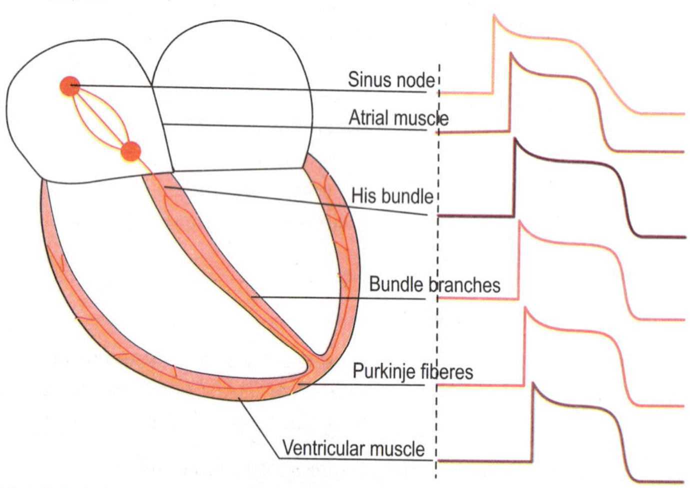

Fig. 29.1: Action potential in different tissues of the heart.

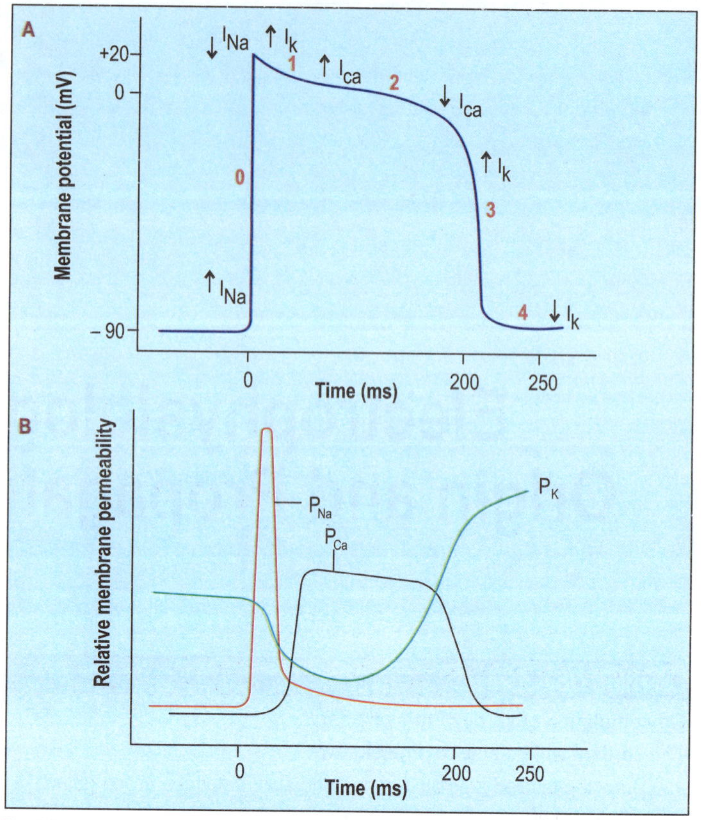

Fig. 29.2: Fast response action potential recorded from ventricular muscle fiber (A), and membrane permeability to different ions during various phases of the action potential (B). Phase 0: Phase of rapid depolarization and overshoot; Phase 1: Phase of initial rapid repolarization; Phase 2: Plateau phase; Phase 3: Phase of final repolarization; Phase 4: Phase of restoration of membrane potential; P_{Na}: permeability to sodium; P_{Ca}: permeability to calcium; and P_K: permeability to potassium.

- In fact, immediately above the threshold level of the membrane potential, sodium channels that were activated initially activate other sodium channels (hence called, **autoactivation of sodium channels**) that results in **manifold opening of the channels.**

Phase 1

This is the **phase of initial rapid repolarization.**

- This phase of partial repolarization is due to **closure of sodium channels** (cessation of sodium influx).
- **Opening of** outward transient **rectifying K^+ channel** that causes transient outflux of K^+ also partly contributes.
- This K^+ current (I_{TO}) is activated by depolarization and is **rapidly inactivated.**

Phase 2

This is known as **plateau phase** as the action potential in this phase remains in a **state of sustained depolarization.**

- This phase is due to **sustained increased permeability** of the membrane to **calcium ions** (through slowly opening calcium channels) that results in **slow calcium influx**, which occurs due to **slower but prolonged opening of voltage-gated calcium channels.**

- **Efflux of potassium ions** contributes to sustained depolarization.
- The plateau phase is of much ***lesser duration in atrial muscle*** than the ventricular muscles.

Phase 3

This is the **phase of final repolarization.**

- This occurs due to **cessation of calcium influx** (*closure of calcium channels*) and increased membrane **permeability to potassium** (***increased potassium efflux***).
- This phase is mainly due to opening of **outward delayed rectifying K^+ channels** (I_{Ks}).

Phase 4

This is the **phase of restoration of membrane potential.**

- The membrane **permeability to K^+ is restored** towards resting value.
- Opening of **inward rectifying K^+ channels** (I_{Kr}) contributes to maintain the restored membrane potential.
- The relative **increase in permeability to K^+** drives the membrane potential towards the equilibrium potential.

Slow Response Action Potential

This type of action potential is seen in **nodal tissues** (SA and AV nodes), **AV junctional tissue, and ischemic or injured myocardium**.

Phases and Ionic Basis

Slow response action potential consists mainly of **three components** (Fig. 29.3): the **phase 0** (depolarization or slow rising upstroke), **phase 3** (phase of repolarization), and **phase 4** (phase of slow depolarization).

- Phase 1 and 2 are usually absent in this type of action potential.

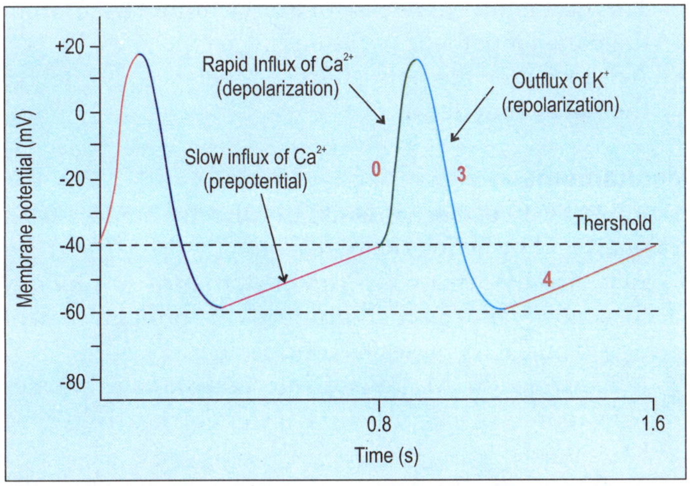

Fig. 29.3: Slow response action potential in cardiac tissues (SA node and AV node). Phase 0: Phase of depolarization; Phase 3: Phase of repolarization; and Phase 4: Phase of slow depolarization to threshold.

- In SA node in the phase 4, instead of restoration of the membrane potential, slow depolarization occurs.

Phase 0

It occurs due to the **opening of calcium channels**.

- This phase is **less steep** in comparison to fast response action potential.
- The depolarization is mainly due to **influx of calcium ions** through the long acting calcium channels (L-calcium channels).
- Therefore, depolarization wave rises slowly.

Phase 3

This phase is due to **closure of calcium channels & opening of the potassium channels** (increased potassium efflux).

Phase 4

This is the phase of **slow diastolic depolarization.**

1. **The early part** of this phase is due to the ***closure of potassium channels*** (decreased potassium conductance).
2. **Later part** is due to ***opening of transient calcium channels*** (T-calcium channels).
3. **Calcium sparks** (release of calcium locally from sarcoplasmic reticulum) also contributes.

Pacemaker Potential PY5.1

The pacemaker of the heart (SA node) discharges rhythmically and automatically.

- The automaticity (the ability of the pacemaker to produce its own impulse) is possible due to **spontaneous diastolic depolarization** of the membrane potential following completion of each action potential.
- The resting (diastolic) membrane potential that depolarizes is called as the **prepotential** as it brings the membrane potential to the threshold level, which then triggers the action potential.

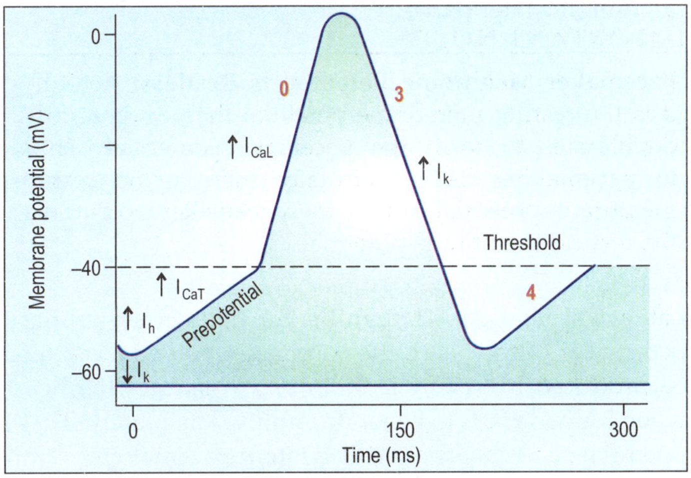

Fig. 29.4: Pacemaker potential. Note that the prepotential of the slow response action potential of SA node is the pacemaker potential.

- The **prepotential** is known as **pacemaker potential** (Fig 29.4).

Ionic Basis

Ionic basis of pacemaker potential has two important components: the ionic basis at initial part of the potential and at the ionic basis at the later part of the potential.

In the Initial Part

The repolarization phase of the action potential in the nodal tissues is due to **efflux of potassium ions**.

- At the peak of each action potential, potassium conductance (I_k) begins.
- Towards the end of repolarization, the I_k declines, which is known as **potassium decay**.
- At this moment, **'f' channels open** (I_f or I_h current) and I_h increases.
- These events allow membrane to depolarize.
- Thus, **K^+ decay and I_h contribute to the initial part of the pacemaker potential**.

In the Later Part

The later part of pacemaker potential is due to the **opening of transient calcium channels (I_{CaT})**.

- The entry of calcium through the T-channels *completes the pacemaker potential* and takes the membrane potential to the threshold level, which then fires to form the action potential.
- The **upstroke** of action potential occurs due to **opening of the long-lasting calcium channels** (I_{CaL}).

Other Ions

It is suggested that the **calcium sparks** (release of calcium locally from sarcoplasmic reticulum) also contribute to the pacemaker potential.

- Contribution of **sodium ion** is linked to the I_h.

Thus, the pacemaker potential is largely due to **decay of the potassium efflux** & I_h (the initial part), and **influx of calcium** (the later part).

IMPORTANT NOTE

Pacemaker Membrane Potential is Restless: Actually, it is the resting membrane potential that automatically depolarizes to form the pacemaker potential. Thus, in pacemaking tissues virtually there is no resting membrane potential, rather the pacemaker potential is the restless membrane potential.

Latent Pacemakers: Though the SA node is the primary pacemaker of the heart, the pacemaker potential can also be produced by ***AV node and other tissues*** of the heart when SA node fails to generate impulse adequately. These potential pacemakers are called **latent pacemakers**.

Rate of Impulse Generation: The rate of impulse generation depends on the ***slope of pacemaker potential***. Sympathetic and parasympathetic stimulation alters heart rate by altering the slope.

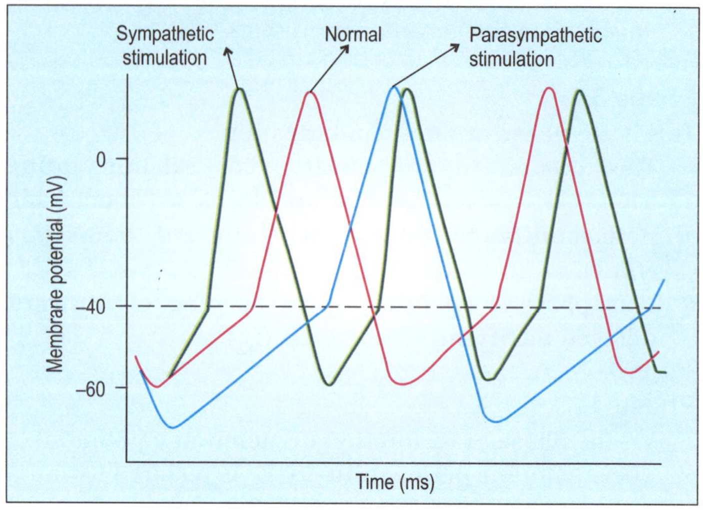

Fig. 29.5: Effects of sympathetic and parasympathetic stimulations on pacemaker potential. These effects on heart rate are mainly due to their influence on the slope of pacemaker potential. Note that sympathetic stimulation increases heart rate by rapidly raising the pacemaker potential so that the slope of prepotential reaches threshold earlier. Parasympathetic stimulation decreases heart rate by slowly raising the pacemaker potential so that slope of prepotential reaches threshold later. Also, parasympathetic stimulation causes hyperpolarization (makes the membrane potential more negative) so that prepotential takes more time to reach threshold from a more negative value. Also note, in the same time scale, the normal discharge pattern of SA node had produced two action potentials, whereas sympathetic stimulation resulted in three and parasympathetic stimulation produced only one action potential.

- **Parasympathetic (vagal) stimulation** makes the slope flat and decreases the heart rate.
- **Sympathetic stimulation** makes the slope steeper and increases the heart rate.

Effect of Vagal Stimulation

The vagal stimulation to the heart **decreases the heart rate**.

- The heart rate decreases because the **membrane is hyperpolarized** and the ***slope of prepotential is decreased*** *(becomes relatively flat)*.
- This occurs due to release of **acetylcholine** (Ach) from the parasympathetic nerve endings.
- Ach increases the potassium conductance and **delays the potassium decay**.

Mechanisms

Ach acts by **two mechanisms**, by directly acting on K^+ channels and by acting on M_2 receptors.

1. Ach directly acts on ***G Protein-Activated K^+ Channel*** (described above) that produces G protein current (I_{KG}). Thus, it increases K^+ conductance.
2. Ach acting on **M_2 muscarinic receptors** stimulates β-γ-subunits of a G protein, which in turn activates the K^+ channels.
   i) It **counters the decay of K^+** and hyperpolarizes the membrane during phase 4 that slows the pacemaker potential.

ii) Ach, also by acting on M_2 muscarinic receptors on the SA node **decreases the concentration of cyclic AMP** in the cells that in turn ***decreases the opening of calcium channels***.

- This **decreases calcium influx** via T-type calcium channels that decreases the slope of prepotential and takes the membrane potential away from threshold level (Fig. 29.5). Therefore, **heart rate decreases**.
- The decrease in intracellular calcium concentration also **decreases the force of contraction**. However, vagal stimulation mainly affects the rate rather than the force of contraction, because ventricles have sparse vagal innervation.

Effect of Sympathetic Stimulation

The sympathetic stimulation to the heart **increases the heart rate** and the **force of contraction**.

Mechanisms

The *slope of prepotential becomes steeper*, so that the **threshold level is reached earlier** than the normal, which increases the heart rate.

- This occurs due to **release of norepinephrine** at the sympathetic nerve endings.
- Norepinephrine binds to β_1 **receptors**, which **increases the intracellular cyclic AMP** that in turn increases the **opening of calcium channels** and causes calcium influx.
- The membrane is **rapidly depolarized** to the firing level and the depolarization phase of the action potential becomes steeper (Fig. 29.5). Thus, **heart rate increases**.
- The **increase in intracellular calcium ion** in the ventricular myocytes **increases the force of contraction**.

CONDUCTING SYSTEM OF HEART

The conducting system of the heart consists of SA node, internodal pathways, AV node, His bundle, bundle branches and Purkinje fibers (Fig. 29.6).

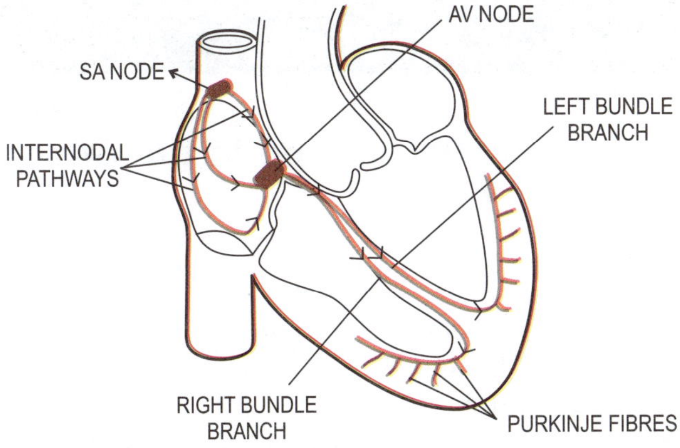

Fig. 29.6: Conducting system of the heart.

SA Node

The sinoatrial (SA) node is the **primary pacemaker** in mammalian heart.

- It is situated in the right atrium close to the opening of superior vena cava.
- It is about 1.5 cm long and 0.5 cm wide in human beings.
- It contains the **pacemaker (P) cells** and few myofilaments.
- The pacemaker cells generate the impulse, which is transmitted in the conducting system for excitation and contraction of heart muscles.
- The **action potentials** generated in SA node are of ***slow response type***.
- The **velocity of conduction** of impulse in SA node is **slow (0.05 m/s).**

Internodal Pathways

There are **three** internodal pathways that connect SA node and AV node (Fig. 29.6).

1. The anterior internodal pathway is called the **tract of Bachman**, the middle internodal pathway is called the **tract of Wenckebach**, and the posterior internodal pathway is called the **tract of Thorel**.
2. There may be few other accessory internodal pathways.
3. The internodal pathways merge into the AV node.
4. The **velocity of conduction** of impulse in internodal pathways is about **1 m/s.**
5. From SA node, a conducting tract arises and directly enters into the left atrium. This is called interatrial tract or **Bachman's bundle**.

AV Node

AV node is situated in the lower part of the right atrium close to the interatrial septum and just above the atrioventricular ring.

- It is 22 mm in length, 10 mm in width and 3 mm in thickness.
- In AV node, the **fiber diameter is small** and there are multiple sub-branches. Therefore, the ***rate of impulse conduction is slow*** in AV node (0.05 m/s).
- Usually, a **delay of about 0.1 second** occurs for the impulse to be transmitted through AV node. This is called **AV nodal delay**.
- This delay is **shortened by sympathetic stimulation** and **lengthened by parasympathetic stimulation** to the heart. The weak impulses may even die out in AV node.
- The ability of the AV node to slow down the transmission of rapid impulses from SA node to the ventricle is also called **decremental conduction** (Application Box 29.1).
- The action potentials generated in AV node are of ***slow response type***.

- Pacemaker **(P) cells** are also present in the AV node but normally AV node is not the pacemaker because the rate of impulse formation is lower in it than that of the SA node. The pacemaker cells of AV node are suppressed by the SA nodal impulses.
- However, when SA node stops producing impulses, AV node becomes the pacemaker of the heart.

Application Box 29.2

Decremental conduction is very useful: The property of AV node to slow down or block rapid impulses that arrive from SA node is the *decremental conduction*. It provides safety to the ventricles. When SA node discharges rapidly and all impulses are allowed to excite ventricles, extreme ventricular tachycardia interferes in ventricular performance. Therefore, nature has provided a safety factor in the form of decremental conduction to check the transmission of rapid impulses to ventricular muscles.

His Bundle

This is a small bundle of fibers that arises from AV node and terminates in the Purkinje system.

- This is situated below the AV node and passes towards the interventricular septum.
- As the fibers are present in the form of a bundle, this is called **bundle of His** (*not the bundle of Her*, as it was described by W. His in 1893).
- The **length of His bundle** is about 1 cm, which on entering the interventricular septum **divides** into right bundle branch and left bundle branch.
- When SA node and AV node are defunct, the bundle of His generates impulses.

Bundle Branches

His bundle **divides into right bundle branch** that conducts impulse to the right ventricle and **left bundle branch** that conducts impulse to the left ventricle.

- The bundle branches enter the ventricular walls and then branch out into very small bundle of fibers in the inner walls of the ventricular muscle.
- These fibers are termed as *Purkinje fibers*.
- Bundle branches also have the potentiality to generate impulses.

Right Bundle Branch (RBB)

RBB is longer and thinner than the left bundle branch. It exclusively supplies right ventricle.

Left Bundle Branch (LBB)

LBB bifurcates into two divisions: the **anterior division** that supplies the anterior portion of the left ventricle, and the **posterior division** that supplies the posterolateral portion of the left ventricle.

Purkinje Fibers

This is a network of small bundles of conducting fibers that are present throughout the sub-endocardial regions of right and left ventricles.

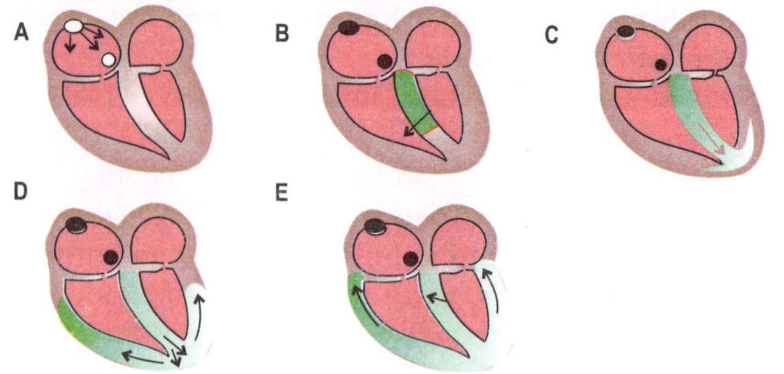

Fig. 29.7: Sequence of spread of electrical activity in cardiac tissues. **A:** atrial depolarization; **B:** Septal depolarization from left to right; **C:** Depolarization of anteroseptal region of myocardium towards apex; **D:** Ventricular depolarization from endocardium to epicardium; **E:** Depolarization of posterior portion of the base of left ventricle and depolarization of the pulmonary conus.

- The cells of the Purkinje system (are also called ***Purkinje cells***) are the **largest cells in the heart**.
- **Numerous gap junctions** (low impedance electrical synapses) are present between the cells.
- Because of the larger diameters of the fiber and presence of low impedance cell-to-cell connections, the **rate of impulse conduction is highest in the Purkinje fibers** (Table 29.2).
- The **conduction rate is almost 4 m/s**.
- The action potentials generated in the Purkinje fibers are of ***fast response type*** and resemble those produced in the ventricular muscles.

Table 29.2 | Conduction velocity in cardiac tissues.

Tissue	Conduction velocity (m/s)
SA node	0.05
Internodal pathways	1
AV node	0.05
His bundle	1
Purkinje fibers	4
Ventricular muscle	1

INITIATION & PROPAGATION OF CARDIAC IMPULSE

PY5.4

Excitation is initiated in the SA Node

Electrical activity in the heart is normally initiated in SA node and spreads in an orderly fashion (Fig. 29.7 A to E).

- The wave of depolarization **spreads in all directions**, to right and left atria directly and to the AV node via internodal pathways.
- However, impulse from atrial muscle cannot directly excite the ventricular muscle because the

atrioventricular ring, a fibrous and non-conductive connective tissue ring separates atria from the ventricles.

- Therefore, transmission of electrical activity from the atria to the ventricles occurs **only from AV node through the bundle of His.**

Conduction Slows in AV Node

For the impulse to excite all regions of the atria, it takes about 60 to 90 msec.

- Conduction of the impulse through the AV node occurs at a much slower velocity (0.05 m/sec).
- Thus, the transmission of impulse is delayed in the AV node for about 0.1 s. This is called the **AV nodal delay.**

The slower conduction velocity in AV node is due **to three factors**:

1. **Small size** of the nodal cells and their **branching patterns**.
2. **Slow upstroke** of the action potential, which occurs due to slow voltage-gated Ca^{2+} channels
3. **Weak electrical coupling** as a result of relatively few gap junctions.

Importance of AV Nodal Delay

There are many physiological and clinical importance of AV nodal delay, as given below:

1. **Allows Ventricular Filling:** Due to AV nodal delay, the **atrial depolarization completes much before** the beginning of ventricular depolarization.
    - Therefore, when atrial systole occurs, ventricle is in diastole. This helps in **ventricular filling to occur**.
    - Otherwise, atria and ventricles *would have contracted simultaneously* resulting in no ventricular filling.
    - Thus, normally the slow AV nodal conduction allows the ventricular filling to occur before the ventricles are excited.

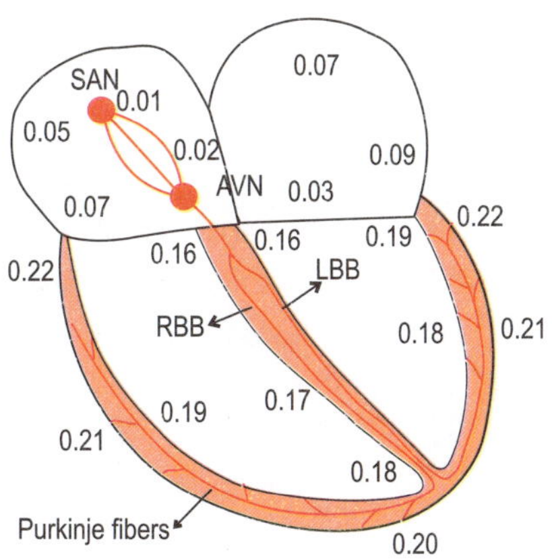

Fig. 29.8: Timing of excitation of different areas of heart by the impulse that originates from SA node (SAN), depicted in fraction of a second. AVN: AV node; LBB: left bundle branch; RBB: right bundle branch. Note, last to be excited are posterobasal portion of left ventricle, pulmonary conus & uppermost portion of septum.

2. **Maintains low ventricular rate in AF:** The slow AV nodal conduction is also beneficial in pathological situations in which rate of atrial depolarization is very high as occurs in **atrial fibrillation** (AF).
    - In such conditions, all the electrical impulses from atria cannot reach the ventricles because of inherent AV nodal delay.
    - Thus, ***ventricles contract at a lower rate than the atria***. This low ventricular rate is helpful as diastolic filling is not severely impaired.
3. **Effects of Drugs:** Many drugs such as digitalis, beta-blockers etc. reduce heart rate partly by promoting AV nodal delay.
4. **Vagal Stimulation:** Also, vagal stimulation causes AV nodal block.

Conduction is Rapid in Ventricles

The impulse spreads rapidly into the ventricular muscles via **His-Purkinje system** (the His bundle, the bundle branches and the Purkinje fibers).

- The Purkinje system is composed of *fibers with large diameter*. The ***slope of depolarization is also very steep*** (refer Fig. 29.1). Therefore, the **conduction velocity is maximum** in Purkinje fibers (4 m/s) in the heart.
    - The wave of depolarization takes about **0.08–0.1 s to spread rapidly** from the top of the septum through the Purkinje fibers to all part of the ventricles (Fig. 29.8).
- The depolarization of the ventricle **starts at the left side of the interventricular septum** and then crosses to the right side through the interventricular septum, and then spreads down to the apex of the heart (Fig. 29.7 B to D).
- Then it depolarizes the muscles in the wall of the ventricle **from endocardial to the epicardial surface**, proceeding from the apex towards the atrioventricular junction.
- In ventricles, the ***endocardial surface depolarizes before the epicardial surface***.
    - The **portions to be depolarized last** are the posterobasal portion of the left ventricle, the pulmonary conus, and the upper most portion of the septum.
- The process of **repolarization of ventricular muscle occurs almost in the reverse direction.**
    - That means, the *epicardial surface repolarizes first* and the septum and endocardial surface repolarize last.
- The conduction velocity through ventricular muscle is 1 m/sec.
    - The complete excitation of both ventricles takes about 75 msec.

- The **rapid and synchronous excitation** of the ventricles ensures almost simultaneous contraction of all ventricular muscles, which is essential for effective ventricular ejection of blood.

Exam Questions

1. With the help of a suitable diagram, describe the phases and ionic basis of ventricular muscle action potential.
2. With the help of a suitable diagram, describe the phases and ionic basis of action potential recorded from SA node.
3. With the help of a suitable diagram explain the mechanism of genesis of pacemaker potential. Briefly describe the effects of sympathetic and parasympathetic stimulation on pacemaker potential.
4. With the help of a schematic diagram, explain the initiation and propagation of cardiac impulse in conducting system of the heart.

Multiple Choice Questions

1. **AV nodal delay helps in:**
   A. Delayed closure of AV valves
   B. Increased ventricular muscle contractility
   C. Faster ventricular depolarization
   D. Adequate filling of ventricle
2. **Long plateau phase of action potential in myocardial fibers is due to:**
   A. Decreased Na^+ conductance
   B. Increased K^+ and Ca^{2+} conductance
   C. Decreased Cl^- conductance
   D. Decreased K^+ conductance
3. **Pacemaker potential is:**
   A. Also called spike potential
   B. Characteristic of atrial muscle fiber
   C. Characterized by unstable RMP
   D. Largely due to increased membrane permeability to K^+
4. **Ventricular repolarization:**
   A. Lasts for about 150 msec
   B. Has the rapid initial fall is due to Ca^{2+} efflux
   C. Starts after the absolute refractory period
   D. Occurs in three phases
5. **Fast response action potential is seen in:**
   A. Atrial muscle
   B. AV junctional tissues
   C. Injured or ischemic myocardium
   D. SA node
6. **Vagal stimulation decreases heart rate by all mechanisms EXCEPT:**
   A. Reducing K^+ conductance in nodal tissue
   B. Hyperpolarization of the membrane in Phase 4
   C. Opposing K^+ decay
   D. Reducing slope of prepotential
7. **The conduction velocity is highest in:**
   A. Ventricular muscle
   B. Purkinje system
   C. His bundle
   D. Internodal pathways
8. **The conduction velocity is lowest in:**
   A. His bundle
   B. SA node
   C. Ventricular muscle
   D. Internodal pathways
9. **Which of the following is NOT true for ventricle?**
   A. Repolarization occurs from epicardial surface to endocardial surface
   B. Depolarization starts at the left side of interventricular septum
   C. Endocardium depolarizes after epicardium
   D. Posterobasal portion gets depolarized in last part
10. **AV nodal delay is due to all EXCEPT:**
   A. More gap junctions in AV node
   B. More sub-branching of fibers in AV node
   C. Small size of AV nodal cells
   D. Slow upstroke of action potential of AV node
11. **Which of the following statement is true for slow response action potential?**
   A. Seen in ventricular muscle
   B. Opening of sodium channels contributes to Phase 0
   C. Opening of calcium channels contributes to Phase 3
   D. Closure of potassium channels contributes to Phase 4
12. **All of the following contribute to the ionic basis of prepotential, EXCEPT:**
   A. Opening of transient calcium channels
   B. Decreased Cl^- conductance
   C. Opening of funny channels
   D. Decreased K^+ conductance

Answers

1. D	**2. B**	**3. C**	**4. D**
5. A	**6. A**	**7. B**	**8. B**
9. C	**10. A**	**11. D**	**12. B**

Chapter 30

Electrocardiogram

Learning Objectives

On completion of study of this chapter:

The student will be able to (must know):

1. Define ECG & list the uses of ECG.
2. Classify ECG leads.
3. Draw a labeled diagram of Lead II ECG and identify the ECG waves, segments and intervals.
4. Define, give normal values & significance of various ECG waves, segments and intervals.
5. Say how the different ECG waveforms are produced.
6. Draw ECG tracings of normal 12 ECG leads.
7. Interpret normal ECG tracings and their physiological application.
8. Determine mean QRS axis, and list the common causes of left and right axis deviations.
9. Identify the ECG changes in arrhythmias, heart blocks, myocardial infarction & electrolyte imbalance.
10. Learn the basics of His bundle electrogram.

The student may also be able to (desirable to know):

1. Explain the mean cardiac vector and its application.
2. Interpret the abnormalities of ECG in different conditions.

Electrocardiogram (ECG) is defined as the ***graphic record of electrical activities of the heart*** obtained by placing electrodes on the surface of the body that records the voltage differences generated by the heart.

- Body is a **volume conductor**, i. e. body fluids are good conductor of electricity. Therefore, electrical changes occurring in the heart with each beat are conducted all over the body and can be picked up from the body surface.
- The **record of these electrical fluctuations during the cardiac cycle** is called electrocardiogram (ECG).
- Thus, ECG recorded at the body surface represents the **algebraic sum of the action potential** of the individual cardiac muscle fibers.

ECG is useful for assessing:

1. Anatomical orientation of the heart.
2. Relative size of the chambers.
3. Disturbances of rhythm and conduction.
4. Ischemia of the myocardium, if present.
5. The location, extent and progress of myocardial infarction.
6. The effects of altered electrolyte concentration.
7. The influence of certain drugs like digitalis.
8. Efficiency of electronic pacemaker function.

TECHNICAL ASPECTS

In modern electrocardiography, **two types of ECG machines** are used: (1) the string galvanometer, and (2) the radio-amplifier.

- ECG is recorded on ECG paper fitted in the machine.
- **ECG paper** is a strip of graph paper that contains ***vertical and horizontal lines*** 1 mm apart.
- The **horizontal axis represents time** whereas the **vertical axis denotes amplitude**.
- There is a heavy line every 5 mm in both the planes.
- Thus, there are **small squares** of 1 mm x 1 mm, and **big squares** of 5 mm x 5 mm. After every 5 big squares the heavy vertical line overshoots the margin.
- The ECG paper is a **heat sensitive plastic-coated paper**. The ECG is inscribed on this paper by a **hot stylus**.
- Conventional ECG is taken at a speed of 25 mm/s.
- One **small square** (1mm) corresponds to ***0.04 second***, while the **big square** (5 mm) is equivalent to ***0.20 second***.

ECG Leads

The ECG leads are of **two categories**: the direct and the indirect leads.

Direct Leads: When a lead is directly applied to the surface of the heart, is called as **direct lead.**

- These leads are used to record cardiac activities during open cardiac surgery.
- Also, used for recording ECG in experimental animals.

Indirect Leads: When the leads are applied away from the heart (usually on the body surface) to record the cardiac activities, they are called as **indirect leads.**

- Conventionally, ECG is recorded using indirect leads.
- Indirect leads are **limb leads, chest leads, and esophageal leads.**

Limb Leads

Limb leads lie in the **frontal plane.** These are of **two types:** the bipolar and the unipolar limb leads.

Bipolar Limb Leads

Three bipolar standard limb leads (**lead I, II, and III**) are the original leads selected by Einthoven to record electrical potential on the frontal plane.

- In the method of recording by bipolar leads, **two electrodes are placed on the body surface** and the *potential difference* between these two electrodes is recorded.
- **Electrodes** are attached to the *right arm, left arm, and left foot* as indicated in the Einthoven triangle (see below).
- Another electrode is applied to the right leg, which acts as a **ground wire** to prevent external disturbances during recording.

Lead I: Between the right arm (negative electrode) and the left arm (positive electrode).
Lead II: Between the right arm (negative electrode) and the left leg (positive electrode).
Lead III: Between the left arm (negative electrode) and the left leg (positive electrode).

Einthoven Triangle

Einthoven triangle is an **equilateral triangle** with each side representing the *axis of one of the bipolar limb leads.*

- It is an inverted triangle with apex pointing towards the groin and the base between two shoulders.
- As body is a volume conductor, electrical attachment to an arm is similar to the connection at the corresponding **shoulder joint,** and attachment to either leg is similar to the connection **at the groin.**
- **Heart** is considered to be present at the *center of Einthoven triangle.*
- Each corner of the triangle serves as the location for an electrode for two leads to the ECG recorder.
- Thus, **three limbs of the triangle represent three leads** (Fig. 30.1).

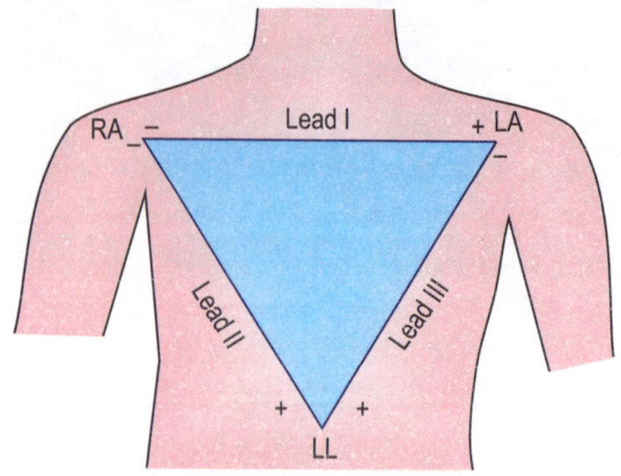

Fig. 30.1: Einthoven's triangle. The heart is considered to be at the center of the triangle. Each corner of the triangle serves as a location for electrode for two leads of the ECG recorder. RA: right arm; LA: left arm; LL: left leg.

Unipolar Limb Leads

In the method of recording by unipolar leads, one electrode is the **active or recording electrode** and the other one is the **indifferent electrode.**

- There are **three** unipolar limb leads: **aVR, aVL, and aVF.** In this, '**a**' stands for ***augmentation*** of the leads.
- The potential recorded in aVL is one and half times more than that recorded in VL, and similarly for aVR and aVF.
    - Therefore, these leads are called **augmented leads.**
    - '**V**' stands for unipolar, and **R, L, and F** indicate that the exploring or active electrode is on the right arm, left arm, and left foot respectively.
- The other electrode, i. e., the ***indifferent electrode*** is connected to the remaining two leads through a resistance coil.

aVR : Between the right arm (positive electrode) and left arm + left leg (negative electrode).
aVL : Between the left arm (positive electrode) and right arm + left leg (negative electrode).
aVF : Between the left foot (positive electrode) and right arm + left arm (negative electrode).
Vector of augmented limb lead = 3/2 vector of unaugmented limb lead.

$$aVR = VR - (VL + VF)/2$$
$$2aVR = 2VR - (VL + VF)$$

Since, VR + VL + VF = zero (Einthoven's triangle),

$$VR = -(VL + VF)$$
$$2aVR = 2VR + VR$$
$$aVR = 3/2VR$$

Chest Leads

Chest leads or **precordial leads** lie in the transverse plane. These are of **two types**: the unipolar and the bipolar chest leads.

Unipolar Chest Leads

There are **six precordial leads** that are used routinely. These are **V_1 to V_6** ('V' stands for unipolar).

- These leads employ an exploring electrode on the chest surface.

- The ***reference or indifferent electrode*** is connected to the right arm, left arm and left leg through the high resistance which is called **Wilson's terminal** that is maintained at zero potential.
- The right leg is connected with a ***grounding electrode*** to avoid electrical interference.

Position of Chest Electrodes:

V_1: In the right fourth intercostal space at the right border of the sternum.

V_2: In the left fourth intercostal space at the left border of the sternum.

V_3: At the midpoint between V_2 and V_4.

V_4: In the left fifth intercostal space on the midclavicular line.

V_5: In the left fifth intercostal space on the anterior axillary line.

V_6: In the left fifth intercostal space on the mid-axillary line.

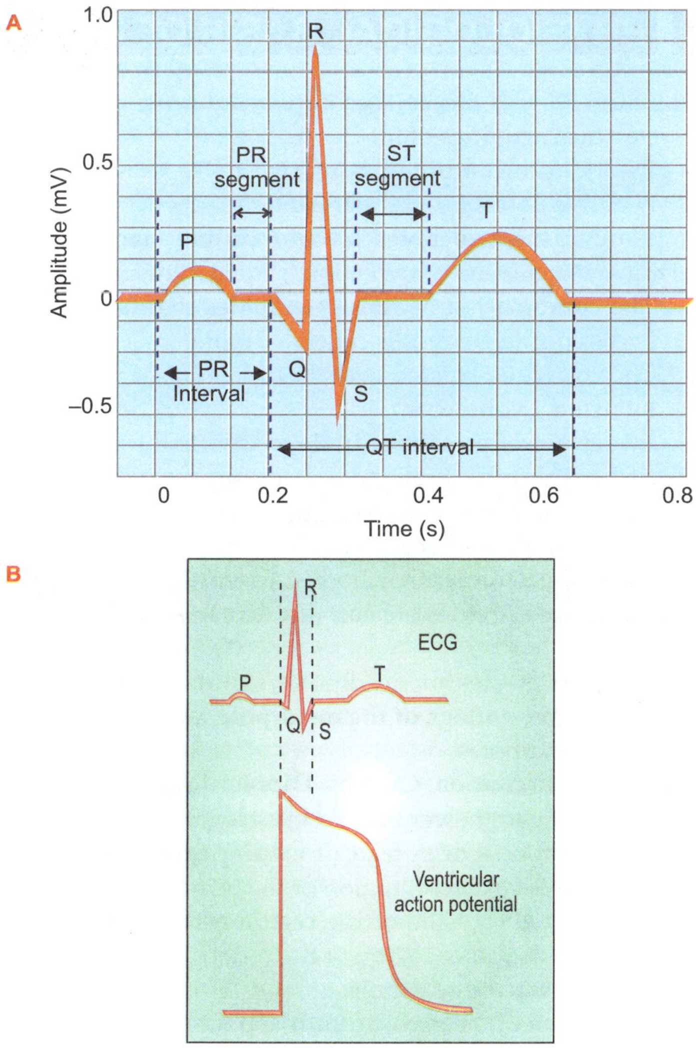

Fig. 30.2: Normal lead II ECG showing different waves, segments and intervals (A) and correlation of ECG with action potential of ventricular muscle (B). Note, QRS complex corresponds to ventricular depolarization.

Bipolar Chest Leads

These leads are used before the discovery of unipolar chest leads.

Lewis Lead: This is a special bipolar chest lead used for recording ECG in ***atrial arrhythmias***. This lead *amplifies the waves of atrial activity.*

Esophageal Leads

In these leads, an **electrode is fixed** on the tip of the **esophageal catheter**, which is positioned in the esophagus close to the heart chambers.

- The leads are designated as E_{18}, E_{20}, etc.
  - E stands for 'esophageal' and the number indicates the distance of the electrode from the incisor teeth expressed in centimeter.

E_{15-25}: Used for recording the activity of the right atrium.

E_{25-35}: Used for recording the activity from the AV groove region.

E_{40-50}: Used for recording the activity from the posterior surface of the left ventricle.

PY5.5

NORMAL ECG

The ECG tracing shows different **waves, segments and intervals** as depicted from a lead II tracing (Fig. 30.2A).

ECG Waves

Waves are positive or negative deflections from baseline. There are four waveforms: P wave, QRS complex, T and U waves.

P Wave

P wave is the ***first positive deflection*** in the ECG, produced by **atrial depolarization**.

QRS Complex

This consists of **Q, R, and S waves**. The QRS complex consists of deflections produced by **ventricular depolarization** (Fig. 30.2B).

Q wave: Is the initial negative deflection in the QRS complex.

R wave: Is the positive deflection in the QRS complex.

S wave: Is the second negative deflection in the QRS complex.

T Wave

T wave is the ***positive deflection***, produced by **ventricular repolarization**.

U Wave

U wave is the ***final positive deflection*** in the ECG.

- Normally, this wave is not always present.
- It occurs due to **slow repolarization of papillary muscle**.

ECG Segments

Segments are **isoelectric lines** in ECG tracing. There are **two segments**: PR segment and ST segment.

PR Segment

This lies between the end of the P wave and the beginning of the QRS complex.

ST Segment

This lies between the end of the QRS complex and the beginning of the T wave.

- The point where the QRS complex ends and the ST segment begins is the **J point.**
- **Elevation of J point** suggests myocardial ischemia or infarction.

ECG Intervals

Intervals usually include **waves and segments**.

PR Interval

Definition: This is the interval between the **beginning of the P wave to the beginning of the QRS complex**.

Normal Duration: The range of PR interval is from **0.12 to 0.20 second** (average 0.18 s).

- PR interval **shortens from 0.18s to 0.14s as the heart rate increases** from 70 to 130.

Significance: This represents **atrial depolarization and conduction through AV node**.

QRS Interval (QRS duration)

Definition: This is the interval of the QRS complex.

- It is measured from the beginning of the Q wave (or R wave if Q wave is absent) to the J point.

Normal Duration: The normal range is from **0.08 to 0.10 second**.

Significance: This represents **ventricular depolarization**. The atrial repolarization also occurs in this period.

QT Interval

Definition: This is the interval for QRS complex, ST segment and T wave. It is measured from the beginning of the QRS complex to the end of the T wave.

Normal Duration: The normal range is between **0.40 to 0.43 second**.

Significance: This represents **ventricular depolarization and ventricular repolarization**.

- It corresponds to the duration of *electrical systole*.

ST Interval

Definition: This is the interval between the J point and the end of T wave.

- It is calculated by deducting QRS interval from QT interval.

Normal Duration: The average duration is **0.32 second**.

Significance: This represents **ventricular repolarization**.

PP Interval

This is the interval measured between either the peak or the beginning of **two successive P waves**.

- PP interval is measured for calculation of the atrial rate.

RR Interval

This is the interval between **two successive R waves**.

- It is measured between the peaks of **two successive R waves**.
- RR interval is measured for calculating the heart rate (the **ventricular rate**).
- RR interval is used for assessment of **heart rate variability** (HRV).

PHYSIOLOGICAL BASIS OF ECG

The ECG records the **voltage between dipoles** produced by electrical activities of the heart.

- Diploes are **combination of two poles** (positive and negative poles) in an **electrical field**.
- Though the **two poles have opposite charges**, they have the currents (flow of ions) equal in magnitude.
- The **combination of these two poles** that have equal and opposite charges is called a **dipole**.
- The voltage associated with the dipole can be measured by using a **voltmeter**.
- In fact, **direction of the dipole** relative to the electrodes and **magnitude (voltage) of the dipole** are the two important factors that affect the recording in voltmeter.
- Thus, **dipole also acts a vector**.

Heart as the Dipole: Our body is a **volume conductor**, and electrical activities of heart create **many dipoles** in the body.

- As heart creates many dipoles simultaneously, **ECG records the voltage of the net dipole**, which is average of all the dipoles.

Spread of Excitation Creates Dipole: Impulse spreads from SA node to the ventricular muscle.

- In this **process of spread of cardiac excitation**, when the impulse excites a region of the heart, ***that region is depolarized*** (outside of the region becomes negative) ahead of the other region of the heart.
- This **generates the dipole**.
- The region of the myocardium depolarized constitutes the **negative pole** and the region ahead of it (yet to be depolarized) constitutes the **positive pole**.
- Likewise, with natural spread of excitation, the **dipole shifts** *from one region to the other*.

- So, heart contains the dipole and the body is the volume conductor.

- The **electrode** located on the volume conductor (on the surface of the body) **records the voltage resulting from the dipole**, which is generated by electrical activity of the heart.

Why has ECG Various Waveforms?

In the myocardium, **many dipoles are formed** as the propagated impulse spreads to various parts of the ventricle (or of the heart) at a time by different branches of the conducting system.

- Thus, **many dipoles are created simultaneously** in the heart.
- The voltage of the **net dipole** (average of many individual dipoles at any given time) is recorded in the voltmeter (electrocardiographic recorder), which is connected to the two points of the volume conductor.

Recording of Lead II ECG

Let us consider the recoding of lead II that records electrical activity between right arm (point B) and left leg (point A) (Fig. 30.3).

- According to the principle of electrophysiology, when point **A is positive** in relation to point B, the ECG ***deflection is upward***, and when **A is negative** in relation to B, the ***deflection is downward***.
    - **Magnitude (strength) of voltage** is indicated by the ***length of the net dipole***.
- When the **net dipole is parallel** to the line AB, the magnitude (strength of voltage) ***is maximal*** and when **it is perpendicular**, ***magnitude is zero***.
- Thus, the magnitude recorded by the electrocardiographic recorder depends on the **direction of the net dipole**, and **the muscle mass of heart** involved in generating the net dipole.
- Accordingly, various **positive & negative deflections** of various magnitudes or **isoelectric lines** are produced in the ECG recordings for various leads ***depending on the position of electrodes*** on the body that records the potential difference at a given instant.

For lead II ECG recording that records the voltage difference between point B (right arm) and point A (left leg), the **following ECG waves** are generated (Fig. 30.3).

P Wave

P wave represents **atrial depolarization.**

- The **magnitude** of the net dipole is proportionate to the **atrial muscle mass and direction of depolarization**.
- Point A is positive in relation to point B that results in an ***upward or positive deflection*** of the ECG (Fig. 30.3-I).
- Thus, the voltage change due to atrial depolarization appears on the ECG as the **P wave**, which is a **positive wave with less height & dome shape**.
    - The **height of P wave is less** because of *less atrial muscle mass* and **dome shape** is due to the *slow nature of depolarization* of atrial muscle.

PR Interval

The PR interval includes the **P wave and PR segment**.

- During PR segment, the wave of depolarization passes **slowly through AV node** and **His bundle.**
- The **net dipole** created by depolarization of these structures **is too small in magnitude** to produce any deflection on the ECG recording.
    - Thus, PR segment is an **isoelectric line.**

QRS Complex

The QRS complex represents **ventricular depolarization**. It consists of **three waves:** Q wave, R wave and S wave.

Q wave: The wave of depolarization passes along the **bundle branches, and Purkinje fibers** to first excite the **interventricular septum**, which depolarizes *from left to right*.

- Thus, Point A becomes negative in relation to point B that results in a **negative wave** (Fig. 30.3-II).
- Therefore, the net dipole of initial depolarization manifests in ECG as Q wave, which is a **small downward sharp wave**.

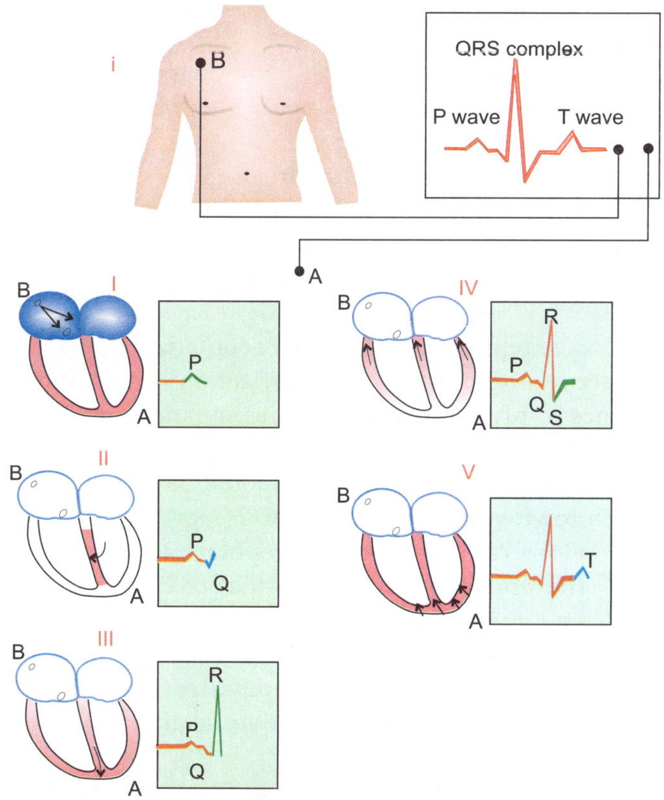

Fig. 30.3: Lead II ECG recording by connecting electrodes that record voltage difference between point B on right arm and point A on left leg (30.3i). Figures 30.3I to 30.3V explain the deflection of ECG waves when sequential depolarization and repolarization occurs in the heart during a cardiac cycle. Note, magnitude and type of (positive or negative) deflection depends on the muscle mass activated and the direction of activation.

- The **small wave** is due to ***less quantity of septal muscle & less time of depolarization*** and **sharpness** is due to the *rapidity of depolarization.*

R wave: The wave of depolarization then spreads from the **sub-endocardial muscle layer to sub-epicardial muscle layer.**

- The ventricular **muscle mass is more,** and the left ventricle is much thicker than the right ventricle.
    - Therefore, the direction and amplitude of the net dipole during this phase is such that point A becomes positive in relation to point B (Fig. 30.3-III; note the bigger length of the arrow, which indicates the magnitude of the dipole).
- The deflection in the ECG appears as R wave, which is **an upward, bigger and sharp wave.**
- The R is **largest wave** in ECG because of the ***greater muscle mass of ventricles.***
- The **sharpness of the wave** represents the ***rapidity of depolarization.***

S wave: The last parts to be depolarized are the **posterobasal portion of left ventricle** and the **pulmonary conus.**

- The direction and duration of depolarization is such that the net dipole has direction with the Point A negative in comparison to point B (Fig. 30.3-IV).
- This appears in ECG as a small downward wave.
- Thus, the S wave is a **small, negative and sharp wave.**

ST Segment

As soon as the ventricular depolarization is completed, all dipoles associated with it disappear and the ECG tracing returns to baseline.

- The ST segment is **an isoelectric line.**
- This indicates that in this phase dipoles are not adequate enough to create any wave in ECG.

T Wave

The T wave represents **ventricular repolarization.**

- Elecrtrophysiologically, repolarization is an **opposite process of depolarization** and repolarization also creates dipoles like that of depolarization.
    - Therefore, repolarization should have produced a downward deflection in ECG.
    - However, **the process of repolarization occurs in the opposite direction** to that of depolarization, i.e., from epicardial to endocardial surface of the ventricular muscle.
- Thus, **sub-epicardial cells repolarize first**, and the sub-epicardium becomes positive relative to the sub-endocardium.
- Therefore, the polarity of the net dipole of repolarization is the **same as the polarity of the dipole of depolarization.**
    - This results in an **upward deflection** in ECG, point A being positive with respect to point B (Fig. 30.3-V).
- This appears in ECG as T wave, which is a **dome shaped positive wave of longer duration.**
    - This indicates that *repolarization is slower than depolarization.*

Cardiac Dipoles as Vectors

As described above, **cardiac dipoles act as vectors** in both direction and magnitude. The net vector (average vector of all cardiac dipoles) can be determined from the ECG recording.

- The **direction of the vectors** is determined from the ECG recorded from leads placed in frontal and horizontal planes of the body.
    - Three **bipolar limb leads** (leads I, II, and III) and **three augmented limb leads** (aVR, aVL, and aVF) give information ***in the frontal plane*** of the body.
- The lead I records the potential differences between the left and right arms and records the electrical vector that is parallel to its axis.
    - The **axis of lead I** passes as a horizontal line through the center of the chest from right to the left arm (Fig. 30.4).
    - Similarly, the **axis of lead II** passes as a 60° line with negative end from right arm to the positive end towards left leg, and **lead III** as a 120° line from left arm to left leg (positive end).
- The **axes of augmented limb leads are interspersed** between the bipolar limb leads as shown in the figure.
    - Thus, the picture of the axis of leads in the frontal plane is called the **hexaxial reference system.**

i) When the net cardiac dipole with its positive charge is directed towards the positive end of the axis of a lead, **upward deflection** occurs in the recording.

ii) If the net cardiac dipole with its positive charge is directed towards the negative end of the axis of a lead, **downward deflection** occurs.

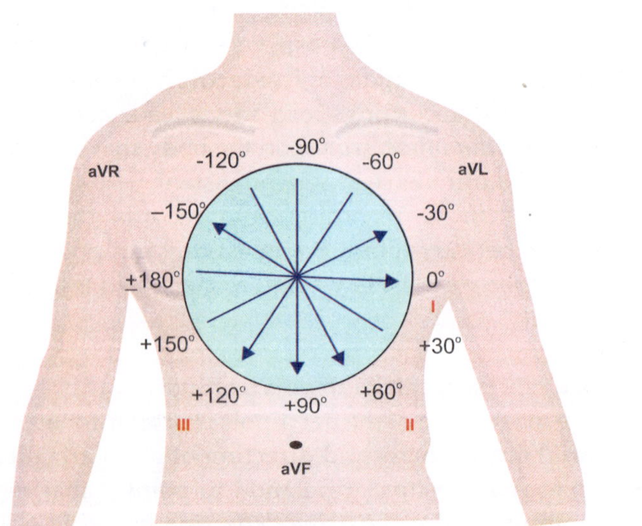

Fig. 30.4: Hexaxial reference system. Six frontal leads pass through the common point providing the views of the heart at 30 degree intervals.

iii) **No deflection occurs**, if positive charge of net cardiac dipole is directed at right angle to the axis of a lead.

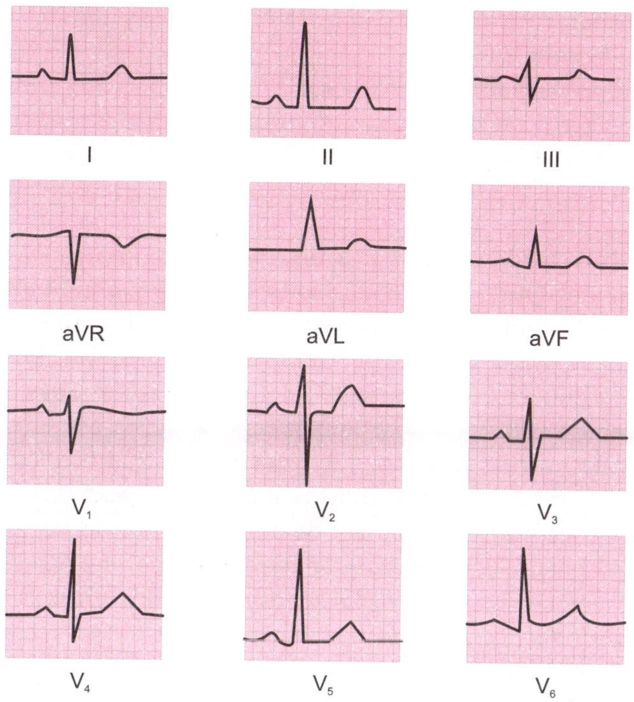

Fig. 30.5: Recoding of normal 12 lead ECG.

This helps us to understand ECG changes in various leads in health and diseases.

Normal 12 Lead ECG

Normally, recording of 12 leads (Fig. 30.5) is considered for complete analysis and interpretation of ECG. The deflection of waves in a particular lead is governed by the basic law of dipole, as described above.

- The **positive or upward deflection** is seen in any lead, if depolarization spreads towards the positive pole of that lead, and a **negative or a downward deflection** is seen in any lead, if depolarization spreads towards the negative pole of that lead.
  - An **isoelectric or biphasic deflection** is seen when the depolarization starts in SA node and spreads downward to the subject's left (towards the positive pole of lead I and away from positive pole of the lead aVR).
- The **P wave is always positive** in lead II and **negative** in lead aVR.
- Ventricular septum depolarizes from left to right (towards lead V_1 and away from lead V_6).
  - This produces small 'q' wave (**septal q wave**) in V_6 and small 'r' wave (**septal r wave**) in lead V_1.
- During ventricular depolarization as the left ventricular mass is more than right ventricular mass; the **net direction of depolarization is towards the left chest leads** (Fig. 30.6).
  - This produces **tall 'R' wave** in leads V_5 and V_6, and a **deep S wave** in leads V_1 and V_2.
  - Chest leads between these two positions show a transitional pattern.
- In extremity lead, the QRS complex varies depending on whether the heart is more horizontal or vertical.
  - **When the heart is more vertical**, leads II, III, and aVF show a 'qR' pattern.
  - When the **heart is more horizontal**, the leads I and aVL show a 'qR' pattern.
- The **T wave** normally follows the direction of the QRS complex deflections.
  - **In chest leads**, the T wave is positive in the left-sided leads (and also in V_2).
  - **In V_1**, T wave may be positive or negative.

SYSTEMATIC INTERPRETATION OF ECG

A routine screening of the ECG needs stepwise examination of the ECG.

1. What is the heart rate? What is the atrial rate and what is the ventricular rate?
2. Is the rhythm regular or irregular?
3. What is the mean cardiac vector?
4. Are the P waves normal? Do the P waves have a fixed relation to the QRS complexes?
5. What is the duration of PR interval? What is the duration, amplitude and configuration of the QRS complex?
6. Is the ST segment isoelectric?
7. Are the T waves normal?
8. What is the duration of QT interval? Is the QTc appropriate for the heart rate (QTc is the QT interval corrected for the rate).

Heart Rate

Though heart rate means the ventricular rate, atrial rate should also be noted.

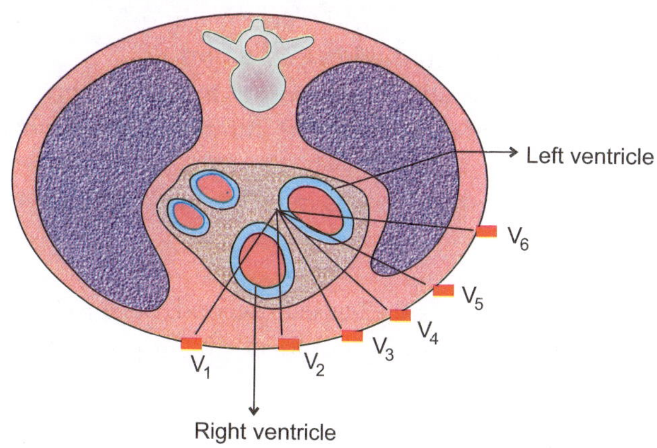

Fig. 30.6: Orientation of precordial ECG leads. Note, leads V_1 and V_2 overlie the right ventricle; leads V_3 and V_4 overlie the precordium that is transitional between right and left ventricles; and leads V_5 and V_6 overlie the left ventricle.

- At a paper speed of 25 mm/s, the **atrial rate** per minute is calculated by dividing 1500 with ***PP interval*** (in mm).
- Similarly, **ventricular rate** per minute is calculated by dividing 1500 with ***RR interval*** (in mm).
- Normally, the RR interval is equal to the PP interval.
  - But, sometimes ventricular rate may be different from the atrial rate.
- The normal heart rate is **60 to 100 per minute**.

Calculation of the ventricular rate when RR interval is irregular: When RR interval is irregular as seen in ***atrial fibrillation***, the number of QRS complexes is counted over 5 second (125 mm) in the rhythm strip and this number is multiplied by 12 to provide the number of QRS complexes in 60 seconds (1minute). This enables the measurement of the average ventricular rate.

Cardiac Rhythm

Normally the rhythm is regular. That means heart normally beats at regular intervals.

- It is observed by calculating the **successive cycle length** (**RR intervals**).
- Sometimes, there may be minor variation of the rhythm in normal conditions.
  - A variation of maximum up to 10% in adjacent cycle length is considered to be normal.
- Abnormalities of cardiac rhythm are called **arrhythmia** (described below).
- An example of physiological arrhythmia is **sinus arrhythmia**.

Waves and Intervals

P Wave

Duration and Amplitude: Normal P wave duration **does not exceed 0.10 s** and P waves are not more than 2.5 mm tall.

Configuration: Usually, P waves are **upright** in lead I to aVF and $V_3 - V_6$; **inverted** in aVR; and **upright, inverted or biphasic** in lead III, aVL, and V_1 and V_6. P wave morphology is best studied in lead II and V_1.

P Wave Abnormalities: P wave may be abnormal due to **atrial enlargement** and intra-atrial ***conduction abnormalities***.

- Atrial enlargement results in **tall & peaked P waves**.

PR Interval

Normal PR interval is 0.12 to 0.20 second, i.e. 3 to 5 small squares. Normally, there should not be any variation in PR intervals.

Short PR Interval:

1. WPW syndrome
2. Nodal rhythm
3. Atrial premature beats

Long PR Interval: (First degree AV block; discussed below)

1. Rheumatic carditis
2. Digitalis effect
3. Coronary artery disease

QRS Complex

Amplitude:

In limb leads (in lead I, II, III, aVR, aVL, and aVF), the total amplitude of QRS should be ***5 mm or more***. **In chest leads**, the amplitude of QRS complex should be ***10 mm or more***.

Duration: Normal duration of QRS complex **does not exceed 0.11 s**.

Configuration: Normally, **R wave is dominant** in lead I, II, V_4-V_6 and **S wave is dominant** in aVR, V_1 and V_2.

- Either R or S wave may be dominant in lead III, aVL, aVF, and V_3 depending on the position of the heart.

Abnormalities: Main QRS abnormalities manifest in the amplitude.

Low amplitude:

1. Marked emphysema
2. Myxedema
3. Pericardial effusion
4. Cardiomyopathy

High amplitude: Seen in ventricular hypertrophy

Q Wave

Normally, Q waves are small in lead I, aVL, V_5 and V_6. A *QS complex* is commonly found in aVR.

- There may be **deep Q waves** in lead III alone in normal individuals and may become less prominent on deep inspiration.
  - Occasionally a deep Q wave is found in V_1 and V_2 normally.
- Depth of Q wave is **less than 25%** of the height of the ensuing R wave in most leads and may be up to 50% in aVL.
  - Any Q wave with amplitude more than 25% is considered to be pathological.

Pathological Q Waves: When the depth of Q wave is ***more than 25%*** of the height of the ensuing R wave, or ***more than 0.04 s*** in duration is considered pathological.

Common causes are:

1. Acute or old myocardial infarction
2. Unstable angina
3. Dilated cardiomyopathy
4. Hypertrophic cardiomyopathy

ST Segment

The normal ST segment is **isoelectric**.

- **ST depression** less than 0.5 mm is not abnormal.

- **ST elevation** up to 1 mm in limb leads and V_5 and V_6 and 2 mm in V_1 - V_4 may be normal.

ST Elevation: Commonly seen in **acute myocardial infarction** and sometimes in acute pericarditis.

ST Depression: Commonly seen in **myocardial ischemia**.

T Wave

T waves are **upright** in lead I, II, V_4-V_6; **inverted** in aVR; and **upright, inverted or biphasic** in lead III, aVL, aVF, and V_1-V_3.

- T wave abnormalities involve either a tall or an inverted T wave.

Tall T wave:

1. Hyperkalemia
2. Acute myocardial infarction

Inverted T wave:

A. Physiological

1. Young children
2. Deep inspiration (sometimes)
3. After heavy meal (sometimes)

B. Pathological

1. Ventricular hypertrophy (strain)
2. Bundle branch block
3. Digitalis effect
4. Myocardial ischemia

QT Interval

The upper limit of normal QT interval is **0.42 s in males** and **0.43 s in females**.

- QT intervals should be measured in the lead where the end of the T wave is best discernible.
- QT interval varies with heart rate.

Therefore, corrected QT interval (QTc) is measured by using **Bazett's formula**.

$$QTc = \frac{QT}{\sqrt{RR}}$$ (QT is QT interval and RR is RR interval)

Abnormal QT Intervals: QT interval may be either prolonged or shortened.

Prolonged QT interval

1. Hereditary
2. Anti-arrhythmic drugs, e.g. quinidine
3. Hypokalemia
4. Acute myocardial infarction

Shortened QT interval

This is of less clinical significance and may be seen in hypercalcemia.

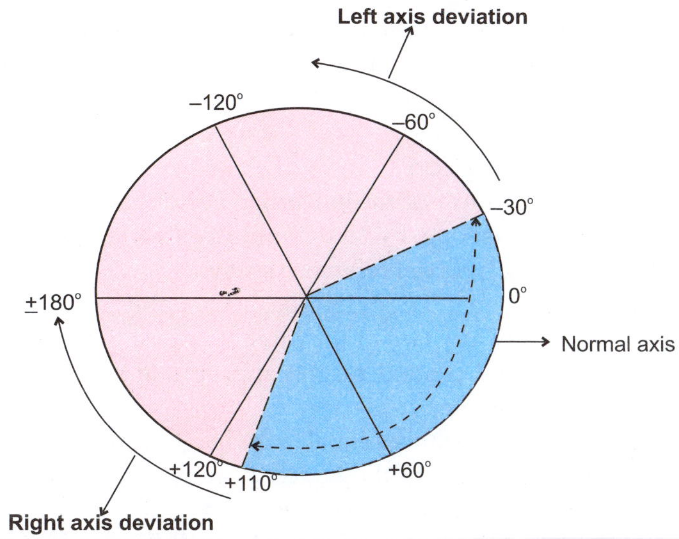

Fig. 30.7: The reference for mean QRS axis. Note, the normal mean QRS axis lies between –30° to +110°.

Mean QRS Axis PY5.5

Mean ORS axis is the **magnitude and direction of the mean cardiac dipole** (the ***mean cardiac vector***).

Normal Value: The normal direction of the mean cardiac vector ranges between –30 to +110 degrees (Fig. 30.7).

- If the axis falls to the left of –30°, **left axis deviation** is said to be present.
- If the axis falls to the right of +110°, the **right axis deviation** is said to be present.

Factors Affecting Mean Cardiac Vector: The mean QRS axis is influenced by four factors:

1. Position of the heart.
2. Properties of the conducting system of the heart.
3. Electrical properties of the ventricular myocardium.
4. Muscle mass of each ventricle.

Thus, the mean QRS axis can provide valuable information about condition of the heart in health and a variety of cardiac diseases.

Measurement of Mean QRS Axis

Mean QRS axis (**mean cardiac vector**) can be measured by approximate and accurate methods.

Rough Estimation

QRS complexes are studied in **leads I and aVF**.

- When the QRS complexes are **predominantly upright** (i.e. there is a dominant R in both leads), the ***axis is said to be normal***.

Right Axis Deviation: If the QRS complex in lead I is predominantly negative (i.e. **dominant S in lead I**) while it is predominantly positive in aVF (i.e. **dominant R in aVF**), there is right axis deviation.

Left Axis Deviation: If the QRS complex is predominantly **positive in lead I**, but **negative in aVF**, left axis deviation is present.

Intermediate Axis: When the QRS complexes in both lead I and aVF are predominantly negative, the axis is intermediate.

Accurate Estimation

Accurate estimation of mean cardiac vector can be done by **two methods**: one, by using Einthoven's triangle, and other, by using hexaxial reference system.

Using Einthoven's Triangle: The net magnitude of the QRS complex of **any two of the three standard limb leads** is measured and plotted on the appropriate axis in the Einthoven's triangle.

- In each lead, **distances** equal to the height of the R wave minus the height of the largest negative deflection in the QRS complex are measured.
  - These **distances are drawn from the midpoint** to the positive or negative side of the triangle representing that lead.
- **Perpendicular lines are drawn** from the midpoint of the arms of triangle to the center. Perpendicular lines are also drawn from the end of the QRS magnitudes drawn on the triangle.
- An **arrow is drawn** from the center of triangle to the point of intersection of perpendiculars extended from the distances measured on the sides. This **arrow represents the magnitude & direction of mean QRS vector**.

For example, as demonstrated in Fig. 30.8, the net magnitude of the QRS complexes of leads I and II are 8 mm and 10 mm respectively. Accordingly, the distances are plotted and perpendicular lines are drawn on Einthoven's triangle. The mean cardiac vector was found to be 40°.

Using Hexaxial Reference System: In this method, first the **six limb leads are examined** to find the one in which the **net deflection QRS complex is close to zero** or R wave has equal upward or downward deflections.

- As we know that when the cardiac dipole is perpendicular to a particular lead, the net deflection of that lead is zero. Thus, it indicates that the **mean cardiac vector is perpendicular to that lead** in which the net QRS deflection is close to zero.
- Now, the **hexaxial reference system is plotted** and referred to estimate the angle of that axis.

For example, the net QRS deflection is closed to zero in lead III (Fig. 30.5). Lead aVR is perpendicular to the axis of lead III in the hexaxial reference system (Fig. 30.4). Thus, the mean QRS axis is estimated to be about +30°.

Abnormal Axis Deviations

Right axis deviation:

1. Right ventricular hypertrophy
2. Left posterior hemiblock
3. WPW syndrome
4. Dextrocardia

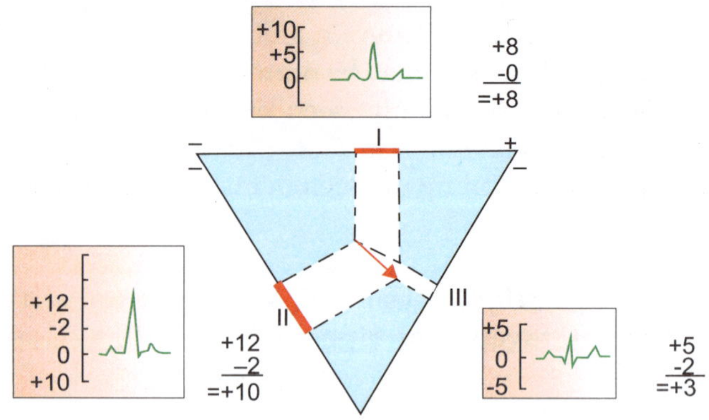

Fig. 30.8: Determination of mean QRS axis. Note, perpendiculars drawn from the midpoint of the limbs of Einthoven's triangle intersect at the center of the electrical activity. From ECG recoding of each lead, a measurement is calculated by subtracting the largest negative deflection of ORS complex from the height of R wave. This measurement in mm is drawn as a distance from the center of the limb to the positive or negative side of the limb according to the positive or negative value obtained. Perpendicular lines are drawn to the interior of the triangle from at least two ends of the distances measured and the point of intersection is noted. An arrow is drawn from the center of the electrical activity to the point of intersection of the perpendiculars drawn from the distances measured. The direction and magnitude of the arrow represent the direction and magnitude of mean QRS vector. For this purpose, the reference axis is given in Fig. 30.7.

Left axis deviation:

1. Left ventricular hypertrophy
2. Left anterior hemiblock
3. WPW syndrome
4. Inferior myocardial infarction
5. Obstructive airway disease

PY5.6

ABNORMAL ECG

ECG is useful in detecting **four types** abnormalities:

1. Abnormal pattern of cardiac excitation resulting in different types of arrhythmias.
2. Abnormalities of myocardium.
3. Cardiac abnormalities due to alteration in plasma electrolytes.
4. Cardiac involvement secondary to other diseases.

Cardiac Arrhythmias

Disorder of the property of rhythmicity of the heart is called arrhythmia. Abnormalities of the rhythm should be better termed as **dysrrhythmia** rather than arrhythmia.

- Clinically, cardiac dysrrhythmias are divided into ***bradyarrhythmias*** (arrhythmias in which cardiac rate is decreased) and ***tachyarrhythmias*** (type of arrhythmias in which cardiac rate is increased).
- Physiologically cardiac dysrrhythmias can be divided into **four categories** depending on the functional sites affected:
  i) Disorders of SA node
  ii) Atrial arrhythmias
  iii) Ventricular arrhythmias
  iv) Conduction disorders.

Disorders of SA Node

The common disorders of SA node are sinus arrhythmia, sick sinus syndrome, sinus tachycardia and sinus bradycardia.

Sinus Arrhythmia

Sinus arrhythmia, a normal physiological phenomenon, referred to **increase in heart rate in inspiration and decrease in heart rate in expiration**.

It is explained by **four mechanisms**:

1. **Alteration in autonomic activity:** Sinus arrhythmia is mostly due to ***alteration in vagal activity*** during inspiration and expiration.
   - **During inspiration**, vagal activity decreases and sympathetic discharge increases. Thus, heart rate increases.
   - **During expiration**, vagal activity increases, which causes a decrease in heart rate.
     - The decrease in heart rate in expiration due to increased vagal discharge is utilized **in pranayamic breathing to improve vagal tone** (Clinical Note 30.1).
2. **Activation of Bainbridge reflex:** During inspiration, ***increased venous return*** to the right atrium increases heart rate.
   - The decrease in intrathoracic pressure during inspiration, increases right atrial filling and stretches the right atrium.
     - Thus, ***atrial tachycardia producing receptors are activated*** that produces tachycardia.
   - Right atrial stretching also stretches SA node, which causes tachycardia.
3. **Irradiation from inspiratory center:** Increased irradiation (spillover) of impulse **from inspiratory center to the vasomotor center** during inspiration increases the heart rate.
4. **Activation of atrial stretch reflex:** Increased venous return during inspiration **stimulates type B atrial stretch receptors**. This increases heart rate.

Clinical Note 30.1

Slow pranayama strengthens vagal tone & decreases heart rate: In normal breathing, duration of inspiration is nearly two-third more than that of expiration. In expiration, vagal discharge increases that decreases heart rate. In slow pranayama, the duration of expiration is prolonged that facilitates vagal activity. Practice of slow pranayamas in which duration of expiration is prolonged, improves vagal tone and promotes cardiovascular health.

Sick Sinus Syndrome

Decrease in heart rate due to disease of SA node is called sick sinus syndrome.

Sinus Tachycardia

When heart rate is **more than 100/min** in adult, it is called sinus tachycardia. Rarely sinus tachycardia is more than 200/min. It is actually not a primary arrhythmia.

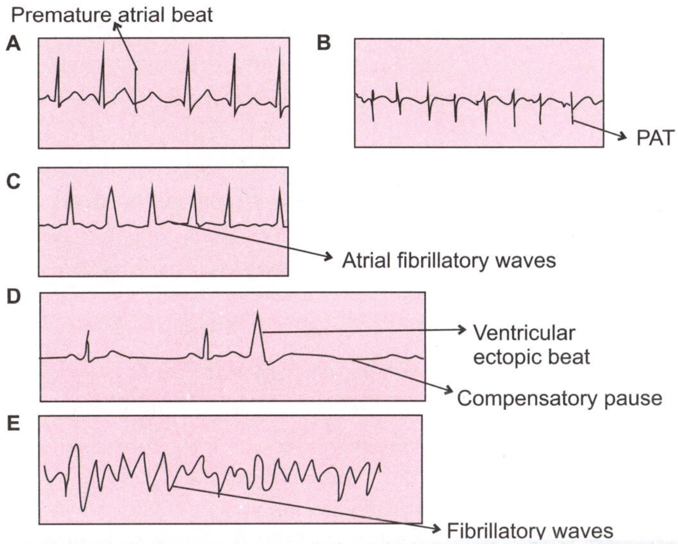

Fig. 30.9: Atrial and ventricular arrhythmias. A: Premature atrial beat (atrial extrasystole); B: Paroxysmal atrial tachycardia (PAT); C: Atrial fibrillation; D: Ventricular extrasystole; E: Ventricular fibrillation.

Causes of sinus tachycardia are:

- Anxiety
- Fever
- Hypoxemia
- Thyrotoxicosis
- Cardiac failure
- Acute carditis
- Drugs like atropine

Sinus Bradycardia

Heart rate **less than 60/min** is called sinus bradycardia. This occurs due to suppression of SA node.

Causes of sinus bradycardia are:

- Strong athletes
- Sick sinus syndrome
- Drugs (e.g. beta blockers)
- Obstructive jaundice
- Raised intracranial pressure
- Myxedema

Atrial Arrhythmias

The common atrial arrhythmias are atrial premature beats, paroxysmal supraventricular tachycardia, atrial flutter and atrial fibrillation.

Atrial Premature Beats

Atrial premature beats occur due to **premature discharge from an ectopic atrial focus**.

- The P wave of premature atrial ectopic beat **appears before the next sinus P wave**.
- The configuration of the ectopic P wave is abnormal.
  - This is also called **atrial extrasystole** (Fig. 30.9A).
- Atrial ectopics are seen in **physiological conditions** like anxiety, consumption of excess tea or coffee, or **in heart diseases** like rheumatic heart disease, coronary artery disease, cardiomyopathies or digitalis toxicity.

Paroxysmal Supraventricular Tachycardia

There are two types of paroxysmal supraventricular tachycardia (PST): Nodal PST and Atrial PST.

Nodal PST: In this condition, tachycardia (heart rate is usually between 170–250/min) occurs due to an **AV nodal reentry**, which occurs due to the presence of **dual AV nodal pathways**.

- It usually **occurs in paroxysm** that lasts for few minutes to hours.
- Identification of P wave becomes difficult as atria and ventricles depolarize almost simultaneously.
- The morphology of QRS complex remains normal and the rhythm is absolutely normal (constant RR intervals).
- It is seen in **normal individuals**.

Atrial Tachycardia (Atrial PST): This occurs when an atrial focus discharges regularly. The atrial rate is usually above 200/min (Fig. 30.9B).

- It is seen in patients **receiving digitalis**.
- Atrial tachycardia may be one of the causes of paroxysmal ventricular tachycardia.

Atrial Flutter

In this condition flutter wave (**F wave**) appears in ECG, which is characterized by undulating baseline resulting in corrugated or **saw tooth appearance**. Usually rhythm is regular.

- All impulses from atria fail to be transmitted to the ventricle. Usually two flutter waves precede one QRS complex (**2:1 AV block**).
  - However, 1:1, 4:1 or rarely 3:1 AV block may occur.
- Heart rate varies between **250– 350 beats per min**.
- Atrial flutter is usually seen in coronary artery disease, mitral valve disease, rheumatic heart disease and thyrotoxicosis.
- Usually it occurs due to intra-atrial reentry.

Atrial Fibrillation

In atrial fibrillation, **atria beat rapidly but irregularly** in a totally disorganized way. Atria beat at a rate of **300 to 500/min** and ventricle beats at 100-180/min.

1. In ECG, the baseline is ***irregular and wavy*** due to the appearance of **fibrillatory waves** (Fig. 30.9C).
2. QRS complexes are normal.
3. It is usually seen in rheumatic heart disease, mitral valvular defects, coronary artery disease, cardiomyopathies, and thyrotoxicosis.
4. It occurs due to the presence of **multiple reentrant excitation** waves in the atria.

Ventricular Arrhythmias

The common ventricular arrhythmias are ventricular extrasystole, paroxysmal ventricular tachycardia, and ventricular fibrillation.

Ventricular Extrasystole

This occurs due to **premature discharge from a ventricular ectopic** focus.

1. The **QRS complex appears early** than anticipated and looks **wide, bizarre and slurred** or notched.
2. The **P wave is not seen** as it is buried in the QRS of the extrasystole.
3. The ventricular premature beats are followed by **compensatory pause** (Fig. 30.9D).
4. It may occur in normal individuals or patients suffering from heart diseases.

Paroxysmal Ventricular Tachycardia

Paroxysmal ventricular tachycardia (PVT) occurs **due to circus movement** (propagation of wave of excitation continuously within a closed circuit) within the ventricle.

1. PVT is distinguished from supraventricular paroxysmal tachycardia (PST) by recording His bundle electrogam (HBE), in which **H deflection** (His bundle deflection) **appears in PST** but not in PVT.
2. PST is usually benign, whereas **PVT could be serious** as it may lead to ventricular fibrillation.

Ventricular Fibrillation

Ventricular fibrillation occurs due to **discharge from multiple ventricular ectopic foci** or due to the presence of **circus movement** in the ventricle, in which **'Reentry' of the impulse** keeps stimulating the ventricle repeatedly in a circuitous manner.

- Ventricular rate is very **high and irregular** (Fig.30.9E).
- **Ventricular contraction** is totally **disorganized and ineffective** due to rapid discharge.
  - Ventricles look like a '**bag of worms**'.
- Pumping of blood by fibrillating ventricle is grossly inadequate.
  - Therefore, **circulation of blood stops**.
  - Thus, ventricular fibrillation is a ***medical emergency***.
- It usually in patients with **acute myocardial infarction** that leads to sudden death.
- Ventricular fibrillation may lead to **ventricular flutter**, which appears as a ***sine wave in ECG*** with a rate between 150 to 300/min.

Conduction Disorders

Conduction disorder may be **conduction block** or **conduction acceleration**.

Conduction Blocks (Heart Blocks)

Defect in transmission of impulses from atria to ventricles is called atrioventricular block (AV block) or heart block. There are **three types** of AV blocks: First degree, second degree and third degree AV blocks.

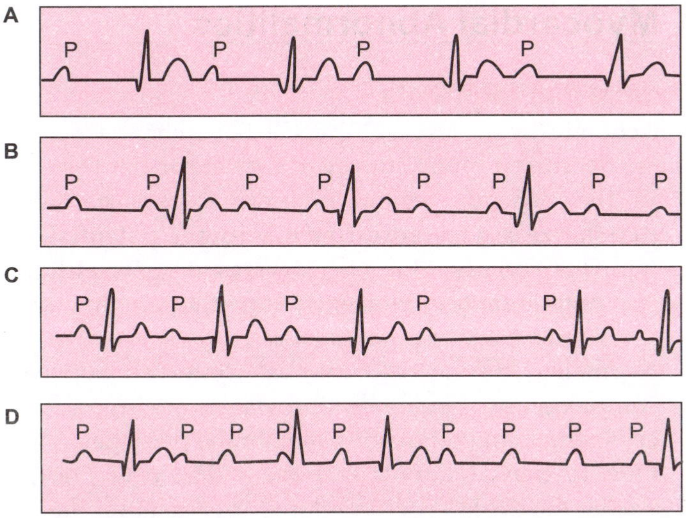

Fig. 30.10: Heart Blocks. A: First degree heart block (note, prolongation of PR interval); B. Second degree heart block of 2 : 1 variety (also called Mobitz Type II block in which for every two P waves one QRS complex is formed); C: Second degree heart block or Mobitz type I in which PR interval progressively lengthens in each cardiac cycle till one QRS complex is dropped, and again the new cycle of progressive prolongation of PR interval starts, this is also called Wenckebach phenomenon; D: Third degree or complete heart block in which atrial impulses do not reach ventricle at all, therefore, atria and ventricles beat separately

- In first and second degree heart blocks, conduction of impulses between atria and ventricles is not completely interrupted. Therefore, they are called **incomplete heart blocks.**
- In third degree heart block, atrioventricular conduction of impulse is completely stopped (**complete heart block**).

First Degree Heart Block

All the atrial impulses reach the ventricle, but the **conduction of impulse is slowed** due to increased delay in AV node.

- Therefore, **PR interval is abnormally prolonged** (Fig. 30.10A).

Second Degree Heart Block

This is further subdivided into Mobitz type I, and Mobitz type II blocks.

Mobitz Type I: In this type of heart block, **PR interval is prolonged progressively** in repeated sequence of beats till a QRS complex (ventricular beat) is dropped.

- PR interval following the dropped beat is usually normal, but in subsequent beats **PR interval progressively prolongs till the next beat is dropped**.
  - This is called **Wenckebach Phenomenon** (Fig. 30.10C).
- This is usually seen in acute inferior myocardial infarction, digitalis toxicity and acute carditis.

Mobitz Type II: In this type of heart block, **all atrial impulses are not conducted** to the ventricles.

- A ventricular beat occurs in **every two or three atrial beats.**
  - Accordingly, it is called **2:1 or 3:1 block** and so on (30.10B).
- This is usually seen in acute anterior myocardial infarction and degenerative disease of the conduction system.

Third Degree Heart Block

This is known as **complete heart block** as conduction of impulses from atria to ventricles is **completely interrupted.**

- **Atria and ventricles beat separately** (atrioventricular dissociation).
  - Therefore, in ECG P waves that appear regularly bear no relationship with QRS complexes (Fig. 30.10D).
- Complete heart block occurs due to **diseases at two locations**: i) At AV node (***AV nodal block***) or, iii) Disease of the conducting system below the AV node (***infranodal block***).

Idioventricular Rhythm: In complete heart block, especially in infranodal block, a portion of ***ventricular muscle becomes the pacemaker.*** This is called *idioventricular rhythm.*

- The rate of idioventricular rhythm is **15–40 beats/min.**
- When the heart rate is as low as 15/min, blood ***circulation decreases*** that results in cerebral ischemia and causes **fainting**.
  - This is called **Stokes-Adam syndrome**.
  - After fainting, blood circulation to brain improves (due to assumption of lying posture of fainting) and patients regains consciousness.
  - But again, he faints after sometimes.

Causes: Common causes of complete heart block are septal myocardial infarction, His bundle injury during surgical procedure for repair of ventricular septal defect, digitalis toxicity and degenerative diseases of the conductive system.

Treatment: Now-a-days, implantation of **electronic pacemaker** is the usual treatment of complete heart block.

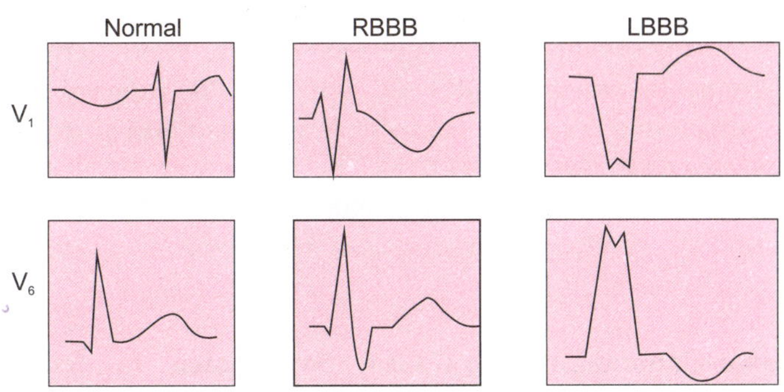

Fig. 30.11: ECG features of right bundle branch block (RBBB) and left bundle branch block (LBBB). Usually right and left bundle branch blocks are better noted in V1 and V6 leads respectively due to their position on precordium. Note, in both conditions there is prolongation of duration of QRS complex; in RBBB, there is depression of ST segment and inversion of T wave in V1 lead; and in LBBB, there is widening of R wave with two peaks in both leads and inversion of T wave in V6.

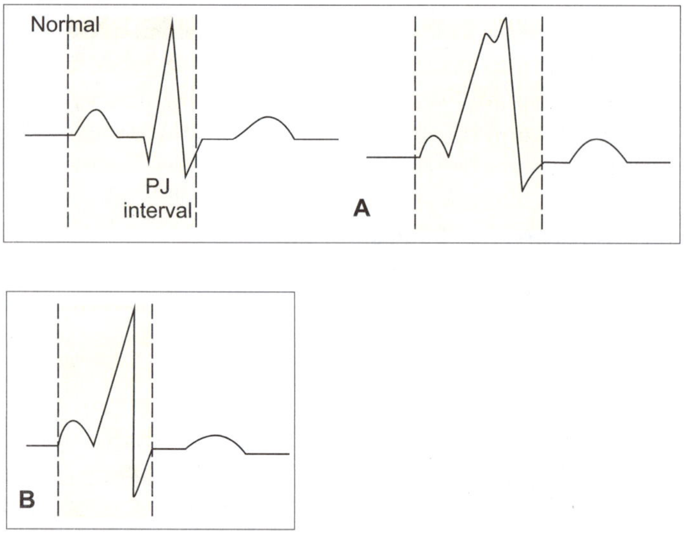

Fig. 30.12: ECG features in WPW **(A)** and LGL **(B)** syndromes. In WPW syndrome, there is shortening of PR interval due to occurrence of premature QRS complex that appears early and merges with normal QRS complex giving rise to the appearance of a bifid QRS. However, the PJ interval remains normal. In LGL syndrome, PR interval shortens due to early onset of a normal QRS complex. The PJ interval is shortened.

Bundle Branch Block

Block of either of the bundle branch results in **prolongation of QRS complex**.

- In **right bundle branch block** (RBBB), depression of ST segment and inversion of T wave occurs (Fig. 30.11).
- In **left bundle branch block** (LBBB), R wave widens with two peaks.

Acceleration of Conduction

There are two important defects of conduction accelerations: WPW syndrome and LGL syndrome.

Wolff-Parkinson-White (WPW) Syndrome: In WPW syndrome, in addition to three normal internodal pathways, an **aberrant pathway** ***(bundle of Kent)*** exists between atria and ventricle.

- This abnormal pathway **transmits impulse faster** than the usual transmission of impulse through the AV node. Therefore, ventricle is **excited early**.
- The QRS complex of this premature activation merges with the normal QRS so that the **PR interval is shortened** and **QRS complex is widened and slurred** in its upstroke (Fig. 30.12A).
- However, PJ interval is normal.
- WPW syndrome predisposes to paroxysmal atrial tachycardia.

Lown-Ganong-Levine (LGL) Syndrome: In LGL syndrome, **impulses from SA node** bypasses the AV node and ***merges with the conducting pathway distal to the AV node*** via aberrant pathways.

- Therefore, **PR interval shortens** in the presence of normal QRS complex (Fig. 30.12B).
- **PJ interval shortens** due to decreased PR interval.

Myocardial Abnormalities

Myocardial Ischemia

In **ischemic heart disease**, myocardial ischemia occurs due to **decreased blood supply** to the ventricular tissue.

- In the ischemic region, myocardial cells **partially depolarize to a lower resting membrane potential**.
  - This occurs due to **decreased gradient of potassium ion concentration** (though they still produce action potentials).
- Normally, during TP interval (interval between completion of T and onset of P wave), the myocardial cells remain in their resting membrane potential.
- **Due to partial depolarization**, a ***dipole is present during the TP interval*** in injured myocardium due to the ***voltage difference*** between **polarized** (normal) and **partially polarized** (ischemic) tissue.
  - However, *no dipole is present during the ST segment* as depolarization is complete and uniform in both normal and ischemic tissues.
- Thus, **ST segment** may be recorded as **either positive or negative** waves.
- The ST segment changes provide major clue for the diagnosis of cardiac ischemic injury.

Myocardial Infarction

ECG changes are very useful in the diagnosis of myocardial infarction and also to assess the location and extent of infarction.

- During the **stage of myocardial ischemia**, *T wave inversion* is seen in ECG.
- The usual changes in AMI are **ST segment elevation** in the leads overlying the infarction and **ST segment depression** in the leads located opposite to infarction (Fig. 30.13).

Physiological basis of ECG changes in AMI

The hallmark of ECG change in AMI is **ST segment elevation**.

This occurs due to **three mechanisms** that operate in sequence:

1. **Rapid repolarization of the infarcted tissue:** Within few seconds of infarction, the infarcted tissue ***rapidly repolarizes*** due to *fast opening of K^+ channels.*
   - Therefore, the ***membrane potential of the infracted area is higher*** than the membrane potential of the normal surrounding area, during the later-part of repolarization.
   - This makes the ***normal region negative*** to the infarcted region.

- As normally **current flows from positive to negative region**, in AMI, the *current flows from infracted area to the surrounding normal areas* and also towards the electrode placed on the infarcted area.

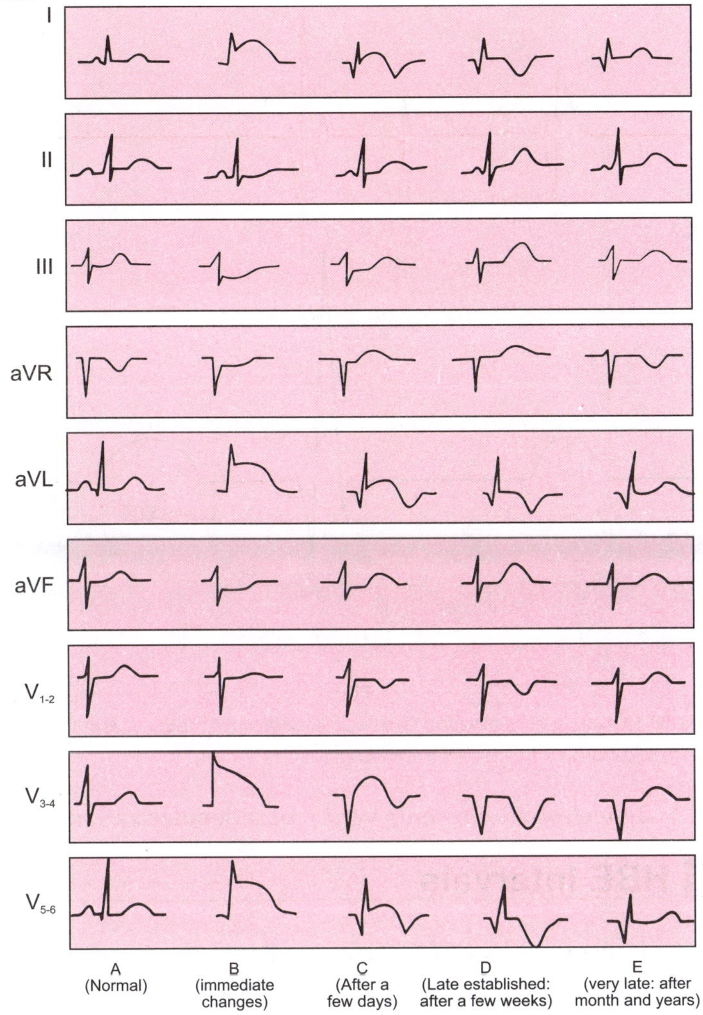

Fig. 30.13: ECG changes in anterior myocardial infarction. Note, in the acute phase, the leads that overlie infarction such as I, aVL, V3–6 show ST elevation, whereas leads that are located opposite to infarction such as III, aVR, aVF show ST depression. The ECG features become almost normal after few years (very late changes).

- This causes **increased positivity** between the S and T wave in ECG and results in ST elevation.

2. **Decreased RMP of infarcted muscle fibers:** Loss of intracellular K^+ *decreases resting membrane potential in the infarcted muscle cell.*
   - This causes *current flow into the infarcted tissue* during diastole, which causes *TQ segment depression* in ECG that manifests as ST elevation.
3. **Delayed depolarization of infarcted cells:** Infarcted muscle fibers **depolarize very slowly** in comparison to the surrounding normal fibers.
   - This makes the *infarcted tissue to be relatively positive* to the normal tissue, especially in early part of repolarization, and causes ST segment elevation.

In CMI

In chronic myocardial infarction, the dead infarcted tissue forms **scar tissue** and becomes **electrically silent**.

- Therefore, the **infarcted tissue becomes negative** relative to the normal tissue.

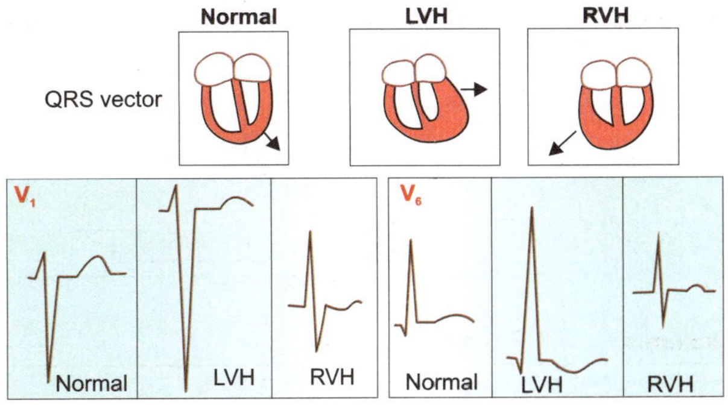

Fig. 30.14: ECG features of right (RVH) and left ventricular hypertrophy (LVH). Usually, RVH & LVH are better diagnosed from mean QRS vector and ECG changes in V1 and V6 leads. In LVH, the mean vector is directed left and posteriorly, and R wave becomes more prominent (more than 25 mm) in both leads with inversion of T wave in V6 lead. In RVH, mean QRS vector shifts to right, and R wave is biphasic in both leads with amplitude of R wave more than 5 mm in V1.

- The ECG manifestations of this negativity of the tissue are many, though the common feature is the **appearance of Q wave** which was not present previously.

Ventricular Hypertrophy

Ventricular hypertrophies are commonly detected by assessing the **deviation of mean QRS axis** of the heart and by observing the **amplitude of R wave** in ECG (Fig. 30.14).

- **In right ventricular hypertrophy**, mean QRS vector deviates to right, and **R wave is high** in amplitude (about 5 mm more than normal) in V1 lead.
- **In left ventricular hypertrophy**, mean QRS vector deviates to left, and **R wave is much higher** in amplitude (about 25 mm more than normal) in V5 and V6 leads.

Myocarditis and Cardiomyopathies

ECG changes are nonspecific in myocarditis and cardiomyopathies.

Effects of Electrolyte Disturbances

Alteration in plasma concentration of K^+, Ca^{++}, and Na^+ usually affect cardiac functions.

Alteration in Plasma K^+

The ECG findings depend upon the concentration of plasma K^+.

Hyperkalemia

Plasma K^+ at about 7 meq/L: Typical ECG feature is **tall and peaked T wave** (Fig.30.15A).

Plasma K^+ at about 8.5 meq/L: Broadening and slurring of QRS complex, and **Tall and slender T wave**.

Plasma K^+ more than 9 meq/L: Ventricular tachycardia and ventricular fibrillation.

Hypokalemia

Plasma K^+ at about 3 meq/L: ST segment depression and appearance of **prominent U wave** immediately following the T wave (Fig.30.15B).

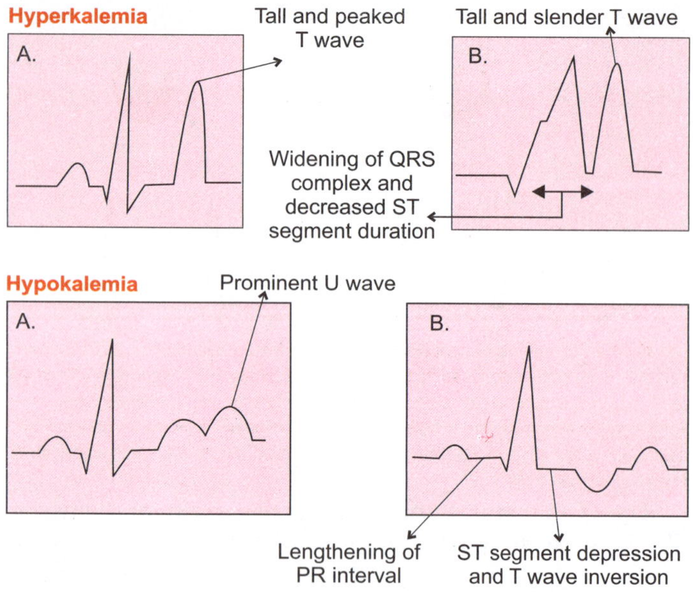

Fig. 30.15: ECG changes in different degrees of hyperkalemia (**A:** plasma K^+ between 5.6 to 8 meq/L; **B:** plasma K^+ more than 8 meq/L) and hypokalemia (**A:** plasma K^+ between 2.5 to 3.5 meq/L; **B:** plasma K^+ less than 2.5 meq/L). Note, the normal plasma K^+ concentration is 3.5 - 5 meq/L.

Plasma K^+ at about 2 meq/L: Prolongation of PR interval, ST segment depression, T wave inversion and prominent U wave.

Alteration in Plasma Ca^{++}

Hypercalcemia: ECG usually remains normal, though hypercalcemia increases the force of contraction and in excess causes calcium rigor. Rarely, QT interval is shortened.

Hypocalcemia: Prolongation of ST segment that causes *lengthening of QT interval*.

Alteration in Plasma Na^+

Hypernatremia: ECG changes are usually **normal** except that *high voltage ECG complexes* appear.

Hyponatremia: *Low voltage* ECG complexes appear.

HIS BUNDLE ELECTROGRAM

Recording of **electrical activities of His bundle** is called His bundle electrogram (HBE).

- HBE is compared with ECG of standard limb leads, especially of lead II to determine few ***electrocardiographic intervals*** that help in better diagnosis of heart blocks.
- For this purpose, a catheter containing an electrode at its tip is inserted through an arm vein **into the right atrium close to the tricuspid valve.**
- The electrode records HBE.

HBE has following **three deflections**:

1. **A deflection:** Represents activation of AV node.
2. **H deflection:** Represents transmission of impulse through His bundle.

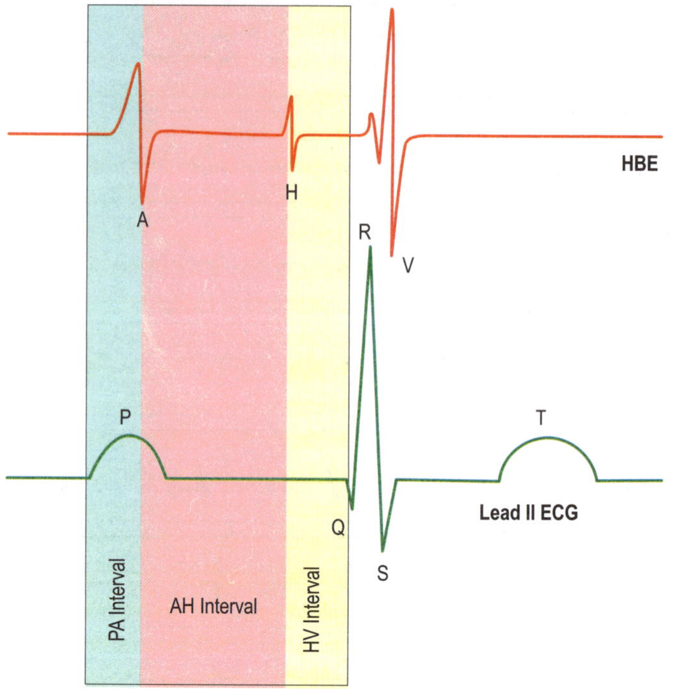

Fig. 30.16: Simultaneous recording of His bundle electrogram (HBE) and lead II ECG. Note the demarcations for PA, AH and HV intervals.

3. **V deflection:** Represents ventricular depolarization.

HBE Intervals

Simultaneously, **lead II ECG** is recoded on the same graph below the HBE on the same time scale. The following **three intervals** are obtained (Fig. 30.16).

PA Interval

This is the interval starting from the beginning of P wave in lead II ECG to the downward deflection of A wave of HBE.

- This represents the time of conduction from SA node to AV node.
- Normally, PA interval is 27 ms.

AH Interval

This is the interval starting from A wave to the H spike of HBE.

- This represents the time of conduction of impulse through AV node.
- Normally, AH interval is 92 ms.

HV Interval

This is the interval starting from H spike of HBE to the start of QRS complex in lead II ECG. This should better be designated as **HQ interval**.

- This represents the time of conduction of impulse through His bundle and bundle branches.
- Normally, HV interval is 43 ms.

Exam Questions

1. With the help of a labeled diagram of lead II ECG, describe the normal duration and physiological significance of various waves and intervals of ECG.
2. With the help of suitable diagrams, explain the electrophysiological basis production of various waveforms of ECG.
3. Define mean QRS axis & give its normal value. List four causes each of right and left axis deviation. Briefly describe the principle of measurements of mean QRS vector.
4. With the help of schematic diagrams of changes in ECG, describe the first, second and third degree heart blocks. Give a note on Stokes-Adam syndrome.
5. What are the ECG changes in acute myocardial infarction? Bridely explain the physiological basis of these changes.
6. Write a short note on His bundle electrocardiogram.

Multiple Choice Questions

1. According to Einthoven's law:
A. I+II=III B. I=II+III=0
C. I+III=II D. I+III=aVL

2. P wave is absent in:
A. Paroxysmal supraventricular tachycardia
B. Atrial fibrillation C. Atrial flutter
D. CCF

3. Electromechanical systole is best defined as:
A. Q wave and R wave
B. Q wave and beginning of T wave
C. Q wave and S1 (QS1 interval)
D. Q wave and S2 (QS2 interval)

4. An ECG gives information about all of the following functions except:
A. Site of pacemaker B. Electrical activity
C. Contractility D. Conductivity

5. An excess A-V nodal delay in conduction will usually cause:
A. Increased heart rate
B. Disappearance of the T-wave
C. The PR interval to decrease
D. The PR interval to increase

6. Which of the following statements about the second-degree heart block is correct?
A. Not all atrial impulses reach the ventricles
B. The PR interval is shortened
C. AV nodal conduction is completely blocked
D. SA nodal conduction is slower

7. Undulating baseline in ECG resulting in saw-tooth appearance is seen in:
A. Atrial flutter B. Atrial fibrillation
C. Ventricular fibrillation D. Sinus arrhythmia

8. The hallmark ECG feature in acute myocardial infarction is:
A. Appearance of Q wave in the leads in which normally it is absent
B. Appearance of Q wave in the leads in which normally it is present
C. Elevation of the ST segment in the leads overlying the area of infarct
D. Depression of the ST segment in the leads overlying the area of infarct

9. Prolongation of PR interval represents increased:
A. Parasympathetic tone to AV node
B. Sympathetic tone to SA node
C. Parasympathetic tone to SA node
D. Sympathetic tone to AV node

10. Ventricular fibrillation is a medical emergency because:
A. QRS complex is abnormal
B. Pumping of blood by fibrillating ventricle is grossly inadequate
C. Ventricles contract at a very high rate
D. Workload on ventricle increases markedly

11. Tall and peaked T wave is seen in:
A. Hypokalemia B. Hypercalcemia
C. Hyperkalemia D. Hypernatremia

12. Which of the following factor does not affect mean cardiac vector?
A. Sodium concentration in ECF
B. Position of heart
C. Properties of conducting system
D. Muscle mass of ventricle

13. Zero potential of indifferent electrodes can be achieved by connecting together the electrodes placed on:
A. Left arm and left foot
B. Left arm and right arm
C. Left arm, Right arm and left foot
D. Right arm and left foot

14. Prominent U wave could be a feature of:
A. Hypernatremia B. Hyperkalemia
C. Hyponatremia D. Hypokalemia

15. First degree heart block differs from second degree heart block in that, in first degree heart block:
A. PR interval is prolonged with atrial-ventricular rate 1:1
B. Atrial-Ventricular ratio is 2:1
C. Gradual lengthening of PR interval till one ventricular beat is dropped
D. All the atrial impulses are not conducted to the ventricle activity

16. Stokes Adams syndrome is the episodes of fainting that happens in:
A. AMI B. Ventricular tachycardia
C. Complete heart block D. Head injury

Answers

1. C	2. B	3. D	4. C	5. D	6. A
7. A	8. C	9. A	10. B	11. C	12. A
13. C	14. D	15. A	16. C		

Chapter 31

Cardiac Cycle

Learning Objectives

On completion of study of this chapter:

The student will be able to (must know):

1. Define cardiac cycle and name the phases of cardiac cycle.
2. Draw a labelled diagram depicting changes in left atrial & ventricular pressures, aortic pressure, left ventricular volume, aortic blood flow, JVP, heart sounds and ECG of a cardiac cycle on the same time scale.
3. Describe various electromechanical events of cardiac cycle.
4. Understand the pressure-volume relationship of left ventricle.
5. Name the waves of JVP & give their causes.
6. Give the causes, characters, and significance of heart sounds.

The student may also be able to (desirable to know):

1. Describe the alterations in pressure-volume loop in systolic and diastolic dysfunctions of ventricle.
2. Explain the common abnormalities in JVP waves.
3. Illustrate the physiological basis of common abnormal heart sounds.

Definition: Cardiac cycle is defined as the **sequence of electrical and mechanical events** occurring in heart during a single beat.

- The resulting changes in volume, pressure, and flow in different chambers and the electrical activities that are recorded in the form of ECG are precisely repeated in each beat.
- The similar electromechanical events occur almost **simultaneously in both left and right sides of the heart**.

PY5.3

PHASES OF CARDIAC CYCLE

Cardiac cycle consists of the **atrial systole and diastole**, and the **ventricular systole and diastole**.

- The atrial diastole is merged in ventricular systole.
- Therefore, events of cardiac cycle are described in **three phases**: atrial systole, ventricular systole and ventricular diastole.

Atrial Systole

The onset of atrial systole coincides with the peak of P wave in the ECG.

- During this period, **blood from atria enters ventricle** due to atrial contraction that ***completes ventricular filling***.
- At rest, it **contributes to less than 20% filling** of the ventricle. Therefore, **ventricular volume curve rises slightly** during this phase (Fig. 31.1).

IMPORTANT NOTE

Ventricular filling is a passive phenomenon: *At rest, atrial systole is not essential for effective ventricular filling* as it contributes to less than 20% filling of the ventricle. In normal conditions, **more than 80% of ventricular filling occurs passively**.

- When there is **significant tachycardia**, the ventricular filling contributed by atrial contraction assumes great importance as the duration of ventricular diastole is reduced.
  - In tachycardia, decreased cardiac cycle length occurs mainly due to the **reduction of the duration of diastole** that decreases diastolic filling of ventricle.
  - As passive ventricular filling is reduced due to decreased duration of diastole, atrial systole contributes significantly to the filling in such conditions.

Major Events: Major changes during atrial systole are as follows:

1. Atrial systole begins from the peak of P wave and ends with the peak of QRS complex as noted in the ECG tracing.
2. **Ventricular volume increases mildly** (Fig31.1).
3. **Atrial pressure rises** due to atrial contraction that

causes genesis of **'a' wave** in the atrial or jugular-venous pressure (JVP) curve.

4. **Atrial pressure exceeds** the ventricular pressure.
5. **Fourth heart sound** is recorded in phonocardiogram.
   - This is produced by ***inrush of blood into ventricle***.
6. **Mitral valve closes** at the end of atrial systole when ventricular pressure exceeds atrial pressure.

Atrial Diastole

Atrial diastole follows atrial systole during which atrial filling occurs.

1. Atrial diastole occurs during ventricular systole.
2. At the beginning of ventricular systole, **bulging of atrioventricular valve** into the atrium results in increase in atrial pressure that produces **'c' wave** in JVP.
3. Venous return **increases atrial volume** and **increases atrial pressure**. This produces **'v' wave** in JVP (discussed below).

Ventricular Systole

The phase of ventricular systole is divided into **two parts**: the phase of isovolumetric contraction, and the phase of ejection.

Phase of Isovolumetric Contraction

Appearance of QRS complex in ECG heralds the onset of systole.

- This phase starts with the closure of mitral valve and ends with the opening of aortic valve (Fig. 31.2).
- Thus, **ventricular volume remains same** throughout this phase.
- Inspite of forceful contraction, ventricular size **(muscle length) apparently remains same** (isometric type of contraction). Therefore, this phase is called as isovolumetric contraction phase.

IMPORTANT NOTE

Atrial systole contributes more in exercise: When increased cardiac output is required to meet the increased need for blood supply to the tissues of the body as happens **during exercise**, contribution by atrial systole assumes importance.

- In exercise, *increased sympathetic activity boosts atrial pump activity*, and increases the contribution by atrial systole to ventricular filling by 30–40%.
- In such conditions, **patients with atrial fibrillation fail to increase their cardiac output** adequately to meet the demand of the body.

Major Events: Major changes in this phase are.

1. This phase starts from the peak of QRS complex in ECG.
2. **First heart sound** appears in PCG (Fig. 31.1).
3. The **ventricular pressure rises abruptly** from zero to 80 mm Hg in left ventricle and to 8 mm Hg in right ventricle.

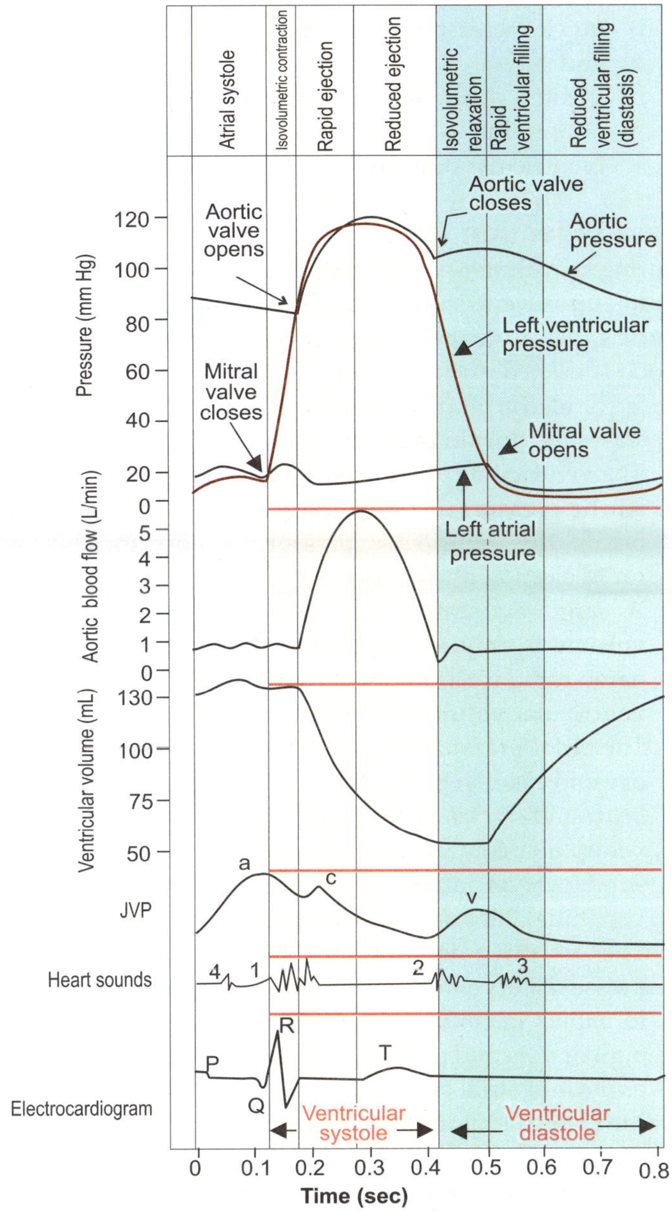

Fig. 31.1: Timing of various electromechanical events in different phases of cardiac cycle at a heart rate of 75 beats per min. (JVP: jugular venous pressure depicting a, c and v waves).

4. The **valves of the heart remain closed**; therefore, rise in ventricular pressure occurs rapidly without change in volume.
5. Ventricular **volume does not change** and **aortic blood flow is nil**.
6. This phase ends with the opening of the semilunar valves when ventricular pressure exceeds aortic pressure.

Phase of Ventricular Ejection

Opening of the aortic valve marks the onset of the phase of ejection. This phase is further divided into **two parts**: a *phase of rapid ejection* (lesser duration), and the *phase of reduced ejection* (longer duration). The phase of rapid ejection is differentiated from the phase of reduced ejection by **two important features**:

i) quick increase in ventricular and aortic pressures, and
ii) greater decrease in ventricular volume that occurs due to abrupt increase in aortic blood flow (ventricular output).

Rapid Ejection Phase

During isovolumetric contraction phase, enough tension builds up in ventricular wall. Therefore, with opening of aortic valve, **aortic blood flow increases abruptly** and the blood is ejected forcefully into the aorta from the left ventricle. Similarly, blood ejected from right ventricle sharply increases the flow in the pulmonary trunk.

- The **ventricular pressure continues to rise** sharply.
- **Aortic pressure also increases sharply**, but it remains below the ventricular pressure almost throughout rapid ejection phase.
- A large amount (about two-third) of **ventricular volume is emptied rapidly** in this phase (hence, the name rapid ejection phase) that causes a **steep fall in ventricular volume curve**.
- The **atrial pressure decreases sharply** at the beginning of rapid ejection phase due to ***descent of the base of the heart*** and ***stretch of the atria*** that occurs due to strong ventricular contraction.
  - However, **atrial pressure rises slowly** after the initial fall due to venous return.
- The **'c' wave is produced** in the jugular venous pressure curve in the early part of rapid ejection due to ***impact of common carotid artery*** with the adjacent jugular vein and also due to ***bulging of closed tricuspid valve*** into atrial chamber.

Major Events: Important events in this phase are:

1. This phase starts with opening of aortic valve.
2. Steep **increase in aortic blood flow**.
3. Steep **fall in ventricular volume**.
4. Ventricular pressure increases further.
5. Aortic pressure also increases but remains just below the ventricular pressure.
6. **Atrial pressure** falls in the early part, but slowly increases thereafter.
7. The **'c' wave** is produced in JVP.
8. This phase corresponds to **ST segment** in the ECG.

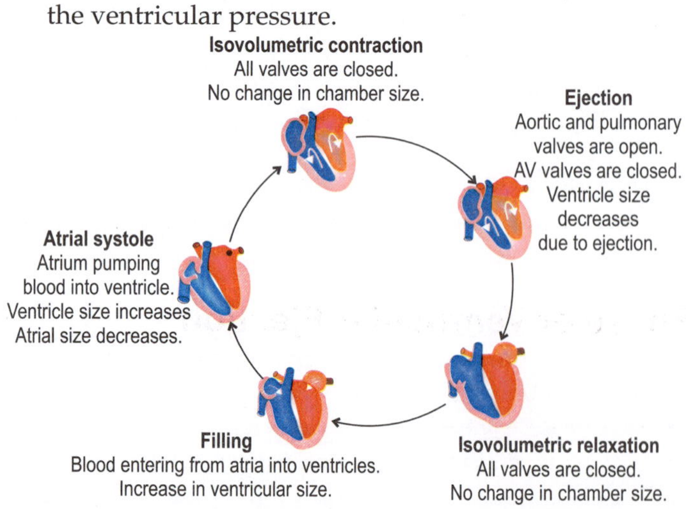

Fig. 31.2: Major changes in the cardiac chambers in five principal steps of cardiac cycle.

Reduced Ejection Phase

This is the **longer phase** of ventricular systole during which **both ventricular and aortic pressures decrease**.

- Aortic pressure declines due to **run-off of blood from the aorta to the periphery** that exceeds ventricular output.
- The ***aortic pressure exceeds*** the left ventricular pressure in this phase.
- In fact, reduced ejection phase begins at about the time when the aortic pressure slowly exceeds the left ventricular pressure.
  - Stored potential energy in the stretched arterial wall contributes to the alteration in ventricular-aortic pressure gradient.
- Inspite of this change in pressure gradient, **blood flow continues** from ventricle into the aorta ***due to the momentum of forward flow*** of blood caused during the rapid ejection phase.
  - This keeps the aortic valve open (Fig. 31.2).
- However, the **aortic flow is significantly reduced** in this phase (hence, the name *reduced ejection phase*).
- **Ventricular volume continues to decrease** and reaches the end-systolic volume at the end of this phase.

Major Events: Important changes in this phase are:

1. **Ventricular & aortic pressure decrease**, but *aortic pressure exceeds* ventricular pressure.
2. **Aortic blood flow** is *greatly decreased*.
3. **Ventricular volume** is further ***decreased***.
4. Atrial pressure continues to increase slowly due to blood returning to atria (atria relax throughout the ventricular systole).
5. **'T' wave** in ECG appears in this phase.
6. The phase ends with closure of aortic valve.

Ventricular Diastole

Ventricular diastole has **two phases**: the phase of ***isovolumetric relaxation*** and the phase of ***ventricular filling***.

Phase of Isovolumetric Relaxation

Ventricle starts relaxing in this phase that results in **steep fall in left ventricular pressure**.

- During this phase, **no change occurs in ventricular volume** as this period is placed between the closure of aortic valve and the opening of mitral valve (Fig. 31.2). Therefore, this phase is known as *isovolumic relaxation* phase.
- This is also called *isovolumetric relaxation phase*, as apparently there is **no change in ventricular muscle length**.

- Due to **closure of the aortic valve**, a characteristic **notch** is produced on the descending limb of the aortic pressure curve at the beginning of this phase.
- Vibrations set up by the closure of aortic valve produce the **second heart sounds** in the phonocardiogram tracing.
- It terminates with the opening of mitral valve.

Major Events: Important events in this phase are as follows.

1. **Rapid fall** in ventricular pressure.
2. No change in ventricular volume.
3. Aortic blood flow is almost nil.
4. **Second heart sound** appears in the first half of this phase.
5. Atrial pressure continues to rise, and the **peak of 'v' wave** of JVP appears towards end of this phase.
6. This phase ends with opening of mitral valve.

Phase of Ventricular Filling

This phase is further divided into **rapid filling** phase and **reduced filling** phase (diastasis).

Rapid Filling Phase

As soon as left ventricular pressure falls below the left atrial pressure, *mitral valve opens*. The blood that accumulates in atria during the ventricular systole rapidly enters into the ventricles as soon as the atrioventricular valves open.

- The major part of the **ventricular filling occurs rapidly** in this phase (hence, called *rapid filling phase*) that ***increases ventricular volume*** to a greater extent.
- Inspite of rapid filling, **ventricular pressure continues to fall** due to ventricular relaxation.
- The rapid flow of blood from left atrium into the left ventricle **decreases left atrial pressure** (Fig. 31.1).
- Vibrations set up due to this rapid inrush of blood into the ventricle produces **third heart sound**, which is recorded in the early part of this phase in the phonocardiogram.

Major Events: Important changes in this phase are:

1. This phase starts with opening of mitral valve, which corresponds to the **peak of 'v' wave** in JVP.
2. **Rapid increase** in ventricular volume.
3. **Decrease in ventricular & atrial pressure** (atrial pressure is just above the ventricular pressure).
4. **Third heart sound** appears in PCG in the initial part.

Diastasis

This is the **phase of slow filling** of the ventricle. During this phase, as filling occurs slowly, **ventricular volume curve also rises slowly**.

- Ventricular pressure and atrial pressure almost remain unchanged.
- It should be noted that (as discussed above) normally the greater part of **ventricular filling occurs passively** in both rapid and slow filling phase, and about *20% filling occurs actively* (by atrial contraction during atrial systole).
- Thus, atrial systole only tops up the ventricular volume.

Major Events: Main events in this phase are:

1. **Slow rise** in *ventricular volume*.
2. No change in left atrial, left ventricular and aortic pressures.
3. In ECG, **'P' wave** begins to appear towards the end of this phase.

Pressure-Volume Relationship

The pressure-volume relationship of the left ventricle plotted in a graphical form forms the **pressure-volume loop** (Fig. 31.3). Pressure-volume loop has **four phases**.

Phase I: Period of Filling (A-B)

Diastolic filling of ventricle starts at 'A' as mitral valve opens and terminates at 'B' as mitral valve closes. During this period, **ventricular volume increases greatly without much change in pressure** as this occurs during the relaxation phase of the ventricle (A–B).

- This phase in the pressure-volume diagram begins at a ventricular volume of about 50 ml and a diastolic pressure of 2 to 3 mm Hg.
- The 50 ml of blood that remains in the ventricle after the previous systole is called the *end-systolic volume.*
    - As venous blood of about 70 ml flows into the ventricle from the left atrium, **ventricular volume increases to about 120 ml**, which is called the *end-diastolic volume.*
- Therefore, the pressure-volume curve during phase I extends from point A to point B, with the volume increasing to 120 ml and the diastolic pressure rising to about 5 mm Hg.

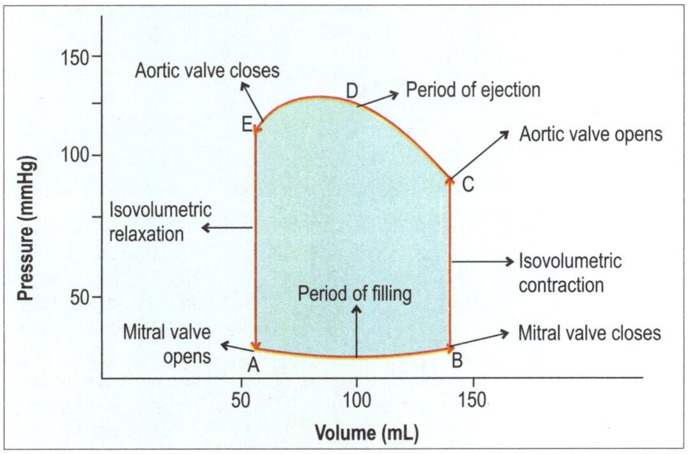

Fig. 31.3: Normal pressure-volume loop of the left ventricle (ABCDE). At point A, mitral valve opens; AB: phase of ventricular filling; at point B, mitral valve closes; BC: phase of isovolumetric contraction; at point C, aortic valve opens; CD: phase of rapid ejection; DE: phase of slow ejection; at point E, aortic valve closes.

Phase II: Period of Isovolumic Contraction (B-C)

During isovolumic contraction, the **volume of the ventricle does not change** because all valves are closed. However, the pressure inside the ventricle increases to equal the pressure in the aorta, at a pressure value of about 80 mm Hg, as depicted by point C.

- With the onset of isovolumetric contraction (B–C), **ventricular pressure rises steeply** without change in volume.
- **Aortic valve opens at point C** that marks the onset of ejection of the ventricle.

Phase III: Period of Ejection (C-E)

During ejection, the **systolic pressure still rises higher** because of more forceful contraction of the ventricle.

- The **volume of the ventricle decreases** because the aortic valve has opened and blood flows out of the ventricle into the aorta.
- The **ventricular pressure** continues to rise, which **reaches a peak** at point D (the rapid ejection phase ends) and then decreases till point E (the end of slow ejection phase).
- The ventricular **volume decreases**.

Phase IV: Period of Isovolumic Relaxation (E-A)

At the end of ejection (point E), the aortic valve closes, and the ventricular pressure falls back to the diastolic pressure level, **without any change in volume**. Thus, the ventricle returns to its starting point, with about 50 ml of blood left in the ventricle and at an atrial pressure of 2 to 3 mm Hg.

- During this isovolumetric relaxation phase, **pressure falls abruptly** (E–A) to meet the point A, which marks the **opening of the mitral valve**.
- This completes one cardiac cycle.

Note the position of diastolic pressure-volume and isovolumic pressure-volume curve in the normal condition.

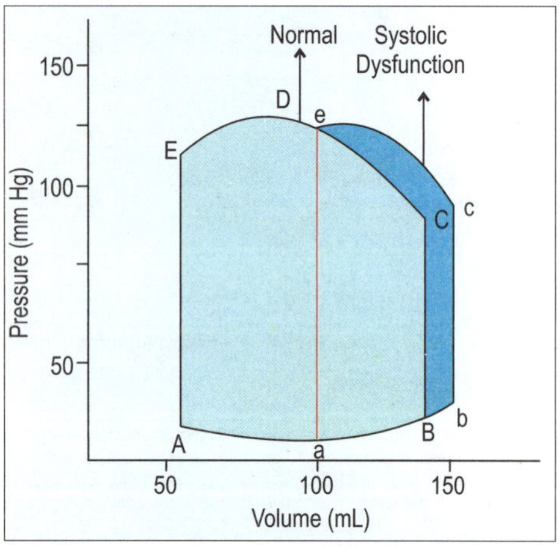

Fig. 31.4: Normal pressure volume loop of the left ventricle (ABCDE). Note, pressure volume loop shifts to right (abce) in systolic dysfunction.

Effects of Ventricular Dysfunctions

Effects of ventricular dysfunction on pressure-volume loop could be due to **systolic dysfunction or diastolic dysfunction.**

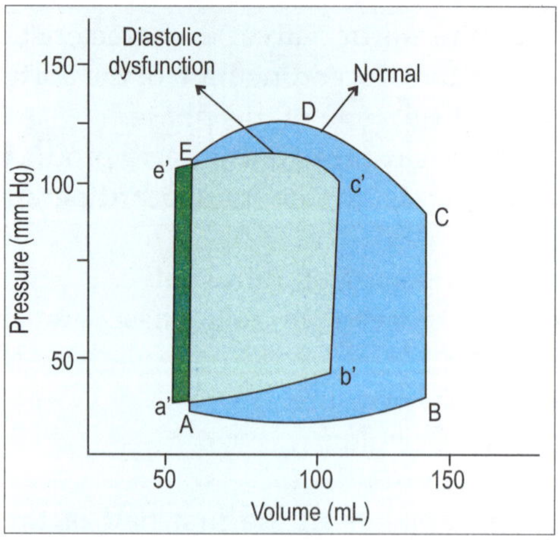

Fig. 31.5: Normal pressure-volume loop of the left ventricle (ABCDE). Note, pressure-volume loop shifts to the left (a' b' c' e') in diastolic dysfunction.

Systolic Dysfunction

Systolic dysfunction is the inability of the ventricle to contract.

- In this condition, **ventricular output is decreased** due to *impaired myocardial contractility*.
- The isovolumic **pressure-volume curve shifts to right** that decreases the stroke volume from **C–E** of the normal curve to **c–e** of the systolic dysfunction curve (Fig. 31.4).

Diastolic Dysfunction

Diastolic dysfunction is the **inability of the ventricle to relax**.

- In this condition, **ventricular output is decreased** due to *impaired end-diastolic volume*.
- The diastolic pressure-volume curve shifts upward and to the left from **A–B** of the normal curve to **a′–b′** of diastolic dysfunction curve (Fig. 31.5).
- This decreases the end-diastolic volume that results in decreased stroke volume.

Duration of Cardiac Cycle

The duration of cardiac cycle is 0.8 s when heart rate is 75/min. The duration of systole is 0.3 s and diastole is about 0.5 s (Fig. 31.6).

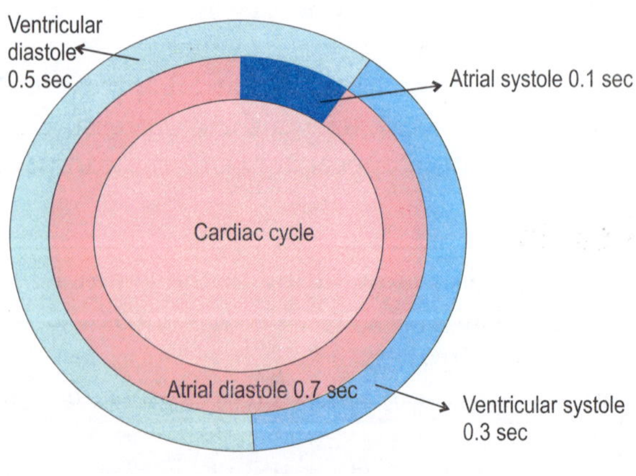

Fig. 31.6: Duration of ventricular systole and diastole, atrial systole and diastole.

In Increased Heart Rate: When heart rate is **increased to about 200/min**, duration of cardiac cycle is 0.3 s with the systole about 0.16 second and diastole about 0.14 second.

- The ***shortening of duration of systole is proportionately very less*** than the duration of diastole. In fact, duration of systole is more than that of diastole.

In Decreased Heart Rate: **When heart rate decreases** to about 40/min, duration of cardiac cycle is 1.5 s with the systole about 0.37 s and diastole about 1.13 s.

- The ***prolongation of systole is proportionately very less*** than the prolongation of diastole. The duration of systole is less than one-fourth of the duration of diastole.

IMPORTANT NOTE

Cardiac cycle length determines duration of diastole: The change in length of cardiac cycle occurs mainly by alteration of duration of diastole.
- Therefore, in tachycardia **ventricular filling is greatly compromised** due to *decreased time of diastole.*
- Resting tachycardia compromises cardiac output

JUGULAR VENOUS PULSE

Pressure change in atrium is directly reflected in internal jugular veins. Therefore, jugular venous pulse (JVP) in the right side of the neck is examined clinically to assess the atrial pressure changes.

Waves of JVP

Jugular venous pulse (JVP) has five waves: **three positive waves and two negative waves** (descents).

The positive waves are ***a*, *c*, and *v* waves**, and two descents are ***x* and *y* descents** (Fig. 31.7).

***a* wave:** This is due to **atrial contraction**.

***c* wave:** This wave coincides with the onset of ventricular systole and results from the **bulging of tricuspid valve ring into the right atrium** as the right ventricular pressure rises.

***v* wave:** indicates the passive **rise in pressure in the right atrium as venous return continues** while the tricuspid valve remains closed.

***x* descent:** caused by a fall of right atrial pressure due to relaxation of the right atrium.

***y* descent:** due to fall in right atrial pressure when blood enters into the right ventricle as tricuspid valve opens.

Abnormal JVP Waves

Conditions of raised JVP:

1. Right-side heart failure
2. Obstruction of superior vena cava
3. Increase in circulating blood volume
   - Pregnancy
   - Acute nephritis
   - Over-enthusiastic treatment with IV fluids
4. Congestive heart failure
5. Constrictive pericarditis
6. Tricuspid incompetence

IMPORTANT NOTE

Increased JVP is an early sign of CCF: Persistent elevation of JVP is one of the earliest signs of congestive cardiac failure (CCF) and it is also a reliable sign of heart failure.

Prominent 'a' Wave

1. Pulmonary stenosis
2. Pulmonary hypertension
3. Tricuspid stenosis (if atrial fibrillation is associated with it, *a* wave may not be seen).
4. Myxoma of right atrium
5. Distended right atrium in atrial septal defect
6. Cardiomyopathy

Physiological Basis: Prominent *'a'* wave occurs due to **increased force of right atrial contraction** associated with right atrial hypertrophy or hypertrophy of right ventricle.

- When ***right atrium contracts against increased resistance***, prominent *a* wave occurs.

Cannon Wave: When amplitude of *'a'* wave is abnormally big, it is called **giant 'a' wave** or **cannon wave** (Fig. 31.8). It occurs when ***right atrium contracts against a closed tricuspid valve.***

Canon wave is seen in:

1. Complete heart block when atrial and ventricular systoles coincide.
2. Nodal rhythm when the atrium and ventricle are activated simultaneously.

Absence of 'a' Wave

The *'a'* wave disappears in **atrial fibrillation**.

Prominent 'v' Wave

It is seen in **tricuspid regurgitation** because when ventricle contracts during systole blood enters into right atrium through the incompetent tricuspid valve.

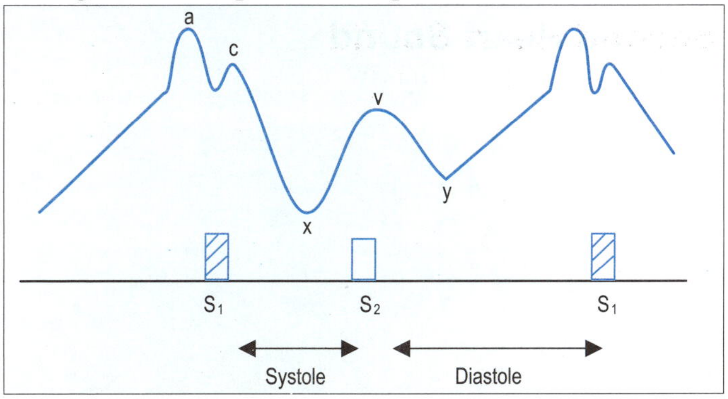

Fig. 31.7: Jugular venous pulse. Note, the a, c, and v waves, and x and y descents, and their relation to the cardiac cycle.

PY5.1

HEART SOUNDS

There are four heart sounds: first heart sound (S1), second heart sound (S2), third heart sound (S3) and fourth heart sound (S4). S1and S2 are heard normally.

First Heart Sound

First heart sound (S1) represents the beginning of systole.

Causes: S1 occurs due to vibration set up by:

1. Sudden ***closure of the AV valve***.
2. **Rapid increase in tension** in the ventricular muscles during isometric contraction acting on filled ventricles.
3. **Turbulence created in the blood** due to ventricular contraction.

Characters: Duration is about 0.15 second

- Frequency is 25 to 45 Hz
- It is a soft sound heard as 'lub'

Significance: It signifies the *beginning of ventricular systole & AV valve closure*.

a) Accentuation of first heart sound occurs in:

- Exercise
- Hyperkinetic circulatory states like anemia, beriberi
- Hypertension

b) Diminution of first heart sound occurs in:

- Shock
- Acute myocardial infarction
- Constrictive pericarditis
- Pericardial effusion
- Cardiomyopathy (in the advanced stage)
- Obesity
- Emphysema

Splitting of S1: First heart sound has ***two components***: the mitral and the tricuspid components.

The **mitral valve closes slightly before the tricuspid valve**. This gives rise to splitting of the first heart sound.

IMPORTANT NOTE

Splitting of S1 is pathological: Normally *splitting is not detected by auscultation*, as both the components are very low pitched and merge into each other. Audible *splitting of the first heart sound is always considered as pathological.*

Second Heart Sound

Causes: This occurs primarily due to closure of semilunar valves.

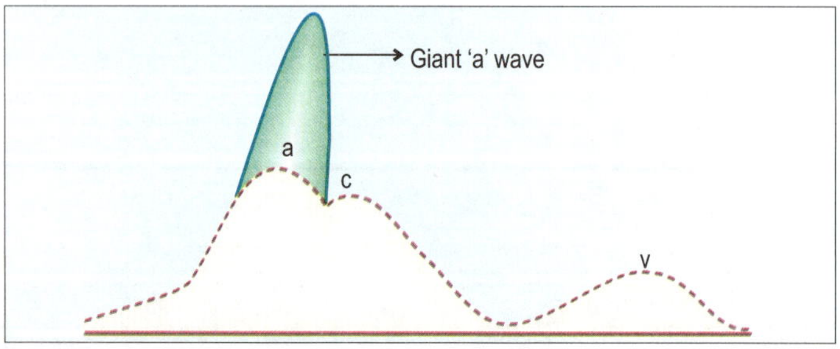

Fig. 31.8: Cannon wave. Note, it is a giant "a" wave in JVP.

- Rush of blood into the ventricles due to opening of the AV valves contributes to it.

Character: Duration is about 0.12 second

- Frequency is 50 Hz
- This is heard as 'dup'

Significance: Second heart sound signifies the end of clinical systole and closure of semilunar valves.

a) **Loud A2** (aortic component) occurs in:

- Systemic hypertension
- Aortic dilatation

b) **Diminished A2** occurs in:

- Aortic stenosis
- Aortic incompetence

c) **Loud P2** (pulmonary component) occurs in:

- Pulmonary hypertension
- Pulmonary artery dilation

d) **Diminished P2** occurs in:

- Pulmonary stenosis

Splitting of S2

Splitting of the second sound is due to the **gap between the aortic and pulmonary components**.

Mechanism of Splitting: The splitting of S2 is due to the separation between the closure of aortic and pulmonary valves. The closure of pulmonary valve always follows the closure of aortic valve (**aortic valve closes first**).

The splitting is ***distinctly heard during inspiration***.

- **During inspiration**, more blood is drawn into the thorax.
  - Therefore, venous return to right atrium increases and **right ventricular stroke volume increases**.
  - This increases the duration of right ventricular systole. Thus, **P2 is slightly delayed**.
- Also, during inspiration, **left ventricular stroke volume decreases**, because blood is pooled in the dilated pulmonary vessels and dilated left atrium, which occurs due to increased negative intrathoracic pressure.
  - Therefore, left ventricular systole is shortened and **A2 arrives earlier**.
- Thus, during inspiration, **A2 occurs earlier and P2 occurs later**.
  - Hence, splitting of the second sound widens during inspiration.
- Opposite mechanisms operate during expiration and splitting narrows.

Reverse Splitting: When **pulmonary valve closes earlier than aortic valve closure**, the condition is called reverse splitting.

- This occurs when the **left ventricle takes more time to empty** than the right ventricle.
- It is seen in **left bundle branch block** (LBBB) and in **left ventricular failure**.

Third Heart Sound

S3 is usually heard in conditions in which the **circulation becomes hyperkinetic**.

- A third sound can arise from either side of the heart, but usually, it arises in the left ventricle.

Causes: It is caused by the vibration setup in the ventricle during the early period of rapid ventricular filling.

- Rebound fencing of the cusp of the valve and chordae of the respective valve due to vigorous elongation of the ventricle caused by rapid inflow of blood.

Character: Duration is 0.1 second

- S3 is low-pitched
- It is best heard in the mitral area.
- It follows the aortic component of the second sound and heard early in the diastole, i.e. just after the second sound.

Significance: It is attributed to rapid ventricular filling and is found in relatively hyperkinetic circulation in young persons.

- It is heard in diseases in which the ***mitral diastolic flow is increased*** as occurs in mitral regurgitation and ventricular septal defect.

IMPORTANT NOTE

S3 is a sign of heart failure: S3 is an **important sign of heart failure** due to any cause. In heart failure, the *atrial pressure is increased*, and the early filling of the ventricle is rapid.

Fourth Heart Sound

This is also called as **atrial sound**, because it is produced during ***atrial contraction***.

- It is never heard in normal individuals.
- Presence of S4 **is always considered abnormal**.

Causes: It is caused by atrial contraction.

- It is produced by the vibration set up within the ventricle due to inflow of blood produced by atrial systole.

Character: It is low-pitched

- Occurs just before the first sound, i.e. late in the diastole.

Significance: It always indicates an increased stiffness or non-compliance of the ventricles.

- Therefore, when the bolus of blood is delivered into the ventricle by atrial contraction, it facilitates a sudden increase in ventricular pressure.
- It is heard in *left ventricular hypertrophy* due to hypertension, myocardial infarction, pulmonary embolism, and pulmonary hypertension.

Triple Heart Sound

This consists of **three heart sounds**: the first and second heart sounds, and the **third sound can be either the third or fourth heart sound**.

- If it is present with cardiac pathology, it may signify the seriousness of the condition.
- When the heart rate increases to more than 100 per minute, the triple rhythm is called **gallop rhythm**, because it produces a typical cadence of the gallop of a horse.

Murmurs

Murmur occurs due to **turbulence in the blood flow** at or near a valve, or an abnormal communication within the heart.

- Depending on the duration, it may be **early diastolic, mid-diastolic, early systolic, pan-systolic**, etc.

Exam Questions

1. Depicting the aortic pressure, left ventricular pressure, left atrial pressure, left ventricular volume, JVP, ECG and phonocardiogram on the same time scale, describe various eleceromechanical events in the different phases of cardiac cycle.
2. With the help of a suitable diagram, describe the phases of the pressure-volume loop of the left ventricle. Explain the effects of systolic and diastolic dysfunctions on pressure-volume loop.
3. What are the waves of JVP and what is their significance? Name the clinical significance and conditions of raised JVP.
4. What are the types of heart sounds? Describe the causes, characters, and significance of each.

Multiple Choice Questions

1. Duration of cardiac cycle at heart rate of 80 beats per minute is:
A. 0.65 sec B. 0.75 sec C. 0.85 sec D. 1 sec

2. The contribution of atrial systole to ventricular filling at rest is about:
A. 50% B. 40% C. 20% D. 5%

3. During isovolumetric ventricular contraction phase of cardiac cycle:
A. It is of 0.05 sec duration
B. A small but short fall in the atrial pressure occurs
C. Sudden opening of semilunar valves occurs
D. Intraventricular pressure rises to its maximum value

4. True statement regarding diastasis is:
A. Dynamic filling of ventricles occurs in this period
B. A-V valve opens at the at the beginning of this period
C. No change in left atrial, left ventricular and aortic pressures
D. Third heart sound coincides with this period

5. Closure of the semilunar valve occurs during:
A. Isovolumetric ventricular contraction phase
B. Rapid ejection phase
C. At the beginning of isovolumetric ventricular relaxation phase
D. At the end of isovolumetric ventricular relaxation phase

Answers: 1. B 2. C 3. A 4. C 5. C

(Remaining MCQs are given in Page 292)

Chapter 32

Cardiac Output

Learning Objectives

On completion of study of this chapter:

The student will be able to (must know):

1. Define cardiac output (CO), stroke volume, EDV, ESV, ejection fraction, cardiac index and cardiac reserve and give their normal values.
2. Appreciate the variation in CO in different physiological conditions.
3. List the methods of measurement of CO and learn the principle of measurement of common methods.
4. List the factors affecting CO.
5. describe the regulation of CO.

The student may also be able to (desirable to know):

1. Describe the measurement of cardiac output.
2. Explain the factors that influence CO..

The **output of each ventricle per minute** provides important information about the working condition of the heart in health and disease.

Therefore, **cardiac output assessment by echocardiography** is a routine investigation in clinical practice.

DEFINITIONS & NORMAL VALUES

Cardiac Output

Definition: Cardiac output is defined as the **volume of blood ejected by each ventricle per minute**.

Cardiac output = stroke volume × heart rate.

Normal Value: Normal cardiac output in adults is **5–6 lit/min** (approximately *8 % of the body weight*)

Stroke Volume

Definition: Stroke volume (SV) is defined as the **volume of blood ejected by each ventricle with each beat**.

Normal Value: Normal stroke volume is *about 70 ml.*

So, if heart rate is 70 per minute, the cardiac output is 70 ml × 70 = 4900 ml (5 lit/min approximately).

Cardiac Index (CI)

Definition: Cardiac index is the cardiac output **per square meter of body surface area**.

Estimation: It is calculated by **dividing cardiac output at rest with body surface area** in m^2.

$$CI = \frac{\text{Cardiac output at rest}}{\text{Body surface area in m}^2}$$

$$= \frac{5\ L / min}{1.7\ m^2}$$

(considering body surface area about 1.7 sq. meter, and cardiac output as 5L/min of an adult)

= 3 L/min/m^2 (approx.)

Normal Value: The normal average cardiac index is **3.2 L.**

Body surface area is calculated by using **Dubois formula**.

Importance: Body size varies greatly in the same age and gender and cardiac output is influenced considerably by the body size.

- Therefore, cardiac index is used to **standardize cardiac output among individuals of different body sizes.**

Effect of Age on Cardiac Index: Cardiac index rises rapidly to a level greater than 4 L/min/ m^2 at age 8 to 10 years, and then it declines steadily to about 2.4 L/min/ m^2 at age 70 years.

- The decrease in cardiac index could be due to **decreased activity and declining muscle mass with age**.

End-diastolic Volume

Definition: The volume of blood **remaining in each ventricle at the end of diastole** is end-diastolic volume (EDV).

Normal Value: 130 ml

Ejection Fraction

Definition: The **percentage of end-diastolic volume ejected with each beat** is the ejection fraction (EF).

- It is the percentage-ratio of stroke volume to end-diastolic volume,

i.e., EF = SV/EDV × 100.

Normal Value: Normally EF is about **65%**. EF is a good index of myocardial performance.

End-systolic Volume

Definition: The volume of blood **remaining in each ventricle at the end of systole** is end-systolic volume (ESV).

Normal Value: It is about 50 ml.

Cardiac Reserve

Definition: It is the amount of blood that can be **pumped by each ventricle in excess of normal cardiac output**.

Normal Value: 15–25 lit/min in non-athletes and 20 to 40 lit/min in trained athletes.

PHYSIOLOGICAL CONDITIONS AFFECTING CARDIAC OUTPUT

A. Conditions that increase cardiac output
1. Exercise
2. Anxiety
3. Emotion and excitement
4. Increased environmental temperature
5. After eating
6. Pregnancy

B. Conditions that decrease cardiac output
1. Standing from lying posture
2. Excessive sweating

C. Conditions that do not change cardiac output
1. Sleep
2. Mild to moderate change in environmental temperature

Effect of Age: Cardiac output is **less in elderly**.

- This occurs due to decrease in heart rate and stroke volume in aged individuals.
- **In children**, though the heart rate is more, cardiac output is less due to less stroke volume.

Effect of Gender: Cardiac output is about **10% less in females**.

Effect of Exercise: Cardiac output **increases in exercise,** due to **sympathetic stimulation.**

- In exercise, cardiac output can be increased upto 700%.
  - It can be increased to **35 liters or even more**.
- Cardiac output increases due to **increased heart rate and stroke volume**.
  - Tachycardia and increased stroke volume occur due to ***increased discharge of noradrenergic sympathetic nerves*** to the heart.
- ***Inhibition of vagal tone*** also contributes to tachycardia.
- **Stroke volume increases** due to increased myocardial contractility by sympathetic stimulation and also due to increased venous return.
- **Venous return increases** due to sympathetic ***venoconstriction and increased skeletal muscle pump*** activity.

Effect of Pregnancy: Cardiac output **increases in pregnancy** due to ***increase in blood volume*** that mainly occurs due to expansion of ECF volume.

- The increase in cardiac output is due to the increase in both stroke volume and heart rate.
- **Stoke volume increases by about 30%**, which peaks at about 24 weeks of pregnancy.
  - Increase in stroke volume is mainly due to increased end-diastolic volume (EDV), which occurs due to increased venous return as a consequence of increased blood volume.
- **Heart rate increases by about 10–15%**, reaching its peak at term.

Effect of Posture: Assuming **standing posture** from lying position ***decreases cardiac output*** due to pooling of blood in veins of lower extremities caused by effect of gravity.

- The effects of a change in posture are **more marked** if it is done passively with the help of a **tilting table**, as the muscular activity of the act of standing is absent in passive tilt.
  - The muscle activity is also lower in passive tilting, as the effect of **Muscle-Heart Reflex is eliminated**.

Effect of Environmental Temperature: Increased environmental temperature **increases cardiac output** by ***two mechanisms***:

1. By activating sympathetic system
2. By increasing body temperature.

Decreased temperature has the opposite effect. However, *mild to moderate change in temperature does not affect cardiac output*.

MEASUREMENT OF CARDIAC OUTPUT

Cardiac output can be measured by **direct and indirect methods**.

Direct Methods

Cardiac output can be measured directly by placing an **electromagnetic flow meter** in the ascending aorta or by using a **cardiometer**.

- These are **accurate methods** of measuring cardiac output.
- They are applicable only in **experimental animals** or in humans (in patients) undergoing **open thoracic surgery**.
- In humans, cardiac output is usually determined by using **Doppler combined with echocardiography**.

Indirect Methods

1. Fick method
2. Indicator dilution method
3. Thermo-dilution method
4. Ballistocardiography
5. Echocardiography
6. X-ray method
7. Pulse-pressure method

Fick Method

Fick Principle: Fick principle **is defined as** the amount of a substance taken up by an organ or by the whole body per unit of time is equal to the arteriovenous difference of the substance times blood flow.

Procedure

Cardiac output can be measured by measuring the **amount of oxygen consumed by the body in a given period** and dividing this value by the **arteriovenous difference of oxygen** across the lungs.

1. The **oxygen consumption** of the body is measured by **spirometry.**
2. As the **arterial content of oxygen** is same in all parts of the body, for measuring oxygen content of the arterial blood, the blood is obtained from **any peripheral artery**.
3. The **venous blood** is collected from the pulmonary artery by placing a catheter into it through the heart.

The cardiac output is calculated as:

$$\text{Output of left ventricle} = \frac{O_2 \text{ consumption (mL/min)}}{(AO_2) - (VO_2)}$$

AO_2: Oxygen content of arterial blood, which is 200 mL/L
VO_2: Oxygen content of venous blood, which is 150 mL/L

$$= \frac{250 \text{ mL/min}}{200 \text{ mL/L} - 150 \text{ mL/L}}$$

$$= \frac{250 \text{ mL/min}}{50 \text{ mL/L}}$$

$$= 5 \text{ L/min}$$

Advantages: i). Result is accurate, and ii). No chemical is injected

Disadvantages:

1. Catheterization should be done by **expert hand.**
2. **Hospitalization** is required for catheterization
3. Patient may be **apprehensive** of catheterization that increases cardiac output.
4. Simultaneous measurement of oxygen consumption makes the process difficult.
5. It is difficult to measure cardiac output by this method in ambulatory patients and during exercise.

Indicator Dilution Method

Principle: In this method, a known amount of an indicator (a dye or a radioactive isotope) is injected into circulation usually through an arm vein and the concentration of the indicator is measured in serial samples of the arterial blood.

- The output of the heart is equal to the amount of indicator injected divided by its average concentration in arterial blood after a single circulation through the heart.

Procedure

This method is popularly known as **Hamilton's dye dilution method** (as described by Hamilton).

- The dye injected is usually the ***Evans' blue* or *indocyanine green*.**
- Before injection of the dye, 10 ml of peripheral venous blood is withdrawn and divided equally into two samples.
    - In one sample of 5 ml, enough quantity of the dye is injected to give a concentration of 0.5 mg/100 ml. (used as standard).
    - The other sample is used as blank.
- One ml of the dye solution containing 5 mg is injected rapidly into the basilic vein.
- From a limb artery, the blood samples are collected at an interval of 2 s in serial tubes.
- The tubes are then centrifuged together with the standard and blank tubes, following which the concentration of dye ***is* determined photocolorimetrically**.
- The concentration of the successive samples is plotted on *a semi-log paper*. The resulting concentration of dye in the arterial blood changes with time.
    i) **First**, the concentration **rises** as the indicator carried by the fast-moving blood reaches the arterial sampling point;
    ii) **Second,** reaches a **peak** as majority of indicator substance arrives at the sampling point; and
    iii) **Finally**, the concentration **falls** as indicator carried by slow moving blood arrives at the point.
- Thus, the result obtained gives a curve with an **ascending limb**, **a peak**, and **a descending limb**. But the descending limb ends with a rise (Fig. 32.1).
- The slope of descending limb is extrapolated to the abscissa.
    - The point on the time scale at which it touches the abscissa, gives the time of first passage of the dye through the artery (t).

Let us say the time of first passage of the dye is 36 s.

Cardiac output is then calculated from the following formula:

$$F = \frac{I}{c \times t}$$

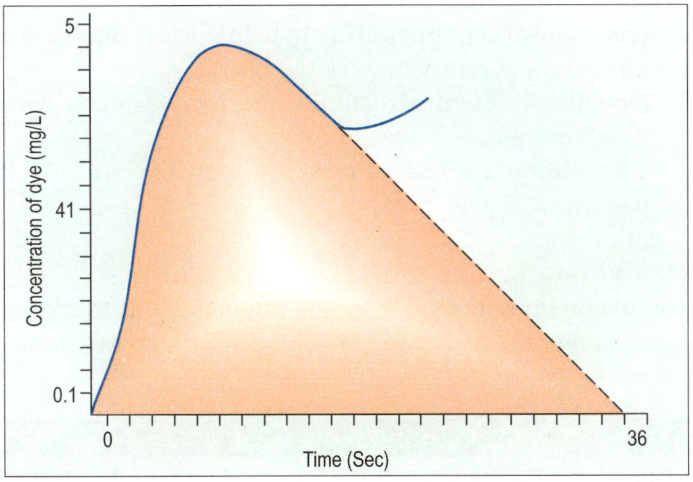

Fig. 32.1: Indicator dilution method of cardiac output measurement. Note, the descending limb of the curve ends with a rise. The slope of descending limb is extrapolated to the time scale in the abscissa and where it touches is the time of first passage of dye through the artery.

'F' is the blood flow in liters per second, 'I' is the total amount of dye injected, 'c' is the mean concentration of the dye, and 't' is the duration of the first passage of the dye through the artery expressed in seconds.

$$F = \frac{5}{1.6} = 3.1 \text{ liters}$$

In one minute, the flow (cardiac output) = 3.1 × 60/36 = 5 liters per minute (approximately)

Advantages: It is an accurate method.

Disadvantages: Should not be repeated in short time as the concentration of the dye of the earlier use may give errors.

Thermodilution Method

Principle: The principle is same as **indicator dilution technique**. In this method, the **cold saline** is used as the indicator. A double lumen catheter is used.

- Following catheterization, the cold saline is injected into the right atrium through one side of the catheter.
- A thermistor is placed in the other end of the other side of the catheter.
- The change in temperature of the blood is recorded in the pulmonary artery through the thermistor placed in the catheter.
- The change in temperature is inversely proportional to the amount of blood flowing through the pulmonary artery.

Advantages:

1. Saline is harmless
2. Cold is dissipated, so recirculation is not a problem
3. Can be repeated many times, if needed
4. Usually preferred for children as saline is nontoxic
5. Useful in severely sick patients (serious patients in intensive care units)

Disadvantages: Cardiac catheterization is required.

Other Methods

Echocardiography

This is a noninvasive technique in which **ultrasonic waves emitted from a transducer detect waves reflected from various parts of the heart**. When it is combined with Doppler technique it determines the velocity and volume of flow of blood through various cardiac valves. Thus, it measures cardiac output. It is useful in detecting valvular lesions and size of the chambers.

Principle: An echocardiogram technique uses **ultrasound waves** to examine the heart.

- **Ultrasound waves are transmitted** into the chest and the reflection of these waves off the various parts of the heart is analyzed.
- A **transducer,** which is a small microphone-like device, is held against the chest.
  - The **transducer sends and receives the ultrasound waves**.
- By moving the transducer to **various positions** on the chest, **different structures of the heart and the blood flow** are analyzed.
- The computer software assembles the reflected ultrasound waves to create an image of the heart.
  - These images appear on a television screen.
- The images may be recorded on videotape or printed on paper for review by the cardiologist.

Parameters Seen

1. **Size and shape of the heart:** The images may be used to measure the size of the heart chambers and thickness of the heart muscle.
2. **Pumping efficiency of the heart:** The images show the efficiency with which the heart pumps blood (***stroke volume and cardiac output***), as well as whether the heart is pumping at full strength or is weakened.
   - The scans may also show whether the **various parts of the heart pump equally** or there are regional hypokinesias.
3. **Valve abnormalities:** An echocardiogram shows the ***shape and motion of the heart valves.***
   - It can reveal if a heart valve is narrowed or leaking and show how severe the problem is.
4. **Other uses:** The test may also detect the presence of ***fluid around the heart; blood clots, or masses*** inside the heart; and ***abnormal holes*** between heart chambers.

Brief Procedure

The subject is asked to remove clothing above the waist, and put on a hospital gown or a sheet to help keep warm and comfortable. Then the subject lies on an examination table.

- The subject will lie on the back or on the left side.

- A colorless gel is applied to the area of the chest where the transducer is placed. Or, jelly is applied to the tip of the transducer.
- The technician or the cardiologist moves the transducer over the chest, to obtain different views of the heart.
- Technician may ask the subject to change positions and breathe slowly or hold his/her breath, in order to get a better picture.

Three Techniques are Used

An echocardiogram study typically involves **three different techniques.**

M-MODE ECHO: The most basic technique, called **M-mode echo**, produces an image that appears as a tracing than an actual heart.

2-D & 3-D ECHO: The **two-dimensional (2-D) echo** shows the actual shape and motion of the different heart structures. This advanced technique provides images that represent "slices" of the heart in motion. **3-D (three-dimensional) echocardiography** technique captures three-dimensional views of the heart structures with greater detail than 2-D echo.

DOPPLER ECHO: The **Doppler** is a third technique that portrays the **flow of blood through the heart**. The images representing the flow of blood through the heart may be displayed as a series of black-and-white tracings or as colour images on the television screen. Doppler is most useful for cardiac output measurements.

Color Doppler: This is an advanced Doppler echocardiography, in which different colors are used to designate the direction of blood flow (Fig. 32.2). This simplifies the interpretation of the Doppler technique.

Advantages

1. A major benefit of the echocardiogram is that it is a **non-invasive test**.
2. The information help to reach at an **accurate diagnosis** and develop a treatment plan.

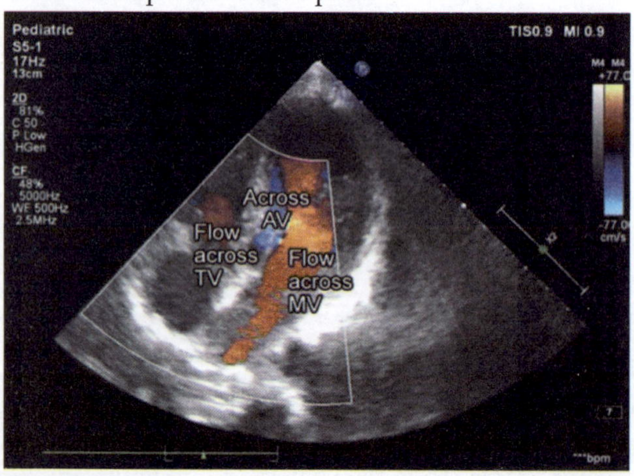

Fig. 32.2: Color Doppler, apical view of four chambers of the heart. Note the view of blood flow across aortic valve (AV), mitral valve (MV) and tricuspid valve (TV)
Courtesy: Dr. Santhosh Satheesh, Professor of Cardiology, JIPMER, Puducherry.

3. it is a **safe and painless** way to help doctors diagnose a number of abnormalities of the heart.
4. Directly, different parts of the heart are seen and their functional status is assessed.
5. **Transthoracic echocardiography** is used in critically ill patients (Clinical Note 32.1)

Limitations

The major limitation is that it is often difficult to obtain good quality images from persons who have broad chests, are obese, or are suffering from chronic lung disease.

Clinical Note 32.1

Transthoracic Echocardiography for critically ill patients: For critically ill patients, transthoracic echocardiography (TTE), a non-invasive means of hemodynamic assessment has been used with accuracy. The method involves measuring the blood flow velocity (using a Doppler technique) at the left ventricular outflow tract (LVOT) and thus obtaining the stroke volume (SV).

Ballistocardiography

In this method, the vibrations generated by each heart-beat are received and **converted into waveforms by a transducer** that records the cardiac activities on an **ink recorder**.

- From the recording, cardiac output is calculated by using a special formula by analyzing the recorded waves.
- However, cardiac output measured by this method is not an accurate one.

X-ray Method

In this method, a **radio-opaque dye** is injected intravenously and then the size of the heart is detected by **serial x-rays** in systole and diastole from which cardiac output is measured using computer programme.

Pulse-Pressure Method

Pulse pressure (difference between systolic and diastolic pressures) provides a rough idea of cardiac output.

FACTORS AFFECTING CARDIAC OUTPUT

Cardiac output is the **product of stroke volume and heart rate** (CO = SV × HR). Therefore, factors that affect stroke volume and heart rate, affect cardiac output.

Factors Affecting Stroke Volume

Stroke volume depends on **three major factors**: the **preload** (degree of ventricular filling or the enddiastolic volume), the **inotropic state** (myocardial contractility), and the **afterload** (resistance offered to the ventricular output).

Preload

End-diastolic filling is the preload to the ventricle and the **end-diastolic volume** (EDV) is the measure of preload.

- **Increase in EDV increases stroke volume** and decrease in EDV decreases stroke volume.
- This is explained by ***Frank-Starling's law*** of the heart.

Frank-Starling's Law: Frank-Starling's law of the heart states that **within the physiological limit, the force of contraction is directly proportional to the initial length of the muscle fiber.**

- The '**initial length**' of the muscle fiber means the fiber length **prior to ventricular contraction** (i.e. just before the onset of systole).
  - The muscle length prior to contraction depends on the **level of stretch of ventricular muscle** at the end of diastole.
- The extent to which ventricle is distended (stretched) depends on the degree of **end-diastolic filling** of the ventricle.
  - Increased ventricular filling **increases the fiber length** that increases the force of contraction. For details of Frank-Starling mechanism, refer 'Cardiac Muscle' in Chapter 28).
- This reflects the relationship between **end-diastolic fiber length & force of contraction** as demonstrated in **Starling curve** (Fig. 32.3).
- This is also known as **heterometric autoregulation** of cardiac output, as the stroke volume varies at various ventricular muscle length.

Factors Affecting Preload

The enddiastolic filling of ventricle depends **on three major factors**: Venous return, atrial pump activity and ventricular compliance

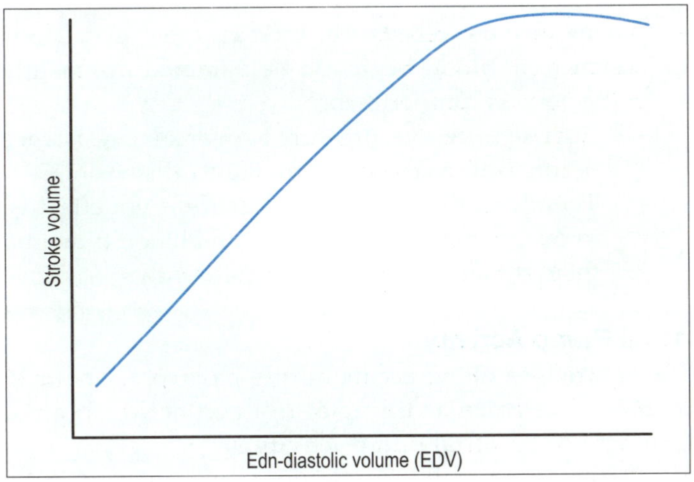

Fig. 32.3: Ventricular function curve (Starling curve). Note, stoke volume increases with increased EDV. EDV represents end-diastolic pressure, which indicates the end-diastolic fiber length. The increase in fiber length increases stroke volume almost linearly till the physiological limit is reached.

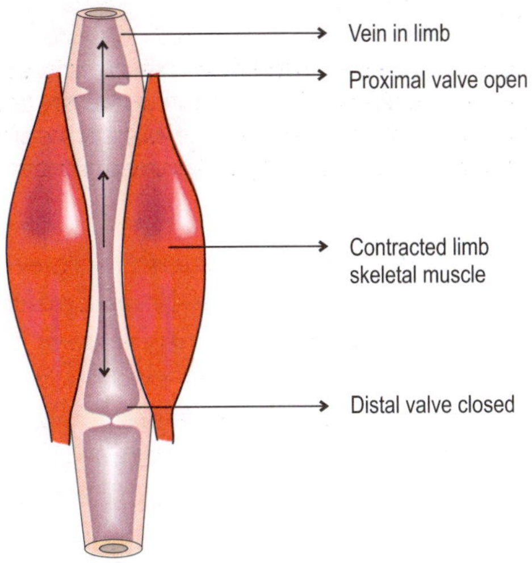

Fig. 32.4: Skeletal muscle pump. Contraction of muscle pumps blood toward the heart through the opened venous valves. Downward flow of blood is prevented by closed venous valves.

Venous Return

Venous return is defined as the **amount of blood that returns to the right atrium** from systemic venous circulation. Venous return depends on many factors. Important among them are:

1. Skeletal muscle pump
2. Thoracic pump
3. Abdominal pump
4. ECF volume
5. Sympathetic activity
6. Right atrial pressure
7. Degree of filling of systemic circulation
8. Resistance to blood flow in venous system.

Skeletal Muscle Pump: In lower limbs, majority of veins are surrounded by skeletal muscles.

- The limb veins contain **valves that open only towards the heart**.
  - Therefore, contraction of skeletal muscle compresses the veins and ***pushes blood towards the heart***. This increases venous return.
  - The back flow of blood in veins is prevented by closed distal valves (Fig. 32.4).
  - Competency of venous valves decreases in varicose veins (Clinical Note 32.2)
- Thus, **cardiac output increases by increased skeletal muscle activities**, as for example, during walking.
- On the contrary, **during quiet standing** for a longer period, pooling of blood occurs in the leg veins due to absence of muscle activity that decreases venous return, which in turn decreases cardiac output.
- Quiet **standing for a longer period** decreases cardiac output, and sometimes may cause fainting. Therefore, the traffic police personnel are usually advised to walk around the traffic or make their limb movements frequently while performing their duties for a longer period.

Clinical Note 32.2

Cardiac output decreases in varicosities: In severe varicosities of veins, venous valves become defunct. This in addition to tortuosity and dilation of veins decrease venous return. Therefore, if the varicosity has affected major veins in both limbs, cardiac output may be decreased to decreased venous return.

Thoracic Pump: Venous return **increases during inspiration**. This occurs due to the thoracic pump activity.

- During inspiration, the **intrathoracic pressure becomes more negative** due to expansion of thoracic cage, which is transmitted to the great veins.
- Therefore, the central venous pressure falls.
- The fall in venous pressure during inspiration facilitates venous return.

Abdominal Pump: During inspiration, **intra-abdominal pressure rises** due to descent of diaphragm.

- The increased abdominal pressure compresses the intra-abdominal blood vessels so that the **blood is pushed towards the heart**.
- Blood is ***not pushed towards the leg veins*** as they are guarded by venous valves. Thus, *venous return increases*.

ECF Volume: Venous return greatly depends on the extracellular fluid volume, especially the plasma volume.

- **Decrease in ECF volume** as occurs in diarrhea, vomiting, etc., ***decreases cardiac output***.
- **Increase in ECF volume** as occurs in pregnancy ***increases cardiac output.***

Sympathetic Activity: Veins are innervated by sympathetic fibers.

- Stimulation of sympathetic system causes **venoconstriction**, which in turn ***increases venous return***. This is one of the mechanisms of increased cardiac output **in exercise**.
- Decreased sympathetic stimulation causes **venodilation** that ***decreases cardiac output*** due to increased venous pooling of blood.

Right Atrial Pressure: Right atrial pressure exerts a backward force on the veins to **impede flow of blood** from the veins into the right atrium. The effect of right atrial pressure on venous return is depicted by **venous return curve** (Fig. 32.5), which demonstrates decrease in venous return due to increased right atrial pressure.

- Within the normal range of right atrial pressure, i.e., 0 – 6 mmHg, with increase in pressure, venous return decreases steadily. Venous return is almost zero above 7mmHg of right atrial pressure.
- With **decrease in right atrial pressure**, there is proportionate ***increase in venous return***. When right atrial pressure falls below zero, increase in venous return is slowed and further increase in venous return does not occur when right atrial pressure falls below –2 mm Hg. There will be a **plateau** in venous return curve.

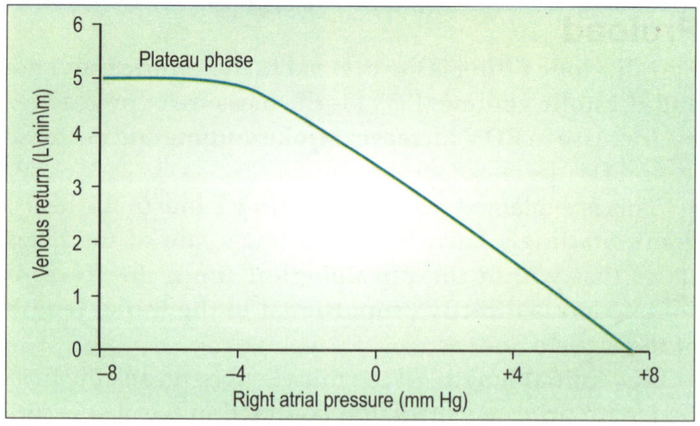

Fig. 32.5: Venous return curve. Note, from 0 mm Hg to – 6 mm Hg of right atrial pressure, venous return decreases steadily.

Degree of Filling of Systemic Circulation: Degree of filling of the systemic circulation **forces the systemic blood toward the heart**.

- This is mainly the **effective blood volume** that fills the circulation and distends the vascular wall.
- This is measured by ***mean systemic filling pressure***.
  - Thus, the effective volume of blood in the entire circulation determines the venous return, as the filling pressure pushes blood from arterial compartment to venous compartment and then to the heart.
- The pressure level that fills the entire circulation is called the ***mean circulatory filling pressure***.
  - The normal mean circulatory pressure is **7 mm Hg**.

Resistance to Venous Return: The resistance to flow of blood between the peripheral vessels and right atrium is called the **venous resistance**, i.e. the *resistance to venous return.*

- Most of the resistance to venous return **occurs in the veins**, although some resistance also occurs in the arterioles and small arteries.
- When **venous resistance increases** as in venous obstruction, **blood begins to be dammed up**, mainly in the venous compartment.
  - But rise in venous pressure to overcome resistance occurs little as the veins are highly distensible.
  - Therefore, rise in venous pressure is not effective in overcoming the resistance, and blood flow into the right atrium decreases significantly.

Atrial Pump Activity

The ventricular filling occurs mostly passively. About **15 to 20% of ventricular filling** at rest occurs due to atrial contraction (the **atrial pump activity**).

- Therefore, normally, atrial pump **does not contribute significantly** to the stroke volume.
- However, in conditions of increased demand for cardiac output as occurs **in exercise**, the atrial systole ***contributes significantly to the enddiastolic filling*** of the ventricle.

- However, in patients with atrial fibrillation, cardiac output does not rise significantly in such conditions (Clinical Note 32.3)

- The *atrial contraction increases* **by sympathetic stimulation**.

Clinical Note 32.3

Cardiac output fails to increase in atrial fibrillation: In atrial fibrillation, cardiac output is not much affected in resting condition as ventricular filling is mostly passive. But in conditions of increased demand for cardiac output, atrial pump fails to increase ventricular filling in patients with atrial fibrillation.

Ventricular Compliance

Normally, the ventricular muscle is compliant (stretchable) enough to accommodate adequate blood during diastole. The normal EDV is 130 ml.

- In pathological conditions like **cardiomyopathies or infiltrative diseases of the heart**, *ventricular filling decreases* due to **decreased compliance** of ventricular muscle (the ability to stretch is decreased).
  - Thus, cardiac output decreases in such conditions.
- Sometimes, the ventricular muscle may be compliant, but there is **restriction to the distention of ventricles** due to pressure from outside as occurs in ***constrictive pericarditis or pericardial effusion***, the enddiastolic volume decreases.
  - In severe **pericardial effusion**, the fluid accumulates in excess in the pericardial cavity, which increases intrapericardial pressure that prevents ventricular expansion and decreases EDV.

Myocardial Contractility

Myocardial contractility exerts a major influence on the cardiac output.

- Factors that increase myocardial contractility are said to be **positively inotropic**, and factors that decrease myocardial contractility are said to be **negatively inotropic**.
- Factors that stimulate contractility ***shift the curve to left*** and factors that inhibit contractility ***shift the curve to right*** (Fig. 32.6).

Myocardial contractility depends on: ventricular muscle mass, state of autonomic activity, concentration of various hormones and chemicals in the blood, drugs, and heart rate.

Ventricular Muscle Mass

Myocardial mass is important in determining stroke volume.

1. **Ventricular muscle mass decreases** either due to loss of myocardium as occurs in myocardial infarction or due to muscle atrophy as seen in some form of cardiomyopathy. In such conditions, ***cardiac output decreases*** significantly.

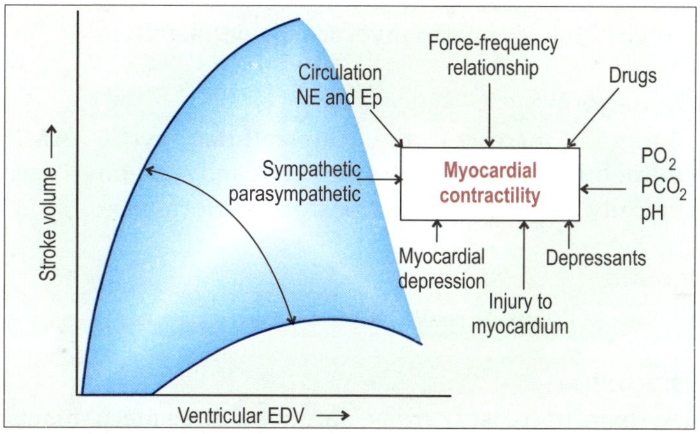

Fig. 32.6: Effects of various factors on ventricular function curve (Starling's curve). Note, factors that stimulate myocardial contractility shift the curve to the left so that greater stroke volume is achieved at lesser EDV, and factors that inhibit myocardial contractility shift the curve to the right so that lesser stroke volume is achieved even at larger EDV.

2. **Increase in myocardial mass increases cardiac output**. The common physiological condition of increased ventricular mass is the *regular practice of physical exercises*.
3. **In strong athletes**, the heart size increases due to physiological hypertrophy of the myocardium. In these individuals, cardiac output increases during exercise by ***mainly increasing the stroke volume*** rather than the heart rate (Application Box 32.1).

Application Box 32.1

Advantage of Training: In fact, the **trained athletes have lower basal heart rate and greater stroke volume.** They achieve a given increase in cardiac output *by increasing their stroke volume* without much increase in heart rate, compared the untrained individuals who increase their cardiac output mainly by increasing heart rate.

Autonomic Activity

Ventricles are supplied by sympathetic fibers.

- **Sympathetic stimulation increases ventricular contractility** and sympathetic inhibition decreases contractility.
- Ventricles are **sparsely innervated by vagal fibers.** Therefore, vagal stimulation has less effect on myocardial contractility.
- However, **vagal stimulation decreases cardiac output** mainly by *decreasing the heart rate.*

Hormonal Factors

Catecholamines

Catecholamines are **positively inotropic**.

- They act on β_1 adrenergic receptors in the ventricle.
- The increased adenylate cyclase activity **increases cyclic AMP** formation in the muscle cell.
- Cyclic AMP ***increases the intracellular calcium*** concentration, which in turn increases myocardial contractility.

Acetylcholine

Acetylcholine acts on **muscarinic receptors** and **decreases intracellular cyclic AMP** concentration. Thus, acetylcholine decreases myocardial contractility.

Glucagon

Glucagon **increases the intracellular cyclic AMP**. Glucagon is a **potent inotropic agent** and sometimes used clinically to enhance the myocardial performance.

Insulin

Insulin is **positively inotropic**.

Thyroxine

Thyroxine increases cardiac output by **three mechanisms**.

1. It increases the **number of β_1 receptors** in the nodal tissues and ventricular muscles.
2. It increases the **sensitivity of these receptors to catecholamines**. Thus, thyroxine produces tachycardia and increases myocardial contractility.
3. Thyroxine also **increases myosin ATPase activity** in the ventricular muscles, which significantly increases myocardial contractility.

Chemical Factors

Xanthines

Xanthines such as **caffeine and theophylline** are positively inotropic.

- They **inhibit intracellular break down of cyclic AMP** so that a high concentration of cyclic AMP is maintained in the ventricular muscle cell.

Inhibiting Factors

The following chemical agents suppress myocardial contractility.

a) Hypercapnia
b) Hypoxia
c) Acidosis (details given below)
d) General anesthetics
e) Toxins

Drugs

Digitalis

Digitalis increases myocardial contractility by **inhibiting the Na^+ - K^+ ATPase activity** on the membrane of myocardial cells (Fig. 32.7).

- This **increases intracellular concentration of sodium** that *opposes sodium gradient* across the membrane from outside to inside the cell.
- Decreased sodium gradient **decreases the activity of sodium-calcium exchanger** on the membrane. As normally, sodium is taken in and calcium is taken out through this exchanger, decreased exchange of these ions leads to ***intracellular accumulation of calcium***.
- Thus, increased cytosolic calcium increases myocardial contractility.

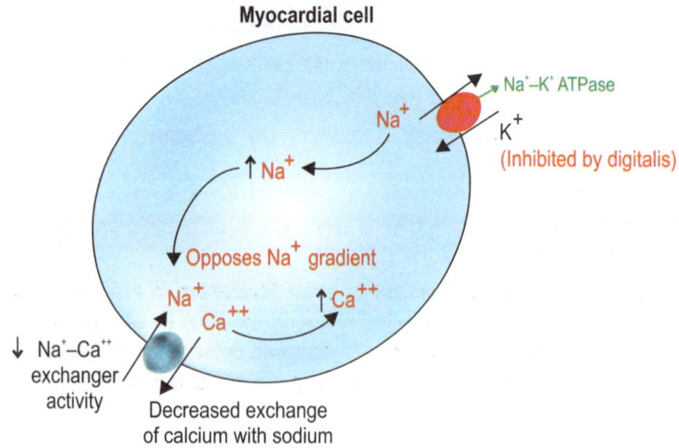

Fig. 32.7: Mechanism of action of digitalis. Inhibition of Na^+-K^+ pump increases Na^+ inside cell that opposes exchange of Ca^{++} with Na^+. Thus, Ca^{++} accumulates in the cell and increases contractility.

Other Drugs

Quinidine, procainamide and barbiturates inhibit myocardial contractility

Afterload

Afterload is the **force against which ventricular muscle fibers shorten**. Essentially, it is the resistance offered against ejection of blood from ventricles. **Peripheral resistance** is considered as the afterload.

- Cardiac output is **inversely proportional to the afterload**.
- Thus, increase in peripheral resistance decreases cardiac output and decrease in peripheral resistance increases cardiac output.
- In this process, cardiac output is altered **without change in ventricular muscle length**.
- Therefore, this type of regulation of cardiac output is called **homometric autoregulation**. This is also known as **Anrep effect** (as described by Anrep in 1974).

Factors Affecting Afterload

Afterload (the peripheral resistance) depends primarily on **two factors**: vessel diameter (vascular hindrance) and viscosity of blood (hematological hindrance).

Vessel Diameter

The decrease in vessel diameter (**vasoconstriction**) increases peripheral resistance that ***decreases stroke volume***.

- Stroke volume increases in **vasodilation** due to decreased afterload.

Viscosity of Blood

Increased viscosity as occurs in polycythemia, increases peripheral resistance and therefore **decreases cardiac output**.

- Cardiac output **increases in anemia** due to decreased viscosity.

Factors Affecting Heart Rate PY5.9

Heart rate is influenced mainly by autonomic activity.

- The **vagal stimulation decreases heart rate** and **sympathetic stimulation increases heart rate**.
- Normally, increase in heart rate should result in increased cardiac output, as cardiac output is the product of heart rate and stroke volume.
  - However, **unless associated with increased venous return** (enddiastolic volume) increase in heart rate may not increase cardiac output proportionately.
- **In severe tachycardia**, the ***duration of diastole shortens*** more than the duration of systole.
  - Therefore, ventricle gets less time to be filled. Thus, enddiastolic volume decreases.
  - Consequently, **cardiac output does not increase proportionately** to that of increase in heart rate.
- Similarly, when **heart rate decreases** (diastole prolongs than systole), diastolic filling of the ventricle increases, which may compensate to maintain cardiac output.

REGULATION OF CARDIAC OUTPUT

Mechanisms regulating cardiac output are broadly divided into **two categories**: a) intrinsic mechanisms, and b) extrinsic mechanisms.

Intrinsic Regulation

The intrinsic regulation is also called as '**Autoregulation' of cardiac output.**

- Two principal intrinsic mechanisms regulate cardiac output.
- These are Frank-Starling mechanism, and rate-induced regulation.

Frank-Starling's Mechanism

The German Physiologist **Otto-Frank** and the English Physiologist **Ernest Starling** described the effect of preload on myocardial performance. This law is therefore known as **Frank-Starling Law** (for details, refer Chapter 28).

- The **increased ventricular volume** (enddiastolic volume) ***increases ventricular contraction*** (stroke volume), and decreased end-diastolic volume decreases stroke volume (details of regulation of EDV is discussed in preceding section).
  - This effect can be demonstrated even in **denervated heart**. Therefore, *regulation by change in preload is **purely an intrinsic mechanism.***
- Such type of regulation of cardiac output by change in ventricular **muscle length at various ventricular volumes** is known as **heterometric autoregulation of the heart**.

Rate-Induced Regulation

Myocardial performance is also regulated by **change in frequency** at which heart muscles contract. With increased frequency the force of contraction increases (**force-frequency relationship**).

This is due to **accumulation of intracellular calcium**, which occurs due to:

1. **Increase in number of depolarizations per minute:** Calcium ions enter the myocardial cells ***during the plateau phase*** (phase 2) of the action potential.
   - Thus, with increase in the number of action potentials (increase in the number of plateau), ***calcium entry into the cell increases*** inspite of decrease in the duration of the action potential.
2. **Increase in the inner calcium current per depolarization:** As the interval between the beats is diminished due to increased frequency, the ***inner calcium current progressively increases*** with each successive beat, which increases the force of contraction.

Extrinsic Regulation

Extrinsic regulation depends on **three major factors**: afterload, neural influences and humoral influences.

Afterload

Change in **peripheral resistance** (afterload) alters cardiac output.

- The increase in afterload decreases cardiac output and decrease in afterload increases cardiac output.
- This type of regulation is known as **homometric regulation of the heart**, as cardiac output is altered without change in muscle length (Application Box 32.2).

Application Box 32.2

Anrep Effect: The homometric regulation of cardiac output is also known as *Anrep effect* as described by Anrep in 1974. It explains the influence of peripheral resistance on cardiac output.

Neural Control

Neural control is primarily by **autonomic influences**.

Sympathetic Influence

Stimulation of sympathetic nerve to the heart **increases heart rate and myocardial contractility** that increases cardiac output.

- Sympathetic stimulation also causes **venoconstriction** and increases the venous return, which also contributes to increase in cardiac output.

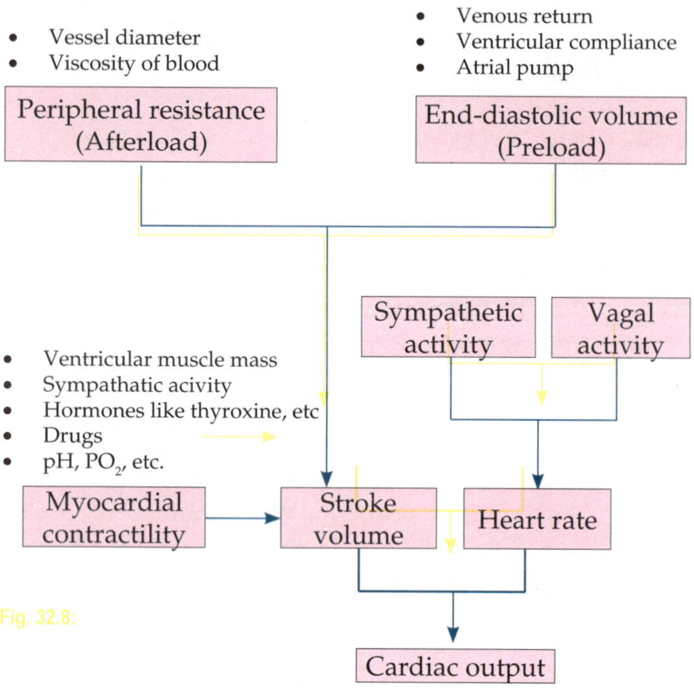

Fig. 32.8: Schematic presentation of major factors regulating cardiac output.

Parasympathetic Influence

Parasympathetic stimulation decreases cardiac output mainly by **decreasing heart rate.**

- Ventricular contractility is marginally decreased, as vagal innervation of ventricle is sparse (Fig. 32.8).

Humoral Control

Humoral control includes regulation by hormones and chemicals.

Hormonal Regulation

Hormonal regulation is mainly by catecholamines, thyroid hormones, insulin, glucagon and growth hormone.

Adrenomedullary Hormones: The hormones secreted by adrenal medulla (epinephrine, norepinephrine and dopamine) **increase myocardial contractility and heart rate** (details, described above). Thus, cardiac output increases.

Thyroid Hormones: Thyroxine increases cardiac output by following **four mechanisms**:

1. By **increasing the myosin ATPase activity**, it increases the excitation-contraction coupling.
2. It **increases the number of receptors** and **sensitivity of the receptors to catecholamines** in the nodal tissues and ventricular muscles. Thus, heart rate and myocardial contractility increases.
3. It **increases protein synthesis** in the myocardial cells that causes ventricular hypertrophy. Increased ventricular mass increases myocardial contractility.
4. It **increases body metabolism**. The increased body temperature causes **vasodilation** that in turn **decreases peripheral resistance**. Decreased afterload increases cardiac output.

Insulin: Insulin has **direct positive inotropic effect** on the heart.

Glucagon: Glucagon has both positive inotropic and chronotropic effects.

- It acts by **increasing intracellular cyclic AMP**.
- Cyclic AMP increases calcium concentration in the myocardial cell by **two mechanisms**.
    i) It increases ***calcium influx*** by opening the calcium channels on the cell membranes.
    ii) It increases ***calcium release*** from the sarcoplasmic reticulum.

Growth Hormone: Growth hormone increases cardiac output by ***increasing the myocardial contractility***.

Chemical Regulation

Chemical regulation is mainly by blood gases and pH.

Oxygen: Mild hypoxia causes **tachycardia**. Moderate to **severe hypoxia decreases cardiac output** by directly *suppressing myocardial contractility* and also by stimulating the peripheral chemoreceptors.

Carbon Dioxide: Carbon dioxide has direct and indirect effects on myocardium.

- Directly it ***depresses the myocardium***.
- The indirect effect is **neurally mediated** through its action on central and peripheral chemoreceptors.

Acidosis: Acidosis **depresses myocardium**.

- The reduced intracellular pH ***diminishes the amount of calcium released*** from the sarcoplasmic reticulum and also ***decreases the sensitivity of the myofilaments*** to the calcium.
- Increase in intracellular pH has the opposite effect.

Exam Questions

1. Describe the methods of measurement of cardiac output (CO).
2. Describe the factors affecting CO.
3. Describe the mechanisms of regulation of CO.
4. List the factors affecting preload. Describe how Frank-Starling mechanism influences CO.
5. List the factors affecting myocardial contractility. Explain how the ventricular muscle mass contributes to CO.
6. What is Anrep effect. Explain its physiological application.

Multiple Choice Questions

1. **If cardiac output is 6 liters/minute and body surface area is 2 m2, cardiac index is:**
   A. 3 liter/min/m^2
   B. 4 liter/min/m^2
   C. 5 liter/min/m^2
   D. 2.5 liter/min/m^2
2. **Ejection fraction is the ratio of:**
   A. End diastolic volume to stroke volume
   B. Stroke volume to end systolic volume
   C. End systolic volume to end diastolic volume
   D. Stroke volume to end diastolic volume
3. **Stroke volume is increased in**
   A. Standing
   B. Decreased muscle tone
   C. Hypovolemia
   D. Lying down
4. **What is the normal left ventricular ejection fraction?**
   A. 65%
   B. 45%
   C. 35%
   D. 25%
5. **Cardiac output in L/min divided by heart rate equals:**
   A. Cardiac index
   B. Cardiac efficiency
   C. Mean stroke volume
   D. Mean arterial pressure
6. **The cardiac output can be determined by all except**
   A. Echocardiography
   B. Indicator-dilution technique
   C. Electrocardiography
   D. Ballistocardiography
7. **Cardiac output decreases during:**
   A. Eating
   B. Standing from lying position
   C. Excitement
   D. High environmental temperature
8. **Cardiac output is increased in:**
   A. Diarrhea
   B. Vomiting
   C. Exercise
   D. Sitting from lying
9. **Frank-Starling's law implies:**
   A. Increased BP increases CO
   B. Increased vagal discharge increased CO
   C. Increased HR causes increased CO
   D. Increased VR increases CO
10. **End diastolic volume increases due to:**
    A. Decrease in total blood volume
    B. Increase in negative intrathoracic pressure
    C. Increase in intrapericardial pressure
    D. Decrease in ventricular compliance
11. **Single most important factor in control of contractility of heart is:**
    A. Myocardial wall thickness
    B. Sympathetic stimulation
    C. Right atrial volume
    D. SA node pacemaker potential
12. **Amount of blood that can be pumped by each ventricle in excess of normal cardiac output is:**
    A. Cardiac efficiency index
    B. Cardiac index
    C. Cardiac diastolic volume
    D. Cardiac reserve
13. **Which of the following statement is NOT true?**
    A. Denervated heart has more heart rate
    B. Vagal stimulation decreases rate of contraction
    C. During exercise systole is shortened more than diastole
    D. Noradrenaline increases force of contraction
14. **Volume determining preload is:**
    A. Stroke volume
    B. End-diastolic volume
    C. End-systolic volume
    D. Total blood volume
15. **Sympathetic stimulation causes all of the following except**
    A. Increase in venous capacitance
    B. Increase in ventricular force of contraction
    C. Increase in heart rate
    D. Increase in total peripheral resistance
16. **Anrep effect represents the regulation of cardiac output by:**
    A. Heart rate
    B. End-diastolic volume
    C. Myocardial contractility
    D. Peripheral resistance
17. **With increase in heart rate, the force of myocardial contraction increases, due to:**
    A. Increase in venous return to heart
    B. Increased effectiveness of the atrial pump
    C. Increase in the inner calcium current per depolarization
    D. Decreased peripheral resistance
18. **Which of the following factor decrease peripheral resistance?**
    A. Fever
    B. Polycythemia
    C. Sympathetic stimulation
    D. Hyperproteinemia
19. **All of the following factors increase myocardial contractility, EXCEPT:**
    A. Insulin
    B. Glucagon
    C. Thyroxine
    D. Acetylcholine
20. **All of the following are needed to calculate CO by Fick method, EXCEPT:**
    A. Pulmonary artery O2 concentration
    B. Radial artery CO2 concentration
    C. Radial artery O2 concentration
    D. Total body O2 consumption

Answers

1. A	2. D	3. D	4. A	5. C	6. C	7. B	8. C	9. D	10. B	11. A
12. D	13. C	14. B	15. A	16. D	17. C	18. A	19. D	20. B		

Chapter 33

Heart Rate and Arterial Pulse

Learning Objectives

On completion of study of this chapter:

The student will be able to (must know):

1. Give normal range of heart rate & physiological variation of heart rate.
2. Understand the mechanisms of regulation of heart rate.
3. Appreciate the graph of arterial pulse tracing.
4. List the causes of bradycardia & tachycardia.
5. Name abnormal pulses and understand their physiological basis.

The student may also be able to (desirable to know):

1. Explain the physiological basis and mechanism of abnormal pulses.

HEART RATE

The normal heart rate is **60 – 100 per minute** in adults.

- Heart rate **less than 60/min** is called ***bradycardia*** and **above 100/min** is called ***tachycardia***.
- Normally, heart rate is more in infants and children and less in geriatric age group.
- As SA node is the natural primary pacemaker, ***heart rate is the rate of discharge of SA node***.

Physiological Variations

Age: Heart rate is **more in infants and children**. After the age of sixty, heart rate decreases.

Gender: Heart rate is *comparatively less in females* due to their relatively high parasympathetic tone and less basal metabolism.

Diurnal Variation: Heart rate is **more in the day**, especially in the afternoon, and **less in the night**, especially during sleep.

- This difference is due to the *less physical activity* and *sympathetic discharge in the night*, and due to the ***low level of stress*** in sleep than in awakened state.

Respiration: Heart rate is **more during inspiration** and less during expiration (**sinus arrhythmia**).

- This is mainly due to alteration in vagal activity, which is more in expiration and less in inspiration.

Body Temperature: Increase in body temperature increases heart rate and decrease in temperature decreases heart rate.

Environmental Temperature: Heart rate is more in summer and less in winter.

Food intake: Food intake increases heart rate by increasing body metabolism.

Posture: Change in posture from **supine to standing increases heart rate** due to decreased stimulation of baroreceptors (for details, see Baroreceptor Reflex).

Exercise: Heart rate increases in exercise **due to sympathetic stimulation**. Heart rate may even increase before starting the exercise due to psychological effects that acts through limbic system.

Regulation of Heart Rate

Mechanisms regulating heart rate can be divided broadly into **two categories**: i) Neural mechanisms, and ii) Humoral mechanisms.

Neural Control Mechanisms

Neural regulating mechanisms are divided into **three categories**:

1. Autonomic regulation
2. Reflex regulation
3. Regulation by higher centers

Autonomic Control

Both parasympathetic and sympathetic divisions of autonomic nervous system influence heart rate.

Normally, **parasympathetic control of SA node dominates** *the sympathetic control*. Therefore, the basal heart rate is less than the intrinsic heart rate.

- The **intrinsic heart rate** is the rate of discharge of SA node when the heart is completely denervated. It is about 110 per minute. This indicates that the *heart rate is more in the absence of neural influences*.
- With intact autonomic innervation, due to ***more vagal influence on SA node*** (as vagus is inhibitory), the normal heart rate is less than the intrinsic heart rate.

Parasympathetic Control

Vagus nerve is the primary regulator of heart rate.

- Stimulation of vagus nerve results in **decrease in heart rate**.
- There is **beat-to-beat control** of SA node by the vagus nerve.

Sympathetic Control

The sympathetic fibers supplying the pacemaker tissue originate from the **lower two cervical and upper six thoracic segments** of spinal cord.

- The stimulation of sympathetic fibers results in **increase in heart rate**.
- The effect of sympathetic stimulation on heart rate remains **for a longer period** than the vagal stimulation.

Reflex Control

Cardiovascular reflexes that regulate blood pressure also control heart rate, as part of the integrated control mechanisms.

- The important reflexes are baroreceptor reflex, chemoreceptor reflex, Cushing's reflex, Bainbridge reflex and other reflexes. (for details, refer Chapter 37)

Control by Higher Centers

Stimulation of motor cortex, frontal lobe, and thalamus increases heart rate.

- **Increase in heart rate in emotional states**, anxiety, and excitement is due to **stimulation of limbic system**.

Humoral Control Mechanisms

- Thyroxine and catecholamines increase heart rate (details are given in previous chapter)
- Hypoxia increases heart rate, which is partly mediated by release of catecholamines from adrenal medulla. Hypercapnia and acidosis decrease heart rate.

ARTERIAL PULSE

Physiological Aspects

Definition: Arterial pulse is defined as the rhythmic expansion of the arterial wall due to transmission of pressure waves along the walls of the arteries that are produced during each systole of the heart.

Clinical Importance: Clinically, **radial pulse** is examined for the assessment of arterial pulse.

- It is an important and essential part of the clinical examination of a patient as pulse is one of the **vital signs** of a living being (other vital signs are BP, respiration and temperature).
- Examination of arterial pulse also provides valuable information regarding the functioning of the heart, condition of hemodynamics like blood pressure, and the condition of blood vessels.

Normal Pulse Rate: Normally, pulse rate is same as heart rate. Thus, the normal pulse rate is 60 to 100 per minute.

- The deficit between pulse rate and heart rate is called **pulse deficit** (Clinical Note 33.1).
  - There is no pulse deficit in normal conditions.
- Pulse rate more than 100 is called ***tachycardia***, and less than 60, is called ***bradycardia***.

Clinical Note 33.1

Pulse Deficit: When the cardiac rhythm is irregular due to some organic heart disease, few contractions of the ventricle may not be sufficient enough to generate pressure waves in the walls of the arteries. Therefore, a deficit occurs between the rate of heart contraction and the pulse rate.

- Pulse deficit is usually seen in atrial fibrillation in which the deficit is more than 10.
- Pulse deficit seen in other arrhythmias and diseases causing heart blocks is usually less than 10.

Normal Pulse Tracing

Arterial pulse tracing shows two waves and one notch.

- The waves are **percussion (p) wave**, also called as tidal wave, and **dicrotic (d) wave** (Fig. 33.1), and the notch is **dicrotic notch** (n).

1. **Percussion wave** occurs due to ejection of blood during ventricular systole.
2. **Dicrotic wave** occurs due to rebound of blood against the closed aortic valve during diastole.
3. **Dicrotic notch** represents closure of aortic valve.

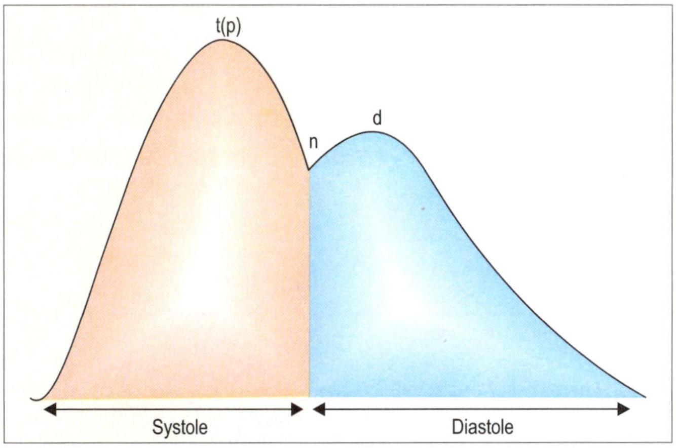

Fig. 33.1: The arterial pulse tracing recorded from a peripheral artery. (t: tidal wave or also called percussion wave (p); d: dicrotic wave; n: dicrotic notch).

Variations in Heart Rate

Tachycardia

Physiological: Exercise, eating, anger, emotion and excitement, infants and children, pregnancy and high environmental temperature

Pathological: Fever, aemia, thyrotoxicosis, beriberi, Paget's disease, arterio-venous fistula, heart failure, paroxysmal atrial tachycardia, ventricular or supra ventricular tachycardia, and other tachyarrhythmias.

Bradycardia

Physiological: Athletes, extreme fear, grief, very old age, and practitioners of yoga.

Pathological: Myxedema, increased intracranial pressure (e.g. brain tumors), obstructive jaundice, different types of heart block, and drugs (e.g. digitalis).

Common Abnormal Pulses

Anacrotic Pulse

This is also called as **anadicrotic pulse**, which means two up beats.

- A *secondary wave* occurs in the upstroke of the pulse.
- It is commonly found in **aortic stenosis**.
- The upstroke is slow and sloping (Fig. 33.2 A).

Dicrotic Pulse

It is also called as twice-beating pulse.

- The **dicrotic wave is prominent** and gives the feeling of two beats (Fig. 33.2 B).

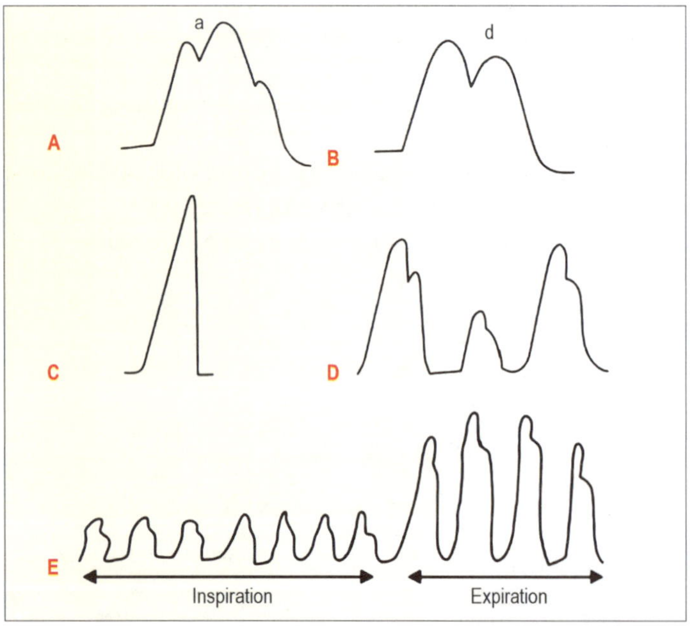

Figs. 33.2A to E: The abnormal arterial pulses. (A) Anacrotic pulse, note that anacrotic wave (a) is abnormally prominent, which is normally not visible; (B) Dicrotic pulse in which dicrotic wave (d) is abnormally large; (C) Water--hammer pulse (note the rapid upstroke and rapid downstroke without a dicrotic notch); D: Pulsus alternans; (E) Pulsus paradoxus (note the gross decrease in amplitude during inspiration.

- It is commonly seen in febrile states, especially in **typhoid fever**.

Water-Hammer Pulse

This is also called as **collapsing pulse or Corrigan's pulse**. It is typically seen in **aortic regurgitation**.

- The collapsing pulse is characterized by **a rapid upstroke** (ascent) and a **rapid down stroke** (descent) of the pulse wave (Fig. 33.2 C).
- The rapid upstroke is due to greatly increased stroke volume and the rapid descent is due to the collapse of the pulse. The collapse of the pulse occurs due to **two factors**:
  i) the **diastolic run-off of blood** into the left ventricle, and
  ii) **rapid run-off of blood** into the periphery because of decreased systemic vascular resistance.
- Therefore, the **pulse pressure is very high**, may be as high as 100 mm of Hg.

Causes:

1. Aortic incompetence
2. Patent ductus arteriosus
3. Arteriovenous fistula
4. Ventricular septal defect (VSD)
5. Hyperkinetic circulatory states e.g. thyrotoxicosis

Physiological Basis: The collapsing pulse is a steep rising, forceful, high amplitude percussion wave which gives a sharp tap to the palpating hand that suddenly disappears. The **steep rise of the ascending limb** of the pulse wave is due to:

- **Increased enddiastolic volume** (EDV) of the left ventricle, as during diastole in addition to the ventricular filling from the left atrium the filling also occurs from the incompetent aortic valve.
- This increases the total EDV, which increases the force of contraction of the left ventricle during systole by ***Frank-Starling mechanism.***
- Thus, steep rise occurs in the percussion wave during systole.

The **steep fall of the descending limb** of the pulse wave is due to **two factors.**

1. ***Diastolic run-off of blood*** into the left ventricle.
2. ***Rapid run-off*** of blood into the periphery due to decreased vascular resistance.

Pulsus Bisferiens

Pulsus bisferiens is a **combination of the low rising pulse (anacrotic pulse) and the collapsing pulse.**

- This is typically seen in **aortic stenosis** associated with **aortic incompetence**.

Pulsus Paradoxus

This is a misnomer. There is nothing paradoxical in this pulse.

1. Actually, this is an accentuation of the normal phenomenon.
2. Normally, the **amplitude of the pulse decreases in inspiration and increases in expiration**.
3. In pulsus paradoxus, in inspiration the **volume of the pulse is grossly decreased**, or may be absent in severe cases (Fig. 33.2 E).

Causes

Common Causes:
1. Constrictive pericarditis
2. Pericardial effusion

Less Common Causes:
1. Emphysema
2. Asthma
3. Massive pleural effusion
4. A mass in the thorax
5. Advanced right ventricular failure

Mechanisms

1. During inspiration, the intrathoracic pressure becomes more negative. Pooling of blood occurs in the pulmonary vascular bed, which **decreases venous return** to the left atrium.
   - Thus, **left atrial filling decreases** that in turn **decreases left ventricular stroke volume**.
   - Therefore, volume of the pulse decreases in inspiration.
   - This is more accentuated in the above-mentioned diseased conditions.
2. During inspiration, the **intrapericardial pressure increases due to the traction from the attachments** put on the pericardium.
   - This ***decreases venous return*** to the heart and results in low stroke volume.
   - This is more accentuated in pericardial effusion and constrictive pericarditis.
3. **In constrictive pericarditis and pericardial effusion**, the filling of the atria and ventricles decreases due to restriction to the expansion of the heart chambers.
   - The ***limitation in the diastolic filling*** of the right atrium and the right ventricle during inspiration results in lowering of left ventricular stroke volume.
4. **In advanced stage of ventricular failure**, increase in lung volume in inspiration *accommodates more blood* than normal due to much decreased pulmonary vascular resistance.
   - As such, there is ***decreased right ventricular output***.
   - These two factors decrease venous return to left atrium that in turn decreases left ventricular stroke volume.
5. **In bronchial asthma**, the increased respiratory effort makes ***intrathoracic pressure more negative*** during inspiration.
   - Hence, there is more pooling of blood in the pulmonary veins that results in decreased ventricular stroke volume.

Pulsus Alternans

The pulse is regular, but the **alternating beats are strong and weak** (Fig. 33.2 D).

- It is difficult to appreciate pulsus alternans by palpating the artery.
  - Diagnosis is confirmed while measuring blood pressure.
- A difference of **5 to 20 mm Hg in the systolic pressure** is marked between two alternate beats.
- When the column of mercury in the manometer is being lowered, the stronger beats are heard first, and on further lowering, the weaker beats also become audible.
  - Thus, suddenly the number of audible beats is doubled.

Causes:

1. Left ventricular failure (commonest cause)
2. Toxic carditis

Physiological Basis: In **left ventricular failure**, due to decreased myocardial contractility the **stroke volume is decreased**. This results in low volume pulse.

- Due to inadequate ejection of blood during systole, the end-systolic volume of the left ventricle increases.
- Therefore, **EDV increases** before the onset of next ventricular contraction.
- This increases the force of contraction of the ventricle in the next beat by **Frank-Starling mechanism**.
- Consequently, the second beat becomes stronger.
- Likewise, the strong and weak beats alternate.

Exam Questions

1. What is the normal heart rate (HR)? What are the physiological variations of HR (tachycardia and bradycardia). Briefly describe the regulation of HR.
2. Draw a schematic diagram to depict the waves of a normal pulse tracing. Describe the waves of arterial pulse tracing.
3. Draw schematic diagram of pulse wave to depict water-hammer pulse, pulsus paradoxus, and pulsus alternans. List 4 causes of each of these abnormal pulses. Describe their physiological basis.

Multiple Choice Questions

1. **Which of the following statement is true?**
   A. HR is the rate of discharge of SA node
   B. Normal pulse rate is 60 – 100 per min
   C. The intrinsic HR is less than the normal HR
   D. The difference between pulse rate and HR is called pulse deficit
2. **Which is true about heart rate?**
   A. Less in female compared to males due to relatively more vagal tone in females
   B. More in night due to less vagal activity
   C. Less in infants and children due to less body size
   D. More in elderly due to more stress of life
3. **All are true about sinus arrhythmia, EXCEPT:**
   A. Irradiation from inspiratory center to vasomotor center contributes to it
   B. It is mostly due to alteration in vagal activity
   C. Bainbridge reflex contributes to it
   D. HR is less in inspiration and more in expiration
4. **Bradycardia is seen in:**
   A. Fever
   B. Hypoxemia
   C. Cardiac failure
   D. Raised intracranial pressure
5. **Stimulation of which of the following medullary center produces tachycardia?**
   A. Dorsal motor nucleus of vagus nerve
   B. Vasomotor center
   C. Nucleus tractus solitarius
   D. Nucleus ambiguous
6. **Water-hammer pulse is seen in all EXCEPT:**
   A. Ventricular septal defect
   B. Hypothyroidism
   C. Aortic incompetence
   D. Arteriovenous fistula
7. **Pulsus alternans is seen in:**
   A. Thyrotoxicosis
   B. Aortic incompetence
   C. Left ventricular failure
   D. Patent ductus arteriosus
8. **Which of the following is NOT true about arterial pulse tracing?**
   A. Tidal wave is due to ventricular diastole
   B. Dicrotic notch is due to closure of aortic valve
   C. Percussion wave is due to ejection of blood during systole
   D. Dicrotic wave is due to rebound of blood against closed aortic valve

Answers

1. C 2. A 3. D 4. D 5. B 6. B 7. C 8. A

Multiple Choice Questions of Chapter 31 (Cardiac Cycle) Contd...

6. **First heart sound (S_1):**
   A. Characterized by high pitch and sharp sound
   B. Marks the onset of ventricular systole
   C. Best heard over aortic and pulmonary areas
   D. Caused by the closure of semilunar valves
7. **The first sound (S_1) occurs due to closure of AV valves during:**
   A. Isotonic ventricular relaxation
   B. Isotonic ventricular contraction
   C. Isovolumetric ventricular contraction
   D. Isovolumetric ventricular relaxation
8. **The second heart sound differs from first heart sound in that:**
   A. Does not split normally
   B. Has higher frequency
   C. Duration greater than first sound
   D. Due partly to turbulence set up by ventricular contraction
9. **Second heart sound (S_2):**
   A. Is due to closure of tricuspid valves
   B. Has frequency greater than first sound
   C. Has duration greater than first sound
   D. Does not split normally
10. **The peak pressure of atrial systole is:**
    A. 7-8mmHg B. 8-15 mmHg
    C. 15-20 mmHg D. 20-25 mmHg
11. **The pulmonary valve opens when right ventricular pressure exceeds:**
    A. 10-12 mmHg B. 12-15 mmHg
    C. 15-20 mmHg D. 20-25 mmHg
12. **The 'a' wave in JVP is absent in:**
    A. Atrial fibrillation B. Ventricular fibrillation
    C. Atrio-ventricular dissociation D. Atrial myxoma
13. **The 'a' wave in JVP becomes very big in:**
    A. Complete heart block with atria and ventricle contracting simultaneously
    B. Atrial hypertrophy
    C. Atrial fibrillation
    D. Atrial asystole
14. **In which of the following condition, contribution of atrial systole to ventricular filling during exercise is not significant:**
    A. Ventricular fibrillation B. Ventricular tachycardia
    C. Atrial fibrillation D. Type II heart block
15. **Semilunar valves open when:**
    A. Pressure in great vessels exceeds the pressure in the corresponding ventricles
    B. Pressure in ventricles exceeds the pressure in the corresponding great vessels
    C. Pressure in left atrium is more than the pressure in the left ventricle
    D. Pressure in right atrium is more than the pressure in the right ventricle
16. **The maximally achievable systolic pressure by left ventricle is:**
    A. 120 B. 150 C. 200 D. 300
17. **Normally, end-diastolic volume to the stroke volume % is:**
    A. 35 B. 50 C. 65 D. 80

Answers

6. B 7. C 8. B 9. B 10. A 11. A
12. A 13. A 14. C 15. B 16. D 17. C

Chapter 34

Principles of Hemodynamics

Learning Objectives

On completion of study of this chapter:

The student will be able to (must know):

1. Apply the basic principles of hemodynamics in cardiovascular functions.
2. Understand the velocity-flow-pressure relationship of blood vessels.
3. List the differences between laminar and turbulent flow.
4. Understand the factors governing peripheral resistance.
5. Learn the application of law of Laplace in cardiovascular functions.

The student may also be able to (desirable to know):

1. Describe the hemodynamic principles and their application in health and disease.

Hemodynamics is the interaction of various physical principles that govern circulation of blood.

- Blood flow is also influenced by **composition and rheological properties** of blood, and **many physico-chemical factors**.
- Blood flow primarily depends on **two important factors**: i) the properties of blood and ii) the diameter of blood vessels.

PY5.7

PHYSICAL PRINCIPLES GOVERNING CIRCULATION

Velocity-Flow-Pressure Relationship

Velocity vs. Blood Flow

Velocity is defined as the **rate of displacement of fluid with respect to time**.

- This is expressed as distance per unit time, for example in cm/s.
- **Flow** is defined as the volume displacement per unit time (cm^3/s).
- The velocity of fluid in a system depends on the **area & the flow**.
- Flow in turn depends on the **pressure gradient, properties of the fluid and dimensions of the hydraulic system** of the tube.

Velocity is the flow divided by the area of the conduit.

$V = \frac{Q}{A}$, V is the velocity, Q is the flow and A is the area.

Effect of Cross-Sectional Area: The average velocity of fluid movement in a system is directly proportional to the flow and **inversely proportional to the total cross-sectional area** of the system.

- Therefore, in vascular system, **velocity gradually decreases** as blood flows from the aorta through arteries and arterioles into capillaries due to ***progressive increase in the cross-sectional area*** (Fig. 34.1).
- Velocity **slowly increases** as blood passes from venules through veins into the vena cava, which occurs due to *gradual decrease in the cross-sectional area* of these vessels as they approach the heart.

Velocity Vs Pressure

Change in pressure in a hydraulic system changes the velocity of fluid movement. The pressure in a hydraulic system has **two components**: the lateral (or the static) pressure component and the dynamic pressure component.

1. **Lateral pressure** is the side pressure that is exerted constantly ***on the wall*** of the tube.
2. **Dynamic pressure** is the component of pressure, which is affected by the ***kinetic energy of flow***; for example, increase in flow increases the dynamic component.

Bernoulli's Principle: Bernoulli's Principle states that the **total pressure** (the static plus the dynamic pressure) in a closed system remains always constant.

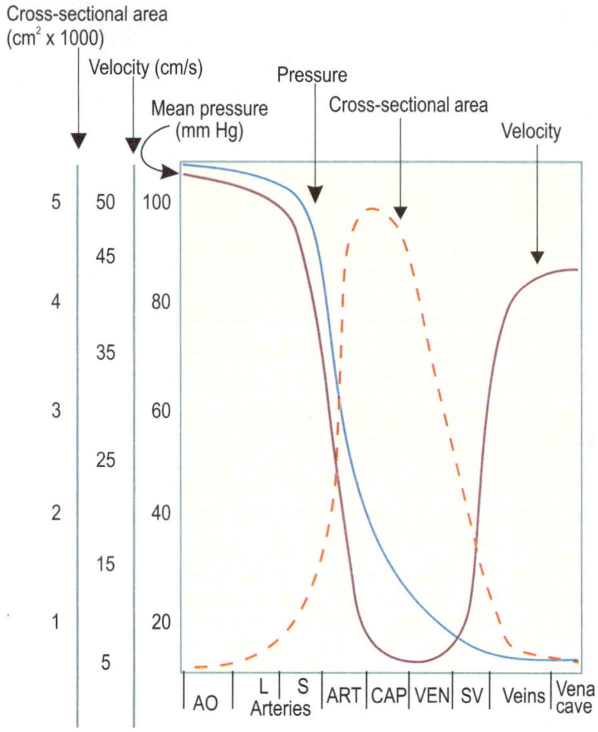

Fig. 34.1: The relationship between pressure, velocity and cross sectional area in circulatory system. Note the inverse relationship between cross-sectional area and velocity of blood flow. Also note that steep fall in pressure occur in the arterioles. (AO: aorta; L: large; S: small; ART: arterioles; CAP: capillaries; VEN: venules; SV: small veins)

- As the total pressure does not change, the **alteration in any component** of pressure occurs at the *cost of the other*. Especially, change in dynamic pressure component that occurs frequently in a hydraulic system *changes the lateral pressure*.
- In circulatory system, at the **sites of narrowing** of blood vessel the **velocity of flow increases**, which in turn increases the dynamic component of the pressure. The increase in dynamic pressure **decreases the lateral pressure** (Fig. 34.2).
- Lateral pressure in the blood vessel **determines the degree of perfusion** of tissues as it decides the amount of blood that enters into the branches from the main vessel.
- Thus, **at the site of constriction** the *perfusion of tissue* ***decreases.*** Therefore, myocardial infarction is common in aortic stenosis (Clinical Note 34.1).

Clinical Note 34.1

AMI is common in aortic stenosis: In aortic stenosis, narrowed aortic valve *increases the velocity of aortic flow*. This increases the dynamic pressure and decreases the lateral pressure. Coronary arteries receive less blood as reduced lateral pressure retards perfusion. This induces myocardial ischemia, which aids to already hypertrophied ventricle pumping blood against a higher resistance. Hence, acute myocardial infarction is common in aortic stenosis.

Flow, Pressure and Resistance

Pressure is one of the principal determinants of the rate of flow. **Increased pressure increases flow** and decreased pressure decreases flow.

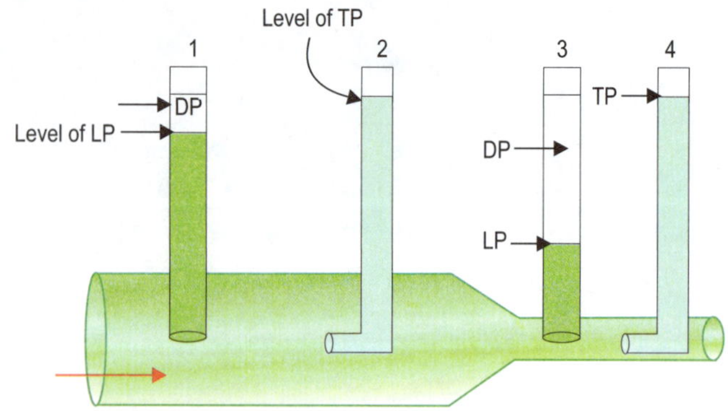

Fig. 34.2: Relationship between dynamic and lateral pressures in vascular system with different diameter (cross-sectional area). The tube with two different diameters represents the wider and narrower regions of vascular system. The red arrow indicates the direction of flow of fluid in the tube. 1, 2, 3 and 4 are pressure probes inserted into the tube for recording pressures. The intraluminal ends of tubes 1 and 3 are present vertically, therefore, they record only lateral pressure (LP) of the fluid, whereas the intraluminal ends of tubes 2 and 4 are present tangentially facing the upstream of flow, therefore, they record the total pressure (TP). Note, the total pressure remains same, but lateral pressure is decreased in the narrow part due to increased dynamic pressure (DP), which is due to increased velocity of flow in this part.

Ohm's Law: The relationship between flow, pressure, and resistance in a hydraulic system is well compared with the relationship between current, electromotive force, and resistance in an electrical circuit. According to **Ohm's Law**:

$$\text{Current (I)} = \frac{\text{Electromotive force (E)}}{\text{Resistance (R)}}$$

$$\text{Similarly, Flow (F)} = \frac{\text{Pressure (P)}}{\text{Resistance (R)}}$$

In vascular system, **pressure** is the ***effective perfusion pressure*** (the mean intraluminal pressure at the arterial end minus the mean pressure at the venous end) and **resistance** is the ***peripheral resistance***.

- Flow is **directly proportional to the pressure** and ***inversely proportional to the resistance***.
- Increase in resistance decreases flow.

Types of Blood Flow

Blood flow is of two types: laminar (streamline) flow and turbulent flow.

Laminar Flow

Normally, flow of blood in the vessels is laminar in nature (laminar means '**in layers**'). That means, the normal blood flow occurs in layers.

- Laminar flow is also called **streamline flow**.
- The layer of the blood, which is in close contact with the wall of the vessel, does not move at all due to the frictional resistance with the vessel wall, the next layer moves with lesser velocity.
  - The **velocity slowly increases towards the center** of the vessel.

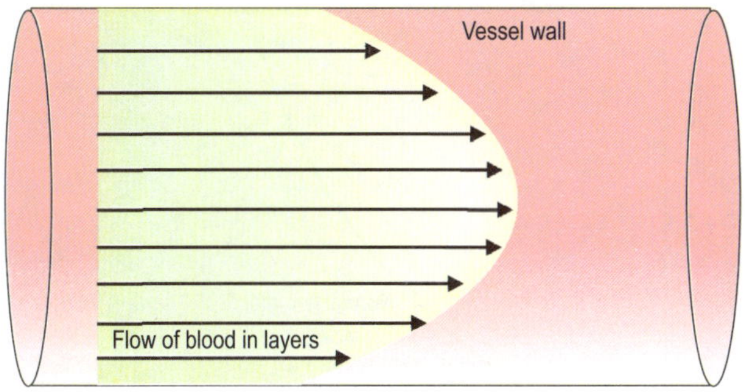

Fig. 34.3: Laminar or streamline flow of blood that occurs in layers. Arrows represent the direction of flow. The length of arrows indicates the velocity of flow in that layer. The velocities have a parabolic distribution with maximum velocity at the center of the stream.

- The velocity of flow is **maximal in the central layer of blood** in the vessel (Fig. 34.3).
  - However, laminar flow occurs *upto a certain velocity* beyond which the flow becomes turbulent.
  - The velocity above which the flow is turbulent is known as **critical velocity**.

Turbulent Flow

The turbulent flow occurs when **velocity is above critical velocity**.

- Turbulence of flow depends on the **diameter of the vessel** and the **viscosity of the blood**.
- The probability of turbulence is expressed in terms of **Reynolds number**, which is calculated as:

$$Re = \frac{\rho DV}{\eta}$$

Where, 'Re' is the Reynolds number, ρ is the density of the fluid, D is the diameter of the tube, V is the velocity of flow and η is the viscosity of the fluid.

- The **probability of turbulence** increases when the value of 'Re' is greater. Usually, when the 'Re' is less than 2000 the flow is laminar and when the ***'Re' is more than 3000 the flow is turbulent***.
- In cardiovascular system, **at the site of constriction**, increase in the velocity of blood flow makes the flow turbulent.

Application Box 34.1

Korotkow sounds are produced by turbulent flow: A better example of sounds produced by turbulence in flow is is the auscultation of Korotkow sounds on the brachial artery in the cubital fossa due to constriction of the artery by inflated BP cuff, during measurement of blood pressure by auscultatory method.

- Turbulence of flow **produces sound** (Table 34.1).
  - Therefore, a murmurish sound is heard on auscultation at the site of constriction of the vessel or cardiac orifice.
- For example, a **bruit** is auscultated over an arterial constriction, or a **murmur** is heard over a stenotic cardiac valve.
  - A better example is the auscultation of *Korotkow sounds* (Application Box 34.1)

Table 34.1 | Differences between laminar flow and turbulent flow.

	Laminar flow	Turbulent flow
1. Nature of flow	Flow occurs in layers (flow is streamline)	No layers (flow is disturbed)
2. Velocity of flow	Below the critical velocity	Above the critical velocity
3. Reynolds number	Below 2000	Above 3000
4. Association of sound	Soundless (silent)	Associated with sound

Poiseuille-Hagen Formula

Poiseuille-Hagen formula denotes the relationship between **viscosity of the fluid with the radius and length of the tube**.

$F = (P_a - P_v) \times \{\pi/8\} \times \{1/\eta\} \times \{r^4/L\}$

Where, F = Flow

$P_a - P_v$ = Pressure difference between the both ends of the tube

η= Viscosity of fluid

r = Radius of tube

L = Length of tube

As discussed above, **flow** is equal to the **pressure difference divided by resistance**.

Therefore, resistance (R) is calculated from the following formula:

$$R = \frac{8\eta L}{\pi r^4}$$

Flow varies directly with the **fourth power of the radius**.

- Therefore, **vessel diameter is most important factor** determining the blood flow and pressure.

Effect of Vessel Diameter: Blood flow is markedly affected by a small change in the diameter of the blood vessel.

- The **flow becomes double** in a vessel by just **increasing the radius to about 20%**.
- Consequently, blood flow is significantly altered by mildly changing the diameter of vessels.
- Flow affects pressure. Thus, change in diameter **changes flow and pressure**.
- **Blood pressure is markedly increased by vasoconstriction** and decreased by vasodilation.
- On the contrary, **resistance is inversely proportional to the radius** (discussed below).

PERIPHERAL RESISTANCE

Resistance offered to the flow of blood in the peripheral circulation is the peripheral resistance.

Factors affecting Peripheral Resistance

Peripheral resistance is determined by **two main factors**: caliber of blood vessel (vascular hindrance) and viscosity of blood (hematological hindrance).

- **Vessel diameter is the most important determinant** of peripheral resistance.

Radius of Blood Vessel

The radius of the blood vessel significantly affects peripheral resistance. This is called **vascular hindrance**.

- Vasoconstriction increases and vasodilation decreases peripheral resistance.
- ***Decrease in radius of vessels to half*** increases peripheral resistance **by 16 times.**
  - This decreases blood flow to organs by 16 times.
- Conversely, when radius is doubled, resistance is reduced to 6% of its previous value.

Viscosity of Blood

Viscosity of blood also affects peripheral resistance. This is called **hematological hindrance**.

- Viscosity mainly depends on the factors like hematocrit, composition of plasma, resistance of red cells to deformation and temperature.

Hematocrit: Hematocrit is the **single most factor** that greatly affects viscosity of blood.

- Hematocrit is the **packed cell volume**, which depends mainly on the number of red cells in the blood.
  - Increase in hematocrit increases viscosity (Fig. 34.4)
- The effect of change in viscosity on resistance is **less in smaller vessels** than in the larger vessels. This is due to the difference in ***nature of flow*** through the small vessels.
- Viscosity increases in polycythemia and decreases in anemia.
- **In anemia,** *circulation is hyperdynamic* due to decreased peripheral resistance.

Composition of Plasma: In plasma, it is mainly the **concentration of plasma proteins** that affects viscosity.

- **Viscosity increases** in conditions in which ***concentration of plasma protein is more***, for example, in paraproteinemia and *multiple myeloma* (increase in myeloma protein).
- Viscosity ***decreases in hypoproteinemia***.

Resistance of red cells to deformation: When the red cells become rigid as seen in ***hereditary spherocytosis***, viscosity increases.

Temperature: Increase in body temperature ***decreases viscosity*** and decrease in temperature increases viscosity.

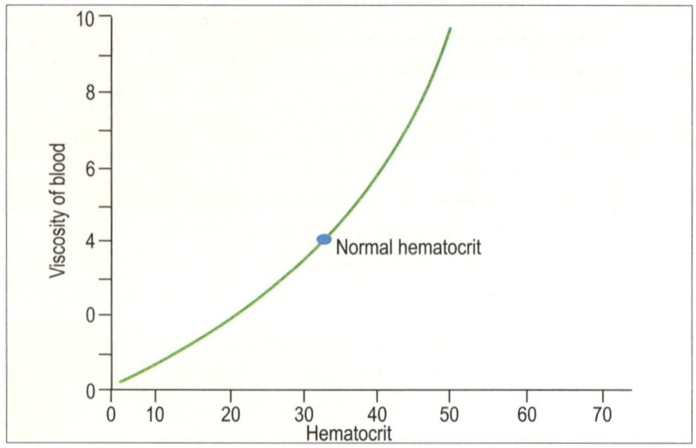

Fig. 34.4: Effect of hematocrit on viscosity of blood.

Plasma Skimming

In blood vessels, **cells mostly accumulate at the center** of the flowing column of blood.

- Therefore, the portion of blood, which is available **at the periphery of blood vessel** (close to the vessel wall) **has low cell content.**
- Blood entering into smaller branches arising from a large vessel mainly comes from the peripheral part of the column of the blood.
  - Thus, **smaller branches receive blood containing less red cell** (Fig. 34.5). This phenomenon is called plasma skimming.
- This explains why the **hematocrit of capillary blood is about 25% less** than the whole-body hematocrit.

Critical Closing Pressure

In a rigid tube, a linear relationship exists between flow and pressure (Fig. 34.6A). With increased flow, the pressure increases. But in blood vessels this relationship is different.

- Especially in capillaries, flow ceases when pressure is reduced beyond a point (but pressure is not zero). The **pressure at which flow stops is called critical closing pressure** (Fig. 34.6B).
- This is explained by **two factors:**
  i) **some pressure is required** to force the red cells to pass through the capillaries which have the smaller diameter than the red cells, and,

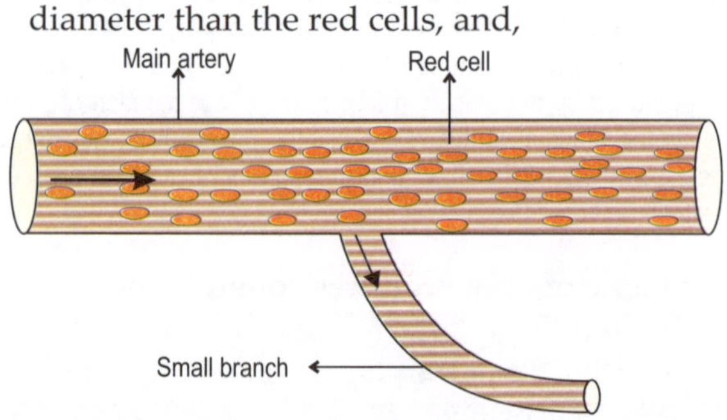

Fig. 34.5: The phenomenon of plasma skimming. The arrows indicate the direction of flow. Note, in the main artery, red cells mainly accumulate at the center of the vessel. Therefore, the smaller branch that receives peripheral blood from the main artery contains less number of cells, which is called as plasma skimming.

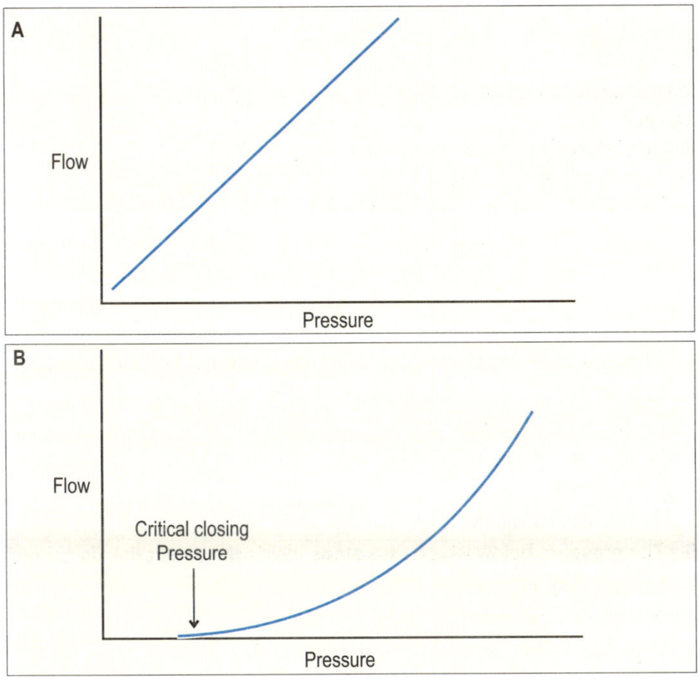

Figs. 34.6A and B: Flow-pressure relationship in a rigid tube (A) and in a blood vessel (B). Note, the relationship is linear in a tube. In a blood vessel, the flow is absent below certain pressure, called as critical closing pressure. Flow-pressure relationship is not totally linear in blood vessel.

ii) blood vessels are surrounded by tissues that exert pressure (**tissue pressure**) on them.

- Thus, intraluminal pressure in capillaries should be more than the tissue pressure for flow to resume.

LAW OF LAPLACE

This law explains the relationship between the **distending pressure (P),** the **tension (T)** in the wall of a structure and **its radius (r).**

$$P = T\left\{\frac{1}{r_1} + \frac{1}{r_2}\right\}$$

Where, r_1 and r_2 are its two principal radii of curvature.

In a sphere, $r_1 = r_2$, so $\quad P = \frac{2T}{r}$

In a cylindrical structure such as a thin-walled blood vessel, the curvature occurs in only one dimension. The other radius is infinite, so,

$$P = \frac{T}{r} \qquad \text{or } T = P \times r$$

So, in a **small diameter blood vessel**, less wall tension is required to balance the distending pressure. This protects small vessels from rupture (Application Box 34.2).

If the **thickness of the vessel wall** (w) is taken into consideration, like in an artery,

$$\text{Wall tension (T)} = P \times \frac{r}{w}$$

Application Box 34.2

Capillaries are less prone to rupture: Smaller the radius of the blood vessel, lesser the tension in the wall needed to balance the distending pressure. Therefore, though the capillaries are thin they are less prone to rupture.

Application of Laplace Law

The Laplace law helps us to understand the physiological mechanisms in altered situations and pathological conditions affecting the functioning of many organs.

- In **hollow viscus** like bladder, ventricle or the alveoli of the lungs, the wall tension depends on the **distending pressure** and its **radius**.
    - That means the **wall tension increases when the organ gets filled** (distending pressure rises) or the cavity size (radius) increases.
- Also, the **wall tension decreases when wall thickness is more** and the wall tension increases when the wall thickness decreases.
- So, in **ventricular hypertrophy** as the wall is thick, ***wall tension is less***.
- On the other hand, in a **dilated heart** as seen in heart failure, more energy is required to pump blood as the wall tension is more (ventricular wall is not thick in dilated heart).
    - Therefore, a **dilated or distended heart pumps blood less efficiently** (Clinical Note 34.2).

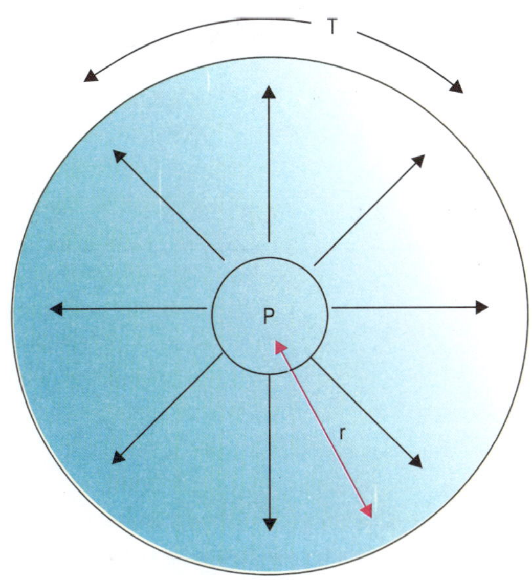

Fig. 34.7: Laplace law. The relationship between intraluminal extending pressure (P) and the tension (T) developed in the wall of a hollow structure. Note, in a spherical structure, the tension in the wall is the product of intra-spherical pressure and the radius (r) of the sphere.

Clinical Note 34.2

Dilated heart fails faster: A dilated heart has to do more work than a non-dilated heart, as with increased radius of the cardiac chamber greater tension must be developed in the myocardium to produce any given pressure (Fig. 34.7).

Exam Questions

1. Describe various principles of hemodynamics that control circulation of blood in the vascular system.
2. Explain the application of Bernoulli principle and Laplace law in blood circulation.
3. List the the differences between laminar flow and turbulent flow. Explain the role of Poiseuille- Hagen formula in hemodynamics.
4. What is plasma skimming? What is critical closing pressure? Briefly describe the role of these two phenomena in the perfusion of organs of the body.

Multiple Choice Questions

1. **Which of the following statement is NOT true?**
   A. Blood vessels are under the influence of humoral factors
   B. Blood flow is not influenced by composition of blood
   C. Blood flow is influenced by rheological properties of blood
   D. Blood flow is influenced by diameter of blood vessels
2. **Hematocrit of capillary blood is 25% less compared to whole-body hematocrit, due to:**
   A. More water in capillary blood
   B. Less proteins in capillary blood
   C. Less blood in capillaries
   D. Less cells in capillary blood due to plasma skimming
3. **All are true for Bernoulli's principle, EXCEPT:**
   A. Increase in dynamic component at the site of narrowing decreases lateral pressure
   B. Dynamic pressure is linked to kinetic energy of flow
   C. Total pressure in a closed system continuously changes
   D. Lateral pressure determines the degree of perfusion of tissues.
4. **Which is NOT true about laminar blood flow?**
   A. Reynold's number is below 2000
   B. Velocity of flow is above the critical velocity
   C. Flow occurs in layers
   D. Velocity of flow is maximal at the central layer of blood in the vessel
5. **Which is not a direct component for calculation of Poiseuille-Hagen formula?**
   A. Temperature of fluid
   B. Flow and pressure
   C. Viscosity of fluid
   D. Radius and length
6. **The pressure below which flow stops inside the capillaries, is called:**
   A. Critical tissue pressure
   B. Capillary distension pressure
   C. Critical closing pressure
   D. Pulse pressure
7. **Which is most important contributor to peripheral resistance?**
   A. Hematocrit
   B. Length of the vessel
   C. Viscosity of blood
   D. Radius of the vessel
8. **Which of the following is not considered for assessing the effect of Laplace in vascular system?**
   A. Composition of blood
   B. Wall thickness and tension
   C. Distending intramural pressure
   D. Radius of the vessel

Answers

1. B 2. D 3. C 4. B 5. A 6. C 7. D 8. A

Chapter 35

Arterial System and Venous System

Learning Objectives

On completion of study of this chapter:

The student will be able to (must know):

1. Learn sympathetic (vasoconstrictor) tone maintains arterial volume and pressure.
2. Name the types of arteries and give their functions.
3. Appreciate the importance of Windkessel effect of larger arteries.
4. Comprehend pattern of pulse pressure in different segment of vascular tree.
5. Understand pressure-volume relationship of venous system.

The student may also be able to (desirable to know):

1. Describe the principle of arterial hemodynamics in in various physiological conditions.

ARTERIAL SYSTEM

The arterial system consists of **aorta, large and small arteries, arterioles and metarterioles**.

- These vessels have all the **three layers** in their walls, namely tunica intima, tunica media and tunica adventitia.
- The tunica media containing smooth muscle is thicker in the arterial compartment than the other compartments of circulatory system.

Innervation

Arterial system is **richly supplied by sympathetic fibers**. Sympathetic fibers originate from thoracic and lumbar segment of spinal cord.

- Normally at rest, there is a **tonic discharge of sympathetic fibers** to arteries in systemic circulation.
    - This is called *sympathetic tone*. Stimulation of sympathetic fibers results in vasoconstriction.
    - Therefore, sympathetic tone is also known as *vasoconstrictor tone*.
- Vasoconstrictor tone is essential for **maintaining normal blood pressure**.
    - Increase in vasoconstrictor tone increases and decrease in vasoconstrictor tone decreases blood pressure.
- There is **no parasympathetic innervation** of blood vessel in general circulation.

Types of Vessels

There are **two types** of vessels in arterial system: elastic vessels and muscular vessels.

Elastic Vessels

Elastic vessels are **aorta and large arteries**.

- In these vessels, the **quantity of elastic component is more** *than the muscle component*.
- Therefore, these arteries are ***more compliant*** (stretchable).
- These are called **Windkessel vessels** (elastic reservoir).

Muscular Vessels

These include **small arteries, arterioles and metarterioles**.

- In these vessels, ***quantity of smooth muscle is more*** *than elastic tissues*.
    - Therefore, these vessels provide maximum resistance to blood flow.
    - These are called **resistance vessels**.
- **Arterioles & metarterioles** are the primary seat of **peripheral resistance**.
- In fact, due to the vascular resistance, a significant fall in blood pressure occurs when blood passes through the arterioles.

Functions of Arteries

1. Arteries **transport blood** from heart to the tissues.
   - Thus, they ***supply oxygen and nutrients*** to the different parts of the body.
2. The **aorta and the large arteries** due to their **elastic recoil property**, maintain *forward movement of blood* during diastole.
3. **Small arteries, arterioles & metarterioles** are *richly innervated by sympathetic fibers* and offer maximum **resistance to blood flow**.
   - They are the seat of **peripheral resistance**.
   - Therefore, these vessels mainly control blood pressure.

Functional Aspects

Arterial Elasticity

Aorta and large arteries have **more compliance** due to the presence of ***more elastic elements*** in their wall.

- When blood is ejected forcefully into the aorta and its major branches during ventricular systole, these vessels are distended.
- **During diastole**, the aortic wall immediately recoils back to its previous position.
  - This *property of recoiling* is known as **Windkessel effect** (Fig. 35.1).
- Due to the Windkessel effect, the vessel wall that recoils back on the blood column **pushes blood to move in forward direction during diastole.**

IMPORTANT NOTE

During systole, forward movement of blood is due to the energy created by forceful ejection of blood that occurs due to ventricular contraction.

- Thus, blood moves continuously during systole and diastole due to the Windkessel effect of elastic arteries.

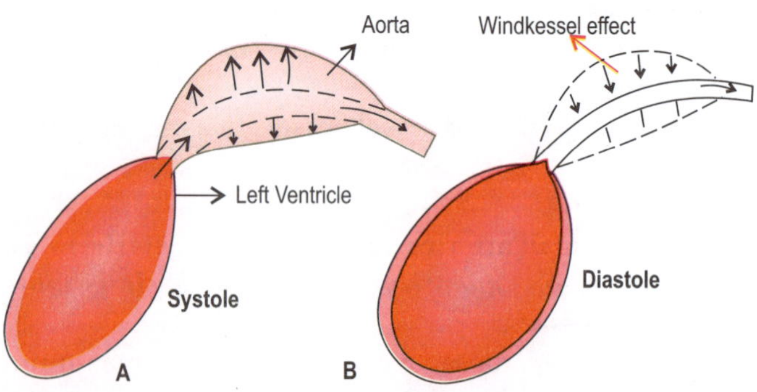

Figs. 35.1A and B: The Windkessel effect. **(A)** During systole, forceful ejection of blood from ventricle into aorta distends the aorta and creates pressure for forward movement of blood in the vessels; **(B)** During diastole, arterial elasticity causes recoiling of the aortic wall that presses on blood in aorta and helps blood to move in forward direction (during diastole). This property of recoiling is called Windkessel phenomenon.

Arterial Pressure Pulse

Arterial pressure pulse is the **pressure wave** that travels along the wall of the arteries created by forceful ejection of blood into the arterial system during ventricular systole. These pressure waves are felt as arterial pulses when clinically examined by the physician.

- The **velocity of transmission of pulse wave** in the wall of the artery is ***fifteen times the velocity of flow of blood*** in the lumen of the artery.
  - For example, in the aorta, the velocity of flow is 0.33 m/s, whereas the velocity of transmission of pressure wave is about 4 m/s.
- The velocity of transmission of pressure wave **increases towards the periphery**.
  - In large arteries, it is about 8 m/s and in small arteries about 20 m/s. Thus, the radial pulse in wrist is felt in 0.1 s from the peak of ventricular ejection.
- The **amplitude & pattern of arterial pulse** also change from central arteries to peripheral arteries. Arterial pulses are recorded (pulse tracing) by a sphygmograph or a physiograph.

Central Arterial Pulse: The central arterial pulse has higher amplitude, steep ascending limb, less sharp peak and incissura in the upper part of the descending limb, which is less steep.

Peripheral Arterial Pulse: The peripheral arterial pulse has steep ascending limb, sharp peak, steep descending limbs, and the dicrotic notch (instead of incissura) present towards the lower part in the descending limb (Fig. 35.2).

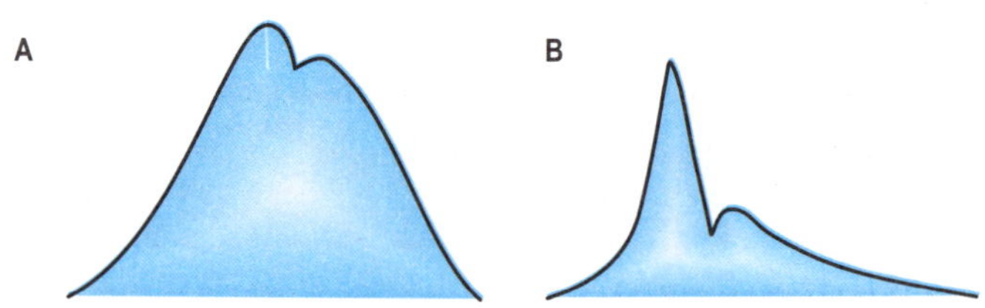

Fig. 35.2: Difference between pulse tracings recorded from central and peripheral arteries. A: The central arterial pulse has high amplitude, steep ascending limb, less sharp peak, incissura present in the upper part of descending limb, and less steep descending limb. B: In peripheral arterial pulse, the amplitude may be less, ascending and descending limbs are steep, peak is sharp, and dicrotic notch (instead of incissura) is present towards the lower part of descending limb.

Arterial Pressure

Arterial pressure is **defined as** the lateral pressure exerted by the column of blood on the walls of the arteries.

- The maximum pressure is recorded during systole (**systolic blood pressure**) and the minimum pressure is recorded during diastole (**diastolic blood pressure**).
- In adults, the normal systolic pressure ranges between 100–119 mm of Hg and diastolic pressure ranges between 60–79 mm Hg.

Pulse Pressure: It is the difference between the systolic and diastolic pressures. Normally it ranges between 20 – 50 mm Hg. Pulse pressure is important for organ perfusion.

- The pulse pressure is high in the aorta and large artery.
- It grossly decreases across the arterioles, almost negligible in capillaries and nil in veins (Fig. 35.3).

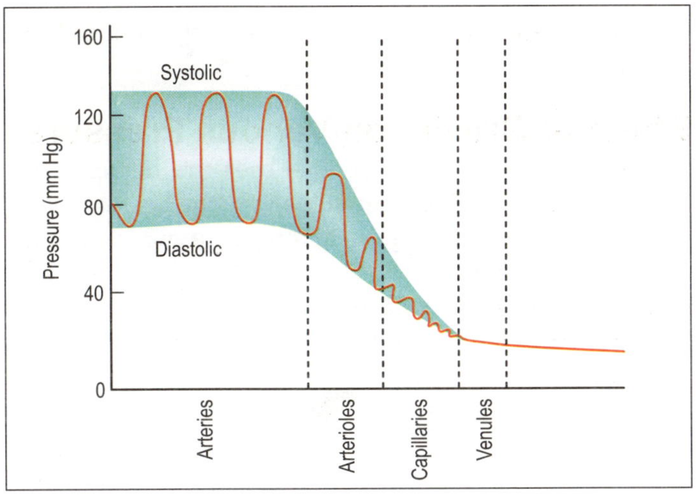

Fig. 35.3: Pattern of pulse pressure (PP) in different segments of circulatory system. Note, PP is high in arterial system, decreases grossly across arterioles and capillaries and nil in venous system.

Measurement of Blood Pressure

Methods of measurement of blood pressure are broadly divided into **two categories**: (1) direct methods, and (2) indirect methods.

Direct Methods

The blood pressure is measured directly by **placing a cannula in the artery** and connecting the cannula to a mercury manometer or a pressure transducer.

- This is the method used for recording blood pressure in *experimental animals*.
- In human beings, blood pressure is usually measured by indirect method.

Indirect Methods

Blood pressure is usually measured with the help of a sphygmomanometer. The procedure is called **sphygmomanometry**.

The blood pressure is usually measured by palpatory and auscultatory methods.

Palpatory Method: In palpatory method, pressure in the cuff is progressively raised and radial artery pulse is palpated simultaneously.

- The **point where the pulsation disappears** is the systolic pressure.
- Diastolic pressure can't be measured by palpatory method.

Auscultatory Method: In auscultatory method, pressure in the cuff is raised by about 20 mm Hg above palpatory level and then progressively lowered during which brachial artery is auscultated for sounds by placing the diaphragm of a stethoscope on it.

- The sounds undergo a ***series of changes in their quality and intensity***. These sounds are known as **Korotkov sounds**.
- **Appearance of the sound** is recorded as systolic blood pressure and **disappearance of sound** is recorded as diastolic blood pressure.

VENOUS SYSTEM

The venous system starts from the capillaries.

- It consists of **venules, small veins, large veins and vena cava.**
- Vena cava drains into right atrium.

Functional Aspect

Wall of Veins

Veins contain **all the three layers** of the blood vessels. However, veins are **significantly thinner** due to the ***thin muscle coat***.

Functions

1. Venous system **transports deoxygenated blood** from tissues to the heart. From heart, blood is pumped into the lungs where carbon dioxide is removed from it.
2. Veins are **capacitance vessels** as they can accommodate a large volume of blood.
   - They act as **reservoir of blood**.
   - In fact, more than 60% of the total blood is present in the venous compartment.

Pressure Volume Relationship of Veins

The veins are thin walled and have **less quantity of smooth muscle**. Therefore, they are **easily distensible and collapsible**.

- The increase in volume of blood in veins ***does not affect significant change*** in pressure upto a point **beyond which the pressure rises steeply** (Fig. 35.4B).
- Normally, veins are **partially collapsed**. Thus, they easily ***accommodate a large amount of blood*** without any change in pressure till they are fully distended.
- However, once the lumen of veins **becomes spherical pressure rises steeply**, whereas in arteries, the pressure-volume relationship is almost linear (Fig. 35.4A).

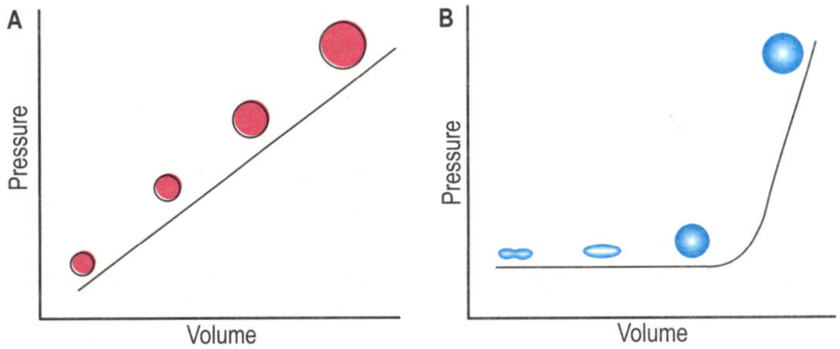

Fig. 35.4: Pressure volume relationship in arteries (A) and veins (B). In arteries, pressure increase is proportionate to increase in volume. In veins, initially there is no appreciable increase in pressure with the volume increase. However, after certain volume that causes almost complete distension of veins, the increase in pressure is rapid and steep.

Innervation

Veins are innervated by **sympathetic fibers.**

- The density of innervation is less in comparison to arteries.
- However, veins **are more sensitive to sympathetic discharge** than arteries due to a greater nerve fiber to muscle fiber ratio.
- Therefore, a significant venoconstriction occurs even at mild sympathetic stimulation that increases venous return adequately.

Venous Return

The amount of blood that drains into the right atrium from the venous compartment is called venous return. It is one of the **major determinants of cardiac output**.

- Details of Venous return are described in Chapter 32.

Venous Valves: Veins are provided with valves that allow forward flow of blood.

- Valves are well developed especially in lower limb veins.
- **Back flow of blood in veins is prevented** by venous valves.

Venous Pressures

Central Venous Pressure

The pressure in the great veins at their entrance into the right atrium is called central venous pressure (CVP).

- CVP is normally about **0 to 5 mm Hg**.
  - But it can be –5 mm Hg when rate and force of contraction of heart increases.
- CVP is measured directly by inserting a catheter into the great veins in the thorax.
- The **right atrial pressure** is also measured to determine CVP.
- Jugular venous pressure (JVP) reflects the right atrial activity.

Peripheral Venous Pressure

Pressure in the venules is about **15 mm Hg**.

- Venous pressure decreases as blood flows into larger veins.
- The pressure in great veins outside the thorax is 5.5 mm Hg.

Effect of Gravity on Venous Pressure

In standing posture, the venous pressure **decreases by 0.77 mm Hg for each centimeter** above the heart.

- Thus, venous pressure is –10 mm Hg in superior sagital sinus (Fig. 35.5).
- Venous pressure increases by **0.77 mm Hg per cm below the right atrium** so that it is as high as *+85 mm Hg at feet*.

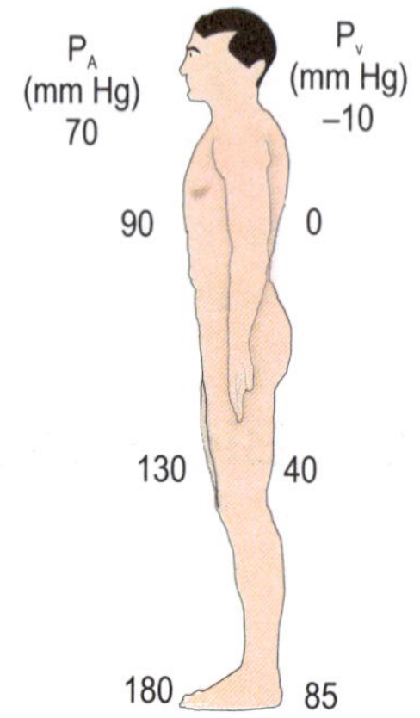

Fig. 35.5: Effect of gravity on arterial and venous pressures. PA: Arterial pressure; PV: Venous pressure. Note, on standing, arterial and venous pressures at heart position are 90 and 0 respectively, at level of head are 70 and –10 respectively, and at feet level 180 and 85 respectively.

Clinical Importance: In upright position, venous pressure above heart level decreases due to effect of gravity so that the **venous pressure in the neck and head is negative**. These veins are therefore normally **collapsed.**

- The pressure in collapsed vein is zero, rather than subatmospheric.
- However, the pressure in dural sinuses in upright or sitting posture is subatmospheric, as sinuses do not collapse due to their rigid walls (Clinical Note 35. 1).

Clinical Note 35.1

Air embolism in neurosurgical procedures: Sometimes, neurosurgical procedures are performed in sitting posture, during which if a sinus is opened accidentally or as part of the surgical procedure, air embolism results as air is sucked into the sinus. A neurosurgeon should be cautious about this possible complication before performing the surgery.

Exam Questions

1. Describe the pattern of autonomic innervation of arterial and venous system and explain their physiological significance.
2. Explain the difference between arterial pressure pulse tracings recorded from central and peripheral arteries. Briefly describe the significance of pulse pressure.
3. With the help of suitable diagrams, describe the difference in pressure volume relationship between arteries and veins.

Chapter 36

Capillary Circulation, Lymphatic Circulation and Edema Formation

Learning Objectives

On completion of study of this chapter:

The student will be able to (must know):

1. Name the types of capillaries and give examples of each category.
2. Correlate the histological difference in capillaries with their functions.
3. List the functional specialties of capillaries.
4. Describe the mechanism of capillary filtration.
5. Define edema and explain the mechanisms of edema formation.
6. Understand the process of lymphatic circulation.

The student may also be able to (desirable to know):

1. Describe the processes of capillary exchange.

PY5.10

CAPILLARY CIRCULATION

Though only about 5% of blood volume circulates in capillaries, the capillary circulation is most important as exchange of nutrients, gases, water and waste products between the blood and tissues occurs in capillaries.

- Capillaries are known as **exchange vessels**.
- The circulation of blood from arterioles to venules through capillaries is called the **microcirculation**.
- Except lens and cornea, all cells in the body are in **direct contact with the microvessels**.
  - Cornea and lens derive their nutrients from the fluids present in the eye.

Functional Morphology

Capillaries form extensive branching networks that increase the surface area for rapid exchange of materials.

- Capillaries are made up of a **single layer of endothelial cells** and **tunica media is completely absent**.
  - Absence of tunica media and the gap in the inter-endothelial junctions contribute to the permeability of the capillaries.

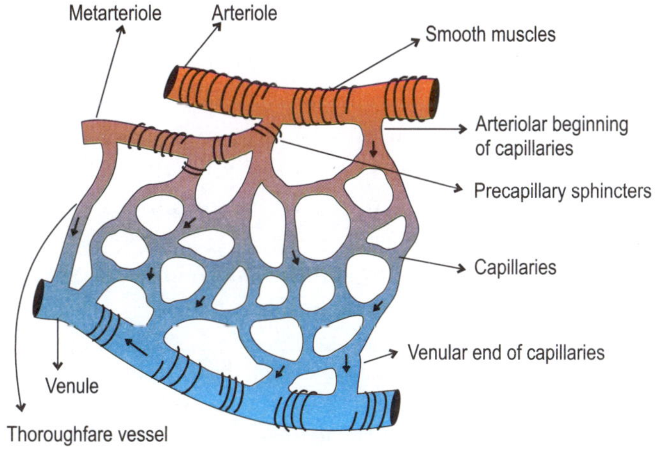

Fig. 36.1: The capillary microcirculation. Capillaries originate either from arterioles or from metarterioles, and their origin is guarded by precapillary sphincter. Note, the quantity of smooth muscle is maximal in arterioles, moderate in venules, less in metarterioles, and absent in capillaries, which determines their responsiveness to sympathetic stimulation. Also note that a capillary thoroughfare vessel directly connects the metarteriole and the venule. Diameter of arteriolar end of capillary is less (about 5 μm) than the venular end (about 8 μm).

- **True capillaries** emerge from the arteriole or metarteriole and form anastomosing network that drain into the venules (Fig. 36.1).
- In many vascular beds, metarteriole is connected directly with venule by a **thoroughfare vessel**.

Types of Capillaries

Capillaries are of three types: **continuous, fenestrated, and sinusoidal**.

Continuous Capillaries

Continuous capillaries are **nonfenestrated** capillaries.

- Endothelial cells form a **continuous ring** around the lumen of capillary except at the gaps (**intercellular clefts**) between endothelial cells.

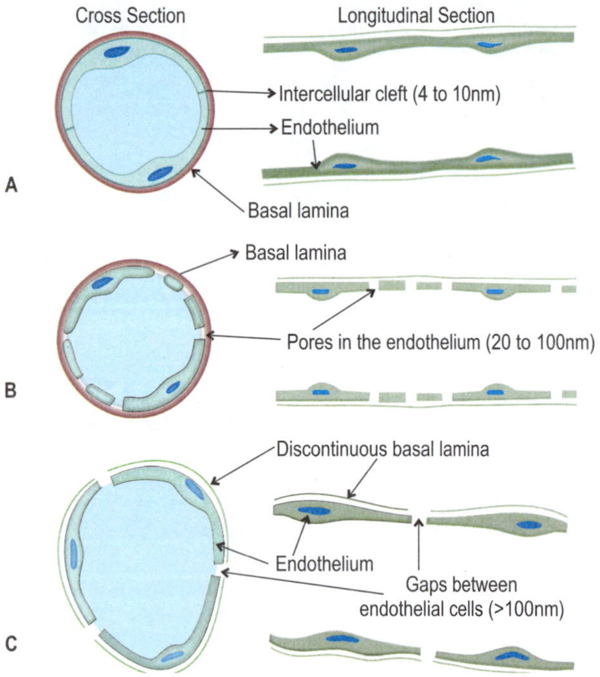

Fig. 36.2: Types of capillaries. Note the size of the gap between endothelial cells in different types. **A:** Continuous capillary; **B:** Fenestrated capillary; **C:** Sinusoidal capillary.

- The **clefts** (gaps at inter-endothelial junctions) are usually **4 to 10 nm** (less than 15 nm) in diameter.
  - There is **no discontinuity** in endothelium of the capillaries (Fig. 36.2A).

This type of capillary is seen in **skeletal and smooth muscles, connective tissues, and lungs**.

IMPORTANT NOTE

Cerebral capillaries have no clefts: The clefts are absent in capillaries of cerebral blood vessels as the inter-endothelial junctions in these vessels are tight junctions to form the blood-brain barrier.

Fenestrated Capillaries

The endothelial cells are **perforated by many fenestrations (pores)**, which are 20 to 100 nm in diameter.
- The cytoplasm of endothelial cells is attenuated to form gaps, which are called **fenestrations** (Fig. 36.2B).

- They are present in **in intestinal villi, choroid plexuses of ventricles** in brain, **cilliary processes of eyes**, exocrine glands and parts of kidneys.

Sinusoidal or Discontinuous Capillaries

They have larger discontinuities between the endothelial cells.

- The **gaps** between the endothelial cells are **more than 400 nm in diameter** (Fig. 36.2C).
  - Some gaps are 600 to 3000 nm in diameter.
- Also, they have multiple **large fenestrae** in their cytoplasm. Therefore, large molecules can easily pass through these capillaries.
- Such capillaries are present in **liver, spleen and bone marrow.**

Active vs. Inactive Capillaries

At rest, most of the capillaries are closed (**inactive capillaries**) and blood flow occurs **mainly by *thoroughfare vessels***.

- **In active tissues**, arterioles and precapillary sphincters dilate that result in flow of blood through the capillaries.
- This **opens up many capillaries** and improves capillary circulation (**active capillaries**).

Capillary Flow: Capillary pressure differs from tissue to tissue, and therefore the capillary blood flow differs.

- Though capillaries are short, the blood flow is **very slow** due to their **large total cross-sectional area**.
  - The flow rate is about **0.07 cm/sec**.
- The **pulse pressure** is about 5 mmHg at the arteriolar end and almost zero at the venular end.
  - Therefore, capillary blood flow **is less pulsatile**.

Functional Specialties of Capillaries

1. The **capillary density** (the ratio of the number of capillaries to the number of cells in the tissue) determines the degree of exchange across the capillary.
   - Capillary density is **high in metabolically active tissues** like cardiac muscle and glands.
   - It is ***low in less active tissues*** like subcutaneous tissue and cartilage.
2. Diameter of a true capillary at arterial end is about 5 *μm and at venualr end is about 8 μm.*

IMPORTANT NOTE

Capillary diameter is less than red cell diameter: Therefore, red cells just squeeze through the lumen of the capillaries in single file. In this process *contact between red cell membrane and capillary membrane becomes maximal that facilitate* capillary exchange.

3. Capillaries **do not have smooth muscle**, hence don't respond to vasoconstrictors or vasodilators.
   - The flow through capillaries is largely regulated by *change in the capacity of precapillary vessels* (arterioles and metarterioles).
   - Capillaries are also **least innervated by sympathetic fibers**.
4. At the origin of capillaries from metarterioles, a flap of smooth muscle forms a cuff, called **precapillary sphincter**.
   - This sphincter is usually ***not innervated*** but responds vasoconstrictors and vasodilators.
   - The capillary circulation **largely depends on** the **contraction or relaxation** of the precapillary sphincter.
5. Endothelial cells of capillaries are surrounded by **pericytes** or **Rouget cells**.

- Rouget cells are *primitive form of vascular smooth muscle* or *myoepithelial cells* that respond to vasoconstrictor agents.
  - They themselves also ***release vasoactive substances***.
  - Therefore, active capillary constriction and dilation do occur to some extent.

6. The **flow of blood is sluggish** in capillaries.
   - Therefore, capillaries are best suited for exchange of materials between the blood and the tissue (**exchange vessels**).
7. The capillaries are weak vessels and surrounded by tissues.
   - Therefore, if the **capillary pressure** *decreases below the tissue pressure*, **capillaries collapse** and the flow in capillaries ceases.
   - The capillary pressure, below which the flow stops, is called **critical closing pressure**.
8. There are few vessels that directly connect the metarterioles and venules, bypassing the capillaries.

These are called **thoroughfare vessels**.

- The **flow of blood mainly occurs** through thoroughfare vessels during resting tissue.
  - However, flow through true capillaries increases during exercise (*active tissue*).

9. The flow of blood through capillaries is **usually intermittent** (not continuous).
   - This is because intermittent contraction and relaxation of the arterioles and metarterioles, which regulate flow through the capillaries.
   - Such intermittent flow (which usually occurs 5–10 times per minute) is called **vasomotion**.
10. **Endothelial cells** of capillaries contain many ***endocytic vesicles*** that contribute to **transcytosis** of water and water-soluble substances across the capillary wall.

Capillary Exchange

Substances are transported across the capillaries by three ways: diffusion, vesicular transport and filtration.

Diffusion

Diffusion is the common method of exchange across the capillary bed in most of the tissues.

- The **gases** (oxygen and carbon dioxide), the **nutrients** (glucose, and amino acids), **hormones**, and other substances are exchanged by means of diffusion.
- **In liver,** because of sinusoidal nature of the capillaries, large molecules like proteins diffuse through capillaries easily.
  - This **transports synthesized proteins** like fibrinogen and albumin to enter circulation.

Vesicular Transport

The transport of substances by means of **endocytosis and exocytosis** is called the vesicular transport.

- **Dissolved proteins** from plasma ***in the form of vesicles*** are taken up by endocytosis, transported across the endothelial cells and then discharged outside by exocytosis.
  - As transport occurs across endothelial cells, the process is also called **transcytosis**.
  - **Transport of large lipid-insoluble substances** that cannot pass through the capillary wall are transported by this process.

Capillary Filtration

This is the major route of transport of fluid between the blood and the interstitial tissue space. Filtration occurs due to the difference in various pressures in the intravascular and extravascular fluid space.

Starling's Forces: The forces that control capillary filtration are named as **Starling's forces** (as described by EH Starling). These are **hydrostatic and osmotic forces**.

Two pressures promote and two pressures oppose filtration.

Pressures promoting filtration are:

1. Hydrostatic pressure of the blood
2. Osmotic pressure of the interstitial fluid

Pressures that oppose filtration are:

1. Oncotic pressure (the osmotic pressure of blood due to the plasma proteins)
2. The tissue hydrostatic pressure

The balance between these pressures determines the net filtration.

Pressure Gradients Across Capillary Wall

Hydrostatic Pressure Gradient

This is the difference between the hydrostatic pressure of **vascular compartment** (i. e. of blood) and the **interstitial tissues compartment** (i. e. of tissue fluid).

- The hydrostatic pressure **pushes fluid out of the compartment**.
  - In skeletal muscle for example, the hydrostatic pressure of blood at the **arteriolar end is 37 mmHg** and at the **venular end is 17 mmHg.**
  - Hydrostatic pressure in the **interstitial tissues space it is negligible**, only 1 mm Hg (Fig. 36.3).
- Therefore, the hydrostatic pressure gradient **favours filtration both at arteriolar and venular end** of the capillaries.
- **At arteriolar end**, the gradient is more i.e, 36 (37–1) mmHg than **at the venular end** of the capillaries, which is 16 (17–1) mmHg.

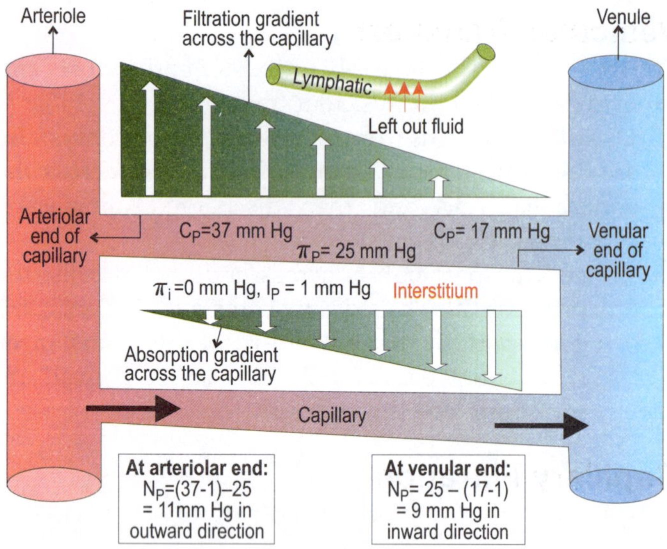

Fig. 36.3: The mechanism of capillary filtration in skeletal muscle capillary bed. C_p: Capillary hydrostatic pressure; π_P: Capillary osmotic pressure or oncotic pressure; I_P: Interstitial hydrostatic pressure; π_i: Osmotic pressure in the interstitium; N_P: Net filtration pressure. Note, at arteriolar end of capillary N_P is 11 mm Hg in outward direction and at venular end N_P is 9 mm Hg in inward direction. The extra unit of fluid left in the interstitium due to 2 mm Hg difference is absorbed by lymphatics. Arrows indicate the direction and magnitude of fluid movement.

Osmotic Pressure Gradient

This is the difference between the **oncotic pressure** (the osmotic pressure of blood), which is **25 mmHg**.

- Osmotic pressure of a fluid compartment withheld fluid (prevents escape of fluid) in the compartment.
  - Therefore, **osmotic pressure opposes filtration**.
- As, **osmotic pressure of tissue space is nil**.
  - Thus, osmotic pressure gradient along the capillary wall **is always inward**.
  - This favours absorption of fluid from the interstitial tissue space into the capillary.

Net Filtration

The net filtration **depends on the difference** between the hydrostatic pressure gradient and the oncotic pressure gradient at arteriolar and venular end of capillaries.

At arteriolar end of the capillary: Net filtration pressure is **11 mmHg** [(37 – 1) – 25] in outward direction.

At venular end of the capillary: Net filtration pressure is **9 mmHg** [25 – (17 – 1)] ***in the inward direction.***

Thus, at the arteriolar end, fluid moves out of the capillaries and at the venular end, fluid moves into the capillaries.

- About **two units of fluid are left in the interstitial tissue space** as the outward filtration at the arteriolar end is 2 mmHg more than the inward filtration at the venular end.
- This amount of fluid is usually **taken up by the lymphatics** in the interstitial space, which is again brought back to the circulation as lymphatics finally drain into the veins.

Role of Capillary Permeability

In addition to the pressure gradients, filtration also depends on **permeability of the capillary membrane**.

- Capillary permeability depends on the integrity of the capillary endothelial membrane.
- Capillary permeability is increased especially in inflammatory conditions.

Arteriovenous Anastomoses

There are short vascular channels that **directly connect arterioles to venules** bypassing capillaries.

1. These are called arteriovenous anastomoses or **arteriovenous shunts.**
2. They have **thick muscular wall** and are ***densely innervated by sympathetic nerves.***
3. AV anastomoses are especially present in the **fingers, palms and ear lobes.**

LYMPHATIC CIRCULATION

Lymphatic System

Lymphatic system consists of **lymphatic vessels and lymphatic tissues.**

Lymphatic Vessels

During circulation of blood through capillaries, part of its fluid remains in the tissues as **tissue fluid**, which returns to the circulation through lymphatics.

The fluid passing through the lymphatic vessel is called **lymph**.

- The smallest lymphatic (or lymph) vessels are **lymphatic capillaries** that join together to form **larger lymphatic vessels**.
- The largest lymphatic vessel in the body is the **thoracic duct**, which drains lymph from the greater part of the body.
- The thoracic duct ends by joining the left subclavian vein at its junction with the internal jugular vein (Fig. 36.4).
- On the right side there is the right lymphatic duct that has a similar termination.

Lymphoid Tissues

Lymphoid tissue may be broadly classified as diffused lymphoid tissue and dense lymphoid tissue.

Diffused Lymphoid Tissue: These tissues consists of **diffusedly arranged lymphocytes and plasma cells** in the mucosa of large intestine, trachea, bronchi, and urinary tract.

Dense Lymphoid Tissue: Dense lymphoid tissue is further calssified as discrete lymphoid organs and mucosa-associated tissue.

- **Discrete lymphoid organs** include **thymus, lymph nodes, spleen, and tonsils.**
- **Mucosa-associated lymphoid tissue (MALT):** Lymphocyte aggregations are seen in mucosa of the

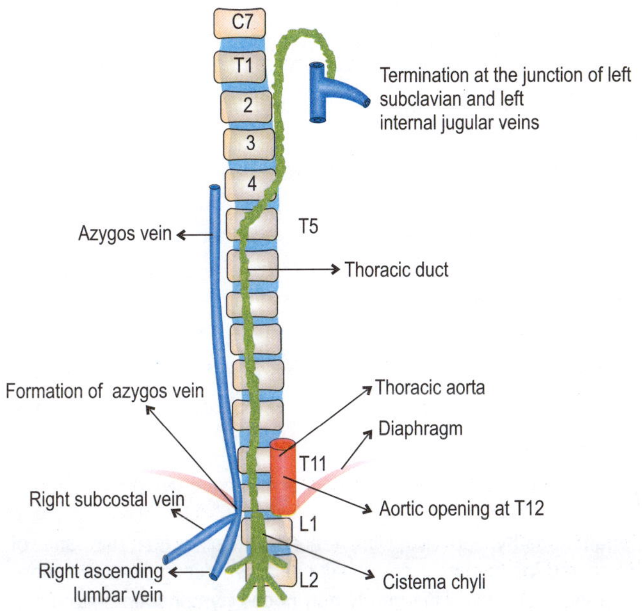

Fig. 36.4: Origin, course, and termination of thoracic duct.

respiratory, alimentary and urogenital tracts. These aggregations are referred to as MALT.

i) Mucosa-associated lymphoid tissues **in the respiratory system** are present in the walls of the trachea and large bronchi. They are termed as **bronchial-associated lymphoid tissue** (BALT).

ii) Mucosa-associated lymphoid tissues **in the alimentary system** is called **gut-associated lymphoid tissue** (GALT) that includes Payer's patches of ileum, adenoids (located in the root of pharynx), lingual tonsils in posterior one-third of tongue, palatine tonsils, and lymphoid nodules in vermiform appendix.

Thymus and bone marrow are **primary lymphoid organs** while others are secondary lymphoid organ.

Mechanism of Lymphatic Circulation

Lymphatics drain lymph from different tissues of the body and **empty the same into the subclavian veins** at their junctions with internal jugular veins.

- Lymphatic vessels typically begin as blind tubular bulbs (**lymphatic bulbs**) that drain into meshwork of interconnected lymph vessels.
- Tissue fluid enters into the bulbs that in turn drain to interconnected lymph vessels and then from these vessels into **tubular lymphatic vessels** and the **larger lymphatic vessels** (Fig. 36.5).
- Lymphatic vessels coalesce into increasingly larger vessels.
- Larger vessels are surrounded by **contractile cells** similar to that of smooth muscles of blood vessels.
- Lymph nodes are interposed in the path of lymphatics.

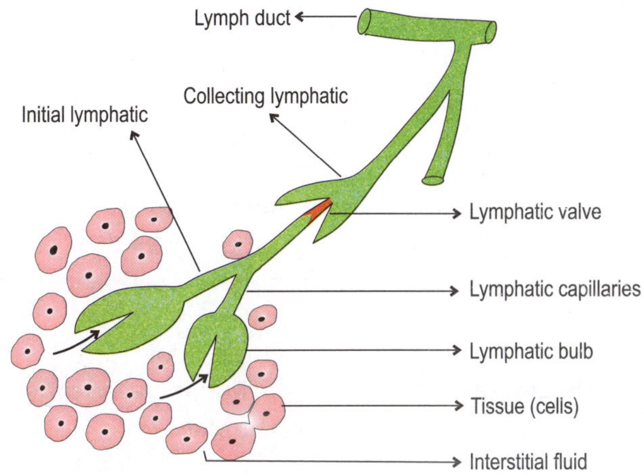

Fig. 36.5: The lymphatic drainage system. Note, there is no valve in initial lymphatics, but the valves are present in collecting lymphatics. Black arrows indicate the direction of flow of fluid movement into lymphatic bulb.

IMPORTANT NOTE

Organs with no lymphatics: Lymphatics are absent in bone, teeth, cartilage, placenta and CNS.

Types of Lymphatics

Lymphatics are of **two types**: Initial lymphatics and collecting lymphatics.

Initial Lymphatics

Initial lymphatics are **lymphatic bulbs** and interconnected vessels (**lymphatic capillaries**).

Specialities of Lymphatic Capillaries: Lymphatic capillaries differ from vascular capillaries in several ways:

1. **No basal lamina** (or scanty basal lamia) under the endothelium.
2. Junctions between endothelial cells are **open**.
3. No fenestrations in endothelium (**non-fenestrated**)
4. **Tight junctions** (tight intercellular connections) **are absent**

Features of Initial Lymphatics:

- Initial lymphatics ***lack valves and smooth muscles*** in their walls.
- Tissue fluid enters into them through gaps or loose junctions between the endothelial cells present in their linings.
- Movement of fluid in them is facilitated by ***contraction of organs*** in which they are present and the ***contraction of arterioles and venules*** with which they are often associated.
- They drain into collecting lymphatics.

Collecting Lymphatics

Collecting lymphatics are **tubular and larger lymphatics**.

- They ***have valves and smooth muscles*** in their walls.
- They **exhibit peristaltic contraction** that propels lymph in forward direction.

- **Lymph flow** in larger lymphatics is further facilitated by:
  i) Skeletal muscle contraction,
  ii) Negative intrathoracic pressure (during inspiration), and
  iii) Suction effect created by higher velocity of flow in veins into which the lymphatics drain.
- **Unidirectional flow** of lymph is maintained by ***presence of valves*** in the larger lymphatic ducts.
- Substances that increase lymph flow are called **lymphagouges**. Usually, agents that increase capillary permeability also act as lymphagogues.

Formation & Composition of Lymph

Composition: Lymph is formed from tissue fluid. Therefore, essentially it is a **modified tissue fluid** (Table 36.1).

- Cells in lymph are cells that are chiefly **lymphocytes**.
- Large **molecules of fat** (chylomicrons) that are absorbed from the intestines enter lymph vessels.
- After a fatty meal these fat globules may be so numerous that lymph become milky (is called **chyle**).
  - Under these conditions the lymph vessels can be seen easily as they pass through mesentery.

Formation: It is formed by **transcapillary exchange** and exchange between tissue fluid and lymphatic ducts.

- Lymph **flow is much slower** (1 ml/min in thoracic duct) than blood.
- Its colloidal **osmotic pressure is less** than that of plasma.
- Presence of more lipid gives milky color to the lymph, hence called **chyle**.

Table 36.1 | Composition of lymph.
1. Proteins: 2–6 mg% (more in liver)
2. Lipids: Intestinal lacteals contain more lipid
3. Carbohydrate: less than plasma
4. Clotting factors: Lymph draining from liver mainly contains clotting factors.
5. Cells: Mainly lymphocytes and few monocytes
6. Ions: Sodium, potassium, calcium, chloride, sulphates, phosphate
7. Water

Functions of Lymphatic Circulation

1. **Prevent Edema Formation: Extra amount of fluid left in the tissue space by capillary filtration is taken up by lymphatics and returned back to circulation.**
   - **Thus, lymphatics prevent accumulation of excess free fluid** in the interstitial space (**prevent edema formation**), and at the same time *contribute to water content of plasma* to some extent.
2. **Maintain Protein Content of Plasma:** In liver and intestine, a significant quantity of protein enters into interstitial space.
   - This **protein is returned to circulation via lymphatics**.
   - This accounts for ***25 to 50% of circulating protein*** in the blood. Thus, lymphatics ***maintain protein content of plasma***.
3. **Long-chain fatty acids, cholesterol and fat-soluble vitamins** absorbed from intestine are transported to circulation via lymphatics.
4. **Mononuclear phagocytes in lymph nodes** remove bacteria and pathogenic organisms from lymph draining from the organ. Thus, they play **protective function** (Clinical Note 36.1).

Clinical Note 36.1

Lymphadenopathy: Specific Lymph nodes draining from the **site of infection and inflammation are usually enlarged** during the active phase of the disease process. **Enlarged lymph nodes (lymphadenopathy)** in a particular part of the body provide clinical clue to the physician to locate the site of infection. For example, enlarged submandibular lymph glands indicate infection in the throat.

EDEMA FORMATION

Definition of Edema: The accumulation of **free fluid in excess** in the interstitial tissues space is called edema.

Mechanisms of Edema Formation

Edema can occur due **two important mechanisms**:

1. Increased filtration of fluid into interstitial tissues space
2. Decreased removal of fluid from interstitial tissues space

Increased Filtration of Fluid into Interstitial Tissues Space

This can occur by **three mechanisms**:

i) increased hydrostatic pressure of capillary blood,
ii) decreased oncotic pressure and
iii) increased capillary permeability.

Increased Hydrostatic Pressure of Capillaries: Capillary hydrostatic pressure increases in following conditions:

1. **Increased venous pressure** that increases capillary pressure, e.g., congestive cardiac failure.
2. **Venular constriction**, e.g., a tumor pressing on a vein causes edema in its territory of drainage.
3. Increased **extracellular fluid volume**, e. g., fluid retention.
4. **Arteriolar dilation**, e.g., local inflammation.

Decreased Oncotic Pressure: The oncotic pressure decreases due to **hypoproteinemia** that occurs in liver diseases (decreased production of plasma proteins), kidney diseases (increased excretion of plasma proteins), malnutrition (decreased intake of proteins), and burns (exudation of protein rich fluid from the burn surface).

Increased Capillary Permeability: The capillary permeability increases by the **action of chemical substances** like histamine, bradykinin, substance P and bacterial toxins.

- Edema that occurs **in inflammation** is due to increased capillary permeability.

Decreased Removal of Fluid from Interstitial Tissues Space

From interstitial space water is removed by lymphatics. Thus, **decreased lymphatic drainage** causes edema formation.

- This can occur either due to **diseases of the lymphatics** (lymphangitis), **surgery** (radical mastectomy that removes lymphatic ducts), or by **infection** (filariasis).
- The decreased lymph flow **decreases the removal of excess fluid** from the interstitial tissues space that results in edema formation.
- Edema due to lymphatic obstruction is **usually non-pitting type**.

Exam Questions

1. With the help of a suitable diagram, explain the mechanism of capillary filtration.
2. What are the types of capillaries? Give a note on functional specialities of capillaries.
3. Describe the mechanism of formation and circulation of lymph in the body.
4. Define edema. Describe the mechanism of formation of edema.

Multiple Choice Questions

1. **Which of the following has maximum density of sympathetic innervation?**
   A. Veins
   B. Venules
   C. Arterioles
   D. Large arteries
2. **Korotkov sounds are heard due to:**
   A. Riva Rocci cuff detects sounds in inflated condition
   B. Heart sounds are transmitted better in the arterial wall
   C. Bell of stethoscope very sensitive to sounds in the circulation
   D. Blood flow becomes turbulent in arteries by constriction produced by inflated cuff
3. **Which of the following is not correct about veins?**
   A. Good sympathetic innervation
   B. As they are collapsible, they accommodate less amount of blood
   C. Pressure-volume curve does not change till veins are distended, then the curve rises steeply
   D. Tunica media layer is most thin in veins
4. **Venous return depends on all EXCEPT:**
   A. Competency of venous valves
   B. Skeletal muscle pump
   C. Parasympathetic stimulation
   D. Degree of venoconstriction
5. **Normal CVP is:**
   A. 25 to 45 mmHg
   B. 15 to 20 mmHg
   C. 8 to 10 mmHg
   D. 0 to 5 mmHg
6. **Sinusoidal capillaries are seen in all the following viscera, EXCEPT:**
   A. Bone marrow
   B. Kidney
   C. Spleen
   D. Liver
7. **The total cross-sectional area is more in which part of circulation?**
   A. Vena cava and bigger veins
   B. Arteries and arterioles
   C. Aorta and bigger arteries
   D. Capillaries
8. **Sympathetic innervation is less to:**
   A. Arterioles
   B. Veins
   C. Capillaries
   D. Arteries
9. **Edema in kidney disease is mostly due to:**
   A. Decreased filtration of fluid in nephrons of kidney
   B. Increased hydrostatic pressure in vessels
   C. Increased capillary permeability
   D. Decreased oncotic pressure
10. **Edema in congestive heart failure is mostly due to:**
    A. Decreased oncotic pressure
    B. Decreased cardiac pumping
    C. Increased capillary permeability
    D. Increased hydrostatic pressure in vessels
11. **All are true of composition of lymph, EXCEPT:**
    A. Cells in lymph are mostly lymphocytes
    B. Intestinal lacteals contain more lipids
    C. Protein content is same as plasma
    D. Carbohydrate is less than plasma
12. **Which of the following is NOT the function of lymph?**
    A. Prevents accumulation of excess fluid in interstitium
    B. Contributes greatly to glucose homeostasis
    C. Helps in maintaining protein content of plasma
    D. Contribute to cholesterol, fatty acids and fat-soluble vitamin level of blood.

Answers

1. C	2. D	3. B	4. C	5. D	6. B
7. D	8. C	9. A	10. D	11. C	12. B

Chapter 37

Regulation of Blood Pressure

Learning Objectives

On completion of study of this chapter:

The student will be able to (must know):

1. Define and give the normal values of systolic BP, diastolic BP, mean arterial pressure and pulse pressure.
2. List the factors affecting BP.
3. Appreciate the physiological variations of BP.
4. Describe the mechanisms of regulation of BP.
5. Draw a schematic diagram of baroreceptor reflex and know the importance of this reflex in BP regulation.
6. Know the importance of sympathetic vasoconstrictor tone in BP regulation.

The student may also be able to (desirable to know):

1. Describe the role of vascular smooth muscle and vascular endothelium in the regulation of BP.
2. Describe the role of medulla in the regulation of BP.

Regulation of blood pressure (BP) is a fundamental physiological process. BP is an important vital sign of clinical examination of a subject or a patient.

DEFINITION & NORMAL VALUES

Blood Pressure

Blood pressure is defined as the **lateral pressure exerted by the column of blood on the wall of arteries**.

- Blood pressure means the **arterial pressure**.
- The arterial pressure fluctuates during systole and diastole of the heart.

Systolic Blood Pressure

Definition: Systolic BP is defined as the **maximum pressure** recorded during the cardiac cycle. As maximum pressure is recorded during systole, the pressure is called systolic pressure.

Normal Value: Normal systolic BP is **100 to 119 mm Hg** in adults.

- Systolic BP 120 to 139 mmHg is classified as **prehypertension** and 140 mm Hg or above is considered as **hypertension**.

Significance: Systolic pressure **depends mainly on the cardiac output**.

- Thus, systolic pressure increases when cardiac output is more and decreases when cardiac output is reduced.
- Systolic pressure is also affected by the **compliance of arteries**.
  - When arteries become stiff as occurs in advanced age, systolic pressure increases.
  - In a stiff vessel, the *ability to accommodate a particular amount of cardiac output decreases* in comparison to a normal vessel.

Diastolic Blood Pressure

Definition: Diastolic blood pressure is defined as the **minimum pressure** recorded during the cardiac cycle. As the minimum pressure is recorded during diastole, the pressure is called diastolic pressure.

Significance: Diastolic blood pressure depends primarily on peripheral resistance.

- Therefore, diastolic pressure changes with alteration in peripheral resistance.
- Peripheral resistance depends mainly on the **diameter of the blood vessels** and **viscosity** of the blood.
- **Vasoconstriction** increases diastolic pressure and **vasodilation** decreases diastolic pressure.

Normal Value: Normal diastolic BP is **60 to 79 mm Hg** in adults.

- Diastolic BP 80 to 89 mmHg is classified as **prehypertension** and 90 mm Hg or above is considered as **hypertension**.

Pulse Pressure

Definition: Pulse pressure (PP) is the **difference between systolic and diastolic** blood pressure.

Normal Value: 20 to 50 mmHg

Significance: This is the pressure that maintains the **normal pulsatile nature** of blood flow in the vascular compartment.

- The pulsatile nature of flow is required for the **perfusion of the tissues**.

Mean Arterial Pressure

Definition: Mean arterial pressure (MAP) is the **average pressure** recorded during the cardiac cycle.

- As the duration of systole is less than the duration of diastole, the MAP is less than the value halfway between systolic and diastolic pressures (Fig. 37.1A).

It is calculated as:

MAP = Diastolic Pressure + 1/3 PP

Normal Value: 75 to 105 mm Hg.

Significance: The MAP is the pressure that helps in **forward movement of blood** in the lumen of blood vessels. It also maintains **perfusion of tissues**.

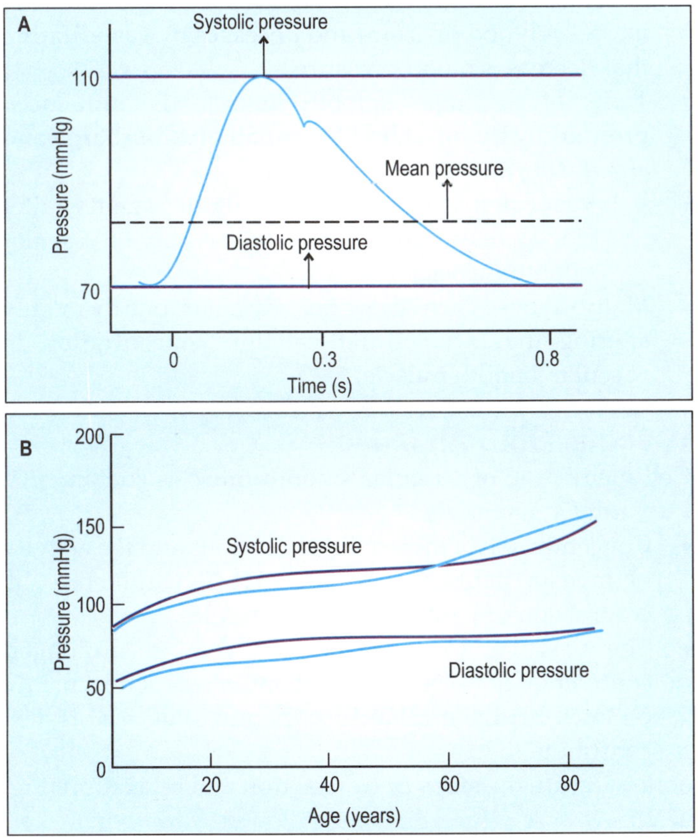

Fig. 37.1: **A:** Normal arterial pressure during a cardiac cycle. Note, the maximum pressure recoded is systolic pressure and the minimum pressure recorded is diastolic pressure. The mean arterial pressure is close towards the diastolic pressure as the duration of diastole is more than the duration of systole. **B:** Effects of age and gender on BP. Note, during the reproductive age, the systolic and diastolic pressure is less in females (blue line) than in males (black line). However, after menopause, in females, diastolic pressure becomes almost equal with males, and systolic pressure may even become more than in males.

Casual Blood Pressure

Blood pressure measured at **any time of the day** or night is known as the casual pressure.

Basal Blood Pressure

Blood pressure recorded **in the basal state** is called basal blood pressure. Usually in clinical practice, basal blood pressure is recorded following physical and mental rest for 10–20 min in supine position **(resting basal BP).**

FACTORS AFFECTING BLOOD PRESSURE

Blood pressure = **cardiac output × peripheral resistance**

- Therefore, factors that influence cardiac output or peripheral resistance affect the blood pressure.
- Alteration in **cardiac output mainly affects systolic pressure** and alteration in **peripheral resistance mainly affects diastolic pressure.**

Factors Affecting Cardiac Output

Cardiac output – **stroke volume** × heart rate

- As cardiac output is the product of stroke volume and heart rate, any factor that affects either of these two parameters, affects cardiac output.
- The stroke volume is affected by preload, afterload and myocardial contractility, and the heart rate is mainly affected by autonomic influences.
- Details of cardiac out are given in Chapter 32.

Factors Affecting Peripheral Resistance

Peripheral resistance depends mainly on **diameter of blood vessel** and **viscosity** of blood (details of peripheral resistance are given in Chapter 34).

Diameter of Blood Vessels: Vasoconstriction increases blood pressure by increasing peripheral resistance and vasodilation decreases blood pressure by decreasing peripheral resistance.

- Diameter of blood vessels depends primarily on the **vasomotor tone**, which is the **sympathetic vasoconstrictor tone.**
- Also, when blood **vessels become stiff** (less compliant), ***peripheral resistance increases*** that increases blood pressure.

Viscosity: Viscosity depends on composition of plasma, total number of cells in the blood, resistance of the cells to deformation and temperature.

Factors that increase viscosity:

1. Polycythemia
2. Hyperproteinemia
3. Hereditary spherocytosis
4. Decreased temperature

Factors that decrease viscosity:

1. Anemia
2. Hypoproteinemia
3. Increased temperature

Physiological Variations

Age: Blood pressure **increases with age.**

In children: Systolic pressure ranges from 90 to 120 mm Hg and diastolic pressure from 50 to 80 mm Hg.

In adults: Systolic pressure ranges from 100 to 119 mm Hg and diastolic pressure from 60 to 89 mm Hg. As per JNC-7 report on hypertension, systolic BP between 120 to 139 mmHg and diastolic BP between 80 to 89 mmHg are classified as prehypertension

In elderly: The upper limit of systolic is considered to be 140 mm Hg. However, ***diastolic pressure above 90 mm Hg*** is always considered to be abnormal.

Gender: Blood pressure is comparatively **less in females** during their reproductive life (Fig. 37.1B).

1. This difference disappears after menopause.
2. Blood pressure is less in females due to the effect of progesterone that relaxes the smooth muscles of the blood vessels and estrogen that prevents atherosclerosis.

Eating: Blood pressure **increases after a meal.** This is due to increased body metabolism that increases circulation and cardiac output following food intake.

Sleep: Blood pressure is **less during sleep** than in the awakened state. When human being is awake, he is under the influence of stress and strain of life.

- Acute stress activates sympathetic activity that increases blood pressure. The level of **stress & sympathetic tone are less** in sleep.
- In addition, **absence of physical activity** during sleep aids to decrease in blood pressure.

Emotion and Excitement: In emotion and excitement, **increased sympathetic discharge** increases blood pressure.

Exercise: During exercise, the **systolic pressure always rises** due to increased cardiac output.

- **Diastolic pressure** depends on the degree of exercise, which increases in mild exercise due to vasoconstriction, but decreases in moderate to severe exercise due to metabolic vasodilation and increased body temperature.
- Thus, **pulse pressure is more** in severe exercise.

Posture: On **immediate standing** from supine posture, **blood pressure decreases** due to venous pooling of blood in the lower limbs.

- However, blood pressure returns to normal or may mildly increase due to the immediate corrections initiated by baroreceptor reflex.
- Baroreceptor reflex controls blood pressure in 15 to 30 seconds.

Temperature: Blood pressure **decreases in hot environment** due to *cutaneous vasodilation* and **increases in cold** environment due to *vasoconstriction*.

Pregnancy: Cardiac output **increases in pregnancy** due to ***increased blood volume*** that increases systolic pressure.

1. **Diastolic pressure falls** due to decreased peripheral resistance, which occurs due to the **effect of progesterone** on blood vessels. Progesterone relaxes smooth muscle and therefore causes **vasodilation.**
2. Thus, **pulse pressure increases** in pregnancy.

Vascular Tone is the Key Factor

Tone of the blood vessel plays a crucial role in the regulation of blood pressure. **Tone of vascular smooth muscle** depends on many neural and humoral actors.

- Smooth muscles of blood vessel like other smooth muscles exhibit tone, **a state of prolonged partial contraction.**
  - Blood pressure is mostly influenced by the **tone of blood vessels**, especially ***of the resistance vessels*** (arterioles and small arteries).
- Vascular tone **increases by vasoconstriction** that increases blood pressure and **deceases by vasodilation** that decreases blood pressure.
- Tone of vascular smooth muscle is influenced profoundly by the **state of sympathetic discharge** and *circulating neurohumoral factors.*
  - **Vasoconstrictor and vasodilator agents** alter blood pressure by altering the activity of vascular smooth muscle.
- Many of these chemicals affect vascular tone by mainly altering the **intracellular calcium concentration** in vascular smooth muscle.

Vascular Smooth Muscle

Cell membrane of vascular smooth muscles contains **K^+, Ca^{++} and Cl^- channels.**

- Concentration of intracellular Ca^{++} ions and the activity of myosin light-chain kinase (**MLCK**) influence the contraction of vascular smooth muscles.
- The vascular tone that occurs due to prolonged contraction of vascular smooth muscle depends mainly on **latch-bridge mechanism,** though other factors also contribute to it.

Following are the **steps of contraction and relaxation** (Fig. 37.2):

1. Opening of **voltage-gated calcium channels** (VGCC).
2. **Influx of calcium** into the muscle cell through VGCC that increases cytosolic calcium.
   - **Calcium activates myosin light chain kinase** that phosphorylates myosin light chain, which in turn causes muscle contraction.
3. Increased cytoplasmic calcium causes **opening of**

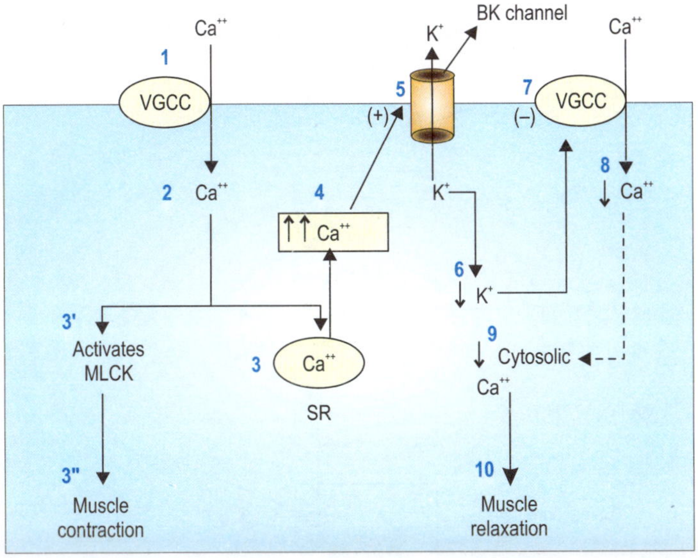

Fig. 37.2: Stepwise depiction of the mechanisms of smooth muscle contraction and relaxation (details of steps are given in the text) BK: Big-K$^+$ channels; Plus sign indicates stimulation and minus sign indicates inhibition.

ryanodine receptor-mediated calcium channels in the sarcoplasmic reticulum.

4. This increases release of calcium from this organelle (**calcium mediated calcium release**).
5. Cytosolic calcium concentration increases to a greater extent that opens up the **calcium-activated K$^+$ channels** on cell membrane.
   - These potassium channels are **BK channels** (Big-K$^+$ channels) as *K$^+$ efflux occurs at a very high rate* through these channels.
   - Calcium acts on **β_1 subunits of BK channels.**
6. Opening of BK channels causes **K$^+$ efflux and reduces cytosolic K$^+$ concentration.**
7. K$^+$ efflux increases the membrane potential that **closes VGCC.**
8. Calcium entry through VGCC decreases.
9. Cytosolic calcium concentration decreases.
10. Decreased calcium produces relaxation.

PY5.9

REGULATION OF BLOOD PRESSURE

The mechanisms involved in regulation of blood pressure can be divided broadly into **two categories**: short-term regulation and long-term regulation.

1. **Short-term regulation** is mainly neural.
2. **Long-term regulation** is mainly hormonal and renal.

SHORT-TERM REGULATION OF BLOOD PRESSURE

Short-term regulation means the regulation of blood pressure **within seconds to minutes,** or in an hour. Short-term regulation occurs mainly by the **neural mechanisms,** though the ***vascular and hormonal mechanisms*** also contribute to it.

Mechanisms of short-term regulation of blood pressure are as follows:

1. **Neural mechanisms**
   i) Autonomic regulation
      – Sympathetic control
      – Parasympathetic control
   ii) Medullary control
   iii) Hypothalamic control
   iv) Cortical control
   v) Reflex regulation
      – Baroreceptor reflex
      – Chemoreceptor reflex
      – Cushing reflex
      – Somatosympathetic reflex
      – Atrial stretch reflex
      – Ventricular and pulmonary stretch reflexes
      – Nonphysiological chemoreflexes (coronary and pulmonary chemoreflexes)
      – Bainbridge reflex
2. **Vascular mechanisms**
   - Capillary fluid-shift
   - Stress relaxation
3. **Hormonal mechanisms**
   - Catecholamines
   - Renin-angiotensin system
   - ADH
   - ANP
   - Kinin-kallikrein system
   - Histamine
   - Endothelins
   - EDRF
   - Adrenomedullin

Neural Mechanisms of BP Regulation

Autonomic Regulation

Autonomic control of blood pressure is **mainly by sympathetic control**, as systemic blood vessels are ***innervated by sympathetic fibers*** and they lack parasympathetic innervation.

Sympathetic Control

Sympathetic regulation is the **main control mechanism** for blood pressure regulation as the sympathetic fibers are the **final pathways** of all neural inputs to the blood vessels. There are **two types of sympathetic systems** for blood vessels:

i) Sympathetic vasoconstrictor system
ii) Sympathetic vasodilator system

Sympathetic Vasoconstrictor System

Noradrenergic fibers supplying blood vessels are **vasoconstrictor in nature**. Therefore, stimulation of these

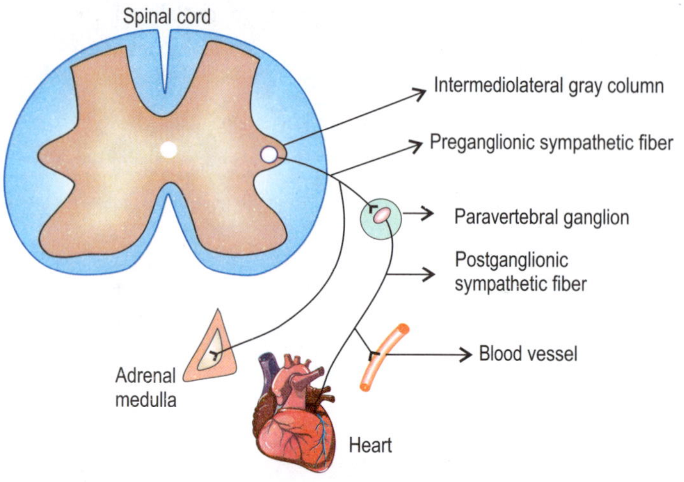

Fig. 37.3: Sympathetic vasoconstrictor system. These fibers originate from ILH of spinal cord. The postganglionic fibers innervate blood vessels and heart, and preganglionic fibers terminate in adrenal medulla.

fibers **increases blood pressure.**

- The sympathetic vasoconstrictor fibers **originate from** the ***intermediolateral horn (ILH) of the spinal cord*** and innervate blood vessels, adrenal medulla and heart (Fig. 37.3).
- Stimulation of these fibers **produces vasoconstriction** and therefore they are called vasoconstrictor fibers.
- It is important to note that the sympathetic vasoconstrictor fibers have the **basal rate of tonic discharge**, which is essential for maintaining the normal **vascular tone**.
  - Thus, the vascular sympathetic tone is also known as **sympathetic vasoconstrictor tone**.
- Sympathetic stimulation also produces **venoconstriction**.
  - Venoconstriction **increases venous return** and cardiac output and shifts blood from the venous compartment to the arterial compartment that aids in increasing blood pressure.
- Sympathetic stimulation also increases blood pressure by its **cardiostimulatory effects** and **effects on catecholamine secretion** from adrenal medulla.

In summary, sympathetic stimulation increases BP by following mechanisms:

1. **Vasoconstriction,** especially constriction of resistance vessels.
2. **Venoconstriction** that increases venous return.
3. **Cardiac stimulation** (increased heart rate and myocardial contractility).

IMPORTANT NOTE

Sympathetic control is critical: Sympathetic regulation is the essential component of blood pressure regulation. Decreased rate of tonic discharge of sympathetic vasoconstrictor nerves produces vasodilation that results in fall in blood pressure. For example, hypotension following spinal transection occurs due to decreased sympathetic outflow.

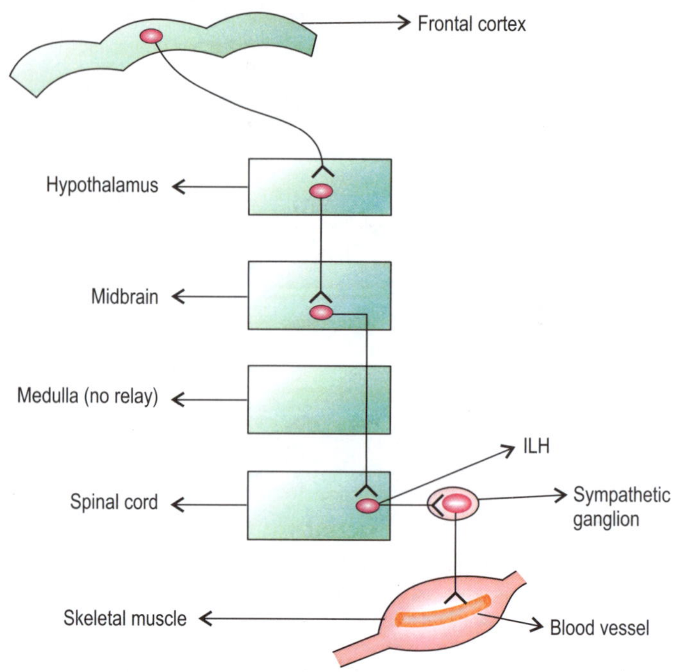

Fig. 37.4: Sympathetic vasodilator system. Fibers originating from frontal cortex relay in hypothalamus and midbrain. From midbrain, fibers descend down to intermediolateral horn (ILH) of spinal cord without contacting neurons in the medullary cardiorespiratory centers. From ILH, sympathetic fibers terminate on blood vessel of skeletal muscle.

4. Increased **secretion of catecholamines** from adrenal medulla.

Sympathetic Vasodilator System

Stimulation of sympathetic fibers supplying arteries and arterioles of skeletal muscles produces vasodilation as they are innervated by sympathetic cholinergic fibers.

- Therefore, this system of sympathetic innervation of blood vessel is called as sympathetic vasodilator system.
- These fibers **originate from frontal cortex** and relay in **hypothalamus & midbrain** (Fig. 37.4).
- Fibers ***pass through medulla without relay*** in medullary cardiovascular centers and ***terminate in intermediolateral gray column*** of spinal cord.
- There is **no basal tonic discharge** of sympathetic vasodilator fibers.

Parasympathetic Control

Systemic blood vessels are not supplied by parasympathetic fibers. However, vagal stimulation *decreases blood pressure* **by decreasing heart rate & cardiac output.**

Medullary Control

Cardiovascular centers are mainly located in the medulla.

- These centers primarily control the **autonomic output** on heart and blood vessels, which is the **major cardiovascular regulatory pathway**.

Medullary cardiovascular centers are broadly divided into two: **vasomotor center and cardioinhibitory centers.**

Vasomotor Center

- Vasomotor centers (VMC) center is present mainly in the rostral ventrolateral medulla.
- VMC has caudal, intermediate and rostral parts; and accordingly they are called caudal ventrolateral medulla (CVLM), intermediate ventrolateral medulla (IVLM) and rostral ventrolateral medulla (RVLM).
    - Though **RVLM is the major area** in these group of neurons, these neuronal groups are collectively known as **vasomotor centers** (VMC), which directly projects to the intermediolateral gray column of the spinal cord via **bulbospinal pathway** from where the sympathetic vasoconstrictor fibers originate (Fig. 37.5).
- Neurons in VMC are *always active* and provide **tonic excitatory drive** to the spinal cord neurons.
    - The **basal tonic sympathetic vasoconstrictor tone** is due to the drive of preganglionic sympathetic neurons by the **tonic discharge of VMC neurons**.
- This **medullary-spinal cord-cardiovascular axis** is the most important pathway for control of blood pressure.
    - As vasomotor center regulates activity of this pathway, control of blood pressure by it is called **Vasomotor Control**.

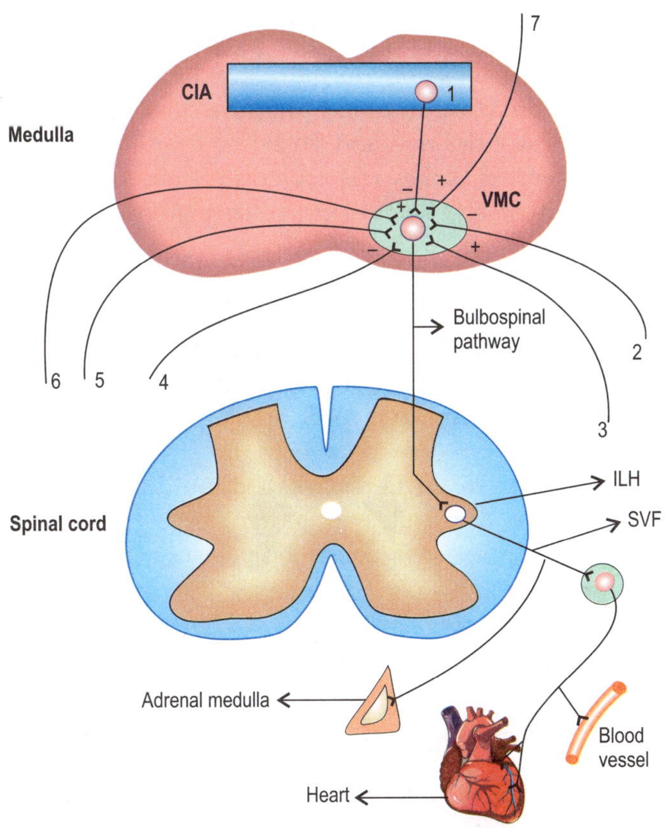

Fig. 37.5: Vasomotor control. VMC receives inhibitory input from cardioinhibitory area (CIA) in the medulla via interneurons (1). VMC also receives inhibitory input from aortic and carotid baroreceptors (2), excitatory input from aortic and carotid chemoreceptors (3), inhibitory input from lungs (4), excitatory input from ascending pain pathways (5), excitatory proprioceptive input (6), and from limbic system (7). Fibers from VMC descend down in the bulbospinal pathway to terminate on the cell bodies in the intermediolateral horn (ILH) of spinal cord and stimulate sympathetic vasoconstrictor fibers (SVF).

- **Stimulation of VMC** causes intense vasoconstriction and cardioacceleration that **increases blood pressure**.
- **Inhibition of VMC** causes vasodilation and cardioinhibition that **decreases blood pressure**.

IMPORTANT NOTE

Lesion of VMC causes severe hypotension: Influence of VMC on control of blood pressure is so crucial that loss of this influence as occurs following transection of spinal cord results in gross *hypotension* in the acute phase of spinal shock.

Vasomotor center **receives inputs** from following structure of the body (Fig. 37.5):

1. Aortic and carotid baroreceptors (inhibitory)
2. Cardiopulmonary baroreceptors (inhibitory)
3. Carotid and aortic chemoreceptors (excitatory)
4. Ascending pain pathways (excitatory)
5. Ascending pathways carrying proprioceptive information (excitatory)
6. Lungs via vagus nerves (inhibitory)
7. Limbic cortex via hypothalamus (usually excitatory, but may be inhibitory)

Following are the **effects of activation** of these inputs:

- **Fibers from limbic cortex** to vasomotor center mediate change in blood pressure during emotion and excitement.
- **Lung inflation** inhibits vasomotor center that produces vasodilation and decreases blood pressure.
- **Pain and proprioceptive stimuli** increase blood pressure by stimulating vasomotor center.
- **Carotid and aortic chemoreceptors** stimulate whereas baroreceptors inhibit vasomotor center.
- **Hypoxia and carbon dioxide** directly stimulate vasomotor center.

Cardioinhibitory Centers

Cardioinhibitory center in the medulla is formed by **nucleus tractus solitarius** (NTS), **nucleus ambiguous** and **dorsal motor nucleus of vagus**.

- Stimulation of these areas results in **bradycardia and decreased cardiac output** by two mechanisms.

1. Vagus nerve originates from cardioinhibitory areas, mainly from NTS, which on stimulation **activates vagal output** that inhibits heart functions (Fig. 37.6).
2. NTS **inhibits vasomotor center** via local inhibitory interneurons that in turn ***decreases sympathetic output***.

Thus, **stimulation of NTS** *increases vagal activity and decreases sympathetic activity* that in turn results in bradycardia, decreased cardiac output, vasodilation and **decreased blood pressure.**

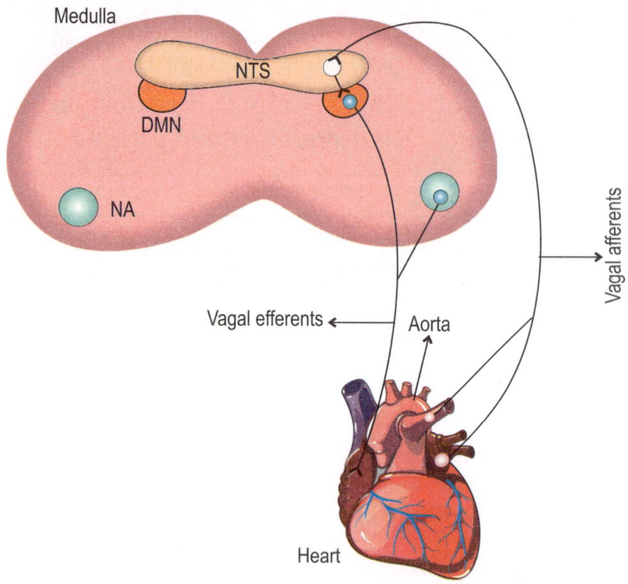

Fig. 37.6: Cardioinhibitory centers (CIC) in the medulla. Nucleus tractus solitarius (NTS) is the major center, others are dorsal motor nucleus (DMN) of vagus and nucleus ambiguous (NA). Sensation from heart and aorta reach NTS vis vagal afferents. NTS projects to dorsal motor nucleus (DMN). DMN is the major efferent nucleus.

Hypothalamic Control

Stimulation of **anterior hypothalamus** produces hypotension and bradycardia and stimulation of **posterolateral part of hypothalamus** produces hypertension and tachycardia.

- Hypothalamus controls **cutaneous blood flow** that affects blood pressure.
- Hypothalamus also mediates the effects of cardiovascular reflexes such as **atrial stretch reflex**.
- A **reciprocal connection** exists between hypothalamus and vasomotor center.
- **Limbic cortex** influences vasomotor center **via hypothalamus**.

Hypothalamus also **secretes ADH** that conserves body water in hypovolemia and hypotension, a mechanism involved in long-term regulation of blood pressure.

Cortical Control

Cortex does not directly influence blood pressure.

- However, stimulation of **motor and premotor cortices** usually *increases blood pressure*.
- **Sympathetic vasodilator system** originates from frontal cortex.

Reflex Regulation of Blood Pressure

Regulation of blood pressure by various cardiovascular reflexes is the most important short-term mechanism as reflexes operate swiftly and effectively in response to change in blood pressure. The important reflexes are baroreceptor reflex, chemoreceptor reflex and Cushing's reflex (the list of other reflexes is given above).

Baroreceptor Reflex

Among all the cardiovascular reflexes, most important is the baroreceptor reflex as it **regulates blood pressure within seconds**.

- This is also called **baroreflex** or **Sino-aortic Reflex**.

Receptors and Stimulus

The receptors are called baroreceptors.

- They detect change in pressure in the blood vessels and chambers of the heart.
- Usually, baroreceptors are classified into two categories: high-pressure and low-pressure receptors.
  - ***High-pressure baroreceptors*** are located in the ventricle and arterial side of circulation, and the ***low-pressure baroreceptors*** are mainly present in the atria and pulmonary circulation (cardiopulmonary baroreceptors).
- Receptors for baroreceptor reflex are **high-pressure baroreceptors** that are present in the wall of the **carotid sinus and aortic arch.**
  - **Carotid sinus** is the initial dilated portion of the internal carotid artery at its origin from common carotid artery (Fig. 37.7).
- These receptors are **branched, knobby and intertwined** terminals of myelinated nerve fibers.
- Baroreceptors **detect change in pressure** in blood vessels in the wall of which they are located.
  - The **increase in blood pressure** causes distension of carotid sinus and aortic arch and ***stimulates receptors*** as they respond to stretch of the organ.
  - Conversely, **decreased pressure** *decreases receptor stimulation*.

Afferent Pathways

Ninth cranial nerve (glossopharyngeal nerve) is the afferent from carotid sinus and tenth cranial nerve (vagus nerve) is the afferent from aortic arch (Fig. 37.8).

- The fibers from carotid sinus in the glossopharyngeal nerve form a distinct branch called carotid sinus nerve.
  - This is also called as buffer nerve as it buffers blood pressure when blood pressure changes.

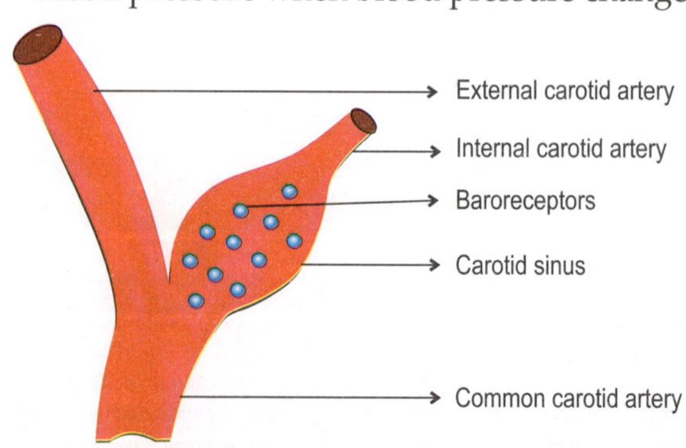

Fig. 37.7: Location of the carotid sinus. Note, it is the initial dilated portion of the internal carotid artery (carotid sinus) at its bifurcation from common carotid. Baroreceptors are located in the wall of the carotid sinus.

- The fibers in the vagus nerve that carry sensation from aortic arch form the aortic nerve.
  - However, aortic nerve forms a *distinct branch* of vagus nerve *only in rabbit*.
- Distension of carotid sinus and aortic arch causes stretching of baroreceptors and increases firing (nerve traffic) in IX and X cranial nerves respectively.

Centers

Centers are located in medulla, called as medullary cardiovascular centers. These include vasomotor center and cardioinhibitory centers.

Vasomotor Center: The vasomotor center (VMC) is the central sympathetic center, as through bulbospinal pathway VMC projects to the intermediolateral horn (ILH) of spinal cord.

- From LIH ***sympathetic fibers originate.***

Cardioinhibitory Center: Nucleus tractus solitarius (NTS) is the major cardioinhibitory center.

- This is the ***main parasympathetic center*** as *vagus nerve originates* from NTS.

IMPORTANT NOTE

NTS stimulates vagus and inhibits VMC: Normally, NTS inhibits vasomotor center via interneurons. Thus, excitation of cardioinhibitory center, i) directly stimulates **vagus** nerve and ii) via inhibition of VMC **inhibits sympathetic fibers.**

Efferent Pathways & Effector Organs

Efferent fibers for baroreceptors are sympathetic fibers and vagus nerve.

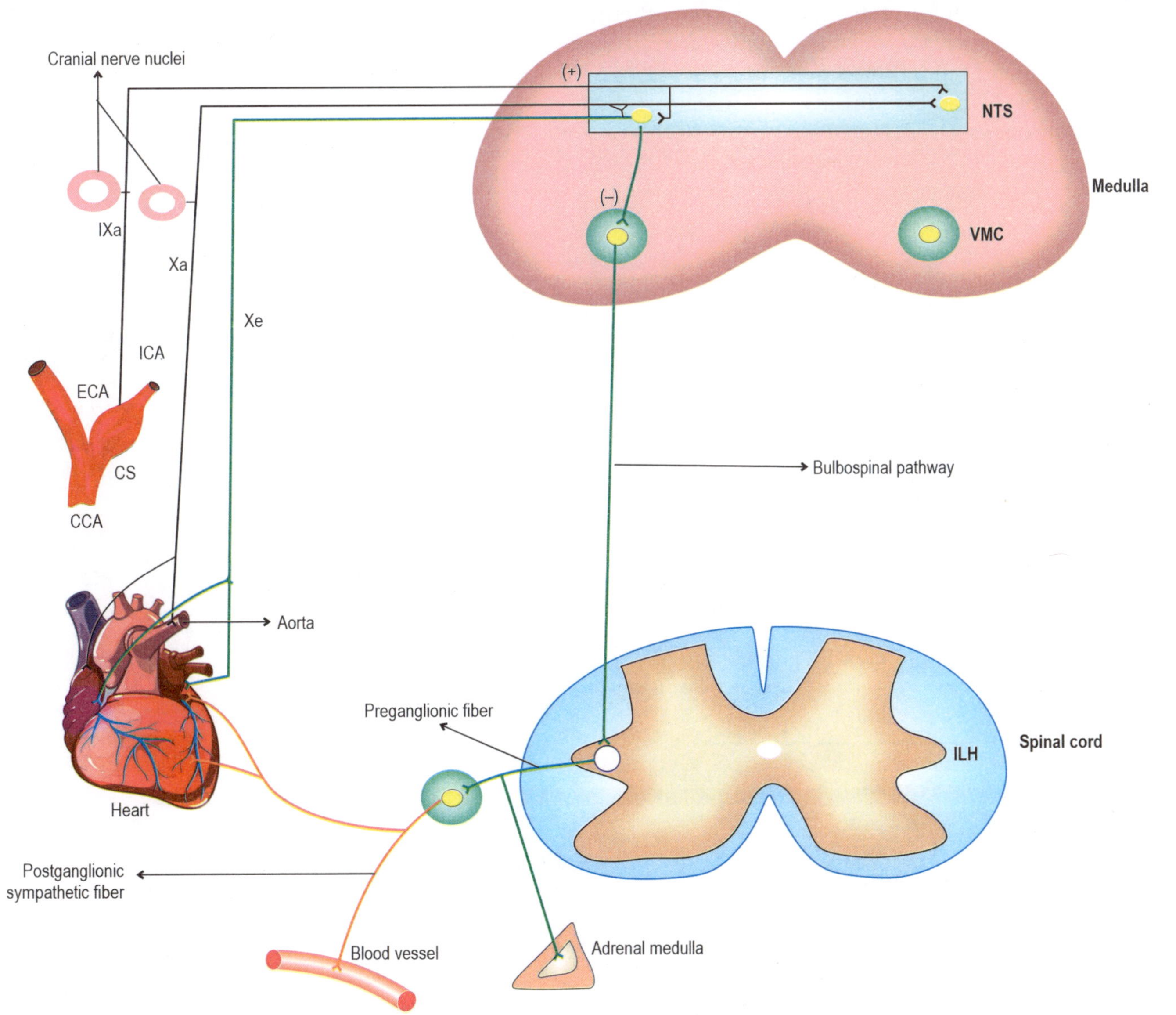

Fig. 37.8: Baroreceptor reflex. Affarent pathway is formed by 9th (IXa) and 10th cranial nerves (Xa) and efferent pathway is by efferent fibers of 10th cranial nerve (Xe) and sympathetic vasoconstrictor system that originates from VMC. CCA: common carotid artery; ICA: internal carotid artery; ECA: external carotid artery; CS: carotid sinus; NTS: nucleus tractus solitarius (NTS); VMC: vasomotor center; +: excitatory neurotransmitter like glutamate; – : inhibitory neurotransmitter like GABA; ILH: intermediolateral horn.

- Sympathetic fibers originate from *ILH of the spinal cord*, which is controlled by vasomotor center.
- Vagus nerve originates from NTS.
- Vagus nerve innervates heart and sympathetic fibers innervate heart and blood vessels.

Responses

Responses depend on the nature of change (increase or decrease) in blood pressure. Responses also depend on degree and rate of change in blood pressure.

When Blood Pressure Increases: Increase in blood pressure **stimulates baroreceptors** in carotid sinus and aortic arch that **increases the nerve traffic** in IX and X cranial nerves.

- This leads to the **excitation of the NTS** in the medulla, which in turn **inhibits vasomotor center** via interneurons.
- Inhibition of vasomotor center **decreases sympathetic output** and causes *vasodilation, bradycardia, decrease in cardiac output* and **fall in blood pressure.**
- Excitation of NTS also directly inhibits heart by ***stimulating vagus nerve*** (Fig. 37.9).

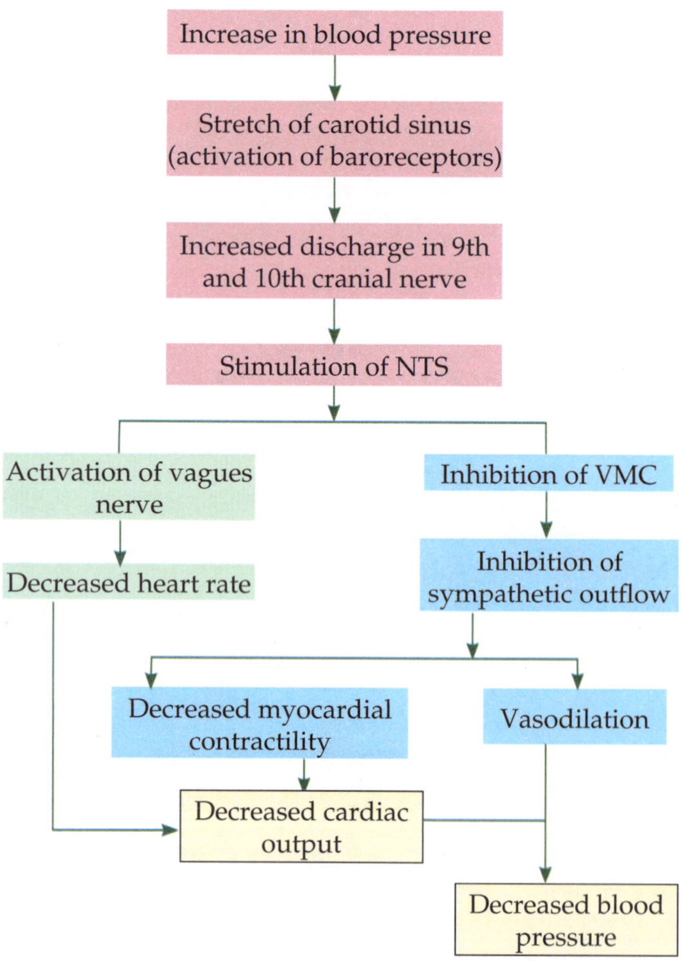

Fig. 37.9: Cardiovascular responses activated by increased blood pressure.

When Blood Pressure Decreases: Fall in blood pressure causes ***less distension*** of carotid sinus and aortic arch that decreases receptor activity and **inhibits discharge rate** in the afferent nerves.

- This **inhibits nucleus tractus solitarius** that in turn causes **disinhibition** of vasomotor center (removal of inhibition of VMC).
  - Thus, vasomotor center is stimulated that **increases sympathetic discharge** and causes *vasoconstriction, tachycardia, increased cardiac output,* and **increase in blood pressure**.
- Inhibition of NTS also stimulates heart by **inhibiting vagus nerve** (Fig. 37.10).
- Sympathetic activation also promotes **release of catecholamines** from adrenal medulla that stimulate heart and cause vasoconstriction.

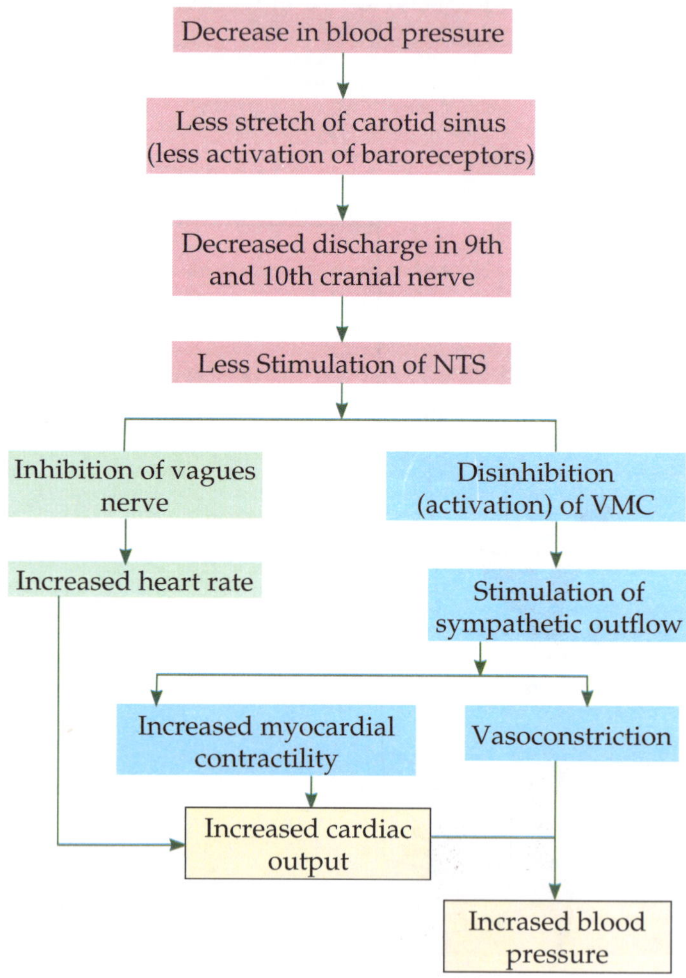

Fig. 37.10: Cardiovascular responses activated by decreased blood pressure.

Pressure Range for Baroreflex Regulation

Baroreceptors regulate blood pressure in the pressure range of **50 to 200 mm Hg**.

- However, a **linear relationship** is observed for the change in blood pressure and the baroreceptor discharge between pressure range of **70 to 140 mm Hg**.
- No response is detected when pressure is less than 50 mm Hg and no further increase in response occurs when pressure is more than 200 mm Hg (Fig. 37.11).

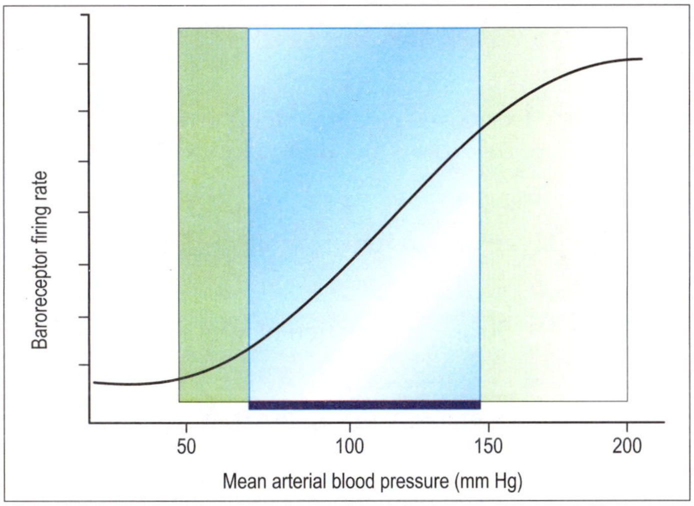

Fig. 37.11: Pressure range of baroreceptor reflex. Note, baroreceptor responds to pressure change between 50 to 200 mm Hg. However, maximum baroreceptor discharge occurs between 70 to 140 mm Hg as indicated by the dark bar below the pressure curve. There is no baroreceptor activation before 50 mm Hg and after 200 mm Hg.

Types of Responses

Baroreceptors respond to change in **pulse pressure** and change in **mean arterial pressure**. Accordingly, there are **two types** of responses: **dynamic response** and **static response**.

- Response mainly to change in pulse pressure is called **phasic or dynamic response** and response mainly to change in sustained pressure (mean pressure) is called **tonic or static response**.
- However, changes in pulse pressure and mean arterial pressure usually occur simultaneously.

Physiological Significance of Baroreceptor Reflex

1. When blood pressure falls, baroreceptor reflex **operates within few seconds** to correct the pressure, which is essential and life-saving in acute hypotension and hemorrhage.
   - This is also **life-saving in day-to-day activities** (Application Box 37.1).
   - For example, blood pressure falls by about 30% on standing from lying posture, which is immediately corrected by baroreceptor reflex.
   - Thus, baroreceptor reflex is the **first and foremost reflex** for regulation of blood pressure.
2. Baroreceptor reflex regulates blood pressure when pressure change is within the **range of 50–200 mm Hg**.
   - Thus, baroreceptors and their reflex pathway constitute a feedback mechanism to stabilize blood pressure **over a wide range of fluctuation** in pressure.
3. Baroreceptor reflex explains the physiological basis for **Marey's Law**, which states that ***heart rate is inversely proportional to blood pressure*** (but not the vice versa).
4. Baroreceptor resetting occurs in chronic hypertension (discussed below).

Application Box 37.1

Baroreflex is life-saving in daily life: Change in posture, especially getting up from supine posture decreases blood pressure due to peripheral pooling of blood that decreases effective blood volume, which may be equivalent to about 15% acute hemorrhage. Such an acute hemorrhage usually leads to shock. However, baroreflex adjusts BP so efficiently and promptly that we never realize we had a situation akin to acute severe hemorrhage.

Chemoreceptor Reflex

Receptors, Stimuli & Afferents: Receptors are **chemoreceptors** that are located in the **carotid bodies and aortic bodies**.

- They respond to change in **chemical composition of blood** that occurs in conditions like hypoxia, hypercapnia and acidosis.
- **Afferents** from carotid body is ***IX cranial nerve*** and from aortic body is ***X cranial nerve***.

Centers: Afferent fibers project to the medullary ***respiratory centers***.

- They also project to the cardiovascular centers, especially to both the **vasomotor and cardioinhibitory centers** (Fig. 37.12).

Effects: Stimulation of chemoreceptors has **two phase effects**: the primary effects and the secondary effects.

1. **Primary effects** of chemoreceptor stimulation are **bradycardia and vasoconstriction**.
   - Stimulation of cardioinhibitory center causes bradycardia and stimulation of vasomotor center causes vasoconstriction.
2. However, hypoxia that stimulates chemoreceptors also causes ***pulmonary hyperventilation*** and increases ***catecholamine secretion*** from adrenal medulla that in turn increases heart rate (**secondary effects**).
3. Therefore, the **net effect** of stimulation of chemoreceptors is no change in heart rate or **mild tachycardia and vasoconstriction** that increases blood pressure.

BP Range: The **range of regulation** of blood pressure by chemoreceptor reflex is **40 to 70 mm Hg**.

CNS Ischemic Response (Cushing's Reflex)

In conditions of **gross hypotension** as seen in acute severe hemorrhage, blood flow is compromised to the vital organs of the body.

- **Decreased cerebral blood flow** produces hypoxia and hypercapnia of vasomotor center.
- Direct hypoxia and hypercapnia stimulate vasomotor center to its maximum, which causes **intense vasoconstriction** so that raised pressure maintains minimum blood flow to important organs.
  - The reflex response is called as **CNS ischemic response**.
- This is activated when *blood pressure falls below 40 mm Hg*.

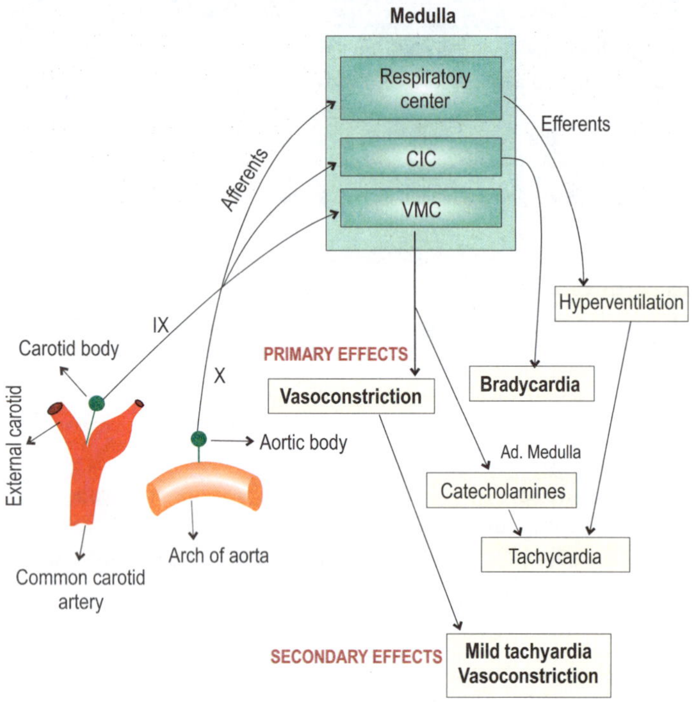

Fig. 37.12: Chemoreceptor reflex. Afferents from carotid and aortic bodies in 9th and 10th cranial nerve respectively stimulate cardioinhibitory center (CIC) to produce bradycardia and vasomotor center (VMC) to produce vasoconstriction. These are primary effects. However, hyperventilation produced by stimulation of respiratory center and catecholamine secretion by stimulation of adrenal medulla result in tachycardia. Thus, net secondary effects are mild tachycardia and vasoconstriction.

- This is the **last physiological reflex to correct blood pressure**, failure of which leads to irreversible shock.

Effects of Raised ICP: When intracranial pressure (ICP) is high, as occurs in **brain tumor**, the blood flow to the vasomotor center decreases due to compression of cerebral blood vessels.

- This causes hypoxic stimulation of vasomotor center and causes intense vasoconstriction that in turn *increases blood pressure*.
  - This is known as **Cushing's Reflex** (Flowchart 37.1).
- The increase in blood pressure in carotid sinus *activates baroreceptor reflex* and causes **reflex bradycardia**.
  - Therefore, bradycardia occurs in brain tumors (Clinical Note 37.1)

Clinical Note 37.1

Bradycardia is a feature of brain tumors: Increased ICP causes reflex bradycardia by activation of Cushing and baroreceptor reflexes. Therefore, *bradycardia is a prominent feature of brain tumors* that increase intracranial pressure.

Somatosympathetic Reflex

The increase in blood pressure in response to **stimulation of somatic afferent nerves** is called somatosympathetic reflex.

1. It is activated usually following stimulation of **ascending pain fibers**.

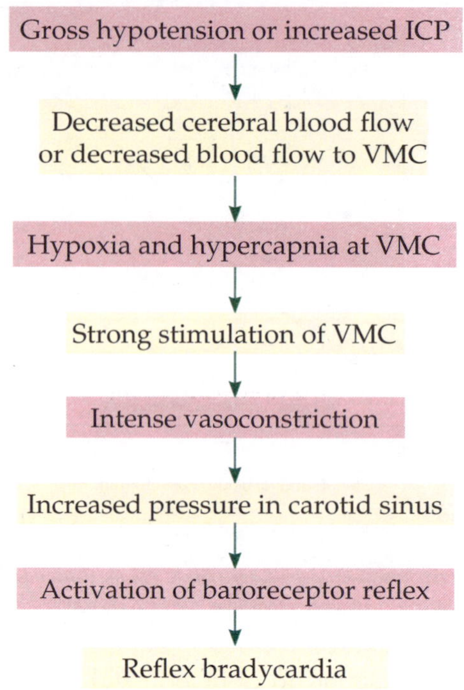

Flowchart 37.1: Cushing reflex (CNS ischemic response).

2. Stimulation of proprioceptive pathway also increases blood pressure.
3. The pressor response is mediated via **vasomotor center** that receives excitatory input from ascending sensory pathway in the brain-stem (Fig. 37.13).

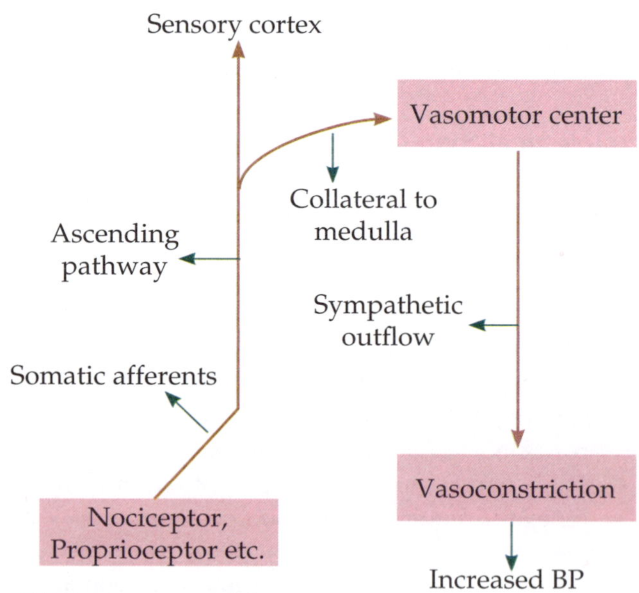

Fig. 37.13: Somatosympathetic reflex.

Atrial Stretch Reflex

Two types of stretch receptors are present in atria: type A and type B receptors.

- **Type A receptors** are stimulated during atrial systole and **type B receptors** are stimulated during peak atrial filling.
- **Increased venous return** as occurs in fluid retention or increased blood volume ***increases atrial filling*** that stimulates **type B receptors**.

- The **responses** to increased atrial filling are **vasodilation, decrease in blood pressure** and **tachycardia**.

- Conversely, decreased ECF volume decreases the activity of atrial stretch receptors that **increase ADH release**. ADH in turn causes water retention and increases blood volume and pressure (Flowchart 37.2).
  - Decreased atrial stretch also **stimulates sympathetic system** that increases renin release, which **activates renin-angiotensin-aldosterone system**.

Increased venous return
↓
Increased atrial filling
↓
stimulation of type-B receptors
↓
Sympathetic inhibition
↓
Vasodilation, ↓BP, but increased heart rate

Flowchart 37.2: Atrial stretch reflex.

Cardio-Pulmonary Stretch Reflexes

Ventricular Stretch Reflex Increased distention of ventricle due to excess ventricular filling as occurs in increased blood volume (*volume overload*) results in bradycardia, vasodilation and hypotension.

- Thus, rise in blood pressure is checked.
- Ventricular stretch reflex also plays a role in maintaining vagal tone that checks the basal heart rate.

Pulmonary Stretch Reflex: Pulmonary baroreceptors are located in pulmonary arteries.

- They are stimulated when ***pulmonary arterial pressure is increased*** as occurs in pulmonary hypertension.
- The responses observed are bradycardia and hypotension.

Nonphysiological Chemoreflexes

Coronary Chemoreflex: Chemoreceptors present in coronary arteries and ventricles are C-fiber endings.

1. The afferents from these chemoreceptors are ***vagal fibers***.
2. Injection of chemicals like capsaicin, veratridine, phenyldiguanide and serotonin into left coronary artery produces hyperventilation, bradycardia and hypotension.
   - This is called coronary chemoreflex or Bezold-Jarisch reflex.

Pulmonary Chemoreflex: Injection of above-mentioned chemical substances into pulmonary arteries produce similar features (hyperventilation, bradycardia and hypotension).

IMPORTANT NOTE

BJR in AMI causes hypotension: In acute myocardial infarction, similar chemical substances are released from the infracted tissue and activate Bezold-Jarisch reflex (BJR). Stimulation of ventricular chemoreceptors and produce bradycardia and hypotension.

The responses are blocked by vagotomy.

- Such responses are observed in ***pulmonary embolism*** that produces pulmonary microinfarction.

Bainbridge Reflex

Infusion of saline or transfusion of blood produces tachycardia **if the initial heart rate is low**. This is called Bainbridge reflex (described by Bainbridge in 1915).

- The receptors are **tachycardia producing atrial receptors** (TPAR) located in the atrial wall where vena cavas open into atria (at venoatrial junction).
- The reflex is **abolished following vagotomy** as the responses are mediated by vagus nerves (Flowchart 37.3).
- The tachycardia produced by this reflex competes with the bradycardia produced by baroreceptor reflex in response to volume expansion.

Infusion of saline or blood (with initial slow heart rate)
↓
Increased venous filling of atria
↓
Stimulation of tachycardia-producing atrial receptor (TPAR)
↓
Tachycardia (afferent & efferent via vagus)

Flowchart 37.3: Bainbridge reflex

Vascular Mechanisms

The vascular mechanisms operate within seconds to minutes. These are **capillary fluid shift** and **stress relaxation**.

Capillary Fluid Shift

When blood pressure decreases rapidly as in acute hemorrhagic shock, the **hydrostatic pressure** in the capillaries **decreases**.

- This causes **shift of fluid** from interstitial tissue space (extravascular compartment) into the intravascular compartment through the capillary membrane.
  - This is called capillary fluid shift.
- In this mechanism, about **300 ml of interstitial fluid** is added to the blood.

- As a result, circulating **blood volume increases** and blood pressure returns to normal.

Reverse Capillary Shift: Reverse mechanism operates when **sudden rise in blood pressure** increases capillary pressure and **facilitates capillary filtration**.

- This decreases blood volume and tends to lower blood pressure.

Stress Relaxation

When blood pressure **increases abruptly**, blood vessels **distend** in response to high pressure.

1. This imparts **acute stretch** on the vessel wall.
2. The **smooth muscles** of the blood vessels **relax in response to sudden stretch**.
3. This decreases vascular tone and **lowers pressure**.

Reverse Stress Relaxation: Reverse stress relaxation occurs when blood pressure decreases.

- Acute fall in blood pressure reduces the normal stretch of the vascular smooth muscle.
- This in turn **causes contraction of smooth muscle** and increases vascular tone, which increases blood pressure.

Hormonal Mechanisms

There are many hormones and chemicals that change blood pressure by causing either vasodilation or vasoconstriction (Table 37.1)

Table 37.1 | Vasodilators & Vasoconstrictors

A. Vasodilators	B. Vasoconstrictors
1. EDRF (nitric oxide)	1. Endothelin-1
2. Bradykinin	2. Angiotensin II
3. Histamine	3. Norepinephrine
4. ANP	4. ADH
5. VIP	5. Serotonin
6. CGRP α	6. Thromboxane A_2
7. Substance P	7. Neuropeptide-Y
8. Prostacyclin	8. Cold
9. Adenosine	
10. K^+	
11. Acidosis	
12. Hypercapnia	
13. Hypoxia	
14. Temperature	

Catecholamines

In acute hypotension, stimulation of **sympathetic fibers to adrenal medulla** releases catecholamines.

- Catecholamines, (especially, norepinephrine) are vasoconstrictors.
  - They also increase heart rate and cardiac output.
- Catecholamines **increase blood pressure** within minutes and injection of catecholamines is life-saving in acute hypotension.

Renin-Angiotensin System

Fall in blood pressure stimulates release of **renin from the JG cells** of the kidney. Renin converts angiotensinogen to angiotensin I, which is further converted to **angiotensin II** by angiotensin-converting enzymes.

- Angiotensin II is a **potent vasoconstrictor** that increases blood pressure.
- Angiotensin II **increases aldosterone secretion**, which increases sodium and water reabsorption from kidney, which is part of long-tern regulation of BP.
  - (for details of Renin-angiotensin-aldosterone system, refer Chapter 86).

Vasopressin

Decrease in blood pressure and blood volume increases the release of vasopressin or antidiuretic hormone (ADH) from posterior pituitary.

- ADH **increases water reabsorption** from kidney that restores blood volume and pressure.
- ADH also **causes vasoconstriction** in higher concentration and increases BP (for details, refer chapter "Posterior Pituitary").

Atrial Natriuretic Peptide

Atrial natriuretic peptide (ANP) is secreted from atrial myocytes in response to stretch. **Increased atrial filling** due to increased venous return stimulates secretion of ANP.

1. ANP produces **diuresis and natriuresis** that decreases blood volume.
2. ANP also causes **vasodilation** that decreases blood pressure (for details of ANP, refer Chapter "Local Hormones").

Kallikrein-Kinin System

Kinins that cause vasodilation are bradykinin and lysylbradykinin. Physiologically, kinins resemble histamine.

Bradykinin: Bradykinin is a potent **vasodilator** and **decreases blood pressure**.

- It relaxes vascular smooth muscle via nitric oxide.
- Bradykinin also **increases capillary permeability**.

Lysylbradykinin: Lysylbradykinin is formed from LMW kininogen by the action of tissue kallikrein. It **increases tissue blood flow**.

Histamine

Histamine is a **potent vasodilator** and therefore, instantaneously **decreases blood pressure**.

- It is involved in short-term regulation of BP.

IMPORTANT NOTE

Histamine causes hypotension in anaphylaxis: Histamine is secreted from mast cells. During **anaphylactic reactions,** histamine is released by degranulation of mast cells that causes **acute hypotension.**

Endothelins

There are 3 different types of endothelins: **endothelin type 1, type 2 and type 3.**

1. **Endothelin 1** is the most **potent vasoconstrictor** known so far.
   - *Veins are more sensitive* to endothelin 1 than arteries.
2. It is also a potent positive chronotropic and inotropic agent (increases heart rate and myocardial contractility).
3. Thus, it **increases blood pressure** by causing vasoconstriction and increasing cardiac output (for details, see "Local Hormones").

Endothelium-Derived Relaxing Factor

Endothelium-derived relaxing factor (EDRF) is the **nitric oxide** (NO) synthesized from arginine in the endothelial cells of blood vessels.

1. NO produces **relaxation of vascular smooth muscle** and **decreases blood pressure.**
2. In fact, NO mediates the action of many vasodilator substances (for details of EDRF, refer chapter "Local Hormones").

NO-Dependent Vasodilators: Histamine (at H_1 receptors), **acetylcholine, bradykinin, VIP and substance P** depend on EDRF for producing vasodilation.

- However, **ANP and adenosine do not depend** on EDRF for their vasorelaxation effect.

Adrenomedullin

Adrenomedullin is secreted from adrenal medulla.

- It **causes vasodilation** by increasing the synthesis of nitric oxide.
- Adrenomedullin decreases blood pressure and **inhibits aldosterone synthesis.**
- Adrenomedullin is formed from **proadrenomedullin,** which also causes vasodilation by decreasing peripheral sympathetic activity.

LONG-TERM REGULATION OF BP

Long-term regulation of blood pressure occurs by **renal and hormonal mechanisms** that primarily involve **change in fluid volume** of the body.

Renal Mechanisms

Kidney controls blood volume by controlling **urinary excretion of salt and water.** With alteration in blood pressure changes the ***rate of excretion of sodium and water*** by kidneys that tend to restore blood pressure over days and weeks.

Pressure Diuresis & Natriuresis: With increase in arterial pressure from 60 to 200 mmHg, there is progressive in water excretion (**pressure diuresis**) and sodium excretion (**pressure natriuresis**) in urine (Fig. 37.14).

- The curve depicting the relationship between arterial pressure and urinary excretion is called **renal output curve.**
  - The renal output curve is less-steep from 60 to 120 mmHg and more-steep from 120 200 mmHg.
- It is suggested that pressure diuresis and natriuresis are **intrinsic property of the kidney** to control blood volume and blood pressure.

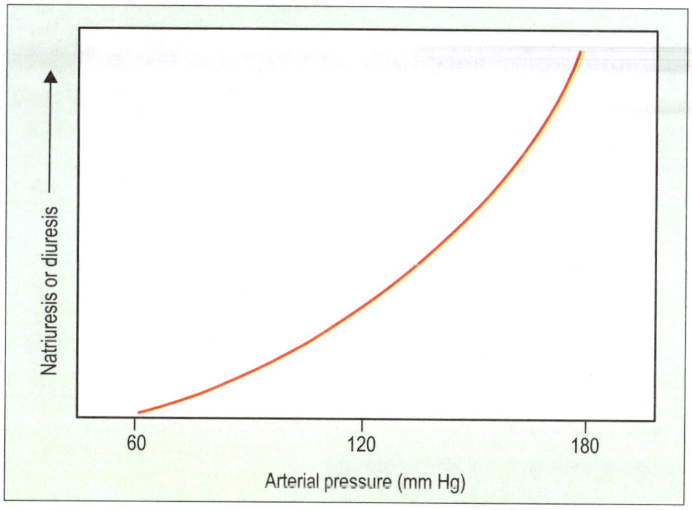

Fig. 37.14: Intrinsic natriuresis and diuresis in response to chronic increase in mean arterial pressure (MAP).

Salt Intake: The major determinant of long-term arterial pressure level in human being is the salt content of plasma.

- More salt intake is the common cause of chronically elevated blood pressure.
- Therefore, salt restriction of salt is the mainstay of treatment of hypertension and heart disease.
- Hypertension is not seen tribes not eating salt (Application Box 37.2).

Hormonal Mechanisms

Hormones that are involved in long-term control of blood pressure are **aldosterone, ADH and ANP.** These hormones act on kidney to regulate water and sodium excretion. These hormones have been discussed above in 'Short-term regulation of BP'. They are also described more in the chpater 'Local Hormones"

Application Box 37.2

Hypertension never occurs in tribes not eating salt: Numidian nomads and certain Bedouins who feed on fish and roasted meat never eat salt with food have reported to be free from hypertension. Eskimos who have not been in contact with Western civilization had a strong dislike for salt. Hypertension is rare in Eskimos.

Neural Mechanisms

Baroreceptor Resetting & Central Adaptation

In chronic hypertension, **baroreceptors are reset** to regulate the elevated blood pressure.

- The firing rate of baroreceptors decreases in response to chronic hypertension.
- Medullary **cardiovascular centers also adapt** to elevated pressure.

Role of Sympathovagal Balance

BP is regulated mainly by sympathetic and parasympathetic systems.

- Though these two systems are physiologically opposite, they are reciprocal to each other in their outflow and functions.
- Therefore, **a state of dynamic balance** between sympathetic and parasympathetic (vagal) systems (**sympathovagal balance**) is essential for long-term BP homeostasis.

Influence of Emotion & Reactivities

Activities and reactivities of both sympathetic and parasympathetic systems are altered in response to **emotional responses and changes in the environment**.

- The **limbic-hypothalamic-autonomic output** governed by emotion and reactivities is the mainstay of long-term regulation of BP.
- Thus, neurohumoral-vascular mechanism, in which autonomic modulation plays a crucial role is the major determinant of the chronic vasomotor tone and BP regulation.

Exam Questions

1. Describe the short-term regulation of blood pressure.
2. Describe the reflex regulation of blood pressure.
3. Describe the role of baroreceptor reflex in regulation of blood pressure.
4. Describe the vascular mechanisms of short-term regulation of blood pressure.
5. Describe the role of cardiovascular medullary centers in control of blood pressure.
6. Describe role of autonomic control mechanisms in the regulation of blood pressure.
7. Describe long-term regulation of blood pressure.

Multiple Choice Questions

1. The normal systolic blood pressure in an adult is:

A. 60-90 mmHg B. 100-119 mmHg
C. 120-140mmHg D. 150-170 mmHg

2. Mean arterial pressure is

A. SBP +1/3rd Pulse pressure
B. SBP + (DBP)/2
C. DBP + 1/3rd Pulse pressure
D. DBP + (SBP)/2

3. Which of the following will be within normal diastolic blood pressure range in an adult?

A. 55 mmHg B. 75mmHg
C. 95 mmHg D. 115 mmHg

4. During diastole, the arterial pressure is maintained by

A. Contraction of left ventricle
B. Musculature of arteries
C. Elastic recoil of aorta
D. Constriction of capillaries

5. Which of the following defines the pressure in the vascular system in the absence of blood flow?

A. Perfusion pressure B. Mean circulatory filling pressure
C. Critical closing pressure D. Pulse pressure

6. Which of the following statement is true regarding arterial BP?

A. Should be measured in both arms
B. Low when taken with small cuff
C. Standing increases both SBP & DBP
D. Diurnal variation present

7. Which is true about measurement of BP with sphygmomanometer versus intra-arterial pressure measurements:

A. Equal to intravascular pressure
B. Less than intravascular pressure
C. Depends upon blood flow
D. More than intravascular pressure

8. Mean circulatory filling pressure is?

A. Mean atrial pressure
B. Difference between central venous pressure and central arterial pressure
C. Arterial pressure taken at the point when heart stops beating
D. Difference between systemic and pulmonary arterial pressure

9. Blood pressure is defined as the product of:

A. SBP × peripheral resistance
B. Cardiac output × peripheral resistance
C. Stroke volume × HR
D. SBP × HR

10. Spuriously high BP is seen in all, EXCEPT:

A. Obesity
B. Thick calcified vessels
C. Auscultatory gap
D. Small cuff

11. Which of the following is for long-term regulation of BP?

A. Diuresis by kidney
B. Baroreceptor reflex
C. Cushing's reflex
D. Chemoreceptor reflex

12. Pressure on carotid sinus cause:
- A. Tachycardia
- B. Dyspnea
- C. Hyperpnea
- D. Reflex bradycardia

13. The first reflex to be activated following rise in BP:
- A. Bezold-Jarisch reflex
- B Bainbridge reflex
- C. Baroreceptor reflex
- D. Chemoreceptor reflex

14. Which reflex on activation primarily produces tachycardia?
- A. Baroreceptor reflex
- B. Chemoreceptor reflex
- C. Bainbridge reflex
- D. Cushing's reflex

15. BP increase in all, EXCEPT:
- A. Immediately standing from lying position
- B. Emotion
- C. Exercise
- D. Pregnancy

16. Shape of the arterial pulse is influenced by:
- A. Cross sectional are of artery
- B. Arterial wall expansion
- C. Viscosity of blood
- D. Velocity of blood

17. Not true about Bainbridge reflex
- A. Was described by Bainbridge
- B. Receptors are located in atrial wall
- C. Abolished by vagotomy
- D. Decreases heart rate on activation

18. Activation of somatosympathetic reflex results in all, EXCEPT:
- A. Stimulation of NTS
- B. Increased secretion of catecholamines
- C. Increase in cardiac output
- D. Increase in heart rate

19. Nitric oxide is produced in:
- A. Platelets
- B. Plasma
- C. Endothelium
- D. Serum

20. Blood pressure is less in all, EXCEPT:
- A. Athletes
- B. Following a meal
- C. Sleep
- D. Yoga

21. A blood loss of about 500 mL over a period of 30 minutes will lead to
- A. Prominent increase in HR
- B. Decrease in HR and BP
- C. Increase in HR, decrease in BP
- D. Slight increase in HR, normal BP

22. Which of the following is NOT synthesized by vascular endothelium?
- A. Angiotensin
- B. Heparin
- C. Prostacyclin
- D. Endothelin

23. SI unit for measuring Blood pressure
- A. Barr B. Torr
- C. mmHg D. $_kP_a$

24. Which of the following is NOT true regarding endothelin-1?
- A. Has inotropic effect B. Bronchodilatation
- C. Decreased GFR D. Vasoconstriction

25. All of the following contribute to long-term regulation of BP, EXCEPT:
- A. Pressure natriuresis
- B. Baroreceptor resetting
- C. Capillary fluid shift
- D. Regulation of renal sodium reabsorption by aldosterone

26. All are true for Cushing reflex, EXCEPT:
- A. Hypoxia inhibits vasomotor center
- B. Last physiological reflex to correct BP
- C. Activated when BP falls below 40 mmHg
- D. Hypercapnea is a stimulus

Answers

1. B	2. C	3. B	4. C	5. A	6. D	7. D	8. A	9. B	10. C	11. A
12. D	13. C	14. C	15. A	16. B	17. D	18. A	19. C	20. B	21. D	22. A
23. D	24. B	25. C	26. A							

Chapter 38

Regulation of Local Blood Flow

Learning Objectives

On completion of study of this chapter:

The student will be able to (must know):

1. Name the local control systems of peripheral blood flow.
2. Explain the mechanism and importance of autoregulation of blood flow.

The student may also be able to (desirable to know):

1. Describe the regulation of local blood flow.

The primary objective of circulation is the supply oxygen and nutrients to various organs and tissues of the body and to remove CO_2 and metabolites from the tissues.

- This is effectively achieved by **distributing the cardiac output** suitably to various organ based their functional and metabolic requirements and controlling the rate of blood flow to these organs.
- Therefore, one of the fundamental functions of circulatory function is the **ability of each tissue to control its blood flow locally** in proportion to its metabolic needs.

PY5.8

TYPES OF REGULATIONS

Regulation of peripheral blood flow is broadly divided into **two categories**: intrinsic and extrinsic regulations.

Intrinsic Regulation

Intrinsic regulation of blood flow is due to operation of two mechanisms: autoregulation and endothelium-mediated regulation.

Autoregulation of Blood Flow

Autoregulation is defined as **capacity of tissues to regulate their own blood flow without any external influence.**

- Under normal conditions, **blood flow to organs remains relatively constant** within the mean arterial pressure range of **60 to 180 mmHg** (Fig. 38.1).
- Autoregulatory mechanisms for blood flow are **well developed in many organs** like kidney, heart, liver, brain and skeletal muscle.

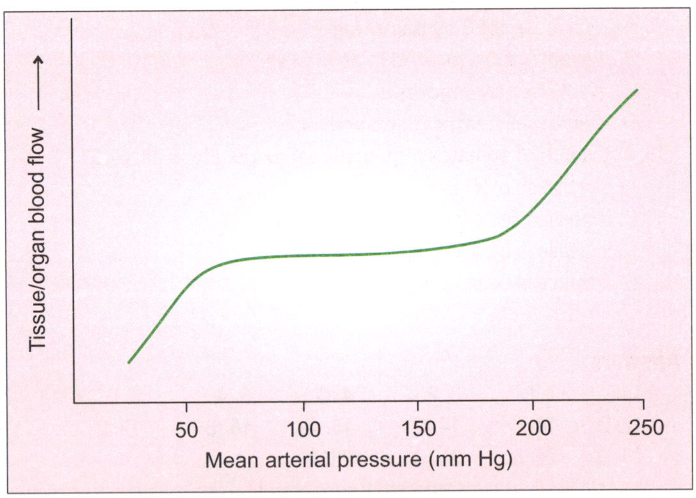

Fig. 38.1: Effect of mean arterial pressure (MAP) on tissue organ blood flow. Note that blood flow is relatively constant between 60–180 mm Hg.

There are **three theories of autoregulation of blood flow:** myogenic theory, metabolic theory and tissue pressure theory.

Myogenic Theory

According to myogenic theory, vascular smooth muscles **contract in response to increased transmural pressure** and relax in response to decreased transmural pressure.

- When perfusion pressure increases abruptly, the *initial blood flow to the organ increases*.
- However, increased pressure distends the vessel that causes **contraction of vascular smooth muscles**.

- **Vasoconstriction decreases the blood flow** and returns blood flow to the previous levels. Degree of constriction is proportional to the degree of distending pressure.

Metabolic Theory

According to metabolic theory, blood flow to an organ or tissue is **controlled by the metabolic activity** of the tissue.

1. When **blood flow decreases** to the tissue, **decreased oxygen supply** results in formation of **vasodilator metabolites** that dilate the blood vessels and restore the flow.
2. The metabolites formed in the tissue act locally to dilate the resistance vessel.
   - **Blood flow proportionately increases** with the increase in the rate of metabolism (Fig. 38.2).
3. Also, when **metabolic activity increases**, the **metabolites** accumulated in the tissue cause vasodilation that increases blood flow.
   - This helps to wash the metabolites from the tissue.

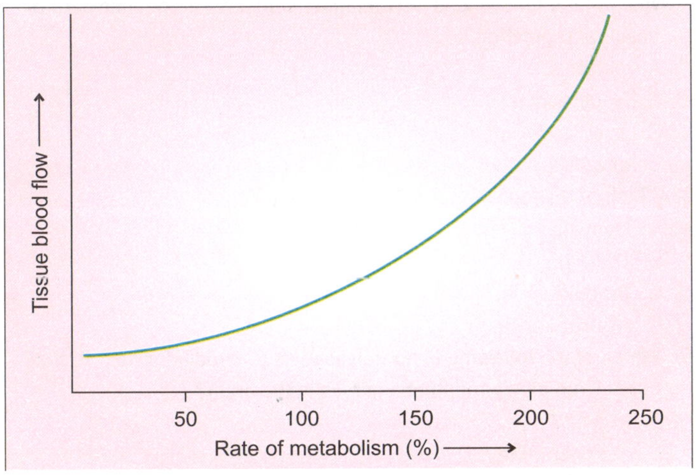

Fig. 38.2: Effect of increase in rate of metabolism on tissue blood flow.

The known **metabolic vasodilators** are:

- Lactic acid
- CO_2
- Hypoxia
- Hydrogen ion
- Potassium ion
- Inorganic phosphate
- Interstitial fluid osmolality
- Adenosine
- Local temperature

Role of Adenosine: Adenosine is an important local vasodilator for controlling regional blood flow.

- For example, **adenosine released from cardiac myocytes** when coronary blood flow is less, causes local vasodilation in the heart and re-establishes coronary blood flow back to normal.
- Also, when metabolic activity is more, **degradation of adenosine triphosphate** (ATP) increases the release of adenosine that in turn causes vasodilation and increased blood supply.

Reactive Hyperemia

Reactive hyperemia occurs when the **blood flow is re-established** to an organ or tissue following a brief period of arterial occlusion, the flow becomes more to the organ or tissue.

- This is typically observed in the arm following blood pressure recording by sphygmomanometer, which is an example of metabolic control of blood flow.

Tissue Pressure Theory

When perfusion pressure increases blood flow increases, which in turn **increases capillary permeability** due to increased hydrostatic pressure.

1. Increased blood flow increases interstitial tissue pressure.
2. When tissue pressure increases significantly, **blood vessel is compressed passively** from outside that decreases blood flow to the tissue and restores normalcy of blood flow.

Endothelium-mediated Regulation of Blood Flow

Endothelium of blood vessels secretes **vasoactive substances** like ***endothelins*** and **vasorelaxing substances** like endothelium-derived relaxing factor (EDRF) or ***nitric oxide*** (NO).

- These chemicals are secreted in various situations to alter blood flow locally according to the need of the organ or tissue.
- Nitric oxide plays a major role in the regulation of local blood flow. Details of endothelins and NO are described in 'Local Hormones'.

Extrinsic Regulation

Extrinsic control of local blood flow is mainly neural and hormonal in nature.

Neural Regulation

Neural control is divided into **sympathetic and parasympathetic** control and **reflex regulation**.

Sympathetic Control

Stimulation of sympathetic fibers supplying the organ or tissue usually causes **vasoconstriction** and decreases blood flow.

Parasympathetic Control

Stimulation of parasympathetic fibers supplying the organ or tissue causes **vasodilation** and increases blood flow.

Vascular Reflexes

Activation of various cardiovascular reflexes like baroreceptor reflex or chemoreceptor reflex control blood flow **by altering the diameter of resistance vessels** (for details, refer Chapter 55)

Hormonal Regulation

- Hormones that **act on β-receptors** like epinephrine ***cause vasodilation*** and increase local blood flow, and hormones that **act on α-receptors** like norepinephrine ***cause vasoconstriction*** and decrease local blood flow.
- Release of **local hormones** such as ***substance P, histamine and bradykinin*** control local blood flow.
- Simulation of cholinergic and histaminergic receptors also causes vasodilation and increases blood flow.

Exam Questions

1. Name the regulating systems for peripheral blood flow. Describe the process of autoregulation of peripheral blood flow.
2. List the mechanisms of intrinsic regulation of peripheral blood flow.

Multiple Choice Questions

1. Which of the following is not a metabolic vasodilator in heart?
A. Lactate
B. Adenosine
C. K+
D. Serotonin

2. Activation of sympathetic fibers caused all except:
A. Increased myocardial contractility
B. Increase in heart rate
C. Increased conduction velocity
D. Decreased coronary blood flow

3. All the following BP regulatory centers are located in medulla, EXCEPT:
A. Center for emotion
B. NTS
C. Vasomotor center
D. Cardioinhibitory center

4. Diameter of blood vessel is affected by all, EXCEPT:
A. Mediators of inflammation
B. Vagal discharge
C. Sympathetic discharge
D. Adrenomedullary hormones

5. Which of the following is not true about vascular smooth muscle?
A. K^+efflux through BK channels opens calcium channels
B. Influx of calcium into the cell occurs by voltage-gated calcium channels
C. Calcium released from sarcoplasmic reticulum is mediated by calcium
D. Calcium-activated K^+ channels cause rapid efflux of K^+

6. Which of the following is not a vasoconstrictor?
A. Endothelin- 1
B. Substance P
C. Thromboxane A_2
D. ADH

7. Which of the following is NOT a higher center for autonomic cardiovascular regulation?
A. Thalamus
B. Hypothalamus
C. Limbic cortex
D. Amygdala

8. Which of the following is NOT a vasodilator?
A. Hypoxia
B. CGRP α
C. Bradykinin
D. Neuropeptide Y

9. Which of the following is not released as a vasodilator neurotransmitter from parasympathetic nerves in the brain?
A. PHM-27
B. Acetylcholine
C. Bradykinin
D. VIP

10. All of the following statements are true, EXCEPT:
A. Profound tachycardia occurs in vasovagal syncope
B. Sympathetic stimulation causes increased skeletal blood flow during exercise
C. Withdrawal of vagal tone occurs during exercise
D. Activation of limbic system often provokes the fight-or flight response

Answers

1. D 2. C 3. A 4. B 5. A 6. B 7. A 8. D 9. C 10. A

Chapter 39

Special Circulations

Learning Objectives

On completion of study of this chapter:

The student will be able to (must know):

1. Understand the importance of regional circulations.
2. Give the normal values of blood flow (expressed in ml/100 gm /min) to important visceral organs.
3. List the special features cerebral, coronary, cutaneous, splanchnic and skeletal muscle circulations.
4. Describe the regulation of all special circulations.
5. Define triple response and explain its mechanism.

The student may also be able to (desirable to know):

1. Describe pathophysiology of stroke & its physiological basis of their treatment.
2. Describe pathophysiology of AMI & its physiological basis of their treatment.

Cardiac output is distributed to different organs of the body according to their metabolic requirements. The blood flow expressed in unit time per unit weight of the tissue is maximum to the carotid body, which is 2000 ml/100 gm/ min, and is minimum to the skeletal muscle, i.e. 2.7 ml/100 gm/ min.

Blood Flow to Different Organs: Among the organs, flow is maximum to kidney (420 ml/100 gm/ min), followed by heart (84 ml/100 gm/ min), liver (58 ml/100 gm/ min) and brain (54 ml/100 gm/ min) (Table 39.1). There are special arrangements of blood vessels and special regulatory mechanisms in these organs to meet their supplies.

PY5.10

CEREBRAL CIRCULATION

Specialities of Cerebral Metabolism

1. Brain tissue is **highly sensitive to hypoxia**.
   - Therefore, adequate blood supply to brain tissue should be continuously maintained.
   - The stoppage of blood flow for more than 15-30 seconds results in unconsciousness, and for more than 5 minutes causes irreparable damage (leads to coma).
2. Brain utilizes **glucose as the main fuel**.
   - *Prolonged hypoglycemia* results in cerebral dysfunction.
   - However, in *conditions of chronic scarcity*, the brain **can utilize ketone bodies**.
3. Utilization of glucose by tissues of the brain is **independent of insulin,** except ventromedial hypothalamus (VMH is insulin-dependent).
4. The metabolic requirements of brain **remain fairly constant** irrespective of activities of the brain tissue.

Table 39.1 | **Blood flow (BF) & O_2 consumption (OC) of visceral organs.**

	Weight (Kg)	BF (ml/min)	BF (ml/100g/min)	% of CO	OC (ml/min)	OC (ml/100g/min)	% of total OC	AV-OD (ml/L)
Kidneys	0.3	1260	420	23.5	18	6	7.2	14
Heart	0.3	250	84	4.7	29	9.7	11.6	114
Liver	2.6	1500	58	27.8	51	2	20.5	34
Brain	1.4	750	54	13.9	46	3.3	18.4	62
Skin	3.5	460	12.8	8.6	12	0.3	4.8	25
Sk. Muscle	31	840	2.7	15.6	50	0.2	20	60
Rest of body	24	340	1.4	6.2	44	0.2	17.6	129
Whole body	63	5400	8.6	100	250	0.4	100	46

CO: Cardiac output; AV-OD: Arteriovenus O_2 difference

Cerebral Blood Flow

Special Features of CBF

1. Cerebral arteries are **end arteries**.
2. Brain is present in the cranium, the rigid cage. The

intracranial contents are incompressible.

- Therefore, a unique feature of cerebral circulation is that **increase in cerebral blood flow** (for example, arteriolar dilation), is usually associated with **comparable increase in venous outflow**.

3. In the brain, volume of blood and extravascular fluid remains relatively constant.

- The change in one component is associated with opposite alteration in the other.

4. The capillaries in brain are mostly **non-fenestrated**.
5. The cerebral blood vessels (especially capillaries) are surrounded by the **end-feet processes of astrocytes** (Fig. 39.1).

- This provides the anatomical basis for the formation of **blood-brain barrier** (BBB).
- Due to the presence of BBB, substances from brain tissue like neurotransmitters cannot easily enter general circulation, and substances from blood also cannot easily enter the brain tissue. BBB provides protection to the brain from the toxic and harmful substances circulating in the blood.
- BBB is also disrupted by inflammation of brain tissue, and brain tumors.

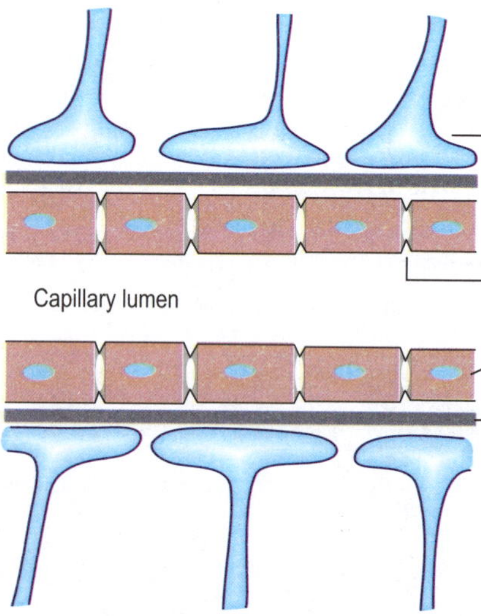

Fig. 39.1: Blood-brain barrier (BBB). Cerebral capillaries are surrounded by end-feet processes of astroglia, which provide anatomical basis for BBB. Note that the tight junctions between endothelial cells of cerebral capillaries are very tight that prevents transfer of substances between blood and the brain tissue. Also note that the basement membrane of capillary is thick.

IMPORTANT NOTE

Kernicterus occurs in children: As BBB is *not well developed in infants and children,* kernicterus (deposition of bilirubin in the basal ganglia) occurs in them in hemolytic jaundice.

6. The *mechanism for vesicular transport* from blood into brain tissue via endothelial wall of the cerebral blood vessels **is less developed.**
7. The **tight junctions** between the endothelial cells of capillaries **are very tight**.

- The **basement membrane of capillaries is also thick**.
- These anatomical modifications contribute to the formation of BBB

Cerebral Blood Vessels

Arterial Supply

The brain receives blood supply from **two major sources**.

1. **Vertebro-Basilar System:** Two vertebral arteries join to from the basilar artery, which finally merges into the circle of Willis.
2. **Internal Carotid Arteries:** Two internal carotid arteries along with basilar artery form the circle of Willis (Fig. 39.2).

Circle of Willis: The circle of Willis, which is formed by basilar artery and two internal carotids, gives rise to **three pairs of large vessels** supplying the brain.

- These are anterior cerebral, middle cerebral and posterior cerebral arteries.
- There is hardly any overlapping of the territories of brain tissues supplied by these cerebral arteries.
  - Thus, functionally, they are **end arteries**.
- Therefore, block in any of the artery results in ischemic damage to the part supplied by the artery.

Venous Drainage

The venous drainage occurs by the **deep veins and dural sinuses**. They drain into the internal jugular veins.

Innervation of Cerebral Vessels

Cerebral blood vessels are innervated by sympathetic, parasympathetic and sensory fibers.

Sympathetic Supply: Sympathetic fibers are **vasoconstrictors**.

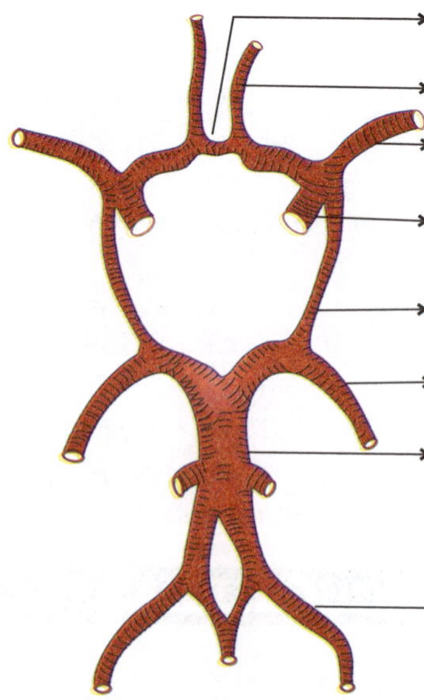

Fig. 39.2: Arterial supply of brain. Note, two vertebral arteries unite to form basilar artery, which along with internal carotids form circle of Wills. From circle of Wills, posterior, middle and anterior cerebral arteries originate.

- Cell bodies of sympathetic neurons are located in *superior cervical ganglia*.
- They release norepinephrine and neuropeptide Y at their nerve endings.
- However, *vasoconstriction effect* of sympathetic stimulation on cerebral blood vessels **is less marked.**

Parasympathetic Supply: The parasympathetic innervation is *not well developed*.

- These fibers secrete acetylcholine, VIP and PHM–27.
- Cell bodies of cholinergic neurons are present in sphenopalatine ganglia.
- Stimulation of parasympathetic fibers **results in vasodilation**.

Sensory Neurons: The sensory nerves contain substance P, CGRP, neurokinin A and VIP.

- These neurotransmitters **cause vasodilation**.
- Cell bodies of sensory neurons are located in trigeminal ganglia.
- The cerebral blood vessels are **highly sensitive to pain**.
  - Pressure on cerebral blood vessels causes pain.
  - But interestingly, the **brain tissues do not receive** pain fibers.

Normal Values of CBF

The brain weighs about 1.4 kg. The total cerebral blood flow is 750 ml per minute, which is about 14% of cardiac output.

- This accounts for about **54 ml of blood per 100 gm of brain tissue per minute**.
- Oxygen consumption of brain is about 45 ml per minute, which is about 3.3 ml per 100 g per minute.

Measurement of CBF

Cerebral blood flow (CBF) can be measured by various methods. The important methods are:

1. Kety method
2. By using radioactive substances
3. By using flow meters
4. Positron emission tomography (PET)
5. Single photon emission computerized tomography (SPECT)

Kety Method: This method uses Fick's principle. In this method, nitrous oxide is used.

- The subject inhales *15% of nitrous oxide* for 10 minutes.
- The arterial sample and the venous sample (from internal jugular bulb) are collected and the arteriovenous difference is measured.

$$\text{CBF} = \frac{\text{Amount of nitrous oxide taken by the brain}}{\text{Arteriovenous difference of nitrous oxide across the brain}}$$

Using Radioactive Substances: Radioactive substance usually used is radioactive Xenon (^{133}Xe).

- The substance is injected into the carotid artery and the radioactivity of different areas of the brain is measured by placing scintillation counters around the skull.
- This is a useful method for studying the regional distribution of CBF in different parts of the brain.

Using Flowmeters: The flowmeters can be directly placed in the cerebral arteries in experimental animals or in patients undergoing neurosurgery and CBF can be measured accurately.

Positron Emission Tomography (PET): This is mainly used for monitoring regional blood flow of various parts of the brain.

- In this method, a short-lived radioisotope is used to label a substance, which is injected.
- Scintillation detectors placed on the head monitor the appearance and clearance of the tracer.
- The information from detectors is processed in a computer that quantifies the flow in a particular region of the brain.
- Single photon emission computerized tomography (SPECT) is also used for the purpose.

Magnetic Resonance Imaging (MRI): This technique is based on detecting resonant signals from different tissues in magnetic field.

- The resolution of MRI is better than the PET.
- Recently, developed functional magnetic resonance imaging (fMRI), measures blood supply to a specific area of the brain.

Regulation of CBF

CBF is affected by alteration in intracranial pressure, neural and metabolic factors, and autoregulatory mechanisms.

Role of Intracranial Pressure

The brain tissue and cerebrospinal fluid (CSF) are essentially incompressible. Thus, at any given time, the total volume of blood, CSF volume and brain tissue in the cranial cavity remains constant. This is called **Monro-Kellie doctrine**.

- Any increase in venous pressure causes similar increase in intracranial pressure (ICP).
- Rise in intracranial pressure results in compression of cerebral arteries that decreases blood flow.
  - This compensates for changes in arterial blood pressure at the level of head.
- Increase in arterial pressure as occurs during downward acceleration, increases arterial pressure in the head.
  - However, ICP also rises simultaneously.
- Increased ICP **prevents rupture of blood vessels** by supporting them.
  - Thus, increased ICP as occurs in downward acceleration or straining (e.g. strenuous defecation

during constipation) helps in protecting cerebral vessels.

IMPORTANT NOTE

Increased ICP activates Cushing's reflex: In brain tumors, compression of cerebral vessels decreases blood flow. Decreased blood flow causes hypoxia at vasomotor center. This activates **Cushing's reflex**, which tries to restore cerebral blood flow.

Neural Regulation

Stimulation of sympathetic fibers causes vasoconstriction, but it is not important, as the *vasoconstrictor system is not well developed* in cerebral vascular bed. Parasympathetic stimulation causes vasodilation.

Metabolic Regulation

CBF is significantly altered by production of local vasodilator metabolites.

- The **vasodilator substances** are usually **potassium, hydrogen, and adenosine**.
- The cerebral vessels also respond to change in carbon dioxide and oxygen.
- Acidosis, hypoxia, and hypercapnia in the brain tissue produce potent vasodilation.
- **70% increase in arterial pCO_2** approximately **doubles the CBF**.
    - A fall in pCO_2 results in cerebral vasoconstriction as seen during hyperventilation.

Role of Astrocytes: With increase in neuronal activity, chemical substances are released in more quantity from astroglia or astrocytes.

- These substances include, nitric oxide, metabolites of arachidonic acid, K^+, adenosine, and few other chemicals.
- These substances contribute significantly to vasodilation and increase in cerebral blood flow.
- Thus, astrocytes greatly influence CBF.

Autoregulation

CBF remains relatively constant within a pressure range of 60 - 140 mmHg (Fig. 39.3). The autoregulation may be due to neural and metabolic factors.

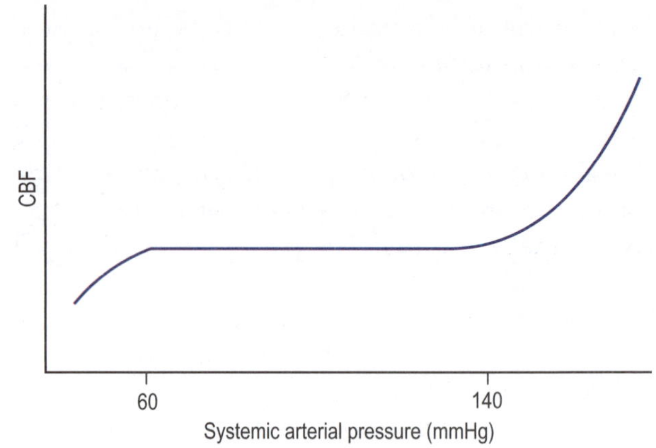

Fig. 39.3: Autoregulation of cerebral blood flow (CBF). CBF remains constant between 60 and 140 mm Hg of systemic pressure.

Clinical Aspects

1. Disruption of BBB occurs at the **site of tumor or inflammation**.
    - Therefore, radioactive study helps in identifying the **site of such lesions**.
2. Cerebral blood vessels do not allow all the substances equally to enter into the brain tissue.
    - Physician must know the **penetrability of a drug** into the brain tissue and accordingly prescribe the drug in proper concentration.
3. **In cerebral infections**, *due to disruption of BBB* the organisms get access into the general circulation and spread to the other parts of the body.
4. **Stroke:** Interruption of blood supply to a part of the brain causes ischemic damage to that part. This is called stroke.

Stroke

Definition: A stroke (cerebrovascular accident) is a syndrome of **rapid onset of neurological deficit** that is attributable to a focal vascular cause.

- As per **WHO definition**, stroke is a rapidly developing clinical signs of focal (or global) disturbance of cerebral function with symptoms lasting for 24 hours or longer or may leading to death with no apparent cause other than of vascular origin.

Types of Strokes

Two main types: **ischemic stroke and hemorrhagic stroke**.

- About 70% is ischemic stroke, 17% is hemorrhagic stroke, and 3% is due to other causes.

Ischemic Stroke

Ischemic stroke occurs due to **blockage of a cerebral artery by thromboembolism**.

- Cerebral infarction is commonly caused by thromboembolic disease secondary to **atherosclerosis in the major extracranial arteries** such as carotid artery and aortic arch.
- 20% of infarctions are caused by **emboli from the heart** *(cardioembolic process)* and about **20% are due to thrombosis in situ** caused by intrinsic disease of small perforating vessels (such as lenticulostriate arteries) producing lacunar infarction.

Pathophysiology: Complete stop of cerebral blood flow causes **death of brain tissue within 4 to 10 min**. The blood flow to ischemic area is usually less than 10ml/100gm/min.

1. Due to thromboembolism, hypoperfusion of the tissue causes **ATP depletion** that in turn causes *activation of enzymes* such as lipid peroxidase, protease, and NO synthase.
2. Activation of these enzymes leads to **destruction of intracellular organelles** and release of **free radicals** that finally causes **liquefactive necrosis** (Flowchart 39.1).
3. Release of free-fatty acids (FFA) activate **procoagulant pathways** that initiates the vicious cycle of further ischemic damage.
4. Usually there will be a rim of **penumbra** (zone of reversible ischemia) surrounding the core infarcted area.

IMPORTANT NOTE

First four hours are crucial in Stroke: If blood flow can be reestablished to this penumbra area within few hours, the area of infarction will be reduced and the penumbra area becomes normal tissue.

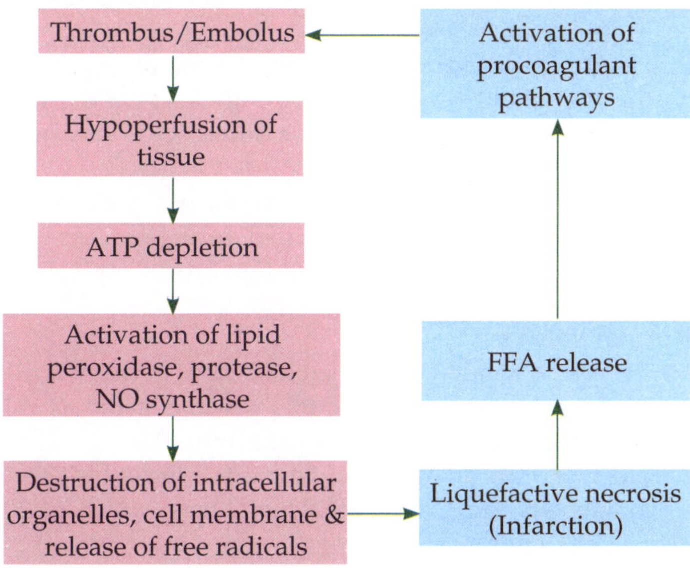

Flowchart 39.1: Pathophysiology of ischemic stroke. FFA: Free fatty acids

Hemorrhagic Stroke

Hemorrhagic stroke is usually caused by **rupture of Charcot's artery** or the **artery of cerebral hemorrhage** i.e. the lenticulostriate branch of middle cerebral artery (at internal capsule) that produces contralateral hemiplegia.

Treatment of Stroke

The treatment of stroke includes intravascular thrombolysis, endovascular mechanical thrombectomy, anticoagulation, antiplatelet therapy, and antiexcitotoxic drugs.

Intravascular Thrombolysis: Fibrinolytic (clot lysing) drugs like **recombinant t-PA** given (0.9mg/kg, i.v.) early in the course of stroke is very useful.

- If t-PA is given within three hours of onset of symptoms, disability and mortality is reduced significantly.
- Therefore, it is important to diagnose and initiate the treatment of stroke at the earliest possible.

Endovascular Mechanical Thrombectomy: Very useful, especially if there is contraindication for thrombolysis.

Anticoagulation therapy for acute ischemic stroke: It is done especially in patients with high risk of early cardiogenic re-embolization, and in cerebral venous thrombosis.

Antiplatelet Therapy: Aspirin, 175mg daily reduces stroke related morbidity and prevents early stroke recurrence.

Antiexcitotoxic Drugs: Normally, brain cells take up and utilize glutamate. Ischemia of brain tissue decreases glutamate uptake that increases local glutamate concentration.

- **Glutamate causes excitotoxic neuronal damage** of the brain tissue (*excitotoxic lesion*).
- Therefore, antiexcitotoxic drugs are quite helpful in the treatment of stroke.

Supportive care: Maintenance of blood pressure, serum glucose, control of ICP, catheterization, prevention of complications and physiotherapy plus other measures of neurorehabilitation.

CORONARY CIRCULATION

Coronary Blood Supply

Arterial Supply

The heart is supplied by **right and left coronary arteries** that originate from the root of the aorta behind right and left cusps of aortic valve respectively.

- The right coronary artery principally supplies the right ventricle and the right atrium, and the left coronary artery supplies the left ventricle and the left atrium (Fig. 39.4).
- Physiologically, **there are no anastomoses** between the right and left coronary arteries.
  - Thus, the coronary arteries are **end arteries** in human beings as the territories of blood supply by these arteries do not overlap.
- The sinuses of Valsalva (small outpouches of the aorta) are present behind the semilunar valves where the **eddy currents** develop which keep the valve leaflets away from the wall of the vessels during systole.
  - In fact, the cusps are not totally pushed to the walls of the aorta during systole; rather they float in the blood in between the wall in their closing position.
- This allows blood to enter into the coronary arteries (these arteries arise from aorta at their origin, behind the cusps of the valve) to some extent, as the coronary ostia are not blocked by the valve cusps

Venous Drainage

The heart has multiple venous drainage systems.

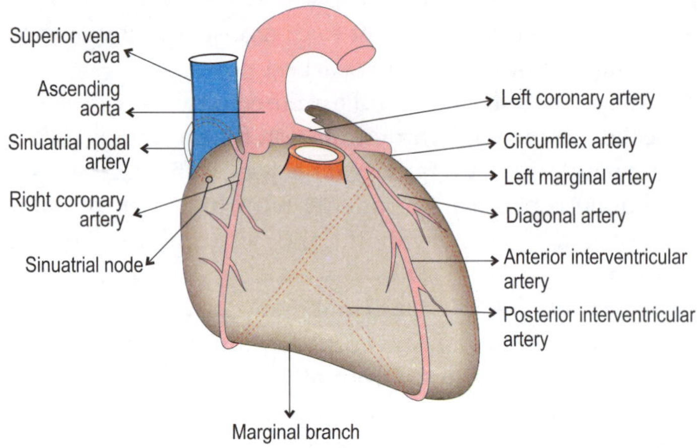

Fig. 39.4: Blood supply of the heart. Note that there is no anastomosis between right and left coronary arteries and territories of blood supply by these arteries do not overlap.

- **The major system** consists of the coronary sinus and the anterior cardiac veins that drain into the right atrium.
- **The minor systems** consist of *arteriosinusoidal vessels* that drain from arterioles to cardiac chambers, *thebesian veins* that drain from capillaries to cardiac chambers, and *arterioluminal vessels* that directly drain from coronary arteries to heart chambers.

Innervation of Coronary Blood Vessels

The coronary blood vessels are supplied by sympathetic and parasympathetic fibers.

Sympathetic Innervation: Sympathetic stimulation to the heart causes **coronary vasodilation** as coronary arteries are rich in β_2 receptors. However, stimulation of α receptors of coronaries causes vasoconstriction.

Parasympathetic Innervation: Parasympathetic stimulation to the heart causes **vasodilation**, which is mediated via cholinergic receptors.

Special Features of Coronary Circulation

1. Heart receives its **major blood supply during diastole.** Coronary blood flow decreases during systole and increases during diastole.
   - The cardiac blood vessels are mechanically compressed during systole due to contraction of the ventricular muscle.
     - Therefore, blood flow during systole decreases to the heart muscle.
   - This vasocompression effect is maximally observed in the deeper layers (**sub-endocardial layers** of the myocardium).
     - The vasocompression during systole is more marked in the left ventricle than right ventricle, as the pressure generated by left ventricle is significantly more.
   - During diastole, relaxation of cardiac muscle increases coronary blood flow.
2. The coronary arteries are **end-arteries.**
   - Therefore, blockage of the coronary arteries results in ischemia and infarction of the cardiac muscles supplied by the artery.
3. The **metabolic regulation** of coronary circulation is well developed.
   - Therefore, coronary blood flow is adjusted according to the metabolic need of the myocardium.
4. Unlike cerebral circulation, significant alteration occurs in the coronary blood flow depending on the cardiac activities.
   - Coronary blood flow can be increased about four to five folds to meet the heart's more oxygen need during exercise.
   - Thus, there is **adequate coronary blood flow reserve.**
5. The heart utilizes wide varieties of substrates for its metabolism. These include free fatty acids, glucose, pyruvate, lactate, ketone bodies, and amino acids.
   - But the major source (about 1/3) of **energy supply is free fatty acids.**
6. Heart muscle **extracts about 80% of the oxygen** from the arterial blood.
   - Thus, arteriovenous oxygen difference is very high in heart even at rest.
   - Therefore, major method to increase the oxygen supply to the heart as required during exercise is to increase the coronary blood flow.

Normal Values

Heart weighs about 300 g. The blood flow to the heart is approximately 250 ml per minute, which is about **84 ml per 100gm of the cardiac tissue per minute.**

- The rate of **coronary blood flow is the second highest** in the body (next to the renal blood flow, which is 420 ml/100g/min).
- The coronary blood flow constitutes about **4.7% of the total cardiac output.**
- However, the rate of **oxygen consumption of heart is highest of all organs of the body,** which is 9.7 ml per 100g of tissue per minute.

Measurement of Coronary Blood Flow

Coronary blood flow is measured by direct method or indirect methods. Indirect methods are Fick method or radionuclide method.

Direct Method: Coronary blood flow can be measured directly by placing an ***electromagnetic flow meter*** in the coronary artery. This is used in experimental animals and in humans undergoing open-heart surgery.

Using Fick Principle: In this method, subject inhales a mixture of air and an inert gas (like **nitrous oxide**) till the gas is distributed in the tissues according to its partition co-efficient.

- Then the arterial blood (from any peripheral artery) and venous samples (from coronary sinus) are collected.
- The coronary blood flow is calculated as the ratio of the amount of the inert gas passing through the coronary arteries in unit time to the average arteriovenous gas concentration difference.

$$\text{Blood flow} = \frac{\text{Amount of inert gas taken up / min}}{\text{Arteriovenous difference of the gas}}$$

Radionuclide Methods: A radioactive substance like **thallium** (^{201}TI) is injected intravenously.

- The gamma camera is placed on the chest to monitor the thallium uptake by the heart.
- Radioactive xenon (^{133}Xe) can also be used for the purpose.
- By this method, the difference in blood supply through individual arteries to different parts of the heart can also be measured.

Regulation of Coronary Blood Flow

Coronary blood flow is regulated by neural factors, metabolic factors, physical factors and autoregulatory mechanisms.

Neural Regulation

Neural regulation is by either sympathetic or parasympathetic fibers.

Sympathetic Control: Stimulation of sympathetic fibers produces vasodilation.

- This is due to the predominance of beta-receptors in the coronary vessels (**stimulation of beta receptors results in vasodilation**).
- Vasodilation also occurs partly due to the **deposition of metabolites** as sympathetic stimulation accelerates cardiac activity that increases myocardial metabolism.

Parasympathetic Control: Parasympathetic (vagal) stimulation **causes vasodilation**, but there is sparse parasympathetic innervation of the coronary blood vessel.

Metabolic Regulation

Metabolic regulation of blood flow is **well developed** in the heart. A close relationship exists between the coronary blood flow and the oxygen consumption of myocardium.

- The **metabolic factors** that cause coronary vasodilation are hypoxia, increased local concentration of carbon dioxide, increased hydrogen and potassium ion concentration, accumulation of lactate, adenosine, and adenine nucleotide, and increased release of prostaglandins locally.
- **Adenosine plays an important role** in regulation of coronary blood flow.
  - Adenosine *mediates reactive hyperemia* of ventricular muscle (increased blood flow to the area supplied by a coronary artery when the flow is re-established following temporary occlusion of the artery).

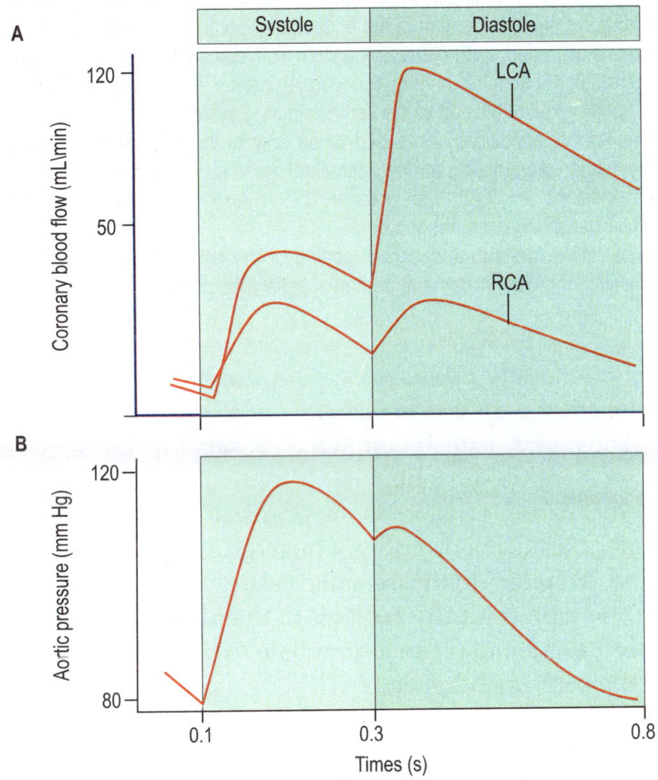

Fig. 39.5: Blood flow into left coronary artery (LCA) and right coronary artery (RCA) during systole and diastole (A). Note that the flow is phasic, being less during systole and significantly more during diastole, especially in the LCA, which is inversely proportional to left ventricular pressure as reflected through aortic pressure recording (B).

Autoregulation

An autoregulatory mechanism exists for the coronary blood flow, which maintains a normal blood flow within the pressure **range of 70–110 mmHg**.

- However, the autoregulation of blood flow in the heart is not so well developed like that in brain.

Physical Factors

The blood flow to the cardiac muscle is dependent on the myocardial tension, the pressure that builds up in the muscle during contraction.

- This is the **primary factor in determining coronary perfusion**.
- The vasocompression during myocardial contraction decreases the coronary blood flow (Application Box 39.1).
- Coronary blood flow increases during diastole (Fig. 39.5).

Clinical Aspects

Coronary Artery Disease

Decreased blood flow to the heart leads to myocardial ischemia (angina pectoris), and if severe and prolonged, results in myocardial infarction (the heart attack).

Application Box 39.1

Subendocardial portion is prone to ischemic damage: The left ventricular muscle tension (the pressure within the ventricular muscle) during systole is maximum in the endocardial portion and minimum in the epicardial portion, as the pressure is more from epicardium to endocardium.
- The high pressure in the endocardial region decreases blood flow significantly to this part of the ventricle during systole.
- In normal conditions, increased blood flow to the endocardium during diastole compensates for the decreased blood supply during systole.
- Conditions in which the coronary blood flow is compromised, the compensation does not occur.
- Therefore, the sub-endocardial portion of the left ventricular muscle is prone for ischemic damage and myocardial infarction.

Angina Pectoris

Angina literally means chest pain. Angina pectoris refers to the **chest pain due to ischemia of the cardiac muscle.**

- The pain is usually felt in the chest below the sternum towards the left side.
- The cause of pain is myocardial ischemia due to decreased blood supply, which results in accumulation of "**P factor**" in the ischemic tissue.
- **The pain typically radiates to the ulnar border of the left hand**, but it can also radiate to the back or even to the neck or abdomen.

Myocardial Infarction

Etiology: Infarction (ischemic cell death) occurs when the **ischemia is prolonged, following more than 75% obstruction** of the coronary arteries (Fig. 39. 6).

- The **factors that precipitate** acute myocardial infarction (AMI) are spasm of the coronary artery at the site of atherosclerosis, platelet aggregation at the site of obstruction, and hemorrhage into the atherosclerotic plaque of the coronary artery.
- **Stress** is known to induce coronary artery spasm.
- AMI causes **severe chest pain** that **radiates along the ulnar border of the upper arm, arm and hand.**

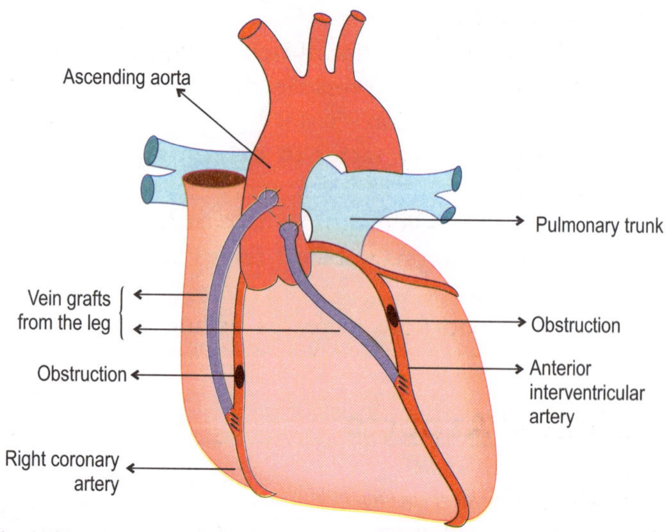

Fig. 39.6: Obstruction of coronary artery causing AMI. Note, in this case there was obstruction in both the coronaries, and the bypass graft (for both coronaries) of veins from the leg was done for treatment.

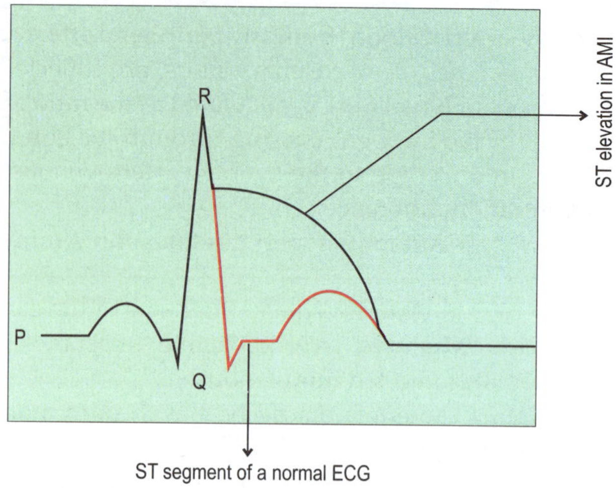

Fig. 39.7: ECG changes in acute myocardial infarction. Note, ST elevation is the prominent feature.

- The chest pain is usually associated with **excessive sweating.**

Diagnosis

Diagnosis of AMI is based on specific electrocardiographic changes, elevation of enzymes specific for myocardial damage, and typical clinical presentation of the patient.

1. **Typical ECG changes:** The ECG is very useful for diagnosing and locating areas of infarction.
   - In acute infarction, the first change to occur is the **ST segment elevation** in the ECG leads recorded with electrodes placed over chest representing the infarcted area (Fig. 39.7).
   - The leads placed on the opposite side of the infarction record **ST segment depression** (for details, refer chapter 30; Abnormal ECG).
2. **Change in enzymes in the plasma:** The damaged myocardium releases enzymes into the circulation.
   - Detection of elevated level of these enzymes plays an important role in the diagnosis.
   - The enzymes most commonly measured are **creatine kinase** (CK) and **lactate dehydrogenase** (LDH), but the most specific is the increased concentration of **CK-MB isoenzyme** of CK, and **fraction 1** of LDH.
3. **Typical clinical presentation:** The **severe chest pain associated with excessive sweating** with (or without) radiation to the ulnar border of the left hand in a person above 40 years is highly suggestive of AMI.
   - If such patients get prompt **relief by nitrate tablets** (or sublingual sorbitrates), diagnosis is almost confirmed.
   - It should be remembered that **chronic diabetic patient** may have **painless AMI**, due to autonomic neuropathy.

Physiological Basis of Treatment

AMI is an emergency condition; treatment should immediately.

1. **Vasodilators: Nitrates like nitroglycerin** produce prompt improvement, as they are potent vasodilators.

- They cause arterial dilation that **decreases the afterload,** and cause venodilation that **decreases the preload** (the venous return).
- This decreases myocardial oxygen consumption and improves heart function.

2. **Streptokinase:** Streptokinase causes **lysis of the intracoronary clot** when injected intravenously. It facilitates conversion of plasminogen to **plasmin that causes fibrinolysis.**
   - If streptokinase is injected in the early part (within 6 hours) of onset of infarction, it removes obstruction (lyses clot) and prevents further progress of infarction.
   - **TPA (tissue plasminogen activator)**, produced in the laboratory by recombinant DNA technology, is another clot lytic agent.
     - It also activates plasmin and causes fibrinolysis.
     - The advantage of using TPA is that **it preferentially causes lysis of clot at the site of thrombosis,** as it activates plasminogen bound to the fibrin clot.
3. **Coronary angioplasty: A catheter containing a balloon** *is inserted into the coronary artery* and then the **balloon is inflated at the site of obstruction** to dilate the constricted artery.
4. **Calcium channel blockers:** Calcium channel blockers like **verapamil** are useful as they produce coronary vasodilation.
5. **Anti-platelet aggregating agents:** The commonly used drug to prevent platelet aggregation is **low dose of aspirin**. Aspirin inhibits platelet aggregation.
6. **Folic acid and vitamin B12:** Increased plasma level of **homocysteine** is strongly correlated with myocardial infarction.

- Homocysteine produces damage to the endothelial cells of blood vessels that becomes the site for platelet aggregation and facilitates atherosclerosis.
- Folic acid and vitamin B12 **convert homocysteine to methionine,** a nontoxic compound.

Surgical Treatment

This definitive treatment is implanting a vein in the heart, taken from other parts of the body (**bypass surgery**) (Fig. 39.6). This is called **coronary artery bypass graft** (CABG).

- The grafted artery bypasses the blocked coronary artery.
- If the artery is directly connected from aorta to the ventricular muscle, it is called **aortic CABG.**

CUTANEOUS CIRCULATION

Circulation of blood through skin is called cutaneous circulation. Cutaneous blood flow plays an important role in temperature regulation.

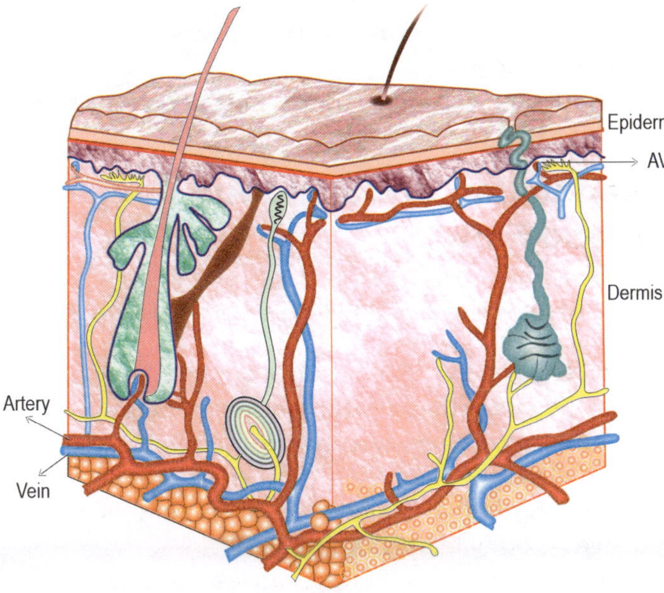

Fig. 39.8: Blood supply to the skin. Note arterioles ascend from deep dermal arcade to superficial layer to form a second arcade and arteriovenous anastomosis (AVA). The capillary loop arises from this AVA and projects to epidermis.

Functional Anatomy

Blood Supply

The blood supply of the skin of **apical regions** (fingers, toes, palm, feet, nose, ear lobes, lips, etc.) is different from the **non-apical regions** (the body torso) of the body.

Apical Areas: In non-apical areas, an **arteriolar arcade** (**network**) exists at the boundary of dermis and the subcutaneous tissue.

- From this arcade, **arterioles ascend** from deep dermis to the superficial layer of the dermis, where they form a **second network** (Fig. 39.8).
- Capillary loops originate from the superficial dermal network and perfuse the dermal papilla and epidermis.
- The dermal arteriolar arcade also provides vessels that supply hair follicles, sebaceous glands and sweat glands.

Non-Apical Areas: In non-apical areas, vascular pattern is modified. The direct vascular connection between arterioles and venules (known as **arteriovenous anastomoses or glomerulus),** mainly occur in the superficial dermal tissue. Arteriovenous anastomoses are absent or very few in deeper demis.

Normal Values

Blood flow to the skin varies from **1 to 150 ml per 100 g** of tissue (skin) per min.

Innervation

The skin blood vessels are supplied by sympathetic fibers. There is **no parasympathetic innervation** of cutaneous vessels.

- **Activation of sympathetic** fibers results in **vasoconstriction**.
- Vasodilation occurs by decreasing the sympathetic activity.

Regulation of Cutaneous Blood Flow

Cutaneous blood flow is regulated by neural, thermal and metabolic factors.

Neural Regulation: The cutaneous blood vessels are supplied by **sympathetic vasoconstrictor fibers**.

- There is **no vasodilator system** supplying the skin blood vessels.

Thermal Regulation: Cutaneous blood flow is mainly regulated by body temperature.

- **Increased body temperature causes vasodilation** and decreased temperature causes vasoconstriction.

Metabolic Regulation: Metabolic regulation is not important for cutaneous circulation.

- However, local production of ***bradykinin*** in the sweat causes *cutaneous vasodilation*.

Applied Physiology

Physiological and applied significance of cutaneous circulation lies in the vascular responses to injury and temporary occlusion.

Vascular Responses to Injury

Two types of responses are observed to injury: **white reaction** in response to light stroke and **triple response** in reaction to firm stroke.

White Reaction

When the skin is stroked lightly with a pointed object, the stroke line becomes pale.

- This is called white reaction.
- This occurs due to decreased blood flow in the capillaries due to **contraction of precapillary sphincter** in response to injury.
- The response is observed in about 15 seconds.

Triple Response

When the skin is stroked firmly with a pointed object, the response to the injury manifests as triple response. This is called triple response as it has **three components**: red reaction, whale, and flare (Fig. 39.9). This is also called **Triple response of Lewis** or Lewis response.

Red Reaction

The skin becomes red in about 10 seconds.

- Redness occurs due to capillary dilation that increases capillary blood flow.
- Capillary dilation occurs due to direct response of capillaries to pressure.

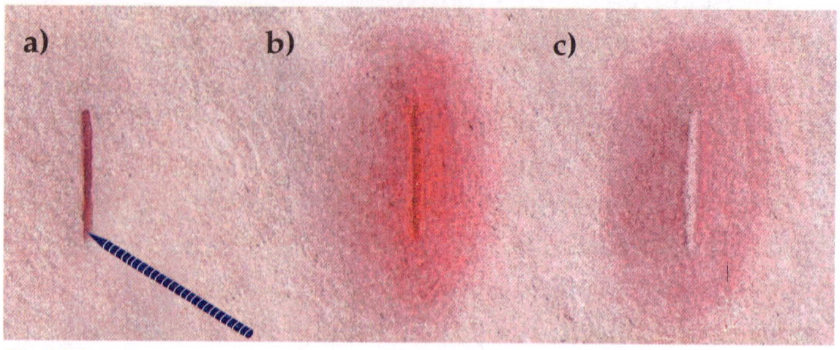

Fig. 39.9: Triple response. Note, a: Red reaction; b: Whale; c: Flare.

Wheal

The swelling (local edema) is called wheal.

- This occurs within few minutes following red reaction.
- Whale occurs due to increased permeability of the capillaries and post capillary venules.
- The histamine released from local mast cells causes vasodilation and increases capillary permeability that results in extravasation of fluid.

Flare

Spreading out of redness from the site of injury to the surrounding area is called flare.

- This occurs due to arteriolar dilation.
- Arteriolar dilation occurs by activation of axon reflex (Fig. 39.10).
    - From the site of injury, the impulse is conducted in the afferent fibers.
    - These sensory neurons give branches to the blood vessels.
    - The impulse, in addition to its conduction to the spinal cord orthodromically, is also relayed antidromically to the blood vessels.
    - Axon reflex is an example of antidromic conduction of the impulse.
- The endings of sensory fibers on the blood vessels release substance P and CGRP that produce arteriolar dilation.
- Thus, redness spreads out from the injury to the surrounding skin in the form of flare.

Vascular Responses to Temporary Occlusion

Reactive hyperemia occurs in response to temporary vascular occlusion.

Reactive Hyperemia

This is defined as **increased blood flow to an area, when blood supply to the area is reestablished** *following a brief period of occlusion*.

- The blood flow to the skin increases when the circulation is reestablished after a **short period of occlusion**.

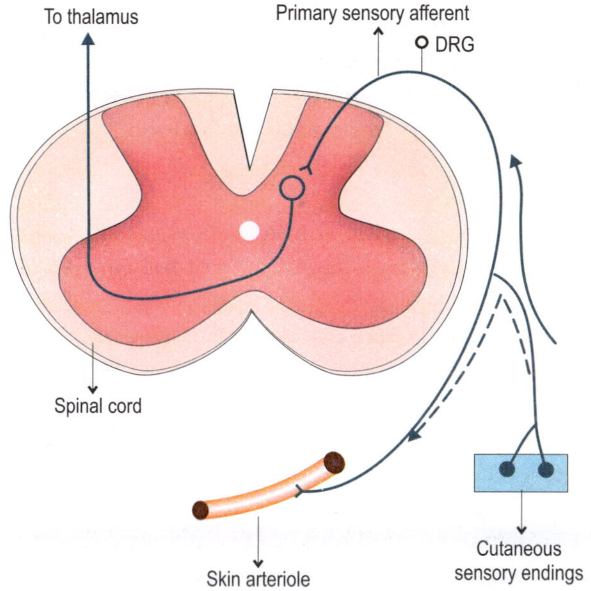

Fig. 39.10: Axon reflex. Note in addition to orthodromic conduction of impulse from sensory organs to the spinal cord (in the direction of solid arrow), the impulse is also conducted antidromically through a branch of the afferent axon to the arteriole (in the direction of dashed arrow) that causes release of vasodilators like CGRP at the nerve ending and produces arteriolar dilation. DRG: dorsal root ganglion.

- The reactive hyperemia **also occurs in visceral organs**.
- It occurs due to **vasodilation produced by hypoxia** during occlusion.
- When circulation is reestablished, blood flow increases through dilated vessels and the skin becomes red.
    - A better example is the *redness of the forearm* of a person immediately following his **blood pressure measurement** by sphygmomanometry.
    - During blood pressure recording, BP cuff is tied around the arm and pressure in the cuff is raised that occludes the forearm arteries.
    - When pressure in the BP cuff is released, the limb becomes red due to reactive hyperemia.

SPLANCHNIC CIRCULATION

Splanchnic circulation means circulation of blood through the abdominal viscera.

It has three components:

1. Circulation through the gastrointestinal tract proper and the mesenteric attachments (**intestinal circulation**).
2. Circulation through the liver (**hepatic circulation**).
3. Circulation through the spleen (**splenic circulation**).

Intestinal Circulation

The normal intestinal blood flow is about **10 – 15% of cardiac output** at rest (**500-750 ml/min**), which increases to 30 – 50 % following a large meal. Without this increase in blood flow, proper digestion and absorption do not occur.

Blood Supply

Arterial Supply: The gastrointestinal tract is supplied by three main arteries: celiac, superior mesenteric, and inferior mesenteric arteries.

- The superior mesenteric artery is the largest branch of the aorta that carries more than 10% of the cardiac output.
    - The branches of the mesenteric arteries (that are called small mesenteric arteries) form an extensive vascular network in the submucosa of the gastrointestinal tract.
- The branches from these arteries penetrate deep into the muscle layers and form the arterioles.
    - The arterioles supply the tip of the villi.
- In resting state, intestinal mucosa receives about 65%, muscularis 25% and submucosa 5% of total intestinal blood flow.

Venous Drainage: The capillaries in the villi drain into the venules that finally drain into the mucosal venules and then into the veins.

- The direction of blood flow in the arterioles and venules in a villus is opposite to each other, which forms a typical counter current exchange system.
- This permits diffusion of oxygen from arterioles to venules directly (Application Box 39.1).
- Therefore, supply of oxygen to the mucosal cells at the tip of the villus (villus capillaries) is reduced.

Normal Blood Flow

The blood flow of gastrointestinal tract can be divided mainly into **three parts.**

1. Gastric blood flow: 40 ml/100 gm of tissue/minute
2. Intestinal blood flow: 60 ml/100 gm of tissue/minute
3. Pancreatic blood flow: 80 ml/100 gm of tissue/minute

Application Box 39.2

Intestinal necrosis is common in shock: In GI tract, oxygen directly diffuses from arterioles to venules in the mucosa bypassing the capillary. Therefore, when intestinal blood flow is reduced as occurs in shock, the shunting of oxygen from the arterioles into the venules is enhanced that causes **extensive necrosis of the intestinal villi.** This facilitates **entry of toxins and bacteria** from intestine **into general circulation.**

Regulation of Intestinal Circulation

Neural Regulation: The neural control of intestinal and mesenteric circulation is mainly achieved by the sympathetic system.

- Stimulation of the sympathetic fibers results in constriction of the mesenteric arteries and arterioles and greatly reduces the blood flow.
    - These effects are mediated via alpha receptors.
- During exercise, the sympathetic vasoconstriction shifts blood from the mesenteric vascular bed to the skeletal muscle.

Autoregulation: Autoregulatory mechanism is **not well developed** in intestinal circulation. The autoregulation of blood flow is mainly due to **metabolic and myogenic** mechanisms.

Metabolic regulation: Metabolic regulation occurs mainly by adenosine, osmolality and potassium.

1. ***Adenosine:*** It plays an important role in regulation of intestinal circulation. It causes **vasodilation** and increases blood flow.
2. ***Osmolality:*** Increased osmolality of the blood passing through the intestine as occurs following ingestion, causes **vasodilation**.
3. ***Potassium:*** K^+ causes **vasodilation**.

Regulation by GI Activity: GI blood flow increases with increase in GI activity as occurs during digestion of food.

- Increased absorption of food also affects intestinal blood flow.
- Several *products of digestion* like chyme, glucose and fatty acids are potent vasodilators.

Physiological Importance

Food intake increases gastrointestinal blood flow. This is known as **functional hyperemia**.

- This is partly due to secretion of ***gastrointestinal hormones*** like gastrin and cholecystokinin and partly to ***products of digestion.***
- Increased blood flow helps in digestion and absorption of food (Application Box 39.2).

Application Box 39.1

Don't do strenuous exercise after meals: Immediately after a meal, one should not perform strenuous physical exercise. During exercise, the sympathetic stimulation causes splanchnic vasoconstriction that diverts blood from GI tract to the exercising muscle. Therefore, the blood will not be adequately available to carry out GI secretion and motility and for assisting in digestion and absorption of food.

Hepatic Circulation

Liver is an important visceral organ as it performs major metabolic activities of the body. Liver requires adequate blood supply to carry out its metabolic functions. Hepatic blood flow constitutes about **28 % of the cardiac output**.

Blood Supply

Blood flow to the liver is derived from two sources: 1) the portal vein, and 2) the hepatic artery.

Portal Vein: It provides about 70% of the blood flow to the liver.

- This blood mainly comes **from the gastrointestinal tract**.
- As the blood has already passed through the capillary bed of the GI tract (oxygen has already been extracted once), the **oxygen concentration is less**.

Hepatic Artery: It provides 30% of the blood to the liver.

- It is **fully saturated with oxygen**.
- Therefore, the **oxygen utilized by the liver** is primarily derived **from the hepatic arterial blood**.

Normal Blood Flow

Liver weighs about 2.6 kg. The blood flow is **1500 ml/min** (58 ml/100gm/min). This is about 28% of the cardiac output.

Regulation of Hepatic Blood Flow

An interactive relationship exists between the regulation of portal venous and hepatic arterial blood flow.

- Normally, alteration in hepatic arterial blood flow occurs reciprocally with portal venous blood flow.
- This is called as **hepatic arterial buffer response**.
- It compensates for change in portal blood flow.

Neural Regulation: Both hepatic artery and portal vein are innervated by **sympathetic vasoconstrictor fibers**.

- These fibers control the hepatic blood flow.

Metabolic Regulation: With increased hepatic activity, the accumulated **metabolites** like carbon dioxide and hydrogen ions **cause vasodilation** and increase hepatic arterial flow.

- Adenosine also causes hepatic vasodilation.

Autoregulation: The portal venous system **does not autoregulate** its blood flow.

- However, autoregulation exists for hepatic arterial blood flow.

Regulation by Intestinal Activity: The activities of the GI tract (increased intestinal movement, splenic contraction, etc.) increase blood flow to the liver via portal system.

Clinical Importance

1. The blood coming out of the GI tract before entering into the systemic circulation **passes through the liver.**
   - Liver therefore, **filters the blood** before allowing it into the general circulation.
   - Toxic substances when absorbed from the GI tract as occurs in poisoning via oral route, are **detoxified in the liver**.
2. The nutrients absorbed from the GI tract **pass through the liver** and are *stored or metabolized* according to the need of the body.
3. When **central venous pressure is elevated** as occurs in congestive heart failure, the ***hydrostatic pressure in hepatic vessels increases.***
   - This results in exudation of fluid into the liver tissue and causes **tender hepatomegaly**.
   - This is an **important feature of heart failure**.
4. Extensive **fibrosis of the liver** as occurs in hepatic cirrhosis causes **increased hepatic vascular resistance**.
   - This increases portal venous pressure, which consequently increases capillary hydrostatic pressure in the splanchnic vascular bed.

- This results in transudation of fluid into the abdominal cavity that causes **ascites**.

5. **In portal hypertension** (increased portal venous pressure), enlargement of the esophageal veins (**esophageal varices**) occurs.
   - These varices may rupture and bleed to cause *hematemesis* (blood vomiting).
   - To prevent this, **portacaval shunt** (anastomosis between portal vein and inferior venacava) is performed surgically to decrease the portal venous pressure.
6. Liver **stores about 15% of the total blood volume** of the body.
   - Therefore, at the time of need as required in hemorrhagic shock, about **60% of the blood from the liver** can be rapidly expelled into the systemic circulation to increase the blood volume.
   - This is achieved by ***constriction of the capacitance vessels*** of the liver by the **sympathetic stimulation**.
     - Hence, liver is an important **reservoir of blood** in humans.
     - **In animals, spleen** (not the liver) acts as an important blood reservoir.

Splenic Circulation

Blood Supply

The main source of blood flow to the spleen is the splenic artery.

Regulation of Splenic Blood Flow

Splenic artery is supplied by the **sympathetic vasoconstrictor fibers**.

- **Sympathetic stimulation** diverts blood from the splenic circulation to the hepatic or systemic circulation.

Clinical importance

Spleen functions as **a reservoir of blood**, especially in animals.

- Stimulation of sympathetic fibers not only causes **vasoconstriction** but also produces **contraction of smooth muscles** present in the ***capsule and trabeculae*** of the spleen.
- The **spleen contracts** as a whole.
- Splenic contraction releases **adequate amount of blood** into the general circulation.
- This serves as a protective mechanism in **exercise and shock**.
- However, spleen is not considered an important reservoir of blood in human being.

SKELETAL MUSCLE CIRCULATION

Skeletal muscles constitute the **largest mass** of the body. In an adult weighing 70 kg, the weight of the skeletal muscle is about 30 kg (**40% of the body weight**), whereas the **blood supply is only about 15%** of the cardiac output.

- However, resistance offered by blood vessels of skeletal muscle accounts for **25 % of systemic vascular resistance**.
- Therefore, caliber of skeletal muscle blood vessels **contributes significantly to blood pressure**.

Normal Blood Flow

At rest, blood flow through the skeletal muscle is very low (**2 - 6 ml /100 gm /min**).

- During **muscular exercise**, blood flow increases 20 - 50 times the resting level (about **100 ml /100 gm /min**).

Blood Supply

The blood supply to skeletal muscle is derived from the skeletal muscle arteries.

- One of the important features of this circulation is the presence of large number of **arteriovenous thoroughfare channels**.
- These blood vessels **short-circuit the blood from the arterial side to the venous side** by bypassing the capillaries (without exchange of fluid or metabolites at the tissue level).

Innervation

Skeletal muscle blood vessels are richly innervated by the sympathetic fibers, which are of two types:

Sympathetic Vasodilator System: The sympathetic fibers supplying the blood vessels of the skeletal muscle **are cholinergic**.

- Therefore, stimulation of these fibers **results in vasodilation** (this is important especially during exercise).

Sympathetic Vasoconstrictor System: There are also sympathetic **noradrenergic fibers** that secrete noradrenaline and cause vasoconstriction.

- **Sympathetic tone at rest restricts muscle blood flow** only during **resting conditions**.

Regulation of Blood Flow

Neural Regulation

At Rest: At rest, the **resistance vessels exhibit a basal tone** that occurs due to *continuous low frequency activity of the* **sympathetic vasoconstrictor system**.

- This tonic activity is greatly influenced by activity of the baroreceptor reflex.
- The muscle resistance vessels **contribute significantly to maintenance of the blood pressure**, as blood vessels

in the skeletal muscle constitute the **largest vascular bed** in the body.

Beginning of Exercise: At the beginning of the exercise, the stimulation of **sympathetic cholinergic fibers increases blood flow** to the skeletal muscle due to vasodilation.

- These vasodilator fibers **supply mainly the thoroughfare (arteriovenous) channels**, not the precapillary sphincters.
- Therefore, this **does not contribute** significantly to the increase in ***oxygen and nutrients supply*** to the skeletal muscle.

During Exercise: But once exercise continues, the **metabolites accumulate** in the exercising muscle and **cause vasodilation.**

- The metabolites and local hypoxia cause dilation of the precapillary sphincters and increase blood flow through the capillaries.
- This increases oxygen and nutrient supply to the skeletal muscle.

Local Regulation

In active muscles, blood flow is regulated by **metabolic factors**.

- **ADP, adenosine, hydrogen ion, carbon dioxide, lactic acid, and hypoxia** cause vasodilation and increase blood flow.
- **Increased temperature** in the active muscles during exercise also contributes to vasodilation.

Regulation by Physical Factors

During exercise, the contraction of skeletal muscle mechanically compresses the blood vessels, therefore, decreases the blood flow.

- Thus, during *active muscle contraction*, ***blood flow is minimal***.
- During strong sustained contraction, blood flow almost ceases temporarily.
- However, **in intermittent contractions**, *blood flow occurs **during the relaxation period*** and venous valves prevent back flow of blood in the veins between the contractions.

Clinical Importance

1. Skeletal vascular bed is the **largest vascular bed** in the body.
   - Therefore, tone of the **resistance vessels** of the skeletal muscle contributes significantly to the **maintenance of systemic blood pressure.**
2. The blood present in the skeletal vascular bed contributes significantly to the **venous return** (the skeletal muscle pump activity).
   - When the **skeletal muscle pump activity** increases, **venous return increases** and therefore, cardiac output increases.
3. When the **venous valves become incompetent**, especially of the superficial leg veins, as seen in pregnancy or in old age, the veins become **dilated and tortuous**.
   - These are called **varicose veins.**
   - **Cardiac output decreases** in such conditions due to **stasis of blood** in dilated & incompetent veins.
   - These conditions are treated by injection of sclerosing agents or by using elastic stockings.

Exam Questions

1. Give the values of blood flow and oxygen consumption of different organs of the body.
2. Describe the structure and functions of blood-brain barrier.
3. List the methods measurement of cerebral blood flow (CBF). Describe the regulation and clinical importance of CBF.
4. List the methods measurement of coronary blood flow (CBF). Describe the regulation and clinical importance of CBF.
5. What is triple response? With the help of a schematic diagram, explain the role of axon reflex in triple response.
6. Give a note on specialities and clinical importance of hepatic circulation.
7. Briefly describe the regulation and clinical importance of skeletal muscle circulation.

Multiple Choice Questions

1. The blood flow per unit gram of tissue/min is highest for:
A. Kidney B. Brain
C. Carotid body D. Heart

2. Which organ has the highest blood flow as % of cardiac output?
A. Kidney B. Heart
C. Carotid body D. Brain

3. Which organ has the highest arterio-venous oxygen difference ?
A. Kidney B. Liver
C. Brain D. Heart

4. Which of the following organs has the maximum amount of blood flow per min?
A. Skeletal muscle B. Brain
C. Kidney D. Liver

5. Which organ has highest oxygen consumption expressed as ml/100gm of tissue/min?
A. Heart B. Brain
C. Kidney D. Liver

6. What is the cerebral blood flow per 100gm of tissue /min?
A. 54 ml B. 80 ml
C. 94 ml D. 420 ml

7. **Which of the following in NOT a feature of cerebral circulation?**
   A. End-feet of astrocytes contribute to BBB
   B. Mechanism of vesicular transport is well developed
   C. Capillaries are mostly non-fenestrated
   D. Arteries are end arteries
8. **Which of the following is NOT true about cerebral metabolism?**
   A. Arteriovenous O2 difference is 62 ml/L
   B. Brain tissues never utilize ketone bodies as fuel
   C. Glucose is the main fuel
   D. Hypoxia more than 5 min to brain tissue causes severe damage
9 **Which of the following method is good for assessing regional blood flow in different parts of the brain?**
   A. Fick method B. Flowmetry
   C. Kety method D. Position Emission Tomography
10. **Which NOT true about regulation of CBF?**
   A. Autoregulation maintains CBF in the MAP range of 60 160mmHg.
   B. Parasympathetic stimulation causes vasodilation
   C. Monro-Kellie doctrine is linked to pressure-flow-velocity relationship of CBF.
   D. Increase in ICP during downward acceleration protects cerebral vessels from rupture
11. **The common artery involved in cerebral hemorrhage is:**
   A. Middle meningeal artery
   B. Anterior cerebral artery
   C. Lenticulostriate branch of middle cerebral artery
   D. Posterior basilar artery
12. **What is the coronary blood flow per 100gm of tissue /min?**
   A. 2.7 ml B. 12.8
   C. 54 ml D. 84 ml
13. **Which of the following is not true about cardiac muscle metabolism?**
   A. Glucose is the main fuel
   B. Arteriovenous O2 difference is 114 ml/L
   C. Extracts 80% of oxygen from arterial blood
   D. Heart utilizesfatty acid for cellular metabolism
14. **Which of the following in not a feature of coronary circulation?**
   A. Heart receives major blood supply during diastole
   B. The coronary blood flow reserve is less
   C. Blood flow is adjusted according to metabolic need
   D. Arteries are end arteries
15. **Which not true about regulation of coronary blood flow?**
   A. Autoregulation is not very well developed like that in the brain
   B. Parasympathetic stimulation causes vasodilation
   C. Subendocardial portion is less prone to ischemia
   D. Depends on myocardial tension built up
16. **The enzyme specific for AMI:**
   A. Muscle phosphatase B. Streptokinase
   C. Creatinine kinase D. Fraction 1 of LDH
17. **What is the total blood flow to heart in a minute?**
   A. 1500 ml B. 1260 ml
   C. 750 ml D. 250 ml
18. **Which of the following method is good for assessing regional blood flow in different parts of the heart?**
   A. Radionuclide method using thallium (201Tl)
   B. Kety-Schmidt method
   C. Fick method
   D. Electromagnetic flowmetry
19. **Which not true about skeletal muscle blood flow?**
   A. Presence of large number of AV thoroughfare channels
   B. Stimulation of sympathetic fibers causes vasoconstriction
   C. Contributes about 25% to systemic vascular resistance
   D. At rest blood flow is 2-6ml/100gm/min
20. **Which of the following in not a feature of cutaneous circulation?**
   A. Vasodilation is due to decreased sympathetic stimulation
   B. No parasympathetic innervation
   C. Arteries are end arteries
   D. Sympathetic stimulation causes vasoconstriction
21. **Axon reflex is an example of:**
   A. Axons controlling the synaptic functions in skin nerve endings
   B. Reflex regulation of blood flow by axons
   C. Antidromic conduction
   D. Orthodromic conduction
22. **Which of the following is not a component of triple response?**
   A. Reactive hyperemia B. Redness
   C. Flare D. Wheal

Answers

1. C	2. A	3. D	4. D	5. A	6. A	7. B	8. B	9. D	10. C	11. C
12. D	13. A	14. B	15. C	16. D	17. D	18. A	19. B	20. C	21. C	22. A

Chapter 40

Fetal and Neonatal Circulation

Learning Objectives

On completion of study of this chapter:

The student will be able to (must know):

1. Appreciate the design of fetal circulation.
1. List the special features of fetal circulation.
2. List the changes in fetal circulation that occur at birth.
3. Correlate the circulatory changes that occur in fetuses due to developmental abnormalities.

The student may also be able to (desirable to know):

1. Describe the arrangement and significance of fetal and neonatal circulation

Circulation in fetus (before birth) differs significantly from circulation in postnatal (neonatal) life. The main difference is that the **fetal lungs are functionally inactive**, and fetus derives oxygen and nutrients from the placenta.

PY5.10

DESIGN OF FETAL CIRCULATION

Fetus receives blood supply from the placenta through umbilical veins (Fig. 40.1). This blood is only **80% saturated with oxygen** as placenta has extracted some of its oxygen.

- The blood **from the umbilical veins enters the liver**, and some amount bypasses the liver and enters the inferior vena cava through the ductus venosus. Blood also comes from other sources.
- The inferior vena cava **drains into right atrium**.
  - About **50% of blood** from the right atrium **enters the left atrium through the foramen ovale**, which is located in the interatrial septum.
  - **Another 50%** of blood from right atrium **enters into the right ventricle**, from where it is *pumped into the pulmonary artery*.
- As the **pulmonary vascular resistance is very high** (because fetal lungs are collapsed), only a **small quantity of blood reaches left atrium** through the pulmonary veins.

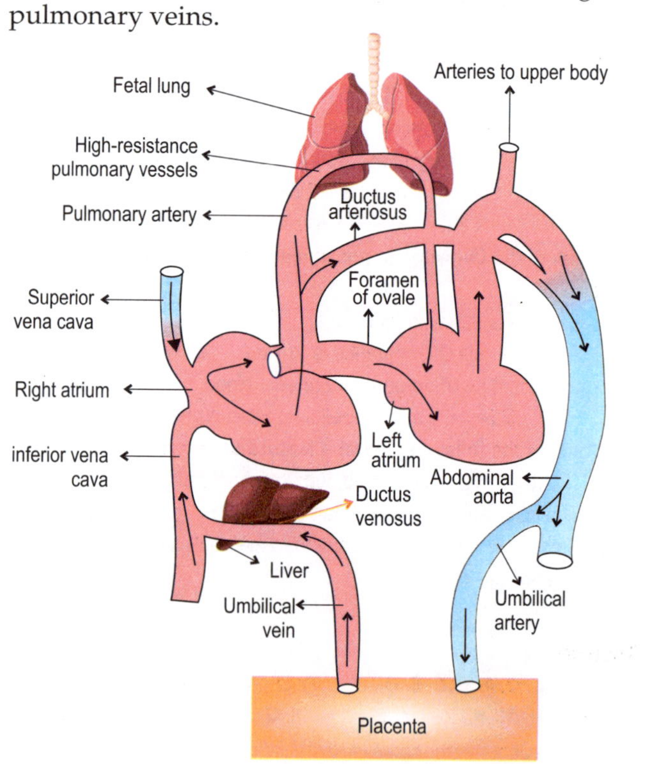

Fig. 40.1: Schematic picture of fetal circulation. Direction of arrows indicates the route of circulation. The oxygenation of blood is roughly indicated by the redness of the fluid in different parts of the fetal vascular tree (more the redness, more is the oxygenation). Umbilical vein supplies more oxygenated blood from placenta to fetus and umbilical artery drains less oxygenated blood from fetus to the placenta.

- The main bulk of the blood from the right ventricle **directly enters the aorta** through ductus arteriosus.
  - The blood in the aorta is then distributed to the whole body.
- **Umbilical artery**, which arises from the aorta, **transports blood to the placenta**, where ***it is oxygenated*** and sent back to the fetus via fetal veins.

- Thus, placenta functions like lungs during fetal life.

Special Features

1. Right ventricle pumps blood into pulmonary artery against higher resistance as the **pulmonary vascular resistance is very high**.
2. Most part of the right ventricular output enters **directly into the aorta through the ductus arteriosus**.
3. The right ventricle receives blood from the placenta and pumps into the aorta from where **about 60% of the blood goes to the placenta for oxygenation** and only 40% is distributed to the different parts of the body.
   - This occurs because peripheral *resistance of the fetal vessels is high*.
   - Whereas resistance of the placenta is relatively low.
4. About 50% of the blood from the right atrium directly enters the left atrium via foramen ovale.
5. **Oxygen saturation of the fetal arterial blood is much lower** than that of the adult.
   - However, **fetal tissues are highly resistant to the effect of hypoxia**.
   - The fetal hemoglobin also has higher affinity to the oxygen.
6. In fetus, the cardiovascular regulatory mechanisms operate **mainly by the local factors**.
   - The baroreceptor and chemoreceptor reflexes develop at about 30th week of intrauterine life.

Changes Occurring at Birth

1. Closure of the umbilical vessel ceases blood flow through the umbilical veins. This results in **closure of ductus venosus**.
2. The clamping of umbilical vessels immediately after birth **causes asphyxia** that activates respiratory center. **Respiratory signal** is generated.
   - This results in expansion of the lungs.
   - As the lung fills with air, the **pulmonary vascular resistance decreases significantly**.
3. Closure of the umbilical vessels **increases the total peripheral resistance** and blood pressure. The **left atrial reserve is raised** above the volume of blood present in inferior vena cava and right atrium. This occurs due to:
   i) The **decreased pulmonary resistance increases blood flow** through the lungs to the left atrium,
   ii) The **decreased flow of blood** to the right atrium occurs due to closure of umbilical vein, and,
   iii) Occlusion of umbilical artery **increases the resistance** to the left ventricular output.

The change in pressure gradient across the atria **abruptly closes the valve of the foramen ovale**, and gradually the interatrial septum closes.

4. The **pulmonary arterial pressure decreases significantly** due to decreased pulmonary vascular resistance.
   - This along with increased aortic pressure **reverses the flow of blood through the ductus arteriosus**.
   - However, constriction of ductus arteriosus begins within few minutes and is completely closed within 1–2 days after birth.
5. Before birth, the thickness of both ventricles is equal.
   - After birth, thickness of the right ventricular wall decreases, whereas *left ventricular thickness increases*.

Clinical Importance

1. If the opening between the two atria (foramen ovale) does not close after birth, the condition is called **atrial septal defect** (patent foramen ovale).
   - This results in mixing of oxygenated blood from the left atrium with that of deoxygenated blood in the right atrium.
   - Thus, oxygen supply decreases to the tissues due to **left to right shunt**.
2. The **failure of the closure of ductus arteriosus** results in flow of blood from the aorta to the pulmonary artery, as the pressure in the aorta is more. This condition is called **patent ductus arteriosus**.
   - This is also an example of **left to right shunt.**
   - Oxygenation of the tissues of the body decreases in this condition.
3. A condition known as **tetralogy of Fallot** occurs rarely in which there are ***four cardiovascular defects***: ventricular septal defect, pulmonary stenosis, right ventricular hypertrophy, and overriding of the aorta.
   - Due to ventricular septal defect and pulmonary stenosis, the **oxygenation of blood is grossly reduced**.
   - Therefore, tissues suffer from severe hypoxia, and cyanosis develops.

Exam Questions

1. Describe the design of fetal circulation. List the changes that occur in fetal circulation at birth.
2. List the special features of fetal circulation. List the changes that occur in fetal circulation at birth. Give a note on clinical aspects of fetal and neonatal circulation.

Chapter 41

Pathophysiology of Hypertension and Hypotension

Learning Objectives

On completion of study of this chapter:

The student will be able to (must know):

1. Define prehypertension and hypertension.
2. List the risk factors for hypertension.
3. Name types of hypertensions and give the important causes of each.
4. Understand the ill effects of hypertension on body systems.
5. Appreciate the physiological basis of treatment of hypertension.
6. Classify hypotension & give their common causes.

The student may also be able to (desirable to know):

1. Describe the physiological changes in the body due to hypertension..

HYPERTENSION

Definition: Hypertension is defined as **sustained elevation of systemic arterial pressure.**

Degrees of Hypertension (in adults): **According to recent report Joint National Committee (JNC-7) on hypertension, systolic blood pressure <120 mmHg and Diastolic blood pressure <80 mmHg are considered normal (Table 41.1).**

Table 41.1 | JNC-7 classification of hypertension.

	SBP (mmHg)	DBP (mmHg)
Normal	100 – 119	60 - 79
Prehypertension	120 – 139	80 – 89
Hypertension:		
Stage 1	140 – 159	90 – 99
Stage 2	160 or more	100 or more

Types of Hypertension

Hypertension is broadly classified into **two categories**: essential and secondary.

Essential Hypertension

Essential hypertension is also called **primary hypertension**. Essential hypertension is a misnomer as it is not essential for health; rather it is nonessential for a healthy life.

- It constitutes about **90% of all types** of hypertension.
- The causes of essential hypertension are **not exactly known**.
- Sympathetic hyperactivity, increased renin secretion, high blood volume, excess salt intake, increased production of salt and water retaining hormones, increased synthesis of vasoconstrictors and decreased synthesis of vasodilators have been implicated in the causation of essential hypertension.

Risk Factors

Followings are the known risk factors for essential hypertension.

Heredity: Hypertension is inherited as **Mendelian dominant**.

- If both parents are hypertensives, chance of children developing hypertension is more than 50%, and when one of the parents is hypertensive, the chance is 25%.

Age: Blood pressure **increases with age**.

- Age related rise in blood pressure is due to **increased arterial wall thickness** and degenerative changes (**decreased compliance**) in the arteries and arterioles.

Gender: Hypertension is less common in females before menopause because of gonadal hormones estrogen and progesterone.

- **Estrogen decreases blood cholesterol** and slows the process of atherosclerosis. Thus, estrogen decreased BP.
- **Progesterone causes relaxation** of smooth muscles and therefore produces vasodilation.

After menopause, the incidence of hypertension in females is equal with males.

Race: Black Africans are more prone to develop hypertension.

Stress: Stress causes **vasospasm by inducing sympathetic activity**.

- Stress also causes hyperlipidemia.
- Stress predisposes to hypertension and heart diseases.

Smoking: Chronic smoking increases **nicotine and carbon monoxide concentration in plasma**.

- Nicotine and carbon monoxide are ***potent vasoconstrictors.***
- Nicotine also increases secretion of catecholamines.

Obesity: Obesity with or without hyperlipidemia increases blood pressure.

- Reduction in body weight by one kg *reduces blood pressure by about 2 mm Hg.*

Hyperlipidemia: Hyperlipidemia facilitates the process of atherosclerosis.

Sedentary Life: Sedentary life is the commonest cause of high blood pressure and coronary artery disease. Lack of exercise is known to produce obesity and hyperlipidemia.

Personality: **Type A personality** (sympathetic overactivity) is more prone to hypertension.

Environmental Factors: Occupation, **family size and crowding** influence blood pressure.

Salt intake & Salt Sensitivity: Increased salt intake and **salt-sensitivity** of the individuals increase blood pressure.

Alcohol: Chronic and excess intake of alcohol increases blood pressure.

Secondary Hypertension

Hypertension that **occurs due to various diseases** is called secondary hypertension. Secondary hypertension is classified into following categories.

A. Renal hypertension

1. Glomerulonephritis
2. Pyelonephritis
3. Polycystic renal disease
4. Renin producing tumors (of JG cells)
5. Renal artery stenosis

B. Endocrinal hypertension

1. Adrenocortical diseases
   - Hyperaldosteronism
   - Cushing's syndrome
   - Hypertensive form of congenital virilizing tumor
2. Pheochromocytoma
3. Acromegaly
4. Myxedema

C. Neurogenic hypertension

1. Acute increase in intracranial pressure
2. Polyneuritis (acute porphyria, lead poisoning)
3. Diencephalic syndrome

D. Miscellaneous forms of hypertension

1. **Pill hypertension** (chronic use of oral contraceptives)
   - Oral contraceptive pills (estrogen-progesterone combination) produce hypertension if taken for many years.
   - Oral contraceptives are known to cause ***sodium and water retention*** from the kidney (expand ECF volume), and also ***increase the release of renin*** (activate renin-angiotensin system).
2. Severe polycythemia
3. **Pregnancy-induced hypertension** (toxemia of pregnancy): Hypertension is not a feature of normal pregnancy, as progesterone produces vasodilation.
   - Pregnancy-induced hypertension is seen in ***complicated and risk pregnancies.***
   - In such conditions, the placenta produces **pressor peptides** (that cause vasoconstriction) or the blood vessels become hypersensitive to the circulating vasoconstrictors.
4. Coarctation of aorta
5. Hypercalcemia
6. Increased blood volume (e.g. excess transfusion, or administration of more i.v. fluid)
7. Glucocorticoid therapy

Experimental Hypertension

Hypertension produced in animal models by various experimental techniques, is called experimental hypertension.

1. **Renal hypertension**: Constriction of renal artery by applying clips produces hypertension (**Goldblatt hypertension**).
   - This type of hypertension is cured by removing the constriction from renal artery.
   - When one renal artery is clipped with other kidney intact (**one-clip, two kidney Goldblatt hypertension**), the hypertension is due to **high renin secretion** that resembles the renal hypertension in human beings.
   - However, *renin concentration remains normal* in **one-clip one-kidney Goldblatt hypertension**.
2. **Neurogenic hypertension**
   - Denervation of carotid sinus and aortic arch
   - Bilateral lesion of NTS
3. Steroid-induced hypertension
4. Partial adrenalectomy
5. Salt-induced hypertension (in salt-sensitive rats)

Effects of Hypertension

Chronic hypertension results in following physiological alterations.

Effects on CVS

On Heart

Peripheral resistance increases in hypertension that **increases afterload** on the heart.

- Compensation for increased excessive workload on heart occurs first by **concentric left ventricular hypertrophy** that increases the wall thickness.
  - Afterwards, **dilatation of the cavity** occurs.
- Ultimately, cardiac function deteriorates and **heart failure** sets in.
- Myocardial *oxygen requirement increases* due to increased ventricular mass.
  - This causes **angina pectoris** and ischemic heart disease.

On Blood Vessels

Hypertension produces **stiffness of the vessel wall** and ***deceases vascular compliance***. Hypertension promotes **atherosclerosis**.

Decreased Vascular Compliance: The blood vessels become stiff (less compliant) due to increased smooth muscles in their wall in response to *chronic wall stress*. This further aggravates hypertension.

Increased Atherosclerosis: Accelerated atherosclerosis is common.

Atherosclerosis and decreased compliance of the vessel wall result in **narrowing of the vessel lumen**.

- Atherosclerosis in the coronary and cerebral arteries is harmful.
- Hypertensive patients are *predisposed to* ***cerebral thromboses and hemorrhage.***

Effects on CNS

Increased cerebral atherosclerosis causes cerebral infarction.

- Hypertension causes the development of cerebral vascular microaneurysm (**Charcot-Bouchard aneurysm**).
- Increased arterial pressure and vascular microaneurysm result in **cerebral hemorrhage**.
- Severe chronic hypertension causes ***hypertensive encephalopathy*** **and** ***retinopathy.***

Effects on Kidney

Arteriosclerosis occurs in afferent and efferent arterioles and glomerular capillaries.

- This *decreases GFR and tubular function*.
- Proteinuria and hematuria are not uncommon.

Physiological Basis of Management

Primary hypertension, in its early phase can be treated *without drugs*. The treatment ***lifestyle modification*** that includes weight reduction, dietary alteration, physical exercise and mental relaxation. However, for **secondary hypertension**, and in chronic or advanced stage of hypertension, ***antihypertensive drugs*** are required for reducing the blood pressure. These include vasodilators, anti-adrenergic drugs, calcium channel blockers, diuretics, ACE inhibitors and angiotensin receptor antagonist.

Lifestyle Modification

Weight Reduction: As hypertension is common in obese persons, reduction of body weight should be an integral part of treatment of all obese hypertensives.

- It has been observed that with ***reduction of 1kg of body weight*** the blood pressure usually **decreases by about 2 mmHg.**

Dietary Modifications: As salt accumulation causes water retention and increases blood volume, ***restriction of salt*** in the diet decreases blood pressure in hypertensive patients.

1. *Salt Restriction:* Salt restriction is advised to ***all hypertensive patients***.
2. *Restriction of fat:* Restriction of fat, especially **animal fat** in the diet decreases the process of atherosclerosis and therefore, reduces blood pressure.
3. *Increased fiber content* of the diet controls obesity and hyperlipidemia. Fibers in the diet ***decrease the absorption of fat*** from the intestine and therefore, prevent hyperlipidemia.

Regular Physical Exercise: practice of isotonic exercise is very effective in reducing blood pressure and body weight. Hypertension and other cardiovascular diseases are common in sedentary individuals.

- The best form of exercise for reducing blood pressure is the **brisk morning walk** (at a speed of 25% more than the normal walk for about 30 - 60 minutes).
- Regular exercise controls blood pressure by **decreasing the sympathetic tone and increasing vagal tone.**
- Exercise decreases heart rate, and improves myocardial performance.

Yoga and relaxation Techniques: **Practice of yoga, change in temperament** (to remain cool or to become less aggressive), and **relaxation exercises** are known to decrease blood pressure in hypertensives.

Mental relaxation through practice of meditation, yogasana or by listening soothing music etc. is known to improve the condition of the patients by reducing sympathetic discharge.

- **Happiness of mind** is the prerequisite for a healthy life and for maintaining normal blood pressure.
- **Slow pranayamas** such as anulom-vilom, chandranadi, sheetali and sheetkari are known improve vagal tone and reduce sympathetic tone, and reduce BP.

Stop Smoking and Alcohol: Smoking **must be stopped completely** and alcohol intake should be *moderated*, as smoking and alcoholism are known risk factors for hypertension.

Antihypertensive Drugs

Antihypertensive drugs include anti-adrenergic drugs, diuretics, calcium-channel blockers, ACE inhibitors, angiotensin receptor antagonists and vasodilators.

Anti-Adrenergic Drugs

These are β receptor blockers and α receptor blockers.

β Receptor Blockers: β receptor blockers are considered to be the first line of drugs in mid to moderate hypertension.

- β blockers like propranolol and atenolol decrease blood pressure by ***blocking sympathetic effects on heart*** that decreases heart rate and cardiac output.
- They also ***reduce adrenergic-nerve mediated release of renin*** from JG cells, which is an important component of lowering blood pressure.

α Receptor Blockers: α receptor blockers like phentolamine decrease blood pressure by *blocking the action of norepinephrine* on blood vessels.

- They also *decrease the release of norepinephrine* at sympathetic nerve endings.
- Usually they are used with β receptor blockers.

Diuretics

Diuretics are mainstay of hypertension management.

Thiazide Diuretics: Thiazide diuretics are frequently used in the treatment of hypertension.

- They produce ***sodium diuresis and volume depletion***.
- They also reduce peripheral vascular resistance.

Loop-Diuretic: Furosemide, a loop-diuretic also decreases blood pressure.

Aldosterone Receptor Blockers: Spironolactone decreases the effect of mineralocorticoid on kidney and causes ***renal sodium loss*** (it is effective, especially in hypertension due to hyperaldosteronism).

ACE Inhibitors

ACE inhibitors like captopril, enalapril etc. are commonly used now-a-days. They **inhibit the action of angiotensin converting enzyme** (ACE).

- Thus, they inhibit the generation of angiotensin II.
- They also **retard the degradation of bradykinin**, a potent vasodilator and also ***reduce the activity of adrenergic nervous system.***
- These drugs are especially useful in the treatment of renal or renovascular hypertension, malignant and accelerated hypertension.

Calcium Channel Blockers

Calcium channel blockers like **verapamil** (a phenylalkylamine derivative), amlodipine, nifedipine and diltiazem (a benzothiazepine) **inhibit calcium entry** into the cells by interacting with specific binding sites on the ***α_1-subunit of*** *L-type of voltage-dependent calcium channel.*

- This decreases vascular tone that in turn decreases blood pressure.
- Verapamil and diltiazem also slow atrioventricular conduction that decreases heart rate.

Angiotensin-II Receptor Blockers

Angiotensin receptor antagonists like losartan, valsartan, telmisartan etc. **block the action of angiotensin II on AT_1 receptor** subtype.

Vasodilators

Vasodilators like hydralazine and minoxidil decrease blood pressure by directly causing **relaxation of vascular smooth muscle**.

HYPOTENSION

Usually, hypotension refers to **decrease in systolic blood pressure**. When systolic pressure is less than 90 mm Hg in adults, the condition is known as hypotension (90 to 99 mm Hg is considered borderline hypotension). However, diastolic pressure is also less when systolic pressure is significantly less.

Clinically, there are **three types of hypotension**: chronic hypotension, acute hypotension, and postural hypotension.

Chronic Hypotension

Chronic hypotension is characterized by **persistent low blood pressure**. Though the patients are usually asymptomatic, they complain lethargy, weakness and giddiness.

Causes of chronic hypotension:

1. Primary adrenocortical insufficiency
2. Hypopituitarism
3. Malnutrition
4. Chronic diarrhea
5. Prolonged bed rest

Acute Hypotension

When blood pressure **falls suddenly**, the condition is called acute hypotension. If severe, it is *associated with fainting*.

Causes of acute hypotension:

1. Acute hemorrhage
2. Acute diarrhea

3. Severe vomiting
4. Acute myocardial infarction
5. Excessive diuresis
6. Acute vasodilation

Postural Hypotension

If systolic blood pressure **falls by 20 mm Hg or more**, when a subject assumes erect posture from the supine posture, the condition is called postural or **orthostatic hypotension**. This usually results from ***autonomic imbalance.***
It may be acute or chronic type.

Acute Postural Hypotension

This is due to temporary fall of blood pressure that may result in transient fainting. It is usually seen in following conditions.

1. Prolonged standing.
2. Getting up from bed after a prolonged illness.
3. Strenuous physical exercise.

Chronic Postural Hypotension

Chronic postural hypotension can be **primary or secondary variety**.

Chronic Primary Postural Hypotension

This is called **idiopathic postural hypotension**. The cause of this hypotension is not known. It usually occurs in elderly and may be due to ***degeneration of peripheral autonomic nerves.***

Chronic Secondary Postural Hypotension

This occurs in following conditions.

1. **Polyneuropathy** as seen in diabetes, amyloidosis and beriberi
2. **Autonomic neuropathy** as seen in syringomyelia, tabes dorsalis, and subacute combined degeneration of spinal cord.
3. Patients receiving **sympatholytic drugs**.
4. Surgical sympathectomy.

Exam Questions

1. Define hypertension and classify hypertension based on JNC-7 Criteria. List the risk factors for essential hypertension. Briefly describe the effects of hypertension on different systems of the body.
2. Briefly describe the etiopathogenesis of primary hypertension. Give the physiological basis of management of hypertension.
3. What is postural hypotension. Briefly describe the etiopathogenesis of postural hypotension.

Multiple Choice Questions

1. **Which of the following is not a cause of hypertension?**
   A. Normal pregnancy
   B. Smoking
   C. Heredity
   D. Stress
2. **Which of the following endocrine disorder does not cause hypertension?**
   A. Pheochromocytoma
   B. Addison's disease
   C. Myxedema
   D. Acromegaly
3. **All the following are neurogenic causes of hypertension, EXCEPT:**
   A. Diencephalic syndrome
   B. Polyneuritis
   C. Pyelonephritis
   D. Raised intracranial pressure
4. **Which of the following is not an effect of hypertension on CVS?**
   A. Increased atherosclerosis
   B. Decreased vascular compliance
   C. Left ventricular hypertrophy
   D. Decreased afterload on the heart
5. **Isolated systolic hypertension is said to be present when the BP is:**
   A. 130/80 mmHg
   B. 140/89 mmHg
   C. 150/95 mmHg
   D. 160/100 mmHg
6. **Severe hypertension is said to be present when the DBP is:**
   A. 95 mmHg
   B. 100 mmHg
   C. 110 mmHg
   D. 120 mmHg
7. **Verapamil acts an antihypertensive by:**
   A. Inhibiting ACE
   B. Blocking beta receptors on heart
   C. Inhibiting calcium entry into the cell
   D. Blocking the action of angiotensin
8. **All of the following are examples of experimental hypertension, EXCEPT:**
   A. Coarctation of aorta
   B. Bilateral lesion of NTS
   C. Denervation of carotid sinus and aortic arch
   D. Goldblatt hypertension

Answers

1. A 2. B 3. C 4. D 5. B 6. D 7. C 8. A

Chapter 42

Pathophysiology of Shock

Learning Objectives

On completion of study of this chapter:

The student will be able to (must know):

1. Define and classify shock and give example for each type of shock.
2. Describe the compensatory mechanisms activated by hemorrhagic shock.
3. Learn the mechanisms of refractory shock.
4. Briefly describe other types of shock.
5. Appreciate physiological basis of treatment of shock.

The student may also be able to (desirable to know):

1. Describe the mechanism of irreversible shock.
2. Explain the management of different types of shock

PY5.11

Shock is **defined** as a syndrome in which there is inadequate tissue perfusion associated with a relative or absolute decrease in cardiac output.

Types of Shock

Shock is classified broadly into **four categories** based on the mechanisms that decrease cardiac output: hypovolemic, distributive, cardiogenic and obstructive.

Hypovolemic Shock

In this type of shock, the inadequate cardiac output is due to **decreased volume of fluid in the vascular system**.

This occurs due to:

1. Acute hemorrhage (hemorrhagic shock)
2. Injury (traumatic shock)
3. Blood loss during surgery (surgical shock)
4. Burn (burn shock)
5. Metabolic diseases like adrenal insufficiency, diabetic ketoacidosis etc.
6. Severe diarrhea or vomiting

Distributive Shock

In this type of shock, blood **volume is normal,** but blood pressure decreases due to ***sudden increase in the capacity of the vascular compartment*** due to **acute marked vasodilation**.

- Cardiac output also decreases in response to decreased venous return due to venodilation.

This may be of following types:

1. Neurogenic shock (as seen in fainting)
2. Anaphylactic shock (due to acute systemic allergy or anaphylaxis)
3. Septic shock (following septicemia)

Cardiogenic Shock

In this type of shock, cardiac output decreases due to **decreased ability of the heart to pump blood**.

It is seen in:

1. Acute myocardial infarction
2. Heart failure
3. Cardiac arrhythmias

Obstructive Shock

In this type of shock, cardiac output is decreased because of **obstruction to the ejection of blood from the ventricle**.

It is seen in:

1. Cardiac temponade
2. Constrictive pericarditis
3. Cardiac tumor
4. Tension pneumothorax

HYPOVOLEMIC SHOCK

Hypovolemic shock is the commonest of all shocks. Common forms of hypovolemic shock are hemorrhagic, traumatic, surgical and burn shocks.

Hemorrhagic Shock

This is the common hypovolemic shock and the commonest of all shocks. **Acute hemorrhage of more than 15 ml/kg** body weight results in shock.

Features

1. Hypotension
2. Tachycardia
3. Rapid and thready pulse
4. Cold and pale skin (***cold shock***)
5. Tachypnea
6. Intense thirst
7. Restlessness
8. Usually, patient is conscious

Stages of Shock

Shock has two stages: reversible stage and irreversible stage.

Reversible Stage

In this stage, with **activation of compensatory mechanisms** the condition of the patient improves.

The **compensatory reactions** are divided into **short-term and long-term mechanisms.**

A. Rapid Compensatory Mechanisms

The rapid compensatory mechanisms are primarily **neural and vascular**, though the **hormonal mechanisms** also play role.

1. **Tachycardia:** Loss of blood decreases blood volume and blood pressure that **decrease stimulation of baroreceptors** (due to decreased stretch), which results in **sympathetic activation** and increases heart rate.
2. **Vasoconstriction:** This also occurs due to decreased stimulation of baroreceptors that **activates sympathetic system**.
   - Vasoconstriction occurs in almost **all parts of the body** *except in the cerebral and the coronary arteries*.
     - Thus, coronary and cerebral blood flow is maintained in shock.
   - The *skin becomes pale and cold* due to intense cutaneous vasoconstriction.
     - Therefore, acute hemorrhagic shock is called **cold shock**.
   - In kidney, the **renal vasoconstriction** decreases renal blood flow and GFR.
     - But efferent arterioles are constricted more than the afferent arterioles.
     - Urine formation is *grossly reduced*.
   - The nitrogenous waste products are retained in the body in prolonged shock that results in uremia (**azotemia**).
3. **Increased Venous Return:** Venous return increases due to **venoconstriction**, which occurs due to sympathetic stimulation.
4. **Increased Thoracic Pumping:** The patients in hemorrhagic shock usually **hyperventilate** (exhibit rapid respiration).
   - This **increases the thoracic pump** and contributes to increased venous return.
5. **Increased Skeletal Muscle Pumping:** The subject is usually **restless**.
   - The skeletal muscle activity is increased due to **active movements** of different body parts.
     - Increases skeletal muscle pumping increases venous return.
6. **Capillary Fluid Shift:** This is the shift of blood from interstitial fluid compartment into capillaries.
   - Due to acute blood loss, the hydrostatic pressure inside the vessel decreases.
     - This **reverses the net filtration pressure gradient,** and fluid from interstitial tissue space enters the capillaries.
     - This contributes to **increase in blood volume**.
7. **Activation of Chemoreceptor Reflex:** When blood loss is severe enough to cause general **hypoxia**, the chemoreceptors are stimulated.
   - Chemoreceptor stimulation results in **intense vasoconstriction** (that restores blood pressure) and stimulates respiratory center (that causes hyperventilation).
8. **Activation of Cushing's Reflex:** When hypotension is severe due to gross hemorrhage, **cerebral hypoxia** directly stimulates vasomotor center.
   - This results in **intense vasoconstriction** that tries to maintain blood pressure and perfusion of vital organs.
9. **Increased Secretion of Catecholamines:** Secretion of catecholamines from the adrenal medulla occurs due to **sympathetic stimulation**.
   - Catecholamines **increase cardiac output** and cause vasoconstriction (**increased blood pressure**).
   - Catecholamines also **stimulate the reticular activating system**, for which patient is often conscious and restless.
10. **Increased Secretion of Vasopressin:** Decreased blood volume stimulates **secretion of ADH** from the posterior pituitary.
    - In higher concentration, ADH causes **vasoconstriction** and increases blood pressure.
    - ADH increases **reabsorption of water** from kidney that restores blood volume.
11. **Increased Secretion of Cortisol:** Glucocorticoid secretion increases due to **increased ACTH secretion**.
    - Glucocorticoid plays a crucial role by **increasing the responsiveness of the blood vessels to**

catecholamines through its *permissive and vasoreactivity* effects.

12. **Activation of Rennin-Angiotensin System:** Hypovolemia and sympathetic stimulation increase the secretion of rennin from JG cells of the kidney that converts angiotensinogen to angiotensin-I, which is then converted to **angiotensin-II.**

Angiotensin-II restores the blood pressure and volume by the following actions:

I. Peripheral actions

- It is a potent vasoconstrictor (increases blood pressure).
- It increases aldosterone secretion (increases water reabsorption from kidney).
- Increases sodium and water reabsorption from proximal convoluted tubule.
- Stimulates release of norepinephrine from sympathetic nerve endings.

II. Central actions

- It stimulates dipsogenesis (increases drinking) by stimulating thirst centers.
- It stimulates vasomotor center and increases sympathetic discharge.
- It increases ADH secretion.
- It also increases ACTH secretion.

13. **Increased Aldosterone Secretion:** Aldosterone secretion increases by angiotensin-II, ACTH, and hypovolemia. Aldosterone **increases water and sodium reabsorption** from kidney.

B. Long-term Compensatory Mechanisms

The long-term mechanisms increase the red cell mass to increase oxygen carrying capacity of the blood.

1. **Increased Synthesis of Erythropoietin:** Erythropoietin secretion from kidney increases within 48 hours.
   - This increases red cells count within 2–6 weeks.
2. **Increased Plasma Protein Synthesis:** Protein synthesis by the liver increases within 2–4 days.
   - This **increases hemoglobin synthesis**.
   - Increased plasma protein also **restores the oncotic pressure** of the plasma.

Irreversible Stage

In this stage, the **compensatory mechanisms fail** to improve body functions.

- **Cardiac output and blood pressure decrease** despite the normal blood volume.
  - This is also called **refractory shock or irreversible shock.**
- Usually, patients die irrespective of judicious treatment to increase the circulatory status.

Refractory Shock

Refractory shock occurs due to the following mechanisms:

1. Initially, **precapillary sphincters constrict** due to unknown mechanisms.
   - This decreases blood flow to the viscera and results in **hypoxic tissue damage**.
   - Free oxygen radicals (released from damaged tissue) and granulocytes adhered to the injured vessel wall facilitate further vessel damage.
2. Later, **precapillary sphincters dilate**, but the venules constrict.
   - This increases capillary hydrostatic pressure, which causes further injury to the vessel wall and increases **transudation of fluid** into the interstitial tissue space.
   - This promotes additional decrease in blood volume and pressure.
3. The **hypoxic damage to GI tract** disrupts the mucosa of the intestine that allows **entry of bacteria into circulation**.
   - This results in bacteremia and septicemia.
   - Release of **endotoxins from bacteria and toxic materials from septic tissues** inhibit cardiorespiratory centers.
4. The hypoxia of the brain for a longer duration **depresses medullary cardio-respiratory centers**, especially the vasomotor center, which further decreases blood pressure and suppresses heart functions.
5. Due to hypotension and tachycardia, **coronary blood flow decreases**.
   - This further **decreases myocardial function**.
6. Damaged blood vessels and damaged tissue **release various coagulants** that trigger **disseminated intravascular coagulation**.
   - This results in **microembolism** in different vascular beds.
7. Severe pulmonary damage occurs due to **pulmonary microembolism**.
   - This finally leads to acute respiratory distress syndrome (**shock lung**).

Other Hypovolemic Shocks

Traumatic Shock

This occurs due to severe injury, especially when **muscles and bones are extensively damaged**. Usually, it occurs in road accidents or in battle casualties.

Mechanisms of Traumatic Shock

1. **Bleeding into the injured muscles** is the main cause of shock.
   - As most part of **bleeding is internal** (occurs in the injured tissue), the degree of external blood loss or injury **does not reflect the actual extent of hemorrhage**.
   - Big muscles like rectus femoris or gluteus maximus can accommodate about one liter of blood without significant increase in their size.

2. **Rhabdomyolysis** (break down of the skeletal muscle) due to **muscle crushing** is another cause of shock.
   - **Myoglobin** released from damaged muscles blocks the renal tubules and causes ***acute renal failure***.
3. In the reperfused areas, **increased accumulation of calcium** (due to exchange of excess sodium for intracellular calcium) also causes tissue damage.

Reperfusion-induced injury: Accumulating in large amount in the muscle compresses muscle blood vessels and decreases blood supply to injured muscle. Free radicals are generated from hypoxic and injured muscles.

- In traumatic shock, blood accumulated in the muscle is collected and then transfused to the patient (**autotransfusion**).
  - However, autotransfusion further complicates the condition.
  - The removal of blood from the injured muscle relieves the pressure on blood vessel.
  - This, plus autotransfusion reestablish the blood supply to the tissue (**reperfusion**).
- When blood supply is reestablished, the free radicals are generated by conversion of tissue xanthine dehydrogenase to xanthine oxidase.
- The **xanthine oxidase** generates free oxygen radicals and hydrogen peroxides that further damage the tissue.
  - This is called **reperfusion-induced injury**.

IMPORTANT NOTE

Allopurinol is useful: Treatment with allopurinol, **a xanthine oxidase inhibitor**, reduces the severity of reperfusion-induced injury.

Surgical Shock

This is seen in surgical procedures **with improper hemostasis** or in prolonged surgeries. It may be due to internal (into the tissue) or external hemorrhage or both.

Burn Shock

In burns, plasma is lost from the burnt surface **as exudate.**

- The exudate is rich in **plasma proteins and fluid** and does not contain red cells.
  - This results in **hemoconcentration**.
  - Therefore, ***hematocrit is high in burn shock***.
- Infection leading to **septic shock** complicates the hypovolemic shock in burns.
- **Hemolytic anemia** also complicates the condition in burns.

OTHER TYPES OF SHOCK

Distributive Shock

In this condition, capacity of the vascular bed is increased suddenly by **marked acute vasodilation**.

- This is also called **warm shock,** as the skin blood flow increases due to cutaneous vasodilation (this is in contrast to the cold shock that occurs in hemorrhagic shock).

The examples of distributive shock are anaphylactic shock, septic shock, endotoxic shock and neurogenic shock.

Anaphylactic Shock: This is seen in acute systemic allergy.

- The antigen-antibody complex ***releases*** **histamine** from the mast cells that causes severe *hypotension due to* ***vasodilation*** and *acute hypovolemia due to* ***increased capillary permeability***.
- Thus, anaphylactic shock is **both distributive and hypovolemic in nature**.

Septic Shock: This is seen in **systemic sepsis** (bacterial infection).

- The bacterial toxins cause vasodilation, suppress myocardial contractility and increase capillary permeability.
- Therefore, septic shock is a **combination of distributive, cardiogenic and hypovolemic shock**.

Endotoxic Shock: This is a special variety of septic shock that occurs due to **infection by gram-negative bacteria**.

- These bacteria release endotoxins that produce **vasodilation**.
- The cell wall of these organisms contains lipopolysaccharides that stimulate macrophages to secrete more **cytokines**.

Neurogenic Shock: In this shock, **sudden vasodilation occurs due to activation of autonomic responses**.

- This causes peripheral **pooling of blood due to vasodilation**.
  - This is frequently seen in emotional outburst, overexcitement and severe fear or grief.
- Fainting or **syncope** (sudden and transient loss of consciousness) occurs in neurogenic shock.

Cardiogenic Shock

Shock occurs due to **decreased myocardial contractility**.

- This may occur due to **extensive myocardial damage** as seen in acute myocardial infarction, or myocardial malfunction as seen in heart failure.
- Cardiac output decreases due to **decreased pumping** of the blood by the heart.

Obstructive Shock

The shock occurs either due to **obstruction to the outflow** of blood from the heart as seen in aortic stenosis or due to the **obstruction to expansion of the heart** as seen in cardiac tamponade (bleeding into the pericardial cavity).

- **In cardiac tamponade**, ventricular muscles cannot relax in diastole due to external pressure that decreases end-diastolic volume; therefore, cardiac output decreases.

TREATMENT OF SHOCK

The aim of shock is to **restore adequate tissue perfusion**. Restoring blood volume in hypovolemic shock, ensuring vasoconstriction in distributive shock and increasing cardiac output in cardiogenic shock achieve this goal.

The common modes of treatment are as follows:

1. **Blood transfusion** is required in hemorrhagic shock to increase blood volume.
2. **Plasma transfusion** is needed in burn shock to increase plasma volume.
   - Administering concentrated human serum albumin that improves plasma volume by drawing fluid from extravascular space can also increase plasma volume.
   - Injection of plasma expanders (sugars of high molecular weight like dextran) is also helpful.
3. **Epinephrine** is injected in anaphylactic shock that increases blood pressure by causing vasoconstriction and by increasing cardiac output.
4. **Dopamine** is the **drug of choice in traumatic and cardiogenic shock** for three reasons:
   i) It produces ***renal vasodilation*** that maintains kidney function.
   ii) It has ***positive inotropic*** effect that increases cardiac output.
   iii) It causes ***vasoconstriction*** in the systemic blood vessels that increases blood pressure.
5. **Sedatives should not be used** in shock as they depress central nervous system.
6. **Over-warming of the body should be prevented** as it causes cutaneous vasodilation and precipitates shock (Clinical Note 42.1).

Clinical Note 42.1

Body should not be covered in shock: In hemorrhagic shock, the skin is usually cold. There is a general practice to cover the body by blankets so that skin remains warm. But, it should never be done, as increased skin temperature causes cutaneous vasodilation and further precipitates shock. Rather, the body should be kept exposed.

Exam Questions

1. Describe the rapid compensatory mechanisms activated by hemorrhagic shock.
2. What is refractory shock. Briefly describe the mechanisms of irreversible shock.
3. What is reperfusion-induced injury. Briefly describe its mechanism and physiological basis of treatment
4. Briefly describe the physiological basis of management of shock.

Multiple Choice Questions

1. **All of the following are compensatory mechanisms of acute hemorrhagic shock, EXCEPT:**
   A. Increased secretion of vasopressin
   B. Increased secretion of cortisol
   C. Increased stimulation of baroreceptors
   D. Increased renal vasoconstriction
2. **The first to be activated as compensatory mechanism of hemorrhagic shock is:**
   A. Cushing reflex
   B. Chemoreceptor reflex
   C. Bainbridge reflex
   D. Baroreceptor reflex
3. **Which of the following is not a hypovolemic shock?**
   A. Blood loss during surgery
   B. Vomitting
   C. Acute myocardial infarction
   D. Adrenal insufficiency
4. **All of the following are features of refractory shock, EXCEPT:**
   A. Precapillary sphincters constrict and cause hypoxia
   B. Stimulation of medullary cardiorespiratory centers
   C. Release of endotoxins from bacteria
   D. Pulmonary microembolism
5. **Which should be avoided in treatment of shock?**
   A. Injection of dopamine
   B. Overwarming of the body
   C. Plasma transfusion
   D. Injection of catecholamines
6. **Which of the following is NOT an obstructive shock?**
   A. Heart failure
   B. Constrictive pericarditis
   C. Tension pneumothorax
   D. Cardiac tamponade
7. **Dopamine is drug of choice in:**
   A. Endotoxic shock
   B. Traumatic shock
   C. Distributive shock
   D. Neurogenic shock
8. **Which of the following is a distributive shock?**
   A. Cardiac arrythmias
   B. Diabetic ketoacidosis
   C. Anaphylaxis
   D. Adrenal insufficiency

Answers

1. C 2. D 3. C 4. B 5. B 6. A 7. B 8. C

Chapter 43

Pathophysiology of Heart Failure

Learning Objectives

On completion of study of this chapter:

The student will be able to (must know):

1. Define heart failure (HF) and classify various types of HF.
2. Understand the physiological basis of cardiac changes in HF due to pressure and volume overload.
3. List the features of heart failure.
4. Explain the physiological basis of orthopnea, paroxysmal nocturnal dyspnea and edema in HF.
5. Appreciate physiological basis of treatment of HF.

The student may also be able to (desirable to know):

1. Describe the cardiovascular changes in HF.

PY5.11

Heart failure **is defined as** a pathophysiologic state in which an abnormality of cardiac function results in inability of the heart to pump blood at a rate adequate for the requirements of the tissues of the body.

- It occurs either due to decreased myocardial contractility or due to an increased pressure or volume overload.

Types of Heart Failure

Heart failure has been classified in various ways.

Acute vs. Chronic Failure: Acute heart failure is seen following acute myocardial infarction or rupture of a heart valve.

- In acute failure, sudden decrease in cardiac output causes severe hypotension (therefore, edema is not a feature).
- In chronic failure, which occurs due to **a slowly progressive disease** like cardiomyopathy, or chronic valvular disease, blood pressure may be maintained (**edema in the dependent parts** is a feature).

Left-sided vs. Right-sided Failure: In left ventricular failure, the congestion occurs in the pulmonary circulation; therefore, ***dyspnea and orthopnea*** are common features.

- In right-sided failure, **congestion occurs in the systemic circulation**, therefore, ***increased JVP, hepatomegaly, and edema*** in the dependent parts are usual features.

High Output vs. Low Output Failure: In high output failure, heart pumps abnormally large quantities of blood to deliver adequate oxygen to the tissues. This occurs in severe anemia, hyperthyroidism, beriberi, arterio-venous fistula and Paget's disease.

- Low output failure occurs due to **failure of the heart to pump blood** (due to decreased myocardial contractility).

Forward vs. Backward Failure: In backward heart failure, the pressure and volume in the atrium and venous compartment behind the failed ventricle are more, therefore, edema occurs.

- In **forward heart failure**, inability of the ventricle to pump blood causes **tissue hypoxia** that increases renin secretion (due to renal hypoxia).
  - This activates **rennin-angiotensin-aldosterone axis**; therefore, edema (due to water retention) may be seen.
  - However, usually both forward as well as backward failures co-exist.

Systolic vs. Diastolic Failure: The systolic heart failure occurs due to the systolic ventricular dysfunction (decreased myocardial contractility).

- It is commonly seen in ischemic heart disease or due to dilated cardiomyopathy.
  - The systolic failure decreases blood supply to the tissues.
- The **diastolic failure** occurs due to the **failure of relaxation of the ventricle**.
  - This is usually seen in restrictive cardiomyopathy as seen in amyloidosis in which the heart muscle is

infiltrated by amyloid proteins.
- Due to inability of the ventricles to relax, the end-diastolic volume and therefore, cardiac output decreases.

Cardiac Changes In Heart Failure

Cardiac changes in heart failure depend on whether the failure is due to **pressure overload**, or **volume overload.**

Pressure Overload

In pressure overload, increased blood pressure **increases the afterload**. Heart pumps blood **against increased resistance**.

Early Stage: Increased afterload results in **concentric hypertrophy of the ventricles.**

- Ventricular wall thickening is more in comparison to cavity size (Fig. 43.1A).
- The ventricular function depends on the **stress exerted on the ventricle**.
  - According to **Laplace law**, stress in the ventricular wall is the product of pressure and radius of ventricular cavity divided by ventricular wall thickness.
  - Thus, ventricular **wall stress increases**.

Stage of Compensation (Concentric Hypertrophy): Wall stress normalizes due to increase in wall thickness and decrease in cavity radius of ventricle (Fig. 43.1B).

- Therefore, ventricular function is maintained.

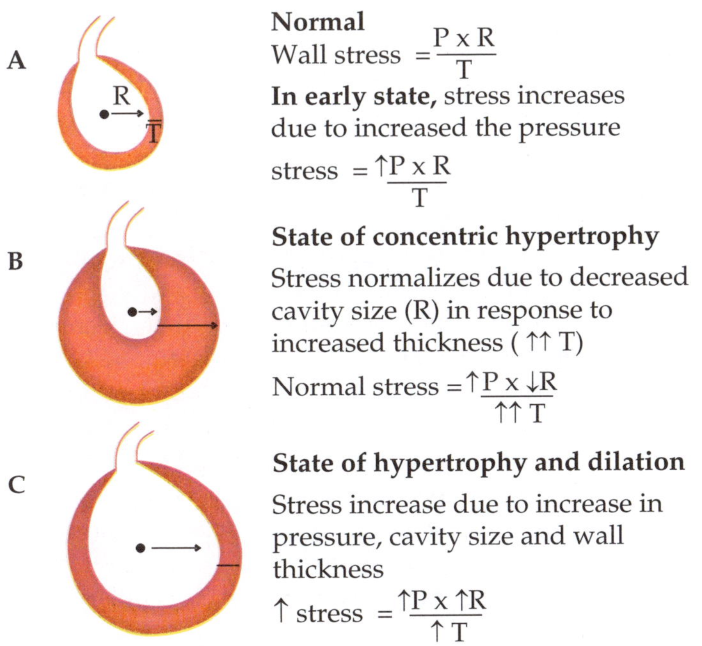

Figs. 43.1: Cardiac changes in heart failure due to pressure overload. **A:** Normal heart: Wall stress is the product of pressure (P) and radius of the ventricular cavity (R) divided by wall thickness (T). In early phase, ventricular pressure increases that increases wall stress. **B:** In later stage (the stage of compensation), wall stress normalizes due to greater increase in wall thickness that decreases cavity radius. **C:** In the stage of hypertrophy and dilation, wall stress increases due to proportionate increase in pressure, thickness, and radius. Thus, dilation of heart that increases wall stress heralds heart failure.

Stage of Hypertrophy & Dilatation: But in the stage of hypertrophy and dilatation, **ventricular stress increases** due to proportionate ***increase in radius*** caused by chamber dilation.

- This leads to failure of the myocardium to pump blood, causing **systolic failure** (Fig. 43.1C).
- *Pressure-volume curve* of left ventricle **shifts to right** (for details, refer Fig. 31.4, Chapter 31) that decreases ventricular ejection.

Volume Overload

In volume overload, due to **increased venous return**, diastolic pressure increases.

- This causes chamber enlargement that mainly results in **eccentric hypertrophy** (Fig. 43.2B).
- In volume overload, dilation of chamber occurs first to accommodate larger end-diastolic volume.

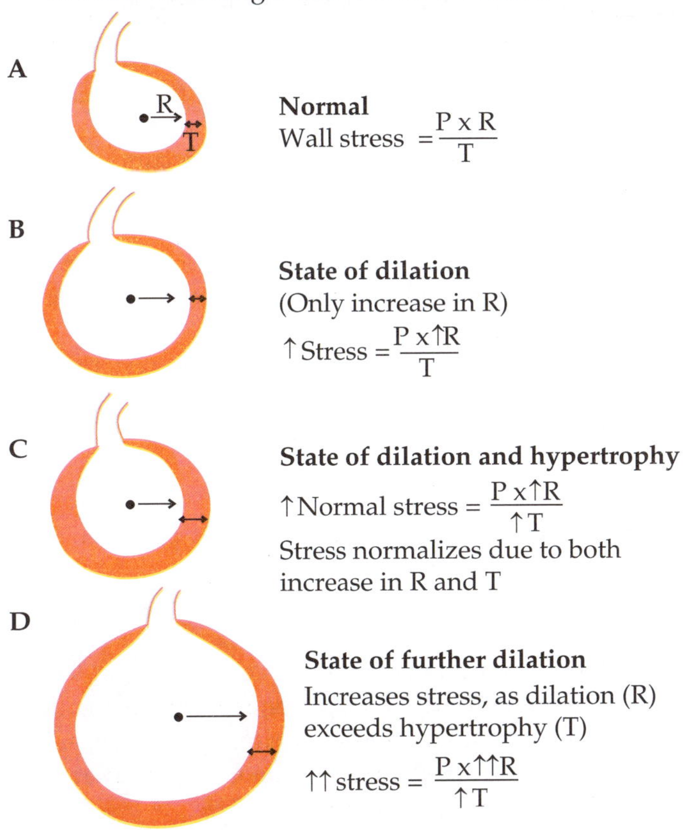

Figs. 43.2: Cardiac changes in heart failure due to volume overload. **A:** Normal heart; **B:** In early phase ventricle dilates to accommodate more blood, which increases wall stress due to increased cavity diameter. **C:** Eccentric hypertrophy (moderate increase in wall thickness) normalizes wall stress due to proportionate increase in radius and thickness. **D:** Due to further dilation (more cavity size), wall stress increases. Thus, increased dilation of heart heralds heart failure.

Early Stage (Stage of Dilation): In the early phase of volume overload, **wall stress increases** due to increased radius (dilation) of the ventricular chamber (Fig. 43.3B).

Stage of Eccentric Hypertrophy: Subsequently, **wall stress is normalized** due to increased wall thickness (eccentric hypertrophy), and decreased radius of the chamber (Fig. 43.2C).

- Thus, ventricular function is maintained in this stage.

- **Stage of Further Dilation:** Later, wall stress becomes more due to increased radius of ventricular chamber (further dilation) that finally causes heart failure (Fig. 43.2D).

A chronically dilated heart may develop ***muscle fibrosis and fail to relax*** properly causing **diastolic dysfunction** that shifts the *pressure-volume curve* of left ventricle **to the left** (for details, refer Fig. 31.5, Chapter 31).

IMPORTANT NOTE

Dilation of chambers causes pump failure: In ventricular failure due to either pressure overload or volume overload, **initially there will be ventricular hypertrophy and compensation**, but later dilatation of chambers occurs that causes heart failure.

- A dilated ventricle works more to pump the same amount of blood than the normal heart, as explained by **Laplace law** (for details, see chapter 34).
- Therefore, heart fails to pump adequate blood.

Clinical Features

Dyspnea

Dyspnea means **breathlessness**. This occurs due to failure of the left ventricle to pump blood effectively that produces tissue hypoxia.

In Early Stage: Dyspnea occurs during exercise (**dyspnea on exertion**) due to failure of left ventricular output to meet oxygen demand during exercise.

In Advanced Stage: **Dyspnea occurs at rest** due to increased pulmonary venous pressure, or due to gross inadequacy of ventricular pumping.

Orthopnea

Orthopnea means **dyspnea in recumbent position**. It is usually **relieved by sitting upright**.

The difficulty in breathing in supine posture occurs due to:

i) **Redistribution of blood** from abdomen and lower extremities into the chest during recumbency causes an increase in pulmonary hydrostatic pressure.
   - Pooling of blood in the pulmonary vascular bed adds to the already congested lungs.

ii) Reduction in vital capacity occurs as **diaphragm is pushed towards lungs** in supine position.
   - This is aggravated by hepatomegaly or ascites.

Paroxysmal Nocturnal Dyspnea

This is defined as **episodes of dyspnea and cough of sudden onset in nights** that usually awaken the patient from sleep.

- This occurs partly due to the **depression of respiratory centers during sleep** and partly to the ***accumulation of excess fluid in the lungs*** in recumbent posture in sleep.
  - During sleep, pulmonary venous pressure and pulmonary capillary pressure increase.
  - This results in **transudation of fluid into the air spaces.**
- Typically, the patient wakes up from sleep frightened with the feeling of breathlessness and choking, and usually sits upright or walks around.
  - He gets immediate relief as the ***pulmonary vascular congestion decreases in upright posture***.
  - He feels comfortable and then sleeps.
- However, after some time the same events are repeated and throughout night many such episodes occur **in paroxysms**.
  - Therefore, it is called paroxysmal dyspnea.
  - As it occurs in the night, it is also called paroxysmal **nocturnal** dyspnea.

Fatigue (Weakness & Exercise Intolerance)

This occurs due to **decreased cardiac output** that causes tissue hypoxia.

- The exercise intolerance occurs due to decreased perfusion of skeletal muscles and decreased oxygen supply to meet the need of the body.

Edema in the Dependent Parts

This is an important feature of congestive cardiac failure. Edema occurs in the lower parts of legs (ankle or **pedal edema**) in ambulatory patients, and in the sacral region (**sacral edema**) in bed-ridden patients.

Edema occurs due to **three mechanisms** (Flowchart 43.1):

1. Decreased cardiac output decreases blood volume. Hypovolemia stimulates **renin secretion**.
   - Renin facilitates **angiotensin II formation** that in turn increases aldosterone synthesis and secretion.
   - **Aldosterone** causes tubular reabsorption of sodium and water.
   - **Retention of water** in the body results in edema formation.
2. Decreased cardiac output also **increases sympathetic activity** that causes renal vasoconstriction.
   - This results in **decreased GFR** that decreases urinary excretion of sodium and water.
   - The **retention of water** causes edema formation.
3. Decreased ability of the heart to pump blood results in venous congestion (due to damming of blood in the venous compartment) and increases venous pressure.
   - This **increases capillary hydrostatic pressure** that increases capillary filtration.
   - Thus, edema results from increased capillary permeability.
   - In the dependent parts of the body, the capillary pressure increases further due to pooling of blood in the parts.

Therefore, dependent edema is a common feature of congestive cardiac failure.

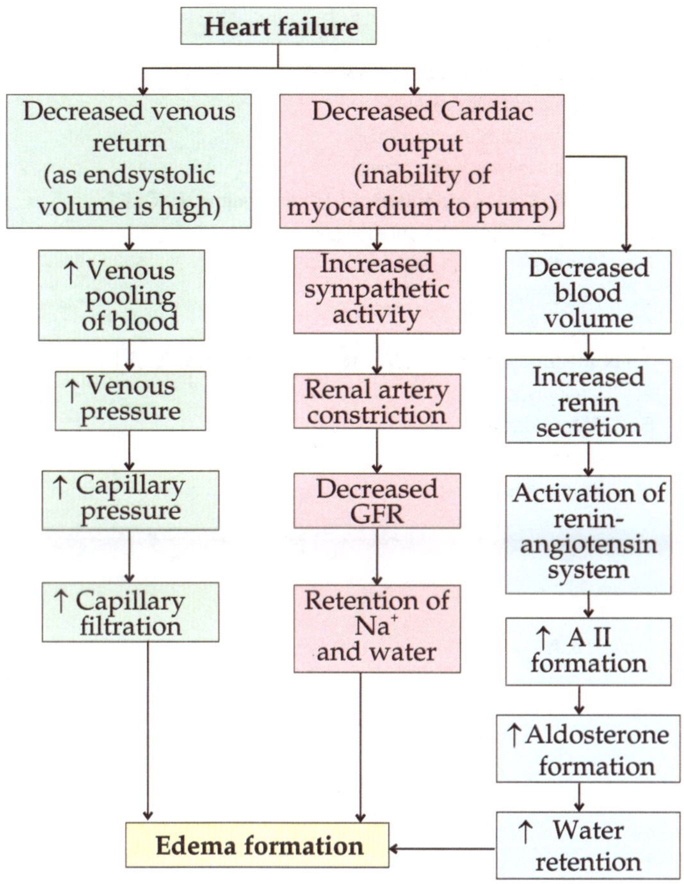

Flowchart 43.1: Mechanisms of edema formation in heart failure.

Hepatomegaly

This occurs due to hepatic congestion. **Tender hepatomegaly** is an important feature of right ventricular failure (and also of congestive cardiac failure).

Increased JVP

Jugular venous pressure is elevated due to increased right atrial pressure. Raised JVP is a reliable sign of congestive cardiac failure.

Ascites

Accumulation of excess of free fluid in peritoneal cavity is called ascites. This occurs in advanced stage of heart failure.

PHYSIOLOGICAL BASIS OF MANAGEMENT

1. **Rest:** Decreased physical activity decreases the demand on the heart.
   - Adequate rest decreases venous pressure and congestion.
2. **Diet:** A **salt restricted**, but a normal caloric diet is prescribed for heart failure patients.
   - Salt restriction decreases water retention.
3. **Digitalis:** Digitalis improves heart function by **its positive inotropic effect.** It increases myocardial contractility and therefore, cardiac output.
   - Digitalis acts by **inhibiting sodium potassium pump activity** on the myocardial cells.
     - Therefore, intracellular sodium increases, which is exchanged with extracellular calcium.
     - This results in increased calcium concentration in the cell that increases myocardial contractility (ref. Fig. 32.7, Chapter 32).
4. **Diuretics:** Diuretics **promote water excretion.**
   - By decreasing ECF volume, diuretics decrease venous return to the heart. This decreases load on the heart.
5. **Vasodilators:** Vasodilators decrease peripheral resistance (afterload).
   - Therefore, cardiac output increases.
6. **ACE inhibitors:** ACE inhibitors prevent the formation of angiotensin II.
7. **Angiotensin receptor antagonists:** Angiotensin antagonist such as losartan prevents the action of angiotensin on blood vessel.
8. **Treatment for the primary cause:** Removal of precipitating factors and correction of underlying cause of heart failure should be initiated along with other modalities.

Exam Questions

1. Briefly describe cardiac changes in heart failure. Explain the physiological basis of management of heart failure.
2. Describe the mechanisms of paroxysmal nocturnal dyspnea and edema formation in heart failure.

Multiple Choice Questions

1. **Which is not a mechanism of edema formation in heart failure?**
   A. Increased aldosterone formation
   B. Retention of sodium and water
   C. Increased capillary hydrostatic pressure
   D. Decreased oncotic pressure

2. **Which of the following is not correct about heart failure?**
   A. JVP is not affected in right-sided heart failure.
   B. Congestion in systemic circulation is the main pathophysiology in right-sided failure
   C. Dyspnea and orthopnea are common in left sided heart failure
   D. Pulmonary congestion is the main pathophysiology in left-sided failure

3. **In volume overload failure:**
   A. Ventricular wall stress is more in the stage of dilation and hypertrophy
   B. Ventricular wall stress is normal in advanced stage of dilation
   C. Dilation of ventricle occurs from the early stage
   D. Venous return is normal
4. **Which of the following is a high output failure?**
   A. Chronic valvular disease
   B. AMI
   C. Beriberi
   D. Cardiac amyloidosis
5. **All are true about pressure overload failure EXCEPT:**
   A. Ventricular wall stress is more in early part
   B. In the phase of dilation, wall stress remains normal
   C. The afterload is high
   D. Concentric hypertrophy normalizes wall stress in the stage of compensation
6. **Digitalis acts by:**
   A. Decreasing hydrostatic pressure
   B. Increasing oncotic pressure
   C. Decreasing capillary permeability
   D. Inhibiting Na+-K+ pump activity
7. **All of the following are treatment of heart failure, EXCEPT:**
   A. Angiotensin receptor antagonists
   B. Diuretics
   C. Vasoconstrictors
   D. Salt-restricted diet
8. **All of the following are high output heart failure, EXCEPT:**
   A. Cardiomyopathy
   B. Paget's disease
   C. Arteriovenous fistula
   D. Severe anemia

Answers

1. D 2. A 3. C 4. C 5. B 6. D 7. C 8. A

Section VI

Respiratory System

"A spiritual atmosphere is more important than outer conditions; if one can get that and also create one's own spiritual air to breathe in and live in it, that is the true condition of progress.

Sri Aurobindo"

Chapter 44

Functional Organization of Respiratory System

Learning Objectives

On completion of study of this chapter:

The student will be able to (must know):

1. Name different phases of respiration and understand their significance.
2. Name the parts of respiratory tract and give their functions.
3. Learn the division of airways and significance of their modifications.
4. Comprehend the reflections and functions of pleura and pleural cavity.
5. Comprehend the concept of a bronchopulmonary segment.
6. List the functions of lungs and the respiratory system.
7. Name the non-respiratory functions of lungs

The student may also be able to (desirable to know):

1. Describe the functions of upper and lower respiratory tract
2. Describe the modifications in respiratory zone and conducting zone

Respiration is defined as the process by which oxygen from atmosphere is delivered to the tissue and carbon dioxide from the tissue is removed into the atmosphere.

Phages of Respiration: Respiration takes place in **four phases** (Fig. 44.1).

Ventilation phase: **Exchange of gases** between the atmosphere and pulmonary capillary blood occurs due to **pulmonary ventilation**.

Transport phase: **Gasses are transported** between the lungs and the tissues.

Exchange phase: **Gases are exchanged** between the systemic blood and the tissue.

Tissue phase: Oxygen delivered to the tissue is **utilized by the mitochondrial enzymes** for metabolism (**cellular respiration**).

PY6.1

COMPONENTS OF RESPIRATORY SYSTEM

Respiratory system is divided **into two parts**: upper respiratory tract and lower respiratory tract (Fig. 44.2).

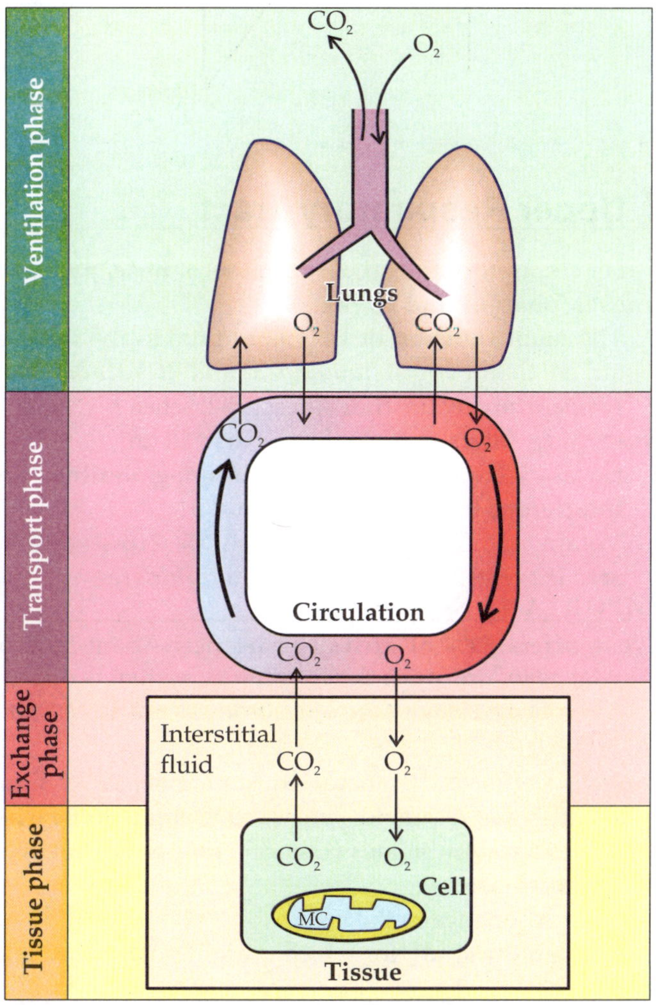

Fig. 44.1: Phases of respiration. Entire process of respiration takes place in four stages. In ventilation stage, gases (O_2 and CO_2) are exchanged with pulmonary capillary blood through lungs. In transport stage, gases are transported between lungs and tissues via circulation. In exchange stage, exchange of O_2 and CO_2 takes between systemic circulation and tissues. In tissue stage, O_2 is taken up by cells and utilized by mitochondria (MC) for oxidation during which CO_2 is produced and released into tissue capillary blood.

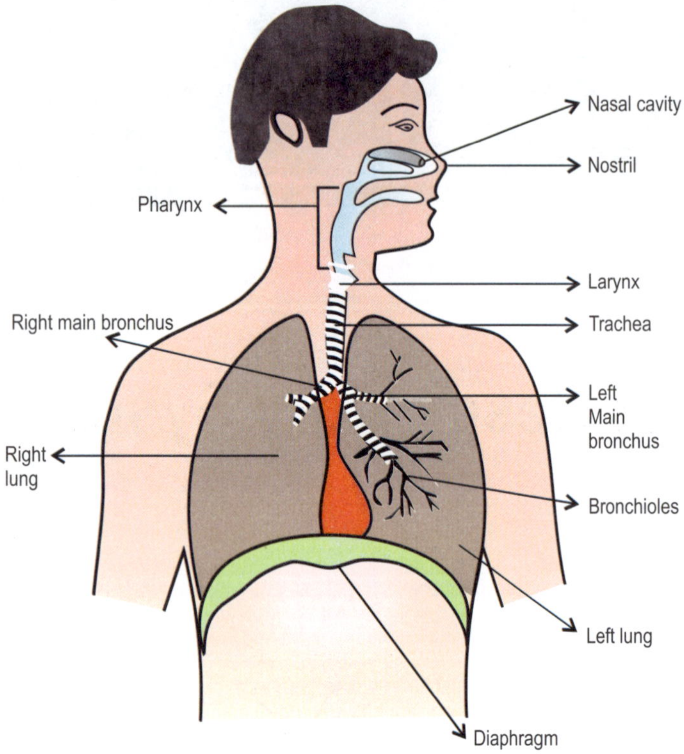

Fig. 44.2: Components of respiratory system.

Upper Respiratory Tract

Upper respiratory tract (URT) consists of **nose, paranasal sinuses, pharynx and larynx**.

- The **main function** of URT is to process the inspired air so that it gets ***humidified and it attains body temperature*** by the time it reaches trachea.

Nose: Nose **filters particle** greater than 10 μm.

- Nasal secretion contains **immunoglobulins and interferons** that kill the organisms.
- Volume of nose is only 20 ml, but the **cross-sectional area is greatly increased** by nasal ***turbinates***.

IMPORTANT NOTE

Nose offers 50% of airway resistance: About 50% of resistance to airflow in the respiratory system is offered by nose. The resistance *increases during viral infections* like common cold.

Paranasal Sinuses: Paranasal sinuses are maxillary sinus, sphenoid sinus, ethmoid sinus and frontal sinus. They open into nasal turbinates (Clinical Note 44.1) They have **three functions**:

1. Offer **resonance** to the voice
2. **Lighten the skull**, for which upright posture becomes easier.

Clinical Note 44.1

Sinusitis: Paranasal sinuses open into the nasal turbinates through their ostia. During inflammation and edema of nasal mucosa, the ostia of sinuses are readily blocked. This results in retention of secretions in the sinuses that in turn causes sinusitis.

3. Provide **protection to brain** during facial trauma.

Pharynx: Pharynx is divided into nasopharynx, oropharynx and laryngopharynx.

1. ***Nasopharynx*** is located behind the nose and extends from posterior nares to the level of soft palate. Eustachian tubes and posterior nares open into nasopharynx. Infection of nasopharynx is common (Clinical Note 44.2).
2. ***Oropharynx*** is located behind the mouth from soft palate above to the level of hyoid bone below.
3. ***Laryngopharynx*** starts from the level of hyoid bone above and opens into esophagus.

Clinical Note 44.2

URTI: Upper respiratory tract infection (URTI) is an acute **nasopharyngitis** manifesting as cold, and usually a self-limiting viral infection. However, secondary bacterial infection may spread to sinuses (sinusitis) and larynx (laryngitis), which warrants antibiotic treatment.

Larynx and Glottis: Larynx consists of **epiglottis, arytenoids and vocal cords**.

- **Epiglottis** and **arytenoids** cover the vocal cord during deglutition that **prevents aspiration of food particles** into the respiratory tract.
  - In children, **arytenoids** enlarge during infections, and cause **obstruction to air flow**.

Muscles of larynx are innervated by ***vagal fibers***.

- The abductor muscles in the larynx contract in the early part of inspiration that pulls vocal cord wide apart and **open the glottis**.
- **During swallowing**, reflex contraction of adductor muscles close the glottis, which ***prevents entry of food materials*** into the respiratory tract.

IMPORTANT NOTE

Aspiration pneumonia in unconscious patients: In unconscious and anesthetized patients, incomplete closure of glottis allows fluid and food particles enter the lungs and cause aspiration pneumonia.

- Paralysis of adductors of larynx produces stridor during inspiration (inspiratory stridor) and produces aspiration pneumonia.

Lower Respiratory Tract

The lower respiratory tract consists of **airway tree and lungs**.

Airway Tree

A series of branching tubes constitute airway tree. The tubes decrease in diameter at each branching.

- **Trachea,** the main airway branches into **two bronchi**.
  - Each bronchus enters a lung and branches many times into progressively smaller bronchi, which in turn form **bronchioles**.
  - This system of tubes is called **tracheobronchial**

tree.

- Trachea and bronchi contain **cartilages**, and their smooth muscle content is relatively less.
    - Trachea and bronchi are lined by a **ciliated epithelium** that contains numerous mucous and serous glands.
    - In respiratory tract, **cilia** are present till respiratory bronchioles, but glands are absent in bronchioles and terminal bronchioles.
- **Bronchioles and terminal bronchioles** have adequate smooth muscles and the **quantity of smooth muscle** as % of wall thickness in respiratory tract is **maximum in terminal bronchiole.**
- Cartilages are absent from bronchioles downward in the airway.

Bronchial Tone: Tone of smooth muscles of bronchi is called bronchial tone. This contributes to **patency of bronchi** and aids in respiration.

- Though bronchial tone is mainly due to neural influence, it is considerably influenced by chemicals and hormones such as inflammatory modulators, cytokines, adenosine, substance P, histamine and VIP.
- **Bronchodilation** is produced by ***sympathetic stimulation*** and **bronchoconstriction** by ***vagal stimulation***.
- There is a **circadian rhythm** for bronchial tone with maximum dilation occurring at 6 PM and maximum constriction occurring at 6 AM.

Generation Numbers: The progressively bifurcating airways are designated by their generation numbers. Trachea is the zero generation. The left and right main bronchi are the first generation.

As the generation number increases, the following changes occur:

1. The airways become smaller, narrower and shorter.
2. The amount of cilia decreases.
3. The number of mucus secreting cells decreases.
4. The quantity of submucosal glands becomes less.
5. The amount of cartilage in the airway wall decreases.
6. The quantity of smooth muscle increases.

Branching of Airways

Airways progressively branch 23 times (23 generations of airways).

- They are broadly divided into ***two categories***: conducting airways that move air by convection into the gas exchange areas of lungs (*conducting zone*) and respiratory airways that participate in gas exchange (*respiratory zone*).

Conducting Zone

The trachea and first 16 generations of airway form the conducting zone (Fig. 44.3).

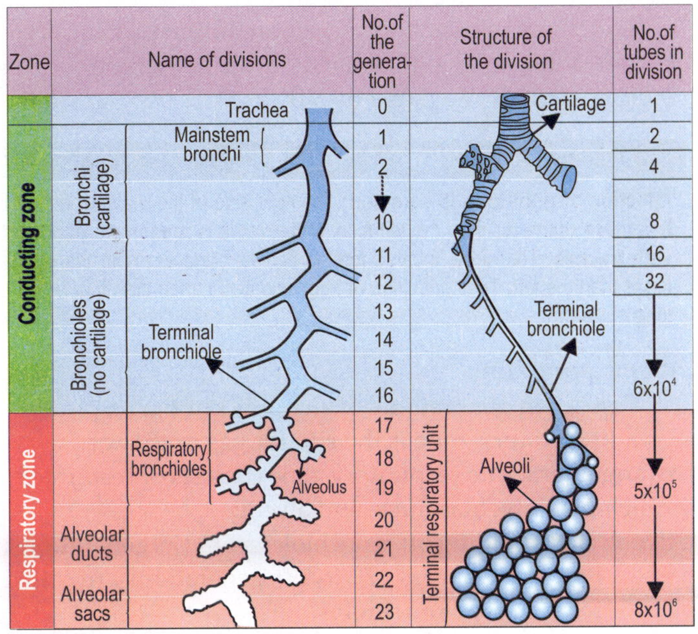

Fig. 44.3: Divisions of airways and their characteristics. Note the differences between conducting and respiratory airways.

Structural Specialization: The considerable amount of **cartilage is present in first four generations** of the conducting zone. This **prevents collapse** of these airways as they are subjected to changes in thoracic pressures.

- Some amount of cartilage is present **upto 10th generation**, upto which the airways are referred to as bronchi.
    - Right side main bronchus is wider (Clinical Note 44.3).
- The **cartilage is absent totally** in the bronchioles and below the level of bronchioles. The smallest airways in the conducting zone are the terminal bronchioles.
    - Though bronchioles lack cartilage, ***elasticity of the lung tissue maintains their patency*** as they are suspended by elastic tissue of the lung parenchyma.
    - However, bronchioles are *susceptible to collapse especially during expiration*.
- As there is no alveoli upto 16th generation, **gas exchange does not occur** in the conducting zone.
    - Therefore, the volume of respiratory tract starting from nose to the generation-16 airways is called anatomic **dead space.**

Nerve Supply: The bronchi and bronchioles are innervated by ANS.

1. **Vagal stimulation** causes **bronchoconstriction** mediated by muscarinic receptors that are plentily available in bronchial tree.
2. **Sympathetic stimulation** causes **bronchodilation**, mediated by **β_2 receptors** that are present in bronchial epithelium and smooth muscle.
    - Activation of β_2 receptors increases bronchial secretion and α_2 receptors inhibits secretion.

3. Also, there is **noncholinergic-nonadrenergic innervation** of bronchiole that causes bronchodilation, which is most likely mediated by VIP.

Clinical Note 44.3

Infection of right lung is common: The right side of the main bronchus has **more diameter** than the left side. Moreover, it is **present in parallel with trachea**. Therefore, inhaled foreign bodies lodge easily in the right lungs than the left. Thus, infection of right lung is common than that of left lung.

Respiratory Zone

The last seven generations of airway form the respiratory zone. Respiratory zone is the **site for gas exchange**.

Arrangement: The respiratory zone consists of respiratory bronchioles, alveolar ducts and alveoli.

Alveoli start budding off bronchioles from 17th generations.

- Bronchioles from 17th to 19th generations are called **respiratory bronchioles**.
- With each descending generation, number of alveoli increases.

Generations 20–22 are the **alveolar ducts** that finally terminate in the alveolar sac (generation 23).

Alveolus: Alveolus is the **functional unit of gas exchange**. There are about **300 million of alveoli** present in both the lungs in adults (Application Box 44.1). Diameter of alveoli ranges from 75 to 300 μm.

- The **total surface area** of all alveoli of both lungs is between **50 to 100 m²**, which is roughly **the size of a tennis court**.
- Thus, alveoli are amongst the **largest biological membranes** in the body.
- The alveoli are surrounded by capillaries that remain in close contact with each other forming **alveolar-capillary membrane** through which gas exchange takes place.

Alveolar epithelium is lined by **epithelial cells** that are of *two types*: Type I and Type II.

- **Type I epithelial cells** are present in more numbers and cover 95% of epithelial surface area of alveoli.
- **Type II cells** secrete **surfactant** and play important role in alveolar repair.

Application Box 44.1

Alveolar damage should be checked: Alveoli increase in number and size during childhood. However, **after adolescence, alveoli increase only in size**, but not in number. Therefore, destruction of alveoli results in permanent damage to lungs as they have limited ability to repair themselves in adults.

The Lungs

Pleura

Pleura is the covering of lungs. There are **two layers** of pleura: parietal pleura and visceral pleura (Fig. 44.4).

1. The **parietal pleura** is the outer layer of pleural sac that contains blood vessels.
2. The **visceral pleura** lies directly on the lung.
3. Normally, about **10–20 ml** of fluid is present in the **pleural cavity**, the space between the parietal pleura and visceral pleura (Clinical Note 44.4).

Pleural Fluid: The viscous pleural fluid forms a lining of about 10 μm thick between the two layers of pleura, which **functions as a lubricant** so that lungs can slide against the chest wall.

- Thus, pleural fluid **facilitates the change in size and shape** of lungs during respiration.
- It also **protects lungs** from external damage.

Clinical Note 44.4

Pleural effusion: Accumulation of pleural fluid in excess in the pleural cavity is called as **pleural effusion**. Significant pleural effusion limits lung expansion and decreases gas exchange. Entry of air into the pleural cavity that occurs either due to trauma or rupture of alveoli results in **pneumothorax**, and entry of blood is called **hemothorax**.

Lobes of Lungs

Lungs are divided into lobes. There are **three lobes in right lung** and **two lobes in left lung**.

- The right lung constitutes about 55% of the total lung mass and function.
- Lungs consist of vascular tree and airway tree that are embedded in elastic connective tissue, the lung parenchyma.

Bronchopulmonary Segments

Bronchopulmonary segment is the **part of the lungs supplied by a segmental bronchus**.

1. There are 10 bronchopulmonary segments in right lung and nine segments in left lung.
   - These are apical, posterior, anterior, lateral, medial (inferior), superior, medial-basal, anterior-basal, lateral-basal, and posterior-basal.

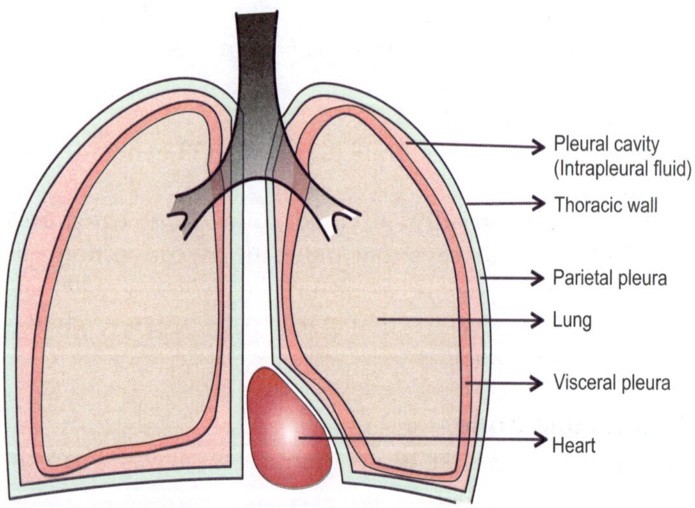

Fig. 44.4: Layers of pleura, and pleural cavity.

2. Each bronchopulmonary segment **is anatomically a single functional unit**.
   - Therefore, normally a disease process involves a bronchopulmonary segment at a time.

FUNCTIONS OF RESPIRATORY SYSTEM

Functions of respiratory system including lungs can be broadly divided into **respiratory and nonrespiratory functions**.

Respiratory Functions

1. **Gas exchange:** Lungs are the central structures in respiration. Inhalation of oxygen into the body and removal of carbon dioxide from the body take place through lungs.
2. **Regulation of blood pH:** By controlling carbon dioxide output from the body, lungs control plasma bicarbonate concentration. Therefore, lungs play an important **role in acid-base balance**.

Non-respiratory Functions

1. **Left ventricular reservoir:** The entire cardiac output from right ventricle is pumped into pulmonary circulation.
   - Due to their high compliance, pulmonary vessels normally accommodate about ***0.5 liter of blood*** at any given time.
   - This serves as reservoir for left ventricular filling.
2. **Filtering small emboli from blood:** Venous blood normally contains microemboli of blood clots, fats or air bubbles. These emboli escape into systemic arterial circulation, tissue damage may occur.
   - Pulmonary vasculature **traps and removes these emboli** before they get the chance to enter the systemic circulation.
3. **Biochemical functions:** Many chemical substances are **removed in the lungs**.
   - Substances that are removed by lungs are: ***PGE_1, PGE_2, $PGF_{2\alpha}$, leukotrienes, serotonin and bradykinin.***
4. **Olfactory function:** Breathing is essential for **delivering odorants** from the environment to the olfactory epithelium.
   - Olfaction is required for *many physiological activities* including **limbic functions**.
5. **Processing of inhaled air:** **Filtration of inhaled air** in the conducting airways is a respiratory function. This prevents entry of toxic substances and infective organisms into the body.
   - Conducting airways filter these particles and expel them in expired air.
   - **Warming and moisturizing of inhaled** air by the conducting airways help to prevent alveolar damage.
6. **Endocrine Functions:** **Angiotensin converting enzyme** is mainly secreted by endothelium of pulmonary blood vessels that converts angiotensin I to angiotensin II, which occurs in pulmonary circulation.
   - Few **local hormones** such as **prostaglandins and histamine** are also synthesized by lungs.
7. **Defense functions:** Defence functions are carried out by following mechanisms:
   i) Organisms that enter the lungs are phagocytosed by **pulmonary alveolar macrophages (dust cells)** or ***interstitial macrophages*** in the lung.
   - Particles less than 2 μm diameter reach alveoli where they are phagocytosed by alveolar macrophages.
   - Particles with 2-10 μm diameter are generally removed by conducting airways.
   - Particles more than 10 μm diameter are removed by hairs in the nostrils.

   ii) **Ig A** present in bronchial secretions provide resistance to infection.
   iii) Epithelium of lungs contains **protease activated receptors** that on activation releases PGE_2, which in turn protects pulmonary epithelial cells.
8. **Metabolic functions:** Lungs perform several metabolic functions.
   i) ***Synthesis:*** Synthesize surfactant
   ii) ***Lysis:*** Lyse clot (local fibrinolytic system)
   iii) ***Synthesis & release***: Synthesize and release following chemicals (local hormones) into systemic circulation:
   - Histamine
   - Kallikrein
   - Prostaglandins

   iv) ***Removal from blood:*** Lungs *do not metabolize* epinephrine, dopamine, oxytocin, gastrin, ADH & angiotensin II.
   - However, lungs **partially remove** prostaglandins, bradykinin, adenosine, serotonin, acetylcholine and norepinephrine from blood.
9. **Speech:** **Phonation** is achieved by larynx.
   - **Larynx acts as a vibrator** and the vibrating elements are the vocal folds.
   - During phonation, vocal cords move together so that passage of air between them will cause vibration.
   - Movement of air in the respiratory passage helps in the improvement of voice.

IMPORTANT NOTE

Voice Paralysis in Acute Laryngitis: Voice becomes thick with nasal intonation in nasopharyngitis and nasal obstruction. Paralysis of voice occurs in acute laryngitis.

Symbols used in Respiratory Physiology

Symbols widely accepted and commonly used in respiratory physiology are:

A : Alveolar
a : Arterial (systemic)
aw : airway
B : Barometric
C : Concentration or content in a liquid
c : Pulmonary capillary
D : Diffusion capacity
E : Expired
F : Fraction
f : Respiratory frequency
I : Inspired
P : Pressure
Q : Flow of blood
R : Resistance
S : Saturation of hemoglobin
V : Volume of gas
$\dot{V}$: Rate of ventilation (volume of gas/unit time)
v : Venous (systemic)
V : Mixed systemic venous

Exam Questions

1. Describe functions of paranasal sinuses, nasopharynx, oropharynx and laryngopharynx.
2. Which parts of the airway are known as conducting zone and respiratory zone and what are their functions?
3. What is bronchial tone and how is it controlled?
4. Describe the nonrespiratory functions of lungs.

Multiple Choice Questions

1. All of the following are stages of respiration, EXCEPT:
A. Tissue stage
B. Transport stage
C. Exchange sage
D. Dynamic stage

2. Which of the following is not a part of upper respiratory tract?
A. Pharynx
B. Larynx
C. Trachea
D. Glottis

3. Which of the following is not a function of nose?
A. Offers about 50% of resistance to airflow
B. The volume of nose is about 20 ml
C. Nose filters particles more than 10μm
D. Nasal secretion does not contain immunoglobulins and interferons

4. All are functions of paranasal sinuses EXCEPT:
A. Offer resonance to the voice
B. Lighten the skull
C. Purifies inhaling air
D. Protection to brain during facial trauma

5. Which of the following is not correct about larynx?
A. Larynx is part of upper respiratory tract
B. Laryngeal muscles are supplied by vagal fibers
C. Contraction of abductor muscle of larynx in early part of inspiration pulls vocal cord wide apart and open the glottis
D. Paralysis of abductor muscles produces aspiration pneumonia

6. Which of the following is not true about bronchial tone?
A. Circadian rhythm causes maximum bronchodilation at 6AM
B. Sympathetic stimulation produces bronchodilation
C. Bronchoconstriction is produced by vagal stimulation
D. Entry of cool air into bronchus during exercise may induce bronchoconstriction

7. All are true about airways EXCEPT:
A. There is considerable cartilage in first four zones.
B. Cartilage totally absent in bronchioles
C. Amount of cilia increases with the increase in generation number of airways
D. Number of mucus secreting cells decreases with the increase in generation number of airways

8. Which of the following is not true about alveoli?
A. Type II alveolar epithelial cells secrete surfactant
B. Diameter of alveoli is less than 50μm
C. Type I alveolar epithelial cells are more in number than Type II alveolar epithelial cells
D. Alveolar macrophages are phagocytes in lungs

9. Which of the following is not a function of respiratory system?
A. Reservoir of blood for right ventricle
B. Assist in phonation
C. Help in conversion of Angiotensin I to Angiotensin II
D. Synthesis and release of some quantity of histamine

10. All of the following statements are true for respiratory zone, EXCEPT:
A. Formed by last seven generations of airways
B. Consists of the respiratory bronchioles, alveolar ducts and alveoli
C. Generations 18-20 are alveolar ducts that terminate in alveolar sac
D. It is the site of gas exchange

Answers

1. D 2. B 3. D 4. C 5. D 6. A 7. C 8. B 9. A 10. C

Chapter 45

PY6.2

Mechanics of Breathing

Learning Objectives

On completion of study of this chapter:

The student will be able to (must know):

1. List the muscles of inspiration and expiration and give their mechanism of action.
2. Explain the alveolar and intrapleural pressure changes during quiet inspiration and expiration.
3. Define lung volumes and capacities and give their normal values.
4. Define lung compliance and describe the factors affecting it.
5. Understand the mechanical properties of lungs and chest wall.
6. List the composition and functions of lung surfactant and name factors affecting its synthesis.
7. Understand the factors affecting airway resistance.
8. Draw pressure-volume curve of lung during forced expiration and inspiration.
9. Define timed-vital capacity and explain its difference in obstructive and restrictive lung diseases.
10. Define and give normal values of various dynamic lung volumes and capacities.

The student may also be able to (desirable to know):

1. Draw relaxation pressure-volume curve of the lung, chest wall and respiratory system and explain its application in lung mechanics.
2. Describe the regulation of surfactant synthesis and explain the role of surfactant in functions and dysfunction of the lung.
3. Explain the factors affecting airway resistance and the application of flow-volume curve.

Mechanics of breathing is study of physical properties of the lungs, airways, and chest wall involved in the physiology of respiration.

- Normally during quiet breathing, **inspiration is an active process**, which occurs due to contraction of inspiratory muscles and **expiration is a passive phenomenon** that occurs due to elastic recoil of the lungs.
- However, **forced expiration is assisted by contraction of expiratory muscles**.

MUSCLES OF RESPIRATION

Muscles of Inspiration

Muscles of inspiration cause expansion of chest and increase the elastic recoil of chest wall. This makes the **intrapleural pressure more negative** that helps in expansion of the lungs due to which the air is sucked in. The inspiratory muscles are divided into **two categories**: primary and secondary (accessory).

Primary Muscles of Inspiration

The **diaphragm and external intercostal muscles** are primary muscles of inspiration.

Diaphragm

The diaphragm is the main muscle of inspiration, which is a skeletal muscle. Inflation of the lungs is caused primarily by contraction of the diaphragm.

Mechanism of Action of Diaphragm

Contraction of diaphragm expands thoracic cavity in two ways.

1. The diaphragm is dome shaped and attached to the lower six ribs & the xiphoid process of the sternum.
   - Thus, when it contracts, the dome is flattened, and abdominal contents are pushed downward so that the *thoracic cavity enlarges* in its rostro-caudal extent.

IMPORTANT NOTE

Diaphragm can descend > 10 cm: During quiet respiration, the diaphragm moves towards abdomen by about 1 to 2 cm. However, **during forced inspiration,** descent of diaphragm occurs by about 10 to 12 cm that greatly increases the thoracic volume.

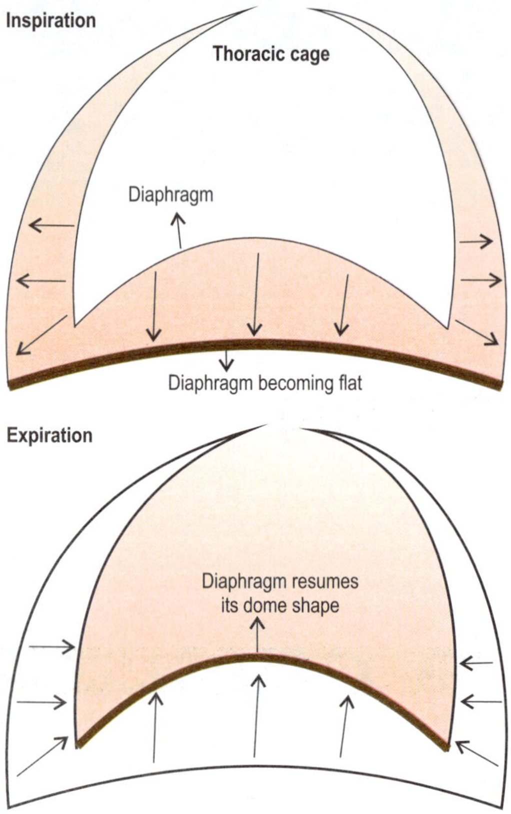

Fig. 45.1: Enlargement of thoracic cage in both vertical and lateral diameters during inspiration occurs due to contraction of diaphragm. Note dome of diaphragm becomes flat during inspiration that pushes abdominal content downward and increases rostro-caudal diameter of thorax. During expiration, relaxation of diaphragm brings back its dome shape and decreases thoracic cage capacity.

- Thus, the vertical diameter of thoracic cage increases (Fig. 45.1).

2. Contraction of diaphragm also pushes the rib cage outward that enlarges the thoracic cavity in its antero-posterior and lateral planes.

Clinical Significance

Inspiration is **significantly compromised** in following conditions.

1. Moderate to **severe obesity, pregnancy** (in third trimester), and **tight clothing** around thoracic and abdominal walls decrease lung expansion by reducing the effectiveness of diaphragm in enlarging the thoracic cage.
2. **Lesion of phrenic nerve** (C_3–C_5) results in paralysis of part of diaphragm of that side.

- In phrenic nerve damage, the portion of **diaphragm of that side moves up** rather than coming down during inspiration. This grossly impairs ventilation.

IMPORTANT NOTE

Pranayama increases thoracic cage expansion: By practice of controlled breathing (pranayamic breathing), magnitude of diaphragmatic contraction and expansion of rib cage are greatly increased. Pranayama considerably increases vital capacity.

External Intercostals

External intercostal muscles are present obliquely between ribs in forward and downward direction.

- Their attachment to lower ribs is more forward from the axis of rotation.
- Therefore, contraction of external intercostal muscles **raises the lower ribs adequately**.

Contraction of external intercostal muscles has **two effects**:

1. The **transverse and antero-posterior diameters of the thorax increase**. This occurs by following ***two mechanisms***.
   i) The 2nd to 10th ribs rotate upward and outward by a movement similar to the movement of the handle of a bucket (**bucket-handle effect**).
   - This increases the **transverse diameter** of the thoracic cavity (Fig. 45.2A).

   ii) The upper 4 ribs rotate the sternum in upward and outward direction by a movement similar to the handle of a water-pump (**pump-handle effect)** (Fig. 45.2B).
   - This mainly **increases the vertical diameter** of thoracic cage though antero-posterior diameter also increases to some extent.
2. The rib cage and the tissues between the ribs **become stiff**. This helps the thoracic cage to withstand better the increasingly negative intrapleural pressure.

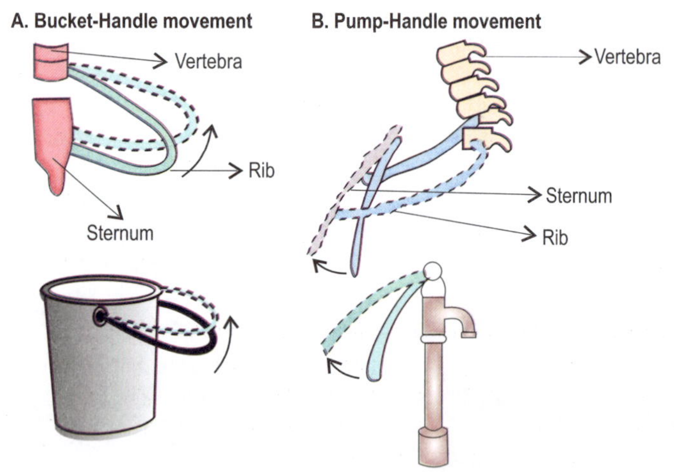

Figs. 45.2: Mechanism of bucket-handle (A) and pump-handle (B) movements of ribs of thoracic cage. Note bucket-handle effect increases transverse diameter and pump-handle effect increases vertical diameter of thoracic cage.

Accessory Muscles of Inspiration

Accessory muscles assist in forced inspiration. These are:

1. **Scalenes:** The scalene muscles of the neck are *inserted into the upper two ribs*.
   - They are brought into play during deep breathing.
   - They **elevate the upper part of rib cage** to further increase the thoracic volume.
2. **Sternocleidomastoids:** Sternocleidomastoids are inserted *into the upper two ribs and top of the sternum*.

- These muscles lift the sternum outward and elevate the rib cage.
- This **contributes to the pump-handle effect** and increases the thoracic volume.

3. **Neck and back muscles:** Contraction of neck and back muscles during forced respiration increase thoracic volume in *two ways*.
   i) They **elevate the pectoral girdle** that increases the cross-sectional area of the thorax.
   ii) They **extend the back** that increases the vertical length of the thorax.

Some important muscles of neck and back that assist forced respiration are posterior muscles of the neck, digastric muscles, mylohyoid, and posterior muscles of the upper back.

4. **Muscles of upper respiratory tract:** Contraction of **alae nasi, levator palati, cheek muscles** and other muscles of upper respiratory passage **decrease airway resistance**. Thus, they facilitate inspiration.

Muscles of Expiration

No Primary Muscles of Expiration: Expiration is a simpler process. During inspiration, lungs undergo elastic expansion.

- At the end of inspiration, the **elastic recoil of the lungs** helps lungs deflate, which results in expiration.
- Thus, quiet expiration is purely a passive process.
- Therefore, there are **no primary muscles of expiration**.

Accessory Muscles of Expiration: Muscles come into play **during forced expiration**, and they are called **accessory muscles of expiration** that include abdominal muscles, internal intercostals, and neck and back muscles.

1. ***Abdominal muscles:*** Muscles of abdominal wall that take part in expiration are **internal oblique, external oblique, and transverse abdominis.**
   - Contraction of these muscles **increases intra-abdominal pressure** and pushes diaphragm upward into the chest cavity.
   - This *decreases rostro-caudal diameter* of thorax and **increases intrapleural pressure**.
2. ***Internal intercostals:*** Internal intercostal muscles **pull the rib cage downward** and *decrease thoracic volume* both in antero-posterior and transverse diameter (opposite actions of external intercostal muscles).
   - These muscles are especially helpful for forced expiration during coughing, vomiting, and strenuous-defecation.
3. ***Neck and back muscles:*** Muscles of neck and back that lower the pectoral girdle **decrease cross-sectional area** of the thorax, and muscles that flex the trunk **decrease rostro-caudal diameter** of the chest cavity.

IMPORTANT NOTE

Few important points should be noted for muscles of expiration.

During forced inspiration, accessory muscles are used to **increase lung volume** rather than to overcome the resistance to airflow, whereas **during forced expiration** accessory muscles are used mainly **to overcome the resistance to airflow**.

1. Quiet expiration is purely passive. However, exception to this is the **individuals suffering from lung diseases like bronchial asthma** in whom airway resistance is high. They require active participation of expiratory muscles even in normal expiration.
2. The strength of expiratory muscles is important in **endurance trainings** like running etc. Therefore, for long-distance runners, physical exercises are advocated **to strengthen their abdominal and chest muscles** as part of their training programmes.
3. **Pranayamas** (yogic breathings) primary enhance the functions of expiratory muscles.

PRESSURE CHANGES DURING BREATHING

Pressures in the Thoracic Cavity

Changes in different pressures in the thoracic cavity that result in breathing are:

1. Intrapleural pressure
2. Transmural pressures
3. Alveolar pressure

Intrapleural Pressure

The pressure **in the pleural space** is the intrapleural pressure.

How is Intrapleural Pressure created & why is it negative? The lungs have the tendency to collapse and the chest wall has the tendency to expand (Fig. 45.3).

- Therefore, **lungs recoil inwardly** and **chest wall recoil outwardly**.

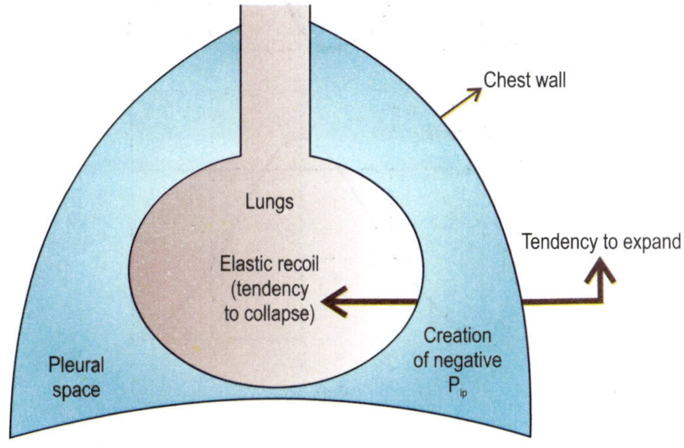

Fig. 45.3: Generation of negative intrapleural pressure (P_{ip}). Note tendency of lungs to collapse and chest wall to expand creates negative pressure in pleural space.

- These equal and opposing forces cause the intrapleural pressure to be negative (less than atmospheric pressure).

Normal Value

In Quiet Breathing: In quiet breathing, intrapleural pressure (relative to atmospheric pressure) **during expiration** is about ***–2.5 to –4 mm of Hg*** (approximately, –5 cm of H_2O) and **during inspiration** is about ***–6 mmHg*** (approximately, –8 cm of H_2O) (Fig. 45.4).

In Forced Breathing: **During forced expiration,** intrapleural pressure becomes ***positive*** and during **forced inspiration** it becomes ***further negative***, may be upto – 30 mm of Hg.

Measurement of Intrapleural Pressure

For measuring intrapleural pressure a catheter is not inserted into the intrapleural space, as it may result in pneumothorax.

- Intrapleural pressure **reflects esophageal pressure.**

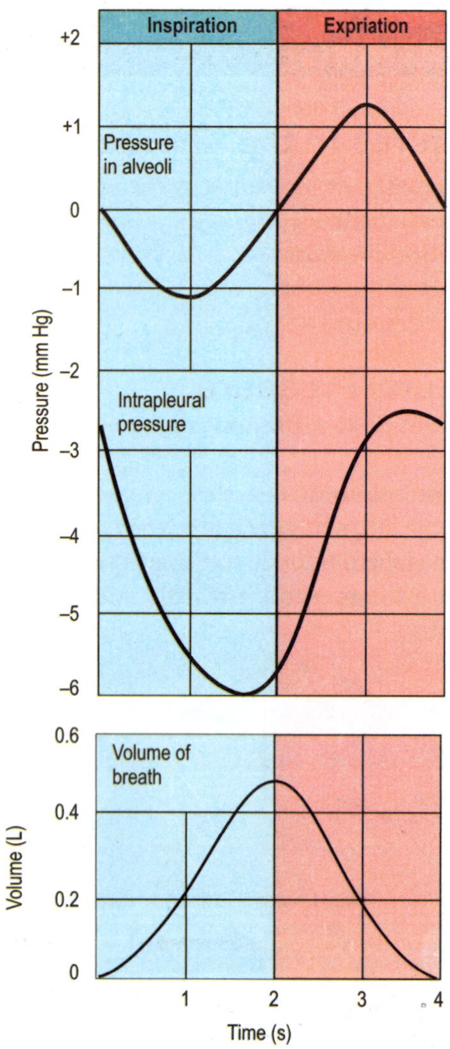

Fig. 45.4: Alveolar and intrapleural pressure during quiet inspiration and expiration. Note intrapleural pressure is negative in both the phases of respiration, and alveolar pressure is negative during inspiration and positive during expiration.

- Therefore, it is measured **by recording intra-esophageal pressure** by introducing a balloon catheter through mouth into the esophagus.

Effects of Posture and Gravity

Upright Posture

In upright posture, intrapleural pressure is about **–2.5 cm H_2O at the base** of the lung and **–10 cm H_2O at the apex** of the lung.

- This **apex to base *increasing negative gradient*** of intrapleural pressure is **due to the effect of gravity.**
- In standing position, the vacuum in intrapleural space is greater in the apex and less in the base of the lung as gravity pulls the lungs downward (away from the apex of the thoracic cage).
- This creates the intrapleural pressure gradient in vertical direction.

Supine Posture

In supine posture, this **difference does not exist.**

- However, **lying on one's side** creates the intrapleural pressure gradient **in transverse direction.**
- As there is no gravitational force in the **outer space,** intrapleural pressure gradient is absent.

Significance of Intrapleural Pressure

Physiological Significance:

1. ***Facilitates Inspiration:*** Expansion of the thoracic cage during inspiration causes the intrapleural pressure to become more negative.
    - A **decrease in intrapleural pressure helps the lungs to expand,** which in turn results in inflow of air into the lungs.
2. ***Maintains shape of chest & size of lungs:*** Intrapleural pressure **maintains normal shape of chest wall** as it resists the recoiling of these structures.
    - *Loss of normal intrapleural pressure* results in lung collapse and **barrel shaped chest.**

Clinical Significance: The clinical significance of intrapleural pressure is observed when the chest wall is perforated and **air enters the pleural space.**

- The normal **pleural pressure is subatmospheric.** When a connection is made between the atmosphere and the pleural space, air moves in and intrapleural pressure becomes atmospheric.
    - This results in **pneumothorax.**
- Due to loss of intrapleural pressure, the **lungs collapse** by inward recoiling, and the **rib cage expands** outward by outward recoiling (Fig. 45.5).
    - The trans-pulmonary pressure becomes zero because the pressure difference across the lung is eliminated.

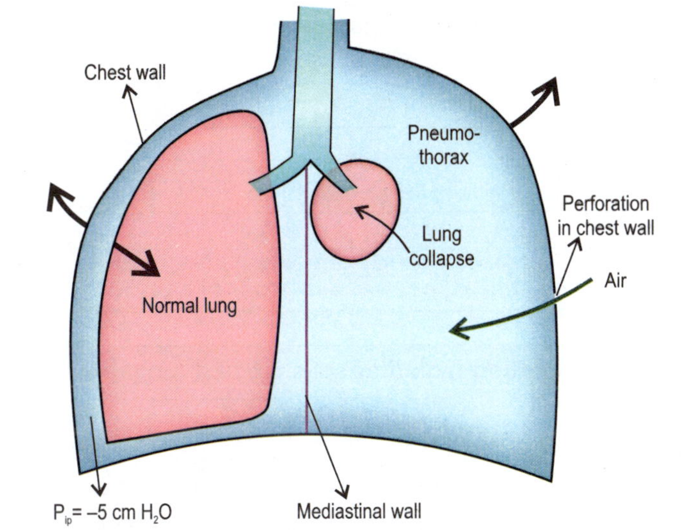

Fig. 45.5: Mechanism of development of pneumothorax. A perforation in the chest wall connects atmosphere to the pleural space. Intrapleural pressure (P_{ip}), which is normally negative becomes zero and lung collapses on the affected side. Air accumulates in pleural cavity. Note the outward recoiling force of chest wall is unopposed; therefore, chest wall is expanded more than that on the normal side. On the normal side, the balance between outward recoiling of chest wall and inward recoiling of lungs (as indicated by equally thick opposite arrows) maintains negative P_{ip} and the normal shape of chest.

Causes of pneumothorax:

1. A gunshot **wound that perforates** the chest wall.
2. Injury with a knife in which the **chest wall is punctured**.
3. In diseases in which the **lung ruptures into the pleural cavity**, e. g., rupture of a lung abscess or rupture of a parenchymal bulla by severe coughing.
4. **During aspiration** of pleural fluid for analysis, *air enters into the pleural cavity* due to faulty technique that may result in pneumothorax.

IMPORTANT NOTE

Therapeutic Pneumothorax: As part of therapy for some lung diseases, for example, for treatment of tuberculosis, pneumothorax is **purposefully created** by inserting a sterile needle into the pleural cavity. For such purposes, **nitrogen is injected** into the pleural space to *provide rest to the diseased lung*.

Transmural Pressures

Transmural pressure is the **pressure difference across an airway or across the lung wall**. There are **two** major transmural pressures: trans-pulmonary pressure, and trans-airway pressure.

Trans-pulmonary pressure: Transpulmonary pressure is the **pressure difference across the lung wall** (Fig. 45.6).

- This is measured by **subtracting pleural pressure from alveolar pressure**.
- Trans-pulmonary pressure is the pressure that **keeps the lungs inflated and prevents the lungs from collapsing**.
- An increase in trans-pulmonary pressure causes the inflation of lungs above the resting volume.

Trans-airway pressure: Trans-airway pressure is the **pressure difference across the airway**, which is the *difference between the pressure inside and outside the airway* (Fig. 45.6).

- Trans-airway pressure is important in ***keeping the airways open*** during forced expiration.

Alveolar Pressure

The alveolar pressure is the pressure inside the alveoli.

1. Change in alveolar pressure moves air in and out of the lungs.
2. During inspiration, alveolar pressure decreases (*becomes subatmospheric*) that sucks air into the lungs, and during expiration the *alveolar pressure increases* that removes air from the lungs (Fig. 45.4).

Normal Value: During inspiration it is approximately –1 mmHg, and during expiration +1 mmHg.

Physiological Significance of Transmural Pressure & Alveolar Pressures

At the end of expiration, when there is no flow of air into airways, the alveolar pressure is zero i. e., equal to atmospheric pressure. Trans-pulmonary pressure, which is the difference in alveolar pressure and pleural pressure, is therefore **+5 $cm\,H_2O$** [0–(–5) = +5] at the end of expiration.

1. Trans-pulmonary pressure **is always positive** in normal breathing.
2. Trans-pulmonary pressure is also referred to as **distending pressure** as it helps in inflation of lungs.
3. When trans-pulmonary pressure becomes more positive, the lungs are **more inflated**.

Summary of Mechanics of Inspiration and Expiration

Sequence of events leading to inspiration

1. Diaphragm and other inspiratory muscles contract that cause expansion of thoracic cage which in turn makes intrapleural pressure more negative.

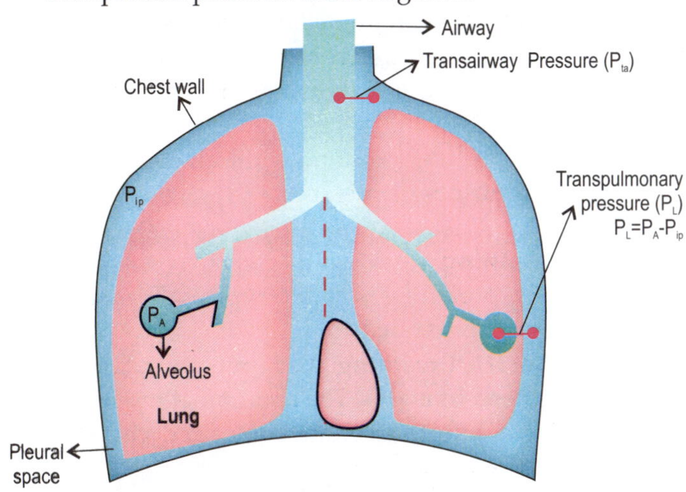

Fig. 45.6: Alveolar (P_A), transairway (P_{ta}), and transpulmonary (P_L) pressures. Note, P_{ta} is the pressure difference across the airway and P_L is the pressure difference between alveolar (P_A) and intrapleural pressure (P_{ip}).

2. This increases transpulmonary pressure as a result of which inflation of lungs occurs.
3. Alveolar pressure decreases (becomes subatmospheric) and therefore, air flows into airways and lungs.
4. Inflow of air stops when alveolar pressure equalizes with atmospheric pressure (Flowchart 45.1).
5. The cessation of contraction of inspiratory muscles ends inspiration.

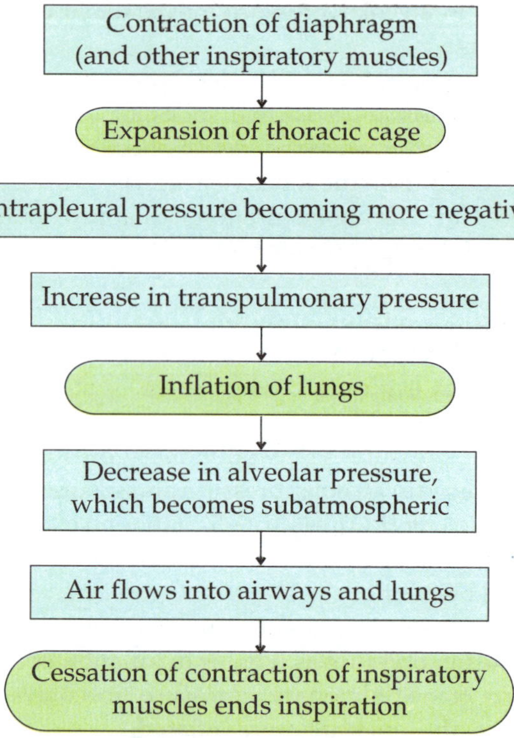

Flowchart 45.1: Sequence of events during inspiration.

Sequence of events leading to expiration

1. Due to relaxation of inspiratory muscles, rib cage drops.
2. Intrapleural pressure becomes less negative which decreases the transpulmonary pressure.
3. Lungs that were stretched in inspiration start deflating, due to which alveolar diameter decreases.
4. The alveolar pressure becomes greater than the atmospheric pressure that pushes air out of the lungs (Flowchart 45.2).
5. Airflow out of lungs continues till alveolar pressure equalizes atmospheric pressure.

Types of Breathing

Physiologically, breathing is of two types: Abdominothoracic and thoracoabdominal.

Abdominothoracic Breathing: Abdominothoracic breathing is usually **seen in males**. The abdominal movement is more prominent. Effective contraction of abdominal muscles facilitates breathing

Thoracoabdominal Breathing: This is predominant **in females and children**. The chest wall movement is more prominent.

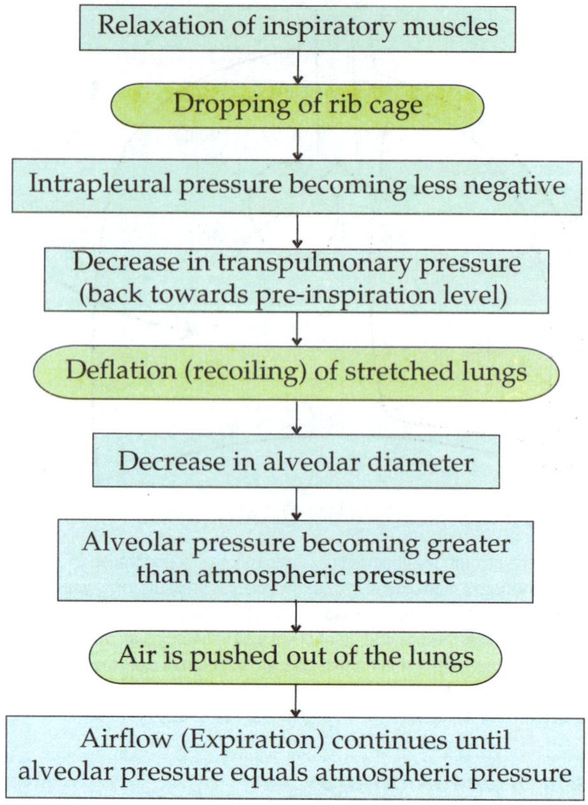

Flowchart 45.2: Sequence of events during expiration.

- In females, descent of diaphragm is less, the exact cause of which is not known.
  - One contributing factor may be the free mobility of the ribs at sternocostal and costovertebral joints in females compared to males.
  - Also, diaphragm is more powerful in males that contributes to abdominothoracic breathing in males.

LUNG VOLUMES AND CAPACITIES

Classification

There are **four lung volumes** and **four lung capacities** (Fig. 45.7).

Lung Volumes

Tidal Volume

Tidal volume (TV) is the volume of gas **inspired or expired during quiet breathing**.

- This is about 500 ml in adults.
- About 150 ml of this volume fills the airways from the nose and mouth down to the respiratory bronchioles and this volume does not take part in gas exchange.
  - This is called ***anatomical dead space***.

- The remaining volume i.e. 350 ml is available for alveolar ventilation.

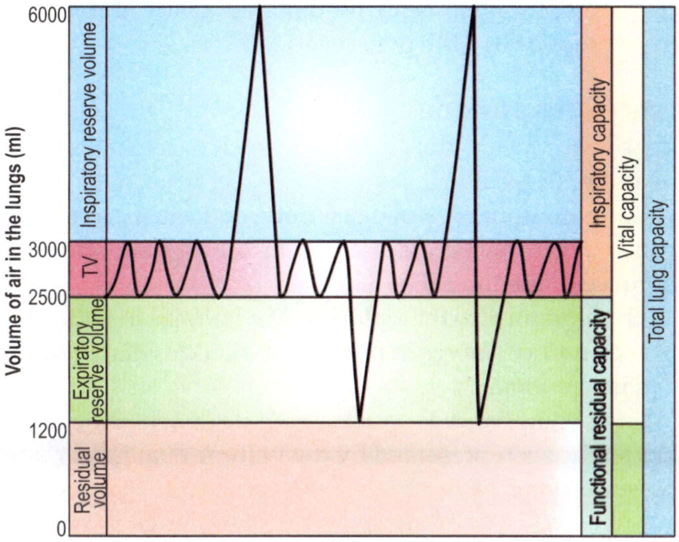

Fig. 45.7: Lung volumes and capacities: TV: tidal volume

Inspiratory Reserve Volume

The volume of **air inspired with a maximal inspiratory effort** in excess of the normal tidal inspiratory volume is called inspiratory reserve volume (IRV).

- The normal IRV is 3.3 liters in men and 1.9 liters in women.

Expiratory Reserve Volume

The volume of air that can be **expired with a maximum expiratory effort** after the normal tidal expiration is called expiratory reserve volume (ERV).

- The normal ERV is 1.2 liter in men and 0.7 liter in women.

Residual Volume

The volume of air **left in the lungs at the end of maximal expiratory effort** is the residual volume (RV).

- The normal value of RV in men is 1.2 liter and in women is 1.1 liter.

Lung Capacities

Vital Capacity

The maximum volume of air that can be **expired after a maximal inspiratory effort** is called the vital capacity (VC).

- The normal value of VC in men is about 4 liters and in women, about 3 liters.

Forced Vital Capacity (FVC)

The total volume of air that can be **expired with greatest force and speed after a maximal inspiration** is the FVC.

- FVC differs very little from VC in the normal subject, but it is proportionately more reduced when there is airway obstruction with air trapping.

Physiological Importance of FVC: From FVC, two other important lung functions are obtained: the **forced expiratory volume of air exhaled in 1 second** (FEV_1), and the **forced expiratory flow** (FEF_{25-75}) that represents the expiratory flow rate over the middle half of the forced vital capacity i.e. between 25 and 75%.

Inspiratory Capacity

This is the maximum volume of air that can be **inspired after tidal expiration.**

- This is the sum of tidal volume and inspiratory reserve volume (TV+IRV).
- Normally, it is about 3.5 liter.

Functional Residual Capacity

This is the volume of air **remaining in the lungs at the end of each tidal expiration.**

- This is the sum of expiratory reserve volume and residual volume (ERV+RV).
- Normally, it is about 2.2–2.5 liters.

Physiological Importance of FRC: FRC is important for **maintaining stable gas tension in the lung**, so that at all times, enough air is available for gas exchange along the alveolocapillary membrane.

- It **prevents sudden alteration in gas tension** due to any brief interruption of respiration. Reduction in FRC may result in hypoxia.
- **FRC increases when there is air trapping** in lungs as seen in asthma or emphysema.

Total Lung Capacity

The volume of the air present in the lungs ***at* the end of maximal inspiration** is the total lung capacity (TLC).

- The normal value in men is about 6 liters and in women is about 4.2 liters.

Measurement

The lung volume and capacities are measured directly by **simple spirometry**.

- RV and FRC can't be measured directly by simple spirometry.
- **RV and FRC** are measured indirectly using a **dilution technique** involving helium (**helium dilution technique**).

Helium Dilution Technique: In this procedure, the subject is connected to a spirometer filled with **10% helium in oxygen** (helium-oxygen mixture) and subject breathes from the spirometer. After the subject rebreathes helium-oxygen mixture and equilibrates with the spirometer, the helium concentration in the lungs becomes same as in spirometer.

Applying the conservation of mass principle, we derive that:

$C_1 \times V_1 = C_2 \times (V_1 + V_2)$; where C_1 is the initial concentration of helium in the spirometer, V_1 is the initial volume of helium-oxygen mixture in the spirometer, C_2 is helium concentration after equilibrium, and V_2 is unknown volume in the lungs.

Thus, $V_2 = \dfrac{V_1 (C_1 - C_2)}{C_2}$

1. **If the test begins at the end of a normal tidal volume** (end of expiration), the volume of air remaining in the lungs represents functional residual capacity.
2. **If the test begins at the end of a forced vital capacity**, then the test will measure residual volume.
3. If the **test starts after a maximal inspiration**, then V_2 would equal total lung capacity.

FRC can also be measured by **body plethysmography**.

Dynamic lung volumes and capacities are FEV_1, PEFR, MMEFR, MVV, MEFVC etc. (discussed below).

Factors Affecting

Lung volumes and capacities are influenced by various factors such as age, gender, built, height, level of physical training, etc. (for details, refer chapter 55 "Pulmonary Function Tests").

MECHANICAL PROPERTIES OF LUNGS & CHEST WALL

Elastic Properties of Lungs & Chest Wall

Elastic Properties of Lungs

Lungs are **elastic tissues.** An elastic tissue once stretched **recoils back** to its un-stretched position like a spring. Similarly, lungs recoil when stretched.

- The ability of the lungs to be inflated is called its **stretchability** or **distensibility**.
  - Distensibility and elastic recoil are opposite to each other.
  - Overstretching of the lungs causes loss of elastic recoil.
- Lung elasticity **depends on the presence of the amount of elastin and collagen fibers** enmeshed in its parenchyma.
  - **Elastin fibers** are highly distensible and can be stretched easily, but **collagen fibers** resist stretch and limit lung expansion.
- The **arrangement of elastin fiber networks** in the lung parenchyma is similar to the arrangement of fibers of a nylon stocking.
  - When the stocking is stretched to fit into the leg, the length of individual fibers does not change much.
  - If the nylon stocking is overstretched, it loses its elasticity and becomes loose (baggy). Similarly, **an overstretched lung** (baggy lung) as seen in emphysema, **can't be deflated easily due to the loss of its ability to recoil.**

Lung Compliance

Compliance means the ability to stretch (stretchability) or the ability to recoil.

- Lung compliance (distensibility and elastic recoil of the lung) can be assessed from the pressure-volume curve of the lung (Fig. 45.8).
- This is similar to the ***inflation of a balloon*** in which for ***each unit of change*** in pressure, balloon is ***distended to a new volume.***
- Lung compliance is a measure of its distensibility.

Compliance is represented by the volume change per unit pressure change, i. e.;

Compliance = $\Delta V/\Delta P$, where ΔV is the change in volume and ΔP is the change in pressure.

Measurement of Lung Compliance

Two types of lung compliances are measured: static lung compliance and dynamic lung compliance.

Static Lung Compliance Measurement: The lung compliance is assessed by analyzing the the pressure-volume relationship.

Pressure-Volume Relationship: The pressure-volume relationship graph is obtained for human lungs by simultaneously measuring ***changes in lung volume*** (with the help of a spirometer) and ***changes in pleural pressure*** (by measuring pressure changes in the esophagus with the help of a balloon catheter).

- For recording pressure-volume curve, the individual inspires maximally to total long capacity (TLC) and then expires slowly (Fig. 45.8).

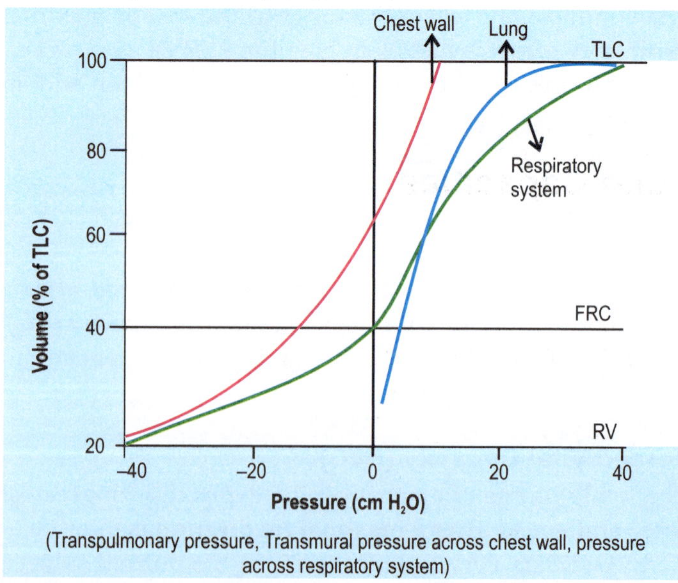

Fig. 45.8: Relaxation pressure-volume curve of lung, chest wall and respiratory system.

Note that at functional residual capacity (FRC), the transmural pressure across the respiratory system is zero, and at total lung capacity (TLC), both lung and chest wall pressures are positive. RV: residual volume.

- During the process of slow expiration, airflow is periodically interrupted (so that alveolar pressure is zero), and lung volume and pleural pressure are measured.
- Lung volume is recorded as % of TLC.
- The compliance (volume change per unit pressure change) recorded in these conditions is called ***static lung compliance***, as airflow does not occur during the recording.
- As lung is deflated from TLC, the deflation pressure-volume curve is obtained by this procedure.
- To obtain the inflation pressure-volume curve, lung is inflated from functional residual capacity (FRC) to the TLC.

Stages of Pressure-Volume Curve: There are four stages in the inflation pressure-volume curve (Fig. 45.9):

1. **Stage 1 (Stage of stable lung volume):** The initial change in intrapleural pressure has ***no effect on lung volume***. This is because a decrease in intrapleural pressure increases transpulmonary pressure and unless transpulmonary pressure is large enough to overcome the collapsing effect of surface tension created by the air-water interface in the airways, the decrease in intrapleural pressure has no effect on lung volume.
2. **Stage 2 (Stage of opening of airways):** When intrapleural pressure decreases above –8 cm H_2O, ***lung volume increases*** first due to opening of proximal airways and then by opening of distal airways.
3. **Stage 3 (Stage of linear increase in lung volume):** When intrapleural pressure decreases further (becomes more negative) opening and expansion of all airways occur. This results in ***steep but linear increase in lung volume***.
4. **Stage 4 (Stage of cessation of inflation):** As increase in lung volume approaches TLC, further ***increase in the volume becomes less***, and finally ceases. This occurs due to decrease in airway and chest wall compliance and limitation of muscle strength.

Hysteresis Loop: The difference between the inflation and deflation pressure-volume curves (Fig. 45.9) is known as *hysteresis*.

1. The **hysteresis loop** occurs because a **greater pressure difference is needed to open an already closed airway than to keep airway open** that has already been opened (to maintain airway opening, i. e. to prevent open-airway from closing).
2. For example, to keep open a previously opened airway at FRC requires a pressure of only about –5 cm H_2O (as noted in the deflation limb of pressure-volume curve), whereas to inflate a collapsed lung at FRC requires a pressure of about –15 cm H_2O (as noted in the inflation limb of pressure-volume curve).
   - However, the **hysteresis loop is much smaller** during normal breathing and is located close to the deflation limb of the pressure-volume curve.

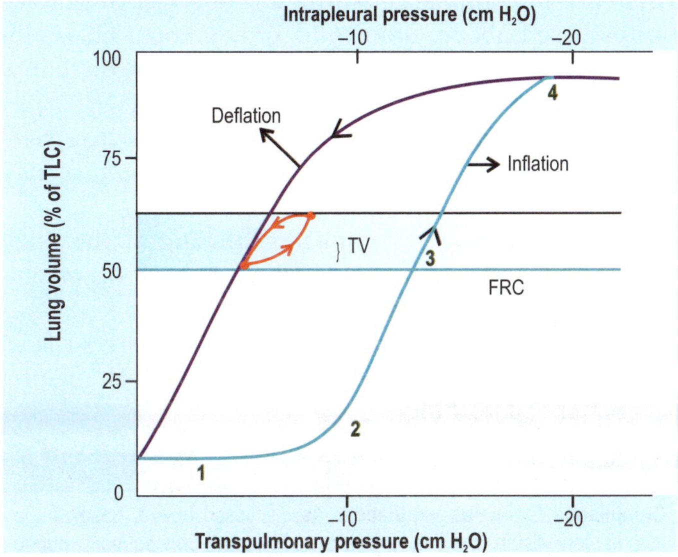

Fig. 45.9: Inflation and deflation of pressure-volume curves. Note, at normal breathing (at tidal volume), pressure volume loop has less hysteresis. TLC: Total lung capacity; TV: Tidal volume; FRC: Functional residual capacity.

3. The slope of pressure-volume curve is the compliance and is the **measure of distensibility of lungs**.

Dynamic Lung Compliance Measurement: Dynamic lung mechanics are the mechanics in play when the lungs are in motion.

1. Dynamic lung compliance is measured by continuously recording the change in intrapleural pressure and lung volume.
2. In pressure-volume loop of dynamic record, the rise in volume in inspiration is in the form of a curve and returning to the starting point during inspiration is another curve.
3. The difference in inflation and deflation limbs of the curve produces a hysteresis, which is much similar to the pattern obtained in pressure-volume curve of static lungs, but the difference is that *dynamic compliance of lung is less than its static compliance*.
4. Dynamic lung compliance increases during exercise (Application Box 45.1).

Application Box 45.1

Exercise, Sighing and Yawning increase dynamic lung compliance: Dynamic lung compliance during exercise is more than during the resting state.

- In resting state, alveolar surface area changes less due to tidal respiration. Therefore, smaller change in alveolar surface area, which is not adequate to bring more surfactant molecules to the surface, makes the lung less compliant.
- During exercise, a larger change in tidal volume causes greater change in alveolar surface area, which incorporates more surfactant molecule to the air-liquid interface of the alveoli. Therefore, the lung is more compliant during exercise, which ensures better ventilation.
- Sighing and yawning also increase dynamic lung compliance.

Regional Variation of Lung Compliance

In upright posture, the lung compliance is **less at the top portion of the lungs than at the base.** This regional difference in compliance is **due to the effect of gravity**. As discussed above, due to the gravitational effect, the pleural pressure is less (more negative) at the apex than at the base of the lungs.

1. At the apex, *trans-pulmonary pressure is therefore more*, which causes the *alveoli in the apical region to be more distended*.
   - This decreases compliance of lung at the apex. Thus, the apex of the lung is less distensible (Application Box 45.2).
2. Thus, at the base of the lung, there is a *larger change in volume for the same pressure change*, which ensures greater expansibility.

Application Box 45.2

Compliance facilitates ventilation: As discussed above, base of the lung is more distensible due to greater compliance. Consequently, during inspiration, a larger share of tidal volume goes to the base of the lungs. This is a major factor for greater ventilation at the base of the lungs in comparison to the apex.

Factors Affecting Lung Compliance

1. **Distensibility and elastic recoil:** More the lung is distensible and elastic more is the compliance. A stiff lung has less compliance.
2. **Lung volume:** The pressure-volume curve of the lung is nonlinear, which indicates that the compliance is not equal at all lung volumes.
   - The compliance is high at low lung volumes and low at high lung volumes.
3. **Lung size:** In general, compliance is **proportionate to the size of the lung**. Thus, the lung of rat has less compliance than the lung of elephant. Children lung is less compliant than the adult lung.
4. **Surface tension inside the alveoli:** Surface tension mainly affects lung compliance (discussed below). Surface tension at the air-water interface of airways accounts for more than half of the lung compliance.

Clinical Significance of Lung Compliance

Diseases of lung alter the lung compliance.

Low Compliance: The low lung compliance indicates **less distensibility**. This means **more work is required** in a lung with low compliance to inflate the lungs to achieve the normal tidal volume.

1. In **restrictive lung diseases**, the compliance of the lungs is significantly low.
   - For example, in pulmonary fibrosis, fibrous tissue is deposited in the lungs, which makes **lungs stiff and difficult to inflate.**
2. **In a normal lung,** tidal volume of 500 ml is achieved at about 2.5 cm H_2O of transpulmonary pressure.
3. **In lung fibrosis,** the same change in pressure produces a much less increase in lung volume (Fig. 45.10). This indicates that in this condition the ***static lung compliance is much less***.

High Compliance: High compliance is also equally bad as low compliance. High compliance is seen in **obstructive lung diseases** like emphysema.

1. In **emphysema**, which occurs in chronic habitual smokers, the lung tissue (extracellular matrix including elastin) is destroyed by elastase released from macrophages.
   - In this disease, it is much ***easy to inflate lung***, since a higher lung volume is obtained at any particular pressure (Fig. 45.9).
   - The ***static lung compliance is higher***.
2. However, the **elastic recoil of lungs is much less,** due to which *getting air out of lung is severely impaired***.** Therefore, emphysematous lungs have **abnormally high residual volume**.

Elastic Properties of Chest Wall

Like lungs, chest wall has elastic properties, but the **elastic recoil of the chest wall is in outward direction**. Thus, chest wall has the intrinsic tendency to expand.

1. The outward recoil of chest wall balances the inward recoil of lungs.
   - Therefore, **if the elastic recoil of the chest wall is unopposed**, as occurs in lung collapse, **chest wall expands to about 70% of total lung capacity** (TLC).
2. That means, when the volume is less than 70% of TLC, the chest wall starts recoiling outward.

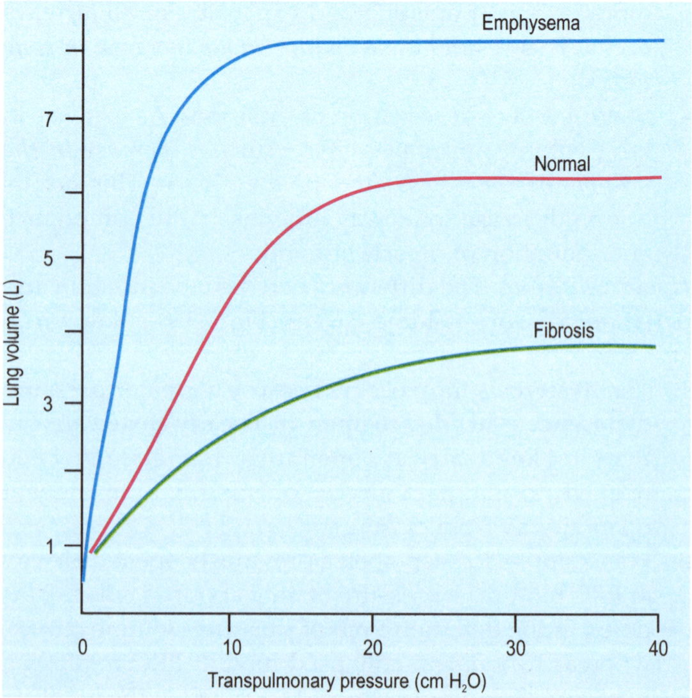

Fig. 45.10: Static pressure-volume curve of lung in normal and disease states.

3. It should be noted that, the outward elastic recoil of the chest wall is maximum at residual volume (and the inward elastic recoil of the lung is maximum at TLC).

At FRC (functional residual capacity), the elastic ***recoil of lung and chest wall balance*** each other.

- That means **for the lung volumes at FRC,** *chest wall and lung have equal elastic recoil forces* in opposite directions.
- Alterations in these elastic forces significantly affect FRC.

Measurement of Thoracic Wall Compliance

To measure thoracic wall compliance, first the compliance of **thoracic cage and lungs are measured combinely**.

- Intrapulmonary pressure (which is the total pressure of lungs and thoracic wall) is measured for each lung volume inhaled.
- Then, lung compliance is measured separately (as described above).

Thoracic wall compliance is then determined from the following formula:

$$\frac{1}{\text{Thoracic wall compliance}} = \text{Total compliance} - \frac{1}{\text{Lung compliance}}$$

$$\text{So, thoracic wall compliance} = \frac{\text{Lung compliance}}{\text{Total compliance x Lung compliance} - 1}$$

Lung-Chest Wall Interaction

During respiration, **lung and chest wall move simultaneously in opposite direction**. The pressures change across the lung and chest wall during the respiratory movements are called **transmural pressures**. The transmural pressures are: transpulmonary pressure, transmural pressure across the chest wall and pressure across the respiratory system.

Transpulmonary Pressure: This is the **pressure difference between the alveolar pressure and the intrapleural pressure** (refer Fig. 45.6).

- To increase its volume, lung requires positive transpulmonary pressure.
- When transpulmonary pressure is zero, the size of the lung is minimum.
  - At zero transpulmonary pressure, though the lung is smallest in size, alveoli are not fully collapsed due to surface tension lowering property of surfactant.

Transmural Pressure Across the Chest Wall: This is the **difference between intrapleural pressure and the pressure surrounding the chest wall** (the body surface pressure or the barometric pressure).

- Transmural pressure across chest wall is **usually negative** as the intrapleural pressure is negative relative to the atmospheric pressure.

Pressure Across the Respiratory System: This is the **sum of the pressure across the lung and across the chest wall.**

- This is calculated as the difference between alveolar pressure and the barometric pressure.

Relaxation Pressure-Volume Curves

Interaction between these transmural pressures determines the lung-volumes and capacities, which can be studied by analyzing the **relaxation pressure-volume curves** of lung, chest wall and respiratory system (Fig. 45.8).

1. **At functional residual capacity** (FRC), *transmural pressure across the respiratory system is zero*, and **at total lung capacity** (TLC), both lung and chest wall *pressures are positive*.
   - This indicates that both lung and chest need positive transmural distending pressures.
2. The **resting volume for chest wall** is the 60% of TLC.
   - This (resting volume for chest wall) is the volume at which the ***transmural pressure for the chest wall is zero***.
3. This means that **at volumes less than 60% of TLC,** *chest wall tends to recoil outward* and at **volumes more than 60% of TLC,** *chest wall recoils inward*.
4. It should be noted that **at transpulmonary pressure of 20 cm of H_2O,** *lung reaches its elastic limit*; therefore, the pressure curve flattens beyond this pressure.
5. The increase in transpulmonary pressure **above 20 cm of H_2O** does not increase lung volume much, as the distension of lung is *limited by the connective tissues of the lung*.
6. **Further increase in pressure** results in **rupture of alveoli** near the lung surface that can lead to **pneumothorax** (escape of air into the pleural space).

ROLE OF SURFACE TENSION

The **force that pulls the surface molecules together** of a liquid at an ***air-liquid interface*** is called surface tension. There is a thin layer of surfactant (a liquid film) lining the inner surface of the alveoli and the alveoli is filled with air; this forms the **air-liquid interface**.

- Surface tension at the air-liquid interface in the lung alveoli **is a major factor that influences lung compliance**, which **accounts for more than half of the elastic recoil of lungs**.
- The surface tension in the alveoli is **directed inward**, and therefore, it **favours collapse of alveoli**.

Pressure-Volume Curves: The importance of surface tension in lung functions is best studied by analyzing the **pressure-volume curves of lungs filled with air and liquid** (Fig. 45.11).

- In this experiment, lungs are removed from chest and inflated or deflated at various pressures separately, first filled with air and then with saline.

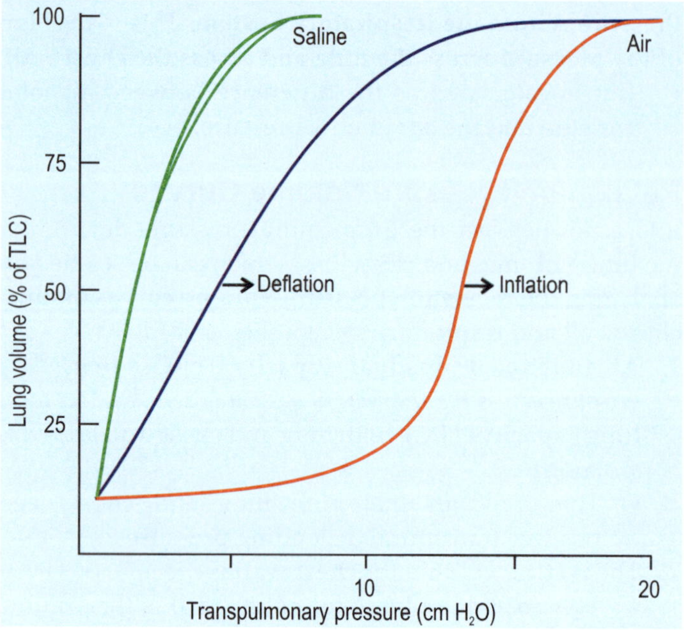

Fig. 45.11: Comparison of pressure-volume relationship in a lung inflated with air and saline separately. Hysteresis is very less in saline lung than in air-lung indicating that in saline-lung, pressure needed to inflate was almost same as to deflate. Also, the slope of inflation limb of saline-lung was steeper than air-lung since static compliance is very high in saline-lung (as lung was inflated with much less pressure) indicating that the lung was more compliant due to elimination of surface tension. These evidences indicate that surface tension significantly affects compliance.

  - Surface tension is generated in the *lung filled with air* as **air-liquid interface is created**, whereas, **surface tension is absent** in the *lung filled with saline* as air-liquid interface is eliminated.
- **Hysteresis** (difference between inflation and deflation limbs) ***is very less*** in saline-lung than air-lung.
  - This indicates that **in saline-lung,** *pressure needed to inflate the lung is almost same as to deflate the lung.*
- The **slope of inflation limb of saline-lung is much steeper** than the inflation limb of air-lung.
  - This is because the *static compliance is very high in saline-lung* as lung was **more compliant** due to *elimination of surface tension.*

Thus, surface tension significantly affects compliance and work of breathing. In the lung, surfactant decreases surface tension and maintains compliance.

Application of Laplace Law

Surface tension also **maintains alveolar stability**. The Laplace law explains the relationship of surface tension with pressure inside a sphere like alveolus. The Laplace law states that the pressure in a spherical structure is equal to twice the wall tension divided by the radius.

i. e. $P = \frac{2T}{r}$, where, P is the pressure, T is surface tension and *r* is radius.

Importance of Alveolar Size: In lungs, all alveoli do not have same diameter, alveoli size also changes during inspiration and expiration, and alveoli are interconnected with each other.

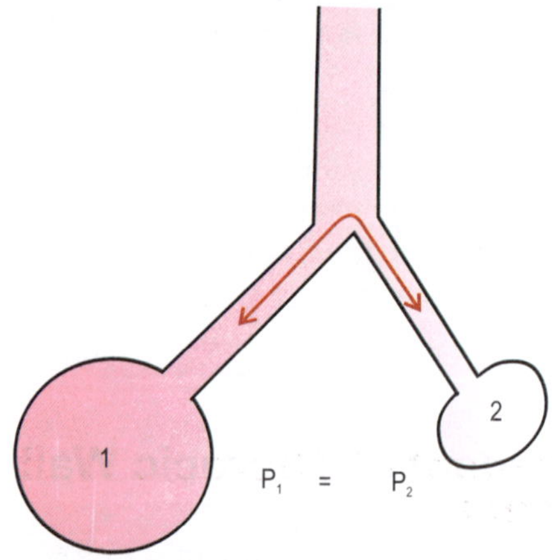

Fig. 45.12: Maintenance of alveolar stability inspite of difference in size of alveoli. As surface tension is constant per unit surface area, surface tension of the alveoli decreases with the decrease in surface area. Thus, distending pressure (2T/r) remains same and smaller alveoli do not collapse.

1. According to the Law of Laplace, pressure would be greater in smaller alveoli than in bigger alveoli and they would empty into the larger alveoli (Fig. 45.12).
2. Thus, one can presume that **larger alveoli tend to distend more** and **smaller alveoli tend to collapse.** But this does not happen.
   - Surface tension ***is constant per unit surface area*** (i.e., 50 dyne/cm^2).
   - So, the ***surface tension of alveoli decreases with decrease in surface area.***
3. Therefore, as the **alveoli become smaller,** *the surface tension also reduces* and as the **alveoli distends** (becomes larger), *surface tension increases.*
4. Thus, the **smaller alveoli do not collapse** as pressure (2T/r) within the alveoli remains same and therefore, volume of interconnected alveoli remains almost same.

Role of Pulmonary Surfactant

The pulmonary surfactant is a **thin liquid film of alveolar lining** that decreases surface tension at the gas-liquid interface of alveoli and alters surface tension with change in alveolar diameter.

Structure and Composition

Pulmonary surfactant is a mixture of lipoprotein rich in phospholipid. The principal surface tension-lowering agent in surfactant is **dipalmitoylphosphatidylcho -line** (DPPC), which is also called **dipalmitoyl-lecithin** (DPL).

1. Phospholipids of surfactant have a hydrophilic head and a hydrophobic tail. The **hydrophobic tail** consists of fatty acids. The tail of phospholipids faces towards the alveolar lumen (Fig. 45.13).
2. The **alveolar surface tension is inversely proportional to the concentration of phospholipids** in the surfactant.

Composition: Surfactant consists of:

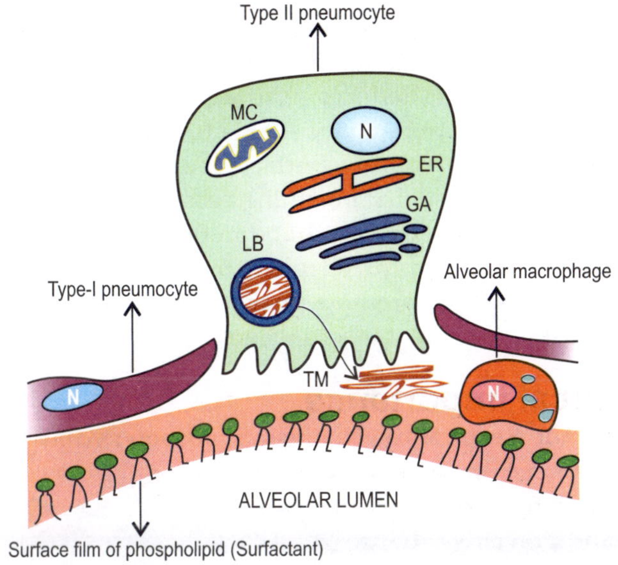

Fig. 45.13: Arrangement of type I and type II pneumocytes and phospholipid surface film (surfactant) in epithelium of alveoli. Note the presence of lamellar bodies (LB) in type II pneumocyte, which stores and secretes tubular myelins (TM) that are released into epithelial surface by exocytosis and act as source of phospholipids. N: nucleus; MC: mitochondria; ER: endoplasmic reticulum; GA: Golgi apparatus.

1. **Lipids:** 90%
   - Dipalmitoylphosphatidylcholine (62%)
   - Phosphatidylglycerol (5%)
   - Other phospholipids (10%)
   - Neutral lipids (13%)
2. **Proteins :** 8%
   - Albumin
   - Immunoglobulin A (Ig A)
   - Apoproteins (SP-A, -B, -C, - D)
3. **Carbohydrates:** 2%

Source

Surfactant is synthesized in Type II pneumocytes.

- There are ***two types of cells*** in alveolar epithelium: type I and type II alveolar epithelial cells.
- Alveolar type II cells are called type II pneumocytes that *are* metabolically active and contain more number of mitochondria.
  - The special histological feature of type II cells is the presence of electron-dense lamellar inclusion bodies (Fig. 45.13).
  - Lamellar inclusion bodies *store surfactant in type II cell*.

Synthesis and Secretion

Palmitate, choline and glucose are substrate molecules for surfactant synthesis. The substrate molecules are taken up by alveolar type II cells from the circulating blood.

- In mitochondria, they are synthesized into DPPC.
- The surfactant is then stored in the lamellar inclusion bodies.
  - Lamellar inclusion bodies are continuously discharged onto the alveolar surface by constitutive exocytosis (exocytosis which is continuous and unregulated).
- The released lamellar body-materials are converted into tubular myelin that forms the film of surfactant on the alveolar surface (steps of surfactant synthesis are summarized in Flowchart 45.3).

Substrate molecules (palmitate, choline, glucose etc) are picked up from blood by type II pneumocytes
↓
Substrate molecules are synthesized into DPPC in mitochondria

Protein component is formed in endoplasmic reticulum

↓
DPCC and proteins are packaged in Golgi apparatus
↓
Materials are stored in lamellar bodies (LBs)
↓
LBs from type II pneumocytes are discharged towards the surface of alveolar epithelium by constitutive exocytosis
↓
LB materials are converted to tubular myelin (TM)
↓
TM forms phospholipid film (surfactant) on alveolar epithelial surface

Flowchart 45.3: Steps of surfactant synthesis.

Time of Surfactant Synthesis in Fetal Life

Lungs are among the last organs to develop during intrauterine life. Therefore, synthesis of surfactant occurs towards later part of pregnancy.

- Surfactant synthesis **starts at about 34 weeks of pregnancy,** which is completed by about **90% at term** (38–40 weeks). Surfactant production continues to the perinatal period.
  - Therefore, **inadequate surfactant synthesis** resulting in lung collapse is among the *major causes of death in premature deliveries*.

Regulation of Synthesis & Secretion

Surfactant synthesis is regulated by hormones, concentration of protein in the surfactant, stretching of lung and various pharmacological agents.

A. Hormonal factors

1. ***Glucocorticoid hormones:*** Cortisol **stimulates surfactant synthesis**. Secretion of glucocorticoids increases towards term. Number of *glucocorticoid*

receptors in lungs also increases in third trimester of pregnancy.

2. ***Thyroxine:*** Thyroxine **promotes surfactant synthesis.** Maternal thyroid deficiency and cretinism decrease surfactant secretion.
3. ***Insulin:*** Insulin **facilitates surfactant synthesis.** Therefore, diabetes during pregnancy decreases surfactant secretion.

B. Quantity and quality of proteins in surfactant

Formation of phospholipid film of surfactant is greatly facilitated by proteins present in the surfactant. Surfactant proteins are albumin, immunoglobulin (Ig A) and apoproteins (surfactant proteins).

Types of surfactant proteins: There are 4 types of surfactant proteins (SP): SP-A, SP-B, SP-C, and SP-D.

- SP-B and SP-C control synthesis of monomolecular film of phospholipid.
- SP-A controls reuptake of surfactant by type II cells.
- The protein content of surfactant depends on concentration of protein in the plasma.

C. Stretching of lungs

Hyperinflation of lungs like yawning ***enhances surfactant synthesis***.

- **Yawning and sighing** during infancy are effective stimuli for surfactant synthesis.

D. Pharmacological agents

- **β adrenergic agonists enhance** surfactant secretion
- **Calcium stimulates** surfactant secretion.

E. Exercise

Practice of **regular physical exercise** stimulates surfactant synthesis in both children and adults.

Functions of Surfactant

1. **Prevents lung collapse:** Surfactant **decreases surface tension** at the air-liquid interface of alveoli. By decreasing surface tension, **it prevents lung collapse**.
   - **During lung deflation**, compression of surfactant molecules decreases surface tension. Especially at low lung volumes, the molecules are tightly compressed.
   - **During lung inflation**, new surfactant is extruded onto the alveolar surface that forms a new film on the alveolar epithelial lining.
2. **Promotes alveolar stability:** In lungs, alveoli of different diameters are connected in parallel to each other. By law of Laplace, smaller alveoli could drain into larger alveoli and collapse. However, that does not happen and alveoli remain patent.
   - This alveolar stability is maintained by surfactant.
   - Surfactant achieves this by **lowering surface tension proportionately more in the smaller alveoli**.
3. **Helps to prevent edema in the lung:** The inward force of surface tension that tends to collapse alveoli also tends to **decrease interstitial pressure** in the lungs, and facilitates pulmonary edema formation.
   - Surfactant reduces surface forces and thus **prevents pulmonary edema formation.**
4. **On work of breathing:** Surfactant **decreases the work of breathing**, so that breathing becomes easier.
5. **On immunity: Ig A and apoproteins** (SP-A and SP-D) in surfactant provide innate immunity by **acting as opsonins**. They **promote phagocytosis** of bacteria and viruses by alveolar macrophages.

Clinical Importance

1. **Infant Respiratory Distress Syndrome:** After birth, the newborn makes strong inspiratory effort so that the lungs expand. **Surfactant helps in lung inflation and prevents collapse.**
   - Lung maturation is incomplete in **premature infants.**
     - Also, hormonal disturbances like **diabetes during pregnancy** interfere with lung maturation.
   - Breathing becomes extremely labored due to high surface tension. This is called *infant respiratory distress syndrome* (IRDS) or **hyaline membrane disease**.
   - Pulmonary edema and atelectasis develop.

   Treatment: Administration of **phospholipid by inhalation**.
   - Inhalation of ***synthetic surfactant*** (or a surfactant preparation derived from bovine lungs)
   - ***Glucocorticoid therapy*** (glucocorticoid promotes surfactant synthesis)
2. **Atelectasis following surgery: Patients recovering from anesthesia** after surgery may develop breathing problem. They are often **encouraged to breathe deeply** to enhance the proper spreading of surfactant on the alveolar surface (Clinical Note 45.1).

Clinical Note 45.1

Deep breathing after surgery improves lung functions: It is difficult to practice deep breathing for patients who have undergone abdominal or thoracic surgery as *pain restricts movement of thoraco-abdominal walls.* Such patients prefer to take shallow breathing for which surfactant spreading becomes inadequate that makes the lungs atelectatic. Therefore, these patients are encouraged to practice deep breathing inspite of pain.

Alveolar Stability

Alveolar stability is maintained by two factors:

1. **Pulmonary surfactant** (discussed above)
2. Principle of Interdependence

Interdependence: Interdependence is the mutual support among adjacent alveoli. Normally, alveoli are interconnected with surrounding alveoli. They support each other because of their ***structural arrangement*** (with many interconnecting links).

- When one alveolus collapses, **it prevents the collapse of adjacent alveoli.**

  - This is because, when alveoli tend to collapse, **surrounding alveoli develop greater expanding forces**. Thus, interdependence not only prevents atelectasis but also ***opens up alveoli*** that have already collapsed.
- **Alveolar interdependence** is the *major factor* **in adult lungs** that maintain alveolar stability.
  - This is so not important in newborns, as **newborn lungs have fewer interconnecting links**.
- **Surfactant** is the *major factor* for maintaining alveolar stability **in newborns and infants**.

PROPERTIES OF THE DYNAMIC LUNG

Properties of dynamic lung are studied when the **lungs are in motion**, associated with ***flow of air in and out*** of the respiratory tract.

Airflow in Airways: Two types of airflow occur in the lung: laminar flow and turbulent flow.

1. ***Laminar Flow*:** When airflow is slow, laminar flow occurs.
   - This is characterized by a **streamlined flow**. The flow is silent because layers of air molecules slide over each other.
   - Normally, this type of flow occurs **in small peripheral airways**.
2. ***Turbulent Flow*:** Turbulent flow occurs **at high flow rates**.
   - This is normally observed **in large airways**, especially in the trachea and large bronchi.
   - It consists of a disorganized pattern of airflow that produces sound.

Airway Resistance

The **air flow causes resistance** to air moving in the airways.

- It is defined as the **ratio of driving pressure (ΔP) to airflow (V)**.
- Airway resistance (Raw) is expressed in cm H_2O/L per second.

For total airway resistance (Raw), the driving pressure is the pressure difference between the mouth (P_{mouth}) and the alveoli (P_A).

$$\text{Raw} = \frac{(P_{mouth}) - (P_A)}{V}$$

Normal Value: In healthy individuals, the airway resistance is about 1–3 cm H_2O/L per second (with lungs at FRC). Airway resistance is more in children due to their smaller airways.

Site of Resistance

The primary site of airway resistance is the **medium**

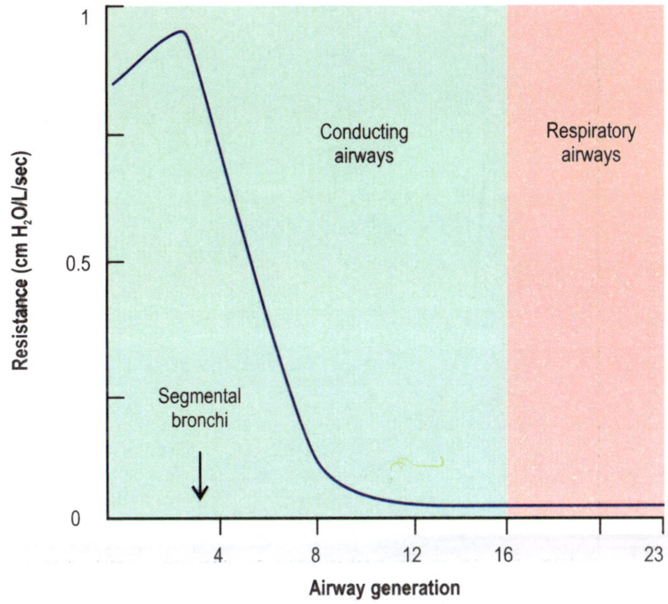

Fig. 45.14: Site of generation of airway resistance in airways. Note, highest resistance is offered by segmental bronchi.

bronchi (lobar and segmental) and bronchi down to about the seventh generation (Fig. 45.14).

- As per **Poiseuille's law**, the airway resistance **increases with the fourth power of airway radius**. Thus, one would expect that the small airways would offer more resistance to airflow.
- However, contribution of **by small airways** to the total airway resistance is **only about 10 to 15%**.
  - This is because most of the small airways are **aligned in parallel** and the ***total surface area*** of small airways (like capillaries in vascular system) is more.

IMPORTANT NOTE

Airways diseases are diagnosed in late stage: Airway diseases, in the early stage mainly affect small airways. However, diagnosing diseases in the initial stage becomes difficult because small airways contribute less to the total airway resistance. Airways diseases are diagnosed usually in their advanced stage.

Factors Affecting Airway Resistance

1. Diameter of airways

Caliber of the airway is the most important factor affecting airway resistance. **Bronchodilation decreases** and **bronchoconstriction increases** resistance.

2. Lung volume

Lung volume is among the major factors affecting airway resistance because **caliber of airways is directly proportionate to the lung volumes.** Bronchi and small airways are embedded in lung tissue. Therefore, airway diameter increases with lung expansion. Thus, airway resistance **decreases during inspiration and increases during expiration.** It should be noted that airway resistance rises sharply at low lung volumes (Fig. 45.15).

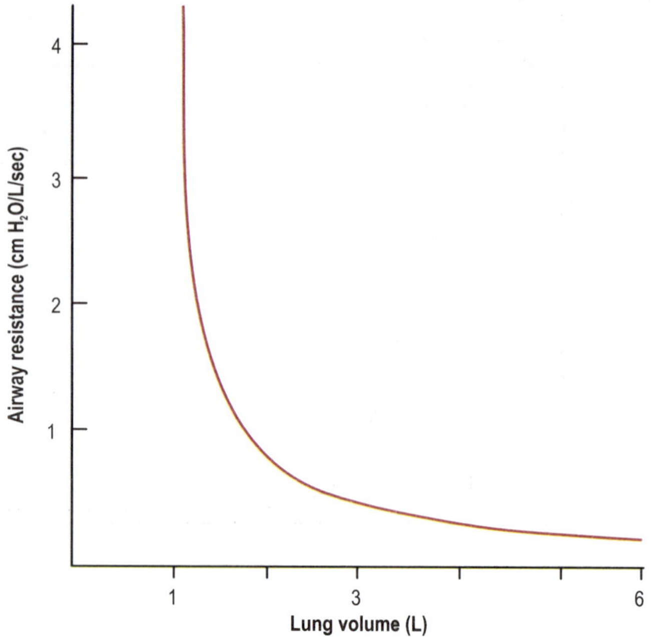

Fig. 45.15: Relation of airway resistance with lung volumes. Note at low lung volumes, resistance is more.

3. Bronchial smooth muscle tone

Bronchial smooth muscle tone also affects airway resistance as it controls airway diameter. The smooth muscle tone of the airway is influenced by following factors:

i) ***Autonomic control:***

a. Parasympathetic: Parasympathetic (vagal cholinergic fibers) stimulation causes ***bronchial constriction*** and increases mucus secretion. These effects are mediated by muscarinic receptors.

b. Sympathetic: Sympathetic Stimulation (adrenergic fibers) ***causes bronchodilation*** and inhibits glandular secretion. Activation of β_2 receptors *causes bronchodilation* increases bronchial secretion, whereas activation of α_2 receptors *inhibits secretion*.

c. **Noncholinergic-nonadrenergic innervation:** Also, there is noncholinergic-nonadrenergic innervation of bronchiole that *causes bronchodilation*, most likely mediated by VIP

ii) ***Humoral factors:*** Epinephrine, norepinephrine and other hormones that stimulate ***β_2-adrenergic receptors cause dilation of airways***.

- Histamine causes constriction of alveolar duct and increases airway resistance.

iii) ***Drugs:*** Drugs such as isoproterenol (***β_2-adrenergic receptor agonists***) produce bronchodilation.

- These drugs are usually used in the treatment of asthmatic attacks as they alleviate bronchial constriction.

iv) ***Environmental factors:*** Breathing chemical irritants, dusts and smoke particles cause reflex constriction of airways.

v) ***PCO_2 in breathing air:*** Increased PCO_2 in the conducting airways causes local bronchodilation.

- However, bronchoconstriction caused by the decreased PCO_2 is of more importance.

4. Viscosity and density of inspired gas

Increase in gas density as occurs in **deep-sea diving increases airway viscosity**. The air density increases because of increased barometric pressure.

- Gas mixture containing **oxygen-helium has low density**.
  - Therefore, a helium-oxygen mixture is often used during dive to make breathing easier.
  - Oxygen-helium mixture is also used in the treatment of status asthmaticus.

5. Phases of respiration

Airway resistance is not significantly altered during quiet breathing. However, during forced expiration as seen in severe exercise, resistance is significantly increased.

- This effect is well demonstrated by a flow-volume curve that depicts the relationship between airflow and lung volume during a forced inspiratory and expiratory effort (Fig. 45.16).

Flow-Volume Curve

A small loop of flow-volume curve is seen during tidal breathing, whereas, a large loop is observed during forced breathing.

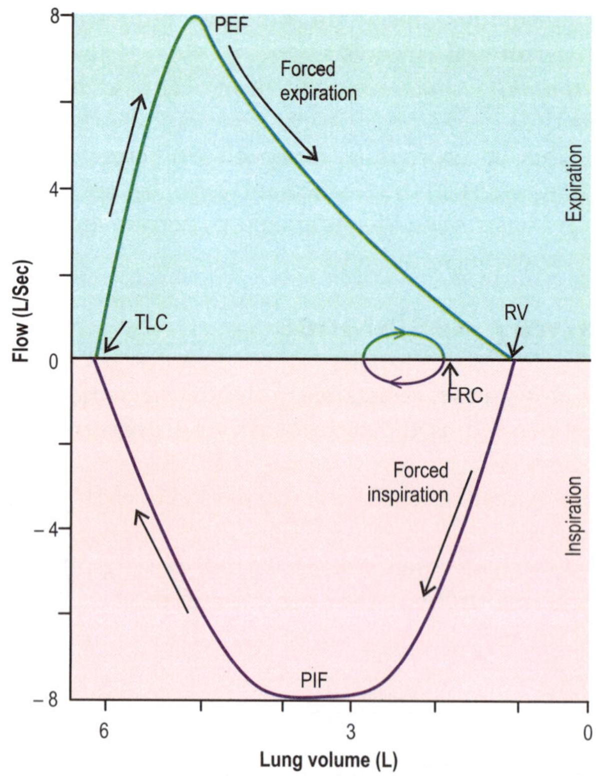

Fig. 45.16: Flow-volume curve. During forced expiration, airflow increases steeply to reach PEF (peak expiratory flow), which is achieved before there is much change in lung volume. Form PEF, flow rate decreases as lung volume decreases to residual volume (RV). The last part of expiratory flow is effort independent due to dynamic airway compression. During forced inspiration, PIF (peak inspiratory flow) is achieved little later (in comparison to PEF) and is maintained over a large change in lung volume as airways are distended (and not compressed). TLC: total lung capacity; FRC: functional residue capacity.

1. During forced inspiration, inspiratory flow is limited only by effort; that means the force with which the individual inspires.
2. During forced expiration (forced vital capacity), flow rises sharply to a peak (peak expiratory flow) and then decreases linearly over most part of expiration as lung volume decreases (Fig. 45.16).
    - The first phase of expiratory flow-volume curve is dependent on effort, but after the peak expiratory flow is reached, flow becomes independent of effort.
    - Thus, during forced expiration, flow is mostly independent of effort. This indicates the importance of dynamic airway compression during expiration.

Dynamic airway compression increases airways resistance, which effectively limits the forced expiratory flow (Clinical Note 45.2).

Dynamic Lung Volumes and Capacities

Timed Vital Capacity (FEV_1)

This is also called **forced expiratory volume in 1 second** (FEV_1).

This is defined as the ***percentage of FVC expired in the specified time***, e.g. FEV_1 the percentage of air expired in 1st second; FEV_2 in 2nd second and so on.

- This is an **index of air-flow rate**.

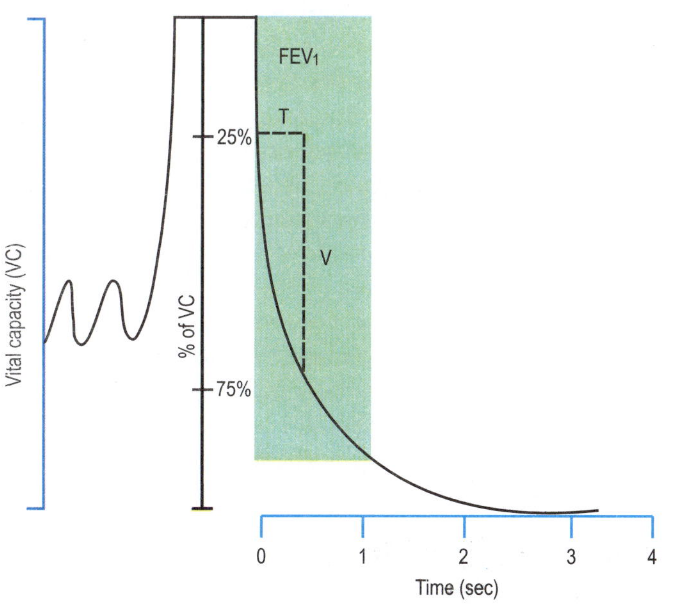

Fig. 45.17: Calculation of timed vital capacity (FEV_1) in physiological spirogram. Forced expiratory volume in first second (FEV_1) is calculated in spirometric recording. After recording of few normal tidal respirations, subject inhales to total lung capacity (deep inspiration with maximum effort) and holds his breath. Immediately, speed of recording is increased and subject exhales forcefully as maximum as possible. The graph gives the expiratory flow over time in seconds. The percentage of vital capacity (VC) expired in 1st second, 2nd second, etc. are calculated as FEV_1, FEV_2, and so on. From the same recording $FEF_{25-75\%}$ (forced expiratory flow in 25–75% of VC) can also be calculated for which T as time and V as volume are drawn in FEV_1 curve

Clinical Note 45.2

Deep breathing after surgery improves lung functions: It is difficult to practice deep breathing for patients who have undergone abdominal or thoracic surgery as *pain restricts movement of thoraco-abdominal walls.* Such patients prefer to take shallow breathing for which surfactant spreading becomes inadequate that makes the lungs atelectatic. Therefore, these patients are encouraged to practice deep breathing inspite of pain.

- In normal conditions, **72 to 85%** of the forced vital capacity is expired in the first second, 95% in two seconds and 97% in three seconds (Fig. 45.17).
- It is one of the most useful tests to **detect generalized airway obstruction**.

The ratio of **FEV_1 to FVC is more important** clinically than their individual measurements, which is normally **about 0.8** as calculated from clinical spirogram (Fig. 45.18).

Clinical Importance of FEV_1

- FEV_1 is the single most useful test to detect generalized airway obstruction.

1. FEV_1 less than 72% indicates difficulty in exhaling air from the lungs due to obstruction.
    - This is a **hallmark of obstructive lung disease** like bronchial asthma.
2. **In restrictive lung disease** like emphysema though FVC is decreased, FEV_1 as percentage of FVC remains normal (Fig. 45.19).
3. Thus, FEV_1 curve **differentiates obstructive from restrictive lung diseases**.

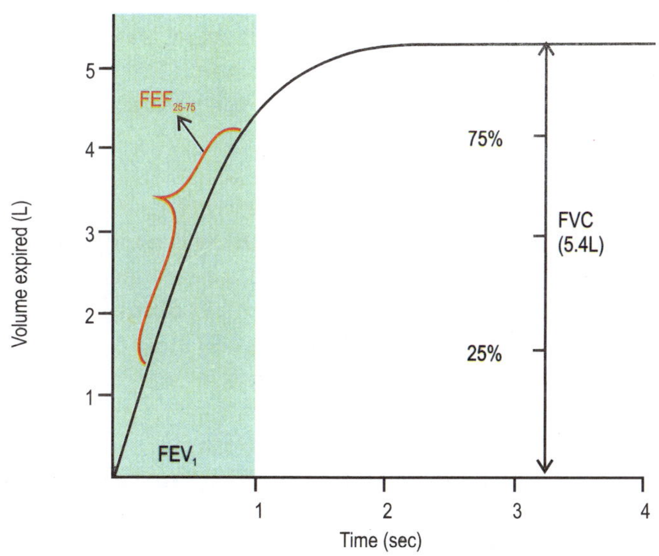

$$FEF_{25-75} = \frac{3L}{0.9s} = 3.3\ L/sec$$

$$FEV_1/FVC = \frac{4.3}{5.4} = 0.79$$

Fig. 45.18: The clinical spirogram. In this, forced expiratory volume (FEV) is plotted as function of time expressed in seconds. This differs from physiological spirogram only in its pattern of curve, as physiological spirogram records FEV_1 from top to bottom. Note, forced expiratory flow (FEF_{25-75}) is calculated as 3.3 L per second and ratio of FEV_1 to forced vital capacity (FVC) as 0.79.

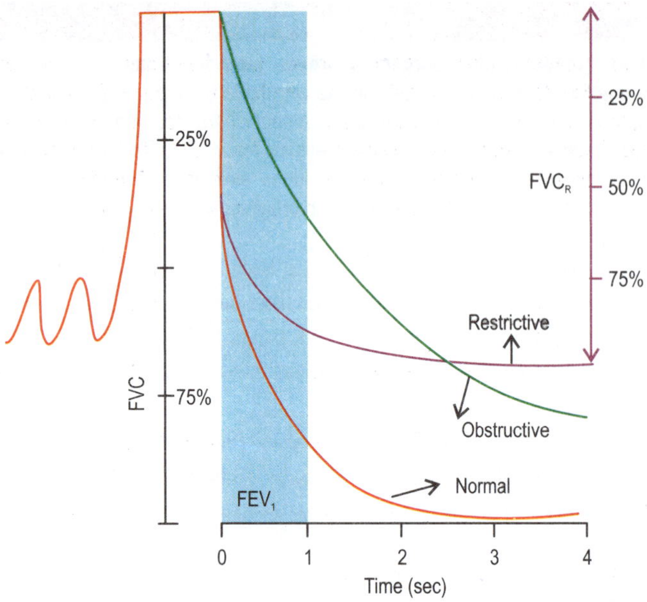

Fig. 45.19: Pattern of FEV1 curve in obstructive and restrictive lung disease. In obstructive disease, forced expiratory volume in first second (FEV_1) is less than 50% and even FEV_4 is less than 80% of forced vital capacity (FVC). In fact, FVC in obstructive disease is not significantly different from the normal, but FEV_1 as percentage of FVC is grossly reduced as there is obstruction to flow of air in respiratory tract. In restrictive disease, the pattern of FEV_1 curve is same as the normal curve and FEV1 as percentage of its own FVC (FVC_R) is normal. However, FVC in restrictive disease (FVC_R) is considerably less than the normal FVC.

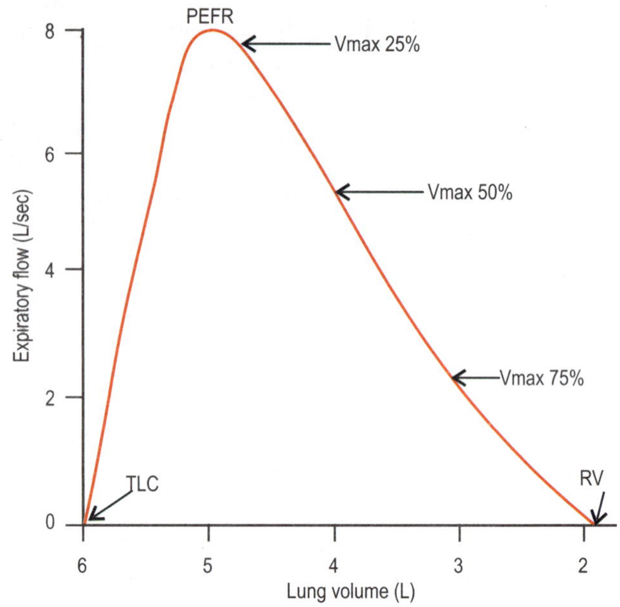

Fig. 45.20: In maximum expiratory flow volume curve (MEFVC), flow is plotted against volume exhaled. Vmax 75% is the flow rate at which 75% of the total FVC has been exhaled, Vmax 50% is the flow rate at which 50% of FVC remains to be exhaled and Vmax 25% is the flow rate at which 25% of the FVC has been exhaled. TLC: total lung capacity; RV: residual volume; PEFR: peak expiratory flow rate.

Maximum Mid-expiratory Flow Rate (MMEFR)

This is the maximum flow achieved during the **middle third of the total expired volume**.

- This is expressed as forced expiratory flow at 25% to 75% of the lung volume (**$FEF_{25\text{-}75}$%**).
- $FEF_{25\text{-}75}$% **indicates the patency of small airways**.

Normal Value: MMEFR between 200 and 1200 ml (**$FEF_{200\text{-}1200}$ ml**) in liters per second **indicates the patency of larger airways**.

Maximum Voluntary Ventilation (MVV)

This is also called as **maximum breathing capacity** (MBC).

- MVV indicates the **maximum volume of gas that can be breathed per minute by maximal voluntary effort**.

Normal Value: MVV in adult male is 150 liters per minute and in female is 125 liters per minute.

Peak Expiratory Flow Rate (PEFR)

PEFR is the **maximum velocity of flow in liters per minute** with which air is forced out of the lungs. PEFR is recorded by using peak-flow meter.

- PEFR is **an index of patency of airways**.
- However, MMEFR is a more sensitive indicator than PEFR.

Normal Value: PEFR is 400 to 600 L/min or 6 to 10 L/s.

Maximum Expiratory Flow Volume Curve (MEFVC)

Because of the limitation of FEV_1, certain other tests are performed to detect airways obstruction in its early phase.

- These include **Vmax 75%, Vmax 50% and Vmax 25%** responses of maximum expiratory flow, which are studied by plotting maximum expiratory flow volume curve (MEFVC) by inhalation of helium.
  - In MEFVC, flow is plotted against volume exhaled (Fig. 45.20).
- **Vmax 75%** is the flow rate at which 75% of the total FVC has been exhaled, **Vmax 50%** is the flow rate at which 50% of FVC remains to be exhaled and **Vmax 25%** is the flow rate at which 25% of the FVC has been exhaled. The maximum flow occurs early (in the first 20%) and decreases progressively thereafter.

When the individual performs at three different efforts (maximum, moderate and minimum), the MEFVC curves indicate that **peak expiratory flow rate (PEFR) increases with effort**.

- However, at lower lung volumes (towards residual volume) the effort has no impact on flow rate as all the three curves merge in the later part (Fig. 45.21).
- This indicates that in expiratory maneuver, the **early part is effort dependent** and the **later part is effort independent**.

Work of Breathing

During breathing, work is done to expand the lungs and overcome the airway resistance. The work done is expressed as a change in lung volume multiplied by the change in trans-pulmonary pressure.

- Thus, work (W) is equal to the product of pressure (P) and volume (V).

$W = P \times \Delta V$, where P is trans-pulmonary pressure and ΔV is change in lung volume.

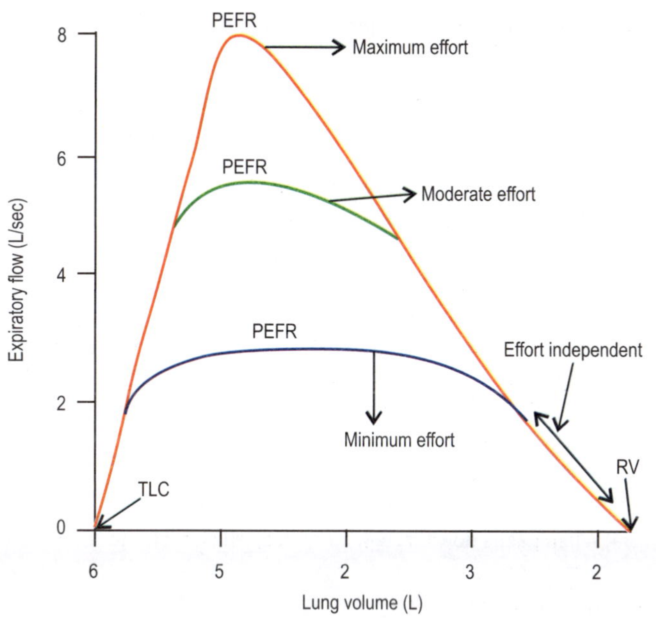

Fig. 45.21: Effect of different degrees of effort (maximum, moderate, and minimum) on expiratory flow-volume curve. Note, peak expiratory flow rate (PEFR) increases with effort. However, at lower lung volumes, i.e. toward residual volume (RV), the effort has no impact on flow rate as all the three curves merge in their terminal part (effort independent region of the curve). TLC: total lung capacity

Energy is spent with muscular contraction **to create a force** (trans-pulmonary pressure) **to increase lung volume** (inflate the lungs).

- The **pressure-volume curve** depicts the work required for breathing in normal lung that spends about 5% of the body's total energy expenditure (Fig. 45.22A).
- **In restrictive lung disease,** work of breathing is increased, as *greater inspiratory effort is required due to marked decrease in lung compliance* (Fig. 45.22B).
  - Therefore, patients with a restrictive disorder economize their ventilation by taking **rapid and shallow breaths.**
- **In obstructive lung disease**, work of breathing increases due to *more expenditure of energy to overcome increased airway resistance* (Fig. 45.22C).
  - Patients with obstructive disorders economize their ventilation by taking **slow and deep breaths.**

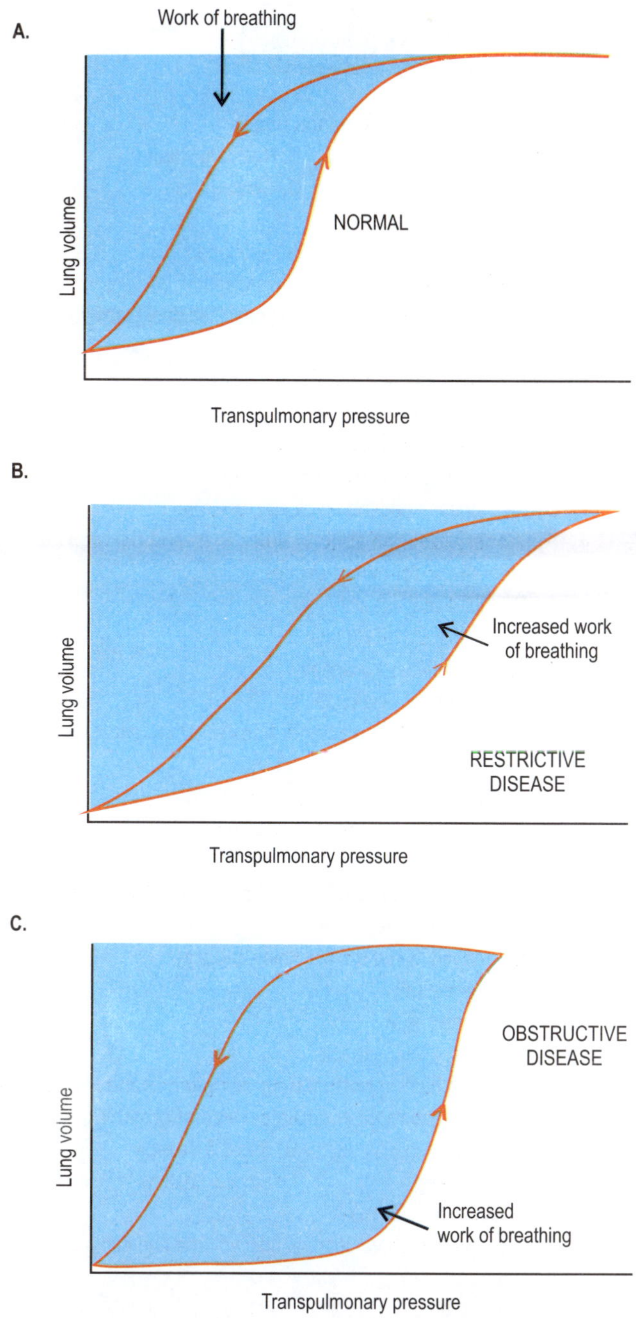

Fig. 45.22: Pressure-volume curve depicting work of breathing. The shaded area represents work of breathing **(A)**. Note work of breathing is increased in both restrictive **(B)** and obstructive **(C)** disorders though the pattern of change in energy spent is different in both conditions.

Exam Questions

1. Describe the mechanics of breathing with reference to the relaxation pressure-volume curve of the lung, chest wall and respiratory system.
2. Name the muscles of inspiration and expiration. With the help of a suitable diagram, depict alveolar and intrapleural pressure during quiet inspiration and expiration. Briefly describe the significance of intrapleural pressure.
3. Draw a labeled diagram to depict lung volume and capacities. Briefly describe how FRC can be measured.
4. Define lung compliance. List the factors affecting lung compliance. Give brief note on clinical significance of lung compliance.
5. List the composition and functions of surfactant. Briefly describe the regulation of surfactant synthesis and secretion.
6. Define airway resistance. List the factors affecting airway resistance.
7. List the dynamic lung volume and capacities. Draw a schematic diagram of FEV1 curve and explain how it is different in restrictive and obstructive lung disease.

Multiple Choice Questions

1. **Total lung capacity depends upon:**
   A. Lung compliance B. Residual volume
   C. Size of airway D. Closing volume
2. **Critical closing volume is:**
   A. Volume at the end of forceful expiration
   B. Volume at the end of forceful inspiration
   C. Volume remaining after Functional Residual Capacity is measured
   D. Close to residual Volume
3. **True about Hyaline membrane disease:**
   A. FRC above the closing volume
   B. FRC below the closing volume
   C. FRC is equal to closing volume
   D. FRC doesn't depend on closing volume
4. **Pulmonary function abnormalities in interstitial lung diseases include all the following except:**
   A. Reduced vital capacity
   B. Reduced FEV1/FVC ratio
   C. Reduced diffusion capacity
   D. Reduced total lung capacity
5. **Set of data which correctly defines restrictive lung disease is**
   A. ↑FRC, ↑compliance of lung tissue
   B. ↑FEV1/FVC, ↓compliance of lung tissue
   C. ↓ FEV1/FVC, ↓compliance of lung tissue
   D. ↑TLC , RV is ↓
6. **In upper air way obstruction, all of the following changes are seen except:**
   A. Decreased Maximum breathing capacity
   B. RV decreased
   C. Decreased FEV
   D. Decreased vital capacity
7. **A person is having normal lung compliance and increased airway resistance. The most economical way of breathing for him**
   A. Rapid & deep B. Rapid & shallow
   C. Slow & deep D. Slow & shallow
8. **Vital capacity is sum of:**
   A. Inspiratory reserve volume, tidal volume and expiratory reserve volume
   B. Tidal volume, Inspiratory reserve volume and Residual volume
   C. Expiratory reserve volume, Inspiratory reserve volume and Residual volume
   D. Residual volume, Inspiratory volume, and Expiratory volume
9. **Routine spirometry can't estimate:**
   A. FRC B. VC
   C. RV D. ERV
10. **The intrapleural pressure is negative both during inspiration and expiration because:**
    A. Intrapulmonary pressure is always negative
    B. Thoracic cage and lungs are elastic structure
    C. Transpulmonary pressure determines the negativity
    D. Surfactant prevents the lungs to collapse
11. **Increased airway resistance is caused by all EXCEPT:**
    A. Forced expiration
    B. Dense air
    C. Low lung volume
    D. High lung volume
12. **More resistance in expiration is due to:**
    A. Increased compression of airway
    B. Due to change from linear to turbulent flow
    C. Saturation with moisture
    D. Increased rate of flow during expiration
13. **Respiration stops in the last stage of expiration, in forced expiration because of:**
    A. Respiratory muscle fatigue
    B. Collapse of alveoli
    C. Dynamic compression of airways
    D. Breaking effect of inspiratory muscles
14. **When gases flow through an orifice, which factor to least likely to effect turbulence:**
    A. Density of gas
    B. Viscosity of gas
    C. Pressure of gas
    D. Diameter of orifice
15. **Specific lung compliance is decreased in all except:**
    A. Pulmonary congestion
    B. Chronic bronchitis
    C. Pulmonary fibrosis
    D. Decreased surfactant
16. **Compliance of lung is measured by**
    A. Elasticity
    B. Amount of air
    C. Blood flow
    D. Presence of fluid
17. **Compliance of lung is:**
    A. 200ml/cm water
    B. 500ml/cm water
    C. 800ml/cm water
    D. 1000ml/cm water
18. **Stability of alveoli is maintained by:**
    A. Lung compliance
    B. Negative intrapleural pressure
    C. Increase in alveolar surface by the surfactant
    D. Residual air in alveoli
19. **An important non-respiratory function of Lungs:**
    A. Anion balance
    B. Sodium balance
    C. Potassium balance
    D. Calcium balance
20. **FEV1 is less than 70% in:**
    A. Pulmonary fibrosis
    B. Lung collapse
    C. Bronchitis
    D. Bronchial asthma

Answers

1. A	2. D	3. B	4. B	5. B	6. B	7. C	8. A	9. A	10. B	11. D
12. A	13. C	14. C	15. B	16. A	17. A	18. C	19. B	20. D		

Chapter 46

Pulmonary Ventilation and Gas Exchange in Lungs

Learning Objectives

On completion of study of this chapter:

The student will be able to (must know):

1. Define minute ventilation, expired minute ventilation and alveolar ventilation and give their normal values.
2. Define physiological and anatomical dead space, give their normal values and understand their principle of measurement.
3. Understand the significance of alveolar ventilation and the principle of its measurement.
4. Name the layers of alveolocapillary membrane and the factors affecting diffusion of gases through it.

The student may also be able to (desirable to know):

1. Describe the procedure of measurement of dead space.
2. Describe the measurement and factors affecting diffusion capacity.

PY6.2

PULMONARY VENTILATION

Definitions

Ventilation: Ventilation is a dynamic process that moves air in and out of the lungs.

Minute Ventilation: Minute ventilation is the volume of air that enters lungs each minute.

- This is the **product of tidal volume and respiratory rate**. This is also called **minute respiratory volume**.
- If tidal volume is 500 ml, and respiratory rate is 12 per minute, the minute ventilation is 6 liters.

Minute ventilation = tidal volume × respiratory rate
= 500 (ml) × 12 (per/min)
= 6000 ml/min

Normally, minute ventilation in adult is **5 L to 10 L per/min**

Expired Minute Ventilation: Expired minute ventilation is the **amount of expired air per minute.**

- At rest is same as minute ventilation as the inspired and expired tidal volume (the amount of air inspired in or expired out in quiet breathing) is same.

Alveolar Ventilation: The **volume of air that actually reaches the alveoli per minute** is known as alveolar ventilation (V_A).

Dead Space

Definition: Dead space is **defined** as space within the airways that do not allow gas exchange with pulmonary capillary blood to occur.

Anatomical Dead Space: The volume of air present within the conducting airways does not take part in the gas exchange with pulmonary capillary blood and this is called dead space volume. Since, the dead space is due to the structural (anatomical) arrangement of the airways, it is referred to as anatomical dead space.

- Due to the anatomical dead space, out of 500 ml of tidal inspiration, **350 ml of air enters the alveoli**. Thus, the **normal dead space volume is 150 ml**.
- The **ratio of dead space volume to tidal volume** in normal health is 25 to 30%.
  - Thus, normally **30% of the minute ventilation does not participate** in gas exchange.

Physiological Dead Space

Alveolar Dead Space: Some amount of inspired air in the alveoli does not participate in gas exchange. This happens as some alveoli due to various reasons **have little or no blood supply**. Therefore, air in these alveoli also becomes part of the wasted air. The volume of air in these alveoli is referred to as **alveolar dead space**.

The sum of the anatomical dead space and alveolar dead space is called **physiological dead space**.

Physiological dead space = anatomic dead space + alveolar dead space

- Alveolar dead space is very negligible in normal individuals.
- Therefore, in normal healthy individuals, **anatomical dead space is almost equal with the physiological dead space**.

However, in various lung diseases, alveolar dead space volume becomes high, in which the physiological dead space is more than anatomical dead space.

Measurement of Dead Space

The volume of dead space is estimated by three methods: the Radford's formula, and the single-breath CO_2 technique, and single breath N_2 techniques.

Radford's Formula

Radford's formula predicts the **anatomical dead space** of the individual. The anatomical dead space of an individual in milliliters is equal to **his weight in pounds**.

- Thus, for a person with body weight of 150 lbs (70 kg), the dead space is 150 ml.
- However, this prediction is **fairly reliable for healthy individuals**, but not in patients with respiratory problems.

Single-Breath CO_2 Technique

The volume of dead space (V_D) is usually measured by the single-breath technique that **uses Bohr's equation** in the form of a gas such as CO_2. **CO_2 used** because it is almost **absent in the inspired air**, and its *alveolar concentration is same as in systemic arterial blood*.

According to Bohr's equation:

$$\text{Then, } V_D = (F_{AX} - F_{EX}) \frac{V_E}{F_{AX}}$$

When, V_D is the volume of dead space, V_E is the volume of expired air, F_{AX} and F_{EX} represent the concentration of gas in the alveolar air and mixed expired air respectively. As alveolar concentration of gas is same as arterial blood, F_{ax} (concentration of substance in arterial blood) replaces F_{AX}.

By using CO_2 as the gas for this estimation,

$$V_D = (P_aCO_2 - P_ECO_2) \frac{V_E}{P_aCO_2}$$

When, P_aCO_2 and P_ECO_2 represent the PCO_2 in the arterial blood and mixed expired air respectively. However, alveolar concentration of CO_2 can be obtained from PCO_2 of last 10 ml of expired air.

Single Breath Nitrogen Technique

Brief Procedure: The subject sitting comfortably breathes room air calmly for few breaths. Then, he is instructed to take a deep breath **from a normal mid-inspiration** during which he is switched over to a pure oxygen source (**takes deep breath with pure oxygen**).

- The subject is then asked to expire slowly and steadily to the maximum, so that the volume expired is his vital capacity.
- As he expires, a simultaneous record is made of the **volume flow rate** and the **percentage concentration of N_2 in the expired air**, which is plotted as a graph (Fig. 46.1).

The graph depicts four phases:

1. When the subject takes deep breath of pure oxygen, all the air in the dead space is replaced with oxygen, while the oxygen in the alveoli mixes with N_2 (and CO_2) in the residual volume. The initial gas exhaled is the **phase I**, which fills the dead space and therefore does not contain N_2.
2. The **phase II** is the mixture of dead space and alveolar gas, and **phase III** is the alveolar gas.
3. **Phase III** ends at closing volume, which is the lung volume above residual volume when airways in the lower parts of the lungs starts closing due to less transmural pressure in these dependent regions.
4. In **phase IV**, content of expired air increases, which ends at residual volume.

Dead space volume is the volume of gas **expired in phase I** and the volume **expired till mid-portion of phase II**.

Calculation of Dead Space

Dead space can be **calculated from the N_2 curve** obtained from the single-breath N_2 test in ***two ways:***

i) By constructing the equivalent dead space-alveolar air boundary
ii) By planimetry measurement

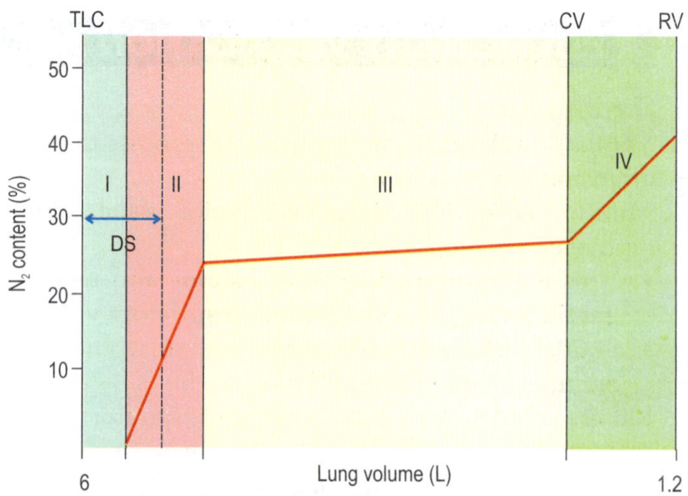

Fig. 46.1: Single-breath nitrogen curve. Expired air of **phase I** does not contain N_2 as it comes out of dead space (DS). **Phase II** contains mixture of dead space and alveolar air. **Phase III** is the alveolar air. As gas in the upper portion of the lung is richer in N_2 than the lower portion of lungs, **phase II** has a sharp rise in N_2 content and phase III has very slow rise in N_2. **Phase IV** has positive slope indicating that air comes again from the upper portion of the lungs toward later part of expiration. Note dead space air constitutes volume of phase I and half of phase II. TLC: Total lung capacity; CV: Closing volume; RV: Residual volume.

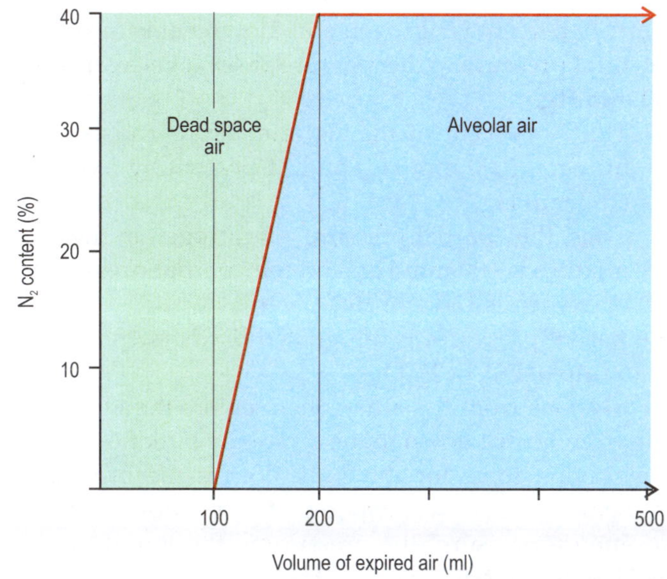

Fig. 46.2: Measurement of dead space by single-breath nitrogen test. Total volume is estimated and equivalent dead space volume is proportionately calculated from the total. Alveolar volume is more than the volume shown in the picture.

Construction of Equivalent Dead Space-Alveolar Air Boundary: Dead space is filled with pure oxygen prior to expiration. Therefore, appearance of N_2 in the curve indicates the air coming from alveoli.

- The boundary between dead space air and alveolar air is **S-shaped** because of some degree of mixing of alveolar gas with dead space air.
- However, an equivalent sharp boundary is constructed in such a way that the amount of N_2 in the dead space area is equal to the amount of N_2 in the alveolar air section.
- The dead space volume is then calculated as the volume expired up to this line and is read from the volume recording.

Planimetry Measurement The area representing dead space volume and the area representing total volume expired (V_E) are estimated with the help of a planimeter. The total area in the graph represents V_E (Fig. 46.2). Hence, the dead space volume from the corresponding area is determined by simple proportion.

Alveolar Ventilation

The **volume of air that fills the alveoli per minute** and takes part in gas exchange is known as alveolar ventilation (V_A).

To know the volume of air that takes part in alveolar ventilation, first the **dead space volume** is subtracted from the tidal volume and then the volume is **multiplied by breathing (respiratory) frequency**.

If the tidal volume is 500 ml, dead space volume is 150 ml and respiratory rate is 15 /min:

Alveolar ventilation is = (500 ml –150 ml) × 15
= 350 ml × 15 = 5250 ml / min

Clinical Importance

If anatomic dead space volume is increased due to any cause, **alveolar ventilation decreases.**

- For example, a patient **on mechanical ventilator**, alveolar ventilation decreases due to increased dead space volume (**by tubing** etc.). In such patients, if minute ventilation remains constant, alveolar gas exchange suffers.

Physiological Significance

Shallow Breathing: In **rapid and shallow breathing,** though minute ventilation does not change much, **alveolar ventilation is grossly impaired** because most of the air inhaled is utilized to occupy the anatomic dead space and the air available to enter into alveoli is less.

- Therefore, patients with rapid and shallow breathing **develop hypoxia and hypercapnia.**

Deep Breathing: The **deep and slow breathing** will have adequate alveolar ventilation though the minute ventilation does not change much. Such subjects have alveolar ventilation even greater than subjects with normal breathing.

- Thus, **to improve alveolar ventilation**, *the depth of breathing* should be increased.
- During moderate to severe exercise, a **trained athlete** achieves the target alveolar ventilation by *mainly increasing the depth rather than the frequency of breathing* (Application Box 46.1).

Application Box 46.1

Pranayama increases alveolar ventilation: In most of yogic breathing exercises like pranayama (controlled breathing), emphasis is given to practice slow and deep breathing, which aims at increasing alveolar ventilation.

Measurement of Alveolar Ventilation

Alveolar ventilation is easy to calculate if dead space volume is known.

- Alveolar ventilation is calculated in the pulmonary function laboratory from the **volume of expired carbon dioxide** per minute and fractional concentration of carbon dioxide in the alveolar gas.
- Because no gas exchange occurs in the conducting airways and the inspired air contains essentially no carbon dioxide, **all of the expired carbon dioxide originates from alveoli**.

Thus, $V_ECO_2 = V_A \times F_ACO_2$

Where, V_ECO_2 is the volume of carbon dioxide expired per minute and F_ACO_2 is the fractional concentration of carbon dioxide in alveolar gas.

Rearrangement of this provides the alveolar ventilation equation:

$$V_A = V_ECO_2 / F_ACO_2$$

The carbon dioxide concentration in the alveoli can be obtained by sampling the last portion of the tidal volume during expiration, the end-tidal volume, which contains alveolar gas.

Alveolar Ventilation reflects P_aCO_2: It is important to note an **inverse relationship exists between V_A and P_aCO_2**. If alveolar ventilation is halved, alveolar PCO_2 will double.

1. Clinically, the ***adequacy of alveolar ventilation is an index of arterial PCO_2***.
2. An **increase in P_aCO_2** reflects hypoventilation and a **decrease in P_aCO_2** reflects hyperventilation.

Clinical Abnormalities of Ventilation

Hypoventilation

Causes of hypoventilation are categorized into depression of respiratory centers by diseases or drugs (**central hypoventilation**), and failure of the ventilatory apparatus (**peripheral hypoventilation**). Hypoventilation leads to decreased P_aO_2 and increased P_aCO_2.

Alveolar hypoventilation occurs commonly in:

1. **Exacerbation of chronic lung disease** such as asthma, chronic bronchitis and emphysema.
2. **Depression of respiratory centers** as occurs in head injuries or by drugs such as barbiturates and opiates.
3. **Neuromuscular disorders** that weaken the respiratory muscles e.g. myasthenia gravis, poliomyelitis, acute polyneuritis, and tetanus.

In hypoventilation, **hypoxia** occurs due to decreased oxygen supply and **hypercapnia** occurs due to decreased CO_2 removal.

Hyperventilation

Hyperventilation usually occurs due to **stimulation of respiratory centers**.

- However, voluntary hyperventilation and exercise induced hyperventilation are common physiological causes of hyperventilation.
- Excess removal of CO_2 in hyperventilation results in **respiratory alkalosis**.

GAS EXCHANGE IN LUNGS

Physiological Aspects

The gases are simple molecules that are free to move among one another by diffusion. The net diffusion of a gas is in the direction of concentration gradient. The partial pressures of individual gas in a mixture of gases are directly proportional to the concentration of the gas molecules.

- Air in atmosphere is mainly the mixture of *oxygen and nitrogen*. The rate of diffusion of each of them is directly proportional to the pressure caused by that gas alone, which is called the **partial pressure** of that gas.
- In air, 79 percent is nitrogen and 21 percent is oxygen. The **total pressure** of this mixture at sea level averages **760 mm Hg**.
  - The 79 percent of the 760 mm Hg is caused by nitrogen (600 mm Hg) and 21 percent by oxygen (160 mm Hg).
  - Thus, the "partial pressure" of nitrogen in the air mixture is 600 mm Hg, and the "partial pressure" of oxygen is 160 mm Hg.
- The partial pressures is designated by the symbols P, for example, PO_2 or PCO_2 .

Bulk Flow: Gas from the atmosphere enters the airways starting from nostril down to the alveoli by bulk flow.

1. The driving force for this bulk flow is the pressure gradient, which is created due to the difference in barometric pressure (the pressure at the mouth) and the alveolar pressure.
2. Exchange of gas between the alveoli and the capillary blood occurs across the alveolar-capillary membrane by diffusion in response to partial pressure gradients of the gases.

Factors Contributing to Gas Exchange

Gas uptake from alveoli is determined by four factors:

1. Diffusion properties of the alveolar-capillary membrane
2. Partial pressure gradient for the gas
3. Pulmonary capillary blood flow
4. **Diffusing capacity** of the gas through the membrane

Alveolar-Capillary Membrane

Alveolar-capillary membrane (also called **Respiratory Membrane**) forms the **blood-gas interface** that separates blood in the pulmonary capillaries from the gas in the alveoli. This membrane is exceedingly thin and is mainly composed of alveolar epithelium, interstitial fluid layer, and capillary endothelium.

Layers of Alveolar-Capillary Membrane

From interior of the alveoli to the capillary blood, the alveolar-capillary membrane is made up of six layers. However, O_2 from hemoglobin molecule in the red cells of pulmonary capillaries to enter into alveolar lumen (or the transport in the reverse direction), passes through **10 layers** (Fig. 46.3):

1. Alveolar surfactant
2. Layer of alveolar epithelial cells
3. Basement membrane of alveolar epithelium
4. A thin layer of interstitial fluid
5. Basement membrane of capillary endothelium
6. Layer of capillary endothelial cells
7. Plasma

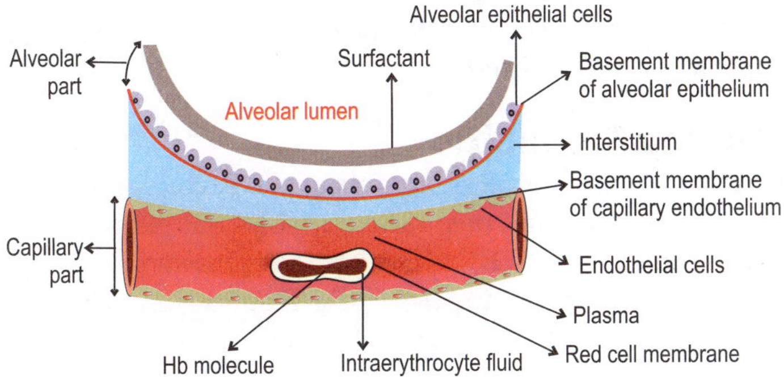

Fig. 46.3: Layers of alveolar-capillary membrane.

8. Red cell membrane
9. Intra-erythrocyte fluid
10. Hemoglobin molecule

Thickness of alveolar-capillary membrane: The thickness of alveolar-capillary membrane is normally **0.2 to 0.5μ**. The thinness of the membrane allows easy diffusion of gasses through it.

Factors Affecting Diffusion of Gasses

Diffusion of gasses through alveolar-capillary membrane depends mainly on ***six factors***.

1. **Difference in partial pressure** of gas on both side of the membrane, i. e. partial pressure gradient for the gas (discussed below)
2. **Diffusing capacity** of the membrane for the gas (discussed below)
3. **Surface area of the membrane:** Surface area for diffusion decreases in conditions like emphysema and increases in conditions in which there is more opening of number of capillaries as occurs in exercise.
4. **Solubility of the gas:** Solubility of the gas in the membrane is an important factor for diffusion. For example, CO_2 being more soluble diffuses easily.
5. **Thickness of the membrane:** Diffusion is **inversely proportional to the thickness** of the alveolar-capillary membrane. When thickness is doubled the diffusion is halved.
6. **Molecular weight of the gas:** Diffusion is **inversely proportional to the molecular weight of the gas**. Thus, gas with smaller molecule diffuses easily through the membrane.

Clinical Significance

Though the alveolar-capillary membrane is thin and does not interfere with gas exchange, diffusion is disturbed in diseased conditions due to some membrane pathology. This is called as *alveolar-capillary obstruction syndrome*.

Alveolar-Capillary Obstruction Syndrome: This syndrome occurs in **two** important types of defects.

1. **Thickening of the alveolar-capillary membrane,** as seen in diffuse interstitial fibrosis, asbestosis etc.
2. **Increased distance between alveolar and capillary membrane** due to ***interstitial edema*** as seen in heart failure etc.

In this syndrome, **diffusion of oxygen is decreased** but not the carbon dioxide, as **CO_2 is 20 times more soluble** in water than oxygen. Hypoxemia develops **without significant change in PCO_2**.

Partial Pressure Gradients

Diffusion Gradient

The diffusion of gases depends on the **difference of partial pressure** of the individual gas across the alveolar-capillary membrane. This is also called as the **diffusion gradient** for the gas.

- For example, **oxygen diffusion gradient** is **about 60 mm Hg**, which is the difference between the PO_2 of the alveolar air (160 mm Hg) and the arterial blood (100 mm Hg).
- **Diffusion gradient for carbon dioxide** across alveolar-capillary membrane ($P_{VCO2} - P_{ACO2}$) **is about 6 mm Hg**, which is much lower than that of oxygen.

Gasses are dissolved plasma and they exert a partial pressure, as governed by two laws.

Henry's Law: Henry's law states that the amount of gas dissolved in a liquid at a given temperature is directly ***proportional to the partial pressure and the solubility*** of the gas.

Fick's Law: Fick's law states that the volume of gas diffusing per minute across a membrane is **directly proportional** to the membrane surface area, the diffusion coefficient of the gas, and the partial pressure difference of the gas, and **inversely proportional** to membrane thickness.

Partial pressure of gasses in different parts of respiratory systems is depicted in Table 46.1.

Table 46.1 | Partial pressure of gases (mm Hg) in different parts of respiratory system:

	O_2	CO_2	N_2	H_2O
Inspired air	158	0.3	596	5.7
Expired air	116	32	565	47
Alveolar air	100	40	573	47
Venous blood	40	46	573	47
Arterial blood	95	40	573	47
Capillary blood	40	46	573	47

Diffusion Coefficient

The diffusion coefficient of a gas is **directly proportional to its solubility** and **inversely proportional to the square root of its molecular weight**.

- Therefore, *a highly soluble molecule or a smaller molecule diffuses rapidly*.
- For example, the diffusion coefficient of carbon dioxide in aqueous solutions is about 20 times greater than that

of oxygen because of its higher solubility, even though it is a larger molecule than O_2.

Capillary Blood Flow

Flow of blood in the pulmonary capillary is important for oxygen uptake. Normally, the **transit time** (time taken by the red cells to pass through the capillary), is approximately **0.75 sec**, during which the gas tension in the blood equilibrates with the gas tension in the alveoli.

Uptake of N_2O is flow-limited: With increase in cardiac output, blood flow through the pulmonary capillaries increases that decreases the transit time. For example, **nitrous oxide** (N_2O), an anesthetic gas easily diffuses across the alveolar-capillary membrane and equilibrates in 0.1 s.

- The **only way to increase the transfer of N_2O** from alveolar air into the blood is by increasing the blood flow, as **N_2O uptake is flow-limited.**

CO transfer is diffusion-limited: Carbon monoxide (CO) readily diffuses across the alveolar-capillary membrane, but due to its high affinity for hemoglobin it rapidly binds to hemoglobin.

- This binding decreases the partial pressure of CO in blood, for which the equilibrium for CO across the alveolar-capillary membrane is never reached in 0.75 s (transit time).
- Therefore, **CO transfer is diffusion-limited** (not limited by the blood flow).

Oxygen uptake is flow limited: The capillary oxygen tension equilibrates with alveolar oxygen tension well within the transit time, normally in one third of the available time, i.e. in 0.3 s.

- Thus, a **wide safety margin** is available for oxygen to ensure that the end-capillary PO_2 is fully equilibrated with alveolar PO_2.
- **During severe exercise**, though the transit is reduced but still time is adequate to fully oxygenate the blood.
- Though, oxygen binds with hemoglobin less avidly than CO, oxygen equilibrates fast. Thus, **oxygen uptake is flow limited.**

Diffusing Capacity PY6.2

The ability of the respiratory membrane to exchange a gas between the alveoli and the pulmonary blood is expressed as **diffusing capacity (DC)** *of the respiratory membrane.* DC is defined as the *volume of a gas that will diffuse through the membrane each minute for a partial pressure difference of 1 mm Hg.*

The diffusing capacity (DC) provides a **measure of the rate of gas transfer** in the lungs as per their partial-pressure gradient.

Measurement of DC

Carbon monoxide (CO) is used to determine the lung diffusing capacity because of **several advantages**:

1. Its uptake is **limited by diffusion** and not by blood flow.
2. There is essentially **no CO in the venous blood.**
3. The **affinity of CO for hemoglobin is 210 times** greater than that of oxygen, which causes the partial pressure of carbon monoxide to remain essentially zero in the pulmonary capillaries.

To measure the diffusing capacity (DC) with CO, the equation is:

D_C = , where V_{CO} is CO uptake in ml/min and P_{ACO} is alveolar partial pressure of CO.

The most common technique for making this measurement is called the **single-breath test.**

Factors affecting DC : **Hemoglobin and capillary blood volume** affect lung diffusing capacity.

- Diffusing capacity not only depends on the **diffusion properties** of the alveolocapillary membrane, but also on **hematocrit and capillary blood volume.**
- A decrease in either the hematocrit or capillary blood volume decreases the diffusing capacity.

Exam Questions

1. What is physiological dead space? Briefly describe the methods of measurement of dead space.
2. List the layers of alveolocapillary membrane. Beefily explain various factors affecting diffusion across the alveolocapillary membrane.
3. List the factors affecting gas exchange in lungs and briefly describe the role of each factor in gas exchange.

Multiple Choice Questions

1. **Calculate the Alveolar ventilation per minute of a patient with respiratory rate 14/min, tidal volume of 500 ml, with a vital capacity 7000 ml:**
   A. 4900 mL B. 2000 mL
   C. 7700 mL D. 7000 mL
2. **Measurement of anatomic dead space is by:**
   A. O2 breath test B. Helium dilution test
   C. N2 breath test D. PCO2
3. **The content of which of the following gas is maximum in inspired air?**
   A. Oxygen B. Nitrogen
   C. Carbon dioxide D. Carbon monoxide
4. **Which of the following is not an important factor for diffusion of gasses through alveolo-capillary membrane?**
   A. Difference in partial pressure of gas across the membrane
   B. Diffusing capacity of the membrane for the gas
   C. Thickness of the membrane
   D. Hemoglobin content of the blood

Answers : 1. A 2. C 3. B 4. D

Chapter 47

Pulmonary Circulation and Ventilation-Perfusion Ratio

Learning Objectives

On completion of study of this chapter:

The student will be able to (must know):

1. Appreciate the arrangement of blood supply to the lung and list the functions of pulmonary circulation.
2. List the special features of pulmonary circulation.
3. List the factors affecting pulmonary blood flow and pulmonary vascular resistance.
3. Understand the basis of difference in pulmonary blood flow in upper, middle and lower zones of the lung.
4. Explain the mechanism of filtration across pulmonary capillaries and genesis of pulmonary edema.
5. Learn the importance of ventilation-perfusion ratio in lung functions.
6. Understand the basis of difference in ventilation-perfusion ratio in apex and base of the lungs and its physiological and clinical importance.

The student may also be able to (desirable to know):

1. Describe the regulation of pulmonary circulation
2. Learn the physiology of bronchial circulation.

PY5.10

PULMONARY CIRCULATION

Functional Organization

The pulmonary arteries branch like that of airways so that each airway branch and arterial branch **run parallel to each other**.

- Pulmonary capillaries are **large in diameter and have multiple anastomoses**. The arrangement of capillaries is such that **each alveolus is surrounded by a capillary basket** (Fig. 47.1).
- A branch of pulmonary artery divides further to form arterioles that in turn form **extensive capillary lattice** around a single alveolus, which drains into a branch of pulmonary veins.

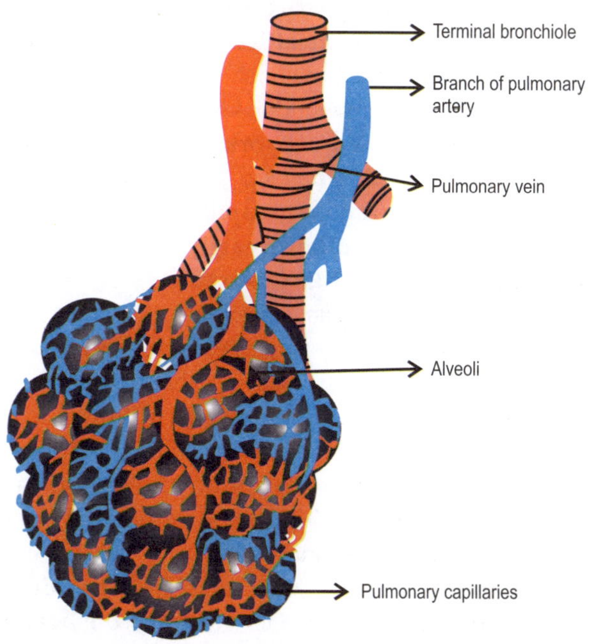

Fig. 47.1: Arrangement of blood supply to alveoli.

Functions of Pulmonary Circulation

1. **Gas exchange:** The primary function of the pulmonary circulation is **exchange of gases**, where CO_2 is removed from pulmonary capillary into alveoli and O_2 is added from alveoli into the capillary blood.
2. **Serves as a filter:** Pulmonary vessels **filter thrombi and emboli** that originate from venous compartment and right side of the heart.
   - Endothelial cells of pulmonary vessels release **fibrinolytic agents** that lyse blood clots (thrombi) and thus **prevent the entry of these thrombi and emboli** into coronary, cerebral, and other important vessels.
3. **Metabolic functions:** Angiotensin I is converted to **angiotensin II** in the lungs by *angiotensin-converting enzyme* (ACE) located in capillary endothelial cells.

- Pulmonary endothelial cells **inactivate bradykinin, serotonin, and prostaglandins E_1, E_2, and $F_{2\alpha}$.**

4. **Serves as a blood reservoir:** About 500 ml of circulating blood is present in the pulmonary circulation at any point of time.

Special Features of Pulmonary Circulation

The pulmonary circulation is a **low-pressure** (mean pulmonary arterial pressure is 15 mm Hg), and **low resistance system**.

1. As pulmonary artery and its branches **have thin walls**, and less smooth muscle in the walls they are **more compliant**. They are much shorter and wider.
   - The pulmonary veins are also **thin-walled and highly compliant.**
   - Therefore, pulmonary vessels can **accommodate a relatively large amount of blood**.
2. Due to thin-wall and less smooth muscle, **ability of pulmonary vessels to constrict is less**.
3. Pulmonary capillaries form **lattice in the alveolar wall** so that blood flows as a thin sheet.
   - Though, they comprise a dense capillary bed, they are not arranged as a network of tubular vessels, and they *do not form a capillary network*.
   - The walls of the pulmonary capillaries are very thin and therefore, **they collapse easily if local alveolar pressure exceeds capillary pressure**.
4. Change in *pulmonary venous and left atrial pressures* profoundly affects gas exchange. The pulmonary **wedge pressure** indirectly measures these pressures.
   - The **wedge pressure** is recorded by introducing a Swan-Ganz catheter percutaneously through the right side of the heart into the pulmonary circulation, where the tip of the catheter literally wedges in small pulmonary artery.
   - A continuous and close column of blood connects the probe's end and the left atrium; the **wedge pressure reflects left atrial pressure**.
5. **Low pulmonary vascular resistance:** Pulmonary vascular resistance is about one-tenth of systemic vascular resistance, which is due to **two factors**:
   i) Pulmonary resistance vessels (arterioles) are **thin, short and wide**. Thus, they have **high compliance**.
   ii) The **resting vasoconstrictor tone is very low or absent** for which the arterioles are mostly dilated (in contrast to systemic arterioles and precapillary sphincters that are partially constricted because of their resting sympathetic tone).
6. A **unique feature** of the pulmonary circulation is that the **pulmonary vascular resistance (PVR) falls with increased pulmonary arterial pressure** as occurs in increased cardiac output. This occurs due to *two mechanisms:*

Capillary Recruitment: Normally, many capillaries are partially closed, and they open when blood flow increases. This is called the **capillary recruitment** and is the primary mechanism of fall in PVR to increased cardiac output.

Capillary Distension: As pulmonary capillaries are exceedingly thin and highly compliant **capillary distension** occurs in response to increased pressure.

Physiological Significance of low PVR with increased Cardiac Output: The decrease in PVR with increased cardiac output has three beneficial effects.

a. The decreased resistance decreases the flow velocity especially when the flow rate is high, which provides more time for pulmonary capillary blood to take up oxygen and dispose of carbon dioxide.
b. The capillary distension increases the capillary surface area, which facilitates diffusion of gases along the alveolar-capillary membrane.
c. The pulmonary capillary pressure remains low that **prevents pulmonary edema**. This also decreases the load on the right ventricle.

IMPORTANT NOTE

Pulmonary edema does not occur during exercise: During vigorous exercise cardiac output increases enormously that increases blood flow and pressure in pulmonary circulation, but due to low PVR, pulmonary edema does not occur.

Pulmonary Blood Flow

There is approximately 500 ml of blood present in pulmonary circulation at any given time, which is about **10% of the total circulating blood volume**. The distribution of 500 ml of blood is as follows:

In pulmonary arteries : 150 ml
In pulmonary veins : 270 ml
In pulmonary capillaries : 80 ml

Distribution of Pulmonary Blood Flow: In upright posture, blood flow **increases from apex to the base of the lungs**. This difference is due to the **effect of gravity**.

Factors Affecting Pulmonary Blood Flow

Factors that affect pulmonary blood flow are:

1. Pulmonary vascular resistance (PVR)
2. Gravity
3. Alveolar pressure
4. Arterial to venous pressure gradient

Factors Affecting PVR

Pulmonary vascular resistance (PVR) is affected by lung volumes, hormones and oxygen tension.

Lung Volumes

Functionally, pulmonary vessels are of two types: alveolar vessels (arterioles, capillaries, and venules), and extra-

alveolar vessels (pulmonary arteries and veins).
- The extra-alveolar vessels are subjected to pleural pressure and alveolar vessels are subjected to alveolar pressure.

High Lung Volumes: At high lung volumes, the pleural **pressure is more negative**. This increases transmural pressure (pressure inside the vessel minus pressure outside the vessel) in the extra-alveolar vessels and vessels are distended.
- However, increased alveolar diameter at high lung volumes decreases transmural pressure in alveolar vessels.
- As a result, the *alveolar vessels are compressed*, and **PVR is increased**.

Low Lung Volumes: At low lung volumes, **pleural pressure is positive**, which compresses the extra-alveolar vessels.
- This **increases PVR**. Thus, PVR also increases at low lung volumes.
- PVR is **lowest at functional residual capacity** and ***increases at both higher and lower lung volumes***.

Hormones

Serotonin, norepinephrine, histamine, thromboxane A_2, and leukotrienes are **potent vasoconstrictors**.
- They **increase PVR**, particularly at low lung volumes when the vessels are already compressed.
- Adenosine, acetylcholine, prostacyclin (PG-I_2), and isoproterenol relax smooth muscle of blood vessel and **decrease PVR**.

Oxygen Tension

Low oxygen tension increases PVR by causing vasoconstriction.

Effects of Gravity

Due to effect of gravity, in **upright posture pulmonary blood flow increases from apex to base of the lungs**.
- Apex of the lungs remains above, and base remains below the **level of the heart**.
  - With 1 cm increase in height above the heart, the hydrostatic pressure ***falls by 0.74 mm Hg*** and with 1 cm decrease in height below the heart, the hydrostatic pressure ***increases by 0.74 mm Hg***.
  - Thus, pressure in the pulmonary artery **at apex**, which is about 10 cm above the heart, **is 7.4 mm Hg less**.

IMPORTANT NOTE

The arterial pressures in lungs at various levels are:

At the level of the heart	: 14 mm Hg
At the apex of the lung	: 6.6 mm Hg (10 cm above; 7.4 mm Hg less)
At the base of the lung	: 17.7 mm Hg (5 cm below: 3.4 mm Hg more)

Gravity Divides Lung into 3 Zones

- Gravity influences **both arterial and venous pressures, and ventilation-perfusion ratio.**
- As gravity causes change in lung vascular pressures and perfusion from apex to base, physiologically, lung is divided into **three zones**: Zone 1 (upper zone), Zone 2 (middle zone) and Zone 3 (lower zone).

In the Upper Zone: The **capillary pressure** in the apex of the lungs is **close to alveolar pressure**. The **arterial pressure** is just sufficient to maintain perfusion.
- If due to any reason the arterial pressure is decreased or the alveolar pressure is increased, capillaries collapse, and no gas exchange occurs.
- Gravity causes capillary beds to be **under-perfused in the apex of the lungs.**
  - The upper zone (zone 1) is **well ventilated but not well perfused**.
  - Therefore, this **increases alveolar dead space.**
  - However, *zone 1 is usually very small or* ***nonexistent*** *in healthy individuals.*

IMPORTANT NOTE

Zone 1 increases in hypotension: The **area of zone 1 increases** in conditions in which alveolar pressure is increased or pulmonary arterial pressure is decreased. For example, ***in hemorrhagic shock***, zone 1 is increased due to low blood pressure.

In the Middle Zone: The arterial and capillary pressures **exceed alveolar pressure**.
- However, as **pulmonary venous pressure is less than alveolar pressure**,
  - Hence, **veins are mechanically constricted** due to the pressure from outside.
  - This results in damming of blood in capillaries.
- But pulmonary veins are compliant.
  - Therefore, veins collect the amount of blood that escapes into them through the constriction.
  - This is called **Water-Fall Effect**.

The middle zone (zone 2) **is present in the middle of the lungs**, where blood flow is determined not by the arterial-venous pressure difference, but by the **difference between arterial pressure and alveolar pressure**.

In the Lower Zone: **Alveolar pressure is lower than the pressure in all vessels** (arteries, capillaries and venules), especially the venous pressure.
- Thus, blood flows by arterio-venous pressure difference.
- The **increase in blood flow** in this region is mainly due to **capillary distension**.

Effects of Alveolar Pressure

Alveolar pressure depends on lung volume.
- Alteration in alveolar pressure due to change in lung volume changes pulmonary blood flow.

Arterio-Venous Pressure Gradient

The difference between the pressure at arterial and venous compartment of pulmonary circulation determines the rate of blood flow.

- Arterial to venous pressure gradient is affected by alveolar pressure.

Regulation of Pulmonary Blood Flow

Pulmonary blood flow is regulated by **active and passive factors**.

Active Factors

Active factors are **neural, hormonal and chemical.**

Neural Regulation: Though the pulmonary circulation is richly innervated with sympathetic nerves, the **resting sympathetic tone of pulmonary circulation is almost absent**.

- However, **sympathetic stimulation** causes *mild vasoconstriction* and **parasympathetic stimulation** causes *mild vasodilation*.

Hormonal Regulation: **Major vasoconstrictors** in pulmonary bed are serotonin, norepinephrine, endothelin, angiotensin, thromboxane A_2, and leukotrienes. They decrease pulmonary blood flow.

- **Vasodilators** that increase blood flow are adenosine, acetylcholine, prostacyclin (PG-I_2), bradykinin and nitric oxide.

Chemical Regulation: Hypoxemia or alveolar **hypoxia causes vasoconstriction** of small pulmonary arteries (in other body parts hypoxia produces vasodilation).

- The mechanism of this unique phenomenon of **hypoxia-induced pulmonary vasoconstriction** is that hypoxia directly causes ***contraction of pulmonary vascular smooth muscles***.

Mechanism: Hypoxia **inhibits K^+ channels** that depolarize the muscle cells. This **opens the voltage-gated Ca^{++} channels**. **Influx of Ca^{++}** causes vasoconstriction.

The hypoxia-induced vasoconstriction is accentuated by high carbon dioxide and low blood pH.

Passive Factors

Passive factors that regulate pulmonary blood flow are **cardiac output, gravity and lung volumes**. Increase in cardiac output increases pulmonary blood flow.

Filtration across Pulmonary Capillaries

Filtration of fluid across capillary walls in the pulmonary circulation is governed by **Starling forces**. In addition, **surface tension and alveolar pressure contribute to filtration**.

- **Alveolar surface tension** pulls alveolar wall inward (facilitates alveolar collapse) that decreases interstitial pressure and therefore draws fluid into the interstitial space (**favours filtration**),
- **Alveolar pressure** compresses the interstitial space and increases the interstitial pressure (**opposes filtration**).

1. **Hydrostatic and osmotic pressure gradients:** The hydrostatic pressure in pulmonary capillaries is about 8 to 10 mm Hg. As it is ***significantly less than the oncotic pressure***, which is 25 mm Hg, this ***favors the net absorption of fluid*** from interstitial space into capillary blood.
2. **Role of alveolar surface tension:** Alveolar surface tension ***favours filtration*** and counteracts the advantage of low hydrostatic pressure.
   - The net result is that a small quantity of fluid fluxes out of the capillaries into the interstitial space, which passes into the lymphatic channels.
3. **Role of lymphatics:** The lymphatic system is **extensive and well developed** in lungs. The lymphatics **drain excess fluid** from peribronchial space.

Pulmonary Edema

Pulmonary edema develops when excess of free fluid accumulates in interstitial spaces and alveoli (Clinical Note 47.1).

Pulmonary edema is caused by **following mechanisms**:

1. **Increased capillary hydrostatic pressure:** This is the **commonest cause** of pulmonary edema. Most frequently it results from an abnormally **high pulmonary venous pressure** as occurs in mitral stenosis or left heart failure.

IMPORTANT NOTE

Pulmonary edema safety factor: Pulmonary capillary pressure should rise to a value equal to or more than the colloid osmotic pressure of the plasma inside the pulmonary capillaries before significant pulmonary edema occurs. The oncotic pressure is 25 mm Hg, therefore pulmonary capillary pressure, which is 7 mm Hg, should be more than 25 mm Hg to cause pulmonary edema. Thus, **safety factor against pulmonary edema** is of 18 mm Hg.

1. **Increased alveolar surface tension:** High surface tension **lowers interstitial hydrostatic pressure** that favours filtration. **Decreased surfactant synthesis** increases the surface tension and causes pulmonary edema as *occurs in ARDS*.
2. **Decreased oncotic pressure:** Plasma colloid osmotic pressure decreases **in conditions of hypoproteinemia**.
3. **Increased capillary permeability:** This is a **major cause** of pulmonary edema. Increased capillary permeability occurs with pulmonary vascular injury as occurs in:
   - **oxidant damage** e.g. oxygen therapy, ozone toxicity

- **inflammatory reactions** e. g. by the action of endotoxins
- **neurogenic shock** e.g. head injury is a major cause of pulmonary edema.

Clinical Note 47.1

Effects of pulmonary edema: Pulmonary edema decreases gas exchange, which results in hypoxemia and hypercapnia.

1. Pulmonary edema **obstructs small airways**, which in turn increases airway resistance.
2. **Lung compliance decreases** in pulmonary edema because of interstitial swelling and increased alveolar surface tension.
3. **Work of breathing increases** due to decreased compliance and airway obstruction.

Physiological Basis of Treatment of Pulmonary Edema

The aim of treatment of pulmonary edema is to **reduce pulmonary capillary hydrostatic pressure**. This is achieved by:

1. **Diuretics** that decrease blood volume
2. **Digitalis** that increases left ventricular function (usually the inability of left ventricle to pump blood effectively produces pulmonary edema)
3. **Vasodilators** that cause relaxation of systemic blood vessels.

Drowning PY6.6

Fresh-Water Drowning

In fresh water drowning, though aspiration of water occurs into the lungs, **death does not occur due to pulmonary edema**.

1. Death in drowning is usually **due to ventricular fibrillation**.
2. The aspirated water enters the alveoli and from there into the pulmonary capillary blood because of low capillary hydrostatic pressure and high oncotic pressure.
3. Entry of water into blood dilutes the plasma and produces hypotonic environment for red cells. This results in **hemolysis**.
4. Hemolysis in turn causes **hyperkalemia and hyponatremia**.
5. Ventricular fibrillation occurs due to hyperkalemia and hypoxemia.

Salt Water Drowning

In salt-water drowning, the **aspirated water is hypertonic** due to high Na^+ and Cl^- content of sea water.

1. Hypertonic fluid in alveoli **produces pulmonary edema**.
2. The cause of death in sea water drowning is **asphyxia**.

VENTILATION-PERFUSION RATIO

PY6.2

Ventilation-perfusion ratio is the ratio of alveolar ventilation to blood flow in lung. As discussed above, there are regions in the lung where ventilation and blood flow are not properly matched.

Normal value: In a normal individual at rest, the alveolar ventilation (V_A) is 4 L/min and pulmonary blood flow (Q) or perfusion (which is same as cardiac output or strictly speaking the right ventricular output) is 5 L/min. Thus, the **normal ventilation-perfusion ratio (V_A/Q ratio) is 0.8**. However, due to effect of gravity, **regional differences** in blood flow and alveolar ventilation exist in the lung.

In upright posture, blood flow is proportionately greater than ventilation at the base, and ventilation is proportionately greater than blood flow at the apex (Fig. 47.2).

1. In fact, the **blood flow exhibits about a 5-fold difference** between the apex and base of the lung, whereas **ventilation exhibits about a 2-fold difference**.
   - This variation in the differences in ventilation and blood flow, results in regional difference the V_A/Q ratio.
2. The V_A/Q ratio is **0.6 at the base** and about **3.6 at the apex** of the lungs.

Importance of V_A/Q ratio

Physiological Importance

The ventilation-perfusion ratio is important for gas exchange in lungs.

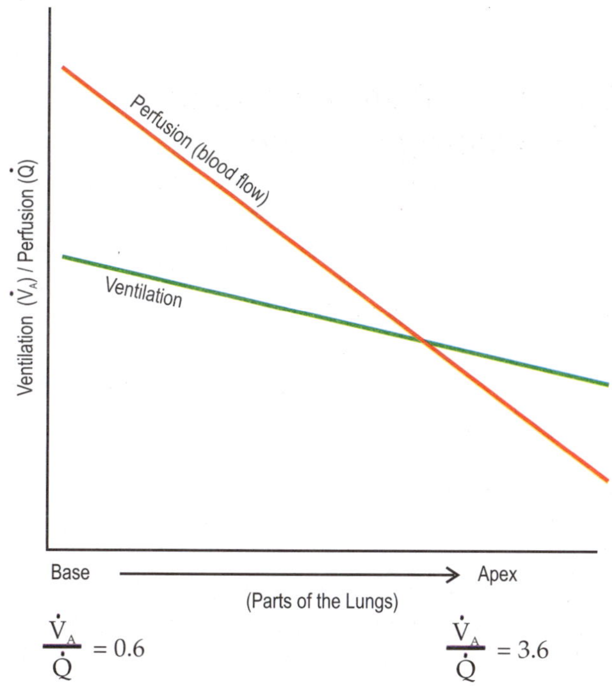

Fig. 47.2: Variation in difference in ventilation and perfusion at bases and apices of the lungs. This contributes to the difference in ventilation-perfusion ratio at base (0.6) and at apex (3.6). Average, ventilation-perfusion ratio is 0.8.

- **At the apex**, the V_A/Q ***ratio is high*** because there is more ventilation relative to blood flow.
  - Therefore, alveolar oxygen tension (P_AO_2) is high and carbon dioxide tension (P_ACO_2) is low at the apex of the lungs.
- **At the base**, the ***ratio is low*** as there is more perfusion relative to ventilation.
  - Thus, some amount of the blood circulates through the base of the lungs without becoming fully oxygenated.

Clinical Importance

Due to differences in regional V_A/Q ratios, some diseases are more localized to a part of the lungs.

IMPORTANT NOTE

Tuberculosis is common in apex: Tuberculosis occurs *more commonly in the apex* because of favorable environment for *Mycobacterium tuberculosis*. The higher oxygen level facilitates growth of tubercular bacilli.

Effects of Change in V_A/Q Ratio

Decreased V_A/Q Ratio: When ventilation to an alveolus is reduced relative to its perfusion, the V_A/Q ratio becomes less.

- In this situation, due to delivery of less oxygen, **alveolar PO_2 falls** and due to removal of less carbon dioxide **PCO_2 rises** (Fig. 47.3).

Increased V_A/Q Ratio: When perfusion is reduced relative to ventilation, V_A/Q ratio increases.

- **Alveolar PCO_2 falls** due to less carbon dioxide delivered into alveoli from blood and **PO_2 increases** as less oxygen is transferred from alveoli into the blood.

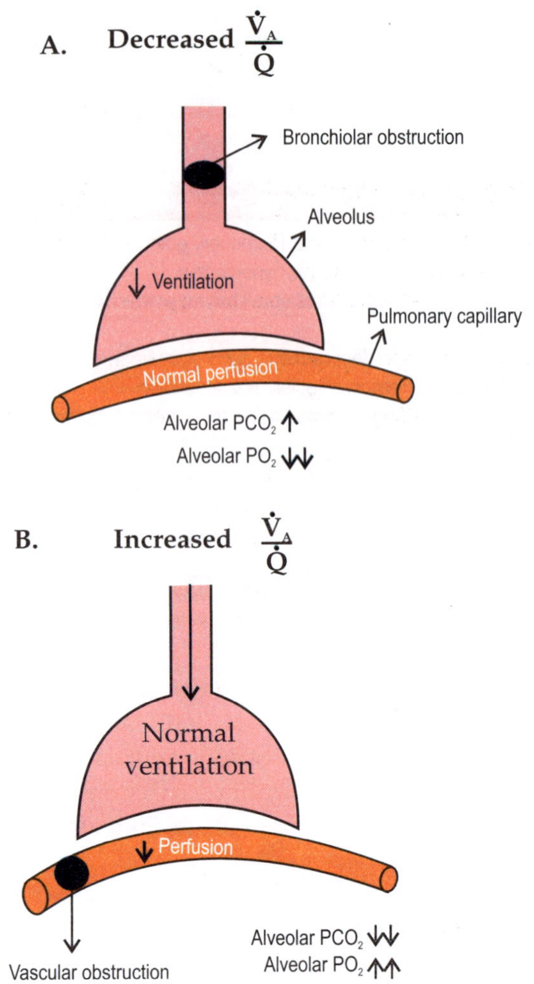

Fig. 47.3: Effects of change in ventilation-perfusion ratio on alveolar PCO_2 and PO_2.

Venous Admixture and Physiologic Shunt

Like physiological dead space that causes wasted ventilation, there is wasted perfusion.

- **Wasted perfusion** refers to the quantity of the venous blood, which is not fully oxygenated. The mixing of unoxygenated blood with oxygenated blood is known as **venous admixture**.

Venous admixture occurs either due to a **shunt** or to a **low ventilation perfusion ratio**.

Shunt

A shunt is a channel in which blood bypasses the lungs. There are two types of shunts.

Anatomical Shunt: In anatomical shunt, blood **bypasses lungs through an anatomical defect**. For example, in **right to left shunt**, admixture of blood occurs through the atrial or ventricular septal defect (Application Box 47.1).

- This also occurs from a **branch of the pulmonary artery connecting directly to the pulmonary vein**.

Physiological Shunt: In bronchial circulation, **deoxygenated bronchial venous blood drains directly into the oxygenated blood of pulmonary veins** that accounts for physiologic shunt.

- Normally, there is physiological dead space as well as physiological shunt in the lungs.

Application Box 47.1

Anatomical shunt causes hypoxia: In normal healthy individuals, the maximum venous admixture *(physiological shunt)* is about 2% of cardiac output. However, in some bronchial diseases this amount can *increase up to 20%* of cardiac output and in congenital disorders with a right-to-left shunt it can *increase up to 50%* of cardiac output. In these conditions, gas exchange is grossly impaired that lowers oxygen tension in the arterial blood.

Low Ventilation-Perfusion Ratio

Low V_A/Q ratio occurs when a **fraction of pulmonary capillary blood is not oxygenated** due to low alveolar ventilation. Normally, this **occurs at the base of the lung**.

- This can also occur if an **airway is partially obstructed** that causes hypoventilation.
- The fraction of the blood that passes through a *hypoventilated part of lung* is not fully oxygenated.
- This results in **venous admixture**.

BRONCHIAL CIRCULATION

The bronchial circulation is the circulation that supplies blood to the walls of the conducting airways and surrounding tissues.

- Bronchial circulation **perfuses the upper respiratory tract**. It does not supply the respiratory bronchiole or alveoli.
- **The venous return** from the bronchial circulation is either by bronchial veins or by bronchopulmonary veins.
- Bronchial circulation **receives only 1% of the cardiac output**. However, in some inflammatory disorders of the airways such as chronic bronchitis, it can be increased to 10% of cardiac output.
- **Bronchial arterial pressure is almost the same as the aortic pressure** and bronchial vascular resistance is much higher than the resistance in the pulmonary circulation.

Physiological Importance

The bronchial circulation (not pulmonary circulation) is capable of undergoing **angiogenesis** (the formation of new vessels).

- This is very crucial to provide **collaterals to the lung parenchyma**, when the pulmonary circulation is compromised.
- When pulmonary blood flow is obstructed by a clot or embolus, the lung parenchyma supplied by these vessels survives due to perfusion by newly formed blood vessels.

Exam Questions

1. List special features of pulmonary circulation. Describe briefly the factors affecting pulmonary blood flow and give a note on regulation of pulmonary blood flow.
2. List the factors that affect pulmonary vascular resistance. Briefly explain the causes and the physiological significance of low pulmonary vascular resistance.
3. Describe the effect of gravity on pulmonary blood flow and ventilation–perfusion ratio.
4. What are the factors that regulate filtration across the pulmonary capillaries, What is the effect of hydrostatic and osmotic pressure gradients on filtration across the pulmonary capillaries. Briefly explain the effects of alveolar surface tension on filtration across the pulmonary capillaries.
5. What is ventilation –perfusion ratio. What is the physiological importance of ventilation–perfusion ratio. Write a note on anatomical and physiological shunt.

Multiple Choice Questions

1. Which of the following is not true about pulmonary circulation?
A. It is a low pressure circulation having MAP of about 15 mmHg
B. It is a low-resistance circulation having less vascular resistance
C. The resting sympathetic tone is high
D. Pulmonary arterioles are thin walled having less smooth muscle in intima media

2. High Oxygen tension in alveoli is due to:
A. Right to left shunt
B. Ventilation perfusion mismatch
C. Bronchial Asthma
D. Inappropriate gas exchange

3. PO_2 is maximum
A. Base of lung B. Posterior lobe of lung
C. Apex of lung D. Middle lobe of lung

4. Ventilation perfusion ratio is maximum at:
A. Apex of lung B. Base of lung
C. Posterior lobe of lung D. Middle of the lung

5. Ventilation perfusion ratio is least at:
A. Apex B. Middle lobe
C. Base D. None

6. True statement regarding Pulmonary ventilation is
A. PaO_2 is maximum at the apex
B. V/Q is maximum at the base
C. Ventilation per unit lung volume is maximum at the apex
D. Blood circulation is minimum at the base

7. Not a stimulus for pulmonary vasoconstriction:
A. Hypoxemia B. Hypercapnia (Hypercarbia)
C. PGI2 D. Thromboxane A_2

8. Normal V-P ratio is about:
A. 0.8 B. 1.2
C. 0.5 D. 2.5

9. Which of the following is not a vasodilator for pulmonary circulation?
A. CGRP B. Angiotensin II at AT_2 receptor
C. Adenosine at A_1 receptor D. VIP

10. Which of the following is a vasoconstrictor for pulmonary circulation?
A. Serotonin at 5HT-1 receptor
B. Tachykinin at NK-1 receptor
C. Endothelin at ET-B receptor
D. Vasopressin at V-1 receptor

Answers

1. C 2. C 3. D 4. C 5. B 6. A 7. A 8. A 9. C 10. A

Chapter 48

Transport of Gases in Blood

Learning Objectives

On completion of study of this chapter:

The student will be able to (must know):

1. Remember the methods of O_2 transport of from lungs to tissue and quantity of O_2 is transported in each method.
2. Describe the processes of O_2 transport in blood.
3. Draw a labeled diagram of O_2-hemoglobin dissociation curve, and explain the factors that shift the dissociation curve to the right and to the left.
5. Appreciate the importance of P_{50}
6. Describe the CO_2 transport in blood
7. Know the importance of Bohr effect and Haldane effect.
8. Understand the mechanism of oxygen delivery to the tissue.

The student may also be able to (desirable to know):

1. Explain the effects of 2,3-DPG, temperature, pH, CO_2 on O_2-hemoglobin dissociation curve.

PY6.3

OXYGEN TRANSPORT

Oxygen is transported from lungs to the tissues in **two methods**: **physically dissolved** in the plasma, and in **combination with hemoglobin** (Hb) in the red cell.

In Physically Dissolved Form

In the physically dissolved form in plasma, only about **2% of oxygen is transported**. The amount of physically dissolved oxygen in the blood can be predicted from **Henry's law**.

- Henry's law states that the amount of gas that dissolves in a liquid at a given temperature is **proportional to the partial pressure of the gas**.
- Thus, the quantity of dissolved oxygen in arterial blood is calculated from the following equation:

Dissolved O_2 (ml/dl) = oxygen solubility × partial pressure of O_2 in arterial blood (PaO_2).

= 0.003 (ml /dl of blood per mm Hg) × 95 mm Hg (normal PaO_2 is 95 mm Hg)

= 0.3 ml/dl of blood

Thus, at PaO_2 of 95 mm Hg, the **dissolved O_2 is 0.3 ml/dl**.

- That means, in a normal healthy adult, **0.3 ml of O_2 is transported in dissolved form in 100 ml of blood** (Application Box 48.1).
- As cardiac output is 5 liters /min at rest, oxygen transported in dissolved form at rest is **about 15 ml/min**.

Application Box 48.1

Hyperbaric O_2 therapy improves tissue oxygenation: Though, 0.3 ml of O_2 is transported in dissolved form in 100 ml of blood, when 100% oxygen is inhaled in hyperbaric chamber, the dissolved oxygen is about 6 ml/dl of blood that accounts for supply of about 300 ml/min, which is adequate for tissue oxygenation.

In Combination with Hemoglobin

More than **98% of O_2** is transported in combination with Hb.

- This becomes possible due to the **binding affinity of hemoglobin for oxygen**.
- Hemoglobin that binds with oxygen is called **oxyhemoglobin** (HbO_2) and the hemoglobin that does not bind with O_2 is called ***deoxyhemoglobin*** (deoxy-Hb) or **reduced-hemoglobin**.

Oxyhemoglobin Formation

The **hemoglobin molecule** is a protein made up of **four subunits** that are bound together. Each subunit consists of a molecular group known as **heme** and a polypeptide attached to the heme. The four polypeptides of a Hb molecule are combinely known as **globin.**

- Each heme group contains one atom of iron (Fe^{++}) to which oxygen binds.
- Since each iron atom can bind one molecule of oxygen, **a single Hb molecule can bind four molecules of oxygen**.
- Hb binds with oxygen **only when the iron is in ferrous (Fe^{++}) state**.
  - The Fe^{++} iron in Hb is oxidized to ferric (Fe^{+++}) iron to form **methemoglobin**.
  - Thus, methemoglobin *can't bind oxygen*.
  - Methemoglobin formation occurs under the influence of various compounds like nitrites or sulfonamides.
  - Methemoglobin is also formed spontaneously.
- However, the enzyme ***methemoglobin reductase*** is present in red cell that reduces methemoglobin to Hb. Therefore, normally only about **1.5% of total Hb is methemoglobin.**
- **Deficiency of methemoglobin reductase** (a genetic defect) increases the methemoglobin concentration and decreases oxygen carrying capacity.

Oxygen binds ***rapidly and reversibly*** to hemoglobin to form **oxyhemoglobin** (HbO_2):

$O_2 + Hb \leftrightarrows HbO_2$

R & T States of Hb: During this process of HbO_2 formation, the heme remains in ferrous state. Thus, this **process is oxygenation**, *not oxidation*.

- As there are four subunits in Hb molecule, Hb reacts rapidly (in less than 0.01 s) with four molecules of oxygen to form HbO_8.
  - When oxygen is not bound with Hb (deoxyhemoglobin), the four subunits of Hb are tightly bound with each other.
  - This configuration of Hb is called **Tense or T state**.
  - In this T configuration, **affinity of Hb for oxygen is less**.
- When, first oxygen molecule binds with Hb, the four subunits enter into the **relaxed or R state** that exposes more oxygen binding sites.
  - Therefore, in R configuration, **affinity of Hb for oxygen is greatly increased** by 200 to 500 times.
- **When PO_2 is very less**, most of Hb molecules are in *T state* and have low oxygen affinity.
- **When PO_2 is very high**, the Hb molecules are in *R state* and have high oxygen affinity.
- Thus, the **quantity of oxyhemoglobin formation** is a function of ***partial pressure of oxygen in the blood***.

In pulmonary capillaries, where PO_2 is high, the reaction *favours to form more oxyhemoglobin*, and **in tissue capillaries**, where PO_2 is low, the reaction *favours formation of deoxyhemoglobin* that helps oxygen to be unloaded from hemoglobin and becomes available to the cells.

O_2 Carrying Capacity of Hb

Each gram of hemoglobin **binds with 1.34 ml of oxygen**. The maximum amount of oxygen that can be carried by hemoglobin is called the **oxygen carrying capacity**.

- In a healthy individual, the oxygen carrying capacity of arterial blood is about **20 ml of O_2 per 100 ml of blood**, considering the hemoglobin concentration of 15 g% (1.34 ml × 15 g = 20.1 ml O_2/dl blood).
  - **Oxygen Content** of Hb (**HbO_2 content**) is the amount of oxygen actually bound to hemoglobin, whereas **Oxygen Capacity** of Hb (**HbO_2 capacity**) is the amount of oxygen that can potentially bind with Hb.
- The **percentage saturation** of hemoglobin with oxygen (SO_2) is the ratio of the quantity of oxygen actually bound (oxygen content) to the quantity that can be potentially bound (oxygen capacity) multiplied by 100.

$$SO_2 = \frac{HbO_2 \text{ content}}{HbO_2 \text{ capacity}} \times 100$$

For example, if oxygen content is 15 ml O_2 per dl blood and oxygen capacity is 20 ml O_2 per dl of blood, then the SO_2 of blood is 75%.

- Normally, in arterial blood, **the percentage saturation of hemoglobin with oxygen is about 98%**.
- Blood PO_2 and O_2 saturation are important indices of oxygen transport, which are best studied by analyzing oxyhemoglobin dissociation curve.

Oxygen-Hemoglobin Dissociation Curve

Oxygen-hemoglobin (Oxy-Hb) equilibrium curve (dissociation or association curve) explains the relationship between ***partial pressure of oxygen*** (PO_2) in blood with ***oxygen saturation of Hb***.

Shape of the Curve: Oxy-Hb equilibrium curve is an **S-shaped curve** over the range of PO_2 from 0 to 100 mm Hg (Fig. 48.1).

- The **sigmoid shape** of the curve results from hemoglobin affinity for oxygen at various PO_2 levels.
- As **PO_2 rises**, the ***Hb saturation progressively increases***.
  - However, the **saturation is not linear** with increase in PO_2 for which the curve becomes sigmoid shaped.
- The S-shaped oxyhemoglobin equilibrium curve enables oxygen **to saturate hemoglobin under high partial pressures** in the lungs and to give up large amounts of oxygen with small changes in PO_2 at the tissue level.

Phases of the Curve: The curve is divided into **two major phases**: the steep phase and the plateau phase.

Steep Phase

The curve has a **steep slope between PO_2 of 10 and 60 mm Hg**.

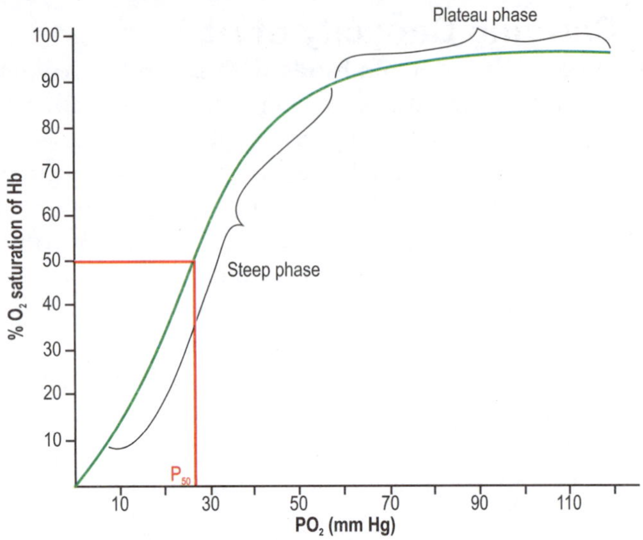

Fig. 48.1: Oxygen-hemoglobin dissociation curve. Note, at PO_2 of 27 mm Hg, Hb saturation of oxygen is 50% (P_{50}). Hb is 89% saturated with oxygen at PO_2 of 60 mm Hg, above which increase in Hb saturation is marginal that results in plateau phase of the curve.

- During this phase of the curve, combination of oxygen with Hb increases very rapidly as the PO_2 increases from 10 to 60 mm Hg.
- Oxygen saturation of Hb is about **90% at PO_2 60 mm Hg**.

Significance of Steep Phase

In the steep phase, ***oxygen saturation of Hb is very high***.

- Less increase in PO_2 leads to greater percentage saturation of Hb and therefore, **facilitates oxygen loading**.
- Also, change in steep portion of the curve in reverse direction (that is, from 60 to 10 mm Hg) causes **unloading of oxygen in the tissues**.
- A small decrease in PO_2 in the tissue results in ***unloading of large amount of oxygen*** to the tissues.
- The steep phase allows **large quantities of oxygen to be released** from hemoglobin in the tissue capillaries where a lower capillary PO_2 prevails.
  - This is especially achieved by **shifting the curve to right** (shift occurs mainly on the steep phase) by increased H^+ or by increased CO_2.

Plateau Phase

The curve begins to plateau at PO_2 around 60 mm Hg and flattens at PO_2 of 70 mm Hg.

- The increase in PO_2 above 60 mm Hg produces **only a small increase in oxygen binding**.
- Increase in PO_2 from 60 to 100 mm Hg in the plateau region of the curve illustrates that ***oxygen saturation and content remain apparently constant*** over a wide alteration in alveolar PO_2.

Significance of Plateau Phase

There are **two significances** of plateau phase:

1. In different situations, like at high altitude or in pulmonary diseases in which a moderate hypoxia (decrease in PO_2 from 95 to 60 mm Hg) occurs, the **total amount of oxygen carried by Hb decreases only by 5–10%**, since Hb saturation is about 90% at PO_2 of 60 mm Hg.
   - Thus, plateau in the curve **provides a safety factor** through which even ***a significant decrease in lung function can allow normal saturation of Hb.***
2. Oxygen saturation and content remain **fairly constant inspite of wide fluctuations in alveolar PO_2** (PAO_2).
   - For example, if PAO_2 rises from 100 to 120 mm Hg, hemoglobin saturation increases only slightly (97 to 98%).
   - This is the reason why **oxygen content cannot be raised appreciably** by hyperventilation or by breathing 100% oxygen because Hb is already completely saturated with oxygen at PO_2 of 100 mm Hg.
     - This is true only for **normal people at sea level.**
     - If a person has **low arterial PO_2 due to lung disease or for his ascension to high altitude,** hyperventilation or breathing 100% oxygen *increases Hb saturation with oxygen* as they have more deoxy-Hb initially.

The P_{50}

The P_{50} is the level of PO_2 at which **50% of the hemoglobin is saturated** with oxygen.

- P_{50} assesses the **binding affinity of hemoglobin** for oxygen.
- In adults at sea level, the normal P_{50} occurs at a **PO_2 of 27 mm Hg.**
- Alteration in the P_{50} value has a greater impact on the steep phase of the curve.

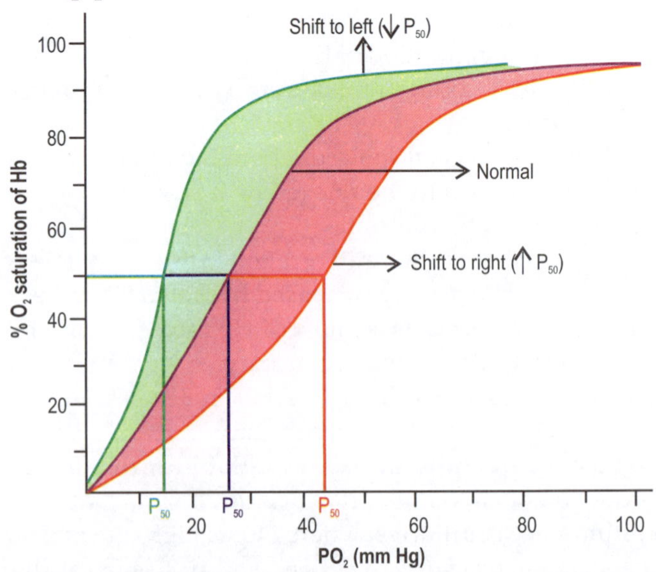

Fig. 48.2: Effect of P_{50} on Oxy-Hb dissociation curve. When P_{50} is reduced (shift of the curve to left) affinity of Hb for oxygen is increased that promotes loading of oxygen to Hb in the pulmonary blood. When P_{50} is increased (shift of the curve to right) affinity of Hb for oxygen is reduced that facilitates release of oxygen from Hb in the tissue.

- If the P_{50} is high, it signifies the *decrease in affinity of Hb for oxygen,* which is seen in right-shift of the oxygen-hemoglobin equilibrium curve.
- Conversely, **if P_{50} is low**, it signifies shift of the curve to the left, in which *affinity of Hb for oxygen is more* (Fig. 48.2).

Factors Affecting Affinity of Hb-Binding with Oxygen

Several factors influence the affinity of hemoglobin for O_2.

- The important factors are **temperature, arterial PCO_2, arterial pH and 2,3-DPG.**
  - A rise in PCO_2, a fall in pH, and a rise in temperature all **shift the curve to the right.**

Advantages of Shift to Right: A shift of the oxyhemoglobin equilibrium curve to the right is **physiologically advantageous at the tissue level**, as affinity of O_2 for Hb is lowered (increased P_{50}).

- A rightward shift **enhances the unloading of oxygen** for a given PO_2 in the tissue.
  - ***A leftward shift*** increases the affinity of hemoglobin for oxygen, thereby lowering the ability to release oxygen to the tissues.

IMPORTANT NOTE

Shift to right is helpful in exercise: The functional importance of this shift is that an **exercising muscle** is warm and acidic and produces **large amounts of carbon dioxide** (high PCO_2). All these factors favor the unloading of more oxygen to metabolically active muscles.

Temperature

Increase in temperature shifts the Oxy-Hb dissociation *curve to right* and **decrease in temperature** shifts the *curve to the left* (Fig. 48.3).

- In other words, high temperature decreases the affinity of Hb for oxygen.
- This helps in *release of oxygen in metabolically active tissues* in which temperature is more.

pH

Alteration in blood pH shifts the Oxy-Hb dissociation curve. Christian Bohr and Neils Bohr in 1904 demonstrated that **respiratory acidosis shifts oxy-Hb dissociation curve to right**. Since then, the decrease in oxygen affinity for Hb in acidosis is known as **Bohr effect.**

- A **decrease in pH shifts the curve to right** and **increase in pH shifts the curve to left** (Fig. 48.4).
- When **blood passes through capillaries**, CO_2 enters red cell that decreases intracellular pH and shifts the Oxy-Hb dissociation **curve to right.**
  - Under normal physiological conditions, **binding of about 0.7 mole of H^+ causes Hb to release 1 mole of oxygen**.

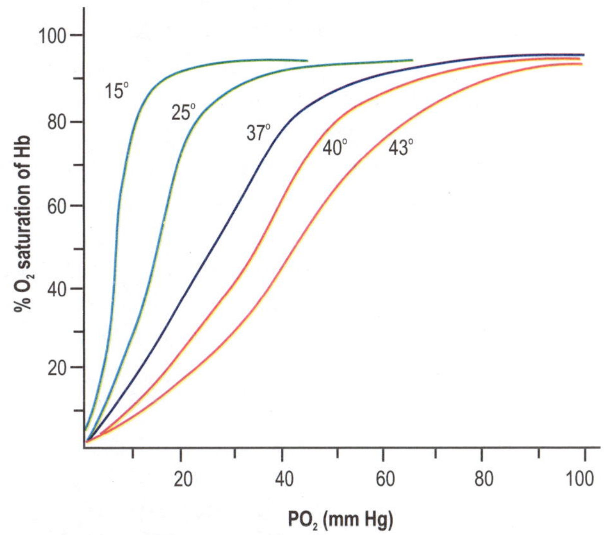

Fig. 48.3: Effect of temperature on Oxy-Hb dissociation curve. Decreased temperature shifts the curve to the left that decreases oxygen release in the tissue, and increased temperature shifts the curve to the right that promotes oxygen release in the tissue. During exercise, increased skeletal muscle temperature facilitates oxygen delivery to the exercising muscle.

  - Thus, when **blood passes through tissue capillaries**, the acidic environment **facilitates release of oxygen** from Hb into the tissues.

Carbon Dioxide

During cellular metabolism, CO_2 is released into circulation that increases generation of H^+ and decreases pH. This **shifts the curve to right**. This helps in release of oxygen from Hb.

- The shift to right in acidosis (**Bohr effect**) is partly due to **effect of decrease in pH** and partly to the **direct effect of CO_2 on Hb**.
- CO_2 combines with unprotonated amino groups on Hb ($Hb\text{-}NH_2$) to **form carbamino groups**.

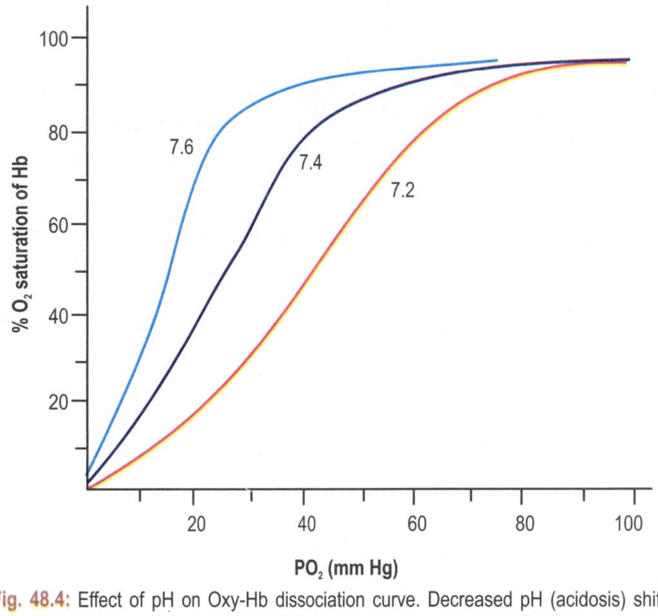

Fig. 48.4: Effect of pH on Oxy-Hb dissociation curve. Decreased pH (acidosis) shifts the curve to right and increased pH (alkalosis) shifts the curve to left. During exercise, metabolic acidosis in the tissue facilitates oxygen delivery to the active skeletal muscle.

- The formation of carbamino group causes negative shift in the charge on one amino acid side chain that changes the conformation of Hb.
- This results in **decrease in oxygen affinity of Hb**.

- In metabolically active tissues, ***metabolic vasodilation*** increases blood flow to the tissue increasing the oxygen transport to the area.
- In the area, already persisting local hypercapnia and acidosis ***shift the curve to the right*** (decrease oxygen affinity for Hb) that **facilitates oxygen delivery** to the tissue.

2,3-DPG

Red blood cells lack mitochondria. Therefore, anerobic glycolysis occurs in red cells. **During glycolysis**, large quantities of **2,3-diphosphoglycerate** (2,3-DPG), It is also called 2,3-bisphosphoglycerate **(2,3-BPG)** which is technically more correct. It is an organic phosphate compound is produced as the metabolic intermediary. Thus, 2,3-DPG level is **much higher in red cells** than in other cells.

- 2,3-DPG significantly affects affinity of hemoglobin for oxygen.
- In red cells, concentration of 2,3-DPG is almost same as that of Hb. In fact, 2,3-DPG binds to Hb in 1:1 stoichiometry, interacting with a central cavity formed by two β chains.
- 2,3-DPG has about **3.5 negative charges** that interact with eight positively charged amino acids in the central cavity. This destabilizes the interaction of Hb with oxygen.
  - Thus, **binding of 2,3-DPG with Hb shifts the Oxy-Hb dissociation curve to right** (Fig. 48.5) and *facilitates the release of oxygen*.
- **At the tissue level,** an increase in 2,3-DPG **facilitates unloading of oxygen** from the red cell.

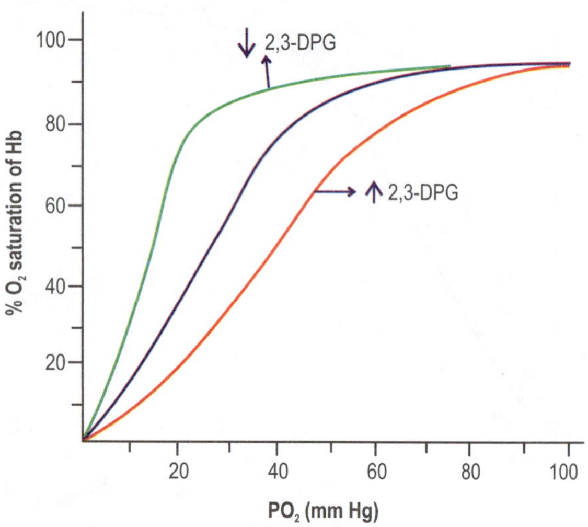

Fig. 48.5: Effect of 2,3-diphosphoglycerate (2,3-DPG) on Oxy-Hb dissociation curve. Decreased 2,3-DPG shifts the curve to the left and increased 2,3-DPG shifts the curve to the right

- Hypoxia stimulates glycolysis resulting in increased production of 2,3-DPG.

- Red cell 2,3-DPG increases in **anemia, exercise and hypoxic conditions** like high altitude, chronic lung disease etc.
  - Therefore, in these conditions, Oxy-Hb dissociation curve shifts to right.

Factors that affect 2,3-DPG in Red Cells:

1. **pH:** Acidosis inhibits red cell glycolysis and therefore decreases 2,3-DPG concentration.
2. **Type of Hb:** The γ chains of **fetal Hb** have less avidity for 2,3-DPG than β chains of adult Hb. Therefore, fetal Hb has higher oxygen affinity. This provides an ***advantage to fetus to extract oxygen*** from maternal blood in the placenta.
3. **Fetal Hb** shifts Oxy-Hb dissociation curve to left (Fig. 48.6)
4. **Hormones:** Growth hormone, thyroxine and testosterone stimulate the synthesis of 2,3-DPG.
5. **Altitude:** At **high altitude**, 2,3-DPG concentration ***increases substantially*** in red cells. This increases the availability of oxygen to the tissues.
6. **PO_2: Hypoxia** increases 2,3-DPG production.

IMPORTANT NOTE

Blood stored with citrate-dextrose-phosphate solution preserves 2,3-DPG level: The 2,3-DPG concentration in red cells of blood stored in blood bank decreases. Therefore, transfusion of stored blood decreases oxygen transport, especially when transfused into hypoxic patients. However, if blood is stored in citrate-dextrose-phosphate solution this effect is less than when stored in acid-citrate-dextrose solution.

Myoglobin

Myoglobin is the Hb pigment in muscle.

- Though it is similar to Hb in structure, myoglobin binds one molecule of O_2 per mole.
- It shifts Oxy-Hb dissociation **curve to left** and the curve becomes **hyperbolic** (loses sigmoid shape) (Fig. 48.6).
- This helps in **picking up of O_2 from blood.**
- Myoglobin is more in regularly **exercising muscles** especially that are trained in isometric exercise.
  - This helps the muscle to **draw oxygen from myoglobin**, especially when blood flow ceases for a longer duration during sustained muscle contraction.
- Myoglobin **facilitates transfer of O_2** from blood to mitochondria.

Effect of Carbon Monoxide (CO)

The binding **affinity of CO with Hb is 210 times more** than oxygen. Moreover, CO interferes with oxygen transport by competing for the same binding sites on hemoglobin.

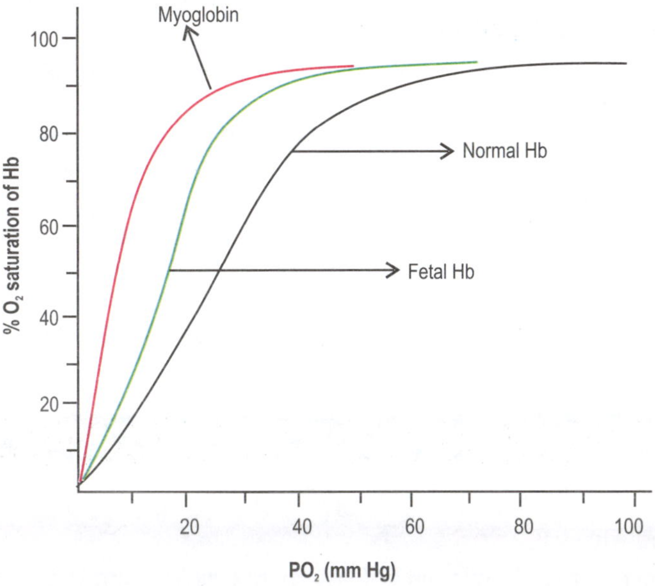

Fig. 48.6: Effects of myoglobin and fetal hemoglobin (Hb) on Oxy-Hb dissociation curve. Note myoglobin makes the curve hyperbolic.

- CO binds to hemoglobin to form **carboxyhemoglobin** (HbCO).
- When the blood is 60% saturated with CO (carboxyhemoglobin) the **oxygen content is reduced to less than 10 ml/dl.**
  - As the partial pressure of CO approaches 1 mm Hg, Hb is fully saturated with CO.
  - But, **oxygen content is greatly reduced** as it can't bind to Hb.
  - This grossly **decreases the oxygen carrying capacity**.
- Moreover, CO also **shifts the Oxy-Hb dissociation curve to the left,** which decreases oxygen release to the tissues.
  - Therefore, **severe tissue hypoxia** occurs in CO poisoning, which is fatal if not treated immediately (Clinical Note 48.1).
- Normally, in healthy individuals, CO occupies 1–2% of Hb binding sites.

IMPORTANT NOTE

CO is high in Smokers: In chronic cigarette smokers, and in traffic personnel or residents of crowded traffic areas (passive smokers), CO concentration increases in plasma and CO occupies about 10% of Hb. Tissue oxygenation in these subjects is less.

Clinical Note 48.1

CO poisoning produces anemic hypoxia: CO has a strong affinity for hemoglobin, which forms carboxyhemoglobin. Therefore, Hb is practically not available for oxygen transport. Hence, it is often classified as **anemic hypoxia.**

- PaO_2 remains normal in CO poisoning. Hence, **feedback mechanism** of hypoxia for corrective measures is absent. Thus, CO produces severe hypoxia without manifesting danger signals of it.
- **Treatment** for CO poisoning is **breathing 100%** oxygen. As O_2 and CO compete for binding with hemoglobin molecule, breathing a high oxygen concentration displaces CO from Hb and favors formation of oxyhemoglobin.

Factors that Shift Oxy-Hb Dissociation Curve

A. Factors that shift the curve to right:

1. Increased temperature
2. Decreased pH
3. Increased PCO_2
4. Increased 2,3-DPG
5. Hypoxia

Shift of the curve to right **increases P_{50}** (decreased affinity of Hb for oxygen), which facilitates oxygen release.

B. Factors that shift the curve to left:

1. Decreased temperature
2. Increased pH
3. Decreased PCO_2
4. Decreased 2,3-DPG
5. Fetal Hb
6. Carbon monoxide

Shift of the curve to left **decreases P_{50}** (increases affinity of Hb for oxygen) that facilitates oxygen uptake and prevents oxygen release.

O_2 Delivery to Tissue

Diffusion of O_2 from Capillaries to Tissue Fluid

When the arterial blood reaches the peripheral tissues, diffusion of oxygen occurs from the peripheral capillary blood into the tissue fluid.

- This occurs along the concentration gradient of oxygen from area of higher level to lower level. The **PO_2 in systemic capillary blood is 95 mm Hg,** whereas **PO_2 in the interstitial fluid** that surrounds the tissue cells is about **40 mmHg**.
  - Thus, there is a great pressure gradient due to considerably **large pressure difference** of O_2 between the systemic capillary blood and the tissue fluid that causes oxygen to diffuse rapidly from the capillary blood into the interstitial fluid.
- Therefore, **PO_2 falls rapidly in the capillary to about 40 mm Hg**.
  - Thus, the PO_2 of the blood leaving the tissue capillaries (PO_2 at venous end of capillary) and entering the systemic veins is 40 mm Hg (Fig. 48.7).
- From tissue fluid, oxygen rapidly enters the cell as in the intracellular fluid the PO_2 is about 23 mmHg (ranges between 7 to 40 mmHg), as oxygen is constantly utilized by cell.
  - Especially in metabolically active tissues, this gradient is more as mitochondrial oxygen utilization is more.
- Diffusion of oxygen to tissues depend on two important factors:
  i) rate of blood flow to the tissue and
  ii) the rate of tissue metabolism.

Oxygen delivery is more if the blood flow is more and the metabolic activity is more.

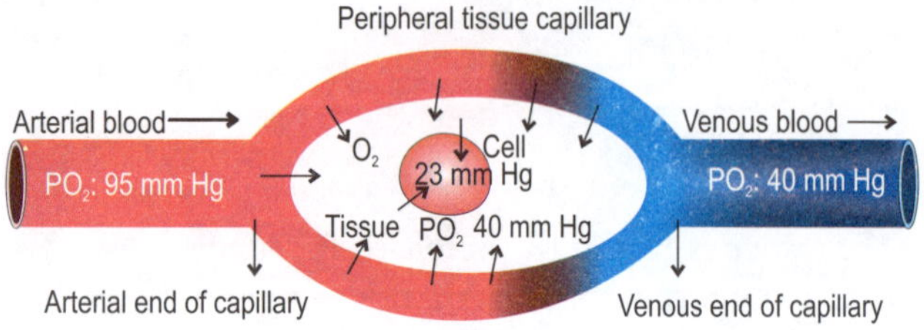

Fig. 48.7: Delivery of oxygen from capillary blood to tissue. Arrows indicate the delivery of oxygen from capillary into tissue fluid and from tissue fluid into the cell. Oxygen delivery is rapid in tissue, hence PO_2 at venous end of capillary is 40 mm Hg.

Bohr Effect

At the tissue level, CO_2 enters the blood and shifts the curve to right. This helps in **unloading of oxygen from Hb and facilitates tissue oxygenation**. This phenomenon is called **Bohr Effect.**

- This occurs mainly due to decreased pH in the tissue. Increased temperature of blood in the tissue also contributes.
  - In tissue, acidification of blood decreases affinity of O_2 to Hb, as deoxygenated Hb binds H^+ more actively than that of oxyhemoglobin.
- The PCO_2 level in the tissue rises, the curve shifts to right and P_{50} rises.
  - Thus, Bohr's effect helps in unloading of O_2 and loading of CO_2.

Significant contribution of Scientist

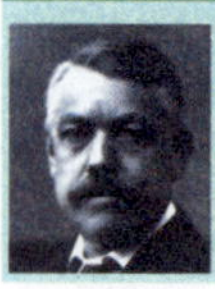

Christian H. L. P. Emil Bohr (1855–1911) was a Danish physician & Physiologist, *father of the physicist and Nobel laureate* Niels Bohr, as well as the *grandfather of another physicist and Nobel laureate* Aage Bohr. In 1903, Christian Bohr described that H^+ and CO_2 decrease hemoglobin's oxygen-binding affinity, called as **Bohr effect.**

Importance of Oxygen Saturation and Content

Oxygen Saturation: The Oxygen saturation is the **ratio of the amount of oxygen bound to Hb to the maximum amount of oxygen that can bind Hb** (100% oxygen capacity). At 100% oxygen capacity, heme groups of Hb are fully saturated with oxygen.

Oxygen Content: The oxygen content of blood is the **volume of oxygen contained in unit volume of blood,** which includes the oxygen bound to Hb and also dissolved in plasma. As the dissolved oxygen is negligible, the oxygen content depends on concentration of Hb and oxygen binding capacity of Hb (Clinical Note 48.2).

Clinical Note 48.2

Oxygen content is important in anemic patients: Oxygen content is more important than PO_2 and oxygen saturation for oxygenation of tissues, when the patient is anemic. A patient with Hb concentration 7 g% or less may have a normal arterial PO_2 and Hb saturation, but oxygen content will be grossly reduced. Oxygen saturation remains normal because oxygen content and capacity are proportionately reduced. Tissue suffers from hypoxia due to decreased oxygen content inspite of normal oxygen saturation.

Oxygen Extraction

Oxygen extraction is the **amount of oxygen taken up by the tissues from the blood**.

- This is an index of oxygen consumption of the tissue.
  - It is better quantified in terms of **Oxygen Extraction Ratio** (OER).
- OER is also called as **oxygen coefficient ratio**, is the amount of oxygen extracted by the tissue divided by the amount of oxygen delivered.
- In metabolically more active tissues like cardiac muscle, **OER is as high as 85% at rest.**

CARBON DIOXIDE TRANSPORT

Diffusion of CO_2 from Tissue Fluid into Capillary Blood

CO_2 produced by metabolism **increases the content of CO_2 in the cell.** CO_2 diffuses from cell into tissue fluid and then from interstitial fluid into the tissue capillaries.

- CO_2 can **diffuse about 20 times as rapidly than oxygen**.
  - Therefore, the **pressure difference required** to cause carbon dioxide diffusion **is much less** compared to the pressure difference required for oxygen diffusion.
- The **PCO_2 in the cell is 46 mmHg**, in the **tissue fluid is 45 mmHg**.
  - Therefore, from cell CO_2 diffuses into the tissue fluid.
- The **arterial blood** that reaches capillary has **PCO_2 40 mmHg**.
  - Hence, ***CO_2 rapidly diffuses*** from tissue fluid into the capillary blood (Fig. 48.8).

Factors Affecting: Two factors influence diffusion of CO_2 from tissues into capillary blood: i) the ***rate of tissue metabolism*** and, ii) the ***rate of tissue blood flow***.

1. **Increased tissue metabolism greatly increases interstitial tissue fluid PCO_2** irrespective of the rate of blood flow.
   - Decrease in the metabolism causes fall in interstitial fluid PCO_2.
2. **Decreased blood flow** from normal to one quarter-normal ***increases tissue PCO_2*** from the normal value of **45 mm Hg to 60 mm Hg**.
   - And conversely, increasing blood flow to six times the normal decreases the interstitial PCO_2 from the normal value of 45 mm Hg to 41 mm Hg.

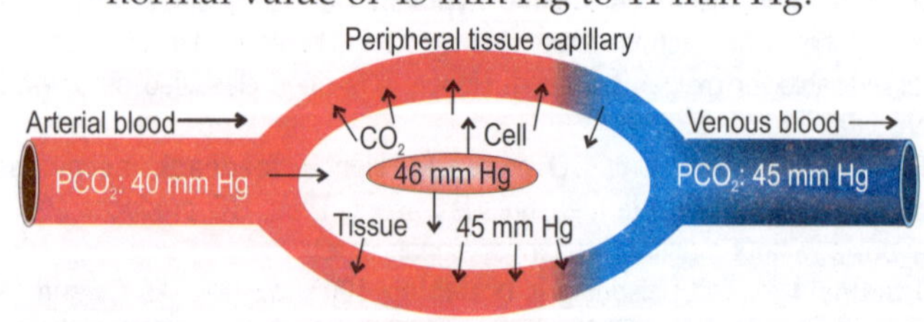

Fig. 48.8: Diffusion of CO_2 from tissue fluid into capillaries. Arrows indicate diffusion of CO_2 from cell into tissue fluid and then rapidly into the capillary blood.

Modes of CO_2 Transport

CO_2 is transported in blood in **three forms:**

1. Physically dissolved in the plasma (7%)
2. As bicarbonate ions in plasma and in red cells (70%)
3. As carbamino protein complexes (23%).
   - Carbamino compounds with plasma proteins
   - Carbamino-Hb in red cells

In Dissolved Form in Plasma

The amount of CO_2 dissolved in plasma is proportional to the partial pressure of CO_2 (PCO_2) as per the principle of Henry's law.

- The **solubility coefficient of CO_2 is 20 times that of oxygen,** i. e. 0.06 ml/dl/mmHg.
- Thus, in venous blood, **2.76 ml/dl** (46 mmHg PCO_2 in venous blood × 0.06) is carried in simple solution. Due to absence of carbonic anhydrase in plasma, **carbonic acid formation is less in plasma**.
- A small amount of CO_2 combines with plasma proteins to form **carbamino-protein complexes**.

As Bicarbonate Ions

About 70% of CO_2 is transported in the form of ***bicarbonate ions in the red cells***. This becomes possible due to presence of *large quantity of carbonic anhydrase in red cells.*

- From tissue, as soon as CO_2 is released into plasma, a bulk of it diffuses into the red cell.
- In red cells, it forms either **carbonic acid** (H_2CO_3) or **carbaminohemoglobin**. CO_2 combines with water to form H_2CO_3 (carbonic acid) by carbonic anhydrase.
- H_2CO_3 is then spontaneously converted into H^+ and bicarbonate (HCO_3^-).

$$CO_2 + H_2O \leftrightharpoons H_2CO_3 \leftrightharpoons H^+ + HCO_3^-$$

Chloride Shift

As carbonic acid readily dissociates to HCO_3^- and H^+, bicarbonate concentration increases in red cells. HCO_3^- leaves the red blood cells and in exchange chloride (Cl^-) enters the cell from the plasma to maintain electrical neutrality.

- The exchange of HCO_3^- for Cl^- occurs by **chloride-bicarbonate exchanger** (anion exchanger) present in the red cell membrane (Fig. 48.9).
  - This exchanger is known as **anion-exchanger 1 (AE1)**, which was previously known as band-3 exchanger.
- The **chloride movement in exchange for HCO_3^-** is known as the *chloride shift*.
  - As this phenomenon was described by Hamburger, chloride shift is also known as **Hamburger Shift.**
- Cl^- accumulate in red cells and increases red cell size (Application Box 48.2).

Application Box 48.2

Hematocrit of venous blood is more: Due to release of chloride from red cells in venous blood its level is about 20% higher than the arterial blood. Chloride is osmotically active and therefore, red cells imbibe water. This increases the size of red cells of venous blood. Thus, hematocrit of venous blood is about 3% more than that of the hematocrit of arterial blood.

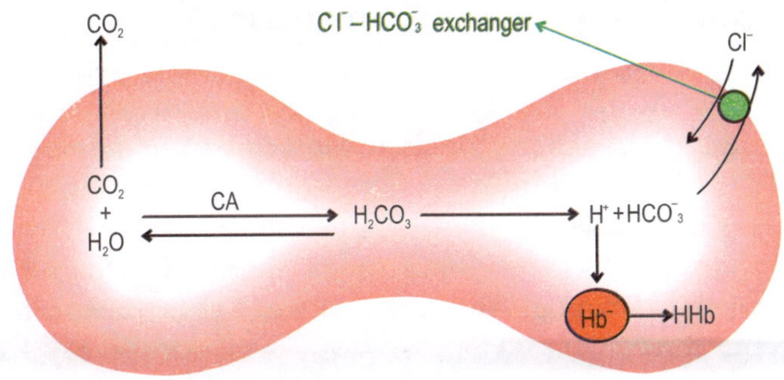

Fig. 48.9: Mechanism of chloride shift. CA: carbonic anhydrase.

The H^+ formed during reaction, cannot easily diffuse out of the cell because of the low permeability of the membrane to H^+. Most of the H^+ produced by the dissociation of bicarbonate **is buffered by hemoglobin**:

$$H^+ + HbO_2^- \leftrightharpoons HHb + O_2$$

- As **H^+ binds to hemoglobin,** it decreases oxygen binding of Hb and shifts the **Oxy-Hb dissociation curve to the right.**
  - This **facilitates release of oxygen from hemoglobin** into the tissue.
  - This also favors transport of carbon dioxide.

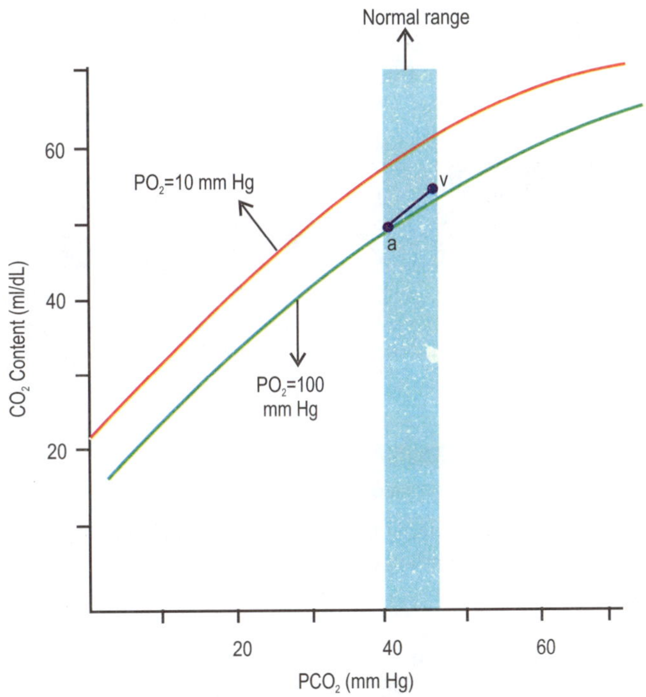

Fig. 48.10: Carbon dioxide dissociation curve. This is relatively a linear curve than Oxy-Hb dissociation curve. Especially, within the normal range of CO_2 i,e, 40–46 mm Hg, the curve is linear, whereas in Oxy-Hb dissociation curve, within normal range of O_2 the curve is mostly flat. Increase in PO_2 causes rightward and downwards shift of carbon dioxide dissociation curve. a: CO_2 content of arterial blood; v: CO_2 content of venous blood.

- Reverse process operates in pulmonary capillaries, where the oxygenation of hemoglobin favors the unloading of carbon dioxide.

The major reactions of CO_2 transport occur in the red cells. However, a large quantity of CO_2 is actually carried in the plasma in the form of bicarbonate.

As Carbamino Compound

Carbon dioxide in red cells also reacts with free amine groups (NH_2) of hemoglobin to form **carbaminohemoglobin** (HbNHCOOH):

$CO_2 + HbNH_2 \leftrightarrows HbNHCOOH$

Deoxygenated hemoglobin binds more CO_2 than the oxygenated hemoglobin. About **23% of CO_2 is transported** in this form.

CO_2 Dissociation Curve

Dissociation of CO_2 from blood is directly related to PCO_2. Therefore, CO_2 dissociation curve is relatively a straight line in the normal arterial PCO_2 range (Fig. 48.10).

The **major features** of CO_2 dissociation curve are:

1. **Linear relationship between CO_2 content and PCO_2:** Within the physiological range of PCO_2 (40–46 mm Hg) the curve is **more linear and steeper** (whereas, Oxy-Hb dissociation curve is neither linear nor steeper within the physiological of PO_2, i. e. from 40 to 100 mm Hg).
2. **Transfer of large quantity of CO_2:** Because of the shape of the CO_2 dissociation curve, **large amounts of CO_2 can be loaded or unloaded** from the blood with a small change in PCO_2. Also, blood can hold much more carbon dioxide than oxygen.
3. **Inverse relationship between PO_2 & CO_2 content:** The CO_2 dissociation curve **shifts downward and to the right at a higher PO_2**. The effect of change in PO_2 (or oxyhemoglobin saturation) on CO_2 content is known as the **Haldane effect.**

- The relationship between PO_2 and CO_2 content is inverse. At any level of PCO_2, the **total CO_2 content increases as PO_2 falls.**
- The advantage of this inverse relationship (**the Haldane effect**) is that it allows the blood to **load more CO_2 in the tissues and unload more CO_2 in the lungs.**
- Thus, when blood enters capillaries in the tissues and releases O_2, the CO_2 carrying capacity increases, and conversely, when blood enters capillaries in the lungs and picks up oxygen, the CO_2-carrying capacity decreases.

Haldane Effect

When blood passes through pulmonary capillaries, oxygen diffuses into the blood and forms Oxy-Hb.

1. **Oxygenation of Hb shifts the CO_2 dissociation curve to right** and Hb begins to lose CO_2.
   - Thus, in the lungs **loading of O_2 facilitates unloading of CO_2.**
   - This is called Haldane effect, as it is named after great ancient respiratory physiologist **John Scott Haldane.**
2. As **deoxyhemoglobin binds H^+ more actively** than that of oxyhemoglobin, binding of O_2 with hemoglobin decreases its affinity for CO_2.

Exam Questions

1. Describe the process of oxygen transport in the blood from lungs to tissues.
2. Draw a labeled diagram of oxygen-hemoglobin dissociation curve. Briefly describe various factors that shift this curve to the right and to the left.
3. What is P_{50}. Briefly describe the effects of P_{50} on oxygen-hemoglobin dissociation curve.
4. With the help of a schematic diagram of carbon dioxide dissociation curve, describe the process of transport of CO_2 from tissues to the lungs.
5. With the help of a schematic diagram, briefly describe the mechanism and significance of chloride shift. Write brief notes on Bohr effect and Haldane effect.

Multiple Choice Questions

1. **At rest, with cardiac output of 5L/min, the amount of oxygen transported in dissolved form in plasma is:**
   A. 0.3 ml/min B. 15 ml/min
   C. 21 ml/min D. 30 ml/min
2. **With hyperbaric O2 therapy, the amount of oxygen transported in dissolved form in plasma in 100 ml of blood is:**
   A. 0.3 ml B. 3 ml
   C. 6 ml D. 15 ml
3. **All of the following statements are true, EXCEPT:**
   A. Hb binds to O_2 only when the iron is in ferric state
   B. About 1.5% of total Hb is methemoglobin
   C. In relaxed state of Hb, the affinity of O_2 for Hb increases 200 times
   D. About 98% of O_2 is transported in combination with Hb
4. **How much oxygen is transported in dissolved form in plasma in 100 ml of blood?**
   A. 0.3 ml B. 15 ml
   C. 21 ml D. 30 ml
5. **The oxygen carrying capacity per 100 ml of arterial blood is:**
   A. 2 ml O_2 B. 20 ml O_2
   C. 50 ml O_2 D. 250 ml O_2

(MCQs continued to Page 423)

Chapter 49

Regulation of Respiration

Learning Objectives

On completion of study of this chapter:

The student will be able to (must know):

1. Name the respiratory centers in medulla and pons and give their functions.
2. Describe the neural regulation of respiration.
3. Understand the structure and functions of peripheral and central chemoreceptors.
4. Illustrate the structure, and functions of carotid body.
5. Describe the chemical control of respiration.
6. Explain the effects of hypoxia, hypercapnia and acidosis on ventilation.
7. Define Hering-Breuer inflation and deflation reflexes and give their role in regulation of respiration.

The student may also be able to (desirable to know):

1. Describe the non-chemical mechanisms respiration.
2. Understand the respiratory changes in metabolic and respiratory acidosis.

Regulation of respiration has both automatic and voluntary control mechanisms. Automatic breathing is produced by **rhythmic discharge of neurons** in the brainstem.

Overview of Control of Breathing: Neurons in the medulla generate appropriate motor signals that drive the cranial and spinal motor neurons innervating respiratory muscles.

1. The area in the medulla that generates this respiratory rhythm is called as **Central Pattern Generator** (CPG) of respiration (Fig. 49.1).
2. The neural control of breathing depends on coordinated cyclical changes in the activity of cells primarily located in **respiratory centers in the medulla** in the brain.
   - The **medullary neurons drive the respiratory motor neurons** that in turn alter the activity of chest wall, diaphragm and conducting airways.
3. Change in ventilation alters **chemical composition of blood** (PO_2, PCO_2 and pH) that provides **feedback signal via peripheral and central chemoreceptors** to the CPG and other pontomedullary respiratory centers.
4. **Alteration in ventilation** also provides ***feedback signals*** via vagus nerve, spinal nerves and proprioceptive pathways.

The neural signals, chemical signals and the feedback signals in turn appropriately modify the output signals from respiratory centers to adjust ventilation according to the need of the body.

Thus, control of breathing is broadly divided into **three categories**:

- Neural control
- Chemical control
- Nonchemical (reflexes from lungs and chest wall) control

NEURAL CONTROL OF RESPIRATION

There are ***two separate neural control mechanisms***: the voluntary control and the automatic control.

Voluntary Control: The centers for **voluntary control** system are located in the cerebral cortex. The cortex controls respiratory muscles via corticospinal tract.

Automatic Control: The centers for **automatic control** are located in brainstem. The neurons of ***brainstem respiratory areas*** converge on spinal cord motor neurons.

1. The **neurons that control inspiration** converge on ***C_3–C_5 motor neurons*** (phrenic nerve) and ***thoracic motor neurons*** that supply external intercostal muscles.
2. The **neurons that control expiration** converge mainly on ***thoracic motor neurons*** that supply internal intercostal muscles.

Medullary Respiratory Centers

Medulla controls the basic rhythm of respiration. Two different groups of neurons have been well defined in medulla.

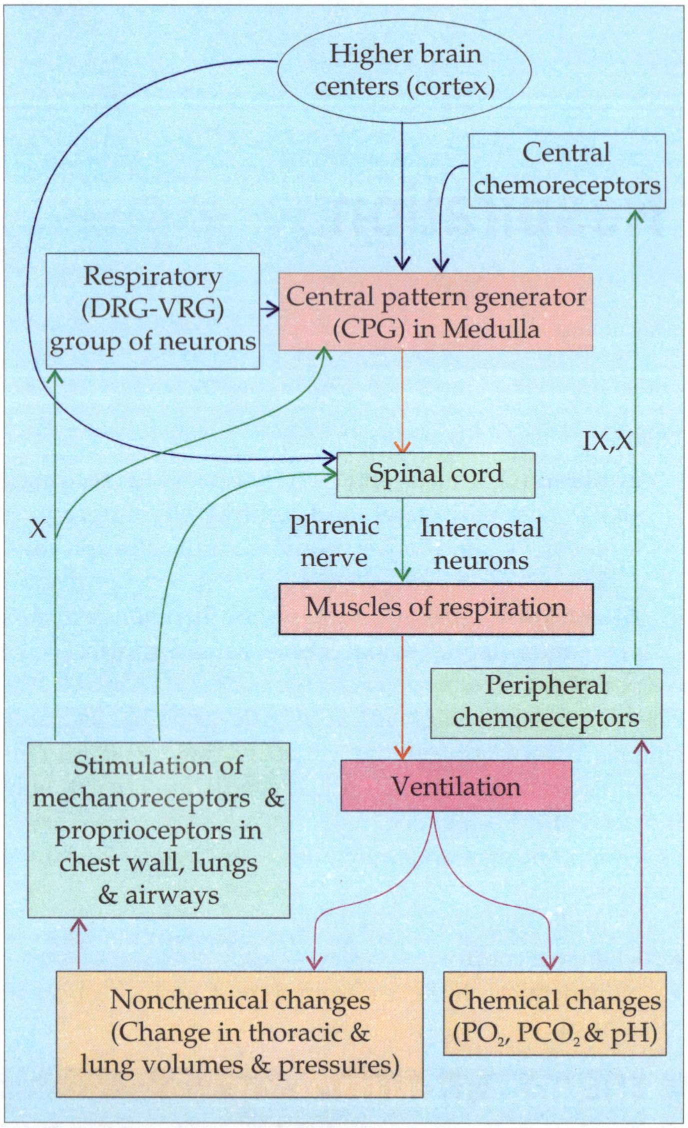

Fig. 49.1: General organization of respiratory control mechanisms. Note, central pattern generator (CPG), which is located in and around DRG-VRG complex receives inputs from different brain centers including cortical and central chemoreceptor inputs, and medullary respiratory neurons. CPG generates basic respiratory rhythm and drives spinal cord motor neurons that innervate respiratory muscles, which on appropriate stimulation produce ventilation. Chemical and nonchemical changes induced by ventilation provide feedback signals to CNS for regulation of respiration.

- According to their anatomic locations they are called as dorsal respiratory group and ventral respiratory group of neurons (Fig. 49.2).
- In addition, CPG is located in the medulla in and around dorsal and ventral group of neurons.

Dorsal Respiratory Group

Dorsal respiratory group (DRG) is named for its dorsal location in the medulla.

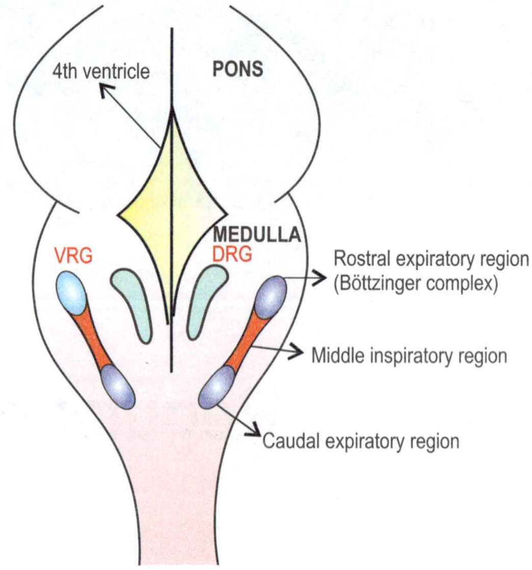

Fig. 49.2: Respiratory centers in medulla. Note the location of dorsal respiratory group (DRG) and ventral respiratory group (VRG) of neurons. Also note the three segments of VRG.

- It is located bilaterally in and around the nucleus tractus solitarius (NTS).
- DRG primarily contains inspiratory neurons.
- NTS receives sensory inputs *from all thoracic and abdominal viscera*.
  - DRG neurons receive sensory inputs from different parts of respiratory system including peripheral chemoreceptors and related respiratory structures via 10th and 9th cranial nerves.
- DRG is primarily responsible for inspiration and for integration of sensory information that originates from respiratory system.
- Neurons from DRG directly project to the cell bodies of phrenic nerve motor neurons in the spinal cord.

Ventral Respiratory Group

Ventral respiratory group (VRG) of cells are located in the ventrolateral medulla in the region of the nucleus ambiguous (retroambiguous and paraambiguous) and retrofacialis.

- VRG has a larger collection of neurons that extends almost the entire length of medulla.
- The VRG contains both inspiratory and expiratory neurons.
- The cells in the nucleus retrofacialis and retroambiguous are active during expiration and cells in the nucleus paraambiguous are active during inspiration.

Parts of VRG: VRG has three regions: rostral expiratory, middle inspiratory and caudal expiratory regions.

i) The rostral expiratory region of VRG (also called as Bötzinger complex) drives the *expiratory activity* of caudal region.
ii) The caudal expiratory region in turn projects to the spinal motor neurons that innervate *muscles of expiration*.

ii) The middle inspiratory region projects to the spinal motor neurons that *innervate inspiratory muscles*, and also to cell bodies of neurons that innervate muscles of pharynx and larynx.

- Thus, the middle region not only controls inspiration, but also ***increases the caliber*** of the upper respiratory tract during inspiration.

Interaction between DRG & VRG: The DRG and VRG are located on both sides and control activities of respiratory apparatus of their respective sides. However, cross-communication between the centers of both sides helps them to work synchronously and harmoniously. Thus, respiratory movements of both sides of chest occur simultaneously and symmetrically.

Central Pattern Generator

Central pattern generator (CPG) is reported to be present within and closely surrounding the area of DRG-VRG complex.

1. CPG is present in the **pre-Bötzinger complex**, a group of **pacemaker cells** located bilaterally between nucleus ambiguous and lateral reticular nucleus (Fig. 49.3).
   - CPG is responsible for **generating normal respiratory rhythm**.
2. The neurons (pacemaker cells) in the pre-Bötzinger complex *discharge rhythmically to* ***activate phrenic motor neuron*** in the spinal cord.

Role of an Integrator: It appears that CPG is influenced by an **integrator**, which is located within the **medullary reticular formation**. Integrator ***receives and processes inputs*** from chemoreceptors and higher brain centers like cortex, hypothalamus and limbic system. The integrator in turn controls mainly the frequency and amplitude of respiratory pattern.

Pontine Respiratory Centers

In pons, there are **two respiratory centers**: pneumotaxic and apneustic.

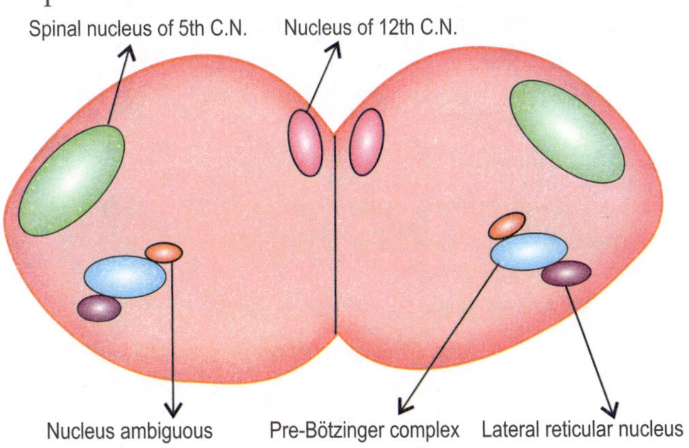

Fig. 49.3: Location of central pattern generator (CPG) of respiration. CPG is located in pre-Bötzinger complex, which is situated between nucleus ambiguous and lateral reticular nucleus in medulla. C.N.: cranial nerve.

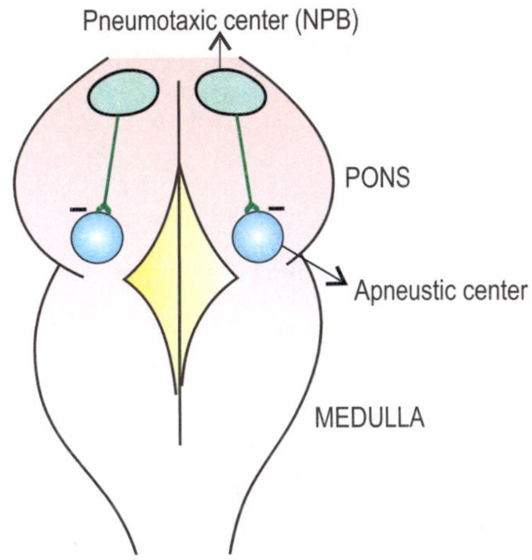

Fig. 49.4: Respiratory centers in pons. Note the location of pneumotaxic and apneustic centers. Nucleus parabrachialis (NPB), the pneumotaxic center located in rostral pons, inhibits apneustic center.

Pneumotaxic Center

Pneumotaxic center is located in **nucleus parabrachialis medialis** and **Kölliker-Fuse nucleus** that are present in the rostral pons (Fig. 49.4).

- Neurons in pneumotaxic center are **active during both inspiration and expiration**.
- Pneumotaxic center **coordinates respiration by switching between inspiration and expiration**.
- Normally, pneumotaxic center **inhibits apneustic center**.
- **Suprapontine lesion** in experimental animals ***does not change*** respiratory rhythm indicating that brain centers above pons do not appreciably influence basic rhythm of respiration.

Apneustic Center

Apneustic center is present in the **caudal pons**.

- Stimulation of apneustic center results in **prolonged inspiratory effort** interrupted by brief expiration (**apneusis**).
- This indicates that apneustic center **strongly activates medullary inspiratory center**.
- However, apneustic center is tonically **inhibited by pneumotaxic center**, and therefore, inspiratory drive originating in apneustic center is checked (Fig. 49.5).

Role of Vagus Nerve

Vagus nerve carries **afferent fibers from lung and airways**. During inspiration, stretching of lung parenchyma increases discharge of afferent fibers in vagus nerve originating from lung.

1. The afferent vagal impulse **inhibits medullary inspiratory neurons**.
   - Therefore, magnitude of inspiration increases following vagotomy and vagal stimulation results in inhibition of respiration.
   - However, **disruption of vagal afferents** (abolition of vagal feedback) **prolongs the activity of motor neurons** supplying inspiratory muscles

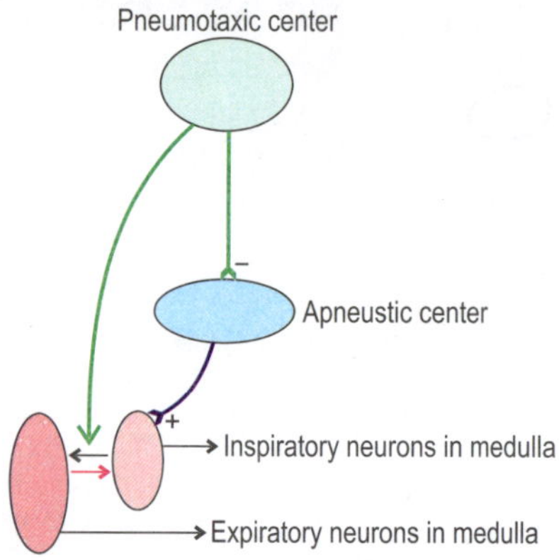

Fig. 49.5: Interaction between pontine (pneumotaxic and apneustic) and medullary (inspiratory and expiratory) respiratory centers. Apneustic center stimulates medullary inspiratory neurons. Pneumotaxic center inhibits apneustic center to check its output, and switches between inspiratory and expiratory neurons in medulla.

i.e., efferent activity in phrenic nerve, without affecting their magnitude.

2. Vagus nerve and pneumotaxic center **keep the activity of apneustic center in check.**
   - As apneustic center normally activates inspiratory drive, which is inhibited by vagus nerve, **vagotomy stimulates inspiration.**
   - Further, **vagotomy following lesion** of pneumotaxic center results in **apneusis** (Fig. 49.6)

Control by Higher Centers

Control of respiration by higher centers in the brain is more complex. Influences from **reticular activating system** (RAS) and **limbic system** are more prominent.

- RAS exerts a **tonic drive on CPG**, which is increased during arousal from sleep.
- The drive **from limbic system** increases during *emotional reactions.*

Integration of Neural Mechanisms

The **basic rhythm generator** for respiration is located **in medulla**. Lesion above pons does not affect respiration, which indicates that the **controlling centers are located mainly in pons** (Fig. 49.6).

- **CPG** located in the DRG-VRG complex, is responsible for **generating normal respiratory rhythm**.
- The pacemaker cells in the pre-Bötzinger complex discharge rhythmically to **activate phrenic motor neurons** in the spinal cord that ***initiate and generate inspiratory breathing patterns.***

Inspiration: During inspiratory phase, **phrenic nerve activity** increases gradually in two seconds that stops suddenly just at the onset of expiration.

1. The **inspiratory neurons** exhibit constant discharge throughout inspiration (***constant inspiratory neurons***) or ramp like discharge during inspiration (***inspiratory ramp neurons***).

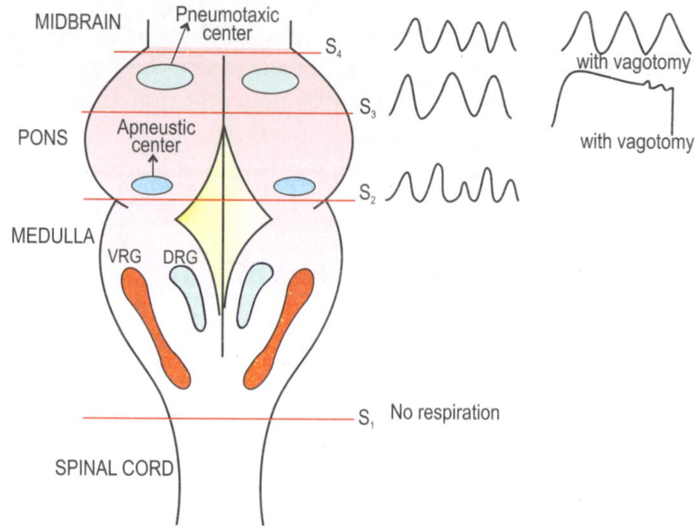

Fig. 49.6: Effects of transection of brainstem at various levels on pattern, rate and depth of respiration. Section below medulla (**S_1**) completely abolishes respiration, which indicates that respiratory rhythm is generated in and above medulla in the brain. In section below pons, i.e., below apneustic center (**S_2**), basic rhythm of respiration occurs, but respiration is irregular indicating that respiratory rhythm is generated in medulla. In section below the pneumotaxic center (**S_3**), amplitude of respiration increases indicating that normally pneumotaxic center inhibits apneustic center. If bilateral vagotomy is combined with S_3, apneusis occurs, which indicates that normally vagus nerve inhibit the output of apneustic center on medullary inspiratory center. Section above pons (**S_4**), does not affect respiration, which indicates that centers for generation and regulation of respiratory rhythm are located in pons and medulla. When bilateral vagotomy is combined with S_4, amplitude of respiration increases, which indicates that vagus nerve inhibits output of pneumotaxic center on respiratory centers.

2. Inspiratory ramp activity **correlates with phasic activity in the phrenic nerve.**
   - Increase in ramp activity ensures smooth increase in lung volume in inspiration.
3. Phrenic nerve activity becomes **silent during expiration** except in the very early part of it when some burst activity occurs.

Expiration: Expiration has **two phases.**

1. In the **very early phase** of expiration, some inspiratory muscle activity persists that serves to control initial part of expiratory airflow.
2. In the **second phase** of expiration, inspiratory muscle activity totally ceases, during which expiratory airflow occurs due to **passive recoil of lungs.**
3. The duration of expiration depends on the **degree of inhibition of inspiratory neurons** in DRG-VRG complex, which is **maximal at the beginning of expiration** that slowly declines as expiration continues.
4. Finally, inhibitory effect becomes inadequate to prevent the onset of inspiration.

Control Mechanisms of Breathing

The essential **pattern of breathing is generated in CPG,** which is located in the medulla. The CPG is extensively influenced by numerous control mechanisms.

1. It is proposed that an **integrator (or controller)** is also located in the medulla that projects to and influences the activity of CPG.

2. Inputs arriving from different **brain areas** (especially from cortex and limbic system), ***proprioceptors, intrapulmonary receptors and changes in blood gases*** influence the controller of respiration.
   - By sensing the magnitude of the **carbon dioxide load** in the systemic blood, medullary pattern generator drives ventilation.
   - **Intrapulmonary receptors** provide feedback signal to respiratory control centers to regulate the degree of breathing.
   - **Proprioceptive inputs** from joints (as during exercise) also provide feedback control of breathing.
3. The controller also **adjusts rate and depth of breathing** to reduce the work expenditure for ventilation of a given magnitude.
   - To achieve this, the controller utilizes **afferent neural signals** about lung volume, rate of change of lung volume, and change in trans-pulmonary pressures, which are provided by ***lung and chest wall mechanoreceptors***.

CHEMICAL CONTROL OF BREATHING

This is the control by chemical composition of blood, especially by PO_2, PCO_2 and H^+. Peripheral and central chemoreceptors detect these chemical changes in blood. Responses to carbon dioxide and blood pH depend mainly on the central chemoreceptors and responses to hypoxia depend mainly on peripheral chemoreceptors.

Peripheral Chemoreceptors

Peripheral chemoreceptors are located in the **carotid** and **aortic bodies**.

- Though they respond to changes in PO_2, PCO_2 and pH, they are **more sensitive to decreased arterial PO_2** (hypoxia).

Carotid Bodies

Carotid bodies are very **small chemosensitive organs** having width of about 2 mm and weight of about 2 mg, located at the **bifurcations of the common carotid arteries** (Fig. 49.7).

- Afferent nerves from the carotid bodies travel to the brainstem in the **glossopharyngeal nerves**.

Two special features of carotid bodies are:

1. The **blood flow is highest** in the body per unit-weight of the tissue.
   - The blood flow is about ***2 L per 100 g of tissue/min***, which is approximately 40 times the blood flow to the brain.
   - Due to the greater blood flow, they **easily detect minor changes in PO_2, PCO_2 and pH** of blood.

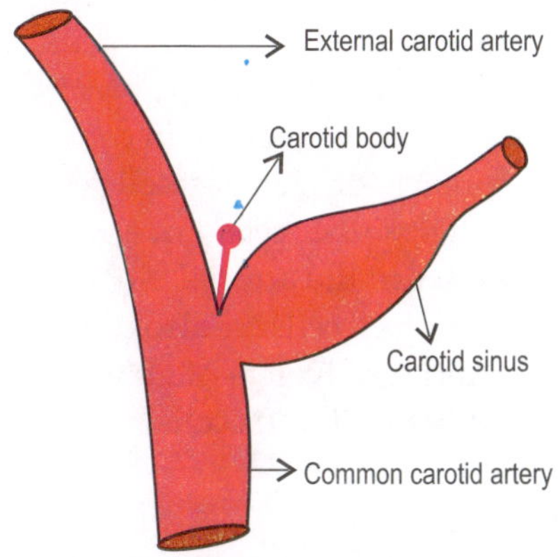

Fig. 49.7: Location of carotid body. It is located at bifurcation of common carotid into internal and external carotids. Carotid sinus is the initial dilated portion of internal carotid artery.

2. They have a **high metabolic rate**, which is about three times greater than that of brain.

Cell Types

Carotid body consists of **two types of cells**: Type I and Type II. These cells are surrounded by **fenestrated sinusoidal capillaries** (Fig. 49.8).

Type I Cells: The type I cells are the **chemosensitive cells;** also called as **glomus cells**.

1. Glomus cells **neuroectodermal in origin** and structurally resemble chromaffin cells of adrenal medulla.
2. They contain **voltage-gated ion channels** on their membrane and **many granules** in their cytoplasm containing catecholamines (norepinephrine, dopamine), substance P, met-enkephalin and acetylcholine.
   - These chemical substances, especially **dopamine** is released from glomus cells **in response to hypoxia.**

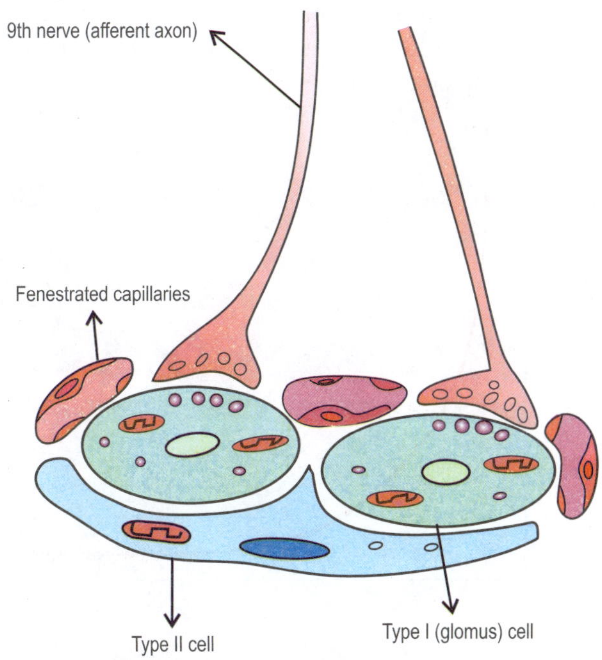

Fig. 49.8: Histology of carotid body. Note, glomus (type I) cells are supported by type II cells and closely surrounded by fenestrated capillaries. Release of neurotransmitter from glomus cell triggers action potential in 9th cranial nerve.

3. **Dopamine** released by glomus cells **acts on D_2 receptors** present on membrane of 9th nerve ending and triggers the action potential in carotid sinus nerve.
4. The close contact of **fenestrated capillaries** with glomus cells helps the cells to **easily monitor the changes of gasses** in the arterial blood.

Type II Cells: The type II cells are also called **sustentacular cells**. They surround the clusters of glomus cells. They are the **supporting cells** for glomus cells.

Aortic Bodies

Aortic bodies are located along the **ascending aorta and arch of the aorta**. They are innervated by **vagal afferents**. They **also contain glomus cells**.

Sensitivity of Chemoreceptors

The chemoreceptors respond to **hypoxia, hypercapnia and acidosis**. The **sensor** for chemical stimuli is the **glomus cell**, which responds to all three chemical changes in blood.

Hypoxia

Hypoxia is the **major stimulus** for activation of peripheral chemoreceptors.

- **Decrease in PaO_2 less than 100 mm of Hg** results in ***progressive increase in the firing rate*** of afferent nerves (Fig. 49.9) that increases ventilation.
  - The *response becomes prominent* when alveolar **PO_2 falls below 80 mm Hg.**
- The **response is most effective at PO_2 less than 60 mm Hg** (Fig. 49.10).
  - Below this level, ventilatory response curve is **steep and almost linear.**

Two mechanisms for less rise in ventilation when PO_2 falls from 100 to 60 mmHg:

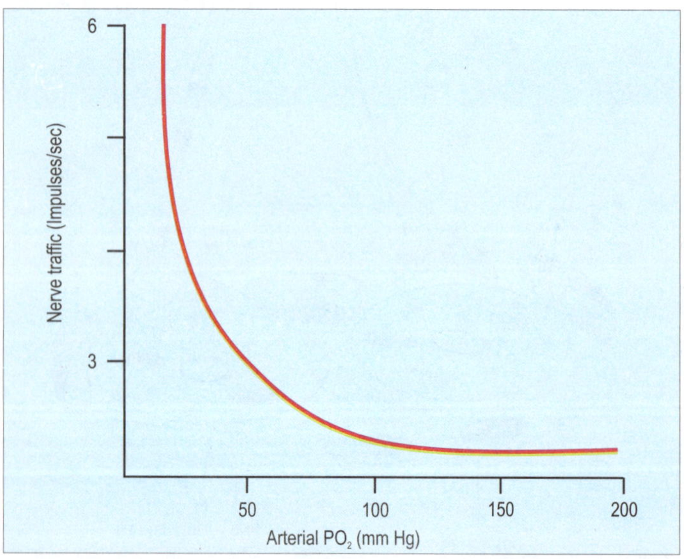

Fig. 49.9: Nerve traffic in 9th cranial nerve in response to change in arterial PO_2. Discharge rate is maximum at lower level of arterial PO_2, especially when PaO_2 is less than 60 mm Hg.

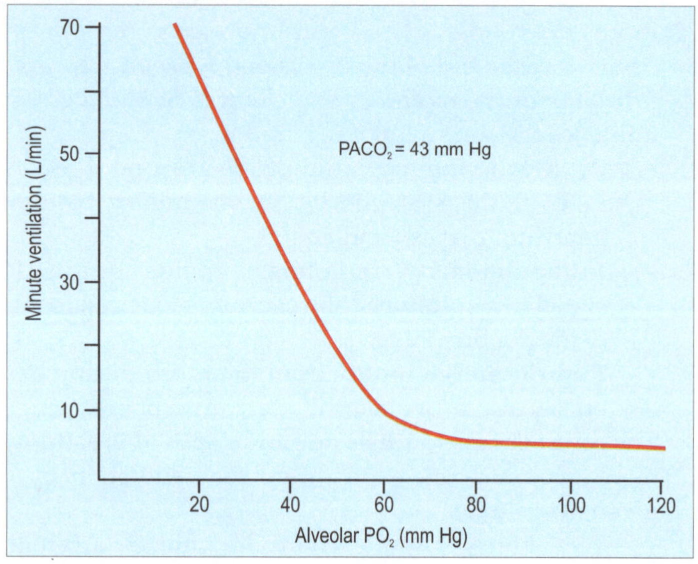

Fig. 49.10: Ventilatory response to hypoxia (alveolar PCO_2 was maintained at 43 mm Hg by adding CO_2 to inspired air to avoid the suppression of ventilation by hypocapnia that occurs secondary to hypoxia-induced hyperventilation). Note, steep increase in ventilation occurs when alveolar PO_2 decreases below 60 mm Hg.

1. In hypoxia, hemoglobin (Hb) is less saturated with O_2. ***Oxy-Hb is a stronger acid*** than Hb.
   - Thus, with fall in arterial PO_2, the **H^+ of arterial blood falls** due to less saturation of Hb with O_2.
   - The **fall in H^+ inhibits respiration.**
2. Increased ventilation due to hypoxia **decreases PCO_2** that in turn inhibits ventilation.

Therefore, **unless hypoxia is strong enough** to overcome the inhibitory effect of decreased H^+ and PCO_2 in arterial blood on ventilation, its effect on ventilation is not prominent.

- When **PO_2 is less than 60 mm Hg,** *hypoxic drive becomes strong* enough to override these inhibitory effects.

Significance

The response of peripheral chemoreceptors to oxygen **depends on PaO_2,** and **not the oxygen content.**

- Therefore, in **anemia or carbon monoxide poisoning,** the two conditions that exhibit reduced oxygen content but has normal PaO_2, ***have little effect*** on the ventilation response curve.

Mechanism

Hypoxia **inhibits K^+ channel**. The accumulation of K^+ in the glomus cell results in **depolarization** that activates **voltage gated Ca^{++} channels.** Increased **Ca^{++} influx** causes neurotransmitter secretion that stimulates the afferent nerve and increased ventilation (Fig. 49.11):

Inhibition of K^+ Channel: Inhibition of K^+ channel by hypoxia occurs by **three possible mechanisms**:

1. The oxygen sensor in the glomus cell is a **heme-containing protein**, which is closely **associated with K^+ channel.**
   - This protein is normally bound to O_2.

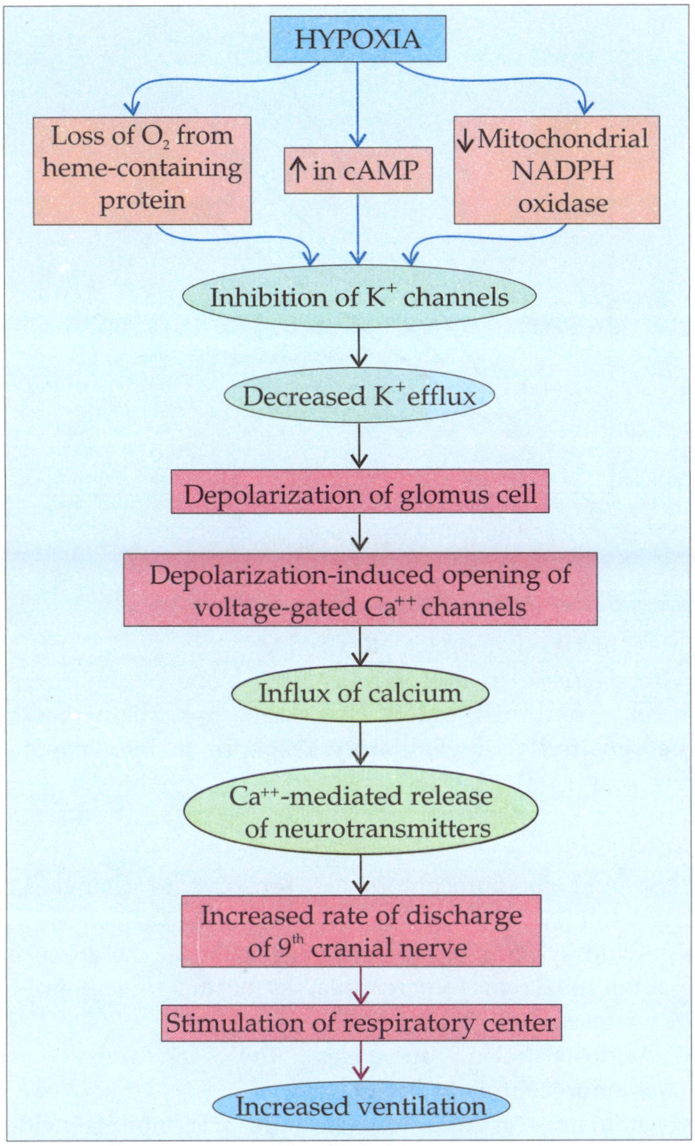

Fig. 49.11: Mechanisms of increased ventilation by hypoxia

- In hypoxia, the heme-containing protein loses its O_2, which leads to inhibition of K^+ channels.

2. Hypoxia **increases cAMP in the glomus cells.** Increased intracellular cAMP **inhibits cAMP-sensitive K^+ channels.**
3. Hypoxia **inhibits mitochondrial NADPH oxidase** in the glomus cells.
   - NADPH oxidase is essential for reduction of glutathione. This increases the ratio of reduced glutathione (GSH) to the oxidized glutathione (GSSG), which directly inhibits K^+ channels.

Effect of Change in $PACO_2$: At lower level of alveolar PCO_2 (37 mm Hg), no stimulation of ventilation occurs by hypoxia *until the alveolar PO_2 is less than 60 mm Hg*, and below this the response curve is steep and linear with progressive decrease in PO_2 (Fig. 49.12).

- **At higher level of alveolar PCO_2** (49 mm Hg), an **inverse relationship** is observed between ventilation and alveolar PO_2, in which ***decrease in PO_2 proportionately increases ventilatory response*** and increase in PO_2 linearly decreases ventilatory response.

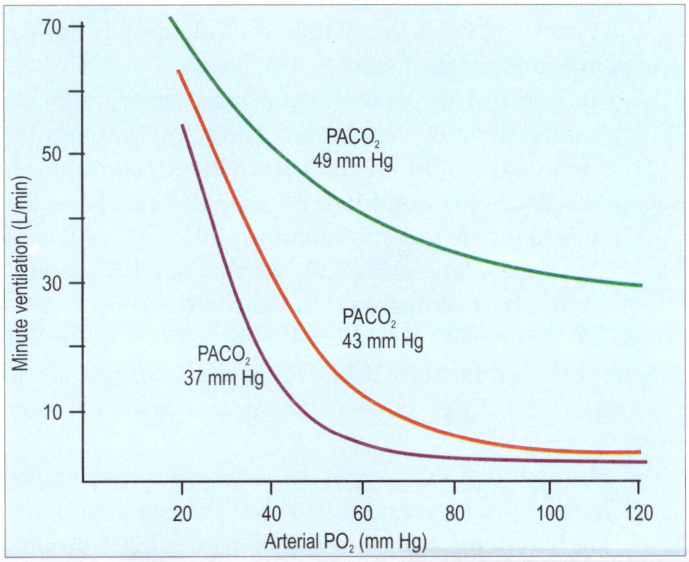

Fig. 49.12: Effect of increased and decreased alveolar PCO_2 ($PaCO_2$) on ventilation response curve produced at different levels of arterial PO_2 ($PaCO_2$).

Hypercapnia

The **rate of discharge** of carotid and aortic chemoreceptors **increases linearly with increase in $PaCO_2$.**

- Increase in $PaCO_2$ stimulates peripheral chemoreceptors by **increasing CO_2 in glomus cells.**
  - In fact, H^+ formed form **H_2CO_3 in the glomus cells is the actual stimulus** rather than the molecular CO_2.
  - Effect of $PaCO_2$ on ventilation is mediated **up to 40%** by peripheral chemoreceptors.
  - **Hypoxia** affects ventilation mainly via ***peripheral chemoreceptors***, whereas **hypercapnia** affects ventilation mainly via ***central chemoreceptors***.

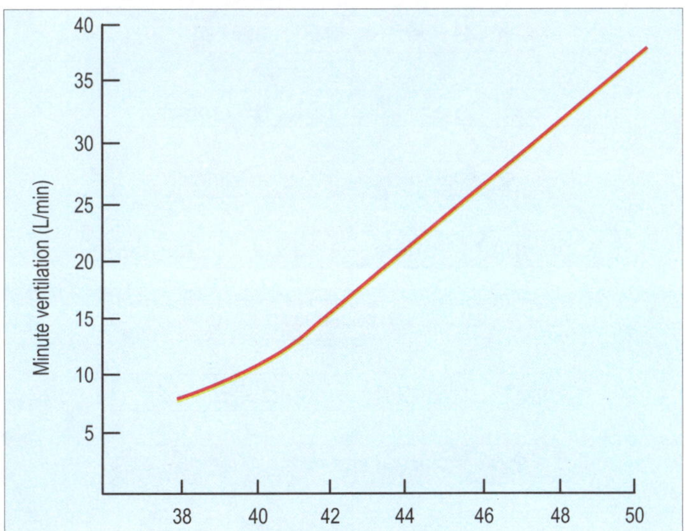

Fig. 49.13: Ventilatory response to hypercapnia (alveolar PO_2 was held at 100 mm Hg). Note that with increase in $PaCO_2$, there was almost a linear increase in minute ventilation.

- The effect of CO_2 on ventilation is studied by **inhaling gas mixture** containing CO_2.
    - Increase in alveolar PCO_2 increases arterial PCO_2 that stimulates ventilation. Though hyperventilation tends to remove CO_2 from blood, stimulation of ventilation continues till the individual continues to inhale CO_2 gas mixture.
    - Increase in alveolar PCO_2 has almost a **linear relationship with increase in ventilation** (Fig. 49.13).

Effect of High CO_2 in Air: When, **CO_2 content of atmospheric air is high** (CO_2 content of inspired air is more than 7%), PCO_2 of alveolar air and arterial blood increase abruptly.

- Elimination of CO_2 from body **becomes ineffective** in this condition and CO_2 accumulates in blood.
- High hypercapnia causes ***CNS depression***. Initially, there will be headache and confusion, which fast leads to coma. The condition is called **CO_2 narcosis**.

Mechanism

Increase in $PaCO_2$ increases entry of CO_2 into the glomus cells.

1. CO_2 forms **H^+ in the cell**. This results in decrease in intracellular pH (increased H^+).
2. Increased cytosolic protons (H^+) block K^+ channels and **inhibit K^+ efflux**.
    - This causes **depolarization** of the cell, which causes opening of voltage-gated calcium channels.
3. **Calcium influx** leads to increased cytosolic Ca^{++} and **Ca^{++}-mediated neurotransmitter release** that leads to increased nerve traffic in 9th nerve (Flowchart 49.1).

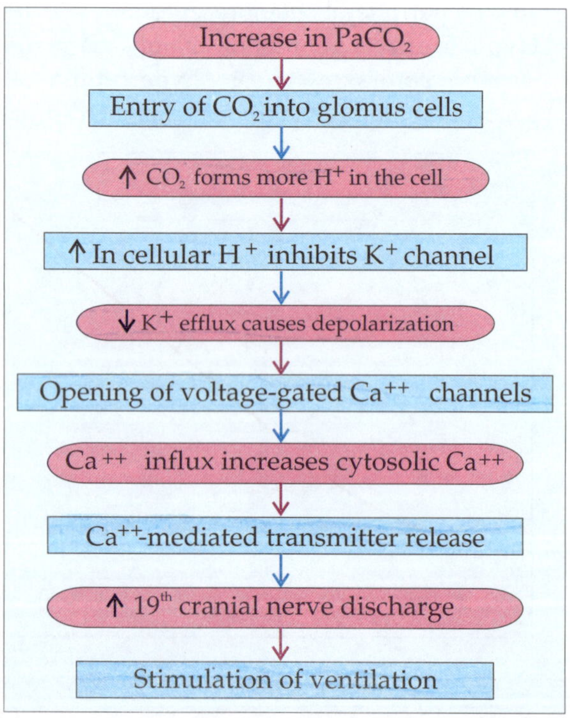

Flowchart 49.1: Mechanism of increase in ventilation by hypercapnia through peripheral chemoreceptors.

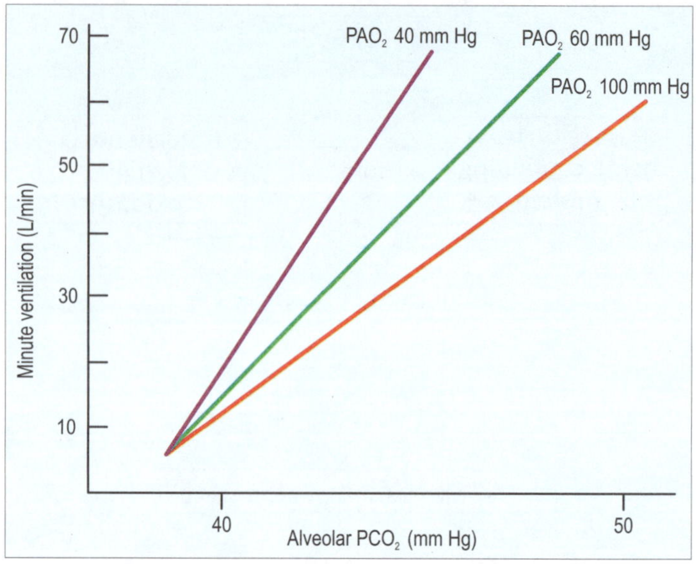

Fig. 49.14: Effects of hypoxia on CO_2 response curve. Note, hypoxia makes the individual more sensitive to PCO_2. The ventilatory response curve becomes steeper.

Effect of Hypoxia on CO_2 Response

With decrease in alveolar PO_2, the slope of the curve increases and **shifts to left.** That means, hypoxia **increases the sensitivity** of ventilatory response to hypercapnia (Fig. 49.14).

Acidosis

Peripheral chemoreceptors are sensitive to change in arterial pH.

- Acidosis **alone stimulates ventilation** in the absence of hypoxia or hypercapnia, as occurs in metabolic acidosis.
- Acidosis also **increases the sensitivity of chemoreceptors to $PaCO_2$.**

Mechanism: Acidosis (decrease in pH) inhibits acid-extruding transporters, like Na-H^+ exchanger.

- This results in increased intracellular acid load (accumulation of H^+ in the cell).
- Increased proton inhibits K^+ channels.

Other Factors

1. **Poisons** that inhibit metabolic respiratory chain like cyanide strongly stimulate peripheral chemoreceptors.
2. **Fall in blood** pressure below 60 mm Hg, with or without change in PaO_2 stimulates chemoreceptor activity.
    - This effect is ***mediated more through aortic bodies***.
    - Afferent impulses from chemoreceptors interact with neural inputs of other reflexes like lung stretch reflex, baroreceptor reflex etc. that especially help in regulation of cardio-respiratory functions.

Central Chemoreceptors

Central chemoreceptors are located as bilaterally paired cell groups just below the surface of the ventrolateral medulla immediately caudal to the ponto-medullay junction. Therefore, they are also called medullary chemoreceptors or chemosensitive areas (Fig. 49.15).

1. On each side, the cell groups are divided into **rostral, intermediate and caudal chemosensitive zones.**
2. The medullary chemosensitive neurons respond to **change in the H^+** of the surrounding interstitial fluid.
   - It should be noted that the cerebral interstitial fluid H^+ concentration is the **function of PCO_2** in the cerebral arterial blood and the **bicarbonate** concentration of cerebrospinal fluid.

Mechanism of Stimulation

Change in H^+ concentration of blood is poorly reflected in CSF, as H^+ penetrates very slowly into the brain. However, **molecular carbon dioxide diffuses readily** into CSF.

1. CO_2 that enters the CSF is immediately hydrated to form H_2CO_3.
   - **H_2CO_3** dissociates to form H^+ and HCO_3^-.
   - Thus, **blood PCO_2 influences the pH of CSF.**
2. In fact, concentration of H^+ in interstitial fluid in the brain parallels the PCO_2 level in arterial blood.
   - The **concentration of H^+** in CSF stimulates central chemoreceptors that increases respiration, and the magnitude of stimulation is proportional to its concentration.

Role of pH of CSF: The pH of CSF is 7.3, which is slightly less than that of blood (7.4). It is primarily **determined by the bicarbonate content** and the **level of PCO_2** in CSF.

- Therefore, the change in CSF pH occurs less than the change of pH of plasma in metabolic acid-base disturbances, whereas in **respiratory acid-base disturbances**, the change in CSF pH ***is same as that of blood.***
  - This happens as in metabolic disturbances the CSF bicarbonate change is about 40% of the change that occurs in blood, whereas in respiratory disturbances the **CSF bicarbonate change is same** as that in blood.

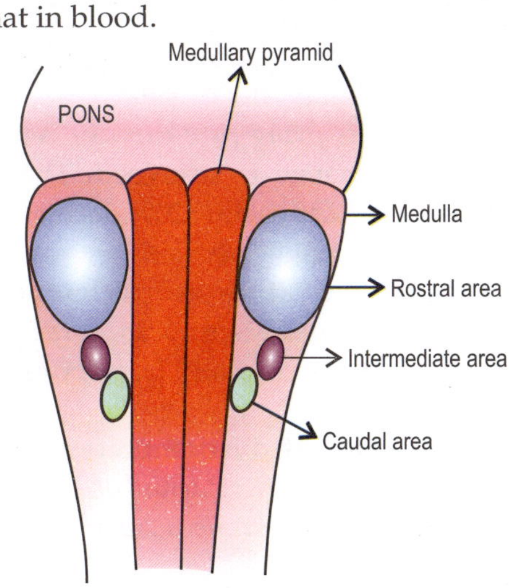

Fig. 49.15: Location of central chemoreceptor areas on ventral surface of medulla. Note the presence of three chemosensitive areas (rostral, intermediate, and caudal).

Integrated Responses to Hypoxia, Hypercapnia and Acidosis

Often hypoxia is associated with hypercapnia and acidosis. Also, the effects are mediated by simultaneous activation of peripheral and central chemoreceptors. Thus, the responses are integrated (Flowchart 49.2).

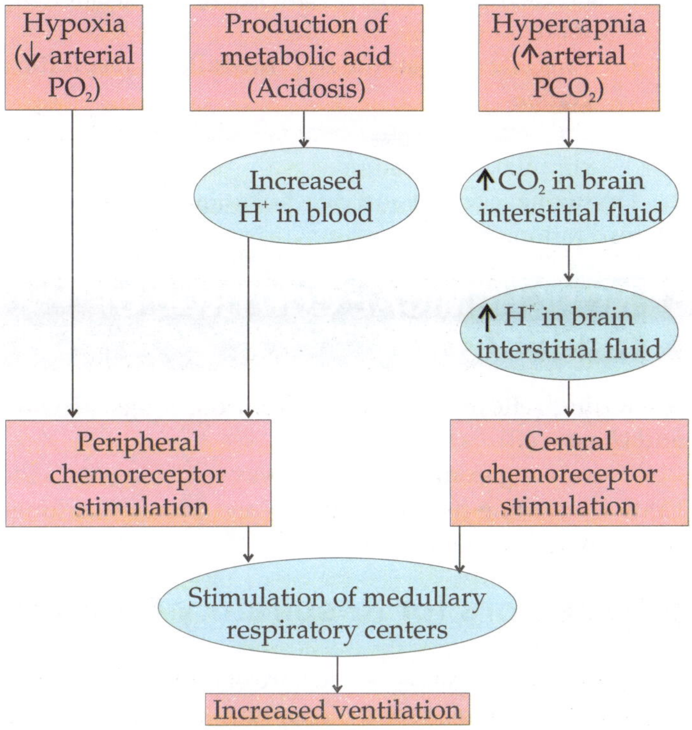

Flowchart 49.2: Integrated effects of hypoxia, hypercapnia, and acidosis on ventilation via peripheral and central chemoreceptors.

1. The **ventilatory response to hypercapnia is more in the presence of hypoxia**, and the degree of increase in ventilation varies with the degree of hypoxia (Fig. 49.14).
2. Similarly, the **ventilatory response to hypoxia increases in the presence of hypercapnia**. Due to this interdependence, the subsequent increased ventilation blunts the response to hypoxia, unless $PaCO_2$ is held constant as $PaCO_2$ decreases due to increased ventilation.
3. The **low $PaCO_2$ blunts the response to hypoxia** mainly by affecting central chemoreceptors.
   - The best example is the hypoxic response at **high altitude.**
   - Hyperventilation occurs due to hypoxic stimulation of peripheral chemoreceptors.
4. Subsequently, **increase in pH** (respiratory alkalosis) created by the hyperventilation allows hypoxic stimulation to be less effective.
5. Also, **H^+ effects on CO_2 response** is additive in nature.
   - The CO_2 response curve shifts to left with decrease in pH as the chemoreceptor sensitivity increases.
   - About **40% of response to CO_2 is abolished** if the decrease in arterial pH by CO_2 is prevented to occur.

Hormonal Control of Respiration

Many hormones influence respiration.

1. **Female gonadal hormones**, especially **progesterone** stimulate ventilation.
   - Therefore, during pregnancy and secretory phase of menstrual cycle, ventilation is considerably more.
   - Progesterone **stimulates medullary respiratory centers**.
   - Progesterone also ***increases body temperature*** that stimulates ventilation.
2. **Thyroxine, cortisol** and catecholamines also influence respiration.

NONCHEMICAL CONTROL OF RESPIRATION

(Including reflexes originating from the lungs, airways and chest wall)

Reflexes arising from the upper airways and lungs provide feedback for fine-tuning breathing and protect the lungs from environmental insults.

Receptors for Respiratory Reflexes

Receptors for respiratory reflexes are of **three types**: slowly adapting receptors, rapidly adapting receptors, and C fiber endings. These receptors are mainly innervated by **myelinated and unmyelinated fibers in vagus nerve**.

Slowly Adapting Receptors

The slowly adapting receptors are located **within the smooth muscle** of conducting airways.

1. They are sensory terminals of **myelinated afferent fibers**.
   - As they ***respond to airway stretch***, they are also known as **pulmonary stretch receptors**.
2. They discharge in response to **increased airway transmural pressure** and sense the **changes in lung volume.**
3. They **adapt slowly to the stretch** imposed on them.
4. When stimulated, they **inhibit inspiration and prolong expiration**.
   - This is called Hering-Breuer reflex.

Hering-Breuer Reflex

This reflex was described by Hering and Breuer in 1868, who found that lung inflation decreases tidal volume and increases respiratory frequency.

There are ***two Hering-Breuer (HB) reflexes***: HB inflation reflex and HB deflation reflex.

Hering-Breuer Inflation Reflex: In HB inflation reflex, steady **increase in lung volume** (lung inflation) results in **increase in duration of expiration.**

- Marked inflation of lungs with sustained pressure may even abruptly terminate inspiration in progress in addition to the prolongation of expiration.

Hering-Breuer Deflation Reflex: In HB deflation reflex, marked **deflation of lung** results in **decrease in duration of expiration**.

- As described above, the receptors are *slowly adapting stretch receptors* in lung parenchyma and airways and *afferent and efferent pathways* are vagus nerve.

Significance of Hering-Breuer Reflex

This is a **protective reflex that protects lung from overinflation** while marinating normal alveolar ventilation.

- It is more **useful in infants** than in adults. It controls tidal volume during eupnea (normal breathing) in infants.
- In adults, this reflex does not operate **unless tidal volume is much greater** than the normal inspiration. Especially in the awake state in adults, this reflex is overwhelmed by more prominent central control.

Other Functions of Slowly Adapting Receptors

Increased lung volume stimulates slowly adapting receptors that excite the inspiratory off-switch.

1. This effect **shortens inspiration** when tidal volume is larger than normal.
2. The slowly adapting receptors are involved in regulating **expiratory time, expiratory muscle activation**, and functional residual capacity.
3. Stimulation of these receptors also **relaxes airway smooth muscle, reduces vasomotor tone** and increases heart rate.

Rapidly Adapting Receptors

The rapidly adapting receptors are **sensory terminals of myelinated afferent fibers** that are found in the larger conducting airways.

1. They respond to a **sudden maintained inflation** with rapid increase in firing rate.
   - However, their ***firing rate rapidly declines*** when the volume change is sustained. The firing rate decreases fast, with about 20% decrease occurring in the first second.
2. They are **very sensitive to different chemical stimuli** like histamine, serotonin, bradykinin and prostaglandins released locally in response to allergy and inflammation.
3. Frequently they are called **irritant receptors,**
   - as they respond to ***irritation of the airways by various noxious substances***, such as smoke, dust, ammonia etc.
4. Receptors are also stimulated by **acute congestion** and inflammation.

Significance of Rapidly Adapting Receptors: Rapidly adapting receptors play important role in detecting pathological processes that involve **irritation, congestion and inflammation** of airways.

- Activity of these receptors is **inversely proportional to lung compliance** and they are considered as the ***sensors of compliance change***, especially in pathological states as they are almost inactive during quiet breathing.
- In general, stimulation of rapidly adapting receptors results in excitatory responses like **coughing, gasping, and prolonged-inspiration**.

C Fiber Endings

C fiber endings are **terminals of unmyelinated nerves**. They innervate the receptors in *alveoli and conducting airways*. They are of ***two types in the lungs***.

1. **Pulmonary C Fibers:** The first category is **pulmonary C fibers** that are located adjacent to alveoli and are accessible from the pulmonary capillary circulation.
   - They are also called as **Juxtapulmonary capillary** receptors or, **J receptors** (described by Indian scientist **A. S. Paintal).**

Significant contribution of Scientist

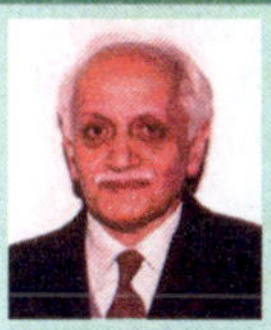

Prof. Autar Singh Paintal (1925 - 2004), was Director of V.P. Chest Institute from 1964 to 1990, and then Director General of ICMR. He studied galvanic skin responses in man (1951), new techniques for recording single nerve fibre conduction velocities (1953), method for locating visceral receptors (1954), discovered Type B atrial receptors (1953), Gastric stretch receptors responsible for the immediate satiation of hunger (1954), Juxtapulmonary capillary (J) receptors in lungs (1955), Ventricular pressure receptors (1955), Mucosal mechanoreceptors of the intestines (1957) and Pressure-pain receptors of muscles (1960). He is **best known for discovery of J receptors** and **J reflex**, that are integral part of non-chemical regulation of respiration. In recognition of his vast contribution to Physiology, the Association of Physiologists of India (ASSOPI) has the "**Professor A. S. Paintal Award**" for the best research publication by a physiologist in the field of Physiology.

2. **Bronchial C Fibers:** The second category is the **bronchial C fibers** that are located in airways and accessible from the bronchial circulation.

Both the categories of receptors are stimulated by lung injury, marked inflation, acute pulmonary vascular congestion, and certain chemical agents.

Significance of C-Fiber Endings

Pulmonary C fibers are more ***sensitive to mechanical processes*** like edema, congestion, and embolism and less sensitive to chemical stimulation like products of inflammation, whereas the **bronchial C fibers** are more ***sensitive to chemical stimulation***.

1. When they are stimulated, they cause rapid shallow breathing, bronchoconstriction, increased airway secretion, and cardiovascular depression. This is called **J reflex** (mediated by J receptor)
2. **Acute stimulation** results in ***apnea and a marked hypotension***. Skeletal muscle tone is also abruptly reduced.

Other Nonchemical Receptors

Chest Wall Proprioceptors

Chest wall proprioceptors provide information about chest movement and muscle tension, especially when the breathing is effortful.

- Intercostal muscles contain plenty of muscle spindles that are rare in the diaphragm. These muscle spindles adjust breathing by *controlling feedback motor neuron activities*.
- Chest wall proprioceptors also play important role in the perception of breathing-effort.

Other Proprioceptors: Joint movements, both active and passive stimulate respiration.

- **Impulses in the ascending fibers** in sensory pathways from proprioceptors in the muscle, tendons, joint ligaments etc. to the thalamus, give **collaterals to brainstem respiratory centers**. Therefore, increased activity in these ascending pathways stimulates respiration.
- This is one of the mechanisms for **hyperventilation that occurs** during exercise.

Receptors in Upper Airways

Receptors from upper part of the airways, especially from **nasopharynx, trachea and bronchi** influence respiration during coughing and sneezing.

Coughing

Coughing could be **voluntary or a reflex** (involuntary) phenomenon to clear the irritants from respiratory tract.

- It occurs with a **deep inspiration**, which is immediately followed by **forced expiration** against a closed glottis.
- The **intrapleural pressure increases to 100 mm Hg** or more and then glottis opens instantaneously causing an explosive outflow of air at a velocity of about ***600 miles per hour***.
- Coughing is intact in individuals with transplanted lungs (Application Box 49. 1).

Application Box 49.1

Coughing remains intact in patients with lung transplant: In transplanted lung, the afferents fibers do not regrow. However, the cough responses to tracheal stimulation remains intact, though cough reflex to stimulation of smaller airways is absent in them.

- Interestingly, pattern of breathing at rest, yawns and sighs in them remain normal, which indicates that these breathing responses do not depend on lung innervation.
- Hering-Breuer reflex is absent in these individuals.

Sneezing

Sneezing is usually an **involuntary phenomenon** to remove the dusts and other irritants from upper part of airways.

- The mechanism is almost same as coughing, but the **glottis remains continuously opened** throughout the reflex act.

Afferents from Viscera

Respiration during swallowing & vomiting

Respiration is **temporarily inhibited,** and **glottis is closed** during swallowing and vomiting that prevents food particle or vomitus to enter the respiratory tract.

- **Afferents from viscera and diaphragm** mediate these responses.

Hiccup

For hiccup reflex, inspiratory muscles including diaphragm contract spasmodically, causing an **instantaneous inspiration.**

- During this process, **glottis closes abruptly**, which produces the typical sound associated with hiccup.
  - The physiologic significance of hiccup is not known, though it **occurs during fetal life** and postnatal life.
- Usually, **holding breath firmly stops hiccup**; but there are intractable hiccups that sometimes respond to centrally acting analgesics and ***dopamine antagonists***.

Yawning

This is a peculiar reflexive respiratory act associated with **deep inspiration and typical prolonged musical sound,** which is often infectious (others start yawning). It is also observed **in fetus, fish, tortoise and mammals.**

The **functions of yawning** are:

1. **Removes excess CO_2 & activates the body:** It is reported that yawning occurs when there is **excess accumulation of CO_2** in the blood.
2. **Heralds sleep:** Just before going to sleep, people often yawn. Yawning occurs frequently in sleeplessness condition.
3. **Improves lung expansion:** It is observed that deep inspiration and stretching of the thorax during yawning **causes expansion of lungs** and improves airflow into underventilated aveoli.
4. **Improves venous return:** Yawning improves venous return by **increasing abdominal and thoracic pump** activities.
5. **Nonverbal communication:** A specific nonverbal message can be delivered to others through yawning, which is true for both animals and human beings.

Afferents from Baroreceptors

Afferent fibers from baroreceptors located in **carotid sinus, aortic arch, ventricles and atria** relay in medullary respiratory centers, in addition to their relay in medullary cardiovascular centers.

- Usually, impulses originating from these baroreceptors **inhibit respiration**, which has temporary and mild effect.
- Hyperventilation that occurs due to chemoreceptor stimulation is not baroreceptor-mediated.

Afferents from Higher Centers

Afferents from **limbic system and hypothalamus** terminate in brainstem respiratory centers.

- They mediate breathing responses during **pain and emotion**.
- Afferents from neocortex to respiratory motor neurons in the spinal cord mediate the **voluntary control respiration**. These cortical neurons do not terminate on brainstem respiratory centers.

Breathing During Sleep

Sleep occurs due to removal of excitatory influences that arise from the brainstem reticular formation.

1. **Reticular activating system** has ***tonic excitatory drive*** on medullary respiratory neurons.
2. In general, during sleep, as the stimulus of wakefulness is removed, **breathing is depressed** with the deepening of sleep and when wakefulness returns as sleep lightens, ***breathing is activated by the carbon dioxide*** accumulated during the interval of sleep.
3. This ***periodic pattern of breathing*** if exaggerated is known as **Cheyne-Stokes breathing**, which usually occurs in slow wave sleep.
   - In **slow-wave sleep,** in stages 1 and 2, there is periodic variation in depth of breathing.
   - However, **in stages 3 and 4**, breathing is *slow, deep and regular*.
4. In **REM sleep**, breathing is *rapid and irregular*.

Responses to CO_2, Hypoxia & Airway Irritation during Sleep

In general, **ventilatory responses to CO_2 are decreased** during sleep.

During Non-REM Sleep: In non-REM sleep, the decreased sensitivity to CO_2 is mainly due to **reduction in wakefulness-stimulus.**

- During slow wave sleep, in the absence of the wake-fulness-stimulus, carbon dioxide-stimulus provides the major background medullary excitation for stable breathing to continue.

During REM Sleep: Breathing is regulated by the behavioral control systems.

- Ventilatory **responses to hypoxia are decreased** during both slow-wave and REM sleep. However, the irregular and rapid breathing of REM sleep remains unaffected by hypoxia.
- During sleep, **hypercapnia is a potent stimulus** than

hypoxia for arousal.

Responses to airway irritation alter during sleep. Stimuli that cause cough, tachypnea, and airway constriction during wakefulness usually cause apnea and airway dilation during sleep.

Upper Airway Obstruction during Sleep

During REM sleep, **skeletal muscle tone is reduced.** Tone of **laryngeal and pharyngeal muscles is also decreased.** Muscles of tongue relax.

- This increases the possibility of obstruction of the upper airways during REM sleep.
- Airway obstruction during sleep **results in snoring.**
- Repeated and prolonged obstruction results in **significant hypercapnia and hypoxemia** that causes repeated arousals from sleep.

Sleep Apnea Syndrome

In **adult sleep apnea syndrome**, marked loss tone of pharyngeal muscles occurs during REM sleep causing **obstruction of airway** during inspiration. This produces apnea. This is called **obstructive sleep apnea.**

- **Obesity** contributes to the obstructive sleep apnea.
- The person wakes up and breathes normally for sometimes, and then sleeps again to have another bout of apnea.
  - Thus, ***repeated apnea occurs during sleep.***
- These people develop morning headache and fatigue due to frequent apnea in the night.
- Sleeplessness occurs during the day (**day somnolence**).

Central Sleep Apnea: In central sleep apnea, the primary cause is the ***decreased neural output*** from medullary respiratory center to the phrenic motor neurons that supply diaphragm.

Exam Questions

1. Describe the neural regulation of respiration.
2. Describe the chemical regulation of respiration.
3. Describe nonchemical regulation of respiration.
4. Name the respiratory centers in brainstem. Describe the effect of transaction of brainstem at various levels on respiration, with or without intact vagus nerve.
5. Describe the role of Hering-Breuer reflex and J reflex in respiratory functions.

Multiple Choice Questions (cont.. from Page 410, Chapter 48)

6 **In an adult, at sea level the normal p50 occur at what level of PO2.**
A. 15 mmHg B. 27mmHg
C. 60 mmHg D. 95 mmHg

7. **Which of the following does not affect oxy-Hb dissociation curve?**
A. Temperature B. 2-3 DPG
C. pH D. Rate of blood flow

8. **All of the following shift the oxy-Hb dissociation curve to right, EXCEPT:**
A. Increased temperature B. Decreased pH
C. Increased 2-3 DPG D. Increased PO2.

9. **All of the following shift the oxy-Hb dissociation curve to left, EXCEPT:**
A. Decreased temperature B. Increased pH
C. Decreased 2-3 DPG D. Increased PCO2.

10. **The volume of oxygen contained in unit volume of blood is called:**
A. Oxygen saturation B. Oxygen content
C. Oxygen extraction D. Oxygen reserve

11. **At the tissue level, CO2 enters the blood and shifts the curve to right. This helps in unloading of oxygen from Hb and facilitates tissue oxygenation. This phenomenon is called:**
A. Bohr effect B. Haldane effect
C. Henry effect D. Dalton effect

12. **What is the PCO2 of venous blood?**
A. 30 mmHg B. 45 mmHg
C. 50 mm Hg D. 60 mmHg

13. **In which form is CO2 transported in more quantity in blood?**
A. Physically dissolved form
B. Bicarbonate ion in plasma and in red cell
C. Carbamino protein complex
D. Carboxyhemoglobin

14. **Chloride shift was described by:**
A. Hamburger B. Haldane
C. Bohr D. Pristley

15. **Oxygenation of Hb shifts the CO2 dissociation curve to right, which facilitates unloading of CO2. This effect is called:**
A. Bohr effect B. Haldane effect
C. Dalton effect D. Henry effect

16. **Hematocrit of venous is about 3% more than arterial blood, due to:**
A. Mechanism of chloride shift
B. Less water content of venous blood
C. Less oxygen content of venous blood
D. Slower dynamics of venous circulation

17. **All of the following statements are true, EXCEPT:**
A. About 7% of CO2 are transported in dissolved form in plasma
B. CO2 can diffuse 20 times more rapidly than O2
C. About 2% of CO2 are transported as carbaminohemoglobin
D. The PCO2 of arterial blood is 40 mmHg

18. **Compared to oxy-Hb dissociation curve, the CO2 dissociation curve:**
A. Is more linear within a PCO2 of 40-46 mmHg
B. Is more steeper within a PCO2 of 40-46 mmHg
C. At higher PO2, the curve shifts to left
D. At higher PO2, the curve shifts downward

Answers : 1. B 2. C 3. A 4. A 5. B 6. B 7. D 8. D 9. D 10. B
11. A 12. B 13. B 14. A 15. B 16. A 17. C 18. C

Multiple Choice Questions of Chapter 49

1. **The center for voluntary control of respiration is present at:**
   A. Pre Botzinger complex
   B. Cerebral cortex
   C. Lateral reticular nucleus
   D. Pnemotaxic centre
2. **Hypoxia inhibits K^+ channels in the glomus cells by all the following mechanisms, EXCEPT:**
   A. Decrease in mitochondrial NADPH oxidase
   B. Increase in cAMP level
   C. Increase in intracellular H^+
   D. Loss of O2 from heme containing protein
3. **The central pattern generator of respiration is present at:**
   A. Dorsal nuclear group
   B. Apneustic centre
   C. Pnemotaxic centre
   D. Pre Botzinger complex
4. **If the apneustic center is destroyed along with the vagi in a cat, which of the following will occur?**
   A. Prolonged inspiratory spasm
   B. Prolonged expiratory spasm
   C. Slow and shallow respiration
   D. Animal will die
5. **Inspiratory depth is halted by:**
   A. Pneumotaxic centre
   B. Apneustic centre
   C. Inspiratory centre
   D. Expiratory centre
6. **Transection of brainstem at the at mid-pons level results in:**
   A. Hyperventilation B. Apneusis
   C. Rapid and shallow breathing D. Hypoxia
7. **What will be the effect on respiration if a transection is made between the pons & medulla?**
   A. Apnoea B. Irregular & gasping
   C. No effect D. Slow & deep
8. **CO2 increases ventilation by acting mainly on receptors of**
   A. Apneustic center
   B. Pneumotaxic center
   C. Ventral surface of medulla
   D. DRG
9. **Central chemoreceptors are most sensitive to following changes in blood:**
   A. Increased PCO_2 B. DecreasedPCO_2
   C. Increased H^+ D. IncreasedPO_2
10. **The primary direct stimulus for excitation of central chemoreceptors regulating ventilation is:**
    A. Increased H^+ B. Increased CO_2
    C. Increased O_2 D. Decreased CO_2
11. **Most important stimulus to peripheral chemoreceptors**
    A. Decreased PO_2
    B. Increased CO_2
    C. Increased pH
    D. Increased HCO_3
12. **Which of the following does not stimulate peripheral chemoreceptors?**
    A. Hypoxia
    B. Hypocapnia
    C. Acidosis
    D. Low perfusion pressure
13. **Administration of pure O_2 to hypoxic patients is dangerous because**
    A. Apnea occurs due to hypostimulation of peripheral chemoreceptors
    B. Pulmonary edema
    C. DPG
    D. Convulsion
14. **Tidal volume excessive load is prevented by activation of which of the following receptors?**
    A. J receptors
    B. Thoracic muscle spindle
    C. Bronchial stretch receptors
    D. Arterial baroreceptor
15. **Herring Breuer inflation reflex causes an increase in:**
    A. Duration of inspiration
    B. Duration of expiration
    C. Depth of inspiration
    D. Depth of expiration
16. **Inflation of lungs induces further inflation, which is explained by:**
    A. Herring-Breuer inflation reflex
    B. Herring-Breuer deflation reflex
    C. Head's paradoxical reflex
    D. J-reflex
17. **All of the following affect resting ventilation except:**
    A. Stretch receptors
    B. J receptor
    C. Oxygen
    D. PCO_2
18. **Depth of inspiration is controlled by:**
    A. Pneumotaxic center
    B. Posterior medulla
    C. Apneustic center
    D. Pons
19. **Which of the following is NOT true about rapidly adapting receptors?**
    A. Stimulated by acute congestion
    B. Stimulation causes prolonged inspiration
    C. Respond to irritation of the airways by noxious substances
    D. Their activity is directly proportional to lung compliance
20. **All of the following are components of pulmonary J reflex, EXCEPT:**
    A. Rapid shallow breathing
    B. Bronchoconstriction
    C. Cardiovascular stimulation
    D. Increased airway secretion

Answers

1. B	2. C	3. D	4. A	5. A	6. B	7. B	8. C	9. A	10. A
11. A	12. B	13. A	14. C	15. B	16. C	17. B	18. C	19. D	20. C

Chapter 50

Physiological Changes at High Altitude

Learning Objectives

On completion of study of this chapter:

The student will be able to (must know):

1. Say the level of altitudes at which different grades of health problems happen.
2. Give the mechanisms of ventilatory adaptation at high altitude.
3. List the respiratory, cardiovascular, hematological and tissue changes at high altitude.
4. Name the high-altitude illnesses and give their physiological basis of treatment.

The student may also be able to (desirable to know):

1. Describe the physiological basis of high altitude illness.

The percentage of oxygen does not alter at high altitude, but the barometric pressure decreases. Therefore, the responses at high altitude are **due to decreased tension of oxygen** (P_IO_2) in inspired gas.

- Hypoxic symptoms appear at 10, 000 feet.
- Symptoms become severe at 15000 to 18000 feet.
- Above 20000 feet, barometric pressure is around 50% of the normal value, and symptom become acute and very severe.

However, normally the effects are not severe when the ascent is slow while camping at different heights.

- **Compensatory mechanisms** develop to adopt to higher altitudes, if the ascension is gradual, in phases with temporary stationing at different heights.

PY6.4

COMPENSATORY MECHNISMS

At high altitude, decrease in P_IO_2 **decreases oxygen supply to the tissues**. To deliver normal quantity of oxygen to the tissues, primary compensatory mechanism is **hyperventilation**, especially when alveolar **PO_2 decreases below 60 mm Hg.**

- Normally drop in alveolar PO_2 to 60 mm Hg occurs at an altitude of approximately 4500 m (14000 feet).

Stages of Compensation

Hyperventilation: The **hyperventilation induced by hypoxia** at high altitude appears in **two stages**:

In First Stage

Immediately on exposure to hypoxia, **ventilation increases instantly.**

- The hyperventilation in first stage is mainly due to **hypoxic stimulation of the carotid bodies**.
- The **magnitude of increase in ventilation is less** because the hypoxic stimulation of peripheral chemoreceptor is **opposed by** the ***decrease in arterial PCO_2*** that occurs due to excess removal of carbon dioxide induced by hyperventilation. This also **increases arterial pH**.
- **Decreased arterial PCO_2 and alkalosis** together blunt the hypoxic response.

In Second Stage

In second stage, ventilation increases slowly in 8 to 10 hours and then remains sustained.

- The **sustained increase** in ventilation is due to the **ventilatory acclimatization** at high altitude.
- **After about 2 weeks**, hyperventilation induced by hypoxia reaches a ***stable plateau***.

Mechanisms: There are **two mechanisms** for ventilatory acclimatization.

1. *Chemoreceptor mechanism:* The pH of CSF is more alkaline in the acute phase.
    - However, ventilation stimulated by hypoxia **brings pH close to normal** by the movement of bicarbonate out of the CSF.

- In prolonged exposure to hypoxia, **sensitivity of carotid body to arterial PO_2 also alters.**

2. ***Renal mechanism:*** The alkaline blood pH that occurs due to hypoxia-induced hyperventilation opposes the hypoxic response that decreases ventilation.
   - However, kidney compensates pH by **excreting more bicarbonate**. This **decreases blood pH** towards normal in about 3 days. Thus, the effects due to alkaline pH are minimized.
   - This allows hypoxic drive **to further increase minute ventilation** and then attain a steady state.

Acclimatization at High Altitude

When a person ascends to high altitude and stays there for longer periods, he slowly gets adapted to the new environment. This process of adaptation is called acclimatization.

- The acclimatization at high altitude **starts within twelve hours** and may take several **days or weeks to complete**.
  - The **maximum height** upto which adaptation occurs is **18000 feet**. Beyond this level, the subject needs O_2 inhalation for survival.
- Adaptive changes mainly occur in **respiratory system, cardiovascular systems, blood and tissues.**
  - The **primary objective** of these changes is to ***increase oxygen supply*** to the tissues.

Respiratory Changes

Hypoxia **stimulates peripheral chemoreceptors.**

1. This **increases pulmonary ventilation** by increasing rate and depth of respiration.
2. Consequently, CO_2 is washed off and **alkalosis develops (respiratory alkalosis).**
   - Alkalosis ***counteracts stimulating effects*** of hypoxia.
3. The kidney corrects blood pH by **excreting HCO_3^-** in urine.
   - Thus, **urine becomes alkaline.**
   - This helps the response of the respiratory center to hypoxia to continue so that **pulmonary ventilation is maintained** at higher levels.
4. Ventilation also steadily increases due to active **transport of H^+ into the CSF.**
   - Though ventilatory response decreases slowly after four days, it remains permanently above the pre-exposure level.
5. After about 4 days of acclimatization, **ventilatory response slowly increases**, which also depends on the level of altitude.
   - As the altitude increases, magnitude of response increases.
   - **Ventilatory equivalent** (VE) increases with increase in height of altitude (Fig. 50.1).
     - VE is a *better index of ventilatory response*. VE is the ratio of expired minute volume (V_E) to the O_2 consumption (VO_2).

Diffusion capacity for O_2 and MVV are more in permanent high-altitude residents.

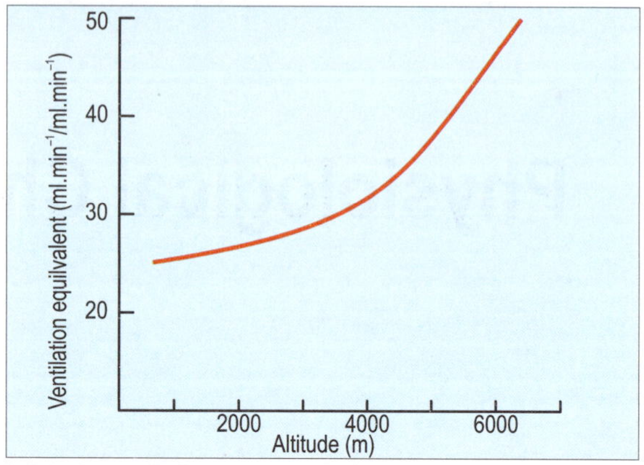

Fig. 50.1: Effect of altitude on ventilatory equivalent (VE). VE is the ratio of expired minute volume (V_E) to the O_2 consumption (VO_2). Note, VE increases with increase in height of altitude.

Hematological Changes

The hematological changes that improve oxygen supply to tissues include **increased red cell production** and **improved oxygen transport.**

1. Hypoxia stimulates **production of erythropoietin** (Ep).
   - Ep-induced erythropoiesis starts in about **three days** and continues till the person remains at high altitude.
   - Increased red cell mass **facilitates oxygen delivery** to the tissues.
2. Oxygen supply to tissues is also favored by **increased concentration of 2,3-DPG** in the red cells.
   - Increased 2,3-DPG **shifts oxyhemoglobin dissociation curve to the right** (though initially oxyhemoglobin dissociation curve shifts to the left due to alkalosis), which **favours release of oxygen** from Hb in the tissues.

Cardiovascular Changes

In the early phase, **heart rate, cardiac output and blood pressure increase.**

1. These changes occur due to activation of **sympathoadrenal axis** by hypoxia.
2. Gradually, **heart rate returns to normal.**
   - **Increased cardiac output** helps to increase blood flow.
3. Hypoxia causes **vasodilation** in the systemic circulation that adds to **increase in blood flow** and oxygen supply to the tissues.
4. Though increased red cell mass improves oxygenation of tissue, significant polycythemia (increased hema-

tocrit) **increases viscosity** of blood, which in turn **increases the workload on the heart**.
- This leads to **cardiac hypertrophy**.

Tissue Changes

Following tissue changes occur, especially in the skeletal muscles:
1. Increase in **number of capillaries**.
2. Increase in the **number of mitochondria** in the cells.
3. Increase in activity of **oxidative enzymes** like cytochrome oxidase.
4. Increase in **myoglobin content**.
5. **Angiogenesis** occurs due to release of chemicals from the hypoxic tissue that stimulate formation of new blood vessels.

HIGH ALTITUDE ILLNESS

High altitude illnesses include acute mountain sickness, chronic mountain sickness, high altitude cerebral edema, and high altitude pulmonary hypertension and edema.

Acute Mountain Sickness

Usually, people develop fatigue, dyspnea, nausea, vomiting, diarrhea, headache, insomnia and palpitations. Loss of co-ordination, memory and judgment are not uncommon. Euphoria and emotional changes are also observed.
- These symptoms **appear within 4 to 8 hours** of arrival at high altitude and may last for several days.
- In severe hypoxia or in susceptible individuals, **pulmonary and pulmonary cerebral edema** develop.

Chronic Mountain Sickness (Monge's Disease)

This is seen in **long-term exposure to high altitude**.
- These people develop malaise, fatigue, hypervolemia, exercise intolerance and polycythemia.
- **Pulmonary hypertension, right ventricular hypertrophy** and **heart failure** are quite common.

Pulmonary Hypertension & Edema

Pulmonary hypertension occurs due to prolonged exposure to hypoxia.
1. Alveolar hypoxia causes **pulmonary vasoconstriction**.
2. **In chronic hypoxia**, smooth muscles in pulmonary arteries undergo ***hypertrophy and hyperplasia*** that cause *narrowing of the arterial lumen.* This increases pulmonary arterial pressure.
3. **In severe hypoxia**, the ***pulmonary veins are also constricted***, that increases capillary pressure.
4. **Increased alveolar capillary pressure** causes transudation of fluid that leads to **pulmonary edema**.
5. Pulmonary hypertension also increases the **workload on the right side of heart**, which may cause *right ventricular hypertrophy*, and in severe cases ***right-sided heart failure***.

Cerebral Edema

The **increased capillary permeability** leads to cerebral edema, which may be associated with disorientation and ataxia. In severe cases, coma may occur due to herniation of brain through tentorium.

Treatment of High Altitude Illness

The individual who does not tolerate high altitude habitation should be **brought back to the low altitude at the earliest**. The condition immediately improves by descent to lower altitude. If the features of sickness still persist, especially **cerebral and pulmonary edema** continues, following treatment should start.
1. **Diuretics:** Diuretics are very useful for the treatment of cerebral and pulmonary edema.
   - *Acetazolamide* is the preferred diuretic.
   - It inhibits carbonic anhydrase and increases bicarbonate excretion in urine, thus **decreases alkali load**.
   - It also decreases the formation of CSF.
2. **Steroids:** Glucocorticoid ***decreses cerebral edema***.
3. **Oxygen therapy:** Hyperbaric oxygen is very useful if pulmonary edema is present.
4. **Nifedipine:** Calcium channel blockers like nifedipine help to ***reduce pulmonary arterial pressure***.
5. **Other drugs:** To improve the general conditions.

Exam Questions

1. Describe the physiological changes following acute ascent to high altitude.
2. List the features of acute mountain sickness and chronic mountain sickness. Briefly describe the physiological basis of their treatment.

Multiple Choice Questions

1. **Which of the following is seen in high altitude?**
   A. Decrease in HR
   B. High SBP
   C. Reduced $PaCO_2$
   D. Hyperventilation

2. **Which of the following is NOT a feature during acclimatization to high altitude?**
   A. Increase in the sensitivity of carotid body to hypoxia
   B. Shift in the oxygen-Hb dissociation curve to the left
   C. Increase in the sensitivity of central chemoreceptors
   D. Increase in minute ventilation

Answers: 1. D 2. B

Chapter 51

Hypoxia, Cyanosis and Oxygen Therapy

Learning Objectives

On completion of study of this chapter:

The student will be able to (must know):

1. Define hypoxia and classify hypoxia and give example for each category.
3. Illustrate the mechanism of each category of hypoxia.
4. Explain why CO poisoning is a type of anemic hypoxia.
5. Define and classify cyanosis and give common causes of each type of cyanosis.
6. List the differences between central and peripheral cyanosis.
7. Name the methods of oxygen therapy.
8. Give physiological basis of treatment of each type of hypoxia.

The student may also be able to (desirable to know):

1. Describe the complications of chronic oxygen therapy.
2. Describe the mechanism of different types of cyanosis.

PY6.6

HYPOXIA

Hypoxia is defined as **deficiency of O_2 at the tissue level.** Tissues suffer from hypoxia when supply of adequate O_2 to them is decreased or when they fail to utilize the available O_2.

Types of Hypoxia

Hypoxia is divided into 4 categories: hypoxic hypoxia, anemic hypoxia, stagnant hypoxia and histotoxic hypoxia.

Hypoxic Hypoxia

Definition: When **PO_2 of arterial blood is reduced**, the hypoxia is called hypoxic hypoxia.

Mechanism of Hypoxia: In hypoxic hypoxia, PO_2 of arterial blood is decreased, due to which the **delivery of O_2 to the tissue is reduced**.

- This occurs either due to **decreased O_2 in the inspired air** or due to *diseases of the respiratory apparatus* that decrease O_2 supply to the tissue.

It is seen in **following conditions**:

1. **Low PO_2 in the inspired air**, e.g., at *high altitude* or in closed chambers. As one ascends rapidly to 3000 m (10,000 ft), hypoxia develops due to decline in alveolar PO_2 to about 60 mmHg. Ascent to more than 5000 m (15,000 ft) produces severe hypoxic symptoms.
2. **Hypoventilation**, e.g. airway obstruction, paralysis of respiratory muscles, and depression of respiratory center, scoliosis etc.
3. **Diffusion defect**, e.g. pulmonary edema, pulmonary fibrosis, lung collapse etc.
4. **Ventilation-perfusion mismatch** (perfusion of poorly ventilated alveoli): Large A-V shunts, atelectasis, lung collapse, cyanotic congenital heart disease.

The last three mechanisms (2 – 4), are also called as **Respiratory Hypoxia**.

Anemic Hypoxia

Definition: When PO_2 of arterial blood is normal, but the **hemoglobin to carry O_2 is not adequate** in amount, anemic hypoxia develops.

Conditions that lead to anemic hypoxia are:

a. **Anemia** (decreased Hb concentration in blood)
b. **Carbon monoxide poisoning**
c. **Altered Hb**, e.g. Methemoglobin

Mechanism of Hypoxia: In anemic hypoxia, as the PO_2 of inspired air is normal and the diffusion capacity of lung is normal, the **PO_2 of arterial blood is normal**.

- But, the O_2 supply to the tissue is reduced, as **adequate Hb is not available** to transport O_2.
- However, in mild to moderate anemia, usually O_2 supply to the tissue is not severely affected, as there is *concomitant increase in 2,3-DPG* in the red cells.
  - Such patients **develop severe hypoxia during exercise** due to their limited ability to deliver O_2

to the tissue.

In CO Poisoning: The **affinity of CO for Hb is about 210 times greater** than the affinity of O_2. CO combines with hemoglobin to form **carbomonoxyhemoglobin or carboxyhemoglobin** (COHb).

- In CO poisoning, release of CO from COHb is very slow due the high affinity of CO to Hb. Therefore, O_2 cannot bind with hemoglobin.
- Thus, in CO poisoning, though the hemoglobin content is normal, **Hb is not available** to deliver O_2 to the tissue.
  - Therefore, *CO poisoning is classified as anemic hypoxia.*
- Moreover, Hb-dissociation curve (for whatever oxy-Hb is available) **shifts to left** that decreases the release of O_2 from Hb.

Stagnant Hypoxia

(Hypoperfusion Hypoxia)

Definition: When hypoxia occurs due to **decreased blood flow** to the tissues, this is called stagnant hypoxia (**stagnation** of flow).

- This is also called *hypoperfusion hypoxia*, as it causes decreased perfusion of tissues due to stagnation of blood flow.
- This is sometimes also called **ischemic hypoxia**.

Causes: Stagnant hypoxia is seen in:

1. Heart failure
2. Shock
3. Vascular obstruction (that causes specific organ hypoxia)

Mechanism: In stagnant hypoxia, O_2 content of arterial blood is normal.

- Hypoxia occurs due to **stagnation of blood** in circulation. Therefore, this is also called **circulatory hypoxia**.
- It occurs either due to **decreased cardiac output** or **decreased blood flow** secondary to some other causes.
- In chronic or complete stagnant hypoxia, local acidosis develops due to accumulation of the lactate that inhibits cellular metabolism.

Histotoxic Hypoxia

Definition: When **tissue cannot utilize oxygen** inspite of normal O_2 supply, the resulting hypoxia is called histotoxic hypoxia.

- As tissue is unable to utilize O_2, the **venous tension of O_2 is high**.
- Usually, hypoxia occurs in **tissue poisoning** as produced by cyanides or similar poisons.

Mechanism: Mechanism of hypoxia depends on the cause of hypoxia.

1. ***Cyanide poisoning:*** Cyanide ***inhibits cytochrome oxidase***. Therefore, tissue oxidation is paralyzed.

Table 51.1 | **Table 51.1: Comparison of different types of hypoxias.**

	Hypoxic Hypoxia	Anemic Hypoxia	Stagnant Hypoxia	Histotoxic Hypoxia
1. Definition based on: i) Arterial PO2 ii) Hemoglobin content iii) Rate of blood flow to tissues	Low arterial PO2 due to decreased oxygen in the environment, when O2 carrying capacity of blood and rate of blood flow to tissue are normal.	Amount of hemoglobin is less available to carry O2 in spite of normal arterial pO2 and normal rate of blood flow to tissues.	Rate of blood flow to tissues reduced so that adequate O2 is not delivered to them in spite of normal arterial pO2 and hemoglobin content.	Normal O2 delivery to tissues but tissue cannot make use of O2 supplied to them due to action of toxic agent.
2. Causes	i) Decreased atmospheric PO_2 ii) Less pulmonary ventilation iii) defective V/P ratio	Total hemoglobin content is less i) Anemia ii) Hemorrhage iii) Presence of abnormal Hb: CO-Hb or methemoglobin	i) Circulatory failure ii) Obstruction to blood flow iii) Heart failure	Cyanide poisoning
3. Arterial PO_2	Decreased	Normal	Normal	Normal
4. Arterial O_2 content	Decreased	Markedly reduced	Normal	Normal
5. Arterial %-O_2 saturation of hemoglobin	Decreased	Decreased	Normal	Normal
6. A-V PO_2 difference	Decreased	Normal	More than Normal	Less than Normal
7. Cyanosis	Present	Absent	Present	Absent (as reduced hemoglobin is produced in small amounts)
8. Stimulation of peripheral chemoreceptors	Present (as dissolved O2 in plasma decreases)	Absent (dissolved O2 in plasma is sufficient to meet receptor demand)	Present (because arterial pCO2 increases and pO2 decreases)	Present (cyanide decreases O2 utilization at tissue level)

2. ***Diphtheria:*** In severe diphtheria, diphtheria toxin inhibits the synthesis of one of the cytochromes and therefore, prevents O_2 utilization.

Treatment: Cyanide poisoning is ***treated by methylene blue or nitrites.***

- They form methemoglobin, which in turn reacts with cyanide to form ***Cyanmethemoglobin***, which is a non-toxic compound. **Hyperbaric O_2 therapy** is also useful in cyanide poisoning.

Differences in types of hypoxias are summarized in Table 51.1

Effects of Hypoxia

Acute & Subacute Hypoxias

Features of acute hypoxia **resemble acute alcoholism.** ***Impaired judgment and motor incoordination*** are major manifestations of acute hypoxia.

1. If hypoxia persists for a longer period, the features are fatigue, drowsiness, nausea, headache, hyperventilation and dyspnea, apathy, inattentiveness, delayed reaction time, reduced work capacity, confusion and disorientation.
   - In severe hypoxia, hypertension occurs.
2. In severe and **prolonged hypoxia**, brainstem is depressed and death results from respiratory failure.
3. **Anerobic glycolysis** results in formation of more lactic acid that leads to **metabolic acidosis**. Stimulation of chemoreceptors by hypoxia produces hyperventilation and causes **respiratory alkalosis.**
   - However, combined with metabolic acidosis, serum bicarbonate level decreases.

Effects on Cells: Transcription factors known as **hypoxia inducible factors (HIFs)** are produced by hypoxia.

1. HIFs have **α and β subunits**. Normally, in the presence of adequate oxygen in the tissues, α subunits are rapidly removed from the cells.
2. In hypoxic conditions, **dimerization of α and β subunits** occurs in the cells. The **α-β dimers cause induction of genes** that produce ***erythropoietin and angiogenic factors.***
3. This is one of the causes of **angiogenesis** or neovascularization in hypoxic tissues.

Effects on Brain: Brain tissue is highly sensitive to hypoxia.

1. Sudden fall in inspired **PO_2 to less than 20 mmHg,** causes ***loss of consciousness in about 15 seconds.*** If hypoxia continues, **death** can occur in **4 to 5 minutes**.
2. This can typically occur in sudden drop in cabin pressure in a plane flying above 16,000 meter.
3. However, **hypoxia of lower intensities**, cause the symptoms similar to that of **acute alcohol intoxication** such as disorientation, impaired judgment, headache, drowsiness etc.

Chronic Hypoxia

In chronic hypoxia, **polycythemia** occurs due to increased erythropoietin production. Local **hypoxic vasodilation** in the tissue increases tissue blood flow.

CYANOSIS

Definition: Cyanosis is the **bluish discolouration of the skin and mucous membranes** of the body due to the presence of reduced hemoglobin or deoxyhemoglobin in more than 5 g% in the blood.

- Cyanosis is normally detected when oxygen saturation is less than 85%.
- It is also seem in excess of abnormal hemoglobin derivatives such as methemoglobin or sulfhemoglobin, etc.

Physiological Basis

When the concentration of **reduced hemoglobin is more than 5 g per cent** in the capillary blood, the skin and mucous membrane become blue because of the **dark colour of reduced hemoglobin.**

- Hemoglobin **in the arterial blood** is 95 per cent saturated with oxygen. Therefore, about 14.25 g (taking 15 g% of hemoglobin as the standard) in the arterial blood is oxyhemoglobin and only **0.75 g is reduced hemoglobin** in a normal adult.
- In **mixed venous blood**, about 70 percent of hemoglobin is saturated with oxygen. Hence, 10.5 g of the 15 g per cent of hemoglobin in the venous blood is oxyhemoglobin and **4.5 g is reduced hemoglobin.**
- The amount of reduced hemoglobin **in capillary blood** is assumed to be the mean of arterial and venous content of the reduced hemoglobin.
  - Thus, in a normal individual at rest, capillary blood contains **3 g% (0.75+ 4.5/2) of reduced hemoglobin.**
  - The colour of normal skin and mucous membrane is therefore pink.
  - When the concentration of reduced hemoglobin is **more than 5 g per cent**, cyanosis appears.
- The presence of **excess of other hemoglobin complexes** like methemoglobin and sulfhemoglobin in the blood also produces cyanosis because of their dark colour.
- Cyanosis is **not seen in severe anemia and CO poisoning** (Clinical Note 51.1)

Clinical Note 51.1

Cyanosis is absent severe anemia and CO poisoning: Patients having severe anemia with hemoglobin content less than 5 g per cent may not show cyanosis (as the total hemoglobin is less than 5 gm per cent). Also, cyanosis may not be seen **in carbon monoxide poisoning**, because carboxyhemoglobin prevents reduction of oxyhemoglobin and the colour of carboxyhemoglobin is cherry red.

Types of Cyanosis

Cyanosis is of **three types**: peripheral, central and mixed. There is another special category of cyanosis, called ***differential cyanosis***. Differences between central and peripheral cyanosis are listed in Table 51.2

Table 51.2 | Differences between central and peripheral cyanosis.

Features	Central cyanosis	Peripheral cyanosis
1. Mechanism	Inadequate oxygenation of systemic arterial blood (hypoxic hypoxia)	Sluggish peripheral circulation (stagnant hypoxia)
2. Sites to look	Tongue and oral mucosa	Acral: Tip of the nose, ear lobules, outer aspects of lip, finger tips, nail bed, extremities
3. Associations	Clubbing, Polycythemia	
4. Extremities	Warm	Cold
5. Warming extremities	No change	Cyanosis disappears
6. Oxygen inhalation	Slight improvement	No change
7. ABG-PaO_2	Low, < 85%	Normal, 85% - 100%
8. Pulse volume	May be high	Usually low
9. Dyspnea	Usually present	Usually absent
10. Exercise	Worsens	May improve

Peripheral Cyanosis

This occurs due to **slowing of the flow of blood** through the tissues that allows more time for removal of oxygen by the tissues.

Causes:

1. Decreased cardiac output, as occurs in heart failure
2. Local vasoconstriction, for example, extreme cold
3. Venous obstruction, for example, superior vena caval syndrome
4. Increased viscosity of blood, as seen in polycythemia, multiple myeloma etc.
5. Arterial obstruction, e.g. peripheral vascular disease (Buerger's disease)

Central Cyanosis

When reduced hemoglobin concentration is more than 5 g% due to mixing of arterial blood with venous blood, or inadequate oxygenation of the arterial blood, central cyanosis results.

- In the early stage, cyanosis manifests in the palate, tongue and lips, but later when reduced hemoglobin becomes very high, it appears in peripheral sites also.

Causes:

I. Due to admixture of venous and arterial blood that occurs in right to left shunt.

1. Congenital heart disease: Fallot's tetralogy
2. Pulmonary arteriovenous fistula
3. Patent truncus arteriosus
4. Transposition of great vessels

II. Due to inadequate oxygenation of arterial blood

1. Low atmospheric oxygen, common example is **high altitude**
2. Inadequate ventilation, for example, lung collapse, airway obstruction
3. Decreased gaseous exchange through the pulmonary membrane, for example, hyaline membrane disease.

Mixed Cyanosis

In this type of cyanosis, both **central and peripheral mechanisms operate**. The most common example is **chronic cor pulmonale** due to emphysema. Also seen in cardiogenic shock with pulmonary edema and CCF due to left sided heart failure,

Other Types

Differential Cyanosis: This is a condition where cyanosis appears only **in one half of the body**. For example, in patent ductus arteriosus with reversal of shunt due to pulmonary hypertension, cyanosis is seen only in the lower limbs; both upper limbs are spared.

Intermittent Cyanosis: Cyanosis seen intermittently (not constantly). Occurs in **Ebstein's anomaly**.

Cyclical Cyanosis: Cyanosis occurs for few days and then disappears and again appears. Seen in **bilateral choanal atresia**.

Orthocyanosis: Cyanosis occurs only in **upright position**. This occurs due to severe hypoxia occurring in erect posture of the body. Seen in **pulmonary arterio-venous malformation.**

OXYGEN THERAPY

Oxygen therapy is **indicated in hypoxia**. It is very useful in acute and severe hypoxia, especially when hypoxia is associated with dyspnea.

Methods

Oxygen is administered by following methods.

1. **Using oxygen tent**: It is very useful in children, as they usually do not tolerate mask or cannula. It is also useful in administering hyperbaric oxygen.
2. **Using oxygen mask**: Oxygen enters the mask at a higher velocity so that oxygen is drawn through the holes in the mask.

3. **Mechanical ventilator**: When patient is semiconscious or comatose, oxygen is administered from a mechanical ventilator through an endotracheal or tracheostomy tube.
4. **Through an intranasal tube**: A cannula is inserted into the nostril, which is connected to the oxygen cylinder. Administration of oxygen through cannula is useful in conditions in which hypoxic drive is essential to drive ventilation, as oxygen content of inspired air never reaches 100% by this method.

O_2 Therapy in Different Forms of Hypoxia

In Hypoxic Hypoxia

As hypoxia is due to decreased PO_2 of arterial blood, oxygen therapy **is very useful**. .

- In such conditions, administration of O_2 increases the pressure gradient between alveoli and the blood that facilitates O_2 entry into the blood.
- However, O_2 therapy is not **beneficial in hypoxic hypoxia due to A-V shunts**, as admixture occurs after oxygenation in the lungs.

IMPORTANT NOTE

O_2 therapy is harmful in states of depressed respiratory centers: Though O_2 therapy is beneficial hypoxic hypoxia, it is harmful to subjects with depressed respiratory centers. In such subjects, blood PCO_2 is high that depresses the respiratory centers, and their breathing is maintained by stimulation due to hypoxia. When 100% O_2 is administered to these subjects, this stimulatory effect by hypoxia is abolished that results in *further respiratory depression*.

In Anemic Hypoxia

Oxygen therapy increases O_2 content of blood by **increasing the quantity of dissolved oxygen** in the blood. Thus, it helps in providing supply of extra O_2 to tissue.

- **In CO poisoning,** ***hyperbaric O_2 is useful*** as it facilitates dissociation of CO from Hb and increases the transport of O_2 in dissolved state.

In Stagnant Hypoxia

O_2 therapy is **not much useful** as blood flow to the tissue is decreased in stagnant hypoxia.

In Histotoxic Hypoxia

Tissue is unable to utilize O_2. Hence, O_2 therapy is not beneficial. But, **hyperbaric O_2 therapy** benefits by displacing the chemical bound to Hb.

Hyperbaric Oxygen Therapy

Hyperbaric O_2 therapy means, administration **of 100% O_2 at increased pressure.**

- When hyperbaric O_2 is administered, the **O_2 transport in the dissolved form** in the plasma increases. The O_2 solubility in plasma is 0.03ml / 100ml / mm Hg.
- Therefore, to achieve the **6 ml/ 100 ml dissolved O_2**, which is adequate to maintain normal metabolic need of the tissues of the body in resting state, **arterial PO_2 should be 2000 mmHg.**
  - This is achieved by administering **100% O_2 at a pressure of 3 atmosphere.**
- Hyperbaric O_2 therapy is very useful in **CO poisoning.**
- However, 100% O_2 at high pressure facilitates the onset of ***oxygen toxicity***.

Effect of 100% O_2 Therapy

The effects depend on the **duration of therapy** with pure O_2, and the **pressure at which O_2 is delivered.**

- When given for **more than 3 days**, 100% O_2 produces side effects.
- When, administered **at 4 atmospheres**, symptoms develop ***in half an hour***, and if administered **at 6 atmospheres**, the features develop ***in just few minutes***.

CNS Effects: Nausea, irritability, dizziness, disorientation, muscle twitching and convulsions. In severe cases person becomes comatose. Hyperbaric therapy **decreases ATP and GABA content** of brain.

Respiratory System: Congestion and irritation of airway **increase tracheobronchial secretion**, and **decrease surfactant** synthesis. This also causes **pulmonary edema** and atelectasis.

Special Sense: Ringing in the ears (tinnitus), blurring of vision, loss of equilibrium, and **retrolental fibroplasia** in newborn that results in premature retinopathy.

- Visual defects also occur due to formation of **opaque vascular tissue** in the eye.
- If given for a longer period, 100% O_2 causes **broncho-pulmopnary dysplasia** and lung cysts, especially in infants treated for respiratory distress syndrome.

Mechanism of Toxicity

With pure O_2 therapy, oxidizing **free radicals** like super oxide anion (O_2^-), and hydrogen peroxide (H_2O_2) accumulate in the body in excess amounts. They oxidize the polyunsaturated fatty acids and **destroy the cellular enzymes**. As a result, toxic effects due to O_2 therapy develop.

Exam Questions

1. Classify hypoxia and list two causes for each category of hypoxia. Briefly describe the mechanism of hypoxia for each type of hypoxia.
2. Define cyanosis. List the differences between central and peripheral cyanosis.
3. List the methods of oxygen therapy. Give a note on oxygen toxicity.

Multiple Choice Questions

1. In severe anemia, cyanosis is not seen as:
A. Oxygen hemoglobin curve shift to the right
B. Oxygen carrying capacity of available Hb is increased
C. Hypoxia stimulates erythropoietin production
D. Critical concentration of Hb required to produce cyanosis is reduced

2. Which of the following variant of hypoxia does not stimulate peripheral chemoreceptors?
A. Hypoxic hypoxia
B. Anemic hypoxia
C. Stagnant hypoxia
D. Histotoxic hypoxia

3. Which of the following conditions leads to tissue hypoxia without alteration of oxygen content of blood?
A. CO poisoning
B. Meth-Hb
C. Cyanide poisoning
D. Respiratory acidosis

4. Which of the following is most prone to hypoxic injury?
A. Thalamus
B. Hippocampus
C. Caudate nucleus
D. Cerebellum

5. Hypoxemia does not depend on:
A. $PaCO_2$
B. Altitude
C. Hb
D. Fraction of inspired O_2

6. Conditions where severe hypoxemia occurs without cyanosis
A. CO poisoning & anemia
B. High altitude
C. Intestinal lung disease
D. Pulmonary A-V malformation

7. Central cyanosis is seen if:
A. Methemoglobin 0.5 gm/dl
B. O_2 saturation <85%
C. O_2 saturation <94%
D. Hb – 4 gm%

8. Concentration of methemoglobin to appears cyanosis
A. 5 gm/dl
B. 2 gm/dl
C. 1.5 gm/dl
D. 12 gm/dl

9. Physiological response to smoking are all, EXCEPT:
A. Decreased HDL
B. Increased hematocrit
C. Increased heart rate and increased catecholamine release
D. Decreased carboxyhemoglobin

10. In which of the following, a reduction in arterial oxygen tension occurs?
A. Anemia
B. CO poisoning
C. Moderate exercise
D. Hypoventilation

11. Which of the following statements about Carbon Monoxide poisoning is not true:
A. Carboxy hemoglobin (COHb) causes left shift of oxyhemoglobin dissociation curve
B. Partial pressure as low as 0.6 mm Hg can be lethal
C. Tissue toxicity plays an important role in clinical CO poisoning
D. Hyperbaric oxygen is used for treatment

12. Toxic effect of high oxygen tension includes all of the following, EXCEPT:
A. Pulmonary edema
B. Decreased cerebral blood flow
C. Retinal damage
D. CNS excitation and convulsion

Answers

1. D **2. B** **3. C** **4. B** **5. C** **6. A** **7. B** **8. C** **9. D** **10. D**
11. C **12. B**

Chapter 52

Hazards of Deep Sea Diving and Effects of Increased Barometric Pressure

Learning Objectives

On completion of study of this chapter:

The student will be able to (must know):

1. List the hazards of deep sea diving.
2. Give the physiological basis of deep sea hazards and the basis of their prevention.
3. Illustrate the mechanism of decompression sickness and the basis of its treatment.

The student may also be able to (desirable to know):

1. Describe the mechanism and prevention of dysbarism.

PY6.4

At sea level, the atmospheric pressure is 760 mmHg (1 atmosphere) and the pressure in the lungs is equal to this pressure. When the individual dives into the sea, he is exposed to a high pressure, which is proportional to the depth to which he dives.

- For **every descent of 33 feet depth (10 meters), there is increase in pressure by 1 atmosphere**.
  - Thus, at 100 feet depth, the pressure is about 4 (3+1) atmospheres.
  - This high pressure in the deep sea causes some hazards.

The **hazards of deep sea diving are** nitrogen narcosis, high pressure nervous syndrome, acute oxygen toxicity, dysbarism and air embolism.

NITROGEN NARCOSIS

During deep sea diving, **gases are inhaled at high pressures**. Inhalation of 100% O_2 at high pressure causes **CNS depression**. Therefore, normally a **mixture of 20% O_2 and 80% N_2** is inhaled at high partial pressures.

- At high pressure, **N_2 produces narcotic effects**.
  - Up to 100 feet (4 atmosphere) the dissolved N_2 produces euphoria.
- However, **narcotic effects of N_2 start at about 120 feet** and become **severe at or below 250 feet** (8.5 atmospheres).
- The **features are similar to alcohol intoxication**. Though the manual agility remains unaffected, intellectual functions are altered.
- The narcotic effects of N_2 are due to its anesthetic effect.

HIGH-PRESSURE NERVOUS SYNDROME

As dissolved N_2 at deeper regions of sea produces narcotic effects, a **mixture of helium and O_2** is preferred for following reasons.

1. The **narcotic effect of helium** is *one-fifth of that of N_2*.
2. **Resistance to air flow is less** as helium is lighter than N_2 (density of helium is 2, whereas density of nitrogen is 14). Thus, the **work of breathing is less with helium mixture**.
3. Helium is **less soluble** in body fluids.

Mechanism and Features: Inhalation of helium mixture during deep dives causes **high-pressure nervous syndrome** (HPNS), due to its **anesthetic effects** at high pressure, which is due to its **lipid solubility** and direct effect on membrane of neurons.

Features: HPNS is characterized by tremors, drowsiness and incoordination. The α activity in EEG is depressed and manual dexterity is impaired.

ACUTE O_2 TOXICITY

Breathing **100% O_2 at a higher-pressure** is toxic. Acute toxicity is due to the **effects on CNS**.

Features: The features of oxygen toxicity are nausea, dizziness, irritability, disorientation, disturbed vision, and convulsions. Pulmonary damage also occurs.

Prevention: The concentration of O_2 is reduced to about 20% to prevent its toxicity.

PY6.5

DYSBARISM (CAISSONS DISEASE)

Dysbarism or **decompression sickness** is a condition, which occurs when the subjects exposed to high atmospheric pressures are **suddenly brought to low atmospheric pressures**.

- For example, deep-sea divers or workers in caisson (**caisson** is a watertight chamber used for performing construction works under water) returning to sea surface rapidly from deep sea level.
  - Rapid ascent to 9000m in an unpressurized cabin of an airplane can also cause this.

Pressure at sea level is 1 atmosphere. Pressure increases by 1 atmosphere for every 10 meter depth of water. Thus, the pressure

at 10 meter depth: 1 + 1 atmosphere,
at 20 meter depth: 2 + 1 atmosphere,
at 50 meter depth: 5 + 1 atmosphere, and so on.

Features and Mechanisms: Deep-sea divers usually breathe **80% N_2 from the gas mixtures**. When the diver descends into the deep sea, **N_2 dissolves in the body fluids**, which is proportional to the depth of descent. N_2 is lipid soluble. Therefore, it also dissolves in the lipid structures of the tissues.

1. **If the return to the surface is slow**, the gases that come out of the solution diffuse into the blood and are eliminated by the lungs.
2. **If the return (decompression) is rapid**, the escape of gases from the solution is quick and bubbles are formed in tissues and blood. This causes damage to the tissues.
   - Bubbles in the tissues cause **severe pain in the tissues**. Pain occurs mainly in *muscles and joints*.
   - This is called **decompression sickness** or **caisson disease**.
3. **In severe cases**, bubbles in the blood vessels **decrease blood flow to brain and spinal cord** resulting in *sensory and motor deficits* in the form of paresthesia, motor weakness paralysis and respiratory failure.
4. **Bubbles in the pulmonary vessels** produce dyspnea and a feeling of *respiratory compression*, and **bubbles in the coronary vessels** produce *myocardial ischemia*.

Features of decompression sickness usually appear **within half an hour** of coming to the surface.

IMPORTANT NOTE

% decrease in pressure is Important: Severity of decompression sickness is not due to the absolute decrease, but the **percentage decrease** in pressure. A rapid decrease upto 50% of the original pressure is safe but decrease below 45% is harmful.

Prevention: Decompression sickness can be prevented by **slow recompression** (gradual ascent to the sea level). Reduction in the pressure should not exceed 50%.

Treatment: As soon as the symptoms develop, the subject should be **recompressed immediately in a pressurized cabin**.

- Quick recompression should be followed by slow decompression.
- Hyperbaric oxygen is also helpful.
- Though recovery is usually complete, some residual neural deficits may persist.

AIR EMBOLISM

When a diver breathing from a tank at increased pressure suddenly ascends to the surface holding his breath, gas in the **lungs expand rapidly and rupture pulmonary veins**. Air escapes into the circulation and causes air embolism.

- Also, **sudden reduction in external pressure** from atmospheric to subatmospheric level can cause rapid expansion of gas in the lungs and produce air embolism, which typically occurs when a **pressurized cabin of an aeroplane or a rocket ruptures at high altitude**.
- Air embolism can also occur during a **rapid ascent from shallow depth of 5 m**. Therefore, to prevent this, a diver can take breath at the surface and then dive into the water holding the breath and come out of it holding the same breath.

SCUBA

Self-contained under-water breathing apparatus (SCUBA) is a **tank and valve system**, used by deep-sea divers.

- It consists of cylinders containing mixture of **compressed helium and oxygen**.
- The valve arrangement helps the subject to inhale and exhale gases.
- **O_2 and helium mixtures** are frequently used as they are less toxic during deep sea diving.

Exam Questions

1. What is decompression sickness. List the features and illustrate the basis of treatment of decompression sickness.
2. Write short notes on nitrogen narcosis, high-pressure nervous syndrome, O_2 toxicity, and Caisson's disease.

(MCQs of this chapter are given in Page 439)

Chapter 53

Respiration in Abnormal Conditions and Abnormal Respirations

Learning Objectives

<u>On completion of study of this chapter:</u>

The student will be able to (must know):

1. Define asphyxia, hypocapnia and hypercapnia and list their causes.
2. Understand the physiological basis of asphyxia, hypocapnia and hypercapnia.
3. Understand the respiratory abnormalities in respiratory acidosis & alkalosis.
4. Define periodic breathing, give its causes and understand its physiological basis.
5. Understand the physiological basis of Kussmaul breathing, Biot's respiration and sleep apnea syndrome.

The student may also be able to (desirable to know):

1. Describe Kussmaul breathing and Biots breathing.

RESPIRATION IN ABNORMAL CONDITIONS

PY6.6

Asphyxia

Asphyxia is a condition in which **hypoxia is combined with hypercapnia**. Usually, asphyxia develops due to **mechanical obstruction of airway** as occurs in suffocation, strangulation, drowning, foreign body impaction in the trachea or larynx, and traumatic compression of the chest.

Stages of Asphyxia

Asphyxia is divided into **three stages**: stage of exaggerated breathing, stage of convulsion, and stage of exhaustion and collapse.

Stage of Exaggerated Breathing: Hypercapnia and hypoxia stimulate respiratory centers strongly. Therefore, breathing becomes **deep and rapid**. Participation of accessory muscles of respiration becomes prominent.

- Patient becomes **severely dyspneic and looks intensely anxious**.
- Cyanosis develops and eyes become prominent.
- This stage **lasts for about 1 or 2 minutes**.

Stage of Convulsions: The respiratory efforts become violent. Generalized muscular convulsions occur.

Increased sympathetic discharge and catecholamine secretion, cause tachycardia and rise in blood pressure.

- This phase **lasts for about a minute**. Consciousness of the patient may be lost.

Stage of Exhaustion and Collapse: Continuation of hypoxia to the vital centers in the brain results in **suppression of cardiorespiratory activities**.

- Convulsions cease abruptly and respirations become gasping. Blood pressure falls, pulse becomes feeble, Reflexes are abolished.
- The pause between respiratory gasps becomes longer, until finally the patient takes his last breath. This stage **lasts for about 5 minutes**.

Hypercapnia

Definition: Hypercapnia is the **retention of CO_2** in the body. CO_2 is a major product of metabolism. Therefore, conditions of **hypermetabolic states** such as fever and excess carbohydrate intake generally produce hypercapnea.

Causes: Hypercapnia is common in conditions of **hypoventilation** in which either the **ventilation is depressed** as seen in ***respiratory failure, brain injury, narcotic poisoning*** etc. or the **ventilation is inadequate** as occurs in *myocardial failure, polyneuropathies, diseases of the chest wall* etc.

1. Hypoxia with normocapnia is termed as **type I respiratory failure** and hypoxia with hypercapnia is

called as **type II respiratory failure**.

2. **In fever**, with rise in body temperature by 1°C, CO_2 production increases by 13%. However, respiration is also stimulated in fever and excess CO_2 is removed from the body.
3. **In high carbohydrate intake**, production of CO_2 is increased due to increase in respiratory quotient.

Effects of Hypercapnia: Hypercapnia **stimulates respiration**. However, **if severe and prolonged**, hypercapnia leads to ***respiratory depression.***

- **Profound hypercapnia** produces **respiratory acidosis**, during which plasma bicarbonate may exceed 40 mEq/L.

Hypocapnia

Definition and Causes: Hypocapnia is **CO_2 washout** from the body that results from hyperventilation. As hyperventilation increases oxygen intake, there is simultaneous increases in PO_2.

1. **Temporary hyperventilation** occurs on sudden exposure to hot environment. Hyperventilation is common in **neurotic patients**.
2. **Voluntary hyperventilation** causes hypocapnia (PCO_2 may fall as low as 15 mm Hg) associated with significant increase in PO_2 in arterial blood, which may rise upto 140 mm Hg.

Effects: Hypocapnia produces **vasoconstriction** and reduces cerebral blood flow by more than 30%.

1. **Cerebral ischemia** may cause dizziness, light headedness and sensory abnormalities mainly in the form of paresthesia.
2. **Depression of vasomotor and respiratory centers** occurs. **Cardiac output is decreased** due to decreased coronary blood blow.
3. **Respiratory alkalosis** results from hyperventilation. Plasma bicarbonate level is decreased.
4. Features of **hypocalcemic tetany** such as Chvostek sign and carpopedal spasm may develop due to decreased ionic calcium level.

Drowning

PY6.6

Drowning is suffocation caused by immersion in water.

1. **In fresh-water drowning**, water enters the lungs and from lungs water is rapidly transferred to blood causing faster hemodilution and hemolysis.
2. **In seawater drowning,** hypertonic water in the lungs draws fluid from vascular space into the lung that causes hemoconcentration.

However, in few cases of drowning, first grasp of water into the respiratory tract causes immediate reflex laryngospasm and water does not enter the lungs. The patient dies of asphyxia.

Respiratory Acidosis

Any condition that **decreases the removal of carbon dioxide** from the body through lungs causes increase in PCO_2. This leads to respiratory acidosis.

1. **Depression of the respiratory centers** as produced by narcotics and barbiturates causes respiratory acidosis.
2. **Diseases that affect respiratory apparatus** like COPD, pneumothorax, pleural effusion, chest wall deformities etc., and **diseases that impair diffusion** of gases through alveolar-capillary membrane like pulmonary fibrosis, pulmonary edema etc. produce respiratory acidosis.

The increase in PCO_2 stimulates respiratory centers and increase rate and depth of respiration. Elimination of CO_2 through lungs restores blood pH.

Respiratory Alkalosis

The basic cause of respiratory alkalosis is **excess elimination of acid** via respiratory tract.

- The decrease in H^+ concentration is due to **hyperventilation** that decreases PCO_2.
- A physiological cause of respiratory alkalosis is ascension to **high altitude.**

ABNORMAL RESPIRATIONS

Periodic Breathing

PY6.6

Cyclical repetition of apnea and shallow breathing (like hyperpnea) in normal individuals is called periodic breathing. This is typically seen following **voluntary hyperventilation** performed for 2 to 3 min.

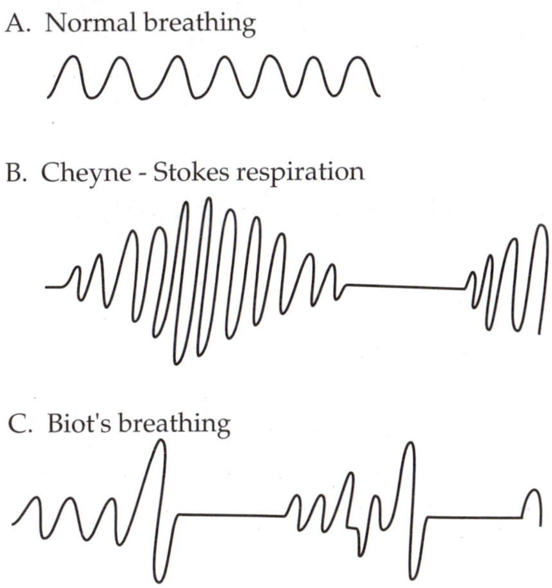

Fig. 53.1: Normal and abnormal breathing patterns.

1. **Apnea** occurs due to removal of CO_2 during hyperventilation that **removes the CO_2 drive on ventilation**.
2. During the period of apnea, **PCO_2 accumulates** and PO_2 falls in the blood that **stimulates ventilation** via chemoreceptor stimulation.
   - This initiates respiration and PO_2 returns to normal.
3. The **elimination of hypoxic drive stops breathing** (apnea), which again leads to **accumulation of PCO_2 and produces hyperventilation.**
   - Thus, cycles of apnea-hyperpnea continue till PCO_2 gradually returns to normal (Fig. 53.1B).

Periodic breathing in abnormal condition is called **Cheyne-Stokes respiration.**

Cheyne-Stokes Respiration

Periodic breathing that occurs in diseases and abnormal conditions is called Cheyne-Stokes respiration. The patients have **increased sensitivity to CO_2** due to disruption of neural pathways.

- Accumulation of CO_2 causes **hyperventilation that lowers PCO_2**.
- Decreased PCO_2 removes the CO_2-drive on ventilation and produces apnea, which consequently **increases the PCO_2 again.**
- The increased sensitivity of respiratory mechanism to PCO_2 produces hyperventilation and the **cycle continues**.

Causes: Cheyne-Stokes respiration is seen in:

1. Premature infants.
2. Unacclimatized persons at high altitude.
3. During deep sleep in some people.
4. Heart failure.
5. Renal failure.

In a normal person periodic breathing is prevented because respiratory center alters the depth of respiration in such a way that arterial PCO_2 does not drop below critical value. If arterial PCO_2 goes below critical level, apnea appears.

Other Abnormal Breathings

Kussmaul Breathing: The pattern of respiration seen in **diabetic ketoacidosis** is called Kussmaul breathing (described by Kussmaul).

- Accumulation of metabolic acids such as acetoacetic acid and β-hydroxy butyric acid produces metabolic acidosis that stimulates respiratory centers.
- This leads to rapid and deep respiration or 'air hunger'.
- **Biot's Respiration:** In this type of abnormal breathing, 3 to 4 cycles of normal respiration is followed by **abrupt onset of apnea** (Fig. 53.1C).
- Before apnea, usually deep gasps occur.
- It is seen in **meningitis**, diseases affecting medulla of the brain, increased intra cranial pressure, morphine poisoning and damage to the brainstem.

Sleep Apnea Syndrome: In adult sleep apnea syndrome, marked loss of tone of pharyngeal muscles occurs during REM sleep causing obstruction of airway during inspiration. This produces apnea.

- The person wakes up and breathes normally for sometimes and sleeps again to have another bout of apnea.
- Thus, **repeated apnea occurs during sleep**.
- These people develop morning headache and fatigue due to frequent apnea in the night. Sleeplessness occurs during the day.

Sudden Infant Death Syndrome: Sudden infant death syndrome (SIDS) is a kind of sleep apnea in premature infants.

- **Loss of rhythmic activity of the respiratory center** leads to apnea in sleep and causes death of the infant.
- The exact cause is not known though it is commonly seen in **premature babies with cardiac arrhythmias** complicating long QT syndrome.
- It is also common in mothers who are **chronic smokers**.

Hysteric Hyperpnea: Spontaneous hyperpnea of sudden onset occurs in patients with hysteria. This results in washing out of CO_2 leading to alkalosis and convulsions. This is treated by allowing the patient to breath into a facial mask till he recovers.

Ondine's Curse: Some patients with brain injury lose their automatic control on breathing but retain voluntary breathing. Such patients require respiratory assistance intermittently.

As depicted in *German mythology*, the unfaithful lover of Ondine, a water nymph was cursed by the king of water nymphs that he will lack automatic breathing and will live till he breathes voluntarily. Ultimately the disloyal lover slept after a long period of sleeplessness and died as he lost the voluntary breathing.

Exam Questions

1. Describe the stages of asphyxia. Give a note on respiratory abnormality in drowning.
2. List the causes of hypercapnia and hypocapnia. Describe briefly the effects of hypercapnia and hypocapnia on the body.
3. Write short notes on periodic breathing, Kussmaul breathing and Biot's respiration.

Multiple Choice Questions of Chapter 52

1. **All of the following are true for high-pressure nervous syndrome, EXCEPT:**
   A. Drowsiness is seen
   B. Alpha activity in EEG is depressed
   C. Manual dexterity is impaired
   D. Is due to anesthetic effect of N_2 at high pressure
2. **In caissons disease pain in joint is because of**
   A. Air in joint
   B. Nitrogen bubble
   C. Carbon monoxide
   D. Oxygen bubble
3. **Caisson's disease**
   A. Gas embolism due to N_2 release from tissue
   B. Amniotic fluid embolism
   C. Tumor embolism
   D. Air embolism due to CO_2 release from tissue
4. **Decompression sickness is seen in all, EXCEPT**
   A. Diver
   B. Pilot
   C. Diver and Pilot
   D. Diver, Pilot and mountaineer
5. **Nitrogen narcosis is caused due to**
   A. Nitrogen inhibits dismutase enzyme
   B. Increase production of nitrous oxide
   C. Increased solubility of nitrogen in nerve cell membrane
   D. Decrease in oxygen free radicals
6. **Which of the following is not a hazard of deep sea diving?**
   A. Acute oxygen toxicity
   B. Respiratory alkalosis
   C. Air embolism
   D. Nitrogen narcosis
7. **Which of the following is not true about Caisson's disease?**
   A. Occurs if the return (decompression) to surface is slow
   B. Deep-sea divers usually breathe 80% nitrogen from gas mixture
   C. Caisson is the water-tight chamber used for performing underwater constructions
   D. Recompression should be done immediately in a pressurized cabin in treatment of dysbarism
8. **All of the following statements are true, EXCEPT:**
   A. For every descent of 33 ft depth, pressure increases by 760 mm Hg
   B. Scuba cylinders contain mixtures of oxygen and helium
   C. The narcotic effect of Helium is twice that of N_2
   D. Air embolism can occur during a rapid ascent from shallow depth of 5 meters

Answers

1. D 2. B 3. A 4. D 5. C 6. B 7. A 8. C

Multiple Choice Questions of Chapter 53

1. **Which of the following is not a feature of hypocapnia?**
   A. Cerebral ischemia
   B. Vasoconstriction
   C. Increased cardiac output
   D. Hypocalcemic tetany
2. **Which of the following is a feature of freshwater drowning?**
   A. Hemolysis
   B. Increased RBC count
   C. Alveoli are distended with fluid
   D. Decreased ESR
3. **All of the following statements are true, EXCEPT:**
   A. Periodic breathing is seen following voluntary hyperventilation
   B. Respiratory alkalosis occurs due to excess elimination of acid via kidney
   C. Narcotics depress the respiratory center and cause acidosis
   D. Severe and prolonged hypercapnea cause respiratory depression
4. **Biot's respiration is NOT seen in :**
   A. Diabetic ketoacidosis
   B. Increased intracranial pressure
   C. Meningitis
   D. Morphine poisoning
5. **Oxygen deficiency combined with CO2 excess is called:**
   A. Hypoxia B. Hypercapnia
   C. Asphyxia D. Hypercarbia
6. **Which of the following is not a feature of hypercapnia?**
   A. Dyspnea
   B. Decreased plasma HCO3- concentration
   C. Headache
   D. Confusion
7. **Which of the following is not a cause of Cheyne-Stokes respiration?**
   A. Heart failure B. Uremia
   C. Premature infant D. Hepatitis
8. **Which of the following is true about Ondine's curse?**
   A. Voluntary control of respiration is disrupted
   B. Automated control of respiration is intact
   C. Seen in spinal poliomyelitis
   D. Patient cannot live by breathing voluntarily
9. **Kussmaul breathing is seen in:**
   A. Diabetic ketoacidosis
   B. Diabetic neuronopathy
   C. Diabetic retinopathy
   D. Diabetic nephropathy
10. **Marked loss of tone of pharyngeal muscles during REM sleep causing obstruction of airway during inspiration is known as:**
    A. Hysteric hypernea
    B. Sudden infant death syndrome
    C. Sleep apnea syndrome
    D. Ondine's curse

Answers

1. C 2. A 3. B 4. A 5. C 6. B 7. D 8. D 9. A 10. C

Chapter 54

Artificial Ventilation and Cardiopulmonary Resuscitation

Learning Objectives

On completion of study of this chapter:

The student will be able to (must know):

1. Name the methods of artificial ventilation.
2. List the indications for CPR.
3. Understand the steps of external cardiac massage.
4. Appreciate the method of CPR.

The student may also be able to (desirable to know):

1. Describe the methods of CPR.

PY6.5

ARTIFICIAL VENTILATION

In respiratory arrest, artificial ventilation is given to the subject till normal rhythmic respiration is restored. Artificial respiration is useful when functions of heart and dynamics of circulation are functional.

Methods of Artificial Ventilation

Two types of artificial ventilatory methods are practiced: the instrumental methods, and the manual methods.

Instrumental (Mechanical) Methods

When artificial ventilation is required for longer period, instrumental methods are used. There are **two types of mechanical methods**: positive pressure and negative pressure methods.

Positive Pressure Method

This is usually used in **operation theaters during surgery**.

- In this method, the lung is inflated by pumping **air or air-O_2 mixture at positive pressure**.
- The **disadvantage** is that it impairs venous return.

Negative Pressure Method

This is achieved by alternate compression and relaxing of chest wall. Some of the **negative pressure methods** are: 1. Drinker's method, 2. Braggpaul method, and 3. Other method using Boyle's apparatus.

Drinker's Method (Iron lung chamber method): The apparatus consists of an **airtight chamber** and the pressure inside the chamber is *alternatively reduced and increased*.

- The patient is placed inside the chamber with his neck and head outside.
- When the pressure inside is increased, expiration takes place due to compression and when the pressure is reduced below atmospheric pressure, inspiration takes place.

Braggpaul Method: This consists of a **hollow elastic rubber bag**, which is wrapped round the chest. When a pump inflates the bag, the chest is compressed and air is expelled out. When the pressure is released the chest passively enlarges and air is drawn in.

Boyle's Apparatus: In the hospitals, this is used for giving artificial ventilation. This is an automatic instrument in which, rate and depth of ventilation and composition of air inhaled can be varied.

Manual Methods

Though there are many manual methods, **Holger-Neilson method** (back pressure–arm lift method), **mouth-to-mouth breathing** and **mouth-to-nose breathing** are usually practiced (described below).

CARDIOPULMONARY RESUSCITATION

The supportive and specific treatment given immediately to patients, in whom for some reasons the cardiac and ventilatory activities have stopped, is called cardiopulmonary resuscitation (CPR).

Indications

CPR is indicated in **conditions of cardio-respiratory arrest**. The common situations that can lead to cardio-respiratory arrest include:

1. Primary cardiac arrhythmias
2. Arrhythmias associated with myocardial infarction
3. Electric shock
4. Poisoning; Drowning
5. Pulmonary embolism
6. Anaphylactic shock
7. Head injury, Accident
8. Cardiac tamponade
9. Acute pulmonary edema
10. Airway obstruction

Objectives of CPR

1. To **provide adequate pulmonary ventilation** so that partial pressure of oxygen in the arterial blood is maintained.
2. To **initiate and facilitate pumping of the heart** so that effective circulation is maintained.

Steps of CPR

CPR has **three steps**: initial evaluation & basic life support, advanced life support and post-resuscitation measures

Initial Evaluation and Basic Life Support

PY11.14

Initial Evaluation

This includes assessment of state of consciousness, respiratory movements, skin color and the state of arterial pulses. If the cardiorespiratory arrest is due to foreign body impaction in the respiratory tract, **Heimlich maneuver** is performed to dislodge the obstructing body.

Basic Life Support

This should start immediately. A clear airway and initiation of breathing are essential parts of successful resuscitative measures. Unless adequate ventilation is achieved, attempts to restore circulation become futile. The steps are:

1. Assess the responsiveness of the patient by gently shaking the subject.
2. Position the patient on a firm and flat surface.
3. Open the mouth of the subject and **remove vomitus, blood, mucus or debris** if present in the oral cavity.
4. **Extend the neck of the subject** to increase the patency of the airway.

- To extend the neck, place the palm of your one hand on the patient's forehead and apply firm pressure to tilt the head backward. At the same time, place the palm of the other hand under the chin to support it (**head tilt-chin lift maneuver**). This raises the tongue away from the spine and opens the airway.
- To ventilate the lungs of the patient, perform any of the following three maneuvers. ***Mouth to mouth breathing*** is performed in adults and ***mouth to nose breathing*** is preferred in infants and children.

1. **Mouth to Mouth Respiration:**
   - Clear the airway and extend the neck
   - Close the nostrils (of the patient) by pinching with the thumb and the index finger of the right hand
   - Take a deep breath
   - Apply your mouth close to the subject's mouth and exhale forcefully into the his mouth
   - Look for chest expansion and abdominal distension
   - Repeat and maintain the breathing at a rate of 10-15 per minute.

- **Mouth to nose respiration:** Usually, it is performed for children. The steps are same as those of mouth-to-mouth respiration except that the mouth of the patient is closed and the rescuer breathes into the nostrils of the subject.

Holger-Nielson Method: (Manual manipulation of the thorax by back pressure-arm lift method):

- Lay down the patient in prone position.
- Abduct the arms at the shoulders and flex the elbows.
- Turn the head to one side testing on the hands.
- Kneel down with one knee near the patient's arm and straighten yourself to raise the subject's arm until resistance is felt (Fig 54.1 A and B). During this maneuver, the thorax of the patient expands and the intrathoracic pressure drops. Thus, inspiration takes place.
- Then, gently drop the patient's arm
- Place your hands with fingers spread apart on the back of the subject in the mid-axillary space, and slightly compress to produce expiration (Fig. 54.1 C and D).
- Repeat the whole cycle 10-12 times per minute.

2. **Palpate the carotid pulse.** Palpation for at least 10 seconds is recommended to ensure that slow, irregular, or very weak pulses are not missed.
3. **External Cardiac Massage:** The hands are positioned about 3 cm above the xiphoid process and to the left with the shoulders of the rescuer vertically above the chest of the subject. With the heel of the hand, and with fingers off the chest, the sternum is compressed 4-5 cm thrusting straight down towards the spine.
   - The recommended compression rate is 80-100 per minute.
   - The rescuer responsible for airway management should assess the adequacy of compression by periodically palpating for the carotid pulse.
   - The **compression-ventilation ratio is 5:1**.

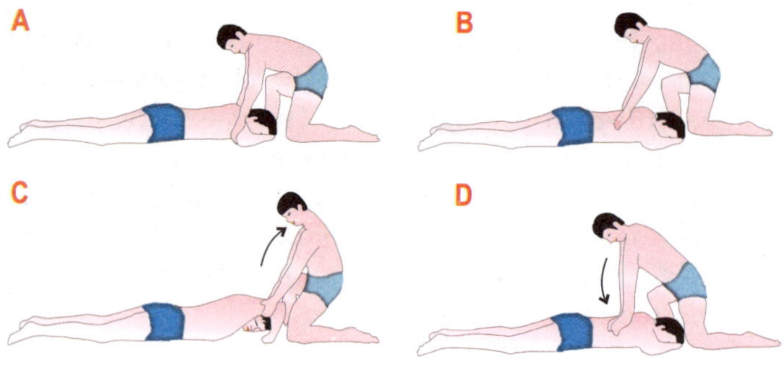

Fig. 54.1 A to D: Holger-Nielson method for artificial respiration. (A and B) For arm lift; (C and D) For back pressure.

4. **If pulses return,** ventilation should be continued as required.

Advanced Life Support

Advanced life support comprises of **primary and adjunctive therapies**.

Primary Therapies

Primary therapy of advanced life support includes defibrillation, and airway management & oxygen therapy

Defibrillation: This is one of the most important modalities of treatment of CPR.

- It should be started **as early as possible**. The time between the onsets of the arrest to the successful defibrillation is the major determinant of survival in cardiac arrest due to ventricular fibrillation.
- A fibrillating heart cannot pump blood, as effective contractions do not occur. Defibrillation converts **fibrillation into flutter or normal rhythm** so that effective ventricular contractions occur and heart pumps blood.
- **Adrenaline and sodium bicarbonate** are administered intravenously.

Airway Management & Oxygen Therapy: ***100 % oxygen*** should be administered and ***endotracheal intubation*** should be carried out by a qualified individual as soon as possible. But, the basic life support ***should not be delayed*** or interrupted for ***more than 30 seconds*** for intubation.

Adjunctive Therapies

Adjunctive therapies include following.

1. **Self-induced Cough:** When the arrest is detected before loss of consciousness, self-induced vigorous coughing can produce minimum blood flow to the brain temporarily until definitive treatment is initiated.
2. **Precordial thump:** A quickly applied solitary precordial thump may convert ventricular fibrillation or asystole to a rhythm.
3. **Atropine sulphates:** Atropine sulphate (0.5 mg) is injected intravenously every 5 minutes for the treatment of bradycardia. It may also help in the treatment of cardiac asystole.
4. **Sodium bicarbonate:** It is given as 1 meq/kg intravenously every 10 minutes for the treatment of cardiac arrest due to hyperkalemia or acidosis.
5. **Pacemakers:** It helps in patients with problems of abnormal impulse formation. Pacing is carried out early during resuscitation in conditions of refractory bradyarrhythmias or persistent asystole.

Other Methods: There are different **methods to assist ventilation** in CPR like **Sylvester-Brosche Method, Drinker's Method, Paul-Bunnel method and Rocking method**. But these methods are not routinely followed.

Post-Resuscitation Care

Post-resuscitation measures aim at **treating the underlying disease** that produced cardiorespiratory arrest. Usually in cardiac arrest for longer period, hypoxic encephalopathy and cerebral edema occur. Recently, **induction of hypothermia** is practiced to reduce metabolic demands and cerebral edema.

Exam Questions

1. List indications of cardiopulmonary resuscitation (CPR). Describe the methods of CPR.
2. Describe the steps of Holger-Nielson method of artificial respiration, and the steps of external cardiac massage.

Multiple Choice Questions

1. **Cardiopulmonary resuscitation is given in all of the following conditions, EXCEPT:**
   A. Drowning B. Poisoning
   C. Fracture of tibia D. Acute pulmonary edema
2. **Which of the following is not a method of artificial ventilation?**
   A. Positive pressure method of ventilation B. Drinker's method
   C. Bragg Paul method D. Priestley method
3. **Which of the following is not part of Holger-Nielson method of artificial respiration?**
   A. Lay the Patient in supine position
   B. Abduct his arm at the shoulder
   C. Turn his head to one side
   D. The CPR giver kneels down to perform the procedure
4. **Which is not done in external cardiac massage?**
   A. Hand is positioned about 3 cm above the xiphoid process and to the left
   B. Sternum is compressed about 4 cm with mainly heel of the hand
   C. Compression rate is 80 to 100 per min
   D. Compression-ventilation ratio is 20:1
5. **Which of the following is not part of mouth to mouth respiration in CPR?**
   A. Clear the airway of the patient B. Flex the neck of the patient
   C. Close the nostril of the patient
   D. Exhale forcefully to patient's mouth at a rate of 10-15 /min

Answers: 1. C 2. D 3. A 4. D 5. B

Chapter 55

Pulmonary Function Tests

PY6.7

Learning Objectives

On completion of study of this chapter:

The student will be able to (must know):

1. Classify PFTs and give the significance of each PFT parameter.
2. Define lung volumes and capacities and give their normal values.
3. Draw FEV1 curves of obstructive and restrictive lung diseases.
4. Understand the application of PFTs.
5. Name common conditions of alteration in PFTs

The student may also be able to (desirable to know):

1. Describe the measurement and application of PFT.

CLASSIFICATION OF PFTs

Classification of pulmonary function tests (PFTs) is based on the kind of lung function assessed by the test. They are of **three broad categories**: tests that assess ventilation, tests that assess gas exchange in the lungs and tests that assess pulmonary circulation.

1. Tests that assess ventilation

a. **Lung volumes and capacities**
b. **Mechanics of breathing:** All dynamic lung volumes and capacities such as FEV1, MMEFR, MVV, PEFR, etc.

2. Tests that assess gas exchange in lungs

a. Assessment of ventilation-perfusion matching
b. Assessment of diffusing capacity
c. Determination of arterial blood gasses

3. Assessment of pulmonary blood flow and pressure

Uses of PFTs: PFTs help in:

1. Diagnosis of respiratory dysfunctions.
2. Monitoring the progress of the disease.
3. Evaluating the efficiency of treatment.
4. Assessing the health status of the person prior to recruitment to military or police services.
5. Determining the efficacy of physical training.
6. Studying the prevalence of respiratory diseases in the community or respiratory industrial hazards.
7. Assessing the respiratory fitness of the patients for general anesthesia prior to surgery.
8. Finalizing medico-legal cases to decide fitness or degree of compensation.

Normal Values of PFTs

Normal values in an adult male:

TV	: 500 ml
IRV	: 3000 ml
ERV	: 1100 ml
FVC	: 4600 ml
FEV_1	: > 80% of FVC
FEV_1/FVC	: 0.75 – 0.80
PEFR	: 400 to 600 L/min
RMV	: 6000 ml
MVV	: 125 to 170 L/min
Breathing reserve (MVV – RMV)	: 115 to 160 L/min
Dyspneic index	: > 90% (< 60% indicates dyspnea at rest).

Values vary greatly for **race, age, gender, height, built and training** of the individual. All lung volumes and capacities are about **15 to 25% less in females**. The values are usually more in athletes and tall persons and less in non-athletes and poorly-built persons.

ASSESSMENT OF VENTILATION

The process of ventilation is assessed by recording lung volumes and capacities that are indices of static dimensions of the lung at various stages of inflation. The mechanics of breathing deal mainly with dynamic properties of the respiratory apparatus.

Lung Volumes & Capacities

Details of "Lung Volumes and Capacities" are described in Chapter 45 (refer, Fig. 45.7)

Mechanics of Breathing

Details of Lung compliance and airway resistance are described in Chapter 45. Also, details of flow-volume curve, FEV_1, MMEFR, MVV, PEFR and MEFVC are described under "Dynamic Lung Volumes and Capacities" in Chapter 45 (refer Fig. 45. 17 to 45.21)

1. **Closing Volume (CV):** This test detects **small airway obstruction** by measuring the volume of gas remaining in the lung after closure of small airways in the gravity dependent lung areas.
2. **Maximal Inspiratory Pressure (MIP):** Patient exhales completely to RV and then tries to inspire maximally against an occluded airway. The pressure generated in this maneuver is the MIP.
   - It assesses the **strength of inspiratory muscles**.
3. **Maximal Expiratory Pressure (MEP):** Patient inhales completely to TLC and then tries to expire maximally against an occluded airway. The pressure generated in this maneuver is the MIP.
   - It assesses the **strength of expiratory muscles**.

Measurement of Ventilatory Functions

Though pulmonary functions are measured by **spirometer**, now-a-days pulmonary functions are measured by **computerized PFT machine**.

- **RV, FRC and TLC can't be measured** by spirometry as they include volume of gases present in the lungs even after maximal expiration.
  - They are measured by **helium dilution technique and total body plethysmography**.

Abnormalities of Ventilation

There are two major types of ventilatory abnormalities: *restrictive and obstructive patterns*. In the obstructive disease, the hallmark of dysfunction is the decrease in expiratory flow rates, particularly the MMFR and FEV_1/FVC and the hallmark of the restrictive disease is the reduction in FVC.

Features of Obstructive Diseases

1. TLC is normal or increased.
2. RV is elevated due to trapping of air during expiration.
3. Ratio of RV/TLC is increased.
4. VC is frequently decreased (not due to decreased lung volumes but due to increased RV).
5. FEV_1 is less than 80% of TLC (refer Fig. 45.19, Chapter 45).
6. FEV_1/FVC decreases.
7. MMEFR decreases.

In the **early phase of obstructive disease** which originates in the small airways, FEV_1/FVC may be normal. However, decreased in MMFR and an abnormal configuration in the terminal portion of forced expiratory flow volume curve may indicate the presence of the disease.

Common obstructive diseases are asthma, COPD (chronic bronchitis, emphysema) and bronchiectasis.

Features of Restrictive Diseases

1. Decreased TLC
2. Decreased VC
3. Decreased RV
4. Preservation of forced expiratory flow rates, especially FEV_1 expressed, as percentage of FVC is normal or supernormal (refer Fig. 45.18, Chapter 45).

The restrictive diseases can be broadly subdivided in to parenchymal and extraparenchymal disease. Extraparenchymal dysfunction is again of two categories, the extraparenchymal dysfunction in inspiration and the extraparenchymal dysfunction in inspiration plus expiration.

Restrictive Parenchymal Dysfunction

Decreased TLC, RV, VC, and normal or increased FEV_1/FVC

Common parenchymal restrictive diseases are pulmonary fibrosis, pneumoconiosis and radiation-induced interstitial lung disease.

Restrictive Extraparenchymal Dysfunction

Inspiratory Dysfunction: In extraparenchymal inspiratory dysfunction, which occurs usually due to either inspiratory muscle weakness or a stiff chest wall, the adequate distending forces are prevented from being exerted on an otherwise normal lung.

- Therefore, TLC is reduced but RV is not affected, and expiratory flow rates are preserved.

Inspiratory plus Expiratory Dysfunction: This usually occurs in expiratory muscle weakness or due to deformed chest wall that is abnormally rigid at lung volumes below FRC.

- Therefore, RV is often significantly elevated. The ratio of FEV_1/FVC may be affected depending on the strength of the expiratory muscles.

Common extraparenchymal restrictive diseases are neuromuscular diseases, myasthenia gravis, paralysis of diaphragm, muscular dystrophy and kyphoscoliosis.

Alterations in Lung Volumes & Capacities

Lung volumes and capacities show a wide range in the normal population depending on the **age, sex, and height of the subject**. Indian population shows significant lower values as compared to their western counter parts.

- **Predicted normograms** are available based on these variable factors.

- Deviation **up to 20%** from the predicted value for a given age, sex, and height is commonly seen in normal subjects.
- However, in a particular individual, even 5% change from his preexisting value may be of significance.
- Therefore, **serial measurement** of these values is of great importance in diagnosis.

Conditions that decrease vital capacity:

1. *Loss of functioning lung tissue*
   - Interstitial pulmonary fibrosis, Chest deformity
   - Neuromuscular disease, Thickened pleura
2. *Loss of distensibility of lung tissues*
   - Atelectasis, Consolidation
   - Pulmonary edema, Pulmonary resection

Conditions that decrease FVC: FVC decreases in conditions in which there is obstruction to the airways **resulting in air trapping**, e.g. bronchial asthma.

Conditions that decrease FEV_1: FEV_1 is an important test to detect **generalized airway obstruction.**

- As it is effort dependent it should be performed properly to get the appropriate result. However, it is not specific for detecting small airway obstruction.
- FEV_1 decreases in **obstructive diseases of the lung**, as in bronchial asthma.

Change in FEV_1/FVC: The ratio of FEV_1/FVC is approximately 0.75 to 0.80. This is a more **sensitive indicator of airway obstruction** than FVC or FEV_1 alone.

Alteration of MMFR ($FEF_{25-75\%}$): This is a sensitive indicator of **patency of the small airways**. This is slowed in small airway obstruction.

Variation in $FEF_{200-1200}$: This is the flow rate between 200 and 1200 ml of FVC.

- A sensitive indicator of **patency of larger airways**.
- It is slowed in large airway obstruction.

Reduction in PEFR: As it measures peak expiratory flow rate during peak of expiration, it **decreases in airway obstruction**. MMFR and $FEF_{200-1200}$ are better indicators than PEFR.

Decline in MVV: The normal value of MVV is **150 liters in males and 125 liters in females**. However, the value can be fallacious if the patient does not cooperate or fails to use maximum effort to carry out the test. MVV **decreases in patients with subjective dyspnea**.

ASSESSMENT OF GAS EXCHANGE

Ventilation-Perfusion Relationship

Ventilation: In erect posture, resting ventilation per unit volume of lung is ***greater at the bases*** than at the apices. The uniformity of distribution of inspired air is measured by **nitrogen washout method**.

- An alveolar gas sample after 7 minutes of breathing oxygen normally contains less than 2.5% of nitrogen.
- The higher the percentage of nitrogen in the alveolar sample, the greater is the degree of non-uniformity of distribution of inspired gas.

Perfusion: The perfusion is also not uniform in erect posture **due to the effect of gravity**.

- The normal ventilation-perfusion ratio is 0.8. But greater degree of non-uniform perfusion occurs in diseases like pulmonary embolism and diseases that destroy lung tissues.

The arterial blood gas tension is primarily affected by the relationship of ventilation with perfusion. Alteration in ventilation-perfusion ratio mainly **affects PaO_2 than $PaCO_2$**.

Diffusion

Diffusion is the physical process by which gas move across a membrane.

- The diffusing capacity of CO_2 is 20 times more than that of O_2. Therefore, diffusion problems usually **do not produce carbon dioxide retention**.
- Measurement of the arterial blood gas tension is essential in the evaluation of pulmonary functions.
- The normal value of **PaO_2 is 90 to 95 mm Hg**, and of **$PaCO_2$ is 36 to 44 mm Hg.**

Hypoxemia: Decrease in PaO_2 is called hypoxemia. It occurs in **four conditions**:

1. Decreased inspired PO_2.
2. Hypoventilation
3. Shunting (when desaturated blood effectively bypasses oxygenation at alveolar-capillary level), common in cyanotic congenital heart disease.
4. Ventilation-perfusion mismatching as occurs in COPD, asthma etc.

Gas Sampling and Analysis

Sampling of Alveolar Air

Sampling of alveolar air is performed by two methods: **Haldane-Priestley Method and Rahn-Otus Method.**

Sampling of Expired Air

Douglas bag is used for this purpose. A two-way valve is fixed to the Douglas bag and then connected to the mouth of the subject. Atmospheric air is inhaled and then exhaled into the bag.

Respiratory Gas Analysis: Samples of inspired air (atmospheric), mixed expired air (from the Douglas bag) and alveolar air (collected by Haldane-Priestley method) are taken for analysis of partial pressure of oxygen, carbon dioxide and nitrogen. Gas analyzers are available to give the partial pressure of different gases.

Blood Gas Analysis: The oxygen content of the blood is determined by **Haldane's gas analyzer.** The venous blood is collected and sent for analysis. The oxygen carrying capacity of the blood is estimated by **Van Slyke gasometric method**. The partial pressure of carbon dioxide is also determined with the help of gasometers.

ASSESSMENT OF PULMONARY CIRCULATION

Pulmonary Blood Flow & Pressure

Assessment of Pulmonary Blood Flow

Assessment of pulmonary circulation depends upon measuring pulmonary vascular pressures and cardiac output. These measurements are usually done in intensive care units with the facilities of invasive monitoring.

- With a flow-directed pulmonary ***arterial (Swan-Ganz) catheter***, the pulmonary arterial and pulmonary capillary **wedge pressures** can be measured directly.
- The cardiac output is obtained by thermodilution method.

The **pulmonary vascular resistance** (PVR) is calculated as:

PVR = 80 (PAP – PCW)/CO

Where, PAP = Mean pulmonary arterial pressure, PCW=Pulmonary capillary wedge pressure and CO is cardiac output)

The normal PVR is 50-150 dynes.s/cm^5

Pulmonary vascular resistance (PVR) increases mainly by pulmonary vasoconstriction and pulmonary thromboembolism.

Conditions that increase PVR

1. **Heart diseases:** Cardiac conditions that elevate left arterial pressure such as mitral stenosis increase PVR.
2. **Lung diseases:** Respiratory conditions that cause chronic pulmonary hypoxemia increase PVR, as seen in, COPD, interstitial lung disease, Kyphoscoliosis, obesity hypoventilation, sleep apnea syndrome
3. **Diseases affecting pulmonary vessels such as** recurrent pulmonary embolism, scleroderma (occludes small pulmonary arteries and arterioles)

Respiratory Causes of Hypoxemia

The causes of hypoxemia are classified into respiratory and non-respiratory. **Respiratory dysfunction** is the most common cause of hypoxemia in adults.

Normal A-aO_2 gradient

Normally, Hb is 100% saturated with oxygen when the blood passes the pulmonary capillaries, so that end-capillary PO_2 is same as alveolar PO_2. But, the blood in the pulmonary veins that returns to the left atrium has a lower PO_2 than pulmonary end-capillary blood. Therefore, the average oxygen tension (PaO_2) in systemic arterial blood is about 95 mm Hg and Hb is 98% saturated.

- The difference between alveolar oxygen tension (P_AO_2) and arterial oxygen tension (P_aO_2) is the **alveolar-arterial oxygen gradient** (A-aO_2 gradient).
- Because alveolar PO_2 is normally 100 to 102 mm Hg and arterial PO_2 is 85 to 95 mm Hg, a **normal A-aO_2 gradient is 5 to 15 mm Hg.**

The respiratory causes of hypoxemia may be due to:

1. Regional hypoventilation
2. Occlusion of a major artery in the lungs by a large blood clot
3. Shunts
4. Generalized hypoventilation
5. Diffusion block.

Exam Questions

1. Classify PFTs and give their normal values. Briefly describe variood PFTs.
2. List the causes of hypercapnia and hypocapnia. Describe briefly the effects of hypercapnia and hypocapnia on the body.
3. Write short notes on periodic breathing, Kussmaul breathing and Biot's respiration.

Multiple Choice Questions

1. **Pulmonary function change seen in Emphysema is:**
   A. ↑TLC B. ↓RV
   C. ↑FEV_1 D. ↑VC
2. **The gradient of alveolar arterial oxygen tension increases in all, EXCEPT;**
   A. Diffusion defect B. Right-left shunt
   C. Hypoventilation D. Ventilation perfusion abnormality
3. **Alveolar hypoventilation is present in all, EXCEPT:**
   A. Bulbar poliomyelitis B. COPD
   C. Kyphoscoliosis D. Lobar pneumonia
4. **CO2 retention is seen in all, EXCEPT:**
   A. Carbon monoxide poisoning and High altitude
   B. Respiratory/ Ventilatory failure
   C. Pulmonary edema
   D. Drowning
5. **Hypercarbia is characterized by:**
   A. Miosis B. Cool extremities
   C. Bradycardia D. Hypertension

Answers

1. A 2. C 3. D 4. A 5. D

Section VII

Gastrointestinal (GI) System

“*Eat for living, but do not live for eating.*

The Mother”
(of Sri Aurobindo Ashram, Pondicherry, INDIA)

Chapter 56

Functional Organization of GI System and Principles of GI Regulations

Learning Objectives

On completion of study of this chapter:

The student will be able to (must know):

1. Name the parts of GI tract and give their functions.
2. Correlate the functional anatomy with functions of GI tract.
3. Name the layers of wall of GI tract, and give their functional importance.
4. Understand the differences in sympathetic and parasympathetic stimulation on GI functions.
5. Appreciate the organization of enteric nervous system.
6. Illustrate the principles of GI regulations.

The student may also be able to (desirable to know):

1. Describe the processes of GI regulations.

FUNCTIONAL ORGANIZATION

Functions of GI Tract

PY4.1

The gastrointestinal (GI) functions are as follows:

1. **Digestion and absorption of food:** The primary functions of GI system are to digest food materials and absorb essential nutrients of digestive products into the bloodstream.
2. **Excretion of waste materials:** Digestive tract excretes waste materials in the form of feces. Fecal matter includes mainly the excretory products of digestion and undigested food particles.
3. **Fluid and electrolyte balance:** On average, an adult consumes **1 kg of food and 1.5 liters of water** per day. An additional amount of **7 liters of fluid is secreted** into GI tract in the form of secretions from various exocrine glands.
   - Thus, intestine is presented with *about* **8.5 liters of fluid per day**.
   - About *99% of this fluid and 90% of solids are absorbed* in small and large intestines along with absorption of various electrolytes, so that only about **100 ml of liquid and 100 g of solids are excreted** in feces per day.
4. **Immunity:** The GI tract is anatomically continuous with the external environment. Consequently, it provides a fine channel for organisms from external world to pass through it.
   - However, the **gut associated lymphoid tissues** (GALTs) protect the body from pathogenic organisms.
   - **Acidic secretion of stomach** kills the organisms.
5. **Intestinal bacterial flora:** Many nonpathogenic bacteria inhabit intestine. They form the normal **bacterial flora of intestine**.
   - This normal flora is essential for **many intestinal functions** like epithelial cell permeability to electrolytes and water, synthesis and absorption of vitamins, stimulation of enzymatic activity, peristalsis and mucus secretion.
   - These bacteria also **detoxify many toxins** present in the chyme and prevent their absorption into the bloodstream.
   - Gut microbiota controls many neural, immunological and other functions of the body through **Gut-Brain Axis** (discussed details in Chapter 62).

Parts of GI System

Gastrointestinal system consists of gastrointestinal tract (GIT) and its associated glandular structures that produce exocrine secretions essential for digestion and absorption of various nutrients. The parts of GIT include **mouth, pharynx, esophagus, stomach, small intestine** (duodenum, jejunum, and ileum), **colon** (ascending, transverse, descending and sigmoid colons), **rectum, and anus** (Fig. 56.1). The major **associated glandular structures**

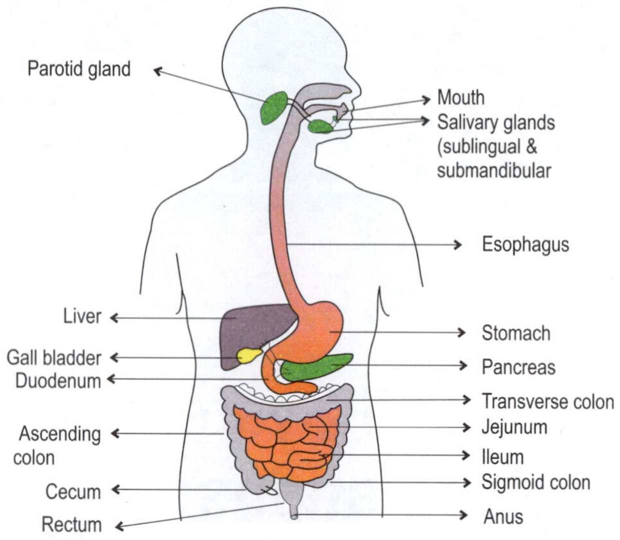

Fig. 56.1: Major parts of the gastrointestinal system.

are salivary glands, liver, exocrine pancreas and intestinal glands.

1. GI tract begins with the **mouth** (oral cavity). **Salivary glands** open into the oral cavity and pour their secretion (saliva) into it.
2. Oral cavity opens into **pharynx** which in turn is continuous with the esophagus.
3. **Esophagus** transmits food from oropharynx into stomach.
4. **Stomach** is a bag like structure that stores and grinds food, and mixes food with gastric juice to form chyme. **Chyme** enters intestine through pyloric sphincter by controlled gastric emptying.
5. **Small intestine** is a 9 feet tube that extends from pyloric sphincter to the ileocecal valve. It consists of ***three parts***: duodenum, jejunum and ileum.
    - **Biliary and pancreatic secretions** are poured into duodenum.
    - Intestinal glands secrete ***succus entericus***.
    - Absorption of most of the nutrients takes place in **jejunum and ileum**.
    - **Small intestinal motility** propels food into large intestine through **ileocecal sphincter**.
6. **Large intestine** absorbs water and electrolyte and temporarily stores the concentrated and undigested material, which then enters the rectum.
7. **Rectum**, the final segment of large intestine stores fecal matter and contracts when distended. *Defecation reflex* relaxes the anal sphincters and expels feces from rectum to outside through **anal canal**.

Structure of the Wall of GI Tract

The basic nature of arrangement of tissues in the wall of GI tract starting from esophagus to the rectum is similar. In general, there are **four layers** from interior to exterior: mucosa, submucosa, muscle layer, and serosa (Fig. 56.2).

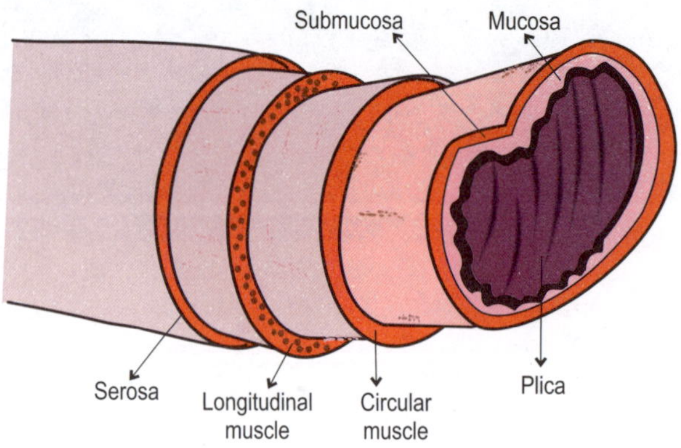

Fig. 56.2: Layers of wall of the gut.

Mucosa

The innermost layer of GI tract is the mucosa, which has an epithelium, lamina propria and muscularis mucosa (Fig. 56.3).

Epithelium: A single layer of epithelial cells lines the mucosa. The cells are tightly bound to each other at their edges by **tight junctions**.

- The epithelium is mainly a **stratified squamous epithelium.**
- In stomach and intestine, the mucosa is lined by **simple columnar epithelium** that facilitates secretion and absorption.
- At places, the epithelium contains endocrine cells (**enterochromaffin cells**) that secrete local hormones.

Lamina Propria: Just below the epithelium is the lamina propria consisting of mainly **loose connective tissue** that contains ***collagen and elastin fibers***.

- This sub-layer is rich in blood vessels, lymph nodes and lymphatic ducts, nerve fibers, and capillaries.
- This layer **supports the epithelium** and also binds epithelium to the muscularis mucosa.
- The **lymphatic tissues** present in this layer form the *local immune system* and prevent the entry of pathogens that try to penetrate mucous membrane to enter into the body.

Muscularis Mucosa: This is the outermost layer of the mucosa and intestinal smooth muscles are present in this part of mucosa. The muscle fibers are arranged in two thin layers, an inner circular and outer longitudinal layer.

- **Contraction of muscularis mucosa** in the stomach and intestine throws the mucous membrane into **folds and ridges**.
- In the intestine, these mucosal folds called **plica** *increase the surface area for absorption* (Fig. 79.4).
- Contraction of muscularis mucosa in small intestine produces ***local movements*** that facilitate the process of digestion and absorption.

Submucosa

Next to the mucosa is the submucosa. It consists mainly of **loose connective tissue** and is **highly vascular**.

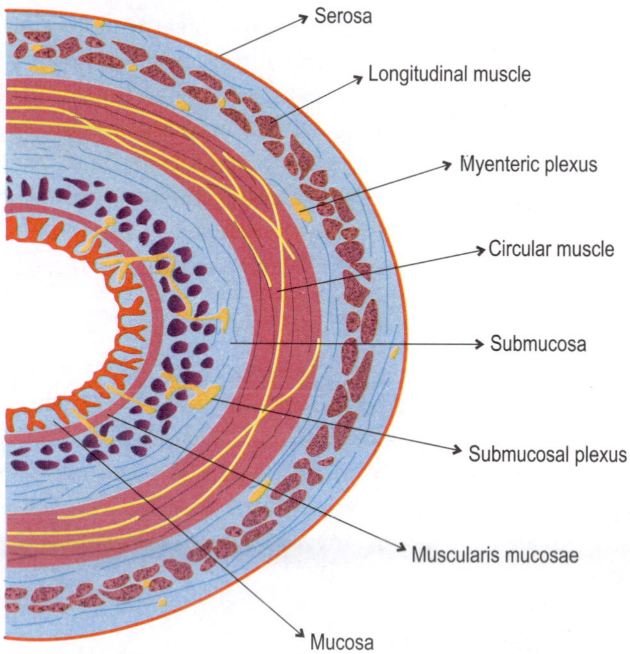

Fig. 56.3: Details of the layers of the gut.

- The submucosal layer contains a **network of nerve fibers** known as *submucosal plexus* or **plexus of Meissner**.
- Autonomic nerve fibers supplying muscles and blood vessels of GI tract closely interact with Meissner's plexus.
- In some regions, especially in intestine, submucosa contains **lymphatic tissue**.

Muscular Layer

This is called **muscularis externa**. It consists of **two layers** of smooth muscles: the **inner circular** and the **outer longitudinal** layers.

- A nerve plexus is located between the muscle layers, called as ***myenteric plexus*** or **plexus of Auerbach**.
- Auerbach's plexus contains fibers from both divisions of ANS.
- Muscularis externa primarily **controls the motility of GI tract** that mixes and circulates the gastrointestinal contents and propels them along the lumen of the tract.

Serosa

This is the outermost layer of the GIT. It consists mainly of a **thin layer of connective tissue** covered with a layer of **squamous mesothelial cells**. It provides **external protection** to the GIT.

Intestinal Modifications

Villi: In small intestine, from the luminal surface, finger like projections extend into the lumen. These are called **villi**. Surface of each villus is covered with an epithelial cell layer.

- Small projections arise from the surface of these epithelial cells, known as **microvilli**.
- Folded mucosa, villi and microvilli increase the surface area of the intestinal luminal epithelium by **600 fold**.

Peyer's Patches: These are the **aggregates of lymphoid tissue** in the mucosal-submucosal regions of the intestinal wall. These are present more in number in ileum. They serve **local immune functions** in the intestine.

Innervation of GI Tract

GI tract is innervated by **sympathetic and parasympathetic fibers**. Also, it has its own neural circuits, the enteric nervous system (ENS).

Sympathetic Innervation

Stimulation of sympathetic fibers to GI tract is **generally inhibitory**.

- Sympathetic innervation is via **noradrenergic fibers** having their cell bodies in the prevertebral and paravertebral chain of ganglia.
  - The postganglionic fibers mainly originate from **celiac, superior and inferior mesenteric ganglia** (refer Fig. 24.5, Chapter 24).
  - Sympathetic fibers don't terminate directly on the GI structures, rather they end on the intrinsic plexuses of enteric ENS (Fig. 56.4).

Sympathetic stimulation results in:

1. Inhibition of motor activity resulting in relaxation of GI smooth muscles.
2. Stimulation or contraction of sphincters.
3. Inhibition of GI secretions.

Parasympathetic Innervation

Stimulation of sympathetic fibers to GI tract is **generally inhibitory**.

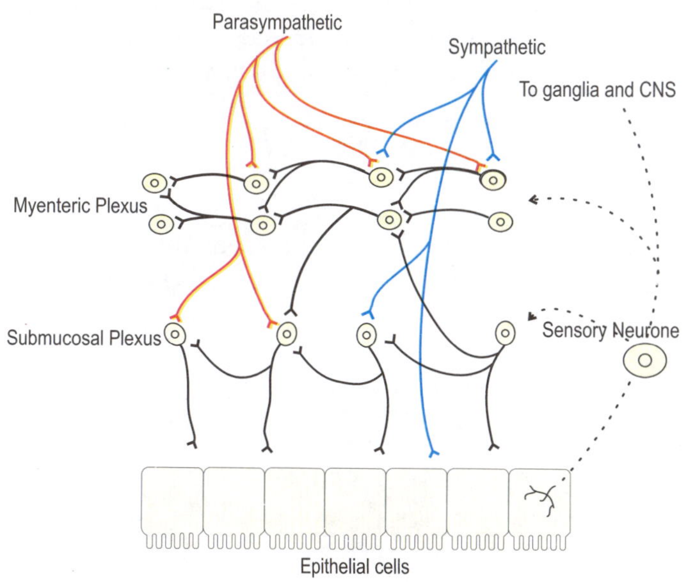

Fig. 56.4: Arrangement of enteric nervous system. Note the sympathetic and parasympathetic neurons ending in the enteric neurons.

- Parasympathetic innervation is **mainly via vagus nerve**, which innervates GI tract from oral cavity upto transverse colon.
- Remaining parts (descending and sigmoid colons, rectum, and anal canal) receive parasympathetic fibers from **pelvic nerves** (refer Fig. 24.7, Chapter 24).
- Parasympathetic fibers don't terminate directly on the GI structures, rather they end on the intrinsic plexuses of enteric ENS (Fig. 56.4).

Parasympathetic stimulation results in:

1. Parasympathetic fibers are **cholinergic** and generally **excitatory**.
2. Parasympathetic stimulation leads to **increased motility and exocrine secretions** of GI tract.

Enteric Nervous System

Enteric nervous system (ENS) is the intrinsic nervous system of the GI tract.

1. This includes **myenteric and submucosal nerve plexuses** in the GI tract (Fig. 56.4). These two plexuses are the network of nerve fibers and ganglion cells.
2. The neurons of these plexuses are **small interneurons** that connect afferent neurons and efferent neurons to smooth muscles, secretory cells and epithelial cells, and they form the ***anatomical basis of local GI reflexes***.
   - Therefore, the reflex arc for local GI reflexes is located within the GI tract. Hence, ENS is capable of coordinating GI activity in the absence of external innervation.
3. The neurons of ENS closely interact with the autonomic nervous system. The sympathetic and parasympathetic fibers project to the neurons of the myenteric and submucosal plexuses, and control GI activities via these neurons (Fig. 56.5).
4. Therefore, ENS is also known as **third division of ANS**. However, it should be remembered that *regulation of GI functions by ENS is independent of autonomic control*.

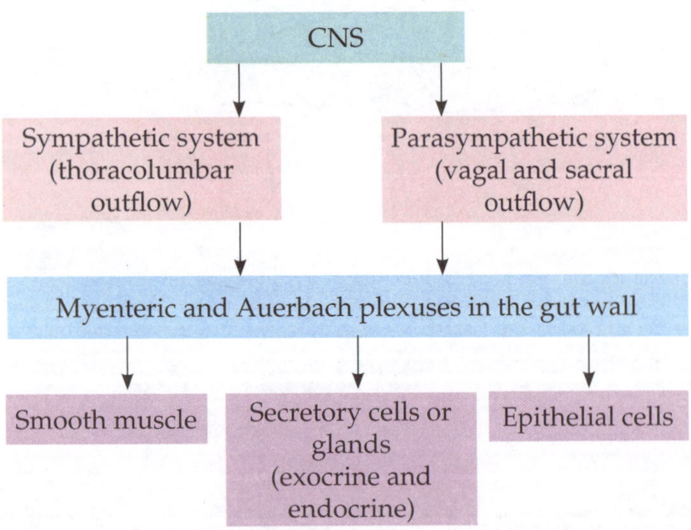

Fig. 56.5: Innervation of the GI tract.

ENS as the Mini-brain of gut: ENS consists approximately of 100 million of neurons, the number of neurons that are roughly present in spinal cord or in entire ANS. These neurons are clustered exclusively in the gut. They have sensory neurons, interneurons and motor neurons. Therefore, ENS is also called the '***mini brain***' for the gut.

Neurotransmitters in ENS: Many neurotransmitters in the ENS have been recently identified.

1. **Acetylcholine** (ACh) is the primary neurotransmitter in preganglionic and postganglionic neurons that regulate secretory and motor activities of GI tract.
2. **VIP, serotonin, enkephalins, substance P, norepinephrine, GABA, ATP, NO and CO** have also been described as neurotransmitters in ENS, and these chemicals play important role in regulation of GI functions.

GI Sphincters

Sphincters are **specialized circular muscles** that are present at the **beginning or at the end of a gut structure.** Sphincters regulate **antegrade (forward) movement** of food and ***prevent retrograde (reverse) expulsion*** of the same.

There are **six sphincters** in GI tract: upper and lower esophageal sphincters, pyloric sphincter, ileocecal sphincter, and internal and external anal sphincters.

GI Immune System

An extensive immune mechanism is developed in GI system, which is called **gastrointestinal immune system**. This system includes:

1. **Mesenteric lymph nodes**
2. **Peyer's patches** (aggregation of lymphatic tissues in the submucosa)
3. **Phagocytic cells and immunocytes** present in the mucosa and submucosa throughout the GI tract.

Immunological Cells in GI System: The **immunological cells** in GI system constitute about **50% of the total immunocytes in the body**. Immunocytes in GI tract are **B and T cells, epithelial lymphocytes, plasma cells**, mast cells and macrophages.

- These cells ***secrete chemicals*** that mediate immunological and inflammatory responses in GI tract.
- They **secrete antibodies** locally in response to antigens that enter through GI tract.
- *Other chemicals* secreted by immunocytes are **leukotrienes, cytokines, prostaglandins and histamine**. These chemicals not only mediate immunological responses, but also influence activities of smooth muscles of GI tract.
- GI immune system plays an important role in the

pathogenesis of inflammatory bowel diseases like ulcerative colitis.

PRINCIPLES OF GI REGULATIONS

The functions of GI tract are regulated mainly by neural and hormonal influences.

Neural Regulation

The digestive system is regulated by the nerves arising locally in the GI tract (**intrinsic neural control**) and the nerves innervating the gut (**extrinsic neural control**).

Intrinsic Neural Regulation

The intrinsic nerves of the GI system form the **enteric nervous system**, sometimes called as *third component of ANS*.

- The nerves are arranged in the submucosal layer as **Meissner's plexus** and in the muscle layer as *Auerbach's plexus*. These nerve plexuses control local secretion and movement of GI tract.
- The Meissner's plexus performs sensory functions and Auerbach's plexus performs motor functions.
- The intrinsic neurons mediate **local or short reflexes**.
- The intrinsic nerve plexuses are connected and controlled by extrinsic nerves.

Extrinsic Neural Regulation

Extrinsic nerves regulating GI functions belong to sympathetic and parasympathetic systems.

- In general, the **sympathetic system to the GI tract is inhibitory** and the **parasympathetic system is stimulatory**.
- Extrinsic nerves **mediate long reflexes**.

Reflex Control

There are **two types of neural reflexes** that operate in GI system: **short or local reflexes** and **long or central reflexes** (Fig. 56.6).

- Afferent pathway in the GIT forms *afferent limb* for both local and central reflexes.
- There are many chemoreceptors and mechanoreceptors in the mucosa and muscularis mucosa that are extensively connected to intrinsic plexuses.
  - Actions of these receptors mediate **local reflex** activity.
  - Enterogastric reflex is an example of a **short reflex**.
- Receptors also provide signals to the CNS that control GI functions via **central reflexes**.
- The *efferent fibers* for central reflexes are present in the autonomic fibers that terminate in enteric nerve plexuses.
  - Reflex secretion of saliva in response to smell of food is an example of a **long reflex**.

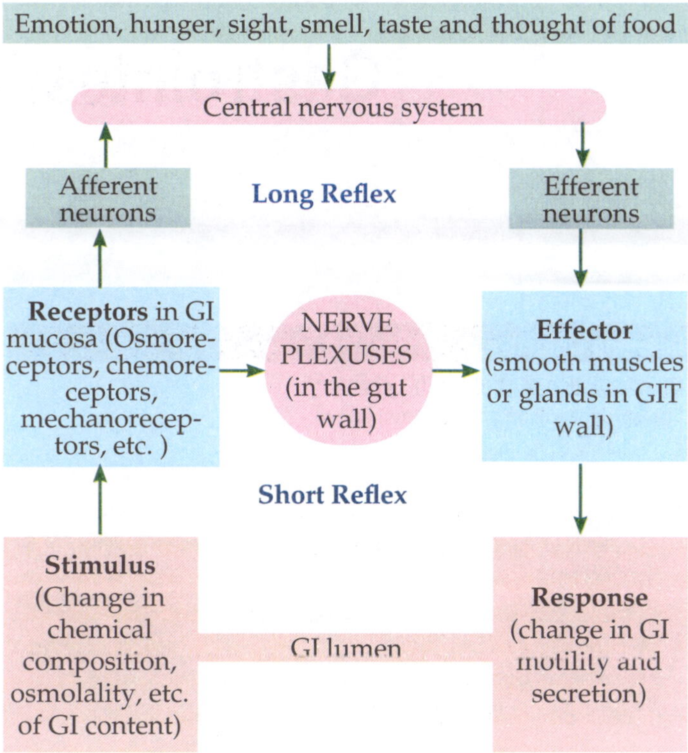

Fig. 56.6: Short and long reflexes in the regulation of GI functions.

Hormonal Regulation

The hormones controlling GI functions are also of two types: intrinsic hormones, and extrinsic hormones.

Intrinsic Hormones: Many hormones are secreted from neuroendocrine cells of GI tract, named are called **GI hormones**. They mainly act in a **paracrine fashion**. They control GI secretion and motility.

Extrinsic Hormones: GI functions are also influenced by hormones secreted from other endocrine glands like thyroxine and cortisol.

Exam Questions

1. With the help of a labelled diagram, describe the different layers of GI tract and briefly decribe their functions.
2. Describe the innervation of GI tract with a special reference to ENS.
3. Briefly describe the organization and importance of short and long reflexes of GIT.

MCQs are given in Page No. 458

Chapter 57

PY4.5

Gastrointestinal Hormones

Learning Objectives

On completion of study of this chapter:

The student will be able to (must know):

1. Classify GI hormones.
2. List the functions of each GI hormone.
3. Understand the role of GI hormones in the regulation of GI functions.
4. Understand the dysfunctions produced by alteration in secretion of GI hormones.

The student may also be able to (desirable to know):

1. Describe the structure, metabolism, mechanism of action, functions and regulation of GI hormones.
2. Explain the role of GI hormones in GI functions and dysfunctions.

The hormones secreted from the **endocrine cells of the GI tract** are collectively known as gastrointestinal hormones (**GI hormones**). Endocrine cells are scattered throughout GI tract, especially in stomach and small intestine.

1. Endocrine cells in GIT are called **enteroendocrine cells**.
2. Cells that secrete serotonin are called **enterochromaffin cells**, and cells that secrete amines and polypeptides are called **APUD cells** (amine precursor uptake and decarboxylation).

Types of GI Hormones: GI hormones are broadly divided into ***three categories***.

1. ***Gastrin family*** that includes cholecystokinin & gastrin.
2. ***Secretin family*** that includes GIP, glucagon, secretin, and VIP.
3. ***Other polypeptides***.

GI HORMONES OF GASTRIN FAMILY

Gastrin

Source

Gastrin is produced by **G cells** in the stomach that are located mainly in the antral region.

- **Gastrin producing cells are also present in** hypothalamus, anterior pituitary, medulla and fetal pancreas.
- Gastrin as a neurotransmitter is also secreted from ***vagus and sciatic nerve***.

Structure

Gastrin is a **polypeptide hormone**.

Types of Gastrin: Though there are different types of gastrins, **three are** are physiologically important.

1. Depending on the number of amino acids, they are named as **G 34, G 17 and G 14.**
2. Other types of gastrins are **C-tetrapeptide** (carboxyl terminal tetrapeptide, which is also called **minigastrin**), and gastrin containing 45 amino acids (**megagastrin**).
3. However, **G 17 is the principal gastrin** *secreted from the stomach* and is the major stimulator of gastric acid secretion.

Metabolism

Gastrin secreted from G cells enters general circulation. In blood, half-life of gastrin is less.

- Half-life of G 14 and G 17 is **2–5 min** and of G 34 is about 15 min.
- Gastrin is inactivated in the intestine and degraded in the kidney.

Functions

1. Primary function of gastrin is the **stimulation of gastric acid and pepsin secretion**.
    - Gastrin is the **most potent natural stimulator of HCl secretion** from parietal cells of stomach.
        - Therefore, hypergastrinemia causes peptic ulcer.
2. Gastrin **stimulates growth of gastric mucosa** and mucosa of intestine.

- This is called **trophic action** of gastrin.

3. It stimulates **gastric motility**.
4. Causes contraction of muscles at the gastro-esophageal junction (lower esophageal sphincter).
   - Therefore, it **prevents reflux esophagitis**.
5. Stimulates exocrine pancreatic secretion.
6. It also **stimulates insulin secretion**.
7. Stimulates **mass movement** of large intestine.
8. Causes colonic contraction that initiates **gastrocolic reflex** after a meal.
   - Therefore, usually defecation is activated after a meal.
9. Stimulates **histamine secretion** from ECL (enterochromaffin like cells) in GI mucosa.

Mechanism of Action: Gastrin acts on gastrin or CCK receptors on parietal cells and increases intracellular calcium concentration via second messenger, IP_3.

- Increased cytosolic calcium ***activates protein kinase*** that **stimulates H^+–K^+ ATPase** to promote acid secretion.

Control of Gastrin Secretion

1. **Stimuli that increase gastrin secretion:** Gastric distention, products of protein digestion (peptides and amino acids) in the stomach, increased vagal discharge via GRP (**non-cholinergic**), epinephrine and calcium (Flowchart 57.1).
   - Hypergastrinemia occurs in **Zollinger-Ellison syndrome** (Clinical Note 57.1).
   - Gastrin secretion is also elevated in **pernicious anemia**, in which acid secretion in the stomach is less as parietal cells are damaged. This causes ***feedback release of gastrin*** from G cells.

Clinical Note 57.1

Gastrinoma: Gastrinoma is a neuroendocrine tumor (NET) that produces gastrin. Though gastrin is not secreted from pancreas after birth, tumor of pancreatic islet (non-α–non-β cell tumor) secretes gastrin. Gastrin secreting tumor causes severe and chronic hypergastrinemia that causes peptic ulcer disease, which is often refractory and severe. This is called Zollinger-Ellison syndrome.

2. **Stimuli that decrease gastrin release:** Acid in the stomach, somatostatin, secretin, GIP, VIP, calcitonin and glucagon.
   - Acid in the antrum inhibits gastric secretion by **negative feedback mechanism**, which is partly by direct action of acid on G cells and partly by release of somatostatin.

Cholecystokinin

Source

Secreted from **I cells** in the mucosa of **upper small intestine**. CCK is present as neurotransmitter in cerebral cortex, in somatic nerves and in nerves of distal ileum and colon.

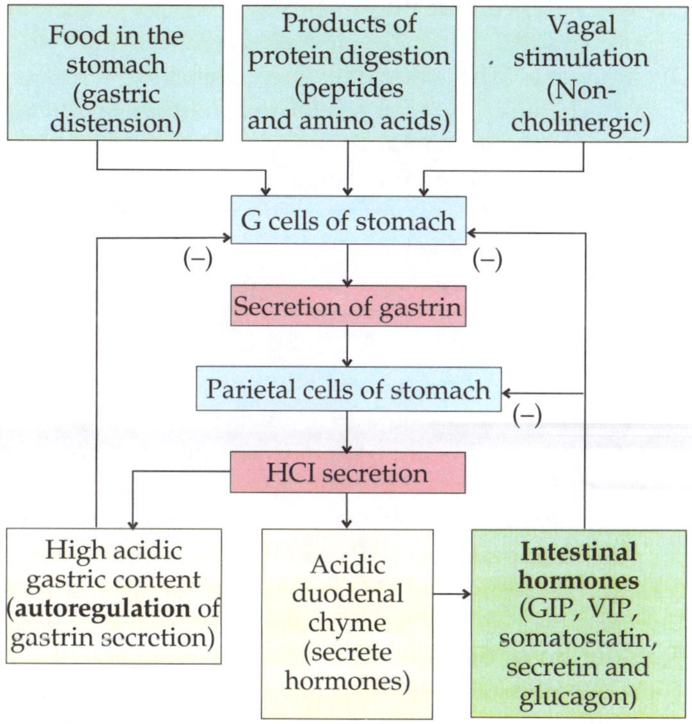

Flowchart 57.1: Regulation of gastrin secretion. Minus sign (–) indicates inhibition.

Structure

Cholecystokinin (CCK) is a polypeptide hormone.

- There are different forms of CCK depending on the number of amino acids present, like **CCK 58, CCK 39, CCK 33, CCK 12, CCK 8, and CCK 4** (carboxyl terminal tetrapeptide).
  - CCK secreted from duodenum and jejunum are usually CCK 12 and CCK 8.
  - CCK in the enteric and pancreatic nerves is mainly CCK 4.
  - The forms of **CCK in brain** are primarily CCK 58 and 8.
- **Half-life** of CCK is about ***5 minutes***.

Functions

1. CCK causes **contraction of gall bladder**. Therefore, CCK **increases bile release** into the intestine following a meal.
2. It stimulates **pancreatic secretion rich in enzymes**.
   - Therefore, CCK is also called *cholecystokinin-pancreozymin* (CCK-PZ).
3. It also **augments the action of secretin** to produce alkaline pancreatic secretion.
4. **Inhibits gastric acid secretion**.
5. **Inhibits gastric motility**, thereby *delays gastric emptying*.
6. Causes **relaxation of sphincter of Oddi** that allows both bile and pancreatic juice to enter duodenum.
7. Stimulates growth of pancreas.

8. Increases secretion of enterokinase.
9. Enhances motility of small intestine.
10. Stimulates **colonic movements.**
    - This action *mediates gastrocolic reflex.*
11. Augments contraction of pyloric sphincter.
    - Therefore, prevents ***reflux of duodenal contents*** into the stomach.
12. Stimulates glucagon secretion.
13. In brain, it acts as an anorexigenic neurotransmitter.
    - It **inhibits food intake.**
14. It also produces analgesia and anxiety.

Mechanism of Action: There are two CCK receptors: CCK A and CCK B.

- **CCK A receptors** are mainly located in the peripheral structures like gall bladder, pancreas, GI tract etc.
- **CCK B receptors** are present in central structures like brain areas.
- CCK acting on both receptors activates membrane **phospholipase–C** and stimulates production of intracellular **IP_3 and DAG.**

Regulation of Secretion

Factors that increase CCK secretion:

1. Contact of intestinal mucosa with products of digestion especially ***fatty acids, peptides and amino acids.***
2. Bile and pancreatic juice: Bile and pancreatic juice facilitate digestion of protein and fat. Therefore, they provide **positive feedback** for CCK secretion (Flowchart 57.2).

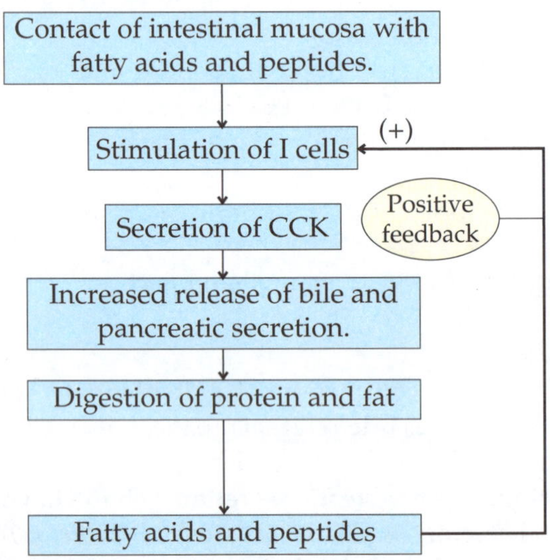

Flowchart 57.2: Regulation of cholecystokinin secretion. Plus sign indicates stimulation.

GI HORMONES OF SECRETIN FAMILY

Secretin

Secretin has an **important place in the history** of endocrine physiology, as it was the **First Hormone to be discovered** (Bayliss and Starling; 1902).

Source

Secretin is secreted from **S cells** located in the mucosa of upper part of small intestine.

Structure

Secretin is a **polypeptide** hormone containing 27 amino acids.

Functions

1. Secretin **increases secretion of pancreatic juice rich in bicarbonate** (watery and alkaline pancreatic secretion).
2. It also increases **alkaline bile secretion.**
3. Augments the action of CCK to produce pancreatic secretion rich in enzymes.
4. Decreases gastric acid secretion and motility.
5. Causes contraction of pyloric sphincter.

Mechanism of Action: Secretin acts on adenylate cyclase on the cell membrane and increases cytosolic formation of cAMP.

Regulation of Secretion

Secretion of secretin is increased by **acidic chyme and products of protein digestion** entering the upper part of intestine.

- Secretin stimulates watery and alkaline pancreatic secretion. When watery and alkaline pancreatic juice enters intestine, the acidic content of upper small intestine is neutralized.
- The increased pH of duodenal and upper jejunal content decreases secretin secretion by **feedback mechanism** (Flowchart 57.3).

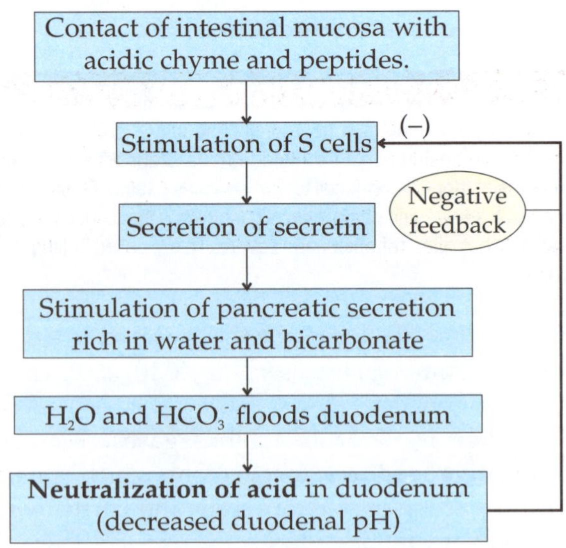

Flowchart 57.3: Regulation of secretin secretion. Minus sign indicates inhibition.

GIP

Structure: Glucose-dependent insulinotropic polypeptide (GIP) is a polypeptide hormone containing 42 amino acids. This is also called gastric inhibitory peptide (GIP).

Significant contribution of Scientist

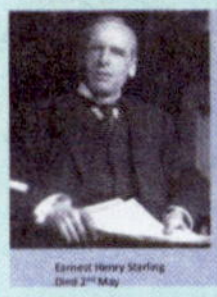

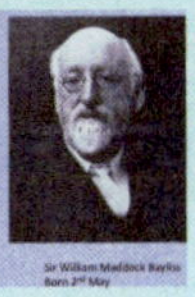

Ernest Henry Starling (1866 –1927) an English physiologist worked with his brother-in-law, **Sir William Maddock Bayliss (1860-1924)**. Both discovered the first hormone, Secretin in 1902. Three years later they introduced the hormone concept with recognition of chemical regulation, and regulatory physiology took a major step forward. To be noted, Bayliss was born on 2nd May and Starling died on 2nd May.

Source: GIP is produced by K cells present in the mucosa of duodenum and jejunum.

Functions: 1. It inhibits gastric secretion and motility.

2. It **stimulates insulin secretion**. For this function, GIP is considered as an important ***physiological regulator of insulin secretion.***
   - Though other hormones like gastrin, CCK, secretin and glucagon also stimulate insulin secretion, plasma ***level of insulin in response to GIP resembles the concentration of insulin*** attained following oral glucose ingestion.
     - Therefore, GIP is called **glucose-like insulinotropic polypeptide**.
- However, **GLP-1,** derived from glucagon appears to be more potent than GIP in promoting insulin secretion.
- Hence, both GIP and GLP-1 are among the important physiological regulator of insulin secretion from beta cells of pancreas.

Regulation of Secretion: Secretion of GIP is increased by glucose and fat in the duodenum.

VIP

Structure: VIP is a polypeptide containing 28 amino acids. It is formed from prepro-VIP that contains both VIP and PHM-27, a closely related peptide.

Source: VIP is secreted from mucosal cells of entire GIT, starting from stomach to colon.

- However, the secretion is more in the colon.
- It is found in the nerves of GIT, other autonomic nerves, blood and also in brain.
- Its half-life is 2 minutes.

Functions:

1. VIP markedly **increases intestinal secretion rich in electrolytes and water**. Therefore, in excess it produces **watery diarrhea**.
2. It causes **vasodilation**. Therefore, it ***decreases blood pressure.***
3. It **decreases GI motility**. It causes relaxation of intestinal smooth muscle including sphincters.
4. It potentiates the action of acetylcholine on salivary glands.
5. It **inhibits gastric acid secretion**.

Clinical Significance: The tumor of VIP secreting cells is called VIPoma. Profuse watery *diarrhea and hypotension* are major features of VIPoma.

Glucagon

This is structurally similar with glucagon secreted from A (α) cells of pancreas. In GIT, it is known as **enteroglucagon**. This produces hyperglycemia.

Source: Glucagon is mainly produced from ***A (α) cells in pancreas*** and ***L cells in intestine.***

A cells: In A cells, preproglucagon is processed to form **glucagon** and **major proglucagon fragments** (MPGF).

L cells: In L cells, it is processed to form **glucagon, glicentin** and **glucagon-like peptides** (GLP).

Both A and L cells also produce oxyntomodulin and glicentin related polypeptide (GRPP)

Glucagon-Like Polypeptides

There are two GLPs: **GLP 1 and GLP 2,** and both are also produced in brain.

1. **GLP 1** is a potent stimulator of insulin secretion.
2. **GLP 2** does not have definitive biological activity.
3. However, GLP 2 produced in the brain inhibits food intake and acts as a neurotransmitter in the neurons that project from NTS to dorsomedial nucleus of hypothalamus.

Oxyntomodulin & GRPP

Both A and L cells also produce oxyntomodulin and **glicentin-related polypeptide** (GRPP).

- **Oxyntomodulin** inhibits gastric acid secretion.
- Exact function of GRPP is not known.

OTHER GI HORMONES

Motilin

Structure & Source: This is a polypeptide hormone containing 22 amino acids. It is secreted from **enterochromaffin cells** and **Mo cells** present in the mucosa of all parts of GIT, except esophagus and rectum. It acts on G-protein coupled receptors on enteric neurons.

Functions:

1. It causes **contraction of intestinal smooth muscle** and therefore, ***increases GI motility***, especially in the interdigestive phase.
2. It is a **major regulator of migrating motor complex** (MMC), that regulates GI motility between meals.

Applied Physiology: Erythromycin can be used in patients having hypomotility of GI tract, as this antibiotic and its derivative bind to motilin receptors and facilitate intestinal motility.

Neurotensin

This is a polypeptide hormone containing 13 amino acids. It is produced by neurons and mucosal cells of intestinal epithelium, mainly in ileum. **It inhibits GI motility** but increases ileal blood flow.

GRP

Gastrin releasing polypeptide (GRP) is a polypeptide containing 27 amino acids.

- It is secreted from non-cholinergic vagal fibers.
- It mediates gastrin release via **non-cholinergic vagal stimulation.**
- The 10 amino acid residues at the carboxyl terminal of GRP is almost similar to the **bombesin** of amphibians.

Somatostatin

This is a polypeptide containing either 14 (*SS* ***14***) or 28 (*SS 28*) amino acids.

- Somatostatin is secreted from **GIT** (starting from stomach to colon), **hypothalamus and D cells of pancreas.**
- It **inhibits gastrin secretion.**
- It also inhibits secretion of VIP, GIP, secretin, and motilin.
- It is an **inhibitory neurotransmitter** in many parts of brain, especially in hypothalamus and pituitary.

Guanylin

Structure and Source: This is a polypeptide hormone containing 15 amino acids. It is produced by **Paneth cells** (endocrine cells located in the crypts of Lieberkuhn) of small intestine.

Mechanism of Action: It acts by stimulating **guanylyl cyclase** (hence called guanylin) which increases the concentration of **cGMP.**

- The cGMP in turn **increases activity of chloride channels** and increases **chloride secretion** into the intestine.

Functions: Guanylin **increases secretion of chloride ions** into the intestinal lumen and therefore **regulates fluid movement** across intestinal tract.

- Guanylin receptors are present in kidney, liver and female reproductive tract.
- In these organs, guanylin appears to control fluid movement and particularly integrates the actions of intestine and kidneys.

Applied Physiology: Enterotoxins of some ***strains of E. coli*** that cause diarrhea have structural similarity with guanylin. They **activate guanylin receptors** in intestine and produce fluid secretion into the intestinal lumen.

TRH

This is structurally similar to the hypothalamic TRH. But, as it does not enter circulation, it does not produce any effect on thyroid. However, it is involved in the regulation of secretory immunity of intestine.

ACTH

Structurally, it is **similar to the ACTH** of anterior-pituitary. The function of intestinal ACTH is not clearly known.

Ghrelin

It is a 28 amino acid polypeptide secreted mainly from stomach. It has more systemic effects than local actions.

- It is a **strong orexigenic** agent that increases food intake by acting on **arcuate nucleus of hypothalamus.**
- It stimulates secretion of growth hormone from anterior pituitary.

Peptide YY

It is a polypeptide hormone secreted from small intestine and colon.

- It **inhibits gastric secretion and motility.** Hence, it is proposed to be an **effective gastric inhibitory peptide.**
- Its secretion is stimulated by presence of fat in jejunum.
- Though, structurally it resembles neuropeptide Y that stimulates food intake, peptide YY inhibits feeding.

Substance P

Substance P is secreted from endocrine cells and neurons of entire GIT starting from stomach to colon. It **increases intestinal motility.** Its role in modulation of pain is discussed in "Physiology of Pain" in Sensory System.

Exam Questions

1. Classify GI hormones and describe their functions.
2. Name the GI hormones of gastrin family. Describe the functions, regulation, and physiological application of gastrin.
3. Name the GI hormones of secretin family. Describe the functions, regulation, and physiological application of secretin.

Multiple Choice Questions of Chapter 56

1. **Which of the following layer of GIT has the the Auerbach plexus?**
   A. Serosa B. Muscular layer
   C. Muscularis mucosa D. Lamina propria
2. **Which of the following is not a layer of the mucosa of GI tract?**
   A. Serosa B. Lamina propria
   C. Muscularis mucosa D. Epithelium
3. **The nerve plexus in the submucosa of GI tract was demonstrated by:**
   A. Auerbach B. Bayliss
   C. Meissner D. Oddi
4. **Which of the following is not correct about submucosa of ileum?**
   A. Highly vascular
   B. Contains many goblet cells
   C. Contains lymphatic tissues
   D. Contains network of nerve fibers

5. **Stimulation of sympathetic fibers to GIT results in all EXCEPT:**
   A. Contraction of smooth muscles
   B. Contraction of sphincters
   C. Decreased motility
   D.Inhibition of secretion
6. **Vagal stimulation to GIT leads to:**
   A. Inhibition of villous contractions
   B. Reduced peristalsis
   C. Reduced segmental contraction
   D. Increased exocrine secretions
7. **Which of the following is not true about immune system in GIT?**
   A. GI immunocytes secrete many cytokines
   B. Peyer's patches are important components
   C. They are not involved in causation of inflammatory bowel disease
   D. Immunological cells of GIT constitute about 50% of total immunocytes in the body
8. **Which of the following is not true about reflexes in GIT?**
   A. The long reflex is known as central reflex
   B. Enterogastric reflex is an example of long reflex
   C. The intrinsic neurons mediate the local reflexes
   D. Chemoreceptors in mucosa mediate the local reflex

Answers

1. B 2. A 3. C 4. B 5. A 6. D 7. C 8. B

Multiple Choice Questions of Chapter 57

1. **The cells in GI tract that secrete serotonin are known as:**
   A. Enterochromaffin cells
   B. APUD cells
   C. Neuroendocrine cells
   D. Myoneural cells
2. **Which of the following cells in GI tract do not participate in secretion of GI hormones?**
   A. Enterochromaffin cells
   B. APUD cells
   C. Neuroendocrine cells
   D. Myoneural cells
3. **Which of the following does not stimulate gastrin secretion?**
   A. Increased acid in the stomach
   B. Gastric distension
   C. Vagal stimulation
   D. Products of protein digestion
4. **Gastrin secretion is inhibited by all EXCEPT:**
   A. Secretin
   B. GIP
   C. VIP
   D. Epinephrine
5. **Which of the following is not a function of cholecystokinin?**
   A. Increased secretion of enterokinase
   B. Decreased colonic motility
   C. Relaxation of sphincter of Oddi
   D. Decreased gastric motility
6. **Gastrin has all the following functions, EXCEPT:**
   A. Stimulates insulin secretion
   B. Increases colonic contractions
   C. Inhibits gastric motility
   D. Stimulates exocrine pancreatic secretions
7. **First hormone to be discovered:**
   A. Gastrin
   B. Cholecystokinin
   C. Insulin
   D. Secretin
8. **Which of the following is true for Ghrelin?**
   A. Secreted from small intestine
   B. Strong anorexigenic agent
   C. Acts on arcuate nucleus of hypothalamus
   D. Inhibits secretion of growth hormone from anterior pituitary
9. **Which of the following is not about GIP?**
   A. Inhibits gastric secretion
   B. Inhibits insulin secretion
   C. Secreted mainly by K cells of duodenum and jejunum
   D. Secretion is increased by glucose
10. **Which of the following is not a function of VIP?**
   A. Increases intestinal secretion rich in electrolytes and water
   B. Causes vasoconstriction
   C. Causes relaxation of intestinal smooth muscle
   D. Inhibits gastric acid secretion
11. **Which of the following is not true about GRP?**
   A. Secreted by vagal cholinergic fibers
   B. Stimulates gastrin secretion
   C. It is a polypeptide hormone
   D. Action on gastrin is noncholinergic
12. **Which of the following statement is NOT true?**
   A. Motilin increases GI motility
   B. Guanylin decreases chloride secretion into the intestine
   C. Somatostatin inhibits GI secretion
   D. Peptide YY inhibits gastric secretion and motility

Answers

1. A 2. D 3. A 4. D 5. B 6. C 7. D 8. C 9. B 10. B
11. A 12. B

Chapter 58

General Principles of GI Secretion and Secretion of Saliva

Learning Objectives

On completion of study of this chapter:

The student will be able to (must know):

1. Name the phases of GI secretion and give their physiological importance.
2. List the general functions of GI secretions.
3. Name the salivary glands, and give the composition and function of saliva.
4. Outline the mechanism and control of salivary secretion.

The student may also be able to (desirable to know):

1. Describe the regulation of salivary secretion.
2. Describe the physiological basis of salivary dysfunctions.

Secretions from exocrine glands associated with GI tract are called **GI secretions**. The major GI secretions include secretion from:

1. Salivary glands (**salivary secretion**)
2. Gastric glands (**gastric secretion**)
3. Exocrine pancreas (**pancreatic secretion**)
4. Liver (**bile secretion**)
5. Intestinal glands (**intestinal secretion**).
6. Colonic secretion

A total of about 7 liters of secretions pour into GI tract from different exocrine glands (Table 58.1).

Table 58.1 | Daily secretion of juices from different parts of GI tract.

Secretions	Daily volume (lit.)	pH
Salivary secretion	1.0-1.5	7.5 -8.0
Gastric secretion	1.5-2.5	0.7-4.0
Pancreatic secretion	1.0-1.5	7.5-8.5
Bile secretion	0.5-1.0	Hepatic bile: 7.5-8.5 Gall bladder bile: 7.0 approx.
Intestinal secretion	1.0-1.5	7.5-8
Colonic secretion	0.5 approx.	7.5 -8

PRINCIPLES OF GI SECRETION

Phases of GI Secretions

Most of the GI secretions occur in **three phases**: cephalic, gastric and intestinal.

Cephalic Phase

When stimuli activate the **brain mechanisms** (*cephalic* means 'head') to alter GI secretions, the phase is called cephalic phase.

- **Sight, smell and thought** of food initiates cephalic phase of secretion.
  - **Taste of food** (food in mouth) and **chewing of food** that increase GI secretions are important stimuli for cephalic phase.
- Various **emotional states** also activate cephalic phase of secretions.

The **efferent pathway is the vagus nerve** that activates neurons in the ENS, which in turn influence gastric secretion and motility.

Importance of Cephalic Phase: Cephalic phase is important for **salivary, gastric, pancreatic and bile secretions**. It accounts for about **90% of volume of salivary secretion**.

- It contributes to about **40% of gastric and pancreatic secretions**.
  - This simply indicates that GI tract *prepares for digestion* even before food enters into stomach and intestine.
  - Therefore, it is desirable to **spend some time in taking soup and starters** before taking a major meal.

Gastric Phase

Gastric phase starts **when food enters stomach**. Stimuli that influence GI secretions when food is present in the stomach are:

1. Distension of stomach
2. Chemical composition (especially, amino acids and peptides) of food in the stomach
3. pH of the gastric content
4. Gastrin secreted from G cells

Importance of Gastric Phase: Distension of stomach is the major mechanical event of gastric phase.

- **Gastric distension** is the primary regulator of satiety.
- Gastric distension along with acidic chyme in the stomach and gastrin secreted from stomach, **activate short and long GI reflexes** to influence gastric, pancreatic, biliary and intestinal secretions.

Intestinal Phase

Intestinal phase is initiated when **chyme enters duodenum.**

- Products of digestion (fatty acids, peptides etc.), presence of acidic chyme, intestinal distension and osmolality of intestinal contents are important stimuli in the intestinal phase of GI secretions.
- They activate various **intestinal reflexes** to alter GI secretions.
- **CCK, secretin, GIP, VIP** and many other hormones are secreted during this phase.

Importance of Intestinal Phase: Chyme in the intestine requires enzymes for digestion of food particles in which the first step is to **hydrolyze macromolecules into their smaller absorbable forms.** This is achieved mainly by pancreatic and intestinal secretions.

1. Acidic chyme in duodenum **stimulates secretion of CCK and secretin.**
2. Through reflex mechanisms, food in intestine **inhibits gastric secretion and motility.**

Principles of Regulation

Regulation of GI secretions occurs mainly by **neural and hormonal factors.**

- **Cephalic phase** is predominantly regulated by **neural mechanisms.**
- **Gastric and intestinal phases** are regulated by **both hormonal and neural mechanisms.**

General Functions of GI Secretion

1. **Digestion:** Enzymes in GI secretion are key elements for digestion. Broadly, amylases digest carbohydrates, peptidases digest proteins and lipases digest lipids.
2. **Protection from infections:** Chemicals present in GI secretions protect the body from infections. Lysozyme in saliva is antibacterial, IgA in saliva provides local immunity and HCl in gastric secretion kills all types of organisms.
3. **Mixing:** The aqueous part of secretions helps in mixing of food with chemicals and enzymes in the secretions.
4. **Lubrication:** Mucus secretions facilitates passage of bolus of food or chyme along the GI tract.
5. **Protection of mucosa:** The mucus and alkaline pH of secretions protect mucosal epithelium of gut from the harmful effects of HCl, bile acids and toxins in the food.
6. **Absorption:** GI secretions present digested food materials to the epithelium of GI tract for absorption.
7. **Appetite regulation:** Chemicals in GI secretions stimulate appetite. For example, bile acids and HCl are appetizers in physiological concentration.

PY4.2

SALIVARY SECRETION

The secretion from salivary glands located in and around the mouth cavity is salivary secretion. It is distinctive for its exclusive neural regulation.

Salivary Glands

There are **major and minor salivary glands.**

1. **Major salivary glands** are three pairs: parotid, sublingual and submandibular glands.
2. Many **minor salivary glands** are located in the mucosa of oral cavity, at the pharyngeal outlet, in the palates and in buccal pouches.

Based on nature of secretion**,** salivary glands may be **serous** that exclusively release watery secretions, **mucous** that secrete viscous secretion mainly containing mucus and **mixed** that secrete moderately viscous secretions.

Parotid Glands: Parotid glands are the **largest salivary glands.**

- They are **entirely serous glands.**
  - Serous cells are usually arranged in the form of **rounded acini.**
- The parotid secretion is rich in **water and electrolytes** and lacks mucins.
- They pour their secretion into the mouth through parotid duct (*duct of Stensen*), which opens at the level of second molar tooth.

Sublingual Glands: These glands are situated below the tongue in the floor of the mouth.

- Secretions drain into the mouth through sublingual ducts (*ducts of Rivinus*).
- They are **predominantly mucous glands.**
- They secrete thick viscous saliva.

Submandibular Glands: Also called **submaxillary glands,** are situated below the inner ramus of mandible on both sides.

1. They pour their secretion through submandibular ducts (*ducts of Wharton*).
2. These glands are **mixed type** (both serous and mucous).

Histology of Salivary Glands

Salivary gland consists of base units called **salivon.**

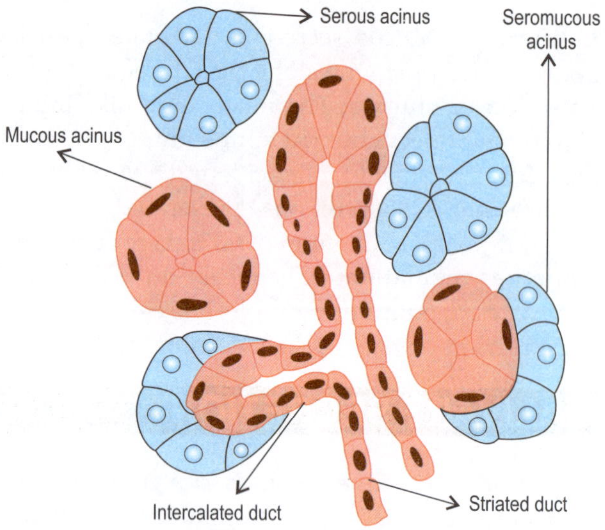

Fig. 58.1: Structure of a salivon (with types of acini in salivary glands).

Each salivon consists of acinus, intercalated duct and striated duct (Fig. 58.1).

Note the location of intercalated and striated ducts in the gland.

Acinus: Acinus is a sac like structure containing many **pyramidal cells**. Myoepithelial cells are present at places surrounding the pyramidal cells.

- **Serous cells** of acinus contain many endoplasmic reticulum and zymogen granules, and secrete digestive enzyme, whereas **mucous cells** contain mucin droplets and secrete mucin (Fig. 58.2).
- The secretion in the acinus is called **primary secretion**. Electrolyte composition of primary secretion is similar to that of plasma.

Intercalated and striated ducts: These ducts are lined by **cuboidal cells**.

- Secretion from these duct epithelial cells modifies the ionic composition of secretion from acinus and determines the final composition of saliva.
- Secretion coming out of duct is called **modified or final secretion.**

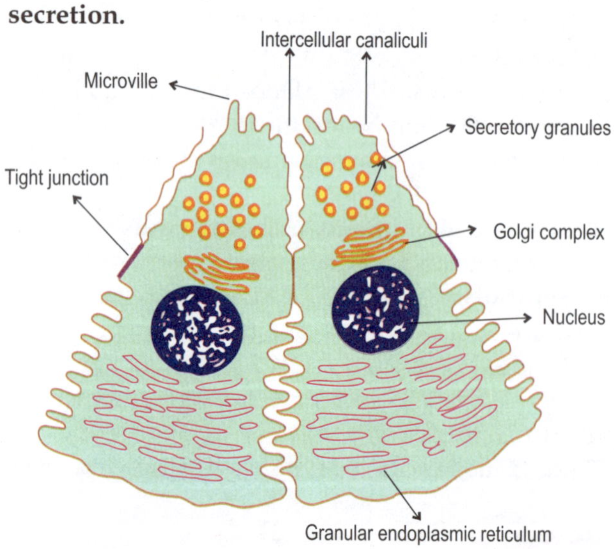

Fig. 58.2: Features of serous cells in a salivary gland.

Innervation of Salivary Glands

Salivary glands are innervated by both the divisions of autonomic nervous system. Parasympathetic activation is the major neural stimulus for salivary secretion.

Parasympathetic Innervation: The centers for parasympathetic fibers are located in medulla.

- Preganglionic fibers **for parotid gland** are present in 9th cranial nerve that originate in **inferior salivary nucleus** and terminate in **otic ganglion** from where postganglionic fibers originate and innervate the gland (refer Fig. 24.7, Chapter 24).
- Fibers for **submandibular and sublingual glands** are present in the 7th cranial nerve.
- In general, **parasympathetic stimulation is excitatory.**

Sympathetic Innervation: Sympathetic fibers originate from upper cervical segments and terminate in **superior cervical ganglion**. Postganglionic fibers leave the ganglion and innervate acini, duct and blood vessels.

- In general, **sympathetic stimulation is inhibitory**.

Salivary Blood Flow

Salivary glands have a high rate of metabolism and a high blood flow. Salivary blood flow is about **50 ml/min/100g** of salivary tissue, which is 10 times the blood flow to that of active skeletal muscles.

1. **Parasympathetic stimulation increases blood flow** by about 10 times by causing vasodilation, which occurs due to secretion of ***VIP, bradykinin and acetylcholine*** at nerve terminals.
2. **Sympathetic stimulation** *decreases blood flow.*

Salivary Secretion

Rate of Secretion: About **1.3 liters** (1000 –1800 ml) of saliva is secreted every day.

- An **orexigenic stimulus**, especially sight, smell or thought of food causes immediate and profuse salivation.
- Salivary secretion **increases in response to feeding**.

Composition of Saliva

Saliva contains mainly water (99.5%) and some solids (0.5%). Solids are organic and inorganic.

Organic Solids: Organic solids are mainly **enzymes** such as ptyalin, lysozyme, lactoperoxidase, carbonic anhydrase, lingual lipase, RNAase and DNAase.

- ***Other organic solids*** include kallikrein, blood group substances, secretory immunoglobulin (IgA), and nerve growth factor.

Inorganic Solids: **Cations** like sodium, calcium, potassium, and magnesium ions, and **anions** like chloride, bicarbonate, phosphate, sulphate and bromide ions constitute the inorganic solids.

Tonicity and pH

Tonicity of Saliva: In human beings, **saliva is always hypotonic to plasma,** about 70% of that of plasma. The tonicity of saliva depends on the rate of secretion. Greater the rate of secretion, higher is the tonicity.

The pH & K^+ content of saliva: The pH of saliva is **alkaline** (about 8).

1. The pH of the **original secretion** in the salivary gland is **slightly acidic**. But as saliva flows down the salivary ducts, it becomes alkaline because of **secretion of bicarbonate from the duct epithelium.**
2. **In increase in flow due to parasympathetic stimulation**, secretion of bicarbonate from duct cells is more that increases salivary content of bicarbonate.
   - Therefore, invariably with increased flow rate, bicarbonate content becomes high.
3. The concentration of **K^+ in saliva is always greater than that in plasma**, but with increase in flow rate, K^+ concentration decreases.

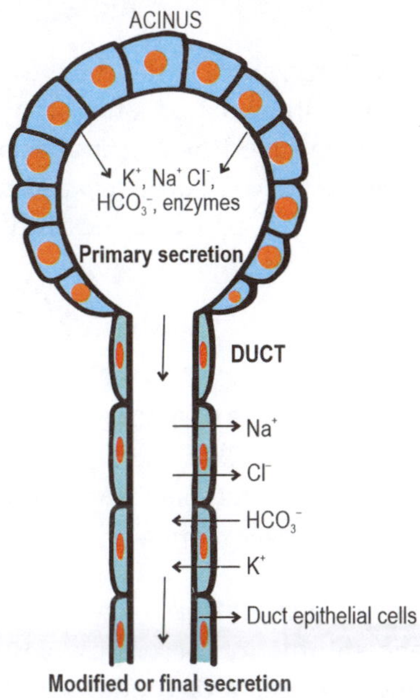

Fig. 58.3: Mechanism of salivary secretion. Note the processes that determine ionic compositions of primary and modified secretions.

Functions of Saliva

Saliva performs many important digestive and non-digestive functions.

1. Saliva contains **ptyalin**. This is an enzyme called *salivary amylase*, which causes **splitting of starch**.
   - Salivary amylase reduces starch to oligosaccharide molecules. However, digestion of starch is not impaired in the absence of salivary amylase (if pancreas is intact).
   - Action of salivary amylase is maximum at pH 6.8. But, digestion by ptyalin takes place in the stomach, as food remains for a short duration in mouth.
   - In the stomach, digestion occurs at the center of food bolus which is still alkaline, until the food is thoroughly mixed with the acidic gastric secretion of the stomach.
2. Saliva has many **protective functions.**
   - Saliva keeps the mouth clean and therefore **prevents oral infection**.
   - Saliva contains **lysozyme**, which is anti-bacterial.
   - **IgA** in saliva provides local immunity and **lactoferrin** in saliva is bacteriostatic.
3. Saliva keeps the mouth cavity and tongue moist, which **facilitates speech**.
   - The importance of this function of saliva is realized when mouth becomes dry due to decreased salivary secretion that impairs speech.
   - Dryness of mouth is usually felt before appearing for an interview, especially for learners.
4. Saliva increases the **taste of food**. Taste is perceived by the taste buds present in the tongue. For taste of food to be well appreciated, food particles should better be present in solution. Saliva dissolves the food and makes the solution of food.
5. Saliva helps in **mastication and swallowing**. This is due to lubricant property of saliva. The mucin in saliva lubricates food. In the absence of saliva, deglutition becomes impossible, especially for dry foods.
6. Saliva contains bicarbonate which **buffers gastric acid** to some extent in the stomach, and therefore reduces heart burn.
7. Proline rich protein in saliva **protects enamel** of the teeth and thus provides them strength. Proline also binds with tannin & reduces its toxicity.
8. Saliva **prevents injury to buccal mucosa** by diluting the hot and irritant food materials.
9. In animals, salivation (panting) is an important process of dissipation of heat and therefore, has contribution in **temperature regulation**.
10. Saliva ***excretes certain heavy metals, thiocyanate and morphine*** from the body.

Mechanism of Secretion

Salivary secretion occurs in **two stages**: secretion in the acinus and secretion in the duct.

Secretion in Acinus of Gland

In the gland acini, the secretion is called **primary secretion** in which ***amylase concentration is more***.

1. The enzyme is produced and stored in the zymogen granules.
2. On stimulation, granules are exocytosed and the enzyme is released.
3. The electrolytes secreted from the epithelial cells of the end pieces are Na^+, K^+, HCO_3^-, and Cl^-.
4. The **fluid of primary secretion is almost isotonic** to that of plasma.

Secretion in Ducts

The composition of secretion in the ducts when the fluid passes through the intercalated and striated ducts, is modified. This is called **modified** or **final secretion**.

1. This is because Na^+ and Cl^- are extracted from the fluid and K^+ and HCO_3^- are added to the fluid.
2. The ducts do not change the volume of saliva but only modify the composition of the primary secretion (Fig. 58.3).

Control of Salivary Secretion

Salivary secretion is controlled exclusively by the **neural mechanisms**. Both sympathetic and parasympathetic stimuli influence salivary secretion.

Parasympathetic Stimulation

Parasympathetic stimulation occurs by **sight, smell and taste** of food, and discussion on food .

1. **Chewing** of food is a potent stimulus for salivary secretion. These factors act through **salivary nucleus** in the medulla (Fig. 58.4).
2. Parasympathetic activation **increases salivary secretion rich in enzymes, and mucin**.
3. It increases secretion by causing *vasodilation* (via bradykinin, VIP, and acetylcholine), and *stimulation of glandular tissue.*

Sympathetic Stimulation

Sympathetic stimulation temporarily increases secretion but **finally decreases it.**

1. The **transient increase** is due to contraction of myoepithelial cells of the glandular tissue.
2. It causes *vasoconstriction* that **decreases saliva formation** and makes the secretion thick.

Reflex Secretion

Saliva is secreted reflexly by contact of food with the mouth cavity. This reflex secretion is **unconditioned** as this is present since birth (does not need learning). However, salivary secretion due to smell or thought of food is a **condition reflex** as these are learnt by social and environmental factors. Conditioned salivary secretion was described by Pavlov.

Hormonal regulation of saliva is negligible.

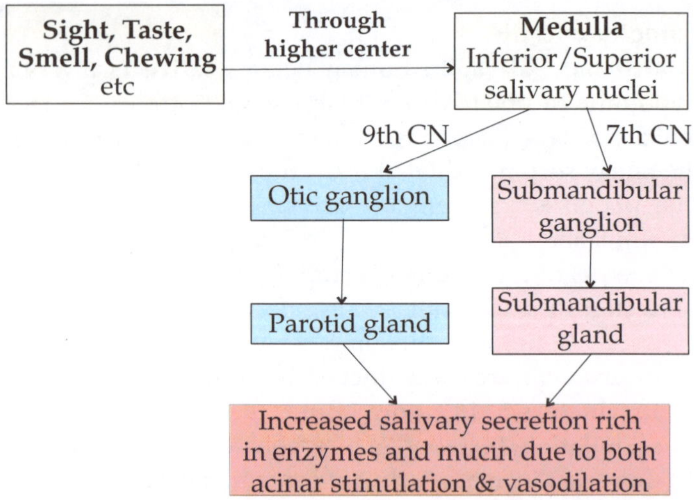

Fig. 58.4: Mechanism of increased salivary secretion by parasympathetic stimulation. CN: cranial nerve.

Applied Physiology

Xerostomia

This is a condition in which there is consistent **decreased secretion of saliva.** This causes dryness of mouth, and predisposes to oral infections. Xerostomia (**dryness of mouth**) is a common in acute **stressful situation** that happens due to sympathetic stimulation

Sjogren's Syndrome: This is an **autoimmune disorder** presents mainly with **xerostomia and xeropthalmia**.

- Main presentations are dry mouth, decreased tear formation, dry skin and joint pain.
- It is more common in women after the age of 40 years.
- May be associated with rheumatoid arthritis or lupus.

Sialorrhoea

In this condition, salivary secretion is increased persistently.

Sialolithiasis

This is the condition in **which stone is formed in the ducts** of salivary gland.

Infections

Viral infection of parotid gland is seen commonly in children (**mumps**).

Exam Questions

1. Describe the composition, mechanism and regulation of salivary secretion,
2. Briefly illustrate the phases of GI secretions and the basic mechanism of secretion in each phase.

MCQs are given in the page no 475

Chapter 59

Gastric Secretion

Learning Objectives

On completion of study of this chapter:

The student will be able to (must know):

1. List the functions of stomach.
2. List the composition and functions of gastric juice.
3. Describe the mechanism of HCl secretion
4. Describe regulation of gastric secretion in different phases.
5. Understand the physiological basis of gastric function tests.
6. Learn the causation of peptic ulcer and the physiological basis of its treatment.

The student may also be able to (desirable to know):

1. Explain the experimental designs to assess each phase of gastric secretion.
2. Describe the structure of gastric glands.
3. Explain the difference in the structure of resting and activated parietal cell

FUNCTIONAL ASPECTS

Functions of Stomach

1. **Temporary storage of food:** The primary function of stomach is the temporary storage of food.
   - It serves as a ***reservoir for food*** so that ingestion of a large meal at a time becomes possible.
   - It is stretchable and can store 1.5 to 4 liters of food, which depends on the habit of eating, age and gender.
2. **Grinding and mixing of food:** Stomach causes grinding and mixing of food.
   - It churns the food and breaks larger food particles (macromolecules) ***into smaller molecules***.
   - It also ***mixes food with gastric juice***.
   - The content of stomach after proper mixing with gastric juice is called **chyme**.
3. **Controlled emptying of food:** Stomach performs its **own controlled emptying (gastric emptying)**.
   - It allows food to enter into duodenum and jejunum ***at a lesser but controlled rate*** so that load on the upper part of the small intestine is not more than the amount that it can handle.
   - This allows intestine to digest and absorb nutrients slowly, steadily and adequately.
4. **Secretion of hydrochloric acid:** Stomach **secretes hydrochloric acid** (HCl), which is essential for digestion of food.
   - Though the exact nature of digestion by HCl is not clearly known, hypochlorohydria decreases the process of digestion and impairs appetite.
5. HCl in the stomach **converts ferric form of iron into ferrous form:** Iron is absorbed from gut only in the ferrous form.
   - Therefore, **HCl deficiency in the stomach results in iron deficiency anemia**.
6. **Kills the microorganism:** Gastric HCl kills the bacteria and other ingested microorganisms.
7. **Activates pepsinogen to pepsin:** HCl activates pepsinogen to pepsin, an *endopeptidase*.
   - Pepsin cleaves protein molecules to form smaller peptides.
   - The optimal pH for endopeptidase activity is 1.8 to 3.5. Thus, HCl not only activates pepsin, but also ***provides acidic environment*** for action of pepsin.
8. **Secretes intrinsic factor:** Stomach secretes intrinsic factor (IF) which is essential for **reabsorption of vitamin B_{12}** (the extrinsic factor) in the terminal ileum.
   - Therefore, gastrectomy or chronic gastric atrophy results in **megaloblastic anemia** (Clinical Note 59.1).

9. Stomach helps in **absorption of water and lipid soluble substances**, such as alcohol and few drugs.
   - Alcohol is absorbed much faster from stomach. Therefore, influence of alcohol appears within few minutes of consumption of alcohol.

Clinical Note 59.1

Dimorphic anemia: When red cell morphologies in an anemia have both microcytic and macrocytic features, the type of anemia is called dimorphic anemia. Anemia following gastrectomy or chronic gastric atrophy results in such type of anemia, as HCl deficiency causes microcytic hypochromic anemia due to iron deficiency and intrinsic factor deficiency causes megaloblastic anemia due to B_{12} deficiency.

Functional Anatomy

Anatomically, stomach is divided into **three major parts**: fundus, body and antrum (Fig. 59.1).

Esophagus opens into stomach through *gastro-esophageal junction* that contains ***lower esophageal sphincter*** (LES). Antrum opens into the duodenum through pylorus which contains **pyloric sphincter**.

1. The **mucous membrane of stomach** is thick and thrown into large folds, called **gastric rugae**. These rugae are more prominent in empty stomach (Fig. 59.2).
2. The mucosal epithelium is formed by ***simple columnar epithelial cells*** that secrete mucous and alkaline fluid.
   - These mucous and alkaline fluids protect gastric epithelium from acidic content and mechanical injury.
3. The mucosal surface of stomach is studded with **gastric pits** (faveola) into which gastric glands empty (Fig. 59.3).
4. The **gastric glands** are situated deep in the mucosal infoldings that open into the pits.

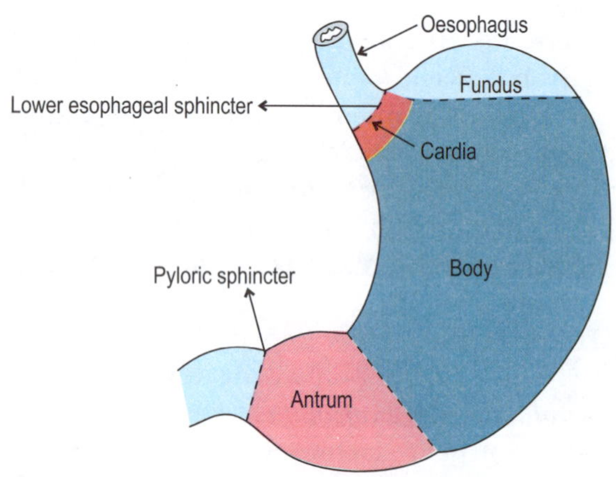

Fig. 59.1: Parts of stomach. LES: lower esophageal sphincter.

Gastric Glands

The mucosal lining of the stomach is a glandular mucosa that contains surface mucous cells in the gastric pit and glands deep in the mucosal infoldings.

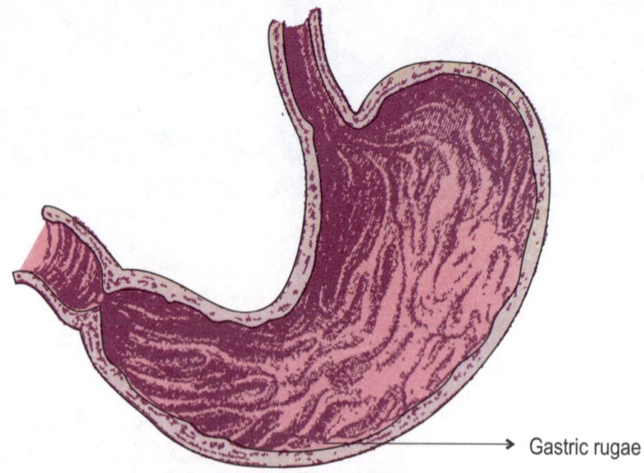

Fig. 59.2: Interior of the stomach. Note that the mucous membrane of stomach is thick and thrown into large folds, called gastric rugae.

There are **three types of gastric glands**:

1. **Cardiac Glands:** Located below the lower esophageal sphincter and contain mainly **mucous secreting cells.** They secrete mucous and bicarbonate ions.
2. **Oxyntic Glands:** Located in the fundus and body of the stomach and contain mainly the **oxyntic cells.**
3. **Pyloric Glands:** Present in the pyloric-antral region and consist mainly of **mucous neck cells** that secrete mucous and G cells that secrete gastrin.

Oxyntic Gland

The acid secreting oxyntic gland is typically a **tubular and straight gland**. It consists of neck, body and base.

Cell Types: Different cell types in the oxyntic glands are:

1. ***Mucous cells:*** They are present in the **neck region** of the gland. The **mucous and bicarbonate ions** secreted by them protect the stomach epithelium from acidic gastric secretion.
2. ***Oxyntic or Parietal cells:*** Oxyntic cells are present mainly in the **body part** of the gland (Fig. 59.3). They secrete **hydrochloric acid and intrinsic factor.**

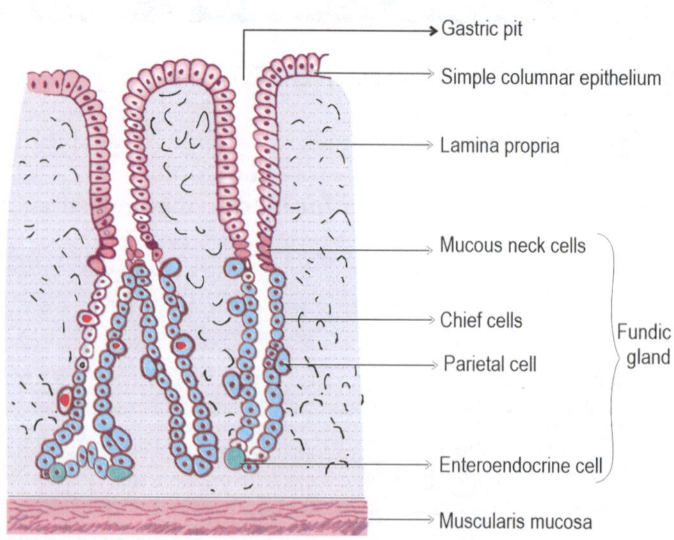

Fig. 59.3: Parts of a general gastric gland in the fundus. Note the location of gland in the deeper part of the mucosal infolding.

3. ***Chief or peptic cells:*** Chief cells are present in the body towards the base of the gland. They **secrete pepsinogen.**
4. ***Endocrine cells:*** The endocrine cells are also called **enterochromaffin or enteroendocrine cells.**They are located in the base of the gland.
   - The major endocrine cells in oxyntic glands are **enterochromaffin-like cells (ECL)** or **mast-like cells** that secrete histamine.
   - There are also other endocrine cells that secrete somatostatin, VIP, glucagon, and enkephalin.
   - **G cells** are present in antral region that secrete gastrin. Antrum also contains **D cells** that secrete somatostatin.

Structure of Oxyntic Cells

Oxyntic cells or parietal cells are present in the body of the oxyntic glands.

1. The apex of the parietal cells faces towards the lumen of the gastric glands.
2. The canaliculi extend from apical surface into the cell.
3. The tubules and vesicles open into the canaliculi.

Resting Cell: In **resting state** of the cells, ***tubules and vesicles*** are present abundantly and microvilli are rudimentary (Fig. 59.4).

- The membrane of these tubulovesicular structures contains **H^+-K^+ATPase**.

Activated Cell: On **activation**, the tubulovesicular membranes fuse with the cell membrane and microvilli that project into the canaliculi (Fig. 59.5), so that the **area of cell membrane** in contact with gastric lumen **is greatly increased**.

- Fusion of tubules and vesicle with microvillar or canalicular membrane ensures **increased H^+-K^+ATPase activity of the membrane** in the active state.

Nerve Supply of Stomach

Stomach is supplied by both divisions of ANS.

1. Parasympathetic innervation is by vagus nerve. **Vagal stimulation facilitates** gastric secretion and motility.
2. **Sympathetic stimulation inhibits** gastric secretion and motility.

Gastric Juice PY4.2

Volume & pH: The amount of gastric secretion per day varies from 1 to 2.5 liters. The gastric juice is highly acidic; having pH 0.7 – 4.

Composition of Gastric Juice

It has following constituents:

1. Water (99.5%)
2. Solids (0.5%)

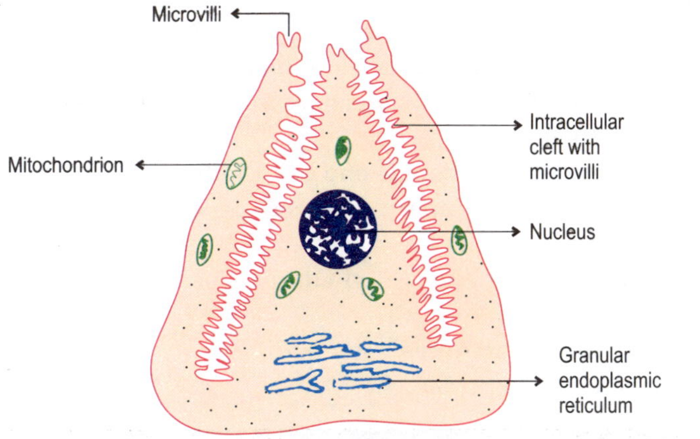

Fig. 59.4: Structure of a parietal cell in the resting state. Note the intracellular cleft contains tubules and vesicles.

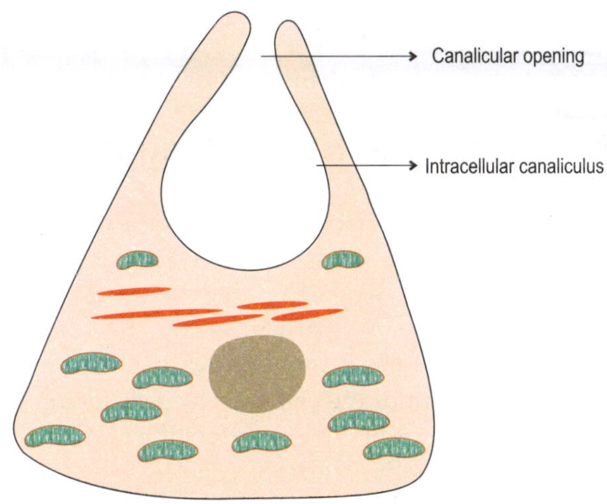

Fig. 59.5: Structure of a parietal cell in the activated state. Note that tubules and vesicles are inserted to the membrane of canaliculus to form big canaliculi, and mitochondria are bigger in size and more in numbers.

Solids contain inorganic and organic substances.

Inorganic Constituents: Anions are Cl^-, PO_4^{3-}, SO_4^{2-}, and HCO_3^-; and cations are H^+, Na^+, K^+, Ca^{2+}, and Mg^{2+}.

Organic Constituents: Pepsinogen, intrinsic factor, mucin, rennin, gastric lipase, gelatinase, carbonic anhydrase, and lysozyme.

Functions of Constituents

Normal concentration of HCl is 40–60 meq/L. The maximum concentration can increase upto 150 meq/L.

1. *Pepsinogen* is secreted from the peptic cells. There are **two types of pepsinogens**:
   - **Type-I pepsinogen** is found in chief cells in fundus and body.
   - **Type-II pepsinogen** is found in the chief cells throughout the stomach.
2. Pepsinogen is **converted into pepsin** by HCl.
   - Pepsin is a ***proteolytic enzyme*** that breaks down protein molecules into peptones. Pepsin acts best at pH of 2 – 4.
   - **Rennin** (also called chymosin) is a proteolytic enzyme.

3. The **mucin** secreted by mucous cells is of *two types*: the ***insoluble mucin***, and the ***soluble mucin.***
   - Mucin forms a *protective layer* on the gastric epithelium.
   - It retains bicarbonate and has **alkaline pH**. Thus, it protects the stomach from acid peptic digestion, as it **buffers HCl**.
4. **Intrinsic factor** helps in **vitamin B_{12} absorption** from terminal ileum.
5. HCl **kills microbes**, in addition to converting pepsinogen to pepsin.

GASTRIC SECRETION

Gastric secretion includes secretion of HCl and other major constituents such as synthesis and secretion of pepsinogen, mucus and intrinsic factor.

Mechanism of HCl Secretion

HCl is secreted from **parietal cells** that are located in the fundus and body of the stomach. H^+ secretion is possible in stomach due to the presence of numerous **H^+-K^+ ATPases** in apical membrane of the parietal cells.

1. **H^+-K^+ pump actively pumps H^+** (against its concentration gradient) out of the cell into the gastric lumen.
   - In exchange for H^+, the **K^+ enters the cell** (Fig. 59.6).
   - As this is an active transport, energy is provided for the process by hydrolysis of ATP.
2. In the cytosol of parietal cell, **H^+ is derived** from the ***breakdown of carbonic acid*** (H_2CO_3).
   - **H_2CO_3 is formed** by combination of CO_2 and H_2O in a reaction catalyzed by **carbonic anhydrase**.
   - This step can be blocked by *acetazolamide*, the carbonic anhydrase inhibitor.
3. **CO_2 utilized** for formation of H_2CO_3 is derived from *intracellular metabolisms* and plasma.
4. **HCO_3^- formed** by break down of H_2CO_3 is **exchanged for Cl^-** on the basolateral membrane of the cell ***by HCO_3^--Cl^- exchanger.***
5. The Cl^- that enters parietal cell is transported into the gastric lumen. In the lumen, Cl^- combines with H^+ to form HCl.
6. The **HCO_3^- enters blood stream** from the interstitial fluid. Thus, ***for each H^+ secreted*** into the gastric lumen, ***one HCO_3^- is reabsorbed*** into the plasma.
7. **Recycling of K^+:** K^+ that enters the oxyntic cell by H^+-K^+ ATPase is ***transported back*** into the gastric lumen, which is ***reutilized*** for further H^+secretion (recycling of K^+).
   - K^+ entering the cell from interstitial fluid through basolateral membrane (by the action of Na^+-K^+ pump located on basolateral membrane) is also secreted into the lumen.

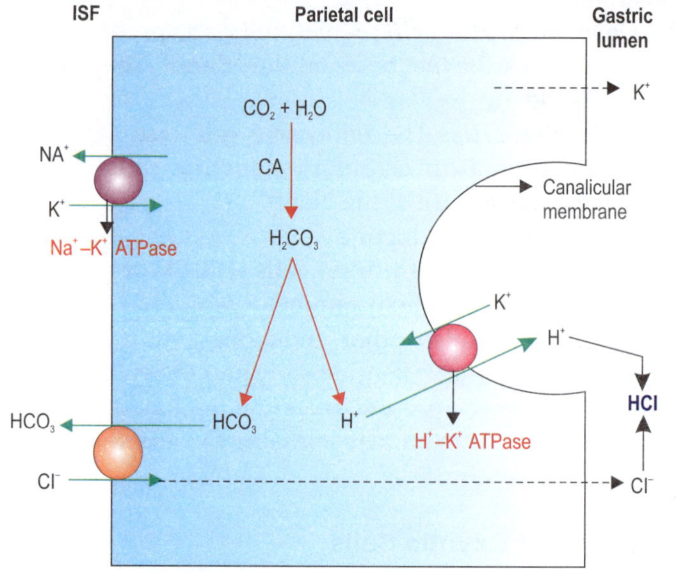

Fig. 59.6: Mechanism of HCl secretion from gastric parietal cell. The dashed lines for K^+ and Cl^- depict their passive diffusion into the gastric lumen. Note the presence of H^+-K^+ ATPase on the canalicular membrane that pumps K^+ into the cell for H^+ into the gastric lumen. ISF: interstitial fluid; CA: Carbonic anhydrase.

   - Thus, **adequate K^+ is available** in the lumen for effective H^+-K^+ pump activity.

Post-Prandial Alkaline Tide: As for each H^+ secreted into the gastric lumen, one HCO_3^- is reabsorbed into the plasma, with **increase in the rate of HCl secretion**, the level of ***HCO_3^- increases in the blood.***

- Consequently, **following a meal** that stimulates gastric acid secretion, **pH of blood increases.**
- As blood becomes alkaline, the **urine becomes alkaline.**
- This alkalinization of urine is called **post-prandial alkaline tide.**

Secretion of Other Constituents

Pepsinogen Secretion: Pepsinogen is secreted from **chief cells.** It is synthesized in the cell like other proteins and **stored in the zymogen granules.**

1. There are two types of pepsinogens: **type-I pepsinogen**, found in chief cells in fundus and body and **type-II pepsinogen** found in the chief cells throughout the stomach.
2. Pepsinogen is **converted into pepsin by HCl**. Pepsin is a strong ***proteolytic enzyme***.
3. Pepsinogen secretion is **stimulated by gastrin and histamine.**

Mucus Secretion: Mucus is secreted by **mucus secreting cells** that are plentily available in the neck region of gastric glands.

1. The **mucin** secreted by mucous cells is of **two types**: the ***insoluble mucin***, which is secreted by mucus secreting cells of entire gastric mucosa and the ***soluble mucin***, secreted from mainly cardiac and pyloric mucosal cells.

- Mucin forms a protective layer on the gastric epithelium.
- It **retains bicarbonate** and has alkaline pH.
- Thus, it **protects** the stomach **from acid peptic digestion**, as it buffers HCl.

2. Mucus secretion is **stimulated by increased blood flow** to the stomach.

Intrinsic Factor Secretion: Intrinsic factor (IF) is secreted from **parietal cells** along with HCl. It is a glycoprotein.

1. It is *synthesized like other glycoproteins* and its **secretion is stimulated by** factors that stimulate HCl secretion like **histamine and gastrin.**
2. IF helps in **vitamin B_{12} absorption** from terminal ileum.

Factors that Influence HCl Secretion

Factors That Stimulate Gastric Acid Secretion

Factors that increase HCl secretion from the parietal cells of stomach mainly act through locally altering the concentration of three hormones: **acetylcholine, gastrin and histamine**. In the parietal cells, there are specific receptors for these hormones (Fig. 59.7)

Acetylcholine: Acetylcholine is an effective stimulator of gastric acid secretion. It is released at the nerve endings of **vagal cholinergic fibers** that innervate parietal cells.

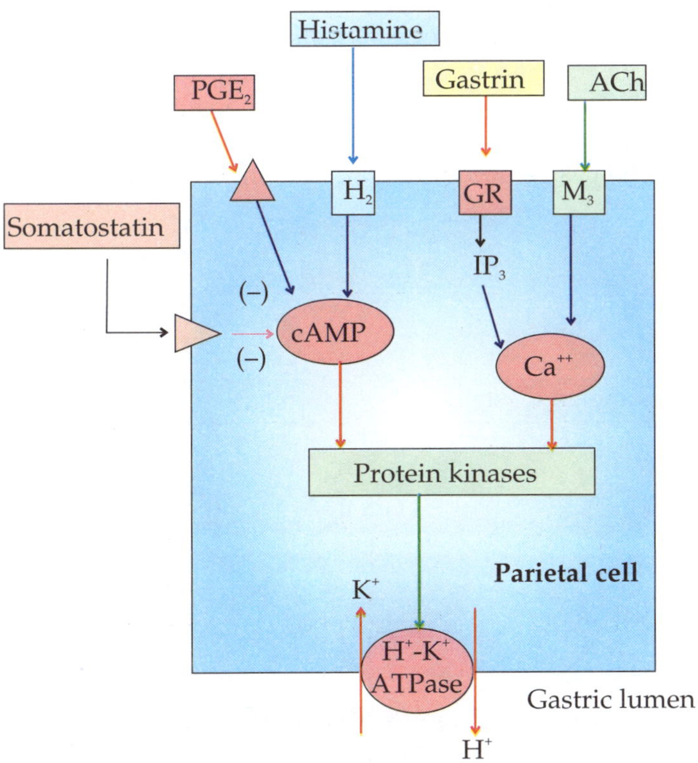

Fig. 59.7: Mechanism of actions of hormones on parietal cell. Note, finally calcium and cAMP act as second messengers for hormones that activate H^+-K^+ ATPase to pump H^+ into the gastric lumen. Minus sign indicates inhibition. GR: gastrin receptor; M_3: muscarinic type 3 receptor; H_2: histamine type 2 receptor; ACh: acetylcholine; PGE_2: prostaglandin E_2.

- Acetylcholine acts on the **M_3 cholinergic receptors** on the parietal cells and **increases intracellular Ca^{++}**.
- It **acts directly** on the parietal cell to increase HCl secretion and **acts indirectly** by secreting histamine and gastrin from ECL cells and G cells respectively that in turn stimulate parietal cells.

Gastrin: Gastrin is the **most potent stimulus** for HCl secretion.

- Gastrin acts on ***gastrin receptors*** on the parietal cells and increases HCl secretion by **increasing intracellular Ca^{++}** (Fig. 59.7).
- Gastrin is secreted from G cells that are present in the antral mucosa of the stomach.
- Vagal fibers innervate G cells and vagal stimulation increases gastrin release.
  - However, vagal fibers that mediate gastrin release are **non-cholinergic** as the neurotransmitter is GRP (**gastrin releasing peptide**).
- Gastrin also ***stimulates histamine release*** from ECL cells that in turn increases secretion of HCl from parietal cells.
- **Gastrin secretion** from stomach is ***increased by*** gastric distension, non-cholinergic vagal stimulation, protein rich food, and catecholamines.
  - **Pentagastrin** is used for assessing gastric acid output (Application Box 59.1)

Histamine: Histamine is a powerful stimulator of HCl secretion from stomach.

- It acts on **H_2 receptors** on the parietal cells and **increases intracellular cyclic AMP** as second messenger. Cyclic AMP stimulates protein kinase, which increases the activity of H^+-K^+ ATPase and HCl secretion.
- Histamine is secreted from enterochromaffin-like **(ECL) cells**.
- **Histamine release** is stimulated by both ***acetylcholine and gastrin***.
- Thus, histamine is considered as a **major mediator of HCl secretion**.
  - Therefore, patients with peptic ulcer are usually first treated with **histamine type-2 receptor antagonists.**

Mechanical and Chemical Factors: Accumulation of food in the stomach increases acid secretion. This mainly occurs due to **mechanical distension that stretches G cells** and stimulates gastrin release. Also, **products of protein digestion** (peptides and amino acids) increase gastrin secretion, and **hot and spicy foods** facilitate HCl secretion from the stomach (Table 59.1).

Application Box 59.1

Pentagastrin test: As gastrin is the most potent stimulator of HCl secretion, exogenously administered synthetic gastrin (pentagastrin) assesses the degree of acid output from parietal cell mass of the stomach. This forms the physiological basis of pentagastrin test.

Factors That Inhibit Gastric Acid Secretion

Increased acid output, somatostatin and acidic content of duodenum decrease gastric acid secretion.

pH of Gastric Luminal Content: Decreased pH of gastric content is an important and natural inhibitor of HCl secretion.

- When secretion of acid is high enough to decrease pH of gastric content to below 2, secretion of HCl is **inhibited by negative feedback mechanism**. Hence, this is called as **autoregulation of acid secretion**.
- The highly acidic gastric pH does not inhibit parietal cell directly; rather inhibition of acid secretion is **mediated by gastrin and somatostatin**.
- The highly acidic chyme **directly inhibits gastrin secretion** from G cells and **stimulates somatostatin secretion** from D cells of stomach.
- Somatostatin inhibits secretion of gastrin from G cells that decreases acid secretion.

Somatostatin: Somatostatin is secreted from the **D cells** of the gastric mucosa.

1. Decreased pH of gastric content (**pH less than 2**) increases the secretion of somatostatin, which **inhibits gastrin release**.
2. As gastrin is the most potent stimulator of acid secretion, decreased gastrin release decreases HCl secretion from the stomach. PGE_2 inhibits gastric secretion.

Chyme in the Duodenum: When **acidic chyme** enters duodenum, **secretin** is secreted from upper intestinal mucosa.

1. **Secretin inhibits gastric secretion** and motility, and gastrin release from G cells.
2. Products of carbohydrate and lipid digestion in the duodenum, and hyperosmolality of duodenal content inhibit acid secretion by increasing the release of an **enterogastrone** called GIP (***gastric inhibitory peptide***).
3. There are **other enterogastrones** also that inhibit gastric secretion.

Table 59.1 | Stimuli that alter gastric acid secretion.

A. Factors that increase HCl secretion
Luminal Factors
1. Distension of stomach
2. Products of protein digestion
Hormonal Factors (locally acting)
1. Acetylcholine
2. Gastrin
3. Histamine
Neural Factors
- Vagal stimulation (cholinergic & noncholinergic)
Blood borne
- Epinephrine
B. Factors that decrease HCl secretion
Luminal Factors
- Increased acid content (highly acidic chyme)
Hormonal Factors (locally acting)
- Somatostatin, PGE_2
Table 59-1 contd..
Blood-borne Factors
- Secretin, GIP, glucagon

Regulation of Gastric Secretion

Gastric secretion occurs in three phases (***cephalic, gastric and intestinal***) and the mechanisms regulating secretion are different for each phase of secretion.

Cephalic Phase

The cephalic phase of gastric secretion is elicited by **smell, sight, thought, taste and chewing of food**. This is called cephalic phase as impulses to increase acid secretion **originate mainly in the brain**.

1. The sensory stimuli **activate dorsal motor nucleus of vagus** in the medulla.
   - Therefore, cephalic phase of gastric secretion is **entirely mediated by vagus nerve** and the fibers are both **cholinergic and noncholinergic** (Fig. 59.8).
2. The vagal fibers that directly contact parietal cells are cholinergic and fibers that contact G cells are **noncholinergic** (**neurotransmitter is GRP**).
3. As **noncholinergic effects are stronger** than cholinergic effects, ***atropine can not effectively prevent*** *vagally mediated acid secretion*.
   - Therefore, *atropine is not prescribed* in the management of peptic ulcer.

The gastric juice secreted in the cephalic phase occurs before food reaches the stomach. Therefore, this is also called **pregastric phase**. This phase accounts for **30–50% of total gastric secretion** (Application Box 59.2).

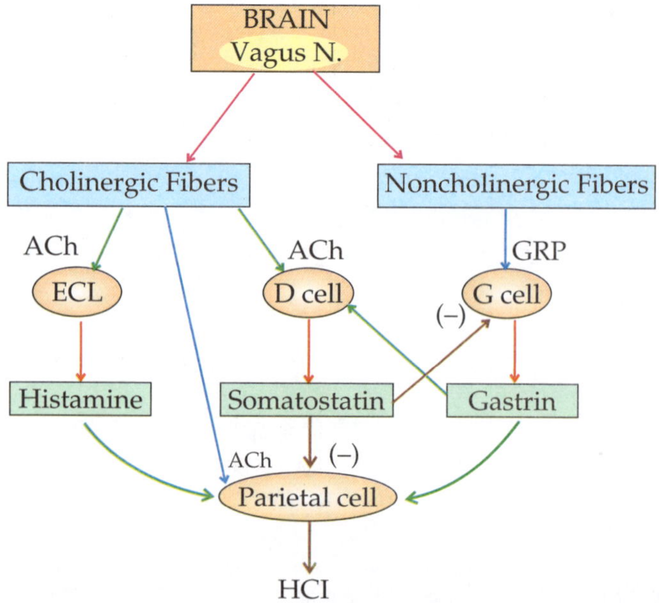

Fig. 59.8: Regulation of gastric secretion by vagus nerve. ECL: enterochromaffin-like cell; GRP: gastrin releasing peptide; ACh: acetylcholine; Minus sign indicates inhibition.

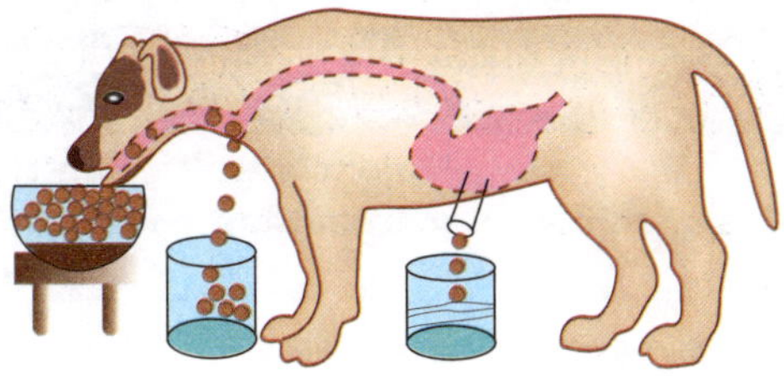

Fig. 59.9: Experiment of sham feeding. Note that food is not allowed to enter into the stomach, which is collected from neck through a fistula. Gastric juice is collected from the stomach through a cannula during the process of eating.

Experimental Design to Study Cephalic Phase

The usual experimental design to assess the integrity of the cephalic phase is the **sham feeding**. In this procedure, a dog is taken as the experimental animal.

1. A **fistula is made in the esophagus** of the dog; so that when animal eats the food comes out of the neck *through the fistula* (food is not allowed to reach stomach).
2. Simultaneously, the **gastric juice is collected** from the stomach by ***placing a cannula*** into it (Fig. 59.9).
   - Gastric juice obtained during the cephalic phase is analyzed for volume and composition.
3. Then, **bilateral vagotomy** is performed and the gastric juice is collected following vagotomy for analysis.
   - **Vagotomy abolishes gastric secretion** during cephalic phase, which proves that this phase is primarily vagally mediated.

Application Box 59.2

Appetite juice: The gastric juice secreted during cephalic phase stimulates the appetite, and therefore, this is called *appetite juice*, as it occurs in anticipation of food. Usually in parties and special dinners, enough time is spent initially in taking soup and appetizers before actual dinner is served. This is meant to stimulate appetite and to ensure enough gastric juice in stomach before food is available to the stomach.

Gastric Phase

The gastric phase of gastric secretion starts when **food enters the stomach**.

- The primary stimulus for secretion in this phase is the **distension of the stomach**.
- Also, **products of digestion** like peptides and amino acids produced by pepsin action that breaks proteins stimulate gastric secretion.
- The distension of the stomach elicits acid secretion by both local as well as central reflexes (Fig. 59.10).
  - **The central reflex** is mediated by vagus nerve (**vagovagal reflex**) and is both cholinergic and noncholinergic.
  - **The local reflex** releases acetylcholine that directly stimulates parietal cell.
  - Distension of stomach *per se* also increases gastrin release from the antral G cells that in turn increases HCl secretion.

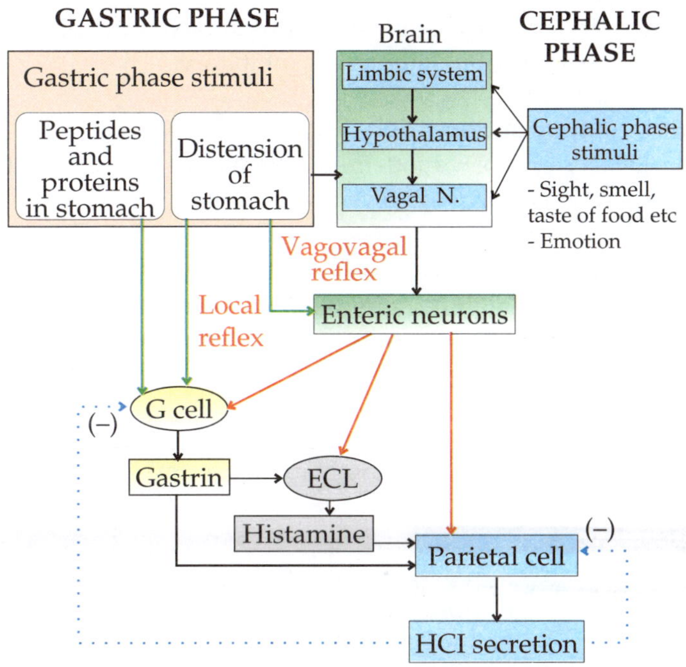

Fig. 59.10: Regulation of HCl secretion in cephalic and gastric phases of gastric secretion. Dotted lines depict HCl inhibition of G cell to reduce gastrin release and direct inhibition of parietal cell by HCl is indicated by minus signs. ECL: enterochromaffin-like cell.

- Amino acid and peptides stimulate G cells to release gastrin.
- Therefore, mechanisms of acid secretion in the gastric phase are **mechanical, neural, and chemical.**
- Gastric phase accounts for **50–60 % of gastric secretion.**

Autoregulation: HCl secretion in this phase is **decreased by the acidic pH** of the chyme bathing in the gastric mucosa. When pH of gastric content becomes less than 2, HCl secretion is effectively reduced. This is called **autoregulation** of gastric acid secretion. HCl **inhibits both G cells and parietal cells.**

Experimental Designs to Study Gastric Phase

Gastric phase of gastric secretion is studied by making five different types of pouches: **Pavlov pouch, Heidenhain pouch, Bickel pouch, Farrell pouch and Ivy pouch.** However, the pouch experiment to study gastric secretion is not performed now-a-days. This is mainly of academic and historical importance.

1. **Pavlov pouch** is a small pouch separated from the main body of the stomach by a double layer of mucous membrane. This gastric pouch of mucous membrane has intact nerve and blood supply. Therefore, it helps to study both neural and chemical factors of gastric acid secretion.
2. **Heidenhain pouch** is a denervated pouch, which helps to study the influence of neural factors on gastric secretion.

Intestinal Phase

When chyme enters the intestine, intestinal phase of gastric secretion starts. This is also called **post-gastric**

phase. Initial part of intestinal phase is stimulatory to gastric secretion, but later part is inhibitory.

Stimulation of Secretion

- Distension of duodenum increases gastric acid secretion by activating **vagovagal reflex**.
- The chemical composition of chyme, especially the products of protein digestion like amino acids and peptide ***stimulate G and other endocrine cells in the duodenum*** and upper jejunum to secrete ***entero-oxyntin***, which in turn stimulates gastric acid secretion (Fig. 59.11).

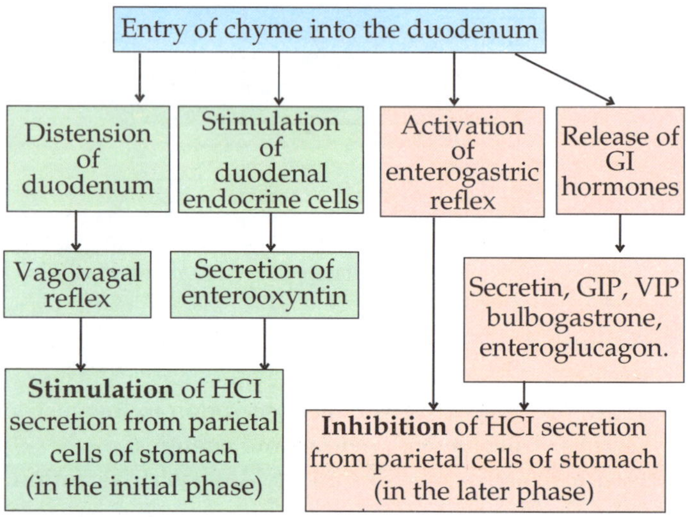

Fig. 59.11: Regulation of HCl secretion in the intestinal phase of gastric secretion. Though initially in the intestinal phase gastric secretion is stimulated, inhibition occurs in the later part of the phase. GIP: gastric inhibitory peptide, VIP: vasoactive intestinal peptide.

Inhibition of Secretion

- Acidic chyme in the duodenum (decreased pH of duodenal content) inhibits gastric secretion via **Enterogastric Reflex**.
- Acid also stimulates release of ***secretin***, which inhibits gastrin secretion from G cells. Secretin also decreases the response of parietal cells to gastrin and histamine.
- Acid in the duodenum and hyperosmolality of duodenal content also secrete a hormone called ***bulbogastrone*** that inhibits acid secretion from parietal cells of the stomach.
- Products of fat digestion especially fatty acids and triglycerides stimulate secretion of ***GIP and CCK*** from upper part of small intestine. These hormones ***inhibit secretion of acid*** from parietal cells.

Thus, the **net effect** of intestinal phase is the **inhibition of gastric secretion**. Hence, intestinal phase accounts for about **10% of gastric secretion**.

The differences between cephalic, gastric and intestinal phase of gastric secretion are summarized in Table 59.2.

Table 59.2 | Mechanisms of gastric secretion in three different phases.

	Major stimuli	Major control mechanisms	Contribution to total gastric secretion
Cephalic phase	It occurs even before the food enters the stomach i.e. psychic stimulation of gastric juice in response to sight, smell, thought or taste of food.	Its influence on gastric juice secretion are vagally mediated responses induced by activity in the CNS.	It accounts for approximately 30-50% of the total gastric juice secretion normally.
Gastric phase	It occurs once food enters the stomach.	Its influence on gastric juice secretion are primarily local reflex responses and response to gastrin	It accounts for upto 50-60% of the total gastric juice secretion normally.
Intestinal phase	It occurs once food enters the duodenum.	Its influence on gastric juice secretion are the reflex and hormonal feedback effects initiated from the mucosa of the small intestine.	Its contribution to gastric juice secretion is much less as compared to cephalic and gastric phase.

PY4.8

GASTRIC FUNCTION TESTS

Gastric function tests (GFTs) include:

1. Examination of gastric contents
2. Test for gastric acid secretion
3. Tests for pepsin, mucous, intrinsic factor
4. Tests for gastrin
5. Visualization of the interior of stomach
6. Tests for gastric motility and electrical activities (gastrography)
7. Obtaining biopsy from the suspected tissue.

Analysis of Gastric Content

Gastric content is examined for the normal and abnormal constituents. The following parameters are looked for in the gastric content sample: Volume of acid (acid output), pH, colour, acidity (total and free), and presence of blood, mucous and food particles.

Examination of gastric contents can be divided into ***three types*** according to the time of examination

1. **At rest:** Gastric juice is collected after the patient awakes in the morning, but still lying on the bed.
2. **After a meal in the post absorptive phase:** A specific diet is provided, which has a fixed composition (also

known as ***fractional test meal analysis***) followed by that gastric content is collected for analysis.

3. **After a specific stimulus:** A specific stimulus for induction of acid secretion is applied following which the gastric content is withdrawn. Mainly the maximum amount of acid output is checked in these types of tests.

Measurement of Acid Output

Two types of acid outputs are assessed: **basal acid output** (BAO), and **maximal acid output** (MAO). Acid output is measured to assess the size of parietal cell mass or the ability of parietal cells to secrete HCl.

Basal Acid Output (BAO)

Gastric juice is collected for about 60 minutes through a Ryle's tube introduced into patient's empty stomach following an overnight fast.

Normal Value: 10–40 meq/L or 0.5–2 meq/hour.

Significance: Increased BAO indicates high gastrin activity as occurs in Zollinger-Ellison syndrome. A pH more than 2.5 for the acid, rules out this syndrome.

Maximal Acid Output (MAO)

This is performed by a **stimulation test** in which a stimulant is injected to increase acid secretion. The chemical is injected and gastric juice is collected by Ryle's tube. Usual tests performed are given below. **Normal Value of** MAO is usually 12–60 meq/hour.

Histamine Test: Historically, histamine was the first standard stimulant used for gastric acid secretion test.

- **0.01mg/kg bodyweight of histamine** phosphate is injected subcutaneously with simultaneous administration of antihistaminic agent to prevent the untoward side effects.
- Then the acid output is measured, **every 10 minutes for 1 hour**. Upto 10 ml of gastric content is aspirated and analyzed.
- It is helpful in the diagnosis of **pernicious anemia, subacute combined degeneration of spinal cord** and assessing the maximum acid output following duodenal surgery.

Histalog (Betazole) Test: Histalog, is a better replacement for histamine as it does not require the simultaneous administration of antihistaminic agent due to its fewer side effects. **1-15mg/kg of histalog** is injected subcutaneously and similar protocol as in histamine test is followed.

Pentagastrin (Peptavlon) Test: Pentagastrin is injected subcutaneously at a **dose of 6µg/kg** and acid output is measured. Being a synthetic analogue of gastrin, it is a potent stimulus for acid secretion.

Insulin Test (Hollander test): Principle of the test is that hypoglycemia produced by insulin causes **vagal stimulation.** Therefore, insulin is used for measuring acid output.

- 15 IU of soluble insulin is injected intravenously, and gastric content is collected every 15 minutes interval for two and half hours.
- Usually, insulin test is performed **to assess the completeness of vagotomy.** No increase in acid production should occur if the vagal resection is complete.

Fractional Test Meal Analysis

Patient is allowed to take a meal that has a particular composition, following which small fractions (10 ml) of gastric content is removed through Ryle's tube every 15 min to estimate the acid secretion for about 3 hours (in 13 samples).

- This test indicates the **acid secretion capacity in the post-absorptive phase.**
- It is useful in the detection of hyperchlorhydria, hypochlorhydria and achlorohydria.

Significance of BAO and MAO

In gastric ulcer, the values of BAO and MAO are usually normal or slightly below normal.

Higher values are found in: Duodenal ulcer and Zollinger-Ellison syndrome (gastrinoma)

Lower values are found in: Pernicious anemia (atrophic gastritis) and Gastric malignancy (Achlorhydria in the presence of gastric ulcer is highly suggestive of gastric malignancy)

Tests for Other Gastric Secretory Products

Test for Pepsin: Pepsin inhibitors are used for analysis of pepsin derived from pepsinogen. The level of pepsin is *low in atrophic gastritis.*

Test for Mucous: Protein content of gastric mucous is measured, normal value being 1.8mg/ml.

- The level is ***increased in chronic hypertrophic gastritis*** (Menetrier disease).

Test for Intrinsic factor: Intrinsic factor (IF) is essential for vitamin B_{12} absorption.

- Schilling test is used for evaluation of patients with suspected ***pernicious anemia***.

Test for Gastrin: The circulating gastrin level is normally 0-200 pg/mL.

1. *Serum gastrin level* estimation by radioimmunoassay (RIA) is commonly used.
   - Normal fasting level of gastrin is 20-150 pg/mL. its levels are higher in
2. *Gastrin provocative tests* are: Secretin test and Calcium infusion test

Other Tests

Barium-Meal X-Ray

A barium-mixed food is swallowed by the subject following which x-rays of upper GI tract are obtained.

- This gives the details of the contour of the lower esophagus, stomach and upper small intestine.
- The **location and size of the ulcer and tumor** can be delineated.

Endoscopy (Gastroscopy)

A fiber-optic gastroscope is introduced into the stomach to study the details of the ulcer or other pathologies. The advantages are:

1. It gives an opportunity to **visualize the lumen** of the stomach, so that the ulcer details can be seen.
2. A **biopsy of the ulcer** can be taken to study the type of ulcer (to exclude malignancy).
3. The tissue is also cultured to study the organism (*to confirm H. pylori infection*).
4. The gastroscope can be introduced into the duodenum and biliary tract to study further details.
5. **Urease test** is performed from the biopsy sample for **H. Pylori confirmation**.

APPLIED ASPECTS

Gastritis

The term gastritis is commonly employed for any clinical condition with upper abdominal discomfort like indigestion or dyspepsia in which the specific clinical signs and radiological abnormalities are absent. Acute gastritis is often due to irregular diet habits, infections, drugs and severe stress. Chronic gastritis, if untreated leads to peptic ulcer.

Peptic Ulcers PY4.9

Peptic ulcer means ulcer in the stomach (**gastric ulcer**) or duodenum (**duodenal ulcer**). Peptic ulcer is called **acid-peptic disease**.

Pathophysiology

Peptic ulcer is caused either by decreased mucosal defense, or by hypersecretion of acid or infection.

Diminished effectiveness of Mucosal Barrier

Mucosal defense barrier is due to the mucus secreted by mucous cells.

- Mucus is a viscous gel that contains mucin, phospholipid, electrolytes (mainly HCO_3^-) and water.
- The **mucous gel layer** is about 0.2 mm thick and effectively separates the bicarbonate rich secretion of epithelial cells from the acidic content of the stomach (Fig. 59.12).
  - This allows the **pH of the epithelial cells to remain alkaline** despite acidic pH of gastric content.
  - It protects mucosal epithelium from injury caused by acidic chyme.

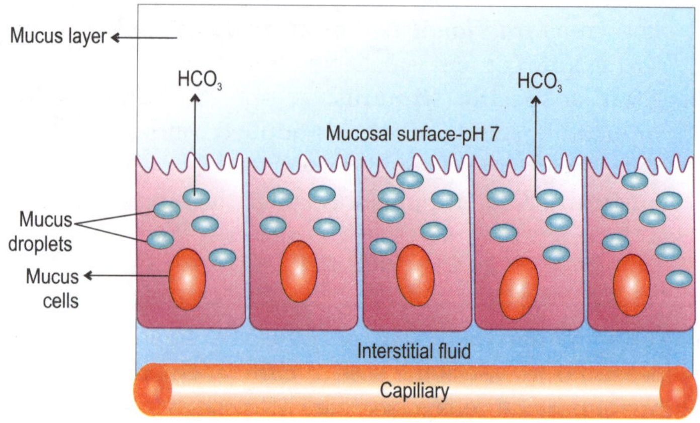

Fig. 59.12: Gastric mucosal defence barrier by mucus and bicarbonate.

- When secretion of mucus is impaired, or bicarbonate production is decreased or when the mucosal coat is mechanically damaged, acid and pepsin cause ulcer formation.

Hypersecretion of Acid

Gastric acid secretion is high in life full of stress. Intake of *more spicy food* is known to increase acid secretion. Therefore, it is stated that **hurry**, **worry**, and **curry** are the causes of peptic ulcer.

Conditions that **cause hyperchlorhydria** are:

- Zollinger-Ellison syndrome
- Gastric outlet obstruction syndrome (as occurs in pyloric stenosis)
- Systemic mastocytosis (histamine secreted from mast cell increases HCl secretion)

Zollinger-Ellison syndrome is a non-α non-β *gastrin secreting tumor of pancreas.*

Helicobacter Pylori Infection

Recently it is reported that **infection by H. pylori** is the major cause of peptic ulcer.

1. This is a **Gram-negative bacillus** that secretes an enzyme called **urease** that converts urea into carbon dioxide and ammonia. Ammonia buffers the acid surrounding the bacteria.
2. H. pylori colonizes the antral mucosa, where it causes **local inflammation** and **disrupts immune responses**. It also **inhibits somatostatin secretion** from D cells that facilitates gastrin release and consequently increased HCl secretion.
3. Therefore, antibiotic therapy to kill H. pylori is frequently successful in the treatment of peptic ulcer.

Clinical Features

In most of the cases ulcer is located in the duodenum, **usually above the ampulla of Vater**, as in this area acidic chyme is not neutralized by alkaline pancreatic juice.

- The main feature of peptic ulcer is **upper abdominal pain** (*epigastric pain*).

- Typically, pain is **experienced in empty stomach** and is **relieved by taking water, food or antacid**.
- If disease is untreated, **hematemesis** (vomiting of blood) or **malena** (dark, tarry stool), **vomiting** (due to pyloric obstruction), and peritonitis due to **perforation of ulcer** into the peritoneal cavity occurs.

Treatment

Specific Treatment

The specific treatment includes use of following drugs.

1. **H_2 receptor antagonists: Ranitidine, cimetidine, famotidine, and nizatidine** are different generations of H_2 receptor blockers.
   - These drugs **block the H_2 receptors** and inhibit histamine secretion.
   - As histamine is a potent stimulator of HCl release from parietal cells, H_2 receptor blockers inhibit HCl secretion.
2. **Proton-pump blocker (H^+-K^+ATPase inhibitor):** This drug inhibits the activity of proton-pump, i. e. the activity of H^+-K^+ATPase. Therefore, the final step of acid secretion is inhibited.
   - This is the most effective medicine for the treatment of peptic ulcer.
   - The usual proton-pump blocker used is **omeprazole**.
3. **Sucralfate:** This is a sucrose octasulfate. It provides a **protective layer** on the ulcer. Therefore, it promotes ulcer healing.
4. **Muscarinic blockers:** Atropine and pirenzepine were used earlier to block the M_1 and M_3 receptors. However, they are not effective and not used.
5. **Gastrin blockers:** A successful gastrin blocker has not yet been used. **Proglumide**, a gastrin blocker is used recently for the purpose.
6. **Antibiotics:** Recently, **high dose of antibiotics** such as amoxicillin to **kill H. pylori** has provided promising result.

Non-specific Measures

Antacids: Antacids give immediate and temporary relief from pain.

Yoga, Relaxation & Other Measures: Yoga, adequate **sleep** and rest, regulation of **diet**, and withdrawal of **drugs** like aspirin and NSAID improve the condition. **Use of cold milk** and **avoidance of spicy food & alcohol** also help in curing the disease.

Surgical Treatment

Inspite of effective use of medicines if the disease is not cured, surgery is advocated. The usual surgical procedures are:

1. **Vagotomy: Truncal vagotomy** (cutting the trunk of vagus nerves in abdomen just below the diaphragm), **selective vagotomy** (cutting vagal branch that supplies stomach), and **highly selective vagotomy** (cutting the vagus fibers that preferentially innervate the parietal cell). *Parietal cell vagotomy is preferred.*
2. **Gastrectomy:** Partial gastrectomy **removes the antral portion of stomach**, as this part contains G cells.
   - **Antrum is the pump** of the stomach that propels food into duodenum. Therefore, *antrectomy results in **stasis of food.***
   - To avoid such complication, usually gastroduodenostomy or **gastrojejunostomy** (the ***drainage procedures***) is performed with gastrectomy.
   - Gastrojejunostomy is also performed with truncal vagotomy.

Exam Questions

1. With the help of a suitable diagram, describe the mechanism of gastric HCl secretion. Briefly describe the regulation of gastric secretion.
2. What are the phases of gastric secretion? Describe the regulation of of gastric secretion in different phases with experimental evidences.
3. Give the composition and functions of gastric secretion. Briefly describe the gastric function tests.
4. Describe the pathophysiology of peptic ulcer. Give note on physiological basis of treatment of peptic ulcer.

Multiple Choice Questions for Chapter 58

1. **Which of the following is NOT true for cephalic phase GI secretion?**
   A. Accounts for 90% of salivary secretion
   B. Thought of food initiates this phase
   C. Efferent pathway is vagus nerve
   D. Accounts for 10% of gastric secretion
2. **Which of the following is not considered as a major salivary gland?**
   A. Parotid gland
   B. Sublingual gland
   C. Pharyngeal gland
   D. Submandibular gland
3. **The quantity of daily salivary secretion is about:**
   A. 1.5 lit B. 3 lit
   C. 0.5 lit D. 5.0 lit
4. **The pH of salivary secretion is about:**
   A. <7 B. 7.5 to 8
   C. >8.5 D. 4 to 6
5. **Lysozyme is present in**
   A. Saliva B. Human milk
   C. Tears D. Mucus
6. **Maximum potassium ions secretion is seen in**
   A. Saliva B. Gastric secretions
   C. Jejunal secretions D. Colonic secretions

7. **Salivary amylase is inactivated by**
   A. Enteropeptidase
   B. Low pH of stomach
   C. High pH of intestine
   D. Intestinal mucus
8. **Stimulation of parasympathetic nerve to salivary gland causes:**
   A. Viscid secretion
   B. Decreased secretion
   C. Increased secretion rich in enzyme and mucin
   D. Secretion is unaffected
9. **Which of the following is NOT true about the salivary gland output in Sjogren's syndrome?**
   A. Decreased output of salivary glands <0.5 ml/min
   B. Increase in IgA concentration
   C. Increase in sodium concentration
   D. Increase in phosphate concentration
10. **Which of the following is NOT true about saliva?**
    A. Excretes morphine from body
    B. Ig G in saliva provides immunity
    C. Increases taste of food
    D. Buffers gastric acid to some extent

Answers

1. D 2. C 3. A 4. B 5. A 6. A 7. B 8. C 9. D 10. B

Multiple Choice Questions of Chapter 59

1. **Cephalic phase of gastric secretion starts:**
   A. On stress B. On food entering intestine
   C. On food entering stomach D. On seeing food
2. **Daily secretion of gastric juice is about:**
   A. 2 liters B. < 1 liter
   C. 5 liters D. 7 liters
3. **Lower esophageal sphincter:**
   A. Has no tonic activity
   B. Has a tone which is provided by the sympathetic system
   C. Relaxes on increasing abdominal pressure
   D. Relaxes ahead of the peristaltic wave
4. **Rennin is present in**
   A. Gastric juice B. Liver
   C. Kidney D. Lung
5. **Pepsinogen is secreted by**
   A. Parietal cells B. Mucus cells
   C. Chief cells D. Oxyntic cells
6. **Intrinsic factor of castle is secreted by which of the following cells in gastric glands:**
   A. Chief cells B. Parietal or Oxyntic cells
   C. Enterochromaffin cells D. B cells
7. **Which of the following enzyme is stable at acidic low pH**
   A. Pepsin/ pepsinogen B. Trypsin
   C. Chymotrypsin D. Carboxypeptidase
8. **Chymotrypsinogen in activated into chymotrypsin by**
   A. Trypsin B. Pepsin
   C. Fatty acids D. Bile salts
9. **Trypsinogen is converted to trypsin by**
   A. Pepsin B. Enterokinase
   C. HCl D. None
10. **All of the following are secreted proenzyme from except**
    A. Trypsin B Chymotrypsin
    C. Pepsin D. Ribonuclease and Amylase
11. **Following are gastrointestinal hormones except**
    A. CCK-PZ B. GIP
    C. Motilin D. Chymotrypsin
12. **What percent of gastric secretion is due to cephalic phase?**
    A. 10% B. 20%
    C. 40% D. 60%
13. **Cephalic phase of gastric secretion is mediated by**
    A. Neurohormones B. Parasympathetic
    C. Sympathetic D. Gastrin
14. **The gastric phase of gastric HCl secretion is brought about by all EXCEPT:**
    A. Neural factors B. Gastrin hormonal factors
    C. Gastric distension D. Presence of proteins in the stomach
15. **Gastric secretion is increased by all except**
    A. Histamine B. Acetylecholine
    C. Gastrin D. HCl
16. **HCl secretion is stimulated by**
    A. Secretin B. Somatostatin
    C. Histamine & Gastrin D. VIP
17. **Gastric secretion is:**
    A. Inhibited by curare
    B. Stimulated by noradrenaline
    C. Increased by stomach antral distention
    D. Stimulated by an increase in tonic activity
18. **Physiological gastrectomy is:**
    A. Ligate all major arteries
    B. Antrectomy
    C. Upper 1/3 of stoma resected
    D. Ligation of 4-out of five arteries
19. **Which of the following is not a gastric function test?**
    A. Histamine test B. Secretin test
    C. Insulin test D. Pentagastrin test
20. **Peptic ulcer can be due to all of the following, EXCEPT:**
    A. Less stressful works B. Bad diet habit
    C. NSAID drugs D. H. Pylori infection

Answers

1. D 2. A 3. D 4. A 5. C 6. B 7. A 8. A 9. B 10. D 11. D
12. C 13. B 14. D 15. D 16. C 17. C 18. A 19. B 20. A

Chapter 60

Pancreatic Secretion

Learning Objectives

On completion of study of this chapter:

The student will be able to (must know):

1. Understand the role of exocrine pancreas in digestion and absorption of nutrients.
2. Give the composition and functions of pancreatic juice.
3. Describe the mechanism of pancreatic secretion.
4. Outline the regulation in different phases of pancreatic secretion.
5. Appreciate the application of pancreatic function tests.

The student may also be able to (desirable to know):

1. Describe pancreatic function tests.
2. Explain the physiological basis of pancreatic abnormalities.

FUNCTIONAL ASPECTS

The exocrine pancreas constitutes about 80% of the total mass of the pancreas (12% by ducts and blood vessels, and 2% by endocrine tissues). This is a unique organ in the body having **both major endocrine and exocrine** tissues in it.

Functional Anatomy

Structure of Exocrine Pancreas

Pancreas forms a major part of the **stomach bed**. The head of pancreas fits into the 'C' curvature of the duodenum.

Pancreatic duct combines with common bile duct to form **hepatopancreatic duct** (form hepatopancreatic ampulla *or* ***ampulla of Vater***) that opens into second part of duodenum as major duodenal papilla via **sphincter of Oddi** (Fig. 60.1).

Often, an **accessory pancreatic duct** opens separately into duodenum as ***minor duodenal papilla***.

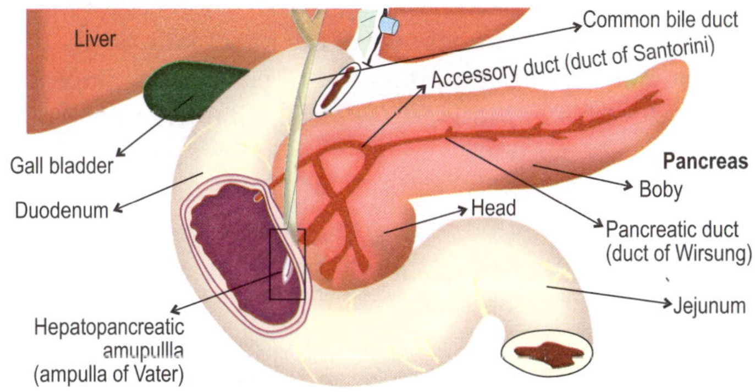

Fig. 60.1: Location and gross structure of pancreas.

Histology & Secretory Apparatus

Histologically, exocrine pancreas *resembles salivary glands*. The exocrine tissue of pancreas consists of **lobules** that contain multiple **acini** (Fig. 60.2).

1. **Acini** are sac like dilatations composed of single layer of pyramidal (acinar) cells. Acinar cells contain multiple endoplasmic reticulum, Golgi apparatus and zymogen granules that are located in the apical region of the acinar cells.
2. A few **centroacinar cells** line the lumen of the acinus.
3. Acini open to **intercalated duct** which in turn empty into **intralobular duct**.
4. Intralobular duct drains into **extralobular duct** that finally open to the main **collecting duct**, the ***duct of Wirsung***.
5. Sometimes an accessory pancreatic duct, the ***duct of Santorini***, drains separately from the head of the pancreas into the duodenum.
6. Collecting ducts combine to form **pancreatic duct** that drains into the common bile duct and form **hepatopancreatic duct** with an ampulla (***Ampulla of Vater***), which opens to the second part of duodenum through the ***sphincter of Oddi***.

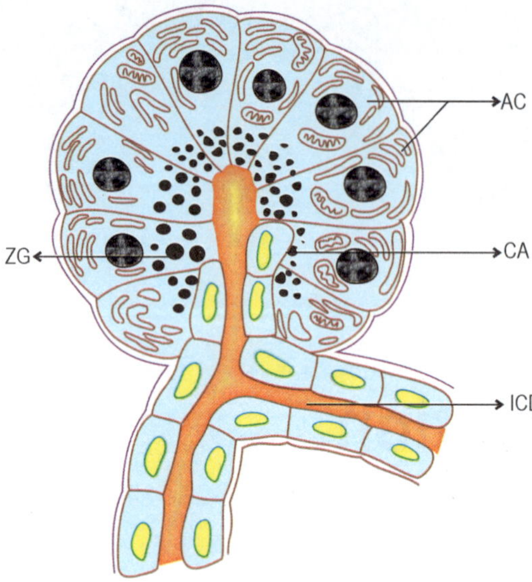

Fig. 60.2: Histology of pancreatic acinus. Note acinar cells are rich in endoplasmic granules at the base and zymogen granules at the apex of the cell. Acinar cells drain into intercalated duct.

7. The **acini secrete enzymes** of the pancreatic juice.
8. The **aqueous component** of pancreatic juice is produced ***by epithelial cells*** that line the pancreatic ducts.

Nerve supply

Pancreas is supplied by both parasympathetic (vagal fibers) and sympathetic fibers.

Vagal Fibers: These fibers innervate both the acinar cells (exocrine tissue) and islet cells (endocrine tissue).

- Stimulation of parasympathetic fibers **increases exocrine pancreatic secretion**.

Sympathetic Fibers: The postganglionic sympathetic fibers from **celiac and superior mesenteric plexuses** innervate pancreatic blood vessel and tissue.

- Stimulation of sympathetic fibers **inhibits pancreatic secretion**.

PY4.2

PANCREATIC SECRETION

VOLUME & pH: The daily secretion of pancreatic juice is 1 to 1.5 liters. Pancreatic juice is alkaline (pH 7.5 – 8.5) as it is rich in bicarbonate. The alkaline nature of pancreatic juice ***protects duodenal mucosa from acidic chyme.***

Composition and Functions

Composition

The pancreatic secretion has **aqueous component** (98%) and **enzyme component** (2%).

Aqueous Component

This contains mainly **water and ions**. The **cations** are Na^+, K^+, Ca^{++}, Mg^{++}, and Zn^{++}, and the **anions** are HCO_3^-, Cl^-, PO_4^{3-}, and SO_4^{3-}.

Enzyme Component

Enzymes for Lipid Digestion: Enzymes for lipid digestion are **pancreatic lipase** (triacylglycerol hydrolase, cholesterol ester hydrolase, and phospholipase A_2), **colipase** and **phospholipases**.

1. The **pancreatic lipase** digests neutral lipids into fatty acids and monoglycerides.
2. The **colipase** facilitates the action of lipase.
3. The **phospholipase** acts on phospholipids.
4. **Cholesterol hydrolase** splits cholesterol esters into cholesterol and fatty acids.

Enzymes for Protein Digestion: Enzymes for protein digestion are trypsin, chymotrypsin, carboxypeptidase, procollagenase, proelastase, and nucleases.

- These proteolytic enzymes are **secreted in the inactive forms** like trypsinogen, chymotrypsinogen, procarboxypeptidase, procollagenases, proelastase, and pronucleases (Table 60.1).
- ***Activation of Enzymes:*** The enzymes are activated in the intestine. The **first step** in the process of activation is the **activation of trypsinogen to trypsin**, which is mediated by the intestinal enzyme **enteropeptidase (*enterokinase*)**.
  - Once trypsin is formed, it converts other proenzymes to their active forms (Flowchart 60.1).
- **Trypsin is strongly proteolytic.**
  - Therefore, once it is activated in the pancreas, it digests the pancreatic tissue (Clinical Note 60.1). However, normally it ***remains inactivated*** in pancreas.

Proenzyme	Activator	Active enzyme
Trypsinogen	Enteropeptidase →	Trypsin
Chymotrypsinogen	Trypsin →	Chymotrypsin
Proelastase	Trypsin →	Elastase
Procarboxypeptidase	Trypsin →	Carboxypeptidase

Flowchart 60.1: Steps of activation of pancreatic proteolytic enzymes.

Factors that normally prevent autodigestion of pancreas are:

1. Enzymes are present in ***inactive form***.
2. ***Trypsin inhibitor in pancreatic tissue*** does not allow active trypsin to be formed *(trypsin remains inhibited)*.
3. The ***wall of acini is thick***, and therefore does not allow pancreatic enzymes to escape into the pancreatic tissue.

Enzymes for Carbohydrate Digestion: Pancreatic amylase splits starch at α-1,4-glycosidic linkage. This is an α-amylase that acts on starch to produce maltose, α-limit dextrin, etc. It differs from salivary amylase by its **action on both boiled and unboiled starch** (*salivary amylase acts only on boiled starch*).

Clinical Note 60.1

Autodigestion of pancreas in acute pancreatitis: Normally, trypsin is not formed in the pancreas due to the presence of **trypsin inhibitor** in the pancreatic juice which prevents the activation of trypsinogen to trypsin. In **acute pancreatitis**, the trypsin inhibitor is deficient. Therefore, activation of trypsin in the pancreas results in *autodigestion* of pancreatic tissue.

Table 60.1 | Functions of pancreatic enzymes.

Enzymes	Functions
A. For lipid digestion	
Lipase	Digests neutral lipids into fatty acids and monoglycerides. Facilitates the action of lipase.
Phospholipase	Acts on phospholipids.
Cholesterol hydrolase	Splits cholesterol esters into cholesterol and fatty acids.
B. For protein digestion	
Trypsin	Cleaves peptide linkages on carboxyl side of basic amino acids
Chymotrypsin	Cleaves peptide linkages on carboxyl side of aromatic amino acids.
Elastase	Cleaves peptide linkages on carboxyl side of aliphatic amino acids.
Carboxypeptidase	Cleaves amino acids from carboxyl end of the peptide.
Ribonuclease	Cleaves deoxyribonucleic acids into mononucleotides
C. For carbohydrate digestion	
Amylase	Splits starch at α-1,4-glycosidic linkage

Functions of Pancreatic Secretion

1. Pancreatic secretion contains enzymes that help in **digestion of fat, protein and carbohydrate** as listed in Table 60.1.
   - Pancreatic enzymes are the primary requirements for digestion and absorption of nutrients.
   - Therefore, **pancreatic deficiency** leads to *severe malabsorption syndrome*.
2. Pancreatic secretion contains **bicarbonate and water** that ***neutralize acidic chyme*** entering intestine from stomach.
   - It protects the duodenal mucosa from damage by acidic chyme.
   - It also neutralizes the effects of bile acids.
   - Thus, it ***prevents causation of duodenal ulcer*** (Clinical Note 60.2).

Clinical Note 60.2

Upper part of duodenum is the commonest site for duodenal ulcer: Acidic chyme from stomach is neutralized by alkaline pancreatic juice. However, as acidic chyme in the 1st part of duodenum (part above the ampulla of Vater, the site of opening of major pancreatic duct) remains mostly unaffected by alkaline pancreatic secretion, it is the commonest site of peptic ulcer. However, if the *duct of Santorini* (accessory pancreatic duct) is present, which opens into 1st part of duodenum, chance of duodenal ulcer is less.

Mechanism of Secretion

Secretion of Aqueous Component

Aqueous component of pancreatic secretion is mainly produced by the **columnar epithelial cells** that line the pancreatic ducts.

- Pancreatic juice is **nearly isotonic with plasma** at any rate of formation and flow. The **ionic composition** includes mainly ***cations*** (Na^+ and K^+) and the ***anions*** (HCO_3^- and Cl^-).
- The **Na^+ and K^+ concentration** of pancreatic juice *is similar to that of plasma*. But, **HCO_3^- and Cl^- concentration** *varies according to the rate of secretion*.
  - **At lower rate of secretion,** concentration of HCO_3^- and Cl^- is about 70% of plasma.
  - **At higher rate of secretion,** their concentration is more than 100% of plasma (Fig. 60.3).
- The aqueous component **secreted by the duct cell** is hypertonic to plasma as it contains more HCO_3^-.
- But, when the secretion passes through the ducts, **water moves into the duct lumen** to make the pancreatic juice ***isotonic***, during which HCO_3^- is partly exchanged with Cl^- by **HCO_3^--Cl^- exchanger** present on the luminal membrane (Fig. 60.4).
  - **HCO_3^-** in epithelial cell is **derived from carbonic acid** (H_2CO_3), which is formed by CO_2 and water in the presence of carbonic anhydrase (CA).
  - The cytosolic H^+ is exchanged by **Na^+-H^+ exchanger**, located on the basolateral membrane.
  - Excess of Na^+ that enters duct epithelial cells, is pumped out of cell by **Na^+-K^+ pump** located on the basolateral surface, which actively pumps K^+ into the cell.
- **In the resting state** (interdigestive phase), the secretion of aqueous component occurs ***mainly from intercalated and intralobular ducts***, but **in the stimulated state** (after eating) the secretion occurs additionally ***from extralobular ducts***, which has higher HCO_3^- concentration.

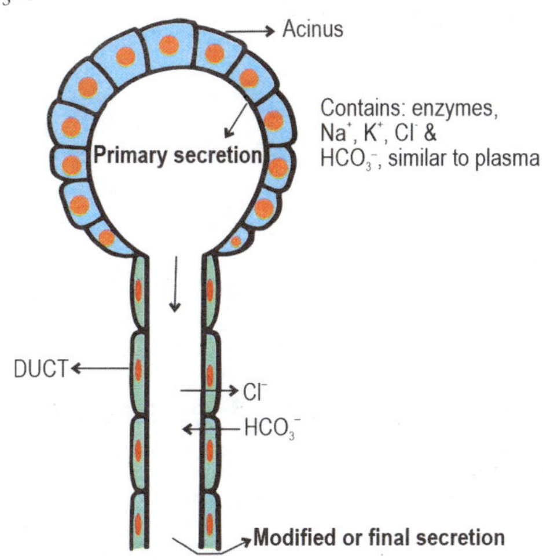

Fig. 60.3: Mechanism of pancreatic secretion.

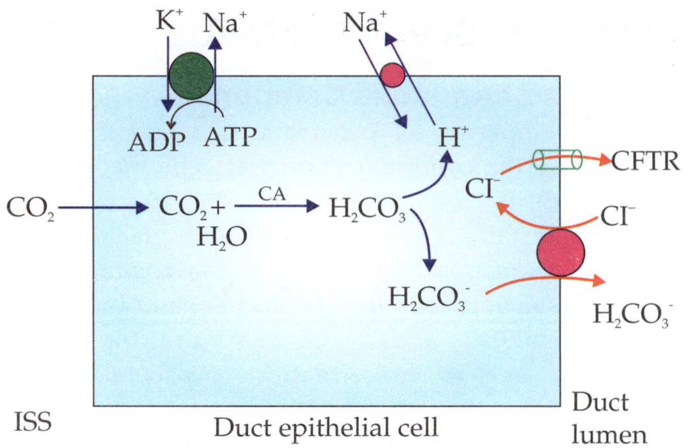

Fig. 60.4: Mechanism of bicarbonate secretion by pancreatic duct epithelial cells. CFTR: cystic fibrosis transmembrane regulator chloride channel; CA: carbonic anhydrase; ISS: interstitial tissue space; ADP: Adenosine diphosphate; ATP: Adenosine triphosphate.

Role of CFTR: Cl^- transport across the acinar cells and duct epithelial cells occurs via **voltage gated Cl^- channels.** The gene that encodes for Cl^- channel is influenced by **cystic fibrosis transmembrane-conductance regulator** (CFTR). CFTR is localized in the apical membrane of epithelial cells in the pancreatic ducts. Alteration of CFTR results in decreased number of Cl^- channel. Therefore, **Cl^- transport into duct lumen is impaired**. Defect in the chloride channel causes **thick exocrine secretion** in the duct (Clinical Note 60.3)

Clinical Note 60.3

Autodigestion of pancreas in acute pancreatitis: Normally, trypsin is not formed in the pancreas due to the presence of **trypsin inhibitor** in the pancreatic juice which prevents the activation of trypsinogen to trypsin. In **acute pancreatitis**, the trypsin inhibitor is deficient. Therefore, activation of trypsin in the pancreas results in *autodigestion* of pancreatic tissue.

- Alteration of CFTR results in decreased number of **Cl^-** channel that **impairs Cl^- transport** into duct lumen. This also **impairs the transport of Na^+ and water**.
- As a result, the **secretion becomes thick** causing **duct obstruction** which in turn causes destruction of acinar cells and duct system.
- This leads to *severe* ***pancreatic deficiency*** causing severe impairment of absorption of important nutrients.
- This is also accompanied by ***progressive pulmonary disease*** causing lung infection, especially in children.

Secretion of Enzyme Components

Pancreatic enzymes are **synthesized in the acinar cells** and stored in the zymogen granules.

- The granules are located towards the apical region of the cells.
- In response to appropriate stimulation, the granules are released by exocytosis into the lumen of acinus.

Factor Influencing Pancreatic Secretion

Pancreatic secretion is influenced by hormonal and neural factors.

1. The **hormonal factors** are mainly cholecystokinin (CCK) and secretin. **Cholecystokinin stimulates enzymatic pancreatic secretion,** whereas **secretin stimulates pancreatic secretion rich in water and bicarbonate.**
2. The **neural factors** are sympathetic and parasympathetic. ***Parasympathetic stimulation increases*** secretion whereas ***sympathetic stimulation decreases*** pancreatic secretion.

However, the control mechanism varies according to the phases of secretion (described below).

Hormonal Factors

1. Cholecystokinin: CCK has two receptors. (CCK-A and CCK B receptors, gastrin acts through CCK B receptors)
2. Secretin
3. Gastrin: Gastrin receptors, CCK B receptors
4. GRP, GIP, and VIP

Cholecystokinin and Secretin: CCK and secretin are natural and primary regulators of pancreatic secretion.

Cholecystokinin: Cholecystokinin (CCK) is a polypeptide hormone. It is **secreted from I cells** located in upper small intestine **in response to fatty foods.**

It has **two receptors**: CCK A and CCK B.

1. **CCK A receptors** are mainly located in the peripheral structures like gall bladder, pancreas, GI tract etc.
2. **CCK B receptors** are present in central structures like brain areas.
3. CCK acting on both receptors **activates membrane phospholipase–C** and stimulates production of intracellular **IP_3 and DAG.** IP_3 and DAG ***increase cytosolic calcium concentration*** (Fig. 60.5).

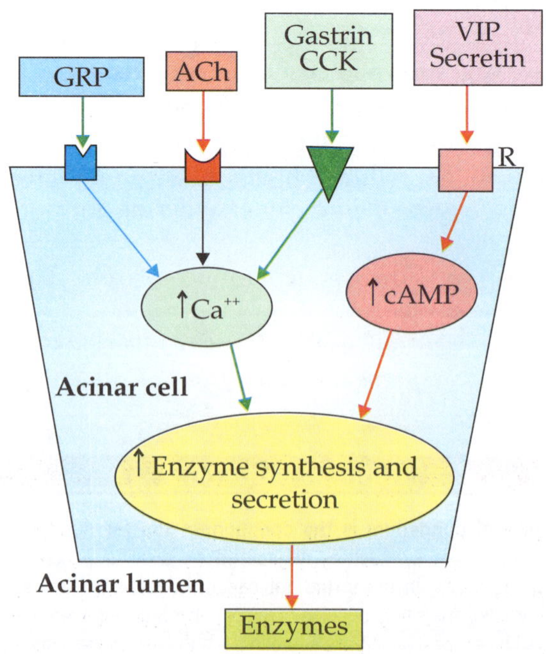

Fig. 60.5: Mechanism of different hormones acting on pancreatic acinar cells. GRP: gastrin-releasing peptide, ACH: acetylcholine; CCK: cholecystokinin; VIP: vasoactive intestinal polypeptide; R: receptors.

4. CCK increases pancreatic secretion **rich in enzymes**.

Secretin: Secretin is **secreted from S cells** of upper small intestine **in response to acidic chyme**.

- It acts on ***adenylate cyclase*** on the cell membrane and increases cytosolic formation of cAMP.
- It increases pancreatic secretion **rich in bicarbonate and water**.

Neural Factors

1. **Parasympathetic:** Stimulates secretion
2. **Sympathetic:** Inhibits secretion

Regulation of Secretion

Phases of Pancreatic Secretion

There are ***three phases*** of pancreatic secretion: **cephalic, gastric, and intestinal**. Mechanisms of pancreatic secretion are different in different phases of secretion (Table 60.2).

Table 60.2 | Mechanisms of pancreatic secretion in its different phases.

	Stimuli	Mechanisms	Effects
Cephalic phase	Sight, smell, thought and taste of food. Chewing & swallowing of food.	Vagal stimulation	Increased secretion containing more enzymes.
Gastric phase	Gastric distension	Vagovagal reflex	Increased secretion containing more enzymes
	Products of protein digestion.	Gastrin	Increased secretion containing more enzymes
Intestinal phase	Acidic chyme in duodenum	Secretin	Increased secretion containing more HCO_3^- and water
	Fatty acids and amino acids	CCK & vagovagal reflex	Increased secretion containing more enzymes.

Cephalic Phase

The cephalic phase is induced by smell, sight, thought and taste of food, and by chewing and swallowing of food.

- Cephalic phase is mediated by **vagus nerve**. The efferent impulses originating from brain directly stimulate pancreatic secretion. The fibers mediating this response are ***cholinergic vagal fibers***.
- Also, **gastrin** released from the stomach in response to vagal stimulation increases pancreatic secretion.
- The pancreatic secretion in cephalic phase is **rich in enzymes** (Fig. 60.6).

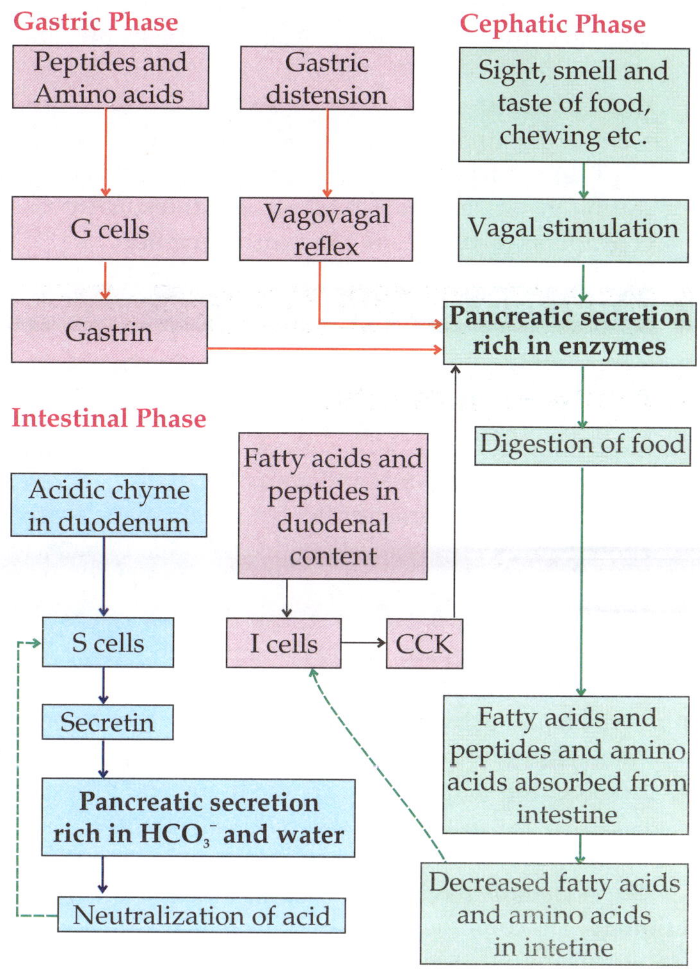

Fig. 60.6: Mechanism of regulation of pancreatic secretion in gastric, cephalic and intestinal phases pf pancreatic secretion. Dotted arrows indicate inhibition.

- Cephalic phase contributes to **15–30%** of pancreatic secretion.

Gastric Phase

When food enters the stomach, gastric phase is initiated.

- Distension of stomach elicits **vagovagal reflex** that stimulates pancreatic secretion.
- Presence of amino acids and peptides in the gastric content stimulate **gastrin** release from stomach that in turn stimulate pancreatic secretion (Fig. 60.6).
- Gastric phase has ***greater effects on enzyme secretion***.
- About **40% of pancreatic secretion** occurs in this phase.

Intestinal Phase

When chyme enters the duodenum, intestinal phase starts.

- **Acidic chyme** increases release of **secretin** from S cells present in the mucosa of upper part of small intestine. Secretin stimulates pancreatic juice **rich in aqueous** (water and bicarbonate) component.
- The presence of **products of protein digestion** like amino acids and peptides, and the **products of fat digestion** like fatty acids and monoglycerides in chyme evoke pancreatic secretion rich in enzymes, which is

mediated by *CCK* secreted from I cells in intestinal mucosa (Fig. 60.6).

- CCK potentiates the effect of secretin on ducts and secretin potentiates the effect of CCK on acinar cells.
- The **vagovagal reflex** also mediates pancreatic secretion during gastric and intestinal phases. Intestinal phase contributes to **40-60% of pancreatic secretion**.

APPLIED PHYSIOLOGY

Acute Pancreatitis

Pathophysiology: This is a serious condition of acute abdomen that occurs due to inflammation of the pancreas.

- The disease is characterized by **severe pain** in the epigastric or periumbilical region that often radiates to back.
- The physiological alteration in the disease is the **activation of trypsin** inside the pancreatic tissue that causes ***autodigestion of the gland.***
- Trypsin also **activates phospholipase-A_2** which forms **lysolecithin** from fatty acid of lecithin.
- **Lysolecithin** damages pancreatic tissue and produces necrosis of surrounding fat.
- In severe case, hemorrhage occurs into abdominal cavity (**hemorrhagic pancreatitis**).

Etiology: The common causes of acute pancreatitis are **gall stone** causing obstruction of sphincter of Oddi, **chronic alcoholism, hypertriglyceridemia,** blunt abdominal trauma and **drugs** like azathioprine, sulphonamides, tetracycline, valproic acid etc.

Diagnosis: Acute pancreatitis is diagnosed by its typical presentation of abdominal pain associated with **increased plasma level of serum amylase**.

Treatment: In 90% of patients, symptoms disappear with **conservative treatment** with i.v. fluid, nil orally, analgesics, antibiotics and nasogastric suction.

- **In severe cases**, especially in hemorrhagic form, abdomen is opened, and blood is collected from abdominal cavity of the patient and filtered, abdomen is thoroughly washed, bleeding points are closed, and the filtered blood is transfused (**autotransfusion**).

Chronic Pancreatitis

Slow and chronic inflammation of pancreas occurs without any definite etiology.

- It may be due to improper recovery from pancreatitis or persistence of low grade acute pancreatitis.
- Patient develops **steatorrhea** due to pancreatic lipase deficiency and **malnutrition** due to indigestion and malabsorption of various nutrients.
- Patient ***may develop diabetes mellitus*** due to associated endocrine deficiency.

Cystic Fibrosis

This is an **autosomal recessive** monogenic disorder, in which the major **defect is in the Cl^- channel**.

- The disease occurs due to **mutation in the CFTR gene** (cystic fibrosis transmembrane-conductance regulator gene), located on **chromosome 7**.
- The disease usually starts in **childhood**.
- **Lung** is the most common organ affected and **decreased nasociliary clearance** is the common pathology.
- **Respiratory features** are chronic sinusitis, nasal obstruction, rinorrhea and cough with expectoration of viscous-purulent sputum.
- Common **gastrointestinal features** are intestinal obstruction and **exocrine pancreatic deficiency**.

PY4.8

PANCREATIC FUNCTION TESTS

Exocrine pancreatic function tests are based on assessment of pancreatic secretion in response to **hormonal stimulation**, or **a meal** or measurement of **production of digestion in the stool** that assesses digestion and absorption of nutrients.

Classification

These are of **two types**: invasive and non-invasive tests.

Invasive Tests

Invasive tests are of **two types**.

1. First type uses ***stimulation of pancreatic secretion by meals*** such as **Lundh meal** or ***duodenal infusion*** of amino acids.
2. Second type makes use of **hormonal injection** intravenously such as secretin, CCK, etc.

Secretin Stimulation Test: Secretin is injected IV at a dose of 1 unit / kg and then the duodenal samples are collected for 80 minutes. It increases rate of formation and flow, and aqueous component of pancreatic juice.

CCK Stimulation Test: CCK increases enzymatic component of pancreatic secretion.

Meal Stimulation Test: The test meal is called Lundh meal (Lundh and Borgstrom, 1962). It consists of milk protein, corn oil, and dextrose. Following ingestion of the meal, duodenal content is aspirated for analysis.

Non-Invasive Tests

These are simpler and cheaper. Therefore, noninvasive tests are preferred to invasive tests. However, they are not as sensitive and specific as the invasive tests.

Visualization of pancreas and scanning by **utrasonography, CT scan, MRI, cholangiopancreatography** etc. are usually performed before opting for biochemical pancreatic function tests. These tests are of **three types**.

1. **First type** includes estimations in stool for food particles that are not absorbed (fecal estimation of fat) and fecal enzymes (trypsin, chymotrypsin and elastase).
2. **Second type** includes estimations in blood, urine and breath for products of digested food due to action of pancreatic enzymes that are absorbed into systemic circulation
3. **Third type** includes estimations in plasma or blood for hormones (Schilling test) and enzymes, amino acids etc.

Fecal Estimation of Fat: Normally, about 5 g of fat is excreted per day in the feces. In pancreatic deficiency, excretion more than 20 g of fat is common. In severe deficiency, fat excretion may be 50 g or more.

Fecal Estimation of Nitrogen: About 7 g of nitrogen is excreted in stool per day in a healthy individual. In pancreatic deficiency, due to decreased proteolytic enzyme activity, nitrogen excretion increases in stool.

D Xylose Absorption Test: A pentose sugar called xylose is administered (25 g, usually) and its recovery in urine is measured over next 5 hours and in blood in next 2 hours.

- This is a test that distinguishes between malabsorption due to pancreatic (normal absorption) and jejunal (low absorption) insufficiencies.
- It also helps evaluate response to therapy.

Schilling Test: It is done to assess the absorption of vitamin B_{12} which requires intrinsic factor.

- Vitamin B_{12} deficiency is seen in chronic pancreatitis because trypsin helps in binding B_{12} to intrinsic factor after which the complex is reabsorbed.

Serum Amylase Estimation: Normal level of serum amylase is 60–120 units per liter.

- In acute pancreatitis, serum amylase concentration becomes very high.
- This differentiates pancreatitis from other conditions of acute abdomen.

Cholangiopancreatography: This is a special radiodiagnostic investigation in which the details of the contour of hepatopancreatic duct system are visualized by introducing an endoscope.

- The procedure is called endoscopic retrograde cholangiopancreatography (ERCP).
- This is the most accurate test for assessing pancreatic structure and function.

Exam Questions

1. Give the composition and function of pancreatic secretion, and describe the mechanism and regulation of pancreatic secretion.
2. What are the phases of pancreatic secretion. Composition and functions of pancreatic secretion, Mechanism of pancreatic secretion. Describe regulation of pancreatic in each phase of secretion.
3. Classify pancreatic function tests. Briefly describe the principle of estimation and application of each test. Write a note on CFTR.

Multiple Choice Questions

1. **Total daily pancreatic secretion is about:**
   A. 0.5L B. 1.5L C. 2.5L D. 5.0L
2. **Secretin causes:**
   A. Increases enzyme rich pancreatic fluid
   B. Gastric hypermotility
   C. Increased gastrin secretion
   D. Secretion of HCO3 rich pancreatic fluid
3. **Most potent stimulus for secretion is**
   A. Dilation of intestine B. Acid chyme
   C. Protein D. Fat
4. **Pancreatic juice rich in water and electrolytes poor in enzymes is secreted in response to:**
   A. Pancreozymin B. Cholecystokinin
   C. Secretin D. Proteins
5. **I cells of upper part of small intestine secrete:**
   A. Secretin B. Gastrin
   C. CCK D. Motilin
6. **Best stimuli for CCK secretion is:**
   A. Acid B. Proteins and fatty acids C. Bile D. Fat
7. **Fat in the duodenum lumen:**
   A. Stimulates gall bladder contraction B. Inhibits gall bladder contraction
   C. Inhibits CCK secretion D. Releases secretion
8. **CCK-PZ causes all of the following, EXCEPT**
   A. Gallbladder contraction
   B. Pancreatic enzyme secretion
   C. Increased gastrin secretion
   D. Decreased lower esophageal sphincter activity
9. **Most important hormone that increased gallbladder contraction after a fatty meal is**
   A. Gastrin B. Secretin C. Vagus D. Cholecystokinin
10. **All the following are true about Cephalic Phase of pancreatic secretion, EXFEPT:**
    A. It is mainly mediated by vagus nerve
    B. Sight, smell and taste of food initiates it
    C. Gastrin released in response to vagal stimulation facilitates it
    D. It caused more than 50% of total secretion
11. **In the intestinal phase of pancreatic secretion:**
    A. Secretin mainly mediates the bicarbonate rich secretion
    B. This phase of secretion constitutes about 50% of total pancreatic secretion
    C. Vagovagal reflex contributes to it
    D. Secretion inhibits pancreatic enzyme secretion
12. **Which of the following is a test for pancreatic exocrine function?**
    A. Barium meal X-ray B. Histalog test
    C. D xylose absorption test D. Hollander test

Answers: 1. B 2. D 3. B 4. C 5. C 6. B 7. A 8. C 9. D 10. D 11. D 12. C

Chapter 61

Hepatobiliary System and Biliary Secretion

Learning Objectives

On completion of study of this chapter:

The student will be able to (must know):

1. Correlate functional anatomy and histology of liver with liver functions.
2. List the functions of liver.
3. Give the composition and functions of bile, and the differences between hepatic and gall bladder bile.
4. Name bile salts and acids and give their functions.
5. Understand the importance of enterohepatic circulation.
6. Outline the mechanism and regulation of bile secretion.

The student may also be able to (desirable to know):

1. Describe the regulation of bile secretion
2. Explain the physiological basis of gall stone formation.

HEPATOBILIARY SYSTEM

Hepatobiliary system consists of liver, gall bladder and biliary tract.

Functional Anatomy PY4.7

Bile is formed in the liver and is excreted through the bile ductules. The **bile canaliculi** start at the space between two hepatocytes, which opens into bile ductules.

- Bile ductules then form the bile duct which leads to **hepatic duct**. The right and left hepatic ducts join to form **common hepatic duct** (Fig. 61.1).
- The **cystic duct** from gall bladder combines with hepatic duct to form **common bile duct**. Common bile duct combines with pancreatic duct and opens to **second part of duodenum** through *sphincter of Oddi*.

Hepatic Circulation

Blood Supply

Liver receives blood supply from **two sources**: portal vein and hepatic artery.

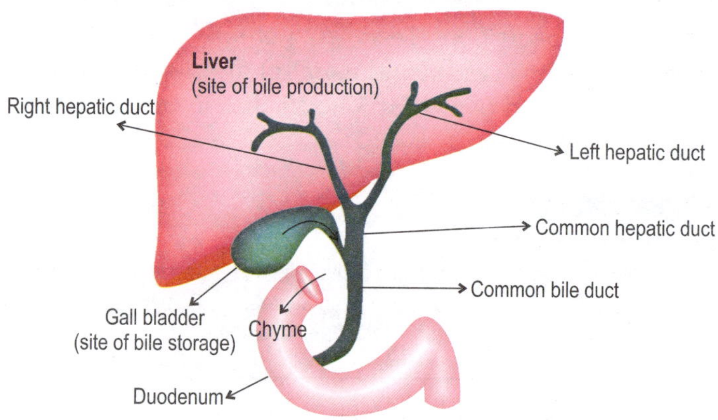

Fig. 61.1: Hepatobiliary system.

Portal Vein: Portal vein is formed by the union of **superior mesenteric vein and splenic vein.**

- As portal vein collects blood from stomach, intestine, spleen, and pancreas, it is **rich in end products of digestion, GI hormones and pancreatic hormones**.
- However, portal blood is comparatively **poor in O_2**.

Hepatic Artery: Hepatic artery contains pure arterial blood and is **rich in oxygen**.

Portal Circulation

The portal vein and hepatic artery break up into **large number of branches.** Blood of these two sets of vessels get mixed up in the **sinusoids** of the liver.

- The hepatic cells receive oxygen and nutrients from the sinusoids.
  - The various substances produced by the liver, products of metabolism, the waste products and the CO_2 are discharged into the sinusoids.
- The **sinusoids drain into central vein** of the lobule.
- Central veins from different lobules unite to form larger veins, which in turn join ultimately and drain into **hepatic vein**, which opens into the inferior vena cava.

Bile Secretion by Liver Cells

The liver cells synthesize bile, which is first secreted to **small canaliculi.** The smaller canaliculi join and ultimately form two **hepatic ducts** (right and left).

Histology of Liver

Liver is formed by large number of **lobules.**

1. The individual lobule is **polygonal in shape** with a central vein at the center.
2. From the central vein, **plates of liver cells radiate** like spokes of a bicycle wheel to the periphery of the lobule (Fig. 61.2).
3. The plates are **one cell thick** and are separated by liver sinusoids.

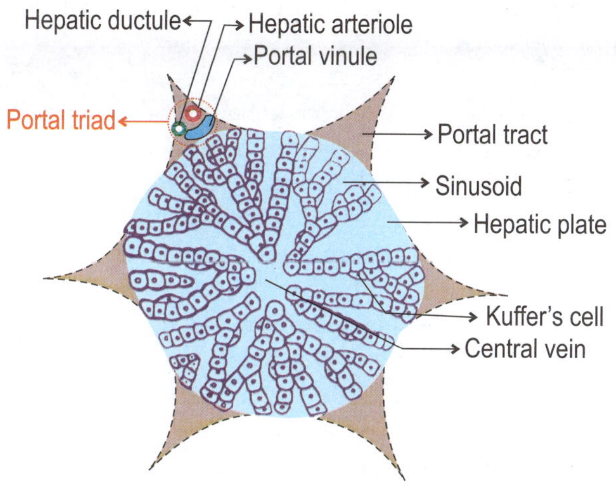

Fig. 61.2: Structure of a hepatic lobule. Note the location of central vein, sinusoids and portal triad consisting of portal venule, hepatic arteriole and hepatic ductule in the portal tract.

Sinusoids and Bile Canaliculi

In a typical lobule, between the plates of hepatic cells, the **sinusoids** are present that carry blood.

1. **Each sinusoid** receives blood from a **branch of portal vein and hepatic artery** of the portal tract and drains into the central vein.
2. Wall of the sinusoids are mostly made up of **endothelial cells**, but at places macrophage cells, called Kupffer cells, are occasionally present.

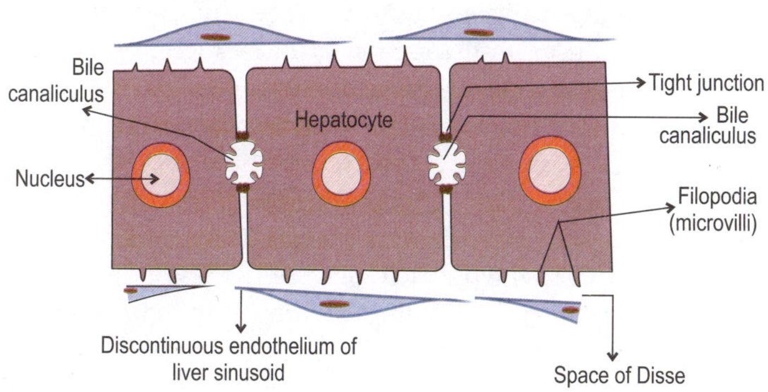

Fig. 61.3: Bile canaliculi. Note the location of space of Disse, and discontinuous endothelium layer in the hepatic sinusoids.

3. The **bile canaliculi** run in between the two layers of cells (layer of cells that make the thickness of each plate) (Fig. 61.3).
   - The **liver cells (hepatocytes) synthesize bile acids** and transfer them into bile canaliculi.
4. The space that lies between sinusoid and hepatocytes is the **space of Disse** (perisinusoidal space).
   - The space of Disse **serves as a route** through which hepatocytes remove certain substances from blood and discharge certain products into the blood.

Portal triad

Portal triads are typically found at the angles of liver lobules. Each portal triad consists of a **branch of portal vein, a branch of hepatic artery and a bile ductule** (Fig. 61.2).

1. The angular space that contains portal triad and its surrounding connective tissue is called **portal canal or tract.**
2. Portal sinusoids originating from portal veins remain in close proximity with bile canaliculi that drain into interlobular bile duct (Fig. 61.4).
3. A small space between hepatocyte and portal canal is called **space of Mall**, the site of origin of lymph in liver.

Functions of Liver PY4.8

Liver is the center metabolism of nutrients. It synthesizes many essential proteins, stores nutrients and detoxifies harmful substances.

1. **Secretory functions:** Liver forms and secretes bile into biliary tract.
2. **Metabolic functions:** Liver is involved in metabolism of major nutrients such as carbohydrate, fat, proteins, and fat soluble and water-soluble vitamins, and urea.
3. **Synthetic functions:** Liver is the major organ for the synthesis of proteins that include clotting factors, acute phase proteins that mediate inflammation, hormone binding proteins, lipids, carbohydrates, vitamins and bile salts.

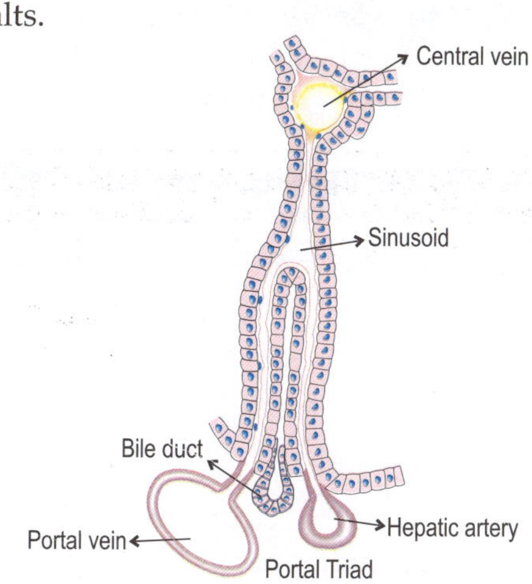

Fig. 61.4: Portal triad in liver. Note the relation of plate of hepatocytes with sinusoids, and sinusoids with bile canaliculi.

4. **Storage functions:** Liver stores glucose, protein, fat, and vitamins.
5. **Detoxifying action:** Liver detoxifies many chemicals and toxins.
6. **Degradation of drugs and chemicals:** Liver is the site of inactivation of many drugs. Liver degrades enzymes, hormones, cytokines and various other chemicals.
7. **Excretory function:** Liver excretes bile pigments, cholesterol, and some metals.
8. **Immunity:** Kupffer cells of liver are part of mononuclear phagocyte system that kill microorganisms.
9. **Endocrine functions:** Liver converts vitamin D_3 to 25-hydroxyvitamin D_3.
   - Liver is a major site for conversion of T_4 to T_3.
   - Somatomedin (insulin-like growth factor) that mediates important functions of growth factor is secreted from liver.
   - Many hormones like insulin, glucagon, growth hormone, GI hormones etc. are degraded in liver.

(Liver Function Tests are given in 'Comprehensive Textbook of Physiology' of Dr. GK Pal).

Bile

PY4.2

About 0.5 to 1 liter of bile is secreted daily. Bile is a greenish yellow fluid formed in the liver and stored in gall bladder.

Composition of Bile

It is composed of water (98%), and solids as given below.

- Bile salts, Bile pigments
- Cholesterol, Fatty acids and fat
- Inorganic salts
- Alkaline phosphatase
- Cations: Na^+, K^+, Ca^{2+} and Mg^{2+}
- Anions: HCO_3^-, Cl^-, SO_4^{2-} and PO_4^{3-}

The colour of bile is greenish yellow due to the presence of **glucuronides of bile pigments**. The bile pigments are **bilirubin and biliverdin.**

Hepatic and Gall Bladder Bile: Hepatic bile (**bile formed in the liver**) differs from gall bladder bile as it is concentrated and acidified in gall bladder (Table 61.1).

Table 61.1 | Differences in hepatic and gall bladder bile.

	Hepatic bile	Gall bladder bile
1. pH	Alkaline (8–8.5)	Acidic (about 7)
2. Water content	98%	85%
3. Solids	2 g%	10–15g%
4. Bile salts & pigments	Less	More

- Water absorption occurs **secondary to Na^+ absorption** by secondary active transport.
  - **Na^+-K^+ ATPase** in the basolateral membrane of epithelial cell lining transports Na^+ actively out of the cell and creates gradient for Na^+ transport into the cell.
  - Water is reabsorbed passively by **osmotic gradient** created by Na^+ movement.
- **H^+ is exchanged with Na^+** that causes acidification of bile.

Bile Acids and Salts

Bile Acids: There are two types of bile acids: primary and secondary.

1. The **primary bile acids** are cholic acid and chenodeoxycholic acid.
   - The primary bile acids are ***formed in the hepatocytes*** from cholesterol.
2. **Secondary bile acids** are deoxycholic acid and lithocholic acid.
   - The secondary bile acids are ***produced in the intestine*** where intestinal bacteria convert primary bile acids into secondary bile acids.

Bile Salts: Bile salts are Na^+ and K^+ salts of bile acids.

- Bile acids are conjugated with taurine or glycine to form **taurocholic acid** or **glycocholic acid**.
- These acids then combine with sodium and potassium salts to form **Na^+-taurocholate, Na^+-glycocholate, K^+-taurocholate and K^+-glycocholate** respectively.

Functions of Bile (of bile salts)

1. **Absorption of fat:** Bile salts are essential for absorption of fat from intestine.
   - This depends on formation of **micelles** by bile salts in the intestine.
     - For their amphipathic (both hydrophilic and hydrophobic domains) property, along with lecithin and cholesterol, bile salts form **cylindrical disks**, called as micelles (for details, refer Chapter 67).
   - **Lipids are transported in micelles** from the lumen to the membrane of intestinal mucosal epithelial cells where micelle dissociates, and lipids are absorbed.
2. **Emulsification of fat:** Bile salts are **surface tension reducing agents.**
   - Along with phospholipids and monoglycerides, they cause emulsification of fat, which is essential for digestion and absorption of fat.
3. **Source of bile acid:** Bile salts are **converted to bile acids** in the intestine, which are then absorbed into portal blood.
   - Thus, bile salts are important sources of bile acids that add to the bile acid pool of the body.
4. **Bile secretion:** Bile salts are important **choleretics.** They are constituent of bile and also, they stimulate bile secretion.
5. **Absorption of fat-soluble vitamins:** Bile salts facilitate absorption of fat-soluble vitamins (**vitamins A, D, E**

and K).

- Hence, in obstructive jaundice, features of deficiencies of fat-soluble vitamins develop.

6. **Activation of pancreatic enzymes:** Bile salts activate **pancreatic lipase**.
7. **Prevention of gall stone formation:** Bile salts along with lecithin **solubilize cholesterol**.
   - Thus, they prevent formation of stones in the gall bladder.
8. **Physiological purgatives:** Bile salts act as physiological purgatives.
   - Constipation occurs in conditions of deficiency of delivery of bile into intestine as occurs in obstructive jaundice.
9. **Stool color:** Bile salts add natural brownish color to the stool.
10. **Prevention of bacterial growth:** Bile maintains pH of intestinal content and prevents overgrowth of bacteria in intestine.

Enterohepatic Circulation

Bile acids and salts are **absorbed from the intestine and re-excreted in the bile**, and this cycle is repeated so many times, which is called enterohepatic circulation of bile acids and salts.

- Bile salts are produced in liver (200 to 500 mg/day) and conjugated. **Conjugated bile salts** (CBS) through biliary tract enter intestine.
- From intestine, they are absorbed into the portal blood to reach liver.
  - Also, in the intestine CBS is deconjugated and **unconjugated bile salt** is absorbed into portal circulation.
- The free bile acids in terminal ileum and colon by the action of bacteria are converted into **secondary bile acids** (SBAs), i. e. *deoxycholic acid and lithocholic acid*.
  - SBAs are also reabsorbed into portal circulation.
  - Thus, from gut, about **95% of secreted bile salts and bile acids are transferred back to liver** via portal circulation, and only 200 to 500 mg/day of bile acids are excreted from stool.
- From liver, again they are **excreted through biliary tract into the intestine**.
  - This forms the **loop-pathway** for enterohepatic circulation (Fig. 61.5).

IMPORTANT NOTE

Enterohepatic circulation preserves body pool of many substances: Enterohepatic circulation ensures **preservation and reutilization of various substances**. For example, bile salts are recirculated 4–12 times a day. The substances that undergo enterohepatic circulation include bile salts, **bile acids, bile pigments, vitamin D, vitamin B12, thyroxine, drugs** etc.

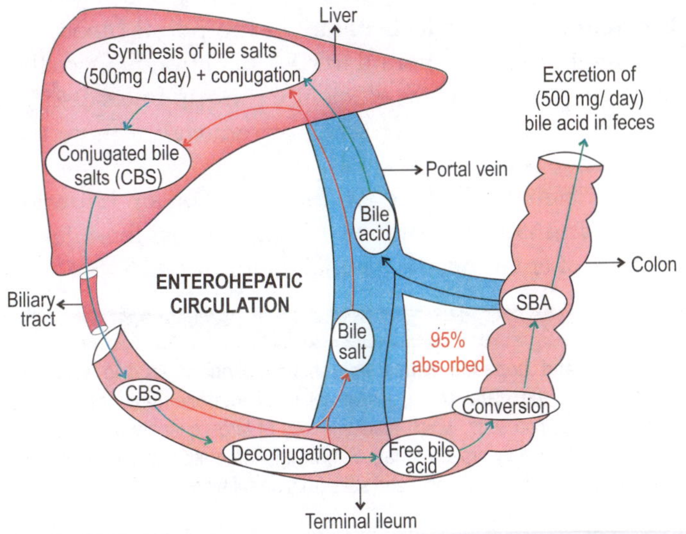

Fig. 61.5: Mechanism of enterohepatic circulation of bile salt and acids. SBA: Secondary bile salt.

Importance of Enterohepatic Circulation

Enterohepatic circulation mainly maintains **the total bile acid pool** of the body.

- **Total amount of bile acids** (conjugated and unconjugated, and primary and secondary) in the body ranges from **2 to 4 g.**
- Bile acid is **cycled several times** a day during meals, so that ***a small pool of bile acid*** can efficiently provide enough bile salts to *facilitate adequate lipid absorption* from small intestine.
  - Some amount is lost with every cycle of passage through intestine, which accounts about ***500 mg of bile acid daily***. But this is replenished by synthesis of new bile acids from cholesterol.
- Thus, **fecal excretion of bile acid** accounts for an efficient medium for **loss of body cholesterol**.

Determinants of Enterohepatic Circulation

The major determinants of enterohepatic circulation are **integrity of intestinal epithelium** to reabsorb them and **efficiency of hepatocytes** to pick them up from portal blood.

Integrity of Intestinal Epithelium: Bile salts are absorbed mainly in the terminal ileum by a **carrier mediated process** so that only a 5% of intestinal bile salts enter the colon.

- Thus, **intestinal absorption of bile acids and salts into portal blood is an important determinant** of enterohepatic circulation of these substances.
- Further, bacteria convert primary bile acids to secondary bile acids that are also absorbed into portal circulation.
  - Therefore, lipid malabsorption occurs in chronic inflammatory conditions of intestine (Clinical Note 61.1).

Efficiency of Hepatic Uptake: In the portal blood, bile salts are transported bound to HDL or albumin. Once they reach liver, hepatocytes efficiently pick-up bile salts from hepatic blood, which accounts for removal of more than 80% of portal bile salts.

1. This **hepatic uptake of bile salts is an important determinant** of secretion of bile salts in the bile and thus of enterohepatic circulation of bile salts.

Clinical Note 61.1

Enteritis and hepatitis cause lipid malabsorption: As bile salts are absorbed in the distal ileum, inflammation of intestine (enteritis) inhibits absorption of bile salts, which results in loss of large quantity of lipid in the stool (due to malabsorption of fat). Similarly, inflammation of liver (hepatitis) impairs the uptake of bile acid and salts from portal blood.

BILE SECRETION

Mechanism of Secretion

The secretion of bile consists of **canalicular flow** and **ductular secretion**.

- In the canaliculi, bile acids and Na^+-K^+ATPase contribute to bile flow.
- In the ducts, epithelial cells secrete HCO_3^- and Cl^- actively into the lumen.

Mechanism of Bile Acid Secretion

Bile is **formed in hepatocytes**. Bile acids are taken up from the sinusoidal blood by transport proteins that are present on the basolateral membrane of the hepatocytes.

- In cytoplasm of hepatocytes, bile acids bind with *bile acid binding proteins*. This **prevents bile acids to accumulate in higher concentration** in cytoplasm. It should be noted that high concentration of free bile acids destroys the organelles of hepatocytes.
- Bile acids are **conjugated with glycine or taurine** and then **secreted into the lumen of hepatic canaliculi by facilitated diffusion.**
- Bile acids move into the bile ***down their electrochemical gradient***. The concentration gradient is maintained by formation of **micelles in the bile** present in the canaliculi.

Mechanism of Water & Electrolyte Secretin

Water and electrolyte concentration of bile in the bile canaliculi is same with that of plasma.

- The bile duct epithelial cells secrete **bicarbonate rich fluid** into the lumen.
- The ions are transported in a way similar to pancreatic extralobular ducts.

Modification of Bile in Gall Bladder

Bile is continuously synthesized and secreted from liver and is stored in the gall bladder. Gall bladder is a small sac like structure with the capacity of 30–60 ml.

Gall bladder performs **three functions**:

1. **Storage of bile**
2. **Acidification of bile:** The ***hydrogen ion is secreted*** from gall bladder epithelial cell into the bile to make the bile acidic.
3. **Concentration of bile:** H^+ is secreted into the lumen of gall bladder in **exchange for Na^+** (Na^+-H^+ exchanger).
   - For Na^+ transport into the cell, the gradient is created by Na^+-K^+ pump located in the basolateral membrane of the epithelial cells.
   - **Water is reabsorbed** from the gall bladder bile so that bile is concentrated (Fig. 61.6).

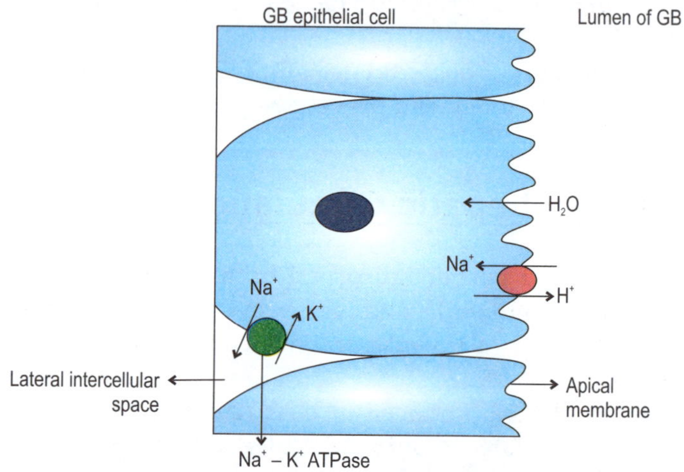

Fig. 61.6: Mechanism of water reabsorption and H+ secretion by epithelial cells of gallbladder (GB) that causes concentration and acidification of GB bile.

Regulation of Bile Secretion

Bile secretion is influenced by **choleretics and cholagogues.**

Choleretics: The substances that enhance the secretion of bile are called choleretics. The important choleretics are:

1. Bile salts
2. Secretin
3. Vagal stimulation.

Secretin increases aqueous component of bile.

Cholagogues: The substances that cause contraction of gall bladder to increase the output of bile from the structure are called cholagogues. The important cholagogues are:

1. Cholecystokinin
2. Fatty acids.

Cholecystokinin causes contraction of smooth muscles of gall bladder and empties its contents.

Composition and functions of bile is given in the early part of this chapter.

Applied Physiology

Gall Stones

Presence of stone in the biliary tract (gall bladder, and

bile ducts) is called gall stone or **cholelithiasis**. Gall stone is commonly associated with **five Fs**: females, forty to fifty age, fair looking individuals, fertile ladies and fat people.

Types

There are **two types** of stones: **cholesterol stones** and **calcium bilirubinate stones**.

In U.S.A. and Europe, 85% of stones are cholesterol stones (***pigment stones***).

- Bile salts along with lecithin solubilize cholesterol. Thus, they prevent formation of stones in the gall bladder.
- When cholesterol concentration is high or bile concentration is less, cholesterol stone develops.

Factors that favor stone formation:

1. ***Bile stasis:*** Decreased bile flow or decreased gall bladder emptying facilitates stone formation.
2. ***Supersaturation of bile*** with cholesterol.
3. ***Nucleation factor*** that favors formation of stones from the supersaturated bile.
   - **Glycoproteins in gall bladder mucus** form the nucleus surrounding which gall stones are formed.

Usually cholesterol stones are big and may be one or two stones are present in gall bladder. The calcium bilirubinate stones are multiple, and more than 50 stones may be present in gall bladder of the patient.

Features

Usually, gallstones are **silent stones**. But, when stones come out of the gall bladder and pass through the biliary ducts, **severe colicky or spasmodic acute abdominal pain** occurs.

1. Chronic gallstones may present with **acute cholecystitis**, bile stasis inducing inflammation of gall bladder.
2. The stone may induce inflammation and edema of gall bladder, resulting in **chronic cholecystitis**.
3. Gall stones may also present with **obstructive jaundice**.

Diagnosis

Diagnosis is usually made by **ultrasound or cholecystography**. Plain x-ray may sometime detect stones.

Treatment

There is no effective medical treatment, though many drugs have been advocated to dissolve stone. Gallstones are **treated surgically** by removal of gall bladder (**cholecystectomy**).

Effects of Cholecystectomy: Gall bladder is not essential for digestive functions. The patients those who have undergone cholecystectomy, maintain normal health and usually their nutrition is not affected.

- They may have steatorrhea if they eat excess of fat food.
- Cholecystectomized patients tolerate fat foods to some extent.
- It decreases body fat and may be beneficial for obese people.

Exam Questions

1. List the functions of liver. Briefly describe intrahepatic bile formation and secretion of bile. Give the physiological basis of the differences between hepatic and gall blabber bile.
2. Describe the mechanism and regulation of bile secretion.
3. List bile salts and bile acids and give functions of bile salts. Add a note on enterohepatic circulation of bile salt.

Multiple Choice Questions

1. **The amount of bile secreted daily is about:**
   A. 1 lit B. 2.5 lit C. 3.5 lit D. 5 lit
2. **Liver synthesizes all, EXCEPT:**
   A. C^3 complement component B. Haptoglobin
   C. Fibrinogen D. Immunoglobulin
3. **Which of the following assay is not for liver disease:**
   A. Alkaline phosphatase B. Aminotransferase
   C. Lactate dehydrogenase D. Creatine kinase
4. **Which of the following is not true for unconjugated bilirubin?**
   A. Serum albumin binding is high
   B. Van dan Bergh reaction is indirect
   C. Renal excretion is absent
   D. Water solubility is high
5. **For conjugated bilirubin, all the following are true, EXCEPT:**
   A. Affinity to lipid (alcohol solubility) is high
   B. Serum albumin binding is low
   C. Van dan Bergh reaction is direct
   D. Renal excretion is significant
6. **Secretion of bile into bile canaliculus is by:**
   A. Osmotic gradient
   B. Facilitated diffusions
   C. Active transport across the membrane
   D. Simple diffusion
7. **Most important stimulant for bile secretion is:**
   A. Cholecystokinin B. Secretin
   C. Bile acid D. Bile salt
8. **Bile acid has a detergent action due to:**
   A. Formation of soap B. Formation of zwitter ion
   C. Amphipathic nature of bile acids
   D. Formation of medium chain triglycerides

Answers : 1. A 2. D 3. D 4. D 5. A 6. C 7. D 8. C

Chapter 62

Intestinal Secretion and Secretion of Large Intestine

Learning Objectives

On completion of study of this chapter:

The student will be able to (must know):

1. Appreciate the role of intestinal secretion in digestion and absorption of nutrients.
2. Understand the significance of mucosal modifications in intestinal epithelium.
3. Give the composition and functions of intestinal secretion.
4. Illustrate the functions of intestinal flora.
5. Learn the physiology of the colon.
6. Give the composition and function of colonic secretion.
7. Outline the physiology of water absorption and secretion through GI tract.
8. Understand the physiology of rectum.

The student may also be able to (desirable to know):

1. Describe the physiological basis of malabsorption syndrome.
2. Explain the mechanism and regulation of intestinal secretion.

SMALL INTESTINE

Small intestine consists of duodenum, jejunum and ileum. It is the longest segment of GI tract, which is about 600 cm (duodenum 25 cm, jejunum 250 cm and ileum 325 cm approx..) in adults.

- Secretion of small intestine is called **succus entericus**, which is about **2–3 liters** of isotonic fluid per day.
- The mucous membrane is thrown into folds or **plicae** which are *more in the jejunum* and less in the ileum. Plicae increases the absorptive surface significantly.

Intestinal Glands

The intestinal wall has all the layers of the gut such as serosa, outer longitudinal and inner circular muscle layers, submucosa, muscularis mucosa, and mucosa. The **mucosa is highly developed** to contain **villi and intestinal glands**.

1. The intestinal glands are called **crypts of Lieberkühn**.
   - These are tubular glands present at the base of the villi.
2. Throughout the length of small intestine, the mucous membrane is covered by **villi**.
   - There are about **20–40 villi per square millimeter of mucosa** (Fig. 62.1).
   - Each villus is a fingerlike projection covered by a ***layer of columnar epithelium*** and contains a network of ***capillaries and lacteals*** (lymphatics).
3. The villi have numerous **microvilli** on their surface that are called **brush border.**
   - Brush border considerably ***increases the surface area*** for absorption.
4. Some quantity of secretion is also added by **Brunner's glands** that are coiled acinotubular glands present **in the duodenum** in addition to crypts of Lieberkühn.
4. The intestinal mucosa is supported externally by thin layer of smooth muscle fibres, **muscularis mucosae**.

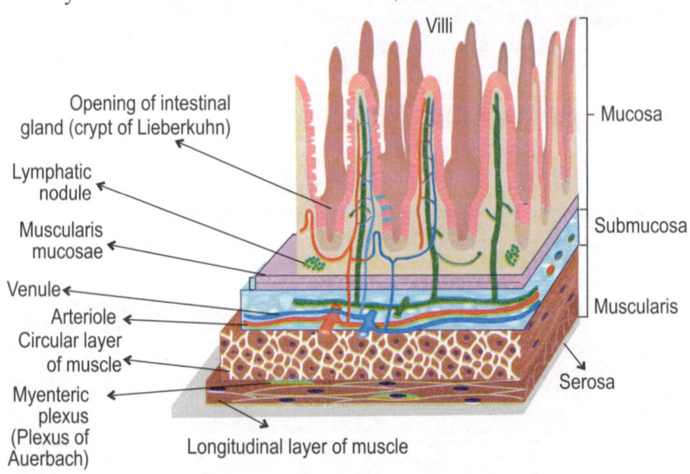

Fig. 62.1: Structure of the wall of small intestine. Note numerous villi projecting from the mucous membrane

Intestinal Mucosa

The mucosa of small intestine contains lymphatic nodules (**Peyer's patches**). In the intestinal mucosa, the cells in the intestinal glands are **enterochromaffin cells, Paneth cells and undifferentiated cells** (Fig. 62.2).

1. The mucous membrane of the intestine contains many valve-like folds called **valvulae conniventes**, which add to the surface area for absorption.
   - In intestine, the surface area for absorption is **increased by about 600 fold** by villi, brush border and valvulae conniventes.
2. The **undifferentiated cells** are the ***progenitor cells*** in the mucosa present in the crypts of Lieberkühn.
   - Progenitor cells ***form new epithelial cells***, which migrate to the surface.
   - The epithelial cells are continuously renewed by progenitor cells.
3. After the life span of about 2–5 days, **enterocytes are sloughed** along with mucosal cells. **Shedding of these epithelial cells** accounts for *daily excretion of about **30 g** of **protein*** as the cells are protein-rich.
4. **Goblet cells** secrete mucins that form a gel solution on the surface of mucosa.

Types of Cells in Villi

Villi contain **4 types of cells** (Fig. 62.2):

1. **Simple Columnar Cells:** They perform absorptive function due to the presence of brush border consisting of large number of villi
2. **Goblet Cells:** These are mucous secreting cells and are interspersed between the columnar cells.
3. **Endocrine Cells:** These are scattered in the villi as well as are widely distributed throughout the gastrointestinal tract. These cells are:
   a) ***Kulchitsky cells:*** after the name of its discoverer
   b) ***Enterochromaffin cells:*** due to their resemblance to chromaffin cells of the adrenal medulla

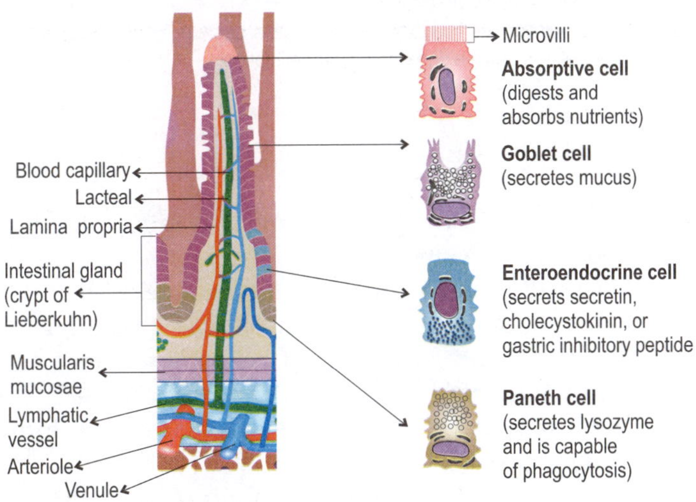

Fig. 62.2: Types of cells in the villi. Note enteroendocrine cells are present in the gland (Crypt of Lieberkühn) and plenty of goblet cells in the mucous membrane.

   c) ***Argentaffin cells:*** as the intracytoplasmic granules stain positively with silver salts by reduction reaction (*agyrophil cells*, on the other hand, require the addition of exogenous reducing substances for staining)
   d) ***Enteroendocrine cells:*** As these specialized cells are considered to be part of **APUD cell system** (having common properties as amine content, **A**mine **P**recursor **U**ptake and **D**ecarboxylation).
   - APUD cells are considered to be ***endodermal*** in origin, while previously they were thought to be neural crest derivative.
   - Endocrine cells are heavily populated in the proximal small bowel as this is the most active site for absorption and secretory activities. They are sparse in the colon which is less active site for such functions.
4. **Paneth Cells:** These are special endocrine cells present in the crypts of Lieberkühn in their deeper part.
   - They secrete ***defensins***, the naturally occurring antibiotics that protect developing enterocytes against infections.
   - Paneth cells also secrete *guanylin*.

IMPORTANT NOTE

APUD Cell System: Other endocrine cells belonging to the APUD cell system are C-cells of the thyroid, chromaffin cells of the adrenal medulla, certain cells of the carotid body, bronchi, hypothalamus, pituitary, and sympathetic ganglia.

Intestinal Secretion

PY4.2

Volume & pH: Daily secretion from small intestine varies from 1–1.7 liters. The pH is 7.5 to 8.

Composition: Intestinal secretion is isotonic, watery and alkaline (pH is about 8).

1. It consists of water (98.5%) and solids (1.5%).
2. The solids contain **anions** (HCO_3^-, Cl^-, PO_4^{3-}, and SO_4^{2-}), **cations** (Na^+, K^+, Ca^{2+} and Mg^{2+}), **enzymes** (Table 62.1), and **mucus**.
3. ***Enterokinase*** is present in the brush border of enterocytes and is extruded with denudation of mucosal epithelium.

Table 62.1 | Actions of Intestinal enzymes.

Enzyme	Substrate	Product
Enterokinase	Trypsinogen	Trypsin
α-dextrinase	α-dextrins	Glucose
Maltase	Maltose	Glucose
Sucrase	Sucrose	Glucose and fructose
Lactase	Lactose	Glucose and galactose
Peptidases	Terminal amino acids	Peptides & amino acids at amino end of peptides
Nucleotidases	Nucleotides	Nitrogenous bases, pentoses, and phosphates.

Mechanism & Regulation of Secretion

Mechanism

The exact mechanism of intestinal secretion is not very clear.

1. The cations are secreted by **active transport** and anions are transported along with cations to maintain electroneutrality.
2. Water follows the ions to **maintain osmotic balance**.
3. **Mucus** *is secreted by surface epithelial cells*, Brunner's gland and goblet cells that are present in the mucosa of the intestine.
   - **Mucin** is the major component of mucous that forms a gel to cover the mucosal epithelium.
   - **Mucus** protects the intestinal epithelium and helps in smooth passage of chyme through the intestinal lumen.
   - Mucus also traps bacteria and holds immunoglobulin.
4. **Secretion of Brunner's gland**, a thick ***alkaline mucus*** protects duodenal mucosa from acidic chyme.

Regulation of Secretion

Intestinal secretion is mainly controlled by **GI hormones and vagus nerve**.

1. **VIP** stimulates watery secretion. Therefore, diarrhea is a major feature of VIPomas.
2. The **vagal stimulation** increases intestinal secretion.
3. Many toxins stimulate intestinal secretion (Clinical Note 62.1).

Clinical Note 62.1

Cholera is a secretory diarrhea: Cholera toxin increases cyclic AMP concentration in the enterocytes that stimulate active secretion of HCO_3^-, and Cl^- into the lumen and produces watery diarrhea.

Functions of Intestinal Secretion

1. **Intestinal secretion helps in proper mixing of chyme.** This provides suitable environment for digestion and absorption of food materials in the intestine.
2. Intestinal secretion contains enzymes for **digestion of various nutrients**.
3. Mucus of intestinal secretion **protects intestinal epithelium** from damage. It also traps and kills bacteria.
4. Mucus in the intestinal secretion contains **immunoglobulins** that play an important role in *local defenses*.
5. The **alkaline secretion of Brunner's gland** protects upper intestinal mucosa from damage by acidic chyme.
6. Intestinal secretion helps in **forward propulsion of chyme** in the intestine.

Absorption of Water

Normally, about **8.5 liters of fluid** is added to GI tract daily. However, only about 100 ml of water is excreted in the stool. Thus, **GI tract absorbs more than 99.5% of water load** presented to it per day. About **75% of water absorption** takes place in the ***distal part of small intestine*** (details given below).

Intestinal Bacteria

Normally, a group of bacteria are present in the intestine. They constitute normal **intestinal flora**. These microorganisms are present **mainly in the ileum** than in upper part of the intestine. This is because the acidic content of duodenum and upper jejunum do not favour growth of bacteria.

1. The **gut microbiota** mainly includes **E. coli, Enterobacter aerogenes and Bacteroids fragilis**.
2. There are also few other bacteria like, ***cocci and bacilli*** of various types.
3. Normally, bacteria **are lost in the stool and replaced** in the intestine by their natural growth.
4. However, excess loss of bacterial flora in diseases like acute diarrhea results in improper digestion and absorption (Clinical Note 62.2).
5. Recent evidence suggests that gut microbiomes through enteric nervous system and autonomic sensory afferent **influence brain functions**, especially the cortical-limbic functions. **PY4.6**

- This is called **gut-brain axis** (GBA) or **gut-microbiota-brain axis**.
- GBA controls many functions that include, learning, memory, neurocognitive faculty, hypothalamo-pituitary endocrine functions, autonomic regulations, and so on.

Clinical Note 62.2

Lactobacilli is used in treatment of diarrhea: Apart from antibiotics, lactobacilli are included as part of the treatment of severe acute diarrhea that causes loss of intestinal flora.

- Bacterial flora is not well developed in infants and is slowly established during early childhood. Therefore, lactobacilli treatment is a must in any acute gastroenteritis in children.
- Many antibiotics interfere in growth of intestinal bacteria. Hence, lactobacilli supplement is given along with higher antibiotics.

Functions of Intestinal Flora

Intestinal bacteria are essential for many gut functions.

1. Normal bacterial flora is essential for **digestion and absorption of essential nutrients** including vitamins, minerals, and water.
2. They **synthesize vitamin K and B complexes**.
3. They produce chemicals that help in formation of short chain fatty acids, which help in **growth of the intestinal mucosa**.
4. Some bacteria species like Salmonella **inhibit inflammatory processes**.
   - They do so by **inhibiting ubiquitination of $I_\kappa B\alpha$**, the step that helps the transcription of factor **$NF_\kappa B$** to initiate inflammation.

- Bacteria also secrete **anti-inflammatory cytokines** like IL-10. Recently, commensal bacteria are genetically programmed to produce IL-10.

5. Some **bacteria utilize** substances like ascorbic acid and cyanocobalamin. Therefore, these vitamins are usually given in higher dosages.
6. **Bile salts are converted to bile acids** by intestinal bacteria, which are then absorbed into portal blood from intestine and colon.
   - Thus, intestinal flora **maintains bile acid pool** of the body.
7. They **impart brown color to the stool** by forming pigments from bile pigments.
   - Therefore, acholic (pale) stool is seen in biliary obstruction.
8. They **produce gases** that cause normal flatus. Normal flatus is required for normal ***distension and motility*** of intestine.
   - Exaggeration or decreased flatus indicates abnormality in intestinal flora.
9. They also contribute to the **odor of the feces**. This occurs due to production of amines like **indole and skatole** by intestinal bacteria.
10. They contribute to **plasma lipid level** by interfering in absorption of LDL and cholesterol.
    - Therefore, poorly absorbable antibiotic like **neomycin that modifies bacterial flora decreases plasma cholesterol.**
11. Through **gut-brain axis**, they control many brain functions.

Though these bacteria are nonpathogenic and beneficial, their entry into systemic circulation can cause systemic sepsis as occurs in ionizing radiation that breaks the intestinal defense barrier. This results in **radiation poisoning**.

Applied Physiology

Malabsorption Syndrome: The commonest abnormality due to inappropriate intestinal secretion is malabsorption syndrome. However, malabsorption also occurs due to gastric, hepatic and pancreatic deficiencies.

- **In malabsorption due to intestinal causes**, the digestive and absorptive functions of small intestine are impaired.
- The common intestinal causes of malabsorption are **sprue** (tropical sprue), **celiac disease** (gluten enteropathy), **Crohn's disease, Whipple's disease** and **radiation enteritis**, surgical resection.

Blind Loop Syndrome: Though normal bacterial flora is essential for health; overgrowth of bacteria is harmful. Such overgrowths occur when there is stasis of intestinal contents.

- This occurs in **surgically created blind loops** of small intestine, which is popularly known as **blind loop syndrome**.
- It causes **macrocytic anemia, malabsorption of vitamin B_{12} and steatorrhea**.

LARGE INTESTINE

Large intestine consists of **cecum, colon and rectum** (Fig. 62.3). the length of large intestine is about 150 cm. Colon forms the major part of the large gut.

Physiology of Colon

Functional Anatomy

Length of colon (ascending, transverse, descending and sigmoid colon) in adult is about 120 cm.

1. The **diameter of large intestine is bigger than small intestine**, which favours *slow passage of chyme* through it and also absorption of maximum quantity of water during its passage.

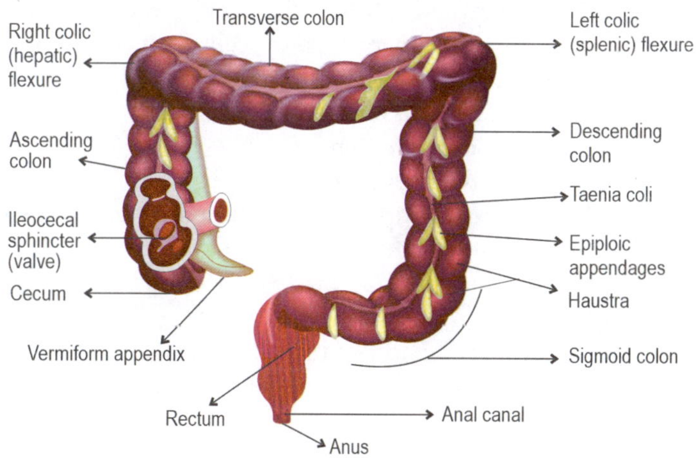

Fig. 62.3: Different parts of the large intestine. Note the presence of tenia coli that makes haustra and demarcates it from other parts of gut.

   - There are **no villi**, though the mucosal epithelium is folded to give villi like appearance to some extent.

2. There are many **crypts of Lieberkühn** in the mucous membrane that secrete a solution isotonic to that of plasma.
3. There are numerous **goblet cells** in the mucosal epithelium that secretes mucus (Fig. 62.4).
4. Lamina propria contains **intestinal glands** and submucosa contains **lymphatic nodules**.
5. No digestive enzymes are secreted in the colon

Colonic Secretion

Volume & pH: Daily secretion from colon is about 0.5 liter. The pH is about 8.

Composition of Secretion

Secretion of large intestine contains mainly **mucous** secreted by goblet cells. It contains **HCO_3^- and K^+** in large amount and some amount of sodium and water.

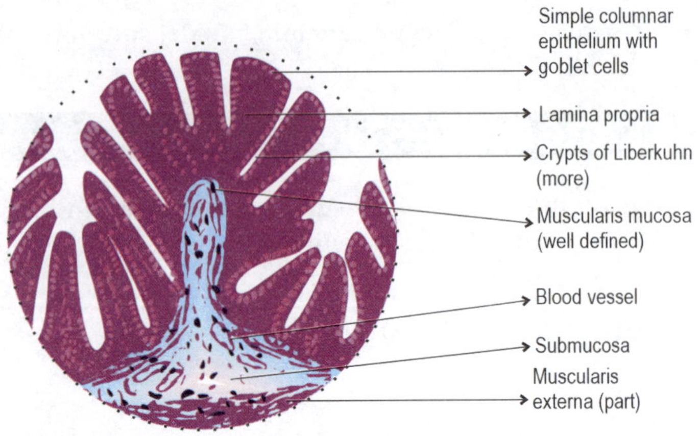

Fig. 62.4: Structure of the wall of large intestine. Note the presence of numerous goblet cells in the mucosa and many crypts of Lieberkühn.

Mechanism of Secretion

There are **crypts** in the mucous membrane that secrete a solution **isotonic to that of plasma**.

1. There are plenty of **goblet cells** that secrete mucous. Mucous secreted from goblet cells has following **functions:**
   - Protects intestinal mucosa
   - Help in stool formation.
   - Lubricate the intestinal mass.
   - Neutralize the acid which is formed by bacteria in the large intestine
2. Water and bicarbonate are secreted in significant amount.
3. Na^+ is reabsorbed and K^+ is secreted in large amount.
4. The **bacterial flora** of large intestine is similar to that of small intestine.
5. About 90% water is reabsorbed from the intestinal contents (both small and large intestine).
   - Therefore, when content of large intestine passes very slowly or there is stagnation, **constipation** occurs due to absorption of more water that causes solidification of stool.
   - Conversely, when the contents pass faster due to increased motility, **diarrhea** occurs.
   - Secretion of water and electrolyte in large quantity can also cause diarrhea.

Transfer of Electrolytes and Water: Large intestine can absorb Na^+, K^+, Cl^-, glucose and certain vitamins.

- However, secretion of K^+ and $HCO3^-$ into the colon is more.
- Colon can't absorb protein, fat or Ca^{2+}.
- Na^+ is actively absorbed from the colon and water follows ***along the osmotic gradient*** generated by absorption of Na^+ and Cl^-.

Colonic Bacteria

Colonic bacteria resemble the intestinal flora inhabiting ileum.

- They produce about **8 liter of gas per day** that contributes to flatus and colonic motility.
- They have **trophic effects** on colonic mucosal growth.
- **Ammonia** is produced by colonic bacteria, which is ***detoxified in the liver***. Hence, in severe liver disease, hepatic encephalopathy (suppression of brain activities) occurs.

Organisms

At birth, the colon is sterile but the colonic bacterial flora becomes established early in life. The micro-organisms habituating the colon are bacilli such as mainly Escherchia coli and Enterobacter aerogens. Gas gangrene bacilli may be present.

Functions of Colonic Bacteria

The physiological role of colonic bacterial flora are:

1. **Synthesis of the vitamins:** Vitamins e.g. ***vitamin K, number of B complex*** vitamins and folic acid are produced by these colonic organisms.
2. **Production of gas:** CO_2, hydrogen sulphide, hydrogen and methane which contribute to the flatus, are produced by bacterial flora (Application Box 62.1)
3. **Smell of stool:** The smell of stool is largely due to sulphides.
4. **Acidic reaction of stool:** Organic acids formed from carbohydrates by bacteria causes slightly acidic reaction of the stool (pH 5 to 7).
5. **Production of amines:** A number of amines are formed in the colon by bacterial enzymes that decarboxylate amino acids.
   - These amines are **histamine and tyramine** which may be harmful if produced in excess quantity.
   - **Indole and skatole** are responsible for the odour of the faeces.
6. **Colour of stool:** Pigments ***biliverdin & stercobilinogen*** formed from the bile pigments by the intestinal bacteria are responsible for the brown colour of the stool.
7. **Decrease blood lipids:** Intestinal bacteria play some role in **cholesterol metabolism** and decrease plasma cholesterol and LDL levels.

Application Box 62.1

Excess gas production causes borborygmi: The volume of gas normally found in the human gut is approximately 200mL, and the daily production is 500-1500mL. In some individuals, more gas is produced in the intestine that causes cramps, borborygmi (rumbling noise) and abdominal discomfort.

Absorption of Water

Normally, about 1.5 liters of water is ingested per day and 7 liters is added from GI secretions per day. However, only about 100 ml of water is excreted in the stool daily. Thus, **GI tract absorbs more than 99.5% of water load** presented to it per day.

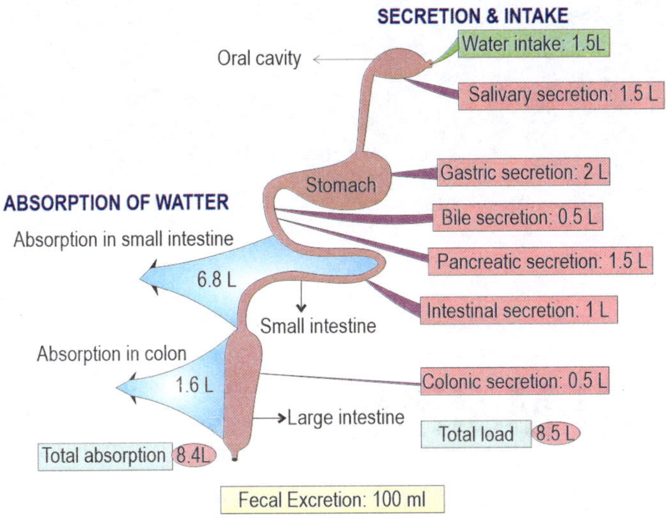

Fig. 62.5: Water absorption in small and large intestines. Note, out of 8.5 liters of load of fluid to the intestine per day, about 75% of absorption takes place in small intestine (6.8 L) and about 25% occurs in large intestine (1.6 L). Thus, total 99.5% of water presented to gut, is absorbed to blood by intestine. Thus, intestine plays an important role in water homeostasis of the body.

1. Water is not absorbed from mouth, esophagus, and stomach.
2. As most of the nutrients are absorbed mainly in the duodenum and jejunum, the osmolality of intestinal content which is about 600 mosm/kg H_2O, decreases to about 200 mosm/kg H_2O in the ileum and colon.
3. Therefore, **water is absorbed mainly from terminal ileum and colon** (Fig. 62.5) by osmotic gradient as osmolality of blood is about 290 mosm/kg H_2O.

Physiology Of Rectum

Rectum stores fecal materials. Role of rectum in **defecation reflex** is discussed in 'Motility of Large Intestine". Though, normally absorption of water from rectum is not significant, the **absorptive capacity is more** (Clinical Note 62.3)

IMPORTANT NOTE

Rectal administration of drugs: The absorptive capacity of mucosa of colon and rectum is large. Therefore, sometimes drugs are administered through rectum. Rectal administration is more preferred in children. Drugs that are administered rectally include purgatives, sedatives, anesthetics, and tranquilizers. However, care should be taken to control the volume of enema introduced into rectum in children as excess water absorption can cause water intoxication.

Exam Questions

1. With the help of labelled schematic diagram, describe the modifications in the intestinal wall. Briefly describe the functions and regulation of intestinal secretion.
2. Describe the role of intestinal bacterial flora in health and disease.
3. List the special features of layers of large intestine. Briefly describe the functions of colonic secretion. Give a note on water reabsorption in small and large intestine.

Multiple Choice Questions

1. Daily secretion of intestinal juice is about:
A. 1.3 lit B. 0.2 lit
C. 2.5 lit D. 3.2 lit

2. The intestinal glands that form intestinal secretion are named as:
A. Brunner's gland B. Crypts of Lieberkuhn
C. Enterooxyntic gland D. Enterochomaffin gland

3. The secretion of intestine is called as:
A. Succus entericus B. Intestinal fluid
C. Intestinal sap D. Intestinal liquid

4. Which of the following is not an important cell in the intestinal gland in the ileum?
A. Panenth cell B. Oxyntic cell
C. Goblet cell D. Enteroendocrine cells

5. All the following cells are endocrine cells in intestine EXCEPT:
A. Kulchitsky cell B. Enterochromaffin cell
C. Argentaffin cell D. Goblet cells

6. Which of the following does not stimulate intestinal secretion?
A. Vagal stimulation B. VIP
C. Guanylin D. Somatostatin

7. What is the experimental design to assess intestinal secretion?
A. Heidenhain pouch B. Bickel pouch
C. Thiry Vella loop D. Pavlov pouch

8. Which of the following is not true about colon?
A. Length is about 120cm
B. There are no villi in mucosa
C. There are many crypts of Lieberkühn
D. There are no goblet cells

9. Which vitamins are synthesized by intestinal bacteria
A. Vit K and D B. Vit K and B
C. Vit A and D D. Vit K and C

10. Which of the following is not the primary function gut flora?
A. Synthesis of short chain fatty acids
B. Decreased proliferation of epithelial cells
C. Production of vit. K
D. Fermentation of mucin

Answers

1. A	2. B	3. A	4. B	5. D
6. D	7. C	8. D	9. B	10. B

Chapter 63

Introduction to GI Motility

Learning Objectives

On completion of study of this chapter:

The student will be able to (must know):

1. Draw a labeled diagram of slow wave of GI smooth muscle.
2. Understand the relation between electrical and mechanical response.
3. Name the GI motilities and give their functions.
4. Mention various GI sphincters and give their functions
5. Appreciate the applied aspects of physiology of GI motility.

The student may also be able to (desirable to know):

1. Describe the electrophysiological properties of GI smooth muscle.

GI SMOOTH MUSCLES

Specialities of GI smooth muscle are:

1. GI smooth muscles are **unitary type** of smooth muscles.
2. They **contract spontaneously** without external neural and humoral influences.
3. They also **contract when stretched** without external innervation.
4. There is **no structured neuromuscular junction.**
5. GI smooth muscles **are long** (about 500 mm) and **slender** (5–20 mm in width).
6. They are arranged in **bundles.**

Electrophysiology of GI Smooth Muscle

Types of Couplings

The smooth muscle cells of the GIT are well coupled (better coordinated). Electrical charge spreads rapidly from cell to cell. This is called **electrical coupling,** which is **better between circular cells than the longitudinal cells** because the circular cells have more gap junctions.

There are **three types** of couplings: electromechanical, pharmacomechanical and mechanomechanical.

Electromechanical Coupling: Like skeletal muscles, smooth muscles have electromechanical coupling.

- That means, depolarization of the membrane causes opening of voltage-gated Ca^{++} channels and increases cytosolic calcium, which leads to muscle contraction.

Pharmacomechanical Coupling: In addition, smooth muscles have an additional mechanism of pharmacomechanical coupling, in which binding of a ligand to its receptor on the muscle membrane leads to opening of Ca^{++} channels and increase in cytosolic calcium without change in membrane potential.

Mechanomechanical Coupling: Stretch of smooth muscle causes muscle contraction, which is known as mechanomechanical coupling.

- Stretch on muscle opens stretch-sensitive calcium channel on the muscle cell membrane.
- Calcium influx causes muscle contraction.

GI Syncytial Tissues & Pacemaker Tissues

GI smooth muscles have numerous **gap junctions** that easily transmit electrical impulse from cell to cell.

- This accounts for the **syncytial nature** of smooth muscle in GI tract.
- Also, there are **pacemaker tissues** in GI tract that generate and spread electrical impulses.

Basic Electrical Rhythm & Slow Waves

Resting membrane potential (RMP) of smooth muscle of GI tract exhibit wide range of fluctuation.

- The electrical **slow waves** are wide spontaneous rhythmic fluctuations in the membrane potential ranging **between –65 to –40 mV** (Fig. 63.1).

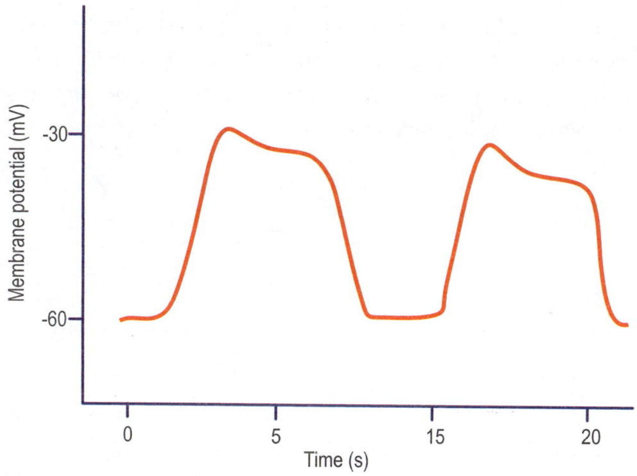

Fig. 63.1: Electrical slow waves of small intestine.

- The slow waves, which oscillate significantly are called **basal electrical rhythm** (BER) that occurs due to wide variation in the RMP of GI smooth muscles.
- The BER is present in all parts of GIT **except in the esophagus.**

Slow Waves

Slow waves in many regions of GI tract represent only as BER, whereas at other places like gastric antrum and intestine, they trigger action potential.

- Slow waves are generated by the **interstitial cells of Cajal** located between the longitudinal and circular muscle layers.
- Interstitial cells have **long processes that form gap junctions** with longitudinal and circular muscle cells. This enables ***easy and rapid conduction of slow waves*** from the interstitial cells into the smooth muscles.
- The slow waves spread throughout the smooth muscles of each segment of GI tract.

Phases of Slow Waves

A typical slow wave has **four phases** (Fig. 63.2).

Phase 1: This is the **rising phase *(depolarization)***, which occurs due to opening of voltage gated Ca^{++} channel.

Phase 2: This is the **plateau phase** that occurs due to balance between inward Ca^{++} current and outward K^{+} current.

Phase 3: This is the **falling phase *(repolarization)*** occurring due to activation of voltage gated K^{+} channel.

Phase 4: Return to membrane potential.

Frequency: The frequency of slow waves is 3/min in stomach, 6 to 10/min in colon, 15/min in jejunum and ileum, and 18/min in duodenum (Fig. 63.3).

- The amplitude and the frequency of slow waves are influenced by the activity of **extrinsic and intrinsic nerves**, and by hormones.
- Usually, **sympathetic stimulation decreases** the amplitude and **parasympathetic stimulation increases** the amplitude of slow waves.

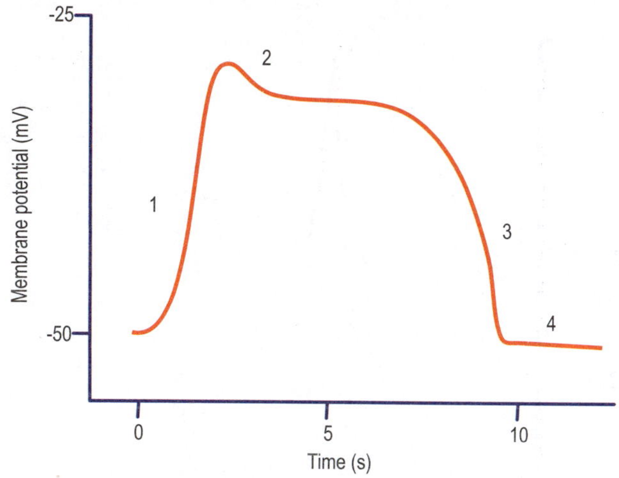

Fig. 63.2: Phases of electrical slow waves of small intestine. When action potential are associated with slow waves, they occur on the plateau phase (phase 2).

Action Potentials

When the peak of a slow wave exceeds the threshold, action potential is **triggered from the peak** (Fig.63.4). These action potentials **facilitate the force of contraction** of smooth muscle.

1. Action potentials have longer duration (10–20 ms). Usually, they do not overshoot.
2. The **rising phase** of the action potential is caused by **influx of Ca^{++} and Na^{+}.**
3. The **repolarization phase** is due to **K^{+} efflux.**
4. The magnitude and frequency of action potential are enhanced by vagal stimulation and inhibited by sympathetic stimulation.

Relationship between Electrical and Mechanical Responses: Slow waves that are not accompanied by action potentials do not elicit contraction, whereas slow waves that are accompanied by action potentials evoke contraction. The **greater the frequency of action potential** (that occur at the peak of slow waves), **the more intense is the contraction** (Fig.63.5).

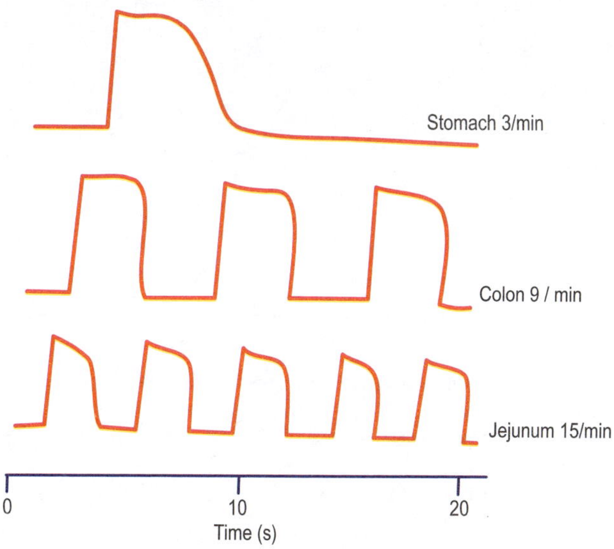

Fig. 63.3: Frequency of slow waves. Note that frequency is least in stomach (3/min) and maximum in intestine (15/min).

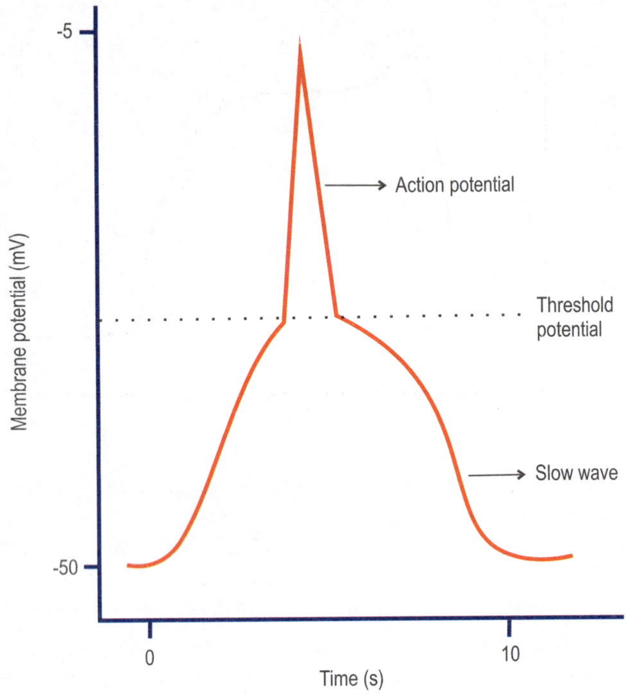

Fig. 63.4: Action potential of GI smooth muscle. Note, once the threshold is reached, action potential is generated on the peak of slow wave.

Enteric Motor Neurons

Organization of enteric nervous system (ENS) has been described in Chapter 56 (refer, Fig. 56.4 and 56.5). Enteric motor neurons **innervate the smooth muscles of GI tract** and are the ***final pathway*** for output of information from autonomic nervous system and ENS to the muscle cells (Fig. 63.6).

1. Cell bodies of enteric motor neurons are present in the myenteric plexus and the axons project aborally to innervate muscle fibers.

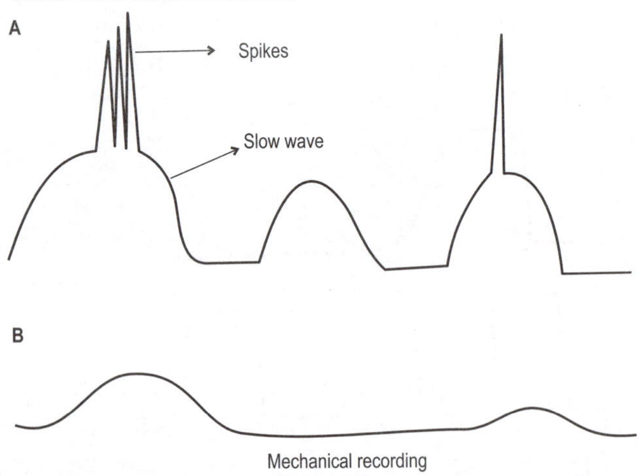

Fig. 63.5: Relationship between electrical (A) and mechanical (B) responses of GI smooth muscle. Note that with increased number of action potential on a slow wave increases the magnitude of contraction and contraction does not occur in the absence of action potential.

- The major **excitatory neurotransmitters** are acetylcholine and substance P, and **inhibitory neurotransmitters** are catecholamines, ATP, VIP and NO.

2. There are also **secretomotor neurons** in the submucosal plexus, that on stimulation release ***histamine during allergic reactions*** and produce **neurogenic secretory diarrhea** during stress.

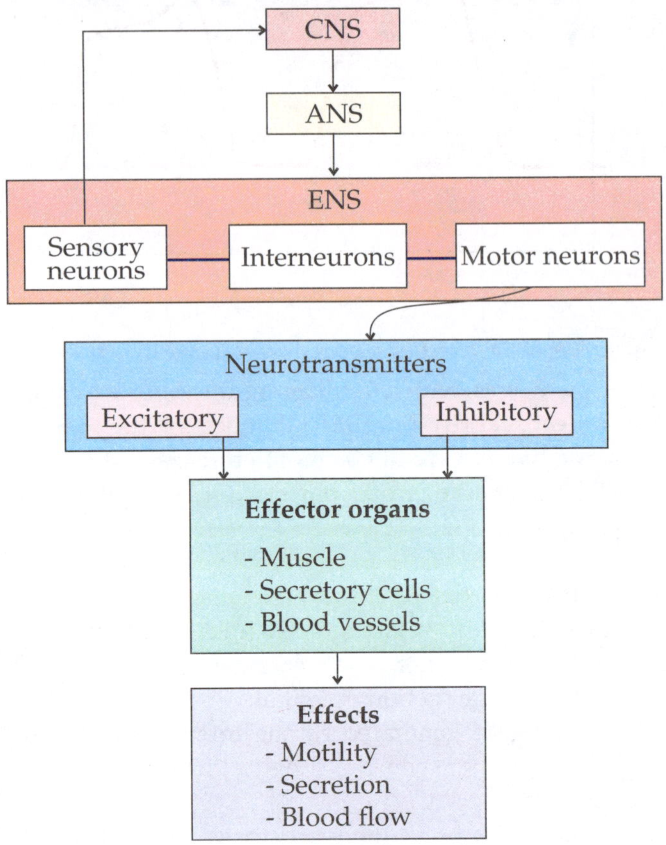

Fig. 63.6: Enteric nervous system (ENS). Note that ENS is the final common pathway for GI effector organs.

BASIC PATTERNS OF GI MOTILITY

GI motility is required for **propulsion, trituration** (crushing and grinding) and **mixing** of food. Propulsion of food is achieved by **peristaltic movement**; trituration and mixing are accomplished by **retropulsive** and **segmental movements**.

Peristalsis

This is a **reflex response of GI tract to stretch**, which results in **organized propulsion of luminal content** of the gut in forward direction.

- This response is present **in all parts of GIT** starting from esophagus to rectum.
- When the **gut wall is stretched** by the contents of its lumen, peristalsis is initiated.

Mechanism

Stretch initiates a circular ring like **contraction behind the stimulus** (i.e. the part before the area of distension) and **relaxation in front of it**.

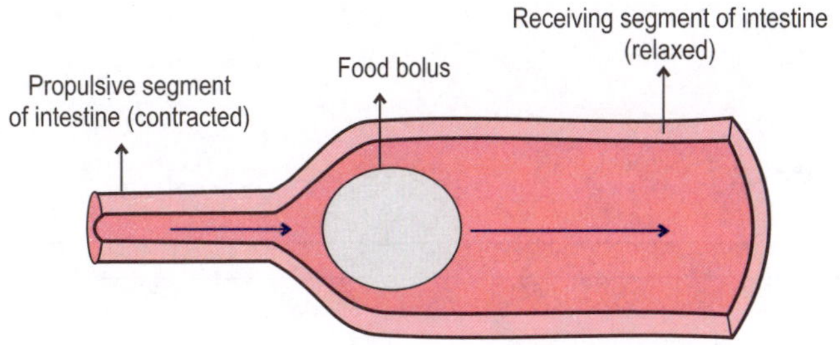

Fig. 63.7: Propulsion of food bolus in gut by peristaltic movement. Direction of arrows indicates the direction of propulsion.

- The part behind the stimulus is called **propulsive segment** as it propels the bolus of food or chyme and the part ahead of the stimulus is called **receiving segment** as it receives the bolus (Fig. 63.7).
  - In the propulsive segment, the **circular muscles contract and longitudinal muscles relax**
  - In receiving segment, the **circular muscles relax and longitudinal muscles contract.**
- The contraction wave then **moves in forward direction**, i.e. from oral to anal direction, **propelling the contents aborally**.

Role of Cholinergic Neurons: The local **cholinergic neurons** play an important role in peristalsis.

1. Cholinergic neurons that are **present in a retrograde direction** (with cell bodies towards anus and terminals towards oral cavity), activate the neurons that release **substance P and acetylcholine**.
   - These neurons **stimulate circular muscle contraction** and help in formation and progression of contractile ring behind the stimulus.
2. Cholinergic neurons that are **present in antegrade direction** (cell bodies towards oral cavity and terminals towards anus) activate the neurons that secrete **VIP and nitric oxide**.
   - These neurons assist in **relaxation of circular muscle** in the portion of the gut ahead of the stimulus.

Factors Influencing Peristalsis

The normal rate of transmission of peristaltic wave varies in different parts of GI tract, ranging between 2–15 cm/s. This is influenced by intrinsic and extrinsic nerve supply.

1. **Sympathetic stimulation** inhibits peristalsis and **parasympathetic stimulation** enhances it.
   - Though the transmission of peristalsis is affected by autonomic influence, its ***genesis is independent of it***.
2. **Serotonin**, secreted by local stretch of gut enhances peristalsis.

Migrating Motor Complex

During the interdigestive period, the electromechanical activity of GI smooth muscles is altered. A cycle of motor activity **migrates from stomach to distal ileum**. This is called migrating motor complex (MMC) or **long peristalsis**.

Phases: MMC has three phases:

Phase-I: The quiescent phase

Phase-II: The period of irregular electrical and mechanical activity.

Phase-III: The period of burst of electrical activities.

Frequency and Duration: Usually, it **originates in the stomach** and transmitted aborally at a **rate of 5 cm/min.** It occurs at an **interval of 90 min**, after which the cycle is repeated.

Significance: MMC occurs in the interdigestive phase.

1. The phase III of MMC results in **long peristalsis**, which starts from stomach and terminates in distal part of the ileum.
   - Therefore, it **sweeps the gastric and intestinal contents** into the large intestine.
   - Consequently, MMC is alternatively called **sweeper of GI tract**.
2. Characteristically, MMC immediately **stops when food is ingested**.

Retroperistalsis

Normally, peristalsis moves in forward direction. However, if there is an obstruction in the lumen, **reverse peristalsis** occurs. This is called retroperistalsis.

1. Vomiting occurs due to retroperistalsis.
2. Retroperistalsis is also initiated by **emotional factors** or due to stimulation of medullary vomiting centers.

Segmentation

This commonly occurs in **small intestine**. It is characterized by **closely spaced contraction** of the circular muscle layer that **divides the small intestine into many segments**. It is primarily **mixes chyme with pancreatic and intestinal secretions,** hence it is called **mixing movement** (details are given in Chapter 66).

Role of Sphincters

Sphincters are rings of smooth muscles that remain in a state of continuous contraction. There are **anatomical and physiological sphincters**.

1. Upper esophageal sphincter is an example of **physiological sphincter**, which prevents esophageal content to regurgitate back into oral cavity.
2. **Anatomical sphincters** are located at gastroesophageal, gastroduodenal, ileocecal junctions, and at the opening of rectum into anus.

Regulate movement of content from upper compartment to lower compartment

They prevent backward movement and regulate **coordinated propulsion of contents aborally**.

Exam Questions

1. Describe the electrical properties of GI smooth muscles.
2. What is migrating motor complex. Describe its mechanisms and physiological importance.
3. Describe the mechanism of peristalsis in the gut. Give a note on retroperistalsis.

Multiple Choice Questions

1. Major regulator of interdigestive myoelectric complexes:
A. GRP
B. Neurotensin
C. GIP
D. Motilin

2. Myenteric plexus is present in:
A. Muscularis externa
B. Submucosa
C. Mucosa
D. Serosa

3. Small intestinal peristalsis is controlled by:
A. Myenteric plexus
B. Meissner plexus
C. Vagus nerve
D. Para sympathetic system

4. Pacemaker of the G.I.T is located in:
A. Fundus of stomach
B. Long muscle of small intestine
C. Pyloric end of stomach
D. Central control of CBD origin

5. Chyme is propelled forward in small intestine by:
A. Segmentation
B. Haustrations
C. Migratory motor complexes (MMC)
D. Peristalsis

6. Major initiating response for peristalsis is
A. Hormonal
B. Local stretching of gut
C. Neural
D. None

7. Migratory motor complexes in the gut reappear after intervals of
A. 90 mins
B. 120 mins
C. 60 mins
D. 150 mins

8. Enterogastric reflex is caused by all, EXCEPT:
A. Duodenum distension
B. Alkaline pH in duodenum & hormones
C. Increased osmolality of chime
D. Products of protein digestion & H+ ions bathing duodenal mucosa

9. Frequency of slow waves (BER) is maximum in:
A. Stomach
B. Ileum
C. Colon
D. Duodenum

10. Maximum postprandial motility is seen in:
A. Ascending colon
B. Sigmoid colon
C. Transverse colon
D. Descending colon

Answers

1. D 2. A 3. A 4. C 5. D 6. B 7. A 8. B 9. D 10. B

Chapter 64

Chewing, Deglutition and Esophageal Motility

Learning Objectives

On completion of study of this chapter:

The student will be able to (must know):

1. List the functions of mastication.
2. Understand the mechanism of different phases of deglutition.
3. Understand the principle of esophageal motility
4. Elucidate the mechanism and importance of esophageal peristalsis.
5. Learn the physiological basis of reflux esophagitis and achalasia cardia.

The student may also be able to (desirable to know):

1. Describe the mechanism of deglutition reflex.
2. Describe the mechanism of esophageal motility.

CHEWING (MASTICATION)

Chewing or mastication is mostly a **voluntary activity**. The process of mastication is **initiated usually reflexly** following the arrival of food in the mouth.

Mastication has following functions:

1. Mastication **cuts and grinds larger food particles** into smaller particles.
2. It **increases salivary secretion** (Application Box 64.1).
3. It **mixes food with saliva**.
4. **Lubricates content** of the oral cavity, so that swallowing becomes easier.
5. **Breaks down starch** and allows saliva to mix with the broken starch particles. Therefore, chewing **improves the taste of starch** containing foods.
6. **Improves dental strength** and hygiene.

Muscles Of Mastication: Chewing occurs due to contraction of **four groups of muscles**.

1. **Masseter** elevates mandible and helps in *clenching of teeth*.
2. **Temporalis** helps in *retracting mandible*.
3. **Pterygoids** (external and internal) protrude mandible and depress chin.
    - This helps in *opening the mouth*.
    - Alternative contractions of right and left pterygoids help in *grinding movements*.
4. **Buccinator** prevents accumulation of food between cheek and mouth.

Application Box 64.1

Food should be chewed adequately before swallowing: Mastication breaks the larger food particles into smaller particles. Mastication is the major stimulus for salivary secretion. More saliva is required for a smooth swallowing. Digestion of salivary amylase takes place in the stomach. Though it has been said to chew 32 times before swallowing, it should be done at least 10 times.

SWALLOWING (DEGLUTITION)

Swallowing or deglutition is the process by which the food material from oral cavity is transported into esophagus. Though it is initiated voluntarily, **most part of it is involuntary** or reflexive. Therefore, this is also called **deglutition reflex**.

Stages of Deglutition

Swallowing is divided into **three stages** (phases): oral, pharyngeal and esophageal phase. Oral phase is voluntary and pharyngeal and esophageal phases are involuntary.

Oral Phase

This is also called **buccal phase**. This is the **voluntary phase** of swallowing.

- It is initiated when the tongue separates a bolus of food from the mass of foodstuff present in the mouth.
- At the beginning, the tip of the **tongue presses against the hard palate** and then the body of tongue presses on

it. This action of the tongue ***moves the food backward*** in the oral cavity. Thus, the food bolus is **forced into the pharynx**.
- Once the food touches the receptors at the pharyngeal opening, swallowing reflex is initiated.

Pharyngeal Phase

The major objective of pharyngeal phase is **to push food bolus into the esophagus** without its entry into respiratory passage.

Reflex Pathway

Receptors: Receptors are present around the pharyngeal opening.

Afferents: Impulses from pharyngeal receptors are transmitted to centers through **trigeminal, glossopharyngeal and vagus nerves**.

Centers: Centers for deglutition are **nucleus tractus solitarius** and **nucleus ambiguous** located in the medulla.

Efferents: Effector organs are muscles of pharynx and tongue that are innervated by **trigeminal, glossopharyngeal, vagus and hypoglossal** nerves.

Events

The events in pharyngeal phase occur in sequence within few milliseconds (Fig. 64.1).

1. The **soft palate is pulled** in upward direction. The **palatopharyngeal folds** move in inward direction.
   - These movements ***prevent entry of food into the nasopharynx.***
   - This also provides a small passage for food to enter the pharynx.
2. Laryngeal opening is closed by vocal cards pulled together.
   - The larynx moves forward and upward against the epiglottis.
   - These events **prevent entry of food into trachea** (Clinical Note 64.1).
3. The **superior constrictor muscles of pharynx** constrict, which forces food to enter deep into the pharynx and then from there into the esophagus.
   - Simultaneously, **relaxation of upper esophageal sphincter** (UES) occurs that allows the food to easily enter the esophagus.
4. During this phase, **respiration is reflexly inhibited** due to inhibition of respiratory centers. This is called **deglutition apnea**.

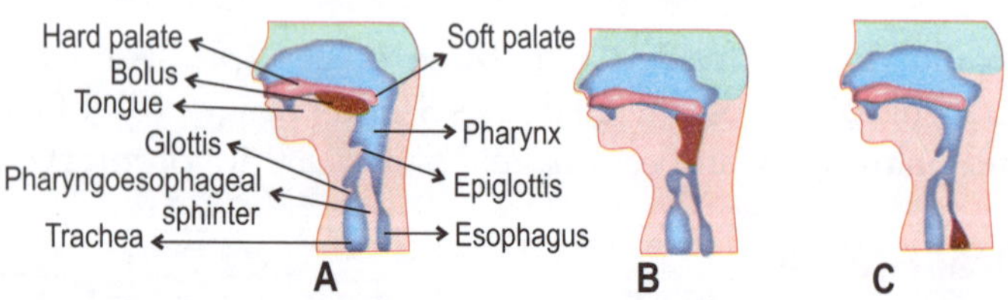

Fig. 64.1: Phases of deglutition. Note the mechanism of deglutition in oral (**A**), pharyngeal (**B**), and esophageal (**C**) stages. In the oral phase, tongue pushes bolus of food into the back of pharynx. In the pharyngeal phase, epiglottis covers the glottis to prevent aspiration of food (prevents food to enter trachea) and soft palate is elevated to prevent food to enter nasal passage. In the esophageal phase, upper esophageal sphincter (UES) relaxes to allow food to descend into esophagus.

Clinical Note 64.1

Do not speak while eating: During deglutition, respiration is temporarily arrested and food does not enter the respiratory passage. Laryngeal opening is closed by vocal cords pulled together. Speaking or coughing during swallowing keeps the laryngeal outlet opened and therefore there is risk of food particle entering into the respiratory passage. Food or water entering respiratory passage may cause choking. One should eat in silently and consciously.

Esophageal Phase

Once food enters the esophagus, which is facilitated by relaxation of UES, the peristaltic wave (**primary peristalsis**) is initiated just below the UES.

1. Reflexly, **UES contracts** that prevent regurgitation of food back into the pharynx.
2. The **peristaltic wave** travels at about 3–5 cm/s. It takes about 10 seconds for food bolus to pass through the entire esophagus.
3. If the primary peristalsis is ineffective, a second peristaltic (**secondary peristalsis**) wave is initiated to push the food bolus.

Disorders of Deglutition

Decreased or absence of deglutition reflex: If deglutition reflex is impaired or abolished, regurgitation of food into the nose or aspiration into the larynx and trachea occurs. It is seen in:
- **IXth or Xth nerve paralysis** in lesions of medulla
- When pharynx is anaesthetized with cocaine. In this deglutition reflex is abolished temporarily.

Dysphagia: Dysphagia is **difficulty in swallowing** due to any cause. Usually, it occurs in **acute and severe pharyngitis**. It can occur due to motor problems in pharynx, upper esophagus or foreign body, acute inflammation in oral cavity.

ESOPHAGEAL MOTILITY

Parts of Esophagus

Esophagus is divided into **three parts**: upper, body and lower.

1. In the **upper part of esophagus**, the **muscles are striated** (like skeletal muscles) muscles.
2. In the **lower part** the muscles are **smooth muscles**
3. In the **middle part**, there is **mixture of smooth and striated muscles** (Fig. 64.2).

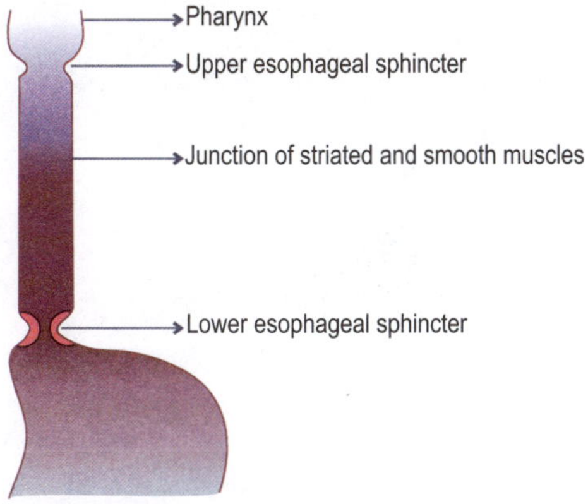

Fig. 64.2: Structure of esophagus. Note that the muscle of upper part of the esophagus is striated and of lower part is smooth. A transitional zone of striated and smooth muscles exists between them.

However, all esophageal muscles are mainly **innervated by vagal fibers**, even the striated esophageal muscles receive vagal motor fibers.

Special Features

1. Esophagus differs from other parts of GI system **for not having electrical slow waves** to trigger contraction. Therefore, **excitability of its muscle is low**.
2. Muscles in the body of the esophagus are **relaxed always**, except during deglutition.
3. **All muscle fibers** including striated fibers are innervated by **vagus nerve**.
4. Activation of deglutition reflex initiates **peristaltic contraction** by neural mechanism ***(primary peristalsis)*** or presence of food bolus locally stimulates peristalsis **(secondary peristalsis).**

Esophageal Sphincters

Upper Esophageal Sphincter: Upper esophageal sphincter is mainly a **physiological sphincter**.

- It ***reflexly relaxes*** to allow the food from pharynx to enter the esophagus.
- However, once food has entered the esophagus, **it constricts to prevent regurgitation of food** back into the pharynx.

Lower Esophageal Sphincter: Lower esophageal sphincter **remains tonically contracted**. It relaxes only when food from the esophagus enters the stomach. Therefore, it always **prevents reflux of food** back into the esophagus from the stomach.

- The significant fraction of **basal tone of lower esophageal sphincter** is contributed by *vagal cholinergic fibers*.
- However, vagal fibers **inhibit circular muscles of the sphincter** in response to primary peristalsis that relaxes the sphincter and allows food to enter the stomach.
- This inhibitory action is mediated by stimulation of other neurons through activation of cholinergic vagal neurons that **secrete VIP and nitric oxide** (NO).

Esophageal Peristalsis

Two types of peristalses occur in esophagus: primary and secondary.

Primary Peristalsis

Primary peristalsis is **initiated by deglutition reflex**.

- In the third phase of deglutition, when food bolus enters esophagus, a ring of contraction appears just cephalad to the bolus, which pushes the bolus towards stomach.
- This is the primary peristalsis, and it appears due to the **act of swallowing whether or not food is present** in the mouth. Even swallowing of saliva activates it.

Secondary Peristalsis

When primary peristalsis fails to push the bolus from the body of the esophagus, secondary peristalsis starts.

- Secondary peristalsis is initiated by **activation of mechanoreceptors** due to presence of food bolus in the esophagus.
- Experimentally, it can be induced by inflating a balloon in the body of the esophagus.

Applied Physiology

Reflux Esophagitis PY4.9

When **LES becomes incompetent**, *reflux of acid gastric content* into esophagus produces esophagitis, known as ***reflux esophagitis***.

- Popularly, it is known as "**heartburn**" as the patient describes the pain in the retrosternal area.
- In chronic cases, it can cause stricture or ulceration of esophagus.
- It is treated by **proton pump blocker** or H_2 receptor blocker.

Fundoplication: Fundoplication may be needed, in which a portion of the fundus of the stomach is wrapped around the lower esophagus so that LES remains inside a narrow tunnel of the stomach.

Barrett's Esophagus

In few cases of chronic reflux esophagitis, the normal squamous epithelium of esophagus is replaced by columnar epithelium.

- This is called columnar metaplasia.
- This is a premalignant condition.

Achalasia Cardia

'Achalasia' means **failure to relax**. In some individuals, **resting tone of LES is high**. Therefore, the **sphincter fails to relax** completely during deglutition. This causes **inadequate emptying of esophagus** and food collects in the esophagus and the **organ is massively dilated**.

Causes: It occurs due to **deficiency of myenteric plexus** at LES in the esophagus. Also, the ***secretion of VIP and NO,*** the neurotransmitters that cause relaxation of GI muscles, *is defective* in this condition. Thus, resting tone of LES becomes high.

Diagnosis: Diagnosis is made by demonstrating **rat tail in barium meal x-ray** (body of esophagus is dilated and lower part is narrowed giving appearance of a rat) (Fig. 64.3) or by demonstrating retained food and fluid in esophagoscopy.

Treatment: Treatment for achalasia is **mechanical pneumatic dilatation** of the sphincter.

1. In severe cases, **surgical weakening** of the sphincter by myotomy (incision of the esophageal muscle) is performed.
2. Also, **administration of drugs** that decrease tone of the sphincter has been successfully tried. For example, **injection of botulinum toxin** into LES that inhibits acetylcholine release produces relaxation of the sphincter.

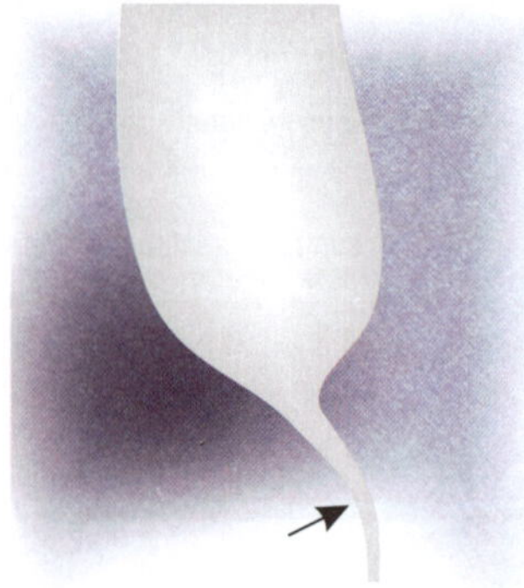

Fig. 64.3: Diagrammatic illustration of 'Rat tail appearance' sign of esophagus as seen in barium meal X-ray. Note, the body of esophagus is dilated and lower part is narrowed giving appearance of a rat tail (arrow mark).

Aerophagia

While eating and drinking, some volume of air is automatically swallowed, which is removed by **belching** (regurgitation) of air. But some individuals have **more aerophagia** and develop ***abdominal discomfort and borborygmi*** (rumbling noises in the intestine and colon). It is seen in nervous individuals who have decreased tone of the upper esophageal sphincter.

Exam Questions

1. List the functions of mastication. Briefly describe the mechanisms in the different phases of deglutition.
2. Briefly describe esophageal peristalsis. Write a note on achalasia cardia.

Multiple Choice Questions

1. **Which of the following is not true about mastication?**
   A. It improves dental strength and hygiene
   B. Masseter helps in clenching of teeth
   C. Temporalis helps in retracting the mandible
   D. Buccinator helps in opening the mouth
2. **All the following are true about deglutition reflex, EXCEPT:**
   A. Oral phase is voluntary
   B. Afferents are present in 5th, 9th and 10th cranial nerves
   C. Constriction of superior constrictor muscles of pharynx pushes food into pharynx and oesophagus
   D. Constriction of upper esophageal sphincter occurs in pharyngeal phase
3. **In the oesophageal phase, bolus of food is pushed down in oesophagus by:**
   A. Heaviness of food B. Effect of gravity on food
   C. Primary peristalsis D. Segmental contraction
4. **Which of the following is not true about esophagus?**
   A. Upper part of esophagus is made up of striated muscle
   B. Lower part is made up of smooth muscles
   C. Esophageal smooth muscles exhibit strong electrical slow waves
   D. Esophageal muscles are mainly innervated by vagal fibers.
5. **Effect of acetylcholine on LES is:**
   A. Contraction B. Relaxation
   C. No effect D. Contraction followed by relaxation
6. **Lower esophageal sphincter**
   A. Has no tonic activity
   B. Has a tone which is provided by the sympathetic system
   C. Relaxes on increasing abdominal pressure
   D. Relaxes ahead of the peristaltic wave
7. **Which of the following neurotransmitter is not released on stimulation of vagal nerve supplying esophageal muscles?**
   A. Acetylcholine B. Nitric oxide
   C. Motilin D. VIP
8. **All of the following are true about achalasia cardia, EXCEPT:**
   A. Deficiency of myenteric plexus at LES is the cause
   B. Neurotransmitter VIP and NO are deficient
   C. Failure of LES to constrict is the is the major problem in this disorder
   D. Rat tail in barium x-ray is a typical finding
9. **Which of the following has both voluntary and involuntary components?**
   A. Mastication B. Deglutition
   C. Gastric emptying D. Reverse peristalsis

Answers

1. D	2. D	3. C	4. C	5. A
6. D	7. C	8. C	9. B	

Chapter 65

Gastric Motility

Learning Objectives

On completion of study of this chapter:

The student will be able to (must know):

1. Name the gastric motilities and give their main functions.
2. Correlate the functional modification in stomach to gastric motor functions.
3. Elucidate the importance of gastric relaxations.
4. Describe the mechanism and regulation of gastric emptying.
5. Understand the link of gastric electrophysiology with gastric motor dysfunctions.
6. Illustrate the mechanism of vomiting.

The student may also be able to (desirable to know):

1. Explain the mechanism, regulation and application of gastric emptying.
2. Describe the vomiting reflex.

Gastric motilities allow stomach to act as a temporary **reservoir of large amount of food** of a single meal, **convert the food into chyme**, and ensure the gastric content **enters the duodenum at a slow but controlled rate** so that duodenum and jejunum being narrower tubes, handle the chyme effectively.

FUNCTIONAL ANATOMY

Parts of Stomach

Stomach is divided into **two parts**: the proximal stomach and distal stomach (Fig. 65.1).

Proximal Stomach

This consists mainly of the fundus and a major part of body of the stomach.

- The proximal part of stomach **accommodates large volume of food** (as large as 2 to 4 liters) without much increase in intragastric pressure.

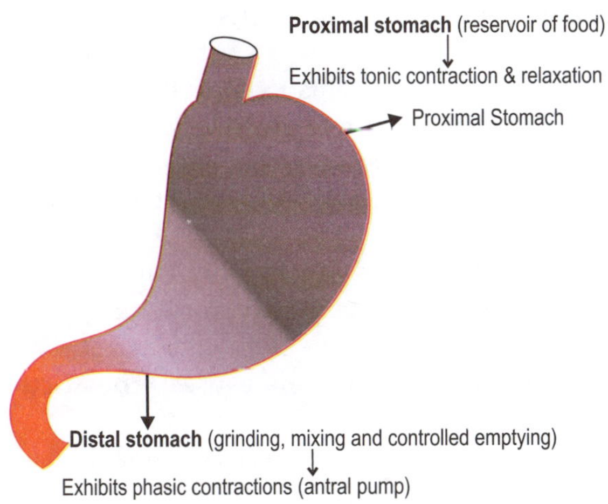

Fig. 65.1: Motor parts of stomach. The proximal stomach is formed by fundus and major portion of the body. The distal stomach is formed by antrum and lower portion of the body.

  - This becomes possible due to the phenomenon of **receptive relaxation**.
- the proximal stomach serves mainly as **reservoir of food**.

Distal Stomach

It consists mainly of the **antrum.**

- The antrum physiologically acts as a **mechanical pump**, which **propels food towards the pylorus** and helps in **grinding and mixing of food**.
- Antral contractions break foodstuff **into smaller particles** and **mix food** thoroughly with gastric juice to form **chyme**.
- **Pyloric sphincter remains partially closed** and does not allow easy entry of gastric contents into the duodenum.
- However, vigorous contractions of gastric antrum help gastric content enter the duodenum at a **slow but controlled rate**.

Structure of Stomach Wall

Stomach wall contains all general components of the wall of the GI tract (refer Fig. 56.3, Chapter 56). However, the muscle coat is more thick, with the **circular muscle layer being more prominent** than the longitudinal and oblique layers.

- **Thickness of muscularis externa increases from body towards pylorus** (Fig. 65.2).
- The highly developed muscle coat helps antrum work as **effective pump**.

Gastroduodenal Junction

The **junction between stomach & duodenum** is called gastroduodenal junction. The pylorus separates antrum and duodenum. There is a sphincter in the pylorus consisting of a ring like thickening of circular muscle fibers, known as **pyloric sphincter**.

Functions: Important functions of gastroduodenal junction are:

1. To allow gastric contents to enter the duodenum at a **slow and controlled rate** (the rate at which duodenum is capable of possessing the chyme).
2. To **prevent regurgitation of duodenal contents** back into the stomach.

Neurohumoral Control of Pyloric Part: The pylorus is richly innervated by parasympathetic (vagal) and sympathetic fibers.

1. **Sympathetic stimulation** causes **constriction of pyloric sphincter**.
2. Activation of **parasympathetic fibers** has both **stimulating and inhibiting effects**.
   - The stimulatory effects are mediated by *cholinergic vagal fibers*.
   - Inhibitory effects are mediated by the vagal fibers that release **VIP or nitric oxide** (NO).

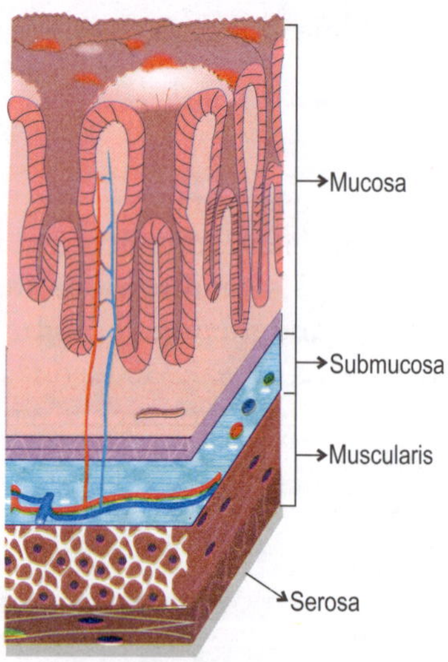

Fig. 65.2: Layers of the stomach wall. Note, muscularis is more developed, especially in pyloric part.

3. **Constriction of pyloric sphincter** also occurs in response to **hormones** like ***CCK, gastrin, GIP, and secretin***. Therefore, these hormones slow gastric emptying.

Innervation of Stomach

Stomach is densely innervated by both the division of ANS and the neurons of the enteric nervous system.

1. **Parasympathetic** innervation (vagal fibers) ***stimulates*** whereas **sympathetic** innervation (fibers originate from celiac plexus) ***inhibits*** gastric motility and secretion.
   - Axons arising from intramural plexuses innervate smooth muscles and secretory cells.
2. **Sensory fibers** provide information about an **intragastric pressure, gastric distention, chemical composition and pH** of gastric content, and ***pain sensation*** originating in the stomach. All these stimuli influence gastric motility

Electrophysiology of Gastric Motility

The **peristaltic waves** in the stomach occur usually at the frequency of **gastric slow waves**.

- The gastric slow wave has **four phases** that resemble the action potentials of cardiac muscle (Fig. 63.2; Chapter 63). However, it ***does not overshoot*** and ***last for a longer period*** (10 times that of cardiac action potential).

1. The smooth muscles of stomach contract when the depolarization of the slow wave *exceeds the threshold for contraction*.
2. The **force of contraction** depends on the **degree, frequency & duration of depolarization.**
   - Greater the depolarization and longer the muscle cells remain depolarized (above threshold), greater is the force of contraction.
   - **In antrum of the stomach**, action potential spikes occur in the plateau phase.
3. **Acetylcholine and gastrin improve gastric contractility** by enhancing the amplitude and duration of the plateau phase of gastric slow waves. **Norepinephrine inhibits** by the opposite mechanism.

TYPES OF GASTRIC MOTILITY

PY4.3

Gastric movements are hunger contractions, receptive relaxation, peristalsis, migrating motor complex and reverse peristalsis.

Hunger Contractions

When, stomach is empty, motility of the stomach increases. If stomach is allowed to **remain empty for a**

longer duration, contractions become **vigorous**. These contractions are called hunger contractions. Usually, hunger contractions are **distressing and painful.**

Gastric Relaxations

Receptive Relaxation

This is the relaxation of the fundus and body of the stomach **in response to chewing and swallowing of food.** Thus, stomach prepares itself to receive food (Fig. 65.3). The relaxation continues till food continues to enter the stomach, so that a large meal is easily accommodated in it.

1. Because of receptive relaxation, the **intragastric pressure does not rise** in spite of accumulation of a large volume of food.
2. The receptive relaxation is **mediated by vagus nerve** (Fig. 65.4).
    - Normally, gastric motility induced by vagal stimulation is mediated by cholinergic fibers.
    - However, receptive relaxation mediated by vagus is due to **release of neurotransmitters like VIP and NO** (*non cholinergic fibers*) at its nerve ending.

Adaptive and Feedback Relaxations

There is other **two types** of gastric relaxations: adaptive and feedback.

Adaptive Relaxation: The **adaptive relaxation** is the relaxation of stomach triggered by distension of stomach.

- Receptive relaxation starts even before food reaches stomach whereas adaptive relaxation occurs **in response to stretching** of stomach wall.
- This is mediated by **vagovagal reflex** (Fig. 65.4) and is meant to accommodate a greater volume of food.

Feedback Relaxation: The **feedback relaxation** of stomach is a **reflexive relaxation** that occurs due to presence of food in proximal segment of small intestine.

- Acidic chyme and fatty acid in intestine inhibit gastric motility by both **hormonal and neural mechanisms** that cause feedback relaxation of stomach (Fig. 65.4).

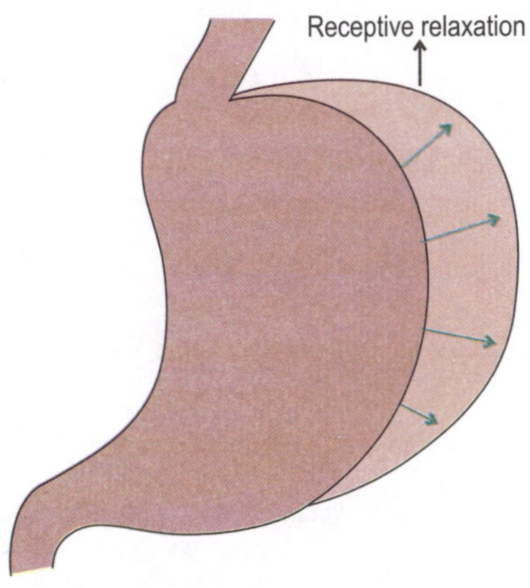

Fig. 65.3: Receptive relaxation of stomach.

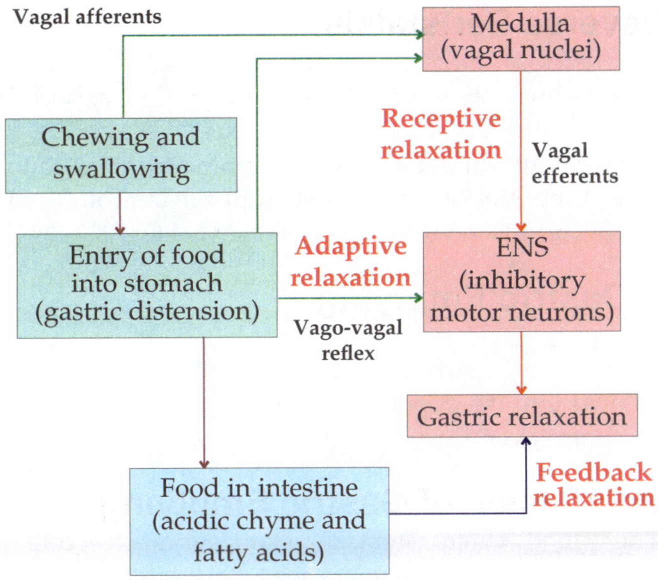

Fig. 65.4: Mechanisms of relaxations (receptive, adaptive and feedback) of stomach. Receptive relaxation is vagally mediated and adaptive relaxation is mainly a vagovagal reflex.

Peristalsis

After about half an hour following gastric filling, gastric peristalsis starts.

- The peristaltic movements are **initiated by gastric slow waves.**
    - The **pacemaker for gastric peristalsis** is located in the middle of the stomach close towards greater curvature.
- It starts as a **ring of contraction** that progress slowly towards antrum.

It usually occurs at the rate of **3 per minute**.

- It helps in **propelling food into the antrum and mixing of food with gastric juice.**
    - During this gastric peristalsis, **pylorus usually remains closed**. Therefore, food does not enter the duodenum, rather is recirculated in the stomach for adequate mixing.

Migrating Motor Complex

During the **interdigestive phase**, antrum of the stomach remains silent for about 75–90 minutes, after which a **burst of electrical and motor activities occurs.**

1. This causes intense antral contraction with **relaxation of pylorus.**
    - Therefore, the **remaining gastric content is emptied** into the duodenum.
2. The wave of contraction progresses from stomach towards terminal ileum.
    - Thus, it helps in **cleaning the stomach and intestine** and keeps the GI tract ready for the next meal.
3. Usually, it is repeated every 90 minutes during interdigestive phase.

Reverse Peristalsis

Sometimes in abnormal situations, peristalsis occurs in reverse direction, which starts in the lower parts of the body and proceeds towards esophagus.

1. **Lower and upper esophageal sphincters relax** so that gastric content is **forced out** of esophagus and oral cavity.
2. This results in **vomiting** (described below).

Gastric Emptying

This is the process by which the content of the stomach is emptied into the duodenum. Usually, it occurs at a slow but controlled rate.

Mechanism of Gastric Emptying

When food enters stomach, stomach relaxes due to receptive and adaptive relaxations. Later, after about half an hour, slowly gastric motility begins.

Gastric emptying occurs by **3 mechanisms**: peristaltic contraction, antral contraction & retropulsion (Fig. 65.5).

Peristaltic Contractions

The peristaltic contractions usually begin in the middle of the stomach and proceed in a ring like fashion towards pylorus (Fig. 65.5A). These contractions mainly push food into the antral part of the stomach.

1. The **velocity and magnitude of contraction** *increase as the contractile waves approach pylorus*.
2. As contractions are ***weak in the fundus and body*** of the stomach, the proximal portion of stomach mainly serves the reservoir function.
   - Therefore, usually proper mixing of food with gastric secretion does not occur in these parts of the stomach.
2. Major amount of **mixing takes place in the antrum**, as antrum contracts vigorously.

Antral Contractions

Antral contractions help **thorough mixing of food with the gastric juice**.

1. The forceful contraction of antrum forces gastric contents towards the pylorus.
   - But, as the pyloric sphincter remains closed, peristaltic wave fails to push food into the duodenum, rather food **returns back into the body of the stomach** (Fig. 65.5B).
2. After few such contractions, **pylorus opens** partially with a ***narrow opening*** at the center.
3. Therefore, stomach ***empties in small squirts*** with each peristaltic wave.

Retropulsion

The terminal part of antrum exhibits rapid and forceful contractions that forces the chyme to be propelled back towards the proximal part of the antrum and body of the stomach (Fig. 65.5C). This movement is called **retropulsion**.

- Retropulsion is very **effective in mixing and grinding** the larger food particles into smaller ones.
- Then, pyloric sphincter partially opens and gastric pump slowly pushes food into duodenum (Fig. 65.5D).

Physiological Significance

As the muscle layers in the fundus and body are thin, contractions in these parts of the stomach are weak. Therefore, gastric content in body of stomach **settles into different layers** based on their density.

1. **Fat content** of the food forms an oily layer on the top of the other gastric contents. This is why **fat is emptied slower than the carbohydrate and protein** (Application Box 65.1).
2. Liquid portion of the food flow around the mass and enter the antrum, and from there into the duodenum. Therefore, **liquid is emptied faster than the solid**.

Application Box 65.1

A cup of fat is taken in cocktail party: As fat decreases gastric emptying, usually a cup of fat is ingested before drinking alcohol in cocktail party. Fat ensures slow gastric emptying and slow absorption of alcohol from intestine.

Regulation of Gastric Emptying

Gastric emptying is regulated by both **neural and hormonal mechanisms.**

1. **Acid in the duodenum:** With decrease in the pH of the duodenal content the rate of gastric emptying decreases.
   - This response is mediated by both *neural and hormonal mechanisms*.
   - The acidic chyme in the duodenum **releases secretin** that decreases gastric emptying by inhibiting contraction of the antrum and by stimulating the contraction of pyloric sphincter.
2. **Products of fat digestion:** Products of fat digestion like **fatty acids** and also some fat molecules in the duodenal

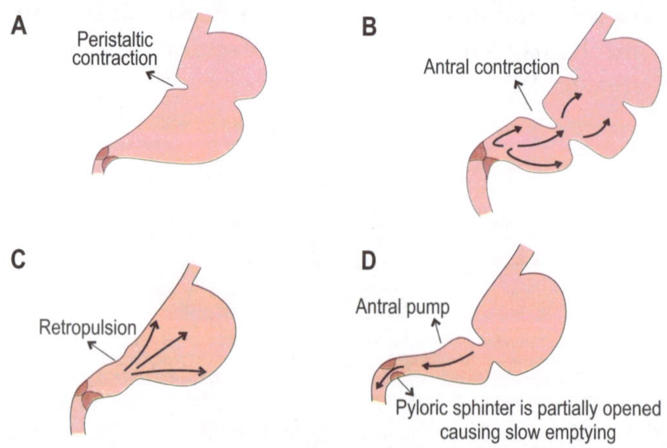

Figs. 65.5: Mechanisms of gastric emptying. Note, pyloric sphincter is closed in stages A, B, and C during which thorough mixing and grinding of food occurs and the food material is converted into chyme. In stage D, sphincter is partially opened that causes slow emptying of gastric content into duodenum.

content **inhibit gastric emptying**. This response is mediated by **CCK and GIP**.

- CCK is secreted from duodenum and jejunum in response to fatty acids and it inhibits gastric emptying.
- GIP, which is released in response to fatty acids also inhibits gastric emptying.

3. **Osmolality of duodenal content:** The chyme entering into duodenum has higher osmolality.
   - There are **osmoreceptors** in the mucosa of duodenum and jejunum that detect change in osmolality of the duodenal content.
   - **Hypertonic solutions in the duodenum** release **hormones that inhibit** the rate of gastric emptying.
4. **Products of protein digestion:** Presence of **peptides and amino acids** in the duodenum release **gastrin** from the G cells located in the duodenum.
   - Gastrin **increases antral contraction** but at the same time also causes **constriction of pyloric sphincter**. Therefore, the net effect is **decreased rate of gastric emptying.**
   - The products of protein digestion also release **CCK and GIP** from duodenum and jejunum that **inhibit gastric emptying.**
5. **Volume of the meal:** Whenever a large amount of food is taken in a meal, the time taken for gastric emptying prolongs. However, if the volume is mainly liquid, the emptying becomes faster.
6. **Stretching of duodenum:** Entry of chyme into the duodenum stretches the wall of duodenum.

- This initiates **enterogastric reflex** that inhibits gastric emptying.
- Enterogastric reflex is also activated by acid in the duodenum.

7. **Neural factors**
   - **Vagal stimulation promotes** gastric emptying.
     - Therefore, **vagotomy produces gastric stasis**.
     - Consequently, whenever vagotomy is performed for the treatment of peptic ulcer, usually a ***drainage procedure*** like pyloroplasty or gastrojejunostomy is also performed to ensure proper passage of food from the stomach into the duodenum (Clinical Note 65.1).
   - **Sympathetic stimulation inhibits** gastric emptying.

Clinical Note 42.1

Drainage procedure is done with vagotomy: As vagotomy decreases gastric motility and produces gastric stasis, whenever vagotomy is performed as done for the treatment of peptic ulcer, usually a drainage procedure like gastrojejunostomy is also performed to ensure proper passage of food from the stomach into the duodenum.

8. **Hormonal factors:** Most of the hormones liberated from duodenum and jejunum like **CCK, GIP, secretin, etc. inhibit gastric emptying**.

APPLIED PHYSIOLOGY

Dysfunctions of Gastric Emptying

Delayed Gastric Emptying

1. Gastric emptying is delayed in **autonomic neuropathy** as occurs in diabetes mellitus.
2. Paralysis of propulsive movements occurs following **vagotomy**, which is called **gastroparesis**.
   - Therefore, a drainage procedure like pyloroplasty is performed to overcome post-vagotomy gastric stasis.
3. **Hypertrophic pyloric stenosis** can cause gastric stasis.

Rapid Gastric Emptying

Normally, vagus stimulation promotes gastric emptying. Therefore, states of **increased vagal activity increase emptying**.

- Conversely, **sympathetic stimulation inhibits emptying**. Therefore, loss of appetite is a feature of acute stress, a state of sympathetic overactivity.
- Hormones like **thyroxine** stimulate gastric emptying and intestinal motility. Hence, increased appetite and hyperdefecation are features of hyperthyroidism.
- Increased liquid content of food increases gastric emptying.

Vomiting

PY4.9

Definition: Vomiting is the **expulsion of gastroduodenal content** from GIT to the external environment via mouth.

Associated Features: Vomiting is usually preceded by the feeling of **nausea, tachycardia, sweating, pallor, dizziness,** and **dilatation of pupils**. It is associated with retching that forces contents of the stomach into the esophagus.

Stimuli and Vomiting Centers: Vomiting is a reflex phenomenon, the center for which is located in the medulla (Fig. 65.6).

- The receptors present in many parts of the body provide inputs to the **vomiting center,** in the brainstem.
- Vomiting center present in the **reticular formation of medulla** consists of various scattered group of neurons that control different aspects of vomiting.
  - **Vestibular nuclei** mediate vomiting in response to motion sickness.
  - Pharyngeal stimulation induces vomiting by activating **nucleus tractus solitarius.**
  - **Area postrema** mediate vomiting activated by drugs (opiates, chemotherapeutic agents etc.) and hormones (as in pregnancy).
- Vomiting activated by emotion influenced by **limbic and diencephalic** inputs.

The **important stimuli** that activate these afferent fibers are:

1. Distension of stomach

2. Tickling the back of throat
3. Painful injury of the genitourinary tract
4. Conditions associated with dizziness and nausea
5. Many chemicals or drugs can elicit vomiting.

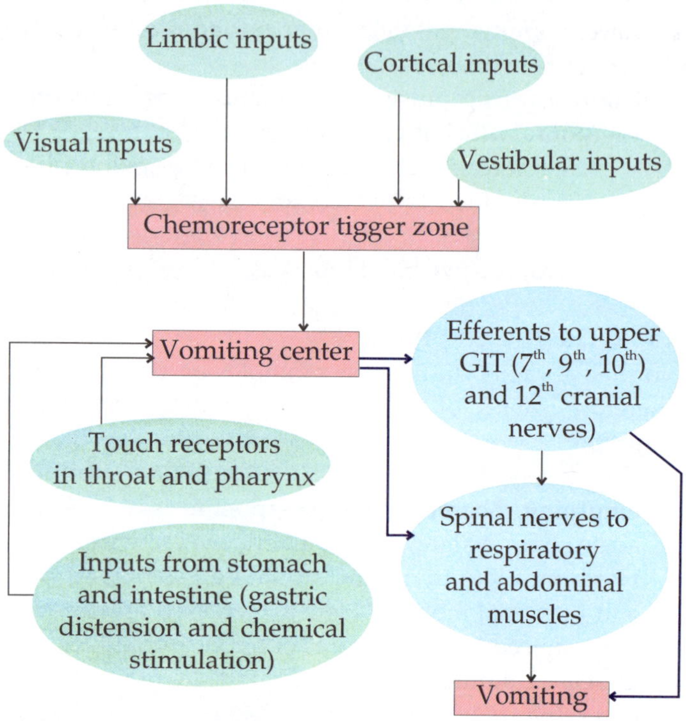

Fig. 65.6: Mechanism of vomiting reflex.

Emetics and Antiemetics: Drugs that induce vomiting are called **emetics**. The common emetics are apomorphine, ipecac, etc.

1. These chemicals stimulate the receptors that are present in the CTZ (**chemoreceptor trigger zone**), located in **area postrema** on the lateral wall of the fourth ventricle.
   - Many **antiemetics** prevent vomiting **by inhibiting CTZ**.
2. There are **5-HT$_3$ and D$_2$ receptors** in area postrema.
   - **Serotonin** stimulates vomiting through **5-HT$_3$ receptors**.
   - **Ondensetron**, a 5-HT$_3$ receptor antagonist is an antiemetic.
3. **Chlorpromazine**, a D$_2$ receptor antagonist and **haloperidol** are also effective antiemetics.

Mechanism of Vomiting: Vomiting reflex is executed in a sequence of events, as given below

1. Genesis of **reverse peristalsis** that starts from the middle of the jejunum. This sweeps the content of intestine and duodenum into the stomach.
2. **Relaxation of the pyloric sphincter** that allows the intestinal content to enter the stomach.
3. Forced inspiration occurs against the closed glottis. Lowering of the diaphragm **increases intra-abdominal pressure**.
4. This is followed by vigorous **contraction of abdominal muscles**.
   - Thus, intra-abdominal pressure sharply increases, which **forces the gastric contents to enter the esophagus**.
5. **Relaxation of the lower esophageal sphincter** allows gastric content to enter the esophagus.
6. Normally, the upper esophageal sphincter remains closed and prevents regurgitation of food into the pharynx.
   - With stronger retching and sharp rise in intra-abdominal pressure, **upper esophageal sphincter relaxes**, which allows chyme to enter the pharynx and then from there into the mouth.

Entry of vomitus into the trachea is prevented by central movement of vocal cards, closure of glottis and inhibition of respiration.

Dumping Syndrome

This is a distressing syndrome consisting mainly of weakness, dizziness and sweating that develop in about **two hours after meal** in persons who have **undergone gastrectomy or gastrojejunostomy** (that bypasses stomach).

This occurs due to **two causes**:

1. **Hypoglycemia:** Rapid entry of food into intestine causes quick absorption of glucose from intestine and produces prompt hyperglycemia, which in turn increases **insulin secretion**.
   - Insulin produces **hypoglycemia** that produces weakness, dizziness and sweating.
2. **Hypovolemia:** The speedy entry of hypertonic meal from esophagus directly into intestine produces **high osmotic load on intestine** *that transfers water from blood into the gut.*
   - This produces hypovolemia, dehydration and hypotension that lead to weakness, dizziness and sweating.

Exam Questions

1. List the factors affecting gastric emptying. Describe the mechanism of gastric emptying.
2. What are the types of gastric relaxations? Write a note on reverse peristalsis of stomach.
3. Describe the mechanism of vomiting. Give a note on dumping syndrome

Multiple Choice Questions

1. **Amount of gas produced daily in GI tract in healthy adult is about:**
   A. 200 ml B. 500 ml
   C. 1 liter D. 2 liters
2. **All of the following statements are true for hunger contractions, EXCEPT:**
   A. Occurs when the stomach is empty
   B. Are distressing and painful
   C. Contraction of pyloric sphincter
   D. Antral contractions are intense
3. **Which of the following is not a relaxation of the stomach?**
   A. Receptive relaxation
   B. Adaptive relaxation
   C. Reciprocal relaxation
   D. Feedback relaxation
4. **Gastro-colic reflex is related to:**
   A. Mass peristalsis B. Segmental movement
   C. Pendular movement D. Colonic cases
5. **Major regulator of interdigestive myoelectric complexes:**
   A. VIP B. GIP
   C. Motilin D. Neurotensin
6. **Motilin secretion decreased in which of the following condition?**
   A. Thirsty B. Starving
   C. Ingested meal D. Interdigestive state
7. **Major initiating response for peristalsis is**
   A. Hormonal B. Local stretching of gut
   C. Neural D. Chemical stimuli
8. **Migratory motor complexes in the gut reappear after intervals of:**
   A. 90 mins B. 120 mins
   C. 60 mins D. 150 mins
9. **Enterogastric reflex is caused by all, EXCEPT:**
   A. Duodenum distension
   B. Alkaline pH in duodenum & hormones
   C. Increased osmolality of chime
   D. Products of protein digestion & H^+ ions bathing duodenal mucosa
10. **All of the following about gastric motility are correct, EXCEPT:**
    A. Fundus and body parts have less contractile efficacy
    B. Antral contractions are very effective
    C. Pacemaker of gastric peristalsis is located in middle of stomach close to greater curvature
    D. Force of contraction is not linked to frequency and duration of slow waves
11. **Frequency of slow waves in stomach is**
    A. 3/min B. 10/min
    C. 15/min D. 18/min
12. **Gastric emptying is faster in all, EXCEPT:**
    A. Vagal stimulation B. Carbohydrate rich meal
    C. Fatty acids D. Gastrin
13. **Which of the following is not a component of dumping syndrome?**
    A. Patient has undergone a bypass procedure of stomach
    B. Rapid absorption of glucose causes insulin-induced hypoglycemia
    C. Hyperosmolality of gut transfers water from blood into gut causing hypovolemia
    D. Symptoms appear at least 8 hours after a meal
14. **Which of the following is NOT true about gastro-ileal reflex?**
    A. Stretching of stomach is the stimulus
    B. Mediated by vagus nerve
    C. Causes constriction of ileocecal valve
    D. Increases motility of terminal part of ileum
15. **All are true about MMC, EXCEPT:**
    A. It occurs every 90 min
    B. Starts in stomach and ends in terminal part of ileum
    C. These are strong propulsive movements
    D. Facilitates migration of colonic bacteria into ileum.
16. **Mass peristalsis is exhibited by:**
    A. Stomach B. Ileum
    C. Jejunum D. Colon
17. **Gastrocolic reflex is mediated by:**
    A. Neural factor B. Hormonal factor
    C. Local intrinsic mechanismD. Composition of gut content
18. **Delayed gastric emptying occurs in:**
    A. Autonomic neuropathy
    B. Hyperthyroidism
    C. Increased liquid content of food
    D. Acute stress
19. **All of the following are true for "vomiting reflex', EXCEPT:**
    A. Vigourous contraction of abdominal muscles
    B. Genesis of reverse peristalsis from the middle of duodenum
    C. Forced inspiration against closed glottis
    D. Relaxation of the pyloric sphincter
20. **Which of the following statements is NOT true?**
    A. Vestibular nucleus mediates vomiting in response to motion sickness
    B. Opiates cause vomiting by activating area postrema
    C. Pharyngeal stimulation cause vomiting by activating NTS
    D. Serotonin inhibits vomiting by inhibiting CTZ

Answers

1. C	2. C	3. C	4. A	5. C	6. C	7. B	8. A	9. B	10. D
11. A	12. C	13. D	14. C	15. D	16. D	17. B	18. A	19. B	20. D

Chapter 66

Intestinal Motility, and Motility of Colon, Rectum and Anal Canal

Learning Objectives

On completion of study of this chapter:

The student will be able to (must know):

1. Understand the modifications in muscle layers of small and large intestines to suit their functions.
2. Elucidate the mechanisms and functions of intestinal movements.
3. Name the intestinal reflexes and give their functions.
4. Name the colonic movements and colonic reflexes and give their functions.
5. Draw the pathway of defecation reflex and explain the reflex mechanism.
6. Name the intestinal motility disorders and give their causes.

The student may also be able to (desirable to know):

1. Describe the electrophysiology of intestinal smooth muscles.
2. Illustrate the physiological basis intestinal motility disorders.

INTESTINAL MOTILITY

Small intestine (duodenum, jejunum and ileum) measures about 600 cm. It takes **3–5 hours** for the chyme to traverse the small intestine.

- The wall of small intestine has all the layers of the gut.
  - However, the **muscularis externa** consisting of outer longitudinal and inner circular muscles is **well developed** in small intestine (refer Fig. 62.2, Chapter 62).
  - This helps in effective intestinal motility.

Electrophysiology of Intestinal Smooth Muscles

The frequency of **slow waves** is maximum in small intestine that occurs regularly.

- The frequency is **highest in duodenum** (about 15 per minute) and decreases slowly towards ileum where it is about 8-10 per minute.
- Slow waves are not always accompanied by bursts of action potential spikes.
  - When slow wave is **associated with spike**, the ***contraction is stronger*** and, in its absence (no spike), contraction is weaker or absent (refer to Fig. 63.5; Chapter 63).
- A **characteristic feature** is that slow waves are ***localized to a short segment*** of the intestine.
  - Therefore, contraction is also localized to the segments.
  - This results in **segmentation type of movement** in the intestine.
- The basic electrical rhythm is **purely intrinsic.**
- The frequency of action potential spike, which determines the strength of muscle contraction, depends on **excitability of the smooth muscles**. The excitability in turn depends on autonomic innervation, activity of the enteric neurons and the circulating hormones.
- **Parasympathetic stimulation enhances** and **sympathetic stimulation inhibits** excitability of intestinal smooth muscles.

Types of Intestinal Movements

PY4.3

Intestinal motilities are segmentation, peristalsis, migrating myoelectric complex, contraction of the muscularis mucosa, villus contractions, and movements due to intestinal reflexes.

Segmentation

This is **mixing movement** and is the **most common** variety of movement of the small intestine.

- It is characterized by **closely spaced contraction of the circular muscle layer**.

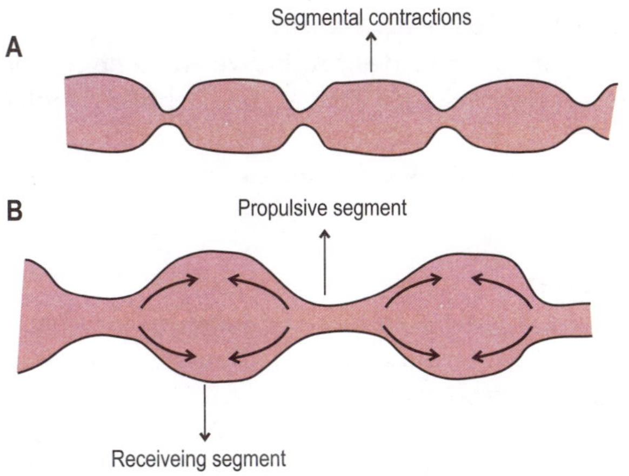

Fig. 66.1: Segmentation movement of small intestine (A). Note the mechanism for mixing of food in segmental contractions (B), in a slightly enlarged view of intestine. The direction of arrows indicates the direction of movement of food particles. Note, in segmental contractions, food is grinded and thoroughly mixed between two propulsive segments.

- These contractions divide the small intestine into many segments (Fig. 66.1A).

- The **rate** of segmental contraction is **same as the frequency of slow waves.**
  - It is about 18/min in duodenum, 15/min in jejunum, and 12/min in ileum.

Mechanism and Function: Segmentation contractions effectively **mix chyme with pancreatic and intestinal secretions.**

- Two nearby propulsive segments force the chyme towards each other into the receiving segment (Fig. 66.1B), which efficiently helps in mixing.
  - They also **bring the fresh chyme into the contact** *with the mucosal surface.*
- Therefore, segmentation movements are also called **mixing movements**. This facilitates digestion and absorption of nutrients.

Peristalsis

Peristalsis is the propelling movement that occurs due to progressive contraction of successive portions of circular smooth muscles of the small intestine.

- The wave of contraction moves in ***orthograde direction*** i.e. towards colon.
  - In fact, peristaltic wave spreads in both directions. However, wave towards oral cavity (oral spread) dies out after a short distance, and wave towards colon (**aboral spread**) continues progressively.
  - This is called '**Law of the Intestine**'.

Mechanism: Peristaltic waves involve a **smaller length of intestine.**

- When chyme enters the intestine, the bolus of the chyme stretches its wall.
- The part of the intestine **behind the chyme contracts** and the part of the intestine **in front of the chyme relaxes** and the ring of contraction proceeds in forward direction (Fig. 66.2).
- Detailed mechanism of peristalsis is described in chapter 63.

Functions: The primary function of peristaltic movements is to **propel chyme in forward direction.**

Rush Peristalsis: Sometimes, the **frequency of peristalsis increases** to an extent that intestinal contents are emptied very fast (with a speed of 20 cm/s) into the colon. This is called **rush peristalsis**. This is typically seen in acute diarrhea.

There are also **anti-peristaltic contractions** of intestine. Antiperistalsis results in **vomiting**.

Short Range Peristalsis

Short range peristalsis occurs less frequently. It occurs for a shorter part of intestine.

1. Short range peristalsis along with segmentation contraction **decreases the net rate of propulsion** of chyme in forward direction.
2. This **allows the chyme to stay longer** in intestine to facilitate digestion and absorption.

Clinical Significance

1. Administration of **codeine** decreases the motility of the intestine, therefore *decreases the frequency of defecation.*
   - The decreased motility also **prolongs the transit time** for the intestinal contents so that more water and nutrients are reabsorbed.
   - Therefore, this also decreases the volume of stool.
2. Administration of **laxative** for example castor oil produces the reverse effect.
   - Laxatives ***increase intestinal motility***, and therefore, **shorten the transit time** of the intestinal content.
   - This **increases the delivery** of chyme and water into the colon that ***causes diarrhea.***

Law of the Intestine

When a bolus of chyme enters the intestine, the part of the intestine behind the bolus contracts and the portion of the intestine ahead of it relaxes.

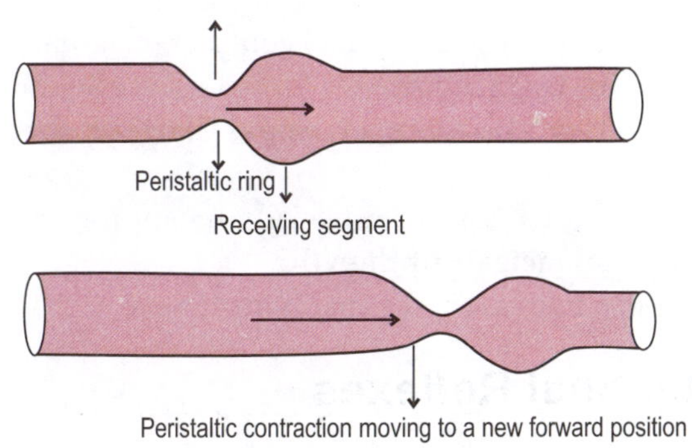

Fig. 66.2: Peristalsis in small intestine. Note, the ring of peristaltic contraction moves from the initial position (upper picture) to a new forward position (lower picture). Thus, peristalsis moves aborally.

- This helps in **propagation of ring of contraction in aboral direction**.
- This response is known as **law of the intestine**.
- This is meant to propel the intestinal content in the forward **aboral direction** as occurs in peristalsis.

Other Motilities

Migrating Motor Complex

In the interdigestive phase, **bursts of intense electrical and contractile activity** occurs once in about every **90 minutes**. This is called migrating motor (myoelectric) complex (MMC).

1. MMC **starts in the stomach** and is propagated throughout the intestine to the terminal part of the ileum.
   - Once, a MMC reaches the distal end of the ileum, a next MMC begins in the stomach.
   - Likewise, MMC is **repeated every 75–90 minutes**.
2. MMC results in vigorous and **strong propulsive contraction**; therefore, this **sweeps** the intestine and empties the remaining contents into the colon.
   - MMC cleans the entire lumen of the stomach and intestine, to keep the house ready for the next meal.
   - Therefore, MMC is known as **housekeeper of small intestine**.
3. MMC also ***inhibits the migration of colonic bacteria*** from colon into the intestine.

Contraction of Muscularis Mucosa

The muscularis mucosa of small intestine contracts irregularly. These contractions **alter the patterns of the mucosal folds**.

- Contractions occur at a frequency of about **3 per minute**.
- Such contractions help in **mixing the luminal contents** and also in **bringing the fresh chyme** *in contact with mucosal surface*.

Villus Contraction

The **villi of small intestine** also contract irregularly. This is called villus contraction.

- This is typically seen in **upper part of the small intestine**.
- These contractions are especially meant for **emptying the central lacteals of the villi**.
- They also increase intestinal **lymph flow**.

Intestinal Reflexes

There are **two reflexes** observed in the intestine: intestino-intestinal reflex and gastroileal reflex.

Intestino-Intestinal Reflex

When a **part of the intestine is over-distended**, the rest of the ***intestine relaxes***. This is called intestino-intestinal reflex.

- It is mediated by **local enteric neurons** and vagovagal pathways.

Gastroileal Reflex

When food enters the stomach (stretching of stomach), the **motility of the terminal part of ileum** is enhanced and **ileocolic sphincter relaxes**.

- This increases entry of contents of ileum into the colon through ileocecal sphincter.
- This reflex is proposed to be mediated **by vagus nerve**.

Function of Ileocecal Sphincter

This is also known as **ileocecal valve**. Normally, the ileocecal sphincter is **tonically contracted**, and therefore the sphincter remains closed most of the time and prevents small intestinal emptying.

1. When a **peristaltic wave reaches the terminal part of the ileum**, the sphincter relaxes so that the ileal content enters the cecum.
2. **Distention of ileum** also causes ***opening of ileocecal sphincter***.
   - On the other hand, **distention of cecum** causes ***closure of ileocecal sphincter***.
3. Ileocecal sphincter is also controlled by **extrinsic nerve fibers**.
   - For example relaxation of the sphincter occurs by vagal stimulation as seen in gastroileal reflex.

Applied Physiology PY4.9

Adynamic Ileus

When the intestine is injured or excessively handled during surgery, the intestinal motility is paralyzed, which is called adynamic ileus or Paralytic Ileus.

- This usually occurs ***following abdominal surgery***.
- Following major abdominal surgeries, GI tract remains paralyzed for few hours to few days.
  - Peristalsis first starts in the small intestine (6–8 hours later) followed by in the stomach (8–12 hours) and finally in the colon (2–3 days).
- Adynamic ileus is also observed in ***peritonitis***.
- This occurs due to **increased discharge of non-adrenergic fibers** in the splanchnic nerves.

Intestinal Colic

Severe abdominal cramps are experienced in **localized obstruction** of small intestine.

- The **segment proximal to the obstruction** dilates and gets filled with fluid and gas.

- This **increases pressure** inside the lumen that causes **compression of blood vessels** in the intestinal wall.
- Resulting **local ischemia** of the intestinal wall produces severe cramping pain.

- Abdominal cramps are also experienced in other diseases that result in distention of the intestine.

MOTILITY OF LARGE INTESTINE

Large intestine consists of cecum, colon, rectum and anal canal. **Colon** (ascending, transverse, descending and sigmoid colon) **constitutes about 90% of large intestine**. The length of large intestine is about **1.5 meters** (5 feet or 150 cm).

Transit Time of Chyme: **Transit time** through different parts of gut is as follows:

1. In small intestine: 4 hours
2. In ascending colon: 6 hours
3. In transverse colon: 8 hours
4. In descending and pelvic colons: 12 hours
5. From pelvic colon to rectum, the transit is very slow, which may even take 1 to 2 days.

However, transit time **depends on the fiber content** of diet. Transit time is less in high fiber diet, sometimes may even be reduced to 6 hours through the entire gut.

Motility of Colon

The **major functions of colon** are storage of chyme that arrives from small intestine, and absorption of salt and water. The **slow movement of the chyme** across the colon, which is about **5–10 cm/hour** allows **maximum absorption of salt and water**.

Modifications in Large Intestine

Structure of the wall of large gut has some **special features**:

1. There are **no villi** on the mucosa (refer to Fig. 62.5; Chapter 62).).
2. There are **many goblet cells.**
3. The colonic glands are small inward projections of the mucosa. They secrete mucus.
4. The **circular muscles usually do not exhibit action potentials**.
5. Outer longitudinal muscle layer is specialized into **tenia coli.**
    - The tenia are shorter than rest of the colon. Therefore, the wall of the colon forms **haustra** (outpouchings) (refer to Fig. 62.4; Chapter 62).

Innervation of Large Intestine

1. **Parasympathetic innervation** to cecum, ascending, transverse and most part of descending colon comes via **vagus nerve**, whereas innervation to the sigmoid colon, rectum, and anal canal comes via **pelvic nerves** that arise from the sacral spinal cord.
    - **Parasympathetic** stimulation ***increases*** colonic movements.
2. **Sympathetic fibers** to large gut come via superior and inferior mesenteric plexuses, and superior and inferior hypogastric plexuses.
    - **Sympathetic** stimulation ***decreases*** colonic movements.

Electrophysiology of Colonic Muscle

Circular Muscle: There are two types of pacemaking (rhythm generating) cells in the colon. They are made up of **interstitial cells**.

1. **The one set** of cells that are present near the inner border of circular muscles produce **regular slow waves of high amplitude** like that of gastric slow waves.
2. **The second set** of interstitial cells is present near outer border of the circular muscle that produces ***waves with low amplitude and high frequency*** oscillations called **myenteric potential oscillations** (MPO).
3. Circular muscles **do not fire action potentials**.

Longitudinal Muscle: These muscles also exhibit myenteric potential oscillations (MPO). However, longitudinal muscles ***sometimes fire action potentials*** at the peak of MPO that elicit contractions of the large intestine.

Colonic Movements

Colonic movements include haustral contractions, propulsive movements, mass peristalsis and colonic reflexes.

Haustral Contractions: These contractions are similar to that of segmentation.

- **Haustra become more prominent** in these contractions. Therefore, they are called haustral contractions.
- They help in **mixing and circulation of chyme** within the large intestine.

Propulsive Movements: These are peristaltic movements that *propel colonic contents* towards the rectum.

- The mechanism of colonic peristalsis is same as intestinal peristalsis.

Mass Colonic Peristalsis: Mass colonic peristalsis is a stronger peristaltic contraction that forcefully pushes the contents from colon into the rectum.

- Activation of mass peristalsis in colon finally leads to the **initiation of defecation reflex**.
- It also **cleans** the large intestine.
- It occurs **3 to 4 times a day** and is initiated ***usually after a meal***.
- Mass peristalsis is not affected after colostomy.

Colonic Reflexes

Colonic reflexes include colonocolonic reflex and gastrocolic reflex.

Colonocolonic Reflex: Colonocolonic reflex is the **relaxation of the entire colon** in response to distention of one part of the colon. This is partly mediated by sympathetic fibers.

Gastrocolic Reflex: Gastrocolic reflex is initiated when food accumulates in the stomach.

1. Distention of the stomach causes **motility of proximal and distal colon**.
2. This pushes colonic content into the rectum, which **stimulates the desire for defecation**.
   - Therefore, usually after taking a large meal, the urge for defecation is enhanced.
   - This reflex is more developed in children.
3. Gastrocolic reflex is **mediated by gastrin** secreted from stomach in response to gastric distension, and not by neural factors.

Motility of Rectum & Anal Canal

Normally, rectum remains empty. **Mass colonic peristalsis** pushes contents in the colon into the rectum. Anal canal **always remains closed** by the tonic contractions of internal and external anal sphincters.

1. The **internal anal sphincter** is made up of thickening of **circular smooth muscle** of the anal canal.
2. The **external anal sphincter** consists of **striated muscle** (Fig. 66.3).
   - Thus, external sphincter is innervated by **somatic motor fibers** via pudendal nerves, which brings it under voluntary control.
3. **With initiation of defecation reflex**, the external sphincter opens, and the person defecates.
   - However, the reflex relaxation of the internal sphincter in response to rectal distention is a temporary phenomenon.

Defecation

PY4.3

Defecation is a **reflex phenomenon with a voluntary control**.

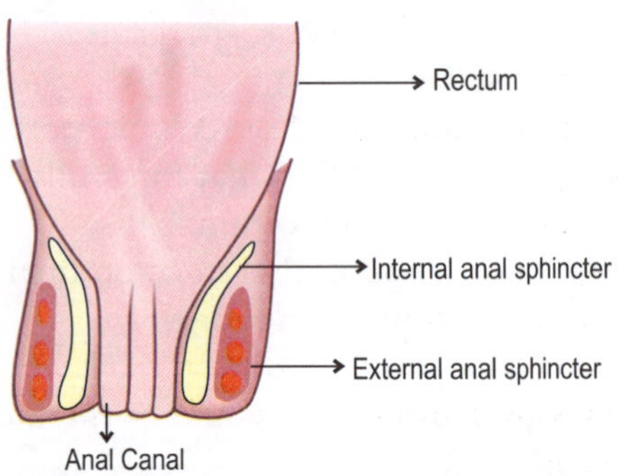

Fig. 66.3: Structure and position of external and internal anal sphincters.

Stimulus: Defecation reflex is initiated when mass peristaltic movement of the descending and sigmoid colons pushes the colonic content into the rectum (filling of the rectum).

1. As the external anal sphincter is innervated by somatic nerves, the **voluntary effort is also important** in initiating defecation.
2. However, normally defecation is inhibited by the **acute anorectal angle**, which is about 90°, and **contraction of external sphincter and puborectalis muscle**.

Pathway: Receptors for defecation reflex are stretch receptors located in the wall of rectal rectum.

1. **Afferent information** from the wall of rectum is conveyed to **sacral segment (S_3) of spinal cord** via pelvic nerve.
2. **Efferent input** from spinal cord to rectum and internal anal sphincter comes via **pelvic nerve** and to external anal sphincter via **somatic nerve** (Fig. 66.4).
3. **Higher center**, especially cortex influences spinal cord center via corticospinal pathway.
4. **Relaxation of internal anal sphincter** is due to inhibitory signals that originate in myenteric plexus in response to peristaltic wave approaching anus. This allows the fecal matter to press onto the anal canal.

Mechanism: The individual sits on toilet and strains. This increases intra-abdominal pressure, which forcefully expels the rectal contents through the anal canal. This is assisted by relaxation of external anal sphincter, decreased anorectal angle and relaxation of puborectalis muscle.

1. Evacuation of bladder is preceded by a **deep breathing that pushes the diaphragm downward.**
2. Contraction of respiratory muscles *increases intrathoracic and intra-abdominal pressures*.
3. Contraction of abdominal wall muscle further increases abdominal pressure.

When all these mechanisms elevate the intra-abdominal **pressure to about 200 cm of H_2O**, the feces is forced out through the external anal sphincter.

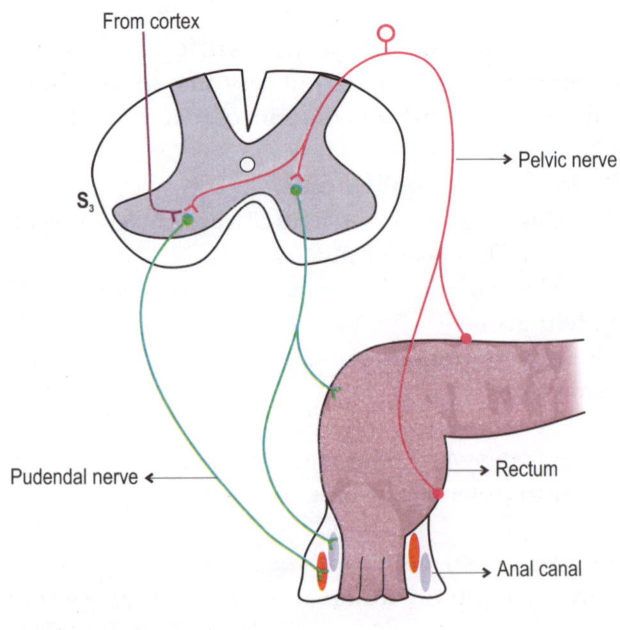

Fig. 66.4: The pathway of defecation reflex.

Applied Aspect: Defecation reflex is a spinal reflex. Therefore, following spinal transection, *defecation is never complete*. However, evacuation of bowel and bladder can be achieved by activating mass reflex in paraplegic patients.

Faeces

Faeces or Stool is a semisolid mass of about 200–250 ml excreted form large gut per day. It contains inorganic material, undigested fibers, bacteria and water.

- Water constitutes 75% and solids 25% of the total volume.
  - The undigested fibers include cellulose and other fibers.
  - **Bacteria and inorganic materials** constitute 30% and 15% of the total solids respectively.
- The composition of feces **is not fully affected by diet** as a large fraction of it comes from **non-dietary origin**.
  - Even in fasting, a good amount of feces is passed.
- The **color of the stool is due to the presence of bile pigments**.
- The **smell of feces is due to presence of indole and skatole**, the amines that are produced by colonic bacterial flora.

Applied Physiology

Hirschsprung Disease PY4.9

Cause: This is also known as **congenital megacolon** or **aganglionosis**. In this condition, the *entire neuronal* **plexuses** in the wall of the colon are *congenitally absent*.

- **Absence of ganglion** *in both myenteric and submucosal plexuses in distal part of colon and rectum*.
- This **prevents relaxation** of rectal outlet and internal anal sphincter in response to rectal filling.
  - Thus, obstruction occurs to the outflow of feces and feces accumulate behind the obstruction.
- Consequently, **distention of the colon** ensues.

Features: Clinically, it manifests as **abdominal distention**, anorexia and lassitude. In severe cases, symptoms appear in newborns as early as third day after birth.

Treatment: Usually, it is treated by **surgical dilation**.

Diarrhea

Diarrhea occurs in many conditions. Physiologically it may be due to either **increased secretion** as occurs in cholera or **increased GI motility** in many gastrenteritis.

Constipation

Constipation occurs due to many causes. However, the physiological basis is the **decreased intestinal motility** that causes stasis of chyme in the large intestine, which facilitates water absorption and dehydration of intestinal contents.

- The chyme hardens and **feces become more solid**.
- Usually, it is treated by distending rectum by inert material.

Irritable Bowel Syndrome (IBS)

IBS is a **functional disorder** of the intestine characterized by alteration of the bowel habits and abdominal pain in the absence of any detectable organic pathology. There is **no morphologic, histologic, microbiologic or biochemical abnormalities** in IBS. Changes in gut motility are observed in several studies though they poorly correlate with the symptoms.

Exam Questions

1. Describe the mechanisms and functions of various motilities of small intestine.
2. Briefly describe the process of mass peristalsis. Give a brief note on colonic reflexes.
3. With the help of a suitable diagram, describe the mechanism of defecation reflex.

Multiple Choice Questions

1. **All of the following statements are true for'intestinal motility, EXCEPT:**
   A. Does not depend on gastric motility B. Increased by distension
   C. Increased by Acetylcholine D. Increased by cholecystokinin
2. **All of the following are true for peristalsis, EXCEPT:**
   A. It occurs for a small length of intestine
   B. Primary function is to propel chyme in aboral direction
   C. This is due to contraction of circular smooth muscles
   D. Ring of contraction wave moves in anterogrde direction
3. **Short range peristalsis along with segmentation:**
   A. Decreases propulsion of chyme
   B. Increases propulsion of chyme
   C. Pushes chyme to move in opposite direction, i.e., towards oral cavity
   D. Inhibits digestion and absorption
4. **Which is not true about colon?**
   A. There are no villi in the mucosa
   B. Circular muscles usually do not exhibit action potentials
   C. Sympathetic stimulation increases colonic motility
   D. Longitudinal muscle fibers specialize into tenia coli
5. **What is not true about mass peristalsis?**
   A. Occurs 3 to 4 times a day B. Severely affected in colostomy
   C. Strong colonic peristaltic contractions D. Initiates defection reflex
6. **All are true about defecation reflex, EXCEPT:**
   A. It has both automatic (reflexive) and voluntary parts
   B. Afferent inputs from rectum is conveyed to S3 segment in spinal cord in pelvic nerve
   C. Efferent to external sphincter comes via somatic nerve
   D. This is a supraspinal reflex with strong cortical regulation

Answers: 1. A 2. D 3. A 4. C 5. B 6. D

Chapter 67

Principles of Digestion and Absorption

Learning Objectives

On completion of study of this chapter:

The student will be able to (must know):

1. Understand the mechanism of digestion and absorption of carbohydrate, protein and fat from intestine.
2. Outline the mechanism of absorption of water, electrolytes, vitamins and minerals from GIT.
3. Learn the physiological basis of common malabsorption syndromes.

The student may also be able to (desirable to know):

1. Describe the mechanism of digestion and absorption of each category of nutrient.
2. Explain the physiological basis of problems in malabsorption syndrome.

PY4.4

Digestion is the process by which foodstuff are broken down into smaller particles that can be absorbed from the GIT. **Absorption** is the process by which the products of digestion, vitamins, minerals, and water are transported from the lumen of the GI tract into the blood and the lymph draining the GI tract.

CARBOHYDRATES

Digestion of Carbohydrate

The dietary carbohydrates are mainly polysaccharides, disaccharides, and monosaccharides. Starch is the polysaccharide that is usually digested in human GI tract.

1. Digestion of carbohydrate begins in the mouth by the action of **salivary amylase** which catalyses the hydrolysis of α-1, 4 linkage (but not α-1, 6 linkage) to form α-dextrins.
2. The **pancreatic amylase** also does the same function.
   - The products of amylase digestion are maltose, maltotriose and α-dextrins.
3. The further digestion of starch is carried out by **oligosaccharidases** that are present in the ***brush border of the intestine***.
   - These membrane enzymes are **α-dextrinase** that causes hydrolysis of α-1, 6 linkage, **maltase** that causes hydrolysis of maltotriose and maltose, **lactase** that causes hydrolysis of lactose into glucose and galactose, **glucoamylase** that splits malto-oligosachharides into single glucose molecules and **sucrase** that causes hydrolysis of sucrose into fructose and glucose.
4. The end-product of these membrane digestions are glucose, galactose, and fructose (monosaccharides).

Absorption of Carbohydrates

The carbohydrate absorption is **maximum in duodenum and jejunum**, which progressively decreases towards the terminal part of ileum. The easily absorbable forms of carbohydrate are monosaccharides that are glucose, galactose, and fructose.

1. They are first transported from the lumen into the epithelial cells. The apical membrane of epithelial cells contains SGLT (**sodium dependent glucose transporter**).
   - The transport is greatly influenced by the concentration of Na^+ in the intestinal lumen. The higher the concentration of Na^+, the greater the degree of glucose absorption.
   - This is because both ***glucose and Na^+ share the same transport protein***, the **SGLT**.
   - The SGLT that transports glucose and Na^+ is SGLT 1.
2. The concentration of Na^+ is less in the enterocytes, which is **created by Na^+-K^+ pump** present on the basolateral membrane of the cells that **pumps Na^+ into**

the lateral intercellular space from the enterocytes in exchange for K^+.
- Therefore, **Na^+ moves into the cells** along the concentration gradient (Fig. 67.1).
- **Glucose enters** along with Na^+ **using the same co-transporter** (SGLT1).

3. From the cell, glucose is transported by GLUT 2 (**glucose transporter**) into the interstitium (ECF).
- From the ECF glucose enters the blood.

As the glucose transport depends on Na^+-K^+ pump present on the basolateral membrane that creates gradient for Na^+, this mechanism of glucose transport is a **secondary active transport**.
- **Galactose uses the same carrier protein** (SGLT 1) for absorption.
- The entry of **fructose** into the enterocytes is facilitated by GLUT 5, which is present only in the brush border of matured enterocytes.

Applied Aspects

Carbohydrate Malabsorption Syndromes

Carbohydrate malabsorption occurs due to **deficiency of oligosaccharidases**, the membrane enzymes of enterocytes.

Lactose Intolerance: This occurs due to **deficiency of lactase** in the brush border of enterocytes.
- Lactose is not digested and enters the colon where it is utilized by colonic bacteria that produce gas, and different metabolites.
- The metabolites increase colonic motility and diarrhea. Excess gas production results in borborygmi (gurgling sounds in the intestine) and abdominal distention.

Sucrase-Isomaltase Deficiency: **Deficiency of sucrase and isomaltase** in the brush border of enterocytes is an *autosomal recessive* disease. Ingestion of fructose in this condition results in diarrhea and flatulence.

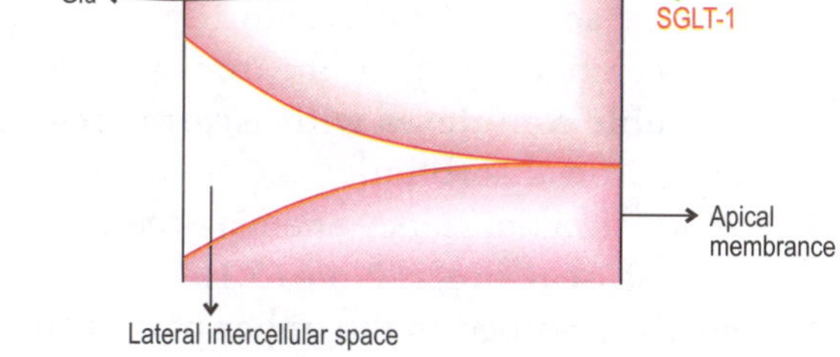

Fig. 67.1: Mechanism of glucose (Glu) absorption in intestine.

Glucose-Galactose Malabsorption Syndrome: This is a rare hereditary disorder due to deficiency of SGLT 1 in the brush border of enterocytes.
- In this condition, ingestion of glucose or galactose or starch produces diarrhea and flatulence.
- Fructose is well tolerated.

PROTEINS

In addition to dietary protein, **10–30g of protein** is added to the intestinal content from the GI secretions and the exfoliated intestinal cells. Normally, all ingested protein is digested and absorbed. However, excess protein intake causes excretion of protein in the stool.

Digestion of Proteins

Digestion of protein starts in the stomach.
1. **Pepsinogen secreted from chief cells** is converted to pepsin by the **action of HCl**.
   - Pepsin hydrolyzes proteins into peptides and amino acids.
2. **In the duodenum and small intestine**, the proteins are **digested by proteases** secreted in the pancreatic secretion.
   - The proteases are trypsin, chymotrypsin, carboxypeptidases and elastase.
3. The **enterokinase** secreted from mucosal cells of duodenum and jejunum converts **trypsinogen into trypsin**, which then ***acts as an enzyme to convert other proteases***.
4. **Peptidases** are also present in the brush border of enterocytes.
   - These enzymes hydrolyze the peptides produced by pancreatic proteases into oligopeptides and amino acids.
   - The **brush border peptidases** are amino peptidases, and dipeptidases.

The **products of protein digestion** are small peptides and amino acids.

Absorption of Proteins

There are many **transport systems** (at least **seven such systems** are known) for absorption of amino acids and peptides.
- The five protein transport systems **require Na^+** like that of Na^+-glucose co-transporter.
- The other two transporters **use Cl^-** (***independent of*** *Na^+*).
- Absorption of amino acid is greater in the **duodenum and jejunum** and slower in ileum.

Defects of Protein Digestion

Hartnup Disease: This is a hereditary disorder in which **absorption of amino acids** in the intestinal and renal epithelial cells is defective.

- The neutral amino acids appear in the stool and urine.

Cystinuria: This is a congenital disease in which the amino acid cystine appears in the urine.

- The **defect is in the protein transporter** in the mucosal cells of intestine and epithelial cells of PCT of kidney.

Prolinuria: This is a rare disorder in which proline is not reabsorbed from intestine and kidney.

- This causes prolinuria and hydroxyprolinuria.

LIPIDS

Digestion of Lipids

Digestion of lipid starts in the mouth.

1. In oral cavity **lingual lipase** is secreted from Ebner's glands in the tongue.
2. **Gastric lipase** also helps in digestion of fat.
    - However, deficiency of lingual and gastric lipase does not result in malabsorption of fat as pancreatic lipase is actually important for lipid digestion.
3. Principal fat digestion starts in the duodenum by the **pancreatic lipase**, which hydrolyses 1 and 3 bonds of triglycerides that results in formation of free fatty acid and 2-monoglycerides (2-monoglycerols).
    - Pancreatic lipase acts on lipids that **have been emulsified** (emulsification by bile acids).
    - Fat digestion is facilitated by ***pancreatic co-lipase.***
4. There is another lipase secreted from pancreas called as **bile salt activated lipase**, which also assists in lipid digestion.
5. The dietary cholesterol is hydrolyzed by **cholesteryl ester hydrolase**.

Absorption of Lipids

Lipids are absorbed by **passive diffusion and carrier mediated transport**. As soon as lipids enter the cell **they are esterified**, therefore a ***gradient is maintained*** for their entry into the cell.

1. For their absorption, fats are **emulsified in the intestine** by detergent action of bile salts, lecithin, and monoglycerides.
    - With the help of bile salt, lipids form micelles.
    - **Micelles** are cylindrical aggregates of lipids like fatty acids, monoglycerides, and cholesterol with their hydrophobic ends at the center.
2. Micelle solubilizes the lipids and provides a medium for their transport to the intestinal epithelial cells.
    - Thus, micelles help in transport of lipids to the enterocytes, where they disintegrate into the individual lipids and passively diffuse into the cells.

Short chain fatty acids are produced in the colon by the colonic bacteria and absorbed there. Short chain fatty acids are absorbed in exchange for H^+, therefore help in acid base balance. They also promote the absorption of Na^+.

Cholesterol is easily absorbed from the intestine in the presence of bile, fatty acid and pancreatic juice. The absorbed cholesterol is incorporated into the chylomicrons that enter circulation via lymphatics.

The **vitamins A, D, E and K** are fat soluble vitamins. Their absorption is facilitated by presence of bile acids and products of lipid digestion in the intestine. Therefore, in the absence of bile acids or malabsorption of fat, deficiency of these vitamins occurs.

Disorders of Fat Digestion

Steatorrhea: This is a condition in which there is passage of **fatty, bulky, and clay colored stool**.

1. This occurs due to **deficiency of exocrine pancreas**.
    - *Pancreatic lipase deficiency* results in impairment of fat digestion.
2. This is also sometimes seen in patients with **excess secretion of gastric acid** in which decreased duodenal pH ***inhibits pancreatic lipase***. Acid also **precipitates bile salt**.
3. Another cause of steatorrhea is **impaired reabsorption of bile salts in the distal ileum**.
4. Steatorrhea can also occur due to **intestinal diseases**.

Tropical Sprue: In this condition, the **enterocytes are distorted** and the **density of microvilli is decreased**. This causes lipid malabsorption probably due to decreased surface area for absorption of lipids.

OTHER NUTRIENTS

Absorption of water, electrolytes (mainly Na+) and minerals has been described elsewhere in this textbook. Absorption of vitamins has been described in Chapter 137 (Physiology of Nutrition).

Absorption of Iron

The normal plasma level of iron is **130 µg/100 ml in males** and **110 µg/100 ml in females**. Normally, absorption of iron ranges from **3–6 % of the iron ingested**. Iron is absorbed in the **ferrous (Fe^{++}) form**.

1. The iron ingested in the diet is present in the ferric (Fe^{+++}) form.
    - In the stomach, *ferric form is converted to ferrous form* by the **action of hydrochloric acid**.
    - Gastric secretion dissolves the iron and allows it to form **soluble complexes with ascorbic acid**, which facilitates iron absorption.
    - Therefore, iron deficiency anemia occurs in chronic gastric disease (Clinical Note 67.1).
2. Iron is mostly absorbed in the **upper part of the small intestine** (mainly in duodenum and jejunum).
    - There is also the enzyme **ferric reductase** in the

brush border of intestine, which converts ferric form of iron to **ferrous form**.
- Iron is absorbed in **heme-ferrous and nonheme-ferrous form**. The heme binds with a transport protein present in the brush border of the enterocytes (Fig. 67.2).
- This transport protein transfers heme into the enterocytes.

3. In the cytoplasm of enterocytes, **heme oxygenase** removes Fe^{++} from the porphyrin.
   - Fe^{++} then is actively transported across the basolateral membrane of the cells to enter the blood where it binds with **transferrin** (the iron bound to transferrin is in the form of Fe^{+++}).
4. Some of the Fe^{++} in the enterocytes is **oxidized to the ferric form**, which bind with **apoferritin** to form **ferritin**.

This serves as **storage of iron in the form of ferritin.**
- Normally, transferrin is only 35% saturated with iron. Therefore, **transport mechanism is usually not exhausted**.

Clinical Note 67.1

Gastrectomy or gastric atrophy causes iron deficiency anemia: Gastric secretion dissolves the iron and allows it to form soluble complexes with ascorbic acid, which facilitates iron absorption. Therefore, though iron is not actually absorbed in the stomach, *gastrectomy or gastric atrophy causes iron deficiency anemia.*

Hemosiderosis & Hemochromatosis

In conditions of ***iron overload***, more ferritin is formed in the enterocytes, which is then excreted in the stool.

1. **Ferritin** is the principal storage form of iron in the tissue. In the tissue, ferritin molecules aggregate in the lysosomal membranes, which is called ***hemosiderin***.
   - Hemosiderin accumulates in the tissue when iron overload is prolonged. The condition is called **hemosiderosis**.
2. Deposition of large of hemosiderin in the tissue causes damage to the tissue. This condition is called **hemochromatosis**, which is characterized by skin pigmentation, diabetes (due to damage to the pancreatic tissue; ***bronze diabetes***), cirrhosis of liver, and ***gonadal atrophy*** (testicular atrophy in males).

Iron present in the body is mainly in the form of **hemoglobin** (70% of the total iron). About 23% is present in the **ferritin** (in the store form) and only 3% is present in the form of myoglobin.

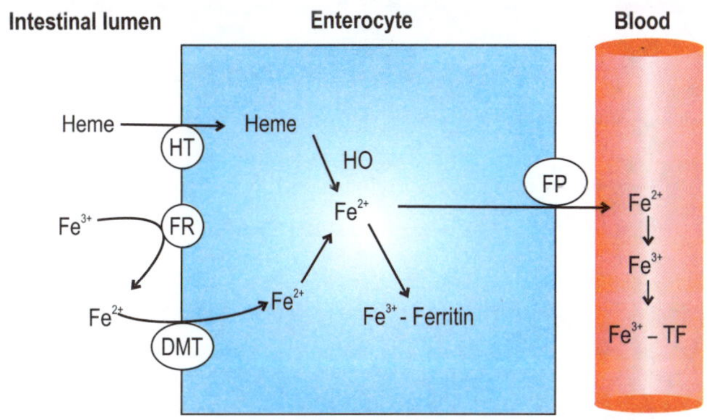

Fig. 67.2: Mechanism of iron reabsorption in intestine. HT: heme transporter; FR: ferric reductase; DMT: membrane iron transporter; HO: heme oxygenase; FP: ferroprotein transporter; TF: transferrin.

Exam Questions

1. Describe the mechanism of digestion and absorption of carbohydrate, fat and proteins from the gut.
2. Describe the mechanism of absorption of iron from the gut.

Multiple Choice Questions

1. **Which of the following is absorbed in the colon?**
   A. Iron B. Proteins
   C. Bile salts D. Electrolytes
2. **Which of the following secretions has a very high pH?**
   A. Gastric juice B. Pancreatic juice
   C. Bile in gall bladder D. Saliva
3. **Short chain fatty acid produced by bacteria are maximally absorbed in:**
   A. Duodenum B. Colon
   C. Ileum D. Jejunum
4. **Gastric secretions are essential for absorption of**
   A. Cobalamin B. Fat
   C. Thiamine D. Folic acid
5. **Vitamin B_{12} is absorbed in:**
   A. Duodenum B. Jejunum
   C. Ileum D. Stomach
6. **Glossitis and chelitis seen with deficiency of:**
   A. Vit. B_2 B. Vit. B_{12}
   C. Vit. K D. Vit. D
7. **Iron absorption is increased by:**
   A. More fibersin diet B. Vitamin C
   C. Phosphate D. Phytic acid
8. **Iron is actively absorbed in:**
   A. Stomach B. Duodenum and proximal jejunum
   C. Large intestine D. Ileum

Answers

1. D 2. B 3. B 4. A 5. C 6. A 7. B 8. B

Section VIII

Endocrine Physiology

"*The future of the earth depends on a change of consciousness.*
The only hope for the future is in a change of man's consciousness and the change is bound to come.
But, it is left to men to decide if they will collaborate for this change or if it will have to be enforced upon them by the power of crushing circumstances.
So, wake up and collaborate!

The Mother"
(of Sri Aurobindo Ashram, Pondicherry, INDIA)

Chapter 68

Introduction to Endocrinology

Learning Objectives
On completion of study of this chapter:
The student will be able to (must know):
1. Name the endocrine glands, name the hormones secreted from each glands and mention their major functions.
2. Classify hormones and give examples of each category.
3. Learn the principles of hormone synthesis.
4. Name the hormone signaling systems and their mechanism of operation.
5. Say the types of intercellular communications outline their mechanisms and give examples for each.
6. Elucidate different types of hormone actions.
7. Outline the mechanisms of regulation of hormone secretion.
8. Describe the feedback control of hormone secretion.
The student may also be able to (desirable to know):
1. Describe the basics of synthesis, secretion, metabolism and degradation of hormones.
2. Understand how the hormones are degraded in the body.
3. Name different methods of hormone estimation.

Endocrine physiology is the branch of physiology that deals with the study of processes involved in regulation and integration of cells and organ systems by specialized chemical substances called hormones. The word '**hormone**' is derived from *"hormaein"* a Greek word, which means 'to excite'.

- **Hormone** is defined as *specialized organic molecules that are synthesized by endocrine glands or tissues in response to specific stimuli and exert their precise effects on particular target cells.*
- An endocrine gland is a **ductless gland** that pours its secretion **directly into general circulation**. Hormones circulate in blood to reach the target tissues on which they act.
- Target cells are conferred with **receptors that are specific in their affinity** for hormones.

ENDOCRINE GLANDS

Endocrine glands (structures) are broadly divided into major endocrine glands and other endocrine organs (Fig. 68.1, and Table 68.1).

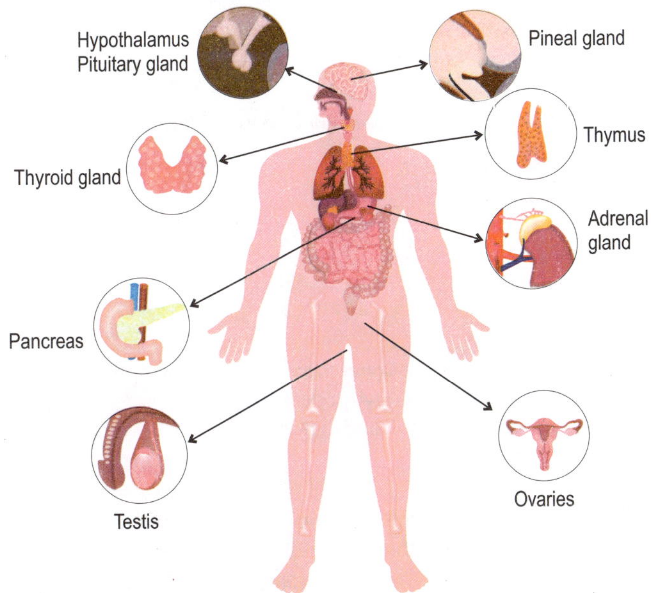

Fig. 68.1: Location of main endocrine glands of the body.

Table 68.1 | Hormones secreted from endocrine glands (organs) and their main functions.

Endocrine organs	Major functions
A. Major glands	
Hypothalamus	
Releasing and release-inhibiting hormones	Control pituitary hormone secretions

Table 68.1: contd...

Anterior pituitary	
1. Growth hormone	1. Growth and development
2. TSH	2. Stimulates thyroid hormone secretion
3. ACTH	3. Stimulates secretion of adrenocortical hormones
4. LH and FSH	4. Control ovarian and testicular functions
5. Prolactin	5. Promotes milk synthesis and secretion
Posterior pituitary	
1. ADH	1. Water reabsorption from kidney & vasoconstriction
2. Oxytocin	2. Milk ejection & Parturition
Thyroid	
1. T3 and T4	Tissue metabolism
Adrenal cortex	
1. Cortisol	1. Metabolism, permissive actions for other hormones, anti-inflammatory and antiallergy function etc.
2. Aldosterone	2. Na^+ & water reabsorption & K^+ secretion in kidney
Adrenal medulla	
1. Catecholamines	Metabolism, sympathetic activation
Pancreas	
1. Insulin	Glucose entry & utilization by cells
Parathyroid	
1. Parathormone	Regulation of plasma calcium & phosphate levels
Testes	
1. Testosterone	Spermatogenesis & male reproductive development
Ovaries	
1. Estrogen & progesterone	Female reproductive functions
Pineal	
1. Melatonin	Inhibits gonadal function, light-dark cycle
B. Others	
Placenta	
1. Human chorionic gonadotropins	1. Growth of corpus luteum
2. Human Somato-mammotropin	2. Fetal development
Kidney	
1. Renin	1. Conversion of angiotensinogen to A-I
2. Erythropoietin	2. Erythropoiesis
3. 1,25- Dihydroxycholecalciferol	3. Bone mineralization
Adipocytes	
1. Leptin	Inhibits food intake & stimulates thermogenesis
Heart	
1. ANP	Natriuresis, diuresis, vasodilation, decreases BP
GI Tract	
1. GI Hormones	GI functions
Lungs	
1. ACE	1. Converts A-I to A-II
2. Local hormones	2. Various functions
Thymus	
1. Thymosin	Immunity

Types of Hormones

Hormones are broadly classified into **three types:** peptides, amino acids and steroids.

Proteins or Peptides

PY8.6

Peptide hormones are made up of peptide chains.

- Depending on the number of amino acids in the chain, they may be **oligopeptides** (less than 10 amino acids) like oxytocin and ADH, and **polypeptides** (10 or more amino acids) like insulin and growth hormone.
- Based on their structure and functions, they are grouped into a **number of families** like insulin, glycoprotein, growth hormone and secretin families (Table 68.2).

Amino acids

These hormones are amines. Many of them are derived from a **common amino acid**, for example dopamine, epinephrine, norepinephrine and thyroxine are derived from tyrosine. They are usually hydrophilic.

Steroids

Steroid hormones are **synthesized from cholesterol**, and are lipid soluble and hydrophobic.

- This group includes hormones of **adrenal cortex and many gonadal hormones**.
- The biological activities of this group are determined by **modification of their side chains, hydroxylation and ring aromatization** at various sites.

Table 68.2 | Classification of hormones.

A. Peptide Hormones	
1. Insulin family - Insulin - Insulin like growth factors - Relaxin	**4. Secretin family** - Secretin - Glucagon - VIP - GIP
2. Glycoproteins - LH - FSH - TSH - hCG **3. Growth hormone family** - GH - Prolactin - Human placental lactogen	**5. Others** - ANP - Calcitonin - CCK - ADH - Inhibin - Somatostatin - ACTH - Parathormone
B. Amino Acid Derivative	
1. Amines - Epinephrine - Norepinephrine - Dopamine - Serotonin	**2. Iodinated amino acid** - Thyroxine (T_4) - Triiodothyronine (T_3)
C. Steroid Hormones	
- Glucocorticoids - Mineralocorticoids - Estrogen - Progesterone - Testosterone - 1,25-dihydroxycholecalciferol	

GENERAL PHYSIOLOGY OF HORMONES

Hormone Signaling

The chemical signaling of hormone occurs through **three pathways**: endocrine, paracrine, and autocrine.

Endocrine Signaling

Hormone secreted from the endocrine gland reaches distant target tissues **via bloodstream**. Most of the hormones signal the target tissues located far away from the gland via this route.

- Thus, cells of hormone secreting tissue communicate with cells of other tissues via endocrine signaling.
- Hence, this type of intercellular communication is called **endocrine communication**.

Paracrine Signaling

Hormone secreted from endocrine tissue diffuses into extracellular space and **signals the neighboring tissue**.

- This is called **paracrine signaling**.
- For example, **somatostatin secreted from D cells** of pancreatic islets influences the secretion of insulin and glucagon from same islet cells (Flowchart 68.1).

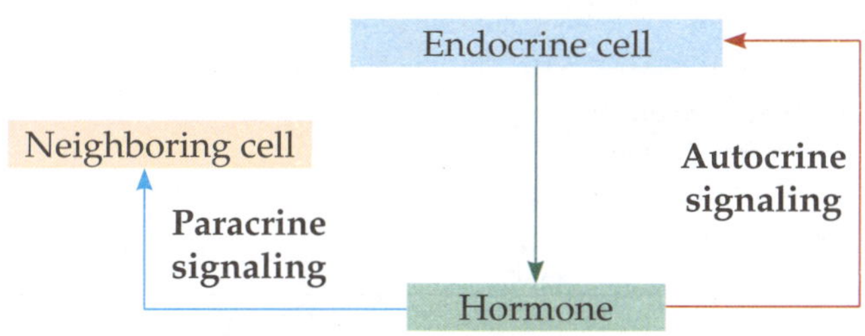

Flowchart 68.1: Paracrine and autocrine hormone signalling.

Autocrine Signaling

Hormone secreted from an endocrine cell binds with the **receptor located in the same cell** that secretes the hormone.

- Thus, hormone modifies the function of its parent cell.
- The example of autocrine **signaling is the platelet activating factor** secreted from platelet, which activates the platelet.

Intercellular Communications

Cells communicate with each other by **five major mechanisms**: direct, neural, endocrine, paracrine and neurocrine (Table 68.3). Autocrine and juxtacrine communications are strictly not part of the intercellular communications, as in these two systems cells influence their own activities or the other cells in the vicinity.

1. **Direct communication:** This occurs between cells **via gap junction** (electrical synapses). Example is rapid transmission of impulse between cardiac myocytes via gap junctions.
2. **Neural communication:** This is the major mechanism of intercellular communication. Examples are neurons communicating through synapses.
3. **Endocrine, paracrine & autocrine communications:** They are described above in 'Hormone signaling'.
4. **Juxtacrine communication:** This is the communication through cell adhesion to growth factors expressed on cell surface.
   - For example, many cells having receptors for ***transforming growth factor*** α (TGFα) interact with each other by attaching themselves to the transforming growth factor α (TGFα) present on their cell surface.
5. **Neurocrine communication:** This is via secretion of chemicals at nerve ending.
   - For example, ***cholinergic vagal fibers*** to oxyntic cells in stomach influence parietal cell function by releasing **acetylcholine** at their terminals, and ***non-cholinergic vagal fibers*** to G cells in the antrum of stomach influence G cell function by releasing gastrin releasing peptide (**GRP**) at their terminals.

Table 68.3 | Intercellular communications.

Types	Mechanism
Direct communication	Via gap junctions between cells
Neural communication	Via synapses (synaptic transmission)
Endocrine communication	Via circulating hormones
Paracrine communication	Via locally released hormones from neighboring endocrine cells
Autocrine communication	Hormone secreted from the same cell
Juxtacrine communication	Through growth factors expressed on the cell surface
Neurocrine communication	Through chemicals released at nerve terminal

Principles of Synthesis & Secretion

Peptide Hormone Synthesis

Protein hormones are first synthesized in rough endoplasmic reticulum as a signal peptide called **preprohormone**, which is then cleaved to form **prohormone**.

1. Prohormone is then transported into the Golgi apparatus, where it is converted into **hormone** (Flowchart 68.2).
2. The hormone is secreted from **stored granules** by ***calcium-mediated exocytosis***.
3. Hormones are also secreted from **neoplastic tissues** (Application Box 68.1).

ok

Preprohormone (Signal peptide)
(in rough endoplasmic reticulum)

↓

Prohormone

↓

Hormone
(Packaged in Golgi apparatus to form secretory granules)

Flowchart 68.2: General outline of peptide hormone synthesis.

Application Box 68.1

Ectopic Hormone Secretion: Sometimes in pathological conditions, non-endocrine tissues secrete hormones. For example, n**eoplastic tissues of lungs** like small cell pulmonary carcinoma produce several hormones. The condition is called **paraneoplastic syndrome**. Hormones are also secreted from gastrointestinal tumors and the condition is called **carcinoid syndrome**.

Pathways of Synthesis

Synthesis and secretion of peptide hormones occur in **two pathways**: the regulated and constitutive pathways.

Regulated Pathway: In regulated pathway, external stimuli trigger release of hormone which is already synthesized and **stored in secretory granules**, and also promote synthesis of some additional hormones. For example, GnRH from hypothalamus stimulates release of gonadotropins and additional synthesis of gonadotropins from anterior pituitary.

Constitutive Pathway: In constitutive pathway, secretion of hormones occurs more directly from endoplasmic reticulum or vesicles formed from the Golgi apparatus, in which additional hormones are formed simultaneously.

Thus, **regulated pathway is capable of secretion of large amount of hormones**, whereas ***constitutive pathway promotes secretory reserve***. In any case, stimuli that trigger secretion also increase synthesis of hormones.

Amine Hormone Synthesis

All amine hormones except serotonin are synthesized from the **amino acid tyrosine** that requires a series of enzymatic reactions. Serotonin is synthesized from 5-HT. Catecholamines are **stored in granules** and secreted by calcium mediated exocytosis of granules in which they are stored.

Steroid Hormone Synthesis

Steroid hormones are synthesized from cholesterol. Many enzymatic reactions are involved in the process of steroid hormone synthesis.

- These hormones are **not stored in the cell as granules**.
- They are usually present in the cytosol **bound to proteins**.
- On stimulation, the hormones become free form intracellular proteins and are transported outside the cell usually by diffusion.

Transport of Hormones

Hormones in the blood either remain **in free form or bind with a specific carrier protein**.

Transport of Amine & Peptide Hormones

Amino acid-derived and peptide hormones **readily dissolve in the plasma** and do not require special mechanism for their transport.

Transport of Steroid Hormones

Thyroxine, steroid hormones and vitamin D are **relatively insoluble in plasma** and circulate in the **bound form**.

- In blood, more than 90% of thyroid and steroid hormones are bound to plasma proteins. The transport proteins are specific for hormones (Table 68.4).
- However, few nonspecific proteins are also involved in the process of hormone transport.

Table 68.4 | Transport proteins for hormones.

A. Specific proteins
1. Thyroxine binding globulin (TBG)
– Transports T3 and T4
2. Corticosteroid binding globulin (CBG)
– Transports cortisol and aldosterone
3. Sex-hormone binding globulin (SHBG)
– Transports testosterone and estrogen
B. Nonspecific proteins
1. Serum albumin
– Transports many steroid and thyroid hormones
2. Prealbumin
- Transports thyroxine

Importance of Hormone Binding

1. **Hormone action:** The intensity of the hormone action depends on the extent to which hormone is bound to the proteins.
   - Usually, hormones that bind to transport proteins remain 1 to 10% only in the free form, which is called as the **biologically active hormone**.
   - Thus, about 90% of these hormones, i. e. the hormone in bound form constitutes the **inactive pool of hormone**.
   - Any condition that **decreases hormone binding** by decreasing the concentration of proteins available for binding or by any other mechanism, **increases the hormone activity** as plasma level of free hormone rises; and conversely, condition that increases binding decreases hormone activity.
2. **Hormone reservoir:** Transport proteins also provide reservoir of hormones that is essential for **buffering rapid change in hormone concentration** in plasma.

3. **Hormone metabolism and clearance:** Binding with carrier protein influences metabolism and removal of hormone from circulation.
   - This **determines the half-life of the hormone**.
   - For example, the plasma half-life of thyroxine is 6 days as it is 99.9% protein bound, whereas half-life of aldosterone is 25 minutes as only 15% of it is bound to protein.
4. **Diagnostic importance:** Form diagnostic viewpoint, it is important to know the both free and bound form of the hormone.
   - **Assay of total hormone concentration** may sometimes be **misleading**.
   - Therefore, free concentration of hormone (**free hormone index**), or the **ratio of free form to bound form** of hormone reflects the actual physiological state of hormone.
   - In the diagnosis of hormonal disorder, **measurement of free hormone index is preferred** to total hormone estimation to evaluate the degree of dysfunction.

Hormone Metabolism

Alteration of Hormone

Some of the hormones are transformed in the peripheral blood, which is **required for their full biological activity**. Examples are the conversion of T_4 to T_3 and testosterone to dihydrotestosterone.

Degradation & Disposal of Hormone

Liver and kidney are the major sites for extraction and degradation of hormones.

- Therefore, diseases of liver and kidney alter hormonal status of the body by impairing removal of hormones from the body.
- Hormone degradation also depends on the rapidity of uptake of the hormone by the target cells like ***receptor-mediated endocytosis*** of peptide hormones.
- Also, metabolic degradation of hormones occurs by various enzymes.

Physiological Importance

1. **Measurement of hormone secretion: Urine is the major route of excretion** for many hormones, and few hormones are excreted in bile.
   - Therefore, for many hormones, measurement of **hormone metabolites in urine** is a better indicator of the rate of production of hormones.
   - For example, **urinary excretion of metanephrine or VMA** *is an index of catecholamine secretion*, which provides a simple and noninvasive test for assessment of adrenomedullary function.
2. **Estimation of metabolic clearance rate (MCR):** Sometimes estimation of rate of metabolism is clinically useful for ***assessing hormone dysfunction***.
   - The rate at which the hormone is removed from the body is one of the indices of MCR.
   - MCR is the hormone removed per unit time divided by the plasma concentration of the hormone.

$$MCR = \frac{\text{Hormone removed per unit time (mg/min)}}{\text{Plasma conc. of hormone (mg/ml)}}$$

MCR is reported as ml of plasma per min. Half-life of hormone and MCR are inversely related. Thus, *shorter the half life, greater is the MCR.*

Estimation of Hormone Concentration

Measurement of concentration of hormone in biological fluids is often performed for confirmation of clinical diagnosis. Hormone estimation can be done by bioassay, radioimmunoassay (RIA) and enzyme-linked immunosorbent assay (ELISA).

Hormone Actions

Most of the hormones have several effects on target tissues that are called as **pleiotropic effects of hormones**.

- As hormones act on different body systems for different actions, some of the actions are **complementary and some are antagonistic**.
- However, both complementary and antagonistic actions of hormones are meant for integration of body functions in normal conditions as well as in different other situations.

Complementary Actions

When actions of different hormones **facilitate a function** of the body in a particular situation, it is called complementary actions of hormone. Complementary actions may be for a **short-term regulation** or for a **long-term modification**.

1. The example for **short-term complimentary action** is the acute physical exercise, during which secretion of epinephrine, cortisol and glucagon contributes to defend plasma glucose concentration.
2. The example of **long-term complementary actions** is the regulation of growth by growth hormone, thyroxine, insulin like growth factors and sex steroids.

Antagonistic Actions

When the action of a hormone on a target organ **is opposed by another hormone**, the process is called antagonistic action.

- The example is the effect of **insulin and glucagon** on liver to regulate plasma glucose concentration.

- *Insulin lowers plasma glucose* by inhibiting hepatic glycogenolysis and gluconeogenesis, whereas *glucagon increases blood glucose* by stimulating glycogenolysis and gluconeogenesis.

- Therefore, antagonistic actions of hormones, is an **important regulatory process** of the nature to fine-tune the physiological activities of the body.

REGULATION OF HORMONE SECRETION

Normally, concentration of a hormone in circulation is maintained within a narrow range. Alteration in hormone concentration is mainly checked by regulation of hormone secretion. Hormone secretion is principally controlled by **four mechanisms**:

1. Feedback control,
2. Neural control,
3. Rhythmic or chronotropic control, and
4. Humoral control.

Of these control processes, **feedback control is the most common and developed** mechanism for regulation of hormone secretion.

Feedback Control

When the change in concentration of a hormone in plasma alters its rate of secretion, the mechanism is called feedback control. There are two feedback mechanisms: The positive and the negative feedbacks.

Negative Feedback

When increased concentration of a hormone and its metabolites provide feedback inhibitory signal to the gland that secretes the hormone, the mechanism is called negative feedback mechanism.

- This is the **common mechanism of hormone homeostasis**.
- Depending on the circuit or the pathway involved in the feedback control, the mechanism may be simple feedback or complex feedback.

Simple Feedback Control

This is the **first order of feedback control** in which the hormone secreted from a gland controls its secretion through the physiological effects. The endocrine cells that secrete the hormone also **sense the biological activity** produced by the hormone.

- When the biological effects are more, the hormone secretion decreases appropriately to maintain normal function of the hormone (Flowchart 68.3).
- For example, β cells of pancreas secrete insulin that acts on liver and skeletal muscles to regulate blood glucose concentration. β cells in turn sense the alteration in plasma glucose and accordingly adjust their insulin secretion to maintain the plasma glucose concentration within normal range.

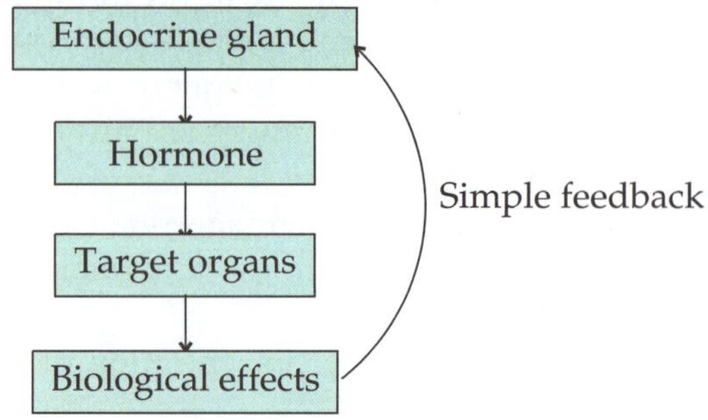

Flowchart 68.3: Simple feedback system in the regulation of hormone secretion. Endocrine gland senses biological activity of the hormone and accordingly modulates its secretion.

Complex or Hierarchical Feedback Control

When the feedback regulation involves **second or third order feedback loop** or both, the control mechanism is called complex or hierarchical control. This multi-order or complex control system is the usual mechanism for regulation of many hormone secretions.

- In this system, the hormone secreted by **first (upper) order gland** stimulates secretion of **second (middle) order gland**.
- Secretion (usually, trophic hormones) of middle order gland stimulates secretion of **final (lower) order gland** or *target gland*.
  - Secretion of target gland (**target gland hormone**) inhibits the secretion of first order or middle order glands (Flowchart 68.4).
  - Also, secretion of middle order gland (**trophic hormone**) inhibits secretion of first order gland.
- This system operates mainly for control of **hypothalamo-pituitary-target endocrine gland axis**.
- As this is an integrated system of control of endocrine functions, disorder at any level of hierarchy influences the function of other levels.

The major hormone axes regulated by **hierarchical system of feedback control** are:

- Hypothalamo-pituitary-thyroid axis
- Hypothalamo-pituitary-adrenal axis
- Hypothalamo-pituitary-gonadal axis

For example, in hypothalamo-pituitary-adrenal axis, excess cortisol in plasma inhibits secretion of adrenal cortex by decreasing ACTH secretion from anterior pituitary or by inhibiting hypothalamic release of CRH.

Loops of Negative Feedback Control

Depending on the distance from which the hormone of the target gland inhibits the upper order glands, the inhibition is classified into **long loop, short loop and ultrashort loop**.

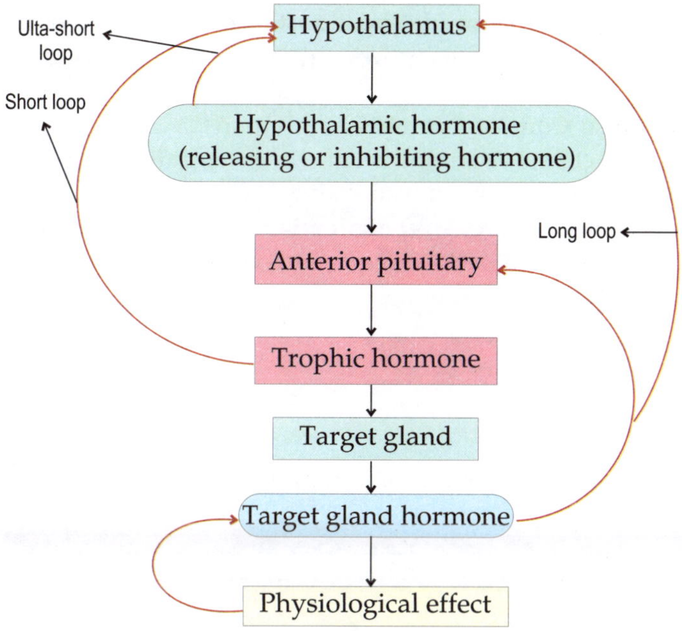

Flowchart 68.4: Hierarchical or complex feedback system in the regulation of endocrine functions. This system operates mainly for control of hypothalamo-pituitary-target endocrine gland axis.

- For example, in the same hypothalamo-pituitary adrenal axis, cortisol inhibiting CRH release is the **long loop** of negative feedback, ACTH inhibiting CRH release is the **short loop** of negative feedback and CRH inhibiting its own release is the **ultrashort loop** of negative feedback (Flowchart 68.4).

Positive Feedback

This is a less common mechanism of regulation of hormone secretion. In this control system, increase in hormone concentration in plasma stimulates further secretion of that hormone so that the hormone concentration **increases steadily to reach a peak plasma level**.

1. The best example of positive feedback regulation is the **LH surge** that occurs just before ovulation.
   - Normally, estrogen inhibits LH secretion; however, just before ovulation, increased estrogen concentration in plasma provides a positive feedback for LH release from anterior pituitary that results in LH surge.
2. Other examples are **oxytocin secretion during parturition**, release of oxytocin **during breast feeding** and release of **melatonin in response to darkness**.

Neural Control

Endocrine glands are usually innervated by both the components of autonomic nervous system.

1. **Stimulation of sympathetic or parasympathetic system** therefore alters the endocrine secretions Secretion of catecholamines from adrenal medulla in response to sympathetic stimulation is an example.
   - However, **the receptor types present in the endocrine tissue determine the final secretion from the gland**.
   - Besides, innervation of the endocrine tissues may also be cholinergic, serotonergic or dopaminergic depending on the neurotransmitter released at the nerve ending.
2. Secretion of hormones in response to various stimuli like visual, olfactory, gustatory, tactile etc. is also neurally mediated.
   - One of the examples is the **milk ejection reflex** in which suckling by the baby increases secretion of oxytocin that causes contraction of myoepithelial cells of the mammary gland.

Rhythmic or Chronotropic Control

Chronotropic control of hormone secretion is the regulatory mechanism operated by **various rhythms of biologic phenomena** that either cycle at regular intervals like **circadian rhythm, sleep-wake cycle, seasonal rhythm and menstrual cycle**, or appear at **different phases of development** like hormonal changes occurring in pre-pubertal children.

Influenced by chronotropic control mechanism, hormones are secreted in a definable and rhythmic pattern, which may be:

- Episodic or **pulsatile** lasting for few minutes to hours
- **Diurnal** lasting for several hours in a light-dark cycle
- **Periodical** lasting for many days
- **Developmental** occurring at different phases of development
- **Seasonal,** in different seasons.

Examples of Chronotropic Control*:*

1. **Example of episodic (pulsatile) hormone secretion** is the secretion of GnRH. Normally, GnRH is secreted in episodic bursts that cause circhoral peaks of LH secretion (for details, refer, "Female Reproduction").
2. **Example of diurnal hormone secretion** is the change in ACTH or cortisol at different times of day and night. Another example of day-night variation is melatonin secretion.
3. **Example of periodical secretion** is alteration in sex hormones or gonadotropins in different phases of menstrual cycle.
4. Alteration in secretion of gonadal hormones at puberty in both boys and girls is the **example of developmental hormonal secretion**.
5. **Example of seasonal variation** is change in hormone concentration in different times in a year that mostly occurs due to environmental changes. This is more prominent in birds.

Mechanisms: The variation in hormone secretion is due to many mechanisms such as change in secretory pattern influenced by photic stimuli (**light-dark variation**), change influenced by sleep (**sleep-wake variation**) or change subjected to environmental alteration (**seasonal variation**).

Humoral Control

Humoral control is the control by hormones and chemicals.

Hormonal Control: Many hormones influence secretion of other hormones.

- Examples are glucagon stimulating insulin secretion, **angiotensin stimulating aldosterone secretion**, somatostatin inhibiting growth hormone secretion and so on.

Chemical Control: Secretion of hormone is influenced by various chemical stimuli such as concentration of blood gasses, acids, ions and osmolality.

- Examples are **hypokalemia inhibiting insulin secretion**, hyperkalemia or hyponatremia stimulating aldosterone secretion etc.

Exam Questions

1. Describe the mechanism of regulation of hormone secretion.
2. What are the types of feedback control of hormone secretion? Describe the significance of each control system with examples.
3. Briefly describe the intercellular communications.
4. Briefly describe the type of hormomone signalling.

Multiple Choice Questions

1. The hormone Leptin is produced from?
A. Myocyte
B. Adipocyte
C. Lymphocyte
D. Thymocyte

2. Example of diurnal hormone secretion is:
A. Melatonin
B. Adiponectin
C. Insulin
D. Dopamine

3. Thyroxine can be transported by all of the following, EXCEPT?
A. Prealbumin
B. Albumin
C. Thyroxine-binding globulin
D. Corticosteroid- binding globulin

4. Activation of platelets by release of platelet activating factor from platelets is an example of?
A. Paracrine signaling
B. Autocrine signaling
C. Juxtacrine signaling
D. Endocrine signaling

5. Which of the following is not considered as an endocrine organ?
A. Heart
B. Kidney
C. Placenta
D. Brain

6. Which of the following is not a protein hormone?
A. Insulin
B. Prolactin
C. Aldosterone
D. Calcitonin

7. Which of the following is not an amine hormone?
A. Serotonin
B. Norepinephrine
C. Epinephrine
D. Relaxin

8. All of the following are examples of positive feedback control of hormone secretion, EXEPT:
A. LH surge
B. Release of ACTH by cortisol level in plasma
C. Release of oxytocin during breast feeding
D. Release of melatonin in response to darkness

9. Regulation of insulin secretion from cells β of islets by somatostatin secreted from D cells of the same islets, is an example of:
E. Paracrine signaling
F. Autocrine signaling
G. Juxtacrine signaling
H. Endocrine signaling

10. Which of the following estimation of hormone level is a better index of physiological state of hormone:
A. Estimation of bound form
B. Estimation of free form
C. Total concentration
D. Ratio of free form to bound form

11. Example of episodic (pulsatile) hormone secretion is secretion of:
A. GH
B. GRH
C. GnRH
D. Insulin

12. All of the following are examples of negative feedback control of hormone secretion, EXEPT:
A. Release of TSH by thyroxine
B. Release of oxytocin during parturition
C. Release of GHRH by GH level in plasma
D. Release of CRH by ACTH level in plasma

Answers

1. B	2. A	3. D	4. B	5. D
6. C	7. D	8. B	9. A	10. D
11. C	12. B			

Chapter 69

Mechanisms of Hormone Action

Learning Objectives

On completion of study of this chapter:

The student will be able to (must know):

1. Understand the role of G proteins in hormone action.
2. List the signal transduction pathways and name the second messengers in each pathway.
3. Name the hormones that act through different second messengers.
4. Describe the mechanism of hormone action via adenylyl cyclase-cyclic AMP system, membrane phospholipid-phospholipase system and transcription of mRNA system.
5. Briefly describe Cyclic-GMP system, Tyrosine Kinase system and Calcium-calmodulin system.

The student may also be able to (desirable to know):

1. Explain the role of G proteins in health and disease.
2. Describe the effects of various second messengers on cells and tissues.

Hormones bind with the **specific receptors** in the target cell and **hormone-receptor complex** (HR complex), activates a series of **signal generating mechanisms** via a cascade of enzymatic reactions.

- The generated signal molecules increase in number in each step leading to manifold increase in final effect of the hormone on the cell. This is called **signal amplification**.
- Normally, concentration of hormones in the body fluid is exceedingly low, which is usually in the range of 10^{-9} to 10^{-12} mol/L. But hormones effectively alter cell functions through the process of signal amplification.

RECEPTOR FUNCTIONS

The receptors located on the membrane are usually **large glycoproteins** with molecular weight of 50,000–2,00,000 dalton. They usually span the membrane seven times.

- Following binding of hormone with the receptor, **HR complex** is formed, which is **internalized by endocytosis**.
- Inside the cell, **HR complex is degraded by lysosomal enzymes.**
- Usually, the receptor molecule is **recycled back to the cell membrane**. However, degradation of the receptor within the cell is not uncommon.
- Mutation of receptors produces receptor diseases (Application box 69.1).

Application Box 69.1

Mutation of Receptors: Receptor diseases are produced by mutation of receptors. Examples are Hirschsprung disease due to mutation of endothelin B receptors, familial hypothyroidism due to mutation of TSH receptors, colour blindness due to mutation of receptors for cone opsins, X-liked nephrogenic diabetes insipidus due to mutation of V_2 vasopressin receptors and so on.

Quantity and Sensitivity of Receptor

The receptor quantity and sensitivity are regulated by the **concentration of the hormone**. Accordingly, there is **up-regulation, down-regulation and desensitization** of receptors.

Up-Regulation: When, concentration of a hormone decreases in plasma for a longer period, the number of hormone receptors for that hormone increases in the target tissue. Also, sensitivity of receptor to the hormone increases. This is called up-regulation.

- Up-regulation of receptors forms the physiological basis of **denervation hypersensitivity**.

Down-Regulation: When, a hormone is present in excess in blood for a longer period, the number of receptors for that hormone decreases in the target tissue. This is called down-regulation.

Desensitization: When cells are *chronically exposed to excess concentration* of a hormone, they become less responsive on subsequent exposures. The process is called desensitization. In this process, the sensitivity of receptors for the hormone decreases.

- Chronic exposure to one hormone can also cause desensitization of receptors ***to other hormones***.
- If desensitization occurs for the same hormone, the effect is called **homologous desensitization**.
- If desensitization occurs for other hormones, the effect is called **heterologous desensitization**.

G Proteins

Receptors are **coupled with G proteins** in the cell membrane.

1. G proteins belong to **several families** of intrinsic membrane proteins that link receptors to the nearby effector molecules in the membrane.
    - Also, there are **different subunits of each family** of G proteins.
    - Specific subunit of G protein of a family relay specific signal from the receptors to the effectors that are usually specific ion channels or enzymes.
2. The effector molecules in turn generate second messengers that produce changes in cell functions when hormone binds with the receptors.
    - Thus, **G proteins convert the signal into biological activities**.

Mechanism: These membrane proteins are called G proteins **as they are attached to GDP**. When the signal binds with the G protein, G protein **exchanges GDP for GTP**.

- The **GTP-protein complex** influences subsequent signal transductions that results in **generation of many intracellular signals**, which mediate physiological effects of the hormone (Fig. 69.1).
- G protein has the **inherent GTPase activity**, which **converts GTP to GDP**. Therefore, once the hormone action is over, resting state of the G protein is restored.

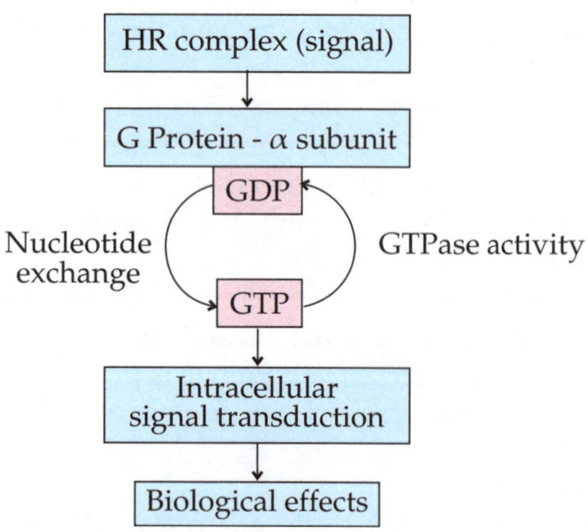

Fig. 69.1: Mechanism of action of G protein.

Significant contribution of Scientist

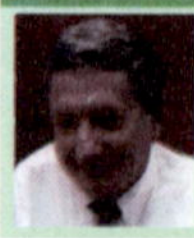

Alfred Goodman Gilman (1941–2015) an American pharmacologist shared **1994 Nobel Prize in Physiology or Medicine** with Martin Rodbell for the **discovery of G-proteins** and the role of these proteins in signal transduction in cells.

Types of G Proteins

G proteins are of 2 types: small G proteins and large G proteins.

Small G Proteins

There are **six different subfamilies** of small G proteins. The major categories among them are **Rab, Rac and Ras families**.

GAPs and GEFs

The **GTPase activating proteins** (GAPs) inactivate small G proteins by facilitating the hydrolysis of GTP to GDP in the central binding site. **Guanine exchange factors** (GEFs) activate small G proteins by facilitating exchange of GDP for GTP in the active site.

Functions of Small G Proteins

The small G proteins **regulate many cellular activities**.

- The **Rab family** regulates rate of vesicle movement between cell organelles and the cell membrane.
- The **Rho/Rac family** mediates interaction between cytoskeleton and the cell membrane.
- The **Ras family** controls growth by regulating transmission of signals from the cell membrane to the nucleus.

Large G Proteins

These are the membrane proteins coupled to the receptors.

- **Five families** of large G proteins have been discovered: G_s, G_i, G_t, G_q and G_{13}.
    - In addition, there are **three genes** for G proteins: 20α, 6β, and 12γ genes.
    - Therefore, a **large number of subunits** of G protein families are produced.
- Usually, G proteins are **trimeric proteins** consisting of ***three subunits***.
    - Therefore, they are called **heterotrimeric G proteins**.
- The subunits are called **α, β, and γ subunits**.
- Normally, α *subunit* is bound to GDP.

Mechanism of Action

When HR complex binds to the **G protein couple receptors** (GPCR), GDP is exchanged for GTP and **α subunit is separated** from β and γ subunits of the G protein.

- This separation of α subunits from β-γ subunits bring about physiological activities (Fig. 69.2).
    - The β and γ subunits do not separate from each other.

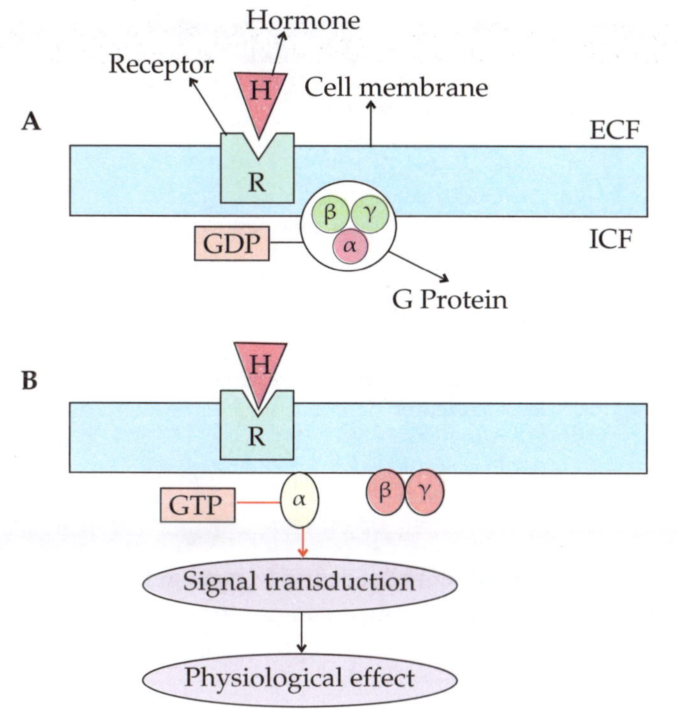

Fig. 69.2: Mechanism of action of hormone through G proteins. A: Note that G protein has three subunits (α, β and γ) and GDP is normally attached to the α subunit of G protein, which is a larger subunit; B: When HR complex is formed (following binding of hormone with receptor), GTP replaces GDP and α subunit is separated from β–γ subunits that remain attached to each other. This separation leads to generation of intracellular signals that in turn mediate hormone action.

- The α **subunit has the intrinsic GTPase activity** that converts GTP to GDP. This results in reassociation of α subunit with the β and γ subunits of the G proteins.
  - The GTPase activity of α subunit can be facilitated by **regulators of G protein signaling (RGS).**

Types of α Subunit: The α subunit of **three types** of G proteins (G_s, G_i, and G_q) are physiologically most important. They are **α_s, α_i and α_q subunits.**

Their activation produces following effects:

1. **Activation of α_s subunit** activates the membrane enzyme adenylyl cyclase that promotes cAMP formation.
2. **Activation of α_i subunit** inhibits the membrane enzyme adenylyl cyclase that decreases cAMP formation.
3. **Activation of α_q subunit** activates membrane bound phospholipases like phospholipase C.

G Protein Coupled Receptors

G protein coupled receptors (GPCRs) are membrane proteins that span the membrane seven times (Fig. 69.3). Hence, they are called serpentine receptors (seven-helix receptors). A large number of GPCR have been cloned recently.

They have diverse way of actions.

1. When a ligand binds with GPCR, conformational change occurs in GPCR that activates the large G protein attached to the cytoplasmic surface of the cell membrane.

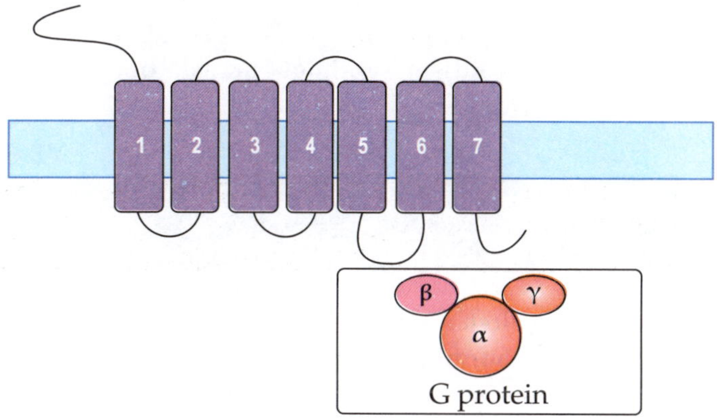

Fig. 69.3: Structure of G coupled protein receptor (GCPR)

2. Activation of a single GPCR can lead to activation of multiple large G proteins that transduces and amplifies the action of first messenger.
3. The GPCR bound to a ligand can be inactivated by phosphorylation of cytoplasmic side of the receptor to limit the process of cellular signaling.

There are many ligands (hormones/chemicals) for receptors coupled to G proteins (Table 69.1).

Table 69.1 | Ligands (hormones/chemicals) that act through G proteins coupled receptors (GPCRs).

A. Neurotransmitters	**B. Other peptides**
1. Catecholamines	1. Angiotensin II
- Epinephrine	2. ADH, Oxytocin
- Norepinephrine	3. GRP, VIP, PTH, TRH
- Dopamine	
2. Acetylcholine	
3. Histamine	
4. Serotonin	
5. Adenosine	
6. Opioids	
C. Glycoprotein hormones	**D. Arachidonic acid derivative**
1. TSH, FSH, LH	- Thromboxane A2
2. hCG	
E. Tachykinins	**F. Other ligands**
1. Neuropeptide K	1. Endothelins
2. Neurokinin A	2. PAF
3. Substance P	3. Testants, Odorants

G Protein Diseases

Mutation of G protein resulting in diseases is not uncommon. G protein responses may be increased or decreased by mutations.

Dysfunction due to Increased G Protein Responses: An example is **somatotroph tumor** causing **acromegaly**, in which mutation of $G\alpha_s$ ***decreases its intrinsic GTPase activity***, therefore G protein activity is prolonged and **more cAMP is produced**. This leads to hyperplasia of somatotrophs of anterior pituitary producing acromegaly in about 40% of patients.

Dysfunction due to Decreased G Protein Responses: An example is **type 1 pseudohypoparathyroidism**, in which **mutation of $G\alpha_s$** leads to failure of G protein to respond to parathyroid hormone. This results in features of **hypoparathyroidism without actual decrease** in parathyroid hormone.

PY8.6

SIGNAL TRANSDUCTION PATHWAYS (Second Messengers)

Hormones are **first messengers** that bind with the receptors to form **hormone-receptor (HR) complex**, which though various intracellular signaling pathways form **second messengers**.

The **processes of second messenger formation** are broadly categorized into **4 types** (Table 69.2):

1. Activation of ion channels
2. Activation of G proteins
3. Activation of intracellular or membrane enzymes
4. Activation of transcription process

Table 69.2 | Broad mechanisms of ligands bringing about change in cell functions.

A. Opening or closure of ion channels
1. Ach on nicotinic receptors
2. NE on K^+ channel in heart
B. Activation of G Proteins
1. Via adenylate cyclase (cAMP formation)
i) NE via β_1 receptor (↑ cAMP)
ii) NE via α_2 receptor (↓ cAMP)
2. Activation of phospholipase C (DAG, IP3 formation)
i) Angiotensin II
ii) NE via α_1 receptor
iii) ADH via V_1 receptor
3. Via cyclic GMP
- ANP, NO
C. Activation of intracellular or membrane enzymes
1. Via tyrosine kinase activity
- Insulin, PDGF, M-CSF, EGF
2. Via serine or threonine kinase
- Inhibin, Activin, TGF-β
D. Via nuclear receptors (m-RNA transcription)
- Steroid hormones
- Thyroid hormones

Role of Phosphorylation: Phosphorylation is an important *post-translational event* in the cell signaling pathway. Phosphorylation is controlled by *two group* of proteins namely **kinases and phosphatases**.

- **Kinases** catalyze the phosphorylation of tyrosine or threonine residues in proteins and **phosphatases** remove phosphates from proteins.
- More than **300 protein kinases** have been described (Table 69.3).
- The process of phosphorylation-dephosphorylation of cellular proteins is important in control of some ligand signaling pathway, which is referred to as **phosphate timer**.

Table 69.3 | Important protein kinases in the cell.

A. Kinases that phosphorylate serine or threonine residues or both
1. Calmodulin-dependent kinases
- Myosin-light chain kinase
- Phosphorylase kinase
- Ca^{++}calmodulin kinase I, II & III
2. Calcium-phospholipid dependent kinases
- Protein kinase C
3. Cyclic nucleotide dependent kinase
- Protein kinase A (cAMP dependent)
- cGMP dependent kinase
B. Kinases that phosphorylate tyrosine residues
- Insulin receptor
- EGF receptor
- PDGF receptor
- M-CSF receptor

Transduction Systems & Second Messengers: Intracellular signal molecules formed by a series of enzymatic reactions after the formation of HR complex are designated as **second messengers**.

1. The **signal transduction pathways** are activated depending on **G protein activation** of membrane enzymes (Table 69.4).
2. **The major second messengers are:** cyclic AMP, diacylglycerol (DAG), inositol triphosphate (IP_3), cyclic GMP, phosphoproteins, transcripted new mRNAs, and intracellular calcium.

There are **four main transduction systems:**

1. Adenylyl cyclase–cyclic AMP system
2. Membrane phospholipase–phospholipid system
3. Guanylyl cyclase–cyclic GMP system
4. Transcription of mRNAs

Table 69.4 | Signal transduction pathways for hormones.

Hormones	Membrane or G proteins	Enzyme activated in the process	Second messenger
PTH, NE (β receptor)	G α_s	Adenylyl cyclase (AC)	cAMP
A II, NE (α_2 receptor)	Gα_i	Inhibition of AC	Decreased cAMP
A II, NE (α_1 receptor), ADH (V_1 receptor), TRH	Gα_q	Phospholipase C	IP_3, DAG
ANP, EDRF	.....	Guanylyl cyclase	cGMP
Insulin, IGF I and II PDGF, EGF, M-CSF	.....	Tyrosine kinase (TK)	Phosphoproteins
GH, Erythropoietin	......	JAK/STAT family of TK	Phosphoproteins
TGF, MAPKs	......	Serine or threonine kinase	Phosphoproteins
T3, T4, steroid hormones	......	Transcription process	mRNAs
NE (on K^+ channels)	Membrane ion channels		K^+ (influx or efflux)
Ach (nicotinic receptor)	Ligand gated Ca^{++} channels		Intracellular Ca^{++}

Adenylyl Cyclase-Cyclic AMP System

Cyclic adenosine monophosphate (cAMP) is an important second messenger **for many peptide and amine hormones**. Formation of cAMP involves a series of events (Fig. 69.4).

Steps of Signal Transduction

1. The hormone binds with the receptor present on the cell membrane and forms hormone-receptor complex (**HR complex formation**).
2. HR complex causes **activation of G proteins** (either α_s or α_i).

a) The membrane enzyme **adenylyl cyclase is activated** (*if α_s is stimulated*).
- When the binding of hormone to receptor **stimulates the stimulatory G protein** (α_s subunit), adenylyl cyclase is activated.

B) If the hormone binding with receptor **stimulates the inhibitory G protein** (α_i subunit), adenylyl cyclase is inhibited.

Accordingly (depending on stimulation or inhibition), in the next step, cAMP formation is either increased or decreased in the cell.

3. Adenylyl cyclase catalyzes the **conversion of ATP to cyclic AMP**.
4. The cAMP **activates protein kinase A** (PKA).
   - **Protein kinase A** (PKA) has two catalytic and two regulatory subunits.
   - cAMP separates catalytic from regulatory subunits. Separation of subunits leads to **activation of PKA**.
5. Free catalytic subunits **phosphorylate the serine and threonine residues** on many cellular enzymes and other proteins.
   - This process of phosphorylation of intracellular proteins results in **formation of various phosphoproteins**.
6. New phosphoproteins **induce cell functions** (mediate the physiological effects of hormone).

IMPORTANT NOTE

cAMP phosphorylates CREB: The PKA also migrates to the nucleus where it **phosphorylates CREB** (cAMP-responsive element-binding protein). CREB binds to DNA and influences **transcription of a number of genes**. Thus, cAMP can also *alter genetic functions* of the cell.

Termination of cAMP Actions: Actions of cAMP in the cell are terminated in two ways.

1. cAMP is **degraded to 5′AMP** in the cell by the cytoplasmic enzyme ***phosphodiesterase*** (PDE).
2. Serine or threonine specific **phosphatases dephosphorylate the proteins** already phosphorylated by PKA.

Clinical Importance

Not only **many hormones** act through cAMP (Table 69.5), but also **toxins** released by various pathogens produce lethal effects by altering cAMP concentration in the cell.

- **Cholera and pertussis toxins** are examples of stimulation and inhibition of cAMP respectively.

Stimulation of cAMP: In cholera, the subunit A_1 of the toxin of Vibrio cholerae **activates adenylate cyclase and increases cAMP production.**

- cAMP **decreases Na^+ absorption and increases Cl^- secretion** in intestinal lumen that produces **isotonic fluid diarrhea**.

Tea and coffee also stimulate cyclic AMP formation (Application Box 69.2)

Inhibition of cAMP: In pertussis (whooping cough), a component of toxin of *Bordetella pertussis* decreases adenylyl cyclase activity **by activating inhibitory G protein**. This impairs the host's defense ability.

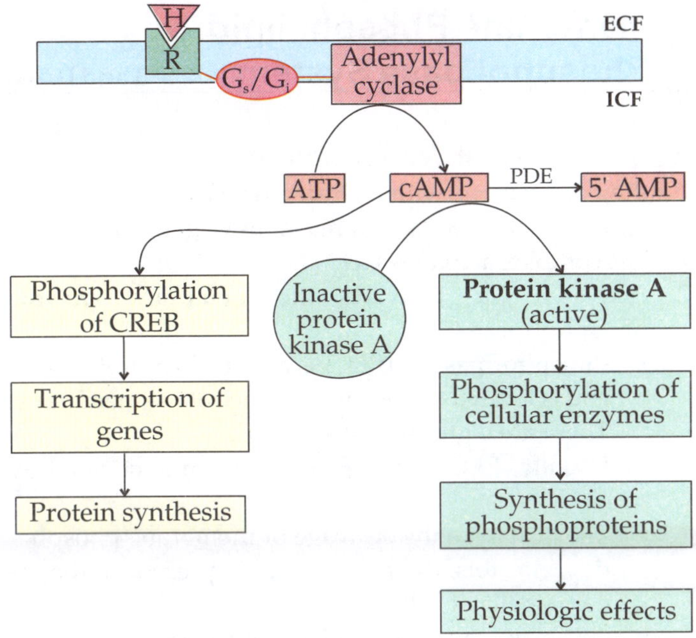

Fig. 69.4: Mechanism of hormone action through adenylyl cyclase-cyclic AMP system. H: hormone; R: receptor; Gs/Gi: stimulatory G protein or inhibitory G protein; PDE: phosphodiesterase; CREB: cAMP-responsive element-binding protein.

Application Box 69.2

Tea and coffee are good for heart: Normally, PDE degrades cAMP in the cells. Therefore, the agents that inhibit the action of PDE like caffeine and theophylline increase the concentration of intracellular cAMP. These chemicals increase myocardial contractility by increasing intracellular cAMP. Hence, moderate intake of tea and coffee is good for heart.

Table 69.5 | Important hormones that act by altering cAMP concentration in the cell.

A. Hormones that act by increasing cAMP formation
1. GHRH 2. CRH 3. GnRH 4. FSH
5. LH 6. Norepinephrine via β1 receptor
7. ADH via V2 receptor
B. Hormones that act by inhibiting cAMP formation
1. Norepinephrine via α_2 receptor
2. Somatostatin

Membrane Phospholipid Phospholipase System (via IP3 and DAG)

Steps of Signal Transduction

Binding of hormone with the receptor (**HR complex**) initiates the following cascade of reactions (Fig. 69.5).

1. HR complex **activates Gα_q**.
2. Activated Gα_q **activates the membrane enzyme phospholipase** C.
   - **Phospholipase C** (PLC) is attached to protein Gα_q and is located on the inner surface of the membrane. There are eight isoforms of PLC.
   - Usually, **PLC β_1 and β_2 isoforms** are activated by Gα_q.
   - They catalyze the cleavage of membrane phosphatidylinositols, the phospholipids present in the inner lamella of cell membrane.
3. PLC β_1 or β_2 causes hydrolysis of phosphatidylinositols 4-5,bisphosphate (PIP_2) that **generates two signal molecules: *inositol 1,4,5-triphosphate (IP_3) and diacylglycerol (DAG).***
   - IP_3 releases calcium from endoplasmic reticulum.
   - DAG stimulates intracellular (submembrane) enzyme protein kinase C.
4. The **increased protein kinase C activity** activates many intracellular enzymes that bring about change in cell functions.

Thus, **two subsystems** are formed in this pathway: the IP_3 subsystem and the DAG subsystem.

In IP_3 Subsystem

5a. IP_3 binds with its receptors located on cytosolic surface of endoplasmic reticulum (ER).
   - This binding facilitates **release of Ca^{++} from ER**, which causes cytosolic Ca^{++} to increase several-fold.

6a. Increased intracellular Ca^{++} facilitates **binding of Ca^{++} with calcium-binding proteins** (CaBP) like calmodulin, and also activates CaBP.
   - Ca^{++}-calmodulin dependent protein kinases are also activated in this process.

7a. CaBP alters cell functions.

In DAG Subsystem

5b. DAG **stimulates the enzyme protein kinase C** (PKC).

6b. PKC causes **phosphorylation of a variety of intracellular proteins** leading to formation of phosphoproteins.

7b. Phosphoproteins alter cell functions.

Examples of hormones that **act via IP_3 and DAG are** norepinephrine acting via α_1 receptors, ADH acting via V_1 receptors, angiotensin II, TRH etc.

Termination of Hormone Effects: When the hormone action is over, **IP_3 is metabolized** by dephosphorylation process to inositol, and **DAG is converted** first to phosphatidic acid and then to cytosine diphosphate (CDP). CDP combines with inositol to form **phosphatidylinositol** to be reused in future for hormone action.

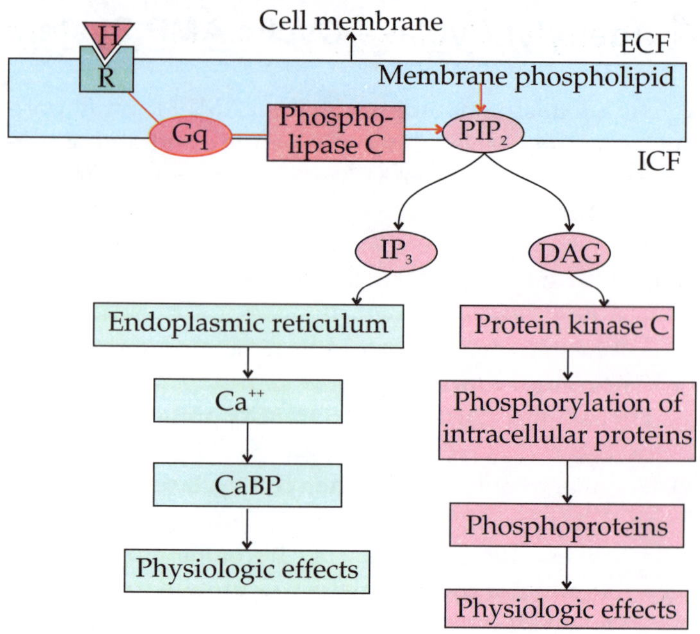

Fig. 69.5: Mechanism of hormone action through membrane phospholipid-phospholipase system. CaBP: calcium-binding protein; DAG: diacylglycerol; Gq: Gαq protein; H: hormone; IP_3: Inositol triphosphate; PIP_2: phosphatidyl inositol biphosphate; R: receptor.

Activation of Phospholipase A_2

Binding of hormone with receptor **activates Gα_q**, which in turn **stimulates DAG production**. DAG and activated Gα_q stimulate membrane bound **phospholipase A_2.**

1. Phospholipase A_2 **converts membrane phospholipid into acrachidonic acid** which in turn is converted by a number of enzymes into **prostaglandins, prostacyclins, thromboxanes and leukotrienes**. These chemicals change cell functions.
2. Few peptide hormones like **TRH** act through activation of phospholipase A_2.

Guanylyl Cyclase-Cyclic GMP System

Steps of Signal Transduction

Binding of hormone with the receptor initiates following cascade of events (Fig. 69.6):

1. The HR complex **activates guanylyl cyclase** in the membrane.
   - **Guanylyl cyclase** is the sub-membrane enzyme that forms part of the receptor.
   - In fact, it is the **cytoplasmic domain of the receptor**. Therefore, binding of hormone with receptor **automatically activates** this enzyme.
   - There are various isoforms of the guanylyl cyclase.

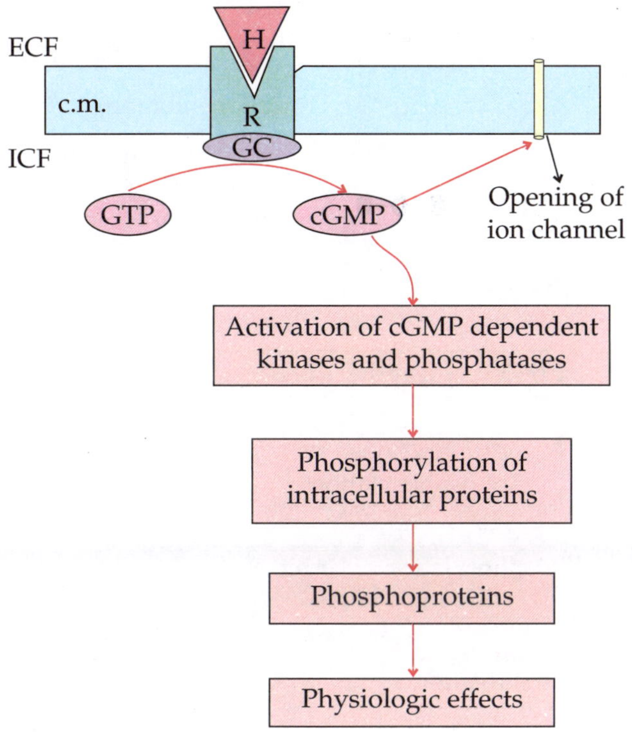

Fig. 69.6: Mechanism of hormone action through GC-cGMP system. c.m.: cell membrane; GC: guanylyl cyclase; H: hormone; R: receptor.

2. Guanylyl cyclase converts cytoplasmic guanosine triphosphate **(GTP) to cGMP.**
3. cGMP activates **cGMP-dependent kinases and phosphatases** that cause phosphorylation of different intracellular proteins.
5. cGMP also **directly opens ion channels.**
   - In **rods and cones**, cGMP operated mechanisms mediate physiologic effects.

Ligands that act through cGMP: The hormones that act through cGMP are **ANP and nitric oxide** (NO). The **enterotoxin of E. Coli** and GI polypeptide hormone **guanylin** also act through cGMP.

Intracellular Receptor (Transcription of mRNA) System

The receptors for **thyroid** and **steroid hormones, 1,25-dihydroxycholecalciferol and retinoids** are located inside the cell.

- The hormone diffuses through cell membrane into the cytoplasm and combines with the receptor, which is present **either in cytoplasm or in nucleus.**
- The receptor for **glucocorticoid is present in cytoplasm**, whereas the receptor for **thyroxine** and other **steroid hormones are located in nucleus.**

Receptors

The receptors for steroid hormones have **five domains** (A to E), and the **homology is mainly seen for the C domain**, especially C1 sub-domain (Fig. 69.7). The *C1 sub-domain* of the receptor is responsible **for binding to DNA.**

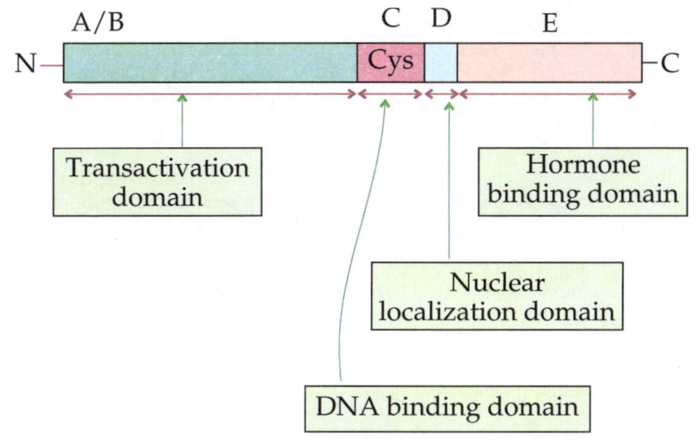

Fig. 69.7: Structure of steroid receptor. C and N at both end of the receptor depict carboxy terminal and amino terminal, respectively.

- The **receptors dimerize** when they bind with DNA, which is essential for gene transcription.
- The receptors have an amino terminal and a carboxy terminal.
  - The **hormone binding domain** is present close to the carboxy terminal.
  - A cysteine-rich **DNA binding domain** is located close to the hormone-binding domain.
- When hormone binds with receptor, C1 DNA binding domain binds with DNA through two zinc fingers.

Steps of Signal Transduction

Binding of hormone with the receptor triggers following series of events:

1. The binding of hormone with the receptor causes **conformational change** in the receptor protein.
   - The DNA binding domain of the receptor is exposed.
2. The hormone and active-receptor complex then moves to the DNA and **binds with the enhancer elements** (also called hormone response elements or steroid response elements; SRE) in the DNA.
   - Normally, steroid receptors are bound to **heat shock protein** (HSP) that covers the DNA binding domain (Fig. 69.8).
   - When hormone binds with receptors, the conformational change in receptor **releases the heat shock protein from it**, which **exposes the DNA binding domain.**
   - Heat shock proteins are intracellular proteins, and they are so named as their concentration increases on exposure of cells to heat and stress.
   - Therefore, they are also called **stress proteins.** They **protect cells** from various stresses.
3. The binding of active HR complex to DNA facilitates **transcription of mRNAs.**

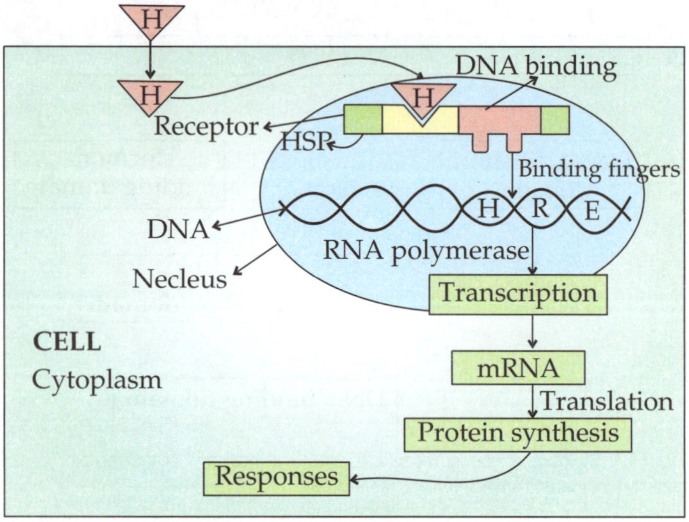

Fig. 69.8: Mechanism of hormone action through intracellular receptor system. The receptor is present either in the cytoplasm or in the nucleus. Note, binding of hormone with receptor exposes DNA binding-domain of the receptor, which interacts with hormone response element (HRE) on DNA. HSP: heat shock protein.

4. The mRNAs are then **translated** in the ribosomes to form **new proteins**.
5. Formation of new proteins in the cell **alters cell function**.

Other Mechanisms of Signal Generation

Tyrosine Kinase Activation

Some peptide hormones do not require G protein for inducing the signal transduction system. The hormone binds with the receptor, which has **intrinsic tyrosine kinase activity**.

- The receptor has three domains: extracellular, membrane and intracellular domains.
- The extracellular domain possesses the binding site for hormone and the intracellular domain possesses tyrosine kinase activity.

Steps of Signal Induction: The steps are as follows:

1. The binding of hormone with the receptor causes **conformational change in the receptor** that exposes the intracellular sites of the receptor for autophosphorylation (Fig. 69.9).
2. The kinase **autophosphorylates** tyrosine residue within the receptor and tyrosine residues on intracellular protein substrates.
3. The phosphorylation of tyrosine residue initiates cascade of phosphorylation reactions that **phosphorylates various enzymes** like serine and threonine kinases, and phosphatases. Phosphorylated enzymes change cellular activities.

The **hormones** that act through tyrosine kinase are **insulin, IGF I, IGF II**, other **growth factors** like PDGF, and EGF, and M-CSF.

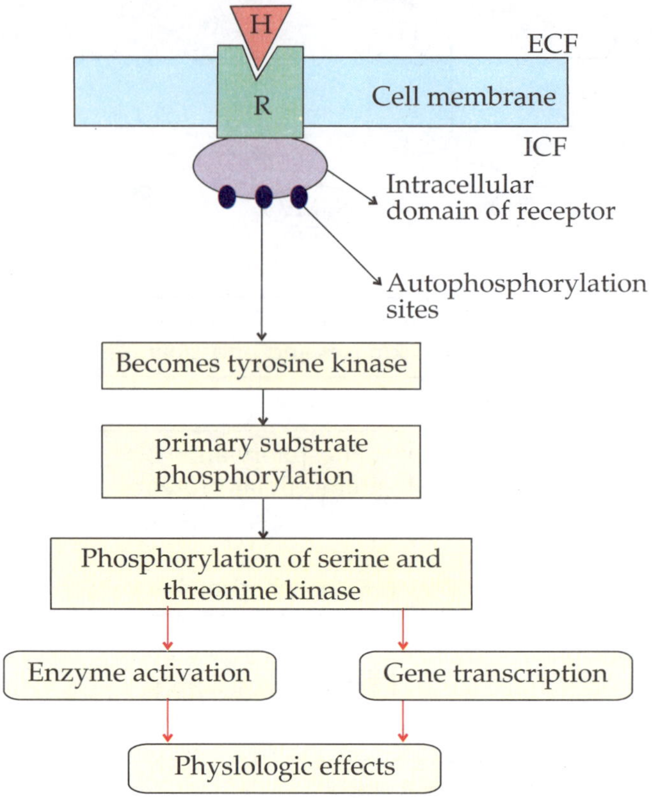

Fig. 69.9: Mechanism of hormone action through tyrosine kinase system. H: hormone; R: receptor.

JAK-STAT Pathway

The other method of tyrosine kinase activation is that the hormone binding causes conformational change in the **intracytoplasmic tip of the receptor** that exposes the sites to which cytoplasmic tyrosine kinase binds.

1. The activation of tyrosine kinase such as Jannus tyrosine kinase (**JAK**) phosphorylates signal transducers and activator of transcription proteins (**STAT proteins**).
2. Activation of **JAK-STAT pathway** further activates intracellular enzymes that change cell function.

Example of the hormone acting through JAK-STAT pathway is the growth hormone (for details, refer "Growth Hormone").

Calcium–Calmodulin System

This is the system binding of hormone to the receptor stimulates G protein to activate **ligand-gated calcium channel** through which ***calcium from the ECF enters into the cell***. Increased intracellular calcium changes cell function by various mechanisms.

1. Thus, in this system, **calcium is the second messenger** for hormone action.
2. Calcium is also **mobilized from the intracellular storage sites** like mitochondria and endoplasmic reticulum (Fig. 69.10).
   - In many tissues, the secretion of calcium from the intracellular storage sites triggers opening of calcium channels in the cell membrane.

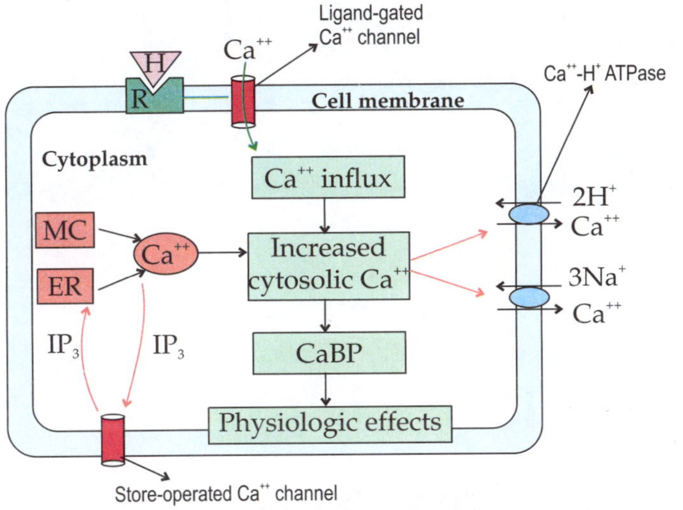

Fig. 69.10: Mechanism of hormone action through calcium-calmodulin system. CaBP: calcium-binding proteins; ER: endoplasmic reticulum; H: hormone; IP3: inositol triphosphate; MC: mitochondria; R: receptor.

- This is called **store-operated calcium influx.**
- This further increases the calcium concentration in the cell and ***replaces calcium in endoplasmic reticulum and mitochondria***.
- Store-operated calcium influx is mediated through IP_3.

4. Calcium then binds with many intracellular **calcium binding proteins**.
   - One of the important calcium binding proteins is the **calmodulin.**

Calmodulin-dependent Kinases: Calmodulin is a polypeptide. Binding of calcium with calmodulin activates calmodulin-dependent kinases. There are various **calmodulin-dependent kinases** in the cell.

The important kinases are:

1. **Myosin light change kinase** that causes phosphorylation of myosin.
2. **Phosphorylase kinase** that causes phosphorylation of many intracellular proteins.
3. Other important kinases are **calcium-calmodulin kinase I, II, and III**. Kinases I and II are concerned with synaptic function and kinase III is involved in protein synthesis.

Calcium Binding Proteins

The calcium binding proteins in the cells are **calmodulin, troponin and calbindin.**

1. The troponin is the calcium binding protein present in the skeletal muscle that is involved in muscle contraction.
2. **Calcineurin**, a calmodulin-activated protein, is a phosphatase, which inactivates calcium channels through dephosphorylation. Calcineurin also participates in immunity by activating T cell.

Rapid Actions of Steroids

Apart from transcription of mRNA (**genomic actions**) by steroids, which is normally time-consuming, some actions of steroid hormones manifest more rapidly through **nongenomic actions**.

1. **For nongenomic actions**, the hormone binds with the surface receptors that either changes membrane permeability to ***calcium or other ions***, or stimulates **formation of second messengers** like cAMP in the cell.
   - An example of nongenomic action is the **rapid neuronal changes induced by steroid.**
2. Thus, steroids also act through **intracellular second messengers** that are activated by other hormones.
3. This forms the physiological basis of interaction of steroid hormones with other hormones.
   - For example, ***estrogen and dopamine*** interact at the second messenger level for nongenomic actions of estrogen.

Exam Questions

1. Describe the mechanisms of hormone action via adenylate cyclase-cyclic AMP and membrane phospholipid-phospholipase pathways.
2. List different hormone signaling pathway. Describe the details of any of the hormone signaling system.
3. List important hoemones that act through G protein coupled receptors. Describe the mechanism of action of hormones through G proteins.
4. Describe the mechanism of action of hormone through the intracellular receptors.
5. Describe the mechanism of hormone action via tyrosine kinase system and calcium-calmodulin system.

Multiple Choice Questions

1. **All of the following are second messengers, EXCEPT:**
   A. Guanylyl cyclase B. cAMP/cGMP
   C. IP3 D. DAG
2. **Which of the following hormone acts on cell membrane receptor?**
   A. TSH B. Thyroxine
   C. Androgen D. Cortisol
3. **Regarding nitric oxide, all the following are true, EXCEPT:**
   A. Derived from endothelium B. Acts by increasing cAMP levels
   C. Potent vasodilator D. Derived from arginine
4. **All the following hormones mediate their action through cAMP as second messenger, EXCEPT:**
   A. Corticotropin B. Dopamine
   C. Glucagon D. Vasopressin

Answers : 1. A 2. A 3. B 4. D

MCQs continued to end of Chapter 70, (Page 545)

Chapter 70

Hypothalamus and Hypothalamopituitary Axis

Learning Objectives

On completion of study of this chapter:

The student will be able to (must know):

1. Appreciate the functions of hypothalamus as an endocrine organ.
2. List the hormones secreted from hypothalamus and mention their functions.
3. Draw a schematic diagram of hypothalamo-pituitary axis (HPA).
4. Understand the functional organization of HPA.
5. Learn the role of HPA in the regulation of pituitary functions.

The student may also be able to (desirable to know):

1. Describe the functions of hypothalamic hormones
2. Explain the differences in HPA for anterior and posterior pituitary.

HYPOTHALAMUS

The hypothalamus through its anterior pituitary influence, controls thyroid functions (**hypothalamo-pituitary-thyroid axis**), adrenocortical secretions (**hypothalamo-pituitary-adrenocortical-axis**), and gonadal functions (**hypothalamo-pituitary-gonadal axis**).

1. Via its influence on sympathetic output, hypothalamus controls secretions of adrenal medulla (**hypothalamo-sympatho-adrenal-axis**).
2. Hypothalamus controls the secretions from posterior pituitary.

Thus, hypothalamus regulates functions of major endocrine glands of the body. Therefore, hypothalamus is designated as the "**master of endocrine orchestra**".

Integration with Neural Structures: Hypothalamus collects and integrates information from various parts of the brain and funnels them through the pituitary gland for modification of endocrine functions. Therefore, hypothalamus is the **primary link between nervous and endocrine systems**.

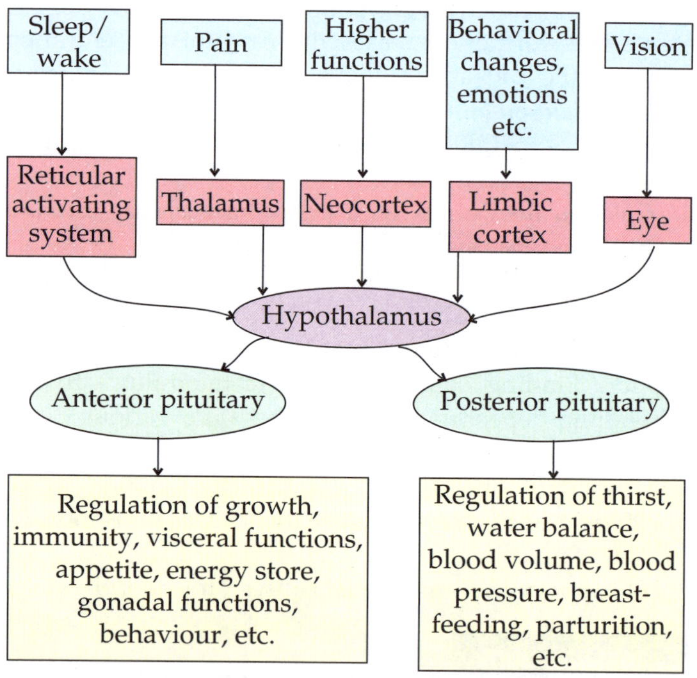

Fig. 70.1: Hypothalamic integration of neural and endocrine functions.

- It receives **afferent signals** from reticular activating system, thalamus, neocortex, eyes and limbic system, especially from amygdala, septum, olfactory bulb, and hippocampus (Fig. 70.1).
- These neural inputs convey the information regarding alertness, application of nociceptive stimuli, sleep-wakefulness, changes in environment, emotion, visual, olfactory and gustatory sensations etc. to hypothalamus, which through its profound influence on endocrine secretions and limbic-autonomic output controls **thirst, appetite, energy store, body fat composition, immunity, behavior and visceral functions**.
- Thus, hypothalamus through its extensive neuroendocrine connections, controls **major body functions**.

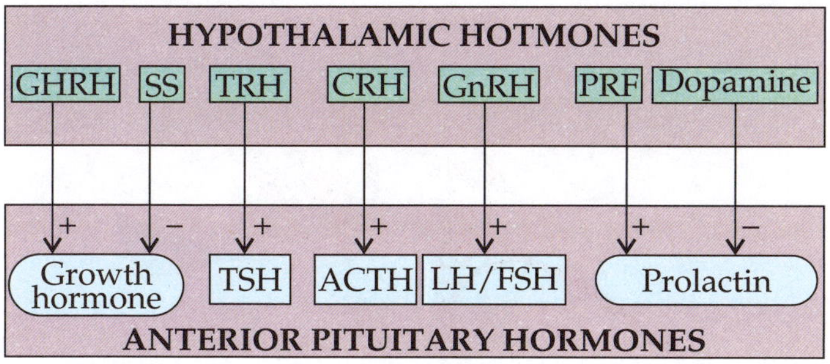

Fig. 70.2: Hypothalamic control of anterior pituitary secretions. PRF: prolactin releasing factor; SS: somatostatin. Plus sign (+) indicates stimulation and minus sign (–) indicates inhibition.

- Hence, diseases affecting hypothalamic nuclei result in **many pathological syndromes.**

Hypothalamic Hormones

PY8.2

Hypothalamic hormones are secreted from various hypothalamic nuclei. They are grouped into **three categories**: anterior pituitary regulating hormones, posterior pituitary hormones and other hormones.

Anterior Pituitary Regulating Hormones

Hypothalamic hormones that regulate anterior pituitary secretions are known as **releasing or release inhibiting hormones** as they stimulate or inhibit the release of various hormones from this part of the pituitary (Fig. 70.2).

- These are **peptide hormones** that act on target cells mostly through **cyclic AMP and IP3 or DAG** as second messengers.

A. Releasing Hormones

Thyrotropin Releasing Hormone (TRH): TRH is an oligopeptide containing 3 amino acids, secreted from paraventricular nucleus of hypothalamus.

Functions:

1. TRH **stimulates secretion of thyroid stimulating hormone** (TSH) or thyrotropin from thyrotrophs of anterior pituitary.
2. It stimulates expression of genes for α and β subunits of TSH in thyrotrophs.
3. It also promotes secretion of prolactin and growth hormone (GH).

Gonadotropin Releasing Hormone (GnRH): GnRH is a peptide containing 10 amino acids, secreted from the arcuate nucleus of hypothalamus.

Functions:

1. GnRH **stimulates secretion of luteinizing hormone** (LH); therefore, GnRH is known as luteinizing hormone releasing hormone (LHRH).
2. It also **stimulates secretion of follicular stimulating hormone** (FSH).
   - Together, it is known as gonadotropins releasing hormone as it stimulates secretion of both LH and FSH.
3. GnRH also stimulates secretion of GH.

Corticotropin Releasing Hormone (CRH): CRH is a polypeptide having 41 amino acids, secreted from paraventricular nucleus of hypothalamus.

Functions:

1. CRH **stimulates the secretion of adrenocorticotropic hormone** (ACTH) or corticotropin from corticotrophs of anterior pituitary.
2. It also stimulates the expression of pro-opiomelanocortin (POMC) gene in corticotrophs.
3. CRH promotes secretion of β- and γ-lipotropin and β-endorphins.

Growth Hormone Releasing Hormone (GHRH): GHRH appears in two forms in humans, one having 40 and the other 44 amino acids. It is secreted from the arcuate nucleus of hypothalamus.

Functions:

1. GHRH stimulates **secretion of growth hormone** from somatotrophs of anterior pituitary.
2. It also stimulates the expression of GH gene in corticotrophs.

Prolactin Releasing Factor (PRF): The source of PRF in hypothalamus is not exactly known.

- It **stimulates prolactin synthesis** and secretion from lactotrophs of anterior pituitary.

B. Release Inhibiting Hormones

Growth Hormone Inhibiting Hormone (Somatostatin): Somatostatin is a peptide having 14 amino acids, secreted from anterior periventricular nucleus of hypothalamus.

- It **inhibits secretion of growth hormone, prolactin and TSH**.

Prolactin Inhibiting Hormone (PIH): PIH is dopamine, which is secreted from arcuate nucleus of hypothalamus.

- It **inhibits secretion of prolactin, TSH, and growth hormone** from anterior pituitary.

Posterior Pituitary Hormones

ADH and oxytocin are synthesized in supraoptic and paraventricular nuclei of hypothalamus and stored in posterior pituitary (for details, refer 'Posterior Pituitary').

Other Hypothalamic Hormones

Other hormones of hypothalamus are **neuropeptide Y, orexins, MCH, ghrelin, MSH and CART**.

Neuropeptide Y (NPY): Cell bodies of neurons that synthesize NPY are present in the arcuate nucleus, and the axons *project to the paraventricular nucleus*. It is the principal neurohormone that stimulates food intake.

Orexins: There are two types of orexins: orexin-A and orexin-B. Orexins are synthesized in the lateral hypothalamus. They stimulate food intake.

Melanin-Concentrating Hormones (MCH): MCH is secreted by pituitary, lateral hypothalamus, and zona incerpta. It increases food intake.

Cocaine and Amphetamine-Regulated Transcript: The hypothalamic hormone CART (cocaine and amphetamine-regulated transcript) inhibits food intake.

Applied Physiology

Endocrine hypothalamic dysfunctions lead to irregularities in anterior and pituitary secretions and many target organ dysfunctions. These are grouped as **hypothalamic syndromes** (for details, refer 'Functions of Hypothalamus' in Section 11).

HYPOTHALAMO-PITUITARY AXIS

The connection between hypothalamus and pituitary is called hypothalamo-pituitary axis. The connection of hypothalamus with anterior pituitary is by means of blood vessels (**portal-hypophyseal vessels**) and with posterior pituitary is through the neurons (**hypothalamo-hypophyseal tract**).

Portal Hypophyseal Vessels

The connection between the anterior pituitary and hypothalamus is vascular. The portal hypophyseal vessels directly connect between hypothalamus and anterior pituitary.

1. The blood vessels **arise from capillaries** on the ventral surface of hypothalamus (***primary capillary plexus***) that derive blood from **superior hypophyseal artery** (Fig. 70.3).
2. The capillaries drain into the sinusoidal **portal hypophyseal vessels**.
   - These **long portal hypophyseal vessels** carry blood down the pituitary stalk to the anterior lobe of the pituitary where they **end in another set of capillaries.**
   - Thus, the system of blood vessels **begins with capillaries and ends with capillaries** without passing through the heart.
   - Therefore, they are examples of **true portal system of blood vessels** (a portal vessel starts and ends with capillaries without traversing through the heart).
3. The releasing hormones secreted from hypothalamus reach anterior pituitary via hypophyseal portal circulation.
   - Therefore, these hormones are also called **hypophysiotropic hormones**.

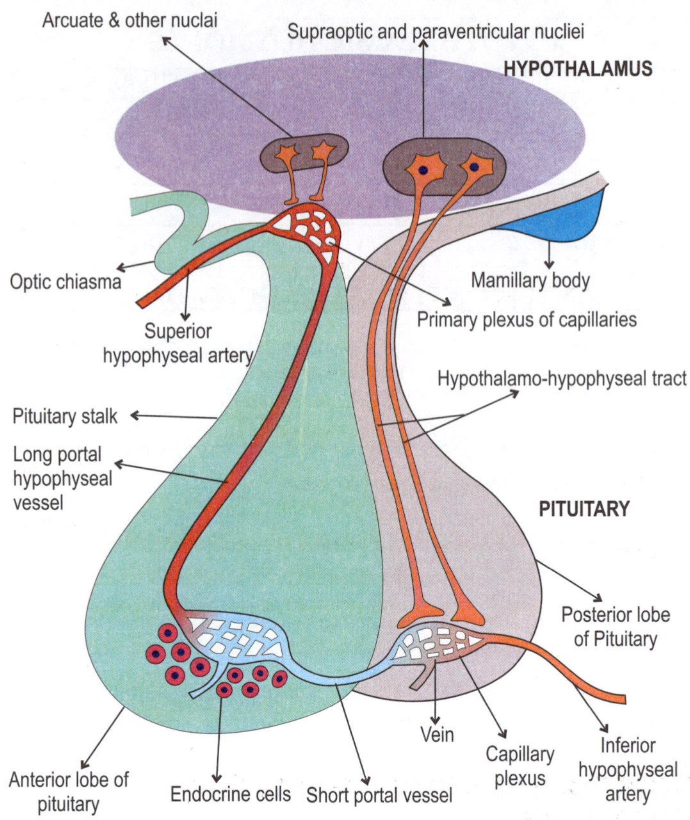

Fig. 70.3: Hypothalamo-pituitary axis. Note, hypothalamus is connected to anterior pituitary via blood vessels (long hypophyseal portal vessel) and to posterior pituitary via neurons (hypothalamo-hypophyseal tract).

4. Hypophysiotropic hormones are synthesized in small hypothalamic neurons (**parvocellular neurons**), the axon terminals of which contact the capillary network in the median eminence and infundibulum in hypothalamus that give rise to long portal vessels in the pituitary stalk.
   - Thus, hypophysiotropic hormones are transported to anterior pituitary via hypophyseal portal blood.
5. **Short portal hypophyseal vessels** communicate the capillaries of anterior pituitary with capillaries of posterior pituitary, which derives blood from **inferior hypophyseal artery**.

Hypothalamo Hypophyseal Tract

The connection between hypothalamus and posterior pituitary is neural. The cell bodies of neurons are present in the **supraoptic and paraventricular nuclei** of hypothalamus.

- The cell bodies of these neurons are larger than the cell bodies of other hypothalamic neurons. Therefore, they are called **magnocellular neurons**.
- The axons arise from these cell bodies and descend down to terminate on the capillary bed in the posterior pituitary.
  - They form the **hypothalamo-hypophyseal tract** (Fig. 70.3).

- Because of its neural origin and connections, posterior pituitary is known as **neurohypophysis**.

- Most of the fibers **originating from supraoptic nucleus** *terminate in the posterior pituitary* whereas some of the fibers **originating from the paraventricular nucleus** in addition to their termination on posterior pituitary *also terminate in the median eminence*.

Exam Questions

1. List hypothalamic hormones. Describe the vascular connection between hypothalamus and anterior pituitary.
2. With the help of a schematic diagram hypothalamo-pituitary axis, describe the connections and functions of hypothalamo-hypophyseal tract.

Multiple Choice Questions of Chapter 69 (Cont...)

5. Cholera toxin acts by which mechanism?
A. Increases the levels of intracellular cyclic GMP
B. Acts through the receptor for opiates
C. Causes continued activation of adenylate cyclase
D. Inhibits the enzyme phosphodiesterase

6. cAMP acts through:
A. Activation of protein kinase
B. Activation of adenylate cyclase
C. Increased Ca^{2+} release
D. PIP-3 pathway

7. Which one of the following acts as second messenger?
A. Mg^{++} B. Cl^{-}
C. Ca^{++} D. $PO43^{-}$

8. Which set of hormones have nuclear receptor?
A. Estrogen, thyroxin & Glucagon
B. Estrogen, Thyroxin & TSH
C. Estrogen, TSH & Gonadotropin releasing hormone
D. Retinoic acid, Thyroxin & Luteinizing hormone (LH)
E. Testosterone, Cortisol & Estrogen

9. Receptors on cell membrane that activate ion channel after binding with agonists are:
A. Nicotinic cholinergic B. Muscarinic cholinergic
C. Optoid μ receptos D. $GABA_B$

10. Action of α-subunit of G protein is:
A. Breakdown of GTP to GDP
B. Conversion of GDP to GTP
C. Internalization of receptors
D. Binding of agonist

11. Following are true about G protein except?
A. G channels B. Phosphorylase formation
C. Made up of 4 units D. Related to ras oncogene

12. All are 'True' about G-protein receptor complex, EXCEPT:
A. It interacts transmembrane domain
B. GTP to GDP
C. Adenyl cyclase activation leads to increased cAMP
D. GPCR has no phosphorylation property
E. Helical structure

13. ANP action is mediated by which of the following second messenger?
A. Inositol phosphate B. DAG
C. cAMP D. cGMP

14. Which of the following act through tyrosine kinase receptor?
A. Insulin B. Glucagons
C. GH D. FSH

15. cAMP mediates action of all except:
A. Glucagon B. FSH
C. LH D. Estrogen

16. Which one of the following molecules is used for cell signaling?
A. CO_2 B. O_2
C. NO D. N_2

Answers : 5. C 6. A 7. C 8. E 9. A 10. A 11. C 12. D 13. D 14. A 15. D 16. C

Multiple Choice Questions of Chapter 70

1. All of the following about hypothalamo-hypophyseal tract are correct, EXEPT:
A. Cell bodies of these neurons are larger, hence called parvocellular neurons
B. Theyoriginatefromsupraopticandparaventricularnucleiofhypothalamus
C. The axons of the neurons form the tract
D. Axons terminate on capillaries in the posterior pituitary

2. Which of the following hypothalamic hormone does NOT stimulate pituitary?
A. TRH B. GnRH
C. Somatostatin D. GRH

3. Hypothalamus is not connected directly with which of the following structure in the brain?
A. Thalamus B. Limbic system
C. Neocortex D. Basal ganglia

4. Food intake is inhibited by:
A. MCH B. CART
C. Orexins D. Neuropeptide

Answers : 1. A 2. C 3. D 4. B

Chapter 71

Anterior Pituitary

PY8.2

Learning Objectives

On completion of study of this chapter:

The student will be able to (must know):

1. List the hormones secreted from anterior pituitary and name the cells producing them.
2. Draw a schematic diagram depicting the mechanism of action of GH.
3. Understand the feedback regulation of GH secretion.
4. Describe the functions GH and functions mediated by IGF-1.
5. Illustrate the dysfunctions of GH excess and deficiency.
6. List the functions of prolactin, TSH, ACTH and gonadotropins.

The student may also be able to (desirable to know):

1. Describe the physiological basis of GH disorders.
2. Describe the functions and dysfunctions of prolactin, TSH, ACTH and gonadotropins.

Pituitary gland consists of **two lobes**: ***anterior and posterior lobes*** (Fig. 70.1). Though, ***intermediate lobe*** of pituitary is present in many species, it is rudimentary in human beings. Anterior and posterior lobes of pituitary are two separate and distinct glands.

1. The anterior pituitary is rich in various ***endocrine cells***. Hence, anterior pituitary is called **adenohypophysis**.
2. The posterior pituitary contains ***neurons that secrete hormones***. Hence, posterior pituitary is called **neurohypophysis**.

The details of vascular and neural connections of hypothalamus with anterior and posterior pituitary respectively (hypothalamo-pituitary axis) are described in previous chapter.

Process of Hormone Secretion: The anterior pituitary has extensive network of **sinusoidal capillaries**. The **endothelium of capillaries is fenestrated**.

1. The endocrine cells contain **numerous granules** that store hormones.

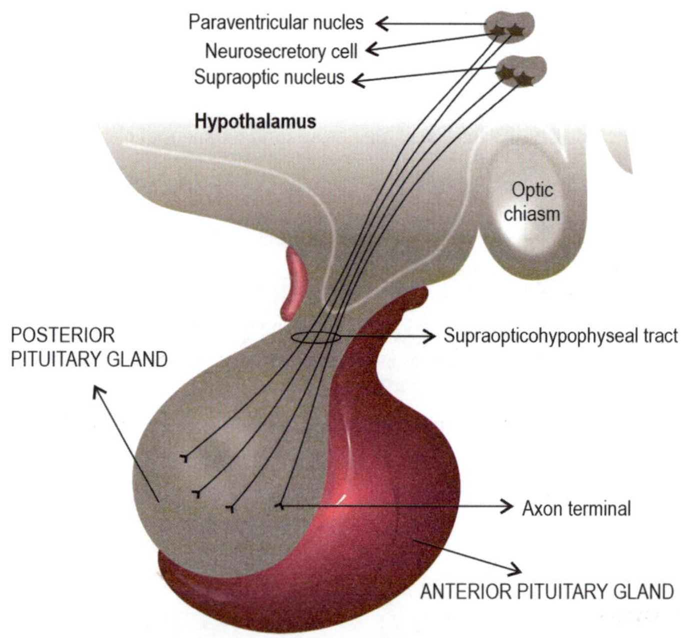

Fig. 71.1: The pituitary gland. The posterior pituitary (pars posterior) is connected to hypothalamus through infundibulum, and anterior pituitary (pars anterior) is connected to hypothalamus through pars tuberalis.

2. Hormones are secreted by **exocytosis of these granules**, following which they immediately enter circulation through the capillaries.

HORMONES OF ANTERIOR PITUITARY

Six important hormones secreted from anterior pituitary are:

1. Growth hormone (GH) or somatotropin
2. Thyroid-stimulating hormone (TSH) or thyrotropin
3. Adrenocorticotropic hormone (ACTH) or corticotropin
4. Follicle-stimulating hormone (FSH) or gonadotropin

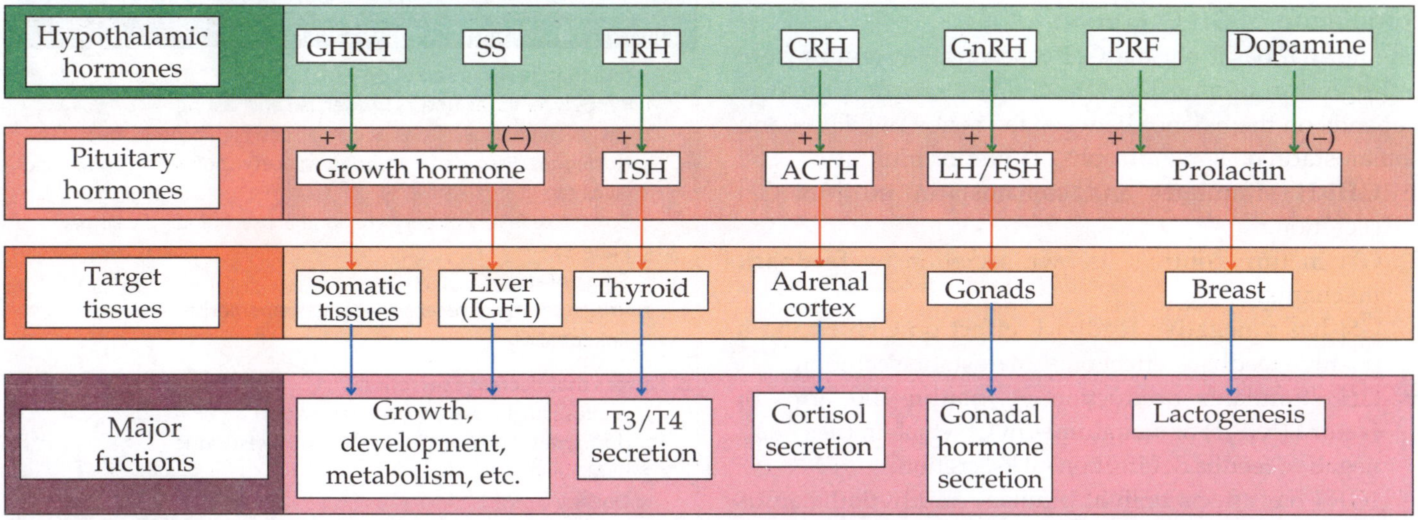

Fig. 71.2: Hypothalamic-pituitary-target organ axis. Plus sign (+) indicates stimulation and minus sign (–) indicates inhibition.

5. Luteinizing hormone (LH) or gonadotropin
6. Prolactin
7. Other hormones are: β–lipotropin (β -LPH), α-melanocyte-stimulating hormone (α-MSH) and interleukins.

Anterior pituitary hormones are **polypeptides**.

- LH, FSH, and TSH are glycoproteins containing two subunits: **the α and β subunits**, similar to that of hCG secreted from placenta.
- The **α subunit** of these hormones have **similar amino acid sequence**.
- Therefore, the β subunit confers specificity to the hormones.

Cell Types of Anterior Pituitary

The cell types of anterior pituitary are divided into two broad categories: **chromophobes and chromophils**.

1. There are **five types of chromophil cells** that secrete hormones (Table 71.1):
2. The **chromophobic cells** are usually *less active* and therefore, have few secretory granules.
3. Recently, **folliculostellate cells** have been identified in the anterior pituitary that secrete cytokines, especially IL-6.

Table 71.1 | Hormone-secreting cells of the human anterior pituitary gland.

Cell type	% of total cells	Staining property	Hormone secreted
Somatotrophs	40–50	Acidophilic	Growth hormone
Lactotrophs	10–25	Acidophilic	Prolactin
Corticotrophs	10–20	Basophilic	ACTH
Thyrotrophs	3–5	Basophilic	TSH
Gonadotrophs	10–15	Basophilic	LH and FSH

The summary of hypothalamic control of pituitary hormones, their target organs and major functions are summarized in Fig. 71.2.

GROWTH HORMONE

Growth hormone (GH) is secreted from **somatotrophs** that constitute about 50% of the total endocrine cells of the anterior pituitary. As GH promotes postnatal somatic growth, it is also known as **somatotropin**. It does not stimulate fetal growth.

Structure

Human GH is a polypeptide containing 191 amino acids. It has structural resemblance with human prolactin and placental lactogen.

Two forms of GH: **22 K GH** (molecular weight of 22000) that constitutes 90%, **20 K GH** (molecular weight of 20000) that constitutes 10% of the total circulating GH.

Synthesis, Secretion & Metabolism

Synthesis of GH

GH is synthesized as a **larger prohormone** in rough endoplasmic reticulum.

- The **prohormone** consists of N-terminal signal peptide and 191 amino acid-peptide hormone.
- Subsequently, the **signal peptide is removed** when the prohormone traverses through the Golgi apparatus.
- Finally, the hormone is packaged and stored in the granules of somatotrophs.

Regulation of GH Synthesis: Two hypothalamic hormones control the synthesis of GH: **GHRH and somatostatin**.

- GHRH stimulates and somatostatin inhibits synthesis of GH.
- GHRH promotes GH synthesis by stimulating expression of *GH gene in the somatotrophs*.

IMPORTANT NOTE

TSH expresses of GH gene: TSH also stimulates expression of GH gene. Therefore, patient with **thyroid hormone gene deficiency also develops GH deficiency**.

Regulation of GH Secretion

The normal basal plasma GH concentration ranges from **0–5 ng/ml** in adults. The rate of GH secretion primarily depends on the balance between the action of GHRH and somatostatin on somatotrophs of anterior pituitary.

1. **GHRH stimulates** and **somatostatin inhibits** GH secretion.
2. GH in turn controls its own secretion by **feedback mechanisms** (Fig. 71.3).

- GH has a **negative feedback effect** on GHRH and a positive feedback effect on somatostatin secretion.
- GH stimulates production of **insulin like growth factor I** (IGF-1) or **somatomedin C**, which in turn has a negative feedback effect on GH secretion.

1. **IGF I** has effects both at pituitary and hypothalamus levels.
2. Various factors regulate GH secretion (Table 71.2) by influencing secretion of GHRH, somatostatin and IGF I.

Recently, a new **growth hormone releasing factor** (GHRF) secreted from hypothalamus has been identified, which profoundly modulates GH secretion. **Ghrelin** is proposed to be the new GHRF.

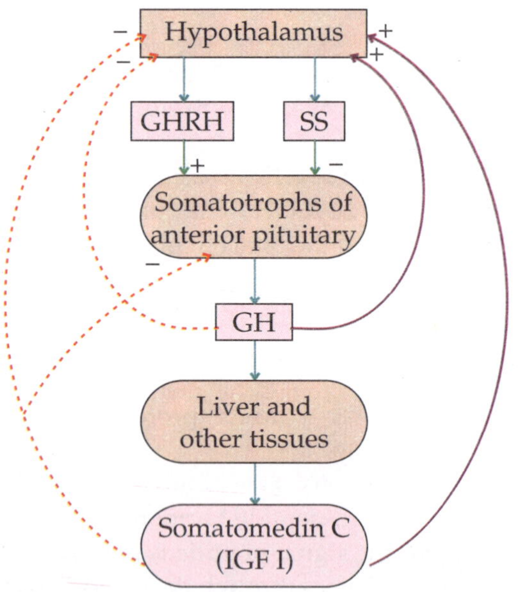

Fig. 71.3: Feedback regulation of GH secretion. Plus sign (+) indicates stimulation and minus sign (–) indicates inhibition. GHRH: Growth hormone releasing hormone; SS: Somatostatin; GH: growth hormone; IGF-I: insulin-like growth factor I.

GH Secretion occurs throughout Life: Exercise, stress, high protein meal and fasting facilitate GH secretion.

1. GH secretion increases during infancy and then the secretion is maintained throughout childhood.
2. GH secretion increases enormously at puberty (Fig. 71.4), which is associated with a sudden increase in height and general growth of the body.
    - The final height of the individual is mainly determined by their ***inherent GH secreting capacity***.

Table 71.2 | Factors affecting GH secretion.

A. Factors that increase secretion
1. Hypoglycemia, as occurs in exercise and fasting
2. Hyperaminoacidemia, as occurs after a high protein meal.
3. Hormones: Estrogens, androgens, acetylcholine, serotonin and glucagon
4. Stress like fever, surgery etc., or any psychological trauma.
5. Puberty
6. Stage IV sleep
7. Drugs: L-dopa, α receptor agonists, apomorphine
8. Enkephalins
B. Factors that decrease secretion
1. Increase in glucose and free fatty acid
2. Hormones: Cortisol, GH, medroxyprogesterone
3. REM sleep
4. Obesity
5. Pregnancy

3. **After puberty**, GH secretion decreases to adult level and maintains till senescence.
4. GH secretion is **less in old age**.

GH Secretion in Sleep: It is not clearly known why GH secretion occurs in episodes or bursts throughout the day when growth occurs slowly over months and years.

- The pulsatile secretion becomes more prominent in the midnight, especially within first few hours of deep sleep (Fig. 71.5).
- Approximately, 70% of total 24 hours GH secretion occurs during slow wave sleep (stages 3 and 4) (Application Box 71.1).

Application Box 71.1

Adequate sleep promotes growth: In a normal sleep, maximum time is spent in slow wave sleep. As GH secretion is maximum in slow wave sleep, individuals who sleep adequate usually remain healthy and those who sleep less do not gain weight. Especially, children (this is the growing phase of life) are advised to sleep more to attain normal growth. Those who have sleeplessness, they do not gain weight.

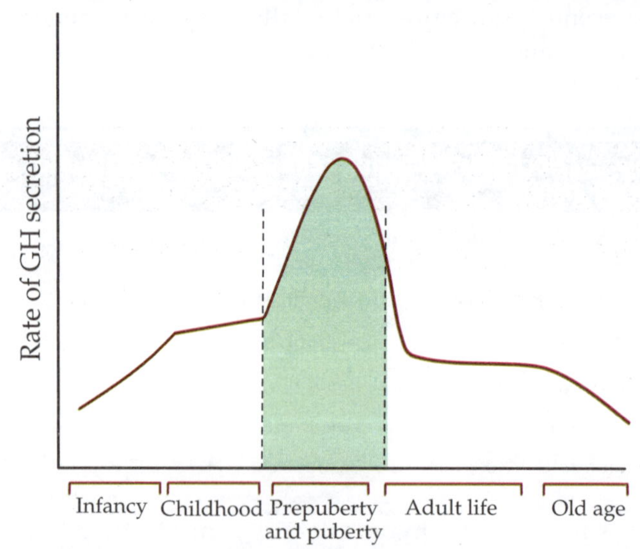

Fig. 71.4: Rate of growth hormone (GH) secretion throughout life. Note that secretion is maximum during pubertal life.

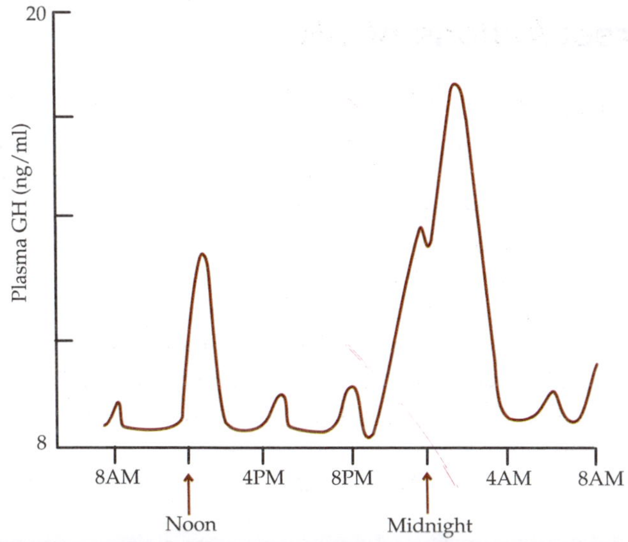

Fig. 71.5: 24-hour fluctuations in plasma growth hormone (GH) level. Note, about two-thirds of secretion occurs in the midnight.

Metabolism

GH binds with a **plasma protein**, which is a **fragment** of the extracellular domain of GH receptor. The concentration of this plasma protein (**GH receptor fragment**) is therefore **an index of the number of GH receptors in the tissue.**

- About **50% of the GH is bound to this protein** that provides a **reservoir of GH** in the plasma.
- GH is metabolized rapidly by the liver.
- The half-life of GH is about **6–20 minutes**.
- Normally, in adult, less than **3 ng/ml** of GH is present in the plasma in basal conditions.
- Though, only a small quantity of GH is excreted unaltered in urine, **daily urinary output of GH reflects its 24 hours profile**.

Mechanisms of Action

GH binds with the receptor called **growth hormone receptor,** which is a membrane polypeptide containing 620 amino acids. This is a **tyrosine kinase associated receptor** that belongs to the member of **cytokine receptor superfamily**.

- It has **three domains**: a large extracellular domain, a transmembrane domain, and a large cytoplasmic domain.
- GH receptor has **two subunits** and there is binding site on each subunit.
- When GH binds to one receptor subunit, the binding site on other subunit is attracted and subunits come close to each other. This produces a **homodimer of GH receptor**.
- This **dimerization is an essential component of receptor activation** as it initiates the activation of a number of enzyme cascades including JAK-STAT pathway of hormone action (Fig. 71.6).

The hormone binding with receptor activates following **four signaling pathways**:

a. **JAK-STAT pathway: JAK-2** is the member of the family of cytoplasmic tyrosine kinases, known as Jannus kinase. It is associated with but not an integral part of GH receptor. **STAT** is the signal transducers and activators of transcription, which belongs to a family of inactive cytoplasmic transcription factor.

- Binding of GH with GH receptor activates cytoplasmic domain of it, which induces JAK kinase.
- STAT on **phosphorylation by JAK kinases** migrate to the nucleus.

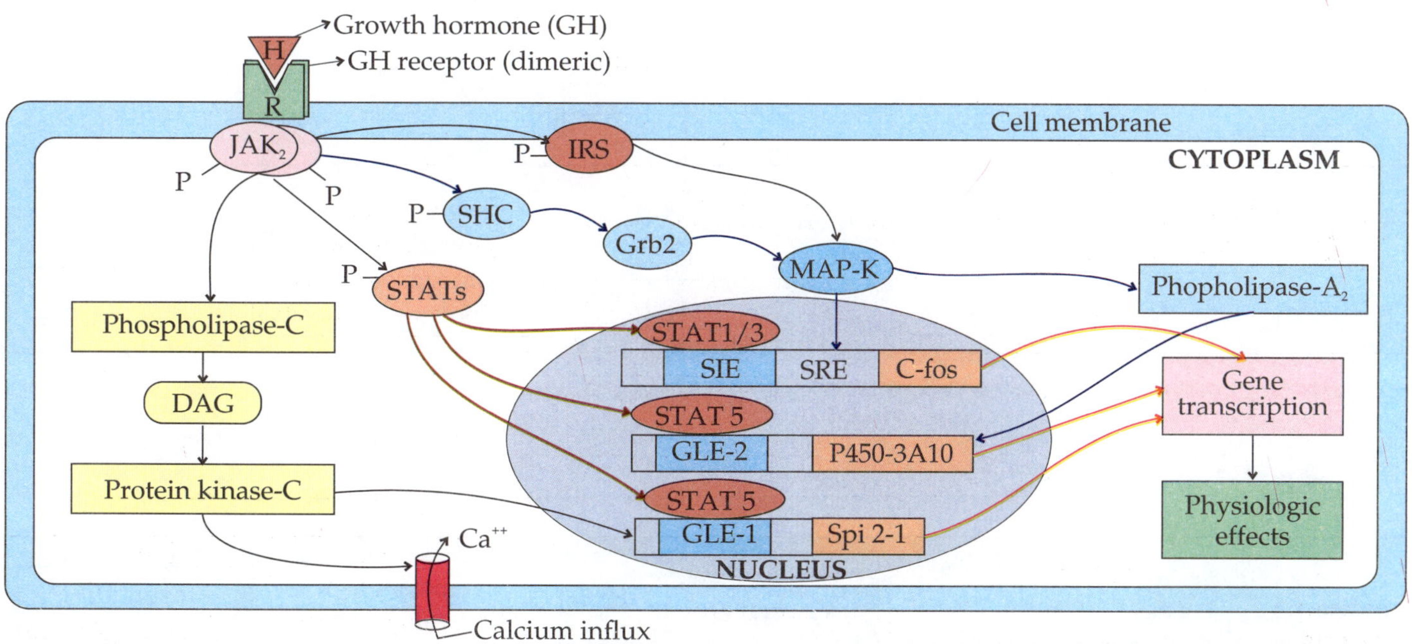

Fig. 71.6: Mechanism of action of GH. Binding of GH with its receptor causes dimerization of the receptor. Dimerization activates JAK 2 (intracellular portion of the receptor), which in turn activates gene transcription via various pathways. JAK: Jannus kinase; STATs: signal transducer and activator of transcription factors; IRS: insulin receptor substrate; SIE: sis-induced element; SRE: serum response element; GLE: interferon -activated response element; SHC and Grb2: intracellular proteins; MAP-K: mitosis activated protein kinase; DAG: diacyl glycerol.

- This results in **induction of various genes** that mediate hormone action.
- Prolactin and other growth factors also act through the JAK-STAT pathway.

b. **SHC-Grb pathway:** JAK 2 phosphorylates intracellular protein SHC which in turn activates Grb2 proteins. **Grb2 proteins** stimulate MAP kinase that induces various gene transcriptions.

c. **TK-IRS pathway:** Activation of JAK-tyrosine kinase causes **phosphorylation of IRS** (insulin receptor substrate) which in turn induces various intracellular enzymes.

d. **Phospholipase-C pathway:** HR complex also stimulates membrane enzyme **phospholipase C**, which results in production of DAG. **DAG initiates calcium influx** into the cell and probably, also initiates gene transcription.

Physiological Actions of GH

Growth hormone is an anabolic hormone with profound **short-term metabolic effects** and **long-term growth promoting effects**.

1. **Acute metabolic effects** of GH like lipolysis in adipose tissue, decreased glucose uptake by muscle and stimulation of gluconeogenesis by hepatocytes are due to its **direct actions** on target tissues.
2. Whereas, many **long-term effects** of GH are mediated by **somatomedins** (IGF-1 and IGF-2) produced by it. Growth promoting effects are also part of the direct effects of GH (Flowchart 71.1).

Direct Actions of GH

Effects on Growth

The most striking and specific effect of GH is the **stimulation of linear growth**, which occurs due to its action **on the epiphyseal cartilage of long bones**. GH stimulates *all aspects of metabolism of chondrocytes* (the cartilage forming cells).

The major actions of GH on chondrocytes include:

1. Incorporation of **proline into collagen** and its conversion into **hydroxyproline** (Application Box 71.2).
2. Incorporation of sulfate into the proteoglycan chondroitin.
   - The hydroxyproline and chondroitin together form the extracellular matrix of cartilage.
   - Thus, GH **promotes cartilage matrix formation**.
3. Increased amino acid uptake and **protein synthesis**, and increased RNA and DNA synthesis in chondrocytes.
4. Increase in **size and number of chondrocytes**.
5. GH also acts directly on progenitor or stem cells such as **prechondrocytes** in growth plates of bone. It facilitates the **differentiation of prechondrocytes to chondrocytes**.

All these actions result in **growth of epiphyseal cartilage** that increases the length of the bone and consequently promotes linear growth of the body. Thus, GH increases the height of the individual before closure of epiphysis.

Other growth promoting effects of GH include:

1. **On bone:** GH stimulates the activity of bone modeling units.
   - It increases activity of both osteoclasts and osteoblasts.

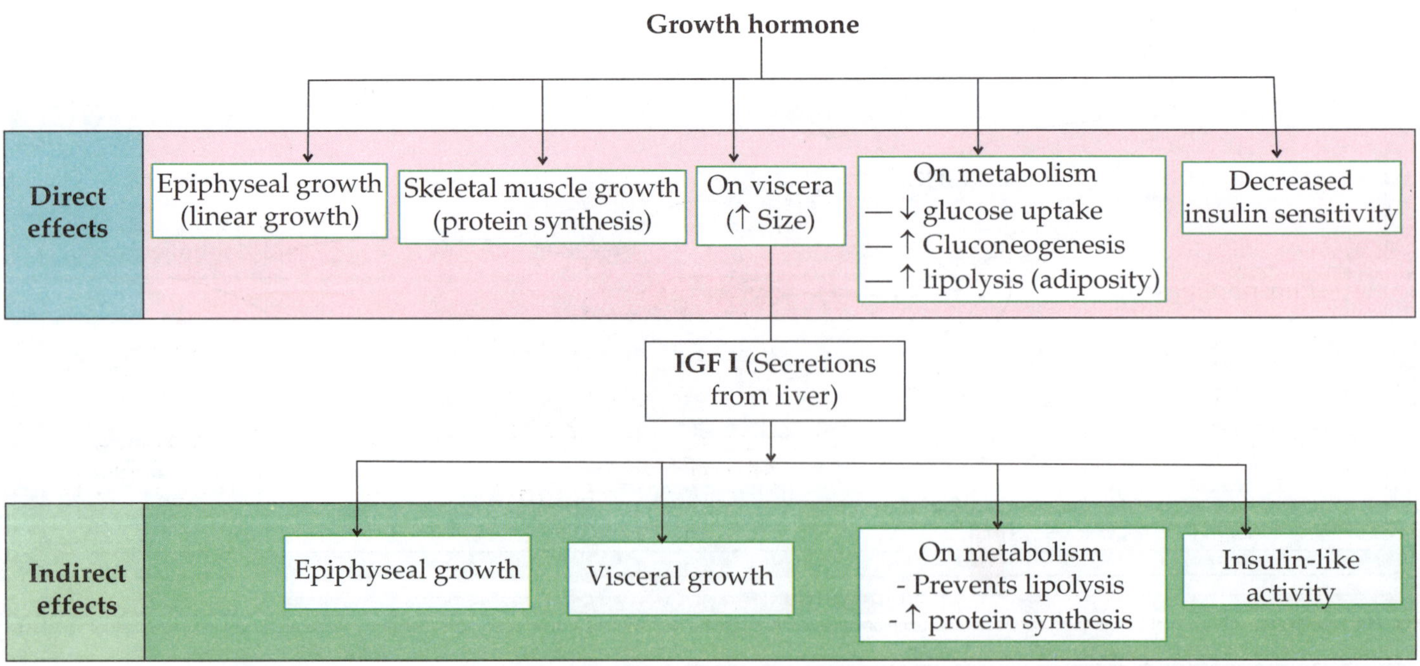

Flowchart 71.1: Direct and indirect (mediated through IGF-I) actions of growth hormone (GH). IGF 1: Insulin-like growth factor 1.

Application Box 71.2

Hydroxyprolinuria reflects GH activity: Increased secretion of GH manifests as hydroxyprolinuria (excretion of hydroxyproline in the urine). Hydroxyproline is derived from collagen. As GH increases the soluble collagen synthesis, hydroxyproline is formed and excreted. Thus, hydroxyprolinuria is an index of GH activity. However, hydroxyprolinuria is also associated with diseases that cause collagen destruction.

- However, **osteoblastic activity predominates**, and therefore bone formation becomes more.
- The total bone mass and mineral content of bone increase.

2. **On skeletal muscle:** GH increases the growth of skeletal muscle by increasing protein synthesis and causing hypertrophy of skeletal muscle cell.
   - It also *promotes activity of satellite cells* of skeletal muscle.
   - **Satellite cells** are progenitor cells in skeletal muscles.
3. **On visceral organs:** GH also **stimulates growth of many visceral organs** like liver, kidney, heart, pancreas, intestine etc., many endocrine organs, skin, and connective tissue. All these organs **increase in size and function** due to *hypertrophy and hyperplasia* in response to GH. Organs grow in size due to:
   - increased protein synthesis,
   - increased RNA and DNA synthesis and
   - increase in cell size and number.
   - The general visceral functions like digestion and specific visceral functions like cardiac output and GFR improve.
4. **Pubertal and gonadal growth:** GH increases height during puberty. It also sensitizes gonads to the actions of LH and FSH. Thus, GH promotes *prepubertal sexual maturation*.

Effects on Protein Metabolism

The effects of GH on general somatic growth are primarily due to the **protein anabolic effects**. These include:

1. Positive nitrogen and phosphorus balance.
2. **Increased amino acid entry** into the cells in many tissues.
3. Increased **RNA and DNA synthesis** in the cell.
4. Increased **protein synthesis**.
5. **Decreased plasma level of amino acid and urea** occur secondary to amino acid entry into the cells and increased protein synthesis.

Effects on Carbohydrate Metabolism

GH is a **prodiabetogenic hormone** as it causes hyperglycemia by following actions.

1. It increases release of glucose from liver by **facilitating hepatic neoglucogenesis**.
2. It **decreases glucose uptake** by skeletal muscle.
3. Decreases insulin sensitivity.

However, GH **stimulates insulin secretion** indirectly by increasing the ability of pancreas to various insulinogenic stimuli. IGF-I, secreted mainly from liver under the influence of GH has insulin like activity.

- Thus, indirectly GH also promotes growth, as insulin is a growth stimulating hormone.

Effects on Fat Metabolism

GH causes **lipolysis and increases plasma level of FFA**.

- By increasing FFA, it **promotes ketogenesis**.
- As it increases FFA and ketoacids in plasma, GH provides energy in various conditions of hypoglycemia and stress.

Effects on Electrolyte and Water Metabolism

GH influences concentration of various electrolytes by following mechanisms.

1. GH **increases plasma Ca^{++}** by increasing its absorption from GI tract. GH also **potentiates the effect of vitamin D** on the intestine.
2. GH causes **Na^+ retention**. It decreases Na^+ and K^+ excretion in urine.
3. It **maintains ECF volume** indirectly by stimulating renin-angiotensin-aldosterone system, and suppressing the action of ANP (atrial natriuretic peptide) on kidney. Thus, GH decreases Na^+ and water excretion.
4. It **increases plasma phosphate level** by increasing its reabsorption from proximal tubules of kidney.

Effects Mediated Through IGFs

The effects of growth hormone on growth, cartilage, and protein metabolism depend partly on the production of **insulin-like growth factors** (IGFs) (Flowchart 71.1). Initially, they were called ***somatomedins***, as they were found to mediate the somatic effects of GH.

- The principal circulating somatomedins are **insulin-like growth factors-I** (IGF-I, which is also called as ***somatomedin C***) and **insulin like growth factors-II** (IGF-II).
- IGF-I and II have similar actions as insulin and therefore, are called insulin like growth factors.
- IGFs are **polypeptide** growth factors synthesized mainly in the liver.
- They are also formed in cartilages and other tissues.

IGF-I

IGF-I is more potent in mediating the effects of GH than IGF-II. It is a **polypeptide** containing 70 amino acids.

- **IGF-I receptor** is very similar to insulin receptor.
- IGF-I is secreted independent of GH before birth. However, after birth, IGF-I secretion and actions are dependent on GH.
  - Its **plasma concentration is 10–700 ng/mL**, which peaks at puberty.

- The concentration of IGF-I rises in childhood, attains peak at puberty and declines in old age.
- It binds with plasma protein called **insulin-growth factor binding proteins** (IGFBP). There are **six IGFBPs.** ***IGFBP-3 is the most prevalent*** IGFBP, which serves as reservoir for IGFs in plasma.
- IGF-I mainly causes **skeletal and cartilage growth.**

IGF-II

IGF-II is independent of GH action and plays an **important role in the fetal growth**. It is a polypeptide containing **67 amino acids.**

- IGF-II receptor is a mannose-6-phosphate receptor.
- In adults, IGF-II genes are expressed only in the choroid plexus and meninges.
- The plasma concentration of IGF II is **300–800 ng/mL.**

Applied Physiology

Hypersecretion of GH

The hypersecretion of GH in adults (after fusion of epiphyses) results in **acromegaly** and in children (before fusion of epiphyses) results in **gigantism.**

Acromegaly

Acromegaly means enlargement of acral (peripheral) parts of the body. 'Acromegaly' is derived from the Greek words, 'akron' means top, and 'megas' means large). Hypersecretion of GH **after the fusion of epiphysis** results in acromegaly.

Etiology: Acromegaly occurs due to tumor of the somatotrophs of anterior pituitary.

1. Usually, tumor of the somatotrophs is associated with ***proliferation of lactotrophs*** also; therefore, prolactin secretion is increased in 20–40% of patients.
2. Acromegaly can also occur due to extra-pituitary causes like increased hypothalamic secretion of GRH (in *hypothalamic tumors*).

Features: Enlargement of acral parts of the body, especially of hands and feet, prognathism (protrusion of lower jaw), acromegalic facies (overgrowth of malar, frontal and facial bones, increased amount body hair, osteoarthritis (due to skeletal changes), glucose intolerance, hirsutism, gynecomastia and lactation, and visual field changes (bitemporal hemianopia) are common features (Fig. 71.7).

1. Visceromegaly increases the size and function of the viscera.
2. Enlargement of acral parts and skeletal deformities occur as ***bones enlarge in width.*** Bones can't grow in length as epiphyses are already closed.
3. The **visual defects** are due to the effect of the pituitary tumor that enlarges the sella turcica and *compresses on optic chiasma*. This also causes **headache.**

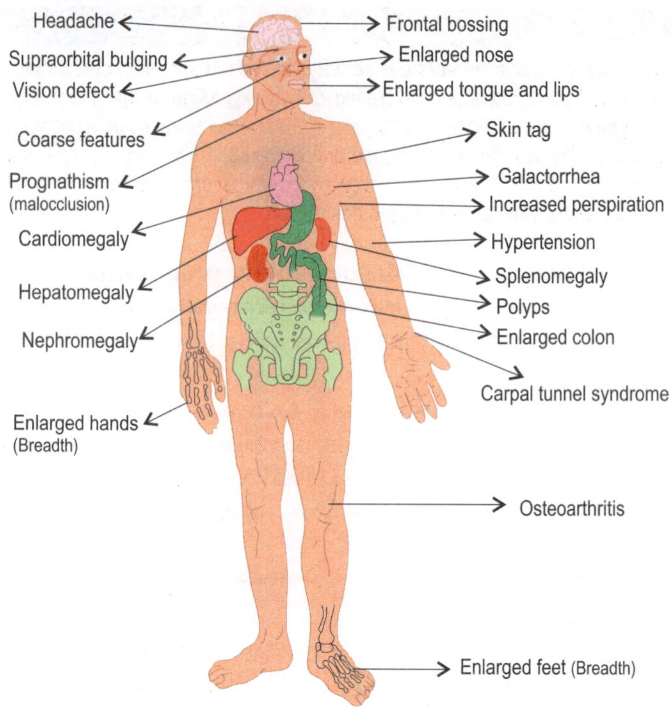

Fig. 71.7: Features of acromegaly. Note the presence of acromegalic facies (malar and frontal prominence) and prognathism (enlarged and protruded mandible), enlarged acral parts of the body (increased hand and finger size), osteoarthritis, macroglossia, increased heel pad thickness and increased size of visceral organs (visceromegaly).

Management: Disease is diagnosed by typical clinical presentation, demonstration of pituitary tumor by CT scan or MRI and demonstration of high GH level in plasma by estimation of the hormone.

- Surgical removal of tumor is the best option to cure the disease.

Gigantism

Hypersecretion of GH before fusion of epiphysis results in gigantism.

Causes: Pituitary tumor (of somatotroph) during childhood resulting in increased GH secretion causes gigantism.

- ***Hypothalamic tumor*** causing excess GHRH secretion can also produce the disease.

Features: Increased GH secretion before closure of epiphysis increases the epiphyseal growth of long bones. Therefore, the patient becomes abnormally tall, with giant stature (Fig. 71.8). Other features are same as acromegaly except the acromegalic facies.

Management: Disease is diagnosed by typical clinical presentation, demonstration of pituitary tumor by CT scan or MRI and demonstration of high GH level in plasma by estimation of the hormone.

- Surgical removal of tumor at the earliest cures the disease.

Hyposecretion of GH

Deficiency of GH results in **dwarfism.**

This may occur due to four causes:

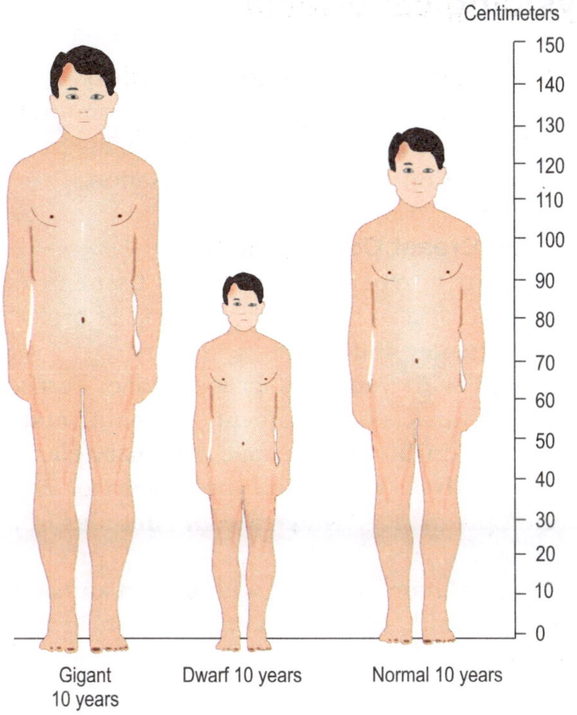

Fig. 71.8: A case of gigantism and pituitary dwarf compared with age and gender-matched normal boy.

1. Decreased GRH deficiency (hypothalamic failure)
2. Decreased GH secretion (pituitary failure)
3. Decreased IGF synthesis by the liver (as seen in African pygmies)
4. Decreased or unresponsive GH receptors (**Laron dwarfism**).

Pituitary Dwarfism

A pituitary dwarf (dwarfism due to **GH deficiency**) is characterized by **short stature** and correspondingly delayed bone and sexual maturation (Fig. 71.8).

1. **Decreased muscle and total body mass**, decreased cardiac function and decreased bone density are common.
2. **Mental power relatively remains normal** in a pituitary dwarf, which helps in differentiating from a **thyroid dwarf** in whom mental retardation is an outstanding feature.
3. It is diagnosed by **low level of GH or IGF-I in plasma**.
4. Pituitary dwarfism is treated by administration of **GH preparations** (Clinical Note 71.1). Details of dwarfisms are discussed in the chapter "Physiology of Growth and Development" in Section XIII.

Clinical Note 71.1

Recombinant human GH: Due to wide species variation in structure, GH extracted from animals does not work in GH deficient patients. Presently, large quantity of human GH is produced by recombinant DNA technology that meets the need of the GH deficient children.

OTHER HORMONES

Prolactin

The term 'prolactin' refers to a hormone that favours lactogenesis ('pro' favouring, and 'lactin' lactogenesis).

Source

Prolactin is secreted from the **lactotrophs of anterior pituitary**, which constitutes 10–25% of the total secreting cells of the gland. The lactotroph population **increases during pregnancy, lactation, and estrogen therapy**.

Structure

This is a polypeptide hormone containing **198 amino acids** with molecular weight of 23,000. It has considerable structural **similarity with human GH**.

Synthesis

Prolactin is synthesized like other peptide hormones, i.e. **preprolactin** that forms **proprolactin**, which finally forms **prolactin**. After synthesis, the hormone is stored in the granules of the lactotrophs and on appropriate stimulation, secreted into circulation.

Regulation of Secretion

Prolactin secretion **increases steadily during later part of pregnancy** and attains peak at term. **Estrogen causes hyperplasia of lactotrophs** and **increases responsiveness of lactotrophs** to other stimuli, though it does not stimulate prolactin synthesis.

Factors that Increase Prolactin Secretion: Prolactin releasing factor, TRH, pregnancy, estrogen therapy, nursing (breast feeding), sleep, stress, angiotensin-II, oxytocin, dopamine antagonists, serotonin, and opioids promote prolactin secretion.

Factors that Decrease Prolactin Secretion: Dopamine and its agonists, somatostatin, prolactin and GABA inhibit prolactin secretion.

Feedback Mechanism: **TRH stimulates prolactin secretion**. Dopamine is **the prolactin inhibiting factor** (PIF) secreted from hypothalamus (Clinical Note 71.2). Somatostatin also inhibits prolactin secretion.

- Prolactin stimulates secretion of dopamine and somatostatin, those in turn inhibit prolactin secretion.
- Thus, prolactin **controls its own secretion** by this **feedback mechanism** (Fig. 71.9)

Clinical Note 71.2

Dopamine is used in Hyperprolactinemia: Dopamine is a potent inhibitor of prolactin secretion. Therefore dopamine is used in the treatment for conditions of hyperprolactinemia and dopamine antagonists are used in conditions of hypoprolactinemia.

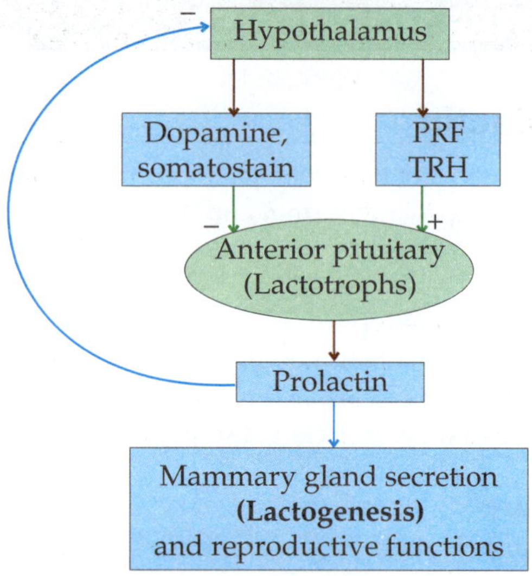

Fig. 71.9: Feedback regulation of prolactin secretion. Plus (+) indicates stimulation and minus (–) indicates inhibition. Note, prolactin stimulates secretion of dopamine and somatostatin from hypothalamus that are known to inhibit prolactin secretion. Thus, prolactin inhibits its own secretion by negative feedback mechanism.

Mechanism of Action

Prolactin binds with the prolactin receptors that are homologous with GH receptors in their extracellular domain. Binding of hormone with the receptor activates the cytoplasmic domain of the receptor, which in turn **activates cytoplasmic tyrosine kinases** (Fig. 71.10).

- Activation of **JAK-STAT signal induction pathway** stimulates formation of transcription factors that induces DNA and mRNA synthesis.
- Increased formation of mRNA promotes **specific protein synthesis** in the ribosomes, which in turn causes formation of casein, lipid and lactose, the ingredient of milk.
- Thus, milk production is stimulated.

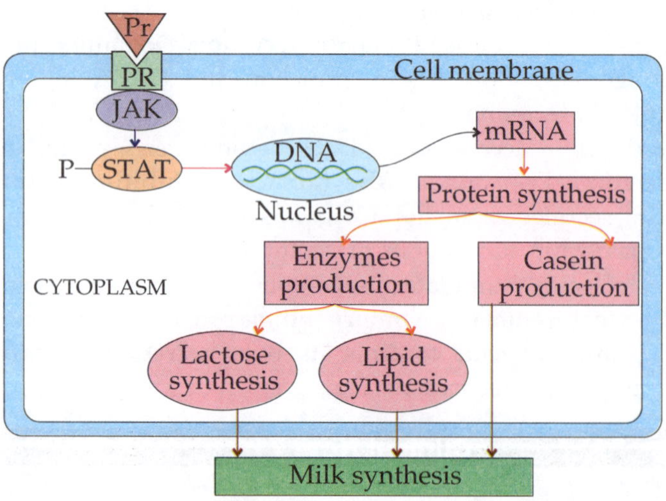

Fig. 71.10: Mechanism of prolactin action. Prolactin (Pr) binds with prolactin receptor (PR) on cell membrane of lobular cells (in which lactogenesis takes place) of alveoli of mammary gland that activates intracellular JAK-STAT pathway for gene transcription. JAK: Jannus kinase; STATs: signal transducer and activator of transcription factors.

Physiological Effects

Effects on Milk Synthesis and Secretion

The primary function of prolactin is to **stimulate milk synthesis and secretion** (therefore, the name pro-lactin). Prolactin secretion increases during lactation.

Effects on Breast Development

Prolactin causes **hyperplasia of breast tissue** before and after puberty. It also causes hyperplasia of breast tissue **during pregnancy and lactation**.

1. Together with estrogen, progesterone, cortisol and GH, it stimulates development (**branching and proliferation of ducts**) of the female mammary gland.
2. Along with estrogen and progesterone, especially during pregnancy, it **increases the lobules of alveoli** of the mammary gland in which milk is produced.
3. During lactation, together with insulin and cortisol, it **increases milk synthesis and secretion** in the mammary gland.

Effects on Reproduction

In Females: Increased prolactin concentration in plasma **inhibits hypothalamic GnRH secretion**. Therefore, the concentration of LH and FSH decreases during lactation.

1. This **prevents ovulation** and causes **amenorrhea in lactating mothers** (Clinical Note 71.3). This is called **lactational amenorrhea**.
2. Prolactin **inhibits libido** and stimulates **maternal behavior** (love, affection and protective behavior of the mother for the newborns).

In Males: In males, prolactin **decreases spermatogenesis**.

> **Clinical Note 71.3**
>
> **Lactation Prevents Pregnancy:** After delivery, pregnancy does not occur till active breast feeding continues. Lactation prevents pregnancy by maintaining high prolactin concentration that in turn inhibits GnRH secretion. Decreased GnRH **inhibits ovulation**. This is **physiological contraception during lactation**.

Effects on Immunity

Prolactin is also synthesized by immunocytes (macrophages, NK cells, T cells and B cells). The immunocytes number increases during pregnancy.

- **Prolactin promotes immunologic balance** required for acceptance of fetal tissue by the mother.
- Prolactin inhibits the negative selection of autoreactive B lymphocytes.

Effects on Liver

Prolactin increases synthesis of **synlactin**, an intermediary growth factor secreted from the liver. Synlactin is structurally analogous to somatomedin and functionally analogous to prolactin. Therefore, prolactin indirectly stimulates growth.

Clinical Correlation

Amenorrhea-Galactorrhea Syndrome

Excess secretion of prolactin occurs in tumors of lactotrophs. **Hyperprolactinemia** causes amenorrhea and infertility. This also causes increased milk secretion in the absence of pregnancy and postpartum lactational state. Therefore, the condition is called **amenorrhea-galactorrhea syndrome**.

- This is seen in **hypothalamic or pituitary tumors** that increase prolactin secretion.
- The **diagnosis is established by detecting high plasma prolactin level** or by demonstrating tumor of lactotroph by CT scan or MRI.
- The disease is treated by **dopaminergic drugs** that inhibit the secretion of prolactin. This restores fertility and libido.

Thyroid Stimulating Hormone

Structure: Thyroid stimulating hormone (TSH) is a glycoprotein. It has two subunits: α and β.

- **The α subunit** is nonspecific as it is similar in structure with that of the LH and FSH because it is derived from the same gene for these hormones. It contains 96 amino acids.
- **The α subunit** contains 110 amino acids and **provides specificity to TSH**.

Source: TSH is secreted from the thyrotrophs of anterior pituitary.

Synthesis: Like other peptide hormones, TSH is synthesized as preprohormone, which is converted to prohormone. The α and β subunits are synthesized separately from separate mRNA molecule.

1. The peptide chains of α and β subunits **undergo glycosylation** in rough endoplasmic reticulum.
2. During packaging in the Golgi apparatus, the carbohydrate unit undergoes modification by **addition of sialic acid and sulphate** to it, which allows two subunits to combine to form TSH molecule.

Regulation of Secretion: The normal plasma concentration of TSH is 0.3 to 5 μU/ml. The secretion of TSH is mainly controlled by two factors:

1. **TRH**, secreted from hypothalamus is the ***major stimulant*** for TSH secretion.
2. **Somatostatin**, released from hypothalamus ***inhibits TSH secretion***.
3. The secretion of TRH is **inhibited by T_3 and T_4** secreted from thyroid gland, by **negative feedback mechanism** (Fig. 71.11).
4. **Dopamine**, another hypothalamic hormone also inhibits TSH secretion.

Mechanism of Action: TSH exerts its effects on thyroid cells by increasing concentration of intracellular cyclic AMP.

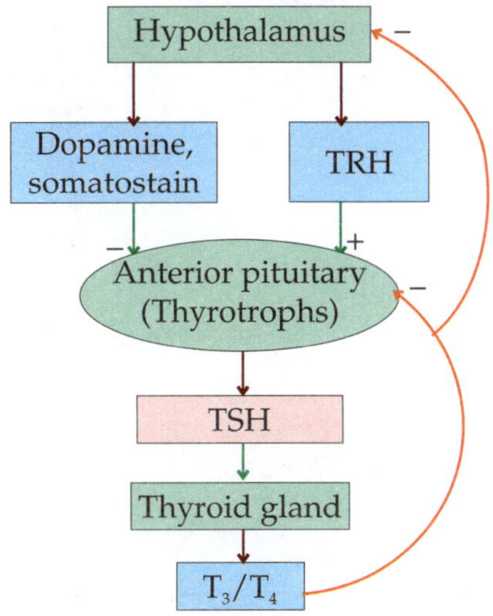

Fig. 71.11: Feedback regulation of TSH secretion. Note, TSH stimulates thyroid gland to secrete T3 and T4 that in turn provide negative feedback to anterior pituitary and hypothalamus to inhibit TSH and TRH secretion respectively. Plus (+) indicates stimulation and minus (–) indicates inhibition.

Functions: TSH promotes growth of the thyroid gland and stimulates thyroid hormone synthesis and secretion.

1. TSH acts almost in all the steps of thyroid hormone synthesis such as iodide uptake and its organification, coupling reaction, thyroglobulin synthesis and secretion into the colloid, and release of thyroid hormones from the gland.
2. TSH **promotes endocytosis** of colloid.
3. It increases blood flow to the thyroid gland.
4. It causes growth and hypertrophy of the thyroid gland.

Applied Physiology: Decreased secretion of TSH due to pituitary diseases results in thyroid atrophy and decreased secretion of thyroid hormones (secondary hypothyroidism *or hypopituitary hypothyroidism*).

- In **primary hypothyroidism**, the blood level of **TSH is high** due to feedback mechanism. Chronic increase in TSH secretion results in hypertrophy of thyroid gland, called goiter.
- In **primary hyperthyroidism**, the blood level of **TSH is low**.
- Estimation of TSH helps in differentiating subclinical hypothyroidism (5 to 10 μU/mL) and clinical hypothyroidism (>10 μU/mL).

Adrenocorticotropic Hormone

Source & Structure: ACTH is secreted from corticotrophs of anterior pituitary. ACTH is the smallest peptide hormone of anterior pituitary containing 39 amino acids.

Synthesis: It is synthesized in the corticotrophs as part of a larger molecule called pro-opiomelanocortin (POMC), which cleaves to form β-lipotropin, and ACTH in human beings.

- ACTH contains **α-MSH sequence** at its N-terminal, and therefore, it possesses **intrinsic α-MSH activity**.

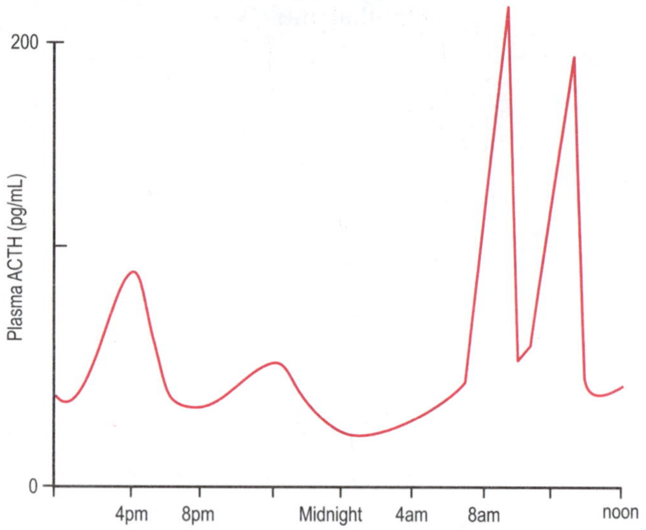

Fig. 71.12: Diurnal variation in secretion of adrenocorticotropic hormone (ACTH). Note, maximum secretion occurs in the early morning between 4 am and 10 am. ACTH secretion is minimum in the midnight when person sleeps.

Circadian Rhythm of ACTH Secretion: There is a prominent diurnal rhythm for ACTH secretion, in which secretion is more in the early morning, which constitutes about 75% of the total 24 hours secretion.

- The secretion **begins to rise at about 4 AM** and reaches a **peak between 7 to 10 AM** and then falls slowly to basal level by noon (Fig. 71.12).
- Another **small peak** occurs in the evening between 4 to 6 PM.

The pattern of secretion is reversed in individuals who sleep in the day and remain awake during night.

Regulation of ACTH Secretion: ACTH secretion from anterior pituitary is controlled by various factors. However, the primary factor controlling the ACTH secretion is CRH (corticotropin releasing hormone) secreted from hypothalamus.

- Many factors influence ACTH secretion by **regulating CRH secretion** from hypothalamus (Fig. 71.13).
- **CRH** in addition to its stimulation of ACTH secretion, also stimulates **sympathetic activity, increases blood pressure** and activates brainstem reticular activating system (**causes arousal**).
- Also, **ADH is an important regulator** of ACTH secretion.

Factors that increase ACTH secretion: CRH, ADH, sleep-wake transition, stress (hypoglycemia, surgery, anesthesia, injury, infection, fever, etc.), anxiety, depression, α receptor agonist, β receptor antagonist, serotonin, acetylcholine, interleukins, and GI hormones.

Factors that inhibit ACTH secretion: Cortisol, ACTH, somatostatin, GABA, brain natriuretic peptide and opioids.

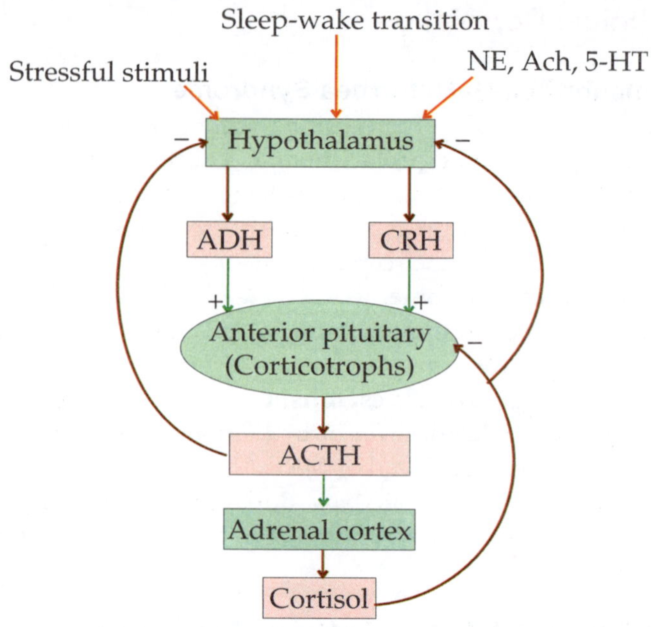

Fig. 71.13: Feedback regulation of adrenocorticotropic hormone (ACTH) secretion. Note, ACTH stimulates adrenal cortex to secrete cortisol that in turn provides negative feedback to anterior pituitary and hypothalamus to inhibit ACTH and CRH secretion respectively. ACTH also inhibits hypothalamic secretion of corticotropin-releasing hormone (CRH). NE: norepinephrine; 5-HT: 5-hydroxytryptamine (serotonin). Plus (+) indicates stimulation and minus (–) indicates inhibition.

ACTH and Stress: Stress profoundly influences hypothalamo-pituitary-adrenocortical axis. Increased ACTH secretion is an immediate response of the body to any form of stress. Therefore, stress is defined as a condition that results in increased ACTH level in plasma.

1. ACTH increases cortisol secretion. In stress, higher brain centers stimulate hypothalamic nucleus to secrete CRH at a higher rate. Thus, **stress induced CRH release overrides the negative feedback control** of cortisol on ACTH secretion.
2. If stress continues, glucocorticoid concentration remains high, and mechanism of negative feedback control operates at a higher set point.

Mechanism of action: ACTH acts primarily by increasing cAMP in the target cells.

Functions: 1. ACTH stimulates synthesis and secretion of cortisol and other steroid hormones from adrenal cortex by stimulating growth of specific zone of the adrenal cortex.

2. ACTH has **intrinsic MSH activity**; therefore, it stimulates growth and activity of melanocytes.
   - This results in **hyperpigmentation of the skin** due to increased synthesis of melanin (Clinical Note 71.4).
3. The receptors for ACTH are also present in the GI tract and brain, where it acts as a **local neurotransmitter**.
4. ACTH influences immunity by controlling **secretion of cytokines from lymphocytes**. Cytokines also stimulate ACTH secretion.

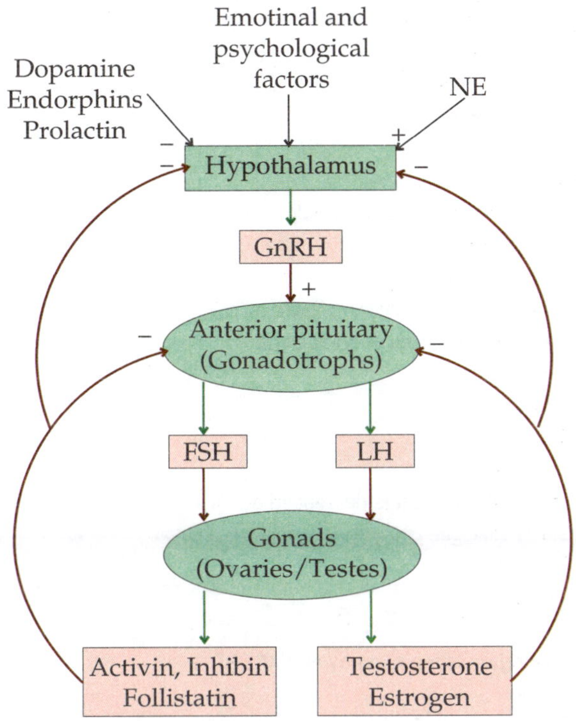

Fig. 71.14: Feedback regulation of luteinizing hormone (LH) and follicle-stimulating hormone (FSH) secretion. Note, LH and FSH stimulate gonads to secrete various gonadal hormones that in turn provide negative feedback to hypothalamus and anterior pituitary to inhibit gonadotropin-releasing hormone (GnRH) and LH/FSH secretions respectively. NE: norepinephrine; Plus (+) indicates stimulation and minus (–) indicates inhibition.

Clinical Note 71.4

High ACTH level causes Hyperpigmentation: Patients with high ACTH level, which may be due to either Addison's disease or ACTH secreting tumor of anterior pituitary, are hyperpigmented (appear black). In Addison's disease, hyposecretion of cortisol increases ACTH production by negative feedback mechanism. ACTH promotes melanocyte activity as it has inherent MSH actions, and therefore causes skin hyperpigmentation.

LH and FSH

Luteinizing hormone (LH) and follicle-stimulating hormone (FSH) are called **gonadotropins** as they regulate growth and development of gonads, pubertal maturation and secretion of sex steroids.

Source & Structure: Gonadotropic hormones are secreted from gonadotrophs of anterior pituitary that constitute 10–15% of cell population of the gland. LH and FSH are glycoproteins. Both of them have α and β subunits.

1. The **α subunit is nonspecific** as it is similar to the α subunit of TSH and hCG.
2. The **β subunit confers specificity** to LH and FSH. The peptide chain of β subunit of FSH contains 111 amino acids and of LH contains 121 amino acids.

Synthesis: There are separate genes that code the synthesis of α and β subunits of gonadotropins. The addition of carbohydrate moiety to the molecules allows variation in biological activity of LH and FSH in different conditions.

Regulation of Secretion: The secretion of gonadotropins is pulsatile, periodic, diurnal, cyclic, and seasonal.

- Secretion of both the hormones is mainly controlled by **gonadotropin releasing hormone** (GnRH) secreted from hypothalamus.
- GnRH secretion is influenced by various **psychological, emotional and chemical factors**.
- Among chemicals, important are **norepinephrine that stimulates**, and **dopamine and endorphins that inhibit** GnRH secretion.

Feedback Control: LH and FSH secretion is regulated by **feedback inhibition through gonadal hormones** such as estrogen, testosterone, activin, inhibin, and follistatin (Clinical Note 71.5).

1. **Testosterone** in males and **estrogen** in females provide ***negative feedback signal*** to inhibit gonadotropin secretion from anterior pituitary (Fig. 71.14).
2. **Inhibin,** a hormone secreted by gonads inhibits GnRH and gonadotropin secretion.
3. **Activin** which is structurally similar to inhibin stimulates FSH synthesis and secretion.
4. **Follistatin** inhibits FSH secretion.
5. **Prolactin** inhibits LH and FSH secretion by inhibiting GnRH secretion from hypothalamus.

Clinical Note 71.5

Oral Contraceptives: Oral contraceptives (estrogen and progesterone preparations) use negative feedback influence of gonadal hormones to interfere with LH and FSH secretion in both timing and concentrations. This prevents ovulation by interfering in balanced action of LH and FSH on ovary.

Functions:

Functions of FSH:

1. FSH stimulates granulosa cells of ovary and Sertoli cells of testis to **synthesize and secrete inhibin-B**.
2. FSH controls **oogenesis and spermatogenesis**.

Functions of LH:

1. LH stimulates theca cells of ovary and Leydig cells of testis to **secrete estrogen and testosterone** respectively.
2. Sudden increase in LH concentration (**LH surge**) in the middle of menstrual cycle is **essential for ovulation**. (For details, refer 'Menstrual cycle').

Exam Questions

1. Describe the mechanism of action and functions growth hormone (GH). Give a note on feedback regulation of GH.
2. Describe the functions of GH. Add a note on hypersecretion of GH.
3. Describe the mechanisms of action, Functions and dysfunctions of prolactin.
4. Describe the regulation of secretion, functions and applied aspects of TSH.
5. Describe the regulation of secretion, functions and applied aspects of TSH.

Multiple Choice Questions

1. **The minimum number of cells in anterior pituitary are:**
   A. Gonadotrophs
   B. Somatotrophs
   C. Corticotrophs
   D. Thyrotrophs
2. **The maximum number of cells in anterior pituitary are:**
   A. Lactotrophs
   B. Corticotrophs
   C. Somatotrophs
   D. Thyrotrophs
3. **Acidophil cells of anterior pituitary secrete:**
   A. GH
   B. TSH
   C. ACTH
   D. FSH
4. **Hypothalamus controls the hormone secretion of**
   A. Anterior hypophysis
   B. Posterior hypophysis
   C. Kidney
   D. Pineal gland
5. **Hypothalamus increases release of all hormones from the pituitary,-EXCEPT the which it can also decrease:**
   A. TSH
   B. FSH
   C. CRH
   D. Prolactin
6. **Basophilic cells of pituitary secretesall, EXEPT:**
   A. Prolactin & GH
   B. TSH
   C. ACTH
   D. LH
7. **Which of the following is NOT a hormone secreted by anterior pituitary?**
   A. Vasopressin
   B. TSH, GH
   C. Gonadotropins
   D. ACTH
8. **ACTH level is highest during:**
   A. Early morning
   B. Evening
   C. Afternoon
   D. Night
9. **Acromegaly is due to excess of:**
   A. Somatomedin
   B. Growth hormone
   C. Somatostatin
   D. Insulin
10. **Somatomedin mediates**
    A. Deposition of chondroitin sulfate in bone for epiphyseal growth
    B. Increased lipolysis
    C. Gluconeogenesis
    D. Decreased rate of glucose uptake by cells
11. **Growth hormone level decreased in:**
    A. Hypoglycemia
    B. Fasting
    C. REM Sleep
    D. Exercise
12. **Secretion of prolactin is decreased by:**
    A. GnRH analogue
    B. Dopamine
    C. Serotonin
    D. FSH
13. **TSH secretion is inhibited by all EXCEPT:**
    A. Cortisol
    B. GH
    C. Dopamine
    D. Thyroxine
14. **Secretion of ACTH is increased by all, EXCEPT:**
    A. Anesthesia
    B. Surgery
    C. GABA
    D. Stress
15. **Secretion of FSH is inhibited by all, EXCEPT:**
    A. Prolactin
    B. Follistatin
    C. Activin
    D. Inhibin
16. **All of the following are functions of prolactin, EXCEPT:**
    A. Inhibits spermatogenesis
    B. Inhibits synlactin synthesis in liver
    C. Inhibits GnRH secretion
    D. Inhibits libido in humans

Answers :

1. D	2. C	3. A	4. A	5. D
6. A	7. A	8. A	9. B	10. A
11. C	12. B	13. D	14. C	15. C
16. B				

Chapter 72

PY8.2

Posterior Pituitary

Learning Objectives

On completion of study of this chapter:

The student will be able to (must know):

1. List the stimuli that increase and decrease ADH secretion.
2. Describe the mechanism of action and physiological effects of ADH.
3. Understand the difference between diabetes insipidus and mellitus.
4. Say what is SIADH and its causes.
5. Describe the physiological effects of oxytocin.
6. Draw a schematic diagram of milk ejection reflex and illustrate the neuro-humoral reflex.
7. Define the role of oxytocin in parturition.

The student may also be able to (desirable to know):

1. Explain the pathophysiology of diabetes insipidus.
2. Describe the synthesis, metabolism and regulation of posterior pituitary hormones.

Posterior pituitary secretes **ADH and oxytocin**. They are called **neurohormones** as they are synthesized and secreted by neurons into the circulation.

ANTI-DIURETIC HORMONE

Structure, Source & Synthesis

ADH, also known as arginine-vasopressin (AVP) or **vasopressin**, is an oligopeptide containing **nine amino acids** (Fig. 72.1).

- It is synthesized in the **magnocellular cells of supraoptic and paraventricular nuclei of hypothalamus.** The synthesis of ADH largely occurs in the supraoptic nucleus.
- It is synthesized as preprohormone which becomes prohormone and then forms the hormone.
  - The genes that cause ADH synthesis are located on **chromosome 20.**

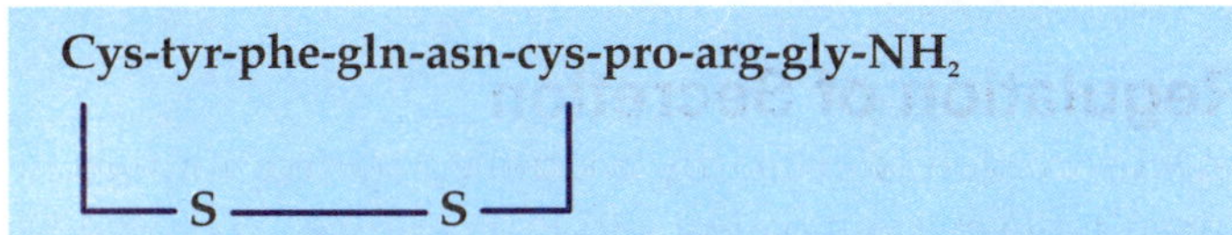

Fig. 72.1: Structure of ADH. Note, it is an oligopeptide containing nine amino acids.

  - They code for synthesis of a larger molecule that includes a distinct larger protein called as **neurophysin.**
- There are two neurophysins: **neurophysin I**, meant for oxytocin, and **neurophysin II**, meant for ADH.
  - The precursor molecule for ADH is **prepropressophysin** having 19 amino acids that contains ADH, neurophysin II and a glycoprotein (Fig. 72.2).
- Prepropressophysin is cleaved enzymatically to **release ADH, neurophysin II and glycoprotein** molecules.
- **Neurophysin serves as carrier protein** to transport the hormone from the cell body to the axon terminals.
  - The secretory granules are called as **Herring bodies** that are transported to axon terminal by slow axoplasmic flow.
  - The axon terminals of the neurons are located in the posterior pituitary.

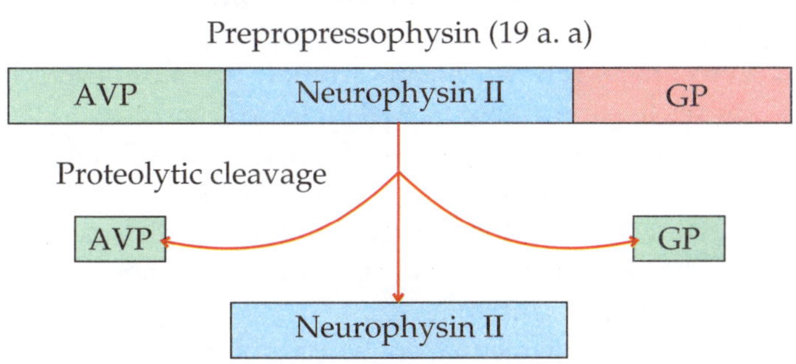

Fig. 72.2: Synthesis of ADH. The other name of ADH is AVP (arginine vasopressin). GP: glycopeptide.

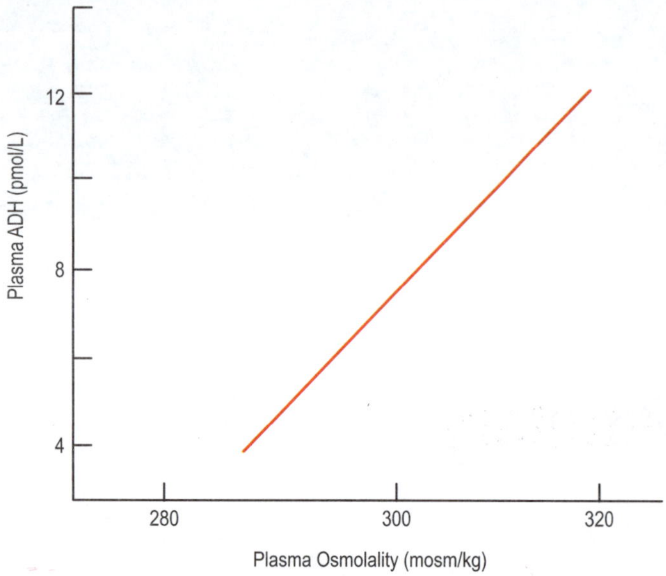

Fig. 72.3: Effect of plasma osmolality on ADH secretion. Note, increase in plasma osmolality above 285 mOsm/kg results in linear increase in plasma ADH concentration. ADH: antidiuretic hormone.

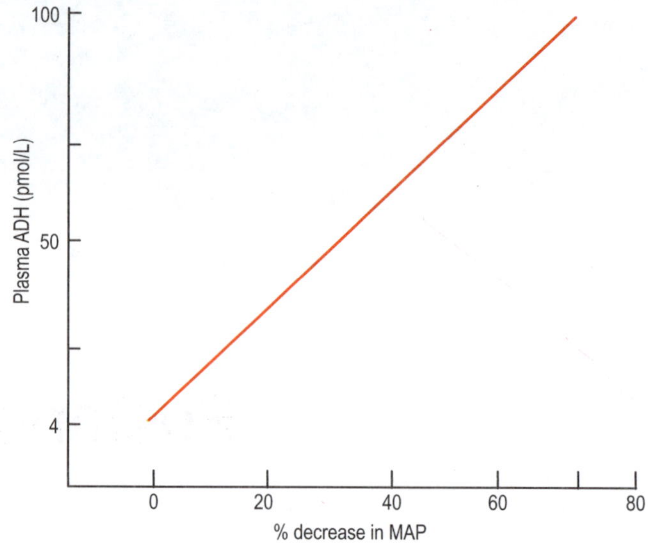

Fig. 72.4: Effect of fall in blood pressure on ADH secretion. Note that % decrease in mean arterial pressure (MAP) results in linear increase in plasma ADH concentration. ADH: antidiuretic hormone.

Regulation of Secretion

ADH secretion is primarily controlled by **two important stimuli**: plasma osmolality and ECF volume.

Plasma Osmolality

Increased plasma **osmolality above 285 mosm/kg** increases ADH secretion proportionate to the osmolality rise (Fig. 72.3).

- The increased osmolality is sensed by **hypothalamic osmoreceptors** that increases the synthesis of ADH in supraoptic and paraventricular nuclei and increase ADH release from posterior pituitary.
  - ADH causes water retention and brings osmolality back to normal.
- Osmolality of plasma is a very **sensitive regulator** of ADH secretion.
  - Even, **change in 1% osmolality** leads to appreciable increase in plasma ADH level.
- The hypothalamic osmoreceptors are **located in the anterior hypothalamus**.

Blood Volume and Pressure

Decrease in blood pressure and blood volume stimulates ADH secretion.

1. Percentage **fall in mean arterial pressure** (MAP) causes linear increase in ADH release (Fig. 72.4).
2. **Decreased ECF volume** also stimulates ADH secretion.
   - However, change in osmolality is a stronger stimulus than the change in volume of plasma.
   - Hypovolemia sensitizes ADH response to hyperosmolality (Fig. 72.5).
3. Effect of hypovolemia on blood volume and blood pressure is partly mediated by activation of ***renin-angiotensin system*** (RAS).

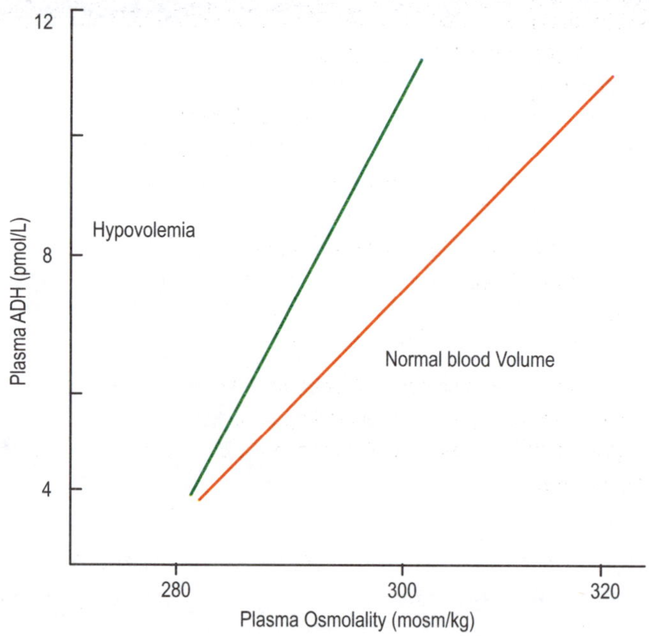

Fig. 72.5: Effect of hypovolemia on osmotically induced change in ADH secretion. Note that hypovolemia potentiates the osmotic effect on plasma ADH level. In hypovolemia, the effect is shifted to left (compared with normal) indicating early and more ADH secretion at the osmolality of plasma. ADH: antidiuretic hormone.

4. Angiotensin II (AII) formed by stimulation of RAS acts on **subfornical organ** (SFO) and **organum vasculosum of lamina terminalis** (OVLT) that are part of thirst center to stimulate thirst and water intake.
   - SFO, OVLT, area postrema and posterior pituitary are called **circum-ventricular organs** (CVO).
   - CVO are located outside blood-brain barrier.

Factors affecting ADH secretion

Factors that increase ADH secretion: Increased plasma osmolality, decreased ECF volume, decreased blood pressure, angiotensin II, pain, nausea and vomiting, emotion, hypoglycemia, standing, increased temperature and stress increase ADH secretion.

Stimuli that inhibit ADH secretion: Decreased plasma osmolality, increased ECF volume, decreased temperature, ethanol, cortisol, ANP, thyroxine and α-adrenergic agonist decrease ADH secretion.

Metabolism

ADH is rapidly inactivated in kidneys and liver. In humans, the biologic half-life of ADH is about 18 min

Mechanism of Action

ADH acts on kidney to conserve water and on blood vessel to regulate blood pressure. There are **receptors for ADH** on these organs.

ADH Receptors

There are **two types of ADH receptors**: V_1 and V_2.

V_2 Receptors

V_2 receptors are located on the **kidney tubules**. ADH increases permeability of the tubular cells by acting on the V_2 receptors.

1. It acts by **increasing the cyclic AMP concentration** on the target cells.
   - Cyclic AMP **activates protein kinase**, which causes **phosphorylation** of different membrane and cellular proteins.
   - This leads to **transport of vesicles or endosomes** by the microfilaments and microtubules from the cytosol to the luminal membrane of the epithelial cells of the tubule.
2. The **endosomes contain water channels** (aquaporins).
   - Thus, *water channels are incorporated into the cell membrane* of epithelial cells on the luminal side of the tubules.
   - This increases the **permeability** of the collecting duct (CD) and distal convoluted tubule (DCT) to water (Flowchart 72.1).
   - The water channels are called **aquaporins**.
3. **Aquaporin 2** is responsible for water reabsorption from DCT by ADH.

Aquaporins: 13 types of aquaporins have been identified till date: AQP0 to AQP12. Aquaporins 1, 2 and 3 are found in kidney, aquaporin 4 is found in brain and aquaporin 5 is present in salivary and lacrimal glands and in respiratory tract.

V_1 Receptors

For its vasoconstriction effect, ADH acts on **V_1 receptors** present in the smooth muscles of blood vessels. There are **two types of V_1 receptors**: V_{1A} and V_{1B}.

- The **V_{1A} receptors** cause *constriction of smooth muscles* of blood vessels. ADH increases calcium concentration in the smooth muscles by activating the membrane enzyme phospholipase C that causes hydrolysis of phosphatidylinositol (increases intracellular Ca^{++} concentration).
- Via its action through **V_{1B} receptors** (that are also called **V_3 receptors**), ADH ***increases CRH and ACTH secretions.***

Release of ADH (from posterior pituitary)
↓
Binding of ADH with receptors on CD and DCT
↓
Activation of adenylyl-cyclase cAMP system
↓
Increased cAMP in cytosol
↓
Activation of protein kinase
↓
Phosphorylation of cytosolic proteins
↓
Transport of endosomes by microfilaments
↓
Incorporation of endosomes (containing water channels of aquaporins) to luminal surface of epithelial cells of DCT and CD
↓
Increased water reabsorption via aquaporins

Flowchart 72.1: Steps of ADH action on kidney tubular cells. ADH: antidiuretic hormone; CD: collecting duct; DCT: distal convoluted tubule.

Functions of ADH

1. **ADH acts mainly on DCT and collecting duct of renal tubule to increase water reabsorption.**
   - It is secreted in conditions of hypovolemia, hypotension and hyperosmolality.
   - It is an important hormone for **restoration of ECF volume** in conditions of depletion like acute diarrhea, vomiting etc. (Flowchart 72.2).
2. Acting on blood vessels, ADH causes **vasoconstriction**.
   - In higher concentration, ADH increases blood pressure.
   - However, water conservation occurs at physiological concentration whereas vasoconstriction occurs at supraphysiological concentration of ADH.
3. ADH **facilitates memory** by acting as a neurotransmitter in memory areas of the brain.

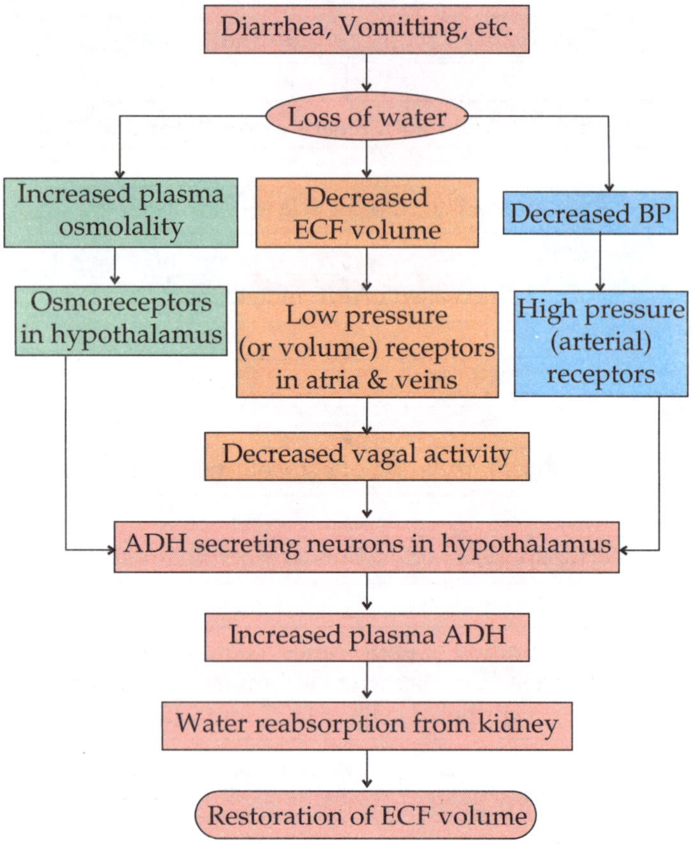

Flowchart 72.2: Restoration of fluid volume of the body by ADH in volume depletion state.

4. It causes **contraction of smooth muscles of spermatic cord**.
   - Therefore, it facilitates ejaculation of sperm.
   - This action is mediated via V_1 receptors.
5. ADH **increases CRH release** and therefore increases **ACTH secretion**.
   - It also directly stimulates corticotrophs to secrete ACTH.
   - This action of ADH is mediated via V_{1B} receptors.
6. ADH acts on area postrema to **decrease cardiac output**.
7. It causes **glycogenolysis in liver**.
8. ADH acts as a **neurotransmitter** in some areas of brain and spinal cord.

Applied Physiology

Diabetes Insipidus

Deficiency of ADH causes diabetes insipidus (DI), a syndrome characterized by production of **abnormally large volume of dilute urine**. Usually, it occurs due to **hypothalamic or posterior pituitary** dysfunctions.

- The main clinical features are **polyuria and polydipsia**.
  - **Polyuria** occurs due to ADH deficiency that promotes water diuresis.
  - **Polydipsia** occurs secondary to dehydration caused by polyuria.
  - Polyuria and polydipsia *are also features of diabetes mellitus*.

IMPORTANT NOTE

Difference in polyuria of DM & DI: The main distinguishing characteristic is the difference in osmolality of the urine; in diabetes insipidus urine is dilute **(pure water loss)** and **urine osmolality is <300 mosm/L, whereas in diabetes mellitus** the urine is hyperosmolal due to loss of glucose in urine (>1200 mosm/L).

- In diabetes insipidus, the urine is tasteless (*insipidus*, means tasteless), whereas in diabetes mellitus urine is tasty due to presence of more glucose in it (*mellitus*, means sweet taste).

Types: There are **two types** of DI: **nephrogenic** (kidneys fail to respond to ADH) and **neurogenic** (deficiency of ADH secretion. Neurogenic DI is also called **central DI**.

Nephrogenic DI

Etiology and Types: In nephrogenic DI, ADH secretion is normal, but **kidney is unresponsive to it** due to receptor deficiency or abnormality. It may be acquired or genetic.

1. **Acquired causes** are **usually due to drugs** such as demeclocycline, rifampicin, aminoglycoside, lithium, cisplantin and amphotericin B.
2. **Genetic disorders** are X-linked recessive defect in which V_2 receptor gene is deficient and autosomal defect in which aquaporin gene is deficient.

Treatment: Chlorpropamide is used for treatment of the disease as it increases the renal response to ADH.

Neurogenic DI

Etiology and Types: This occurs in **diseases of CNS** in which hypothalamus, hypothalamo-hypophyseal tract or posterior pituitary are affected. Accordingly, the disease is referred to as, **central, neurohypophyseal or pituitary DI**.

- It occurs in head injury, tumors such as craniopharyngeoma and suprasellar pituitary tumors, infections such as meningitis and encephalitis, etc.
- ADH secretion is deficient in these conditions.

Treatment: Uncomplicated pituitary DI is cured completely by **treatment with DDAVP**, a synthetic analogue of AVP that acts **selectively on V_2 receptors** to increase water reabsorption from tubular fluid.

- Injection of vasopressin is useful. **Clofibrate therapy** also improves the condition.

Syndrome of Inappropriate ADH Secretion

Excessive secretion of ADH occurs in a clinical syndrome called as SIADH (syndrome of inappropriate ADH secretion). The term SIADH is used as ADH secretion is inappropriately high relative to serum osmolality. **SIADH is seen in:**

1. Head injury
2. **Ectopic production of ADH** by some malignant tumors such as carcinoma of lungs, pancreas, ovary and bladder.

3. **Neurologic diseases** like multiple sclerosis, Guillain-Barré syndrome, brain abscess, meningitis, encephalitis etc.
4. **Drugs** such as desmopressine, chlorpropamide, high dose of oxytocin, vincrisitine, phenothiazine, carbamazepine etc.

In SIADH, not only there is dilutional hyponatremia due to increased absorption of large quantity of water from kidney, but also there is natriuresis (loss of sodium in urine) secondary to decreased aldosterone secretion activated by expansion of ECF (Application Box 72.1).

- If SIADH is due to brain diseases, the condition is called cerebral salt wasting.
- If SIADH is due to lung diseases the condition is called pulmonary salt wasting.

Application Box 72.1

Vasopressin Escape: In lung cancers and other malignant tumors, ADH secretion is very high. In such conditions, the water retaining action of ADH is counteracted by a process called vasopressin escape that limits the degree of hyponatremia. This escape phenomenon occurs due to **down regulation of aquaporins production** in collecting duct. Thus, urine output increases despite high ADH levels in plasma, which indicates that the kidney has escaped from the effects of vasopressin (hence, the term 'vasopressin escape').

OXYTOCIN

Structure, Synthesis & Secretion

Oxytocin is an **oligopeptide** containing **nine amino acids**. The hormone is synthesized in magnocellular neurons of hypothalamus. Oxytocin is mainly synthesized in the **paraventricular cells of hypothalamus** though synthesis also occurs in supraoptic nucleus (refer Fig. 70.3, Chapter 70).

- After synthesis, oxytocin is **secreted into the posterior pituitary** where it is stored.
- The precursor molecule is **prepro-oxyphysin** that contains oxytocin, neurophysin I and a glycoprotein. (Note: Steps of synthesis and secretion of oxytocin are similar to that of ADH, as described above).

Regulation of Secretion

Oxytocin secretion occurs in response to **two important physiological stimuli**:

1. **Suckling** at the time of breast feeding, and
2. **Cervical dilatation** at the time of parturition.

Genital stimulation in females during coitus increases oxytocin release. **Stressful stimuli** facilitate oxytocin release. Oxytocin secretion is inhibited by alcohol.

Functions

Oxytocin mediates two physiological reflexes: 1. Milk ejection reflex and 2. Parturition reflex.

Milk Ejection Reflex

Discharge or **expulsion of milk from the breast** of the mother **into mouth of the baby** when baby suckles during breast feeding, is called milk ejection reflex.

Receptors

Tactile receptors in and around the nipple.

Reflex Arc

Nipple is stimulated by suckling of the baby.

1. The afferent neural impulses are transmitted from the nipple to the spinal cord and from there via **spinothalamic tract to the brainstem** (Fig. 72.6).
2. In the midbrain, the information reaches **paraventricular nucleus** of hypothalamus via collaterals arising **from the ascending sensory pathway**.
   - The neurons terminating on hypothalamus **are cholinergic**.
3. These fibers stimulate oxytocin secreting magnocellular neurons of hypothalamus.
4. Via **hypothalamopituitary axis**, oxytocin is released from posterior pituitary and enters circulation.
5. Oxytocin causes **contraction of myoepithelial cells** of the milk-laden alveoli of the mammary gland.
   - Therefore, **milk is forced** from the alveoli into the ducts and from there to the mouth of the infant.

Effects

Due to initiation of this reflex, milk from the mother's breast *is forcefully discharged* into the mouth of the baby. Therefore, the reflex is called milk ejection reflex.

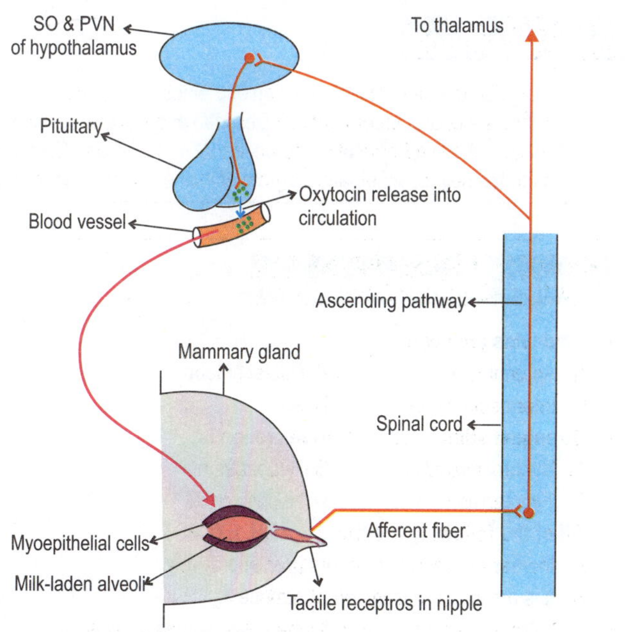

Fig. 72.6: Milk ejection reflex. Note that afferent limb is the ascending spinothalamic tract that gives collateral to supraoptic and paraventricular nuclei (SO and PVN) of hypothalamus. The efferent limb is mainly humoral, in which oxytocin from the posterior pituitary released into circulation causes contraction of myoepithelial cells of alveoli to eject milk into the milk duct.

Physiological Significance

Neurohumoral Reflex: This is an example of ***neurohumoral reflex*** (Application Box 72.2).

- **Ovulation** that occurs ***during mating*** in some animals like rabbit is also an example of neurohumoral reflex.

> **Application Box 72.2**
>
> **A Neurohumoral Reflex:** Normally, a reflex is purely a neural phenomenon, the reflex arc having neurons in both afferent and efferent limbs. When, a hormone forms part of the efferent limb, the reflex becomes a neurohumoral reflex. Thus, the neurohumoral reflex involves both neurons and hormones in the reflex pathway. Therefore, milk ejection by oxytocin is a neurohumoral reflex.

Parturition Reflex

Oxytocin causes **contraction of uterine muscle**.

- Towards term, oxytocin secretion gradually increases and reaches its peak just before parturition. Also, **number of oxytocin receptor** increases in the uterine muscle.
- Due to increased plasma level of oxytocin and **increased sensitivity of uterus to oxytocin**, uterus contracts vigorously leading to expulsion of the fetus.
- Thus, oxytocin **initiates and completes parturition**.
- Parturition reflex is also a **neurohumoral reflex**.

Other Functions of Oxytocin

1. Oxytocin receptors are also present in the ovary. It facilitates **degeneration of corpus luteum** at the end of the menstrual cycle.
2. Oxytocin **secretion increases in males during orgasm**, though the exact physiological significance of it is not known.
   - At the time of ejaculation in male, possibly oxytocin causes **contraction of smooth muscles of vas deferens** that helps in propelling sperms towards the urethra.
3. In females, following ejaculation of sperms into female genital tract, oxytocin **causes contraction of nonpregnant uterus to facilitate sperm transport** into fallopian tubes.
   - Though sperm transport to the fallopian tube for fertilization depends on motility of sperm, ***uterine contraction facilitates*** the process.
4. Oxytocin has recently been reported to contribute to **blood glucose homeostasis** by increasing insulin secretion and sensitivity. Also, oxytocin is reported **to decrease BP** by modulating autonomic regulation.

Applied Physiology

Oxytocics (preparations of oxytocin) are used routinely for:

1. **Induction of labor**, if labor pain does not start effectively at term.
2. Oxytocic infusion is given to **facilitate the progress of labor**.
3. It is routinely injected immediately following delivery of placenta, to **prevent excessive postpartum hemorrhage**, in which uterus contracts severely in response to oxytocic and bleeding vessels are compressed in the contracted uterus that prevents bleeding.

Exam Questions

1. Describe the mechanism of action and function of ADH.
2. What is a neurohumoral reflex? Describe in detail the mechanism of a neurohumoral reflex.
3. What is the syndrome of inappropriate ADH secretion? Give a note on diabetes insipidus.
4. With the help of schematic diagram of milk ejection reflex, describe its mechanism and significance.

Multiple Choice Questions

1. Pituicytes are seen in

A. Anterior lobe B. Posterior lobe
C. Intermediate lobe D. All

2. Strongest stimulator for ADH secretion is:

A. Hyperosmolarity B. Hyponatremia
C. Hypotension D. Hypovolemia

3. All of the following are true for ADH, EXCEPT:

A. Increase in secretion occurs post-operatively
B. It is a neurosecretion/neurohormone
C. Increased secretion occurs when plasma osmolality is low
D. Act on distal tubule and increases permeability

4. All can be caused by accidental transection of pituitary stalk, EXEPT:

A. Diabetes mellitus B. Polyuria
C. Galactorrhea D. Diabetes insipidus

5. Which of the following is not a neurohumoral reflex?

A. Milk ejection
B. Ovulation during mating in rabbit
C. Parturition reflex
D. Deglutition reflex

6. Herring body is seen in

A. Pars intermedia B. Pineal gland
C. Pars nervosa D. Adenohypophysis

Answers :

1. B 2. A 3. C 4. A
5. D 6. C

Chapter 73

Thyroid Gland

Learning Objectives

On completion of study of this chapter:

The student will be able to (must know):

1. Name thyroid hormones and briefly describe the steps of thyroid hormone synthesis.
2. Explain the role of TSH in thyroid hormone synthesis and secretion.
3. Outline the regulation of thyroid hormone secretion.
4. Illustrate the mechanism of action of thyroid hormone.
5. Outline thyroid hormone metabolism, and give the normal serum levels of T3, T4 and TSH.
6. Describe the physiological effects of thyroid hormones.
7. List the features of hyperthyroidism and hypothyroidism and give the physiological basis of thyroid function tests.

The student may also be able to (desirable to know):

1. Describe the synthesis and secretion of thyroid hormones.
2. Describe the regulation of thyroid hormone secretion.
3. Describe the thyroid function tests.

Thyroid hormones primarily govern the rate at which **metabolism occurs in the individual cells**. They profoundly influence **growth and development,** and functions of various body systems of the body They are essential for **mental and psychological development in infancy and early childhood**.

FUNCTIONAL ANATOMY

Thyroid gland is present in the neck **anterior to trachea,** between the cricoid cartilage and the suprasternal notch. It consists of **two lobes** that are connected by a band of thyroid tissue called **isthmus**.

- The weight of thyroid gland in a healthy adult is between **15 to 20 g**.
- Four tiny **parathyroid glands** are located posteriorly at each pole of thyroid gland.
- **Recurrent laryngeal nerves** traverse beneath the lateral borders of the thyroid gland on both sides.

IMPORTANT NOTE

Surgical precautions during thyroid surgery: During thyroidectomy, utmost care is taken not to remove parathyroid glands that are embedded in thyroid tissue posteriorly, to avoid **hypocalcemic tetany**. Also, **recurrent laryngeal nerves** are carefully preserved to prevent **vocal cord paralysis.**

Blood Supply

Thyroid gland has rich blood supply, which is maximal among all endocrine organs. Blood flow per gram is even more than that of kidneys.

- The blood supply to thyroid gland is derived from **superior and inferior thyroid arteries** that originate from ***external carotid and subclavian arteries*** respectively (Fig. 73.1).
- Thyroid veins drain into external jugular and innominate veins.

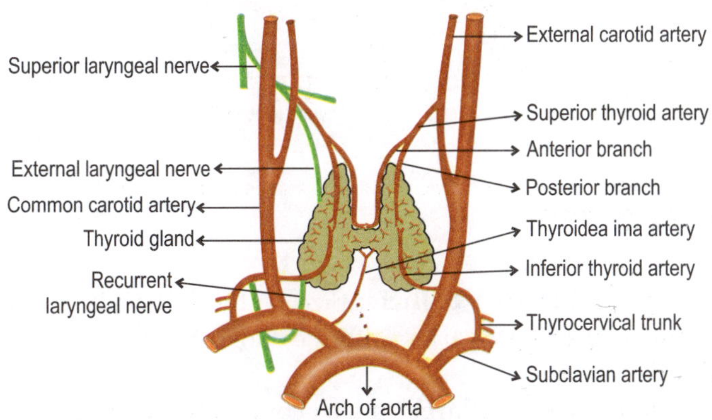

Fig. 73.1: Arterial supply of thyroid gland. Note, anterior and posterior branch of superior thyroid artery (originating from external carotid) and inferior thyroid artery originating from common carotid supply thyroid gland. Also note the recurrent laryngeal nerve embedded posteriorly in the gland.

Innervation

Thyroid gland is innervated by autonomic nerves. The fibers for **sympathetic innervation** originate from cervical ganglia and fibers for **parasympathetic innervation** travel in vagus nerve.

- Autonomic innervation **regulates delivery of TSH and iodide** to the gland by controlling vasomotor tone.
- Sympathetic innervation influences functions of thyroid cells.

Histology

Thyroid gland is formed by aggregates of acini or **follicles**.

- The **thyroid follicles** are spherical in shape and are formed by a single layer of epithelial cells that surround a central thick solution called **colloid**, which is a viscous-gel like substance containing thyroglobulin in it (Fig. 73.2).
- The apical membrane of the follicular cells that face the colloid is covered with **microvilli**. The cells contain numerous granular endoplasmic reticulum, lysosome, Golgi complex.
- The basal membrane of the follicular cells is in close contact with the **numerous capillaries** present in the interfollicular space.
- **Parafollicular cells** or C cells that secrete calcitonin are present close to follicles.

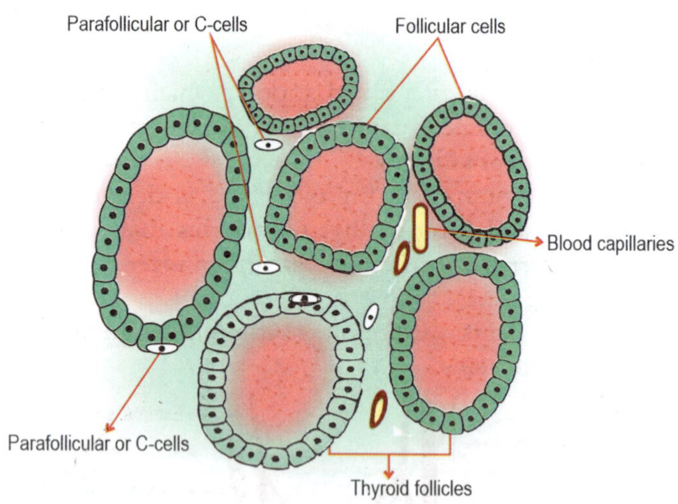

Fig. 73.2: Histology of thyroid gland showing the follicles containing colloid, capillaries and parafollicular cells.

Active vs. Inactive Follicle: Size of the follicle and the quantity of colloid varies with the **state of activity of the gland**.

The follicles are large in size containing more colloid when the **gland is inactive** (resting state).

In the **active gland**, follicles are small, cells are cuboidal, and colloid is present in small quantity (Fig. 73.3).

Resting Follicle

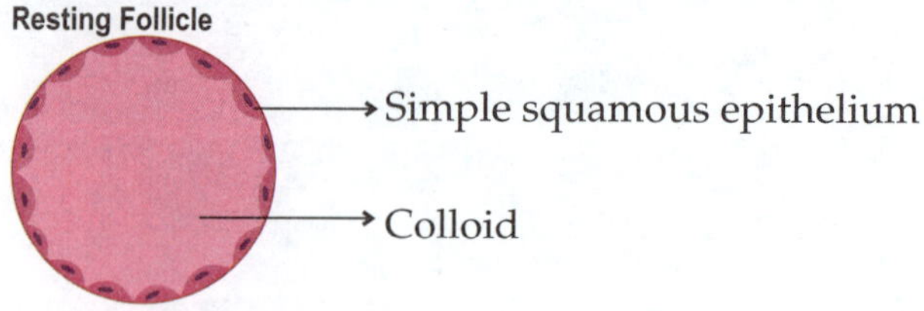

- Follicles are large
- Lined by squamous epithelium with few microville on the luminal surface
- Nucleus of epithelial cell is dark
- Large amount of acidophilic colloid in the lumen

Active Follicle

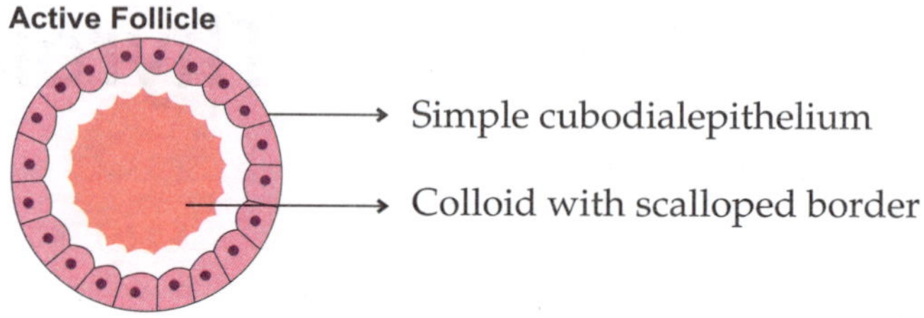

- Follicles are large
- Lined by cuboidal to low columnar epithelium with more microvilli
- Nucleus of epithelial cell is pale
- Little amount of colloid with scalloped border

Fig. 73.3: Differences between inactive (resting) and active follicle.

PY8.2

SYNTHESIS, SECRETION & METABOLISM OF THYROID HORMONES

The **principal hormones** synthesized and secreted by thyroid gland are;

1. T_4 (thyroxine)
2. T_3 (triiodothyronine).
3. RT_3 (reverse-triiodothyronine), secreted in small quantity.
4. Calcitonin

T_4, T_3, and RT_3 are secreted from thyroid follicles and **calcitonin** is secreted from the parafollicular cells (C cells) of thyroid gland.

- Normally, **T_3 is more active** than T_4, though **T_4 is secreted in more quantity** from thyroid gland.
- T_4 is converted to T_3 in the peripheral blood and tissues. Therefore, T_4 is **mainly a prohormone**.
- RT_3 is physiologically inactive.

The raw materials required for thyroid hormone synthesis are the **iodine and tyrosine**. Therefore, iodine deficiency or excess produces thyroid dysfunction.

Iodine Metabolism

Iodide uptake is the first and crucial step in the thyroid hormone synthesis.

- About **500 µg of iodine is ingested daily** in the food, which is converted to iodide and absorbed from GI tract.
- Ingested iodine binds with albumin and unbound iodine is mainly excreted in urine.

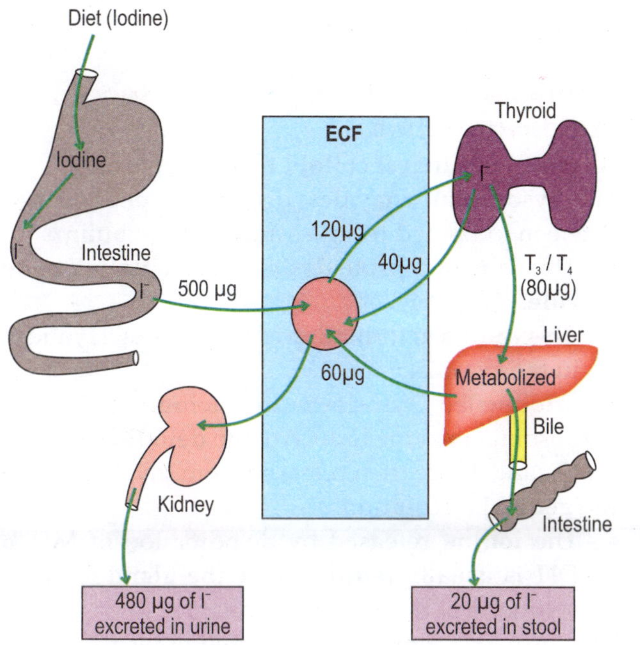

Fig. 73.4: Metabolism of iodine. Note, normally a balance is maintained between the amount of iodide presented to extracellular fluid from intestine and the amount excreted from the body (in urine and stool).

- However, **daily ingestion of 150 µg of iodine** in an adult maintains normal thyroid function.
- The normal plasma concentration of iodide is **0.3µg/dL.**
- Thyroid gland is the principal organ that takes up iodine to form thyroid hormone.
- Normally, about **120 µg of iodide** is taken up by the ***thyroid gland per day*** for thyroid hormone synthesis.
- **Kidney** is the principal organ that *excretes iodide in the urine.*
- The thyroid gland secretes **80 µg of iodine in the form of T_3 and T_4**, and 40µg of iodine directly into ECF per day (Fig. 73.4).
- T_3 and T_4 are primarily **metabolized in liver**. Daily, liver releases about 60µg of iodine into the ECF and 20µg of iodine into bile, which is excreted in stool.
- On average, **480 µg of iodine** is excreted ***in the urine*** and **20 µg** is excreted ***in the stool***.

Iodine deficiency is prevalent in developing countries and ***in mountainous regions*** all over the world. When iodine intake is **less than 50 µg per day**, thyroid hormone synthesis decreases. The consequent increase in TSH results in goiter, hypothyroidism and cretinism.

Thyroid Hormone Synthesis

The thyroid hormone synthesis involves following **five steps**:

1. Iodide trapping
2. Conversion of iodide into iodine
3. Thyroglobulin synthesis
4. Coupling reaction
5. Proteolysis of thyroglobulin and secretion of thyroid hormones

Iodide Trapping

Thyroid gland takes up iodide by **active mechanisms**. The active transport of iodide from circulation into the colloid of the thyroid follicles is known as iodide trapping or **iodide pump**.

1. The transport process is a **secondary active transport**.
   - **Na^+ and I^- are co-transported** into the thyroid cell by means of **Na^+-I^- symporter (NIS)** or cotransporter (Clinical Note 73.2).
   - NIS can cause ***20 to 40 times*** *intracellular iodine accumulation*, compared to the concentration of iodine in plasma.
2. **TSH induces expression and retention of NIS** in the basolateral membrane of thyrocytes where it facilitates sustained iodine uptake.
3. The **Na^+ is pumped back** into the interstitium by Na^+-K^+ pump (Fig. 73.5).
   - The RMP of thyroid cell is –50 mV and iodide is negatively charged.
   - Therefore, iodide is pumped into the cells **against the electrical gradient**.
4. The iodide concentration inside the colloid is usually very high. Therefore, iodide is also pumped **against its own chemical gradient**.
5. **ATP is used** in iodide uptake by thyroid cells.
   - This enables the follicular cells to **accumulate more iodide** than its concentration in blood.
   - The **other tissues that accumulate iodide** are salivary gland, placenta, choroid plexus, mammary gland, gastric mucosa, and ciliary body; however, *they* ***do not form thyroid hormones***.
6. Iodide trapping is **stimulated by TSH**.

Clinical Note 73.1

NIS deficiency: Mutation of NIS (Na^+-iodide symporter) gene, an autosomal recessive condition results in decreased thyroid uptake and causes congenital hypothyroidism.

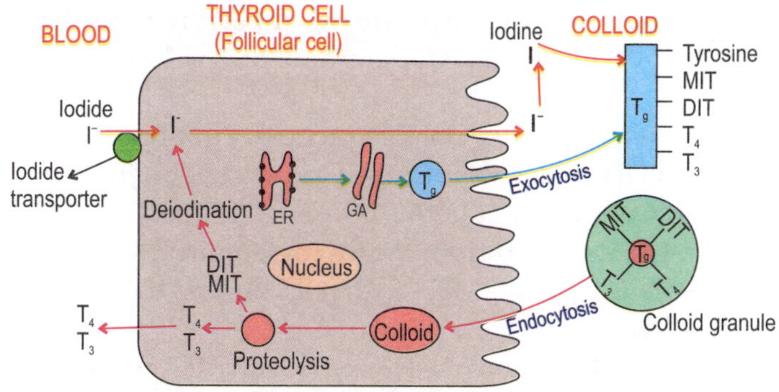

Fig. 73.5: Steps of synthesis of thyroid hormones. Tg: Thyroglobulin; ER: Endoplasmic reticulum; GA: Golgi apparatus; MIT: Monoiodotyrosine; DIT: Diiodotyrosine.

Conversion of Iodide into Iodine

Iodide that is actively transported into the colloids of thyroid follicles is **immediately converted to iodine** by means of oxidation.

- This oxidation of I^- to I, also known as **organification** (Clinical Note 73.2).
- Organification is facilitated by the enzyme **thyroid peroxidase**.

> **Clinical Note 73.2**
>
> **Pendred syndrome:** An iodine transporter called **pendrin** is located on the apical surface of the thyroid cells that transports iodine actively from thyroid cells into the colloid. Pendirn is an **anion exchanger** (Cl^--I^- exchanger). Mutation of pendrin gene leads to **Pendred syndrome**, which is characterized by **defective organification of iodine, goiter and sensorineural deafness.**

Thyroglobulin Synthesis

Thyroglobulin is the glycoprotein with two subunits and the molecular weight of 6,60,000. It contains 123 tyrosine residues.

- It is synthesized in the endoplasmic reticulum of thyroid cells, packaged in Golgi apparatus and then, **secreted into the colloid by exocytosis**.
- This secretion is **facilitated by thyroid peroxidase**.
- The thyroid hormones are synthesized in the thyroglobulin molecule and **remain bound** with the thyroglobulin till they are secreted.

Binding of Iodine to Thyroglobulin: Once reactive iodine is formed (by oxidation of iodide to iodine), it binds immediately with the tyrosine molecule, which is attached to thyroglobulin molecule at 3 position. This binding of iodine to thyroglobulin is facilitated by thyroid peroxidase.

Coupling Reaction

Binding of iodine with tyrosine at 3 positions forms **monoiodotyrosine** (MIT), which is again iodinated in the 5 position to form **diiodotyrosine** (DIT).

- Two DIT molecules undergo oxidative condensation to form **thyroxine** (T_4). This is called ***coupling reaction***.
- The coupling reaction is also **facilitated by thyroid peroxidase**.

Theories of Coupling: There are **two theories of coupling reaction**: intramolecular coupling and intermolecular coupling.

Intramolecular Coupling: In this process, coupling occurs with both DIT molecules attached to thyroglobulin.

Intermolecular Coupling: In this process, DIT that forms the outer ring is detached from the thyroglobulin.

The condensation of MIT with DIT forms **triiodothyronine** (T_3).

- When condensation of DIT occurs with MIT, **reverse-T_3** (RT_3) is formed.
- Normally, distribution of MIT, DIT, T_4, and T_3 in the thyroid cell is 23%, 33%, 35%, and 7% respectively.
- RT_3 is present in very minor quantity.

Proteolysis of Thyroglobulin & Secretion of Thyroid Hormones

The thyroid cells **ingest colloid by endocytosis.**

- The **lysosomal enzymes** digest the peptide bonds between iodinated residues and thyroglobulin.
  - This is called **proteolysis of thyroglobulin molecule.**
  - This results in formation of free T_4, T_3, DIT, and MIT in the cytoplasm.
- The iodinated tyrosines are **deiodinated** by the microsomal enzyme **iodotyrosine deiodinase.**
- The T_3 and T_4 are then **released** from thyroid cells **into the general circulation.**
  - The **iodine released** by deiodination of MIT and DIT is usually **reutilized by the gland** for further synthesis of thyroid hormone.
- This provides ***more supply of iodine*** for thyroid hormone synthesis in comparison to the iodine available by iodide pump.
  - MIT and DIT are not secreted by the thyroid gland.

Functions of Thyroid Cells: Thus, thyroid cells serve **three important functions**:

1. They **actively accumulate iodide** from blood for synthesis of thyroid hormones.
2. They **synthesize thyroglobulin molecules** and secrete them into the colloid.
3. They **digest the colloid** and **free thyroid hormones** from thyroglobulin molecules to secrete them into the circulation.

Structure of T_3 and T_4

Thyroxine contains four iodine atoms, each one at 3, 5, 3′ and 5′ positions, whereas triiodothyronine contains three iodine atoms, each one at 3, 5 and 3′ positions of the thyronine ring structures (Fig. 73.6). For the positions of iodine atoms in thyroid hormones, thyroxine and triiodothyronine are abbreviated as T_3 and T_4 respectively.

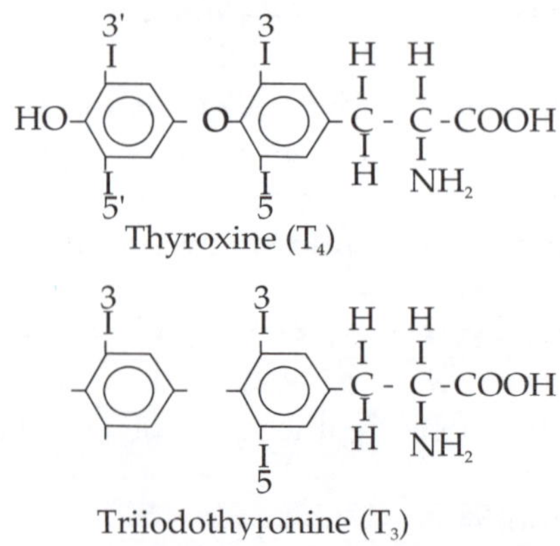

Fig. 73.6: Structure of T_3 and T_4. Note, thyroxine contains four iodine atoms, at 3, 5, 3′, and 5′ positions, and triiodothyronine contains three iodine atoms at 3, 5, and 3′ positions of the thyronine ring structures.

Metabolism of Thyroid Hormones

Normal Concentration

In a normal individual, total plasma T_4 concentration is about **8 µg/dL**, and plasma **T_3 is about 0.15 µg/dL.**

- In circulation, most of the thyroid hormones bind with the plasma proteins.
- About 99.9% of T_4 and 99.8% of T_3 are bound to plasma proteins.
- Therefore, the **free T_4 level in plasma is about 2 ng/dL,** and **free T_3 is about 0.3 ng/dL** (Application Box 73.1).

Application Box 73.1

Measurements of free and bound forms: Concentration of thyroid hormone is measured by RIA. As physiological effects of thyroid hormones **depend on their free-form level in plasma,** and the free hormone component influences feedback control of hypothalamo-pituitary-thyroid axis, in thyroid dysfunctions, mainly the free hormone concentrations are noted. Usually, both total and free level of hormones are measured.

Protein Binding

Thyroid hormones bind with **three types of plasma proteins**:

1. Thyroxine binding globulin (TBG)
2. Thyroxine binding prealbumin (TBPA), also called transthyretin.
3. Albumin.

Normally, T_4 binds mainly with TBG and TBPA, and T_3 binds with albumin and TBG.

TBG

TBG is a glycoprotein synthesized by liver. Its molecular weight is 54000. Each TBG molecule has a single binding site on it for a molecule of thyroid hormone.

- About **70% of T_4 and 45% of T_3 are bound to TBG.**
- TBG level in plasma **increases in pregnancy** and in patients receiving **estrogen, major tranquilizers, clofibrate** etc.
- Plasma **TBG level decreases** in patients receiving glucocorticoids, androgens, danazol and L-asparginase (cancer chemotherapeutic drug).
- Salicylates, phenytoin (anticonvulsant), mitotane (cancer chemotherapeutic drug) and 5-flurouracil **inhibit binding of T_3 and T_4 to TBG.**

TBPA

TBPA, though named as prealbumin is not an albumin, rather a globulin.

- Recently, TBPA has been designated as **transthyretin**.
- The binding of T_3 with TBPA is very less (less than 1%), whereas about 20% of T_4 binds to it.

Albumin

T_3 mainly binds with albumin. About 55% of T_3 and 10% of T_4 bind with albumin.

The concentration of free T_3 and T_4 depends on the concentration of plasma proteins that bind these hormones.

- When, *concentration of thyroid binding proteins increases in plasma*, the ***free level of thyroid hormones decreases***.
    - However, the decreased hormone level provides **feedback signals** to secrete more TSH, which in turn **increases secretion of thyroid hormones.**
- The *opposite phenomenon* occurs when level of plasma binding protein decreases in plasma.
- Thus, initial change observed in thyroid hormones due to change in plasma proteins is a **temporary effect**.
    - Therefore, thyroid activity remains normal (*euthyroid state*) in patients with altered binding proteins.

Importance of Protein Binding

1. Protein-bound forms of T_3 and T_4 **serve as reservoir** of these hormones.
    - This can replenish the circulating hormone, when due to some reasons or the other, the secretion is decreased or metabolism is increased suddenly and temporarily.
2. Protein binding **protects the hormone against metabolic degradation.**
    - Therefore, the half-lives of circulating T_3 and T_4 are more (1 day for T_3 and 7 days for T_4).
3. Circulating free form concentration provides **feedback effect on regulation** of hormone secretion.

Peripheral Conversion

The major product of thyroid gland secretion is T_4.

1. Normally, about **35% of secreted T_4 is converted to T_3** in the circulation by the enzyme **5′-deiodinase** present in liver and kidney, and this accounts for about 85% of circulating T_3 (Fig. 73. 7).
2. **T_3 mainly acts on the target cells.**
    - Therefore, physiologically T_3 is considered as the most **active hormone**.
3. About **45% of T_4 is also converted to RT_3** by the enzyme **5-deiodinase**, which accounts for 95% of circulating RT_3.
    - However, **RT_3 is physiologically inert.**
    - As **5′-deiodinase** is present in **high concentration** *in pituitary and cerebral cortex*, the ratio of T_3/T_4 is very high in these structures.
4. Remaining about 20% is conjugated with sulphates and glucuronides.

Peripheral Degradation

Thyroid hormones are metabolized mainly by enzymes **deiodinases** (Fig. 73. 8).

- There are **three types of deiodinases**: Type 1 (D_1), type 2 (D_2) and type 3 (D_3).
- **D_1 and D_2 are 5′-deiodinase** that convert T_4 to T_3 and ***maintain level of intracellular T_3*** in their target tissues.

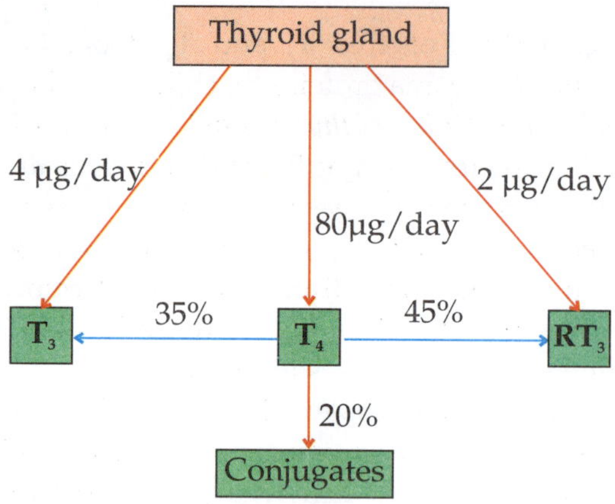

Fig. 73.7: Daily secretion and fate of thyroxine.

- **D_3 promotes** conversion of **T_4 to RT_3**.

- Especially in brain, D_2 maintains the supply of T_3 to the neurons.
  - T_3 is degraded to diiodothyronines by deiodinases that are present in the liver and kidney.
- In liver, T_4 and T_3 are metabolized by **conjugation with sulphates and glucuronic acid**.
  - The conjugated forms are **secreted in the bile into the intestine** to reenter the *enterohepatic circulation*.
  - Thus, iodine is lost minimally, about 4% in stool.
- In many tissues, T_4 is also metabolized to **tetraiodoacetic acid (tetrac)**.

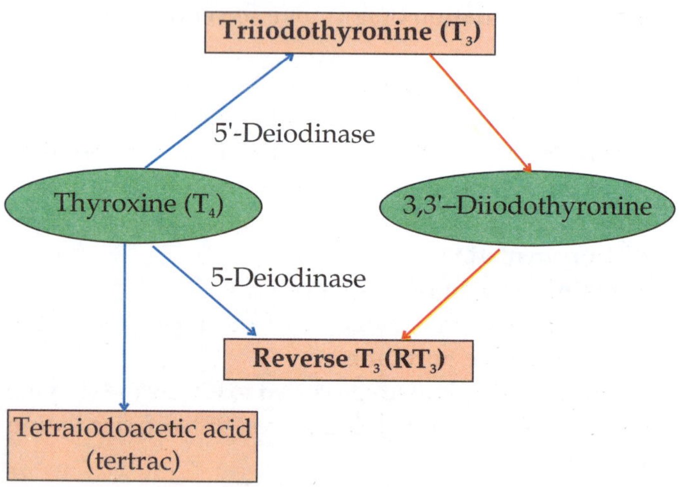

Fig. 73.8: Metabolism of thyroxine.

Regulation of Secretion

Secretion of thyroid hormones is regulated by a **feedback control mechanism** under the influence of **thyrotropin releasing hormone** (TRH) and **TSH. TSH stimulates thyroid gland** to secrete T_3 and T_4.

For details of **feedback control** by TRH and TSH, refer Fig. 71.11, Chapter 71).

TSH: Details of structure, regulation and function of TSH are described in 'Anterior Pituitary', Chapter 71.

MECHANISM OF ACTION

The mechanism of action of thyroid hormones is **similar to that of steroid hormones**. They act by binding with the **intracellular receptors**. With few ***exceptions like adult brain and gonads***, receptors for thyroid hormones are present **in all tissues and organs**. Though the developing neurons in infants and children are highly sensitive to thyroid hormones, it is not clear why the adult neurons are not so sensitive.

The **steps of mechanism** of action are as follows:

1. T_3 and T_4 enter the cells of the target organs by **carrier mediated** (energy dependent) transport.
2. Inside the cell, most of the **T_4 is converted to T_3**, which then binds with the **thyroid-hormone receptors** (TR) present on nucleus.
   - The thyroid receptor protein binds to **thyroid-hormone response elements** (TRE) in the DNA via zinc fingers.
3. Binding of T_3 with thyroid hormone receptor-TRE elements causes **transcription of DNA** that in turn increases the **translation of mRNA** (Fig. 73.9).

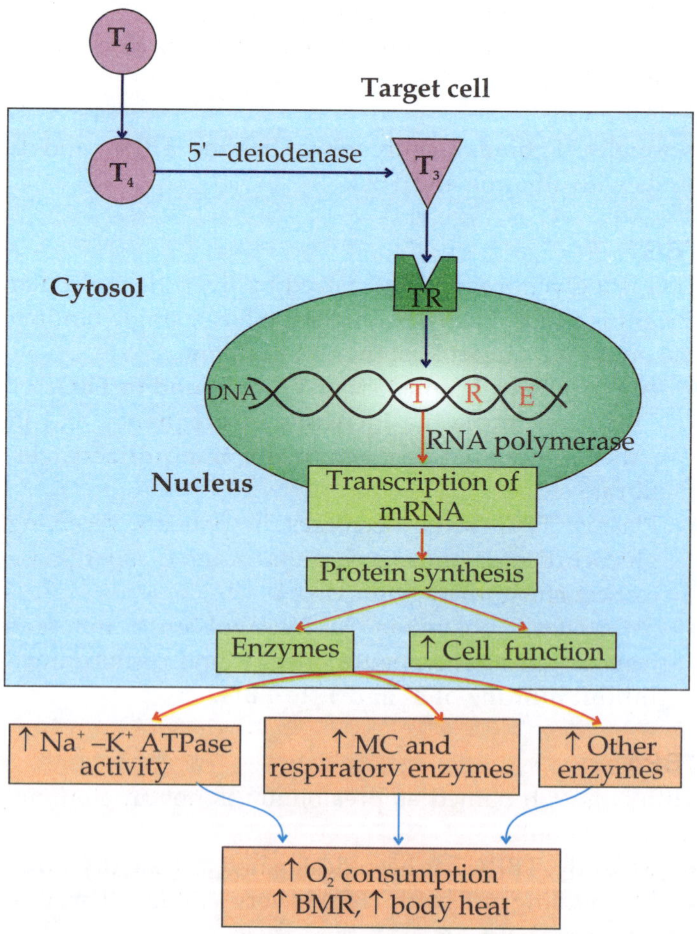

Fig. 73.9: Mechanism of action of thyroxine. Note, the mechanism of thyroxine action is similar to steroid hormones. TR: thyroid-hormone receptor; TRE: thyroid-hormone response element; MC: mitochondrial; BMR: basal metabolic rate; T3: triiodothyronine; T4: thyroxine.

4. Increased mRNA causes increased **intracellular protein synthesis** that stimulates cellular growth and maturation, increases intracellular enzyme synthesis, increases mitochondria formation and respiratory enzyme synthesis, and increases **Na^+-K^+ ATPase activity**.
5. The increased Na^+-K^+ ATPase activity **increases cellular oxygen consumption** and increased **mitochondrial activity** increases general metabolism of the cell.

Thyroid-Hormone Receptors (TR)

There are **two human TR genes**: α and β. The **α receptor gene** is located on chromosome 17 and **β receptor gene** is located on chromosome 3.

- Each of them synthesizes **two different mRNAs.** Therefore, two different receptor proteins are formed: **TRα1, TRα2, TRβ1 and TRβ2.**
- TRα1, TRβ1 and TRβ2 bind with T_3.
  - **TRα1 and TRβ1** are widely distributed in tissues.
  - **TRα2** does not bind with T_3, though widely distributed and its function is not clearly known.
- **TRβ2** is found only in the brain.
- There are many activators and repressors of TR, which makes thyroid hormones, exert their diverse effects in various tissues.
- T_3 binds more rapidly and avidly to TR.
  - Therefore, **T_3 is more potent than T_4.**
- **In myocytes**, especially in heart T_3 is not formed from T_4.
  - However, T_3 directly enters myocyte to combine with nuclear receptors and promotes expression or inhibition of genes.

PHYSIOLOGICAL ACTIONS

General Effects on Basal Metabolism

The metabolism of a cell depends on the rate of its **oxygen consumption**. Oxygen is essential for oxidative **phosphorylation of ADP to ATP** that takes place in mitochondria.

1. Thyroid hormones **increase the basal rate of oxygen consumption** and therefore, the basal metabolism of the tissues.
   - This **increased metabolism increases the rate of heat production**.
   - This is called **calorigenic** or **thermogenic actions** of thyroid hormones.
2. The cellular metabolism is also activated by **increased Na^+-K^+ ATPase activity**.
   - Increased oxygen consumption by the cells **parallels their increase in Na^+-K^+ ATPase activity**.
   - In some of the tissues, inhibition of Na^+-K^+ pump decreases oxygen consumption.
3. T_3 also stimulates the **transcription of genes** for both α and β subunits of Na^+-K^+ pump.

- Therefore, it is strongly perceived that **increased oxygen consumption** stimulated by thyroid hormones is **mediated by Na^+-K^+ ATPase activity**, at least partly.

Target Tissues: The increased consumption of oxygen by thyroid hormone is observed in **all tissues of the body**, which is prominent especially **in skeletal muscle, liver, heart, kidney and connective tissues**.

- However, **EXCEPTIONS are** anterior pituitary, adult brain, gonads (testis and ovary), uterus, lymph nodes, and spleen that show little thermogenic response.
- **Receptors** for thyroid hormones are almost ***absent in adult brain***.

On Basal Metabolic Rate

In the resting stage, oxygen consumption in human is about 250 ml/min.

- In hyperthyroid state, it increases to about 400 ml/min. Therefore, the **basal metabolic rate** (BMR) **increases to about +80%** in hyperthyroidism.
- Conversely, in hypothyroidism BMR decreases to **as low as –40%.**
- Increased BMR increases body temperature.

Mitochondrial Mechanism: Increased metabolism is not only by increased oxygen consumption and Na^+-K^+ ATPase activity, but also by increase in **synthesis of mitochondrial cytochromes** and **cytochrome oxidase activity**.

- Thyroid hormones regulate the number of respiratory unit in each cell and their capacity to carry out **oxidative phosphorylation**.
- Thyroid hormones also stimulate **synthesis of uncoupling protein 1** (**UCP-1**) that contributes significantly to oxidation of nutrients and heat production.
- The tissue expression of **UCP-2 and UCP-3** are also increased by thyroid hormones.

Effects Secondary to Metabolic or Thermogenic Actions

1. Increased body metabolism **increases nitrogen excretion.**
   - Therefore, increased food intake should be associated with hypermetabolic states to prevent catabolism of endogenous protein and fat.
   - Thus, **significant weight loss** occurs promptly in increased thyroid activity, without adequate nutrient supplementation.
2. Increased metabolism **increases body temperature**.
   - This causes thermogenic **vasodilation** that **decreases peripheral resistance** and consequent changes occur in hemodynamics.
3. Increased metabolism also **increases the requirement for vitamins**.
   - Therefore, **vitamin deficiency** is common in increased thyroid activity.

Effects on Nervous System

Thyroid hormones are essential for **development of the central nervous system**, especially **during infancy and early childhood**. Development of brain occurs maximally in last six months of fetal life and first six months of postnatal life. During this period, thyroid hormones initiate and facilitate the process of **differentiation and maturation of brain cells.**

Thyroid hormones are required for **following neural functions**:

1. **Growth of** cerebral and cerebellar cortices, and basal ganglia.
2. Proliferation of **axons** and branching of **dendrites**.
3. Development of **synaptic connections**.
4. Development of **neurotransmitter systems** in CNS.
   - Thyroid hormones induce ***synthesis of enzymes*** essential for production of **neurotransmitters**.
5. Increase in the number of **receptors** for various neurotransmitters in different brain tissues.
6. **Myelination of neurons**.
   - Thyroid hormones stimulate ***galactosyl sialyl transferase activity***, which is essential for myelin formation.
7. **Synthesis of proteins and various enzymes** like succinate dehydrogenase that are required for energy generation in neurons.
8. **Cell migration** during brain development.
9. General **alertness and responsiveness** to various stimuli.
10. Speed and amplitude of **stretch reflexes**.
11. **Memory**, learning and ***intellectual capacities***.

CNS Development in Infancy: Deficiency of thyroid hormones during infancy results in **irreversible retardation** in CNS development (Clinical Note 73.3). Thyroid deficiency in newborn should be detected early and treated promptly.

In Adults: Cerebral blood flow, glucose and oxygen utilization by brain **remains normal** in adult hypothyroidism and hyperthyroidism.

Clinical Note 73.3

Mental retardation in hypothyroid children: Thyroid hormones are essential for normal mentation. Therefore, mental retardation is an important feature of a thyroid deficiency in infancy and early childhood **(thyroid dwarf)**. This differentiates it from a pituitary dwarf in whom mental activities are apparently normal. Decreased stretch reflex activities, especially decreased reaction time of **Achilles tendon reflex** (ankle jerk) is diagnostic in hypothyroidism.

Effects on Growth and Development

Thyroid hormones are essential for **normal growth and musculo-skeletal maturation**.

1. Thyroid hormones promote **expression of gene for growth hormone** (GH) in somatotrophs of anterior pituitary.
   - Stimulate GH secretion
   - Also, they facilitate the effect of GH on tissues.
3. By direct action, thyroid hormones stimulate **linear growth of bones**, and **endochondral ossification and maturation** of epiphyseal bone centers.
   - They enhance the **activity of chondrocytes** in cartilage.
   - They increase **osteoid activity** and bone remodeling.
4. They cause eruption and development of **teeth**.
5. They promote epidermal growth, and growth of **nails and hairs**.
6. They stimulate synthesis of structural and **enzymatic proteins**.

In hypothyroid children, bone growth is slowed and epiphyseal closure is delayed.

On Tissues: Thyroxine causes alteration in the **characteristics of mucopolysaccharides** in the subcutaneous tissue.

- It decreases synthesis and promotes degradation of glycosaminoglycans (mucopolysaccharides).

Effects on Cardiovascular System

Thyroid hormones increase heart rate and myocardial contractility. Therefore, they **increase the cardiac output**.

1. **On Heart Rate:** Thyroid hormones **increase the number of β receptors** on the nodal tissues (SA and AV nodes) of the heart and increase the **sensitivity of β receptors to catecholamines**.
   - Thus, thyroid hormones **increase the heart rate**.
   - Tachycardia is a common feature of hyperthyroidism (Clinical Note 73.4).
2. **On Myocardial Contractility:** Myocardial contractility increases by following mechanisms:
   i) Thyroid hormones induce **myosin heavy chain** (MHC) expression in the cardiac muscle. Especially, the α-MHC activity is increased, which has more actin and calcium-activated ATPase activity.
   ii) Thyroid hormones increase the **expression of β receptors, G proteins and Na^+-K^+ ATPase** in myocardial cells.
   iii) They also increase the **calcium-ATPase activity** of the sarcoplasmic reticulum in cardiac muscle, which facilitates sequestration of calcium.

All these factors increase the force of contraction that in turn **increase stroke volume**.

MHC in Heart Muscle: Normally, heart muscle contains two MHCs: α and β MHCs.

- The α MHC has high myosin ATPase activity, and β MHC has low myosin ATPase activity.
  - Thyroid hormones **stimulate α MHC and inhibit β MHC activities.**
- In hyperthyroidism, expression of α MHC gene is enhanced and of β MHC gene is suppressed.

- Further, in myocytes, thyroid hormones ***inhibit adenylyl cyclase, T_3 nuclear receptor and Na^+-Ca^+ exchanger***, in addition to its inhibition of β MHC.

3. **On Systolic Pressure:** Increased heart rate and stroke volume result in increase in cardiac output (Fig. 73.10).
   - Thus, **systolic blood pressure increases** significantly.
4. **Diastolic Pressure:** Via its calorigenic action, thyroid hormones increase body temperature that causes **thermogenic cutaneous vasodilation** and decreases peripheral resistance.
   - Thus, **diastolic pressure decreases**.
5. **Pulse Pressure and Circulation Time:** The net effect on blood pressure is **increased pulse pressure**.
   - Wide pulse pressure is a prominent feature of hyperthyroidism.
   - Increased cardiac output and vasodilation makes the circulation hyperdynamic.
   - Therefore, **circulation time is shortened**.

Clinical Note 73.4

Tachycardia in sleep: Tachycardia is an important feature of hyperthyroidism. Tachycardia due to other causes (anxiety, tension, etc.) usually disappears during sleep or heart rate falls significantly. In thyroid excess, tachycardia persists even during sleep. **Sleeping tachycardia is an important diagnostic feature of thyrotoxicosis.** Sometimes atrial arrhythmias such as flutter or fibrillation are also seen in hyperthyroidism, especially in elderly people.

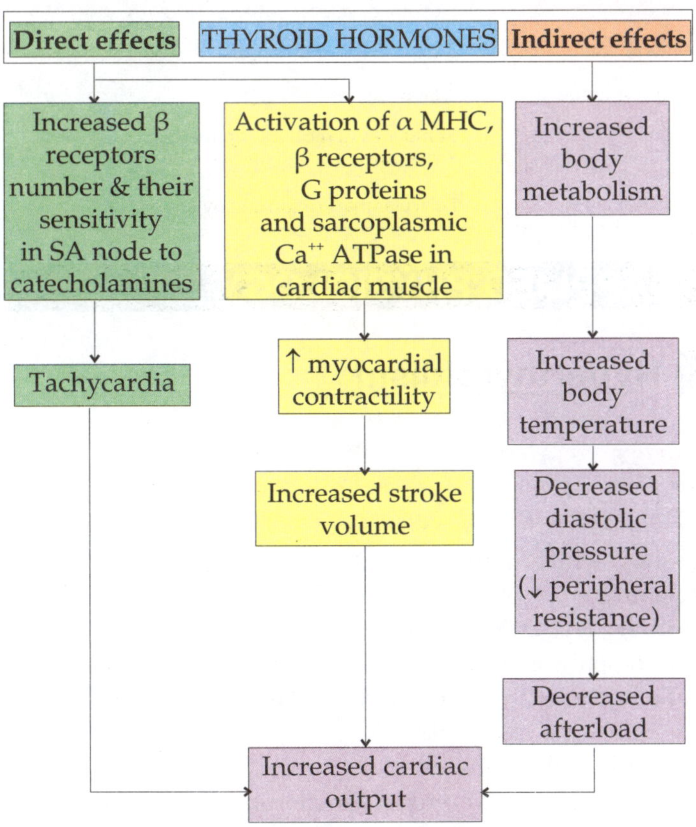

Fig. 73.10: Mechanisms of increased cardiac output by thyroid hormones. MHC: Myosin heavy chain.

Effects on Intermediary Metabolism

On Carbohydrate Metabolism

Thyroid hormones **increase absorption of glucose** from intestine.

- They **increase hepatic glucose output** by inducing **gluconeogenesis**.
  - They also stimulate **hepatic glycogenolysis**.
  - Therefore, plasma glucose level increases.
- However, thyroid hormones **increase the turnover of glucose** by increasing its uptake and oxidation.
  - Therefore, the net effect is **no substantial change** in plasma glucose concentration.
- In hyperthyroidism, though plasma glucose level rises fast after a carbohydrate meal, it **decreases rapidly**.
- Thus, sustained hyperglycemia or **glucose intolerance is not a usual feature** of hyperthyroidism.
  - Some patients develop **glucose intolerance or even diabetes** in the long run.

On Fat Metabolism

Thyroid hormones **stimulate lipolysis**.

- Thus, thyroxine increases **release of free fatty acids and glycerol** from adipose tissues.
  - Glycerol is utilized for gluconeogenesis.
- Thyroid hormones also **increase turnover of lipids**, by facilitating their oxidation.
- They **stimulate synthesis of cholesterol** and simultaneously promote its oxidation and biliary excretion.
  - Hepatic uptake of cholesterol is increased by increased expression of LDL receptors in liver.
- Therefore, the net effect is **significant decrease in plasma cholesterol** and total lipid.

On Protein Metabolism

Thyroid hormones **promote proteolysis** in skeletal muscle, increasing the release of amino acid. They **increase protein turnover** by promoting protein degradation.

On Metabolic Actions of Other Hormones

Thyroid hormones **potentiate the metabolic actions of catecholamines, glucagons, cortisol and growth hormone**, especially their **gluconeogenic and lipolytic** effects.

Effects on Sympathetic Nervous Systems

Thyroid hormones increase the rate of metabolism, heat production, heart rate and neuromuscular functions; the features that are **similar to the effects of sympathetic stimulation** (Clinical Note 73.5).

1. They also synergize the metabolic effects of catecholamines like lipolysis, glycogenolysis, and gluconeogenesis.

3. In fact, they do not increase the release of catecholamines; rather **increase the expression and sensitivity** of β receptors in various tissues like heart, skeletal muscle and adipose tissues to catecholamines.
4. Recently, it has been observed that T_3 **stimulates the production of thermogenin**, a protein in the brown adipose tissue that partly mediates the thermogenic action of catecholamines.

Clinical Note 73.5

Hypersympathetic state: The features of hyperthyroidism mimic the features of sympathetic stimulation like increased metabolism, increased body temperature, nervousness, increased motor activity, and excessive sweating. Use of sympathetic blockers such as **propranolol** alleviates many features of hyperthyroidism.

Effects on Respiratory System

Thyroid hormones **increase oxygen utilization** of tissues. Therefore, the demand for oxygen also increases.

1. Thyroxine meets this demand by **stimulating the rate of respiration, minute ventilation, and ventilatory responses** to hypercapnia and hypoxia.
   - Thus, **arterial PO_2 increases** that increase the *supply of oxygen to tissues*.
2. Thyroid hormones **stimulate erythropoiesis** by increasing the synthesis of erythropoietin.
   - Thus, the supply of oxygen to the tissues is also increased.

Effects on GI tract

Thyroid hormones **enhance the motility** GI tract.

- Therefore, **hyperdefecation** is a feature of hyperthyroidism and **constipation** is a feature of hypothyroidism.
- Thyroid hormones also **increase appetite and food intake, and reabsorption of glucose** from GI tract.

Effects on Skeletal Muscle

Thyroid hormones increase the **expression of MHC genes** in the skeletal muscle. Therefore, hypothyroidism is associated with **muscle cramp and weakness**.

- However, muscle weakness also occurs in hyperthyroidism, which may partly be due to **increased protein catabolism** in the muscle. **Myopathy** occurs in chronic hyperthyroidism (**thyrotoxic myopathy**).

Effects on Reproductive System

In both males and females, thyroid hormones play an important role in the regulation of reproductive functions.

In Females: In women, they facilitate **follicular maturation** and **ovulation**.

- Thyroid abnormalities in woman result in irregularities in menstrual cycle, such as *menorrhagia* (increased menstrual loss) in hypothyroidism and *oligomenorrhea* (decreased menstrual loss) in hyperthyroidism.

In Males: In males, they promote **spermatogenesis**.

- T_3 promotes **differentiation of** prepubertal testicular *Sertoli cells*.

Effects on Kidney

Thyroid hormones increase **kidney size** and promote **growth of renal tubular epithelial cells**.

- They **increase renal blood flow and GFR**.
- Tubular **reabsorption of electrolytes, glucose and water** is also increased by thyroid hormones. Increased water reabsorption increases blood volume.

In summary, thyroid hormones have widespread effects on metabolism, growth and development and control of many systemic functions (Table 73.1)

Table 73.1 | Summary of physiologic effects of thyroid hormones.

Target system	Functions
Metabolism	Increase in BMR (↑ O_2 consumption in all tissues except testes, uterus, lymph node, spleen & anterior pituitary)
CVS	1. Tachycardia (increased no. & sensitivity of β receptors) 2. Increased myocardial contractility (increased MHC & myosin ATPase) 3. Increased SBP (↑cardiac output) 4. Decreased DBP (↓ peripheral resistance)
CNS	Brain development
Bone	Skeletal development and ↑ growth
Muscle	↑ Expression of MHC gene, Protein catabolism
Adipose tissue	↑ Lipolysis
GIT	Stimulates GI motility, ↑ appetite, ↑ Carbohydrate absorption
Reproduction	Follicular maturation and ovulation

APPLIED PHYSIOLOGY

Hyperthyroidism

Types

Hyperthyroidism occurs due to hypersecretion of thyroid hormones from thyroid gland or from extrathyroidal tissues, which may be broadly divided into **primary and secondary** varieties.

Primary Hyperthyroidism: When hyperthyroidism occurs due to pathology of the thyroid gland, the condition is called primary hyperthyroidism. The common causes are:

1. Adenoma of thyroid
2. Multinodular goiter
3. Metastatic carcinoma of functioning thyroid gland
4. Grave's disease
5. Activating mutation of TSH receptors

6. Iodine excess (**Jod-Basedow phenomenon**)

Secondary Hyperthyroidism: When hyperthyroidism occurs due to the pathology outside thyroid gland, the condition is called secondary hyperthyroidism, which may be due to a tumor of the pituitary gland or of extrathyroidal tissue.

Pituitary Causes: Tumor of thyrotrophs of anterior pituitary (secretes excess of TSH)

Extrathyroidal Causes: Chronic excess administration of thyroid hormones (iatrogenic), tumor of ectopic thyroid tissue (lingual thyroid), hCG secreting tumors such as choriocarcinoma.

Features of Hyperthyroidism

Features of hyperthyroidism in descending order of frequency are:

Symptoms: Hyperactivity and irritability, **heat intolerance**, fatigue, **tremor**, sweating, **palpitation**, nervousness, hyperphagia (due to increased appetite), **weight loss inspite of hyperphagia**, **hyperdefecation** (due to increased GI motility), loss of libido, and oligomenorrhea (in females).

Signs: Sinus **tachycardia**, atrial fibrillation, **systolic hypertension** and increased pulse pressure, **fine tremor**, thyroid swelling (goiter), increased body temperature (**warm and moist skin**), muscle weakness (proximal myopathy), protrusion of eyeball with retracted lid (**exophthalmos**) (Fig. 73.11), periorbital edema, and gynecomastia (in males).

Increased BMR to as high as +100 is an important and diagnostic laboratory finding of hyperthyroidism.

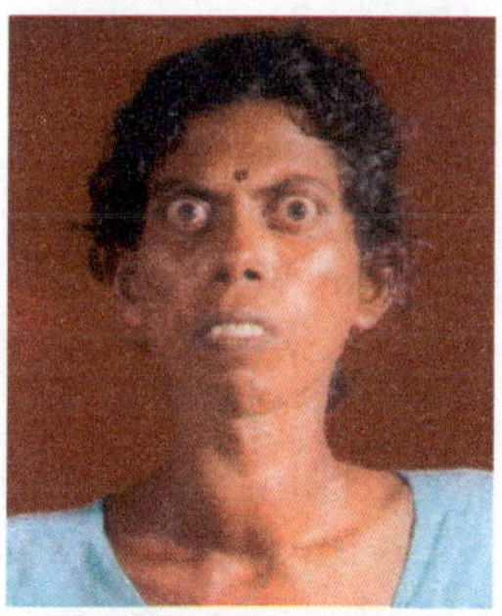

Fig. 73.11: A hyperthyroid patient. Note the presence of exophthalmos and goiter. Courtesy: Dr Abdoul Hamide, Senior Professor of Medicine, JIPMER, Puducherry.

Diagnosis of Hyperthyroidism

Diagnosis is made by estimation of T_3, T_4, and TSH in plasma.

1. Typically, in **primary hyperthyroidism,** *T_3 and T_4 are high* and ***TSH is low***.
2. **In secondary hyperthyroidism** due to pituitary cause, **TSH is high** along with high T_3 and T_4.

Physiological Basis of Treatment

Administration of **antithyroid drugs** is the mainstay of treatment of hyperthyroidism. They usually inhibit iodide trapping mechanism or binding of iodide with the tyrosine molecule.

Antithyroid drugs are thionamides, anions, high dose of iodides, nonspecific beta-blockers and radioiodines.

Thionamides: These are thiourylenes, a group of compounds related to thiourea. The commonly used thionamides are propylthiouracil, carbimazole and methimazole (active metabolite of carbimazole).

The mechanisms of action of thionamides are:

1. They inhibit the function of thyroid peroxidase.
2. They inhibit oxidation and organification of iodide. Thus, they inhibit iodination of monoiodotyrosine and coupling reaction.
3. They reduce the level of thyroid stimulating antibodies.
4. Propylthiouracil reduce the rate of conversion of T_4 to T_3 by inhibiting D_2–deiodinase activity.

The Anions: These are chlorate, perchlorate, pertechnetate, periodate, biiodate, etc. They are monovalent anions that compete with iodide for transport into the thyroid via NIS (Na^+-I symporter).

- Thus, **they prevent iodide trapping**.
- Thiocyanate is also an anion that **inhibits iodide transport**, but is less potent.

High Dose of Iodide: Iodide is essential for thyroid hormone synthesis. However, in very high dose it prevents organic binding by itself, and therefore, prevents thyroid hormone synthesis.

- This inhibition is called **Wolff-Chaikoff effect**.
- High dose of iodide also **inhibits the effect of TSH** on the gland by decreasing cAMP production in the cell, and by inhibiting proteolysis of thyroglobulin.

Propranolol: It is a nonspecific β-blocker. By preventing the action of catecholamines on β receptors, propranolol ameliorates many of the hyperthyroid features.

- It decreases heart rate, cardiac output, nervousness etc.
- Is very helpful in the early stages of the disease.

Radioiodine: It causes progressive destruction of thyroid cells and achieves euthyroid state. The dose should be appropriately adjusted to prevent development of hypothyroidism.

Special States of Hyperthyroidism

Thyrotoxicosis

Thyrotoxicosis is not synonymous with hyperthyroidism. It is a state of thyroid hormone excess that occurs due to **severe hyperthyroidism** as seen in **Grave's disease**, toxic **multinodular goiter** and **toxic adenoma**. This can also occur due to excess administration of thyroid hormones (***thyrotoxicosis factitia***).

Grave's Disease

Grave's disease is a condition in which there is diffuse enlargement of thyroid gland, which is usually associated with **exophthalmos**.

- This is an **autoimmune disease** that occurs due to development of **autoantibodies against TSH receptors**.
  - The antibodies formed against the TSH receptors activate the receptors. Therefore, thyroid gland **becomes hypertrophied and hyperactive**.
- There is marked stimulation of secretion of thyroid hormones. Therefore, plasma level of **T_3 and T_4 is very high.**
- **TSH concentration is less** as excess thyroid hormones inhibit TSH secretion.
- **Exophthalmos** occurs due to swelling of extraocular muscles and proliferation of connecting tissue within the bony walls of the orbit that pushes the eyeball forward.

The disease is treated by using antithyroid drugs, by decreasing thyroid hormone synthesis, or by reducing the amount of thyroid tissue (with treatment of radioactive iodine like ^{131}I or by subtotal thyroidectomy).

Thyroid Storm

A patient suffering from hyperthyroidism becomes **suddenly extremely ill** and sometimes circulatory collapse.

- Seen in a hyperthyroid patient **undergoing major surgery, major trauma or illness.**
- This is a **medical emergency**.

Hypothyroidism

Hypothyroidism in Adult

Hypothyroidism in adult is usually known as **myxedema**.

Etiology

Hypothyroidism, according to the cause may be classified into two categories: Primary and secondary.

Primary Hypothyroidism

When hypothyroidism develops due to the **diseases or causes that primarily affect thyroid gland**, is classified under primary hypothyroidism.

The common causes are:

1. Autoimmune hypothyroidism: for example **Hashimoto's thyroiditis.**
2. Iatrogenic: Excess use of radioiodine (^{131}I), thyroidectomy etc.
3. Iodine deficiency
4. Drugs: Excess of iodine, excess use of antithyroid drugs, lithium etc.
5. Congenital hypothyroidism

Secondary Hypothyroidism

When hypothyroidism develops due to a **defect outside the thyroid gland**, the condition is called secondary hypothyroidism. Usually, it occurs due to a defect either in the pituitary or in the hypothalamus.

1. **Pituitary hypothyroidism:** Pituitary resection, pituitary tumors affecting thyrotrophs, and Sheehan's syndrome (**post-partum necrosis of pituitary**). Hypothyroidism *occurs due to decreased TSH secretion.*
2. **Hypothalamic hypothyroidism:** Brain injury involving hypothalamus, tumors of hypothalamus, etc in which *secretion of TRH is less.*
3. Features of hypometabolism similar to hypothyroidism could occur due to resistance of peripheral tissues to thyroid hormones, called as **thyroid hormone resistance** (Clinical Note 73.6).

Clinical Note 73.6

Thyroid Hormone Resistance: In this condition, the tissues become resistant to the effects of T_3 and T_4. Features of hypothyroidism may not develop. But, **features of hypometabolism** occur in peripheral tissues.

- TSH level of plasma remains inappropriately high, which is not suppressed by exogenous thyroxine.
- The patients with **peripheral tissue resistance** have hypometabolism despite normal levels of T_3 and T_4.
- It has been observed that the attention deficit hyperactive disorder in children is more associated with thyroid hormone resistance.

Features of Hypothyroidism

Following are the features in descending order of frequency:

Symptoms: Cold intolerance, weakness and easy-tiredness, dry-thick skin, loss of hair, poor memory and inability to concentrate, **constipation** (due to decreased GI motility), **weight gain** inspite of poor appetite, **thick and husky voice** (typical hoarse voice that helps physician to **diagnose the disease over phone**), yellow skin (occurs due to carotenemia, as thyroxine causes conversion of carotene to vitamin A; therefore deficiency of it causes deposition of carotene), alopecia, psychosis (myxedema madness) menorrhagia (in females), galactorrhea and infertility .

Signs: Cool extremities with dry coarse skin, dry hair, bradycardia, puffy face (Fig. 73.12), with edematous hands and feet (**myxedema**), diffuse alopecia, goiter, bradycardia, hypertension (diastolic), anemia, decreased reaction time of tendon reflexes (especially, delayed Achilles tendon reflex relaxation), carpal tunnel syndrome and periorbital edema.

BMR decreases to about –40, and plasma cholesterol is usually elevated.

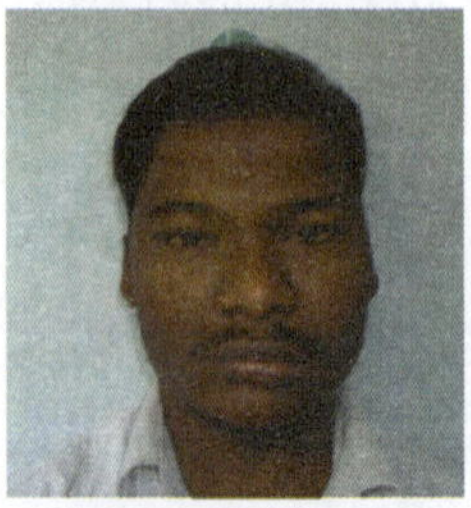

Fig. 73.12: A hypothyroid patient. Note pronounced myxedema in face (puffy face) with coarse hair on head. Courtesy: Dr T Kadhiravan, Professor of Medicine, JIPMER, Puducherry

Diagnosis of Hypothyroidism

- **In primary hypothyroidism**, T_3 and T_4 levels are decreased, but **TSH is increased** by feedback mechanism.
- **In hypopituitary or hypothalamic hypothyroidism**, the TSH concentration is less, in addition to decreased T_3 and T_4.
  - The **TSH response to TRH** is *usually normal* in hypothalamic hypothyroidism, whereas it is *increased* in hypothyroidism caused by thyroid disease.

Treatment of Hypothyroidism

Thyroid hormone replacement is the mainstay of treatment. **T_4 is instituted** at a dose (usually 10 to 15 µg/kg/day) to maintain its normal level in plasma.

Hashimoto's Thyroiditis

It is a chronic form of *autoimmune thyroiditis* in which **antibodies are formed against the thyroglobulin and thyroid peroxidase**. Therefore, thyroid cells are damaged and hypothyroidism develops. Fine needle aspiration cytology (FNAC) demonstrates **sheet of hurthle cells** with *lymphoid infiltrate*.

Hypothyroidism in Children (Cretinism)

Cretinism is the hypothyroidism in children. When hypothyroidism develops from or before birth, the patients are called **cretins**.

Causes: Maternal iodine deficiency during pregnancy, maldevelopment of thyroid gland during fetal life, inborn errors of thyroid hormone synthesis, antithyroid antibodies in mother that crosses placenta and enters fetal circulation, and hypopituitarism in fetal life are usual causes of cretinism.

Features: Patients are dwarf and mentally retarded. Typically, they have potbelly and protrusion of tongue. Other features of hypothyroidism are also present.

Treatment: Hypothyroidism is an important cause of mental retardation, which can be prevented if the disease is diagnosed and treated immediately after birth. Thyroid hormone replacement early in infancy can totally cure the disease. The usual treatment is the *prompt replacement of thyroxine* as soon as the diagnosis is made.

PY8.4

THYROID FUNCTION TESTS

Thyroid function tests include measurement of hormones, TSH, binding proteins, TRH response test, radioactive iodine uptake, thyroid scanning, detection of thyroid antibodies, and determination of cholesterol level in blood.

Measurement of Thyroid Hormones

T_3 and T_4 concentration in plasma are usually measured by RIA or sometimes by ELISA test.

- In **primary hyperthyroidism**, the thyroid hormone levels are increased, but typically the TSH is reduced due to feedback inhibition.
- In **primary hypothyroidism**, T_3 and T_4 are decreased but TSH level is elevated (Table 73.2).
- In **pituitary hypothyroidism** T_3, T_4 and TSH are decreased.

Plasma TSH Estimation

Measurement of plasma TSH is an important diagnostic tool for the detection of thyroid abnormalities.

- In *primary hypothyroidism* TSH label is high but, in secondary hypothyroidism TSH as well as T_3 and T_4 are low.
- In *primary hyperthyroidism*, TSH is low. But, in hyperthyroidism due to pituitary causes the TSH, T_4 and T_3 are high.

Table 73.2 | Thyroid function tests in primary thyroid dysfunctions.

	Hyperthyroidism	Hypothyroidism
Plasma total T_3, T_4	High	Low
Plasma free T_3, T_4 (Normal free-T_3:0.2 – 0.4 ng/dL; Normal free-T_4: 0.8 – 2.7 ng/dL)	High	Low
Plasma TSH (Normal TSH:0.4 – 4.2 µIU/mL)	Low	High

Measurement of Binding Proteins

Usually, T_3 uptake by the resin is measured. The **T_3 resin uptake** indicates the free binding sites on the TBG.

TRH Response Test

This is a useful test for diagnosing both hypo- and hyperthyroidism. Normally, administration of TRH increases TSH production and therefore, the secretion of T_3 and T_4.

Detection of Thyroid Antibodies

Detection of antibodies is essential for diagnosing Grave's disease and Hashimoto's thyroiditis.

Plasma Cholesterol

Cholesterol level in plasma is **high in hypothyroidism** and low in hyperthyroidism.

Estimation of BMR

BMR is **high in hyperthyroidism** and **low in hypothyroidism**.

Thyroid Scintiscanning

Scintiscanning offers a **visual display** of the size and shape of the thyroid gland.

- **Technetium pertechnetate** is used.

Fine-Needle Aspiration Cytology

This biopsy of FNAC is a very **valuable preoperative procedure** done routinely. A correct diagnosis can be obtained in over 80% of cases.

Ultrasound, CT and MRI

- **Ultrasound scanning** provides an accurate indication of the size and is useful for *differentiating cystic from solid lesions*.
- **CT and MRI** are useful in the evaluation of retrosternal and retrotracheal extension of the gland, compression of trachea, extent of intrathoracic extensions of thyroid malignancy and infiltration to adjacent structures.
- **MRI** gives better delineation of soft tissue involvement like infiltration of nerves.

Exam Questions

1. With the help of a suitable diagram, describe the steps of thyroid hormone synthesis. Add a note on regulation of thyroid hormone secretion.
2. With the help of a suitable diagram, describe the mechanism of action of thyroid hormones. Add a note on thyroid hormone receptor resistance.
3. Describe the physiological actions of thyroid hormone.
4. Describe briefly the physiological basis of features of hyperthyroidism, and hypothyroidism Add a note on thyroid function tests.

Multiple Choice Questions

1. Which of the following hormone is secreted in more quantity from thyroid gland?

A. T4 B. T3
C. RT4 D. RT3

2. Which of the following is not secreted from thyroid gland?

A. T_3 B. T_4
C. Calcitonin D. TSH

3. All of the following are steps of thyroid hormone synthesis, EXCEPT:

A. Iodide trapping
B. Conversion of iodide to iodine
C. Thyrotropin synthesis and secretion
D. Coupling reaction

4. In thyroid follicle, for how long thyroxine is stored?

A. 2-3 weeks
B. 2-3 days
C. 2-3 months
D. 2-3 years

5. Thyroid hormones in blood is transported by all of the following, EXCEPT:

A. Albumin
B. Globulin
C. Prealbumin
D. Ceruloplasmin

6. Regarding thyroid hormone all are true, EXCEPT:

A. T_3 is more avidly bound to nuclear receptor than T_4
B. T_4 has the maximum plasma concentration
C. T_3 is more active than T_4
D. T_4 has shorter half-life than T_3

7. Wolf-Chaikoff effect is due to:

A. Suppression of TSH secretion
B. Decreased iodination of MIT
C. Decreased T_3 to T_4 conversion
D. Iodine intake

8. Sodium-iodine symporter is not present in:

A. Pituitary gland
B. Placenta
C. Parotid
D. Thyroid

9. Iodide uptake is seen in all the following organs, EXEPT:

A. Ovary
B. Thyroid
C. Salivary gland
D. Mammary gland

10. Thyroxine injected to rat produced all, EXCEPT:

A. Lipolysis
B. Increased O_2 consumption
C. Decreased BMR
D. Increased myocardial contractility

11. TRH stimulation test is useful in diagnosis of disorders of which of the following hormone?

A. Insulin
B. ACTH
C. Growth hormone
D. PTH

12. In hypothyroidism, all are true, EXCEPT:

A. T3 is less
B. T4 is less
C. TSH is less
D. Concertation of TBG is normal

13. Which of the following is not a feature of hypothyroidism?

A. Cold intolerance
B. Hyperdefecation
C. Thick and husky voice
D. Wait gain

14. Which of the following is not a feature of hyperthyroidism?

A. Tachycardia
B. Heat intolerance
C. Systolic hypertension
D. Wait gain due to hyperphagia

Answers :

1. A	2. D	3. C	4. C	5. D	6. D	7. D	8. A	9. A	10. C
11. C	12. C	13. B	14. D						

Chapter 74

Adrenal Cortex

Learning Objectives

On completion of study of this chapter:

The student will be able to (must know):

1. Correlate the histological specialization of different layers of adrenal gland with their secretion.
2. List the hormones secreted from different layers and their steps of synthesis.
3. Illustrate the feedback regulation of cortisol secretion.
4. Describe the mechanism of action and functions of glucocorticoids.
5. Appreciate indications & contraindication of cortisol use in clinical medicine.
6. Comprehend the physiological basis of dysfunctions caused by excess or deficiency of glucocorticoids and mineralocorticoids.
7. Describe the regulation of secretion, mechanism of action and functions of mineralocorticoids.
8. Outline the functions and dysfunctions of adrenal sex steroids.

The student may also be able to (desirable to know):

1. Describe the deficiency of adrenocortical enzymes causing a specific dysfunction or syndrome.
2. Describe the steps of synthesis and regulation of secretion of adrenocortical hormones.
3. Describe the role of cortisol in stress.
4. Describe the functions and dysfunctions of adrenal sex steroids

The adrenals consist of two distinct endocrine glands, one inside the other. The inner adrenal medulla is surrounded by the outer adrenal cortex that consists of three layers (Fig. 74.1).

- The outer zone of adrenal gland, i.e. the adrenal cortex forms about 80–90% of the total gland, the inner zone, i. e. the adrenal medulla consists of 10–20% of the gland.
- Developmentally and functionally, these glands are **two separate endocrine organs**.
    - Adrenal cortex develops from the mesodermal tissue and secretes steroid hormones.
    - Adrenal medulla develops from neuroectodermal tissue related to sympathetic ganglia, and therefore secretes catecholamines.

PY8.2

FUNCTIONAL ANATOMY

Adrenal cortex secretes **three categories of hormones**: glucocorticoids, mineralocorticoids and sex hormones (Table 74.1).

Table 74.1 | Hormones secreted from adrenal cortex.

Hormones
Mineralocorticoids
i) Aldosterone
ii) Deoxycorticosterone
2. Glucocorticoids
i) Cortisol
ii) Corticosterone
3. Sex steroids
i) Dehydroepiandrosterone
ii) Androstenedione

Histology

Adrenal cortex consists of **three layers:** the outer zona glomerulosa that secretes mineralocorticoids, the middle zona fasciculata that secretes glucocorticoids and sex steroids, and the inner zona reticularis that secretes sex steroids and glucocorticoids (Fig. 74.1).

Zona Glomerulosa: This is the outermost and thinnest layer of the gland.

- It constitutes 20% of the adrenal cortex.
- It consists of **small clumps of cells** that contain numerous mitochondria.
- It **secretes mineralocorticoids**, mainly aldosterone.

Zona Fasciculata: This is the middle and **widest layer** of the adrenal cortex.

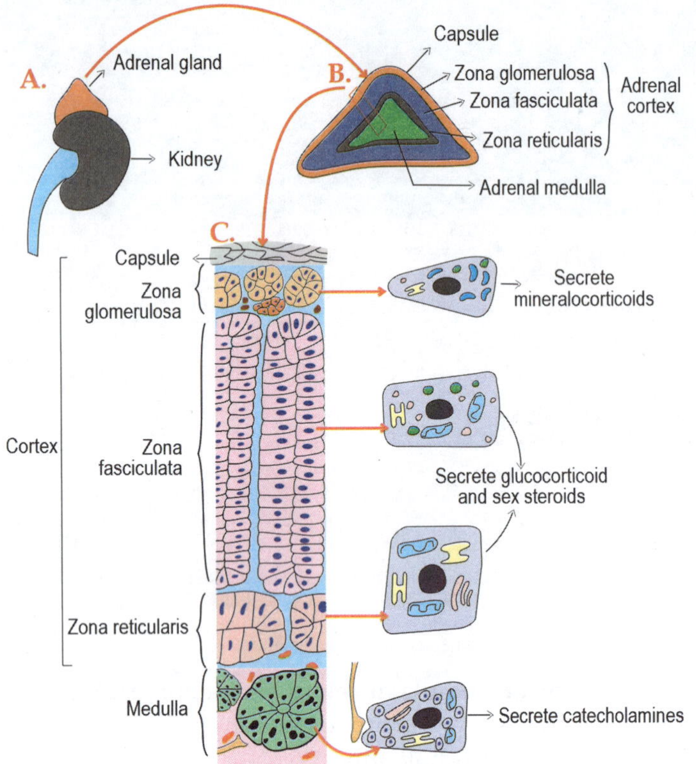

Fig. 74.1 A: Location of adrenal gland; **B:** Parts of adrenal gland as seen in cross section of the gland; **C:** Histology of adrenal gland. Note, zona fasciculata constitutes more than 80% of adrenal cortex

- It constitutes 80% of the adrenocortical mass.
- It consists of **columnar cells that form long cords**.
  - The cytoplasm is loaded with vacuoles and lipid droplets.
  - The ***mitochondria are large*** and contain numerous ***vesicular cristae***.
- Cells of this layer **secrete glucocorticoids** (mainly cortisol and corticosterone) and sex steroids.

Zona Reticularis: This is the innermost layer of the adrenal cortex.

- It constitutes about 10% of its mass.
- It contains **network of intercalated cells**.
  - The mitochondria are large and have vesicular cristae.
  - There are no vacuoles and fat droplets.
- Cells of this layer **secrete sex steroids** like androgens and estrogens, and to some extent also glucocorticoids.

SYNTHESIS & METABOLISM OF ADRENOCORTICAL HORMONES

Adrenocortical steroid hormones are synthesized from **cholesterol**. Cholesterol used for synthesis of steroid hormones in the adrenal cortical cells, are made available from **two sources**: blood, and synthesized de novo.

From Blood: Most of the cholesterol used for biosynthesis of steroid hormones is derived from cholesterol esters attached to the LDL (*LDL-cholesterol*) in circulating blood.

- Cells of adrenal cortex **actively take up cholesterol** from plasma by **endocytosis of LDL molecules**.
- Under basal conditions **plasma cholesterol is the major source** for adrenocortical hormone synthesis.

From Cell Itself (De Novo Synthesis): Cholesterol is synthesized de novo in the cytosol of adrenocortical cells from acetate by the action of the enzyme **HMG CoA reductase**.

- **When hormone synthesis is stimulated by ACTH**, the ***stored cholesterol*** in the cytosol of adrenocortical cells and ***newly formed cholesterol*** in the cytosol become the important source for hormone synthesis.

Role of Cytochrome P-450 Enzymes

The synthesis of hormones from cholesterol involves **cytochrome P-450 enzymes**, also known as CYPs (Table 74.2). These enzymes that **catalyze hydroxylation of steroids**. They are located in the membranes of endoplasmic reticulum and mitochondrial cristae.

- Cytochrome P-450 enzymes for their steroid synthetic actions depend on an extra nuclear receptor, called **steroid factor 1** (SF 1).
- Therefore, when the gene for SF-1 is knocked out, adrenals and gonads do not develop.

Table74.2 | Adrenal steroidogenic enzymes.

Usual name	Old name	New name
Cholesterol side-chain cleaving enzyme	$P450_{SCC}$	CYP11A1
3β hydroxysteroid dehydrogenase	3β-HSD	3β-HSD11
17α-Hydroxylase	$P450_{C17}$	CYP17
21α-Hydroxylase	$P450_{C21}$	CYP21A2
11β –Hydroxylase	$P450_{C11}$	CYP11B1
Aldosterone synthase	$P450_{C11AS}$	CYP11B2

Rate Limiting Step: Once inside mitochondria, cholesterol is converted to **pregnenolone** by cholesterol side-chain cleaving enzyme, also called **cholesterol desmolase** ($P450_{SCC}$) or CYP11A1. This is the **first and rate limiting step** in adrenal steroid synthesis.

Synthesis of Glucocorticoids

Synthesis of glucocorticoids occurs mainly in the **zona fasciculata of adrenal cortex**. Zona reticularis also contributes to this. The main glucocorticoids formed are **cortisol and corticosterone** (Application Box 74.1).

Steps of Cortisol Synthesis

Steps of **cortisol synthesis** are depicted in Flowchart 74.1. **In the mitochondria**, pregnenolone forms **17-hydroxy-pregnenolone** by the enzyme 17α-hydroxylase.

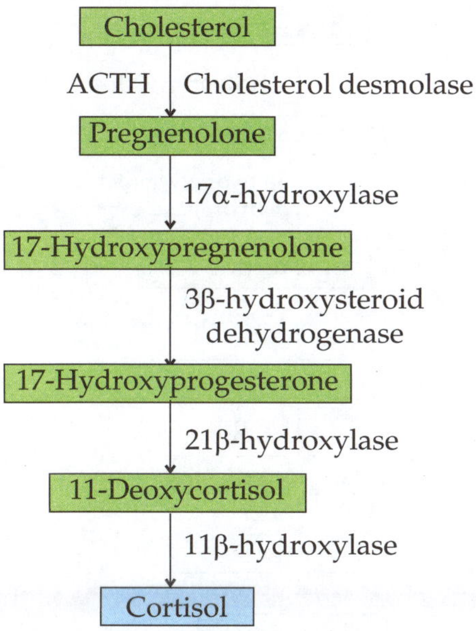

Flowchart 74.1: Steps of cortisol synthesis.

- 17-hydroxypregnenolone then ***moves into endoplasmic reticulum***, where it is converted to **17-hydroxyprogesterone** by 3β-hydroxysteroid dehydrogenase, which in turn is hydroxylated to **11-Deoxycortisol** by 21β-hydroxylase.
- 11-Deoxycortisol then ***moves back to mitochondria*** to be hydroxylated to form cortisol by mitochondrial enzyme 11β-hydroxylase (Fig. 74.2).

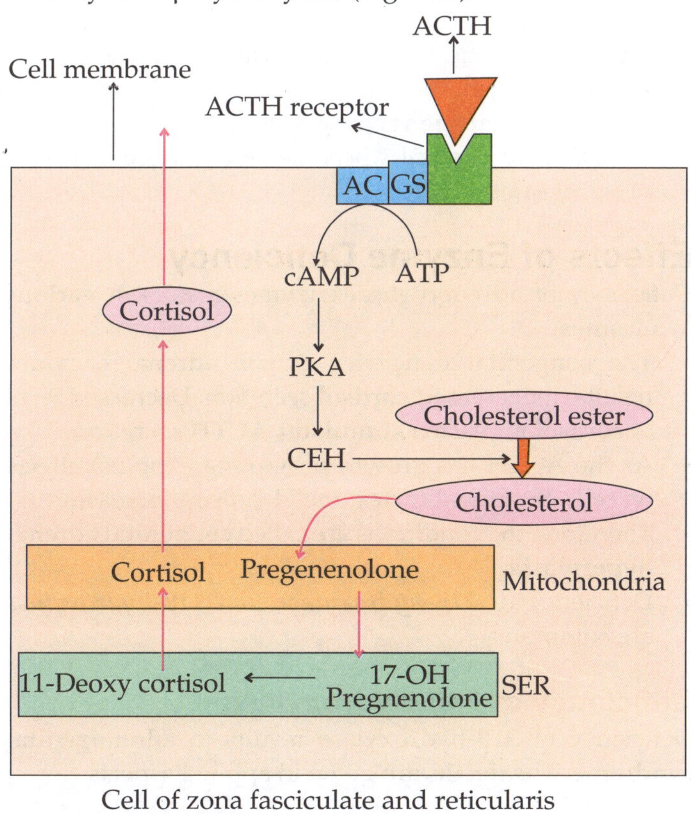

Fig. 74.2: Mechanism of cortisol synthesis. Note, ACTH facilitates cortisol synthesis by activating the enzyme cholesterol ester hydrolase (CEH) that converts cholesterol ester in the cell into cholesterol that enters mitochondria for cortisol synthesis. GS: stimulatory G protein; AC: adenylyl cyclase; PKA: protein kinase A; SER: smooth endoplasmic reticulum.

- ACTH facilitates cortisol synthesis by **increasing the supply of cholesterol** and by converting the **cholesterol to pregnenolone**.

Steps of Corticosterone Synthesis

Steps of **corticosterone synthesis** are depicted in Flowchart 74.2.

The cholesterol is converted to **pregnenolone** by the mitochondrial enzyme cholesterol desmolase.

- Pregnenolone, then moves to endoplasmic reticulum where it is dehydrogenated to form **progesterone** by the enzyme 3β hydroxysteroid dehydrogenase.
- Progesterone is hydroxylated by the 21β-hydroxylase to form **11-deoxycorticosterone**, which then moves back to mitochondria to form **corticosterone** by the enzyme 11β-hydroxylase.

> **Application Box 74.1**
>
> **Glucocorticoid secretion varies in different species:** The **ratio of cortisol to corticosterone** varies from species to species. In rats, mice and birds, corticosterone is the major glucocorticoid. In humans, monkeys and cats, the major glucocorticoid is cortisol. In dogs, cortisol and corticosterone are secreted in equal proportions.

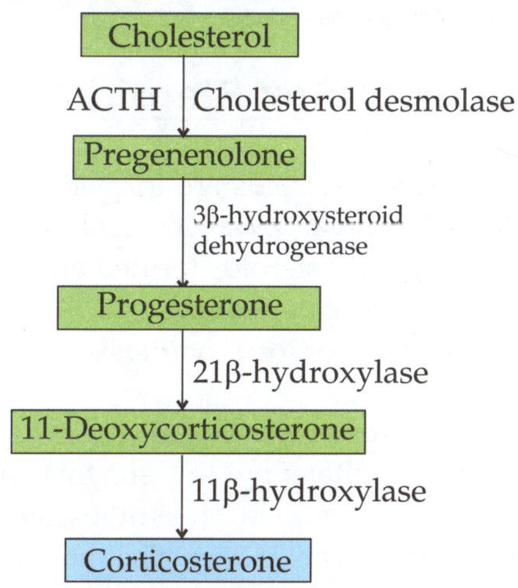

Flowchart 74.2: Steps of corticosterone synthesis.

Synthesis of Mineralocorticoids

Mineralocorticoids are formed in the **zona glomerulosa** of adrenal cortex. Aldosterone is the major mineralocorticoid synthesized in humans.

The steps of **aldosterone synthesis** are depicted in Flowchart 74.3.

The conversion of cholesterol to pregnenolone is **stimulated by ACTH and A II.** The steps till the formation of 11-deoxycorticosterone is same as described above in glucocorticoid synthesis. The rest of the steps of aldosterone synthesis are catalyzed by the enzyme **aldosterone synthase**.

1. *Aldosterone synthase* is found ***only in the cells of zona glomerulosa*** of adrenal cortex. Therefore, aldosterone synthesis is limited to the zona glomerulosa.

2. Zona glomerulosa lacks the enzyme 17α-hydroxylase. Hence, synthesis of glucocorticoid and sex steroid does not occur in this layer of adrenal cortex.

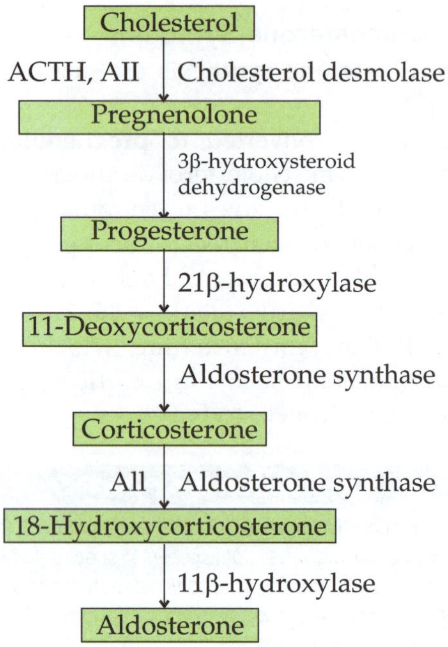

Flowchart 74.3: Steps of aldosterone synthesis.

Synthesis of Sex Steroids

In adrenal cortex, sex steroids are formed mainly in the **zona reticularis**. However, zona glomerulosa also contributes to it. The major sex steroids formed are **dehydroepiandrosterone and androstenedione**.

The steps of **androstenedione synthesis** are depicted in Flowchart 74.4.

1. **Dehydroepiandrosterone** is converted to dehydroepiandrosterone sulfate by the enzyme sulfokinase. Though, androstenedione is synthesized from dehydroepiandrosterone, it can also be formed from **17-OH-progesterone.**
2. Androstenedione is then converted to **testosterone**, which later forms estradiol.

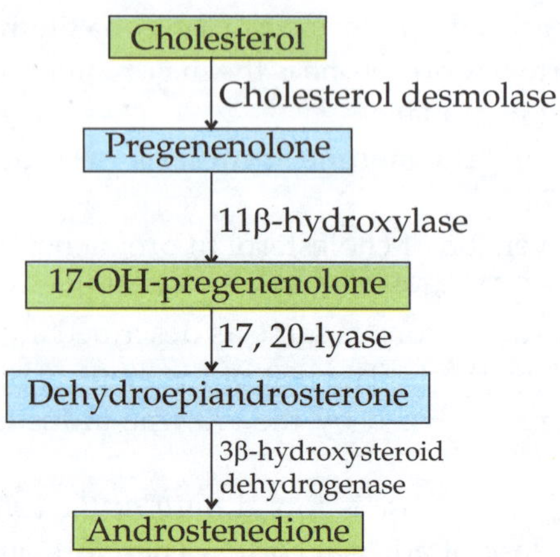

Flowchart 74.4: Steps of androstenedione synthesis.

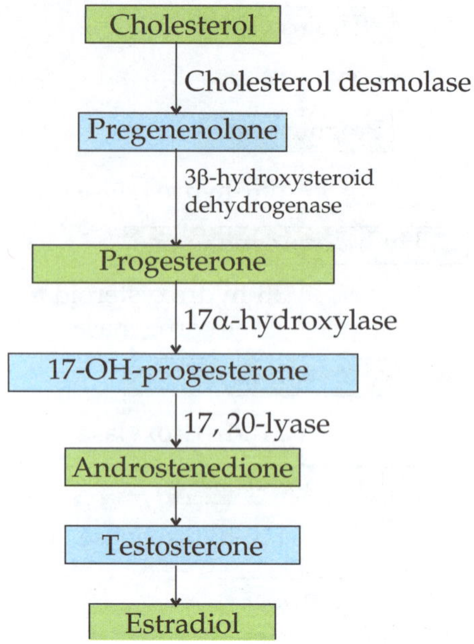

Flowchart 74.5: Steps of estradiol synthesis.

The steps of **estradiol synthesis** are depicted in Flowchart 74.5.

In Woman: In woman, adrenal gland supplies about **50–60% of the androgenic hormones**.

- The **adrenal androgen is not important in males** because the testes produce testosterone. Similarly, the conversion of androgen to estrogen in the adrenal cortex in females is not important because ovaries secrete estrogen.
- However, **after menopause** secretion of *estrogen from adrenal gland in females* becomes the important ***source of estrogenic activity***.

Effects of Enzyme Deficiency

Deficiency of adrenocortical enzymes results in **various syndromes**.

- The congenital deficiency of the adrenal enzymes results in **decreased cortisol** secretion. Decreased level of cortisol in plasma **stimulates ACTH secretion**.
- As the ACTH has growth promoting (trophic) effects on cells of adrenal cortex, the gland size increases.
- Therefore, the conditions are called **congenital adrenal hyperplasia**.
- Deficiency of ***21β-hydroxylase and 11β-hydroxylase*** are common.

Deficiency of 21β-Hydroxylase

Deficiency of 21β-hydroxylase results in **adrenogenital syndrome**. The details are given in applied aspects.

Deficiency of 11β-hydroxylase

In 11β-hydroxylase deficiency, **increased production of androgen** is associated with increased secretion of **11-deoxycortisol and 11-deoxycorticosterone.**

- The 11-deoxycorticosterone is a **mineralocorticoid**.
- Thus, excess mineralocorticoid activity increases **retention of Na^+ and water**.

Hypertensive Congenital Virilizing Adrenal Hyperplasia: Due to retention of Na^+ and water, patient develops **hypertension** in addition to virilization, called as **hypertensive form of congenital virilizing adrenal hyperplasia**.

Treatment: In all virilizing forms of adrenal hyperplasia, **glucocorticoid therapy** is preferred.

- Exogenously administered glucocorticoid fills the endogenous cortisol deficit, and also suppresses the production of ACTH.
- Thus, ACTH induced excess production of sex steroid is decreased.

Deficiency of 17α-hydroxylase

This is a rare condition. It results in **decreased production of sex steroids**.

- Therefore, **female external genitalia** are present.
- However, as the production of aldosterone and corticosterone is normal, elevated level of mineralocorticoids result in **hypertension and hyperkalemia**.

3β-hydroxysteroid dehydrogenase

This is also a rare condition, in which **production of dehydroepiandrosterone is increased**.

- There is some degree of **masculinization in females**.
    - But, as dehydroepiandrosterone is a weak androgen, it does not cause full masculinization of the genitalia in genetic males.
- Therefore, **hypospadias** (urethral opening on the undersurface of the penis) develops.

Cholesterol desmolase deficiency

Deficiency of the cholesterol side-chain cleaving enzyme **decreases production of all adrenocortical hormones** as it converts cholesterol to pregnenolone, the first step in steroidogenesis.

- The condition is **fatal during fetal life**. This condition is very rare.

Metabolism of Adrenocortical Hormones

Normal Secretion

The daily secretion and plasma concentration of adrenocortical hormones are listed in Table 74.3.

Table74.3 | Daily secretion and plasma concentration of adrenocortical steroids.

Hormone	Daily secretion (mg/24h)	Average plasma conc. (μg/dL)
Cortisol	10–15	14
Corticosterone	2–4	0.5
Aldosterone	0.1–0.2	0.0006
Deoxycorticosterone	0.2–0.25	0.0006
Dehydroepiandrosterone	20–25	175

Plasma Protein Binding

Adrenocortical steroids usually bind with proteins such as transcortin and albumin.

Transcortin Binding

About **80% of adrenal steroids**, especially cortisol and corticosterone bind with a plasma protein called **transcortin**, or **corticosteroid binding globulin** (CBG). The transcortin is a glycoprotein produced by liver. The normal plasma concentration of transcortin is **3 mg/dL.**

- The concentration **increases in pregnancy and estrogen therapy**.
    - When transcortin level increases, the quantity of hormone binding to it increases that in turn **decreases free cortisol level**.
- The decreased free hormone **increases ACTH secretion**, which consequently increases cortisol secretion.
    - However, a **new state** is reached at which the bound form is increased, but the **free form remains normal**.
- Thus, the **total hormone concentration increases without changing** *the concentration of the free form*.
    - Therefore, **in pregnancy features of cortisol excess do not appear** inspite of increased total cortisol level.

Albumin Binding

About **10–15% of cortisol** is bound to albumin. Thus, only 5–10% of cortisol is free in the plasma.

IMPORTANT NOTE

Half-life of cortisol is more: Because of its protein (TBG+albumin) binding, the **half-life of cortisol is more** (60–90 min), its concentration as free hormone in plasma is less and its excretion in urine is less.

- As binding of aldosterone to protein is less, the **half-life of aldosterone is less** (about 20 min).

Metabolic Degradation

Cortisol is **metabolized in liver**, where it is reduced to **dihydrocortisol and tetrahydrocortisol glucuronides**. The tetrahydroglucuronide derivative cortisol and corticosterone are **water soluble**, and therefore is **rapidly excreted in urine** (Flowchart 74.6).

IMPORTANT NOTE

Urinary Metabolites are Indices of Cortisol Secretion: The free cortisol circulating in the plasma is filtered by kidney and about 50μg is excreted in the urine. Therefore, measurement of **urinary metabolite of cortisol provides a reliable index of cortisol secretion**.

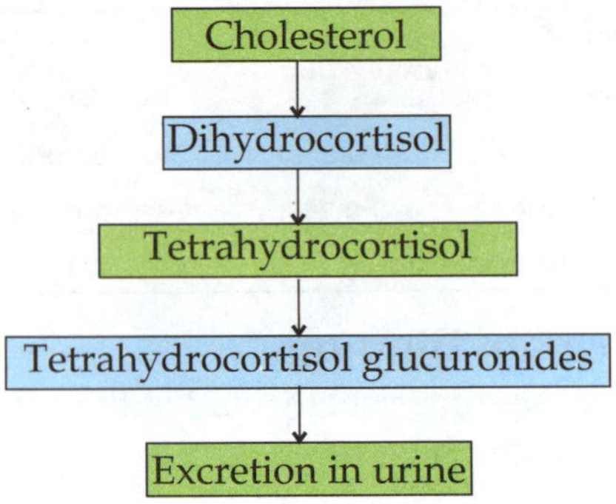

Flowchart 74.6: Steps of metabolic degradation of cortisol

- The excretion of **17-hydroxycorticoids** represents about 50% of the total daily cortisol secretion. Normally 2–12 mg of 17-hydroxycorticoids is excreted per day.
- The precursors of cortisol (progesterone and 17-OH-progesterone) are metabolized to *pregnanediol and pregnanetriol*.
- **In adult females,** urinary excretion of these metabolites reflects the ***activities of ovarian-adrenal axis***. However, their increased urinary concentration **in pre-pubertal girls** indicates specific **congenital defect in cortisol secretion** (due to disease of the adrenal cortex, not the ovary).

17-Ketosteroids

17-Ketosteroid derivative is **formed in the liver from cortisol**. However, corticosterone does not form 17-ketosteroid. **Dehydroepiandrosterone**, the major adrenal androgen is a 17-ketosteroid. **Testosterone** is converted to 17-ketosteroid.

- **Etiocholanolone,** a metabolite of adrenal androgens and testosterone, forms 17-ketosteroid.
- 17-ketosteroid is **excreted in the urine**.
- Normally, 5–10 mg of 17-ketosteroids in women, and 8–20 mg of 17-ketosteroids in men is excreted in urine per day.
- About **70% of this amount** excreted is normally derived ***from adrenal cortex*** and 30% from the gonadal androgens.
- When they accumulate in blood, they cause episodic fever known as **Etiocholanolone Fever**.

GLUCOCORTICOIDS

Regulation of Secretion

Glucocorticoid secretion is controlled mainly by **feedback mechanisms of ACTH secretion**. Angiotensin II and other hormones also contribute.

Role of ACTH

This **circadian rhythm** (the diurnal variation) of ACTH secretion (refer Fig. 71.12, Chapter 71) is an important regulator of cortisol secretion. Therefore, **cortisol secretion**

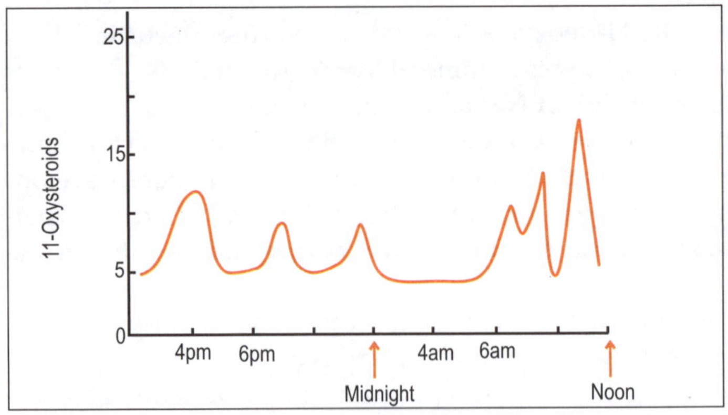

Fig. 74.3: Circadian variation in cortisol secretion. Note, it closely follows the pattern of ACTH secretion as depicted in Fig. 44.11 (in Chapter 70). 11-Oxysteroid is the plasma cortisol estimated (Duration of the night is trauncated in the time scale).

also has a definite pattern that follows the pattern of ACTH secretion (Fig. 74.3).

Feedback Control

Glucocorticoid secretion is controlled by feedback release of **ACTH** from the anterior pituitary.

- ACTH secretion is stimulated by **CRH** (corticotropin releasing hormone) secreted from the hypothalamus CRH secretion is influenced by various stimuli originating from the limbic system, pain pathways, NTS, reticular formation and suprachiasmatic nucleus (Fig. 74.4).

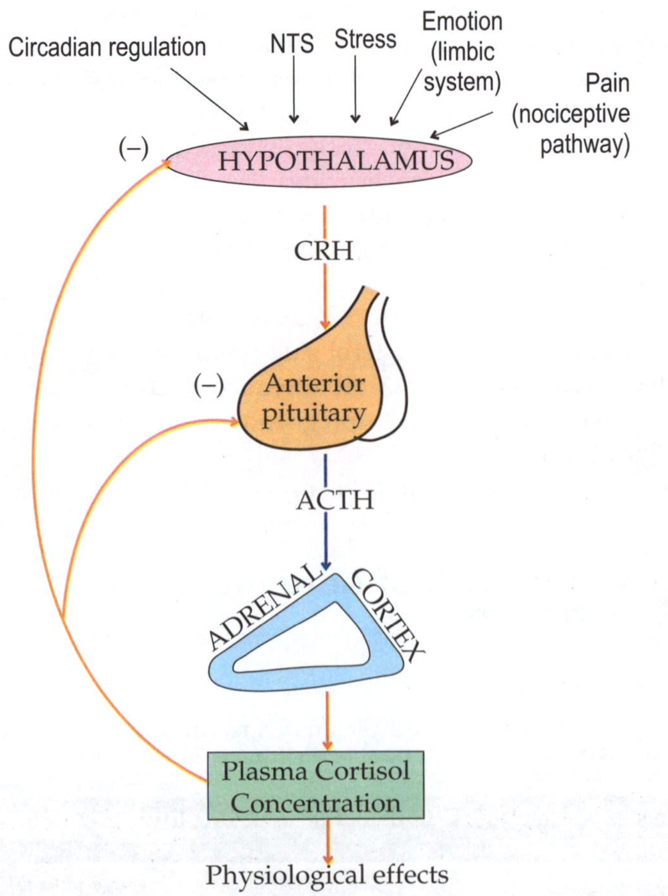

Fig. 74.4: Regulation of cortisol secretion. NTS: nucleus tractus solitarius. Minus sign indicates inhibition.

Clinical Note 74.1

Steroid therapy should not be stopped abruptly: A patient receiving steroid for a long time should not stop the medicine abruptly. After a prolonged treatment with steroid, the adrenal cortex atrophies and becomes unresponsive to the ACTH for about six months. Also, pituitary secretes less ACTH initially, due to its diminished synthesis. However, pituitary recovers and secretes more ACTH thereafter.

- Increased level of ACTH slowly stimulates adrenal cortex to secrete glucocorticoids and it takes about eight to ten months for cortisol level to return to normal plasma level (**Fig. 74.5**).
- ACTH, from its level also returns to normal in about ten months.
- Thus, **pituitary-adrenocortical axis takes about ten months** to recover from the suppressive effect of prolonged steroid therapy.
- During this period, the individual fails to cope with stress and **may succumb to stressful situations.**

To prevent such a dangerous complication, steroids should not be stopped abruptly after a prolonged therapy; rather the dose should be decreased gradually over weeks before finally stopping the treatment.

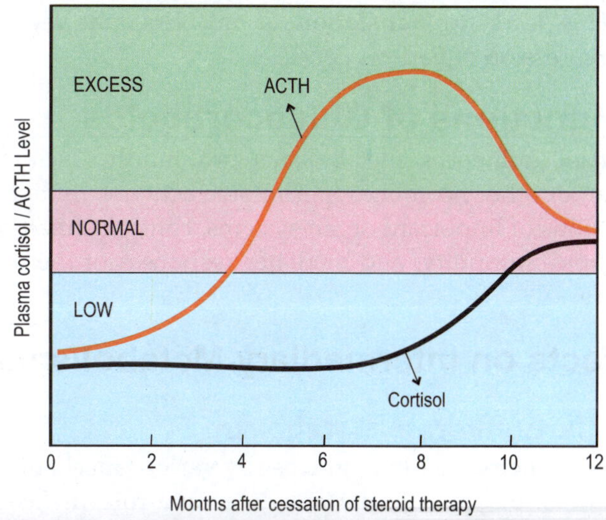

Fig. 74.5: Pattern of plasma level of cortisol and ACTH following cessation of high dose steroid therapy given for a longer duration. Note, cortisol takes about 8 to 10 months to return to normal, though ACTH secretion recovers early. This is the period during which the subject is vulnerable to collapse on exposure to stress; therefore, steroid therapy is advised to be withdrawn slowly over a period of months instead of stopping abruptly.

- **CRH increases ACTH secretion**, which in turn increases glucocorticoid secretion from the adrenal cortex.
- **Increased glucocorticoid** level in plasma provides **negative feedback signal to the hypothalamus and anterior pituitary** to inhibit the secretion of CRH and ACTH respectively.
- Thus, cortisol secretion returns to normal.
- Conversely, **decreased glucocorticoid** secretion increases CRH and ACTH release by feedback mechanisms that tend to increase the secretion of cortisol (Clinical Note 74.1).

In Stress

In stress, increased cortisol secretion occurs mainly due to **increased hypothalamic release of CRH**.

- Fibers projecting from limbic system, especially from amygdala to hypothalamus (amygdalo-hypothalamic pathway) mediate the responses to **emotional stress**, fear, and anxiety.
- Ascending nociceptive fibers give collaterals to hypothalamus and they mediate the **stress response to painful stimuli** or injury.

Angiotensin II

Normally, angiotensin II is an important stimulator for aldosterone secretion. However, it also induces glucocorticoid secretion.

Other Hormones

ADH, serotonin, and VIP also stimulate glucocorticoid secretion. But their role in the physiologic regulation of glucocorticoid secretion is not clearly known.

Mechanism of Action

Cortisol takes few hours to days to exert its effect.

1. It diffuses into the cell and binds with the **glucocorticoid receptors (GR) present in the cytoplasm**.
2. Binding of cortisol with the receptor displaces the inhibitory heat shock protein complex from the receptor.
3. This results in alteration in the receptor configuration and causes **hyperphosphorylation** of the receptor.
4. Then, the hormone-receptor complex enters the nucleus, where it binds with the specific **glucocorticoid regulatory elements** (GRE) on the target DNA molecule (Fig. 74.6).

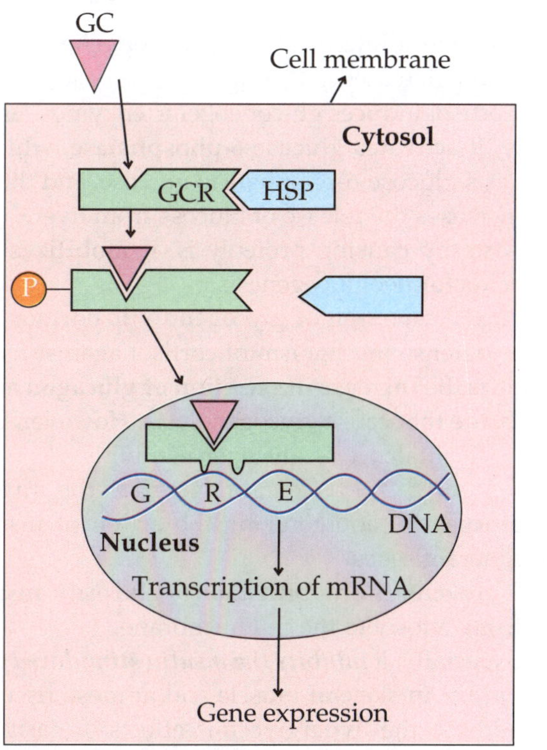

Fig. 74.6: Mechanism of cortisol action. GC: glucocorticoid; GCR: glucocorticoid receptor; HSP: heat shock protein; P: phosphorylation of hormone-receptor complex; GRE: glucocorticoid response element.

5. This leads to **translation of mRNAs** that regulate expression of various genes.

Functions of Glucocorticoids

Cortisol influences metabolisms profoundly, facilitates action of other hormones (permissive actions), influences functions of important organ systems, controls inflammation and immunity, and mediates responses of the body to stress.

Effects on Intermediary Metabolisms

On Carbohydrate Metabolism

Cortisol increases blood glucose by various mechanisms, and thus, plays an **important defensive role in fasting** and against **hypoglycemia induced by insulin.**

- Glucocorticoid is **essential for survival during fasting** (Clinical Note 74.2).
- In prolonged fasting, the liver glycogen store is depleted and unless there is gluconeogenesis, death occurs due to hypoglycemia.

> **Clinical Note 74.2**
>
> **Adrenal-deficient patients should not fast:** In adrenal insufficiency, blood glucose remains normal so long as the food intake is normal. However, fasting induced hypoglycemia becomes fatal in such patients, as cortisol defense of hypoglycemia is lacking. Therefore, patients suffering from adrenocortical insufficiency are advised not to fast.

Cortisol increases plasma glucose by following mechanisms:

1. **Cortisol stimulates hepatic gluconeogenesis:** Cortisol secretion increases in fasting.
   - Cortisol induces gluconeogenic enzymes. Especially, it **activates glucose-6-phosphatase**, which converts glucose-6-phophate to glucose, and therefore, increases the release of glucose from liver.
   - Also, by causing proteolysis, it **mobilizes amino acids** for neoglucogenesis.
2. **Increased secretion of glycogenolytic hormones:** Another defense mechanism of cortisol against hypoglycemia is the **increase in secretion of glucagon and epinephrine** that cause glycogenolysis. However, cortisol per se facilitates liver glycogen synthesis.
3. **Anti-insulin effect:** Cortisol **decreases the utilization of glucose** by antagonizing the action of insulin on peripheral tissues.
   - It **prevents the mobilization of glucose transporters** from cytosol to the cell membrane.
   - Especially, it ***inhibits the insulin stimulated glucose uptake*** in skeletal muscle and adipose tissue. This adds to the hyperglycemic effects of cortisol and makes diabetes worse (Clinical Note 74.3).
   - It also **reverses insulin suppression** of hepatic glucose production.

> **Clinical Note 74.3**
>
> **Cortisol complicates diabetes:** In normal individuals, rise in blood glucose by cortisol increases insulin secretion, which counteracts ketone bodies and lipids raised by the cortisol. In diabetes, cortisol effects on ketone body and lipid remain unaffected as insulin is lacking. Thus, excess cortisol makes the diabetes worse by promoting ketoacidosis.

On Protein Metabolism

Cortisol **facilitates proteolysis**, especially in skeletal muscle, and ***inhibits protein synthesis***.

- It **mobilizes muscle protein** for gluconeogenesis. The overall action is to **facilitate the conversion of protein to glycogen**.
- The chronic administration of cortisol or excess secretion of glucocorticoid causes **depletion of protein storage** in the body, especially in the muscle, bone, skin, and connective tissue.

On Fat Metabolism

Cortisol causes **lipolysis**. In fact, the **lipolytic effect of epinephrine** and growth hormone requires cortisol (permissive action).

- During fasting, by **promoting lipolysis**, cortisol causes rapid release of free fatty acid and glycerol from adipose tissues, which are utilized for gluconeogenesis.
- Increased free fatty acid formation **promotes ketogenesis**, especially in diabetes.

On Food Intake & Fat Distribution

Cortisol **increases appetite** and food intake by *stimulating* ***neuropeptide Y secretion*** from the hypothalamus.

1. It stimulates differentiation of pre-adipocytes to adipocytes in the adipose tissue.
2. It also **stimulates lipogenesis** by activating lipoprotein lipase and glucose-6-phosphate dehydrogenase activity of the adipocytes in some other parts of the body.
   - Therefore, the action of cortisol **varies from tissues to tissues**.
3. Thus, cortisol excess causes **maldistribution of fat** in the body that result in **truncal obesity, moon face and buffalo hump** with thinning of extremities.
   - The exact cause of peculiar distribution of fat is not known, but it is ***associated with insulin resistance*** and/or increase in insulin level.
4. Cortisol also **increases leptin synthesis** in adipose tissue.
   - Therefore, obesity is restricted by the ***negative feedback actions of leptin*** (leptin inhibits feeding).

To summarize the effect of cortisol on metabolisms, it is an important **diabetogenic, ketogenic, and anti-insulin hormone** (Flowchart 74.7).

Permissive Actions of Cortisol

Glucocorticoid is essential (even in small quantity) for some **physiological actions of other hormones to take**

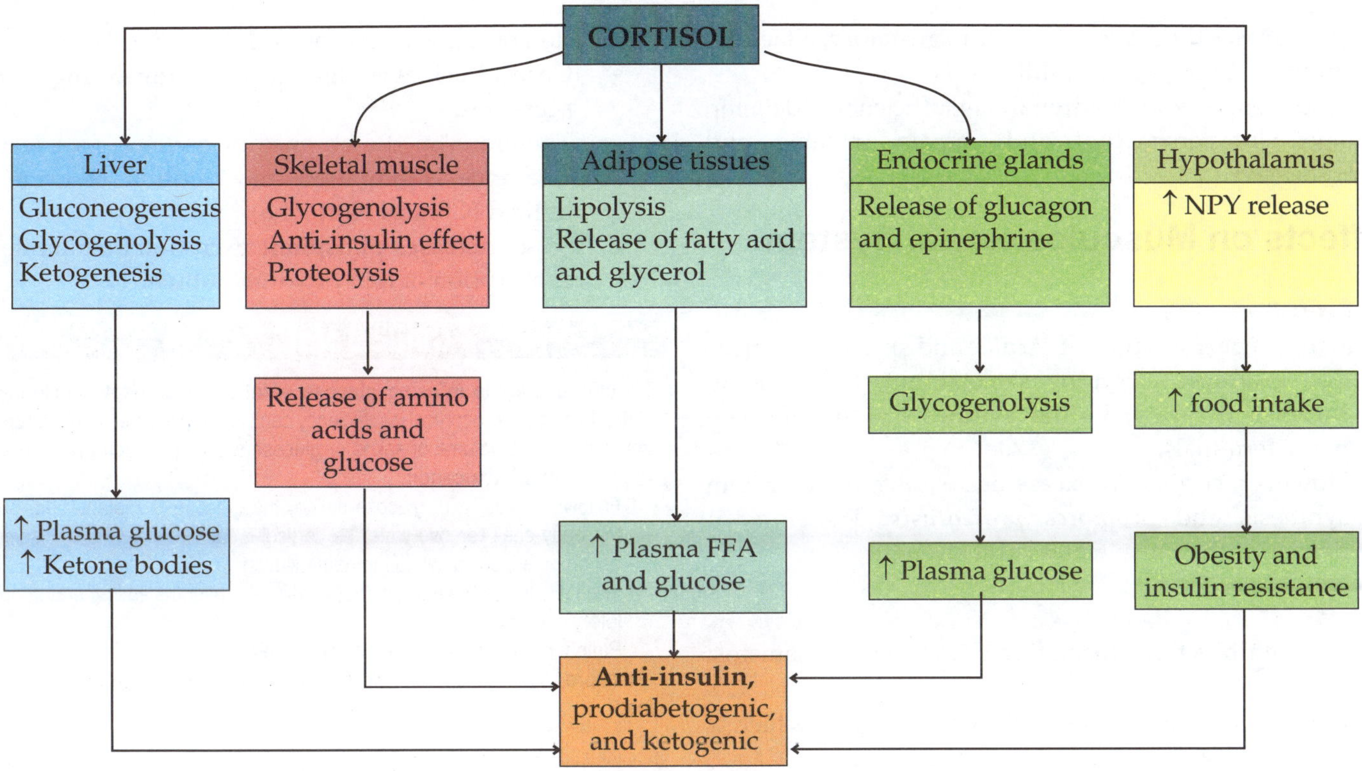

Flowchart 74.7: Summary of metabolic actions of cortisol.

place. This is called *permissive action* (as cortisol permits the specific actions of these hormones to occur, though it does not produce these effects by itself).

Permissive actions of cortisol include:

1. **Vasopressor and bronchodilator effects** of catecholamines.
2. **Calorigenic effects** of glucagon and catecholamines.
3. **Lipolytic effects** of catecholamines.
4. Development of ***mammary gland*** during puberty, in females.
5. Development of **hepatic enzyme systems** during fetal life.
6. **Surfactant synthesis** in the fetal lung and maturation of lungs during intrauterine life.
7. Development of **bacterial flora and enzyme** systems in the intestine.

Effects on Cardiovascular System

On Heart

Cortisol **increases myocardial performance** by increasing **Na^+–K^+ ATPase activity** and also by increasing **expression of β-adrenergic receptors** in the heart.

On Blood Vessels

Cortisol maintains **vascular reactivity**. This is an important action of cortisol. It increases the **responsiveness of arterioles to catecholamines and angiotensin II**.

1. Probably, this action is mediated by **inhibition of Na^+-Ca^{++} exchanger** in the cell membrane so that the Ca^{++} concentration is maintained in the blood vessel smooth muscle cells.
2. Cortisol also **decreases the release of vasodilators** like prostaglandins.

In adrenal insufficiency, blood vessels become unresponsive to catecholamines (Clinical Note 74.4). This **promotes vascular collapse**, as already hypovolemia exists in such patients.

Clinical Note 74.4

Injection of cortisol is a must in shock: Injection of catecholamines in hypovolemic shock is required to restore blood pressure, as they cause vasoconstriction and increase cardiac output. However, it is essential to inject cortisol along with catecholamines as it maintains vascular reactivity.

- Also, cortisol mediates responsiveness of catecholamines to vasoconstrictors by its permissive action.
- Catecholamine injection without administration of cortisol in shock does not ensure adequate vasoconstriction and blood pressure continues to remains low.

Effects on Central Nervous System

Cortisol influences the **mood and behavior of individuals**. There are abundant glucocorticoid receptors (both type I and type II) in limbic system including prefrontal cortex.

1. Cortisol **decreases REM sleep** but increases the slow wave sleep.
   - The increased level of cortisol in plasma can cause insomnia.
2. It causes both elevation and depression of mood, and **impairs memory**.

3. It **decreases the responsiveness** to gustatory, olfactory, auditory, and visual stimuli.

The patients with adrenal insufficiency develop changes in personality, and remain irritable and apprehensive.

Effects on Musculoskeletal System

On Muscle

It **increases performance** of cardiac and skeletal muscle.

- The **inotropic effect** on skeletal muscle is due to **increase in acetylcholine synthesis** at the muscle-nerve terminals.
- However, cortisol **in excess** decreases muscle protein synthesis and ***promotes proteolysis***. Therefore, it **decreases the muscle mass and strength**.

On Bone

Cortisol **inhibits bone formation** by various mechanisms:

1. It **decreases the synthesis of type-I collagen**, which is a fundamental component of bone matrix.
2. It **inhibits the conversion** of *osteoprogenitor cells to the osteoblasts*.
3. It **decreases absorption of Ca^{++}** from GI tract (by inhibiting the effect of vitamin D on GIT). It also ***decreases the synthesis of active vitamin D***.
   - Thus, it decreases supply of Ca^{++} to the bones, which is essential for bone mineralization.
4. Cortisol also **facilitates bone resorption**.

The overall effects are **decreased bone mass and mineralization**. Therefore, prolonged administration of cortisol may cause **osteoporosis** (Clinical Note 74.5).

Clinical Note 74.5

Bone x-ray should be done to check complications: Cortisol decreases bone mass and promotes osteoporosis. Even, vertebral collapse may occur. Therefore, patients receiving steroid for a longer period should be checked for osteoporotic changes by taking bone X-rays or MRI, especially in elderly patients.

Effects on Connective Tissue

Cortisol **inhibits collagen synthesis**. Therefore, it decreases skin thickness and causes **thinning of capillary walls**.

- The **capillaries become fragile** (susceptible to rupture).
- Thus, ***intracutaneous hemorrhage*** occurs in cortisol excess.

Effects on Kidney and Water Metabolism

Cortisol **increases GFR** by increasing glomerular blood flow.

- It is essential for the **rapid clearance of a water load** (fast excretion of water from the body) as happens in infusion of saline or glucose solution.
  - Cortisol achieves this partly by **inhibiting ADH secretion**.
  - Therefore, in the absence of cortisol, **free water clearance is impaired** and dilution of urine is limited (Clinical Note 74.6).
- It also **increases phosphate excretion** by inhibiting reabsorption of it in proximal tubule.

Clinical Note 74.6

Be cautious while infusing glucose solution in cortisol deficiency: Patients with adrenocortical insufficiency can't excrete a water load. Sudden infusion of large volume of saline or glucose solution in such patient may result in **water intoxication**.

- Following infusion of glucose saline, the glucose is metabolized, but the body can't remove water as cortisol is lacking. Therefore, plasma becomes hypoosmolal due to hemodilution.
- The cells in the brain swell, that impairs the hypothalamic thermoregulatory centers.
- Patient develops high fever and collapses.

Therefore, such patients should receive cortisol while receiving a water load.

Apparent Mineralocorticoid Excess

In the absence or deficiency of 11β-OH-steroid dehydrogenase type-2 (that converts cortisol into cortisone), **cortisol has marked mineralocorticoid activity** (Table 74.4), which causes hyperaldosteronism like situation due to action of cortisol on mineralocorticoid receptors.

- The patient develops clinical features of **hyperaldosteronism**, though the **plasma aldosterone and plasma renin activity remain low**.
  - Hence, the condition is called **apparent mineralocorticoid excess.**
- It may occur due to congenital deficiency of the hormone or ingestion of licorice.
- **Licorice** contains glycyrrhetinic acid that inhibits 11β-OH-steroid dehydrogenase type-2. Persons consuming large quantity of licorice may also **develop hypertension** as sodium absorption through ENaC (epithelial sodium channel) in kidney is high.

Table 74.4 | Mineralocorticoid & glucocorticoid activities of various naturally occurring steroids in comparison to cortisol (considering cortisol effect as 1).

Steroid	Mineralocorticoid activity	Glucocorticoid activity
Cortisol	1	1
Corticosterone	15	0.3
Aldosterone	3000	0.3
Deoxycorticosterone	100	0.2
Cortisone	0.8	0.7

Effects on Fetus

Cortisol imparts profound influence on fetal maturation.

1. Cortisol causes **maturation of CNS** during intrauterine life.
2. It causes **growth of retina, GI tract, lungs, and skin** of the fetus.
3. The **intestinal enzyme system** of fetal pattern to the postnatal or adult pattern is altered by cortisol, which is essential for disaccharides to be digested by the infants.
4. Cortisol causes **lung development**.
   - It promotes growth of alveoli and causes flattening of alveolar epithelial cells. Cortisol also facilitates **pulmonary surfactant synthesis**.
   - All these actions allow the fetal lung to satisfactorily expand at the first breath.

Effects on Blood Cells

Though, cortisol influences all the three formed elements of blood, the impact is more on leucocytes.

On Leucocytes

Cortisol causes leucocytosis. Though it causes mild neutrophilia and monocytosis, it causes profound **lymphocytopenia, eosinopenia and basopenia**.

Causes of lymphocytopenia:

1. Cortisol decreases circulating lymphocyte count by **decreasing mitotic activity of lymphocyte precursors.**
2. It decreases the size of lymph nodes and thymus.
3. It **decreases the ability** of lymphocytes and monocytes **to secrete cytokines** that are essential for proliferation of lymphocytes.

Causes of eosinopenia:

1. Cortisol causes eosinopenia by **stimulating apoptosis** (programmed cell death) of eosinophil.
2. By **inhibiting the release of cytokines**, it prevents eosinophil growth.
3. It facilitates **sequestration of eosinophil** in spleen and lungs (thus, decreases the peripheral eosinophil count).

On RBC

It causes **mild erythrocytosis** by stimulating erythropoietin production.

On Platelets

It produces **mild thrombocytosis**.

Effects on Inflammation

Cortisol has profound **anti-inflammatory and anti-allergic actions**. Inflammatory responses (rubor, calor, dolor and tumor) are mediated by various chemicals like prostaglandins, thromboxanes, leukotrienes, kinins, histamine, serotonin, lymphokines, EDRF and PAF (platelet activating factor).

Cortisol interferes in **most of the mechanisms** of inflammation (Flowchart 74.8).

1. **Inhibits Chemical Mediators:** Cortisol **inhibits synthesis** of chemical mediators of inflammation.
   - It stimulates synthesis of **lipocortins** (a family of phosphoproteins) in the target cells.
   - Lipocortin **inhibits the activity of phospholipase** A_2; therefore, **decreases the release of arachidonic acid**, which is the precursor for many mediators of inflammation like prostaglandins, thromboxanes, leukotrienes, etc.
   - Thus, cortisol **prevents the formation of these mediators** of inflammation.
2. **Stabilizes Membrane:** Cortisol **stabilizes the lysosomal membrane**.
   - Therefore, it **decreases release of proteolytic enzymes** *and hyaluronidase* from lysosomes that are required for inflammatory reactions to occur.
3. **Inhibits Mast Cells**: Cortisol inhibits mast cell activity.
   - It **prevents differentiation and proliferation** of mast cells.
   - Consequently, it **decreases the release of histamine**, an important mediator of inflammation (histamine causes vasodilation and increases capillary permeability).
4. **Inhibits Leucocyte Functions**: Cortisol inhibits functions of leucocyte.
   - It **prevents migration** of leucocytes to the site of inflammation or infection.
   - It **prevents the margination of leucocytes and adherence of leucocytes** to the capillary endothelial wall.
   - Cortisol **inhibits the expression of receptors** in the endothelial cells that normally causes chemotactic peptides to interact with leucocytes to stick to the vessel endothelium.
5. **Inhibits Neutrophil Phagocytosis:** Cortisol **inhibits phagocytic and bactericidal** activity of neutrophils.
   - Though cortisol causes mild neutrophilia, it actually decreases the activity of leucocytes.
6. **Inhibits Fibroblasts**: Cortisol **inhibits proliferation of fibroblasts**.
   - Thus, it ***decreases the synthesis and deposition of fibrils*** at the site of inflammation. This forms the basis of chronic anti-inflammatory action of cortisol to injury.
   - Cortisol **prevents walling off in a chronic infection**.
7. **Inhibits NF_kB:** Cortisol inhibits **nuclear factor-$_k$B.**

Recent evidences suggest that a transcription factor, called **nuclear factor-$_k$B** (NF_kB), plays an important role in inflammation.

- Normally, NF-$_k$B is **bound to** another cytoplasmic

protein called I_kB_α, and this binding ***keeps NF-$_k$B in an inactive state.***
  - Viruses and cytokines that induce inflammation **separate NF-$_k$B from I_kB_α** by activating I_KB kinase.
  - NF-$_k$B then **migrates to nucleus** and attaches with the DNA.
  - This induces the **transcription of genes** for formation of various chemicals that participate in inflammation.
- Thus, NF-$_k$B stimulates synthesis and secretion of mediators of inflammation.
- Glucocorticoids **increase the production of I_kB_α** in the cell, and therefore, **prevent the activation of NF-$_k$B.** This is suggested to be the *primary mechanism of anti-inflammatory actions* of cortisol (Flowchart 74.8).

Nevertheless, the physician should be cautious for use of cortisol to prevent inflammation (Clinical Note 74.7)

Effects on Allergy

Cortisol has intense **anti-allergic effects**. Allergy occurs due to antigen-antibody reaction that stimulates the release of histamine from mast cells.

The **antiallergy effects** of cortisol include the following:

Clinical Note 74.7

Cortisol should be given with antibiotics: For its strong anti-inflammatory properties, cortisol is very often prescribed for the treatment of inflammatory diseases. However, it should not be prescribed for treating acute inflammations due to infections.

- If cortisol is given in infections, the toxic features of infection dramatically disappear due to its anti-inflammatory actions. This may give the wrong impression that the infection has subsided.
- But, actually infection spreads as cortisol suppresses immunity (discussed below).
- Thus, cortisol in such conditions masks the actual disease and delays the diagnosis.
- Moreover, it also aggravates the disease, which may become fatal.

Therefore, cortisol is usually not be prescribed in acute infections. However, if situation warrants cortisol treatment in such conditions, it should always be prescribed with appropriate and adequate antibiotics..

1. Cortisol inhibits degranulation of mast cells, and therefore, **prevents release of histamine.**
2. It also **prevents the growth of mast cells.**

Thus, cortisol strongly prevents allergic reactions. Therefore, cortisol is used frequently for the treatment of allergy both locally and systemically.

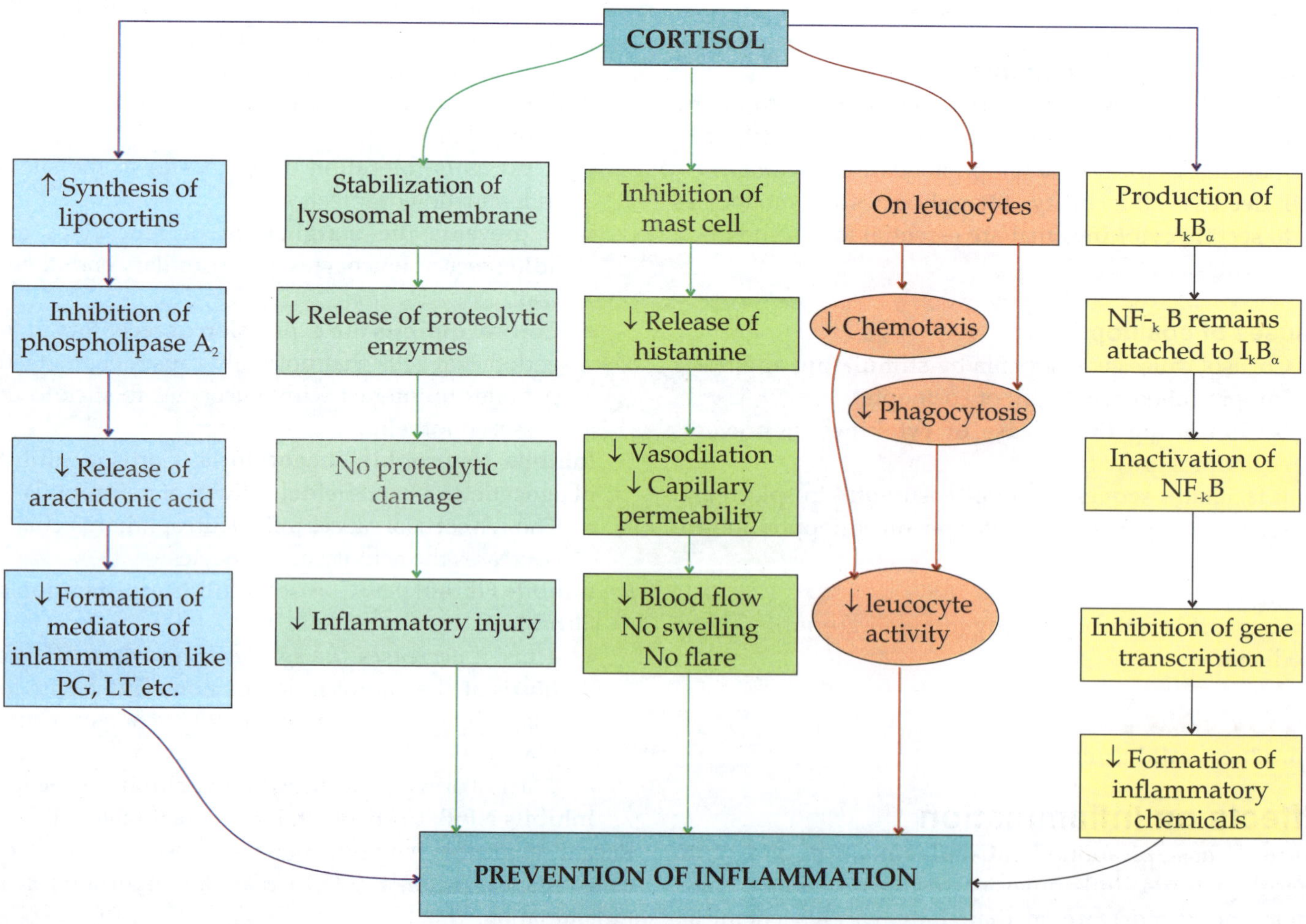

Flowchart 74.8: Mechanism of anti-inflammatory actions of cortisol. PG: prostaglandins, LT: leukotrienes; IkBα: A cytoplasmic protein; NFk-B: Nuclear factor-kB.

IMPORTANT NOTE

Use & Misuse of Steroids: Steroids are used in the treatment of various diseases for their anti-inflammatory, immunosuppressive, antiallergic, metabolic and permissive actions.

However, they are **also misused** by some sportspersons and others.

The usual **synthetic steroids in use** are:

1. **Prednisolone:** It has predominantly glucocorticoid activity and less mineralocorticoid activity. Its glucocorticoid activity is about **four times that of cortisol**.
2. **Dexamethasone:** It has only glucocorticoid activity. Its glucocorticoid activity is about six **times that** of prednisolone.
3. **9α-Flurocortisol:** It has predominantly mineralocorticoid activity and less glucocorticoid activity. Its glucocorticoid activity is about **two-and-half times that of prednisolone**.

Effects on the Immune System

Cortisol has **profound immunosuppressive effects**. The influence is **more on cellular immunity**. Cortisol suppresses immunity by following mechanisms.

1. **Causes Lymphocytopenia**: Cortisol **decreases circulating lymphocytes** by inhibiting lymphocyte mitotic activity.
   - It mainly decreases T cell population, especially ***type-I helper T cells by stimulating their apoptosis.***
   - Immature T cells in thymus and immature B and T cells in lymph nodes are destroyed by high level of plasma cortisol, which in turn decreases the size of thymus and lymph nodes.
2. **Inhibits T_8 cells:** Cortisol **inhibits the cytotoxic effects of T cells** by ***inhibiting the transport of lymphocytes*** to the site of antigenic stimulation and by ***decreasing the production of cytokine***s from them.
   - Cortisol **inhibits cytokine secretion** by ***inhibiting the NF-$_k$B activity*** of the cells.
3. **Inhibits Production of Cytokines**: Cortisol **inhibits production of interleukins** (IL-1, IL-2, and IL-6) from the helper T cells, and inhibits synthesis of γ interferon from macrophage and lymphocytes.
   - IL-2 and γ interferon are essential for cellular immunity.
4. **Inhibits Lymphocytes:** Cortisol **inhibits both resting as well as activated lymphocytes**.
   - It **inhibits lymphocyte proliferation**. It also inhibits differentiation of monocytes to macrophages (Flowchart 74.9).

Prevention of Transplant Rejection: As cortisol has **profound inhibitory effects on cellular immunity**, it is frequently **used for prevention of transplant rejection**.

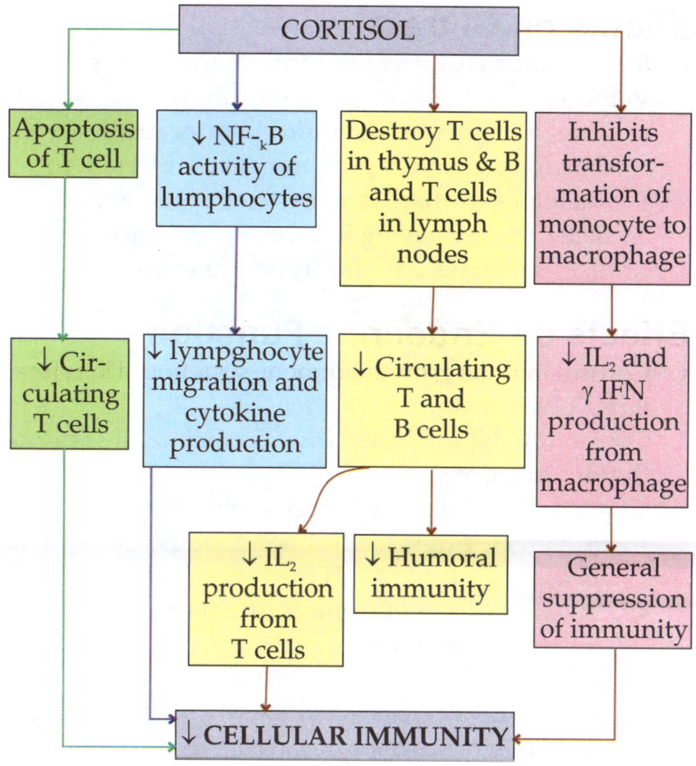

Flowchart 74.9: Immunosuppressive mechanisms of cortisol.

IMPORTANT NOTE

Indications & Contraindications of Cortisol Use: Cortisol is used in the treatment of many diseases and contraindicated in other diseases.

1. Cortisol is used for the treatment of **inflammatory diseases** like rheumatoid arthritis etc. When an inflammatory process is life threatening, administration of cortisol provides immediate relief.
2. Cortisol is frequently used for **prevention of transplant rejection** as it inhibits cellular immunity. However, cortisol given for a long time decreases body immunity, and therefore, increases the susceptibility to various bacterial fungal and viral infections. Therefore, cortisol treatment is supplemented with antibiotics.
3. Cortisol is used in the **treatment of both local and systemic allergy**. For example, in the management of bronchial asthma, to ensure effective bronchodilation, inhalation of both cortisol and sulbutamol is advised. In acute exacerbation of asthma, systemic steroid is very helpful.
4. Cortisol prevents fibroblastic growth. Therefore, it is used in the treatment of **keloid** (the tumor of scar tissue) by local injections.
5. A person suffering from acute infection **should not be treated with steroids without antibiotics**, though it suppresses inflammation and dramatically improves the condition. This is because cortisol suppresses immunity and spreads infection (person may die due to severe infection).

Effects on GI tract

1. **It stimulates HCl secretion** from parietal cells of the stomach.
   - Thus, it causes **hyperacidity and gastritis**. Given for a long period, it produces gastric ulceration.
   - Therefore, cortisol is prescribed cautiously in patients already having history of peptic ulcer.
2. Cortisol **decreases Ca^{++} absorption** from GI tract.

Effects on Endocrine Function

1. **Cortisol inhibits growth hormone secretion. Therefore, it inhibits growth.**
2. Cortisol inhibits TSH secretion. Therefore, it **inhibits thyroid functions.**
3. Glucocorticoids **inhibit ACTH secretion.**
   - In cortisol excess ACTH secretion is less and in cortisol deficiency ACTH secretion is more.
   - This helps in the diagnosis of adrenocortical dysfunction by **estimating plasma ACTH** concentration.
4. Cortisol **induces expression of PNMT** (phenylethanolamine-N-methytransferase), the enzyme that catalyzes the formation of epinephrine from norepinephrine.

Role in Stress

The most important function of cortisol is to protect the body against stress. In absence of glucocorticoids, body can't cope with stress even in its mild intensity.

- The glucocorticoid secretion increases due to **increased ACTH secretion**, which exclusively occurs due to increased **release of CRH from hypothalamus.**
- In fact, stress is defined as the condition in which plasma ACTH secretion is high. The stimuli that increase ACTH secretion are called **stressors.**
- **In stress,** glucocorticoid is essential for catecholamines to **exert their FFA mobilizing action** (FFA is an important source of energy supply in emergency situations) and for **maintenance of vascular reactivity** to catecholamines (Fig. 74.7).
- Therefore, in absence of cortisol, the individual succumbs to stress.

Rapid Actions of Steroid

As steroids act though transcription of genes in the cells, it **takes hours to days** for their full actions to manifest. These are called **genomic actions.**

- However, recently it has been observed that some of the steroid actions occur **within few minutes.**
- These rapid actions of steroid are due to their direct action on the **membrane channels or enzymes.**
  - These are called **nongenomic action** of steroids.
- They ***activate various membrane enzymes*** that lead to formation of **second messengers** like cAMP in the cells, and second messengers in turn change cell functions.

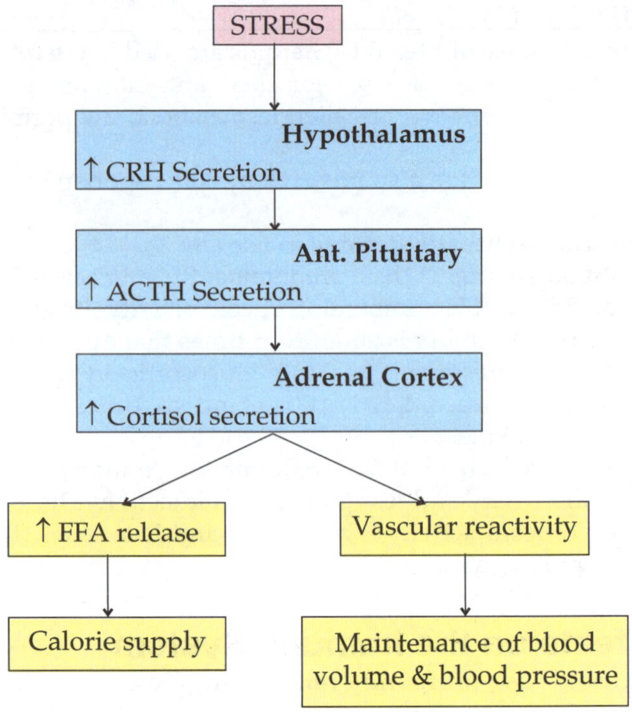

Fig. 74.7: Role of cortisol in stress.

Dysfunctions of Glucocorticoids

Cushing's Syndrome

This is a pathological condition that occurs due to **hypersecretion of glucocorticoids.** This is called Cushing's syndrome as it was described by Harvey Cushing.

Etiology

It occurs due to either a **tumor of the adrenal cortex** that causes cortisol excess or exogenously administered excess steroids (**ACTH independent**) or **due to the tumor of the pituitary** that increases secretion of ACTH (**ACTH dependent**).

Traditionally, **Cushing's disease** refers to the disease that occurs only due to the ACTH producing tumor of pituitary, whereas **Cushing's syndrome** refers to all the causes of cortisol excess.

The **common causes** of Cushing's syndrome are:

1. **Adrenal hyperplasia** secondary to pituitary ACTH producing tumors, hypothalamo-pituitary dysfunctions, and ectopic ACTH or CRH producing tumors such as bronchogenic carcinoma.
2. **Adrenal tumors** (adenoma or carcinoma)
3. Adrenal **macronodular** hyperplasia
4. Familial adrenal dysplasia (**Carney syndrome**)
5. Prolonged and **excess use of ACTH or cortisol** (iatrogenic)

Features

The features of Cushing's syndrome according to their frequency of occurrences are:

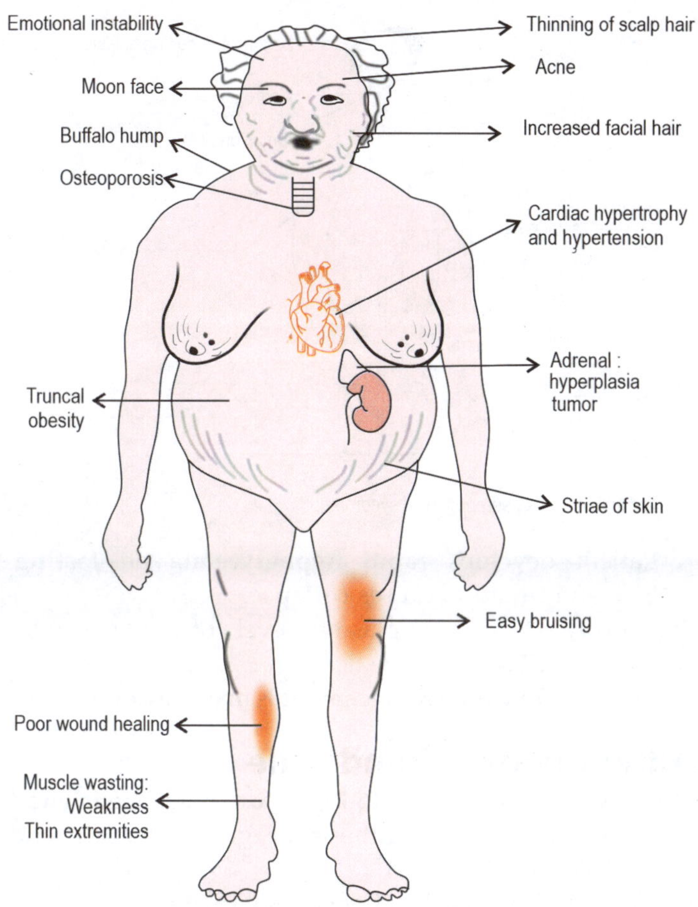

Fig. 74.8: Features of Cushing syndrome.

1. **Centripetal obesity and overweight:** This is due to peculiar distribution of body fat in which fat is deposited more in the abdomen and upper back.
    - Fat pad in lower neck and interscapular region gives the typical appearance of **buffalo hump** (Fig. 74.8).
2. **Moon face:** The face becomes round with red cheeks due to *fat deposition*.
    - Salt and water retention contribute to it.
3. Fatigability and weakness
4. **Hypertension:** Patient develops hypertension due to water accumulation as glucocorticoid in excess has significant *mineralocorticoid activity*.
    - Increased *angiotensinogen secretion* by cortisol and direct action of cortisol *on blood vessel* contribute to it.
5. **Hirsutism and amenorrhea:** Occurs due to associated increased adrenal androgens.
6. **Reddish purple striae**: Striae develop on the abdomen (Fig. 74.9). Excess fat deposition in abdomen causes rapid stretching of the skin that results in formation of striae.
7. **Ecchymoses:** The skin and subcutaneous tissue are thin as a result of protein catabolism.
    - Capillaries of the skin become thin and fragile.
    - Therefore, minor injury causes ecchymoses and bruises (subcutaneous and intracutaneous hemorrhages).
8. **Proximal myopathy:** The *legs become thin* due to proteolysis in the skeletal muscle and reduced bone mass. The muscle development is poor.
9. **Poor wound healing:** Hyperglycemia promotes growth of the organism at the wound site.
    - Also, decreased immunity favours growth of the organism.
    - Cortisol prevents walling off of a chronic infection.
10. Many patients develop **hyperglycemia** and glucose intolerance, and about 20% of patients develop insulin resistant *diabetes mellitus*.
11. **Osteoporosis** develops due to decreased bone mineralization and decreased bone mass.
    - This may cause *collapse of vertebral bodies* and *pathologic fractures* of bones.
12. **Emotional changes** may be profound ranging from irritability to frank **psychosis**.
13. **Hyperacidity** is common. Some patients may develop **peptic ulcer**.
14. The **hairs are thin and scraggly**. Some may have increase in facial hair and acne.

Diagnosis

PY8.4

Diagnosis is based on demonstrating increased cortisol production (**increased plasma level of cortisol**) and failure to suppress cortisol secretion by dexamethasone (**dexamethasone suppression test**).

- **ACTH in plasma** differentiates pituitary (ACTH dependent) causes from adrenal (ACTH independent) causes.
- In general, in ACTH independent cases, ACTH is less, and in ACTH dependent cases, ACTH is high.

Treatment

If the disease is due to tumor of adrenals or pituitary, **surgical resection** of the tumor is required. **Medical adrenalectomy** is done in few patients by inhibiting steroidogenesis with administration of *high dose of ketokonazole or metyrapone* that inhibit cortisol synthesis.

Adrenocortical Insufficiency

Hypofunction of adrenal gland may be **primary or secondary** variety.

Primary adrenal insufficiency: Primary adrenocortical insufficiency is called **Addison's disease.**

1. Idiopathic atrophy of the gland (usually due to an autoimmune process).
2. Surgical removal of the gland
3. Infection (Usually tubercular infection, but fungal and viral infection may also cause)
4. Bilateral hemorrhage into the gland
5. Metastatic invasion of the gland

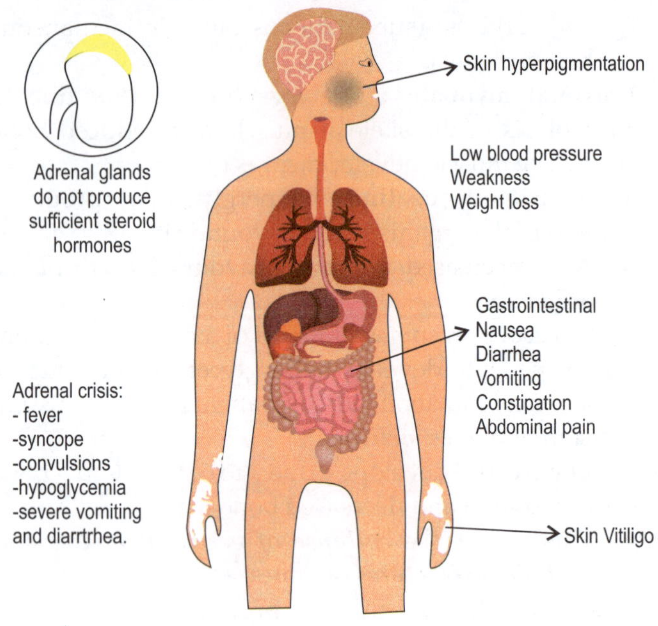

Fig. 74.9: Features of Addison's disease.

6. Drugs: ketokonazole, metyrapone, mitotane etc.

Secondary adrenal insufficiency:

1. Pituitary disease that decreases ACTH secretion
2. Hypothalamic disease that decreases CRH secretion

Addison's Disease

This is the condition of **hyposecretion of glucocorticoid** that results from progressive destruction of the adrenals.

Etiology: The atrophy of the adrenal cortex is **usually idiopathic**. An autoimmune mechanism is thought to be responsible.

- **Tubercular infection** of the adrenal gland, secondary **metastasis, amyloidosis** and cytomegalovirus infection affecting the gland may destroy and produce the disease.

Clinical Features: Features, in order of their frequency are (Fig. 74.9):

1. Loss of weight and easy fatigability
2. ***Pigmentation of skin:*** The most characteristic feature of the disease is **hyperpigmentation** of skin, especially marked over the pressure points, sun-exposed areas and on the scar marks.
   - Less plasma cortisol ***increases ACTH secretion*** by feedback mechanism.
   - As ***ACTH has intrinsic MSH activity***, pigmentation occurs.
3. ***Hypotension:*** Hypotension occurs due to ***decreased mineralocorticoid activity*** and decreased ***vascular reactivity***. In severe cases, ***hypotensive shock*** occurs.
4. Anorexia, nausea and sometimes abdominal pain.
5. Hyponatremia (depletional), hyperkalemia.
6. ***Eosinophilia:*** Cortisol causes eosinopenia. Therefore, deficiency of it produces eosinophilia.

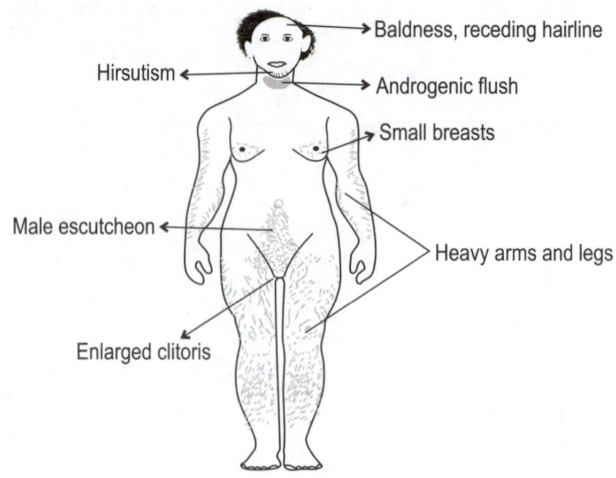

Fig. 74.10: Features of adrenogenital syndrome.

7. Patient develops **rapid hypoglycemia on fasting**. Stressful situation causes **collapse**.

Diagnosis: Decreased plasma level of cortisol with **increased ACTH** is diagnostic.

Treatment: Hormone replacement is mainstay of therapy.

Adrenogenital Syndrome

Etiology: This occurs due to **21β-hydroxylase deficiency**, which decreases the synthesis of glucocorticoids and mineralocorticoids.

- Decreased plasma level of cortisol **increases secretion of ACTH** by feedback mechanism that increases the production of pregnenolone.
- **Excess pregnenolone** is diverted for the production of androgen. Thus, steroids in this syndrome are converted to excess of androgen that produces **virilization**.

Features: Excess androgen secretion in females causes **masculinization** and **precocious pseudopuberty** or **female pseudohermaphroditism** (Fig. 74.10). The usual features are:

1. Hirsutism
2. Small breast
3. Receding hairline
4. Heavy arms and legs
5. Enlarged clitoris (Clitoromegaly)
6. Male escutcheon (male distribution of suprapubic hair)
7. Androgenic flush

MINERALOCORTICOIDS

Aldosterone is the major mineralocorticoid in humans.

Regulation of Aldosterone Secretion

Aldosterone secretion is regulated mainly by ***three important stimuli:*** **angiotensin-II, ACTH, and plasma K$^+$** concentration. Many conditions alter aldosterone secretion (Table 74.5) by influencing these stimuli.

Angiotensin II

Angiotensin II is an **important stimulator of aldosterone synthesis and secretion**. It is formed from angiotensinogen, an α_2-globulin secreted from liver.

1. **Renin**, a circulating protease secreted from JG cells of kidney catalyzes the conversion of angiotensinogen to **angiotensin I** (A I).
2. A I is converted to **angiotensin II** (A II) by the action of angiotensin converting enzyme (ACE), which is further degraded to **angiotensin III** (A III).
3. **A II and A III** stimulate the formation of aldosterone (Flowchart 74.10).
   [Details of renin-angiotensin-aldosterone system is given in Chapter 86, of 'Renal System')].

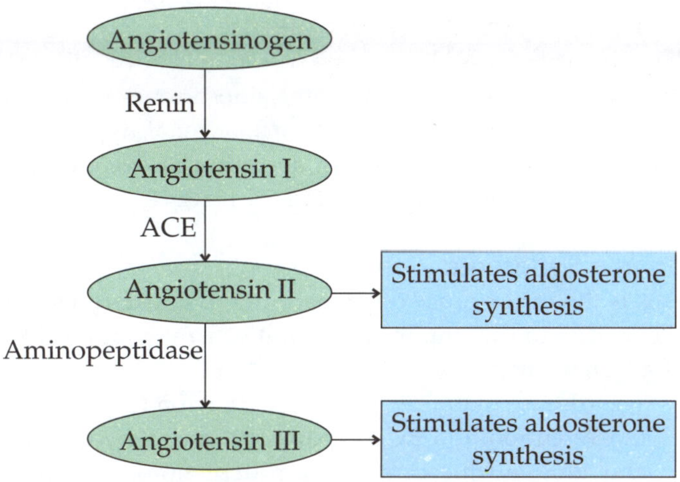

Flowchart 74.10: Renin-angiotensin system controlling aldosterone secretion.

- **A III is as potent as stimulator** of aldosterone synthesis and secretion as A II.

Angiotensin Receptors: There are **two types** of angiotensin receptors: AT_1 and AT_2.

- **AT_1 receptors** are present on the zona glomerulosa cells of adrenal cortex.
- A II binds with AT_1 receptors and increases intracellular **IP_3 and DAG** production that in turn increase intracellular calcium.
- **Rise in calcium** facilitates **aldosterone secretion**

ACTH

Cells of zona glomerulosa of adrenal cortex have ACTH receptors.

1. ACTH stimulates aldosterone synthesis and secretion, **mediated by cyclic AMP and protein kinase**.
   - However, the quantity of ACTH required to stimulate aldosterone secretion is more than the concentration required to stimulate cortisol secretion.
2. The effect of ACTH on aldosterone secretion is **temporary** (Application Box 74.2).
   - **Aldosterone secretion declines**, even if ACTH secretion is elevated, which is partly due to ***decreased renin secretion*** secondary to hypervolemia.
   - Interestingly, deoxycorticosterone (another mineralocorticoid) secretion remains high.

Application Box 74.2

ACTH stimulated aldosterone secretion is not transient in GRA: Though ACTH-mediated aldosterone secretion is a temporary phenomenon, it is persistent in **glucocorticoid-remediable aldosteronism** (GRA).

- GRA is an autosomal dominant disorder, in which ACTH causes persistent hypersecretion of aldosterone that leads to hypertension.
- GRA occurs due to fusion of genes coding for 11β-hydroxylase and aldosterone synthase (as they are 95% identical and remain close together on chromosome 8) forming a **hybrid gene** called **ACTH-sensitive aldosterone synthase**.
- Therefore, ACTH effect on aldosterone secretion becomes a prolonged phenomenon.

Hypertension in GRA is treated by glucocorticoid, as this decreases the production of ACTH, which in turn decreases the synthesis of aldosterone. Hence, this syndrome is called **glucocorticoid-remediable** aldosteronism.

Table 74.5 | Conditions that alter aldosterone secretion.

A. Conditions that increase secretion
1. Hemorrhage
2. Hypovolemia
3. Hyperkalemia
4. Hyponatremia
5. Standing
6. Anxiety
7. Physical trauma and surgery
8. Secondary hyperaldosteronism: Aldosterone secretion may increase in congestive heart failure, cirrhosis of liver, and nephritic syndrome.
B. Conditions that decrease secretion
1. Expansion of ECF volume
2. Hypernatremia
3. Hypokalemia

Hyperkalemia

Aldosterone secretion is stimulated by increase in K^+ in ECF.

1. Rise in ECF K^+ ***activates voltage gated calcium channels*** that increases intracellular calcium.
2. **Increased cytosolic calcium** increases aldosterone synthesis and secretion.
3. Aldosterone, in turn promotes excretion of K^+.
   - Thus, **aldosterone is a natural regulator of K^+ level in ECF**.
   - Also, **acute decrease in plasma Na^+** or increase in plasma K^+ stimulates the aldosterone synthesis and secretion.

Mechanism of Action of Aldosterone

Aldosterone binds with the **cytoplasmic receptor**.

- The HR complex moves to the nucleus where it induces **translation of mRNA**.
- This increases new protein synthesis that alters cell function.

Aldosterone has both genomic and nongenomic actions:

Genomic Action: The gene activated by aldosterone is sgk gene (serum and glucocorticoid regulated kinase gene).

- This is an early response gene that increases **ENaC** (Epithelial Na^+ Channels) activity.
- Aldosterone also **increases mRNA activity** for synthesis of proteins that form subunits of ENaC.
- Aldosterone increases **insertion of these channels** on cell membrane and also **increases their activity**.

Nongenomic Action: Nongenomic action occurs rapidly.

- This is due to stimulation of the activity of Na^+-K^+ exchanger, which increases intracellular accumulation of Na^+.
- The second messenger that mediates this action is IP_3.

Physiological Actions of Aldosterone

Electrolyte and Water Balance

The main function of aldosterone is to **increase Na^+ and water reabsorption** and to **promote K^+ and H^+ excretion** from the kidney.

- Na^+ reabsorption is the primary function, and other effects are mostly secondary to Na^+ reabsorption.
- For Na^+ reabsorption, aldosterone acts primarily on **P cells** (principal cells) of **collecting duct and distal tubule** of kidney.
- In fact, aldosterone controls only 3% of total Na^+ reabsorption from the kidney. However, aldosterone deficiency results in significant hyponatremia.

Mechanisms: Aldosterone increases Na^+ and water reabsorption by following mechanisms:

1. It increases the **number of Na^+ channels** in the epithelial cells of the kidney tubule.
2. It **stimulates Na^+-K^+ ATPase activity**, therefore Na^+ is reabsorbed and K^+ is excreted.
3. It **stimulates enzymes of Krebs cycle** that facilitate ATP generation and provide energy for removal of Na^+ from the interstitial fluid into the capillary.

Thus, aldosterone increases plasma Na^+ concentration and **decreases K^+ concentration**. Therefore, **in aldosterone deficiency**, hyponatremia is associated with ***hyperkalemia***.

- As Na^+ is reabsorbed, **Cl^- is transported** in the same direction to maintain electroneutrality.
- The reabsorption of NaCl causes **osmotic reabsorption of water**.
- Thus, reabsorption of salt and water leads to **ECF expansion**.

Aldosterone Escape Phenomenon

Increased reabsorption of salt and water by aldosterone causes **ECF expansion**.

- Increased ECF volume **increases venous return** to the heart that causes further **distention of atria** during their filling.
- Atrial stretching **increases synthesis and secretion of ANP** from atrial myocytes.
- ANP causes profound **natriuresis and diuresis**.

Therefore, **ECF volume returns back to normal**. This is called aldosterone escape phenomenon as kidney escapes from the effect of aldosterone.

Dysfunctions of Aldosterone

Hypersecretion of Aldosterone

Hyperaldosteronism can be divided broadly into **two categories**: primary and secondary.

Primary Hyperaldosteronism

The cause of excess aldosterone secretion is due to adrenal disease. The usual causes are aldosterone-producing adrenal adenoma (*Conn's syndrome*), adrenal hyperplasia and adrenal carcinoma. **Renin secretion is decreased** in primary hyperaldosteronism (Fig. 74.11A).

Conn's Syndrome

This is the major cause of primary hyperaldosteronism. It occurs due to the **tumor (adenoma) of zona glomerulosa of adrenal cortex**.

1. The disease manifests with **hypertension** (due to sodium retention and ECF expansion), **muscle weakness** and fatigue (due to potassium depletion), and **polyuria** (due to impairment of urinary concentrating ability).
2. Edema is usually not a feature of primary hyperaldosteronism.
3. **Hypokalemia**, hypernatremia and low renin in plasma, and **metabolic alkalosis** are usual laboratory findings.

Secondary Hyperaldosteronism

Increased aldosterone secretion due to **activation of renin-angiotensin system** is called secondary hyperaldosteronism.

- It is associated with **increased renin in plasma** (Fig. 74.11B), as decreased volume is the initiating stimulus for renin secretion. This is a *major differentiating feature* from primary hyperaldosteronism, in which renin secretion is less.
- It occurs in **congestive heart failure, cirrhosis of liver and nephritic syndrome**. Renin secreting tumor (***primary reninism***) can also cause it.
- **Edema is a usual feature** in secondary hyperaldosteronism.
    - However, secondary hyperaldosteronism in **Batter syndrome and Gitelman syndrome** occurs without edema.

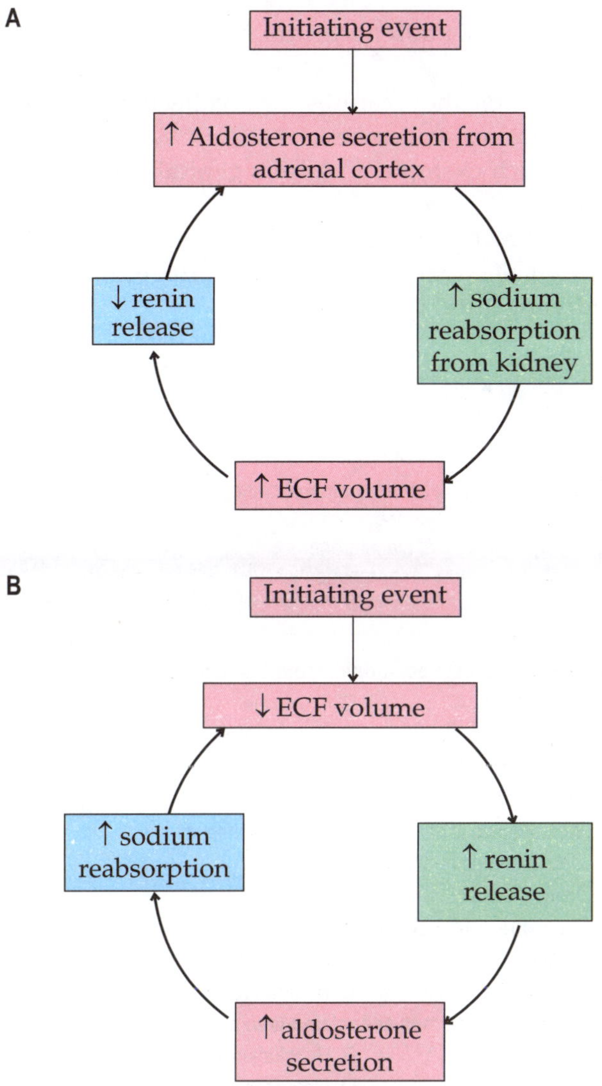

Fig. 74.11: Renin secretion in primary (A) and secondary (B) hyperaldosteronism. Note, decreased renin secretion occurs (hence, no activation of renin-angiotensin-aldosterone axis) in primary aldosteronism; therefore, edema is not a feature. In secondary aldosteronism, renin secretion is more (activation of renin-angiotensin-aldosterone axis) hence, edema is usually a feature.

Batter Syndrome

It is a condition of hyperplasia of JG cells (**Juxtaglomerular hyperplasia**).

- The disease occurs due to **mutation in the Na^+-K^+-$2Cl^-$ cotransporter gene**, which results in ***high renin activity*** and increased aldosterone synthesis.
- Hyperaldosteronism produces **K^+ depletion**.
- Major features are **hypokalemic alkalosis and hypercalciuria**.
- However, **blood pressure remains normal and there is no edema**.

Hyposecretion of Aldosterone

Hyposecretion of mineralocorticoid is usually associated with **adrenal insufficiency**. However, **isolated hypoaldosteronism** with normal cortisol production occurs in following conditions;

1. **Inherited defects** of biosynthesis of aldosterone.
2. Decreased renin production (**hyporeninemic hypoaldosteronism**)
3. Surgical removal of aldosterone secreting adenoma causing **more resection** of normal adrenocortical tissue.
4. During protracted **heparin administration**.
5. Selective unresponsiveness of Zona glomerulosa to angiotensin II (**hyperreninemic hypoaldosteronism**)
6. Pretectal disease of nervous system.
7. Severe postural hypotension.

SEX STEROIDS

Sex steroids secreted from adrenal gland are called **adrenal androgens**. The major adrenal androgens are **dehydroepiandrosterone and androstenedione**.

1. Androstenedione is **converted to estrogen** in the peripheral blood and tissues.
2. The secretion of adrenal androgen increases at puberty, reaches peak at about twenty years of age and then declines slowly to reach a low level in old age. These changes correlate with the change in 17 α–hydroxylase activity.
3. The secretion of adrenal androgen is **controlled by ACTH**, not by gonadotropins.

Functions of Adrenal Androgens

Adrenal androgens have less than 20% of activity of testicular androgen.

1. **Adrenarche:** At the onset of puberty in both boys and girls, in the **stage 1** (before the physical development of puberty), *secretion of adrenal androgen becomes high* before the gonadal secretions are significantly elevated. This is called **adrenarche**.
    - It is reported that adrenarche *initiates the process of puberty* in which **adrenal androgen sensitizes the gonads** to secrete more sex hormones and **sensitizes the sex organs** to the effects of sex hormones.
2. They exert **masculinizing effect**: However, the masculinizing effect is less in normal concentration of adrenal androgens.
    - These effects are prominent only when the hormones are **secreted in excess amount**.
3. **Promote protein synthesis:** They are protein anabolic, **increase protein synthesis**.
4. **Facilitate growth**: They facilitate sexual growth.
    - In **adult males**, they accentuate the already developed sex characteristics.
    - However, **in prepubertal boys**, in excess, they develop secondary sex characteristics precociously. This is called **precocious pseudopuberty**.

5. **Source of estrogen:** Adrenal androgens are converted to estrogen in the peripheral tissue and serve as the ***major source of estrogen*** in males and postmenopausal females.

Dysfunctions of Adrenal Androgens

Excess of adrenal androgens results in **virilization**. However, along with increased secretion of adrenal androgens, other adrenocortical hormones are secreted in larger quantity.

- Therefore, the features are collectively called as **virilization syndromes**.

1. One such example is '**Adrenogenital syndrome**' (Fig. 74.11).
2. In males, they cause **precocious pseudopuberty.**
3. In females they cause **pseudohermaphroditism** and **adrenogenital syndrome**.

Exam Questions

1. Describe the functions of glucocorticoids (or cortisol).
2. Give the steps of cortisol synthesis. Briefly describe the mechanism of action of cortisol and regulation of cortisol secretion.
3. Describe the actions of cortisol on inflammation, immunity and allergy. Give a note on Cushing syndrome.
4. Describe the regulation of secretion, mechanism of action, physiological actions and dysfunctions of aldosterone.
5. Give the steps of synthesis of adrenal sex steroids and briefly describe their functions. Add a note on adrenogenital (Virilization) syndrome.

Multiple Choice Questions

1. Major androgen secreted from adrenal cortex is:
A. Testosterone
B. 11-hydroxy derivative of androstenedione
C. 17-ketosteroid dehydroepiandrosterone
D. Cortisol

2. Destruction of zone glomerulosa will deplete:
A. Aldosterone B. Cortisol
C. Testosterone D. Catecholamines

3. From zona reticularis of adrenal cortex, which hormone is the main secretion?
A. Aldosterone B. Cortisol
C. Androgen D. Corticosterone

4. Mineralocorticoid receptors are present in all of the following organs, EXCEPT:
A. Hippocampus B. Kidney
C. Colon D. Liver

5. What of the following is the effect of cortisol on metabolism?
A. Decreased blood glucose
B. Increased lipogenesis
C. Increased proteolysis
D. Increased ketone body formation

6. Effects of steroids on calcium
A. Increased plasma calcium level
B. Increased absorption from gut
C. Increased excretion from kidney
D. Increased synthesis of calcium

7. Anti-inflammatory action of steroids due to:
A. Inhibition of phospholipase A2
B. Inhibition of cyclooxegenase
C. Increased activity of lipolipase
D. Inhibition of lipooxegenase

8. Diurnal variation in eosinophil count is related to:
A. Cortisol B. Thyroxine
C. Growth hormone D. Testosterone

9. In Cushing syndrome, which of the following is NOT seen?
A. Increased aldosterone
B. Increased vascular reactivity to angiotensin II
C. Decreased epinephrine
D. Truncal obesity

10. Aldosterone synthesis is inhibited by:
A. Renin B. Dopamine
C. Endorphin D. Hypernatremia

11. Hyperaldosteronism is associated with all,EXCEPT:
A. Hypernatremia B. Hypokalemia
C. Hypertension D. Metabolic acidosis

12. Excess and prolonged secretion of aldosterone causes all, EXCEPT:
A. Increased ECF
B. Very high Na+ in plasma
C. Increased BP
D. Natriuresis

13. Least mineralocorticoid activity is seen in
A. Aldosterone B. Deoxycortisone
C. 9 α Flurotisol D. Dexamethasone

14. All of the following are features of Conn's syndrome, EXCEPT:
A. Hyperpigmentation of skin
B. Hypertension
C. Eosinophilia
D. Hyperkalemia

Answers :

1. C 2. A 3. C 4. D 5. C 6. C 7. A 8. A 9. C 10. D
11. D 12. B 13. D 14. B

Chapter 75

Adrenal Medulla

Learning Objectives

On completion of study of this chapter:

The student will be able to (must know):

1. Name the hormones secreted from adrenal medulla and give the steps of their synthesis.
2. Describe the functions of catecholamines.
3. Understand the differences between the functions of epinephrine and norepinephrine.
4. Outline the role of catecholamines in fight or flight response.

The student may also be able to (desirable to know):

1. Describe the synthesis, secretion and regulation of secretion of adrenomedullary hormones.
2. Explain the role of catecholamines in acute and chronic stress.
3. Learn the physiological basis of features of pheochromocytoma.

Essentially, adrenal medulla represents an enlarged and **specialized sympathetic ganglion** in which the postganglionic fibers are embedded and modified to become the endocrine cells. The tissue of adrenal medulla weighs about 1 g in adults.

CELL TYPES

Adrenal medulla is surrounded by adrenal cortex. The gland consists of clumps and strands of **chromaffin cells,** interspersed with venous sinuses (refer Fig. 74.1, previous chapter).

- The cells are called **chromaffin cells** as they have *greater affinity for chromium stains.*
- They contain numerous granules that are present in the vesicles that **store catecholamines** (Fig. 75.1).

Types of Endocrine Cells

There are **two types of endocrine cells** in the adrenal medulla: epinephrine-secreting and norepinephrine-secreting.

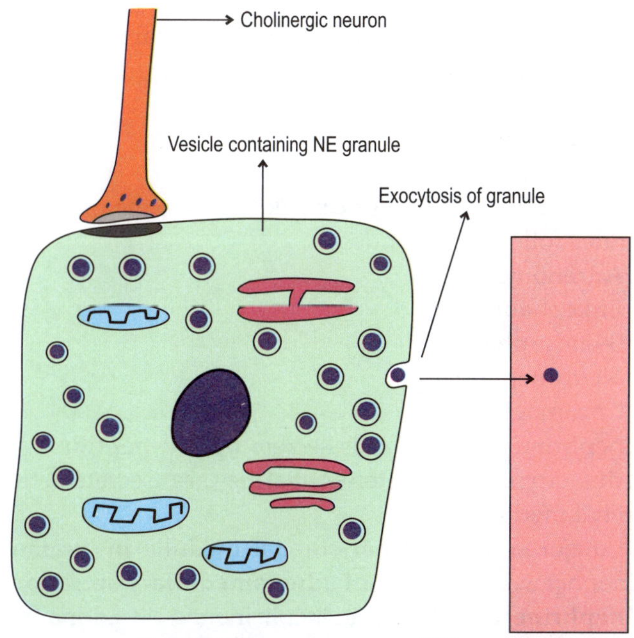

Fig. 75.1: The cell (chromaffin cell) of adrenal medulla. Note, the cell is innervated by sympathetic preganglionic cholinergic neuron. The granules containing hormone is discharged into extracellular space by exocytosis and from there the hormone enters sinusoidal vein. NE: Norepinephrine

1. **Epinephrine-secreting type:** In humans, **90% of cell types** in adrenal medulla are epinephrine-secreting type.
   - The granules in these cells are **lager and less dense**.
   - Granules completely fill the vesicles.
2. **Norepinephrine-secreting type:** They constitute **10% of the cell mass** of adrenal medulla.
   - The granules in these cells are **small and very dense**.
   - The granules do not fill the vesicles in which they are present.

The types of **cells that secrete dopamine** are not clearly known, but are believed to be very less in number.

- Chromaffin cells receive **sympathetic preganglionic cholinergic innervation** and on stimulation discharge their content into venous sinuses.
- Small group of chromaffin cells are present near abdominal sympathetic ganglia. These are called **paraganglia**. They also secrete catecholamines.

Effect of Sympathetic Stimulation

Sympathetic stimulation not only **increases norepinephrine secretion** from its nerve endings that slowly enters circulation, but also **directly increases epinephrine secretion** *from adrenal medulla* that rapidly enters circulation.

- Thus, sympathetic activation increases the level of **both epinephrine and norepinephrine** in blood.

Adrenomedullary Hormones **PY8.2**

The **major hormones** secreted from adrenal medulla are **catecholamines:**

1. Epinephrine
2. Norepinephrine
3. Dopamine.

In addition to secretion of catecholamines, the gland **also secretes** following peptides:

1. Adrenomedullin
2. Enkephalins
3. β-endorphin
4. Neuropeptide-Y
5. Chromogranin

Epinephrine secreting cells secrete **opioid peptide**. Most of the circulating **metenkephalins** are secreted from adrenal medulla.

The major secretion from adrenal medulla in human is epinephrine. About **85% of adrenomedullary secretion is epinephrine,** 10-12% is norepinephrine and 1-3% dopamine, whereas secretion from sympathetic noradrenergic nerve ending is almost entirely norepinephrine.

CATECHOLAMINES

Synthesis and Secretion

Catecholamines are synthesized from the amino acid **phenylalanine and tyrosine** (Flowchart 75.1).

- Conversion of **tyrosine to Dopa** is catalyzed by *tyrosine hydroxylase* and **dopa to dopamine** by *dopa decarboxylase*.
- **Norepinephrine** is formed by hydroxylation and decarboxylation of tyrosine.
- **Epinephrine** is formed by methylation of norepinephrine by *phenylethanolamine-N-methyl-transferase* (PNMT).
- After synthesis, the hormones are **stored in the granules** of chromaffin cells before they are secreted into venous blood.

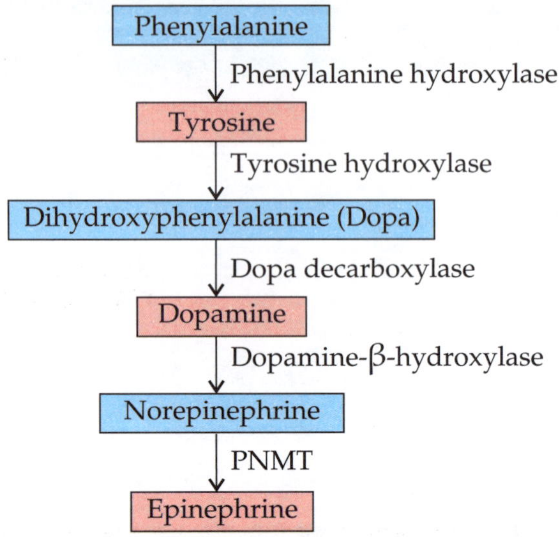

Flowchart 75.1: Synthesis of adrenomedullary hormones. PNMT: phenylethanolamine-N-methyltransferase

Effects of Glucocorticoid: The enzyme **PNMT is induced by glucocorticoid** at higher concentration.

- It may be noted that, the concentration of **glucocorticoids is normally high in blood bathing adrenal medulla** as blood from cortex drains into medulla before entering general circulation.
- Therefore, **in adrenocortical deficiency, epinephrine synthesis is also reduced**. Also, glucocorticoid promotes normal growth of adrenal medulla.

Effects of 21β-hydroxylase: During **fetal life**, the adrenocortical enzyme, 21β-hydroxylase stimulates **development of adrenal medulla**.

- Therefore, **fetal deficiency of 21β-hydroxylase** results in dysplasia of adrenal medulla, and if enzyme deficiency is not corrected promptly after birth, circulating catecholamines remain permanently low.

Regulation of Secretion

Catecholamine secretion from adrenal medulla increases in following conditions.

1. Exercise
2. Hypoglycemia
3. Trauma (Physical injury)
4. Anger and anxiety
5. Pain
6. Cold

The main mechanism of secretion in these conditions is **sympathetic stimulation**.

- **Hypoglycemia** is a strong stimulus for catecholamine release.
- When **blood glucose is less than 60 mg%**, CNS receptors monitoring plasma glucose are activated.

They stimulate the neural pathways that ***activate sympathetic fibers*** to release norepinephrine and adrenal medulla to release mainly epinephrine.

- These catecholamines in turn increase plasma glucose level.

Metabolism

The normal **plasma concentration of free hormone** in recumbent posture is as follows:

Norepinephrine : 300 pg/mL
Epinephrine : 30 pg/mL
Dopamine : 35 pg/mL

About 70% norepinephrine and epinephrine, and 90% of dopamine are **conjugated to sulfate**. They have very short life span. **Half-life** is about **1–3 minutes**.

- **They are metabolized primarily in the liver and kidney.**
  - The **key enzymes** of metabolism are catecholamine-O-methyltransferase (**COMT**), and monoamine oxidase (**MAO**).
- Metabolism of epinephrine forms **metanephrine** and norepinephrine forms **normetanephrine**.
- Epinephrine and norepinephrine are also commonly degraded to form *dihydroxymandelic acid* which is further metabolized to form **vanillylmandelic acid** (**VMA**) and **methoxyhydroxy-phenylglycol** (**MOPG**).

Steps of Degradation: The steps of degradation of epinephrine and norepinephrine are summarized in Flowchart 75.2.

- Only 2–3% of catecholamines are excreted unchanged in urine.
- About 50% of secreted catecholamines appear in urine as **metanephrine and normetanephrinre**, and 35% as 3-methoxy-4-hydroxy-mandelic acid, also called as **VMA** (Application Box 75.1).

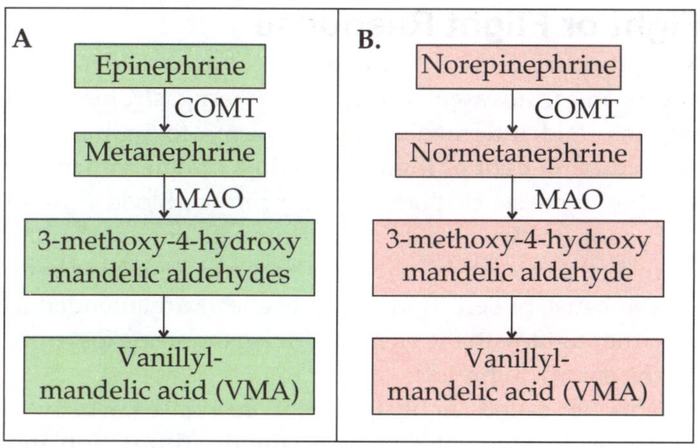

Flowcharts 75.2: Metabolic degradation of epinephrine (A) and norepinephrine (B).

The **steps of degradation of dopamine** are listed in Flowchart 75.3:

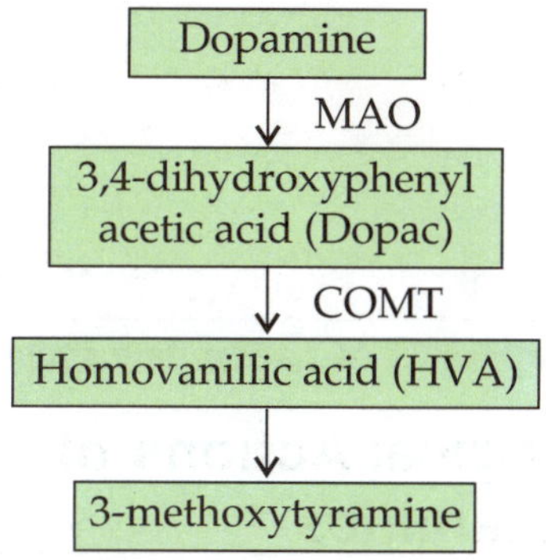

Flowchart 75.3: Steps of metabolic degradation of dopamine.

24 h Urinary Excretion: The normal daily urinary excretion of catecholamines and their metabolites are as follows:

Metanephrine plus normetanephrine : 300 μg
VMA : 400-600 μg
MOPG : 200 μg
Norepinephrine : 30 μg
Epinephrine : 6 μg

Application Box 75.1

VMA is the index of sympathetic activity: Urinary excretion of VMA and MOPG reflect activity of sympathetic nervous system as they are mainly derived from norepinephrine. Epinephrine contributes relatively less to the production of VMA and MOPG. Therefore, the activity of adrenal medulla is assessed primarily by measurement of plasma epinephrine or free urinary epinephrine.

Mechanism of Action

Catecholamines act on **α and β receptors**. There are **three types of β receptors**: β_1, β_2, and β_3, and **two types of α receptors**: α_1 and α_2.

1. The **α_1 and α_2 receptors** have *three subtypes each*.
2. Epinephrine and norepinephrine act on both α and β receptors.
   - However, in general, **epinephrine acts more on β receptors** and **norepinephrine on α receptors**.
   - β_1, β_2, and α_2 are structurally similar.
3. The **β_1, β_2, and β_3 receptors are coupled to adenylyl cyclase**; therefore, catecholamine action through these receptors is mediated by ***increase in cAMP*** in the cell (Table 75.1).
4. The **α_2 receptor is coupled to inhibitory G protein**; therefore, binding of catecholamines with this receptor ***decreases cAMP*** in the cells.
5. The **α_1 receptor is coupled to phosphatidylinositol** in the membrane. Therefore, hormones acting on this receptor exert their action through ***DAG and IP$_3$*** as second messengers.

Table 75.1 | Mechanism of action at various catecholaminergic receptors.

Receptors	G-proteins	Enzyme	2nd Messengers
α_1	$G\alpha_q$	PLC	↑ IP3, DAG, Ca^{++}

Table 75.1: contd...			
α_2	$G\alpha_i$	AC	↓ cAMP
β_1	$G\alpha_s$	AC	↑ cAMP
β_2	$G\alpha_s$	AC	↑ cAMP
β_3	$G\alpha_s$	AC	↑ cAMP

PLC: phospholipase C; AC: adenylate cyclase

Physiological Actions of Catecholamines

Catecholamines have profound effects on carbohydrate and fat metabolisms. They supply energy at the time of emergency and prepare the individual for either fight or flight responses. They also control many autonomic and visceral functions.

Effects on Intermediary Metabolism

On Carbohydrate Metabolism

Catecholamines act on liver to **increase glucose production** by following mechanisms:

1 Catecholamines **stimulate hepatic glycogenolysis** by activating the key enzyme **glycogen phosphorylase**, which causes hydrolysis of stored glycogen.
   - They, also activate ***glycogenolysis in the skeletal muscle***.
2. They **stimulate gluconeogenesis** from lactate and amino acids in the liver.
3. They also **inhibit glycogen synthesis** by inhibiting glycogen synthase enzyme complex.
4. Epinephrine **inhibits insulin mediated glucose uptake** by the skeletal muscle and adipose tissue.
5. Catecholamines also **stimulate glucagon and inhibit insulin** secretion from pancreas.

All these effects are primarily aimed to **increase plasma glucose concentration**.

On Fat Metabolism

Catecholamines **promote lipolysis**.

1. Epinephrine **activates hormone sensitive lipase** in the adipose tissue that causes hydrolysis of triglycerides and **increases plasma FFA**.
   - FFA provides an alternative substrate for energy metabolism.
2. Catecholamines also **promote β oxidation of FFA** in muscle and liver to **form ketone bodies**.

Catecholamines are therefore **prodiabetogenic and proketogenic** hormones.

On Thermogenesis

Epinephrine is more potent than norepinephrine in most of the metabolic effects.

- Epinephrine **increases BMR** by 10–15%.
- It increases **nonshivering thermogenesis** and **diet-induced thermogenesis**.
- Therefore, epinephrine plays an important role in body adjustment mechanisms in response to cold.

During Hypoglycemia

Secretion of catecholamines increases in profound hypoglycemia, as occurs during strenuous exercise or fasting.

- Catecholamines induce **glycogenolysis and gluconeogenesis** to combat hypoglycemia.
- **Lipolysis-induced release of FFA** is used as alternative fuel.
- In such situation, catecholamines also stimulate secretion of glucagon and inhibit insulin release.

Various **metabolic and other effects** of catecholamines mediated though different receptors are summarized in the Table 75.2.

Table 75.2 | Major actions of catecholamines..

Beta receptors (E > NE)	Alpha receptors (NE > E)
↑ glycogenolysis	↑ gluconeogenesis (α_1)
↑ gluconeogenesis (β_2)	↑ glycogenolysis (α_1)
↑ lipolysis (β_3,β_2)	
↑ insulin secretion (β_2)	↓ insulin secretion (α_2)
↑ glucagon secretion (β_2)	
↑ muscle K^+ uptake (β_2)	
↑ cardiac contractility (β_1)	↑ cardiac contractility (α_1)
↑ heart rate (β_1)	
↑ conduction velocity (β_1)	
↑ arteriolar dilation (β_2) (decreased BP)	↑ arteriolar constriction (α_1) (increased BP)
↑ muscle relaxation (β_2) (GI, urinary & bronchial)	↑ sphincter contraction (α_1) Pupillary dilation (α_1)

Fight or Flight Response

Norepinephrine and epinephrine have **widespread effects** on cardiovascular, respiratory and gastrointestinal systems, and intermediary metabolisms to prepare the **individual to fight or flight** at the **time of emergency**.

- They increase cardiac output, promote blood flow to organs, increase ventilation, stimulate energy supply, relax the smooth muscle of GI tract and urinary system, and cause piloerection; all these effects are intended to either fight with the enemy to finish or escape fast from the enemy to protect.
- This is called fight or flight response, which is exclusively mediated by **sympathetic stimulation and catecholamines released** from adrenal medulla.
- For details, refer Chapter 24, 'Sympathetic System').

Effects on Cardiovascular System

Both epinephrine and norepinephrine **increase force**

and rate of contraction of the heart that are mediated by β_1 receptors. Catecholamines also increase cardiac *excitability and conductivity*.

Effects of Epinephrine

1. Epinephrine **increases heart rate and force of myocardial contraction**, and therefore, causes adequate **increase in cardiac output**.
2. Due to increased cardiac output **systolic pressure increases**.
3. It causes ***selective arteriolar constriction*** in renal, splanchnic and cutaneous vascular bed.
   - However, epinephrine **produces vasodilation** in the skeletal and hepatic circulation via β_2 receptors.
4. The ***vasodilation effect of epinephrine overrides the vasoconstriction effect*** and therefore, **total peripheral resistance falls**.
   - Consequently, the **diastolic pressure decreases mildly**.
5. Thus, **pulse pressure widens**.
   - This occurs especially during sympathetic stimulation that takes place **during exercise**.

The primary aim of all these changes is **to divert blood** from splanchnic and cutaneous circulation **to the exercising (active) muscles**, while ***maintaining the cerebral and coronary blood flow***.

- This also occurs **during stress**.
- These changes ensure delivery of substrate for energy production to the vital organs during fight or flight situations (Application Box 75.2).

Application Box 75.2

Chronic catecholamine secretion is not good: In shock or circulatory failure, sympathetic stimulation that causes catecholamine secretion benefits the individual. However, if secretion of catecholamine is prolonged, then the effect on the body is deleterious, because renal vasoconstriction decreases kidney blood flow and compromises kidney function. Decreased splanchnic circulation impairs visceral functions. Chronic sympathetic stimulation may even result in intestinal paresis or hepatic failure.

Effects of Norepinephrine

1. Norepinephrine produces **vasoconstriction** in most of the organs via α_1 receptors.
   - This **increases peripheral resistance** and therefore, **diastolic blood pressure rises**.
2. Norepinephrine also produces some degree of tachycardia and increases myocardial contractility.
   - Therefore, **systolic blood pressure also increases**.
3. Hypertension produced by norepinephrine stimulates baroreceptors in the carotid sinus and aortic arch (activates **baroreceptor reflex**) that causes **reflex bradycardia,** and **overrides cardio-acceleratory effects**.

Therefore, the net effect is **decrease in heart rate and cardiac output** inspite of increased peripheral resistance (Fig. 75.2).

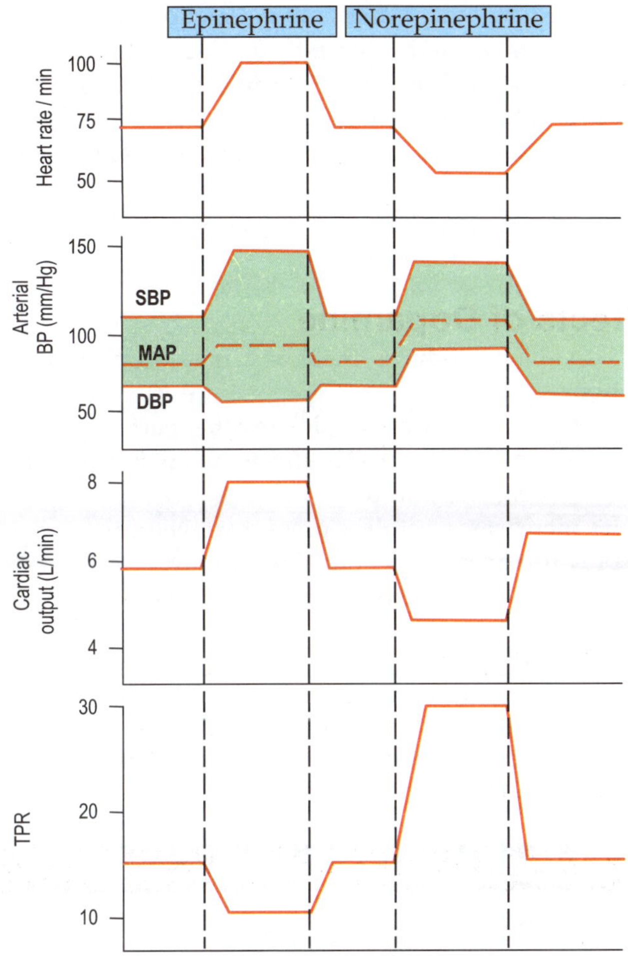

Fig. 75.2: Cardiovascular changes following iv administration of epinephrine and norepinephrine. DBP: diastolic blood pressure; MAP: mean arterial pressure; SBP: systolic blood pressure; TPR: total peripheral resistance.

Effects on Other Systems

GI System: Catecholamines **inhibit gastric secretion** and motility.

Respiratory System: Catecholamines cause **bronchial dilation** (prevent expiratory airway obstruction) so that gas exchange improves. They also stimulate respiration.

On Eye: They cause **pupillary dilation**; therefore, vision for distant objects improves.

- This helps to see the surroundings clearly that helps the endangered individual.

On Endocrine Glands: Catecholamines **stimulate ADH release** through β receptors.

- They also increase **renin secretion** from the JG apparatus of kidney.
- Catecholamines **increase thyroid hormone** secretion and promote peripheral **conversion of T_4 to T_3** which is mediated by β_2 receptors.

On Kidney: Catecholamines **increases Na^+ reabsorption** from kidney.

- Catecholamines also redistribute renal blood flow.
- They **increase renin formation** that causes angiotensin

and aldosterone synthesis and secretion, which in turn increases Na^+ and water retention.

On electrolyte balance: Catecholamines stimulate the entry of K^+ into the muscle cell.

- Therefore, they decrease plasma K^+ (**prevent hyperkalemia**).
- Catecholamines also increase plasma Na^+ concentration.

Effects of Dopamine

1. Dopamine produces **renal and mesenteric vasodilation**.
   - It causes **vasoconstriction in other parts** of the body.
2. It has **positive inotropic effects (via β_1 receptors),** increases cardiac output.
3. It **increases systolic pressure**, whereas diastolic pressure does not change significantly.
4. It causes **natriuresis**, by inhibiting Na^+-K^+ ATPase in proximal tubule.

IMPORTANT NOTE

Dopamine is used cardiogenic shocks: As dopamine increases systolic pressure and at the same time maintains kidney functions, it is very useful for the treatment of **traumatic and cardiogenic shocks.**

APPLIED PHYSIOLOGY

Clinical Uses of Catecholamines

Agonists and antagonists of catecholamines are widely used in clinical practice.

1. The **agonists** are used as ***nasal decongestant***, appetite inhibitor, and for stimulation of general body functions.
2. The **antagonists** (both α and β receptor antagonists) are used for the treatment of ***hypertension***.
3. The antagonists (β receptor blockers) are also used for the treatment ***hyperthyroidism***, especially to prepare the patient ***before thyroid surgery*** to decrease the heart rate.
4. Catecholamines are used for the **treatment of shock**.
5. **Dopamine** is used for treatment of **traumatic and cardiogenic shock**.

Pheochromocytoma

Pheochromocytoma is a tumor of adrenal medulla that occurs due to **hyperplasia of chromaffin cells**. Also, **proliferation of chromaffin cells of paraganglia** is associated with this condition.

- Most of pheochromocytomas produce both epinephrine and norepinephrine.
- Therefore, **concentration of epinephrine and norepinephrine is very high**.
- However, few pheochromocytomas produce either epinephrine or norepinephrine.

Features: The most common feature is **sustained hypertension.**

1. The disease is associated with increased metabolic rate, profuse sweating, extreme tachycardia and high BP, hyperglycemia, and loss of appetite and body weight.
   - In this disease, though there is continuously high secretion of catecholamines, typically there are **episodes of excess catecholamine release**.
   - The burst of catecholamine secretion usually occurs following **rapid change in posture** or the regular physiological events that stimulate sympathetic system.
2. This manifests with **severe headache, tachycardia, palpitation, extreme anxiety, perspiration**, either pallor or flushing, severe rise in blood pressure and a feeling of impending death. PY8.4

Diagnosis: Diagnosis is established by detecting **increased concentration of catecholamines** in blood when the patient is in recumbent and at rest.

- Urinary excretion of **metanephrine and VMA** also increases.

Treatment: Treatment is by **surgical removal** of the tumor.

- The systematic improvement occurs with administration of α blockers.

Role of Catecholamines in Stress

Stress activates **CRH and ADH secreting neurons** of hypothalamus.

- CRH in turn increases **adrenergic discharge**.
  - Adrenergic stimulation **increases plasma catecholamine** concentration.
- All these hormones together **increase glucose concentration** in plasma.
  - Catecholamines increase glycogenolysis and cortisol promotes gluconeogenesis.
- They also shift glucose utilization from peripheral tissues to the neural tissue.
- Epinephrine **increases supply of FFA** to the heart.
- Catecholamines increase **cardiac output and blood pressure** and promote **supply of substrate** to the tissue.

Acute vs. Chronic Stress: During acute stress, a **general state of arousal and vigilance** is maintained by catecholamines.

In chronic stress, reproductive functions, sexual activity, and feeding are suppressed that are also mediated by catecholamines.

- A variety of **cytokines** are secreted during stress.
- The **hypothalamic-pituitary-adrenal axis** works in adaptation to stress. They generally activate the lifesaving mechanisms.

OTHER ADRENOMEDULLARY PEPTIDES

Adrenomedullin

Adrenomedullin is a polypeptide hormone. It is synthesized from **proadrenomedullin**. It is also formed in other tissues like brain and kidney.

Functions:

1. Adrenomedullin **decreases blood pressure** by causing **vasodilation**, which is due to the increased production of EDRF by it.
2. It **inhibits aldosterone secretion**, and therefore, decreases ECF volume.
3. It, along with proadrenomedullin **decreases peripheral sympathetic activity**.

Chromogranin

This is a granular protein present in the secretory granules of chromaffin cells. The protein makes the dense core vesicles denser. The dominant chromogranin in human is **chromogranin B**.

- Chromogranins are secreted along with catecholamines from the granules.
- Therefore, measurement of their concentration in plasma **indicates the secretory activity of chromaffin cells** and indirectly the rate of catecholamine secretions.

Other Hormone

Enkephalins, endorphins and neuropeptide Y are discussed elsewhere in the book.

Exam Questions

1. Describe the synthesis, metabolism and physiological effects of adrenaline and noradrenaline.
2. Explain the difference in the effects of adrenaline and noradrenaline on cardiovascular system. Add a note on Pheochromocytoma.

Multiple Choice Questions

1. **Of the adrenal gland, adrenal medulla consists of about**
   A. 1-2% B. 2-5%
   C. 10-20% D. 30-40%
2. **Which of the following is an enlarged and modified sympathetic ganglion?**
   A. Pineal gland B. Adrenal cortex
   C. Posterior pituitary D. Adrenal medulla
3. **The epinephrine secreting cells in adrenals medulla constitute about:**
   A. 90% B. 50%
   C. 20% D. 10%
4. **In adults, the tissues of adrenals medulla weigh about:**
   A. 0.1g B. 1g
   C. 10g D. 50g
5. **Hormones secreted by adrenal medulla are**
   A. Glucagon B. Cortisol
   C. Catecholamines D. Aldosterone
6. **Which of the following endocrine gland is derived from neuroectodermal tissue?**
   A. Thyroid gland B. Pancreas
   C. Anterior pituitary D. Adrenal medulla
7. **Which of the following cells synthesize and store catecholamines in adrenal medulla?**
   A. Chromaffin cells B. Parafollicular cells
   C. Ganglionic cells D. Mesenchymal-glandular cells
8. **Which of the following is not a measure of increased sympathetic activity?**
   A. Increased catecholamines in plasma
   B. Increased metanephrine and normetanephrine in plasma
   C. Increased VMA in urine
   D. Decreased MOPG in urine
9. **Which of the following is not a function of epinephrine?**
   A. Increased peripheral resistance
   B. Increased heart rate
   C. Increased cardiac output
   D. Increased systolic BP
10. **All the following are metabolic effects of catecholamines, EXCEPT:**
    A. Increased blood glucose
    B. Increased glucagon secretion
    C. Increased lipolysis
    D. Decreased ketone bodies
11. **Which of the following is the function of adrenomedullin?**
    A. Increased cardiac output
    B. Decreased BP due to vasodilation
    C. Increased aldosterone secretion
    D. Increased ECF volume
12. **All of the following are the hormones secreted from adrenal medulla, EXCEPT:**
    A. Neuropeptide Y B. Enkephalin
    C. Serotonin D. Adrenomedullin
13. **Measurement of Chromogranin B in plasma indicates secretory activity of:**
    A. Parafollicular cells B. Chromophil cells
    C. Chromaffin cells D. Folliculostellate cells
14. **The scientist pioneer in studies of secretions of adrenal medulla was:**
    A. John Eccles B. John Jacob Abel
    C. Bernardo Alberto Houssay D. Emil Theodor Kocher

Answers :

1. C	2. D	3. A	4. B	5. C
6. D	7. A	8. D	9. A	10. D
11. B	12. C	13. C	14. B	

Chapter 76

Endocrine Pancreas, Blood Glucose Homeostasis and Diabetes

Learning Objectives

On completion of study of this chapter:

The student will be able to (must know):

1. List the hormones secreted form endocrine pancreas and cells secreting them.
2. Outline synthesis, regulation of secretion and metabolism of insulin.
3. Explain the role of glucose in insulin secretion.
4. Classify GLUTs and give their functions.
5. Illustrate the mechanism of insulin action.
6. Describe the functions of insulin.
7. Understand the basic etiopathogenesis and treatment of diabetes mellitus
8. List the important functions of glucagon, somatostatin and pancreatic polypeptide.
9. Appreciate the importance of insulin-glucagon ratio.

The student may also be able to (desirable to know):

1. Describe the pathophysiology of diabetes mellitus.
2. Describe the process of blood glucose homeostasis.

ISLETS OF LANGERHANS

The endocrine pancreas, which constitutes less than **2% of the total pancreatic tissue**, is formed by **islets of Langerhans** (named after the German medical student Paul Langerhans who first described it in a dog pancreas in 1869).

- Islets are **more abundant in the tail** than the head and body of the pancreas.
- There are about **1 million islets** in the human pancreas.
- Islets are oval in shape with diameter ranging from 50–300 µm. Each islet contains about **2,500 cells**.

Cell Types

PY8.2

Four types of cells present in the islets:

1. **β cells** (B cells): Secrete **insulin**.
2. **α cells** (A cells): Secrete **glucagon**.
3. **δ cells** (D cells): Secrete **somatostatin**.
4. **F cells** (PP cells): Secrete **pancreatic polypeptide**.

β Cells: They constitute **70–80% of islet cells** that **secrete insulin**. The cells are placed centrally in the islet (Fig. 76.1).

- The diameter of each cell is 10-20 µm.
- Packets of insulin are present in the form of **secretory granules** in the cell cytoplasm that measure about 0.25 µm.
- Each **packet of insulin** is present in a vesicle and a **clear space or halo** exists between the wall of the vesicle and the packet.
- A developed system of **microtubules and microfilaments** are present in the cytoplasm that facilitates the exocytosis of vesicles.

α Cells: They constitute 15–20% of islet cells that secrete glucagon. They are present in the periphery of the islet.

δ Cells: They constitute about **10% of islet cells** that **secrete somatostatin**. The cells are typically located towards the periphery between the β and α cells.

F Cells: They constitute **1–2% of islet cells** that **secrete pancreatic polypeptide**. The cells are distributed randomly among the D cells.

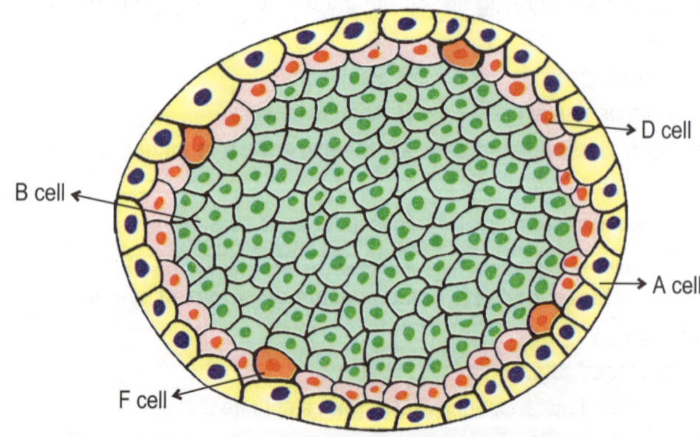

Fig. 76.1: Structure of islet of Langerhans. Note, beta cells constitute majority of cell mass of the islet.

Fate of Islet Hormones

The hormones secreted from islets are released into the *pancreatic vein* from where they are transported into the *portal vein* and from there, they enter general circulation.

- This special arrangement provides **liver the first and maximum access** to the proper concentrations of islet hormones as they are secreted, and then to other tissues in the body.
- Thus, liver being the primary site of substrate metabolism avails maximum **advantage of actions of islet hormones**, especially of insulin and glucagon.

Islet Blood Supply

Islets are **highly vascular**.

- They receive about **10% of the total pancreatic blood** supply though they constitute only about 1% of the pancreatic tissue.
- There is a **portal arrangement** of the blood vessels of pancreas, which allows hormones secreted from a cell group to ***reach the other islet cells***.
    - This arrangement is essential for **paracrine regulation of hormone secretion** from the islet cells.

Innervation

Islet cells are **neuroectodermal in development**. They receive both **parasympathetic and sympathetic** innervations.

1. Stimulation of β adrenergic receptor increases insulin secretion and α adrenergic receptor decreases it.
2. **Vagal (cholinergic) stimulation** *increases insulin secretion*.

INSULIN

Structure

Insulin is a peptide hormone consisting of A chain and B chain that are connected by disulfide bridges. The molecular weight of insulin is 6,000.

1. The **A chain** contains 21 amino acids and **B chain** 30 amino acids (Fig. 76.2).
    - The **final structure** of insulin is ***determined by*** the N-terminal and C-terminal amino acids of A chain, and the hydrophobic character of the amino acids at the C-terminal of B chain.
2. Nevertheless, the **hydrophobic character** of the amino acids at the **C-terminal of B chain** is important for ***biological activity*** of insulin.

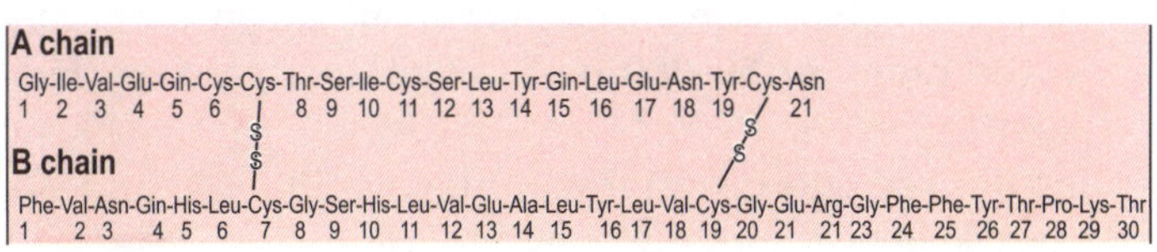

Fig. 76.2: Structure of insulin. Note, A and B chains contains 21 and 30 amino acids respectively, and they are connected by disulphide bridges.

3. Insulin is synthesized as monomers that immediately form the crystalline hexamer unit within two zinc atoms (Application Box 76.1).

Application Box 76.1

Synthetic insulin: Insulin is synthesized in pharmaceuticals usually as crystalline zinc insulin. This preparation is the fast-acting insulin. Usually, insulin is injected subcutaneously as it is absorbed slowly to provide a slow rise in insulin concentration that resembles basal insulin secretion from pancreas.

Significant contribution of Scientist

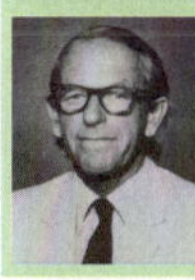

Frederick Sanger (1918-2013) Frederick Sanger, a British biochemist who **won the Nobel Prize twice in Chemistry**. In 1958, he was awarded his 1st **Nobel Prize in Chemistry** for his pioneering work on **amino acid sequencing of insulin**. In 1980, he got 2nd Nobel prize for fundamental studies of nucleic acids, with special regard to **"recombinant DNA"**.

Synthesis of Insulin

Like other peptide hormones, insulin is synthesized as preproinsulin, containing 110 amino acids.

- The **insulin gene** is located on the **short arm of the chromosome 11**.
- Insulin is first formed as **preproinsulin** in the ribosome of rough endoplasmic reticulum.

The **preproinsulin** contains ***four sequential peptides***:

1. An N-terminal signal peptides
2. The B chain of insulin
3. A connecting peptide (C peptide)
4. The A chain of insulin.

The **N-terminal signal peptide** is immediately cleaved from the preproinsulin molecule to form the **proinsulin**, an 86 amino acid peptide, which then enters the Golgi apparatus.

1. **In the Golgi apparatus**, the disulfide bridges are established that allows the proinsulin molecule **to be folded** (Fig. 76.3).
    - The A and B chains of insulin are linked by the **connecting peptide (C peptide)**.
    - The C peptide **not only connects, but also facilitates folding of A and B chains.**
2. During packaging in the Golgi apparatus into the granules, the **proinsulin is cleaved to form insulin** molecules, and **C peptides are retained** in the granules.
    - Therefore, when insulin is secreted, the ***C peptide is also released*** in **equimolar concentration** with insulin.
3. Insulin is associated with zinc as molecule matures. The zinc insulin crystals form the **dense central core** of the granule with a ***clear space around.***
4. The **C peptide is present in the clear space** between the membrane of the granule and the central dense core.
5. Also, during insulin secretion, some amount of **proinsulin is secreted from** the granules.

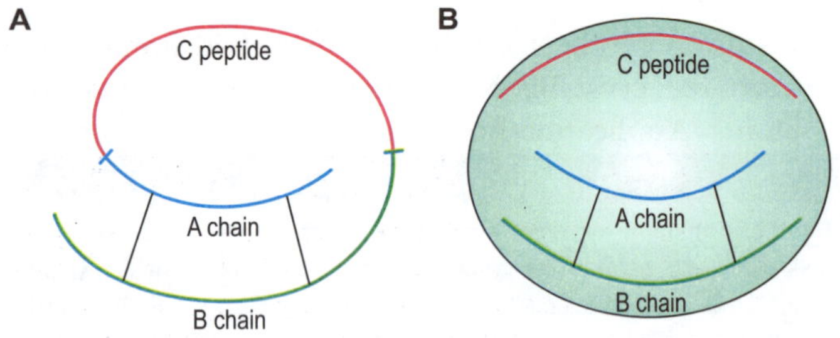

Fig. 76.3 **A:** Structure of proinsulin as formed in endoplasmic reticulum (ER). Note, the molecule containing A and B chains and connecting peptide (C peptide) is folded. The A and B chains are connected by C peptide. B: Insulin molecule in packaged in the granule in Golgi apparatus (GA), after its synthesis. The granules contains insulin and C peptide.

β-cell Secretions

Thus, β-cell granules secrete the following substances:

1. **Insulin:** Insulin constitutes about ***95% of secretion*** from β-cell.
2. **Proinsulin:** Proinsulin is an 86 amino acid peptide.
   - It has about ***10% of biological activity*** of insulin.
   - It is secreted as only **about 3%** of the amount of secreted insulin.
   - However, as plasma clearance is slower (half-life 15-30 min) than insulin, the **plasma concentration** in fasting state is about ***10-15% of insulin*** concentration.
3. **C peptide:** It is a 31 amino acid peptide. The amount of C-peptide secreted is **about 7%** of the insulin secreted from the gland.
   - It has **no biological activity of insulin**.
   - Its importance lies in the fact that it is **secreted in equimolar ratio with insulin**.
   - Measurement of C-peptide has advantages over measurement of insulin. Hepatic metabolism of C-peptide is negligible; therefore, its **concentration in plasma directly reflects the β-cell activity**.
   - Moreover, C-Peptide assay **does not measure exogenous insulin** and do not cross-react with insulin antibodies, whereas insulin measurements have these fallacies.
   - Therefore, C-peptide assay is the **better index of β-cell activity** (Application Box 76.2).

Substances having Insulin like Activity: There are few substances present in human plasma having insulin like activity. Important among them are **nonsuppressible insulin like activities** (NSILAs) that are mainly **somatomedins** (IGF I and II). NSILAs are not suppressed by anti-insulin antibodies.

Following are the **insulin like activities** in human plasma:

1. Insulin
2. Proinsulin
3. NSILA (IGF I, IGF II and IGF bound proteins).

However, their insulin activity is very poor. Therefore, insulin deficiency or insulin resistance leads to diabetes.

Application Box 76.2

C peptide measurement: As C peptide is secreted in equimolar concentration with insulin, and is least degraded in liver, its concentration in plasma provides a good index of beta cell secretory capacity. It is measured by RIA.

The major **regulator** of insulin synthesis is the **plasma glucose concentration**. Glucose increases **insulin synthesis** by increasing **translation of insulin mRNA and transcription of insulin gene**.

Secretion of Insulin

Insulin secretion is greatly influenced by **plasma glucose concentration**. Elevation of glucose level in plasma is an important stimulator of insulin secretion. Factors that control insulin secretion are listed in Table 76.1.

Table 76.1 | Important factors that regulate insulin secretion.

A. Factors that increase insulin secretion
1. Carbohydrates: Glucose, galactose, mannose, and glyceraldehyde (Hyperglycemia is the important stimulator).
2. Amino acids: Arginine, lysine, leucine, alanine.
3. Ketoacids
4. Free fatty acids, especially long chain FFA
5. Hormones: GIP, gastrin, secretin, glucagon, GLP1, cholecystokinin.
6. Increased vagal activity, acetylcholine
7. β adrenergic receptor agonists
8. K^+, Ca^{++}
9. Theophylline
B. Factors that decrease insulin secretion
1. Hypoglycemia as occurs in fasting, exercise
2. Somatostatin
3. Leptin
4. Interleukin I
5. α adrenergic agonists, and β blockers
6. Hypokalemia
7. β cell poisons: Streptozotocin, alloxan
8. Inhibitors of microtubules like colchicine

Regulation of Insulin Secretion

Insulin secretion is mainly regulated by the **feedback control signal** provided by **nutrients level in plasma. When the nutrients are more, insulin secretion increases to facilitate their metabolism and use, and when nutrients are less, insulin secretion is less.**

Plasma Glucose

Glucose is the **most important stimulator** of insulin secretion.

- With the rise in plasma glucose level, there is almost a **linear rise in plasma insulin** concentration **in the range of 50–300 mg%** of plasma glucose (Fig. 76.4).
- Insulin secretion is almost nil below 50 mg% and no extra secretion above 300 mg% of plasma glucose.
- The secretion of insulin in response to rise in plasma glucose concentration occurs in **two phases**.

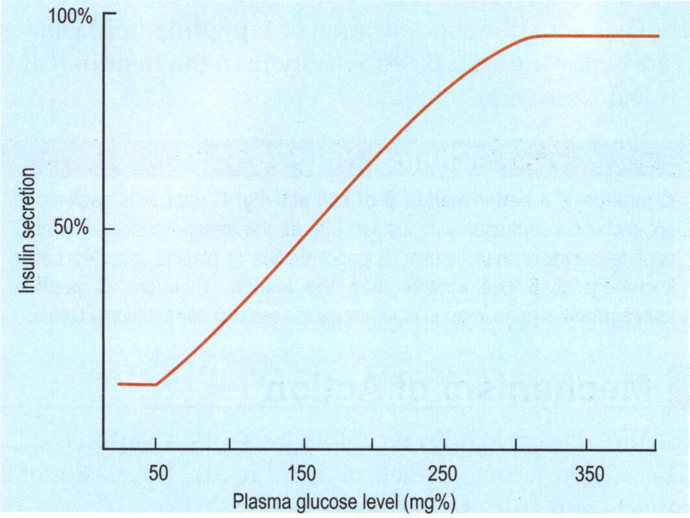

Fig. 76.4: Relationship between plasma glucose and the rate of insulin secretion. Note, a linear relation exists between 50 to 300 mg% of plasma glucose concentration.

First Phase Response: Immediately following the rise in plasma glucose (in response to i.v. glucose infusion), insulin secretion increases rapidly to reach a **peak within 1–2 minutes** and then **decreases to basal level in another 2 to 3 minutes** (Fig. 76.5).

1. This is the ***first and rapid phase*** of insulin secretion in response to sudden increase plasma glucose concentration.
2. The first phase response is due to **release of already synthesized and stored insulin** from granules of β cells.

Second Phase Response: In the next phase, the rise in plasma insulin concentration **occurs slowly** that reaches a **peak in about 60 minutes** and then **remains elevated for 3–5 hours**. The second and slow phase insulin response is due to **stimulation of insulin synthesis and secretion.**

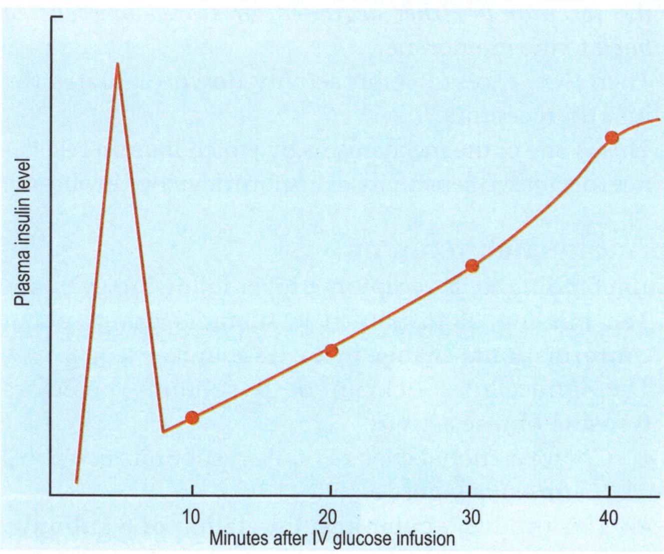

Fig. 76.5: Level of plasma insulin following i.v. infusion of plasma glucose. Note, a biphasic response is observed in which, there is a sharp increase in plasma glucose within five minutes of infusion, which falls immediately, and then a slow rise occurs in the plasma glucose.

Mechanism of Glucose-Induced Insulin Secretion: **Glucose enters β-cells of pancreas via GLUT 2.**

- In the β-cells, glucose is utilized by **glycolytic enzymes** (see below) to pyruvate that enters TCA cycle to **produce ATP.**
- Increased intracellular ATP **inhibits ATP-sensitive K^+ channels**, which ***increases cytosolic K^+*** by decreasing K^+ efflux (Fig. 76.6).
- This depolarizes the β cells, which in turn **opens the Ca^{++} channels.** ***Ca^{++} influx*** increases cytoplasmic Ca^{++} that facilitates **Ca^{++}-mediated exocytosis** of insulin granules.
- Plasma K^+ is a natural regulator of insulin secretion. **Hypokalemia decreases insulin secretion** (Application Box 76.3).

Response depends on route of administration: **The insulin response to plasma glucose depends on the route of glucose administration.**

- The response of insulin secretion **to orally administered glucose is more** than the glucose administered intravenously.

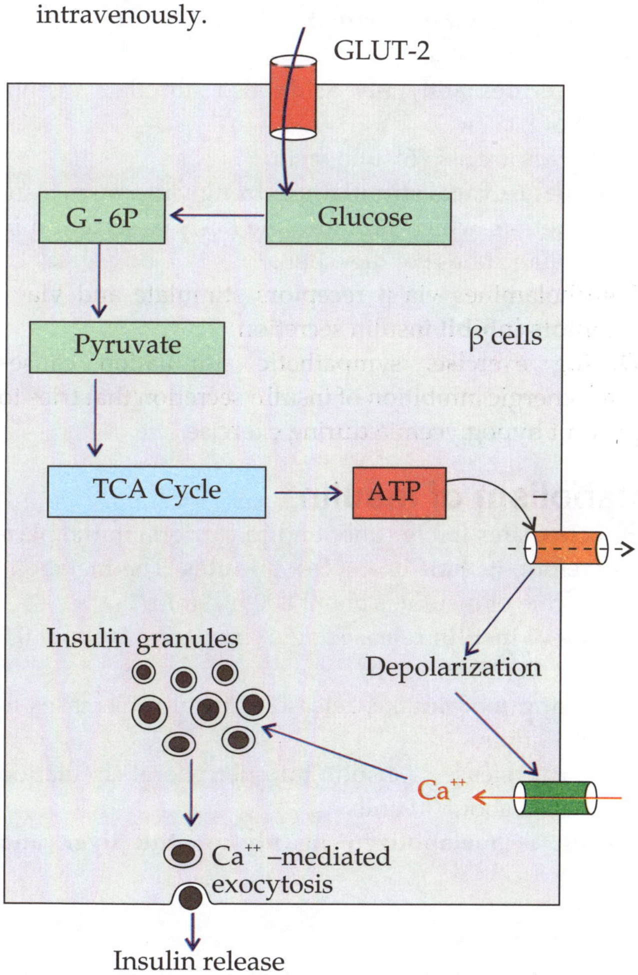

Fig. 76.6: Mechanism of insulin secretion from beta cells in response to glucose. Note, glucose enters the cell through GLUT 2 and is immediately converted to glucose-6-phosphate (G-6P) by glucokinase (GK), which undergo metabolism to generate ATP. ATP inhibits K^+ efflux that causes depolarization of the cell. Voltage gated Ca^{++} channels open and calcium influx increases intracellular Ca^{++} concentration. Ca^{++} mediated exocytosis of insulin granules leads to secretion of insulin.

- When given orally, glucose stimulates **secretion of hormones** from gastrointestinal tracts.
  - Many **GI hormones** such as gastrin, secretin, enteroglucagon, GLP1, and GIP are insulinogenic.
- They stimulate insulin secretion **in addition to its secretion** that occurs due to ***rise in plasma glucose***.
  - Therefore, **insulin response is higher when glucose is given orally than intravenously**.

Application Box 76.3

Effects of Hypokalemia: Hypokalemia decreases insulin secretion. Therefore, patients with hypokalemia as seen in primary hyperaldosteronism develop impaired glucose tolerance. Similarly, patients receiving thiazide diuretics develop glucose intolerance as thiazide causes hypokalemia and may also produce damage to pancreatic islets.

Other Stimuli

Insulin secretion is also stimulated by **products of protein digestion**. Arginine, leucine, lysine and alanine are potent stimulator of insulin release.

1. **Glucose and amino acids** facilitate the insulinogenic action of each other.
2. **Triglycerides and fatty acids** also stimulate insulin secretion.
3. **Ketoacids** are also insulinogenic.
4. **Cholinergic vagal stimulation** strongly increases insulin secretion, which provides the basis of secretion in the cephalic phase of digestion.
5. **Catecholamines via β receptors stimulate and via α receptors inhibit** insulin secretion.
6. **During exercise,** sympathetic stimulation causes α-adrenergic inhibition of insulin secretion that tries to prevent hypoglycemia during exercise.

Metabolism of Insulin

Insulin circulates freely (unbound to carriers) in the plasma; therefore, its **half-life is 5–8 minutes**. The metabolic clearance rate of insulin is about 800 ml/min.

- The **basal insulin release** to the circulation is about 0.5 – 1 unit/h (20–40 μg/h).
- Following food intake, release of insulin increases to about 10 times.
- The total release of insulin into peripheral circulation in a day is about 30 units.
- Insulin is **metabolized mainly in the liver and kidney**.

C peptide Activity

C peptide is secreted in **equimolar concentration** to that of insulin.

1. However, the basal plasma concentration of C peptide is **5 times more than insulin** (1 ng/ml).
   - This is because the **metabolic clearance of C peptide is slower** than insulin.
2. Therefore, the concentration of **C peptide in plasma is a better index of β cell activity than the insulin** (Clinical Note 76.1).

Clinical Note 76.1

C peptide is a better marker β of cell activity: C peptide is secreted in equimolar concentration with insulin. But, as the metabolic clearance of C peptide is slower than insulin, its concentration in plasma provides better knowledge of **β cell activity than the insulin.** Therefore, **C peptide assessment** is done in good laboratories to assess **β** cell functional status.

Mechanism of Action

Insulin acts on insulin receptors present on various cells. The major target tissues of insulin are **liver, skeletal muscle and adipose tissues.**

Insulin Receptor

Insulin receptor (IR) is a **glycoprotein tetramer** consisting of **two α and two β subunits**.

1. The α subunits are present on the membrane extracellularly, whereas the β subunits traverse the membrane (Fig. 76.7).
   - Thus, β subunits have extracellular domain, membrane domain, and intracellular domain.
2. The α and β subunits are glycosylated. They are bound to each other by **disulfide bridges**.
3. The **insulin receptor gene is located on the chromosome 19**, which belongs to the superfamily of genes that code for other growth factors also.

Down Regulation of IR: Insulin binds with α subunits of the insulin receptor, which results in conformational change of the receptor. The **HR complex is then internalized** by endocytosis.

- The hormone is degraded in the cytoplasm, whereas the ***receptor is either degraded, or stored or recycled back*** to the membrane.
- Therefore, excess insulin activity **down-regulates the insulin receptors**.
- This is one of the mechanisms by which **insulin resistance** (decreased sensitivity to insulin) develops in obesity.

Hormone Mechanisms

Insulin binding to its receptors trigger following events:

1. The binding of insulin to α subunits brings about **conformational change** in the β subunits.
2. The intracellular domain of β subunits possesses **tyrosine kinase activity**.
   - Conformational change of the β subunits ***activates its tyrosine kinase*** activity.
   - This produces **autophosphorylation of β subunits** on tyrosine residues.
3. Autophosphorylation triggers **phosphorylation of many intracellular proteins** that alter cell functions. Also, dephosphorylation of proteins occurs.

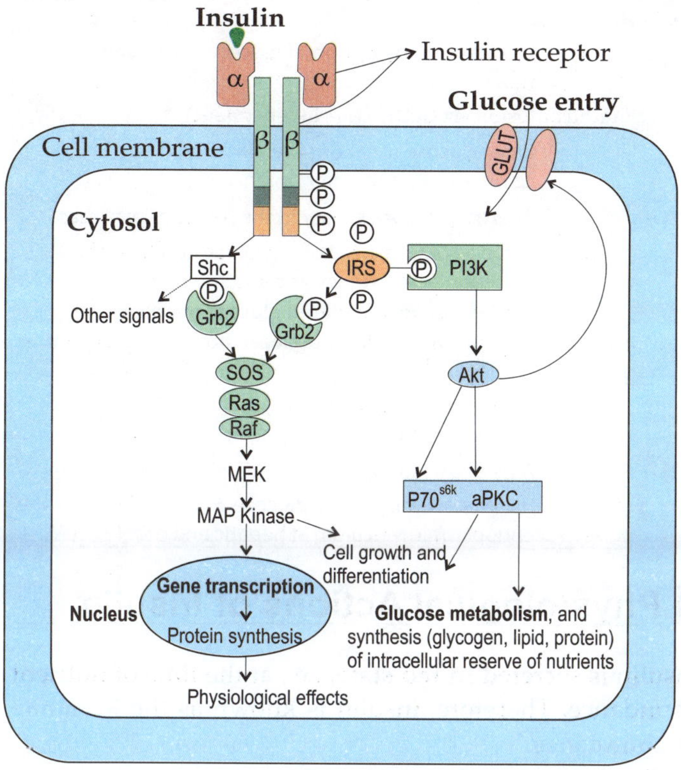

Fig. 76.7: Mechanism of action of insulin. Binding of insulin with α-subunit causes autophosphorylation of intracellular part of β-subunit of the insulin receptor. This causes phosphorylation of intracellular proteins like IRS and Shc that in turn activate phosphorylation cascades and generate other signals. Phosphorylation of Grb 2 proteins activates a series of signals that finally activate mitogen activated protein (MAP) kinase, which induces gene transcription. Phosphorylation of IRS activates intracellular enzymes that alter cell metabolisms, and transfers GLUT from cell to the cell surface. Increased GLUT on cell surface increases glucose uptake of the cell.

4. The active tyrosine kinase ***phosphorylates tyrosines*** on **insulin receptor substrates** (IRS 1 and IRS 2).
   - IRS proteins are **docking proteins** to which a variety of downstream proteins bind.
   - Thus, IRS phophotyrosines serve as **docking site and activating site** for different protein kinases and protein phosphatases (Fig. 76.7).
   - The IRS also serves as **facilitatory proteins** that link to membrane G proteins, phospholipases, and ion channels.
5. Phosphorylation of IRS causes **activation or deactivation** of many ***target enzymes***, **translocation of GLUTs** (glucose transport proteins) to the cell membranes and **induction or suppression of genes** in the nucleus.
   - This results in **synthesis of different intracellular proteins.**
6. The GLUTs that move to the cell membrane **facilitates glucose entry** into the cell.
7. The **insertion of different protein channels** on the plasma membrane increases entry of amino acids, potassium, magnesium, and phosphates into the cell.
8. Activation of mitogenic proteins **increases transcription of various factors** that are essential for stimulation of gene expression, especially concerned with cell growth.
9. IRS also activates **growth receptor binding protein-2** (GRB 2), which stimulates binding of GTP to **ras oncogene** (a proto-oncogene present in plasma membrane).
   - This activates the enzyme ***glycogen synthase***, a key enzyme that modulate the metabolic effects of insulin.

Action through GLUT 4

Binding of insulin with receptors rapidly **mobilizes glucose transport** into the muscle and adipose tissue cells. This process of glucose entry into the cell is **increased by about 20 times** by the activation of a glucose carrier system in the plasma membrane.

- Insulin **rapidly recruits the glucose transporter 4** (GLUT-4), which is specifically meant for insulin-stimulated glucose uptake in skeletal and cardiac muscle, adipose tissue and other tissues.
  - In the basal state, GLUT 4 is **internalized from cell membrane into the endosomes** of the cell and maintained in the cytoplasm in vesicles.
- **On activation** by insulin, the vesicles containing GLUT 4 are **swiftly transported to the cell membrane.**
  - Membrane of vesicles fuses with the membrane of the cell during which **GLUT 4 is inserted** into the cell membrane (Fig. 76.8).
- Insulin facilitates this process of recruitment of GLUT 4 from its intracellular pool to the membrane pool by activating the enzyme **phosphoinositol-3-kinase**, and perhaps this is the **most important function of insulin** (Application Box 76.4).

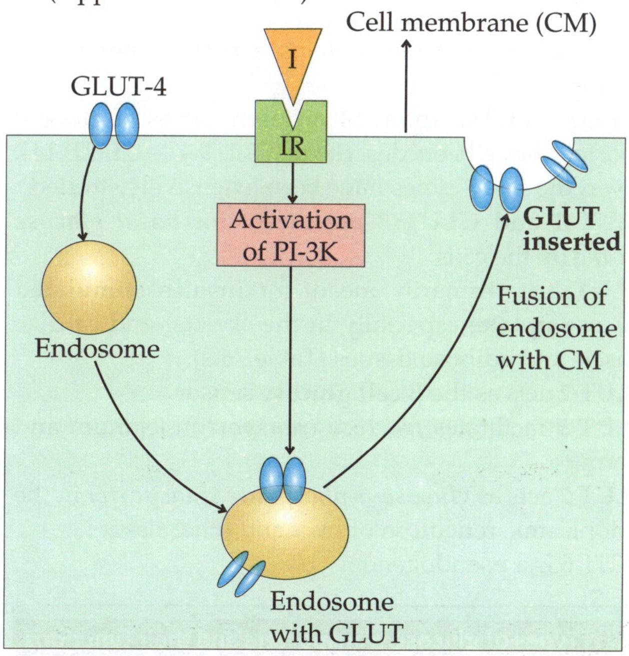

Fig. 76.8: Mechanism of insertion of GLUT into cell membrane by insulin in insulin sensitive cells. Binding of insulin (I) with insulin receptor (IR) activates intracellular enzyme phosphoinositol-3-kinase (PI-3K), which mobilizes endosomes containing GLUT-4 to the membrane. Endosomes fuse with the membrane, and in the process, GLUTs are inserted.

Application Box 76.4

Regular exercise prevents diabetes: Exercise facilitates the recruitment of GLUT 4 from its cytoplasmic pool into the cell membrane in all tissues of the body, especially in the skeletal muscle and adipose tissues. Thus, exercise promotes glucose uptake by the cells and decreases blood glucose level.

- The increased glucose entry into the cell persists for many hours after exercise. Moreover, exercise-induced glucose entry does not **depend on insulin.**
- It is likely that **5′-AMP-activated kinase** facilitates GLUT 4 insertion from endosomes into membrane in exercise.
- Thus, to check the rise in plasma glucose, one should perform regular exercise. Also, regular exercise can cause prolonged increase in insulin sensitivity. .

- Once insulin action is over, again GLUTs are internalized into the vesicles.

In liver, insulin facilitates glucose uptake by **activating the enzyme glucokinase**, not by GLUT 4.

Glucose Transporters

Glucose enters the cell by means of facilitated diffusion or by secondary active transport with sodium in intestine and kidney. In skeletal and cardiac muscle, adipose tissue and other tissues, entry of glucose into the cell is facilitated by insulin by **increasing the number of glucose transporters** (GLUTs) in the cell membrane.

- GLUTs **promote the facilitated diffusion of glucose** into the cell.
- Glucose transporters are **different** from ***sodium dependent glucose transporters*** (SGLT 1 and SGLT 2) that mediate secondary active transport of glucose in the kidney and GIT.
- GLUTs are expressed in different tissues.
- GLUTs are membrane proteins that **span membrane 12 times**.

TYPES OF GLUTs: About **14 different types** of glucose transporters have been described (GLUT 1 – GLUT 14). However, the first 7 types have been extensively studied.

1. **GLUT 1 and GLUT 3** are meant for ***basal glucose uptake*** by the cells.
2. **GLUT 4** is primarily meant for **insulin stimulated glucose uptake** especially in the skeletal and cardiac muscle and adipose tissues (Table 76.2).
3. **GLUT 2** acts as the **β cell glucose sensor**.
4. **GLUT 5** facilitates ***fructose transport*** in jejunum and sperm.
5. **GLUT 7** acts as ***glucose-6-phosphate transporter*** in the endoplasmic reticulum of liver and other tissues.
6. GLUT 6 is a pseudogene.

Table 76.2 | Types of glucose transporters and their functions.

Types of GLUT	Functions
A. Secondary active transport (Na+-Glucose cotransport)	
SGLT 1	Increases absorption of glucose in the intestine and kidney tubules.
SGLT 2	Increases reabsorption of glucose in the kidney tubules
B. Facilitated diffusion via GLUTs (Na+ independent)	
GLUT 1	Basal glucose uptake in the placenta, brain, RBC, colon, kidney and other organs.
GLUT 2	Acts as a glucose sensor in the β cells of pancreas.
GLUT 3	Same as GLUT 1, i.e., basal glucose uptake in the placenta, brain, kidney and in other tissues.
GLUT 4	Causes **insulin stimulated glucose uptake** in the skeletal and cardiac muscle, adipose tissue, and other tissues.
GLUT 5	Facilitates transport of fructose in the jejunum and into the sperm
GLUT 6	Acts as a pseudogene
GLUT 7	Increases transport of glucose 6-phosphate into the endoplasmic reticulum in hepatic and other tissues.

Physiological Actions of Insulin

Insulin is secreted in fed state, i.e., at the time of nutrient abundance. Therefore, insulin is known as the hormone of abundance.

- Insulin ensures **optimum utilization** of nutrients.
- Insulin **facilitates storage of nutrients** when nutrients are present in excess of the energy need.
- It also ***suppresses mobilization of endogenous substrates***. The stored nutrients are made available at the time of need like exercise, fasting, etc.

Insulin produces its target effects by acting mainly on the **liver, adipose tissue, and skeletal muscle**.

On Carbohydrate Metabolism

Insulin **increases glucose entry** into the cell, stimulates its **oxidation** and also promotes its storage. At the same time insulin inhibits glucose production.

- **Therefore, the primary function of insulin is to lower the plasma glucose concentration.**
- It is the **only hormone that decreases plasma glucose level** (decreases basal glucose level and also prevents rise in plasma glucose following feeding).
- Insulin is the **only effective anti-diabetogenic hormone**. The antidiabetogenic functions of insulin are mediated by its action on liver, adipose tissue and muscle.

In general, insulin **increases glucose entry** into cells of almost all tissues of the body **except** brain (excluding ventromedial hypothalamus), RBCs, epithelium of GI tract, and renal tubules.

In Liver

In liver, insulin promotes glucose storage and prevents its production by following mechanisms (Flowchart 76.1):

1. Insulin **facilitates glucose entry** into the hepatic cell by inducing the action of the enzyme ***glucokinase***.

- Glucokinase catalyzes phosphorylation of glucose to **glucose-6-phosphate**.
- Thus, by facilitating glucose entry into the cells and also simultaneously **converting glucose into glucose-6 phosphates**, insulin keeps cytoplasmic glucose concentration at lower level.
- Therefore, **facilitated diffusion** of glucose into the cell **continues**.

2. It **stimulates glycolysis** by activating the enzymes ***phosphofructokinase*** and ***pyruvate kinase***.
   - These actions convert glucose into **pyruvic and lactic acids**.
   - **Pyruvate and lactate are also oxidized** by insulin as it stimulates *pyruvate dehydrogenase* activity.
   - Thus, insulin **decreases the cellular concentration of glucose** and consequently helps in its facilitated diffusion into the cell.
3. It **promotes glycogen synthesis** in liver.
   - In the liver cells, it ***activates the enzyme glycogen synthase complex*** that promotes formation of glycogen.
   - Thus, it promotes storage of glucose in the form of hepatic glycogen.
4. It **inhibits hepatic glycogenolysis**, and therefore it decreases hepatic glucose output.
   - Insulin achieves it by inhibiting the activity of the enzymes *glycogen phosphorylase* and *glucose-6-phosphatase*.
5. It also **inhibits gluconeogenesis**.
   - This is achieved by ***two mechanisms***: 1) insulin **inhibits gluconeogenic enzymes** (*pyruvate carboxylase, phosphoenolpyruvate carboxykinase, and fructose-1, 6-diphosphatase*), and, 2) **insulin decreases hepatic uptake** of gluconeogenic amino acids.

In Adipose Tissue

Insulin **stimulates entry of glucose** into the adipose tissue cells by ***activating GLUT 4 and hexokinase activity***.

1. In fat cells, glucose is then **converted into α-glycerophosphate** (α-GP).
2. The α-GP is used for the **esterification of fatty acids**.
3. It also promotes storage of fatty acids as triglycerides.

In Skeletal Muscle

Insulin **facilitates transport of glucose** into the muscle cells by ***activating GLUT 4 and hexokinase activity***.

1. In muscle cell, **glucose is oxidized** by activation of the enzyme ***pyruvate dehydrogenase***.
2. Glucose is also **stored as muscle glycogen**, which is stimulated by insulin.

On Fat Metabolism

Actions of insulin on fat metabolism are as profound as its influences on carbohydrate metabolism.

- **Insulin increases storage of fat** and **inhibits mobilization and oxidation** of fatty acids from fat depots. It decreases the level of free fatty acids and ketoacids in the plasma.
- Insulin is the **only anti-ketogenic hormone** in the body.

The functions of insulin on fat metabolism are achieved by its actions on **adipose tissue and liver**.

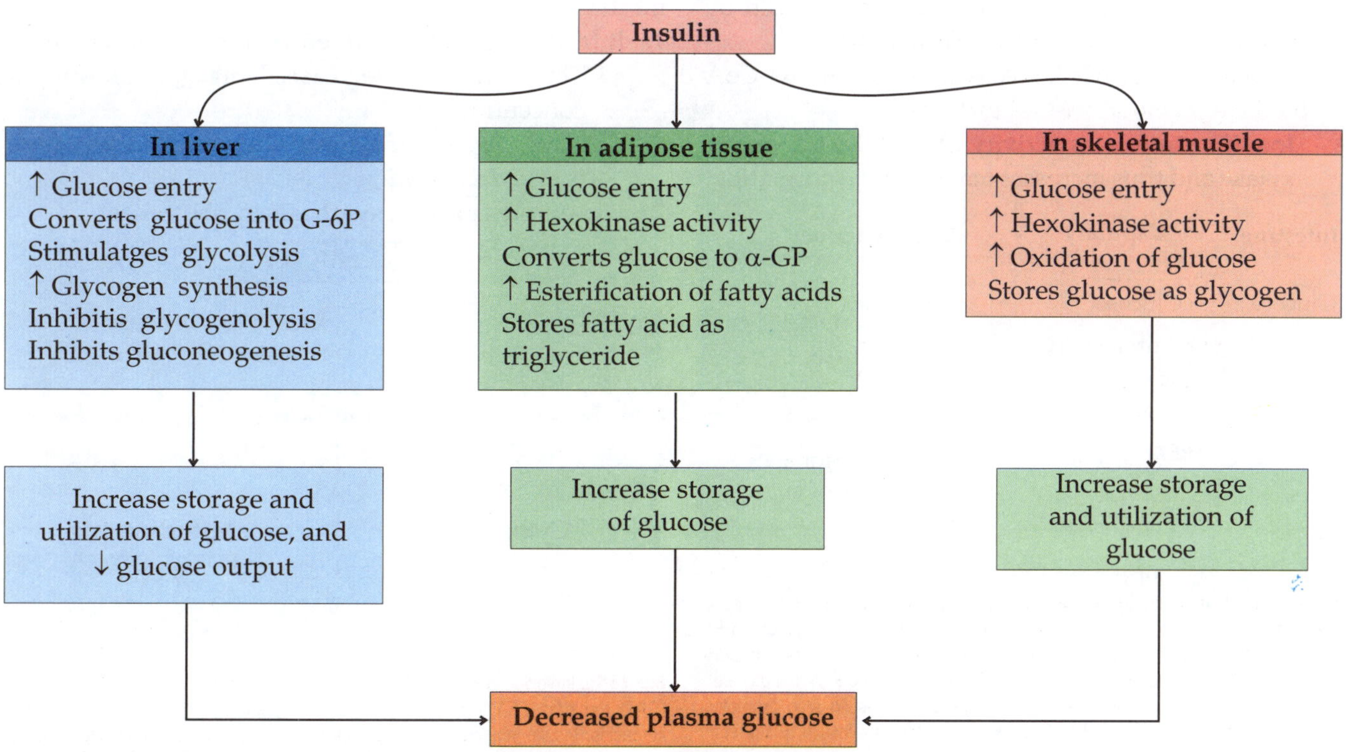

Flowchart 76.1: Summary of insulin actions on carbohydrate metabolism. G-6P: glucose-6-phosphate; α-GP: α-glycerophosphate.

In Adipose Tissue

Insulin **promotes storage of fat** in the adipose tissues in various ways.

1. **By inhibiting lipolysis:** Insulin **inhibits the activity of hormone sensitive lipase** (HSL) in adipose tissues.
   - HSL causes breakdown of triglycerides into free-fatty acids (FFA) and glycerol. Thus, insulin inhibits lipolysis and **decreases release of stored FFA**.
   - Decreased plasma FFA **decreases the formation of ketoacids**.
   - Insulin also **facilitates the use of ketoacids** by peripheral tissues.
   - Thus, insulin **profoundly decreases ketoacid level** in the plasma (see below).
2. **By promoting lipogenesis:** Lipids absorbed from intestine circulate in plasma in the form of triglycerides. Triglycerides can't enter adipose tissue as such. They must be split by lipoprotein lipase, which is present in the vascular endothelium to FFA and glycerol. Then, FFA can enter adipose tissue and form TG there.
   - Insulin **promotes the enzyme lipoprotein lipase**, therefore makes FFA available from blood stream for formation of triglyceride in the adipose tissue cell (Fig. 76.9).
   - FFA is immediately **esterified to α-glycerophosphate** in adipose tissue, which is also induced by insulin.

In Liver

Insulin is **anti-ketogenic and lipogenic** in liver.

1. The **anti-ketogenic** function of insulin is achieved by *its* **stimulation of malonyl-CoA formation**.
   - Normally, acetyl-CoA is converted to malonyl-CoA by the enzyme *acetyl-CoA carboxylase*.
     - **Insulin stimulates activity of acetyl-CoA carboxylase** and thus increases malonyl-CoA formation.

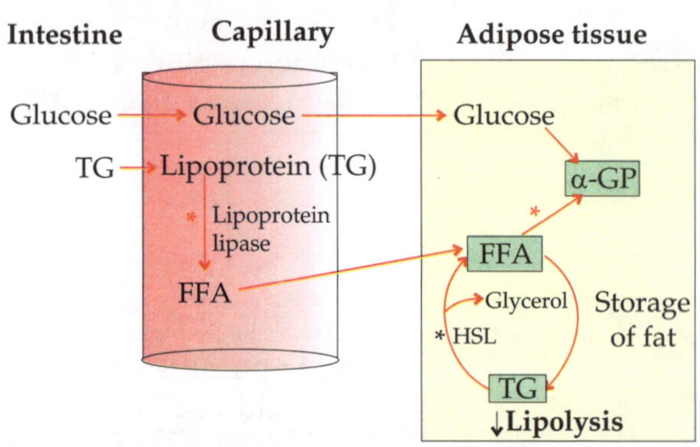

Fig. 76.9: Actions of insulin on adipose tissue. Note, insulin activates lipoprotein lipase in capillary and therefore, splits triglyceride into free fatty acid (FFA) and glycerol. FFA enters adipose tissue and form TG there. In adipose tissue, insulin inhibits hormone-sensitive lipase (HSL) and therefore, prevents breakdown of TG into FFA and glycerol. Thus, insulin prevents lipolysis and promote storage of fat. Insulin also promotes formation of α-glycerophosphate (α-GP). Red star: stimulation by insulin; Black star: inhibition by insulin.

   - **Malonyl-CoA inhibits** the enzyme *carnitine-acyl transferase* (CAT).
     - CAT transfers FFA from cytoplasm into mitochondria for oxidation and then conversion into ketoacids.
   - Thus, insulin by inhibiting CAT through malonyl-CoA **prevents ketoacid formation** (Fig. 76.10).
2. **Fatty acid is synthesized** from glucose by insulin. Insulin achieves this by **three mechanisms**:
   i) The rate-limiting step in fatty acids synthesis is the **conversion of acetyl-CoA to malonyl-CoA** by the action of *acetyl-CoA carboxylase*, which is activated by insulin.
     - **Malonyl-CoA** is used as **substrate for FFA synthesis**.
   ii) Insulin also ***induces fatty acids synthase***, the final step in fatty acid synthesis.
   iii) Insulin **activates the HMP shunt** by activating the enzyme *glucose-6-phosphate dehydrogenase*. HMP shunt increases the supply of reduced triphosphopyridine nucleotide, which is required for fatty acid synthesis.

Thus, from circulation, FFA is shunted away from oxidation and ketogenesis to be stored in the liver.

3. Insulin **facilitates synthesis of cholesterol** in the liver from acetyl-CoA by activating the enzyme ***HMG-CoA reductase***, the rate-limiting step in the process.

On Protein Metabolism

Insulin is an anabolic hormone. It **facilitates protein synthesis** in the muscles and liver by following mechanisms:

1. It **facilitates amino acid entry** into the muscle cells.
   - Therefore, it **decreases plasma amino acid** concentration.
   - Thus, **supply of amino acids** for gluconeogenesis is also ***decreased***.
2. It promotes **protein synthesis** in ribosomes.

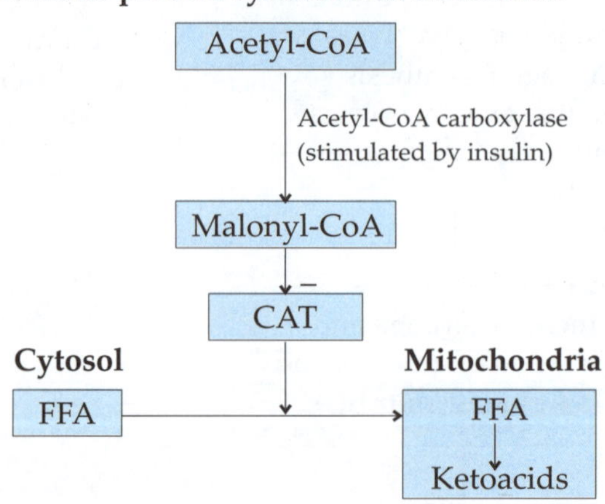

Fig. 76.10: Inhibition of ketoacid formation by insulin. Normally, carnitine acyl transferase (CAT) transfers FFA from cytoplasm to mitochondria, where FFA is converted to ketoacids. Insulin inhibits CAT (as depicted by minus sign) by promoting formation of malonyl CoA. Thus, insulin inhibits ketogenesis.

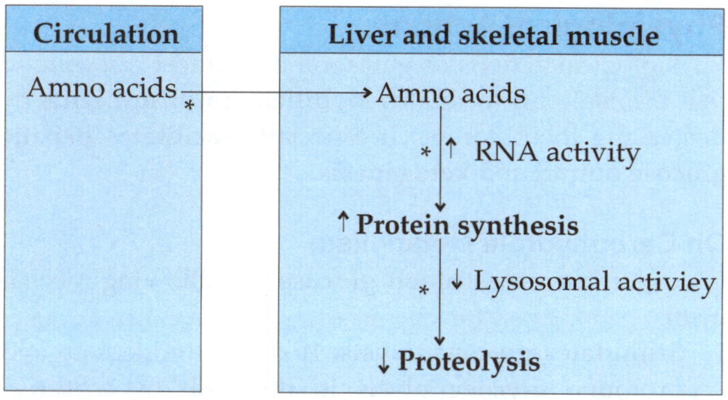

Fig. 76.11: Effects of insulin on protein metabolism. Note, insulin promotes transfer of amino acids into the cells and increases protein synthesis. Insulin also inhibits proteolysis. Star indicates site of action of insulin.

- This is achieved by **induction of gene transcription** for various proteins by insulin (Fig. 76.11).

3. Insulin also **decreases degradation of RNA.**
4. Insulin **inhibits proteolysis** by decreasing lysosomal activity.
   - Thus, it **decreases release of amino acid** from muscle and inhibits their oxidation.

On Plasma K^+ Concentration

Insulin facilitates the rapid entry of K^+ into the cell by stimulating Na^+-K^+ ATPase activity in the membrane. Thus, it **decreases plasma K^+ level**.

1. Insulin is considered as a **physiological regulator of plasma K^+ concentration**.
2. Infusion of insulin in glucose solution markedly decreases plasma K^+ level; and therefore, is very useful in the **management of acute renal failure** (Clinical Note 76.2).
3. This is the reason why diabetic patients receiving insulin sometimes develop hypokalemia.

Clinical Note 76.1

Insulin is given with glucose in the treatment of hyperkalemia: Hyperkalemia is a feature of acute renal failure (ARF) and it is dangerous if remains untreated for a longer time. Insulin for its rapid and profound hypokalemic effect may be prescribed in the treatment of hyperkalemia as seen in acute renal failure, for prompt relief. Glucose is administered simultaneously, as insulin induces hypoglycemia.

Other Actions of Insulin

1. Insulin increases **entry of phosphate and magnesium into the cell.**
2. It also **increases reabsorption of K^+, Na^+,** and phosphate from the kidney.
3. Insulin **decreases food intake**. This action is partly mediated by its inhibitory effect on neuropeptide Y release from hypothalamus.
4. Chronic insulin excess **increases body weight and adipose tissue mass**. The leptin level in plasma increases that promotes satiety (decreases food intake).
5. **Growth promoting actions:** Insulin stimulates synthesis of macromolecules in cartilage and bone that promotes their growth. Insulin stimulates ***transcription of genes for growth factors*** such as IGF-I and II. Thus, insulin facilitates growth of the individual, in addition to its stimulation of protein synthesis. Therefore, deficiency of insulin in childhood (as in diabetic children) decreases their height, growth, and maturation.

Summary of Insulin Actions

In summary, insulin by acting on liver, adipose tissue and muscle **increases glucose uptake and utilization** and also

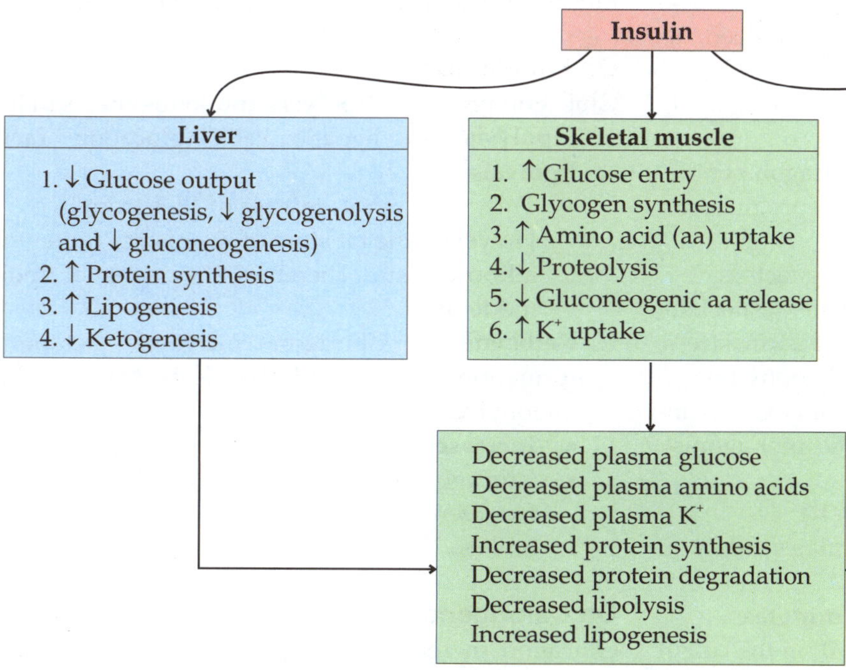

Flowchart 76.2: Summary of insulin actions. GP: glycerophosphate; HSL: hormone sensitive lipase; LL: lipoprotein lipase.

its storage, **decreases lipolysis**, promotes lipogenesis and **stimulates protein synthesis** (Flowchart 76.2).

Applied Aspects

Insulin Deficiency: Deficiency of insulin results in diabetes mellitus (DM). details of DM are discussed below.

Insulin Excess: Insulin excess occurs in **insulin secreting tumor** of pancreas **(insulinoma)**. This causes hypoglycemia.

1. **Chronic hypoglycemia** causes incoordination of movement and slurring of speech.
   - This is usually ***misdiagnosed as drunkenness***.
   - It is typically most common in the morning, as towards the early morning blood glucose concentration decreases and hepatic glycogen store is depleted.
2. Hypoglycemia also occurs in **excess administration of insulin** in the treatment of diabetes.
   - But in this condition **hypoglycemia is acute** and manifest in the form of ***sweating, palpitation, anxiety***, and other autonomic functions.

OTHER PANCREATIC HORMONES

Glucagon

Source & Structure

Glucagon is secreted from **α-cells of pancreas,** which constitutes about **20-25% of the islet cell mass**. It is a **polypeptide hormone** containing 29 amino acids.

Synthesis and Secretion

Like other peptide hormones, it is synthesized as **preproglucagon** that has 179 amino acids.

- Preproglucagon forms **proglucagon** that finally forms **glucagon**.
- Both glucose and insulin inhibit glucagon synthesis by suppressing transcription of preproglucagon gene.

Glucagon secretion is **regulated by** following factors.

Factors that increase secretion: Amino acids (especially gluconeogenic amino acids), cortisol, CCK, gastrin, stress, exercise, infection, β receptor agonist and theophylline.

Factors that decrease secretion: Glucose, somatostatin, insulin, secretin, ketone bodies, FFA and α receptor agonist.

Metabolism & Mechanism of Action

It is mainly degraded in the **liver**. It circulates **freely in blood**.

- Its half-life in circulation is about **5–10 minutes**.
- Glucagon acts by **increasing cyclic AMP** in the cell. It also **increases IP_3** in the cell.

Physiological Actions

Physiological actions of glucagon are almost opposite to that of insulin. It facilitates **mobilization of nutrients** by decreasing their storage. It especially **facilitates hepatic glucose output** and **ketogenesis**.

On Carbohydrate Metabolism

Glucagon **increases blood glucose** by following mechanisms:

1. **Stimulates glycogenolysis:** It causes immediate and profound **glycogenolysis in the liver** by *activating glycogen phosphorylase*. This causes release of **glucose 6-phosphate**.
   - Glucagon **increases cAMP** in the cell. cAMP **stimulates protein kinase A** that in turn activates **phosphorylase** and other enzymes.
   - Activated protein kinase A also **inhibits conversion** of fructose-6-phosphate to fructose 1,6-biphosphate, which helps in **increasing glucose 6-phosphate** in the cell.
   - Accumulated glucose 6-phophate is **converted to glucose**. Thus, more glucose is released from liver.
   - It does not cause glycogenolysis in muscle.
2. **Gluconeogenesis:** It also ***stimulates gluconeogenesis*** by activating ***gluconeogenic enzymes***, especially *phosphoenolpyruvate carboxykinase*.
   - It also promotes hepatic proteolysis and supplies more **amino acids for gluconeogenesis**.
3. **Inhibition of glycogenesis:** Glucagon ***inhibits glycogen synthase***. Therefore, conversion of glucose to glycogen is inhibited.

All these actions result in increased output of glucose from the liver. Normally, the metabolic actions of glucagon on muscle and adipose tissue are not significant.

On Fat Metabolism

Glucagon promotes **lipolysis and ketogenesis** in liver.

1. **Lipolysis:** In hepatic cells, glucagon **facilitates lipolysis**.
   - Thus, it increases **release of FFA** from liver.
   - However, the fat store of liver is not more unlike in adipose tissue. Therefore, the degree of lipolysis is moderate.
2. **Ketogenesis:** Glucagon increases ketone body formation in liver cells by decreasing the level of malonyl-CoA.
   - **Increased FFA** also promotes ketogenesis.
   - Glucagon facilitates **entry of FFA** into mitochondria for their β-oxidation and production of ketone bodies.

On Calorigenesis

Glucagon increases calorigenesis. Calorigenic action of glucagon is not due to increased blood glucose, rather to the **hepatic deamination** of amino acids.

On Heart

Glucagon in supraphysiological concentration **increases myocardial contractility** by increasing cyclic AMP level in myocardial cells. Therefore, glucagon is advocated for the ***treatment of heart diseases.***

On Other Hormones

Glucagon stimulates secretion of **growth hormone, insulin, and pancreatic polypeptide**.

Insulin-Glucagon Ratio

Insulin is the hormone of energy storage and glucagon is the hormone of energy release. Body maintains a balance between the secretion of insulin and glucagons for maintaining normal metabolic functions. Therefore, insulin-glucagon molar ratio (I/G ratio) in plasma is more important than their individual concentration.

- Normally, the **I/G ratio following a balance diet is approximately 3**.
- Following overnight **fasting, it decreases to 1,** and after prolonged fasting the ratio may be as low as 0.4.
- Following **glucose infusion**, the ratio may **rise up to 30**.

Physiological Significance

1. **During starvation**, the ***low I/G ratio*** favors glycogen breakdown and gluconeogenesis that increases nutrient supply.
2. During **high-fed state,** the ***ratio is high*** favoring deposition of nutrients in the form glycogen, protein and fat.
3. **During neonatal period** (immediately after birth), a ***low I/G ratio is critical for the survival*** of the neonate.
   - In first few hours to days, the abrupt cessation of maternal fuel supply during which neonate does not receive required amount of fuel from its own GI tract, a ***low I/G ration maintains internal supply*** of nutrients.
4. **In diabetes,** inappropriate I/G ratio influences metabolic status.
   - Secretion of ***glucagon is inappropriately elevated*** in insulin deficiency.
   - The metabolic derangements are affected by this abnormal ratio.

Applied Physiology

Glucagon excess is produced by tumor of α**-cells** of pancreas. This is called **glucagonoma**. It causes ***hyperglycemia, ketosis*** and other metabolic derangements that mimic diabetes mellitus. In fact, insulin deficiency in diabetes is associated with glucagons excess. **Glucagon deficiency** occurs rarely.

Somatostatin

Source and Structure: Somatostatin is secreted from **D cells of pancreas**. It is also secreted in **hypothalamus and gastrointestinal tract**. Somatostatin is a **peptide hormone**.

- It has **two forms**. One contains 14 amino acids and the other 28 amino acids.
- The **14 amino acid somatostatin** is mostly synthesized in *pancreas* and 28 amino acid peptide in GI tract.

Synthesis and Secretion: Like other pancreatic hormones it is synthesized as **preprosomatostatin**, which becomes **prosomatostatin**. Prosomatostatin is converted to **somatostatin**.

- Somatostatin **secretion is stimulated by** glucose, amino acids, free fatty acids, GI hormones, glucagon, vagal stimulation and sympathetic stimulation via β receptors.

Functions: Somatostatin **profoundly inhibits the secretion of insulin and glucagon** from pancreas, by neurocrine and paracrine fashions.

- It **decreases the rate of assimilation** of all nutrients from GI tract.
- It **inhibits** gastric, duodenal and gallbladder motility.
- It **inhibits HCl & pepsin secretions** from stomach, and intestinal secretions.
- It inhibits secretion of secretin and gastrin.
- It inhibits pancreatic exocrine secretion.
- It **inhibits absorption of glucose, and triglycerides** from the mucosal epithelial cells of intestine.
- It regulates **feedback control of gastric emptying** (entry of food from stomach into the intestine).
  - When food enters intestine, somatostatin inhibits gastric emptying.
  - Therefore, it **prevents rapid overload of intestine** by gastric content.

Clinical significance:

Treatment of Diarrhea: Somatostatin preparations are used in medical practice for the **treatment of diarrhea** as somatostatin inhibits GI motility.

Somatostatinoma: In **tumor of D cells of pancreas** (somatostatinoma), excess somatostatin secretion ***decreases nutrient absorption*** from GI tract.

- Excess of **undigested food appears in the stool**. This causes weight loss.
- Moderate hyperglycemia is observed due to low insulin level in the plasma.
- These patients also develop **dyspepsia** due to decreased gastric emptying and decreased gastric secretion.
- They also develop **gall stone,** which is precipitated by decreased gall bladder contraction as somatostatin inhibits CCK secretion.

Pancreatic Polypeptide

Source & Structure: Pancreatic polypeptide is secreted from **F cells of pancreas.** It is a **polypeptide** containing **36 amino acids**.

- It has a characteristic C terminal tyrosine-amide residue.
- Structurally, it is similar to the **neuropeptide Y** (NPY) secreted from hypothalamus and polypeptide YY, a GI hormone. However, in functions, it is not very similar to them.

Synthesis and Secretion: It is synthesized like other peptide hormones.

1. It is secreted **primarily in response to food intake**.
   - When food is ingested and food passes through the GI tract, the ***GI hormones and vagal stimulation*** stimulate the secretion of pancreatic polypeptide.
2. It is also **stimulated by hypoglycemia and inhibited by hyperglycemia**.
3. Its secretion is also **inhibited by somatostatin**.
4. Its secretion is stimulated by **protein rich food, fasting and exercise**.

Functions: 1. It **inhibits exocrine pancreatic secretion**. This is partly due to its inhibition of uptake of precursor amino acids by the acinar cells.
2. It **slows the absorption of food** from the GI tract.
3. Recent research suggests that it **inhibits food intake**.

Clinical Significance:

1. Increased secretion of pancreatic polypeptide is invariably **associated with islet cell tumors**. Therefore, its increased level in plasma serves a **tumor marker** for the tumors of endocrine pancreas.
2. Failure of pancreatic polypeptide concentration in plasma to rise in response to hypoglycemia suggests loss of cholinergic innervation of pancreatic islets.

BLOOD GLUCOSE HOMEOSTASIS

Blood Glucose Levels

Normal fasting plasma glucose is 70-99 mg/dL. After food intake, this value increases but remains within 200 mg/dL range. Therefore, random blood glucose when < 200 mg/dL is considered normal. The normal postprandial 2 hours blood glucose level is < 140 mg/dL (Table 76.3).

Table76.3 | Blood glucose levels (mg%) in normal (euglycemic), state of impaired fasting glucose (IFG), impaired glucose tolerance (IGT) and diabetes mellitus.

	Normal	IFG	IGT	Diabetes
Fasting	70-99	100-125	-----	≥ 126
Postprandial	< 140	-----	140-199	≥ 200
Random	< 200	-----	-----	≥ 200

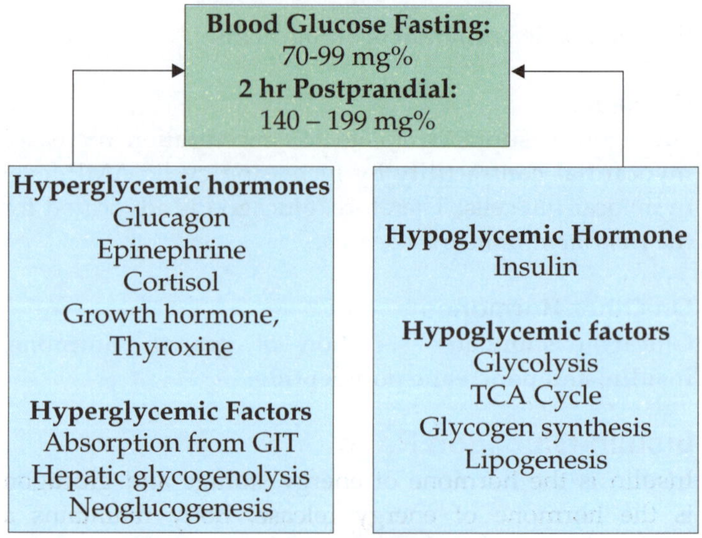

Fig. 76.12: Regulation of blood glucose concentration.

Regulation of Blood Glucose

Blood glucose is regulated by hormones, autonomic influences and calories intake.

Hormonal Regulation

Regulation of blood glucose is the interplay between hyperglycemic and hypoglycemic hormones (Fig. 76.12). Details of these hormones are described in this chapters and in the preceding chapters.

Autonomic Regulation

Increased **vagal activity** (cholinergic innervation) increases insulin secretion and sensitivity. Therefore, yoga, pranayamic breathing and exercises that improve vagal tone are known to check blood glucose and prevent diabetes.

Sympathetic stimulation (through α receptors) decreases insulin secretion. Therefore, chronic stress that increases sympathetic drive is known to increase blood glucose and cause diabetes.

Calorie Intake

Excess calorie intake (excess eating, fast food, junk food) increases blood glucose. Restriction of calorie intake (or utilization of calorie) by adopting to balanced diet maintains blood glucose in the normal range. Details of this topic is discussed in 'Nutrition".

DIABETES MELLITUS

Causes and Types

Etiology

In human beings, diabetes mellitus (DM) occurs usually due to **destruction of β cells of pancreas** or due to **decreased sensitivity of insulin receptors** to insulin. In animal models, diabetes is produced experimentally by administration of alloxan or streptozotocin (**experimental diabetes**).

Diabetes is state of starvation in the midst of plenty: In diabetes, inspite of hyperglycemia, the **tissue cannot utilize glucose** either due to insulin deficiency or due to insulin resistance. Thus, cells can't utilize glucose though they are surrounded by a high concentration of glucose. Therefore, diabetes is called a disease of "**starvation in the midst of plenty**".

INSULIN IS PRIMARY: Though there are few more chemical factors (**insulin like substances**) in the body having insulin activity, they are *don't adequate metabolic actions of insulin*. Therefore, insulin deficiency leads to DM.

Etiological Classification

Etiologically, diabetes has been traditionally classified into two:

1. **Type 1 DM:** Is it is associated with profound **insulin deficiency** and requires insulin replacement therapy. Earlier this was called **insulin-dependent DM** (IDDM).
2. **Type 2 DM:** Is it is associated with **normal insulin level** in plasma and patient is usually treated without insulin replacement therapy. Earlier this was called **non-insulin-dependent DM** (NIDDM).

Recently it has been observed that more than 25% of type 2 DM **ultimately develop insulin deficiency** requiring insulin replacement therapy. Therefore, the classification of **IDDM and NIDDM has become obsolete**. Etiological classification of diabetes is depicted in Table 76.4.

Table 76.4 | Etiological classification of diabetes.

I. Insulin deficient (Type 1 diabetes)
- Immune mediated (Type 1a)
- Nonimmune mediated (Type 1b)
II. Insulin Resistant or Deficient
A. Polygenic (Type 2 diabetes)
- Insulin resistance
- Pancreatic β cell failure
B. Monogenic (MODY, LADA, PNDM)
(Genetic defects of β cell function or of insulin action)
- Maturity Onset Diabetes Mellitus (MODY)
- Latent Autoimmune Diabetes of Adult (LADA)
- Permanent Neonatal Diabetes Mellitus (PNDM)
III. Other specific types of diabetes
1. Pancreatic diseases (pancreatitis, pancreatectomy cystic fibrosis, hemochromatosis, neoplasia)
2. Excess endogenous production insulin antagonists, for example GH (acromegaly), cortisol (Cushing syndrome), NE (pheochromocytoma), thyroxine (thyrotoxicosis), glucagon (glucagonoma), etc.
5. Drug-induced (corticosteroids, thiazide diuretics phenytoin)
6. Viral infections (congenital rubella, mumps, etc.)
7. Genetic syndromes (Turner, Klinefelter, Down etc.)
IV. Gestational Diabetes
- Diabetes induced by pregnancy

Major Types of DM

Diabetes is primarily classified into two types: type-1 and type-2.

Type-1 Diabetes Mellitus

Type 1 DM is characterized by insulin deficiency, which is usually caused by selective **autoimmune destruction of β-cells** of pancreas. Therefore, the disease has traditionally been called ***insulin dependent diabetes mellitus*** (IDDM).

1. The disease starts with insulitis. Many patients demonstrate **antibodies against β-cell surface antigens**.
2. If one of the twins develops the disease the other twin has more chance of developing the disease than people in the general population (the concordance rate is < 50%).
3. The disease usually **starts early in childhood**, and **ketoacidosis is common** (Table 76.5).
4. The disease is treated by insulin replacement.
5. Sometimes it occurs due to **mutation of proinsulin gene** that decreases insulin synthesis.

Type-2 Diabetes Mellitus

Type 2 DM is characterized by impaired ability of the target cells to respond to insulin. This is usually caused by **insulin receptor resistance**. The insulin secretion may be normal or even more. Therefore, the disease has traditionally been called ***non-insulin dependent diabetes mellitus*** (NIDDM).

1. The chance of identical twin developing the disease (concordance rate) is 100%.
2. The disease **usually starts late**, in third or fourth decade of life.
3. The patients are **usually overweight** and sedentary in their habit.
4. Feeding habit and environment also contribute.
5. **Chronic stress** is usually associated with it.

Table 76.5 | Major differences between Type 1 and Type 2 diabetes mellitus.

	Type 1 DM	Type 2 DM
1. Age of onset	Before the age of 40 (Juvenile onset diabetes)	After the age of 40 (Maturity onset diabetes)
2. Body fat mass	Not obese	Obese
3. Incidence	10% of the total diabetes	90% of the total diabetes
4. Genetic susceptibility	Concordance rate is < 50%	Concordance rate is > 50%
5. Incidence of ketoacidosis	High	Low
6. B cell mass of pancreas	B cells destroyed	B cells morphology is normal.
7. Nature of onset	Rapid	Gradual
8. Usual complication	Ketoacidotic coma	Hyperosmolal coma

6. Usual complication is hyperosmolal coma.
7. Oral antidiabetic drugs are usually preferred for treatment. However, insulin may also be prescribed.

Mechanism of Insulin Resistance

The exact mechanism of insulin resistance in type II DM is not known. However, insulin resistance has been highly correlated with body weight gain and few other factors. The ***following factors contribute*** to insulin resistance.

1. **Obesity:** In obesity, insulin fails to transport glucose into the tissues.
   - Obesity eventually leads to hyperinsulinemia, hyperlipidemia and accelerated atherosclerosis that are part of metabolic syndrome (Clinical Note 76.3). These are combinely called as **metabolic syndrome** of obesity.
   - With reduction in body weight, insulin resistance and dyslipidemia decrease.
2. **Adipokines:** The chemical signals originating from adipose tissue are recently proposed to be contributing factors for insulin resistance. Fat cells secrete a group of hormones called ***adipokines*** that influence insulin resistance. The **known adipokines** are:
   i) Leptin
   ii) Adiponectin
   iii) Resistin
   iv) Tumor necrosis factor (TNF α)

Usually, leptin and adiponectin decrease, and resistin and TNF α increase insulin resistance. ***Resistin and TNF*** *α* ***are increased significantly*** in NIDDM.

3. **Decreased second messengers:** Knockout of intracellular second messengers that are usually formed following autophosphorylation of tyrosine kinase has been recently reported to be the major factor in insulin resistance.
4. **Decreased GLUT:** Knock out of glucose transporters in skeletal muscles and adipose tissue has been suggested as a contributing factor.
5. **Free fatty acids:** Increased FFA contributes to insulin resistance

Clinical Note 76.3

Metabolic Syndrome: The constellation of abnormalities classified as metabolic syndrome include: hyperinsulinemia/insulin resistance, low HDL cholesterol, elevated triglyceride, central obesity and hypertension. Metabolic syndrome is also called **Raven syndrome**, and **Syndrome X**, and is strongly associated with macrovascular disease such as coronary artery and cerebral artery disease.

Maturity Onset Diabetes of the Young (MODY)

MODY constitutes about 5% of all cases of diabetes. This is a **form of Type 2** (maturity-onset) DM in younger individuals.

- **Eleven types of MODY have recently been described, MODY 1 to MODY 11.**
- Commonest is **MODY 3** (20 – 75% of all MODYs) and **MODY 2** is the next common (10 – 65%).
- **MODY 3** occurs due to **mutation of HNF1-α gene** (gene for hepatocyte nuclear factor 1 alpha), and **MODY 2** occurs due to ***mutation of glucokinase gene.***

Secondary Diabetes Mellitus

Diabetes occurs due to the **diseases of pancreas** like pancreatitis or following pancreatectomy. Diabetes can also occur in **Cushing's syndrome** (cortisol increases plasma glucose) and **acromegaly** (growth hormone increases plasma glucose). These forms of diabetes are included under the category of *secondary diabetes mellitus*. This category constitutes about **5% of the total diabetes.**

Gestational DM

This refers to the **hyperglycemia occurring for the first-time during pregnancy**. 80% of women with gestational diabetes develop diabetes postpartum.

Features of DM

Diabetes mellitus is characterized by **polyphagia, polyuria, polydipsia, weight loss in spite of increased food intake, hyperglycemia, and glycosuria.** If not treated, the disease leads to ketosis, acidosis, and coma. In chronic cases, there may be diabetic retinopathy, neuropathy and nephropathy.

Polyphagia

Glucose entry into cells of brain except in ventromedial hypothalamus (VMH) is independent of insulin. Thus, VMH depends on insulin for its glucose uptake.

1. VMH is the *satiety center* that normally inhibits the lateral hypothalamus (LH), the *feeding center*.
2. As VMH depends on insulin for glucose uptake and utilization, **insulin deficiency in diabetes decreases the activity of VMH.**
3. Decreased VMH activity **removes its inhibitory effect on LH** (Fig. 76.13).
4. Therefore, LH activity increases due to **disinhibition** (abolition of inhibition from VMH).
5. **Facilitation of feeding center** (increased LH activity) increases feeding (polyphagia).

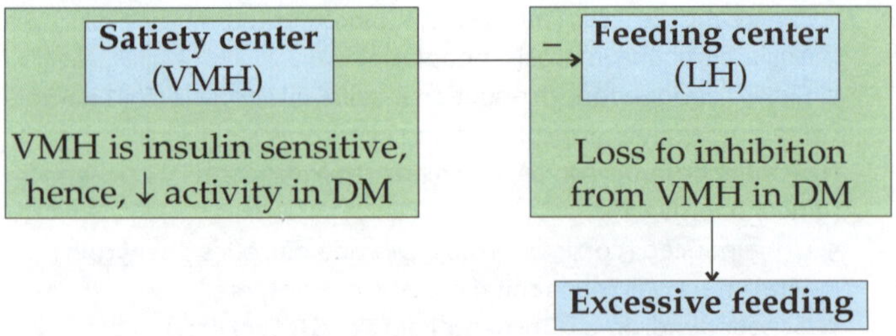

Fig. 76.13: Mechanism of polyphagia in diabetes. Normally, VMH inhibits LH. In diabetes, loss of inhibitory control of VMH on LH leads to excessive feeding. VMH: ventromedial hypothalamus; LH: lateral hypothalamus; DM: diabetes mellitus.

Polyuria

In diabetes, when plasma glucose concentration increases **above renal threshold** (above 180 mg%), glucose appears in urine.

- Filtration of more glucose increases its tubular load.
- Increased concentration of glucose in the tubular fluid causes **osmotic diuresis** that result in polyuria.

Polydipsia

In diabetes, because of polyuria water is lost in excess from the body. This decreases plasma and ECF volumes. **Dehydration stimulates thirst center** that causes polydipsia.

Other Features

Weight Loss: In diabetes, inspite of more food intake, **glucose is not utilized by the cells** due to deficiency of insulin. Therefore, weight loss occurs.

Hyperglycemia and Glycosuria: Deficiency of insulin results in hyperglycemia. When plasma glucose concentration **exceeds renal threshold** (180 mg%) glucose appears in urine (glycosuria).

Ketosis: Insulin **prevents lipolysis** and decreases release of free fatty acids into the circulation.

- Insulin also facilitates **utilization of ketone bodies** (acetoacetate, acetone, and β-hydroxybutyrate) by the tissue. Therefore, ketosis occurs in insulin deficiency diabetes (IDDM).
- Presence of **excess acetyl-CoA** also facilitates conversion of acetoacetyl-CoA to acetoacetate in the liver.

Acidosis: The **hydrogen ions liberated from ketone bodies** (acetoacetate and β-hydroxybutyrate) are usually buffered.

- When ketosis becomes severe, the **buffering capacity decreases**. This causes plasma acidic.
  - Decreased pH of plasma stimulates respiration (**Kussmaul breathing**).
  - Urine also becomes highly acidic.
- Normally, insulin increases Na^+, K^+ and phosphate reabsorption from kidney.
  - Therefore, in diabetes, there is **loss of electrolyte and water**.
- This causes **dehydration, hypovolemia, and hypotension**.

Diabetic acidosis is a **medical emergency** that requires immediate and appropriate replacement of electrolyte and fluid.

Coma: Coma in diabetes is of two types: **Acidotic coma** (due to acidosis) and **hyperosmolar coma** (due to hyperosmolality of plasma).

1. **In acidosis**, loss of water and electrolyte ***causes dehydration*** that results in coma (Fig. Flowchart 76.3). Accumulation of lactate (lactic acidosis) also causes coma.

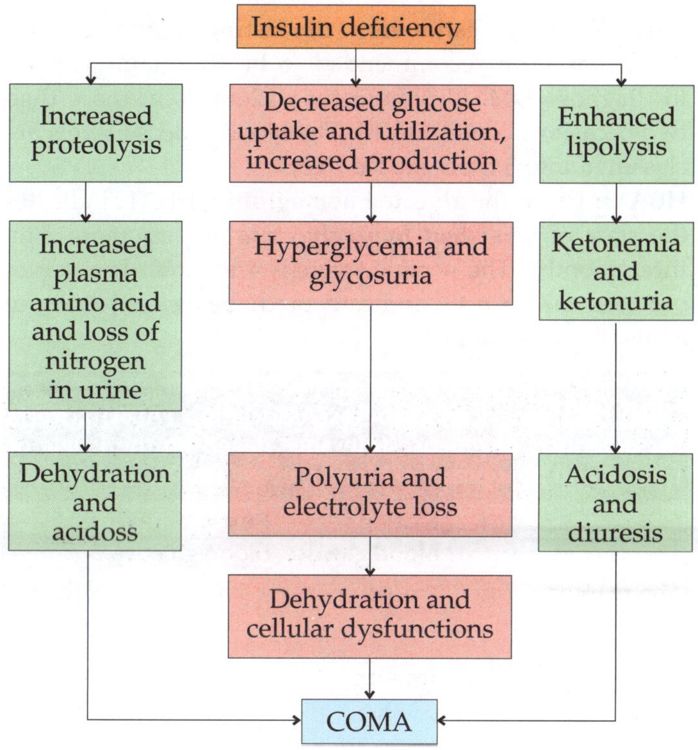

Flowchart 76.3: Mechanism of development of coma in diabetes mellitus.

2. **Increased glucose concentration** in plasma to a very high level increases its osmolality to the extent that it causes ***dehydration of brain cells*** that results in coma without affecting pH.

Diagnosis

PY8.4

Diagnosis of diabetes is done by **demonstrating persistent hyperglycemia** and glycosuria. This is done by GTT, estimation of fasting blood glucose (FBG), and estimation of glycated hemoglobin (HbA1c).

The ***GTT curve in diabetes*** typically exhibits persistent rise in blood glucose above the normal value (Fig. 76.14).

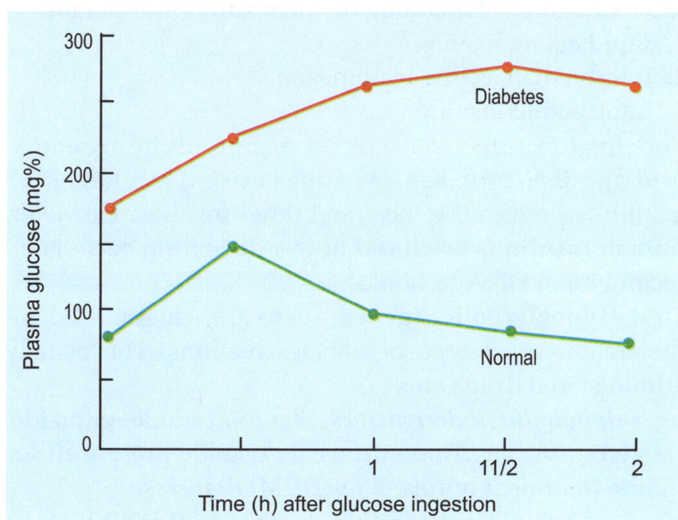

Fig. 76.14: Plasma glucose response to oral glucose tolerance test (GTT). Note, plasma glucose level remains always above the normal GTT value in diabetic patients and does not come into the normal range of plasma glucose (60 to 90 mg%).

FBG: Recently, **estimation of fasting blood glucose** (FBG) has been recommended to be the main criterion to diagnose DM. FBS more than 126mg% in more than two occasions confirms DM. The blood glucose levels are classified into 3 types (Table 76.6).

HbA1c: This is the **glycated hemoglobin**. HbA1c indicates the state of ***persistent hyperglycemia*** at least more than three months. The normal range is 4 to 5.6%. The values between 5.7 to 6.4% indicate prediabetes, and 6.5% or above indicates diabetes.

Table 76.6 | American Diabetes Association (ADA) criteria for diagnosis of glucose tolerance based on the levels of fasting and post-prandial blood glucose (mg%), and HbA1c.

	Fasting blood glucose	Post-prandial blood glucose	HbA1c
Normal blood glucose	70 – 99	< 140	4 to 5.6%
Impaired fasting glucose or Impaired glucose tolerance (Prediabetes)	100 – 125	140 – 199	5.7 to 6.4%
Diabetes	126 or more	200 or more	6.5% or high

Treatment

Diabetes is usually treated by insulin and oral hypoglycemic agents.

Insulin Therapy: Insulin replacement is the cornerstone of **treatment of type 1 DM**. The *maximum decline* in plasma glucose occurs ***following 30 minutes*** after IV injection of crystalline insulin. Insulin is also injected **subcutaneously**, but decrease in plasma glucose concentration occurs in **2–3 hours**.

Different types of insulin preparations are commercially available. Generally, **insulin preparations** are divided into three categories depending on their duration of action:

1. Rapid acting insulin,
2. Intermediate acting insulin, and
3. Long acting insulin.

Pork insulin differs from human insulin only by ***one amino acid*** and therefore, has low antigenicity. Therefore, pork insulin is preferred to beef and other insulins. However, **human insulin** is produced now-a-days from bacteria by recombinant DNA technology.

Oral Hypoglycemic Agents: These are usually used for the treatment of type II diabetes mellitus. The usually administered drugs are:

1. ***Sulphonylurea derivatives*****,** like tolazamide, glipizide, glyburide, etc. These drugs are usually prescribed for the ***treatment of type-2 (NIDDM) diabetes***.
   - They act by **binding to the ATP-inhibited K^+ channels** in the membrane of B cells of pancreas.
   - This **increases Ca^{++} influx and increases insulin secretion**.
2. ***Biguanides*** (phenformin and metformin) are other oral hypoglycemic agents are.
   - **Metformin** acts mainly by decreasing gluconeogenesis; therefore, it decreases hepatic glucose output.
3. ***Thiazolidine-diones*** (***troglitazone*** is an example of this group) are also used. They increase insulin mediated peripheral glucose disposal. Hence, they decrease insulin resistance (used in NIDDM).
   - Troglitazone also binds with peroxisomes proliferator-activated receptor γ (**PPAR** γ) in the nucleus of the cell.
   - It **activates PPAR** γ, which induces nuclear transcription that in turn regulate metabolic functions of the cell.

Change in Lifestyle: In addition to drugs, it is important to assure lifestyle modification and proper calorie intake in the long-term management of DM:

1. ***Calorie Intake:*** Food intake should be adjusted to ensure appropriate nutritional requirements. Excess intake should be avoided. Diet should have less carbohydrate and fat, more fibers and adequate proteins and vitamins.
2. ***Regular Exercise:*** Morning walk and freehand exercises improve insulin release and decreases insulin resistance.
3. ***Relaxation of body and mind:*** Healthy body and mind without stress will not only cure diabetes, but also prevent other diseases.
4. ***Practice of yoga.*** Yoga is very helpful in reducing the intensity of diabetes, and reducing the complications.

Complications

Microangiopathy causes retinal edema and scarring, which is often associated with hard exudates in retina, the condition known as **diabetic retinopathy,** which also occurs due to neovascularization. (Fig. 76.15).

1. The microangiopathy in kidney is known as **diabetic nephropathy**.
2. The macrovascular complications lead to **heart attack** (myocardial infarction) and **stroke**.

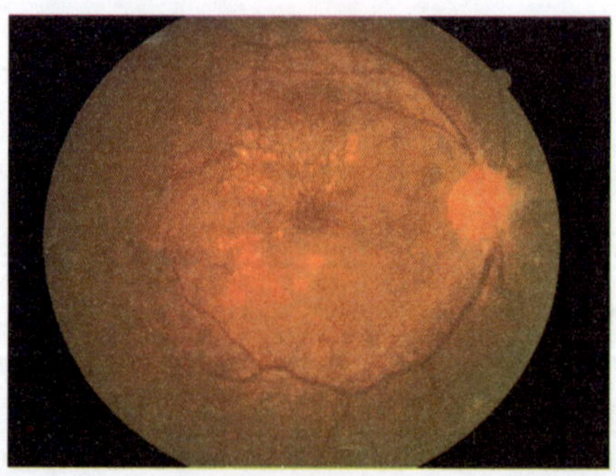

Fig. 76.15: Funduscopic view of proliferative diabetic retinopathy in chronic diabetes. Note the prominent neovascularization of retina, dot-blot hemorrhages, and hard exudates in macula.

Courtesy: Dr Subashini Kaliaperumal, Professor of Ophthalmology, JIPMER, Puducherry.

3. **Autonomic neuropathy** (diabetic neuropathy) is common.
4. Hyperglycemia and neuropathy.

- Results in **chronic ulcer and gangrene** formation especially in the foot, called as diabetic foot.

Exam Questions

1. Describe the functions of insulin.
2. With the help of a schematic diagram, explain the mechanism of action of insulin. Add a note on GLUTs.
3. List the factors affecting insulin secretion. Describe how blood glucose level controls insulin secretion.
4. Classify diabetes. Briefly describe the physiological basis of four cardinal features of diabetes.

Multiple Choice Questions

1. Glucose mediated insulin release is mediated through:
A. ATP-dependent K^+ channels B. cAMP
C. Carrier modulators D. Receptor phosphorylation

2. Insulin secretion is inhibited by
A. Secretin B. Epinephrine
C. Growth hormone D. Gastrin

3. Insulin secretion is increased by all, EXCEPT:
A. Gastrin B. Secretin
C. VIP D. GIP

4. Rapid infusion of insulin causes which of the following?
A. Hyperkalemia B. Hypokalemia
C. Hypernatremia D. Hyponatremia

5. In fetus, the insulin secretion begins by:
A. 3rd month B. 5rd month
C. 7rd month D. 9rd month

6. All are actions of insulin, EXCEPT:
A. Gluconeogenesis B. Glycolysis
C. Glycogenesis D. Lipogenesis

7. Which of the following is NOT done by insulin?
A. Glycogen synthesis B. Glycolysis
C. Lipogenesis D. Ketogenesis

8. What is not the role of insulin in lipid metabolism?
A. Activates lipoprotein lipase
B. Increases lipolysis
C. Activates hormone sensitive lipase
D. Decrease free fatty acid level

9. Insulin increases the activities of all of the following enzymes, EXCEPT:
A. Glucokinase B. Pyruvate carboxylase
C. Glycogen synthase D. Acetyl-CoA carboxylase

10. GLUT-2 is present mainly in:
A. Beta cells of pancreases B. Placenta
C. Skeletal muscle D. Cardiac muscle

11. Insulin-mediated glucose uptake occurs through:
A. GLUT-1 B. GLUT-2
C. GLUT-3 D. GLUT-4

12. Insulin mediated glucose uptake occurs in:
A. Adipose tissue & Skeletal muscle
B. Kidney
C. Brain
D. Intestine

13. Insulin does not facilitate glucose uptake in all the following, EXCEPT:
A. Epithelium of GI tract
B. Ventromedian hypothalamus
C. RBC
D. Kidney

14. First response to hypoglycemia:
A. Decreased insulin
B. Increased glucagon
C. Increased cortisol
D. Increased nor epinephrine

15. Glucagon causes all, EXCEPT:
A. Hepatic glycogenolysis
B. Gluconeogenesis
C. Lipolysis
D. Glycogenesis

16. Which of the following is not a known hyperglycemic hormone?
A. Glucagon
B. Cortisol
C. Growth hormone
D. Prolactin

17. Polyphagia in diabetes is mainly due to:
A. Decreased glucose utilization in the most of the tissues of the body
B. Decreased glucose uptake by whole brain
C. Decreased glucose utilization by entire hypothalamic nuclei
D. Decreased glucose utilization of VMH causing less VMH activity

18. Chronic hyperglycemia in diabetes is better assessed by estimation of:
A. Fasting blood glucose
B. HbA1C
C. Postprandial blood glucose
D. Fundus examination of the eye

Answers :

1. A	2. B	3. C	4. B	5. A	6. A	7. D	8. C	9. B	10. A
11. D	12. A	13. B	14. A	15. D	16. D	17. D	18. B		

Chapter 77

Calcium and Phosphate Metabolism, Physiology of Bone and Parathyroid Gland

Learning Objectives

On completion of study of this chapter:

The student will be able to (must know):

1. Learn the basics of calcium and phosphate metabolism and list the functions of calcium and phosphate.
2. Outline the hormonal regulation of calcium metabolism.
3. List the constituents of bone, cell types of bone and give their functions.
4. Describe bone formation and resorption & give the functions of osteoblasts and osteoclasts.
5. Mechanism of action and functions of parathormone.
6. Mechanism of action and functions of calcitonin and vit D.

The student may also be able to (desirable to know):

1. Describe the role of calcium and phosphate in bone physiology.
2. Learn the physiological basis of osteoporosis and ostepetrosis.
3. Describe the physiological basis of hypoparathyroidism and hyperparathyroidism.

CALCIUM AND PHOSPHATE METABOLISM

Calcium Metabolism PY8.1

The normal **plasma calcium concentration is 9–11 mg%** (average 10 mg%).

Functions of Calcium

Calcium ion is involved in many key functions:

1. Genesis and **maintenance of action potentials**, especially in cardiac and smooth muscles.
2. Genesis of **pacemaker potential** in various pacemaking tissues.
3. **Excitation-contraction coupling** during muscle contractions.
4. **Excitability of nerve and muscle:** Calcium influences ***sodium permeability and*** therefore, influences the ease with which action potentials are triggered.
5. Controls **cell division**.
6. Bone formation (**mineralization of bone**).
7. Secretion of endocrine and exocrine glands (**calcium-mediated exocytosis** causes release of hormones from gland cells).
8. **Neurotransmitter release** from nerve terminals.
9. **Blood coagulation:** Calcium is coagulation *factor IV* and is highly essential for clotting of blood. Many ***anticoagulants*** chelate calcium to prevent clotting.
10. Modulation of various **enzyme activities** (enzymes use calcium as cofactor).
11. Calcium acts as a **second or third messenger** in various intracellular signaling pathways for hormone actions.
12. **GI motility** and motility of many other structures.

Distribution of Calcium in the Body

In the cell, calcium is **stored in mitochondria and endoplasmic reticulum**. The total **intracellular free calcium is about 0.2 mg**, whereas about 9 g is present in the bound form or in the storage sites such as in mitochondria and endoplasmic reticulum.

- Normally, a healthy adult contains 1 to 1.5 kg of calcium in his body.
  - About 99% of the total calcium is present in **bones and teeth** (Table 77.1).
- The total extracellular pool of calcium is about 1 to 1.5 g and intracellular pool is about 10 – 15 g.
  - The half of total plasma calcium (about **50%) is ionized** and present in the *biologically active form*.

- About **10% of the plasma calcium is in the non-ionized form** like calcium bicarbonate, and about 40% is bound to albumin.
  - The **pH of blood affects ionization of calcium**.
  - ***In alkalosis***, ionized calcium concentration decreases, and ***in acidosis***, it increases.

Table 77.1 | Distribution of calcium in the body.
Total body content : 1200 g (average)
In bones and teeth : 99% of total
In intracellular fluid : 0.9% (11 g approx.)
In extracellular fluid : 0.1% (1 g approx)

Metabolism

Daily dietary intake of calcium ranges from **200 mg to 2 g.** In an adult, the ***recommended daily intake*** is about 800 mg.

- Calcium absorption from the intestine is **inversely proportional to its intake**.
  - This **prevents calcium overload** *when intake is high* or maintains calcium concentration even with low intake.
- With a daily intake of 1 g of calcium, generally 30% (300 mg) of it is absorbed in the intestine and about **70% (700 mg) is excreted in the stool**.
- About 150 mg of calcium is secreted into the intestine, which makes a total of about **850 mg excreted daily in the stool**.

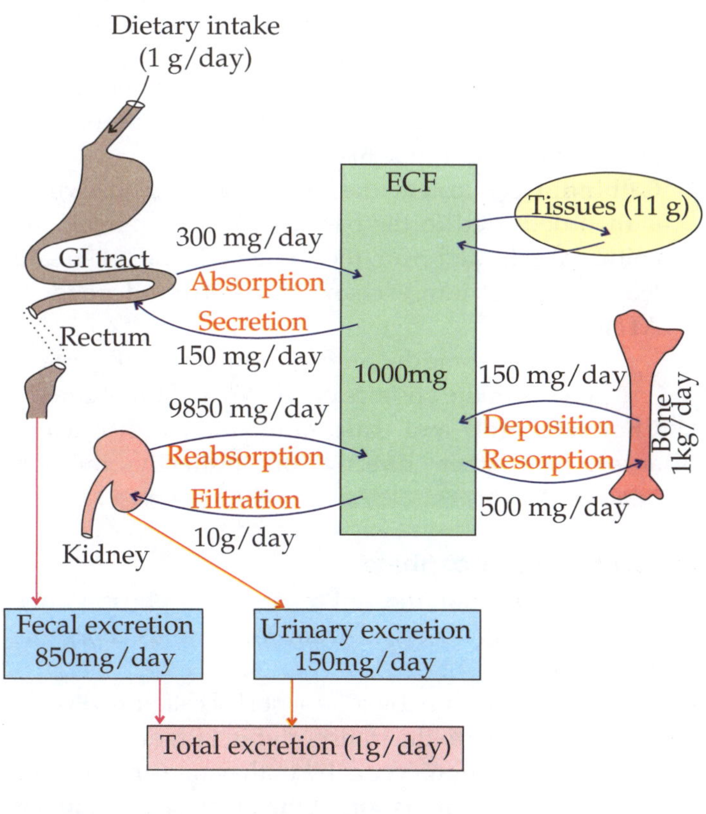

Fig. 77.1: Summary of calcium metabolism.

  - About 150 mg is excreted in the urine.
  - Thus, about 1 g of calcium is excreted daily from the body to maintain the balance between input and output (Fig. 77.1).
- Calcium absorbed from intestine enters the **ECF pool** of calcium which is about **1000 mg**.
  - This is in equilibrium with the **rapidly exchangeable pool** (4000 mg) of the body.
- From the rapidly exchangeable pool of plasma, **500 mg of calcium enters bones** for normal bone remodeling and from bone about 500 mg of calcium extrudes back into the plasma.

Phosphate Metabolism

The normal **plasma phosphate concentration *is* 2.5 to 4.5 mg%**.

Functions of Phosphorous

Phosphorous (usually as phosphate has biological activities.

1. Phosphate is present in the ATP, creatine phosphate, various co-factors like NAD, NADP, and thiamine pyrophosphate.
2. Phosphate is an **integral part of second messengers** in the cells like cyclic AMP and inositol triphosphate.
3. It is also found in **DNA and RNA**.
4. Phosphate is required for **phosphorylation of many intracellular proteins**, for formation of phosphoproteins.
   - Phosphoproteins mediate many intracellular metabolic activities.
5. Phosphate acts as **covalent modifier** of many enzymes.
6. It is a **major constituent of the bone and teeth** like that of calcium.
7. Phosphate serves as an important component of **intracellular pH buffering system**.

Distribution of Phosphate in the Body

Total body phosphate content is roughly half of the calcium content. Out of 600 g of total phosphate in the body, about **86% is present in the bones**, 14% in intracellular fluid and 0.08% in extracellular fluid (Table 77.2). About 6% is present in the muscle and 8% in other cells.

Table 77.2 | Distribution of phosphate in the body
Total body content: 600 g (average)
In bones and teeth : 86% of total
In intracellular fluid : 14% (about 84 g)
In extracellular fluid : 0.08% (1.2 g)

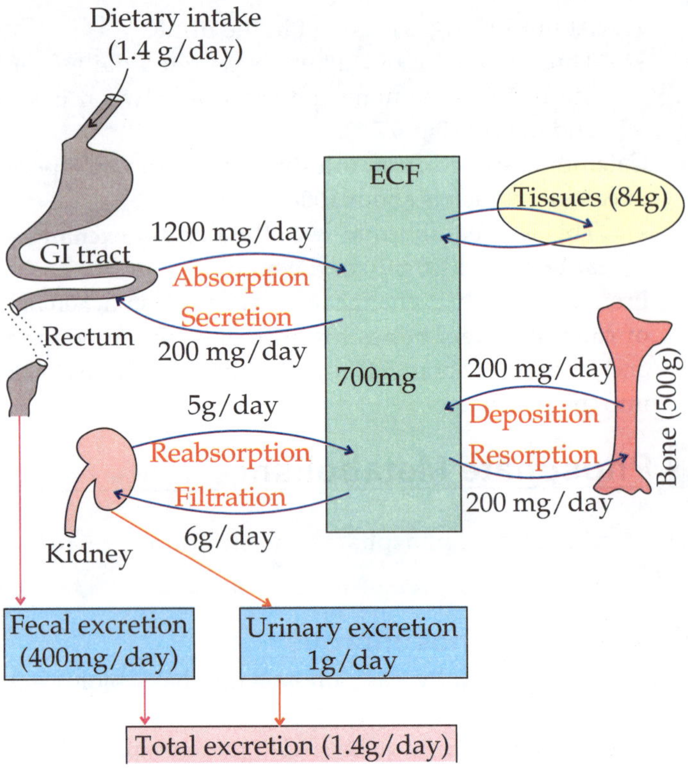

Fig. 77.2: Summary of phosphorus metabolism.

Metabolism

The daily phosphate intake is about 1400 mg, of which **75% is absorbed from the intestine** and 25% is excreted in the stool.

- The phosphate pool in the ECF is about 700 mg, from where about **200 mg is exchanged** with the bones for bone remodeling.
- Normally, about 1000 mg is excreted in urine.
  - Regulation of **renal excretion** of phosphate mainly controls the concentration of plasma phosphate.
- Renal (1 g) and fecal (0.4 g) excretion balances the daily intake with daily output of phosphate (Fig. 77.2).

Phosphate deficiency results in muscle weakness, cardiac and respiratory dysfunction, abnormal bone formation, and loss of red cell membrane integrity.

Magnesium

Magnesium is closely related with the calcium and phosphate metabolisms.

- It is essential for **neuromuscular transmission** and it serves as **cofactor for many enzymatic activities.**
- The **normal plasma level** of magnesium is **1.5–2.5 mg%.**
  - About 35% of it is bound to protein.
- There is about 25 g of magnesium in our body of which about 50% is present in the bones and rest 50% in the intracellular fluid.

The magnesium depletion causes **neuromuscular dysfunction** and **ventricular arrhythmias**.

Regulation of Calcium & Phosphate Homeostasis

Homeostasis of calcium and phosphate is influenced mainly by **exchange** of these ions **between plasma and bone**. Also, **absorption** of calcium and phosphate from intestine and kidney that determines their fecal and urinary **excretion** respectively greatly contributes to their homeostasis.

- In general, **calcium is excreted more in the stool** (850 mg/day) and **less in urine** (150 mg/day), whereas **phosphate is excreted more in urine** (1000 mg/day) and **less in stool** (400 mg/day).

Intestinal Control of Calcium and Phosphate

Absorption of calcium and phosphate from intestine significantly contributes to their plasma concentration.

Absorption of Calcium

About one third of ingested calcium is absorbed from GI tract and remaining two-third is excreted. About 150 mg of calcium enters intestine in the form of various **GI secretions**, and from **sloughing of mucosal cells.**

1. Calcium absorption occurs by **active transport in duodenum and jejunum**, and **passive diffusion in ileum**.
   - Active transport is **facilitated by 1,25-dihydroxy-cholecalciferol** (metabolite of vitamin D), which increases the ***expression of calcium binding proteins*** in the intestinal epithelial cells increasing their capacity to transport more calcium.
2. Calcium is transported across the brush border of intestinal epithelial cells via **TRPV6** (transient receptor potential vanilloid type 6) channels.
3. **Calbindin** sequesters the absorbed calcium, which is then delivered to the basolateral membrane of the epithelial cells and from there enters the blood stream via sodium-calcium exchanger or calcium-dependent ATPase.
   - However, some degree of intestinal calcium uptake persists in the absence of TRPV6 and calbindin.
4. **Cholecalciferol and calcitonin** influence calcium absorption either directly or indirectly through vitamin D.

Absorption of Phosphate

In contrast to calcium, most of the ingested phosphorous (about 75–85%) is absorbed from intestine as inorganic phosphate (Pi).

1. Pi absorption occurs by a transporter called **NaPi-IIb**, which is related to the transporter in kidney.
2. Though absorption occurs by both active and passive processes, **active transport is the primary mechanism** of absorption.

- However, the regulatory mechanism for phosphate absorption is not well developed. To some extent, it is **coupled to calcium absorption**.

Renal Control of Calcium and Phosphate

Reabsorption of calcium and phosphate from kidney contributes significantly to their plasma concentration.

Reabsorption of Calcium

About **60% of plasma calcium is filtered** in the glomeruli and 40% is bound to plasma proteins.

1. Of the filtered calcium, 1–5% is excreted in urine and about **95% is reabsorbed back into the plasma**. Therefore, the total urinary excretion is less.
2. Of the filtered load of calcium, about **65% is reabsorbed in proximal tubule**, 25% in loop of Henle and 8% in distal tubule.
   - In proximal tubule, the transport process is active that involves two **sodium-dependent Pi co-transporters** such as **NaPi-IIa and NaPi-IIc**.
3. **Parathyroid hormone** (PTH) ***inhibits NaPi-IIa***. PTH regulates plasma calcium by also acting on the distal tubule.

Reabsorption of Phosphate

Phosphate is mainly excreted in urine.

1. Usually, **75–85% of filtered phosphate** is reabsorbed.
2. The **major site of reabsorption is proximal tubule**, where about ***70% of the filtered load*** of phosphate is reabsorbed.
3. **Parathyroid hormone** controls phosphate excretion by mainly **inhibiting its reabsorption in the proximal tubule**.

BONE PHYSIOLOGY

Bone is a compact living connective tissue, which is well vascularized.

The **major functions** of bones are as follows:

1. They form the **skeletal framework of the body**, which is crucial for changing and maintaining various body postures.
2. By providing stable postural background, bones allow **movements** to occur.
3. They play important role in metabolism of various minerals, especially, contribute to **calcium, phosphate and magnesium homeostasis**.
4. Bones **protect important structures** and viscera in the thoracic and pelvic cavities and in the skull.
5. Bone (bone marrow) is the primary **site of hemopoiesis**. They produce and supply formed elements of blood.

Composition of Bone

Bone is simply a **collagen framework** in which inorganic minerals are deposited on an organic matrix.

Inorganic Components

Inorganic component consists of various minerals such as calcium, phosphate, carbonate, magnesium and sodium. Minerals constitute about 25% of the bone volume, but they comprise half the bone weight because of their high density.

- Bone is the major reservoir of these minerals in the body.
- About **99% of calcium, 86% of phosphate, 80% of carbonate and 50% of magnesium** of their total body content are present in bones (Table 77.3).

Organic Matrix

Organic matrix of the bone is called **osteoid**.

1. It is formed mainly by the **Type I Collagen**, which forms 95% of the matrix.
2. The remaining 5% noncollagen part is called the **ground substance**, which is a mixture of various proteoglycans and high molecular weight compounds, consisting mainly of polysaccharides.
3. **In compact bone**, the collagen is arranged in concentric layers around **haversian canals** forming cylinder like structures called **osteons** or **haversian systems** (Fig. 77.3).

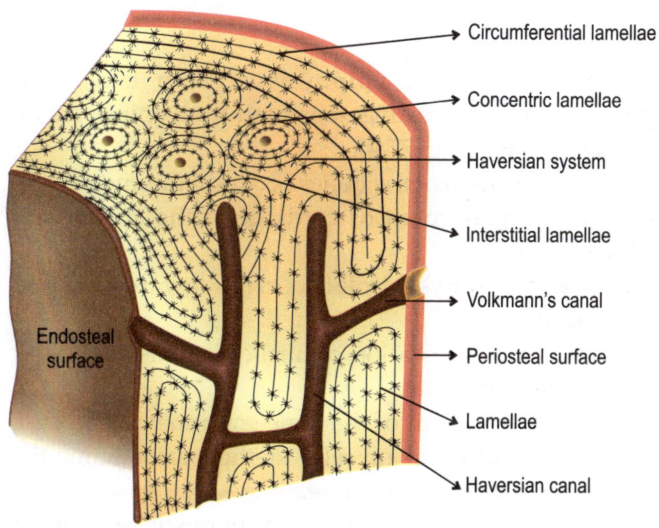

Fig. 77.3: Transverse section and longitudinal section through a compact bone. Note the arrangement of concentric lamellae and Haversian system.

Hydroxyapatite Crystals: The mineral component of calcium and phosphate in the bone forms **hydroxyapatite crystals**.

- The hydroxyapatite crystals are microscopic needle like structures that lie in parallel alongside the collagen fibers and this arrangement provides strength and hardness to the bone.

- **Demineralization of bone** causes loss of hydroxyapatite crystals and makes the organic matrix (collagen framework) weak, and loss of organic matrix makes the bone brittle.

Table 77.3 | Constituent of bone

A. Inorganic components
Calcium : 99% of total body content
Phosphate : 86% of total body content
Carbonate : 80% of total body content
Magnesium : 50% of total body content
Sodium : 35% of total body content
Water : 8% of total body content
B. Organic components
Type I collagen (95% of the bone matrix)
Ground substance (5% of the bone matrix)
– Proteoglycans
– High molecular weight substance

Structure of Bone

Bone consists of **two parts**: the outer cortex and the inner trabeculae.

1. **The cortical bone**, also called ***compact bone*** constitutes 80% of the total bone mass of the body. It consists of **dense concentric outer layers of the long bones** and a ***thinner outer layer of the flat bones***.
2. The **trabecular bone**, also called ***spongy bone*** constitutes 20% of the bone mass. It consists of **bone spicules** that make up the inner part of the axial skeletons and the smaller interior of the long bones.

Parts of Bone

Long bones consist of **epiphysis** at both ends, and **diaphysis**, the shaft which is separated from epiphyses by **epiphyseal plates** (Fig. 77.4).

- The linear growth of the bones occurs at the end of long bones by **replacement of cartilage at the epiphyseal plates**.
- **Closure of epiphyseal plates** occurs towards the end of puberty.
  - This causes cessation of further increase in height of the individual.
  - However, width of the bone continues to increase due to addition of cells to the **periosteum**, the outer surface of the bone.

Remodeling of Bone: Bone is continuously remodeled throughout the life, which is synchronized by bone formation and resorption (bone destruction).

1. **During the growth period**, bone formation exceeds bone resorption so that the bone mass increases.
2. **During the adulthood**, rate of formation and resorption is almost balanced so that the bone mass remains unchanged.
3. **After the age of 40 to 50**, bone resorption exceeds formation so that bone mass slowly decreases.

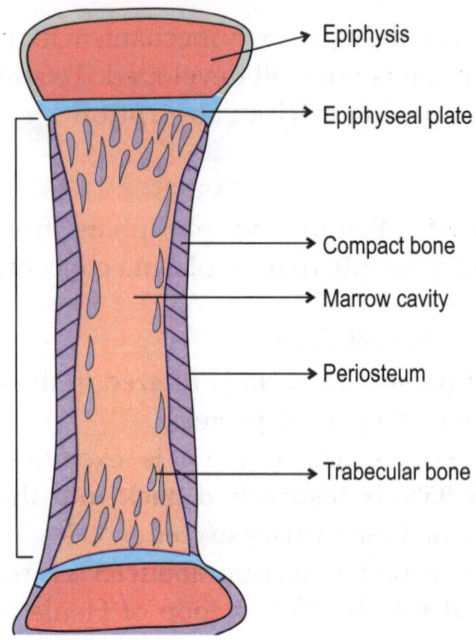

Fig. 77.4: Structure of a bone.

4. The process of bone turnover is known as **remodeling** and this is a *major mechanism of maintaining calcium homeostasis* in the body.
5. Normally, turnover of about 10% of the total bone mass occurs in a year in adults.

Cell types in Bone

There are **three types of cells** in the bone: these are **osteoblasts, osteoclasts,** and **osteocytes** (Fig.77.5). Osteoblasts and osteocytes are called **osteoprogenitor cells** as they develop from primitive cells. Osteoclasts develop from the precursors such as monocytes and tissue macrophages.

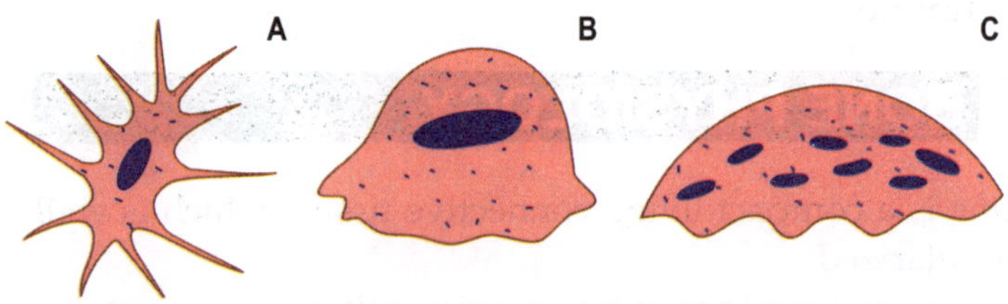

Figs. 77.5: Bone cells. A: Osteocytes; B: Osteoblast; C: Osteoclast.

Osteoblasts and Osteocytes

Osteoblasts are bone forming cells. They are modified fibroblasts.

- **Osteoblasts** synthesize **osteoid**, the organic matrix of the bone.
  - They have numerous endoplasmic reticulum and Golgi apparatus.
  - They are present towards the periphery of the bone and their cytoplasmic processes connect osteocytes that are present deeper in the bone.
- Osteoid produced by osteoblasts is **secreted towards the interior** of the bone.
  - Slowly the osteoblasts are surrounded by osteoid and **osteoid is mineralized**.

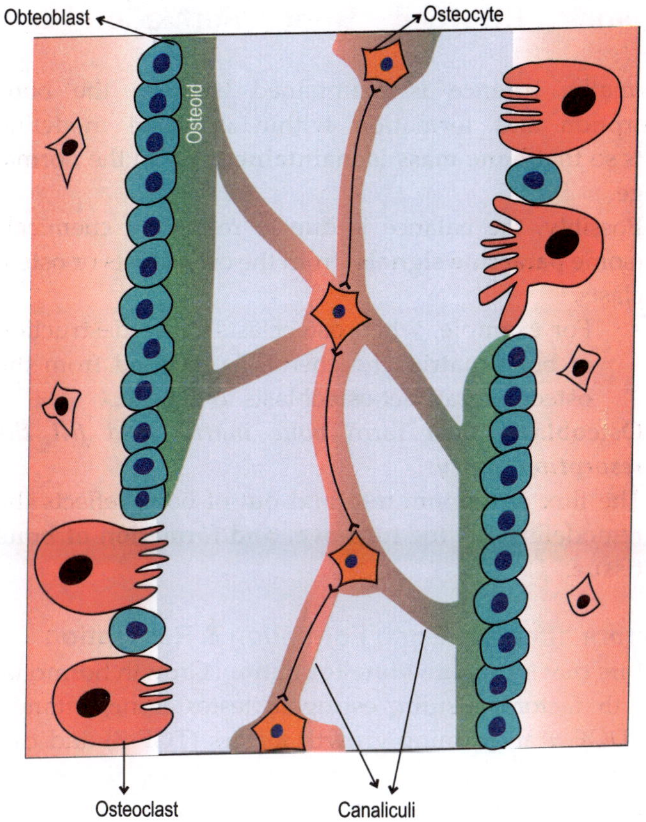

Fig. 77.6: Arrangement of cells in the bone. Note that canaliculi connect between osteocytes and osteocytes with osteoblast.

- Osteoblasts surrounded by mineralized osteoid gradually **lose their ability to form bones** and they become **osteocytes**.
- The cytoplasmic connection between osteoblasts and osteocytes become **canaliculi** (Fig. 77.6).
- The canaliculi are the anatomical link for transfer of nutrients, chemicals and waste products between the surface and interior of the bone.

Osteoclasts

Osteoclasts are **cells of mononuclear phagocyte system** in the bone. Therefore, they are large, multinucleated cells located towards the periphery of the bone.

- They **cause bone resorption** by secreting proteolytic enzymes into the surroundings.
- The chemicals secreted by osteoclasts make the **environment acidic** that enhances the solubility of bone minerals and the enzymes secreted cause *degradation of the organic matrix*.

Mechanism of Bone Formation

Formation of bone is the **function of osteoblasts**.

1. Osteoblasts synthesize **collagen** and extrude it into the adjacent extracellular space.
   - The *collagen fibrils* form the organic matrix of the bone, which is called as **osteoid**.
2. In the osteoid, calcium-phosphate is deposited which is called as **mineralization** of bone.
   - Thereafter, to the organic matrix, hydroxides and bicarbonates are added to form the **hydroxyapatite crystals** (the *complete mineralization*).
3. Osteoid converted into lamella of the bone.
4. The mineralized matrix **slowly accumulates and surrounds the osteoblasts** (Fig. 77.7-**1**).
   - As this process of mineralization of matrix continues, the osteoblasts decrease their synthetic activity and become **osteocytes**.
5. **Osteoblastic activity** is seen ***along the surface*** of the bones.
   - Lamellae of the bones are formed with osteocytes remaining inside the lamellae.
   - **Vitamin D** is essential for bone mineralization. It profoundly influences the availability of calcium and phosphate to the bone matrix.
6. The canaliculi that connect osteocytes from bone interior to the surface ***transfer calcium from the interior to the exterior bone units*** and then from there to the ECF.
   - This process of transfer of calcium carried out by osteocytes is known as **osteocytic osteolysis**.
   - Normally, this process **does not decrease the bone mass** rather ***removes calcium*** from the recently formed bone crystals.

Role of Chondrocytes & Endochondral Ossification

Before epiphyseal closure, the leading edge of the epiphyseal plate contains **chondrocytes**.

1. The **active chondrocytes synthesize cartilage** that gradually embeds the chondrocytes.
   - The ***embedded chondrocytes die*** and are **replaced** by new chondrocytes and the formation of cartilage continues.
2. The cartilage is **slowly calcified,** and **osteoblasts migrate** into it.
3. **Osteoblasts secrete osteoid** that ultimately **mineralize** and the ***new bone is formed***.
   - Thus, the bone increases in length as the **epiphyseal plate lays down new bone** on the end of the shaft.
   - This is called **endochondral ossification** (Fig. 77.7-**4**).
4. **IGF I, insulin and thyroid hormones** stimulate chondrocyte activity.
   - Within few years from the onset of puberty, the **chondrocytes become unresponsive** to hormonal stimuli and lose their activity.
5. Finally, the **epiphyses unite with the shaft** and this process is called **closure of epiphysis** (Clinical Note 77.1).
   - This is also called **ossification**.
   - This stops the linear growth of the bone.

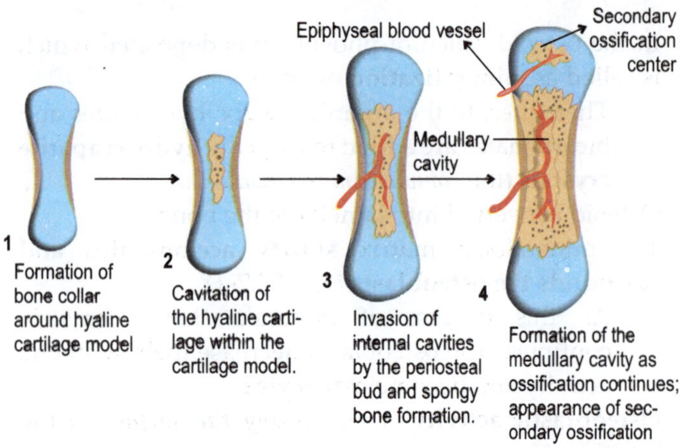

Fig. 77.7: Stages of endochondral bone formation.

Clinical Note 77.1

Epiphyseal closure determines age: The epiphyses of various bones close in an orderly fashion in sequence and the age at which they close is known. Therefore, the age of an individual especially in adolescents and young adults can be determined easily by taking x-rays of bones by determining whether the epiphysis is closed or still open..

Bone Resorption

This is process of **destruction of the bone matrix.**

Phases of Bone Resorption

Bone resorption occurs **in two phases.**

First Phase: In the first phase, **H^+ is secreted** by osteoclasts. There are proton pumps (**H^+-dependent ATPases**) in the endosomes present in the cytosol of the osteoclasts.

- When osteoclasts are activated, **proton pumps migrate** to the cell surface and are **inserted into the osteoclast membrane.**
- Secretion of H^+ makes the **environment acidic;** pH decreases to about 4. The **acidic pH dissolves the hydroxyapatite** and favors action of acidic enzymes.

Second Phase: In the second phase, the **acid protease enzyme** secreted by osteoclasts **destroys the collagen,** the organic matrix.

- The collagen breakdown products have **pyridinoline** structures. One such important product is **hydroxyproline.**
- Therefore, **hydroxyprolinuria is an index of bone resorption.**

IMPORTANT NOTE

Level of hydroxyproline indicates the rate of bone resorption: During the process of resorption, the **calcium, phosphate, hydroxyproline,** and **hydroxylysine** are released into ECF. The rate of excretion of these organic compounds, especially hydroxyproline indicates the rate of bone resorption.

Balance Between Bone Formation and Resorption

Normally, balance is maintained between the bone resorption and formation within its bone modeling units so that **bone mass is maintained** within the normal range.

- Possibly, the balance is due to release of chemicals (some **paracrine signals**) from the osteoblasts or osteoclasts.
  - For example, when osteoclasts cause destruction of bone matrix, the chemicals released from the osteoclasts attract osteoblasts to the site.
- **Osteoblasts** then form ***bone matrix and fill the resorption cavity.***
- The flux of calcium into and out of bone reflects the remodeling, i.e. the **turn-over and formation of bone tissue.**

Factors affecting Bone Formation & Resorption

Factors that stimulate bone formation: Growth hormone, growth factors, insulin, estrogen, testosterone, vitamin D, PDGF, transforming growth factors (TGF-β) and calcitonin.

Factors that inhibit bone formation: Cortisol

Factors that stimulate bone resorption: Parathormone, cortisol, thyroxine, prostaglandins, interleukin 1 and 6, and TNF.

Factors that inhibit resorption: Estrogen, androgen, calcitonin, γ interferon, and TGF-β.

Applied Physiology

Osteoporosis

Postmenopausal Osteoporosis: **In females,** the process of bone resorption is facilitated at the time of menopause due to cessation of estrogen secretion. This is postmenopausal osteoporosis.

Involutional Osteoporosis: Osteoporosis is **decrease in bone mass and density.** Usually, **after the age of 40,** bone mass ***gradually decreases.*** This is called involutional osteoporosis.

In fact, the rate of bone remodeling increases with age. However, **with increased osteclastic activity,** bone matrix is lost and ***more cavities are formed,*** which is not refilled by the osteoblastic activity.

- Also, the mineralization decreases.
- This causes **reduction in bone density and bone mass.** The process is known as **osteoporosis.**
- Osteoporosis increases the **susceptibility of bones to fractures,** especially in elderly.

Treatment: The **treatment is by administration of calcium** and **vitamin D** tablets. In severe case in females, estrogen therapy may be instituted.

Osteopetrosis

Defective increase in bone formation is called osteopetrosis.

- The bone resorption is defective due to **decreased osteoclastic activity**. Therefore, **osteoblastic activity is unopposed**. This results in unusual increase in bone formation.
- **Bone density is increased** and bones are deformed.

PY8.2

Parathyroid Gland

Physiological Anatomy

In human beings, there are **four parathyroid glands** present in the anterior aspect of the neck embedded posteriorly at four poles in the thyroid tissue (Fig. 77.8). The total weight of the four glands is about 200 mg, each gland weighing approximately 50 mg. Parathyroid glands derive **blood supply from the thyroid arteries**.

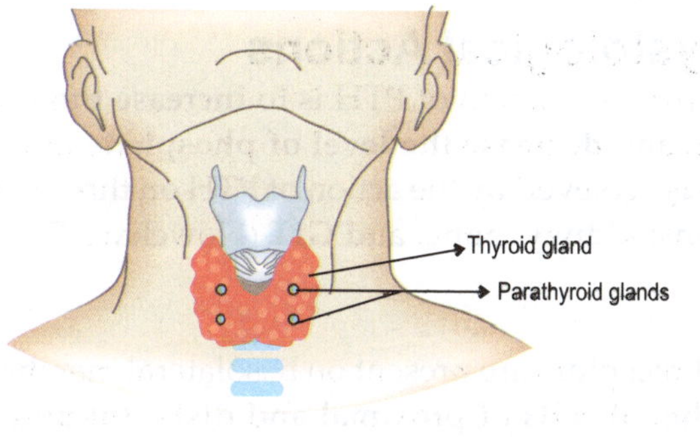

Fig. 77.8: Location of the parathyroid glands. Note that there are four small glands (two superior parathyroids and two inferior parathyroids) located behind the thyroid gland.

Cell Types

Parathyroid glands contain **two types of cells**: chief cells and oxyphil cells (Fig. 77.9).

Chief Cells: The chief cells are the **predominant cells** in the parathyroid gland that are present throughout life.

1. They have **bigger Golgi apparatus** in their cytoplasm.
2. They also contain **numerous vesicles and endoplasmic reticulum**.
3. Chief cells **secrete PTH.**

Oxyphil Cells: Oxyphil cells are less plentiful in parathyroid gland. They **appear in the glands during puberty** and then the number increases with the advancement of age. They contain numerous **oxyphil granules**. Normally, they do not secrete PTH.

Parathyroid Hormone (PTH)

PTH is polypeptide containing **84 amino acids**. The biological activity, especially the calcium regulating ability of PTH **resides in the N-terminal portion** of the molecule (within amino acids 1–27).

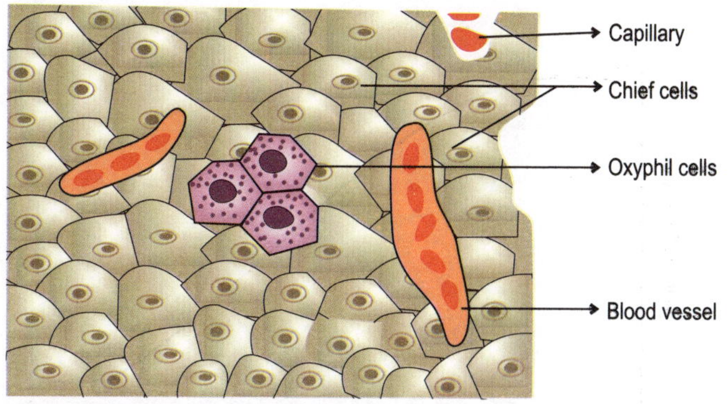

Fig. 77.9: Histology picture of parathyroid glands. Note the presence of chief cells and oxyphil cells.

Synthesis, Secretion and Metabolism

Like other peptide hormones, PTH is synthesized from the larger precursor molecule called **prepro-PTH** that contains 115 amino acids.

- The leader sequence containing 25 amino acids is removed from amino terminal in endoplasmic reticulum to form **pro-PTH**, which contains 90 amino acids.
- In the Golgi apparatus, another six amino acids are removed from the amino terminal to from **PTH** containing ***86 amino acids.***
- PTH is then packaged and stored in the granules of chief cells.

Regulation of Secretion

PTH secretion is regulated mainly by **plasma calcium and vitamin D. Other factors** also influence PTH secretion.

Plasma Calcium Level

The **major regulator** of PTH secretion is the plasma calcium level and they have **inverse relationship**.

- With **increased** plasma concentration of **ionized calcium,** ***PTH secretion decreases.***
  - The relationship is **linear** between 3–6 mg% of the ionized plasma calcium (Fig. 77.10).
  - It may be remembered that about 50% of the total plasma calcium is present in the ionized form.
  - Conversely, with decreased plasma calcium, PTH secretion increases.
- Recently, the receptors for sensing plasma calcium, the **calcium sensing receptors** (**CaSR**) have been identified on the membrane of chief cells.
  - The CaSR is a **G-protein coupled receptor** attached to **phospholipase C** and on binding with calcium generates **IP_3 and DAG.**
- IP_3 and DAG **release calcium** from cytosolic stores and activate protein kinase C that inhibits PTH secretion.
- Another example of increase in calcium inhibiting hormone secretion is **decreased renin release** from JG cells of kidney.

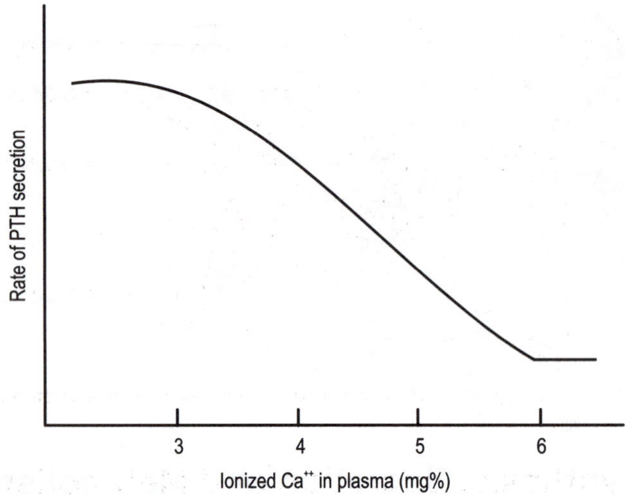

Fig. 77.10: Relation of plasma-ionized calcium with the rate of PTH secretion. Note that from 3 mg% to 6 mg%, the relationship is linear.

Vitamin D

Vitamin D **inhibits PTH secretion** by decreasing the formation of prepro PTH mRNA.

Other Factors

1. **Plasma phosphate:** Usually phosphate does not affect parathormone secretion.
   - However, a **rise in plasma phosphate stimulates PTH secretion** by lowering plasma calcium and inhibiting formation of 1,25-dihydroxycholecalciferol.
2. **Cyclic AMP, β receptor agonists, dopamine, magnesium, and histamine** (H_2 receptor) *stimulate* PTH secretion.
   - **Prostaglandins and α receptor agonists** *inhibit* PTH secretion by decreasing cyclic AMP.

Metabolism of PTH

The normal plasma PTH level is **10-60 pg/mL.**

- As PTH is **rapidly degraded by Kupffer cells** in liver to carboxy terminal and mid-region fragments, the **half-life of PTH is about 10 minutes.**
- The fragments are cleared by kidneys.
- However, the **synthetic PTH** which has only 34 amino acid sequence of amino terminal of the natural PTH, possesses all the biological effects of the hormone.

Mechanism of Action

PTH Receptors

There are **three types of PTH receptors**.

Type 1 Receptor (PTH 1R): It binds to PTH and **PTH related proteins** (PTHrP). The action of PTH to regulate plasma calcium is **mediated via PTH 1R.**

Type 2 Receptors (PTH 2R): It **binds to PTH,** but not to PTHrP. It is found in brain, pancreas and placenta.

Type 3 Receptor (CPTH): It reacts only with carboxy terminal of PTH (therefore called **CPTH**) and not with the amino terminal of the hormone.

G Proteins for PTH

PTH 1R and 2R are coupled to two types of G proteins **G_s and G_q**. Therefore, the binding of PTH with the receptors activates both adenylate cyclase and phospholipase C in the membrane.

This results in activation of **two signaling systems** (Fig. 77.11):

1. Activation of **adenylate cyclase-cyclic AMP system** that increases cAMP. cAMP activates protein kinase A that causes phosporylation of intracellular proteins. Formation of phospoproteins increases transport of calcium and other ions.
2. Activation of phospholipase C that **increases IP_3 and DAG** in the cell. IP_3 causes intracellular calcium mobilization and DAG causes activation of protein kinase C.

Physiological Actions

The primary action of PTH is to **increase the level of calcium** and **decrease the level of phosphate** in the plasma. This is achieved by the action of PTH on three major target organs: **kidney, bone, and GIT** (Flowchart 77.1).

Actions on Kidney

PTH receptors are present on basolateral membrane of the **epithelial cells of proximal and distal tubules**. PTH has **three major effects** on kidney:

1. Increased reabsorption of calcium.
2. Decreased reabsorption of phosphate.
3. Stimulation of 1, 25-dihydroxycholecalciferol formation.

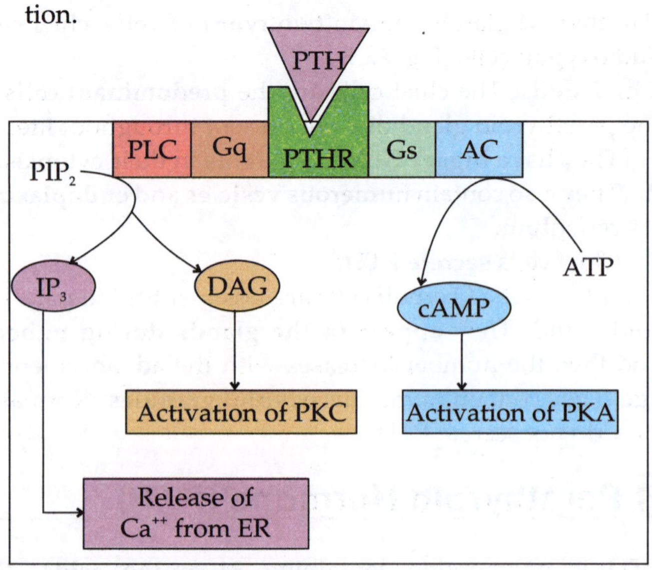

Fig. 77.11: Mechanism of action of PTH. Note that binding of PTH with its receptor (PTHR) activates two signalling pathways (cAMP and IP3-DAG) in the cell. PK: protein kinase; PLC: phospholipase C; AC: adenylyl cyclase.

Increased Reabsorption of Calcium: Normally, 65% of filtered calcium is reabsorbed in proximal tubule, 25% in thick ascending limb of loop of Henle and 5-10% in distal tubule. About 1-2% of filtered load is excreted in urine.

- PTH increases calcium reabsorption from kidney by **mainly acting on distal tubule and thick ascending limb of loop of Henle**. Thus, PTH action on kidney *decreases the calcium excretion to a very minimal quantity*.
- PTH action on kidney is relatively rapid which increases plasma calcium within minutes following its injections.
- PTH also increases the formation of **1, 25-dihydroxycholecalciferol**, which in turn increases calcium absorption from distal tubule of kidney.

Decreased Reabsorption of Phosphate: PTH decreases reabsorption of phosphate by **mainly acting on proximal tubule**.

- This causes **phosphaturia**.
- By decreasing plasma phosphate concentration, PTH prevents calcium-phosphate salts to precipitate.

Stimulation of 1, 25-Dihydroxycholecalciferol Formation: In kidney, in the mitochondria of proximal tubule, PTH **facilitates the hydroxylation** of 25-hydroxycholecalciferol to **1,25-dihydroxycholecalciferol**, the active form of vitamin D. 1,25-dihydroxycholecalciferol increases calcium reabsorption from kidney, calcium absorption from intestine and calcium mobilization from bone.

Actions on Bone

PTH acts on the **receptors present in osteoblasts and osteoclasts**. Thus, it activates both bone synthesis and resorption. However, the **net effect is increased bone resorption** and excess mobilization of calcium and phosphates from bones into plasma.

1. **Stimulation of osteoclastic activity:** This is a slower effect of PTH in which **it stimulates osteoclasts** to resorp mineralized bones. In this process both calcium and phosphate are transferred into the ECF. The bone matrix is hydrolyzed by the collagenase and lysosomal enzymes.

- PTH increases the number and size of osteoclasts and also the synthesis of RNA in the osteoclast.
- PTH also stimulates the **differentiation of precursor cells** (monocytes, macrophages, etc.) into the osteoclasts. Under the influence of PTH **giant osteoclasts** (osteoclasts of bigger size) are formed that cause resorption of the larger areas of bone (creates large resorption cavity).
- The **products of bone resorption** are released into the plasma. These include *calcium, phosphate, hydroxyproline and hydroxylysine*.
- Excretion of these substances in the urine especially that of **hydroxyproline is an index of osteoclastic activity**.

2. **Stimulation of osteolysis:** PTH activates the process of **osteocytic osteolysis**.

- In this process, calcium is transferred from the bone fluid into the osteocyte and then from osteocytes into osteoblasts.
- Osteoblasts then pump calcium into the extracellular matrix.
- Calcium is also pumped into the ECF.

3. **PTH also acts on osteoblasts:** PTH **inhibits the synthesis of collagen** by osteoblasts at higher concentration.

- However, **at lower doses**, *PTH increases osteoblastic activity* and increases collagen synthesis. Especially, **trabecular bone mass is increased**.
- This anabolic effect is mediated by increased secretion of insulin like growth factors and transforming growth factors.
- Therefore, the **net effect** of PTH on bone is ***increase in the bone mass in lower concentration*** and ***decrease in bone mass in higher concentration***.

In primary hyperparathyroidism (due to parathyroid adenoma), hypercalcemia, hypophosphatemia, hypercalciuria (due to increased filtered load of calcium), and renal calculi are usually seen. Areas of ***osteoclastic hyperactivity*** and ***bone resorption*** are present along with excessive and ***disorganized trabecular bone formation***. In hypoparathyroidism, generally bone mass is increased.

Actions on GI tract

Acting on intestine, PTH **increases absorption of calcium.** However, this effect is **mostly indirect**, mediated through *1,25-dihydroxycholecalciferol*, which is formed in kidney by PTH.

Thus, the overall effects of PTH are to **increase plasma level of calcium and decrease plasma level of phosphate** (Flowchart 77.1).

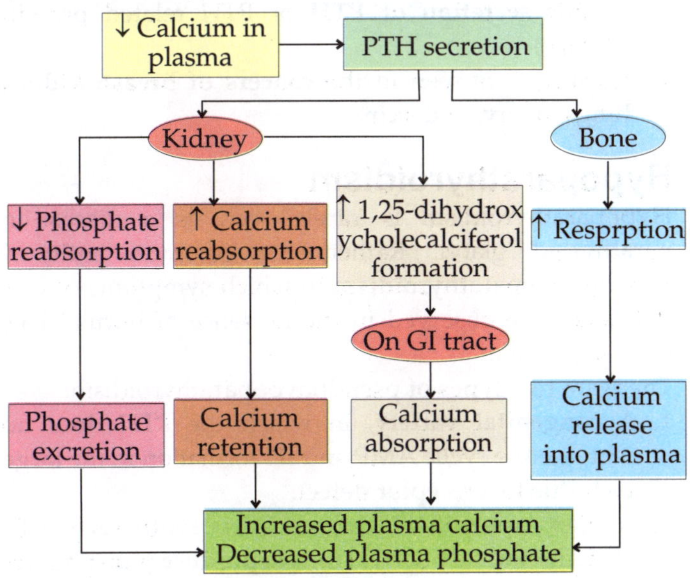

Flowchart 77.1: Summary of effects of PTH.

Applied Physiology

Hyperparathyroidism

Hyperparathyroidism or PTH excess is divided into **two main categories**:

1. Primary hyperparathyroidism
2. Secondary hyperparathyroidism.

Primary Hyperparathyroidism

Primary hyperparathyroidism occurs due to the tumor of parathyroid gland such as parathyroid adenoma that secretes excess PTH. It may be part of multiple endocrine neoplasia (MEN) syndrome. It is common in MEN type-1.

- The disease is characterized by hypercalcemia, hypophosphatemia, demineralization of bone, hypercalciuria, and renal stone formation.
- The chronic effect of parathyroid excess results in the bone disease called osteitis fibrosa. There will be features of osteopenia and fracture.
- In this disease, the bone marrow is fibrosed and bone resorption exceeds the bone formation.

Secondary Hyperparathyroidism

Secondary hyperparathyroidism occurs in chronic renal disease and rickets.

- In these diseases, the chronic hypocalcemia causes increased secretion of PTH.
- This results in secondary hypertrophy of parathyroid glands.
- Neonatal primary hyperparathyroidism has also been described that occurs due to a genetic defect.

In Malignancy: *Hypercalcemia* occurs in malignancies.

- This is mainly due to the **bone metastases** by the cancer cells that cause **local osteolysis** which results in hypercalcemia.
- Hypercalcemia also occurs in malignancy due to **ectopic secretion of PTH** or PTH related proteins (PTHrP).
- Usually, it is seen in the **cancers of breast, kidney, lungs, ovary, and skin.**

Hypoparathyroidism

Hypoparathyroidism is rarely seen as a disease of parathyroid gland. Rather, the common entity is **pseudohypoparathyroidism** in which symptoms of PTH deficiency are observed in the presence of normal PTH level in plasma.

There are **two types** of pseudohypoparathyroidism:

1. A **congenital variety**, in which the PTH does not increase the cyclic AMP and IP_3 formation in the target cells due to a receptor defect.
2. Another variety in which cyclic AMP synthesis by PTH remains normal but PTH **fails to produce phosphaturic effect.**

In hypoparathyroidism, hypocalcemia and increased bone density are main feature.

Hypocalcemic Tetany

Hyposecretion of parathyroid is rather common **following thyroid surgery** in which parathyroid glands are **usually removed by mistake** along with thyroid tissue. This causes severe hypoparathyroidism that leads to acute hypocalcemic tetany.

Effects of Parathyroidectomy

The symptoms of tetany following thyroid surgery develop in 24 to 48 hours postoperatively.

The features of tetany are:

1. **Chvostek's sign:** This is the quick contraction of facial muscles of the same side by tapping over the facial nerve at the angle of jaw.
2. **Trousseau's sign:** The spasm of the muscles of the upper extremity that causes flexion of the wrist and thumb (i. e. flexion at metacarpophalangeal joints) with extension of fingers (i.e. extension of interphalangeal joints) (Fig. 77.12).
3. **Carpopedal spasm:** There is also spasm of muscles at the wrist joints (***carpal spasm***). The changes at wrist and ankle joints together called as carpopedal spasm.
4. **Laryngospasm:** In hypocalcemic tetany, usually patients die due to hypoxia that occurs due to laryngospasm. The muscles of larynx contract and occlude the laryngeal passage.
5. **Hypocalcemia:** Significant hypocalcemia occurs.
6. Hyperphosphatemia.

The **treatment** of hypocalcemic tetany includes immediate administration of ionized calcium and parathormone.

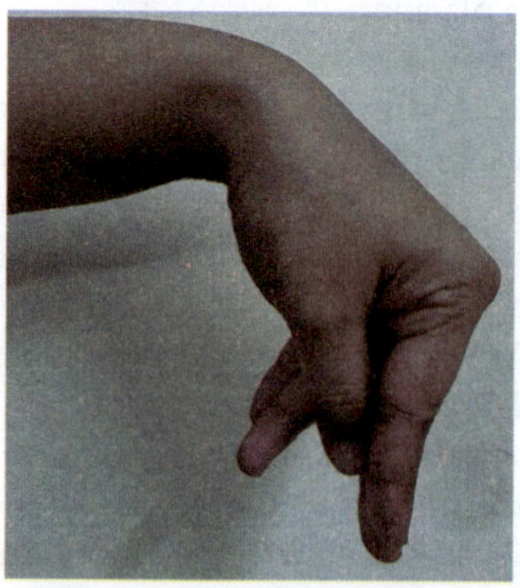

Fig. 77.12: Trousseau's sign. Flexion of the wrist and thumb and flexion at metacarpophalangeal joints with extension of fingers.

Parathyroid Hormone Related Protein

The parathyroid hormone related protein (**PTHrP**) is produced by many tissues in the body. It is a **polypeptide containing 140 amino acids**. The gene that encodes the formation of PTHrP is present on the human **chromosome 12** (it should be noted that the gene for PTH is present on chromosome 11). PTHrP has marked homology with the PTH.

Functions of PTHrP:

1. PTHrP stimulates **proliferation of chondrocytes** in developing cartilage and inhibits their mineralization.
2. It also **acts as a growth factor** for the development of skin, hair follicle, and breast.
3. PTHrP is produced in large quantities in the lactating breast tissue and secreted in the milk. However, the plasma concentration of PTHrP does not increase during lactation.
4. PTHrP has also been described in kidney (renal glomeruli) and in the brain (cortex, hippocampus and cerebellum). But, functions of PTHrP in these organs are not clearly known.
5. It also causes calcium transport in placenta.
6. PTHrP is elevated in hypercalcemia of malignancy (Clinical Note 77.2)

Clinical Note 77.2

Hypercalcemia of Malignancy: Hypercalcemia is common in malignancy. In 80% cases, it is due to elevated PTHrP. This is known as **humoral hypercalcemia of malignancy.** That commonly occurs in malignancy of ovary, breast, kidney and skin. In rest 20% cases, hypercalcemia is due to secondary metastasis of bones that erodes the bone and release calcium. This is called **local osteolytic hypercalcemia**.

ROLE OF CALCITONIN, VITAMIN D & OTHER HORMONES

Calcitonin

Source and Structure

Calcitonin is secreted from **parafollicular cells (C cells)** of the thyroid gland. The parafollicular cells develop from ultimobranchial bodies, a pair of glands that develop from 5th branchial pouch.

1. Calcitonin is a polypeptide hormone containing **32 amino acids**. The molecular weight is 3,500.
2. The **calcitonin gene** that transcribes mRNA to form calcitonin is processed to form a different mRNA in the nervous system where it forms **calcitonin gene-related peptides** (CGRP).
3. CGRP is a potent vasodilator.

Synthesis and Secretion

The **major stimulus** for calcitonin secretion is the **rise in plasma calcium level**. Above the concentration of 9 mg% of plasma calcium, the secretion of calcium becomes directly proportional to the calcium concentration.

Other Stimuli: The β receptor agonists, dopamine, GI hormones (CCK, glucagons, gastrin, secretin), and estrogen stimulate calcitonin secretion. ***Gastrin*** is a strong stimulus for calcitonin release (Clinical Note 77.3).

Clinical Note 77.3

Calcitonin is more in Zollinger-Ellison syndrome and in pernicious anemia: Gastrin stimulates calcitonin secretion. Therefore, plasma calcitonin concentration is raised in Zollinger-Ellison syndrome and in pernicious anemia as gastrin concentration increases in these diseases.

Metabolism

The concentration of calcitonin in plasma is 10–20 pg/ml. The concentration increases to almost 10 fold in hypercalcemia. The hormone is degraded in the liver. The half-life of calcitonin is 5–10 minutes.

Mechanism of Action

Calcitonin acts on calcitonin receptors present on the target cells. The receptors are coupled to G_s proteins and therefore, stimulate the **adenylate cyclase–cyclic AMP system**.

Physiological Actions

Calcitonin decreases the plasma calcium level by acting mainly on bones and kidney (Flowchart 77.2).

Effects on Bone

Calcitonin mainly acts on the osteoclasts.

- It **decreases osteoclastic activity**. Thus, it **inhibits the bone resorption**. The number and size of osteoclasts decrease.
- The action of calcitonin on bone is just opposite to that of PTH with respect to the calcium turnover in the bone.
- However, the effect on phosphate turnover is same as that of PTH. It **decreases plasma phosphate level**. This is due to inhibition of bone resorption, facilitation of phosphate entry into the bone, and also mild increase in urinary phosphate excretion.
- Thus, the hypophosphatemic effect of calcitonin is independent of hypocalcemic effect.

Effects on Kidney

It **decreases calcium reabsorption** from kidney. Therefore, it produces calciuria. It also causes mild phosphaturia by acting on proximal tubule.

Calcitonin Escape: Injection of calcitonin produces hypocalcemia mainly by antiosteoclastic activity. However, this antiresorptive action of calcitonin begins to wane within hours.

- The body escapes from hypocalcemic effects of calcitonin. This is called **calcitonin escape**, the exact mechanism of which is not known.
- It is probably due to **rapid down regulation of calcium receptors**. Therefore, calcitonin is effective in decreasing plasma calcium only for a short duration.
- This **limits the use of calcitonin** in long-term management of hypercalcemia.

Physiological Significance:

1. Due to calcitonin escape phenomenon, the **bones remain essentially normal** in conditions of hypersecretion of calcitonin like medullary carcinoma of thyroid.
2. Calcitonin is **secreted more in young individuals,** which is believed to play some role in skeletal development.
3. **Feeding** increases calcitonin secretion by releasing GI hormones. Calcitonin escape **protects against postprandial hypercalcemia.**
4. During and after pregnancy, **calcitonin protects bone loss in pregnant and lactating mother.**
   - During pregnancy maternal calcium is used for bone **formation in fetus** and after pregnancy calcium is utilized for **lactogenesis.**
   - To maintain maternal plasma calcium, 1,25-dihydroxycholecalciferol level is increased, which causes bone resorption.
   - Therefore, increased calcitonin level in pregnancy **prevents bone loss by opposing osteoclastic activity.**
5. Calcitonin and CGRP are found together in some brain regions like pituitary, hypothalamus, limbic system etc, where they **act as co-transmitters.** They inhibit transmission of pain impulses in CNS independent of opioid system.

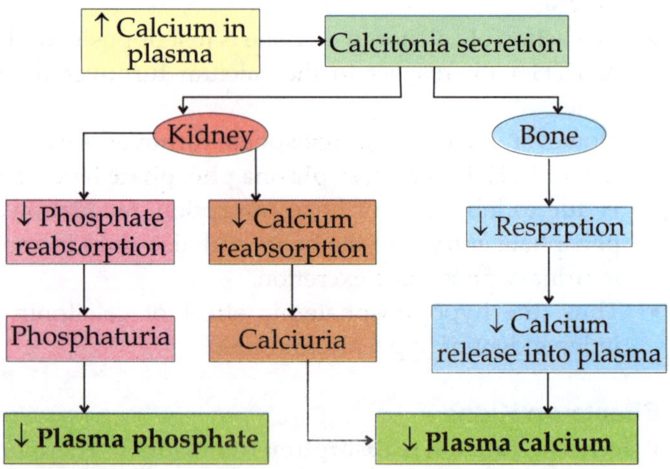

Flowchart 77.2: Summary of effects of calcitonin.

Applied Aspects

Clinical Use of Calcitonin

Calcitonin is used in the treatment of hypercalcemia, and in the diseases in which osteoclastic activity needs to be reduced, for example in **Paget's disease.** Calcitonin is sometimes used as a **central analgesic** as it blocks the transmission of pain impulses in CNS.

Paget's Disease

In this disease, increased osteoclastic activity of unknown etiology results in **localized regions of bone resorption** followed by a compensatory osteoblastic activity causing **patchy new bone formations.**

- Thus, pagetic bones are structurally **disorganized and susceptible to deformities.**
- **X-ray** pictures show areas of increased density and resorptive cavities.
- Though most of the patients are initially asymptomatic, bone deformities resulting in compressive neuropathy and subsequent neuromuscular dysfunctions are not uncommon.
- The disease is **treated by daily injections of calcitonin.**
- **Bisphosphonates** like ***etidronate and pamidronate*** are more useful in preventing bone resorption.

Vitamin D

Vitamin D **increases plasma calcium** level by increasing **calcium absorption from GI tract, calcium reabsorption from kidney** and mobilization of calcium from bone. It has similar effects on phosphate.

Synthesis of Vitamin D

Vitamin D is acquired from **two sources** in human being. 1. Skin (ultraviolet irradiation of skin produces vitamin D), and 2. Diet.

- Vitamin D_3 is **synthesized in** the skin on exposure to sunlight (Flowchart 77.3).

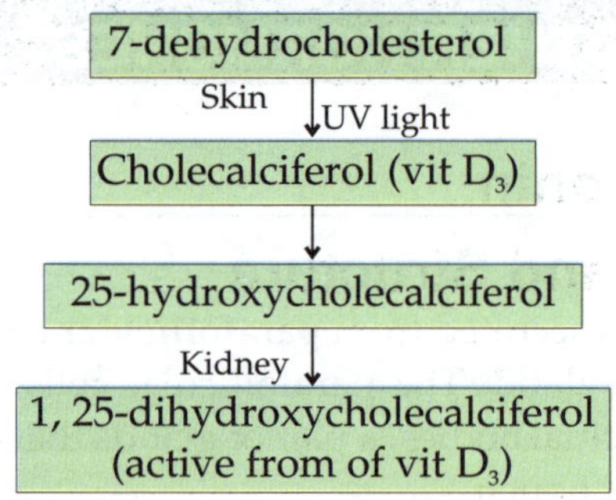

Flowchart 77.3: Steps of synthesis of active Vitamin D_3.

Physiological Actions

Vitamin D increases plasma calcium level by acting on intestine, kidney and bone, summarized in Flowchart 77.4 **Anti-aging protein:** Anti-aging protein exerts effects partly via 1,25-dihydroxycholecalciferol (Application Box 77.1).

Application Box 7.1

α-Klotho partly acts through Vit. D: The anti-aging protein α-Klotho that plays a major role in calcium and phosphate metabolism has been observed to act partly through 1,25-dihydroxycholecalciferol. .

- α-Klotho facilitates membrane localization of proteins that are involved in calcium and phosphate reabsorption, such as **TRPV5** and **Na^+-K^+ ATPase.**
- It enhances the activity of **FGF-23** (fibroblast growth factor) by acting at the receptor level.
- FGF-23 **decreases the renal NaPi-IIc activity** and **inhibits synthesis of 1α-hydroxylase** that reduces the level of 1,25-dihydroxycholecalciferol.

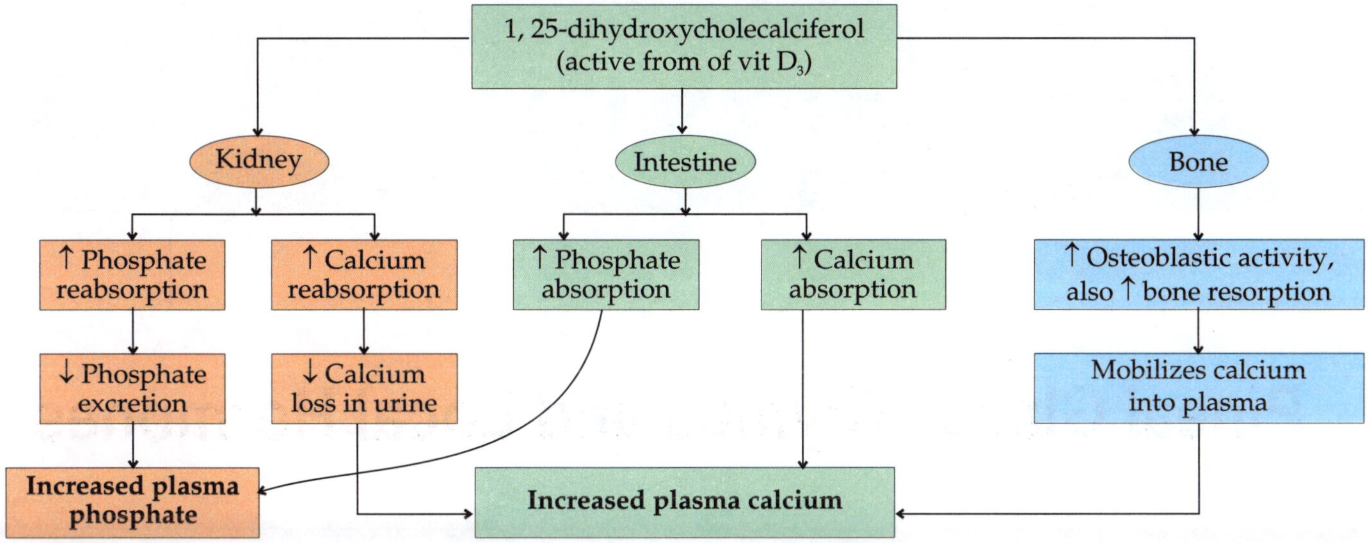

Flowchart 77.4: Summary of physiological effects of vitamin D.

Other Hormones

Glucocorticoids: Glucocorticoid decrease plasma calcium level by inhibiting osteoclastic activity and decreasing calcium absorption from intestine.

Growth Hormone: Stimulates osteoblastic activity and bone formation.

Growth Factors: Promote protein synthesis in bone. Bone formation is increased.

Insulin: Promotes bone formation.

Thyroid Hormones: In excess, cause hypercalcemia and hypercalciuria.

Estrogen: Inhibits osteoclastic activity and prevents osteoporosis.

Testosterone: Maintains normal bone mass and promotes bone development.

Exam Questions

1. Describe the hormones regulating calcium and bone metabolism.
2. Describe the mechanism of action, regulation of secretion and physiological actions of parathormone.
3. Describe the regulation of secretion and physiological actions of calcitonin.
4. Describe the mechanisms and regulation of bone formation and bone resorption.

Multiple Choice Questions

1. In bone, H+ is secreted by:
A. Osteoblast B. Osteoclast
C. Osteocyte D. Lamellar cells

2. Calcium absorption occurs mainly from:
A. Proximal small intestine
B. Distal ileum
C. Middle small intestine
D. Ascending colon

3. Calcium absorption from gut is increased by all except:
A. Phytate B. Vitamin D
C. Alkaline pH in gut D. Protein in diet

4. Which of the following inhibits bone resorption?
A. Estrogen B. Thyroxine
C. Cortisol D. Parathormone

5. Which of the following inhibits bone formation?
A. Vitamin D B. Estrogen
C. Testosterone D. Cortisol

6. Parathyroid hormone is responsible for all actions except:
A. Increased absorption of phosphorous
B. Increased Vit D absorption
C. Mobilizes calcium from bone
D. Increase intestinal absorption of calcium

7. True about parathyroid hormone are:
A. It is steroidal in nature
B. Decrease 1, 25 D3 formation
C. Inhibits Ca2+ absorption from the intestine
D. Increases the resorption of bone

8. Acute hypocalcemia is characterized by all, EXCEPT:
A. Numbness and tingling of circumoral region
B. Hyperactive tendon reflexes and positive Chvostek's sign.
C. Shortening of QT interval in ECG
D. Carpopedal spasm

9. All of the following are true aout Paget's disease, EXCEPT:
A. Increased osteoclastic activity
B. Increased density and resorptive cavities in bone x-ray
C. Calcitonin is not useful
D. Compensatory osteoblastic activity makes patches of new bone formation

Answers : 1. B 2. A 3. C 4. A 5. D 6. A 7. D 8. C 9. C

Chapter 78

Pineal Gland, Thymus and Local Hormones

Learning Objectives

On completion of study of this chapter:

The student will be able to (must know):

1. Name hormones secreted from pineal gland, give the steps of melatonin synthesis, list List the functions of pineal gland.
2. Correlate melatonin secretion with the diurnal rhythms.
3. Understand thymus as an endocrine organ and the role of thymus in immunity.
4. List the local hormones and give functions of each.
5. Illustrate the role of histamine, serotonin and prostaglandins in health and disease.

The student may also be able to (desirable to know):

1. Describe the functions of pineal gland.
2. Describe the histology and functions of thymus gland
3. Describe the synthesis and functions of various prostaglandins. .

PY8.3

PINEAL GLAND

Physiological Anatomy

Pineal gland is known as **epiphysis.** Along with habenular and posterior commissures, it makes up the **epithalamus.** It is connected by a stalk to the posterior and habenular commissures (Fig. 78.1).

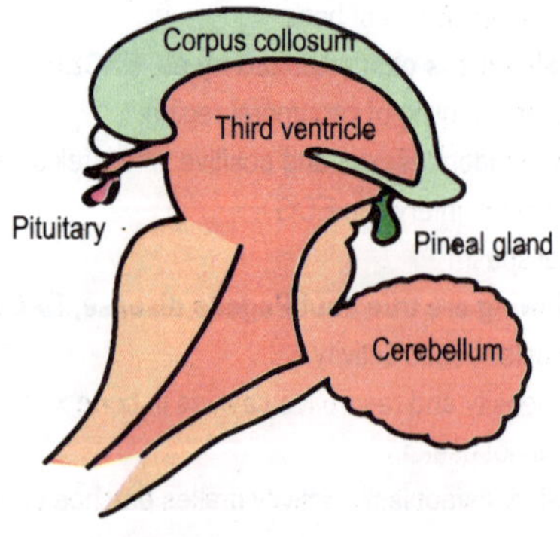

Fig. 78.1: Location of pineal in the brain.

- It is **larger in size during infancy and childhood.** It regresses at the time of puberty and is **small in size in adults.**
- The stroma of the pineal gland consists of **neuroglial cells, pinealocytes, and parenchymal tissue.**

Hormones of the Pineal Gland

Pineal gland secretes the hormone **melatonin.**

- Recently, other peptides that have been identified in pineal are **arginine vasotocin, arginine vasopressin, oxytocin, pro-opiomelanocortin** derived peptides like ACTH, α-MSH and β-endorphin, **angiotensin II, renin like activity, and TRH and GnRH** like peptides.
- Thus, it appears that pineal gland might be involved in control of many endocrinal functions of the body.

Melatonin

Melatonin is N-acetyl-5-methoxytryptamine, which is synthesized from the amino acid tryptamine (Flowchart 78.1).

It is synthesized by the parenchymal cells of the pineal gland and then released into circulation and CSF.

- The plasma level of **melatonin,** which is secreted from pineal gland, **in children is about 250 pg/ml,** which is much higher than the level **in adults, i.e. about 70 pg/ml.**
- Melatonin secretion exhibits a remarkable **diurnal variation.**
  - The secretion is ***maximum in the night,*** especially between 11 PM to 7AM (Fig. 78.2).
  - It is reported that this **diurnal variation** is due to the ***alteration in sympathetic discharge*** to the pineal gland, mediated by **norepinephrine via β** receptors.

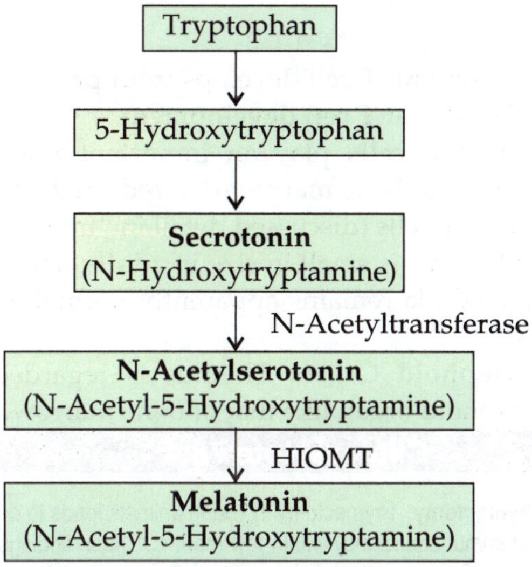

Flowchart 78.1: Synthesis of melatonin. HIOMT: hydroxyindole-O-methyltransferase.

- The **pineal sympathetic output** synchronized with light dark cycle is controlled by **inputs from retinohypothalamic pathway** that projects to suprachiasmatic nucleus.
- Fibers from **suprachiasmatic nucleus** terminate in intermediolateral gray column of the thoracic spinal cord that in turn projects to *superior cervical ganglion* from where fibers originate to end in the pineal gland (Flowchart 78.2).

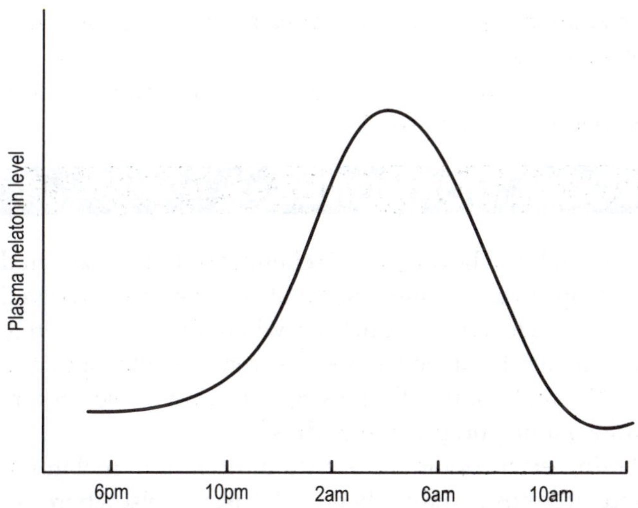

Fig. 78.2: Diurnal variation in melatonin secretion. Note, secretion is maximum between 11 PM and 7 AM.

Melatonin Receptors

Two types of melatonin receptors have been described: **ML 1 and ML 2.**

1. Melatonin at **ML 1 receptor** subtype acts ***by increasing cAMP***. ML 1 receptor has **two sub types:** Mel 1a, and Mel 1b.
2. **ML 2 receptor** subtype acts by increasing IP_3 and DAG in the target cells.

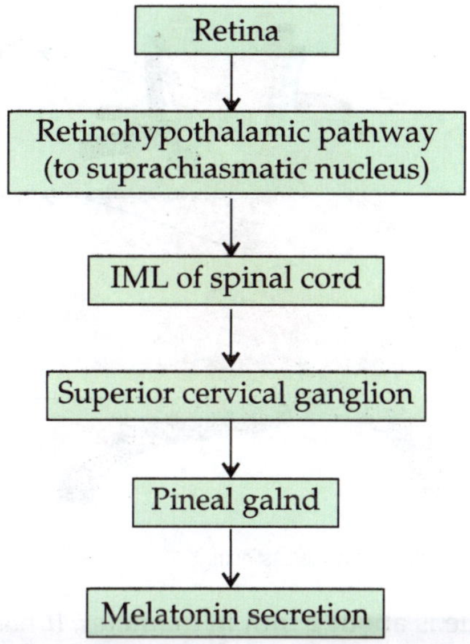

Flowchart 78.2: Pathway from retina that causes melatonin secretion during night. IML: intermediolateral horn.

Functions of Pineal Gland

Melatonin has following functions:

1. Melatonin secreted from pineal has a definite **diurnal pattern**.
   - This diurnal change in melatonin level is believed to coordinate the **endocrinal responses** of the body with the light-dark cycle in the environment.
2. Melatonin secreted from pineal **inhibits gonadal function**.
   - Pineal secretion **inhibits the onset of puberty**.
     - Therefore, regression of pineal stimulates the beginning of pubertal changes.
     - It has been observed that ***precocious puberty and sexual precocity are associated with pineal abnormalities***.
3. In lower animals, melatonin influences the activity of melanophores and thereby controls **skin colour**. However, such function in human appears to be uncertain.

THYMUS

The thymus is located in the superior mediastinum (Fig. 78.3).

- **At birth**, the thymus weighs 10-15 grams, which increases to 30-40 grams at puberty.
- Subsequently, much of the organ is replaced by fat and is **atrophied in adults**.
- The thymus is important as it processes T lymphocytes throughout life.

Structure

The thymus consists of right and left lobes that are joined together by fibrous tissue. Each lobe has a connective tissue capsule, which has septa passing inwards from the capsule that subdivide the lobe into a larger number of **lobules**.

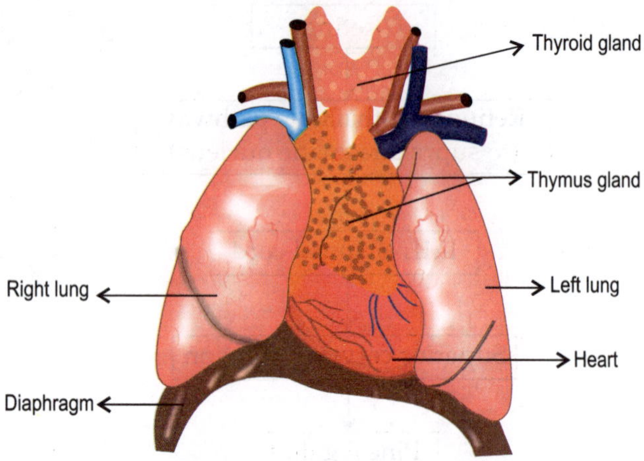

Fig. 78.3: Location of thymus in the mediastinum.

1. Each lobule is about 2 mm in diameter. It has an outer **cortex** and an inner **medulla** (Fig. 78.4).
   - Both the cortex and medulla contain cells of two distinct lineages.
   - The medulla of adjoining lobule is continuous.
2. The thymus has a rich blood supply. It does not receive any lymph vessels, but gives off efferent vessels.
3. Epithelial cells are called **epitheliocytes**. Seven types of epitheliocytes are recognized.
4. Lymphocytes of thymus are called **thymocytes**.
5. Thymus contains a fair number of **macrophages** that are part of mononuclear phagocyte system (MPS).
   - The **subcapsular macrophages** are highly phagocytic.
   - Macrophages present more deeply are **dendritic cells**.

Hassall's Corpuscle: These are small rounded structures present in the medulla of the thymus.

- Each corpuscle has a central core formed by epithelial cells that have undergone degeneration.
- - These cells ultimately form a pink staining **hyaline mass**.
- Around this mass there is a wall formed by concentrically arranged epithelial cells.

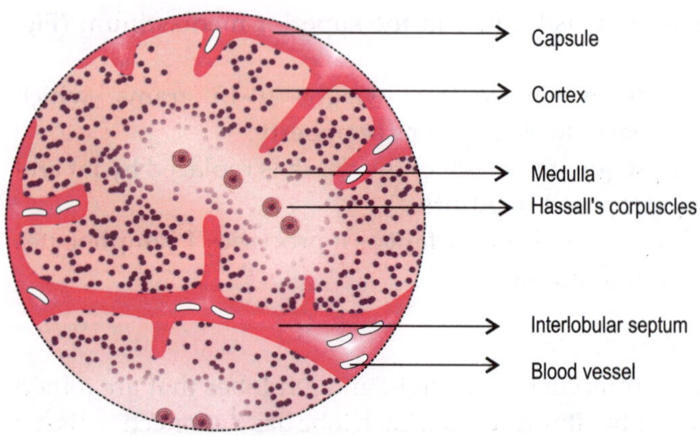

Fig. 78.4: Histology of thymus. Note the presence of Hassall's corpuscle in medulla.

Functions of the Thymus

T cell Development: T cell develops from pre-T cell. The thymus is the **site for T cell development**.

- The **epithelial cells** play an important role in the development of bone marrow-derived prethymic cells into mature T cells (discussed detail in "Immunity").
- Though thymus is small in size in adults, and the less cellular medulla remains apparently normal (Clinical Note 78.1).

Primary Lymphoid Organ: Thymus is regarded as a primary lymphoid organ like that of bone marrow.

Clinical Note 78.1

Effects of thymectomy: Thymectomy in young animals leads to depletion of T cells and immunodeficiency within few months. These findings depict the importance of thymus in development of T cells in childhood and maintenance of T cells in adult life.

Thymic Hormones

A number of hormones produced by the thymus have now been identified as follows:

1. **Thymulin:** Thymulin enhances the function of various types of T cell, specially that of suppressor cells.
2. **Thymopoietin**: Thymopoietin stimulates the production of cytotoxic T cells. The combined action of thymulin and thymopoietin allows precise balance of the activity of cytotoxic and suppressor cells.
3. **Thymosin:** **Thymosin α-1** stimulates lymphocyte production and also the production of antibodies. **Thymosin β-4** is produced by mononuclear phagocytes.
4. **Thymic humoral factor** controls the multiplication of helper and suppressor T cells.

LOCAL HORMONES

Definition: Local hormones are chemicals that are secreted locally from an endocrine tissue that are primarily involved in control of local tissue functions where they are secreted.

- The major local hormones are renin, erythropoietin, ANP, melatonin, thymosin, histamine, serotonin, bradykinin, and prostaglandins.
- Renin, erythropoietin, ANP, bradykinin, melatonin and thymosin have been discussed elsewhere in different chapters in the book.

Histamine

Source, Synthesis & Metabolism

Histamine is secreted from **mast cells and basophils**. It is widely distributed in mammalian tissues.

- It has highest concentration in the skin, gastric mucosa, pituitary and lungs.
- Histamine is synthesized from the amino acid **histidine** by the action of enzyme *histidine decarboxylase*.

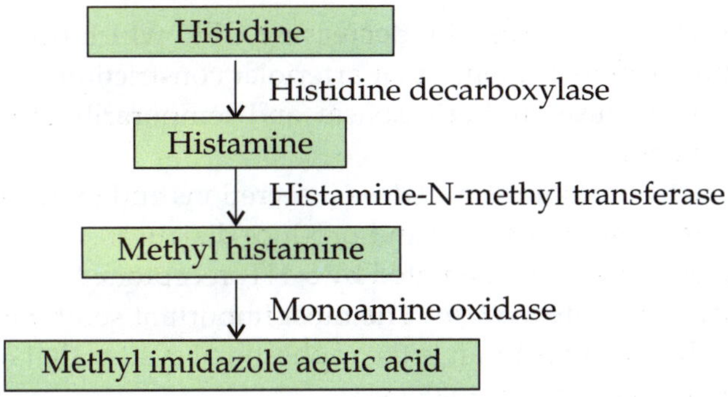

Flowchart 78.3: Synthesis and metabolism of histamine.

- Histamine is converted to **methylhistamine** by *histamine-N-methyltransferase,* which is further converted to **methyl-imidazole-acetic acid** (Flowchart 78.3).

Histamine Receptors

Three types of histamine receptors have been described so far. They are: **H_1, H_2 and H_3** receptors. All are found in brain and peripheral tissues.

H_1 Receptors: They are attached to phospholipase C. On activation, they produce **IP_3 and DAG** in the cell. These receptors mediate inflammation and allergy.

H_2 Receptors: Histamine at H_2 receptors acts by **increasing intracellular cAMP**. They are found in gastric mucosa and mediate gastric acid secretion.

H_3 Receptors: They are found in CNS, especially in presynaptic membrane and are coupled to G proteins. They inhibit release of histamine and other neurotransmitters from presynaptic nerve terminals.

Physiological Actions

Histamine acts mainly on the cardiovascular system, smooth muscles, and exocrine secretions. It mediates inflammation and allergy.

On CVS: Histamine is a potent vasodilator.

- It decreases blood pressure (causes hypotension).
- It also decreases the cardiac output.

On Smooth Muscles: Histamine increases tone of most of the smooth muscles.

- It increases intestinal motility and causes bronchoconstriction.

On Exocrine Secretions: Histamine is a powerful stimulator of HCl secretion from parietal cells stomach. It also potentiates salivary, pancreatic, and intestinal secretions.

Role in Inflammation: It is an important mediator of inflammation.

- Histamine, by causing local vasodilation increases blood flow at the site of inflammation and by increasing capillary permeability causes local swelling.
- It mediates responses (triple response) to local injury.

Role in Allergy: Allergic reactions are mostly mediated via histamine.

1. **In acute systemic allergy** (anaphylaxis), hypotension occurs due to release of histamine from mast cell that produces acute vasodilation.
   - Histamine is released from mast cells in response to the antibody Ig E (the **reagin antibody**).
   - The antigen-antibody complex causes **degranulation of mast cells** and release histamine.
2. **Local allergic reactions** like urticaria, allergic rhinitis, hay fever, etc. are also due to the release of histamine at the local sites.
3. **Bronchial asthma** is precipitated or induced by histamine.
4. Histamine is released from mast cell along with **slow reacting substance for anaphylaxis** (SRS-A).
   - **Histamine and SRS-A** mediate allergic reactions.
   - Hence, **antihistaminics** are mainstay of treatment for allergies.

Relation with Itch: Histamine acts as a neurotransmitter for itch sensation.

- Itching associated with skin allergy (urticaria) is cured by antihistaminics.

On CNS: Histaminergic neurons project from tuberomamillary nucleus to all parts of the brain.

- These histaminergic fibers are involved in the control of blood pressure, sexual and ingestive behaviours, arousal and alertness, pain and secretion of anterior pituitary hormones.

Antihistaminic Drugs

Antihistaminics are used for the treatment of allergy and inflammations.

H_1 Receptor Antagonists: H_1 antagonists like **mepyramine and promethazine** are used to prevent histamine induced contractions of smooth muscles of intestine and bronchi.

- They are also used frequently in the treatment of allergies.

H_2 Receptor Antagonists: H_2 antagonists like **cimetidine, ranitidine, and famotidine** are used to inhibit histamine induced HCl secretion in the stomach.

- These drugs are frequently used in the treatment of peptic ulcer.

Serotonin

Source

Serotonin is **5-hydroxytryptamine** (5-HT). It is distributed in various tissues. It is present in high concentration in GI tract, CNS, especially in the hypothalamus and brainstem, and skin.

- Due to its higher concentration in the intestine, it is also known as **enteramine**.
- It is also present in platelets and basophils.

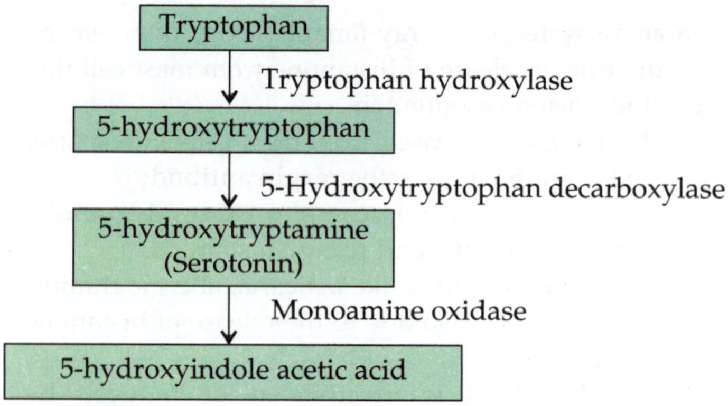

Flowchart 78.4: Synthesis and metabolism of serotonin.

Synthesis and Metabolism

Serotonin is synthesized from the amino acid **tryptophan**.

- Tryptophan is converted to **5-hydroxytryptophan** by the action of enzyme tryptophan hydroxylase.
- 5-hydroxytryptophan is then decarboxylated to form 5-hydroxytryptamine (serotonin) catalyzed by the enzyme 5-hydroxytryptophan decarboxylase (Flowchart 78.4).

Metabolism: Serotonin is metabolized by the enzyme monoamine oxidase to form 5-hydroxyindole acetic acid (5-HIAA), which is excreted in urine.

- 5-HIAA is physiologically inactive.
- However, the level of it in urine is an index of serotonin secretion in the body.

Serotonin Receptors

There are **seven types of serotonin receptors**. They are 5-HT_1, 5-HT_2, 5-HT_3, 5-HT_4, 5-HT_5, 5-HT_6, 5-HT_7.

- The 5-HT_1 is further subdivided into 5-HT_{1A}, 5-HT_{1B}, 5-HT_{1D}, 5-HT_{1E}, and 5-HT_{1F}.
- Also, 5-HT_2 is further subdivided into 5-HT_{2A}, 5-HT_{2B} and 5-HT_{2C}.
- The 5-HT_5 has two subtypes: 5-HT_{5A} and 5-HT_{5B}.

Physiological Actions

Serotonin mainly acts on cardiovascular system, respiratory system, kidney, smooth muscle, and nervous system.

Cardiovascular System: Serotonin, acting locally produces vasoconstriction. It facilitates platelet aggregation.

- These two functions of platelets are mediated via **5-HT_{2A} receptors** and are essential for **temporary hemostasis.**
- Serotonin also produces **tachycardia.**

Respiratory System: Serotonin increases bronchial tone (causes bronchoconstriction), which is mediated via 5-HT_{2A} receptors.

- In asthmatic patients, it **induces the acute attack** of asthma.
- It also **stimulates rate of respiration.**

Kidney: Serotonin has mild antidiuretic effect.

- It prevents diuresis by decreasing GFR, which occurs due to afferent glomerular arteriolar constriction.
- It also causes ureteric spasm and temporarily stops urination.

GI Tract: Serotonin stimulates GI secretions and motility.

- It promotes peristalsis and produce diarrhea.
- These effects are mediated by 5-HT_4 receptors.

Central Nervous System: The most important serotonergic pathway in the brain is the raphespinal system that on stimulation produces analgesia.

- 5-HT_3 receptors are present in area postrema that on activation induces vomiting. 5-HT_6 and 5-HT_7 receptors are distributed throughout the limbic system, neocortex, cerebellum and spinal cord.

It has following central functions:

1. ***Inhibits transmission of pain impulses*** in dorsal horn of spinal cord, and thus, it is an important component of **endogenous analgesia system.**
2. Stimulates **prolactin secretion** from anterior pituitary.
3. Regulates **circadian rhythm** (suprachiasmatic nucleus receives heavy serotonergic innervation).
4. Serotonin is a strong **antidepressant.**
   - Hallucinogens produce euphoria by releasing serotonin in the brain.
   - Antidepressant drugs such as fluoxetine act by inhibiting serotonin reuptake in the brain.
5. Serotonin is a strong **anorectic agent.** It *inhibits feeding* by acting on hypothalamic and other feeding areas in the brain.
6. Serotonin **suppresses sleep** and serotonin antagonists enhance slow wave sleep.

Clinical Correlation

Increased serotonin activity is seen in some endocrine tumors, which is detected by estimation of urinary 5-HIAA. This is usually observed in **carcinoid syndrome.**

Prostaglandins

Prostaglandin was first described by **Von Euler** in 1937. It was named prostaglandin for its enumeration in the secretion from prostate gland. Afterwards, prostaglandins were found to be synthesized in various tissues of the body.

- They are **20-carbon unsaturated fatty acids** containing a cyclopentane ring.

Types

The commonest prostaglandins are PGE, PGF, PGI, PFH and PGA.

- Further, each has subcategories like are PGA_1, PGA_2, PGE_1, PGE_2, $PGF_{1\alpha}$, and $PGF_{2\alpha}$ etc.

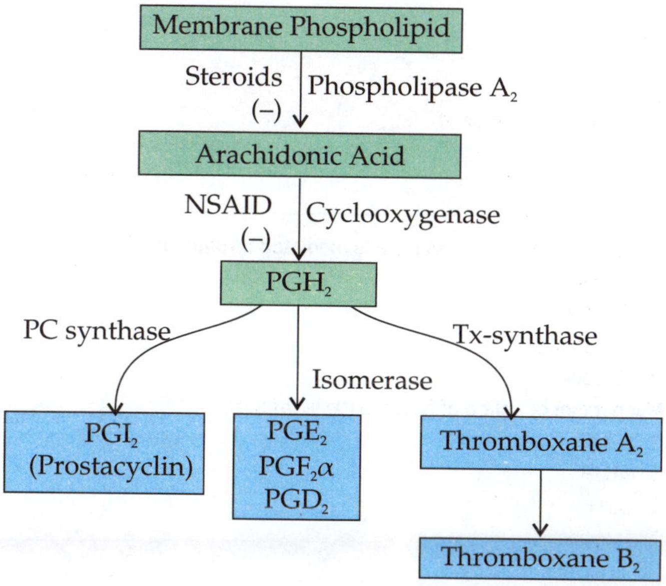

Flowchart 78.5: Prostaglandin synthesis. NSAID: nonsteroidal antiinflamatory drugs; PC: prostacyclin; T_X: thromboxane; (–): indicates inhibition.

Synthesis

Prostaglandins are synthesized from **arachidonic acid**, which is formed from membrane phospholipid by the enzyme **phospholipase A_2**.

- Arachidonic acid is then converted to cyclic endoperoxides (PGH_2) by the action of enzyme **cyclooxygenase** (prostaglandin synthase).
- PGH_2 is then converted to prostacyclin by the enzyme prostacyclin synthase or thromboxane A_2 by the enzyme thromboxane synthase (Flowchart 78.5).
- PGH_2 is also converted to PGE_2, $PGF_{2\alpha}$ etc. by various isomerases.

Physiological Actions

Prostaglandins are present in almost **all the tissues of the body**. They are mainly involved in the control of functions of various organ systems, hemostasis, and metabolisms and play an important role in inflammation.

Cardiovascular System: PGA_1 and PGA_2 cause peripheral arteriolar dilation.

- **Prostacyclin** produces ***vasodilation*** and **thromboxane A_2** causes ***vasoconstriction***.

Reproductive System: 1. $PGF_{2\alpha}$ produces contraction of gravid uterus.

- The concentration of this chemical increases in the maternal blood during parturition.
- It is reported that the increase in **$PGF_{2\alpha}$ initiates labor** in the presence of high concentration of oxytocin.

2. Prostaglandins facilitate **luteolysis** (regression of corpus luteum).
   - They decrease the secretion of progesterone.
4. Prostaglandins **increase in uterine fluid** and cause necrosis of blood vessels of the uterus just before the bleeding starts during menstrual cycle.
   - It is observed that prostaglandins **initiate the process of bleeding**.
5. It increases **secretion of GnRH** from hypothalamus.

Hemostasis: Prostacyclin inhibits platelet aggregation and produces vasodilation whereas thromboxane A_2 and endoperoxides *promote platelet aggregation and cause vasoconstriction*.

- The balance between the prostacyclin and thromboxane A_2 determines the degree of **platelet plug** formation (for details, refer to Chapter 16).
- Thus, prostaglandins greatly influence temporary hemostasis.

Respiratory System: Prostaglandin E causes bronchodilation whereas $PGF_{2\alpha}$ produces *bronchoconstriction*.

- $PGF_{2\alpha}$ is implicated in the genesis of bronchial asthma.

GI System: Prostaglandin E and $F_{2\alpha}$ *inhibit absorption of sodium and water*.

- The **watery diarrhea** produced in cholera is mediated by prostaglandins.
- They also stimulate **intestinal motility**.

Central Nervous System: Prostaglandins act as neurotransmitters in various parts of the brain. PGE inhibits release of norepinephrine from the nerve endings.

Inflammation: Prostaglandin E and A increase capillary permeability during inflammation.

- PGE sensitizes the nerve endings to bradykinin and produces pain.

Metabolisms: PGE_1 inhibits lipolysis, induced by ACTH, GH, glucagons, and epinephrine.

Clinical Correlation

Prostaglandin preparations are used in the treatment of different diseases.

1. **Steroidal anti-inflammatory drugs** such as cortisol inhibit prostaglandin production by inhibiting the enzyme phospholipase A_2.
2. **Nonsteroidal anti-inflammatory drugs** (NSAID) such as ibuprofen inhibit prostaglandin synthesis by inhibiting the enzyme cyclooxygenase (Flowchart 120.3).

Carcinoid Syndrome

These are tumors of **enterochromaffin cells** of the GI tract or bronchus or pancreas.

- A characteristic feature of carcinoid syndrome is the **episodic flushing** of the skin, associated with hypertension, abdominal pain, diarrhea, and bronchoconstriction.
  - These episodic attacks occur due to secretion of various chemicals from the tumor enterochromaffin cells.
- Usually, these tumors secrete **excess of serotonin and histamine**.
  - Therefore, the disease is diagnosed by the **excretion of increased amount of 5-HIAA** in the urine.

Exam Questions

1. Describe the steps of melatonin synthesis and briefly describe its regulation of secretion.
2. Give a brief note on functional histology of thymus gland. Briefly describe the functions of thymus gland.
3. Briefly describe the synthesis, mechanism of action and functions of histamine, serotonin and prostaglandins. Add a note on carcinoid syndrome.

Multiple Choice Questions

1. **The plasma melatonin level in an adult is about:**
   A. 450 pg/mL B. 250 pg/mL
   C. 170 pg/mL D. 70 pg/mL
2. **The plasma melatonin level in adults is Which of the following gland is called epiphysis?**
   A. Anterior pituitary B. Posterior pituitary
   C. Pineal gland D. Hypothalamus
3. **Melatonin is secreted by:**
   A. Hypothalamus B. Adrenal cortex
   C. Pineal gland D. Melanocytes
4. **Exposure to darkness leads to increased melatonin secretion. It is brought about by:**
   A. Decreasing the activity of suprachiasmatic nuclei
   B. Increasing the activity of serotonin N-acetyl transferase
   C. Decreasing the hydroxyl-indole-o-methyl transferase activity
   D. Blocking the release of norepinephrine from sympathetic nerve terminals
5. **Melatonin secretion is maximum during:**
   A. 5 PM to 10 PM B. 7 PM to 1 AM
   C. 11 PM to 7 AM D. 4 AM to 10 AM
6. **Melatonin acting on ML-1 receptor causes which of the following?**
   A. Increase in cAMP B. Increase in DAG
   C. Increase in calcium D. Increase in IP3
7. **Which of the following is not true about pineal gland?**
   A. Melatonin is secreted from pinealocytes
   B. Pineal gland size increases after puberty
   C. Secretion f pineal gland is more in the night, during sleep
   D. Sympathetic innervation of pineal gland is the major neural control
8. **Which of the following is not the function of histamine?**
   A. Vasodilation
   B. Decreased cardiac output
   C. Decreased GI motility
   D. Bronchoconstriction
9. **All of the following are functions of serotonin, EXCEPT:**
   A. Platelet aggregation
   B. Bronchoconstriction
   C. Increased GI secretion and motility
   D. Increased appetite
10. **Bradykinin causes all, EXCEPT:**
    A. Contraction of visceral smooth muscle
    B. Increased capillary permeability
    C. Vasodilation
    D. Decreased pancreatic and salivary secretion
11. **Stress induced hyperglycemia is mediated through all, EXCEPT:**
    A. Glucagon
    B. Thyroxine
    C. Epinephrine
    D. Cortisol
12. **Mechanism of action of Nitric oxide is through**
    A. cGMP
    B. cAMP
    C. Ca++
    D. Tyrosine
13. **NO is synthesized by:**
    A. Uracil
    B. Aspartate
    C. Guanosine
    D. Arginine
14. **Nitric oxide synthase:**
    A. Is inhibited by Ca++
    B. Catalyzes a dioxygenase reaction
    C. Accepts electrons from NADH
    D. Requires NADPH, FAD, FMN & Heme iron
15. **All the statements about nitric oxide are true, EXCEPT:**
    A. Vasodilator
    B. Oxidizing agent
    C. Catalyst
    D. Platelet aggregator
16. **The primary action of nitric oxide on gastrointestinal tract is:**
    A. Vasodilatation
    B. Vasoconstriction
    C. Gastrointestinal smooth muscle relaxation
    D. Gastrointestinal slow smooth muscle contraction
17. **ANP produces all, EXCEPT:**
    A. Diuresis
    B. Decreased capillary permeability
    C. Decreased sensitivity of blood vessel to vasoconstrictors
    D. Vasodilation
18. **All of the following are features of carcinoid syndrome, EXCEPT:**
    A. Episodic flushing
    B. Bronchodialtion
    C. Excess secretion of histamine
    D. Increased secretion of 5-HIAA in urine

Answers: 1. D 2. C 3. C 4. B 5. C 6. A 7. B 8. C 9. D 10. D 11. B 12. A 13. D 14. D 15. D 16. C 17. B 18. B

Section IX

Reproductive System

“ *To conquer a desire brings more joy than to satisfy it.*

The Mother ”
(of Sri Aurobindo Ashram, Pondicherry, INDIA)

Chapter 79

Sex Differentiation and Physiology of Puberty and Menopause

Learning Objectives

On completion of study of this chapter:

The student will be able to (must know):

1. Understand the mechanism of sex differentiation and development in males and females.
2. Outline the regulation of sex differentiation.
3. List the abnormalities of sex differentiation and understand the physiological basis of their causation.
4. Name the common developmental anomalies and differentiate between male and female pseudohermaphroditism.
5. Describe the physiological changes of puberty in girls and boys.
6. Explain the physiological changes during menopause.

The student may also be able to (desirable to know):

1. Describe the regulation of sex differentiation.
2. Describe the mechanisms of dysfunctions of sex differentiation

PY9.1

SEX DIFFERENTIATION

Normal Chromosomal Pattern

In a normal human being, there are 46 (23 pairs) chromosomes: 22 pairs are autosomes and one pair is sex chromosome (Fig. 79.1).

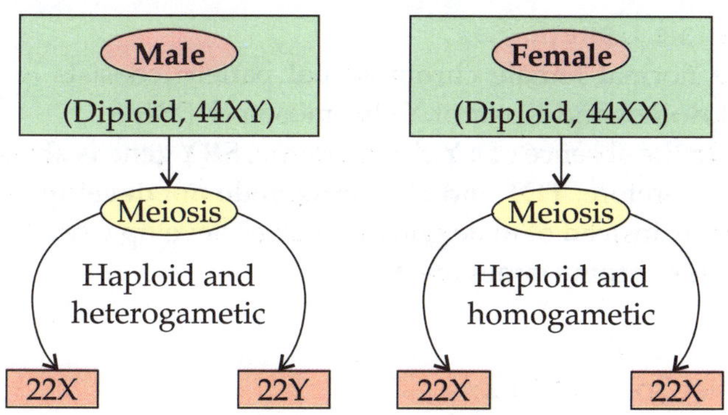

Fig. 79.1: Chromosomal pattern in males (44 XY) and females (44 XX).

In Males: The pattern is 22 pairs of autosomes, and **one X and one Y** chromosomes (44 XY).

In Females: The pattern is 22 pairs of autosomes and **two X chromosomes** (44 XX).

Sex Chromosomes

Gender is determined by the genetic inheritance of two chromosomes, called sex chromosomes. The two sex chromosomes are the **X chromosome**, the larger one, and the **Y chromosome**, the smaller one.

Females possess **two X** chromosomes and **males** have **one X and one Y** chromosome.

- Thus, ovum always contributes only one X chromosome, whereas half of the sperms contribute X and another half Y.

2. Generally, the **male births are slightly more than the female births**.
   - This difference in sex ratio could be because the sperms that contain **Y chromosomes are lighter** than the sperm that contain X chromosome as **Y chromosome is smaller in size** than X chromosome.
   - Therefore, **sperms with Y chromosomes swim faster** in female genital tract and reach ovum earlier.
   - Thus, the opportunity for these chromosomes to fertilize ovum is more than the sperm with X chromosomes.

Genetic Male: When a sperm containing Y chromosome fertilizes an ovum, the resultant zygote develops into a **genetic male** having XY pattern of sex chromosomes. The karyotype is **44 XY.**

Genetic Female: When a sperm containing X chromosome fertilizes an ovum, the resultant zygote develops into a **genetic female** having XX pattern of sex chromosomes. The karyotype is **44 XX.**

Sex Determination

Karyotyping

Sex determination is usually done by **karyotyping**, a technique used for ***determining sex chromosome composition*** by employing tissue culture visualization of all chromosomes. The differences in shape and size of chromosomes in males and females help in concrete determination of sex.

Demonstration of Sex Chromatin: This is a relatively easy method to demonstrate sex chromatin **(Barr body)** in leucocytes or mucosal cells of the oral cavity.

- Barr bodies are usually formed in females as they have two X chromosomes.
- When two X chromosomes are present, one X chromosome is functional and other X chromosome which is nonfunctional condenses to form sex chromatin.
- Thus, presence of **Barr body generally indicates female sex.**

Sex Differentiation

The process of sex differentiation includes the pattern of development of the gonads, genital ducts, and the external genitalia.

- During pregnancy, no differences in the gonads of male and female fetuses occur during the first five weeks of gestation. This is called the **stage of indifferent gonads.**
- The differentiation of gender starts **from sixth week** of intrauterine life and continues even after birth till the complete maturation of the gonad of either gender is achieved.

Cell Lines of Development: Following fertilization, two different cell lines develop in the indifferent gonad.

1. The **one cell line** forms the ***granulosa cells*** of the ovarian follicle and the ***Sertoli cells*** of the testicular seminiferous tubules.
    - The cells of this cell line **nurse the germ cells** and promote their maturation, and finally guide their development into the ***genital duct system***.
    - These cells in females **produce estrogen.**
2. The **other cell line** of the indifferent gonad (the interstitial cells) forms ***theca cells*** in the ovary and ***Leydig cells*** in the testis.
    - These cells mainly **secrete androgen,** which is essential for the development of ***male sexual characteristics*** and spermatogenesis.
    - In females, they form the **precursors for estrogen synthesis.**

Differentiation of the Genetic Sex, Gonadal Sex & Phenotypic Sex

Genetic Sex

Male Genetic Sex

The male chromosomal pattern is 44 autosomes and a pair of sex chromosomes. The sex chromosomes in a normal male are X and Y. The presence of **Y chromosomes determines the maleness** of the individual, without which neither testis nor the male genital pattern develop.

1. The Y chromosome contains the **SRY gene** (sex-determining region of the Y) which is located on the distal part of its short arm (Fig. 79.2).
2. This gene encodes the **testis determining factor** (TDF). The
    - TDF is a ***transcription factor*** that binds to DNA molecules.
3. A gene identical to SRY gene encodes a histocompatibility antigen known as **H-Y antigen.**
    - These are glycoprotein antigens present on the surface of all male cells.
    - Both these antigens are ***involved in rejection of male tissue*** by the female recipients.
    - This H-Y antigen helps in **development of male gonads,** and masculinization.
4. Though SRY gene is essential for masculinization, ***it is not adequate*** for the complete maleness.
5. Virilization of the genital duct and external genitalia requires the presence of an **androgen hormone receptor.**
    - This receptor is encoded by the gene present on the X chromosomes.
    - Therefore, *X chromosomal gene* also contributes to the *development of maleness.*

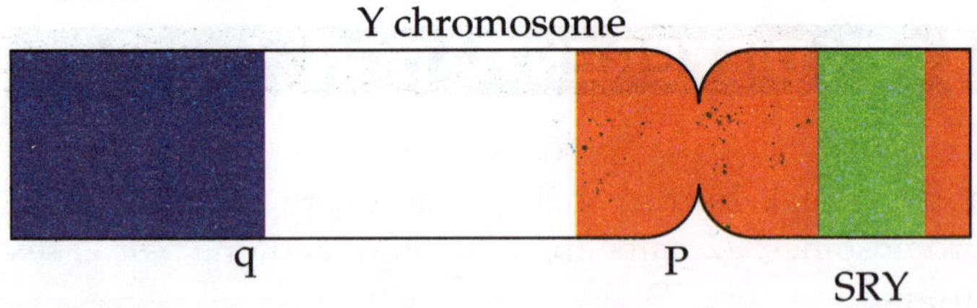

Fig. 79.2: Sex-determining region of Y (SRY) chromosome.

Female Genetic Sex

The normal female chromosomal pattern consists of 44 autosomes and a pair of X chromosomes (XX).

1. In the absence of a Y chromosome, **SRY gene is absent.**
2. Therefore, **TDF and H-Y antigen do not develop.**

Hence, instead of male gonads ovaries develop when both the sex chromosomes are X.

Gonadal Sex

Male Gonadal Sex

In a normal genetic male, the seminiferous tubule starts to form at 6–7 weeks of gestation.

- The Sertoli cells enclose the germ cells.
- The **Leydig cells appear at 8–9 weeks**. The testis starts **secreting testosterone** during this period. This helps in development of male sex.
- The **SRY gene prevents synthesis of estrogen** and **inhibits** the enzyme ***aromatase***, which inhibits the development of female systems.

Female Gonadal Sex

In a normal genetic female, the differentiation of indifferent gonad into the female gonads (ovaries) starts after nine weeks of gestation.

- Both the X chromosomes in the **germ cells are activated**.
- The germ cells then undergo divisions to **form oogonia** that continue to proliferate.
    - Immediately after the start of meiosis, oogonia are surrounded by granulosa cells.
    - Stroma appears inside it, which gives rise to interstitial cells.
    - Now the germ cells are known as primary oocytes.
- The female gonad remains in this stage (***primary oocyte stage***), i.e. in the stage of diplotene or late prophase of meiosis **for many years** until ovulation occurs.

Estrogen secreted from the granulosa cells help in the female development.

Phenotypic (Genital) Sex

Under the direction of a positive hormonal influence, the male gonadal system develops, and in the absence of any hormonal control, female genitals develop. The development of brain is also linked to the phenotypic sex (Application Box 79. 1).

Application Box 79.1

Phenotypic sex development influences brain development: Development of brain is linked to the development of the external genitalia in the early part of life, which is influenced by exposures to androgens. The pattern of hypothalamic control of gonadotropin release that starts with the onset of puberty is determined earlier by the exposure to androgen in first few days of life. In the absence of androgen exposure, female pattern develops.

In Males

In males, at about 9–10 weeks **Wolffian** or **mesonephric ducts** develop which gives rise to epididymis, vas deferens, seminal vesicles, and ejaculatory ducts.

1. Development of this system is presided by the appearance of Leydig cells in the testis that secrete testosterone.
2. Testosterone stimulates growth and differentiation of Wolffian duct into the male genital system (Flowchart 79.1).

In Females

In females, the Wolffian duct degenerates at about 10–11 weeks as ovary does not secrete testosterone. From Wolffian ducts on each side, the **Müllerian ducts** arise, which develops into fallopian tubes and uterus.

Role of MIS: In males, müllerian ducts regress at about 8 weeks of gestation, the time during which Sertoli cells appear in the testis. The Sertoli cells produce a hormone called **müllerian inhibiting substance** (MIS). This is also known as *antimüllerian hormone* or *müllerian regression factor*.

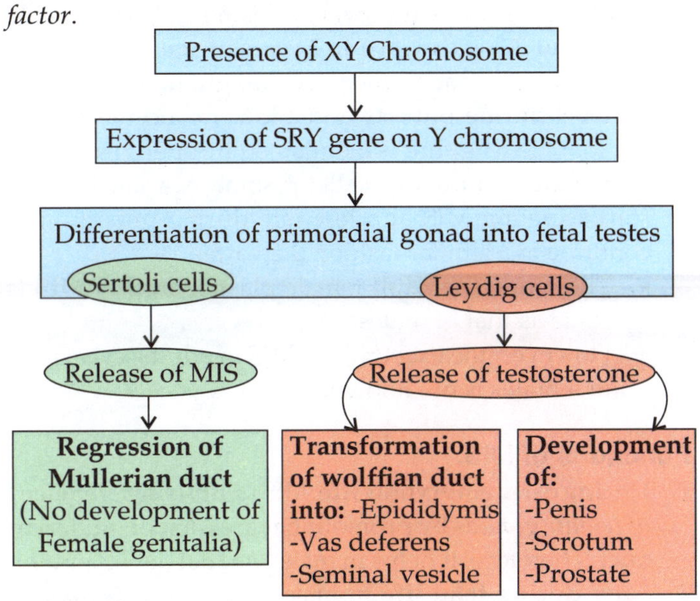

Flowchart 79.1: Mechanism of sex differentiation in male.

- MIS causes degeneration of müllerian duct by facilitating its apoptosis.
- The SRY gene promotes the synthesis of MIS.
- In females who **lack MIS**, ***müllerian duct continues to grow*** and form fallopian tubes, uterus, cervix, and vagina (Flowchart 79.2). This differentiation is completed by 18–20 weeks of gestation.

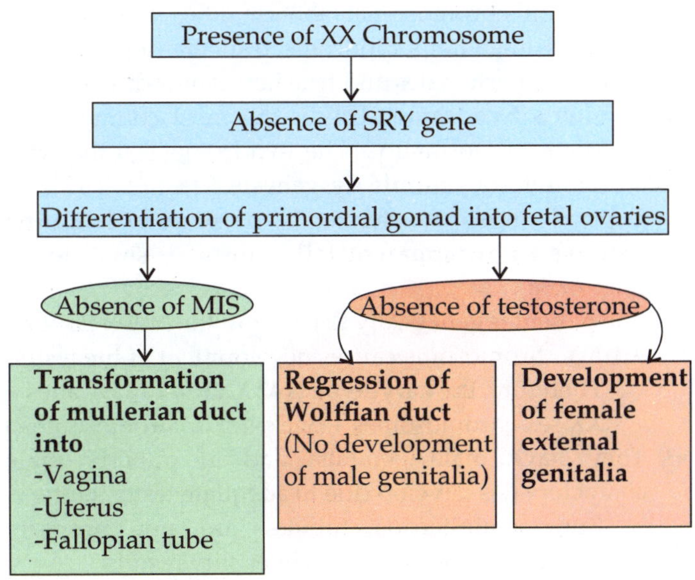

Flowchart 79.2: Mechanism of sex differentiation in female.

Müllerian Inhibiting Substance (MIS)

Also known as **antimüllerian hormone** or **müllerian regression factor**, MIS is a polypeptide hormone containing 536 amino acids **secreted by the Sertoli cells** of testis. It belongs to the **TGF β superfamily** of growth factors that includes activin and inhibin.

1. **In males**, though the secretion of MIS starts at 8–10 weeks of gestation, the level in plasma reaches its peak, i.e., about 50 ng/mL at 1 to 2 years of age.
   - The concentration then declines gradually to a low-level during puberty and a lower concentration of about 2–5 ng/mL is maintained through rest of life.
2. **In females**, granulosa cells of some ovarian follicles start secreting MIS at a low rate during puberty and continue in a similar fashion thereafter.
   - Therefore, the adult female plasma level of MIS is same as that of males.
   - However, the exact role of MIS in adults, especially in females is not known.

Functions of MIS:

1. **During early embryonic life**, MIS ***inhibits development of female gonads*** by promoting regression of müllerian duct. Therefore, it helps in male gonadal development.
2. Later **during fetal life** in males, it helps in ***testicular descent***.
3. In both sexes, it helps in **maturation of germ cells**.

Abnormalities of Sex Differentiation

The abnormalities of sex differentiation can be broadly divided into **two categories**: chromosomal and developmental abnormalities.

Chromosomal Abnormalities

The common chromosomal abnormalities are Turner's syndrome, Klinefelter's syndrome, testicular feminization syndrome, superfemales and true hermaphroditism.

Klinefelter's Syndrome: This is the most common sex chromosome abnormality. The syndrome is otherwise called seminiferous **tubule dysgenesis**.

- Typically, it is characterized by presence of **feminine features in an apparent tall male** with small testes (Fig. 79.3a).
- The patient is genetically female, but the presence of an extra Y chromosome causes development of the testis.
  - Therefore, the **karyotype is 47 XXY** (44 autosomes + XX sex chromosomes + one extra Y chromosomes).
- They have male genitalia and at puberty male characteristics develop due to adequate testosterone.
  - But, seminiferous tubules are not properly developed and therefore, infertility results.
- Thus, the syndrome usually presents with **primary hypogonadism and infertility** in male.
- Mental retardation is common.

Turner's Syndrome: This is otherwise known as **gonadal or ovarian dysgenesis**.

- It is characterized by diminished sexual development, dwarfism, multiple nevi on skin and webbing of the neck in patients with no gonadal tissue or rudimentary gonads (Fig. 79.3b).
- The chromosomal **pattern of sex chromosomes is XO**, which means there are 44 autosomes and one X chromosomes (total 45 chromosomes).
  - It results from nondisjunction of one of the X chromosomes during oogenesis.
- Usually, it presents with *primary amenorrhea*. No sexual maturation occurs at puberty.

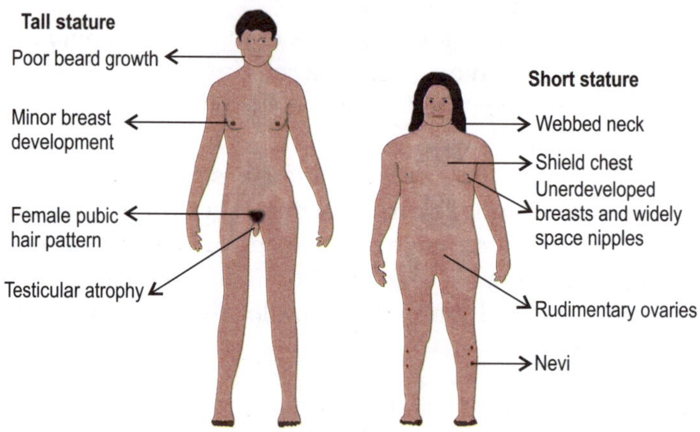

Fig. 79.3: Salient clinical features of Klinefelter (a) and Turner (b) syndrome.

Superfemales: This is a **common aberration** of sexual differentiation.

- Usually, it is ***not associated with*** any characteristic abnormalities and therefore remains undetected.
- The abnormality is commonly diagnosed while performing **chromosomal analysis** for some other causes.
- The karyotype is XXX.

Testicular Feminization Syndrome: The patients appear **normal females externally.** At puberty though breasts develop normally, the growth of pubic and axillary hairs is scanty. It causes primary amenorrhea.

- Though the external genitalia are of female type, there is **no development of uterus**.
  - The vagina ends in a blind pouch.
- The **gonads are testis**, with immature seminiferous tubules.
  - Therefore, it is called testicular feminization syndrome.
  - Though testes are present, **spermatogenesis does not occur**.
- The patients are **genetic males** (XY karyotype).

True Hermaphroditism: This is a rare condition in which **both testes and ovaries are present**. Sometimes, ovary is present on one side and the testis on the opposite side.

- Both male and female sex differentiations occur with the development of combined **female and male external and internal genitalia.**
- Usually, the **karyotype pattern is 46 XX-XY.**

Trisomy 21: This is nondisjunction of chromosome 21 (an autosome). This is associated with **Down's syndrome or mongolism**. It is not an aberration of sex chromosome, rather an **autosomal abnormality**.

Developmental Abnormalities

The developmental abnormalities are mainly hormonal disorders that are broadly divided into **pseudohermaphroditisms** (both female and male patterns) and **enzyme deficiencies**.

Pseudohermaphroditisms

A **pseudohermaphrodite** is an individual with **genetic constitution and gonad of one sex**, but the **external genitalia of the other sex**.

Female Pseudohermaphroditisms: Male external genital development occurs in **genetic females** exposed to androgen during 8th to 13th week of gestation.

- Source of androgen is usually **congenital virilizing adrenal hyperplasia** of fetus or **virilizing ovarian tumor** of the mother.
  - Sometimes it may be **iatrogenically-induced** following treatment of mother with androgens or progestational drugs.
- In a typical female pseudohermaphrodite, the individual **possesses ovaries, oviducts**, but there is varying degrees of **masculine differentiation of external genitalia.**
- The **chromosomal sex is female.**

Male Pseudohermaphroditisms: Development of female external genitalia in a **genetic male** is called male pseudohermaphroditism.

- It is usually due to **defective testicular development**.
- As MIS secreted from testis during early embryonic life prevents development of female gonads, in defective testicular development the internal genitalia are also of female pattern.
  - Male pseudohermaphroditism could also be due to **androgen resistance** that usually occurs in ***deficiency of 5α-reductase***, the enzyme that forms dehydroepiandrosterone or due to defects in androgen receptors.
- In **complete androgen resistance syndrome** (testicular feminizing syndrome), MIS is secreted as testes are normal; therefore, vagina ends blindly due to absence of internal genitalia.

Enzyme Deficiencies

Congenital **17α-hydroxylase deficiency** causes **male pseudohermaphroditism**. This also occurs in **congenital adrenal hyperplasia** in which enzyme defects block the formation of pregnenolone (for details, refer to Chapter 'Adrenal Cortex')

PY9.2

PHYSIOLOGY OF PUBERTY

Definition & Concept

The period of **transition from the non-reproductive state to the state of reproductive functions that allows procreation** is defined as puberty.

- This period of maturation is known as puberty or **adolescence**.
- During this period the endocrine and gametogenic functions of the gonads first develop to the point where the reproduction becomes possible.

Age of Onset of Puberty: Puberty occurs between the age of 8–13 in girls and 9–14 in boys. In developing nations, the age of onset of puberty is **11–16 years in girls** and **13–18 years in boys**.

Initiating Stimulus: The increased secretion of adrenal androgen, called **adrenarche**, occurs about one to two years before the onset of puberty.

- This **increased adrenal androgen** ***stimulates the production of gonadal hormones*** that cause maturation of reproductive organs.
- As increase in adrenal androgen at this stage occurs ***without any alteration in ACTH or cortisol secretion***, it is proposed that this is the **primary and sole stimulus that heralds puberty**.

Stages of Puberty

In Boys

The pubertal development in males occurs in **five stages** (by **Tanner method**, modified) (Fig. 79.4.1 I-V). Usually, it is ***completed within two to four years*** from its onset.

Stage I: This is the **preadolescent stage**. There is no enlargement of external genitalia (penis, scrotum and testes).

- No pubic hair is present.
- However, secretion of adrenal androgen is increased (**adrenarche**).

Stage II: Testes enlarge to more than 2.5 cm, which occurs due to growth of seminiferous tubules.

- Though this occurs due to the secretion of **adrenal androgen** (adrenarche), **testicular androgen** also contributes.
- Testicular testosterone secretion increases significantly.
- **Pubic hairs appear** in scanty at the root of the penis.

Stage III: Penis enlarges in length. Scrotum and testes are further enlarged.

- Pubic hairs **become darker and coarser** above the pubis.
- **Sperm first appears** in the morning sample of urine (**spermarche**).

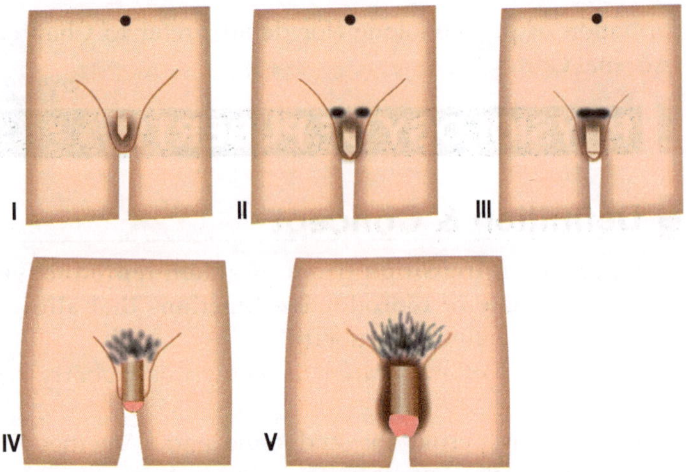

Figs. 79.4: Stages (I to V) of pubertal development in males.

Stage IV: Penis enlarges in width and further in length.

- Scrotal and testicular enlargement continues.
- Pubic hair becomes adult type.
- **Ejaculation of sperm** occurs either in dreams, or on masturbation or by sexual act.

Stage V: Full adult pattern of sexual features develops.

In Girls

The pubertal development in females also described in **five stages** (by **Tanner method**, modified) (Fig. 79.5 I-V). Usually, it is completed within two to five years from its onset.

Stage I: This is **the preadolescent stage**. There is no breast development.

- No pubic hair is present.
- However, secretion of adrenal androgen is increased (**adrenarche**).

Stage II: Breast development starts (**thelarche**). **Breast paillae is elevated** and the diameter of areola is increased.

- Secretion of estrogen from ovary increases significantly.
- Sparse hairs appear along the labia majora.

Stage III: Breast enlarges with enlargement of areola.

- **Pubic hairs develop**, grow and become dark (**pubarche**).
- Hairs appear in axilla.

Stage IV: Breast further enlarges with areola and papillae projecting out of it.

- Pubic hair becomes adult type but covers smaller area.
- **Menstrual cycle starts** (**menarche**), but irregular at the beginning.

Stage V: Full adult pattern of breasts and pubic hairs develop. Menstrual cycle occurs regularly.

Mechanism of Onset of Puberty

The **hypothalamic neurons** gradually mature to **secrete more GnRH**. This maturational process is genetically preprogrammed.

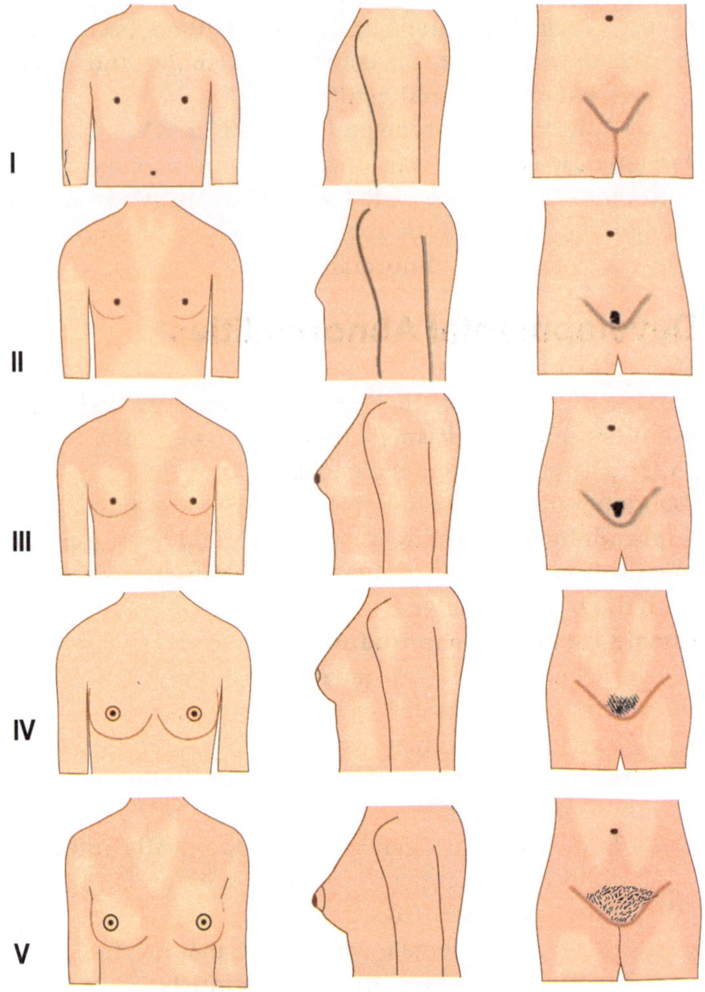

Figs. 79.5: Stages (I to V) of pubertal development in females.

- Dehydroepiandrosterone secreted from adrenal gland plays some role in the **maturation of hypothalamic neurons**.
- The adipose tissue via secretion of **leptin** also plays some role in the determination of the time of onset of puberty (see below).
- Normally, the **secretion of GnRH, LH and FSH** is not pulsatile before the onset of puberty.
  - It is clear that **until puberty the release of GnRH is non-pulsatile**, which prevents puberty to occur.
  - It is not known what mechanism inhibits the **GnRH pulse generator** till puberty.
  - However, before puberty, the GnRH is secreted in a **pulsatile pattern** that stimulates **pulsatile secretion of LH and FSH**.
- It is proposed that this **pulsatile secretion of GnRH** brings about the onset of puberty.

Role of Leptin: It has been observed that **body weight increases to a critical level** before the onset of puberty, especially in females. It is also observed that the onset of puberty is **delayed in girls with lower body weight**.

- Leptin, the hormone secreted from adipose tissue cell is believed to help in the **maturation of hypothalamo-gonadal axis**.

- But the exact role of leptin in the control of puberty is not known.

Abnormalities of Puberty

Abnormalities of puberty can be broadly classified into precocious puberty and delayed puberty.

Precocious Puberty

Precocious puberty may be of **two types**: true precocious puberty and precocious pseudopuberty.

True Precocious Puberty

Early development of **secondary sexual characteristics** may be associated *with premature development of gonads* is known as true precocious puberty. Precocious puberty can occur in both girls and boys. This occurs due to early pubertal pattern of secretion of gonadotropin from pituitary.

True precocious puberty occurs due to **following causes:**

1. **Hypothalamic precocity:** usually occurs due to tumor or infection of hypothalamus that causes premature increased secretion of GnRH.
2. **Gonadotropin independent precocity:** Precocious gametogenesis without increase in gonadotropin secretion. Usually, it occurs due to increased sensitivity of LH receptors to gonadotropins.
3. **Constitutional precocity:** when the actual cause of precocity can't be ascertained.
4. **Tumor** of pineal gland.

Precocious Pseudopuberty

The development of secondary sexual characteristics **without gametogenesis** is called as precocious pseudopuberty. This occurs due to exposure of immature males to abnormal quantity of androgen, and in immature females the abnormal exposure to estrogen.

Precocious pseudopuberty occurs due to following causes:

1. **Adrenal causes:** ***Congenital virilizing adrenal hyperplasia*** can lead to precocious pseudopuberty. ***Androgen secreting or estrogen secreting tumors*** of adrenal gland resulting in precocious pseudopuberty are not uncommon.
2. **Gonadal causes:** ***Leydig cell tumor*** of testis in male or ***granulosa cell tumor*** of ovary in females can cause precocious pseudopuberty.

Delayed Puberty

When onset of puberty is **delayed beyond the age of 17 in girls** and **20 in boys**, the condition is called delayed puberty.

- It occurs usually due to **panhypopituitarism** that causes failure of maturation of gonads.
- It is also associated with chromosomal abnormality of **XO pattern** or **gonadal dysgenesis**.
- Puberty may be delayed in spite of presence of normal gonads, which is called **eunuchoidism** in males and **primary amenorrhea** in girls.

PY9.11

PHYSIOLOGY OF MENOPAUSE

With advancement of age, gonadal functions gradually decrease. In females, **ovaries become unresponsive** to the gonadotropins. The functions of gonads slowly decrease finally resulting in complete cessation of menstrual cycle. This is called menopause or **climacteric**.

Mechanism & Features

Mechanism of Menopause

The mechanism and purpose of menopause are not clear. The **female gonads progressively become unresponsive to gonadotropins** with advancing age. The mechanism by which ovarian responsiveness decreases is not known. Ovaries stop secreting progesterone and estrogen in appreciable amount. The *negative feedback effect* of ovarian hormones causes **increased secretion of LH and FSH**. The uterus and vagina become atrophic.

Age at Menopause

In Women: The onset of menopause occurs between the age of 45–55 years. In recent years, the age at menopause has gradually increased.

In Males: Though there is some decline in reproductive capacity from 5th decade of life, **climacteric does not occur.**

- Testicular functions and potency persist till 8th decade.
- Thus, in males, there is no **andropause** (male menopause).
- However, decline in reproductive functions in males after the age of 60, is apparently referred to as **male menopause**.

Features of Menopause

Hot flushes (sensation of warmth spreading from trunk to the face) occur frequently. Night sweating, tachycardia, mental symptoms are also observed.

- The mechanism of hot flushes is not exactly known but it coincides with the **surges of LH secretion**.
    - With the onset of menopause, **LH secretion is increased**, which occurs in episodes of 30–60 minutes.
    - This is called **circhoral secretion of LH.**
    - Each hot flush **coincides with an episode of LH surge**, through experimental evidences indicate that hot flushes are not due to episodic secretion of LH per se.

- The decreased secretion of estrogen triggering some **hypothalamic mechanism** is proposed to cause both episodic secretion of LH and hot flushes.
- There is a tendency to become obese, develop hypertension and CV risks.

Management of Menopause

The fear that the women will lose her womanhood may cause **psychological depression**.

1. It needs proper **care, counseling and assurance** of the spouse to make her understand and adjust to this physiological phenomenon of the nature.
2. In some cases, hot flushes and psychological symptoms become more problematic. In such women, **hormonal supplementation** of estrogen is usually helpful.
   - However, metabolic and other complications of estrogen should be kept in mind while continuing estrogen therapy for a longer period.

Exam Questions

1. Describe the mechanism of regulation of hormone secretion.
2. What are the types of feedback control of hormone secretion? Describe the significance of each control system with examples.
3. Briefly describe the intercellular communications.
4. Briefly describe the type of hormomone signalling.

Multiple Choice Questions

1. Sex of the individual is determined by:
A. Genotype and phenotype both
B. Genotype only
C. Hormones
D. FSH and LH

2. Upto to what intrauterine life, primitive gonads are identical in both the sexes?
A. 2nd week B. 4th week
C. 6th week D. 8th week

3. Which of the following is not correct about Klinefelter syndrome?
A. Common sex chromosome disorder
B. Seminiferous tubule dysgenesis occurs
C. Tall patient with muscular body
D. XXY pattern with genetic female

4. Which of the following is not true about Turner syndrome?
A. Common feature is amenorrhea
B. Tall patients with webbed neck
C. Female type of sexual development
D. Associated with female phenotype

5. Which of the following statement about Barr body is correct?
A. Chromatin material seen as small drumstick appearance projecting from nuclei of leucocytes
B. Inactivated X chromosome forms
C. Seen in nuclei of somatic cells in females
D. Represents inactivation of Y chromosome forms

6. Number of males born is slightly more than females, due to all EXCEPT:
A. Y chromosome is smaller in size compared to X chromosome
B. Y chromosome is absent in females
C. Sperm with Y chromosomes swim faster in female genital tract
D. Sperm with Y chromosomes are lighter

7. What is true about development of genital duct from primordial genital tract?
A. External genitalia develop in both sexes by second month
B. Wolffian duct form uterus, fallopian tubes and upper part of vagina
C. Mullerian duct form epididymis, vas deferens and seminal vesicle
D. Upto 7th week of gestation, there is no sex difference in the genital duct

8. Congenital 17-α-hydroxylase deficiency causes:
A. Male pseudohermaphroditism
B. Female pseudohermaphroditism
C. Male hermaphroditism
D. Female hermaphroditism

9. Development of puberty was staged by:
A. Tanner B. Harris
C. Edward D. Graafian

10. The first to happen in puberty in male is:
A. Pubarche B. Adrenarche
C. Spermarche D. Receding hairline in head

11. The first to happen in puberty in female is:
A. Pubarche B. Thelarche
C. Menarche D. Axillary hair

12. Which of the following hormone is reported to promote maturation of hypothalamo-gonadal axis during pubery?
A. Insulin B. LH
C. Testosterone D. Leptin

13. Which of the following is not true about true precocious puberty?
A. Early development of secondary sexual characteristics
B. Associated with premature development of gonad
C. Early pubertal pattern of secretion of gonadotropin from anterior pituitary
D. Never happens in boys

14. All of the following are true about menopause in females, EXCEPT:
A. Gonads become progressively unresponsive to gonadotropins
B. Ovaries stop secreting estrogen and progesterone
C. Hot flushes have no link with LH level
D. LH secretion is increased

Answers

1. B	2. C	3. C	4. B	5. A	6. B	7. D	8. A	9. A	10. B
11. B	12. D	13. D	14. C						

Chapter 80

Male Reproductive System

PY9.3

Learning Objectives

On completion of study of this chapter:

The student will be able to (must know):

1. Name the different parts of male reproductive system and give the functions of each.
2. List the functions of Sertoli cells and Leydig cells.
3. Understand the importance of blood-testis barrier in testicular functions.
4. Illustrate the steps and regulation of spermatogenesis.
5. Appreciate the importance of semen analysis.
6. List the functions of testosterone and describe regulation of testicular functions.
7. List the secondary sex characteristics in males.

The student may also be able to (desirable to know):

1. Describe the cellular organization, functions and regulation of functions of Sertoli cells and Leydig cells.
2. Describe the physiological basis of testicular abnormalities.

FUNCTIONAL ANATOMY

The male reproductive system consists of testes, epididymis, vas deferens, ejaculatory ducts, prostate, urethra, and penis (Fig. 80.1).

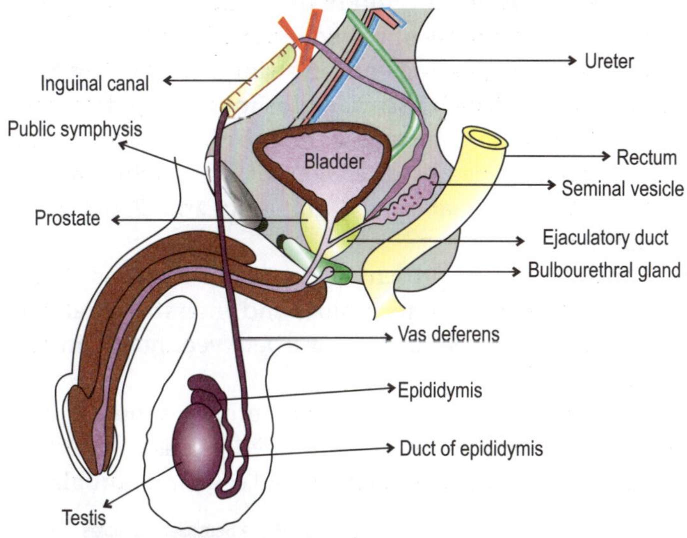

Fig. 80.1: Parts of male reproductive system

Testes

During intrauterine life, testes **descend** from abdominal cavity **to the inguinal canal** during mid-pregnancy and descend into the scrotum two months before term (Application Box 80.1).

- Weight of each testis is about 10–15 grams, length 5 cm and width 2.5 cm in adults.
- Testes receive blood supply from the spermatic arteries that originate directly from the aorta.
- **Scrotal temperature is less** than the core body temperature that facilitates spermatogenesis.

The **scrotal is cooler for following reasons**:

1. **Anatomical location:** Scrotum forms sacs that are like **outpouching from the body**, which has **less transmission of the inner body temperature** into it.
2. **Pampiniform plexus of the blood vessels:** These plexuses of blood vessels **serve as counter-current exchanger** between warm arterial blood entering the testes and cooler venous blood leaving the testes.
3. **Role of cremasteric & dartus muscles:** Cremaster muscle is a small band of skeletal muscle present in the spermatic cord that contracts or relaxes in response to change in environmental temperature.

- It **contracts on exposure to sever cold** and elevates the testis and **relaxes in warm environment** and lowers the testis.
- Also, a flap of smooth muscle is present in the fascial layer of scrotum, called **dartus muscle**, which contracts on exposure to cold.

- This increases **wrinkling of scrotal skin** and facilitates lifting of the testis.
- Thus, cremasteric and dartus muscles on exposure to cold push testes close to the pelvic cavity where they can absorb body heat, and pull them away from the body in hot environment.

Application Box 80.1

Separate domicile for male gonad: Testes are the male gonads that are placed in separate sacs almost hanging away from the body. In female, the gonads (ovaries) are well preserved in the abdominal cavity. Then, why has the nature provided separate external compartments for male gonads? Scrotum is the sac, which keeps testes at about 2 – 3°C below the core body temperature and this cooler environment is highly essential for spermatogenesis.

Functional Histology of Testis

Testes are covered by thick connective tissue membrane called **tunica albuginea**. Each testis is made up of **seminiferous tubules**. Hundreds of tubules are tightly packed to from a **mass of coiled loops** (Fig. 80.2).

- Each loop begins and ends in a single duct called **tubulus rectus**, which in turn drains into the epididymis.
  - Tubules are **arranged in lobules** separated by septa formed by extensions of tunica albuginea.
- Each tubule is about 50 cm long and 250 µm in diameter.
- **Myoid cells** are present surrounding the basal lamina of the seminiferous tubules and **interstitial cells of Leydig** are present in the space between the seminiferous tubules.

Thus, testis consists of seminiferous tubules and interstitium that mainly contains Leydig cells, connective tissues and capillaries, and few myoid cells and fibroblasts.

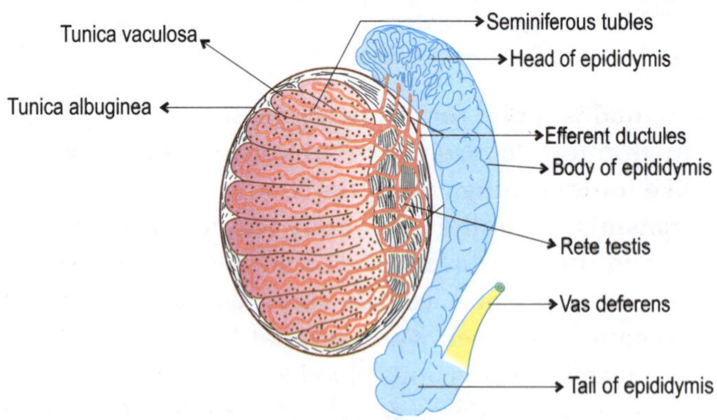

Fig. 80.2: Arrangement of seminiferous tubule in in the lobules of testis. Also note the position and parts of epididymis.

Seminiferous Tubule

Each seminiferous tubule has a basement membrane that separates it from the surrounding **Leydig cells**, the **peritubular cells (myoid cells)** and the connective tissue.

- Spermatogonia and **Sertoli cells** are located in the wall of the tubule just beneath the basement membrane (Fig. 80.3).

There are **two principal cell types** in seminiferous tubules: somatic cells (**Sertoli cells**) and **germ cells**.

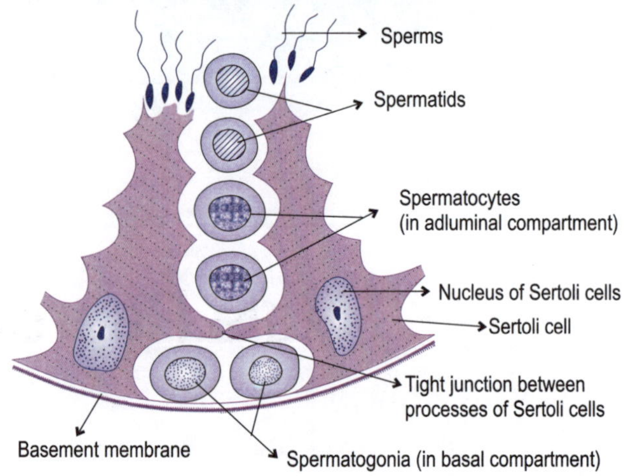

Fig. 80.3: Arrangement of Sertoli cells and germ cells in seminiferous tubule. Also note the germ cells undergoing spermatogenesis (spermatogonia, spermatocytes, spermatids, and sperms).

Sertoli Cells

Sertoli cells are the sustentacular cells in seminiferous tubules, which form the major cell mass in them.

Structure of Sertoli cells

They are irregularly shaped cells that are extended from the basement membrane into the lumen of seminiferous tubule. Sperms are attached to the apical membrane of the Sertoli cells (Fig. 80.3).

- At their bases, Sertoli cells are attached to each other by tight junctions.
- Tight junctions divide tubules into **two compartments:** basal compartment and adluminal compartment (Fig. 80.4).

Basal Compartment: The basal compartment is the *outer compartment* that mainly consists of **spermatogonium**.

- It is **exposed to circulating substances** as the capillaries are in close contact with it and substances from blood can easily be exchanged.

Adluminal Compartment: Adluminal compartment is the *inner compartment* that consists of **primary and secondary spermatocytes and spermatids**.

- It is *separated from blood-borne agents* by the tight junctions between the Sertoli cells close to basal lamina.

Blood-Testis Barrier

Because the tight junctions between Sertoli cells are too tight, they do not allow substances from interstitial space and blood to pass through them except steroids and few proteins. Thus, ***tight junction between Sertoli cells near the basal lamina*** forms the **blood-testis barrier** (BTB) (Fig. 80.4). It is a misnomer, as strictly it is not a blood-organ(testis) barrier; it is actually Sertoli cell-barrier.

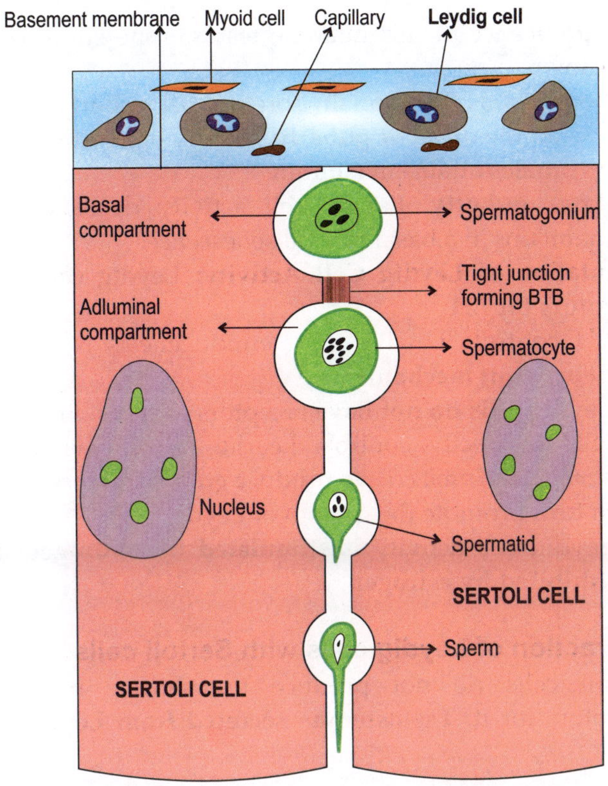

Fig. 80.4: Relationship (arrangement) of Sertoli cells with Leydig cells and germ cells. Note, tight junction between Sertoli cells that forms the blood-testis barrier (BTB) separates basal compartment containing spermatogonium from adluminal compartment containing spermatocytes, spermatid and sperm.

- Though large molecules are not transported through BTB, **maturing germ cells pass through it** to enter into adluminal compartment.
- When spermatocytes attempt to penetrate the barrier, the tight junction in front of them dislocate and allow them and after they pass through, the tight junctions immediately form re-form behind them.
- Thus, physiologically, maturing germ cells pass through BTB without actually disrupting it.

Functions of BTB:

1. BTB **protects germ cells** in the seminiferous tubules from harmful elements in blood.
2. BTB **prevents these antigenic products to escape into circulation** from tubule and thus prevents autoimmune reactions.
3. BTB maintains the composition of the fluid in the lumen **of seminiferous tubules, which is rich in androgens, estrogens, K^+, inositol, glutamic and aspartic acids.**
4. BTB maintains higher osmolality of luminal content of the seminiferous tubules, which favours the osmotic movement of fluid into the tubular lumen.

Functions of Sertoli Cells

Sertoli cells have multiple functions. Important among them are:

1. **Germ cell development:** Sertoli cells are critical to germ cell development.
    - They provide structural support and nutrition to germ cells.
    - Sertoli cells are rich in glycoproteins that nourish the germ cells.
2. **Phagocytosis:** Sertoli cells phagocytose residual bodies and damaged germ cells from the seminiferous tubules.
    - **Residual bodies** are cytoplasmic fragments formed by excess cytoplasm resulting from transformation of spermatids to spermatozoa.
3. **Nourishment and growth of spermatids:** They nourish the developing spermatids.
    - About 10 to 12 spermatids are attached to each Sertoli cells.
    - Sertoli cells synthesize **transferrin**, an iron-transport protein that helps in development of sperms.
4. **Formation of tubular fluid:** They secrete fluid into the lumen of seminiferous tubule. This fluid later forms the major components of seminal fluid.
5. **Support spermiation:** This is the process of detachment of mature sperms from Sertoli cells into the lumen.
    - In this process, **plasmin**, the proteolytic enzyme assists in release of sperms from Sertoli cells.
    - Sertoli cells produce plasminogen activator that causes formation of plasmin.
6. **FSH and testosterone sensitivity:** Sertoli cells have receptors for FSH and testosterone.
    - FSH receptors are present on the cell membrane and testosterone receptors are present within the nucleus.
    - During puberty, receptors for these hormones on Sertoli cell increase.
    - FSH **increases cAMP** in Sertoli cells and induces **production of androgen-binding protein** (see below) and plasminogen activator in Sertoli cells. These chemicals help in **sperm development**.
7. **Endocrine functions of Sertoli cells:** Sertoli cells secrete many hormones. These are;
    i) Inhibin: Inhibin suppresses FSH release from pituitary.
    ii) Activin: Activin stimulates release of FSH.
    iii) Follistatin: It decreases FSH secretion stimulated by activin.
    iv) Müllerian regression substance: During 8th week of gestation MIS is secreted from fetal Sertoli cells. MIS causes regression of müllerian duct in fetuses destined to become males.
    v) Estrogens: Sertoli cells contain the enzyme aromatase that converts androgen into estrogen.
8. **Secretory functions:** Sertoli cells secrete *androgen binding proteins* (ABP) and ***H-Y antigen***.
    - ABP maintains ***concentration of androgen*** in Sertoli cells, which is essential for maturation of spermatozoa.

- H-Y antigen is secreted by Sertoli cells during fetal life that controls development of testis.

Androgen Binding Proteins (ABP): Sertoli cells secrete and synthesize ABP, a protein having molecular weight 90,000 into the luminal fluid.

i) ABP has *high affinity for binding dihydrotestosterone* and *testosterone*.

ii It is present in high concentration in luminal fluid. A high concentration of androgen in luminal fluid is **essential for production and maturation of spermatozoa**.

iii) ABP maintains this concentration of androgen in luminal fluid.

iv) It helps in *storage of androgen* in seminiferous tubule and facilitates transport of testosterone from testis to epididymis.

9. **Blood-testis barrier:** Sertoli cells provide the blood-testis barrier (BTB) for the seminiferous tubules. Thus, they **protect developing sperms** from harmful effects of blood-borne toxins. Other functions of BTB are discussed above.

Germ Cells

Germ cells are **germinal epithelial cells** of seminiferous tubules. Each germ cell is a spermatogonium that forms spermatocytes and spermatozoa in the process of its development, i.e., spermatogenesis (see below).

Leydig Cells

Leydig cells are **primary cells of steroidogenesis**. They produce testosterone.

Location and Structure

Leydig cells are present near the capillaries **in the interstitial space between seminiferous tubules**. They are rich in mitochondria and endoplasmic reticulum. The activity of Leydig cells is different in different phases of life.

Functions

Leydig cells mainly **secrete testosterone**. However, dehydroepiandrosterone and androstenedione are also secreted to some extent.

Leydig Cells Activity in Different Phases of Life:

1. During **8-15 weeks of intrauterine life**, Leydig cells are active and prominent as ***steroidogenesis*** is essential for differentiation of male genital ducts.
   - During this period, as hypothalamo-pituitary gonadal axis is not fully formed, steroidogenesis is controlled by hCG, not by LH.
   - Thereafter, Leydig cell activity decreases.
2. **In male infants**, during **3-5 months of postnatal life**, Leydig cell activity *increases significantly* that results in increased testosterone secretion. The physiological significance of this infantile testosterone surge is not known.
3. Leydig cells then remain **dormant till puberty**.
   - At the **onset of puberty**, activity of Leydig cells in males attains maximum.
4. **After puberty**, Leydig cell activity decreases, but maintains at a basal rate till senescence.

Regulation of Leydig Cell Activity: Leydig cells have **receptors for LH**.

- LH controls Leydig cell steroidogenesis by **cAMP-dependent mechanism**.
- Leydig cells **do not have** receptors for FSH. However, FSH indirectly controls Leydig cells activity. FSH *stimulates Sertoli cells* to produce ***growth factors***, which in turn promote the growth of Leydig cells.
- Leydig cell activity is **stimulated by androgen and inhibited by estrogen**.

Interaction of Leydig cells with Sertoli cells

Sertoli cells do not produce testosterone but have receptors for it. **Testosterone secreted from Leydig cell**

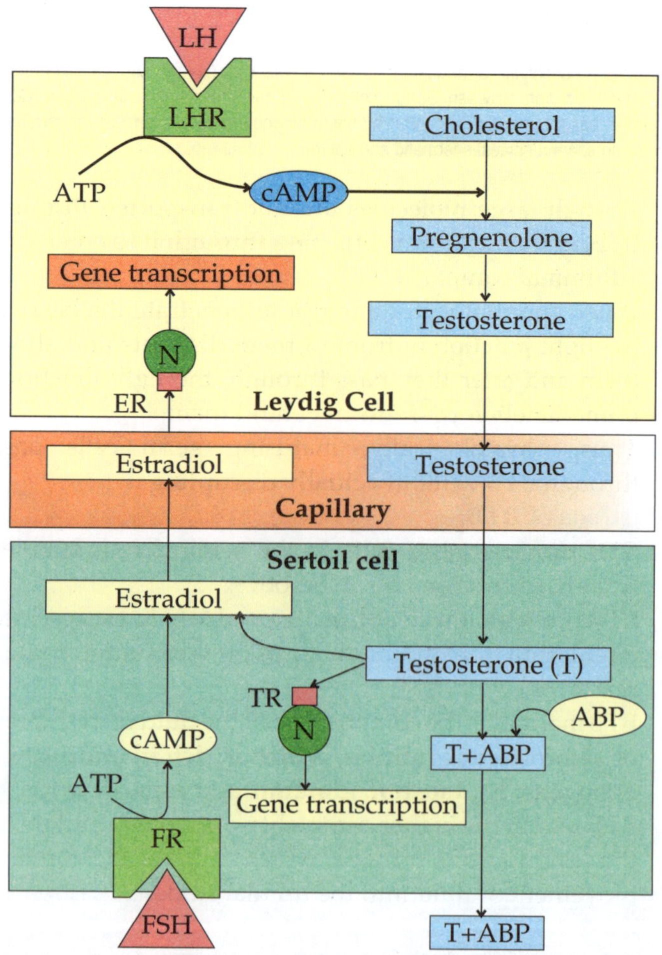

Fig. 80.5: Interaction between Leydig and Sertoli cells. Note that testosterone secreted from Leydig cells enters Sertoli cell and influences Sertoli cell functions. Similarly, estradiol produced in Sertoli cells enters Leydig cell and control Leydig cell functions. ABP: androgen binding protein; ER: estrogen receptor; FR: FSH receptor; FSH: follicle stimulating hormone; LH: luteinizing hormone; LHR: LH receptors; N: nucleus; TR: testosterone receptor.

enters **Sertoli** cells where it binds with the ABP. This **testosterone** is essential for three important functions:

1. Spermatogenesis
2. Functioning of Sertoli cells
3. **Estrogen production** in Sertoli cells.

Estrogen produced in Sertoli cells ***diffuses back into the Leydig*** cells and **regulates Leydig cell function** (Fig. 80.5).

Functions of Testis

Testis serves **three important functions**.

1. **Spermatogenesis**, i.e., production of sperms (see below)
2. **Steroidogenesis**, i.e., synthesis of steroid hormones, mainly testosterone, which is later, converted to dihydrotestosterone and estradiol (see below).
3. Testis **secretes other hormones** like ***activin, inhibin and follistatin*** that influence many other reproductive functions.

Epididymis

Seminiferous tubules open into a network of tubules, called **rete testis**. Rete testis opens into epididymis via *efferent ductules.*

Structure

Epididymis is located on the posterior aspect of the testis. It contains a **highly convoluted long duct**, which is about 5 meter in length. Epididymis is divided into **three parts**: head (the part close to testis), body and tail (Fig. 80.2).

Function

The function of epididymis is the **storage and maturation of spermatozoa** (Application Box 80.2).

1. About 99% of testicular fluid is reabsorbed in the epididymis and rete testis. Spermatozoa from tubular fluid and rete testis are transferred to epididymis almost passively as they are essentially immotile.
2. In epididymis, they **acquire the capacity for progressive forward movement** and the ability to attach to zona pellucida of ovum and penetrate into it.
3. Thus, the sperms obtained directly from testis are functionally immature, whereas **sperms obtained from body of the epididymis or further down in the male genital tract are fertile.**

Application Box 80.2

Fate of stored spermatozoa: Spermatozoa are carried from epididymis via vas deferens and ejaculatory duct into the urethra in penis to be removed out of it at the time of ejaculation. The sperms that are not voided are ultimately phagocytosed by macrophages in the epididymis or voided slowly in urine.

Fate of stored spermatozoa: Spermatozoa are carried from epididymis via vas deferens and ejaculatory duct into the urethra in penis to be removed out of it at the time of ejaculation. The sperms that are not voided are ultimately phagocytosed by macrophages in the epididymis or voided slowly in urine.

Vas Deferens

Epididymis empties its content into the vas deferens, which *transfers sperms* further down in the duct.

- Proximal part of vas deferens like epididymis **stores the sperms.**
- Vas deferens joins with the duct arising from seminal vesicle to from the **ejaculatory duct**.
- The movement of sperm in vas deferens is active as they are capable of motility. Also, **contraction of muscle** in the wall of vas deferens facilitates the process of ***sperm movement***.

Seminal Vesicle

There are two seminal vesicles located close to the prostate. They secrete a viscid and alkaline fluid called **seminal vesicular fluid.**

- Seminal vesicular fluid contributes to **70% of the total volume** of the semen.
- Rest 20% of the volume is contributed by epididymal fluid and fluid secreted from accessory sex glands, and 10% is contributed by sperms.
- The seminal vesicles **secrete vitamin C and fructose**.
- The fluid appears light yellowish as it contains **flavins**.
- Most of the **prostaglandins** found in semen are contributed by seminal vesicle.

Accessory Sex Glands

Accessory male sex glands are **prostate gland and bulbourethral glands** of Cowper.

Prostate Gland

The ejaculatory duct enters the prostatic portion of the urethra after passing through the prostate.

1. Prostate gland consists of 30-50 **branched tubulo-alveolar glands** whose secretions empty into prostatic urethra.
2. The prostatic fluid contains **fibrinolysin, fibrinogenase** and large quantity of **acid phosphatase**.
    - Fibrinolysin ***prevents sperm heads to clump***.
3. Prostate gland also releases **a factor**, which contains sugar, sulfate and vitamin E derivative that also ***prevents sperm head to cluster***.

Bulbourethral Glands

They secrete mucus and alkaline fluid. They also secrete the enzyme **hyaluronidase** that *facilitates penetrability of* *oocytes by sperms.*

SPERMATOGENESIS

The process of **development of male germ cells into spermatozoa** is known as spermatogenesis.

Course of Spermatogenesis in Life: Spermatogenesis begins at puberty. The germ cells remain inactive throughout childhood.

1. **At puberty**, under the influence of increasing level of gonadotropins and testosterone, the germ cells are activated, and spermatogenesis is initiated.
2. From puberty onwards, spermatogenesis **continues throughout life**, though the process declines at old age.

Steps of Spermatogenesis

The process of spermatogenesis can be divided into **three distinct phases**: Mitosis, meiosis and spermiogenesis (Fig. 80.6). **Spermatogonium** undergoes ***mitosis*** to produce **primary spermatocytes** that undergo two ***meiotic divisions*** to form **spermatids** (refer Fig. 80.3, depicted above). Spermatids, by the process of **spermiogenesis** become mature spermatozoa.

Mitosis

The primitive germ cells (spermatogonia) that are present in the basal lamina of seminiferous tubules undergo mitotic divisions to from **primary spermatocytes** (Fig. 80.6). This is called **spermatocytogenesis**. In fact, the spermatogonia undergo many mitotic divisions to produce two types of **spermatogonia:** spermatogonia A and spermatogonia B.

Spermatogonia A: Spermatogonia A formed by mitotic divisions resemble the original spermatogonia and are the source of subsequent spermatogonia in the testis. Thus, they form the **spermatogonia reserve pool** in the testis.

Spermatogonia B: Spermatogonia B grow and enter adluminal compartment where they develop into primary spermatocytes.

Meiosis

- The primary spermatocytes (diploid 4N DNA) undergo **two meiotic divisions**.
- The first meiotic division forms **secondary spermatocytes** (haploid 2N DNA)) and the second meiotic division forms **spermatids** (haploid 1N DNA).
- Spermatids contain half of the number of chromosomes (23 chromosomes, i.e., 22 autosomes and 1 sex chromosome, which is either an X or a Y chromosome).
- Of every four spermatids formed from primary spermatocytes, two of them contain X chromosome and two Y chromosomes.

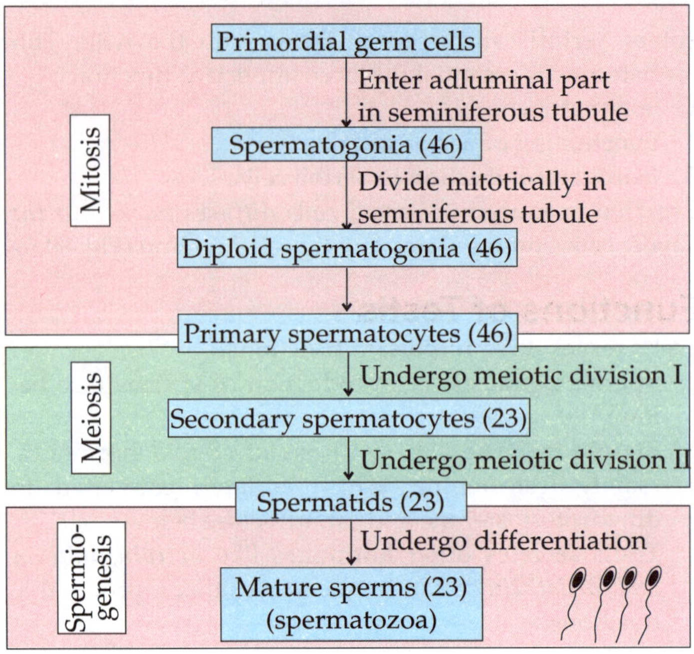

Fig. 80.6: Steps of spermatogenesis. Note that, till the stage of primary spermatocyte, each cell contains 46 chromosomes and from secondary spermatocyte to spermatozoa, each cell contains 23 chromosomes (number indicated against each category of cells as 46 chromosomes and 23 chromosomes in brackets).

- Normally after undergoing several mitotic and two meiotic divisions in the process of spermatogenesis, *each spermatogonium yields 512 spermatids.*

Spermiogenesis

The process of **development of spermatids into matured spermatozoa** is called spermiogenesis. Spermatids are small, round and less characteristic cells. They undergo many **structural changes** to form spermatozoa. The major changes are:

1. **Massive reduction in cytoplasm.** Cytoplasmic fragments are discarded as residual bodies.
2. **Elongation of the nucleus** to become head of spermatozoa.
3. Acquirement of an upper covering for the head called **acrosomal cap**.
4. Formation of a **middle piece and a tail piece** with the ability to move efficiently and swiftly.

- All these changes occur in mature sperms to enable them to survive in a foreign and even hostile environment (**acidic vaginal pH**) in the female genital tract and to recognize and fertilize the ovum.
- These changes mainly help the sperm to move forward towards the ovum in the female genital tract, the movement known as **progressive motility** of the sperm.

Spermiation

Spermatozoa, after they are formed, remain in the lumen of the seminiferous tubule sticking to the apical membrane of the Sertoli cells.

- They **adhere tightly to the Sertoli cells**.
- The process of **detachment of head of spermatozoa and their free release** into the luminal fluid is called spermiation.

Capacitation

When spermatozoa are ejaculated into the female genital tract, they undergo further maturation called capacitation.

- This includes **increase in further motility of sperms** and **preparation for acrosomal reaction**.
- However, capacitation is not so much essential for fertilization as fertilization can also occur in vitro.

Structure of Spermatozoa

A matured sperm is a motile cell rich in DNA, consisting of head, middle peace and tail (Fig. 80.7). A human sperm is about 65 µm long with average diameter of 2 µm.

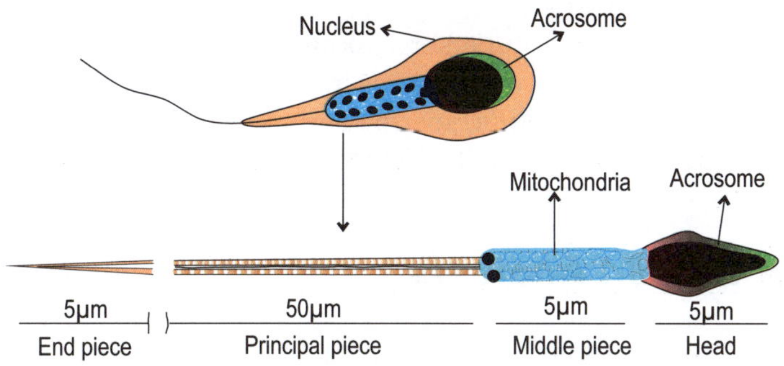

Fig. 80.7: Structure of immature (A) and mature spermatozoa (B).

Head: Head contains a prominent nucleus at the center, which is condensed with chromatin. The head is covered by a cap called acrosome, which is formed as a big vesicle from Golgi apparatus.

- Acrosome is a special primary lysosome **rich in proteolytic enzymes** such as hyaluronidase, acrosin, neuraminidase and esterases that are activated during **acrosomal reaction** and help in sperm penetration of the ovum at the time of fertilization.
- The ***nucleus decondenses*** and becomes **a pronucleus** at the time of fertilization.

Middle Piece: The middle piece of sperm contains numerous mitochondria in the form of a spiral sheath surrounding a long **axial filament made up of microtubules** (9+2 arrangement; i. e., nine peripheral doublet microtubules surrounding a central pair).

- The long axial filament **becomes axoneme in the tail**.
- The mitochondria **provide energy** for sperm metabolism and motility.

Tail Piece: The tail piece is divided into **a principal piece and an end piece**.

- They contain a central **axoneme** consisting of microtubules. The axial filament arrangement in microtubules (9+2 arrangement; i. e., nine peripheral doublet surrounding a central pair) is typical that of cilia and flagella. Therefore, the **tail portion is highly motile**.
- The tail of the sperm exhibits **a twisting movement** by which it propels the body of the sperm in forward direction. The twisting movement occurs due to the interaction between tubulin fibers and dyenin side arms, which requires ATP.
- The axoneme is surrounded by a **fibrous sheath** that provides strength to the tail. The membrane of the sheath contains **germinal angiotensin converting enzyme**. The exact function of this enzyme is not known but reduction of this enzyme concentration is suggested to be associated with decreased fertility.

Role of CatSper protein: The principal piece of tail contains a protein called **CatSper protein**, which is a calcium channel. This allows cAMP mediated ***calcium influx*** and **facilitates sperm motility**.

Duration of Spermatogenesis

In human beings, the process of formation of sperm from the spermatogonium takes **65–74 days**. Sometimes, the stages of development of sperms are collectively called as **spermatogenic cycle.** Each stage has a relatively constant duration:

1. Spermatogonia to primary spermatocytes is 16–20 days.
2. Primary spermatocytes to secondary spermatocytes is 23–25 days.
3. Secondary spermatocytes to spermatids is approximately 1 day.
4. Spermatids to spermatozoa is about 25 days.

Hormones like gonadotropins or androgen influence the number of spermatozoa produced, but not the duration of the cycle.

- Thus, the **duration of spermatogenesis remains virtually constant.**
- Normally, new cycles are initiated in every 2 to 4 weeks before the completion of old cycle.
  - Therefore, in the tubules, **cells of different stages** are seen at any particular time.
  - This ensures uninterrupted supply of spermatozoa throughout life.

Rate of Production of Sperms

A single spermatogonium **forms 512 spermatids**, if all of them remain alive.

- Approximately, **200 million of sperms are produced daily** in an adult testis in humans. This is roughly same as the number of sperms in an ejaculate in a normal healthy adult. Expressed per unit weight of testicular tissue, about **6–7 million sperms are produced per gram per day**.

- The rate of production of sperms **falls progressively in old age**. After the age of 50, the rate of sperm production is 3.5–4 million per gram of tissue.
- The decrease in production in elderly is due to **degeneration of germ cells** during meiotic prophase. However, appreciable spermatogenesis continues even at the age of 90.

Differences between Spermatogenesis & Oogenesis

There are few basic differences in the process of gametogenesis in females and males. These are:

1. **In females,** mitotic proliferation of germ cells completes ***before birth***, whereas **in males**, spermatogonia grow only at the time of puberty and then continue to proliferate throughout life,
2. **In female**, the meiotic division of primary oocyte produces ***only one ovum***, whereas **in males** one primary spermatocyte produces ***four spermatozoa.***
3. **In female**, second meiotic division is completed ***only upon fertilization***, whereas **in males** second meiotic division is completed during spermatogenesis.

Regulation of Spermatogenesis

Factors controlling spermatogenesis can be broadly divided into ***two categories***: hormonal and environmental.

Hormonal Factors

Androgen, estrogen and gonadotropins mainly control spermatogenesis.

1. **Androgen:** Androgens **stimulate spermatogenesis.** LH creates an elevated local concentration of androgen in the testis by stimulating Leydig cells to secrete testosterone, and this **high intertesticular testosterone is essential for spermatogenesis**.
   - Testosterone secreted from Leydig cells diffuse into the seminiferous tubule. In tubule, only the Sertoli cells (not spermatogenic cells), have receptors for testosterone.
   - **Testosterone binds with ABP in the Sertoli cells** (as given above in Fig. 80.5), which maintains a high concentration of testosterone in the cell. However, it is not clearly known how testosterone promotes spermatogenesis.
   - It appears that, till the formation of spermatid does not depend on androgen, rather **spermiogenesis** (spermatids developing to spermatozoa) **is androgen dependent**.
2. **Estrogen:** Estrogen content of the fluid in the rete testis is high and there are **estrogen receptors in the rete testis**.
   - Rete testis reabsorbs fluid and makes the spermatozoa concentrated, which is required for sperm maturation. The diluted volume of large fluid that enters rete testis and epididymis unless absorbed adequately results in infertility.
   - **Estrogen concentrates the fluid** by facilitating fluid reabsorption.
3. **LH and FSH:** LH helps in spermatogenesis by **producing a high local concentration of androgen**.
   - FSH maintains ***gametogenic functions*** of testis.
   - It appears that FSH is required for initiation of spermatogenesis at the time of puberty, and then LH maintains it.

Environmental Factors

It is mainly the **temperature** that influences spermatogenesis.

- Lower environmental temperature facilitates spermatogenesis. Spermatogenesis **best occurs at 30 to 35°C**. However, very low temperature inhibits it.
- Conversely, **increased temperature inhibits spermatogenesis**.
  - Therefore, in persons taking repeated hot bath or those who regularly use insulated athletic support for the scrotum, sperm count is invariably less.

Generally, sperm count is **more in comfortable winter** and less in intense summer.

Semen Analysis — PY9.9

Semen analysis is one of the important tests **for assessment of male fertility**. It is performed to know if the sterility is related to sperm production. It is also performed after vasectomy, to check its completeness. It reflects the activity of the testes and accessory sex organs in males.

Analysis of freshly collected sample of semen gives the knowledge about the male fertility which is detected by examining the sample under microscope. Usually, the sample is collected after a period of sexual abstinence for 2 days.

Composition of Normal Semen

Volume	: 2 to 5 ml
Colour	: White, opalescent
Specific gravity	: 1.028
Motility	: > 60% should be actively motile within 3 h of collection
Count	: > 40 millions / ml is considered normal (usually, 100millions/ml is seen normally)
Liquefaction	: Should liquefy within half-an-hour
Morphology	: > 80% should have normal morphology
pH	: 7.3 to 7.5
Fructose content	: Fructose concentration is 2–7 mg/ml

Other biochemical constituents:

1. Prostaglandins

2. Ascorbic acid
3. Flavins
4. Phosphorylcholine
5. Ergotheoneine
6. Fibrinolysin, fibrinogenase
7. Acid phosphatase
8. Zinc
9. Phospholipids
10. Cholesterol
11. Spermin
12. Citric acid
13. Phosphate
14. Bicarbonate
15. Hyaluronidase

Fructose and other biochemical compositions as noted above from serial **No. 1 to 5 are synthesized and secreted from seminal vesicles**. The secretion from seminal vesicle constitutes 60% of the semen volume. Other biochemical compositions from serial **No. 6 to 11 are released from prostate.** Secretion from prostate contributes to 20% of the total semen volume.

- Bicarbonate and phosphates are buffers in the seminal fluid.
- Normally, sperm motility is facilitated by **prostate specific antigen** (PSA) (Clinical Note 80.1).

Clinical Note 80.1

PSA is a marker of prostate cancer: Prostate specific antigen (PSA) is 30 kDa serine protease formed and secreted from the prostate into the seminal fluid. **Semenogelin**, the sperm motility inhibitor is hydrolyzed by PSA. Thus, PSA facilitates sperm motility. The PSA gene has two androgen response elements.

- Though PSA is elevated in BHP (benign hyperplasia of prostate) and prostatitis, it is markedly increased in malignancy of prostate.
- Hence, elevated plasma PSA is used as a screening test for detection of prostate cancer.

Abnormalities

Volume: A low volume might suggest an anatomical or functional defect or an inflammatory condition of the genital tract. Volume decreases with advancing age.

Motility: In a normal sample, at least 60% of the sperms should exhibit forward motility within the first 3 hours of collection of the specimen.

- Motility **less than 40% is associated with sterility**.
- The speed of normal human sperm in female genital tract is **3mm/min**.
- Within one hour of ejaculation in the vagina, the sperms reach fallopian tube where they fertilize the ovum.

Count: Sperm count below 20 millions/ml results in sterility.

- A count between 20 to 40 millions/ml indicates borderline infertility.

Liquefaction: Delayed liquefaction of more than 2 hours suggests inflammation of accessory glands or enzyme defects in the secretory products of the glands.

Morphology: Normally 70% of the sperms should have normal morphology.

- Abnormalities more than 30% indicate serious pathology.
- The abnormalities include abnormal shapes, and poorly formed head or tail. The abnormal sperms may have bifurcated tail, bifid head, spirally coiled tail, or absence of head (Fig. 80.8).

pH: pH below 7.0 indicates semen content is mainly prostatic fluid, which may be due to congenital absence of seminal vesicle.

Fructose Content: The normal fructose content of semen is 2–7 mg/ml. Its absence indicates obstruction or absence of the ejaculatory ducts or seminal vesicle.

Effects of Vasectomy

Vasectomy is the bilateral ligation of vas deferens. This is the permanent contraceptive procedure for males. This is a safe and convenient contraceptive procedure.

1. About 50% of vasectomized males **develop antibodies against sperms**. However, the incidence is more following restoration of patency of the vas deferens in males those who wish to restore their fertility.
2. As such, restoration of patency of the vas (**recanalization**) is a difficult procedure. The antisperm antibodies further reduce the fertility.

PY9.5

TESTICULAR HORMONES

Testosterone

Testosterone is synthesized by the **Leydig cells of testis**. Testosterone (androgen) is also secreted from **adrenal cortex, ovaries and placenta**. Thus, a small amount of testosterone is secreted in females.

Synthesis and Secretion

It is a C_{19} **steroid hormone** with an OH group at 17 position.

- It is **synthesized from cholesterol** in Leydig cells of the testis.
  - It is also formed from **androstenedione** secreted from **adrenal cortex**.
  - Though, the biosynthetic pathways in the endocrine tissue that form steroid hormones are similar, minor **differences exist among the enzymes** that are involved in the process.
  - For example, the **17α-hydroxylase is found in testis**, whereas 11– and 21–β hydroxylases are found in adrenal cortex.
- Therefore, in testis, pregnenolone is hydroxylated at 17 position.

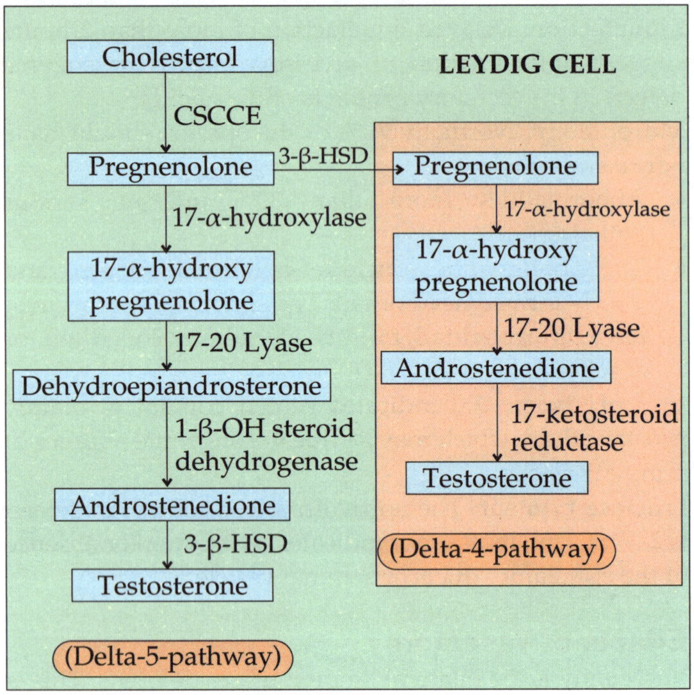

Fig. 80.8: Steps of testosterone synthesis. CSCCE: cholesterol side chain cleavage enzyme HSD: hydroxy steroid dehydrogenase.

- Pregnenolone is converted to testosterone in two pathways: **delta 5** and **delta 4 pathways.**
  - Major steps of **these pathways are** summarized in Fig. 80.8.
- Pregnenolone also forms progesterone, which forms 17α-hydroxyprogesterone, which in turn forms androstenedione and testosterone by **delta-4-pathway**.

Normal Level: The normal secretion rate of testosterone from testes is 4–10 mg per day. The normal plasma concentration of testosterone is **300–1000 ng/dL in adult males** and ***30–70 ng/dL in females***.

Metabolism

About 98% of testosterone binds with plasma proteins and only 2% is free in plasma.

1. The free testosterone enters the target tissues in which it is converted to its active form **dihydrotestosterone** (DHT) by 5α-reductase and **estradiol** (17β-estradiol) by *aromatase*.
   - Thus, testosterone acts as prohormone and **DHT is the biologically active** hormone (Clinical Note 80.2).

Clinical Note 80.2

Penis-at-14 syndrome: Normally, DHT which is formed from testosterone is essential for the development of male genitalia during early embryonic life. In the absence of DHT, female genitalia predominate in genetic male (**male pseudohermaphroditism**) at birth.

- Undescended testis is a common feature in this condition, and they are born as female children.
- At the time of puberty, testosterone secretion increases, and they develop male figure with enlargement of clitoris to become a penis like structure.
- At this point in their life, they become boys and change their name and sex.
- They may even develop full male libido and do intercourse with women.
- As it occurs around the age of 14, syndrome is called penis-at-14-syndrome. It is common in Dominican Republic.

2. DHT has 2–3 times more affinity than testosterone for **binding with androgen receptors.**
3. DHT causes **hypertrophy of prostate** (Clinical Note 80.3)

Clinical Note 80.3

Treatment for prostate hypertrophy: DHT induces hypertrophy of prostate. Therefore, drugs that inhibit 5α-reductase are currently used in the treatment of benign hypertrophy of prostate (BHP). If it is androgen dependent BHP or malignant neoplasia, GnRH antagonists are used that inhibit LH secretion which in turn inhibits estrogen secretion from Leydig cells.

17-Ketosteroids

About 65% binding of testosterone in plasma occurs with **gonadal steroid binding globulin** (GBG) and 33% with *sex steroid binding globulin* (SBG).

- Most of the circulating testosterone is converted into **17–ketosteroids** by the enzyme 17β-dehydrogenase and a small amount into **estrogen**.
- 17–ketosteroids possess about **20% of androgen activity**.
  - The **principal ketosteroids** are androsterone and etiocholanolone.
- Ketosteroids are **excreted in urine**.
  - However, ***two-thirds*** of urinary ketosteroid is of **adrenal origin** and ***one-third of testicular origin***.

Testicular Estrogen

Circulating estrogens are **estradiol and estrone**. Estradiol is the major estrogen.

- **In men**, the plasma estradiol level is 20 – 50 pg/ml. The **production of estrogen increases** with advancement of age **in males**, whereas estrogen production decreases with age in female.
- In males, only **15% of circulating estradiol** and 5% of circulating estrone comes from testes (Clinical Note 80.4).
- Rest is produced by ***aromatization of estrogen*** from testosterone outside the testes and secreted from adrenal cortex.

Clinical Note 80.4

Gynecomastia in males: In adipose tissues, skin, liver and brain, testosterone is aromatized to estrogen, which is then released into circulation. Therefore, in men, circulating level of estrogen (estradiol and estrone) is almost close to the level of estrogen in follicular phase in females.

- But men are protected from feminization due to high level of androgens and high responsiveness of tissues to androgens.
- Therefore, use of anabolic steroids or testosterone analogues (as athletes use), decreased testosterone secretion, estrogen producing testicular tumors, and tissue insensitivity to androgens result in gynecomastia.

Mechanism of Action

Testosterone like other steroid hormones acts by binding with the cytoplasmic nuclear receptors. In the cell, two pathways are activated: DHT pathway, and testosterone pathway (Fig. 80.9).

DHT Pathway

This pathway is mainly active in **prostate, scrotum, penis, skin and bones**. The testosterone is converted to DHT by **5α-reductase**. DHT then binds with androgen receptors in the nucleus and induces RNA transcription to form various proteins.

- This causes **sexual maturation at puberty and external virilization**.
- Thus, DHT is mainly responsible for **development of facial hair, skin changes, recession of hair line**, and enlargement of prostate, scrotum, penis and bone.

Testosterone Pathway

Testosterone directly binds with testosterone receptors in the nucleus that induces m RNA activity.

- This pathway **mainly regulates gonadotropin secretion**, causes muscle development, **controls spermatogenesis**, and influences male **sex drive and libido**.

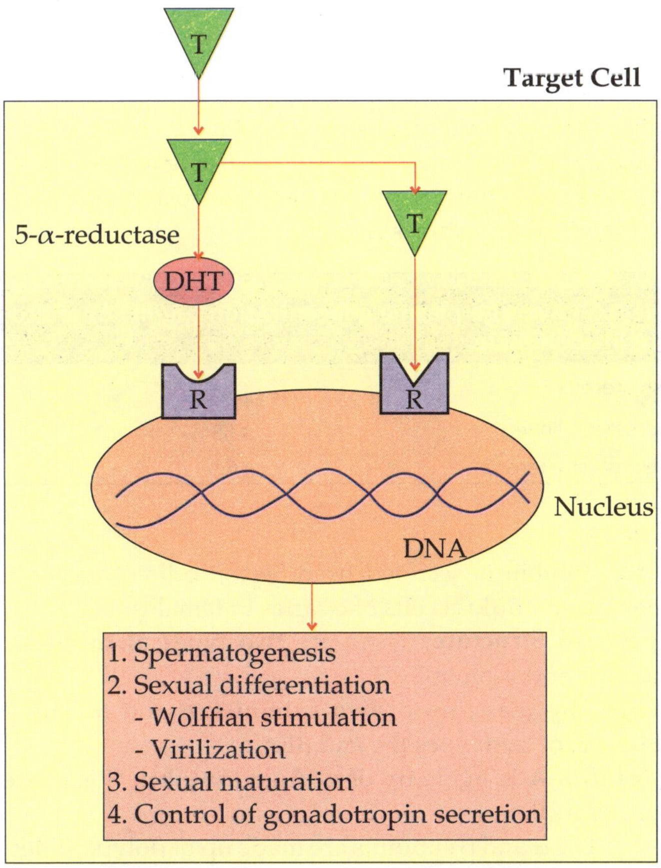

Fig. 80.9: Mechanisms of testosterone action. Note that testosterone (T) is converted to dihydrotestosterone (DHT) in the cell. There are separate receptors (R) for both testosterone and DHT in the nucleus. Therefore, two separate mechanisms exist in different cells for testosterone actions.

Physiological Actions

Testosterone is an **anabolic hormone**. It promotes growth of male reproductive system and causes development of secondary sex characters. Among various androgens, the potency in order of sequence is as follows:

DHT > testosterone > androstenedione > DHEA*

*DHEA is dehydroepiandrosterone.

Development of Secondary Sex Characteristics

Testosterone develops and maintains male secondary sex characteristics. These features are:

1. **Changes in external genitalia:** Penis enlarges **in length and width**. The scrotum becomes more rugose and pigmented.
2. **Changes in internal genitalia:** Seminal vesicles increase in size and start secreting fructose. Prostate gland enlarges and secretion increases from prostate and bulbourethral gland.
3. **Growth and distribution of body hairs:** Hair growth is classified into **three groups** depending on their sensitivity to androgens: nonsexual, ambisexual and sexual.
   - **Nonsexual hairs** are hairs of eyebrows and extremities.
   - **Ambisexual hairs** are the hairs in the axilla, and **sexual hairs** are the hairs in the face, chest and upper pubic triangle.
   - Androgen ***stimulates growth of all types of hairs***, though the effects are more on sexual and ambisexual hairs.
   - It promotes hair growth in axilla, on the chest and pubic triangle, and around the anus. In the face, hairs grow in the form of moustache and beard.
   - Pubic hairs grow with male pattern (in the *shape of a triangle of which the apex is upward*).
   - The hair line on the scalp recedes in males. Therefore, it is believed that **baldness is a sign of maleness**.
4. **Skin changes:** In general, skin becomes tough. Secretion of sebaceous gland increases and becomes thick.
   - This leads to **acne formation**. Sometimes *acne vulgaris* appears.
   - Skin derived from urogenital sinus, i.e., the prepuce, clitoris, labia majora and scrotum becomes **more sensitive**.
   - Skin in and around genitalia becomes **more pigmented**.
5. **Mental changes:** The individual becomes more **active and aggressive**. He takes more **interest in opposite sex**.
6. **Voice change:** Enlargement of larynx and thickening of vocal cord occur. Therefore, **voice becomes thick and deep**.

7. **Body configuration:** General increase in body height and girth occurs (growth spurt).
    - Especially, **broadening of the shoulder** occurs with general increase in size of skeletal muscles.
    - These changes impart masculine phenotypic expression.
8. **Musculoskeletal changes:** Growth of long bones, pectoral girdle and vertebral bones occurs at puberty.
    - Testosterone causes **closure of epiphysis** of long bone, ultimately ***limiting increase in height*** of the individual.
    - It causes ***muscle hypertrophy***, increases muscle protein synthesis and **increases muscle mass**.

Effects on Spermatogenesis

Testosterone **stimulates spermatogenesis**, the exact mechanism of which is not known. It is essential for sperm production and maturation.

1. It mainly **facilitates the process of spermiogenesis**.
2. It initiates spermatogenesis at puberty and then maintains it throughout adulthood and also in old age.

Effects during Embryonic Life

In male fetus, between 8th and 18th week testosterone causes the **differentiation of male genitalia**.

1. The **development of Wolffian duct** into epididymis, vas deferens and seminal vesicles depends directly on the effects of androgen.
2. Also, the **differentiation of urogenital sinus and genital tubercle** into penis, scrotum and testis is mediated by testosterone and DHT.
3. Further, **descent of testis** into scrotum is promoted by testosterone.

Anabolic Effects

Testosterone **increases the synthesis of proteins** and decreases its catabolism. This results in increased growth and development of bones and muscles.

1. It **causes sodium, potassium, calcium, phosphate, and water retention** from kidney.
2. It is used as an **anabolic drug** in patients suffering from wasting diseases. Athletes use it as anabolic steroids.

Effects on Brain

Many areas in the brain have androgen receptors. However, the receptors are **densely located in limbic areas**, especially in amygdala and septum, and in hypothalamus, pituitary and preoptic area.

- In these areas, testosterone is **aromatized to estrogen** (Fig. 80.10).
- **Sexual dimorphism of neurons** in the brain with respect to their distribution, size, number and activity has been reported in preoptic area and amygdala.

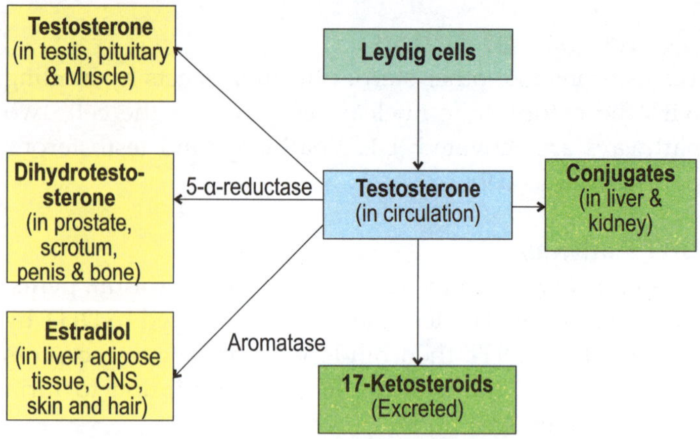

Fig. 80.10: Fate of testosterone secreted from Leydig cells.

Other Effects

Testosterone, by its negative feedback effects, **inhibits GnRH secretion** from hypothalamus and **inhibits LH and FSH secretion** from anterior pituitary. It **stimulates erythropoiesis**.

Other Testicular Hormones

Other testicular hormones are androgens other than testosterone, inhibin, activin and follistatin. Estrogen is also produced in testis by aromatization of androgen in Sertoli cells.

Other Androgens

Testis secretes androgens. Testicular androgens are testosterone (described above), **androstenedione** and **dihydrotestosterone**. Among them, testosterone is the major androgen (Table 80.1).

Table 80.1 | **Average plasma concentration (μg/lit) of androgens in adult male.**

Androgen	Concentration
Testosterone	: 6.5
Androstenedione	: 1.5
Dihydrotestosterone	: 0.5

Inhibin

Source: Inhibin is secreted from Sertoli cells of testes in males and granulosa cells of ovaries in females.

Types and Structure: There are **two types of inhibins**: inhibin A and inhibin B.

Inhibins are made up of **two subunits**: **α** and **β**. **The β subunit** is of two types βA and βB.

- **Inhibin A** is made up of αβA and **inhibin B** is made up of **αβ**B.
    - The α and β subunits are made up of polypeptides.
- **Inhibin B** is the FSH regulating peptide.

The homodimers and heterodimers of β subunits are formed.

This results in formation of βAβB, βBβB, and βA**B**A.

- These are called **activins**.

- **Activins and inhibins** are found in the gonads, brain, and many other tissues.
  - In bone marrow, activins stimulate leucopoiesis.

Functions: The main function of inhibin is to **provide feedback signal to inhibit FSH secretion** from anterior pituitary. Inhibin B mainly inhibits FSH secretion.

Activin

It is a polypeptide hormone **produced by Sertoli cells.**

1. It stimulates **secretion of FSH**.
2. Activin results from various combinations of **β**A and **β**B subunits of inhibin that forms βA**β**B, **β**B**β**B, and **β**A**β**A.
3. They stimulate WBC development in the bone marrow, formation of mesoderm during embryonic life and also gonadal development.

Follistatin

Follistatin is a single chain protein having molecular weight of about 40, 000. It has various isoforms that binds and **inactivates activin**.

1. When activins bind with follistatin they lose their functions.
2. Thus, FSH secretion is reduced from pituitary cells.
3. Follistatin **influences developing spermatogenic cells** by a paracrine mechanism.

Regulation of Testicular Functions

Testicular functions are controlled by hypothalamic and pituitary inputs.

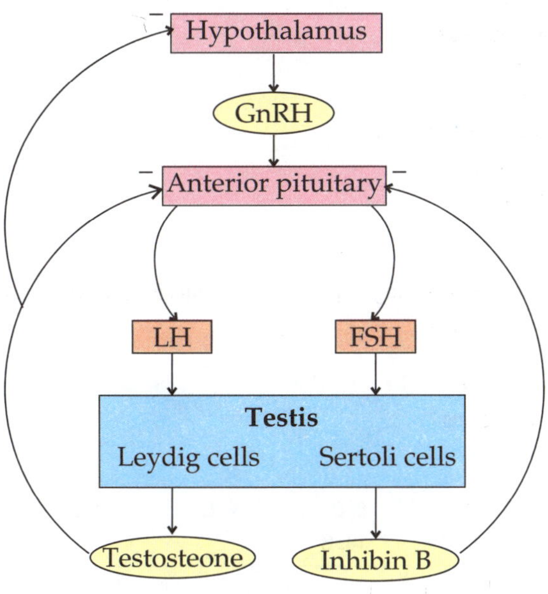

Fig. 80.11: Feedback regulation of gonadal hormone secretion. Minus (–) sign indicates inhibition]. (GnRH: gonadotropin-releasing hormone; LH: luteinizing hormone; FSH: follicle stimulating hormone).

Hypothalamic Control: Hypothalamus secretes GnRH.

- **GnRH stimulates LH and FSH secretion** from anterior pituitary that in turn influences testicular steroidogenesis.

Pituitary Control: Anterior pituitary controls testicular functions by secreting LH and FSH.

- **FSH stimulates Sertoli cells to produce inhibin** that maintains the gametogenic functions of the testis. FSH also stimulates secretion of androgen binding protein.
- **LH stimulates Leydig cells to secrete testosterone,** which controls gametogenesis.

Steroid Feedback: Testosterone provides negative feedback signal to hypothalamus to inhibit the secretion of GnRH, and to gonadotrophs of anterior pituitary to inhibit secretion of LH (Fig. 80.11).

Inhibin provides negative feedback effect on anterior pituitary to inhibit the secretion of FSH.

PY9.7

TESTICULAR ABNORMALITIES

Cryptorchidism

The **failure of migration** of testis from abdominal cavity into the scrotum during fetal development is called **undescended testis** or cryptorchidism. The usual site of undescended testis is inguinal rings.

Treatment: Treatment with **gonadotropin hormones** facilitates the descent of testis. Surgical correction is required when the hormonal treatment fails.

Complications: Undescended testis **decreases sperm production**, as temperature is high in the abdomen. The **incidence of malignant tumors** is significantly more in undescended testis.

Male Hypogonadism

There are mainly **two types**: Hypergonadotropic hypogonadism and hypogonadotropic hypogonadism.

Hypergonadotropic Hypogonadism: If this occurs due to testicular dysfunctions, plasma level of gonadotropin is increased.

Hypogonadotropic Hypogonadism: This occurs mainly due to tumor of hypothalamus or pituitary. Gonadotropin level in plasma is depressed.

1. If hypogonadism **occurs after puberty**, the secondary sex characteristics regress slowly as androgenic maintenance of these features is less essential. However, loss of libido is common.
2. If loss of Leydig cells **occurs from childhood**, ***eunuchoidism*** results.

Enuchoids are usually **tall, with narrow shoulders** and less muscular development.

- The genitalia are small.
- Though **pubic hairs** are present they are usually sparse and exhibit ***female pattern***, i.e. triangle with base up.

Androgen Secreting Tumors

Hypersecretion of testis is usually due to a **tumor in the testis**.

- **Leydig cell tumors** secrete androgen and result in **precocious puberty** in prepubertal boys.

Exam Questions

1. What is blood-testis barrier and what are its functions. Describe the functions of Sertoli cells.
2. Describe the steps of spermatogenesis. Give a note on factors regulating spermatogenesis.
3. Give the composition of semen and draw the structure of a normal sperm. Briefly describe common sperm abnormalities.
4. With the help of schematic diagram, describe the mechanism of action of testosterone. Describe the functions of testosterone.
5. Describe the steps of synthesis and metabolism of testosterone. Give a note on secondary sexual characteristics in males.

Multiple Choice Questions

1. Before the onset of puberty, the GnRH neurons are under the inhibitory control of:
   A. Glycine B. Glutamate
   C. Gamma amino butyric acid (GABA) D. Beta-endorphin

2. The gene coding for androgen receptor is located on:
   A. Short arm of X –chromosome
   B. Short arm of Y-chromosome
   C. Long arm of X-chromosome
   D. Long arm of Y-chromosome

3. Sertoli cells play a key role in which of the following process:
   A. Spermiogenesis B. Testosterone secretion
   C. Secretion of seminal fluid D. Production of germ cells

4. Sertoli cells secrete:
   A. Testosterone B. Estrogen
   C. Androstenedione D. Inhibin

5. Sertoli cells have receptors for
   A. Inhibin B. Luteinizing hormone (LH)
   C. Follicle stimulating hormone (FSH) D. Melatonin

6. Blood testes barrier is located between
   A. Sertoli and Sertoli cells
   B. Leydig and myoid cells
   C. Sertoli cell and germ cells
   D. Sertoli cells and spermatid developing cell

7. Testosterone production is mainly controlled by
   A. Leydig cells B. Sertolie cells
   C. Seminiferous tubules D. Epididymis

8. Which of the following is the primary action of inhibin?
   A. Inhibits secretion of prolactin
   B. Stimulates synthesis of estradiol
   C. Stimulates secretion of TSH
   D. Inhibits secretion of FSH

9. Semen is released by:
   A. Epididymis B. Testes
   C. Vas deferens D. Prolactin

10. Sperms become motile in:
   A. Prostate B. Seminal vesicle
   C. Epididymis D. Vas deference

11. Capacitance of sperms takes place in:
   A. Seminiferous tubules B. Epididymis
   C. Vas deference D. Uterus

12. Dihydrotestosterone acts on:
   A. Pituitary B. External genitalia
   C. Internal genitalia D. Testis

13. Negative feedback in spermatogenesis by
   A. ABP B. Inhibin
   C. Progesterone D. None

14. Prolonged administration of testosterone in a man causes:
   A. Azoospermia
   B. Increased GnRH
   C. Increased sperm mobility
   D. Increased spermiogenesis

15. Velocity of human sperm
   A. 1-3 mm/min
   B. 4-6 mim/min
   C. 6-9 mm/min
   D. 10-13 mm/min

16. Prostaglandins in semen are mainly secreted by:
   A. Prostate
   B. Seminal vesicle
   C. Sperms
   D. Testes

17. Not found in seminal fluid
   A. Prostaglandins
   B. Spermine
   C. Citric acid
   D. Inositol

18. Which of the following organs secretes zinc in large amount in man?
   A. Seminal vesicle
   B. Prostate
   C. Epididymis
   D. Vas deferens

Answers

1. C	2. C	3. A	4. D	5. C	6. A	7. A	8. D	9. C	10. C
11. D	12. B	13. B	14. A	15. A	16. B	17. E	18. B		

Chapter 81

PY9.4

Female Reproductive System

Learning Objectives

On completion of study of this chapter:

The student will be able to (must know):

1. Name different parts of female reproductive tract and give their functions.
2. Describe the steps of Oogenesis.
3. Explain the mechanism and regulation of different phases of ovarian follicle.
4. Describe (with the help of a schematic diagram) the uterine, ovarian and hormonal changes in menstrual cycle.
5. List the indicators of ovulation and give the mechanism and importance of ovulation.
6. List the ovarian hormones and give their functions.
7. List the secondary sexual characteristics in females.
8. Illustrate the mechanisms of control of ovarian functions.
9. Define common abnormalities of female reproductive functions reproduction.

The student may also be able to (desirable to know):

1. Describe the process and regulation of oogenesis.
2. Describe the regulation of ovarian functions
3. Describe synthesis, regulation and functions of ovarian hormones

FUNCTIONAL ANATOMY

External Genitalia

Female external genitalia include labia majora, labia minora, clitoris, vestibule of vagina and vestibular glands (Fig. 81.1). These structures are collectively called as vulva.

Labia Majora: Labia majora are analogous to scrotum in males. These are two major skin folds that form the outer lips of vaginal vestibule, which include **vaginal and urethral openings.**

Labia Minora: Labia minora are two minor skin folds present between labia majora and form inner lips of vaginal and urethral openings.

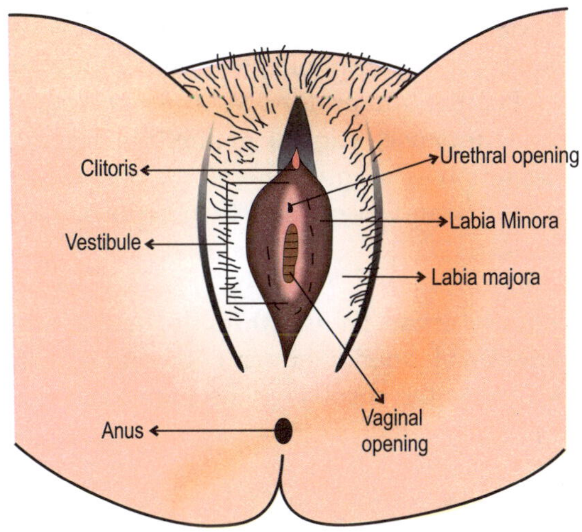

Fig. 81.1: Female external genitalia.

Clitoris: Clitoris is located at the anterior pole of vaginal vestibule. This is the *female analogue of penis*.

It consists of erectile tissue.

The tip of the clitoris is the **glans clitoris** similar to glans penis.

Vaginal Vestibule: Vaginal vestibule contains **two openings:** vaginal and urethral openings.

- Vaginal opening lies below and posterior to urethral opening.
- In virgins, vaginal opening is partially closed by **hymen**, a thin fold of mucous membrane.
- Vestibular glands empty their secretion into the vaginal vestibule.

Internal Genitalia

The female internal reproductive organs are present in the pelvis and consist of vagina, uterus, fallopian tubes and ovaries (Fig. 81.2).

Vagina

This is a tubular canal which is present anterior to rectum and posterior to the urethra and bladder. It connects vaginal opening in the vestibule to the uterine cervix.

- The length of vagina in adult is about 8 cm, but it is highly stretchable as its wall is folded normally. It can ***elongate to more than double of its length*** during sexual act.
- Under the action of relaxin, it **widens and stretches further during parturition**.
- **Vaginal wall** contains muscle and contraction of vagina during sexual act facilitates the transportation of sperm into the uterus.
- **Vaginal epithelium** changes during different *phases of menstrual cycle*.
    - **In proliferative phase**, under the influence of estrogen, **cornification** (keratinization) of vaginal epithelium occurs that secretes thin mucus.
    - **In the luteal phase**, under the influence of progesterone, cornification of epithelium is reduced; rather, polymorphonuclear leucocytes infiltrate and epithelium proliferates to ***secrete thick mucus.***
- **After menopause**, vaginal epithelium becomes thin and secretion is scanty. Therefore, post-menopausal vagina is dry and susceptible to infections.

Uterus

This is hollow organ having **thick muscular wall**. It is placed between bladder anteriorly and rectum posteriorly. It has **two parts**: the corpus (or the body) and the cervix (Fig. 81.3).

Body of Uterus

Uterus consists mainly of **two layers** (myometrium and endometrium) and uterine cavity.

Myometrium: The myometrium consists of multiple layers of smooth muscle.

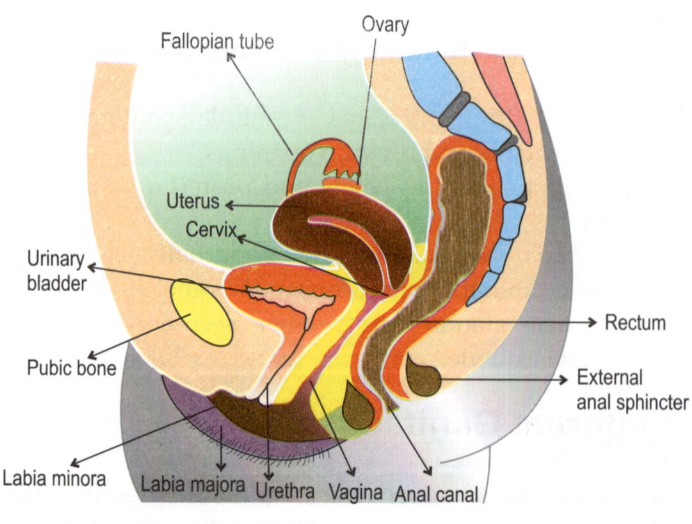

Fig. 81.2: Reproductive organs in female.

Endometrium: The endometrium has **two layers**: a stromal layer close to myometrium and an epithelium.

- **The stroma** is penetrated by spiral arteries and contains adequate connective tissue.
- **The epithelium** contains uterine glands that are lined by columnar secretory cells. The glands also infiltrate into stroma. The ***arterial and glandular changes*** occur in different phases of menstrual cycle (see below).
- **Shedding of endometrial tissue** at the end of luteal phase results in menstrual bleeding. Uterus enlarges during pregnancy to accommodate the growing fetus and expels the fetus at the time of parturition.

Uterine Cervix: The cervix is a narrow muscular tube that connects vagina with body of the uterus. It has internal os, cervical canal and external os.

- Cervical mucus changes from thick and viscous liquid to profuse, watery and highly elastic liquid, which forms the physiological basis of '**spinnbarkeit test**' for ovulation (spinnbarkeit refers to a highly elastic substance).
- Under the influence of estrogen, cervical mucous forms typical '**fern pattern**', which disappears following ovulation.
- **Cervical dilation** is done for uterine investigations (Clinical Note 81.1). Cervical dilation is the initial event in the initiation of parturition.

Clinical Note 81.1

D and C: Dilation of cervix is performed routinely in gynecological practice to obtain endometrial tissue from cervix or body of the uterus for diagnosis of various uterine pathologies. This is called dilatation and curettage (D and C). D and C are also performed therapeutically for treatment of few uterine diseases. Cervical dilation is done to evacuate the uterine content (conceptus) for abortion.

Fallopian Tubes

Two fallopian tubes (also called **oviducts**) arise from both sides of upper poles of uterus. Oviducts are 10–15 cm in length. They have **three parts**: isthmus, ampulla and infundibulum (Fig. 81.3).

- **Infundibulum** opens into pelvic cavity close to ovaries.

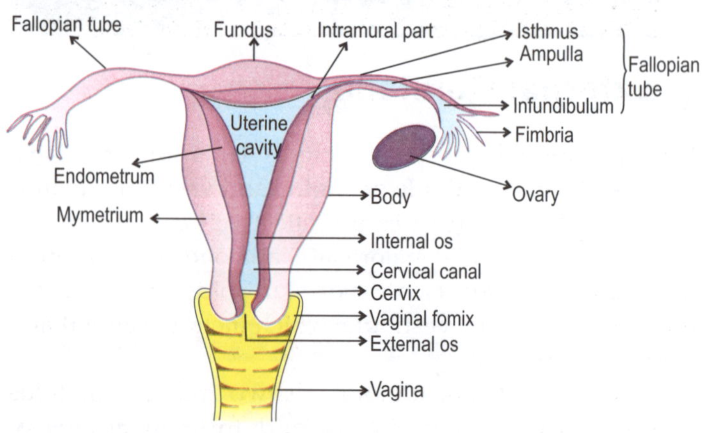

Fig. 81.3: Parts of uterus and fallopian tube.

- Infundibular openings have **fimbriae** (finger like projections lined by ciliated epithelium) that help in grasping ovum at the time of ovulation.
- Normally, **fertilization takes place in ampullary part** of the oviduct and then fertilized ovum is transported to uterine cavity for implantation.
  - Thus, maldevelopment or diseases of fallopian tubes result in infertilization (Clinical Note 81.2).

Clinical Note 81.2

BTL: Bilateral tubal ligation (BTL) is the commonest and permanent method of sterilization in parous women. Tubal ligation is preferred to tubectomy, when the parents keep the option for recanalization of the tubes if necessity arises in future.

Ovaries

There are two ovaries each weighing about 10 g in adults. Each one present on both sides of uterus and are attached by ovarian ligaments. Ovary consists of **two zones**: the cortex, and medulla.

Cortex of Ovary: The cortex is the outer and the major zone lined by the germinal epithelium. It is surrounded by a layer of fibrous tissue called **tunica albuginea**.

1. Cortex contains oocytes. Each oocyte is enclosed within a follicle, the **ovarian follicle.**
   - Ovarian follicles are present in their **various stages of development** (Fig. 81.4).
   - The matured ovarian follicle is called **Graafian follicle**.
2. The **stroma** of the ovary is present in between the follicles, which consists of supporting connective tissue and interstitial cells.

Medulla of Ovary: The inner zone of the ovary forms the medulla that contains different types of interstitial and connective tissue cells. Blood vessels and lymphatics enter the ovary through its hilum.

Functions of Ovary:

1. Oogenesis during fetal life.
2. Maturation of oocyte.
3. Ovulation
4. Secretion of female sex hormones and peptide hormones.

The primary function of ovary is to **develop ovarian follicles** and **release ovum at the time of ovulation**, and to **secrete steroid hormones** that control various reproductive and metabolic functions.

OOGENESIS

Unlike spermatogenesis that starts at puberty and continues throughout life, the process of oogenesis starts in fetal life and ceases at menopause. Also, the process of development of each spermatocyte is completed in few days, whereas **development of each oocyte that begins in intrauterine life is completed with ovulation** that occurs during menstrual cycle.

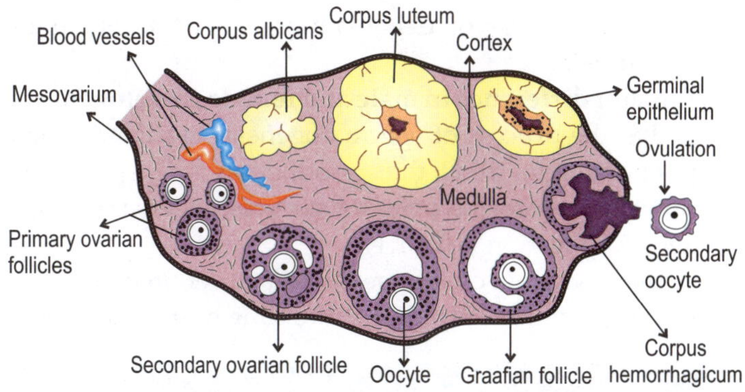

Fig. 81.4: Structure of ovary. Note the development of ovarian follicle in different stages

Stages of Development: The stages of development of oocytes occur in three stages: Oogonium becoming primary oocyte, primary oocyte converted to secondary oocyte, and finally secondary oocyte developing to mature ovum.

Oogonia Becoming Primary Oocyte

Oogonia

The primordial germ cells (oogonia) migrate from the **yolk sac of embryo** to the genital ridge at about 6th week of gestation.

- The, oogonia undergo **many mitotic divisions** and the number of oogonia reaches to about 7 million.
- When mitosis cease, the oogonia are called **oocytes**.

Primary Oocytes

The oocytes undergo **two meiotic divisions** (the meiotic cycle) at different stages of development to produce a haploid ovum. Oocytes in their preliminary stage of development are called primary oocytes.

First Meiotic Division: The first meiotic division starts in primary oocytes **during fetal life**, which occurs at about **8th week of pregnancy, is arrested in prophase**. The oocytes then grow in size.

- However, the first meiotic division is not completed in fetal life, ***not even till puberty***; in fact, it is **completed just prior to ovulation**.
- Therefore, the **life span of a primary oocyte** can be upto ***50 years***, as ovulation can continue upto this age.
- The suspension of oocyte division in prophase for such a long period depends on the internal hormonal environment provided by the surrounding supporting cells.

Oocyte Degeneration: The oocyte degeneration, however, **starts from the intrauterine life** so that only about 1 million primary oocytes remain at the time of birth.

- By the time of **puberty about 200,000** and by the age of 30 only about 26,000 oocytes remain in the ovary.
  - At menopause, ovaries are virtually devoid of oocytes.
  - During a woman's life, only **about 400 oocytes are ovulated** and the other oocytes degenerate.

- The process of degeneration of oocyte is called **atresia**.

- A **major difference in male and female gametogenesis** is that the process of spermatogenesis is a continuous phenomenon and the production of sperm is unlimited, whereas primary oocytes degenerate with age (Application Box 81.1).
- As new oogonia cannot be manufactured in ovary, the **oocytes totally disappear at the time of menopause**.

Application Box 81.1

Age of oocyte contribute to health of children: Because of the peculiar pattern of development of oocyte in females, the life span of an oocyte may be as old as 50 years.
- The oocyte that ovulates at about 40 years of age is about 25 years older than the oocyte that ovulates at the age of 15.
- This one of the important factors that contribute to the anomalies in children born to older woman as the aged-eggs oocyte have degenerative changes and therefore their fertilization may result in defective embryo.

Primary Oocyte Converted to Secondary Oocyte

In fetus, oogonia develop into primary oocyte, which undergo first meiotic division. However, the first meiotic division is not completed in fetus. This is called as **meiotic arrest**. Thus, all eggs present at birth are **primary oocytes** in meiotic arrest containing 46 chromosomes. This state continues until puberty.

- The primary oocyte that is destined for ovulation **completes the first meiotic division just before the ovulation**.
- This division results in production of two structures: one is the daughter cell, called **secondary oocyte** containing 23 chromosomes, and the other is the **first polar body** (Fig. 81.5).
- However, the **cytoplasmic division is grossly unequal** in this process in which the secondary oocyte retains nearly all the cytoplasm with polar body containing very little of it. Thus, the polar body becomes completely nonfunctional.

Secondary Oocyte Forming Ovum

Second Meiotic Division: The second meiotic division **occurs in the secondary oocyte** after ovulation, and is **arrested in metaphase**.

- The second meiotic division is **completed when the egg is penetrated by a sperm**. Thus, **meiotic cycle is completed only on fertilization**.
- As a result of this meiotic division, **the ovum** containing 23 chromosomes and the **second polar body** are formed (Fig. 81.5). The polar body is extruded.
- Thus, in the process of oogenesis, **each primary oocyte produces only one ovum**.

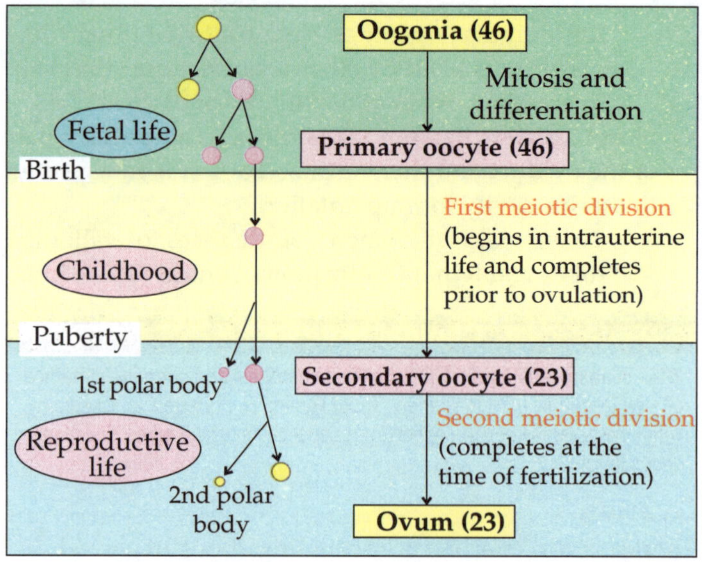

Fig. 81.5: Stages of oogenesis. Note first meiotic division of oocyte begins during fetal life and completes prior to ovulation, whereas second meiotic division completes at the time of fertilization.

DEVELOPMENT OF OVARIAN FOLLICLE

Stages of Folliculogenesis

Follicular development is called **folliculogenesis**, which occurs in four stages (Fig. 81.6).

Stage 1 (Primordial Follicular Stage)

The ovarian follicle, also called **Graafian follicle** begins as a **primordial follicle** (Fig. 81.1A).

- The primordial follicle consists of a **primary oocyte** at the centre surrounded by a **layer of spindle cells** (flattened **pregranulosa cells**) that form granulosa cells later.
  - A basal lamina is formed outside the spindle cells. The size of oocyte in primordial follicle is about 25 μm.
- Primordial follicles form the **resting pool of follicles** in the ovary.
  - However, they *degenerate progressively from fetal life to menopause*.
- The oocyte enters into **first meiotic division** and the division is **arrested in prophase**. This prophase of oocyte is maintained till just prior to ovulation.

Stage 2 (Primary Follicular Stage)

The primordial follicles grow into the **primary follicles**.

- During this process the flattened pregranulosa cells (spindle cells) become **cuboidal granulosa cells** that further proliferate to form a continuous cell layer surrounding the oocyte (Fig. 81.6B). The size of oocyte increases to about 80-140 μm.

- A type of ***glassy material*** consisting of mucopolysaccharide is secreted from granulosa cells, which forms a thick layer between the oocyte and the granulosa cell layer, called as **zona pellucida**.

- The primordial follicle becomes primary follicle at about 28th weeks of gestation.
- The **prophase of first meiotic division** of oocyte is maintained.

Stage 3 (Secondary Follicular Stage)

The primary follicle becomes **secondary follicle** in this stage during which the granulosa cells divide and form several layers of cells around the oocyte. Thus, the size of follicle increases enormously in this stage to about 500 µm. At this, stage, follicle is called **preantral follicle.** However, small antrum may develop (Fig. 81.6C).

A layer of spindle cells (**pre or early theca cells**) is formed at the periphery of the basal lamina, which forms the **theca cell layer** in the next stage.

- All these developments occur slowly in the **prepubertal ovary**.

- The oocyte is maintained in **prophase of its first meiotic division**.

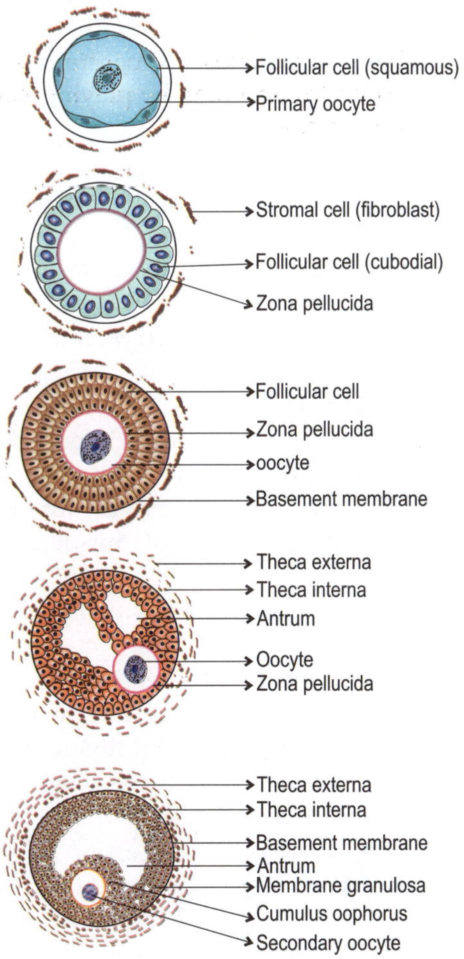

Figs. 81.6: Stages of development of ovarian follicle. A: Primordial follicular stage; B: Primary follicular stage; C: Secondary follicular stage; D: Tertiary follicular stage E: Matured follicle.

Stage 4 (Tertiary Follicular Stage)

This is the final stage of follicular development. It occurs in **two sub-stages**: the early tertiary stage and the Graafian follicular stage.

Early Tertiary or Antral Follicular Stage: In this stage, the spindle cell layer surrounding the basement membrane proliferates and differentiates into inner theca interna and outer theca externa.

- **Theca interna cells** multiply to form multiple cell layers and become steroidogenic.
- **Theca externa cell** lie in a single layer and provide mechanical support to the follicle from outside.
  - Theca cells receive blood, lymphatic and nerve supply whereas **granulosa cells remain avascular** as blood vessel can't penetrate the basement membrane.
- Along with the expansion of theca cell layer, a ***fluid-filled space*** is created in the midst of granulosa cells, called as **antrum** (Fig. 81.6D).
  - Therefore, the follicle in this stage is also called **early antral follicle** and the stage also as early ***antral follicular stage***.

The granulosa cells increase in number and **acquire receptors for FSH** and start secreting estrogen. In fact, the progression of early tertiary stage to the next stage of follicular development is **FSH dependent**.

Late Tertiary or Graafian Follicular Stage: This is the most **rapid stage of development.** It occurs only **in the post-pubertal ovary**.

1. After 5–7 days of onset of menses, a single follicle becomes **dominant follicle** for that cycle.
   - The follicle in this stage is called **Graafian follicle** (Fig. 81.6E) and the stage is called *Graafian follicular stage*.
   - It occurs in one ovary during each cycle.
2. The size of the **antrum and the amount of antral fluid** are increased significantly. This ***pushes the oocyte to the periphery*** of the follicle.
   - The mucopolysaccharide, which is present in the antral fluid, is ***depolymerized*** to increase the osmotic pressure of the fluid.
   - However, the total *intrafollicular pressure* remains within 20 mmHg.
   - The antral fluid **contains many hormones** such as estrogen, progesterone, FSH, LH, prolactin, androstenedione and growth factors, inhibin, activin, GnRH, CRH, opioid peptides and oxytocin.
   - It also contains plasminogen activator, mucopolysaccharide, proteins, electrolytes, gycosaminoglycans and proteoglycans.
3. The **vascularity** of theca increases.
4. The **granulosa cells in this stage** are anatomically divided into **three compartments**: antral, cumulus and mural granulosa cells.

Antral Granulosa Cells: Granulosa cells lining the antral cavity are called antral granulosa cells (**Discus proligerous**).

- Antral granulosa cells are **highly steroidogenic**.

Cumulus Granulosa Cells: Granulosa cells surrounding the oocyte are cumulus granulosa cells (**cumulus oophoricus**).

- Therefore, the granulosa cells that project into the antrum like a mound are collectively called as **cumulus oophorus**.
- Cumulus granulosa cells are **less steroidogenic**.

Mural Granulosa Cells: Granulosa cells that are attached to the basement membrane are called mural granulosa cells (Membrana granulosa).

Mural granulosa cells are **highly steroidogenic**.

1. The diameter of the follicle in this stage is about 2.5 cm. The follicle is called **pre-ovulatory follicle** as it is ready for ovulation at this stage.
   - The ***basement membrane*** close to the surface of the ovary undergoes **proteolysis** that slowly *leads to rupture of the follicle* resulting in release of oocyte from the follicle, the process called **ovulation**.
2. Just prior to ovulation, **the first meiotic division is completed**.
3. The oocyte is **taken up by the fallopian tube**.
4. **If fertilization occurs**, the penetration of ovum by the sperm **completes the second meiotic division**, which results in **functional ovum** (fertilized egg).
   - If fertilization **does not occur**, the oocyte begins to degenerate in 24 to 48 hours.

Corpus Luteum Formation

Luteinization

After ovulation, the ruptured follicle is quickly filled with blood, and at this time, the follicle is called **corpus hemorrhagicum**. However, the cells lining the follicle rapidly proliferate to replace blood with luteal cells that are rich in lipid. Now, the follicle is called **corpus luteum** and its appearance heralds the beginning of luteal phase of the cycle.

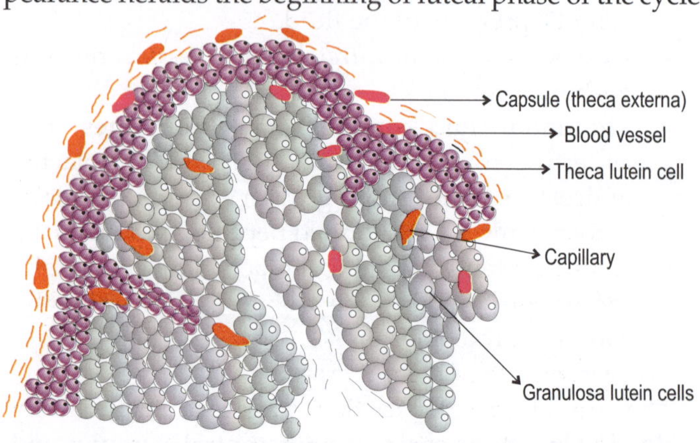

Fig. 81.7: Structure of corpus luteum. Note the abundance of theca lutein cells and granulosa lutein cells. Also, the presence of more capillaries indicates high vascularity.

1. The corpus luteum is a yellow body made up of **endocrine tissue** that consists of **granulosa luteal cells, theca luteal cells and fibroblasts.**
   - The number of mitochondria, lipid droplets and the endoplasmic reticulum increase in the granulosa cells of corpus luteum.
   - These morphological changes are collectively known as **luteinization**, which is ***essential for synthesis of more steroid hormones***.
2. The granulosa and theca cells of matured corpus luteum are respectively called as **granulosa lutein cells** and **theca lutein cells** (Fig. 81.7).
3. **Luteal granulosa cells are vascular** unlike the follicular granulosa cells that are nonvascular.
4. Vascularity of luteal cells **facilitates the synthesis of steroid hormones** by promoting the supply of cholesterol from plasma to these cells.

Regulation of Luteinization

Progesterone, estrogen and androgen are formed in corpus luteum.

1. **Progesterone secretion** reaches its peak in menstrual cycle at about 7 days after ovulation, which ***correlates with the full maturity*** of corpus luteum.
   - **These hormones (Progesterone, estrogen and androgen) may be playing some role in luteinization.**
2. **LH is the major stimulator of luteinization**. LH maintains the functions of corpus luteum by **promoting luteinization** of its cells, and therefore, LH is referred to as luteinizing hormone.
3. **FSH increases** the number of ***LH receptors*** on the cells.

Luteal Regression

If **fertilization does not occur**, corpus luteum **degenerates in about 13 days** after ovulation.

- The endocrine cells of corpus luteum become necrotic and are invaded by leucocytes and fibroblasts.
  - This process is called **luteolysis** or luteal regression.
- The exact mechanism of luteolysis is not known. However, it is proposed to be due to the action of **luteolysins** that are produced locally in the ovary.
  - The proposed luteolysins are **oxytocin, prostaglandins and GnRH.**
- Luteolysins promote luteal regression by **preventing the action of LH** on corpus luteum.
- The degenerated corpus luteum is replaced by avascular and nonfunctional fibrous tissue, known as **corpus albicans**.

If **fertilization occurs**, the implanted fertilized ovum secretes hCG from its embryonic trophoblast, which has

LH-like activity. Therefore, **hCG maintains luteinization** and promotes the functions of the **corpus luteum of pregnancy**.

Functions of Corpus Luteum:

1. The corpus luteum **secretes hormones**. During luteal phase, increased ***secretion of progesterone, estrogen and inhibin A*** occurs from corpus luteum. It also secretes androgen.
2. It provides endocrinal **environment for implantation of fertilized ovum**.
3. It **maintains the early part of pregnancy** by secreting progesterone in adequate concentration till the placenta becomes functional.

Infertility occurs due to luteal deficiency (Clinical Note 81.3)

Clinical Note 81.3

Luteal deficiency: One of the common causes of infertility is the luteal deficiency, also called luteal insufficiency, in which either luteinization of granulosa cells of corpus luteum is deficient due to less number LH receptors on luteal cells, or due to ovulation of prematurely developed follicle that contains less number of luteinized granulosa cells. FSH also promotes expression of LH receptors in the follicular cells. Therefore, FSH deficiency can also cause luteal insufficiency.

Atresia of Follicle

During the entire reproductive period of a woman, about 400 oocytes grow to culminate in ovulation. The follicles that do not become dominant undergo a ***process of degeneration*** called atresia.

- Atresia starts in fetal ovary soon after the appearance of primordial follicles.
- It occurs due to **apoptosis**, a process of programmed cell death.

Regulation of Follicular Development

Factors affecting development of follicles are different in different phases of follicular growth.

Primordial Follicular Stage

The growth of primordial follicle is **not affected by gonadotropins**. It is purely a local phenomenon.

Primary Follicular Stage

The **chemical substances secreted by oocyte** stimulate the transformation of pregranulosa cells to granulosa cells.

- The **products of granulosa cells** stimulate the formation of spindle (pre-theca) cells.
- **FSH and LH** stimulate the development of follicle towards the later part of gestation.
- During early childhood, though LH and FSH are secreted in low concentration, they are essential to maintain follicular growth.
- Follicular growth is impaired without gonadotropins.

Secondary Follicular Stage

At the time of puberty, secondary follicles start developing. The granulosa cells of secondary follicles **acquire FSH receptors** and secrete estrogen in less concentration. This **follicular estrogen** promotes further follicular development.

Early Tertiary Stage: Immediately after menarche (the first menstrual bleeding), in the early luteal phase of the same first cycle, usually the secondary follicles enter the tertiary follicular stage of development. The granulosa cells respond to FSH in the follicular phase of the next cycle.

1. The **FSH stimulates the granulosa cell** and increases the aromatase activity, which increases the synthesis of estrogen from androgen. The follicular concentration of estrogen increases.
2. **Estrogen** along with FSH induces expression of LH receptors on granulosa cells. Estrogen also conditions hypothalamo-anterior pituitary axis that maintains LH activity in the plasma.
3. **LH synthesis is increased** by estrogen at this point of time, which is essential for **pre-ovulatory surge of LH.**
4. **Estrogen** also *increases the number and sensitivity of LH receptors in the theca cells*. Therefore, **LH stimulates androgen synthesis** in theca cells that becomes substrate for estrogen production in the granulosa cells (Fig. 81.8).
5. LH also stimulates granulosa cells to produce progesterone. Therefore, progesterone concentration also increases.

Late Tertiary Stage: Between 5th to 7th days of follicular phase, only one follicle grows sufficiently to become **the dominant follicle**.

The aromatase activity and number of FSH receptors increase in the granulosa cells of dominant follicle.

- This increases the **synthesis of estrogen**, and more concentration of estrogen allows the dominant follicles to prime the hypothalamo-pituitary axis to generate LH surge just prior to ovulation.
- Under normal conditions, estrogen inhibits LH secretion.

1. But, when the plasma concentration of estrogen reaches about 200 pg/ml and maintains that high concentration for about 36 hours, estrogen stimulates LH secretion.
   - Thus, the **positive feedback effect on LH** increases more secretion of LH. This leads to **LH surge**, which causes ovulation (see below).
   - This positive feedback on LH secretion is due to the effect of estrogen both at the levels of hypothalamus and pituitary.
2. LH **increases progesterone secretion**, which increases the **proteolytic enzyme activity** and causes the distention of follicle due to rapid **increase in follicular fluid volume**.

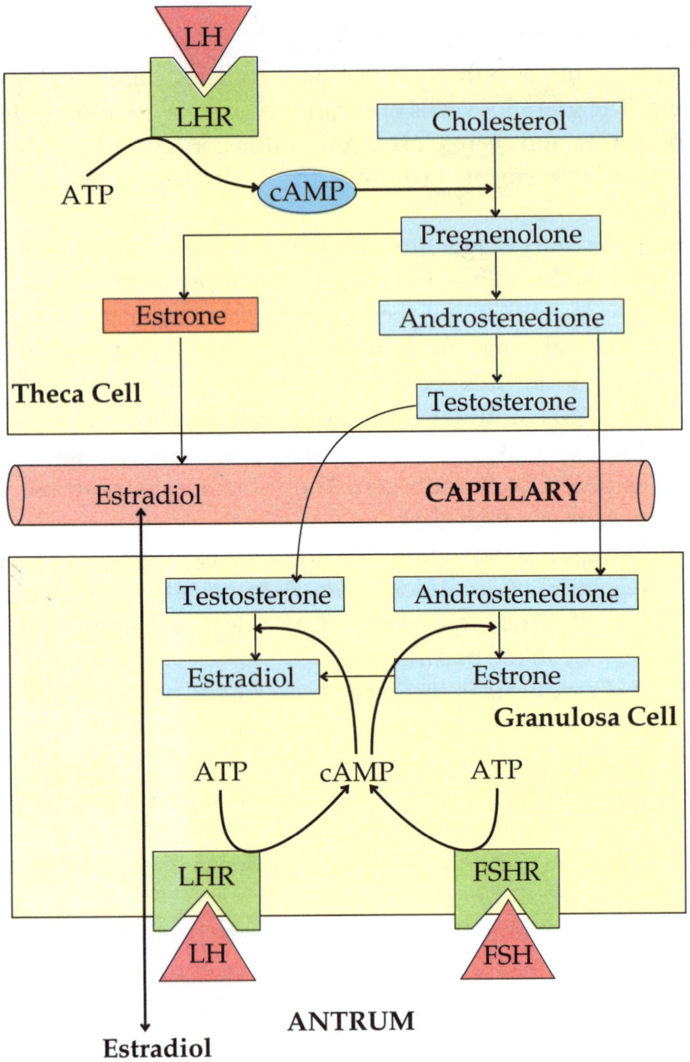

Fig. 81.8: Interaction of theca cell with granulosa cells. LHR: Luteinizing hormone receptor; FSHR: FSH receptor.

- LH also stimulates the activity of endoperoxide synthase that increases **synthesis of prostaglandins** and leukotrienes.

2. **Prostaglandins cause lysis of follicular wall** leading to rupture of follicle.
    - Breaking down of follicular wall is facilitated by the proteolytic enzyme **plasmin**.
    - FSH, by stimulating the **activity of plasminogen activator** facilitates the formation of plasmin.
3. **Oxytocin causes contraction of follicular wall** and extrudes the oocyte. This is called **ovulation**.
    - Immediately after LH surge, the number of LH receptors decreases.
    - This desensitizes granulosa and theca cells to LH.

OVULATION

Ovulation is the **process of release of ovum** (oocyte) from the ovary that results from rupture of Graafian follicle at the end of the follicular phase of the menstrual cycle.

- Usually, ovulation **occurs on 14th day** in a 28 days cycle.
- However, if the cycle length is altered, ovulation occurs 14 days before the onset of menstrual bleeding as the **duration of luteal phase (which is 14 days) always remains constant.**

Mechanism of Ovulation

Ovulation occurs due to midcycle **LH surge.**

1. LH surge occurs due to high rise in estrogen concentration towards the later part of follicular phase that provides a **positive feedback effect on LH secretion** from pituitary.
    - Normally, a mild to moderate increase in estrogen for a brief period is inhibitory on LH secretion.
2. **Two-days prior to ovulation**, ***estrogen concentration increases*** to a higher level and when this high concentration is maintained for about 36 hours, the process of ovulation is initiated.
    - A series of biochemical and morphological changes occur in ovarian follicle that culminates in **follicular rupture**.
3. **Three chemical substances** are involved in rupture of ovarian follicle: **prostaglandins, cyclin D_2** (a protein that regulates cell cycle) and **C-EBP** (CCAAT-enhancer binding protein).
    - Decreased formation of these chemicals in ovary has been demonstrated to prevent ovulation in mice.

Steps of Follicular Rupture

1. LH surge increases release of **prostaglandins and bradykinin** that increase the ovarian blood flow. Thus, **follicular blood flow increases**.
    - The dominant follicle becomes **highly vascularized** and edematous.
    - This **increases the size** of the follicle **to about 25 mm**.
3. Follicular blood flow also **increases antral fluid volume**, which in turn exerts pressure on the surrounding granulosa cells. The **cumulus-oophorus complex gets detached** from the follicular wall.
4. The **basement membrane** that separates granulosa cells and theca cells **disintegrates** due to intrafollicular pressure and the effects of proteolytic enzymes.
5. LH promotes **synthesis of plasminogen activator** by granulosa and theca cells, which causes conversion of plasminogen to plasmin.
    - Plasmin causes **proteolysis of follicular wall**.
    - Plasmin also activates the **synthesis of collagenase** that causes destruction of connective tissue matrix of the follicular wall and adjacent ovarian capsule.
6. Increased **intrafollicular pressure** and **degeneration of follicular wall** facilitate the rupture of the follicle,

which results in expulsion of oocyte from the follicle and the ovary.

FSH surge is not essential for ovulation (Application Box 81.2)

Application Box 81.2

FSH surge occurs simultaneously: It should be noted that though midcycle FSH surge also occurs almost simultaneously along with LH surge, FSH surge is not essential for ovulation. However, FSH primes the follicular cells to express adequate number of LH receptors.

Indicators of Ovulation

It is important to know the day of ovulation for its physiological and clinical significance. The indicators of ovulation are as follows:

1. **Rise in of basal body temperature:** The basal body temperature (BBT) increases during ovulation by about 0.5°C. Accurate charting of this temperature can exactly detect the day of ovulation.
   - It is recorded orally, early in the morning before getting up of the bed, and before taking any drink or washing the mouth.
   - The increase in body temperature is due to the **influence of progesterone** that starts increasing with the beginning of secretory phase. Progesterone is thermogenic.
2. **Fleeting lower abdominal pain (Mittelschmerz):** With ovulation, bleeding occurs into the antrum of the follicle.
   - Small amount of **blood also escapes into the abdominal cavity**, which causes peritoneal irritation and produces fleeting (short-lived) lower abdominal pain.
   - This is called as **mittelschmerz**.
3. **Vaginal discharge (spotting):** There may be **transitory increase in vaginal discharge** during ovulation.
   - When rise in BBT is associated with mittelschmerz and spotting, they are collectively called as **ovulation cascade**.
   - If all the three features are present, occurrence of ovulation is almost confirmed.
4. **Spinnbarkeit:** In the proliferative phase, estrogen makes the cervical mucous thin and alkaline.
   - With the beginning of secretory phase, progesterone secreted from corpus luteum makes the cervical mucous thick and tenacious. Thus, **uterine mucous is thinnest at the time of ovulation and its elasticity is maximal**.
   - Therefore, a drop of cervical mucous collected at the time of ovulation can be **stretched to as long as 10 cm or more** like a thread. This elastic nature of the mucous is called **spinnbarkeit.**
   - **Decreased elasticity indicates ovulation** has already taken place.
5. **Fern test:** Under the effect of estrogen, the cervical mucous **before ovulation forms an arborizing fern like pattern**, when the mucous is spread on a slide.
   - This is confirmed by microscopic examination of the mucous smear (Fig. 81.9).
   - Following ovulation, due to progesterone effect, the mucous become thick and fern pattern is not observed in smear of the mucous.
6. **Laparoscopic observation:** Demonstrating ovum in the abdominal cavity by laparoscopy confirms ovulation.
7. **Demonstration of LH peak:** LH surge occurs just prior to ovulation. Therefore, daily estimation of plasma LH in the periovulatory period will accurately detect the day of ovulation.

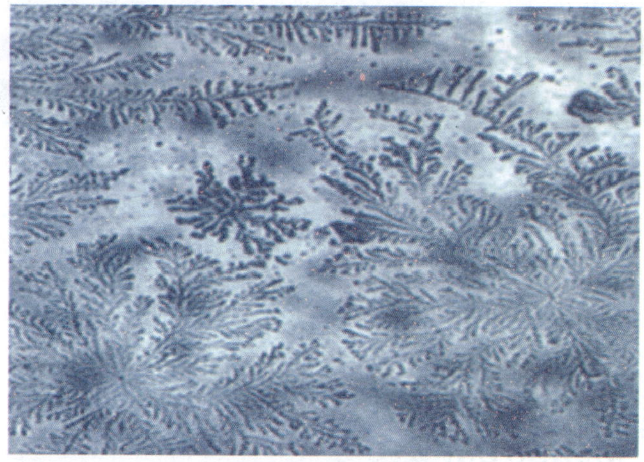

Fig. 81.9: Microscopic view of fern pattern of cervical mucus.

Physiological Importance

Determination of day of ovulation **helps in family planning.**

1. The life span of ovum is about 72 hours.
2. Therefore, those who are **desirous of a child**, should have regular sexual act in the periovulatory period (day of ovulation, and two days before and after the ovulation)
3. **Those who want to avoid pregnancy**, should not have unprotected sexual act during the unsafe period (day of ovulation, four days before and after ovulation) of the cycle (Fig. 81.10).
4. Thus, it helps in **planning both conception and contraception** (for details, see "Female Contraceptives").

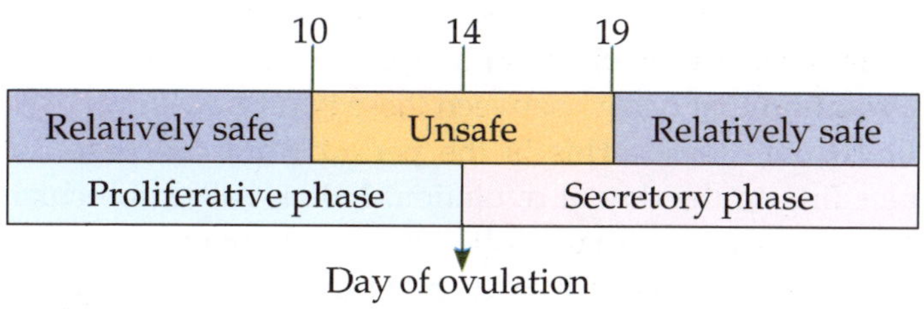

Fig. 81.10: Unsafe and safe periods in menstrual cycle. In regular cycles of 28 days, ovulation occurs on 14th day. Four days before and after ovulation (10th to 19th day of the cycle) is called unsafe period as unprotected sex leads to conception. Rest of the period is considered relatively safe, as chance of conception is minimal during these days.

Anovulation

Absence of ovulation during a menstrual cycle is called anovulatory cycle.

1. **Following menarche**, menstrual cycles may be anovulatory for first 1 to 2 years.
2. Few cycles may also be anovulatory in **lactating woman**, and about six months **before menopause**.
3. Anovulation also occurs in severe strenuous exercise or severer job-related stress.
4. Except these physiological situations, anovulation is abnormal and occurs mainly due to **hormonal deficiencies**.

Treatment of anovulation: Clomiphene, that binds with estrogen receptors and blocks estrogen action, induces ovulation. Clomiphene increases LH and FSH secretion by *reducing the negative effects of estrogen*.

MENSTRUAL CYCLE

The reproductive functions in women exhibit cyclical changes that occur regularly over a period of about one month. In human beings and primates, the reproductive cycle externally manifests by periodic vaginal bleeding, called as **menstruation**. Therefore, the cycle is called menstrual cycle.

Duration & Phases of Menstrual Cycle

Duration

The length of menstrual cycle usually averages at about 28 days. However, the duration of cycles is never fixed in all women. Also, the duration of all cycles is not same in one woman. This is because menstrual cycle is frequently influenced by psychological, environmental, nutritional and social factors.

1. Normally, it ranges from 21 to 35 days.
   - The cycle is described by number of days, the first day being the ***day of beginning of menstrual bleeding***.
2. Physiologically, menstrual cycle temporarily ceases during pregnancy and lactation.

Phases of Menstrual Cycle

Characteristically, the menstrual cycle is divided into two phases: **follicular phase and luteal phase**, separated by **ovulation** that occurs between these two phases.

Follicular Phase: This is the period from the onset of bleeding to the day of ovulation. This is called follicular phase as the **dominant follicle** in ovary matures in this phase to terminate in ovulation at the end of the phase.

- This phase has **two parts**: the ***menstrual phase*** (the phase of menstrual bleeding), and the ***proliferative phase*** (phase of proliferation of the uterine endometrium).
- Follicular phase is also called **preovulatory phase**.

Luteal Phase: This is the part of menstrual cycle between **ovulation and the onset of the next menstrual bleeding.**

- This is called **luteal phase** as corpus luteum is formed in the ovary, which mainly controls activities of this phase.
  - This is also called the **secretory phase** as uterine endometrium is highly secretory during this phase.
- Luteal phase is also called **postovulatory phase**

Length of Each Phase of Cycle

In a 28 days cycle, the follicular phase is of 14 days (1–14 days) and the luteal phase is of 14 days (15 to 28 days).

- However, **alteration of the length** of menstrual cycle occurs due to **alteration in the duration of follicular phase**.
- Once ovulation occurs, **menstrual bleeding starts after 14 days** of ovulation.
- Thus, the **length of the luteal phase remains constant** irrespective of the cycle length.

Menstrual cycle is sometimes loosely divided into ***four phases***: bleeding phase, follicular phase, ovulatory phase and luteal phase.

- However, it should be remembered that *bleeding phase is part of the follicular phase* and ovulation is not a separate phase, but an event that occurs at the junction between proliferative and secretory phases of the cycle.

Changes in Reproductive Organs in Menstrual Cycle

Changes in the Follicular Phase

(Menstrual & Proliferative Phase)

Ovarian Changes

In the follicular phase, one follicle is selected to become the **dominant follicle** by 4th day. The ***mechanism of selection of a follicle*** to grow is not known.

1. The dominant follicle **develops into mature follicle** (details follicular development, described earlier in this chapter).
2. The **granulosa and theca interna cells** of the follicle proliferate and **secrete estrogen**.
3. The **antrum increases in size** and **stromal fluid increases in volume**.
4. The distended **follicle ruptures** at about 14th day resulting in **ovulation**.

Uterine Changes

In the early part of the follicular phase, along with the menstrual bleeding, layers of the uterine endometrium are sloughed. Under the influence of estrogen secreted from the developing follicle, **thickness of endometrium rapidly increases** from 5th to 14th day of the cycle.

During this process, ***following uterine changes*** occur (Fig. 81.11 C):

1. The uterine **endometrium undergoes hyperplasia and hypertrophy** and increases in size and thickness.
2. The **endometrial glands lengthen and glands are drawn out**. The glands are lined with columnar epithelium.
3. The endometrium is vascularized with **formation of more number of spiral arteries** that increase blood supply to the deeper layers. Increased blood supply further promotes growth of uterine mucosa.
4. Endometrial veins also grow in size.
5. **Myometrial excitability increases** due to the effect of estrogen.

As proliferation of endometrium is the major feature in this phase of the cycle, this is called proliferative phase. This is also called **preovulatory phase** as the changes occur before ovulation.

Change in Uterine Cervix

Under the effects of estrogen, **volume of cervical mucous increases**.

1. The **alkalinity and elasticity** of cervical mucous also increase.
2. This forms the physiological basis for **spinnbarkeit.**
3. The cervical epithelium becomes more **secretory**. Sperm easily passes through the estrogen-dependent cervical mucous.

Vaginal Changes

During this phase, under the influence of estrogen, vaginal **epithelial cells become cornified** (keratinized). The **cornification index increases** from almost zero on day 1 to about 100 on 14th day.

Changes in the Luteal Phase

(Secretory Phase)

Ovarian Changes

Luteal phase starts after ovulation. Following ovulation, follicle is **rapidly filled with blood**. Therefore, the follicle is called **corpus hemorrhagicum**. The blood clot inside the follicle is replaced by proliferation of granulosa cells.

- The granulosa and theca cells of the follicle undergo **luteinization** to become granulosa lutein cells and theca lutein cells. Thus, the follicle develops into **corpus luteum** (Fig. 81.11 D).
- The luteal cells secrete progesterone and estrogen.
- If pregnancy occurs, corpus luteum persists; otherwise, it degenerates between 26th to 28th days, and forms **corpus albicans**.

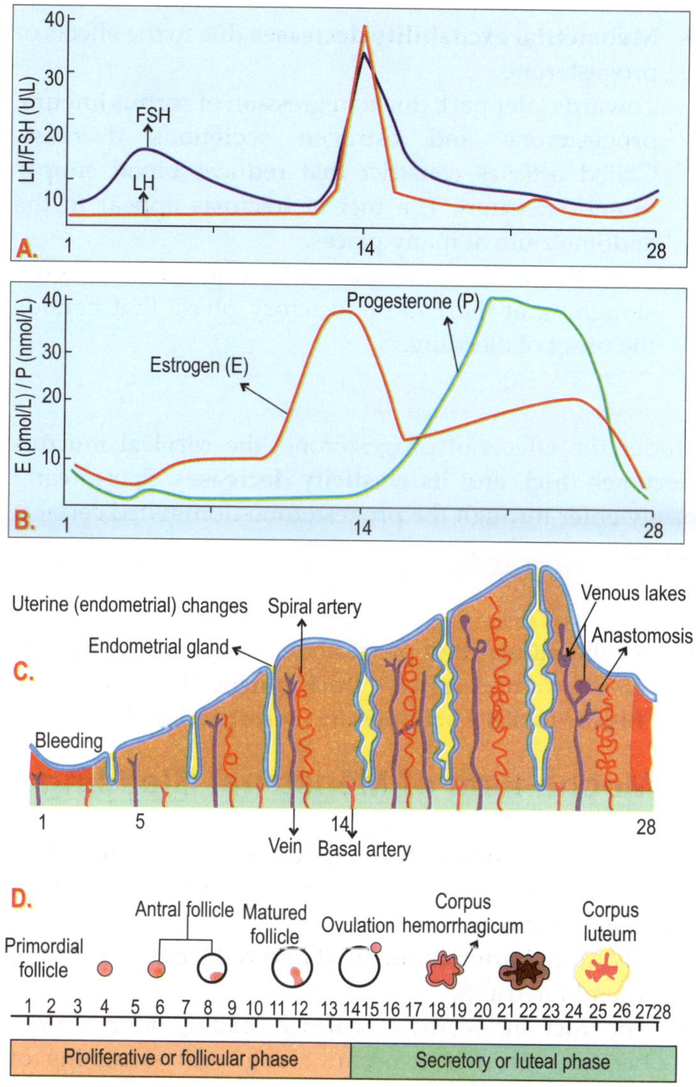

Figs. 81.11: Changes in reproductive organs and secretion of hormones in menstrual cycle. **A:** Changes in LH and FSH level; **B:** Changes in estrogen and progesterone level; **C:** Endometrial changes; **D:** Follicular changes. LH: luteinizing hormone; FSH: follicle-stimulating hormone.

Uterine Changes

During the luteal phase, progesterone secretion increases significantly. Estrogen secretion also increases to some extent. Therefore, following uterine changes occur under the combined effects of estrogen and progesterone. However, major changes are due to the effects of progesterone.

1. The uterine glands become **coiled and tortuous.**
2. The glandular cells store glycogen and secrete **large quantity of carbohydrate-rich mucous and fluid.** Therefore, this phase is called **secretory phase.**
3. The **vascularity of endometrium increases further** due to combined effects of estrogen and progesterone secreted from corpus luteum. **Spiral arteries become tortuous** (Fig. 81.11 C).
4. Due to increased blood supply and increased secretion, the endometrium becomes edematous and thick.
5. Endometrial veins form **venous lakes and anastomoses.**

6. **Myometrial excitability decreases** due to the effects of progesterone.
7. Towards later part, due to regression of corpus luteum, progesterone and estrogen secretions decrease. Coiled arteries constrict that reduces blood supply to endometrium. The **foci of necrosis** appear in the endometrium at many places.
8. **Necrotic areas coalesce** and endometrium starts sloughing at the end of secretory phase that heralds the onset of bleeding.

Change in Cervical Mucous

Under the effects of progesterone, the **cervical mucous becomes thick and its elasticity decreases**. Sperm can't easily enter through the progesterone-dominated cervical mucous.

Vaginal Changes

Under the influence of progesterone, **vaginal epithelium proliferates** and secretes a **thick mucus**. The epithelium is infiltrated with leucocytes and **cornification decreases**.

Mechanism of Menstrual Bleeding

When **corpus luteum degenerates**, hormonal support of endometrium is withdrawn. This causes the ***endometrium to become necrotic***.

- The **coiled arteries constrict** and reduce blood supply to endometrium.
- The **foci of necrosis coalesce** leading to confluent hemorrhage, which occurs along with sloughing of endometrium.
- This results in menstrual bleeding.

Mechanism: The mechanism is **initiated by decreased secretion of steroid hormones**.

1. Reduction in steroids causes **destabilization of lysosomal membranes** in the endometrial cells, which leads to release of **proteolytic enzymes** and **production of prostaglandins**, especially **$PGF_{2\alpha}$**.
2. The proteolytic enzymes cause **lysis of the endometrial tissue** and $PGF_{2\alpha}$ causes vasospasm producing **endometrial ischemia** (Application Box 81.3). The ischemic changes result in **areas of local necrosis**, which is facilitated by proteolytic damage.
3. The **foci of necrosis join with each other** that result in sloughing of the uterine endometrium.

Application Box 81.3

Prostaglandins cause menstrual cramps: Vasoconstriction and uterine contractions are mediated by prostaglandins formed in the endometrium in response to the decrease in plasma estrogen and progesterone. The main mechanism of dysmenorrhea (menstrual cramps) is overproduction of prostaglandins causing excessive uterine contractions. Prostaglandins also cause smooth muscle contraction in other parts of body that accounts for nausea, vomiting, and headache associated with dysmenorrhea.

Amount of Loss

During a normal menstruation, about **30–130 ml of blood** is lost. The menstrual blood contains tissue debris, prostaglandins and fibrinolysin. Increased menstrual loss is known as **menorrhagia** and decreased loss as **hypomenorrhea**.

Hormonal Changes in Menstrual Cycle

Estrogen

Estrogen has **two peaks** in the menstrual cycle.

1. **The fist peak**, which is the major peak, occurs about 48 hours before ovulation and **the second peak**, which the minor peak, occurs in the post-midluteal phase (Fig. 81.11 B).
2. With the growth of ovarian follicle, estrogen concentration slowly increases in the early part of follicular phase. The concentration **rises rapidly** from 8th day of cycle to **reach the peak about one or two days before ovulation**. The concentration decreases thereafter and decreases further after ovulation.
3. About two days after ovulation, (after the formation of corpus luteum), again ***estrogen concentration increases*** slowly to reach a **smaller peak** that occurs just after the midsecretory phase.

Progesterone

Progesterone concentration is minimal in the proliferative phase.

1. It starts rising following ovulation and reaches **peak in 4 to 5 days after ovulation**.
2. The **peak is maintained till corpus luteum is active**.
3. With regression of corpus luteum, progesterone concentration decreases towards the end of luteal phase.

LH

The concentration of LH remains low almost throughout the proliferative phase. However, about a day before ovulation, the **secretion of LH increases sharply** to reach the peak about 8–10 hours before ovulation.

- This is called **LH surge**.
- Then, it declines fast in 24–48 hours and remains low in rest of the secretory phase (Fig. 81.11 A).

FSH

FSH secretion **increases in the early part of the follicular phase** (during menstrual bleeding), and then declines slowly.

- Synchronous with the rise in LH, secretion of FSH **rises towards ovulation** and thereafter the pattern of change in FSH is similar with LH pattern.

Inhibins

The pattern of change in concentration of **inhibin B coincides with the change in concentration of FSH**, whereas the concentration of **inhibin A coincides with the pattern of progesterone**.

Disorders of Menstrual Cycle

Amenorrhea

Absence of menstrual cycle is referred to as amenorrhea. Amenorrhea is broadly classified into two categories: **primary and secondary**, and each category subdivided into ***physiological and pathological***.

Primary Amenorrhea

When menstruation has never occurred, the condition is called primary amenorrhea. There are physiological and pathological causes.

Physiological Primary Amenorrhea: Physiological amenorrhea is more common.

1. *Before puberty:* Amenorrhea is normal in childhood and prepubertal age. Usually, menstruation starts at the age of 12–14 years.
2. *Constitutional amenorrhea:* Though menstrual cycle starts normally before the age of 16 years, sometimes it may not occur even at the age of 18 years or more, without there being any abnormality. This is called *constitutional amenorrhea*.

Pathological Primary Amenorrhea: It is pathological when menstrual cycle *does not start till the age of 18 years*.

1. **Congenital and genetic defects,** such as Turner syndrome, Kallman syndrome etc.
2. **Congenital malformations** of reproductive tract like absence of uterus.

Secondary Amenorrhea

When menstrual cycle stops in a woman ***who had normal cycles before***, the condition is called secondary amenorrhea.

Physiological Secondary Amenorrhea: Physiological causes are more common than pathological causes.

1. *Peri-pubertal amenorrhea:* In first one to two years of onset of menarche, menstrual cycles are often anovulatory and therefore irregular.
2. *Pregnancy:* Pregnancy is the ***commonest cause of secondary amenorrhea***.
3. *Lactation:* In a lactating mother, high prolactin inhibits the secretion of GnRH, and therefore, ovulation is prevented. This is called **lactational amenorrhea**. This causes physiological contraception.
4. *Emotional disturbance:* Psychological trauma frequently causes amenorrhea by disrupting hypothalamic release of GnRH via limbic-hypothalamic connections.
5. *Change in environment:* Sudden change of place, especially exposure to extremes of climates produces amenorrhea during the acclimatization period.
6. *Menopause:* Menstrual cycle ceases at menopause.

Pathological Secondary Amenorrhea: Pathological secondary amenorrhea occurs due to a defect in hypothalamus, pituitary, ovary and uterus or due to a systemic disease or chronic use of some drugs.

1. *Hypothalamic disorders:* Hypothalamic diseases resulting in **decreased secretion of GnRH** leads to amenorrhea.
2. *Pituitary disorders:* Tumors and other diseases of pituitary (**hypopituitarism**) resulting in decreased secretion of gonadotropins leads to amenorrhea.
3. *Ovarian diseases:* Diseases that ***decrease the production of estrogen and progesterone***, frequently lead to amenorrhea. Example, Stein-Leventhal syndrome (a polycystic ovarian disease).
4. *Uterine pathology:* Congenital absence of uterus, underdeveloped uterus and severe infective or non-infective endometritis produce amenorrhea.
5. **Systemic illness:** Amenorrhea occurs in chronic illnesses like chronic hypothyroidism, chronic renal failure and cirrhosis of liver.
6. *Drugs:* Phenothiazine derivatives, reserpine, ganglion blocking agents and estrogen-progesterone preparations (pill contraceptives) are common drugs that prevent menstrual cycles.

Hypomenorrhea and Oligomenorrhea

Hypomenorrhea: **Decreased menstrual bleeding** in duration or amount or both is called hypomenorrhea. It may be constitutional, or due to uterine pathology or due to hormonal disorders.

Oligomenorrhea: **Decreased frequency** (cycle more than 35 days) of menstrual cycle is called **oligomenorrhea.** Usually, oligomenorrhea occurs in ***ovarian diseases*** in which menstruation is irregular and infrequent.

Dysmenorrhea

Dysmenorrhea means **painful menstrual bleeding**. It is classified into two categories:

1. **Primary dysmenorrhea** in which there is no visible pelvic pathology, and
2. **Secondary dysmenorrhea** in which a uterine or pelvic pathology is associated with it. Usually, it occurs due to passage of clots in flow.

Other Menstrual Problems

Menorrhagia: ***Increased menstrual bleeding*** in amount, duration or both is called menorrhagia.

1. It is generally caused by conditions that affect **uterus and its vascular apparatus** rather than any ovarian dysfunction.

2. Or, sometimes it may be a manifestation of **coagulation disorder**.

Metrorrhagia: Bleeding occurring **between the periods** (acyclical and irregular) is called metrorrhagia. It usually indicates a *surface lesion in the genital tract*, which may be benign or malignant.

Polymenorrhea: When menstrual cycle **occurs frequently** (less than 21 days), it is called polymenorrhea. Usually, the amount and duration of bleeding remain normal.

Premenstrual Syndrome

Few women develop some nonspecific features about a week before the onset of menstrual bleeding that are combinely called as premenstrual syndrome (PMS) or **premenstrual dysphoric disorder** (PMDD).

Features: The usual features are edema, painful or swollen breasts, depression, loss of concentration, irritability, headache, behavioral changes and emotional disturbances. These features disappear within 1–3 days after the start of menstruation.

Etiology: Though the salt and water retention has mainly been attributed to PMS, the exact cause of it is not known.

Treatment: Treatment with alprazolam (**minor tranquilizer**), prozac (**serotonin uptake inhibitor**) and **GnRH agonist** gives some relief.

Anorexia Nervosa

It is a complex behavioral disorder in women which manifests as severe anorexia (loss of food intake) associated with functional abnormalities.

1. **Amenorrhea** is seen in 30–40% of cases.
2. Patient is grossly **emaciated.**
3. Emaciation (low body fat) and stress **inhibit LH secretion** through endorphins.
4. Pubic hair development and breast development usually remain unaffected.

PY9.5

OVARIAN HORMONES

Ovary secretes **estrogens, progesterone, inhibins and relaxin**.

Estrogens

The naturally synthesized estrogens are **17β-estradiol, estrone, and estriol**. Estradiol is 15 and 80 times more potent than estrone and estriol respectively.

Source

Estrogen is secreted from **granulosa cells of ovarian follicles, corpus luteum, and placenta**.

- Estrogen is not directly secreted from **adrenal gland**, but adrenal androgen is converted to estrogen by the enzyme aromatase.

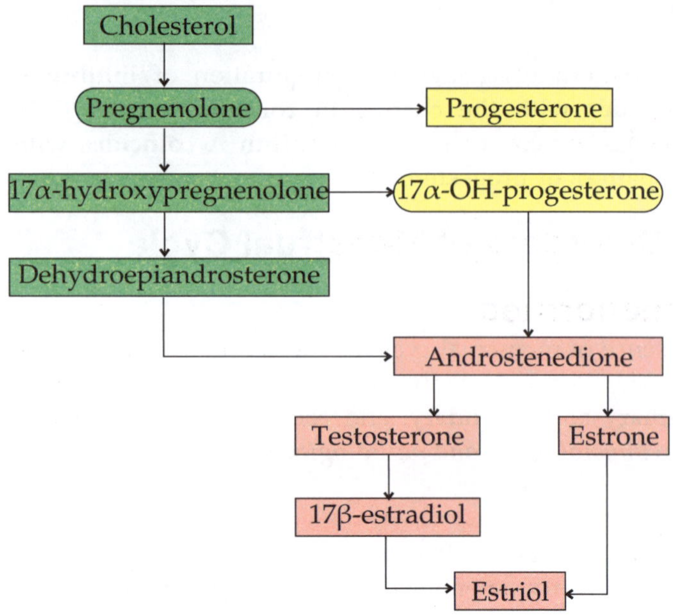

Fig. 81.12: Synthesis of estrogens.

Synthesis

Estrogen is a steroid hormone, synthesized from cholesterol (Fig. 81.12). **LH, acting on LH receptors** located on **theca interna cells** converts cholesterol to androstenedione.

- **In theca cells**, some androstenedione is converted into estradiol, but **most of it is supplied to granulosa cells to be converted into estrogen** in those cells.
- **FSH acting on the FSH receptors** on the granulosa cells facilitates the *conversion of androgen to estrogen* by activating the activity of the enzyme aromatase.
- However, mature **granulosa cells** also acquire LH receptors and **directly form estrogen**.

Secretion and Metabolism

Estrogen secretion occurs in **two peaks** during the menstrual cycle.

- A **larger peak** occurs during proliferative phase just before ovulation and a **smaller peak** in the midsecretory phase.
- The rate of secretion of estradiol is about 35 μg per day in the early follicular phase, **400 μg per day just before ovulation** and 250 μg per day in the midluteal phase.

About **98% of circulating estrogen is bound to proteins.** In liver, estrogens are metabolized through oxidation or are converted to their **glucuronide and sulfate derivatives** that are excreted in urine.

Mechanism of Action

Like other steroid hormones, estrogen binds with the receptor in the nucleus and increases the formation of mRNA.

- There are **two types of estrogen receptors**: ERα and ERβ.

- ERα are present mainly on uterus, liver, kidney and heart, and ERβ are present in ovaries, brain, GI tract, hemopoietic tissues, lungs and prostate.

- Estrogens have both **genomic and nongenomic actions**.
- **Most of the actions are genomic** that are mediated via production of mRNA.

Physiological Actions

Effects on Female Reproductive System

Estrogen promotes growth of all components of female reproductive system. In general, it causes growth of smooth muscle and proliferation of epithelial lining of reproductive tract.

On Ovary: Estrogen stimulates **growth of ovary and ovarian follicles**. Role of estrogen on follicular growth has been described in Chapter 128 'Follicular development'.

On Fallopian Tubes: Estrogen stimulates smooth muscle **contraction of fallopian tubes** and therefore increases ***fallopian tube motility***. It also increases ***ciliary activity*** of the tubes.

On Uterus: Estrogen has wide ranging effects on uterus.

1. It **increases uterine size**. Therefore, in prepubertal girls the uterus is small with thin myometrium.
2. During the follicular phase of menstrual cycle, estrogen causes **proliferation of uterine endometrium**.
3. During luteal phase, along with progesterone, it **increases uterine fluid secretion**. It also increases progesterone receptor on uterine endometrium.
   - Thus, estrogen prepares endometrium for progesterone action.
4. It **increases uterine blood flow**. Therefore, it increases myometrial size (Application Box 81.4).
5. It increases the **content of contractile proteins** in uterine smooth muscles. It increases the activity and **excitability of uterine muscle**.
   - It also increases the **sensitivity of uterus to oxytocin**.
   - Estrogen secretion increases towards term and all these uterine changes prepare the uterus for **parturition**.

Application Box 81.4

Withdrawal bleeding and breakthrough bleeding: Chronic estrogen treatment causes excessive endometrial hypertrophy. In such patients, discontinuation of therapy causes sloughing of the uterine endometrium that produces bleeding. This is called withdrawal bleeding. Sometimes, bleeding also occurs during the course of treatment of estrogen over a longer period. This is called breakthrough bleeding.

Effects on Cervical Mucus: Under the influence of estrogen, cervical mucus becomes **abundant, clear, and watery**. These characteristics become more pronounced at the *time of ovulation* to allow sperm to easily pass through the cervical mucus barrier on their way to the uterus and fallopian tubes.

Effects on Breast: Estrogen causes **breast enlargement** during puberty. Therefore, it is known as **"growth hormone of the breast"**.

- It causes growth of ducts of the mammary gland.
- It also causes pigmentation of the areola.

Effects on Secondary Sexual Characteristics

At the time of puberty, secondary sexual characteristics develop in girls due to the effects of estrogen.

1. ***Female body configuration:*** Narrow shoulders and broad hips.
2. ***Wide carrying angle:*** Thighs that converge and arms that diverge.
3. ***Female distribution of fat:*** Fat deposition in the hips and breast (breast enlargement).
4. Voice remains **high pitched**, as no change in larynx occurs.
5. Less hair on the body and more hair on the scalp.
6. ***Pubic Hair:*** Female escutcheon of pubic hair. Pubic hair distribution in females forms a triangle with **base upward and apex downward**.
7. ***Internal Genitalia:*** Vagina, uterus, ovary, fallopian tube grow in size and functions (as described above).

It is reported that growth of pubic and axillary hairs occurs due to androgen in females rather than estrogen.

Effects on Endocrine Organs

Estrogen has wide ranging endocrine effects.

1. Estrogen **inhibits LH secretion** by its negative feedback effects directly on pituitary and by indirectly inhibiting GnRH secretion from hypothalamus. However, before ovulation, the feedback becomes positive that results in LH surge.
2. Estrogen **inhibits FSH secretion**.
3. It **stimulates prolactin secretion**. However, it inhibits the milk producing action of prolactin on breast.
4. It **promotes the synthesis of angiotensinogen** from liver.
   - Thus, it **activates renin-angiotensin system**.
   - By increasing the formation of angiotensin II, it **increases blood pressure**, especially when estrogen is taken for a longer period; for example as ***contraceptive pill***.
5. Estrogen **increases the formation of thyroxine-binding globulin**.
   - Therefore, the **free thyroxine concentration decreases** in estrogen therapy and also in later part of pregnancy when estrogen concentration is high.
6. It **stimulates androgen secretion** from adrenal cortex (Application Box 81.5).

Application Box 81.5

Estrogen stimulates growth of animals: In farm animals, commercially available estrogen injections are given to increase the body weight of the animal. This occurs due to the **protein anabolic effect** of estrogen, which is **induced by increased androgen** secretion from adrenal cortex. Estrogen injection is known to promote growth of chickens and cattle.

Effects on CNS

By **activating neurons in the limbic system**, estrogen stimulates **libido**. Especially, acting on the suprachiasmatic area of hypothalamus, it produces **sexual behaviors**.

Effects on Musculoskeletal System

Estrogen **stimulates bone growth**.

1. It **prevents osteoclastic activity**.
   - Therefore, estrogen **prevents osteoporotic activity**.
2. Estrogen causes **epiphyseal closure**.
   - Hence, it causes ***cessation of longitudinal growth*** of bone and therefore, **determines the height** of the female.
3. Estrogen has *no direct effect* on growth of skeletal muscle. However, by stimulating ***androgen secretion***, it **facilitates skeletal muscle development**.

Effects on Water and Electrolyte Metabolisms

Estrogen promotes **salt and water retention** to some extent by directly acting on kidney tubules.

- This contributes to **ECF expansion and hypertension** in chronic estrogen therapy, in addition to its activation of renin-angiotensin system.

Effects on Lipid Profile

Estrogen is a strong **cholesterol lowering agent**, and therefore, it **prevents atherosclerosis**. Estrogen also increases HDL concentration in plasma.

Effects on Sebaceous Secretion & Skin

From sebaceous gland, estrogen promotes more fluid secretions. This antagonizes the thick sebaceous secretion of androgen. Thus, estrogen **inhibits the formation of acne.** Chronic high estrogen levels may produce cutaneous angiomas (Clinical Note 81.4)

Clinical Note 81.4

Hyperestrogenemia in liver diseases: Androstenedione is metabolized in liver. Therefore, in advanced liver diseases, circulating androstenedione concentration increases, that facilitates their conversion into estrogen. Hence, spider angiomas and breast enlargement are features of advanced stage of liver diseases.

Estrogen Preparations

Synthetic estrogens are selective estrogen receptor modulators. Examples are tamoxifen and raloxifene.

Progesterone

Source, Synthesis and Metabolism

Progesterone is secreted from **corpus luteum, placenta and ovarian follicle**. It is also an intermediate product in many steroid biosynthesis.

- It is formed from pregnenolone. The plasma concentration of progesterone in **follicular phase** is about **0.9 ng/mL**, and in **luteal phase** at its peak is **18 ng/mL**.
- Progesterone is mainly **bound to plasma proteins**. Only 2% circulates freely in plasma.
- In the liver, it is converted to **pregnanediol**, which forms **glucuronide conjugates** and excreted in urine (Flowchart 81.1).

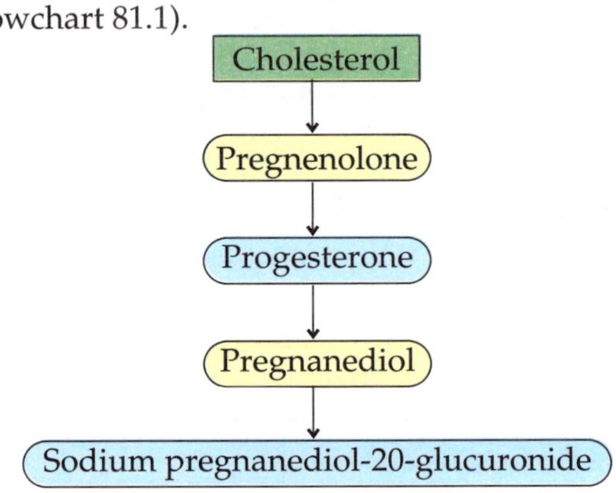

Flowchart 81.1: Synthesis and metabolism of progesterone.

Mechanism of Action

Like other steroid hormones, progesterone acts on the receptors located in the nucleus, and the biochemical mechanism of action is through increased **gene transcription**.

Physiological Actions

Effects on Reproductive Organs

Progesterone **inhibits uterine myometrial contractions**, by following mechanisms:

1. It **opposes the stimulatory actions of estrogen** and locally generated prostaglandins.
   - This is very important for **implantation of fertilized egg** and ***continuation of pregnancy***.
2. It increases the **rate of conversion** of 17β-estradiol to less-active estrogens.
3. Progesterone also directly **causes relaxation of uterine smooth muscles**.
4. It also **decreases excitability of myometrium** and the sensitivity of myometrium to oxytocin. Progesterone increases the membrane potential and decreases the spontaneous electrical activity of myometrial cells.
   - Uterine quiescence is maintained throughout pregnancy by progesterone, which is crucial

to **prevent premature expulsion of the fetus** (abortion).

5. It causes the **cervical mucus to become thick and sticky**; in essence, this **acts as a plug** that prevents infective organisms from vagina to enter the uterus.
   - This antibacterial blockage **protects the growing embryo** if conception has occurred.
6. Progesterone acts on estrogen-primed endometrium and **increases secretions from endometrial glands**. It inhibits proliferation of the cells lining the vagina.

Effects on Breast

It promotes growth of the breast, especially the **growth of the glandular tissue** (lobules and alveoli).

- It supports the differentiation of estrogen-prime ductal tissue.
- It also supports the **secretory functions** of breast during lactation.

Effects on Body Temperature

Immediately after ovulation, there is a small increase (approximately 0.5°C) in body temperature that occurs due to an action of progesterone on temperature regulatory centers in the brain. **Progesterone is thermogenic**.

Effects on Hypothalamo-Pituitary Axis

Progesterone has **negative feedback effects** on hypothalamo-pituitary axis.

- It **decreases LH secretion**.
- In large doses, it also potentiates the ***inhibitory effects*** of estrogen. Therefore, **it prevents ovulation**. Hence, it is used as a *contraceptive agent*.

Effects on Respiration

Progesterone **stimulates respiration and produces tachypnea**. Therefore, the PCO_2 decreases in pregnancy.

Effects on Blood Pressure

Progesterone **causes vasodilation** (relaxation of vascular smooth muscle). Therefore, **diastolic pressure decreases in pregnancy**.

- Thus, hypertension is never a feature of normal pregnancy.
- This also contributes to **wide pulse pressure in pregnancy** as systolic pressure increases due to ECF expansion.

On Electrolyte and Water Metabolisms

In large doses, progesterone produces **natriuresis and diuresis** by blocking the effects of aldosterone on kidney tubules.

Other Ovarian Hormones

Relaxin

Relaxin is a **polypeptide hormone**. Structurally it is similar to insulin and insulin like growth factors. The gene for relaxin is located on chromosome 9.

Source: Relaxin is secreted from **corpus luteum, placenta, uterus and breast** in females, and **prostate glands** in males. The secretion of relaxin increases towards later part of pregnancy reaching a peak just before term.

Functions:

1. It **relaxes pubic symphysis** and **pelvic joints and ligaments**.
2. It causes **softening and dilation of uterine cervix**. Thus it facilitates parturition.
3. It **inhibits uterine contraction**.
4. It promotes development of mammary gland.
5. In nonpregnant woman, it is secreted from corpus luteum in the secretory phase of menstrual cycle. However, its physiological significance is not known.
6. In males, it is secreted from prostate. It **facilitates sperm motility** and penetration of ovum by sperm.

Inhibins

Inhibins are secreted from granulosa cells of ovary. Inhibin **inhibits the secretion of FSH** from anterior pituitary (for details, refer 'Testicular Hormones').

Androgens

Androgens are secreted in women from **adrenal glands and ovaries**.

1. These androgens play some role in the female reproductive functions.
2. They **stimulate the growth of pubic and axillary hairs** and possibly they also promote **growth of skeletal muscle**.
3. They also help **maintain sexual desire**.
4. However, excess production leads to male body hair distribution, abnormal skeletal muscle growth, enlargement of clitoris and reduction in breast size.

CONTROL OF OVARIAN FUNCTIONS

Functions of ovaries:

1. Synthesis and **secretion of gonadal hormones**.
2. Release of oocyte (**ovulation**) at the end of proliferative phase of the menstrual cycle.
3. Nourishment and **development of resident oocytes**.
4. Preparation of fallopian tube to **facilitate fertilization**.
5. Preparation of uterus for **implantation** of fertilized ovum.
6. Providing **hormonal support** to the embryo till placenta starts functioning.

The ovarian functions are controlled by hormones secreted from **hypothalamus, anterior pituitary and ovary**.

Hypothalamic Control

Hypothalamus plays an important role in regulating ovarian functions by controlling the secretion of gonadotropins from anterior pituitary.

1. Hypothalamus secretes GnRH, which is released in **episodic bursts**.
   - This **episodic secretion of GnRH** determines circhoral peaks of LH secretion. A constant and steady release of GnRH inhibits, whereas episodic and pulsatile injection of GnRH stimulates LH secretion (Clinical Note 81.5).
2. Episodic secretion of GnRH not only stimulates LH secretion, but also regulates secretion of other hormones that **control menstrual cycle**.
   - The **frequency of GnRH burst** is important in **bringing the LH surge.**
3. Also, the sensitivity of gonadotrophs of anterior pituitary to the GnRH burst is important in bringing **LH surge**, which increases towards ovulation.
4. The higher concentration of **estrogen stimulates this frequency towards the later part of follicular phase** that finally culminates in LH surge.
5. However, the exact site of **GnRH pulse generator** in the hypothalamus is not known.
6. Progesterone, androgen, catecholamines, enkephalins and endorphins inhibit frequency of GnRH pulses.

Clinical Note 81.5

Long-acting GnRH analogs: As described above, a constantly elevated GnRH level in plasma inhibits LH secretion by down-regulating receptors on gonadotrophs. Therefore, long-acting GnRH analogs are used in treatment of precocious puberty as it inhibits LH secretion by chronically maintaining a GnRH level. It is also used in therapy of prostate cancer.

Pituitary Control

The anterior pituitary secretes LH and FSH. The major target organs of these hormones are gonads. Therefore they are called **gonadotropins**. Primarily, they control ovarian functions in both the phases of menstrual cycle. Ovarian control by gonadotropins has a similar analogy with testicular control (Clinical Note 81.6).

Clinical Note 81.6

Analogy with testis: The granulosa and theca cells of ovarian follicle are similar to the Sertoli and Leydig cells of testis.
Granulosa cells resemble Sertoli cells in their function by providing environment for development of oocyte, and for their control by FSH. Like Sertoli cells granulosa cells also secrete inhibin-B that controls FSH secretion from pituitary. The theca cells are like the Leydig cells in that they produce androgens and are stimulated mainly by LH.

Pattern of Secretion of Gonadotropins

Regulation by FSH: Ovarian follicle development requires stimulation by FSH.

1. **Before puberty,** the concentration of FSH in the plasma is too low to bring such development.
2. **After puberty**, during first half of each menstrual cycle, increase in FSH secretion stimulates follicular growth. FSH stimulates **proliferation of granulosa** cells to produce estrogen, and stimulates **enlargement of the antrum**.
3. FSH also primes the granulosa and theca cells to the effect of LH.

Regulation by LH: LH acts on the theca and granulosa cells.

- These cells are converted to luteal cells as follicle becomes corpus luteum after ovulation.
- LH **causes luteinization** of these cells.
- LH surge is responsible for ovulation to occur

Ovarian Control

Ovary controls its own functions by secreting hormones that directly influence granulosa cell function or indirectly influence **hypothalamic-pituitary-ovarian axis** (feedback control).

Pattern of Secretion of Gonadal Hormones

Estrogen: Estrogen secretion increases in the second week of cycle as the dominant ovarian follicle grows and secretes more estrogen.

1. **Estrogen peak occurs about two days before ovulation** and then decreases rapidly in next two days.
2. The second but **slow and small peak** of estrogen occurs in luteal phase due to its secretion from corpus luteum.

Progesterone: Progesterone release is low during the follicular phase.

1. But, soon after ovulation, progesterone concentration **increases rapidly in luteal phase** due to its release in large amount from corpus luteum.
2. Inhibin-B secretion resembles the secretory pattern of FSH.

Direct Regulation

Theca cells secrete androgen, which facilitates secretion of estrogen by the granulosa cells.

Feedback Regulation

The dominant follicle secretes estrogen that inhibits gonadotropins (the **negative feedback effect**) from pituitary and GnRH secretion from hypothalamus (Fig. 81.13).

1. When plasma concentration of estrogen is very high the secretion of gonadotropin increases (the **positive feedback effect**).
   - But, how exactly low concentration of estrogen exerts negative feedback inhibition and high

concentration provides positive feedback effect on the secretion of gonadotropins is not clearly known.

- However, the effect is partly mediated via hypothalamus.

2. Large dose of **progesterone inhibits LH secretion** and **potentiates the usual inhibitory effect of estrogen**. Therefore, **combination of estrogen and progesterone** is used in the prevention of ovulation.
3. The **increase in plasma inhibin** concentration in the luteal phase also contributes to the ***suppression of FSH secretion***.
   - Therefore, in the luteal phase, plasma concentrations of the gonadotropins are very low.

Thus, ovarian events via hormonal feedback mechanisms **control hypothalamus and anterior pituitary** secretions.

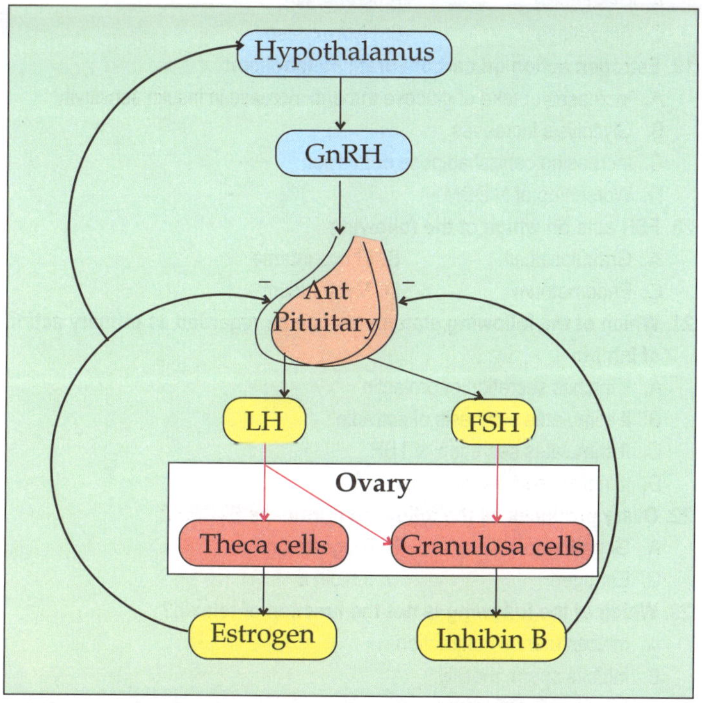

Fig. 81.13: Feedback regulation of ovarian functions. Minus sign is inhibition.

PY9.7

APPLIED ASPECTS

Reproductive abnormalities that either lead to or occur due to ovarian dysfunctions can broadly be classified into two categories: genetic and hormonal abnormalities.

Genetic & Hormonal Abnormalities

Following genetic abnormalities are common in women, and are associated with hormonal dysfunctions:

GnRH Resistance: This occurs due **to decreased number and sensitivity of GnRH receptors** on gonadotrophs of pituitary.

FSH Resistance: This occurs due to **decreased number and sensitivity of FSH receptors** on granulosa cells of pituitary.

LH Resistance: This occurs due to **decreased number and sensitivity of LH receptors** on granulosa and theca cells of ovarian follicles.

Aromatase Deficiency: Aromatase (CYP 19) converts testosterone to estradiol and androstenedione to estrone. Therefore, its deficiency leads to **estrogen deficiency and amenorrhea**.

McCune-Albright Syndrome: This is an example of **receptor protein (G protein) abnormality** in which $G_{S\alpha}$ is active in some cells and defective in others.

- It causes endocrine dysfunctions associated with **precocious puberty, amenorrhea and galactorrhea.** Common in Lina Medina of Peru.

Kallmann's Syndrome: This is a hypogonadal form of **deficiency of LH and FSH neurons** that occurs due to failure of migration of these neurons from the olfactory bulb.

- The GnRH secretion from hypothalamus is less and therefore deficiency occurs in secretion of LH and FSH.
- Pubertal maturation of testes in males and ovaries in females fail to occur (**hypogonadotropic hypogonadism**).

Exam Questions

1. Describe the stages and regulation of oogenesis.
2. With schematic diagram of ovarian follicle in stages, describe the steps and regulation of follicular development.
3. Describe the structure and functions of corpus luteum.
4. With a schematic diagram of ovarian, uterine and hormonal changes on the same time scale, describe the ovarian, uterine and hormonal changes in menstrual cycle.
5. Describe the mechanism of ovulation. Give a note on indicators of ovulation.
6. Describe the synthesis, regulation of secretion and functions of estrogen.
7. Describe the synthesis and regulation of secretion and functions of progesterone.
8. With the help of a suitable schematic diagram, describe the regulation of ovarian function.

Multiple Choice Questions

1. **The commonest cause of primary amenorrhea with ambiguous genitalia in a female with 46XX chromosome**
   A. 21 hydroxylase deficiency B. 17 hydroxylase deficiency
   C. 11 hydroxylase deficiency D. Desmolase hydrolase deficiency

2. **Which of the following hormone is not secreted from ovary?**
   A. Inhibin B. Relaxin
   C. Follicular stimulating hormone D. Progesterone

3. **Which of the following is the most potent naturally synthesized estrogen?**
   A. Estradiol B. Estrione
   C. Estrone D. Estriol
4. **Beta HCG is secreted by**
   A. Ovary B. Pituitary
   C. Corpus luteum D. Placenta
5. Which of the following is not seen in humans
   A. Estrous cycle **B.** Menstrual cycle
   C. Endometrial cycle **D.** Ovarian cycle
6. Ovulation is associated with sudden preovulatory (surge) rise in
   A. GnRH and FSH B. Testosterone
   C. LH D. Oxygen
7. Ovulation in a woman with normal health and cycle, occurs at:
   A. 14 days prior to start of menstrual bleeding
   B. Just before LH surge
   C. Just after corpus leuteal maturation
   D. During progesterone rise
8. **Positive feedback action of estrogen for inducing LH surge is associated with which of the following steroid hormone ratios in peripheral circulation**
   A. High estrogen : low progesterone
   B. Low estrogen : high progesterone
   C. Low estrogen: low progesterone
   D. High estrogen : high progesterone
9. **Corpus luteum is maintained in pregnancy by:**
   A. Progesterone B. LH
   X. FSH Δ. Estrogen
10. **Follicular stimulating hormone receptors are present on:**
    A. Theca cells B. Granulose cells
    X. Leydig cells Δ. Basement membrane of ovarian follicle
11. **Ovarian reserve is best indicated by:**
    A. LH B. FSH
    C. LH/FSH ratio D. Estrogen
12. **Main hormone in luteal phase is:**
    A. Estrogen *B.* Progesterone
    C. Prolactin *D.* Oxytocin
13. **The laboratory report shows values of gonadotropin and ovarian hormones of the blood sample taken, on day 20 of the menstrual cycle of a young women whether her cycle was ovulatory or not may be validly assessed by the reported serum level of:**
    A. FSH B. LH
    C. Oestradiol D. Progesterone
14. **Estrogen is secreted during pregnancy, mostly by:**
    A. Maternal ovary B. Fetal ovary
    X. Pituitary Δ. Hypothalamus
15. **Most common end product of progesterone metabolism found in urine is**
    A. Pregnanetriol B. Pregnenolone
    X. Pregnanediol Δ. 17 hydroxypregnenolone
16. **There is a mid-cycle increase in the basal body temperature (BBT) after ovulation in women. This is caused by:**
    A. FSH-peak B. LH-peak
    C. Oestradiol D. Progesterone
17. **In post-ovulary phase thickness of endometrium is because of:**
    A. Progesterone B. Oestrogen
    C. FSH D. LH
18. **The enzyme associated with the conversion of androgen to estrogen in the growing ovarian follicle is:**
    A. Desmolase B. Isomerase
    C. Aromatase D. Hydroxylase
19. **Estrogen action on carbohydrate metabolism:**
    A. Increases uptake of glucose through increase in insulin sensitivity
    B. Glycolysis increases
    C. Increasing central adipose deposition
    D. Worsening of NIDDM
20. **FSH acts on which of the following**
    A. Granulosa cell B. Theca interna
    C. Endometrium D. Myometrium
21. **Which of the following statements can be regarded as primary action of inhibin**
    A. It inhibits secretion of prolactin
    B. It stimulates synthesis of estradiol
    C. It stimulates secretion of TSH
    D. It inhibits secretion of FSH
22. **Ovary produces all the following hormones EXCEPT:**
    A. Gonadotropin B. Progesterone
    C. Estrogen D. Inhibin B
23. **Which of the following is not the function of relaxin?**
    A. Inhibits uterine contraction
    B. Inhibits sperm motility
    C. Dilation of uterine cervix
    D. Relaxation of pubic symphysis
24. **Relaxin is secreted by all the following organs, EXCEPT:**
    A. Corpus luteum B. Placenta
    C. Prostate gland in males D. Liver

Answers

1. A	2. C	3. A	4. D	5. A	6. C	7. A	8. A	9. B	10. B	11. B
12. B	13. D	14. A	15. C	16. D	17. A	18. C	19. B	20. A	21. D	22. A
23. B	24. D									

Chapter 82

Physiology of Copulation

Learning Objectives

On completion of study of this chapter:

The student will be able to (must know):

1. Give the blood supply and innervation of the erectile tissues of the penis and describe the mechanism of erection of penis.
2. Outline the process of emission and ejaculation.
3. Describe the sexual responses in males and females
4. Appreciate the mechanism and significance of orgasm.

The student may also be able to (desirable to know):

1. Define impotence and premature ejaculation and give their physiological basis.
2. Say the physiological basis of use of Viagra in the management of impotence.

Copulation is the process of mating that occurs in human being by coitus (sexual intercourse). Though the physiology of mating is similar in primates, the sexual responses of male and female are different in human being.

MALE SEXUAL ACT

In sexual intercourse, male is the active partner. The major events of male sexual act include:

- Erection of penis,
- Penetration of penis into the vagina, and
- Ejaculation.

These are the **series of reflexes that are integrated in the spinal cord** and mediated via ***autonomic and somatic nerves***.

1. Male genital tract receives both **sympathetic and parasympathetic** innervation, and in addition, penis receives the **somatic innervation**.
2. Though the sexual act per se is *mainly a neural process*, its overall integration is a **behavioral phenomenon** that includes hormonal, biochemical and psychological interactions.

Erection

Blood Supply: Penis is supplied by **internal pudendal arteries** that enter the organ as **dorsal artery of penis** from its dorsal surface.

- Dorsal artery penetrates deeply into the erectile tissues of penis as **deep artery** (Fig. 82.1).
- **Venous drainage** from penis occurs by ***dorsal vein***.

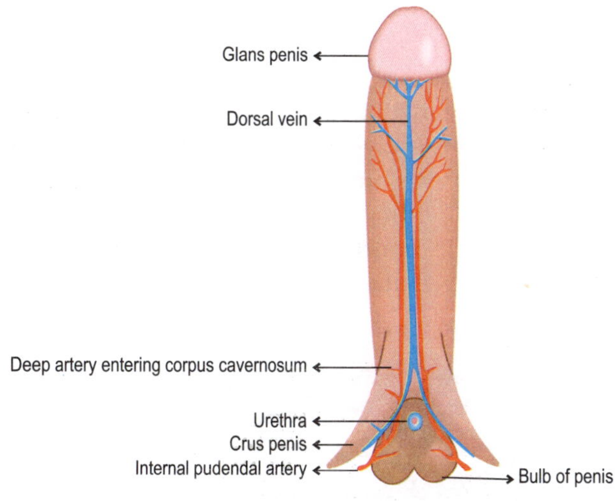

Fig. 82.1: Blood supply of penis. Blood supply to penis is from internal pudendal artery that enters penis from its dorsal surface as dorsal artery and penetrate deep into the organ as deep artery.

Mechanism

Erection occurs due to dilatation of **the penile arterioles filling the erectile tissues** of the penis by blood. The erectile tissues of penis are **three in numbers**: **two corpora cavernosa** and **a corpus spongiosum** (Fig. 82.2).

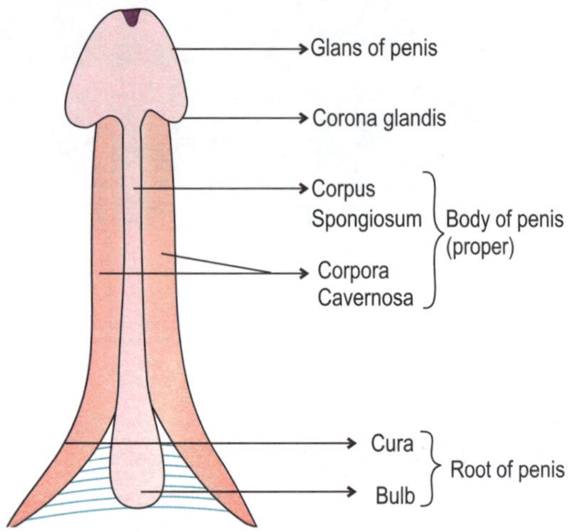

Fig. 82.2: Muscle of the penis.

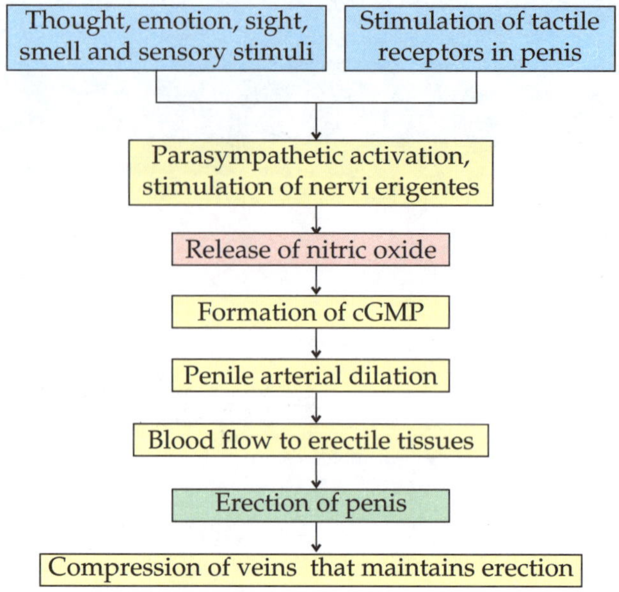

Flowchart 82.1: Mechanism of penile rection.

- In normal state, penis is flaccid due to paucity of blood in the spaces of these erectile tissues.
- **Upon arousal,** mainly the spaces in **cavernous erectile tissue fill with blood** and penis becomes **turgid** (Fig. 82.3).
- Relaxation of the **smooth muscles of corpora** allows increased flow of blood into corporal interstices (cavernous spaces) that increases the volume and rigidity of the penis.
- As **veins are compressed** by the erectile tissues filled with blood, engorgement of penis **inhibits venous return** and keeps the interstices filled with blood, which maintains erection.

Parasympathetic Control

Penile erection is mainly achieved by **parasympathetic activity** that relaxes smooth muscles of corpora, causes vasodilation and increases blood flow to the corporal interstices.

- The effects are mediated via parasympathetic fibers in **nervi erigentes** (pelvic splanchnic nerves) that release ***acetylcholine, VIP and nitric oxide*** (NO) (Flowchart 82.1).
- Nonadrenergic noncholinergic fibers are present in nervi erigentes that are **rich in NO**.

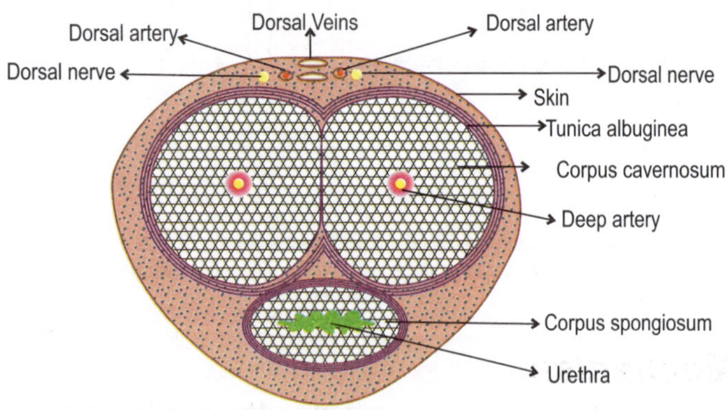

Fig. 82.3: Transverse section of penis. Note, the major erectile tissues are two corpora cavernosa that are separated by median septum and penetrated by deep artery of penis at their center. Increased blood flow into the cavernous spaces in these erectile tissues makes the penis turgid.

- **NO plays an important role** in causing **erection** of the penis.
- **NO activates guanylyl cyclase** that increases the **production of cGMP**, which is a **potent vasodilator**.
  - The drugs that **inhibit the breakdown of cGMP** such as tadalafil, vardenafil and sildenafil are very useful in the treatment of erectile dysfunctions.

Impotency

Impotency is the **erectile dysfunction in males**. It is the inability to keep the penis adequately erected to be penetrated into the female genital tract.

- **Erectile dysfunction** (ED) or impotence is the sexual dysfunction characterized by the **inability to develop or maintain the erection** of penis during sexual activity in humans.
  - It can temporarily happen due to psychosocial disturbances or acute illness.
- But it can regularly happen due to physical problems and neural deficits that causes deficit in sexual reflexes.
  - It may be treated by appropriate use of Viagra (Clinical Note 82.1)

Clinical Note 82.1

Use of Viagra: Spinal cord diseases, peripheral neuropathies, spinal cord injuries, psychological trauma, chronic physical stress and aging cause erectile dysfunction. Sildenafil (Viagra) is used for the treatment of erectile dysfunction. It prevents the breakdown of cGMP by inhibiting phosphodiesterase. Thus, it potentiates the action of NO. It is used worldwide for the treatment of impotence.

- It produces side effects like visual problems by inhibiting cGMP specific phosphodiesterase V1 (PDE V1) in the retina, transient inability to differentiate blue and green color, and hypotension (by aggravating vasodilation).
- Viagra should be taken one hour before planned intercourse. For chronic use, it should be used cautiously for its known side effects.

Ejaculation

Ejaculation is the **emission of semen** from the male genital tract and **its propulsion** out of the urethra at the time of orgasm. Thus, it is a **two-part reflex response**: the emission and the ejaculation *per se*.

Emission

Normally, sperms are stored in epididymis and proximal part of vas deferens.

1. Emission is the process in which sperms move into the urethra.
2. It is a **sympathetic response** that occurs due to **contraction of smooth muscle of vas deferens and seminal vesicles.**
3. The fibers travel in hypogastric nerve.

Ejaculation

This is the **propulsion of semen out of urethra** at the time of orgasm.

1. This occurs due to **contraction of bulbocavernosus muscle,** a skeletal muscle.
2. This is a **spinal reflex** integrated at lower lumbar and upper sacral segments of spinal cord (L_5, S_{1-3}). The efferent fibers traverse in pudendal nerve.
3. It is proposed that the **carbon monoxide (CO) is the transmitter** in the neural circuit of ejaculation as evidenced from the fact that the ejaculatory performance is diminished when the gene responsible for the enzyme **HO_2 (heme oxygenase)** is knocked out.
   - HO_2 normally catalyzes the formation of CO.
   - Retrograde ejaculation occurs in diabetes (Application Box 82.1).

Application Box 82.1

Retrograde ejaculation: The internal urethral sphincter constricts at the time of emission. When this sphincter fails to constrict, the sperms instead of passing down the urethra enter the urinary bladder. The quantity of ejaculate decreases and sperms appear in urine (more than 15 sperms per high power field). Usually it occurs in diabetic neuropathy, multiple sclerosis and use of sympatholytic drugs.

Premature Ejaculation

Premature ejaculation (PE) occurs when a man ejaculates sooner during sexual intercourse. Though the prevalence of PE vary, as many as 1 out of 3 men say they experience this problem at some time. As long as it happens infrequently, it's of no much concern. But if it occurs often, investigations should be done to detect its cause.

Diagnostic Criteria: The diagnostic criteria for premature ejaculation are:

1. Always or nearly always ejaculate **within one minute of penetration.**
2. Are **unable to delay ejaculation** during intercourse all or nearly all of the time
3. Feel **distressed and frustrated,** and tend to avoid sexual intimacy as a result of it.

Causes and Treatment; Both **psychological and biological factors** can play a role in premature ejaculation. Although many men feel embarrassed to talk about it, premature ejaculation is a common and treatable condition.

1. **Regular counseling, learning the proper sexual techniques** and few medications can delay ejaculation.
2. Physical, mental and psychosocial **stress should be reduced.**
3. As penile ***erection is a parasympathetic*** and ***ejaculation is a sympathetic*** mechanism, the male partner has to learn to delay the sympathetic activation during sex to avoid early ejaculation.
4. Practice of **Yoga** that improves **sympathovagal (sympatho-parasympathetic) balance** helps a lot to improve sex life.

FEMALE SEXUAL ACT

Normally, during sexual intercourse, female is the **passive partner.** However, the responses to intercourse in females are not passive.

- The female responses are characterized by **marked increase in blood flow and muscular activities** in many parts of the body.
- Increased sexual excitement is accompanied by **engorgement of the breasts** and **erection of the nipples, increased diameter and length of clitoris** due to increased blood flow into these structures.
- **Nipple and clitoris** have rich sensory innervation.
  - Therefore, **clitorial and nipple stimulations** during sexual act add to sexual excitement.
- Blood flow also increases to vagina due to release of VIP from vaginal nerves and **increased fluid secretion from vagina** lubricates vaginal epithelium.
- **Mucus secretion** is also increased from vestibular glands.

Sexual desire in women is possibly ***dependent on androgens***, because sex drive is maintained long after the menopause, when estrogen level in plasma is very low. Therefore, it is believed that androgens secreted by the adrenal glands maintain sexual appetite in females.

Vaginal Changes

Vaginal secretion increases during sexual excitation and intercourse.

1. This occurs mostly due to **release of VIP** from vaginal nerves.
2. **Vestibular glands** secrete mucus that also helps in lubrication.
3. The **stimuli** for vaginal secretion are tactile stimulation of clitoris, labia minora, breast and sexual excitement.

Visual, olfactory and auditory stimuli aid to the excitement.

The sexual gratification in females culminates in **orgasm** that manifests as ***rhythmic vaginal contractions*** mediated by autonomic influences (Application Box 82.2).

Application Box 82.2

Male orgasm should coincide with the female orgasm: For the best conjugal life, the orgasms of male and female should appear concurrently. As female is the passive partner, orgasm in females comes usually later. The male partner should learn to excite the female partner so that orgasm in both arrives together.

- In males, orgasm occurs with ejaculation, following which the penis becomes flaccid. Therefore, the male should understand the time of orgasm of the partner and maintain erection till then.
- Usually, after marriage it takes a year or more for both to adjust to each other's' physical and emotional needs to bring at once their orgasms.
- Moreover, if the male can further maintain erection and continue the act after the female orgasm, subsequent multiple orgasms can occur in female.
- Thus, sexual act is more of an art than a science.

Orgasm

It is the **climax of sexual excitement and pleasure** that occurs with satisfactory intercourse. The natural sexual act culminates with orgasm.

- **Orgasm** (climax) in female is associated with a **pleasurable feeling** accompanied by sudden increase in skeletal muscle activity, heart rate and blood pressure, and ***rhythmic contraction of the vaginal wall,*** rapid breathing, flushing of face and sweating.
  - Though, **vaginal contraction** during orgasm facilitates sperm transport, it is **not essential for fertilization** since conception can occur in the absence of orgasm.
- All these changes are due to increased **epinephrine secretion** into the circulation.

Fate of Sperms in Female Genital Tract

Normally 10^8 to 5×10^8 motile sperms are released into the female vagina on ejaculation. The sperms move at the rate of **1-3 mm/min** and only about **100 sperms reach the oviduct within 30 minutes**. Vaginal contraction during mating facilitates sperm movement.

1. The fluid medium in the uterus is favourable for sperms.
   - **Uterine muscular movements** and ciliary activity may aid in migration of sperms within the uterus.
2. Some **spermatozoa can survive** in a viable state within the slightly alkaline medium of the cervical mucus for upto **48 hours**.
3. Finally, only one sperm fertilizes the ovum.
   - The initial process is called **capacitation** which makes the sperm (spermatozoon) able to adhere to the ovum.
   - It is followed by the **acrosomal reaction** in which one spermatozoon releases enough lytic enzymes locally to penetrate the cumulus cells and the zona pellucida that surrounds the ovum.
4. The remaining **sperms disintegrate** and liquefy in the female genital tract.

Exam Questions

1. Describe the mechanisms of male and female sexual responses. Adda note on orgasm.
2. Describe the mechanism of erection of penis. Add a note on erectile dysfunction.

Multiple Choice Questions

1. **Given that a) Compression of veins; b) Increased formation of cGMP; c) Release of NO; d) Penile arterial dilatation; which of the following is the correct sequence of events in penile erection?**
   A. a b c d B. a c b d
   C. c b a d D. c b d a
2. **Which of the following is NOT true about erectile dysfunction in male?**
   A. Inability to develop or maintain penile erection
   B. Can happen due to psychosocial disturbances
   C. Cannot happen due to neural deficits
   D. Can be treated by viagra
3. **Which of the following is NOT true about erection of penis?**
   A. Sympathetic stimulation causes vasodilation and maintain erection
   B. Dorsal artery of penis that supplies blood deep into erectile tissues is the branch of internal pudendal artery
   C. Erection occurs due to dilation of penile arterioles filling the erectile tissue by blood
   D. Erection is maintained by compression of veins that keep the interstices filed with blood
4. **Which of the following is NOT true?**
   A. Retrograde ejaculation occurs in diabetes
   B. Ejaculation is the sympathetic function
   C. Nervi erigentes is involved in ejaculation
   D. Emission is the process during which sperms move into the urethra
5. **All of the following are true about sexual reflex EXCEPT:**
   A. This is a spinal reflex integrated at L5 and S1-3 spinal segments
   B. Contraction of bulbocavernosus muscle causes propulsion of semen
   C. Carbon monoxide is the likely transmitter in the neural circuit
   D. If ejaculation occurs within 10 min of erection, is called premature ejaculation
6. **All of the following are true about fate of sperm in female genital tract, EXCEPT:**
   A. About 100 sperms reach the oviduct within 30 minutes
   B. Capacitation is release of lytic enzymes to penetrate the cumulus cells
   C. The uterine fluid is favorable for sperms
   D. Only one sperm fertilizes the ovum

Answers

1. D 2. C 3. A 4. C
5. D 6. B

Chapter 83

PY9.8

Physiology of Pregnancy and Parturition

Learning Objectives

On completion of study of this chapter:

The student will be able to (must know):

1. Understand the physiology of fertilization and fetal maturation.
2. Name the placental hormones and mention their functions.
3. List the causes of female infertility and give outline the concept of IVF.
4. Describe the systemic maternal changes in pregnancy.
5. Briefly explain the mechanism of parturition and the role of oxytocin in it.

The student may also be able to (desirable to know):

1. Describe the process of fertilization and fetal development.
2. Explain the fetomaternal changes in pregnancy.

PHYSIOLOGY OF PREGNANCY

Transport of Gametes

Transport of Egg

Following ovulation, the oocyte is extruded onto the surface of the ovary or into the abdominal cavity. The fimbriae located at the end of the fallopian tube **actively pick up** the oocyte.

1. These **ciliary motions** sweep the egg into the fallopian tube as the egg emerges from follicle to the ovarian surface.
   - Inside the fallopian tube, egg movement is driven by fallopian-tube cilia, which is a normally a **slow process**.
2. Fertilization occurs **in the distal portion of fallopian tube** (within a day of ovulation) because of the short viability of the unfertilized egg (Fig. 83.1).

Transport of Sperm

Though usual **transit time** of sperm to reach fallopian tube is 4–6 hours, within few minutes of ejaculation, sperms have been detected in the uterus and tubes.

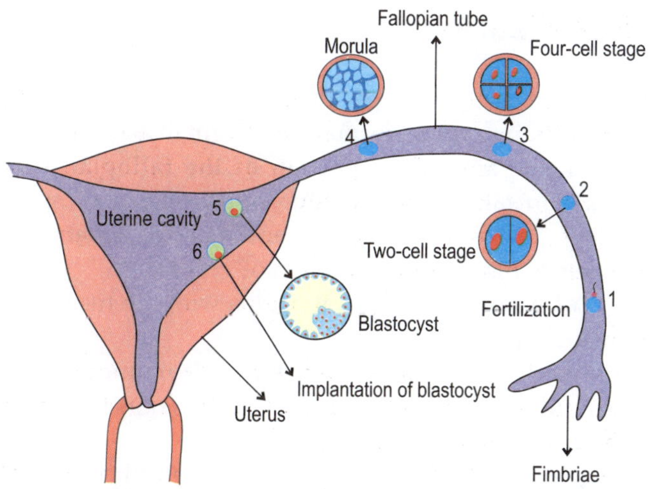

Fig. 83.1: Fertilization and implantation of fertilized ovum. **1:** Site of fertilization, which takes place in ampullary portion of the tube; **2:** Two-cell stage; **3:** Four-cell stage; **4:** Morula formation; **5:** Formation of blastocyst, which is floating in uterine cavity; **6:** Implantation of blastocyst on endometrium.

Transport of Sperm in the Cervix: Passage of sperms through cervix is favoured by:

1. ***Nature of cervical mucous:*** Sperm transport is **favoured by estrogen-induced changes** in consistency and orientation of the mucous. Estrogen makes the mucous **thin and elastic**.
2. ***Orientation of the mucous:*** Also, under the influence of estrogen, **cervical mucous is oriented in parallel** that favours the transport of sperm.

Transport of Sperm in the Uterus: Transport of the sperm through the entire length of the uterus and then into the fallopian tubes occurs due to sperm's own motility and uterine contractions.

Transport of Sperm in the Fallopian Tube: In the fallopian tube, sperm motility is facilitated by three factors:

1. Ciliary movement in the tube
2. Peristaltic activity of the tube
3. Flow of fluid in the tube

IMPORTANT NOTE

Sperm count must be very high: Though several millions of sperms are deposited in the vagina, only **about 50–100 reach the fallopian tube.** This is the major reasons that **there must be many millions of motile sperms** in the seminal fluid for fertilization to occur. Thus, decreased count and motility of sperms lead to infertility in males.

Changes in Sperm in Female Genital Tract

Sperms undergo changes in the female genital tract that make them able to fertilize the egg. These changes are collectively called **capacitation**.

Capacitation includes **two major changes** in sperms:

1. The wavelike beating of the tail of the sperms is replaced by **whip-like movements** that propel the sperm forward in strong lurches.
2. **Alteration in the plasma membrane** (modification of surface proteins) of sperms that makes them capable of fusing with the surface of the egg.

Fertilization

Fertilization is the process of union of sperm with egg that **results in zygote formation**. Normally, fertilization occurs in the **ampullary portion of the fallopian tube**. Fertilization takes place in **four steps**: Fusion of sperm with egg, acrosome reaction and sperm penetration, polyspermy block, and formation of zygote.

Fusion of Sperm with Egg: It begins with the fusion of a sperm and egg.

- Many sperms move between the cumulus cells (granulosa cells still surrounding the egg) to bind to the *zona pellucida* of the egg.

Acrosome Reaction & sperm penetration: The binding sperm to the zona pellucida triggers *acrosome reaction* in the bound sperm.

The steps of acrosome reaction and penetration of the sperm are as follows:

1. ***Change in membrane of sperm head:*** Redistribution of constituents of the plasma membrane of the sperm head at the site of the attachment results in alteration in the membrane.
2. ***Increased fluidity*** of the membrane of the sperm head.
3. ***Increased calcium permeability*** of the sperm membrane.
4. ***Digestion of a part of zona pellucida:*** The membrane-bound acrosomal enzymes in the sperm head is exposed to the zona pellucida.
   - These are *proteolytic enzymes* that include ***acrosin***, a trypsin-like protease.
   - They digest a portion of the zona pellucida at the site of binding.
5. ***Penetration of sperm through perivitalline space:*** As the zona pellucida gives way, sperm advances through this coating using its propulsive force of the tail.
   - Then, sperm penetrates the ***perivitalline space*** (the space surrounding the egg membrane) to reach the egg's plasma membrane.
6. ***Fusion of sperm head with egg membrane:*** The sperm head fuses with the egg's membrane, which is facilitated by sperm surface protein, called **fertilin**. Then, sperm slowly enters the egg's cytoplasm (ooplasm).

Polyspermy Block: Only one sperm penetrates the egg.

- As soon as the sperm penetration starts, immediately **a series of changes** occur in the egg that prevent the entry of additional sperms. This is called *polyspermy block*.

There are **two mechanisms** of polyspermy block:

1. The initial fusion of the sperm with egg plasma membranes triggers a reaction that **changes the membrane potential** of the egg, which prevents additional sperm binding.
2. The enzymes released from egg cytoplasm enter zona pellucida and cause **inactivation of sperm-binding sites** and **hardening of the entire zona pellucida**. Thus, binding of additional sperms to the zona pellucida is prevented.

Zygote Formation: The sperm penetration of egg is called fertilization.

- The fertilized egg **completes its second meiotic division in next few hours**.
- Second polar body is formed, which is extruded from ooplasm.
- The remaining haploid nucleus containing 23 chromosomes is transformed into **female pronucleus** in two to three hours.
  - The two sets of chromosomes (23 from the egg and 23 from the sperm) each surrounded by distinct membranes known as **pronuclei** (the male pronucleus and the female pronucleus) **migrate to the center** of the cell by contraction of microfilaments and microtubules.
- Simultaneously, the DNA of chromosomes in both pro-nuclei is replicated and **pronuclei fuse**.
  - Then the pro-nuclear membranes break down. Now, the cell is ready to undergo a mitotic division.
- This completes the process of fertilization, and the **fertilized egg is called zygote**.

Cleavage

The fertilized egg (zygote) remains in the fallopian tube for three to four days. While in the fallopian tube, a **number of mitotic cell divisions** take place. This process of mitotic cell divisions is known as **cleavage**.

- The first cell division takes place in 24 hours to produce two unequal sized cells, the structure called **blastomere**.

- Then each cell divides to form a four-cell conceptus, eight cell conceptus and **morula** (16 to 32 cell conceptus) in 48, 72 and 96 hours respectively.
  - **Twin is formed** if dividing cells grow into two independent cell masses (Application Box 83. 1)

Application Box 83.1

Development of twins: Each of the cells of blastomere is a totipotent cell. They have the capacity to develop into an entire individual. Therefore, identical (monozygotic) twins result when, at the time of cleavage, the dividing cells are completely separated into two independently growing cell masses. And, fraternal or dizygotic twins result when, two eggs being ovulated and fertilized simultaneously.

Blastocyst Formation & Implantation

The morula enters uterus about **four days of fertilization**. After reaching the uterus, the conceptus **floats free** in the intrauterine fluid **for three days**, during which it further undergoes cell divisions.

- Now, the conceptus is known as a **blastocyst**, the stage which the cells have lost their totipotentiality and have begun to differentiate.
- Blastocyst derives nourishment from the uterine fluid.

The blastocyst consists of **three components** (Fig. 83.2):

1. **Trophoblast:** An outer layer of cells of blastocyst is called **trophoblast**. The trophoblast consists of extraembryonic ectodermal cells present on embryonic membrane. It helps in implantation of the conceptus and contributes to placenta formation. Trophoblast and its membrane secrete hCG.
2. **Embryoblast:** An inner cell mass called **embryoblast** that gives rise to fetus.
3. **Blastocele:** A central fluid-filled cavity of blastocyst is called **blastocele**. It forms amniotic cavity.

Implantation and Early Development

Implantation is the **attachment of the blastocyst to the endometrial surface** of the uterine wall.

- It occurs about 7–8 days after fertilization. Implantation occurs in estrogen and progesterone primed uterus.
- Progesterone prepares the endometrium for implantation of blastocyst.
- The **trophoblast cells are very sticky**, especially at the **region that overlie the inner cell mass** and this part of blastocyst adheres to the uterine wall for implantation.

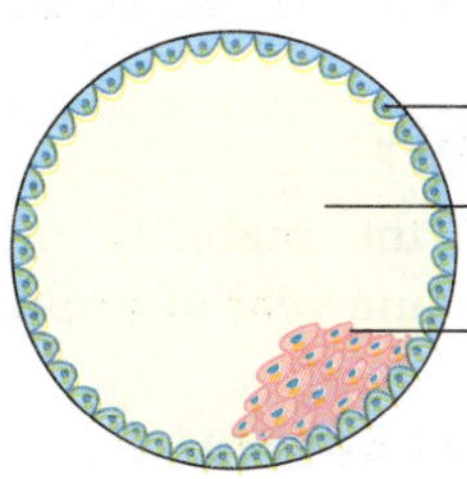

Fig. 83.2: Structure of blastocyst.

  - Implantation outside uterus leads to ectopic pregnancy (Clinical Note 83.1)

Mechanism of Implantation: Implantation occurs due to changes in blastocyst, in endometrium and interaction of blastocyst with endometrium.

Changes in Blastocyst: Enlargement of blastocyst (before implantation) results in **rupture of zona pellucida**.

- The trophoblast cells are denuded and become **negatively charged**. This facilitates the **blastocyst attachment** to endometrium via surface glycoprotein.
- The initial contact between blastocyst and endometrium induces **rapid proliferation of the trophoblast**.

Interaction of Blastocyst with Endometrium: The proteolytic enzymes secreted by the trophoblast allow the **blastocyst to bury in the endometrium**.

- Microvilli of trophoblast cells interdigitate with endometrial cells and **form junctional complexes**.

Changes in Endometrium: At the site of contact, endometrium also undergoes changes. By the influence of progesterone, endometrium undergoes **decidualization**.

- In this process, the endometrial cells are hypertrophied and their glycogen and lipid content increase.
- The endometrium at the site of implantation is called **decidua**.

As soon as the implantation is completed, the nutrient-rich endometrial cells **supply the nutrients required for early growth of the embryo**, which is adequate for the embryo in the first few weeks. Later, this function is taken over by the placenta.

Clinical Note 83.1

Ectopic pregnancy: The usual site of implantation is the dorsal wall in the body of uterus. Sometimes, a fertilized egg remains in the fallopian tube and gets implanted in the wall of the tube. This is called **tubal ectopic pregnancy.** Rarely, implantation can occur in abdominal cavity causing **abdominal ectopic pregnancy**. Usually, in ectopic pregnancy as there is risk of rupture and maternal hemorrhage.

Fertilization Placentation & Amnion Formation

Placenta Formation

Implantation is completed in about 10–12 days after ovulation. The trophoblast cells become **cytotrophoblasts** (large polyhedral cells) that are surrounded by **syncytiotrobhobalsts** (cells with no boundaries).

- The blood vessels in the endometrium dilate and form lacunae. **Chorionic villi**, the functional unit of placenta begins to form at about 12th day from fertilization.
- **Placenta** is the combination of interdigitating fetal and maternal tissues that serves as the organ of exchange between mother and fetus during pregnancy.
- The **fetal part of the placenta** is formed by the outermost layers of trophoblast cells, **the chorion**,

and the **maternal part** is formed by the endometrium underlying the chorion.

Formation of Amnion

Once placenta is well formed, the **fetal heart begins to pump blood at about 5th week of gestation**. A space is formed between the inner cell mass and the chorion, called the **amniotic cavity** (Fig. 83.3A).

1. The cavity enlarges and is slowly lined by epithelial cells layer derived from the inner cell mass called the **amnion**, or **amniotic sac**.
2. Amnion finally fuses with the chorion to form a single combined membrane that surrounds the fetus (Fig. 83.3B).
   - The fluid in the amniotic cavity is the **amniotic fluid** (Clinical Note 83.2) that buffers mechanical stress and temperature variations.
   - The fetus floats in the amniotic cavity.
3. Fetus is attached to the placenta by the umbilical cord (Fig. 83.3C).
   - Eventually, it is only the amniotic sac that separates the fetus from the uterine lumen.

Clinical Note 83.2

Amniocentesis: Aspiration of fluid from the amniotic sac is called amniocentesis. Amniocentesis can be done as early as the sixteenth week of pregnancy by inserting a needle into the amniotic cavity. Few genetic diseases can be diagnosed by the demonstrating certain chemicals in the amniotic fluid or in sloughed fetal cells in the fluid. Amniocentesis for diagnosis of fetal sex has been banned in India.

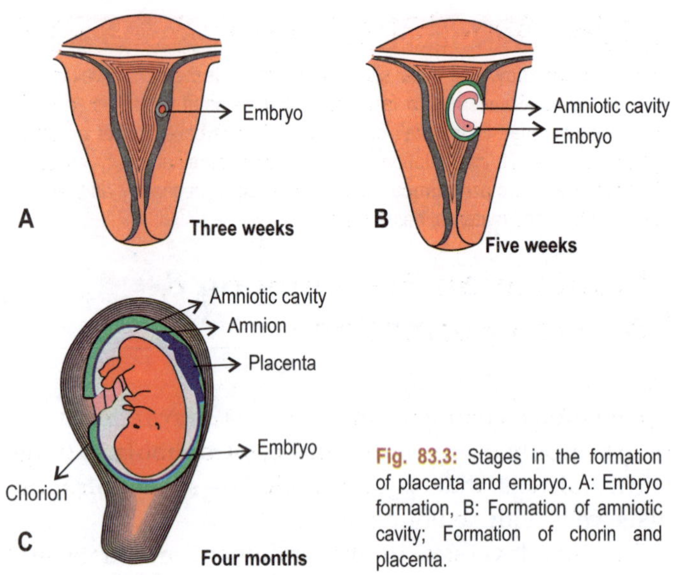

Fig. 83.3: Stages in the formation of placenta and embryo. A: Embryo formation, B: Formation of amniotic cavity; Formation of chorin and placenta.

Organogenesis & Fetal Nutrition

Once placenta is formed, fetus derives nutrition directly from the mother's blood. Therefore, **maternal nutrition is crucial** for the fetal development. Malnutrition in mother causes fetal growth retardation.

- Organogenesis starts **as early as 5th to 8th weeks** of pregnancy.
- If mother takes drugs (like aspirin etc.), alcohol and does smoking during this period, defects in the fetus occur. These chemicals are known **teratogens**.

Fetoplacental Unit

For steroidogenesis, fetus and placenta interact closely. This is called fetoplacental unit. Placenta forms pregnenolone from cholesterol, which in turn forms progesterone.

1. **Placental pregnenolone** enters fetal circulation and become substrate for synthesis of **dehydroepiandrosterone** (DHEA) and **16-hydroxydehydroepiandrosterone** (16-OHDHEA) in fetal adrenal.
2. Formation of 16-OHDHEA also occurs in the fetal liver. DHEA and 16-OHDHEA formed in fetus are taken back into the placenta, where DHEA forms estradiol and 16-OHDHEA forms estriol.
3. **The placental progesterone** also enters fetal adrenal and forms cortisol, corticosterone and androgen in adrenal cortex of fetus (Fig. 83.4).

IMPORTANT NOTE

Estriol in maternal urine indicates fetal health: The major estrogen formed by placenta is estriol for which the substrate is fetal adrenal 16-OH-DHEA. Therefore, **excretion of estriol in maternal urine is a good index of health of the fetus.**

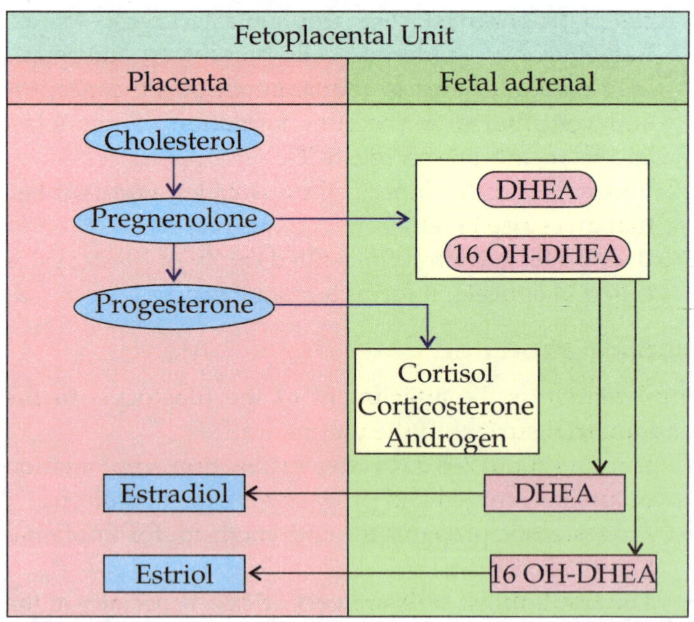

Fig. 83.4: Interaction between placenta and fetal adrenal gland for steroidogenesis. DHEA: dehydroepiandrosterone; OHDHEA: hydroxydehydroepiandrosterone.

Female Infertility

PY9.12

Infertility is defined as the **inability of a couple to achieve conception after one year of unprotected sexual intercourse**.

In females, infertility may be due to following causes.

1. **Ovarian factors:** Anovulation (absence of release of

ovum from the ovary) causes infertility. For details of anovulation, refer previous chapter.

2. **Peritoneal factor:** Pelvic adhesion or pelvic peritonitis prevents fallopian tube to pick up the ovum from pelvic cavity.
3. **Tubal factors:** Partial or complete bilateral tubal obstruction resulting from infective or noninfective salpingitis prevents fertilization to occur.
4. **Uterine factors:** Endometritis, intrauterine adhesions, or anatomical defects can prevent implantation of the fertilized ovum.
5. **Cervical factors:** Thick cervical mucus or presence of sperm antibodies in the mucus makes the sperm impenetrable.
6. **Vaginal factors:** Infections in the vagina or anatomical defects in the vagina prevent sperm to reach cervix.

In-Vitro Fertilization and Transfer (IVF-ET)

IVF-ET is done for infertile women. It is done in three steps: oocyte retrieval, fertilization in vitro and transfer of gametes of embryos.

Oocyte Retrieval: Oocyte retrieval is done aseptically through **vaginal route** under ultrasound guidance.

1. With the development of vaginal transducers, **vaginal needle aspiration** is done about **36 hours after hCG administration** but before ovulation occurs. Intravenous analgesia and sedation (propofol) is adequate in most of the cases.
2. The oocyte is easily recognizable as a single cell surrounded by a mass cumulus cell. After recovery, the oocytes are maintained in culture in vitro for 4-6 hours.

Fertilization in Vitro: The sperm used for insemination in vitro is prepared by the **wash and swim up or density gradient centrifugation** (preferred) technique.

1. Approximately 50,000 to 1,00,000 capacitated sperm are **placed in the culture media** containing the oocyte within 4-6 hours of retrieval. The eggs may demonstrate signs of fertilization when examined 16-18 hours after insemination (presence of two pronuclei in the presence of a second polar body).
2. Sperm **density and motility** are two most important criteria for successful IVF. The semen is collected just prior to ovum retrieval.

Embryo Transfer: The fertilized ova at the **6-8 blastomere stage** are placed into the uterine cavity close to the fundus about 3 days after fertilization through a fine flexible soft catheter transcervically. Not more than three embryos are transferred per cycle to minimize multiple pregnancy.

PLACENTAL HORMONES

Placenta is an endocrine organ as it secretes many hormones (Table 83.1).

Table 83.1 | Hormones secreted from placenta

A. Steroid hormones	B. Protein hormones
1. Estriol	1. hCG
2. 17-β estradiol	2. hCS
3. Estrone	3. Relaxin
4. Progesterone	4. Prolactin
	5. CRH
	6. GnRH
	7. β-endorphin
	8. α-MSH
	9. Dynorphin-A
	10. Insulin like growth factors
	11. ACTH

hCG

The **human chorionic gonadotropin** (hCG) is the gonadotropin secreted from syncytiotrophoblast of placenta. The **syncytiotrophoblast cells** start producing hCG between 6–8 days after fertilization.

Structure: It is a glycoprotein hormone containing galactose and hexosamine. It is made up of two subunits: α and **β.**

- The α subunit contains 92 amino acids and has molecular weight 18,000 whereas as the β subunit contains 145 amino acids and has molecular weight 28,000.
- The α subunit of hCG is similar to the α subunit of LH, FSH and TSH.

Secretion: hCG secretion is ***more in the early pregnancy***. It appears in maternal plasma as early as sixth day after fertilization.

- Its concentration increases rapidly to reach a **peak in about 10–12 weeks** of gestation, when the concentration is about 5mg/ml.
    - Then, the concentration decreases to 75% at about 25th weeks and remains at that level till term (Fig. 83.5).
- Associated with the decline of hCG secretion, the *placenta begins to secrete estrogen and progesterone in large amount*.

Functions: hCG binds to LH receptors in corpus luteum. Therefore, it has mainly luteinizing and luteotropic activities. It has very less FSH activity.

1. It **stimulates progesterone production** from corpus luteum.
2. hCG plays a critical role in **placental steroidogenesis**.
3. hCG also helps in **sexual differentiation** in male fetus.
4. hCG **stimulates vomiting centers** in the brain. Therefore, morning sickness (sense of nausea and vomiting in the morning) is an early feature of pregnancy. Morning sickness is common in the first pregnancy, and usually disappears after first trimester. **PY9.10**

Clinical Significance: hCG is detected in plasma as early as 6 days after conception. Therefore, demonstrating hCG in plasma by RIA is a pregnancy diagnostic test.

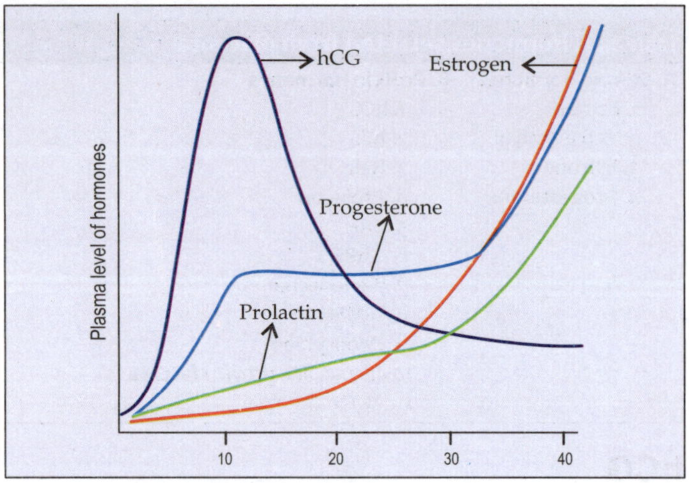

Fig. 83.5: Level of various hormones in maternal plasma throughout pregnancy. hCG: human chorionic gonadotropin.

- hCG appears **in urine from 14th day** of conception onwards. Detection of hCG in urine is easier, as blood collection is avoided.
- However, hCG is **not specific for pregnancy** as it is secreted from *many gastrointestinal and chorionic tumors*. It is also secreted in some amount from ***fetal kidney and liver***.

hCS

The **human chorionic somatotropin** (hCS) is also called human chorionic somatomammotropin or **human placental lactogen** (hPL) or chorionic growth hormone.

Source: hCS is secreted from syncytiotrophoblast of placenta.

Structure and Secretion: Structurally, it is similar to human growth hormone.

- hCS, GH and prolactin are formed from common precursor hormone. It contains 191 amino acids and has molecular weight 22,000.
- Secretion of hCS starts from **third week of pregnancy** and slowly rises till term.
- The peak concentration in plasma is achieved at term when it is about 15mg/ml.

Functions: hCS has functions similar to growth hormone and prolactin.

1. It promotes growth of mammary gland and **stimulates production of milk**. Therefore, it is also called **human placental lactogen**. However, hCS is less potent in milk production than prolactin secreted from anterior pituitary.
2. It **stimulates somatic growth of the fetus**. Therefore, it is also called growth hormone of pregnancy.
3. It causes **maternal lipolysis** and releases FFA from fat tissues.
4. It **decreases glucose utilization** in mother. It induces maternal insulin resistance and glucose intolerance.
5. It alters fuel availability for the fetus by antagonizing maternal glucose consumption and enhancing fat mobilization. This ensures **adequate supply of fuel for the fetus**.

Clinical Significance: The quantity of hCS secreted is proportional to size of the placenta. Therefore, a low **hCS level in third trimester** indicates placental adequacy or insufficiency.

Other Hormones

1. **Relaxin** secreted from placenta causes ***uterine relaxation*** in the early part of pregnancy like progesterone to facilitate implantation and prevent expulsion of fetus. Its concentration in plasma is highest (1 ng/ml) in first trimester of pregnancy. Towards term, it causes relaxation of pubic symphysis and pelvic ligaments to facilitate delivery of fetus.
2. **Progesterone** causes myometrial quiescence and promotes continuation of pregnancy (Fig. 131.7).
3. **Estrogen** secretion increases slowly in third trimester and reaches peak at term. The major estrogen secreted in pregnancy is **estriol**, which normally secreted in very less amount from the ovary of a nonpregnant woman. Estrogen facilitates parturition (discussed below).

MATERNAL CHANGES DURING PREGNANCY

The maternal changes are primarily meant to supply adequate oxygen and nutrients to fetus for its growth and development, and remove CO_2 and waste products from the fetal circulation.

Changes in Blood Volume

There is rapid and significant increase in total blood volume in pregnancy. The increase is about 40% of the prepregnant stage, which occurs due to increase in both plasma and cell components (Fig. 83.6).

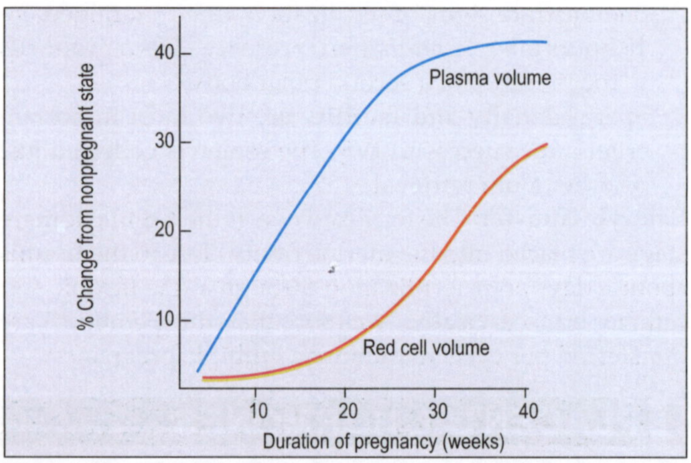

Fig. 83.6: Changes in plasma volume and red cell volume in pregnancy. Note, plasma volume increases early and attains about 40% increase, whereas, red cell volume increases gradually and attains about 30% increase.

1. The **increase in plasma volume** is primarily due to the **expansion of ECF volume.**
2. **Increase in red cell mass** occurs slowly after 16 weeks of gestation and the increase is usually about 20–30%.

However, **due to hemodilution** the red cell count remain low, which is called **physiological anemia of pregnancy**.

Hematological Changes

Hematological changes are primarily designed to increase oxygen supply to the fetus and protect the fetus against infections.

1. **Red cell count increases** to about 20–30%, which is slower than the increase in plasma volume (as described above).
2. There is **moderate leucocytosis.** Leucocytosis occurs mainly due to **neutrophilia.** Moreover, **shift occurs to left in Arneth count.**
3. *Platelet count remains almost normal* in normal pregnancy.
4. The **increase in procoagulant activity** is among the striking hematological changes in third trimester of pregnancy.
   - This occurs due to increased **hepatic synthesis of clotting factors by estrogen.**
   - Fibrinogen concentration increases 2–4 times.
   - In abnormal pregnancies, **DIC** (disseminated intravascular coagulation) occurs due acceleration of procoagulant activities.

Changes in Cardiovascular System

Cardiac Output: Cardiac output starts increasing in the early phase of pregnancy and is significantly high by the end of first trimester (Fig. 83.7).

- The increase in cardiac output reaches its maximum, i. e. about 40% increase in mid-pregnancy and then remains elevated at that level till term.

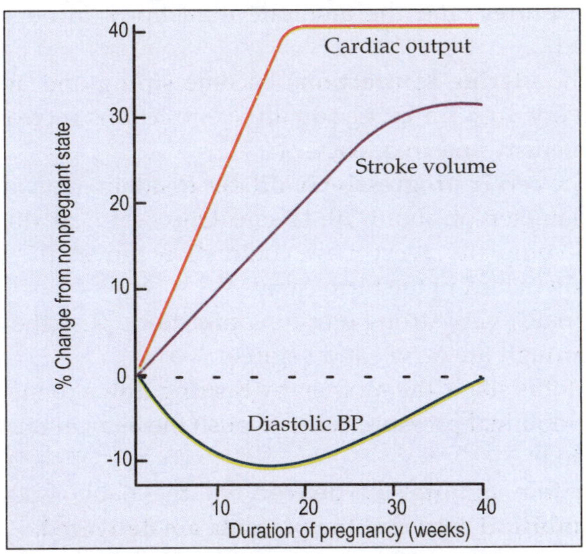

Fig. 83.7: Changes in cardiac output, stroke volume, and diastolic pressure in pregnancy. Cardiac output increases by about 40%, and stroke volume increases by about 30%, whereas diastolic pressure decreases by about 10%. BP: blood pressure

- The increase in cardiac output is due to the increase in both stroke volume and heart rate.

Stroke Volume: Stoke volume **increases by about 30%,** which peaks at about 24 weeks of pregnancy. Increase in stroke volume is mainly due to increased end-diastolic volume (EDV), which occurs due to increased venous return as a consequence of increased blood volume.

Heart Rate: Heart rate **increases by about 10–15%,** reaching its peak at term.

Systolic BP: Systolic pressure **increases in pregnancy,** which is mainly due to increased cardiac output. The increase occurs more in the second and third trimester.

Diastolic BP: Diastolic pressure **falls slowly,** reaching a nadir at about 20th week, which then slowly increases to normal by term.

- Fall in diastolic pressure is due to the **vasodilation effect of progesterone. Pulse pressure** is wide due to increase in systolic and decrease in diastolic pressures.

Changes in Respiratory System

Respiratory changes aim to improve supply of oxygen to the fetus and removal of carbon dioxide from the fetus.

1. The most striking effect is the **increase in minute ventilation.**
2. Respiratory rate does not increase significantly. The increase in ventilation is mainly due to the **increase in tidal volume** (TV).
3. Residual volume **(RV) decreases by 20%.**
4. Expiratory reserve volume (ERV) decreases by 15%.
   - Due to decrease in RV and ERV, **functional residual capacity decreases.**
5. Inspiratory reserve volume (IRV) increases.
   - Increase in TV and IRV, **increases inspiratory capacity.**
6. Diffusing capacity of alveolar membrane does not change significantly.

In third trimester, inspite of elevation of diaphragm due to increase in size of uterus, ventilation is not impaired significantly.

Changes in Kidney Functions

1. **Renal blood flow increases** by 35% that parallels the increase in blood volume and cardiac output.
2. There is remarkable **increase in glomerular filtration rate** (GFR). Significant increase in GFR to about 40% occurs by midpregnancy and continues at that level till term.
3. The **load of filtered glucose increases** without increase in tubular capacity to reabsorb glucose. Therefore, **glycosuria** is common in pregnant woman. Aminoaciduria also occurs.

Changes in GI System

GI **motility is decreased.** As a result, gastric emptying

time is increased.

1. Due to increased transit time for chyme to pass though intestinal lumen, more water is absorbed that leads to **constipation**.
2. Towards term, enlarged uterus presses on the stomach, which increases intragastric pressure.
3. This results in propulsion of acid-gastric content into the esophagus leading to **reflux esophagitis**.

Changes in Endocrine System

Pituitary Secretions: The size of **anterior lobe increases two to three times** during gestation, which is mainly due to increase in size and number of prolactin secreting cells.

1. **Prolactin** secretion starts increasing from end of first trimester and at term it is almost 10 times more than the pre-pregnant level.
2. The **hypothalamo-pituitary-ovarian axis is suppressed** by high level of sex steroids. This **decreases LH and FSH secretion**, and therefore **ovulation does not occur** during pregnancy.
3. **Growth hormone** secretion decreases and ***TSH secretion remains normal*** in pregnancy.
4. ACTH secretion is usually **suppressed**.

Thyroid Secretion: Increase in GFR increases the renal clearance of iodine. **Depletion of iodine leads to moderate increase in size of the thyroid gland**, unless dietary intake of iodine increases in pregnancy.

1. High level of circulating estrogen in the later part of pregnancy **increases TBG** (thyroxine binding globulin) production.
2. Therefore, though secretion of T_3 and T_4 is increased, **euthyroid state is maintained in pregnancy**.

Adrenocortical Secretion: Secretion of glucocorticoid and mineralocorticoid is **increased in pregnancy.**

- The plasma free cortisol concentration increases due to its displacement from CBG (cortisol binding globulin). However, clinical hypercortisolism is not encountered.

Calcium Metabolism: The demand for calcium increases in pregnancy to facilitate fetal bone formation.

- This is achieved partly by **increased absorption of calcium** from GI tract by vitamin D and partly by the **increase in parathyroid hormone secretion**.
- Calcium supplementation is invariably given in the later part of pregnancy.

Body Weight Gain

A major external change in the pregnant woman is the increase in body weight.

- In the first and second trimesters, it occurs mainly due to **fat deposition** induced by progesterone that stimulates food intake and diverts glucose for fat formation. In the third trimester, it is mainly due to increase in **size of fetus and uterus**.

Clinical Note 83.3

Toxemia of Pregnancy: About 5–10% of pregnant women develop edema, proteinuria and hypertension, known as **pregnancy-induced hypertension** (PIH). When all these features are present, the condition is called **pre-eclampsia**. If convulsion is associated, the condition is termed **eclampsia**. These two syndromes are collectively called toxemia of pregnancy.

- However, **fluid retention** significantly contributes to it. Body weight gain is usually more in eclampsia (Clinical Note 83.3)

PARTURITION

Pregnancy terminates either in abortion or in parturition. The **duration of normal pregnancy** in human is approximately **40 weeks from the first day of last menstrual cycle**, or 38 weeks from the day of ovulation. Delivery of the fetus at term through vaginal route is called parturition (as fetus can also be delivered by cesarean section). When fetus is delivered after 28th week and before 37th complete week of gestation, is called **premature infant**.

1. In last few weeks of pregnancy, due to **increased level of estrogen**, uterine muscle cells **synthesize more connexin**, the protein that form gap junctions. This facilitates coordinated **contractions of myometrium**.
   - However, the cervix of the uterus becomes soft due to enzymatic lysis of its collagen fibers.
   - **Relaxin** secreted from placenta and ovaries **facilitate cervical softening and dilation**.
2. Estrogen induces the synthesis of **oxytocin receptors**, which enhances uterine smooth muscle contraction.

Mechanism of Parturition

Parturition is produced by **strong contractions of the myometrium**. At the **onset of parturition**, the **amniotic sac ruptures**, and the amniotic fluid flows through the vagina.

1. The **uterine contractions** become strong and appear every 10–15 min. Gradually, contractions increase in intensity and frequency.
2. The **cervix progressively dilates** to attain a maximum diameter of about 10–12 cm. Once cervical dilation is complete, every new contraction moves the fetus downward in the birth canal.
3. Finally, very strong uterine contractions push the fetus through the cervix and vagina.
4. At this stage, the mother, by **bearing down** to increase abdominal pressure, adds to push the baby in the birth canal.
5. Within minutes of delivery of the baby, both the **umbilical cord and the placenta are delivered**.
   - Placenta, which remains tightly adhered to uterine wall throughout pregnancy, is separated from it by a series of waves of uterine contractions and

delivered after the delivery of the baby (hence, called **after birth**).

Parturition Reflex

Parturition is a reflex phenomenon.

1. Towards term, the pregnant uterus synthesizes and secretes **prostaglandins** (PGE_2 and $PGF_{2\alpha}$) that area potent stimulators of uterine muscle contraction (Flowchart 83.1).
2. **Oxytocin** causes stronger uterine muscle contraction and also stimulates uterus to synthesize more prostaglandins.
3. **Estrogen** increases uterine muscle excitability and contractility.

Under the effect of estrogen, the **number and sensitivity of oxytocin receptors in uterine muscle cells increase** during the last few weeks of pregnancy.

Role of Oxytocin and parturition reflex has been described in Chapter 72.

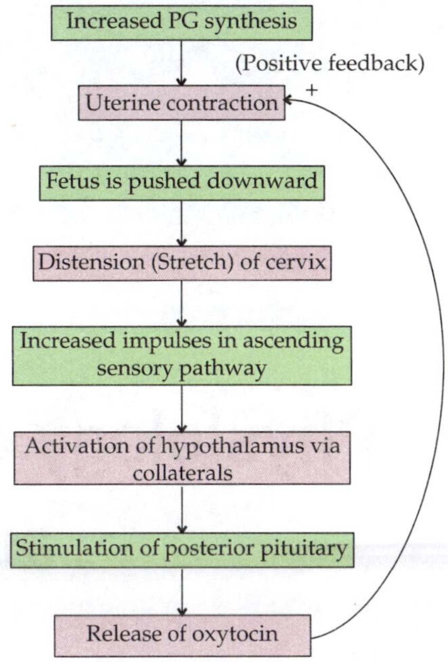

Flowchart 83.1: The mechanism of parturition reflex. Note the positive feedback regulation in this reflex.

Exam Questions

1. Describe the process of fertilization and development of embryo. Give a note on In-Vitro Fertilization.
2. Describe the changes in maternal functions of various systems during pregnancy.

Multiple Choice Questions

1. What is not true about transport of egg in female reproductive system?
A. Contraction of smooth muscle of fimbriae help them to pick up egg
B. Cilia in fallopian tube facilitate the movement of egg in the tube
C. Normally ovum remains in ampullary portion of the tube where fertilization takes place
D. Egg takes four days to reach uterus and fertilization takes place in uterus

2. All of the following are true about zygote formation EXCEPT:
A. The fertilized egg completes its second meiotic division within few hours of fertilization
B. Second polar body is formed and extruded from ooplasm
C. Remaining haploid nucleus containing 23 chromosomes is transformed into pronucleus in 2 to 3 hours
D. Only one pronucleus participates in zygote formation

3. Which of the following is not true about implantation of fertilized egg?
A. The 1st cell division in 24 hours results in two unequal sized cells and the structure is called blastomere
B. Series of divisions result in 16 to 32 cell structure called morula
C. Morula enters uterus in 4 days and forms blastocyst
D. On 4th day blastocyst is implanted on uterine wall at the cervical opening

4. All are true about placentation and amnion formation, EXCEPT:
A. Implantation is completed in 10-12 days after fertilization and formation of chorionic villi starts from 12th day
B. Chorionic villi originate from endothelial cells of blood vessel in the endometrium
C. Fetal part of placenta is formed by outermost layers of trophoblast cells called chorion
D. Maternal part of placenta is formed by endometrium underlying the chorion

5. Which of the following placental hormone is secreted more in quantity in early part of pregnancy?
A. hCG B. Estrogen
C. Prolactin D. Relaxin

6. On which day after fertilization hCG appears in maternal plasma?
A. 2nd day B. 6th day
C. 12th day D. 21st day

7. Which of the following is not true about CV maternal changes in pregnancy?
A. Stroke volume increases
B. Diastolic pressure increases
C. Systolic pressure increases
D. Heart rate increases

8. Which of the following is not true about parturition reflex?
A. It is a neurohumoral reflex
B. Oxytocin is the main hormone to induce uterine contraction
C. Control of uterine contraction by oxytocin is an example of negative feedback regulation
D. Estrogen increases umber and sensitivity of oxytocin receptors in uterine muscle

Answers

1. D	2. D	3. D	4. B	5.A
6. B	7. B	8. C		

Chapter 84

Physiology of Breast Development and Lactation

Learning Objectives

On completion of study of this chapter:

The student will be able to (must know):

1. Outline the process of development of breast in different phases of life of women.
2. Describe the role of various hormones in breast development.
3. Illustrate the mechanism of lactogenesis.
4. List the composition of human milk.

The student may also be able to (desirable to know):

1. Describe the mechanisms and regulation of breast development.
2. Describe the mechanisms of lactogenesis and lactation.

BREAST DEVELOPMENT

Structure of Breast

Breast is a mass of fibrofatty tissue containing **alveoli and ducts**.

1. Ducts in breast branch all through the mammary tissue and converge at the nipples.
   - Ducts begin in saclike glands called **alveoli**.
   - Alveoli are the sites of milk secretion and they look like bunches of grapes with stems terminating in the ducts (Fig. 84.1).
2. **Ductules** originate from alveoli. Ductules open to ducts that in turn drain to **lactiferous ducts**.
3. Lactiferous duct terminates in dilated **lactiferous sinus**.
4. Sinuses open to nipple through **nipple-pores**.

The alveoli and ducts are surrounded by specialized contractile cells called **myoepithelial cells**.

Contraction of myoepithelial cells causes **milk ejection** into the lactiferous sinuses.

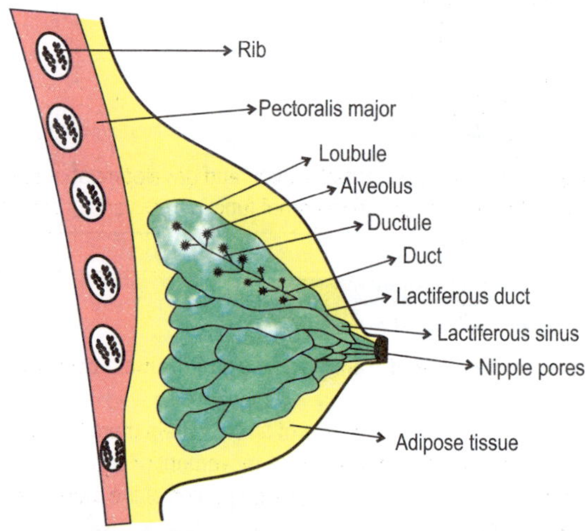

Fig. 84.1: Structure of breast of nonpregnant adult female. Note the arrangement of alveoli and ducts in the mammary gland.

Breast Development in Different Phases of Life

During Intrauterine Life: After 5th month of gestation, the primitive mammary bud forms about 20 secondary buds that form ductal system in the mature gland.

- These ducts undergo proliferation in third trimester of pregnancy in response to various hormones.
- **At birth**, mammary gland is rudimentary.
- In some newborns, small quantity of milk is secreted due to high prolactin concentration in them at that time. This is called *'witch milk'*.

During Childhood: After birth, breast regresses due to lack of hormonal support and remains in a quiescent stage.

During Puberty: With the onset of puberty in girls, marked enlargement of breast occurs **due to the effects of estrogen.**

1. The breast development is mainly due to **enhancement of duct growth and branching of ducts** with relatively little growth of the alveoli.

- The breast enlargement is significantly contributed by **fat deposition**.
2. When menstrual cycle starts at puberty, **progesterone** secretion commences in the luteal phase of each cycle, which contributes to breast enlargement by stimulating the **growth of alveoli**.
3. The areola enlarges and becomes more pigmented.

During each Menstrual Cycle: During each menstrual cycle, **in the late luteal phase, breast size increases** due to alveolar growth in response to progesterone and ductal growth in response to estrogen.

During Pregnancy: Breast enlargement occurs due to the stimulatory effects of high plasma concentrations of **estrogen, progesterone, prolactin, and hCS**.

1. Appreciable breast enlargement occurs after second month of gestation.
2. The **areola and nipple increase in size and become more pigmented**.
   - **Montgomery tubercles** appear in the areola.
3. **Alveoli, ducts and glands** gradually increase in size.
4. In the last trimester, acini differentiate into **secretory glands**.
5. Parenchymal cells of **alveoli undergo hypertrophy** increasing the size of the breast.

All these changes are meant to prepare breasts for lactogenesis and lactation.

During Lactation: A lactating breast is large in size with nipple projecting about 2 cm beyond the areola.

- Breast changes during lactation occur mainly due to the **action of prolactin** secreted from anterior pituitary.
- Prolactin also stimulates the production of milk.

PY9.8

LACTOGENESIS AND LACTATION

Though prolactin level is high in later part of pregnancy, milk production does not occur due to the **inhibitory effects of estrogen and progesterone** at their high concentrations on lactogenesis.

1. **Estrogen increases secretion of prolactin** and along with prolactin promotes breast growth and differentiation.
   - But, along with progesterone, it **antagonizes prolactin action on milk production** and secretion.
2. **Following parturition**, estrogen and progesterone concentration falls appreciably and **milk production by prolactin is unopposed**.
3. The role of prolactin in lactogenesis has been described in the Chapter 71 (Anterior Pituitary).

Role of hypothalamus

Prolactin level **still remains very high** till the mother continues to nurse the breast milk.

1. **Large secretory bursts of prolactin** occur during each nursing period.
   - This **episodic burst of prolactin** signals the breasts for maintenance of milk production.
   - These **prolactin pulses** continue for several days after the mother completely stops nursing her infant.
2. The mechanism mediating prolactin pulses is initiated by **stimulation of nipple receptors by suckling** that sends afferent input to the hypothalamus.
3. This input **inhibits hypothalamic release of dopamine**.
   - As normally dopamine inhibits prolactin secretion, decreased dopamine release stimulates prolactin secretion.
4. **Prolactin also inhibits GnRH secretion** from hypothalamus that **prevents ovulation**.
   - Therefore, till mother continues to nurse the baby, normally ***pregnancy does not occur***.

Suckling also initiates **milk-ejection reflex** (for details, refer Chapter 72, Posterior Pituitary).

Breast Milk

Immediately after delivery, a watery fluid is secreted from breasts called **colostrum**, which is rich in protein. Colostrum secretion is replaced by milk in about 24 to 48 hours.

1. **Mother's milk contains all nutrients in adequate quantity**: carbohydrate in the form of lactose (milk sugar), protein (casein), fat, minerals, vitamins and water (Table 84.1).
2. Milk contains **antibodies** meant for protecting the newborn from various infections.
3. Milk also contains **growth factors and hormones** that help in physical development and maturation, and large number of **neuropeptides and endogenous opioids** that facilitate the development of brain and behaviour of infant.
   - The milk proteins are not destroyed in the GI tract as low gastric acidity in newborn fails to denature them.
   - Also, the intestinal epithelium in infant is **more permeable to proteins** than in the adult, which facilitates their absorption.

Thus, mother's **milk proteins easily enter into blood of the infant**.

Table 84.1 | Composition of human milk.

Component	Average Quantity
Water	87%
Solids	13%
Proteins (gm%)	2.5
Carbohydrate (gm%)	6
Fats (gm%)	5

Table 84-1: Contd...	
Calcium (mg%)	40
Phosphorous (mg%)	30
Magnesium (mg%)	5
Sodium (mg%)	15
Potassium (mg%)	60
Vitamin C (mg%)	4.5
Vitamin A (μg%)	5
Vitamin D (IU)	5
Vitamin B1 (μg%)	15
Riboflavin (μg%)	45
Niacin (μg%)	180
Vitamin B6 (μg%)	10
Pantothenic acid (μg%)	200
Calories/100 g	67

Abnormalities of Breast Development & Lactation

Small Breasts: Small breast may be constitutional, genetic and familial.

Polythelia: Polythelia is condition in which there are more than two number of breasts.

- More number of breasts can develop in the **milk line starting from axilla to the groin**.

Deficient Lactation: Deficiency of lactation can occur due to following causes.

1. *Poor breast development:* A small breast, and flat or inverted nipple may impede suckling.
2. *Generalized illness:* A chronic illness during pregnancy or lactation may decrease lactogenesis.
3. *Hypothalamo-pituitary disorder:* Decreased prolactin secretion due either due to hypothalamic or to pituitary dysfunctions result in deficient lactation
4. *Failure of baby to suckle:* Prematurity, congenital anomalies of mouth and neonatal illness can cause inefficient suckling.

Breast Engorgement: Failure of the baby to empty the breast sufficiently results in breast engorgement.

- Breast becomes hard, tense and painful.
- Treatment consists of **drawing off milk using breast pump** or expressing milk from the breast manually.

Galactorrhea

Galactorrhea is the continuous secretion of milk in the absence of recent pregnancy. When it is associated with amenorrhea, the condition is called **galactorrhea-amenorrhea syndrome**.

1. The tumor of pituitary gland causing excess secretion of prolactin can cause this syndrome (**hyperprolactinemia-galactorrhea syndrome**).
2. It is also seen in **Chiari-Frommel syndrome**, which is characterized by excess lactation, amenorrhea, and super-involution of uterus dating from pregnancy.
   - It occurs due to persistent prolactin secretion without secretion of FSH and LH.
3. Galactorrhea may occur **due to some drugs** such as reserpine, phenothiazine derivatives, α-methyldopa and tricyclic antidepressants.

Exam Questions

1. Describe the mechanism of development of breast in different phases of life. Explain the role of prolactin in breast development.
2. Describe the process of lactogenesis. Give the composition and specialities of breast milk.

Multiple Choice Questions

1. **Which of the following hormone does not participate in breast development?**
   A. Progesterone B. Prolactin
   C. GnRH D. hCS
2. **Estrogen mainly causes development of component of the breast?**
   A. Duct system B. Lobulo-alveolar system
   C. Parenchyma of breast D. Myoepithelial cells of breast
3. **Progesterone mainly causes development of which component of the breast?**
   A. Duct system B. Lobulo-alveolar system
   C. Parenchyma of breast D. Myoepithelial cells of breast
4. **Among electrolytes, which of the following is the highest content of human breast milk expressed in %?**
   A. Calcium B. Potassium
   C. Sodium D. Magnesium
5. **Which of the following is the main hormone for milk synthesis and secretion?**
   A. Estrogen B. Oxytocin
   C. Prolactin D. Progesterone
6. **Which hormone causes milk ejection from breast during breast feeding?**
   A. Oxytocin B. Prolactin
   C. GnRH D. Progesterone

Answers

1. C 2. A 3. B 4. B 5. C 6. A

Chapter 85

Physiology of Contraception

Learning Objectives

<u>On completion of study of this chapter:</u>

The student will be able to (must know):

1. Classify male and female contraceptives and list the merits and demerits of each.
2. Explain the mechanism of action of OCP and IUCD.
3. Say which contraceptive will be ideal for which category of couple.

PY9.6

CONTRACEPTIVE METHODS

Contraceptive methods may also be **classified as** temporary and permanent methods.

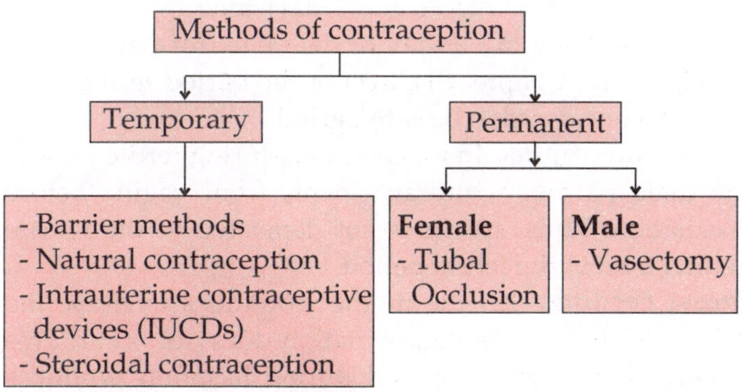

Physical Methods

In Males: Condom is the most widely used barrier device in male.

- It prevents sperm to be deposited in the vagina.
- The biggest advantage is that it provides protection against sexually transmitted diseases.

In Females: Diaphragm is the most commonly used vaginal barrier. **A spermicidal jelly** is usually used along with the diaphragm.

- Another female barrier device is **vaginal sponge**.

Chemical Methods

Various spermicidal agents like **foams, creams and suppositories** are inserted manually into vagina before intercourse. These act as 'surface active agents' that attach themselves to sperms and decrease their oxygen uptake and kill them. They have high failure rate.

Intrauterine Devices

Intrauterine devices (IUDs) are **most effective contraceptive devices for a parous lady** (who has borne at least one child).

Types: The IUD are of **three generations**:

1. First generation IUD
- Lippes Loop

2. Second generation IUD
- Earlier devices: Copper–7; Copper T–200
- Newer devices: Copper T variants (T–Cu 220C; T–Cu 380A; T–Cu 380Ag)

3. Third generation IUD (with hormonal preparation)

Progestasert: a T shaped device filled with 38 mg of progesterone.

Levonorgestrel–20 (LNG-20): a T shaped IUD releasing 20 mcg of levonorgestrel, a synthetic steroid.

Mechanism of Action: IUD works by several mechanisms.

1. Usually, they work after fertilization has occurred but before implantation is completed. The presence of these small objects in the uterus brings about uterine changes that **interfere with the endometrial preparation** for acceptance of the blastocyst. Thus, implantation is prevented.
2. They also act as **foreign body** in the uterine cavity causing cellular and biochemical changes in the endometrium and the uterine fluid that impair the viability of the gamete. Therefore, the chance of fertilization is reduced.

3. **Copper facilitates cellular reaction** in endometrium, composition of cervical mucus, impairs sperm motility and impairs capacitation of sperm.
4. Hormone releasing devices increase the viscosity of cervical mucus by releasing progesterone. They **make mucous thick**, so that sperm can not enter uterus. They also make the endometrium unfavorable for implantation.

Hormonal Contraceptives

1. **Oral contraceptive pills:** Combined pill, Progestogen only pill, post-coital pill, once-a-moth pill.
2. **Depots** (slow releasing formulations): Injectable preparations, subcutaneous implants & vaginal rings.

Oral Contraceptive Pills (OCPs)

Presently, OCPs contain 30-35 mcg of estrogen and 0.5 to 1 mg of progesterone. The pill is given for 21 days from 5th day of the cycle.

- Oral contraceptives are based on the principle that estrogen and progesterone **inhibit pituitary gonadotropin release**, thereby *preventing ovulation.*
- Progesterone only pill affects the composition of the cervical mucus, reducing the ability of the sperm to pass through the cervix, and inhibit the estrogen-induced proliferation of the endometrium, making it inhospitable for implantation.

Side effects of OCP

Though OCPs are 100% effective in preventing pregnancy, there are risks of few side effects, especially when consumed for many years.

Cardiovascular Side Effects: Myocardial infarction, cerebral thrombosis, venous thrombosis and **hypertension** have been reported. These side effects are more seen in aged (more than 35 years) woman and in smokers.

- *Hypertension* occurs due to fluid retention and increased angiotensin level.
- Estrogen ***increases renin-angiotensin activity*** and thereby increases angiotensin II production which is a potent vasoconstrictor.

Carcinogenesis: Increased risks of cervical cancer and breast neoplasia have been reported. Hepatic tumors occur rarely.

Metabolic Side Effects: OCPs **decrease HDL** and alter blood coagulability.

- These two factors ***facilitate atherosclerosis*** and proneness to myocardial infarction and stroke.
- They also cause *glucose intolerance* and insulin resistance.

Miscellaneous: Other side effects include cholestatic jaundice, breast tenderness, weight gain and migraine.

Depots

Subcutaneous implants are contraceptive (progestogen) capsules (Norplant) implanted beneath the skin that releases hormone slowly and last for five years. **Injectable forms** (intra-muscular injection of progestogen substance like Depo-Provera every three months) are also available.

Post-Conceptional Pills

Contraceptives can be used **within 72 h** after intercourse (post-coital contraception).

1. These pills interfere with ovulation, transport of the conceptus to the uterus, or implantation.
   - Usually, **high dose of estrogen**, or two large doses (12 h apart) of a **combined estrogen-progestin** oral preparations are prescribed.
2. Most effective with fewer side effects is the **pill RU 486** (mifepristone), which antagonizes progesterone activity by binding competitively with progesterone receptors in the uterus.

Other Methods

Rhythm (Safe Period) Method: The rhythm method is the a**bstinence from sexual intercourse during the fertile period of the cycle (near the time of ovulation).**

1. In 28 days regular cycles, normally ovulation occurs between 12th and 16th day (usually on 14th day). Functionally sperm can survive for two days and ovum for 3 days.
2. Therefore, unprotected intercourse should be avoided during the **fertile period** of the cycle, which will fall between 2 days before and 3 days after ovulation i. e. from 10th day to 19th day of the cycle (for details refer Fig. 81.10; Chapter 81). Rest of the period in the cycle may considered to be **safe period**.

Coitus Interruptus: In this method, during fertile period, the male partner withdraws penis from vagina before ejaculation. Thus, sperm is not deposited in the female genital tract in the fertile period.

Breast Feeding: Till the mother continues to nurse the baby with breast feeding, ovulation does not occur. This is because prolactin secreted during lactation **produces lactational amenorrhe**a by inhibiting GnRH secretion.

Family Planning Operations

Male Sterilization: Male sterilization is performed by **vasectomy** or bilateral **ligation of vas deferens**

Female Sterilization: Female sterilization is performed by **bilateral tubal ligation**.

Exam Questions

1. Classify contraceptives, describe the mechanism, merits and demerits of various contraceptive methods used in females and males.
2. Describe mechanisms of action of intrauterine devices (IUDs) and oral contraceptive pills (OCPs)

Section X

Renal System

"*No life can be successful without self-discipline.*

The Mother"
(of Sri Aurobindo Ashram, Pondicherry, INDIA)

Chapter 86

PY7.1

Introduction to Renal System and Functional Anatomy of Kidney

Learning Objectives

On completion of study of this chapter:

The student will be able to (must know):

1. List the functions of kidney.
2. Name the parts of a nephron, and correlate histological modification at different parts with their functions.
3. List the differences between cortical and juxtamedullary nephrons.
4. Outline the ultrastructure of glomerulo-capsular filtration barrier.
5. Illustrate the structure and functions of JG apparatus.
6. Elucidate the pathway of renin-angiotensin system and list the functions of angiotensin II.

The student may also be able to (desirable to know):

1. Describe the structural and functional organization of different parts of the nephron.
2. Explain the role of JG apparatus in health and disease. .

RENAL SYSTEM

Renal system consists of kidney, ureter, urinary bladder, and urethra (Fig. 86.1). Kidneys play vital role in volume and electrolyte homeostasis and urinary system is crucial for excretion of waste products of metabolism from the body.

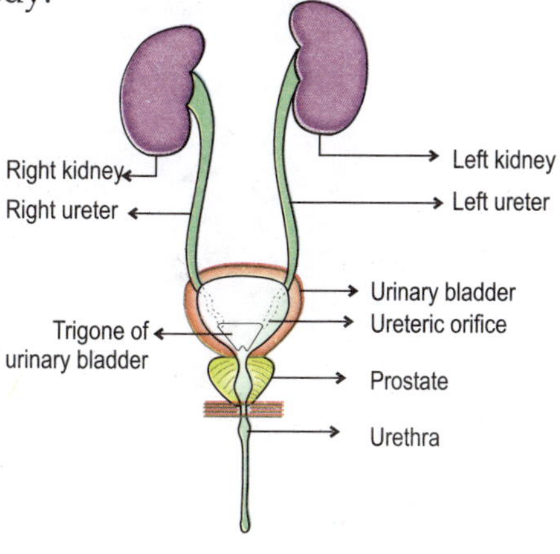

Fig. 86.1: Components of urinary system

Functions of Kidney

1. **Urine formation and excretion of waste products:** The primary function of the kidneys is to **excrete waste products of metabolisms** from the body such as urea, creatinine, uric acid etc. dissolved in urine.
   - Kidneys form urine and excrete many toxic waste products from the body dissolved in urine.
   - Thus, kidneys prevent their accumulation to a dangerous level in the body.
2. **Regulation of ECF volume:** Kidneys play an important role in regulation of ECF volume of the body.
   - Many hormones such as aldosterone, ADH, ANP, angiotensin etc. involved in regulation of ECF volume act on kidney tubules to achieve this function.
   - These hormones modify reabsorption of sodium and water from kidneys to control ECF volume.
3. **Regulation of blood pressure (BP):** Kidneys contribute mainly to **long-term regulation of arterial volume and pressure**.
   - Renin secreted from kidney activates renin-angiotensin-aldosterone axis that plays an important role in regulation of BP.
   - Many hormones act on kidney to regulate blood volume and pressure.
   - Kidneys have also their intrinsic mechanisms to alter sodium and water excretion to regulate BP.
4. **Regulation of electrolyte composition of body fluids:** Composition of electrolytes in ECF is mainly the function of kidney.
   - **Excretion and reabsorption of electrolytes** from kidneys directly influence their concentration in ECF.
   - Kidneys also contribute to vitamin D synthesis that controls plasma calcium concentration.

5. **Acid-base balance:** Kidneys contribute significantly to acid-base balance by controlling **bicarbonate excretion and H^+ secretion.**
   - Thus, it controls blood pH and pH of other body fluids.
   - Therefore, kidney abnormalities may cause metabolic acidosis or alkalosis.
6. **Regulation of plasma osmolality:** By controlling **NaCl and water reabsorption,** kidneys control plasma osmolality.
   - Change in plasma osmolality provides feedback signal for secretion of ADH that acts on kidney to regulate the osmolality.
7. **Regulation of erythropoiesis:** ***Erythropoietin***, the major regulator of erythropoiesis is secreted from interstitial cells in the peritubular capillary bed of kidney.
   - Therefore, kidney diseases result in **anemia.**
8. **Endocrine functions:** Kidney secretes **thromboxane A_2** and **prostaglandins,** in addition to the secretion of erythropoietin.
   - Kidneys secrete **renin** that activates renin-angiotensin system.
   - Kidneys also form **calcitriol** (1,25-dihydroxycholecalciferol), the active form of vitamin D_3 from 25-hydroxycholecalciferol.
9. **Gluconeogenesis:** Though kidneys are not the primary site of gluconeogenesis, in starvations, synthesis of glucose from noncarbohydrate sources, especially from glutamine occurs in these organs.

FUNCTIONAL ANATOMY OF KIDNEY

Size of **each kidney** in adult is roughly about the size of ***one's fist*** **(11cm in length and 6 cm in width),** and the weight is about **150g**. Kidneys are covered by a thick capsule called **renal capsule.**

- Internally, **two distinct regions** are seen: the ***outer cortex*** and the ***inner medulla.***

Cortex: The cortex is **granular in appearance** and contains all glomeruli, convoluted tubules and cortical portion of collecting ducts.

Medulla: The medulla is **striated in appearance** due to presence of loop of Henle, medullary portion of collecting duct and blood vessels that are arranged in parallel.

- The medulla is divided into 8–12 conical masses, called the **renal pyramids** that appear in a radiating pattern.
- Medullary pyramids originate at the corticomedullary junctions and terminate into a **papilla,** which is present within the **minor calyx.** Minor calyces unite to form **major calyx.**
- The major calyces open into **renal pelvis,** which is the upper expanded portion of the ureter (Fig. 86.2).

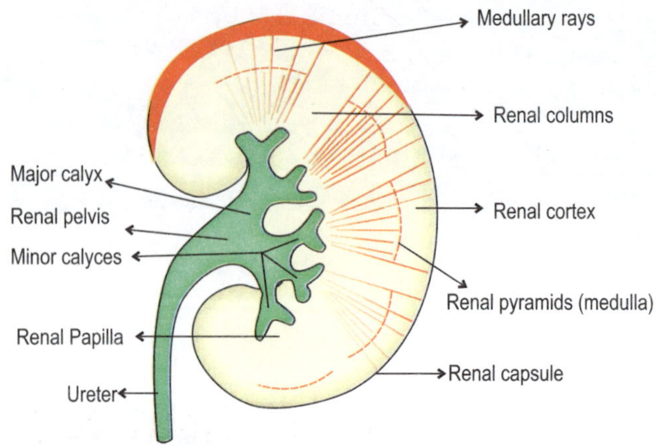

Fig. 86.2: Gross histological structure of kidney in sagittal section.

Parts of the Nephron

Nephron is the **basic structural and functional unit** of the kidney. There are about **1.2 millions** of nephrons in each kidney in human beings.

- A **nephron consists of** renal corpuscle, proximal convoluted tubule (PCT), loop of Henle, distal convoluted tubule (DCT), and collecting duct system (Fig. 86.3).
- The **total length** of the nephron ranges from **45 to 65 mm.**

Renal Corpuscle

The renal corpuscle, also called Bowman's capsule, contains the **glomerulus,** a tuft of capillaries. **Bowman's capsule** filters blood from glomerular capillaries to form the **ultrafiltrate,** which is delivered into proximal tubule.

Proximal Tubule

This is the **initial segment** of the nephron, hence called proximal tubule (PT).

- As **most part of it is coiled,** proximal tubule is also called ***proximal convoluted tubule*** (PCT).
- It ends in a **small straight segment** that continues to form loop of Henle.
- The PT is about **15 mm long and 40 μm in diameter.**

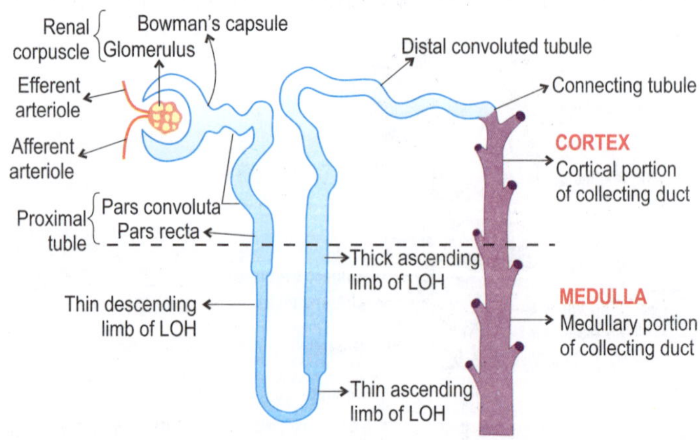

Fig. 86.3: Parts of a nephron. LOH: loop of Henle

- PT **recovers most of the filtrate** for its considerable capacity of reabsorption.

Features of PT Cells: The tubular cells of PT exhibit features that correlate with their functions of extensive reabsorption (Fig. 86.4A).

1. The proximal tubular epithelial cells have **extensive folding of the apical membrane**. Also, apical membrane contains **microvilli (brush border)** that further increase the luminal surface area for transport of ions and water.
2. The basolateral membrane of epithelial cells has multiple infoldings.
3. The epithelial cells **contain many mitochondria** that are present towards the basal part of the cells.
4. The adjoining epithelial cells are **bound to each other by tight junctions** at their luminal ends creating **paracellular and basolateral spaces** that help in transport of solutes and water.

Parts of PT: The PT is divided into **two parts**; the initial major convoluted portion (**pars convoluta**) and the distal smaller straight portion (**pars recta**) that opens into loop of Henle.

- Pars convoluta constitutes about **70% of the PT**.
- The number of infoldings of luminal border and the number of mitochondria in pars recta are less than in pars convoluta.

Loop of Henle (LOH)

LOH is the continuation of pars recta of PT. It consists of **descending and ascending limbs**.

1. The **descending limb** is thin throughout in all nephrons, whereas the **ascending limb** has ***thin and thick portions*** in a typical juxtamedullary nephron.
   - Thus, LOH ***in juxtamedullary nephrons*** has **three parts**: thin descending, thin ascending and thick ascending limbs.
   - In a ***cortical nephron***, thin ascending part of LOH is almost absent.
2. The **total length** of LOH varies from **14 to 26 mm** depending on the type of nephrons (see below).
   - The thin limb is about 2 to 14 mm long and the thick limb is about 12 mm long.
3. About **15% of filtrate is reabsorbed in LOH**.
   - The LOH of juxtamedullary nephrons plays an important role in **counter-current mechanism of urine concentration**.

Thin Limb of LOH: The length of hairpin loop depends mainly on the **length of thin part**, which varies from 2 mm in superficial or cortical nephrons to 14 mm in juxtamedullary nephrons (Fig. 86.3).

- **In cortical nephrons**, thin segment is very short and has no ascending portion and barely penetrates medulla.
- **In juxtamedullary nephrons**, the thin segment is long, has an ascending portion and penetrates deep into the medulla.
- The **diameter** of thin limb of LOH is about **15 μm**.

The cell structure of thin segment of LOH is simple suggesting the passive nature of exchange of solutes and water in this part.

1. The **epithelial cells are flat** with relatively **smooth apical and basolateral membranes**.
2. Cells contain **few mitochondria** (Fig. 86.4B).

Thick Limb of LOH: The transition between thin and thick parts of ascending limb is abrupt. The **tubular diameter** increases from 15 μm to **30 μm**. Changes also occur in histology that suits for active transport of solutes and water.

1. Epithelial cells are small and cuboidal.
2. The basolateral membrane of cells has **extensive infoldings**.
3. The luminal surface of cells has less infoldings.
4. Cells contain **numerous mitochondria** that are mainly located towards basal part (Fig. 86.4C).

The thick ascending limb of LOH terminates in DCT. The junction between the thick ascending limb and DCT comes in contact with the afferent or efferent arteriole **to form JG apparatus** (described below). The tubular epithelial cells at this junction are histologically modified **to form macula densa**.

Distal Convoluted Tubule

The distal convoluted tubule (DCT) begins immediately after the macula densa. It is **5 mm** in length.

1. The epithelial cells of DCT are somewhat larger than those of thick ascending limb; otherwise they closely resemble them (Fig. 86.4D).
2. They have **extensive infoldings of basolateral membrane** of cells that contain abundant mitochondria.
3. The luminal surface of cells has less infoldings.

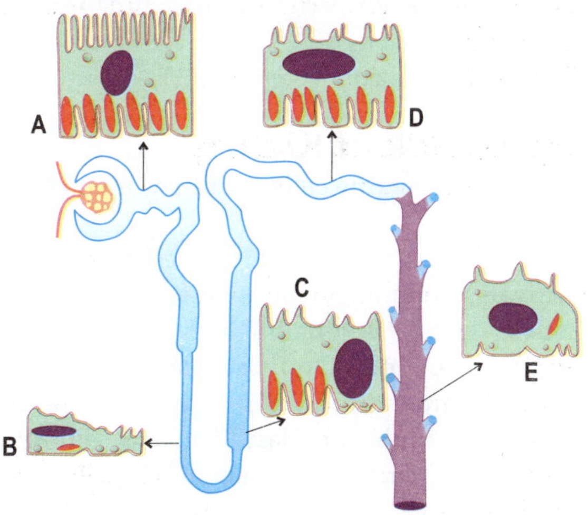

Fig. 86.4: Histological specialties of different parts of nephron. Note the structural differences in epithelial cells of different parts (as described in the text) such as in PCT **(A)**; thin descending limb of LOH **(B)**; thick ascending limb of LOH **(C)**; DCT **(D)**; collecting duct **(E)**.

Though, DCT is **relatively impermeable to water**, hormones like aldosterone and ADH facilitate its absorption in this segment.

Connecting Segment

The DCT empties into collecting duct through the connecting segment or tubule. This is a **small and relatively straight tubule** with morphological and transport characteristics similar to that of collecting duct.

Collecting Duct

Several DCTs empty into collecting duct. The collecting duct is **20 mm** long.

- It passes through the cortex and medulla to empty into the pelvis of the kidney at the apex of medullary pyramids. Thus, it is divided into **two parts**: cortical and the medullary portions.
- The **medullary portion** of the collecting duct is further divided into **outer medullary** and **inner medullary parts**.
- The epithelial cells of collecting duct are modified to participate in transport of ions and water. The water permeability is controlled mainly by ADH whereas Na^+ transport is controlled by aldosterone.

Histological modifications are as follows:

1. Epithelial cells are cuboidal with **minimal infoldings of basolateral and apical membrane**.
2. Mitochondria are few in number (Fig. 86.4E).
3. The epithelium of collecting duct contains ***two types of cells***: **principal cells** (P cells) and **intercalated cells** (I cells). P cells are more in number than I cells.

P Cells: The P cells have moderate basolateral infoldings and **few mitochondria**. They are involved in sodium reabsorption and **ADH-induced water reabsorption**.

I Cells: The I cells contain **more microvilli**, more basolateral infoldings and **more mitochondria**.

- They are involved in **acid secretion and bicarbonate transport**.
- Few I cells are also present in DCT.

Secretory Cells of Kidney

The secretory or **endocrine cells** in kidney are mainly **two types**:

1. **Juxtaglomerular (JG cells) cells:** JG cells **secrete renin** that activates renin-angiotensin system.
2. **Interstitial cells (IS cells):** Three are **two types** of interstitial cells; cortical and medullary.
   - **Cortical interstitial cells** are of two types: phagocytic and fibroblast-like cells. **Fibroblast-like cells** (peritubular interstitial cells) ***secrete erythropoietin***.
   - **Medullary interstitial cells** are of two types: type-I and type-II. **Type-I medullary interstitial cells** secrete prostaglandins, especially PGE_2.

Types of Nephron

Anatomically, there are **three types of nephrons**: superficial nephrons, mid-cortical nephrons and juxtamedullary nephrons. Physiologically, superficial and midcortical nephrons are considered as **cortical nephrons** due to their similarity in histological morphologies and functions.

Cortical Nephrons

The renal corpuscle of cortical nephrons is located in superficial region of the cortex. The glomerulus is usually smaller. LOH of these nephrons is short. LOH **does not have a thin ascending limb** (Fig. 86.5).

- However, the total length of the nephron is almost same as the juxtamedullary nephron, as the DCT is longer.
- Efferent arteriole supplying cortical nephron **branches into peritubular capillaries** that surround the segments of the nephron of its own and of adjacent ones.

Juxtamedullary Nephrons

The renal corpuscle of juxtamedullary nephrons is located in the juxtamedullary region of the cortex, i.e. the inner region of the cortex close to medulla (Table 86.1).

1. The glomerulus is usually larger.
2. They **have long loop of Henle** that extends deep into the medulla. They also have a thin ascending part of LOH.
3. The efferent arterioles form peritubular capillaries and a series of vascular loops called **vasa recta** (for details, see next chapter).

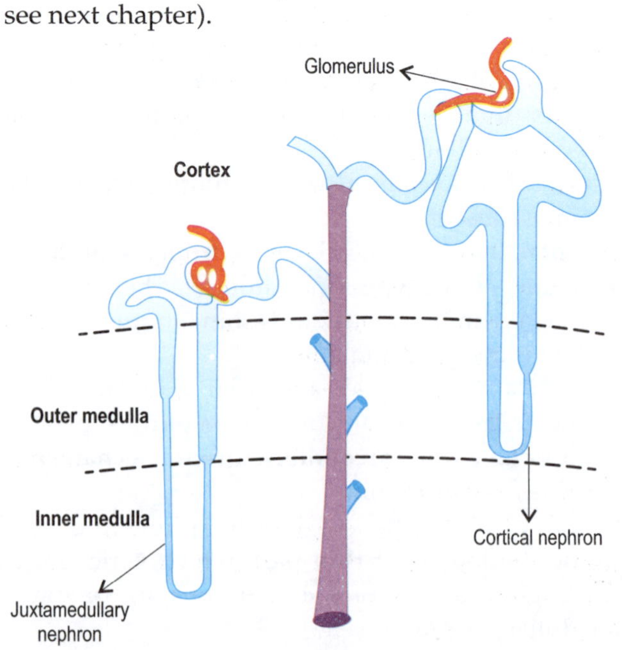

Fig. 86.5: Differences between cortical and juxtamedullary nephrons. Note that the renal corpuscle is located in superficial layers of cortex, glomerulus is small, and the loop of Henle is small in cortical nephron. In juxtamedullary nephron, corpuscle is close to corticomedullary junction, glomerulus is big, and the loop of Henle is long.

Table 86.1 | Differences between cortical and juxtamedullary nephrons.

	Cortical nephrons	Juxtamedullary nephrons
1. Location of renal corpuscle	In the superficial region of cortex	In the juxtamedullary region of the cortex
2. Number	85% of total	15% of total
3. Length of LOH	Shorter	Longer
4. Length of thin limb of LOH	Shorter, and thin ascending is almost absent	Longer, and thin limb has ascending & descending parts
5. Size of glomerulus	Usually small	Usually large
6. Tubular function	Filtration & reabsorption	Filtration, reabsorption, & creation of medullary osmolar gradient
7. Rate of filtration	Slow	High
8. Efferent arteriole	Forms peritubular capillaries.	Forms peritubular capillaries and vasa recta.
9. Vasa recta	Absent	Present, dipping into medulla
10. Efficiency in concentrating urine	Less	More
11 Renin content	More	Less
12. Main function	Urine formation & excretion of waste products	Urine concentration

Ultrastructure of Renal Corpuscle

Renal corpuscle consists of **Bowman's capsule** that contains **glomerulus** and **mesangium**.

Glomerulus

Glomerulus, a **tuft of capillaries** located in the initial dilated and cup like portion of the tubule, called Bowman's capsule.

- Glomerulus is formed by the capillaries that arise from **afferent arterioles.**
- The glomerular capillaries drain into the **efferent arteriole** (Fig. 86.6).
- The glomerular capillaries are the **only capillaries in the body that start with arterioles and end in arterioles.**
- The capillaries are covered by epithelial cells called **podocytes.**

Bowman's Capsule

Bowman's capsule is the initial cup like dilated portion of the nephron that accommodates glomerulus.

1. The capsule has two layers: **visceral layer** that remains in close contact with glomerulus and the **parietal layer** that forms the outer portion of the capsule.
2. The **podocytes** form the visceral layer of Bowman's capsule.

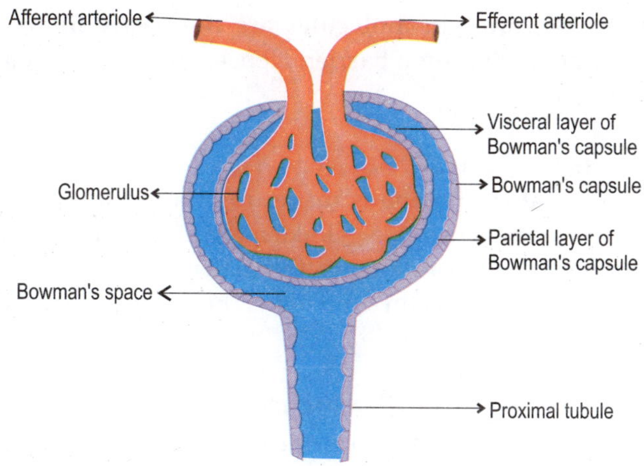

Fig. 86.6: Structure of renal corpuscle

3. The parietal layer of the Bowman's capsule is formed by **parietal epithelial cells** (Fig. 86.7A). The space between visceral and parietal layers is called **Bowman's space.**

Filtration Barrier

The **endothelial cells** of glomerular capillaries are covered by basement membrane. **Podocytes** surround this basement membrane. The ***capillary endothelial cells, basement membrane, and foot process*** of podocytes form the filtration barrier (Fig. 86.7B) through which blood from glomerular capillaries is filtered to form the tubular fluid.

Capillary Endothelium

The endothelium of glomerular capillaries is of **fenestrated type** as it contains fenestra (**pores** or windows).

- These pores are large in diameter (50 to 100 nm in diameter) and therefore, they freely allow passage of large molecules through them. This allows water and small solutes like sodium, urea, and glucose to pass through the capillary endothelium.
- The endothelial cells are **negatively charged** due to presence of anionic glycoproteins on their surface. The proteins in plasma are also anionic.

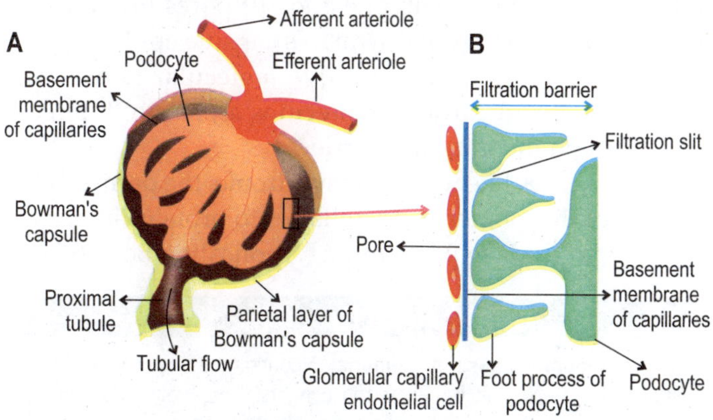

Fig. 86.7 A: Ultrastructure of renal corpuscle; B: structure of glomerulo-capsular filtering membrane.

- Therefore, **protein molecules are not easily filtered** through the filtration barrier. Hence, normally protein is absent in urine.

Basement Membrane

The basement membrane is made up of a **meshwork of fine fibrils** entrenched in a gel like matrix. It is an important **barrier for the proteins** as the matrix contains collagen, laminin, fibronectin, and other negatively charged proteins.

Foot Processes of Podocytes

The podocytes (**foot cells**) form the third or the **inner layer of the filtration barrier**.

1. **Podocytes** constitute the **visceral layer of Bowman's capsule**. They are the **epithelial cells**.
2. Their extensions terminate as **foot processes** that lie on the outer layer of the basement membrane (Fig. 86.7B).
   - The foot processes of podocytes interdigitate to cover the basement membrane.
   - The interdigitating processes are separated by gaps (the space between adjacent foot processes) called **slit pores** or **filtration slits,** having width of 20 nm.
3. The filtration slits are bridged by a ***thin diaphragm*** called **filtration slit diaphragm** that contains small rectangular pores, which ***do not allow free passage*** of molecules.
4. The filtration slit diaphragm is made up of a key molecule called **nephrin.**
   - The nephrin molecules form a zipper-like structure.
   - Minute rectangular pores with dimensions of 40 x 140 Å are formed between the prongs of the zipper.
5. Thus, filtration, especially of protein molecules is **greatly restricted by nephrins**.
6. Filtration slit diaphragm also contains negatively charged particles that prevent passage of proteins.

Restricted Permeability: As we understand from the anatomy of filtration barrier, filtration through glomerulo-capsular filtration barrier occurs **mostly through extracellular route** that consists of **pores** in the capillary endothelial cell layer, basement membrane and slit pores in the foot processes of podocytes of Bowman's capsule epithelium.

- The molecules with effective **molecular radius 20 to 45 Å** and **cationic molecules** are easily filtered through the filtration barrier.
- In diseases like nephrotic syndrome, the permeability of the glomerular capillaries to proteins increases that leads to proteinuria (Application Box 86.1).

Application Box 86.1

Nephrin mutation causes proteinuria: Nephrin, the key component of filtration slit diaphragm is mutated in congenital nephrotic syndrome. Abnormality of nephrin molecules allows free filtration of protein molecules resulting in massive proteinuria, the outstanding feature of the disease.

Mesangium

This is an important component of renal corpuscle. It consists of **mesangial cells** and **mesangial matrix**.

Mesangial Cells

Mesangial cells are derived from blood monocytes and are the components of **mononuclear phagocyte system**. Mesangial cells are present in the mesangium, close to the glomerular capillaries (Fig. 86.8). The function of mesangial cells are:

1. They provide **structural support** for the glomerular capillaries.
2. They **secrete extracellular matrix** (the glomerular or **mesangial matrix**).
3. They secrete **prostaglandins and cytokines.**
4. They are **phagocytic** in nature.
   - They are part of mononuclear phagocytic system.
   - They kill and remove the foreign organisms and debris in the kidney by phagocytosis.
5. The mesangial cells contain **contractile units** that are present in close contact with glomerular capillaries.
   - Therefore, ***contraction or relaxation*** of mesangial cells influences **alteration in GFR** by changing blood flow through glomerular capillaries or by **changing capillary surface area.**
6. Mesangial cells that are present outside the glomerulus are called **extraglomerular mesangial cells.**
   - They are also called **lacis cells** or **Goormaghtigh cells.**
   - They are mainly located between the afferent and efferent arterioles.
   - They secrete some quantity of **renin and erythropoietin**, and also possess phagocytic activity.
7. Mesangial cells are involved in the development of **immune complex-mediated glomerular disease**.

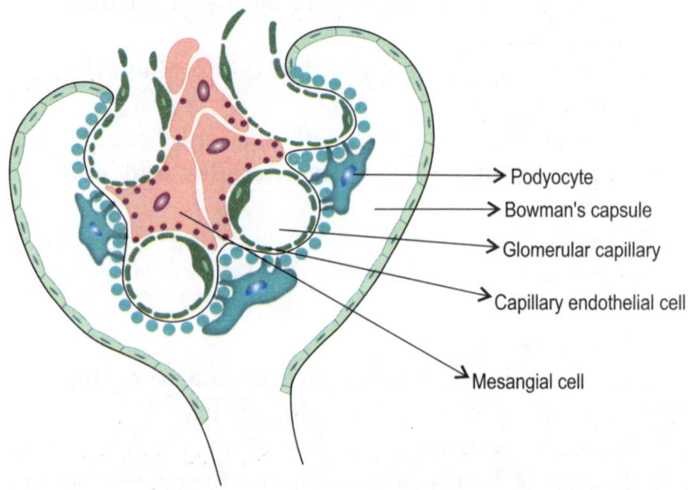

Fig. 86.8: Location of mesangial cells in the renal corpuscle. Also note the placement of podocytes along the glomerular capillary.

JUXTAGLOMERULAR APPARATUS

PY7.2

Structure

The **thick ascending limb** of loop of Henle when comes in contact with the **glomerulus** of the same renal corpuscle, structural modifications occur in the tubule and afferent and efferent arterioles (Fig. 86.9). The entire modified structure (**tubular & vascular components, and cells** between them) is called juxtaglomerular apparatus (JGA). JGA has **3 components**:

1. **Macula densa** of the thick ascending limb of LOH,
2. **Juxtaglomerular cells** (the modified muscle cells mainly of afferent arterioles), and
3. **Lacis cells** (extraglomerular mesangial cells).

Macula Densa: Macula densa cells are **modified epithelial cells** of the thick ascending limb of LOH when it comes in contact with the afferent and efferent arterioles.

- The terminal portion of the thick ascending limb of LOH that passes through the angle formed by afferent and efferent arterioles of the same nephron possesses this tubular epithelial modification. This appears as a **dense area** (hence, called **macula densa**) in the tubule as epithelial cells are ***densely packed*** in this region (Fig. 86.10).
- Macula densa **acts as the sensor** that monitors the **change in ionic composition** and **rate of flow of the tubular fluid** in the lumen of the tubule.
- It provides appropriate **feedback signal to renal corpuscle** to change the rate of filtration so as to meet the need of the kidney functions.
- Therefore, this is an important component in the ***tubuloglomerular feedback*** circuit (see below).

Juxtaglomerular (JG) Cells: JG cells are the granular **epitheloid cells** present mainly in the tunica media of the afferent arteriole (few are also present in efferent arteriole) that come in contact with the terminal part of thick ascending limb of LOH.

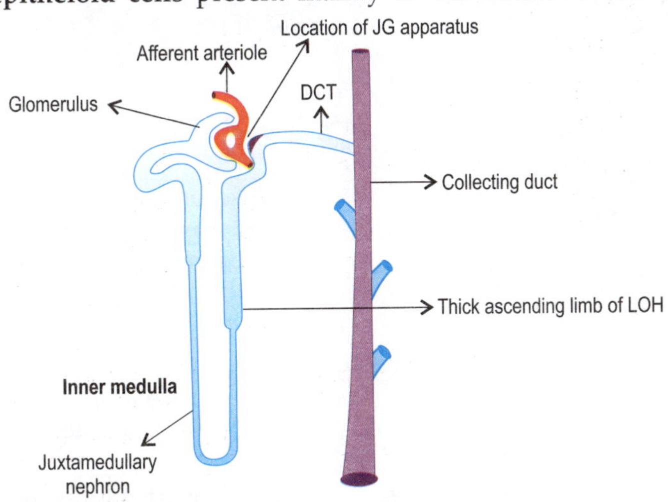

Fig. 86.9: Location of JG apparatus. When terminal part of thick ascending limb of LOH comes in contact with glomerulus and afferent and efferent arterioles, modifications in vascular and tubular cells form JG apparatus.

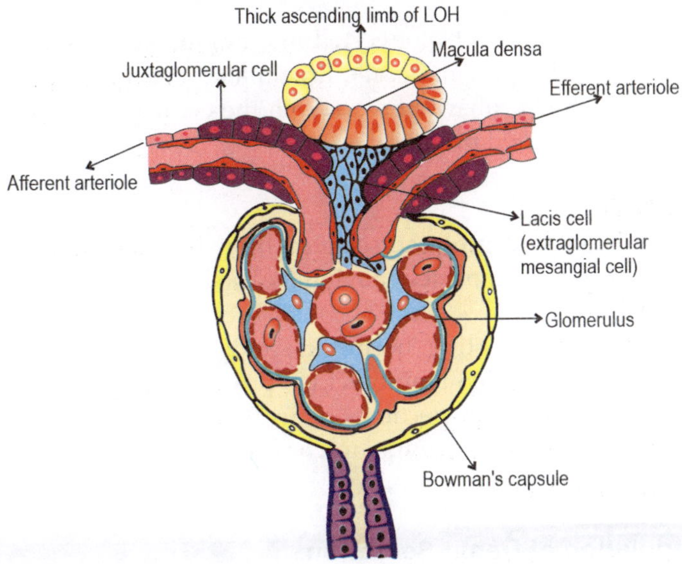

Fig. 86.10: Ultrastructure of JG apparatus. JG apparatus is formed by modified smooth muscle cells mainly of afferent arteriole (JG cell), modified epithelial cells of ascending limb of LOH (macula densa) and extraglomerular mesangial cell (Lacis cell).

1. In fact, these granular cells are **modified vascular smooth muscle cells** with an epitheloid appearance.
2. The cells are highly granular as they **contain many secretory granules**.
3. They are also called **Polkissen cells**.
4. JG cells **secrete renin** that activates renin-angiotensin system.

Lacis Cells: Lacis cells are present in the triangular space formed by efferent and afferent arterioles and the macula densa. Lacis cells are the **mesangial cells present outside the glomerulus**; hence called **extraglomerular mesangial cells**. These are agranular cells that secrete some quantity of renin and erythropoietin.

Functions of JG Apparatus

1. JG cells secrete renin that activates **renin-angiotensin system**, which is involved primarily in the **regulation of blood volume and pressure**.
2. Macula densa cells act as sensor that detects the change in rate of flow and volume of flow in the tubule, and composition of tubular fluid.
   - This provides feedback signal to the glomerulus to change the rate of filtration, which forms the physiological basis of **tubuloglomerular feedback**.
   - Thus, they **control glomerular filtration**.
3. Lacis cells **secrete renin and erythropoietin**.

Renin-Angiotensin System

Renin secreted from JG cells of kidney activates **angiotensinogen to angiotensin I**, which on further enzymatic action gets converted into **angiotensin II and III**. Hence, this system is called renin-angiotensin system (RAS). RAS is primarily involved in the control of blood volume and blood pressure.

Renin

Renin is an **acid protease** secreted from JG cells of kidney. This is a **glycoprotein** having the molecular weight of 37,326.

- Like other peptide hormones, it is synthesized as **preprorenin** (406 amino acids), **prorenin** (383 amino acids), that finally becomes **renin** (340 amino acids).
- Renin acts as an enzyme to **convert angiotensinogen to angiotensin I**.

Regulation of Renin Secretion

Renin activates the renin-angiotensin system, which is essential for regulation of ECF volume, blood volume and blood pressure. Control of ECF volume is closely related to control of **plasma electrolyte** concentration, especially Na^+, Cl^- and K^+. Therefore, change in plasma concentration of these solutes affects renin secretion. **Blood volume** and **blood pressure** are also affected by sympathetic activity, circulating catecholamine and ADH. Therefore, alteration in these factors alters renin-secretion.

Factors that increase renin secretion:

1. Decreased blood volume and/or pressure
2. Decreased plasma Na^+ concentration, increased K^+ concentration
3. Increased sympathetic activity (stimulation of JG cells via renal nerve)
4. Increased circulating catecholamines
5. Prostaglandins

Factors that decrease renin secretion:

1. Increased plasma Na^+ concentration (increased sodium reabsorption via macula densa)
2. Increased blood pressure (increased afferent arteriolar pressure)
3. ADH
4. Angiotensin II

Conditions in which secretion of renin is high:

1. Hypotension
2. Hyponatremia
3. Hyperkalemia
4. Hypovolemia (like hemorrhage)
5. Dehydration
6. Constriction of renal artery (renal artery stenosis)
7. Cardiac failure
8. Standing
9. Cirrhosis of liver
10. Psychological depression

Role of Sodium in Renin Secretion: Plasma sodium is an important electrolyte that controls renin secretion.

- **Decreased plasma sodium** *decreases the filtration of sodium* through the renal corpuscle (glomerular filtering membrane). This **decreases Na^+ concentration in the tubular fluid**.
  - The decreased Na^+ load is **sensed by the cells of macula densa**, which immediately provides feedback information to the JG cells to secrete renin.
- Renin **activates RAS** that results in angiotensin II formation.
- **Angiotensin II increases sodium and water reabsorption** that restores ECF volume.
- The opposite mechanism operates when sodium concentration increases in plasma.

Angiotensinogen

This is a **glycoprotein synthesized in liver**. It contains 453 amino acids. The concentration of angiotensinogen in the plasma **increases by following hormones**:

1. Glucocorticoids
2. Thyroid hormones
3. Estrogen
4. Cytokines
5. Angiotensin II.

Angiotensin II provides a **positive feedback** for further synthesis of angiotensinogen. Angiotensinogen is *physiologically inactive*. It **acts as precursor for the formation of angiotensin I**. Angiotensin I is converted to angiotensin II by angiotensin converting enzyme.

Angiotensin Converting Enzyme

Angiotensin converting enzyme (ACE) is a **carboxypeptidase** that acts on angiotensin I to **convert it to angiotensin II** (Flowchart 86.1).

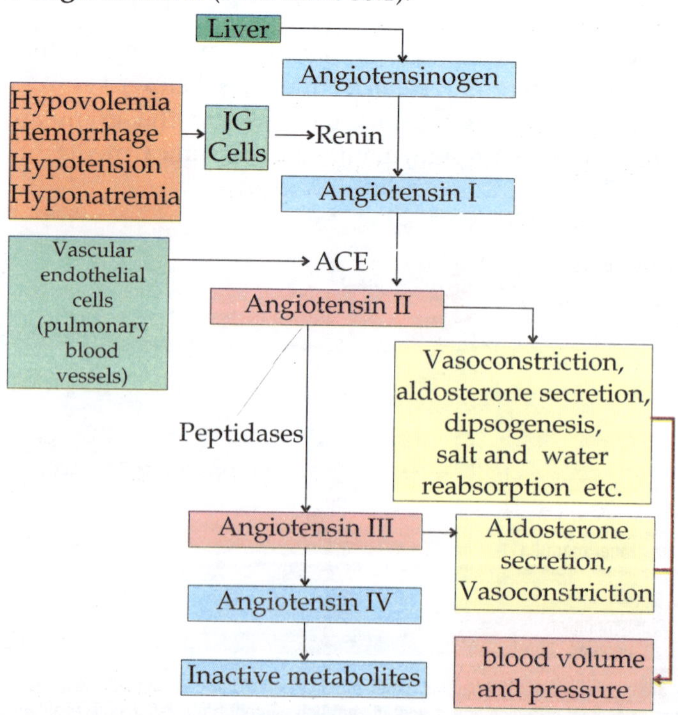

Flowchart 86.1: Renin-angiotensin system. ACE: Angiotensin converting enzyme.

- Though ACE is synthesized and secreted by the endothelial cells of blood vessels throughout the body, it is more formed in **blood vessels of lungs**. Hence, major conversion of angiotensin I to angiotensin II occurs in the lungs.
- ACE exists in **two forms**: somatic form and general form. However, physiological significance of existence in two forms is not known.
- ACE also **inactivates bradykinin**.

Angiotensin II, III and IV

Angiotensin II is formed from angiotensin I by the action of ACE.

- Angiotensin II has **short plasma half-life of 1–2 min** as it is rapidly metabolized by various peptidases and is rapidly converted to form **angiotensin III**.
- Angiotensin III is converted to **angiotensin IV**.
- Physiologically, **angiotensin II is the most active angiotensin**. Angiotensin III and IV are also physiologically active.
- **Plasma renin concentration** is measured to determine the ***angiotensin activity*** in the body.

Physiological Actions of Angiotensins

Angiotensin I

It acts as **precursor for angiotensin II**. Otherwise, it is physiologically inactive.

Angiotensin II

This is the most important among all angiotensins. All of its actions are aimed at **increasing the blood volume and pressure**. The functions of angiotensin II can be divided into **central and peripheral functions.**

Peripheral Actions:

1. It is one of the **most potent vasoconstrictors**. The vasoconstriction potency of A II is about 8 times more than that of norepinephrine. Thus, when injected, it increases blood pressure drastically.
    - However, the vasoconstrictor activity of angiotensin II ***decreases in cirrhosis of liver and in patients with hyponatremia***.
    - A chronic increase in angiotensin II level in plasma in these conditions ***decreases the angiotensin II receptors*** on the smooth muscle of blood vessels. Therefore, the vasopressor activity of angiotensin II **is less in hepatic cirrhosis and hyponatremic conditions**.
2. It **increases the synthesis and secretion of aldosterone** from adrenal cortex.
    - In fact, angiotensin II is the major regulator of aldosterone secretion. Therefore, the RAS is also called ***renin-angiotensin-aldosterone axis***.
    - Aldosterone increases sodium and water reabsorption from kidney that *increases ECF volume*.
3. Angiotensin II directly increases the **release of norepinephrine (NE)** *from the post-ganglionic sympathetic neurons*.
    - Thus, it also **potentiates vasoconstriction** through NE release.
4. Angiotensin II causes **contraction of mesangial cells** that decreases the glomerular filtration.
    - Therefore, angiotensin II ***decreases GFR***.
5. Angiotensin II increases **sodium, and water reabsorption** from proximal convoluted tubules of kidney.

Central Actions:

1. Angiotensin II acts on the **brain centers to decrease the sensitivity of the baroreflex**. This potentiates the pressure effect of angiotensin II.
2. It **stimulates the thirst centers** in the brain to increase water intake. It does not penetrate the blood brain barrier.
    - It acts on the **circumventricular organs** (the structures present outside the blood brain barrier) that include subfornical organ (SFO), organum vasculosum of lamina terminalis (OVLT), area postrema (AP) and the posterior pituitary.
    - SFO and OVLT are amongst the **thirst centers** in the brain.
3. Angiotensin II **increases the secretion of ADH** from posterior pituitary.
4. It **increases the secretion of ACTH** from anterior pituitary.
5. It **acts as neurotransmitters** in some areas of the brain.

Angiotensin III

Angiotensin III possesses about **40% vasopressor activity of angiotensin II**.

- However, it has **100% aldosterone secreting activity** of angiotensin II.
- Thus, angiotensin II and III are involved in aldosterone secretion, whereas angiotensin II in primarily involved in the **regulation of blood volume and pressure**.

Angiotensin IV

This is the recently discovered angiotensin. It has some biological activities in the brain. Probably, it **stimulates vasomotor center.**

Angiotensin II receptors

There are ***two types of angiotensin II receptors***: angiotensin 1 (AT_1), and angiotensin 2 (AT_2).

AT_1 Receptors: These receptors are present in the **arteries and adrenal cortex**.

- Acting on AT_1 receptors, angiotensin increases intracellular calcium level via phospholipase C that forms **diacylglycerol and IP_3**.
- There are **two sub-types of AT_1 receptors**, AT_{1A}, and AT_{1B}. **AT_{1A} receptors** are present in blood vessels, and

brain, and AT_{1B} **receptors** are present in adrenal cortex and anterior pituitary.

AT_2 Receptors: These receptors are attached to G proteins that **increase the intracellular cGMP**. These receptors are mainly present in fetuses and neonates. However, they are also present in **brains** in adults.

Clinical Importance of RAS

RAS is implicated in the **genesis of hypertension**. Renin increases angiotensin formation that causes intense vasoconstriction, which in turn increases blood pressure. Therefore, the conditions in which renin secretion is high, blood pressure is invariably high. This is the important physiological basis of **renal hypertension**.

1. In experimental animals, hypertension is produced by constricting the renal artery (producing renal ischemia). This is called **Goldblatt hypertension** (for details, refer Chapter 41, Pathophysiology of Hypertension).
2. Etiologically, hypertension is classified into three categories depending on the concentration of renin in the plasma: **hyper-renin hypertension, normo-renin hypertension, and hypo-renin hypertension**.
3. In the treatment of hypertension, the drugs that inhibit ACE (**ACE blockers**) are very effective in controlling blood pressure than other group of drugs.
4. The commonly administered ACE blockers are **captopril** and **enalapril**. Angiotensin II receptor blockers like **losartan** have been recently tried.

INNERVATION OF KIDNEY

Renal nerve controls renal blood flow, glomerular filtration rate, and electrolyte and water reabsorption from the kidney.

1. Renal nerve contains **sympathetic noradrenergic fibers**.
   - There is **no parasympathetic innervation of kidney**.
2. Sympathetic fibers also secrete **dopamine**.
3. Stimulation of sympathetic fibers causes constriction of both afferent and efferent arterioles. However, afferent arteriolar constriction is more.
   - This **decreases renal blood flow and glomerular filtration rate**.
4. The JG cells are innervated by sympathetic fibers.
   - Activation of sympathetic fibers results in **increased renin secretion**.

Exam Questions

1. Describe the structural modification of tubular epithelial cells in different parts of the kidney tubules and their physiological significance.
2. List differences between cortical and juxtamedullary nephrons. Add a note on glomerulo-capsular filtering barrier.
3. Describe the structure and functions of JG apparatus. Add a note on glomerular mesangial cells.
4. Describe the role of renin-angiotensin system in the regulation of kidney functions.

Multiple Choice Questions

1. Angiotensin II causes all of the following, EXCEPT :
A. Stimulation of thirst
B. Increased ADH secretion
C. Vasodilatation
D. Aldosterone secretion

2. Renin is secreted by:
A. PCT
B. DCT
C. Collecting duct
D. Juxtaglomerular apparatus

3. Macula densa in kidney is located in:
A. PCT
B. DCT
C. Afferent arteriole
D. Efferent arteriole

4. Lacis cells are located at :
A. JGA
B. Proximal tubule
C. Distal tubule
D. Loop of henle

5. All are true about juxta-glomerular apparatus of kidney, EXCEPT:
A. Important source of angiotensinogen
B. Important source of renin
C. Consists of macula densa
D. Consist of of lacis cell

6. Which is true about juxtamedullary nephrons?
A. Accounts for 85% of total nephrons
B. Length of LoH is short
C. Efferent arteriole form vasa recta
D. Renin content is less

7. Which of the following is not a function of kidney?
A. Regulation of erythropoiesis
B. Control of plasma volume and osmolality
C. Gluconeogenesis
D. Metabolism of fat

8. Which is true about renin?
A. It converts angiotensinogen to angiotensin-I
B. Secreted by PCT
C. Increased GFR causes increased secretion of renin
D. Decreases plasma Na^+ & H_2O

Answers

1. C	2. D	3. B	4. A	5. A
6. C	7. D	8. A		

Chapter 87

Renal Blood Flow and Glomerular Filtration

Learning Objectives

On completion of study of this chapter:

The student will be able to (must know):

1. Appreciate the arrangement of arterial supply and peritubular capillaries and vasa recta in nephrons.
2. Know the basic principles of measurement of renal blood flow (RBF).
3. Describe the mechanisms of regulation of RBF.
4. List the hormones that cause renal vasoconstriction and vasodilation.
5. Define GFR, give its normal value, and explain the mechanism of glomerular filtration.
6. List the factors that affect GFR.
7. Name the chemicals that cause contraction, & relaxation of mesangial cells of kidney.
8. Understand the basic principle of measurement of GFR.
9. Elucidate the mechanisms of regulation of GFR.

The student may also be able to (desirable to know):

1. Describe the measurement and regulation of RBF.
2. Describe the measurement and regulation of GFR. .

RENAL CIRCULATION

Kidneys receive about **23.5% of the cardiac output**. The blood flow to kidneys is about 1260 ml/min or **420 ml/100g of tissue/min**.

Renal blood flow is maximum in cortex and minimum in medulla.

- Average blood flow **in the cortex is about 5 ml/min/g** of tissue and **in medulla, about 0.5 ml/min/g** of tissue (Fig. 87.1).

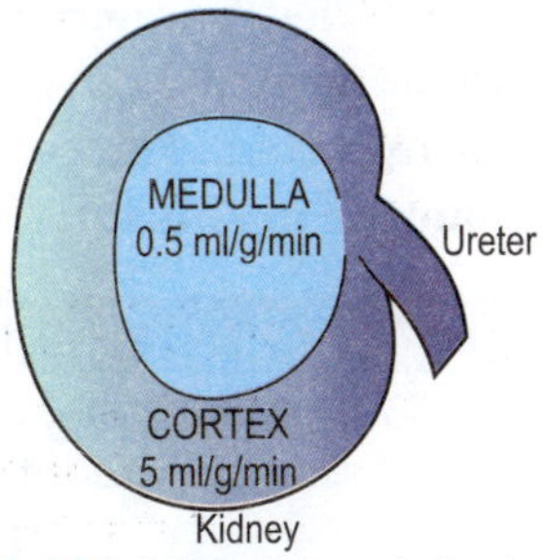

Fig. 87.1: Difference in cortical and medullary blood flows in kidney.

- The low blood flow in medulla **helps to maintain hyperosmolality in the medullary interstitium** that plays an important role in counter-current mechanism of urine concentration.

Functional Anatomy

Arterial Supply

Each kidney is supplied by a single **renal artery** that originates from aorta.

- Renal artery branches to form **anterior and posterior divisions** that form total five **segmental arteries**.
  - Each segmental artery branches into **interlobar artery**, which in successive divisions forms **arcuate artery**, **interlobular artery** (cortical radial artery) and **afferent arteriole**.
- Afferent arteriole gives rise to **glomerular capillary** network (glomerulus) that finally drains to **efferent arteriole**.
- Efferent arterioles lead to a second capillary network, which is formed around the renal tubules (hence called **peritubular capillaries**) (Fig. 87.2).

Venous Drainage

The venous system of kidney parallels the arterial system.

1. Efferent arterioles form peritubular capillaries or vasa recta which drain into interlobular veins. The subsequent sequence of drainage is arcuate veins, interlobar veins, segmental veins and finally the renal vein (Flowchart 87.1).
2. In the medulla of kidney, blood supply is derived from efferent arteriole of juxtamedullary glomeruli. These efferent arterioles in juxtaglomerular nephrons, in addition to formation of **peritubular capillaries**, form an extra set of capillaries called **vasa recta** (Fig. 87.2).
3. Vasa recta are straight and long capillaries that run deep into the medulla. Thus, there are **descending**

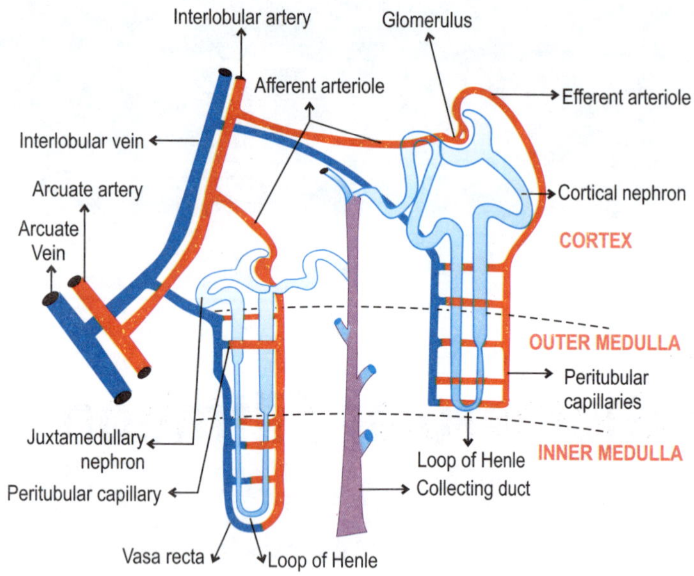

Fig. 87.2: Blood supply to kidney. Note the arrangement of peritubular capillaries in cortical nephron, and peritubular capillaries and vasa recta in juxtamedullary nephrons.

and **ascending limbs** of vasa recta that remain in close contact with each other.

4. This arrangement of vasa recta helps it to function as the **counter exchanger** in urine concentrating mechanism by exchanging substances between blood flowing into and out of medulla.
5. The blood from the inner medulla returns to the cortex in the ascending limb of vasa recta.

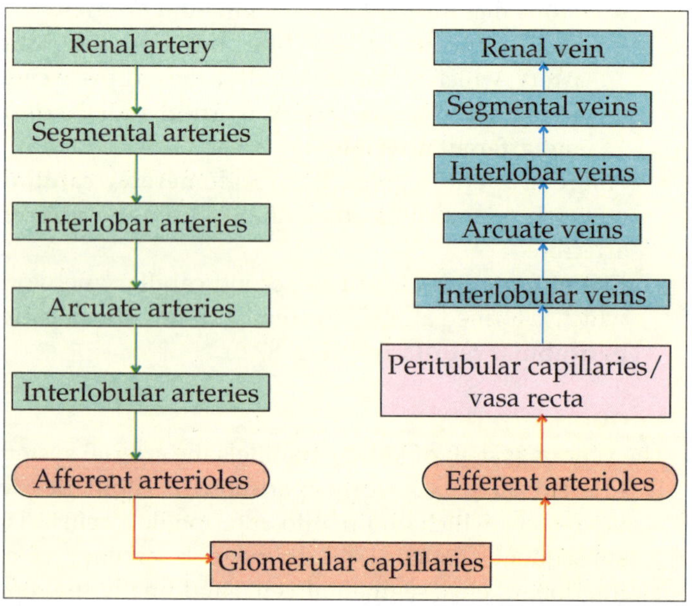

Flowchart 87.1: Sequence of arterial supply and venous drainage in kidney.

Functions Vasa Recta

1. It provides oxygen and nutrients to the nephron segments.
2. It delivers substances to the nephron for secretion into the tubular lumen.
3. It serves as a pathway for the return of reabsorbed water and solutes to the circulatory system.
4. It participates in concentration (as counter current exchange) and dilution of urine.

Importance of Renal Blood Flow (RBF)

The flow of blood through kidneys serves following important functions.

1. Supplies **oxygen, nutrients**, and hormones that control kidney functions.
2. **Delivers metabolites and waste products** to the kidney for their excretion in the urine.
3. Controls **concentration and dilution of urine**.
4. Influences solute and water reabsorption from kidney.
5. **Determines GFR** (RBF is the main determinant of GFR).

Oxygen Consumption of Kidneys

Kidneys are metabolically active organs. Therefore, the oxygen consumption by kidneys per unit tissue (**6 ml per 100g** of tissue per min) is **more than other metabolically active organs** like liver (2 ml per 100g of tissue per min) and brain (3.3 ml per 100g of tissue per min). A greater blood flow to kidneys (**23.5% of the cardiac output**) ensures a higher oxygen supply to the organs.

- However, oxygen supply to kidneys is more than they normally need. The oxygen consumption by kidneys as a whole is much less, which is about 18 ml per min, in comparison to 52 ml per min for liver, 50 ml per min for skeletal muscles, 45 ml per min for brain and 30 ml per min for heart.
  - Therefore, the **arteriovenous oxygen difference across the kidney is considerably less** than the other organs (Application Box 87.1).
  - This ensures **adequate oxygen reserve** for kidneys in various physiological conditions.
- Nevertheless, inspite of adequate oxygen supply to kidneys, damage to renal tissues occurs in hypoxic conditions as in shock.

Physiological Significance: The vascular arrangement in most part of kidney tissue permits **shunting of a greater fraction of oxygen** in the arterial blood to the venous blood before blood passes through the capillaries. Therefore, inspite of adequate oxygen supply to kidneys, the oxygenation of renal tissue is not as high as expected. Hence, kidney is **susceptible to hypoxic damage in shock**.

Application Box 87.1

Venous blood of kidney is bright red: The venous blood of kidney has a bright red color as the red cells in it have **high oxyhemoglobin content**. This is due to the **low renal extraction of oxygen**, as kidneys receive much more oxygen than they utilize.

Measurement of RBF

Principle of Measurement

RBF can be measured by **Fick principle**. Also, **electromagnetic flow-meter** and other flow-meters measure RBF.

Fick Principle: With the application of Fick principle, RBF is detected by measuring the **amount of a given substance** taken up by the organ per unit time and dividing this value with the **arterio-venous (AV) difference** of the substance across the organ (kidney).

- Kidney filters blood to form urine. Therefore, renal blood flow equals the amount of a substance **excreted per unit time divided by its renal AV difference**.

The substance used for measurement of RBF should have **following properties**:

1. The substance used should be measurable in the arterial and venous blood
2. Should not be metabolized
3. Should not be stored
4. Should not be produced by the kidney, and
5. By itself, should not affect the blood flow.

Usually the substance used for RBF measurement is **para-aminohippuric acid** (PAH), as it possesses all the above-mentioned properties. RBF is measured by using the appropriate formula that uses renal plasma flow (RPF) and hematocrit (see below). Renal blood flow is renal plasma flow (RPF) divided by 1 minus hematocrit (Hct).

$$\text{Renal blood flow} = \text{RPF} \times \frac{1}{1 - \text{Hct}}$$

Thus, first RPF and hematocrit are estimated. Hematocrit is determined by centrifuging a blood sample. RPF is measured by clearance of PAH infused intravenously.

Measurement of Renal Plasma Flow

RPF is measured by **injecting PAH** and then determining the concentration of PAH **in urine and plasma**. The **extraction ratio** (i.e. arterial concentration minus renal venous concentration divided by arterial concentration) for PAH is high, because PAH is filtered from the glomerulus and secreted by tubular cells.

- Following its injection, 90% of PAH from the arterial blood is removed in the kidney through its single circulation.
- Therefore, usually renal plasma flow is calculated by **dividing the amount of PAH in urine by the plasma level of PAH** (concentration of PAH in renal venous blood is ignored).
  - Peripheral venous plasma is used as the concentration of PAH in peripheral plasma is essentially identical to that in the arterial plasma reaching the kidney.
- The value obtained is called **effective renal plasma flow** (ERPF) to emphasize that the level in the renal venous plasma is not measured.
- In human being, **ERPF is about 625 ml/min** in average.

$$\text{ERPF} = \frac{U_{PAH} \times V}{P_{PAH}} = \text{Clearance of PAH } (C_{PAH})$$

For example, when concentration of PAH in urine (U_{PAH}) is 12.4 mg/ml, urine flow (V) is 1 ml/min, and concentration of PAH in plasma (P_{PAH}) is 0.02 mg/ml, ERPF is calculated as follows:

$$\text{ERPF} = \frac{12.4 \times 1}{0.02} = 620 \text{ ml/min}$$

ERPF is converted to actual renal plasma flow by the following method:

As the average PAH extraction ratio is 0.9,

$$\text{Actual RPF} = \frac{\text{ERPF}}{\text{Extraction ratio}} = \frac{620}{0.9} = 689 \text{ ml/min.}$$

If hematocrit (Hct) is 47%, then RBF will be:

$$\text{RBF} = \text{RPF} \times \frac{1}{1 - \text{Hct}} = 689 \times \frac{1}{1 - 0.47}$$

$$= 689 \times \frac{1}{0.53} = 1300 \text{ ml/min}$$

Thus, renal blood flow, as calculated from the above equations is 1300 ml/min

Regulation of RBF

Renal blood flow is regulated by neural, hormonal, and local factors, and by autoregulatory mechanisms.

Neural Factors

Sympathetic Control: Stimulation of renal sympathetic fibers causes **vasoconstriction that decreases renal blood flow.**

1. Therefore, conditions that activate renal sympathetic fibers such as hemorrhage, cold, pain, exercise, anesthesia etc. decrease blood flow to kidney.
2. Sympathetic stimulation also **increases renin secretion** from JG cells that **activates renin-angiotensin system**. Formation of **angiotensin II** causes renal vasoconstriction and further decreases blood flow.
3. However, angiotensin II and sympathetic stimulation to kidneys stimulate the production of **local prostaglandins** (PG E_2 and I_2) that produce vasodilation and oppose the vasoconstriction effects.
   - Therefore, sympathetic stimulation unless intense and longstanding, can't ordinarily compromise renal functions.

Hormonal Factors

Circulating **catecholamines** and other vasoactive peptides like **angiotensin II** cause renal vasoconstriction (Table 87.1).

- However, **dopamine** in high dose causes ***renal vasodilation***.
- Therefore, **dopamine is preferred for the treatment of cardiogenic shock**, as its systemic effect increases blood pressure and its renal vasodilation effect maintains renal perfusion.

Table 87.1 | Hormones affecting renal blood flow.

A. Vasoconstrictors	B. Vasodilators
Epinephrine	ANF
Norepinephrine	Dopamine
Angiotensin II	Histamine
Adenosine (A1 receptor)	Kinins
Endothelin	EDRF
Vasopressin	PG E_2
Thromboxane A2	PG I_2 Acetylcholine Adenosine (A_2 receptor)

Local Factors

Locally produced **metabolites and chemicals** like ***CO_2 and prostaglandins*** cause renal vasodilation and maintain renal blood flow. Though **adenosine** is a potent vasodilator in coronary and cerebral circulations, it causes constriction in renal vascular bed.

Autoregulation

Blood flow to kidney is maintained at a relatively constant level despite the change in systemic pressure range between **80 to 180 mmHg**. This is called autoregulation of renal blood flow (Fig. 87.3).

Myogenic Mechanism of Autoregulation: The renal autoregulatory mechanism is an **intrinsic phenomenon** as it is also observed in isolated and denervated kidney.

- However, it is absent when renal vascular smooth muscle is paralyzed by drug administration. This indicates that the autoregulation is mainly due to direct contractile response of renal smooth muscle (of afferent arteriole) to stretch. This is called the **myogenic mechanism of autoregulation**.
- In this process, increased pressure in the blood vessel causes stretch of the vessel wall that **opens cation channels resulting in depolarization**. This leads to **voltage-dependent opening of calcium channel** causing calcium influx. **Increased intracellular calcium** causes vasoconstriction.
- Opposite changes occur when blood pressure decreases.

Metabolic Mechanism: Local **metabolic mechanism** also contributes to autoregulation of blood flow, in which NO, prostaglandins, adenosine and other metabolites produced in the tissue influence blood flow.

Glomerulotubular Feedback Mechanism: Glomerulotubular feedback mechanism also plays role in autoregulation of blood flow, in which composition and flow of tubular fluid determine RBF and glomerular filtration.

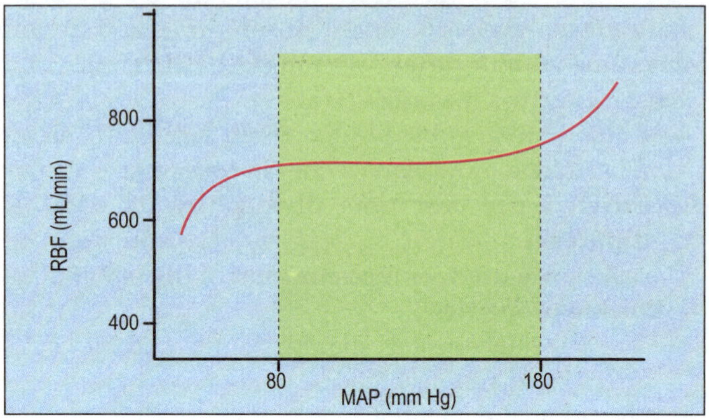

Fig. 87.3: Autoregulation of renal blood flow (RBF). Note, within the mean arterial pressure (MAP) range of 80–180 mm Hg, renal blood flow almost remains constant.

PY7.3

GLOMERULAR FILTRATION

The glomerular filtration is the **first step** in urine formation. This involves **ultrafiltration of plasma** that takes place through the *glomerulocapsular filtering membrane*. The product of filtration is called **filtrate** (the ultrafiltrate of plasma) that flows down the tubular lumen.

Mechanism of Glomerular Filtration

Glomerular filtration occurs through the **glomerulocapsular filtration barrier** that consists of fenestrated capillary endothelium, the basement membrane and podocytes of capsular epithelium. This is governed by ***two major factors***: **pressure gradients** or starling forces (hydrostatic and osmotic pressure gradients) across the glomerular capillary wall and **filtration coefficient** (size of the capillary bed and permeability of the capillaries).

Glomerular filtration = $K_f [(P_{GC} - P_T) - (\Pi_{GC} - \Pi_T)]$

When, K_f is filtration coefficient (the product of glomerular capillary wall permeability and the effective filtration surface area), P_{GC} is the mean hydrostatic pressure in glomerular capillaries, P_T is mean hydrostatic pressure in tubule, Π_{GC} is glomerular capillary oncotic pressure, and Π_T is osmotic pressure of the filtrate in the tubule.

Pressure Gradients

The pressure gradients across glomerular capillary wall are different from the pressure gradients along the capillaries of other vascular beds.

- Therefore, quality and degree of filtration are different through the filtration barrier.

- Like other capillary beds, the pressure gradients are due to operation of **Starling forces** that are **hydrostatic and oncotic pressures.**

Hydrostatic Pressure Gradient

The hydrostatic pressure in glomerular capillary is **considerably higher** than the capillary pressure in other parts of the body. This is because the afferent arterioles directly arise from interlobular arteries and they are short and straight.

- The glomerular capillary pressure at the afferent arteriolar end is same as **at efferent arteriolar end**, i.e. 45 mmHg.
- This pressure is *opposed by* the hydrostatic pressure **in Bowman's capsule**, which is 10 mmHg.
  - Therefore, the hydrostatic pressure gradient across the filtering membrane is 35 mmHg (45–10 mmHg) towards the capsule.
- Thus, hydrostatic pressure **strongly favors filtration** across the entire glomerular capillary membrane from its afferent end to efferent end (Fig. 87.4).

Osmotic Pressure Gradient

The hydrostatic pressure gradient is opposed by the osmotic pressure gradient. Osmotic pressure gradient depends on the glomerular capillary **oncotic pressure** and the **osmotic pressure of the filtrate in the tubular fluid.**

- Oncotic pressure at the afferent arteriolar end is 20 mmHg and at the efferent arteriolar end is 35 mmHg.
- This pressure is **opposed by tubular fluid osmotic pressure.** However, the osmotic pressure of the tubular fluid is negligible.
  - Therefore, the **osmotic pressure gradient is towards capillary lumen** and the magnitude is more at efferent end than at afferent end.

The Net Filtration Pressure: The net filtration pressure (P_{UF}) across the glomerular membrane depends on the **difference between the hydrostatic pressure gradient and the glomerular capillary oncotic pressure** (as the oncotic pressure of tubular fluid is negligible).

$P_{UF} = (P_{GC} - P_T) - \Pi_{GC}$

At the afferent end of glomerular capillary, the net filtration pressure is:

Afferent P_{UF} = 35mmHg – 20 mmHg
= 15 mm Hg outward

At efferent end of glomerular capillary, the net filtration pressure is:

Efferent P_{UF} = 35mmHg – 35 mmHg
= 0 mm Hg

Thus, the net filtration gradient is **always from glomerular capillaries towards the tubule,** which is high at afferent arteriolar end that slowly declines to almost nil at efferent arteriolar end.

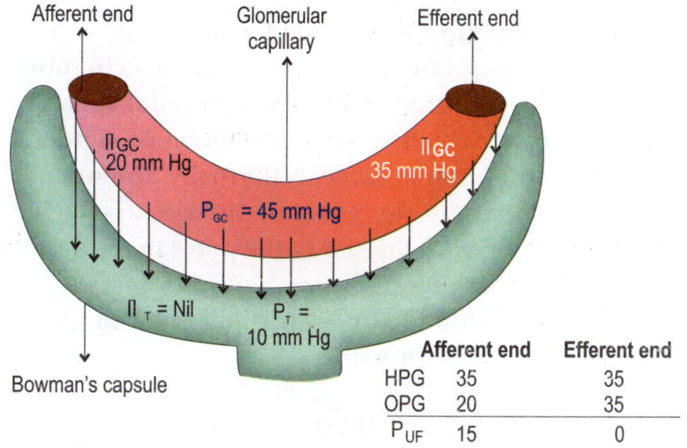

Fig. 87.4: Mechanism of filtration along the glomerular capillary membrane. Note that filtration occurs almost along the entire length of capillary membrane. However, the degree of filtration is maximum at afferent arteriolar end, which gradually decreases to almost zero at the extreme efferent end of the capillary. The magnitude of arrow indicates the degree of filtration. P_{GC}: Mean hydrostatic pressure in glomerular capillaries; P_T: Mean hydrostatic pressure in tubule; Π_{GC}: Glomerular capillary oncotic pressure; Π_T: Osmotic pressure of the filtrate in the tubule; HPG: hydrostatic pressure gradient; OPG: Osmotic pressure gradient.

Filtration Coefficient

Filtration coefficient (K_f) is the product of **glomerular capillary wall permeability** and the **effective filtration surface area** (size of the capillary bed).

Capillary Permeability

Glomerular capillaries are **highly permeable,** i.e. about 50 times that of capillaries in skeletal muscle. However, **filtration depends on** the size and shape of the molecules and the electrostatic charge they carry.

Molecular Size: Molecular size is an important determining factor of filterability of the substance. Neutral substances with molecular diameter of less than 4 nm are freely filtered and substances with **diameter of more than 8 nm are not filtered.**

Shape: The elongated particle with large molecular weight can pass easily, whereas globular particle of same molecular weight cannot pass through.

Electrostatic Charge: The particles with **positive charge can easily pass** through the glomerular filtering membrane than the negatively charged particles.

1. This is because the glomerular capillary wall is negatively charged due to the presence of **sialoproteins.**
2. Therefore, **permeability of cationic molecules is more** than neutral and anionic molecules.
3. The effective diameter of circulating albumin is less than 8 nm, but **albumin is anionic.** Therefore, normally **albumin is not filtered** through the glomerular capillaries.
4. However, in **diseases in which the charge of glomerular capillaries is lost** as occurs in glomerular nephritis, albumin appears in urine.

Clinical Significance: Normally, about less than 100 mg of protein is excreted in urine per day. This is not due to the filtration of proteins by the glomerular membrane, rather **due to secretion** by the tubular cells.

1. In fact, protein is not secreted, but it appears in tubular fluid due to **shedding of tubular epithelial cells.**
2. **Albuminuria**, which refers to excretion of significant amount of albumin in urine, is normally absent.
3. However, albuminuria is seen in diseases in which:
    - There is increase the size of the pores in the glomerular membrane, or,
    - There is disruption of electrostatic force of glomerular membrane proteins.

Size of the Capillary Bed

The surface area for filtration of the capillary bed depends on the size of **mesangial cells**. The *contraction of mesangial cells decreases the area* available for filtration and *relaxation of mesangial cells increases the area* for filtration. Thus, **mesangial cell contraction impairs and relaxation facilitates GFR**. The factors that alter mesangial cell activity are listed in Table 87.2.

Table 87.2 | Factors that alter mesangial cell activity.

A. Factors that produce contraction of mesangial cells
- Angiotensin II
- Norepinephrine
- Endothelins
- ADH
- PDGF (platelet derived growth factor)
- PAF (platelet activating factor)
- Histamine
- Thromboxane A_2
- PGF_2
- Leukotrienes
B. Factors that produce relaxation of mesangial cells
- Dopamine
- ANP (atrial natriuretic peptide)
- cAMP
- PGE2
- Nitric oxide
- Bradykinin

Glomerular Filtration Rate

Definition and Normal Value: Glomerular filtration rate (GFR) is defined as the amount of filtrate formed by glomerular filtering membrane of both the kidneys in a unit time. Normally, it is **125 ml/min** (7.5 L/h or 180 L/day).

Factors Affecting GFR

GFR is influenced by factors that alter renal blood flow, pressure gradients, glomerular capillary permeability and surface area for filtration.

1. **Change in renal blood flow:** Increased blood flow to kidney increases the delivery of blood to glomerulus that promotes filtration and conversely decreased flow decreases filtration. Thus, renal vasodilation maintains GFR.
2. **Glomerular capillary hydrostatic pressure:** Hydrostatic pressure in glomerular capillary depends on the **amount of blood delivered** to and the **amount of blood drained** from the glomerulus.
    - Afferent arteriolar dilation or efferent arteriolar constriction increases capillary hydrostatic pressure and therefore, increases GFR.
    - Conversely, afferent arteriolar constriction or efferent arteriolar dilation decreases GFR.
3. **Change in capsular hydrostatic pressure:** Hydrostatic pressure in the Bowman's capsule and tubule opposes filtration.
    - **Tubular obstruction increases tubular hydrostatic pressure** and therefore decreases GFR.
4. **Oncotic pressure:** Osmotic pressure in glomerular capillaries due to plasma proteins opposes filtration.
    - Therefore, **hypoproteinemia results in more GFR**.
    - Conversely, dehydration decreases GFR and urine formation.
5. **Glomerular capillary permeability:** Integrity of glomerular capillary is an important determinant of GFR. Increased capillary permeability increases GFR as occurs in glomerulonephritis.
6. **Effective filtration surface area:** Size of filtration area depends on mesangial cells.
    - Mesangial cell contraction distorts the capillary lumen and decreases the area available for filtration.
    - Conversely, relaxation of mesangial cells increases filtration.
    - Many hormones and chemicals control GFR by altering mesangial cell activity.
7. **Size, shape and electrical charge of the macromolecules**

Molecular size determines the filterability of the substance.

- Any substance having molecular weight less than 10,000 can be freely filtered by the glomerular filtration barrier and molecules with weight more than 10,000 have restricted filterability (Table 87.3).

Table 87.3 | Filterability of some common substances through glomerular filtration barrier.

Substance	Mol. Wt.	Mol. Diameter	Filterability (%)
Water	18	0.20	100
Glucose	180	0.70	100
Inulin	5,000	2.8	100
Myoglobin	17,000	4.0	75
Hb	68,000	6.6	3
Albumin	69,000	7.2	0.01

- Most of the proteins in plasma are larger molecules and therefore can't be filtered. Also, the molecular shape influences filterability.

- **Slender and supple molecules can easily pass through** than the spherical and rigid molecules.
- Due to the presence of negatively charged particles in all the three layers of glomerular filtration barrier, **molecules with negative charges can't easily be filtered**, whereas neutral and cationic substances can do so.

Filtration Fraction

Filtration fraction (FF) is the **ratio of the GFR to renal plasma flow**.

1. Normal FF ranges between **0.16 to 0.20**. This is a better **index of glomerular activity**. For example, decreased blood pressure increases FF without much change in GFR.
2. **In hypotension**, renal plasma flow decreases. However, GFR decrease is less than the decrease in renal plasma flow as efferent arteriolar constriction maintains GFR. Thus, *FF remains elevated*.

Measurement of GFR PY7.4

Concept of Renal Clearance: Measurement of GFR and RBF is based on the principle of renal clearance.

Renal clearance of a substance is defined *as the volume of plasma from which that substance is completely cleared (removed) per unit time*.

- When a substance is removed in urine, a certain volume of plasma is cleared (freed) of that substance.
- Therefore, clearance assesses an important aspect of kidney function as normally kidney is capable of clearing the substance from the plasma.

The clearance of a substance can easily be assessed by determining the concentrations of the substance in plasma and urine, and by estimating the urine flow rate. The formula is as follows:

$$C_X = \frac{U_X \times V}{P_X}$$

When, C_X is the clearance of the substance, U_X is the concentration of substance in urine, V is the urine flow in unit time, and P_X is the concentration of substance in the plasma.

Inulin Clearance Test

Inulin clearance test is commonly used for the assessment of glomerular filtration.

- It can be measured by measuring the concentration of the substance in urine and the plasma concentration of the substance.
- The substance **should be freely filtered through the glomeruli and should neither be secreted nor be reabsorbed** by the tubules.

GFR is equal to the concentration of the substance (x) in urine times the urine flow per unit time divided by the plasma concentration of the substance.

$$GFR = \frac{U_X \times V}{P_X}$$

When, U_X is the concentration of substance in urine, V is the urine flow in unit time, and P_X is the concentration of substance in the plasma. As the substance is not metabolized in the body the concentration in the venous plasma can be taken for the concentration in plasma. This value of GFR is called the *clearance of the substance* (C_X).

Criteria of the substance used:

1. It should be freely filtered by the glomeruli.
2. It should neither be reabsorbed from nor secreted in the renal tubules.
3. It should not be synthesized or stored or altered in the kidney.
4. It should not be metabolized in the body.
5. It should be non-toxic to the body.
6. Its concentration in plasma and urine should be easily measured.

The substance usually used is **inulin**, a polymer of fructose, as it meets all the criteria of an ideal substance for measuring GFR.

It is injected intravenously initially as a bolus dose and then through the continuous infusion to maintain a constant concentration in the arterial plasma. Once, inulin equilibrates with body fluids, the urine and plasma sample are collected for its estimation.

For example, if urine concentration is 40 mg/ml, plasma concentration is 0.25 mg/ml and rate of urine flow is 0.8 ml/min. Then:

$$C_{IN} = \frac{U_{IN} \times V}{P_{IN}} = \frac{40 \times 0.8}{0.25}$$

C_{IN} = 128 ml/min

As inulin is neither reabsorbed nor formed, altered and stored in kidney, the *filtered load of inulin equals the rate of inulin excretion*. Therefore, **inulin clearance equals the GFR**.

Creatinine Clearance Test

Endogenous creatinine clearance is used clinically to estimate GFR.

- Creatinine is the **end product of creatine phosphate**, a skeletal muscle derivative. It is produced continuously in the body and excreted continuously in urine.
- Therefore, the concentration of creatinine in plasma and urine are normally stable. Its concentrations are measured in plasma and urine and the urine flow rate is (volume of urine formed per unit time) determined.

Then, creatinine clearance is calculated as:

$$C_{Creatinine} = \frac{U_{Creatinine} \times V}{P_{Creatinine}}$$

The **advantages** are that no infusion of creatinine is required; neither there is need for catheterization of bladder.

Conditions that Alter GFR

GFR changes in different physiological and non-physiological conditions. The changes are due to the change in renal blood flow, glomerular oncotic pressure, glomerular hydrostatic pressure, change in plasma protein concentration, etc.

Exercise: GFR decreases in exercise ***due to sympathetic stimulation*** that causes more afferent arteriolar constriction than constriction of efferent arteriole.

Pregnancy: In pregnancy, RBF and **GFR increase**. RBF increases due to increase in blood volume, cardiac output and decreased renal vascular resistance.

- GFR increases mostly secondary to increase in RBF.
- However, hormonal changes also a play a role. About 40–50% increase of GFR occurs in second and third trimesters of pregnancy.

Posture: Maintaining body in ***standing position for a longer duration decreases GFR*** due to sympathetic stimulation and decreased effective blood volume (pooling of blood in veins of lower limbs and abdomen). Conversely, **supine posture increases GFR**.

Sleep: GFR is usually less during sleep due to decreased circulatory activity. However, supine position maintains GFR.

Weather: GFR is ***more in rainy season and less in summer***. In summer, decreased ECF volume decreases GFR. In winter and rainy season, GFR is more due to decreased loss of water from the body and less humidity.

Gender: GFR is ***less in females*** than in males.

Age: GFR decreases in geriatric age group due to ***functional loss of nephrons***. GFR is also less in children.

Food Intake: Diet rich in proteins increases GFR.

Regulation of GFR

Usually, factors that affect RBF also affect GFR. Thus, regulation of glomerular filtration involves neural mechanisms, hormonal mechanisms, myogenic mechanism and tubuloglomerular feedback.

Neural Mechanism

Both the afferent and efferent arterioles are innervated by sympathetic fibers.

- The sympathetic activity in the renal nerve is less when the blood volume is normal. When blood volume decreases, increased renal sympathetic activity and increased circulating catecholamines cause renal vasoconstriction that in turn decreases RBF and GFR.
- ***Activation of sympathetic fibers causes constriction of afferent arteriole*** that decreases blood flow to glomerulus and therefore, decreases GFR.
  - Thus, sympathetic stimulation as occurs in emotion, fear, pain, etc. decreases GFR.

Hormonal Mechanism

Various hormones affect GFR. These include angiotensin, histamine, dopamine, ANP, endothelin, bradykinin, nitric oxide, adenosine, glucocorticoids and prostaglandins.

Angiotensin: Angiotensin II causes constriction of afferent and efferent arterioles. However, the ***effect on* afferent arteriole is more** than that on the efferent arteriole. Therefore, it decreases GFR.

Histamine: The release of histamine locally plays an important role in the control of GFR. Though, histamine causes arterial dilation and increases renal blood flow. However, by causing **contraction of mesangial cells** it decreases GFR.

Dopamine: Dopamine causes **renal vasodilation**.

- Thus, it increases renal blood flow and GFR.
- Dopamine also **relaxes mesangial cells** and therefore, increases GFR.
- Dopamine is produced by proximal tubular cells.
  - Acting locally, it **inhibits renin secretion** from JG cells that decreases angiotensin II production.
- This also contributes to increase in GFR.

ANP: Increased blood volume increases ANP secretion.

- ANP causes **dilation of the afferent arteriole** and constriction of the efferent arteriole.
  - Therefore, it **considerably increases GFR**.
- This contributes to decrease in blood volume by increasing urine formation (diuresis).

Endothelin: Endothelin is a **potent vasoconstrictor**.

- It is secreted from the endothelial cells of the renal blood vessels, mesangial cells, and cells of the distal tubules.
- It produces significant **vasoconstriction of both afferent and efferent arterioles**.
  - Therefore, it appreciably decreases GFR.

Nitric Oxide: The endothelial derived relaxing factor **(EDRF)** is the nitric oxide.

- EDRF causes significant renal **vasodilation** and **dilation of both afferent and efferent arterioles**.
  - This also opposes the vasoconstriction effect of angiotensin II and catecholamines.
- Thus, EDRF causes **profound increase in GFR**.

Bradykinin: Bradykinin is synthesized from kininogen.

- It is a **potent vasodilator**.
- It stimulates release of NO and prostaglandins.
  - Thus, it **increases GFR**.

Adenosine: Adenosine is produced by the kidney tissue.

1. It causes **constriction of the afferent arteriole** and therefore **decreases GFR**.
2. It also plays a role in tubuloglomerular feedback.

Glucocorticoids: Glucocorticoids **increase RBF and GFR**. But the mechanism of alteration of GFR by glucocorticoids is not clearly known.

Prostaglandins: Prostaglandins are formed and secreted by kidney.

1. They increase RBF by **decreasing the vasoconstrictor effects of catecholamines and angiotensin II.**
2. PGE_2 causes **relaxation of mesangial cells** that contributes to increases in GFR.
   - In conditions like hypotension and shock, prostaglandins play important role in regulation of GFR.
3. **In hypovolemic shock**, sympathetic activation causes renal vasoconstriction, which deteriorates kidney functions.
   - However, renal vasodilation effect of prostaglandins in shock *protects kidney by opposing the sympathetic constrictor activity* and maintaining renal blood flow.

Autoregulatory Mechanisms

Similar to autoregulation of RBF, GFR is also autoregulated. The autoregulation of GFR maintains a constant rate of glomerular filtration despite change in systemic arterial pressure within the **range of 80–180 mmHg** (Fig. 87.5). This is mainly due to the myogenic theory and theory of tubuloglomerular feedback.

Myogenic Theory: Myogenic mechanism controls renal blood flow and GFR.

- When arterial pressure increases, the afferent arteriole is stretched and stretch-induced contraction of the smooth muscles of afferent arteriole decreases GFR.
- Opposite mechanism operates in hypotension.

Tubuloglomerular Feedback: Increased renal arterial pressure increases pressure in the glomerular capillaries.

- This increases GFR and flow of fluid in the tubule, which is **sensed by macula densa cells.**
- Tubular cells provide **signal to the glomerular apparatus** that causes **afferent arteriolar constriction** to decrease GFR and bring it back to normal and maintain the constancy of load delivered to the tubule. This is called *tubuloglomerular feedback*.

Detailed mechanism of tubuloglomerular feedback is described in next chapter.

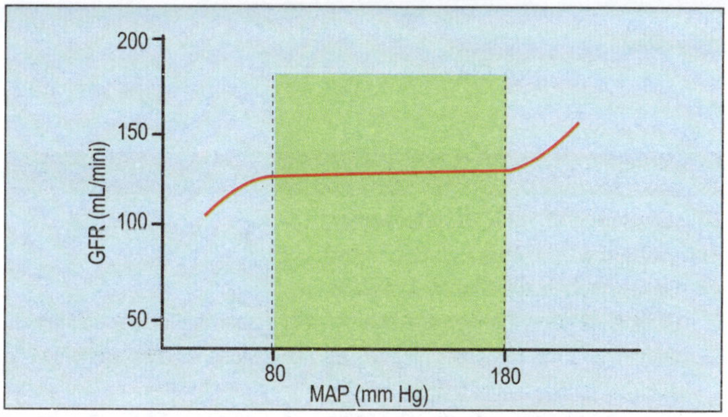

Fig. 87.5: Autoregulation of glomerular filtration rate (GFR). Note, that within the mean arterial pressure (MAP) range of 80–180 mm Hg, GFR almost remains constant.

Exam Questions

1. With the help of a schematic diagram of arrangement of capillaries for the nephrons, describe the design of renal circulation. Add a note on regulation of renal blood flow.
2. With the help of a suitable diagram, describe the mechanism of glomerular filtration.
3. Define glomerular filtration rate (GFR) and give its normal value. List the factors affecting glomerular filtration rate (GFR). Briefly describe the regulation of GFR..

Multiple Choice Questions

1. **Renal blood flow per 100 gm of tissue per min is:**
   A. 250 B. 420
   C. 600 D. 120
2. **Why is kidney more susceptible to hypoxic damage in shock?**
   A. Oxygen supply to renal tissue is low
   B. Shunting of greater fraction of O_2 from arterial blood to venous blood
   C. Blood supply to cortex of kidney is less than the medulla
   D. Kidney is located away from the heart
3. **Which substance is usually used for measuring renal blood flow?**
   A. PAH B. Creatinine
   C. Urea D. Inulin
4. **Autoregulation of RBF occurs within the mean arterial pressure range of:**
   A. 30 – 90 mmHg B. 50 – 100 mmHg
   C. 60 – 110 mmHg D. 80 – 180 mmHg
5. **Which of the following is a renal vasodilator?**
   A. Epinephrine B. Dopamine
   C. Endothelin D. ADH
6. **All are correct about glomerular filtration, except:**
   A. Glucose concentration of glomerular filtrate is same as plasma
   B. Glomerular oncotic pressure is less than of filtrate
   C. Constriction of afferent arteriole decreases glomerular hydrostatic pressure
   D. Ureteric obstruction increases the hydrostatic pressure of Bowman's space
7. **Relaxation of mesangial cells of kidney is brought about by:**
   A. cAMP & Dopamine B. Endothelin
   C. PGF_2 D. Vasopressin & Angiotensin II
8. **Which of the following cell is responsible for acid secretion in kidney?**
   A. I cells B. P cells
   C. Mesangial cells D. Pericycles
9. **Which of the following does not participate in filtration barrier in nephrons?**
   A. Podocytes B. Mesangium
   C. Endothelial cells D. Basement membrane
10. **Best test for GFR measurement is done with:**
    A. Inulin B. Hippuric acid
    C. Creatinine D. PAH

Answers: 1. B 2. B 3. A 4. D 5. B 6. B 7. A 8. A 9. B 10. A

Chapter 88

Tubular Functions

Learning Objectives

On completion of study of this chapter:

The student will be able to (must know):

1. Define major steps of urine formation.
2. Outline transport mechanisms that operate across the tubular epithelium.
3. Understand the transport mechanisms of various solutes and water in different parts of renal tubule.
4. Elucidate functions of PCT, LoH, DCT and collecting duct.
5. Describe the mechanism of reabsorption of sodium and glucose from kidney tubules.
6. Define tubular load, transport maximum, renal threshold and renal splay and enumerate their significance.
7. Understand the mechanism of water reabsorption in different parts of nephron.
8. Learn the importance of tubuloglomerular feedback and glomerulotubular balance.

The student may also be able to (desirable to know):

1. Explain the role of proximal tubule, loop of Henle, and distal tubule in urine formation.
2. Correlate tubular functions with its dysfunctions.

Steps of Urine Formation:

Formation of urine occurs in three steps: ultrafiltration of plasma through renal corpuscle, reabsorption of water and solutes from the tubular fluid, and secretion of selected solutes into the tubular fluid (Fig. 88.1).

Extent of Reabsorption: The glomerular filtration is 180 liters/day and the volume of urine formed is about 1.5 liters/day, which is less than 1% of the filtrate. Thus, the renal tubules have **vast capacity to reabsorb water and solutes**. Glucose and HCO_3^- are almost reabsorbed completely (Table 88.1).

Table 88.1 | 24 h filtration and reabsorption of various substances in nephrons (in order of % reabsorption).

Substance	Filtered	Reabsorbed	% reabsorption
Glucose (mmol)	800	800	100
HCO_3^- (meq)	4,500	4,500	100
Na^+ (meq)	26,000	25,850	99.4
Cl^- (meq)	18,000	17,850	99.2
Water (L)	180	178.5	99.2
*K^+ (meq)	600	560	99.3
Urea (g)	56	29	51.7

* Among the solutes, K^+ is also secreted in the tubule

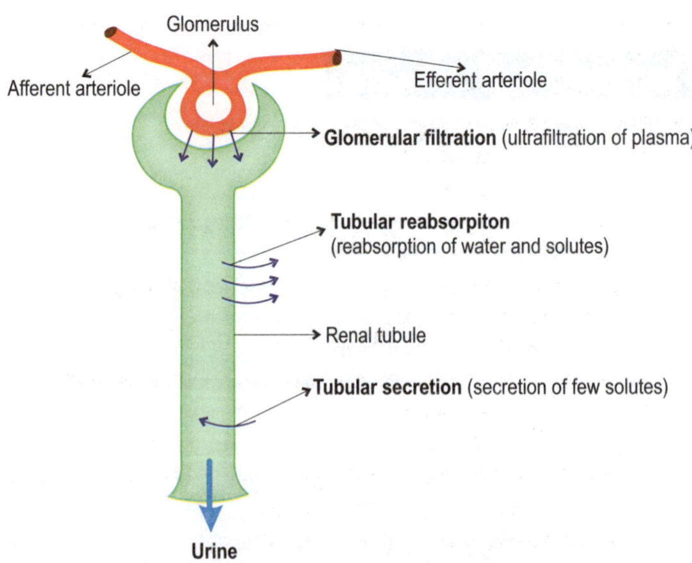

Fig. 88.1: Major steps of urine formation. Note, glomerular filtration, tubular reabsorption, and tubular secretion are three main processes in formation of urine. Number of arrows indicates the magnitude of the process.

COMMON PRINCIPLES OF TUBULAR FUNCTIONS

Transport Mechanisms

Processes of transport across tubular epithelium can be broadly divided into **two categories**: *passive and active.*

Passive Transport Mechanisms

The passive transport mechanisms include diffusion, facilitated diffusion, solvent drag and osmosis.

Diffusion

The solutes are transported by means of diffusion from their area of higher concentration to the area of lower concentration. This is the transport **along the chemical gradient**.

- Especially, **uncharged solutes like glucose** are transported by this mechanism.
- However, though charged solutes especially ions are also transported by diffusion, their electrical gradient greatly influences this passive transport.

Facilitated Diffusion

In this transport mechanism, a **specific carrier protein** in the membrane facilitates the process of diffusion. **Reabsorption of glucose via glucose transporter** is an example of facilitated diffusion.

- **Sodium and potassium ions** are also reabsorbed from kidney tubule through the water filled channels created by the carrier proteins.
  - Transport of glucose, proteins and urea from the tubular fluid are other examples of facilitated diffusion.
- **Coupled transport**, which is a form of facilitated diffusion, serves as major mechanism of transport of solutes in the tubules.

There are **two mechanisms of coupled transports**: symport mechanism, and antiport mechanisms.

Symport Mechanism: The symport mechanism is the process of coupled transport of **two or more solutes in same direction** by a carrier protein. The examples are the transport of ***Na^+-glucose, Na^+-amino acid,*** etc.

Antiport Mechanism: Antiport mechanism is the process of coupled transport of **two or more solutes in opposite direction** by a carrier protein.

- An example is the **Na^+-H^+ exchange** in the proximal tubule that reabsorbs Na^+ from the tubular fluid in exchange for secretion of H^+ into it.

Solvent Drag

When bulk amount of water is reabsorbed, the **solutes dissolved in water are also transported** along with water across the tubular epithelium. This process is called solvent drag. This contributes to **reabsorption of substantial quantity of solutes** in the proximal tubule.

Osmosis

When a considerable amount of osmotically active solute is transported, water is reabsorbed along with it **to maintain the osmotic balance**.

- This is the major mechanism for **reabsorption of water** from the tubular lumen. For example, water reabsorption follows reabsorption of Na^+ and Cl^- from the tubular fluid.
- Conversely, increased osmolality of tubular fluid increases water excretion, known as **osmotic diuresis** (Application Box 88.1).

Application Box 88.1

Glycosuria causes osmotic diuresis in diabetes: Osmotic diuresis typically occurs in diabetes mellitus. In diabetes, when plasma glucose is more than renal threshold, glucose appears in urine (glycosuria). More glucose in tubular fluid causes water retention that leads to polyuria. This differentiates from water diuresis seen in diabetes insipidus that occurs due to ADH deficiency.

Active Transport Mechanisms

Transport of solutes is considered to be active when **ATP is utilized in the process**. In this mechanism, solutes are transported from the ***area of lower concentration to the area of higher concentration***. The best example of active transport mechanism is the **Na^+-K^+ pump**.

- The **Na^+-K^+ ATPase** is mainly located in the basolateral membrane of the tubular epithelial cells. This pumps sodium out of the tubular epithelial cells and potassium into the cell.
- The other examples include **H^+-ATPase, H^+-K^+ ATPase, Ca^{++}-ATPase** etc.

Various transporters in different segment of tubule are listed in Table 88.2

Secondary Active Transport

This is the major mechanism by which **Na^+, glucose and associated solutes are reabsorbed** from kidney tubules.

1. The active transport mechanism, i.e. **Na^+-K^+ ATPase** located in the basolateral membrane of epithelial cells pumps Na^+ out of the cell. This creates a **low concentration of Na^+ in the tubular cells**. Therefore, Na^+ is reabsorbed from the tubular fluid along its concentration gradient into the tubular cells.
2. The carrier protein for Na^+ facilitates reabsorption of Na^+ into the tubular cells. **Glucose is reabsorbed by the same carrier protein** that reabsorbs Na^+. Therefore, reabsorption of glucose by this mechanism is an example of secondary active transport (details given below).
3. The similar mechanism operates in the epithelial cells of intestine.

Table 88.2 | Various transporters in apical membrane of epithelial cells in different segment of kidney tubule.

Site	Transporter	Function
PCT	Na^+-Glucose CT Na^+-Pi CT Na^+-AA CT Na^+-lactate CT Na^+-H^+ exchanger	Na^+ and glucose uptake Na^+ and Pi uptake Na^+ and AA uptake Na^+ and lactate uptake Na^+ uptake & H^+ secretion
Thick limb of LOH	Na^+-K^+- Cl^- CT Na^+-H^+ exchanger K^+ channel	Na^+, K^+, & Cl^- uptake Na+ uptake & H^+ secretion K^+ secretion
DCT	NaCl CT	Na^+ and Cl^- uptake
CD	ENaC	Na^+ uptake

CT: cotransporter; Pi: inorganic phosphate; AA: amino acids; PCT: proximal tubule, DCT: distal tubule; CD: collecting duct.

Key Concepts in Transport Mechanisms

Paracellular Pathway of Transport

Close to apical membrane, tubular epithelial cells have **tight junctions** between them. Immediately after the tight junctions between the epithelial cells, the **lateral intercellular space** starts. However, these tight junctions are not very tight and they have **leaky channels**.

Paracellular Pathway: When transport of solutes and water occurs **between the cells through tight junctions and lateral intercellular space**, the process is called transport across the paracellular pathway.

- A considerable quantity of **Ca^{++} and K^+ are reabsorbed** in proximal tubule via paracellular pathway.
- Some amount of Na^+ and water is also reabsorbed via this route.

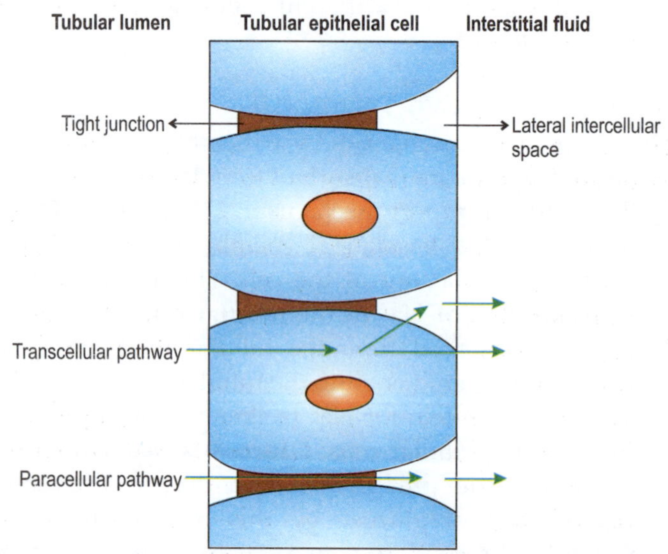

Fig. 88.2: Mechanisms of transcellular and paracellular transports across the renal tubular epithelium. Note that paracellular transport occurs through the tight junction between epithelial cells.

Transcellular Pathway: This is to differentiate from the transcellular pathway of transport in which transport occurs through the cell.

- Transport of **sodium and glucose** from tubular fluid into the tubular cells and from there into the ECF is the example of transport via transcellular pathway (Fig. 88.2).

Transport Maximum

The transport systems in the renal tubule like transport systems in other parts of the body have their maximal rate (capacity), which is called as the **transport maximum (Tm).**

- This is the rate at which the **tubule maximally transports a particular solute.**
  - That means, the amount of a particular solute transported depends on the amount of the solute in tubular fluid present upto the Tm for the solute.
- Tm is the amount of the substance **delivered to the tubule per minute.**
- When the concentration of the solute in tubular fluid is more than the Tm concentration, the mechanism of transport is **said to be saturated**, and beyond this there will be no appreciable increase in transport of the solute.
  - For example, the **Tm for glucose** is *375 mg/min. in males* and *300 mg/min. in females*.

Tubular Load

The quantity of a **solute filtered** by the glomerulo-capsular filtering barrier and **presented to the tubular fluid** is the tubular load.

- Tubular load contributes to **glomerulotubular balance.**
  - Tubular load determines the amount of the substance to be reabsorbed from the tubule, as normally, a **constant fraction of the load is reabsorbed** by the kidney tubules, which is called *glomerulotubular balance*.
- Tubular load also **determines the Tm for the substance.**
  - The amount of the substance delivered to the tubular fluid per unit time (tubular load of the substance) greatly **contributes to the maximum quantity of the substance** that can be reabsorbed.
- However, Tm depends on **plasma concentration of the substance** and the **rate of filtration** of the substance, i. e. plasma concentration × GFR.
- For example, **Tm for glucose is 375 mg/min**, which indicates that plasma concentration of glucose upto 300 gm%, tubule can transport glucose totally from the tubular fluid (300 mg/100ml × 125 ml/min).
- However, normally, **glucose appears in urine above 200 mg%** (more accurately, above 180 mg% of venous blood) of plasma level. This is due to the **mechanism of renal splay** for glucose (details given below)

Renal Threshold

This is the **concentration of the solute in the plasma at or above which the solute first appears in urine** or appears in more amount than its normal concentration.

- For example, normally **glucose** is not present in urine and its **renal threshold is 180 mg%** in venous plasma (200 mg% in arterial plasma).
- Therefore, glycosuria occurs when plasma concentration of glucose is above 180 mg%.

PY7.3

TUBULAR FUNCTIONS

Proximal Tubular Functions

The proximal tubule is the most important part of the nephron as it reabsorbs **about 67% of the filtered water, Na^+, Cl^-, K^+, and HCO_3^-** and **almost all the filtered glucose and amino acids.**

- The proximal tubule has convoluted and straight portions. Though the convoluted part (PCT) comprises 70% of the tubule, **functionally both the parts are similar** with few minor differences.
- The primary focus of reabsorption process in the proximal tubule is directed at the **Na^+ reabsorption**, which is usually **secondary to electrochemical gradient created by Na^+-K^+ pump** located on the basolateral membrane of the epithelial cells.
- Reabsorption of **water and most of the solutes** is directly or indirectly linked with Na^+-K^+ pump. Therefore, abnormalities of this pump (i. e. Na^+ reabsorption process in the tubule) results in many renal dysfunctions.

Important Facts: The fluid in the early part of proximal tubule is almost **isosmotic to plasma**.

1. **Na^+** and its two major anions **Cl^- and HCO_3^-** are the major solute in plasma and glomerular filtrate.
2. **HCO_3^- is reabsorbed** mainly in the convoluted portion of the proximal tubule leading to its drastic fall in rest of the tubule.
3. **Cl^- is reabsorbed** in the second half of the proximal tubule (later part of convoluted portion and straight portion) which creates a lumen positive transepithelial potential difference that favours passive reabsorption of Na^+.
4. About of 67% of filtered **K^+ is reabsorbed** along with 67% of water.
5. **Glucose and amino acids are almost completely reabsorbed** in proximal tubule resulting in their steep fall in rest of the tubule.
6. Thus, at the end of proximal tubule, only **one-third of** Na^+, Cl^- and K^+ remain with almost **absence of glucose, amino acid and bicarbonate** in the tubular fluid.
7. However, **urea concentration is increased** as it is not at all absorbed in this part of the tubule.

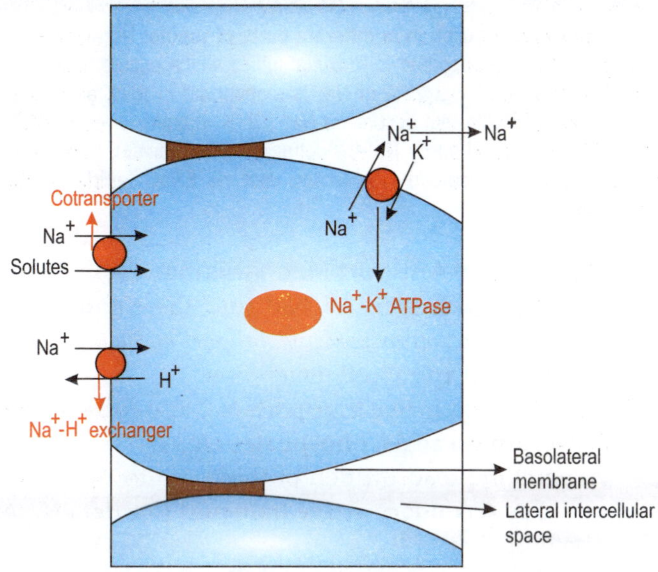

Fig. 88.3: Mechanism of Na^+ reabsorption in proximal tubule. Note that Na^+ pumped out of the cell by Na^+-K^+ ATPase located on the basolateral membrane creates the gradient for Na^+ transport from tubular fluid into the tubular cells. Na^+-K^+ antiport located on the apical membrane contributes considerably for transfer of Na^+ from tubular fluid into the cell.

Na^+ Reabsorption

In proximal tubule, reabsorption of Na^+ is important among all transport processes as it generates the **major driving force for reabsorption of water and other solutes.**

- From tubular fluid, Na^+ enters the tubular epithelial cells along the electrochemical gradient.
  - Inside the **tubular cells**, concentration of Na^+ is about **35 meq/L** in comparison to about ***140 meq/L in the tubular fluid.***
- The lower intracellular concentration of Na^+ is due to the activity of **Na^+-K^+ pump located on the basolateral surface of the cells.**
  - Vigorous activity of Na^+-K^+ ATPase constantly removes three Na^+ out of the cell for bringing in two K^+ for each cycle of the pump.
  - This active transport mechanism **constantly creates a low concentration of Na^+ in the cell.**
- The Na^+ removed from the cell into the lateral intercellular space enters interstitial fluid, and the K^+ pumped into the cell diffuses out of it through basolateral membrane mostly via K^+ channels.
- Thus, the **net effect** is the **decreased Na^+ level in tubular cells.**
  - This causes Na^+ from tubular fluid to enter the tubular cells (Fig. 88.3).

As the Na^+ entry from the luminal surface into the cells utilizes the energy generated by Na^+-K^+ pump on the basolateral surface, the process of **Na^+ reabsorption is an active transport mechanism.**

- About 67% of filtered Na^+ is reabsorbed in proximal tubule (Application Box 88.2).

Application Box 98.2

The % of Na^+ reabsorption in different parts of tubule: Normally, 67% of filtered Na^+ is reabsorbed in proximal tubule which occurs mainly by Na^+-H^+ exchange. About 25% of Na^+ is reabsorbed in thick ascending limb of loop of Henle that occurs via Na^+-$2Cl^-$-K^+ cotransporter. In DCT, about 5% is reabsorbed by Na^+-Cl^- cotransport mechanism. Remaining of about 3% is reabsorbed in collecting duct via **ENaC (epithelial Na channels)**.

Cotransport and Antiport Mechanisms

From tubular fluid, entry of Na^+ into the tubular cells occurs via various *cotransport and antiport mechanisms* that are located on the apical cell membrane.

1. The carrier protein that transports Na^+ also **cotransports glucose, amino acids, phosphates** etc.
   - Therefore, reabsorption of these solutes is considered as **secondary active transport** (for details, see below).
2. Na^+ is also transported from tubular fluid by antiport, especially by **Na^+–H^+ exchanger** which reabsorbs Na^+ into the cell in exchange for secretion of H^+ into the luminal fluid.
   - Normally, **Na^+–H^+ exchanger is the primary mechanism** of entry of Na^+ into the epithelial cells, which accounts for about **60% of the total Na^+ entry**.

Associated Anion Reabsorption

Na^+ reabsorption is accompanied by **reabsorption of anions** such as HCO_3^- and Cl^- to maintain electroneutrality. However, process of anion absorption along with Na^+ is **different in first and second half of proximal tubule.**

In First Half of Proximal Tubule: In first half of proximal tubule, Na^+ reabsorption is mainly **associated with HCO_3^- and organic solutes** like glucose, amino acids, phosphates, etc.

- Thus, Na^+ and HCO_3^- reabsorption in the first part of PCT is **coupled to the transport of organic molecules**.
- Therefore, simultaneous reabsorption of Na^+, bicarbonate, and organic solutes from the proximal tubular fluid **establishes an osmotic gradient** that results in reabsorption of water.

In Second Half of Proximal Tubule: In second half of proximal tubule, Na^+ reabsorption is mainly **associated with Cl^- reabsorption via transcellular and paracellular pathway**. In the later part of proximal tubule, Na^+ reabsorption is coupled with the Cl^- rather than bicarbonate or organic solutes because of **two reasons**.

1. In distal part of proximal tubule, **concentration of Cl^- is very high,** whereas the concentration of glucose and amino acid is less in this region as Na^+ and bicarbonate are preferentially reabsorbed in the first half of PCT.
2. Also, presence of more **chloride-anion antiporter** in the distal part of the proximal tubule facilitates transport of Cl^- into the cell.
   - Na^+ that enters cell is pumped out of it to enter ECF via Na^+-K^+ pump located on the basolateral membrane. The Cl^- leaves the cell by means of **K^+-Cl^- symporter** located on the basolateral membrane.
   - Thus, Na^+ and Cl^- are reabsorbed from tubular fluid into the interstitial fluid via tubular cells. This is called **transcellular pathway of reabsorption** of solutes.

- Increased concentration Na^+ in lateral-interstitial space creates **an electrical gradient for Cl^- ions** also to move through the paracellular pathway.
  - This is because the *tight junctions* between the tubular cells at their apical margin contain ***leaky channels that transport Cl^-*** along its electrical concentration gradient from the tubular fluid into the interstitial space.
  - This is called **paracellular pathway of reabsorption** solutes.

This paracellular pathway of solute reabsorption constitutes about **25% *of NaCl reabsorption*** in the proximal tubule.

Creates Osmotic Gradient: Thus, Na^+ reabsorption helps in reabsorption of **Cl^-, HCO_3^-, other cations and anions** and various **organic solutes.**

- Transfer of organic and inorganic solutes from tubular fluid into the interstitial space **creates the transcellular osmotic gradient** for the reabsorption of water in the proximal tubule.

Water Reabsorption

Normally, **65% of the filtered water** is reabsorbed in the PCT. The driving force for water reabsorption is the **transcellular osmotic gradient**, which is established by reabsorption of Na^+ and accompanying solutes.

- **Transcellular and paracellular reabsorption** of NaCl and other solutes from tubular fluid into the lateral intercellular and interstitial spaces **increases the osmolality of fluid in these spaces.**
  - **Permeability** of epithelium of proximal tubule *to water is extremely high*.
  - Water passes through the epithelial cells **via water channels (aquaporin 1)** present in the cell membranes and also through the water channels present in the paracellular route (in tight junctions between the cells).
- Therefore, even a smaller osmotic gradient (osmolality of **interstitial fluid of about 293 mosm/L** against osmolality of **tubular fluid of about 285 mosm/L**) result in adequate movement of water.
  - Thus, water flows along the osmotic gradient **via the transcellular and paracellular pathways** (Fig. 88.4).

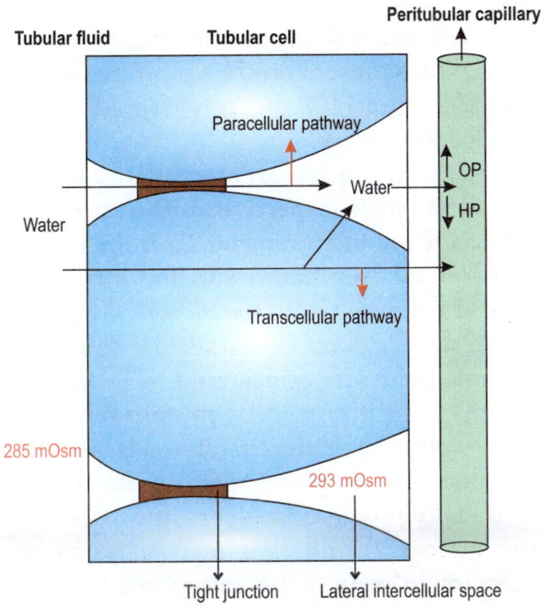

Fig. 88.4: Mechanism of water reabsorption in proximal tubule. Note, water reabsorption is efficient inspite of small difference between osmolality of tubular and interstitial fluids. Water is reabsorbed via both transcellular and paracellular pathways. High oncotic pressure (OP) and low hydrostatic pressure (HP) in peritubular capillary favour reabsorption of water.

- Thus, reabsorption of water is **coupled with the reabsorption of solutes**, especially with that of Na^+ and Cl^- (that creates osmotic gradient as NaCl is osmotically most active).
- The transfer of large amount of water (**bulk flow**) helps in **transport of ions like K^+ and Ca^{++}** that are carried along with water.
  - This process is called **solvent drag**.

Accumulation of water in the interstitial space **increases the hydrostatic pressure** that favors ***transfer of water*** from there into the ECF.

Role of Peritubular Capillaries

The peritubular capillaries play **important role in absorption of solutes and water** from the tubule. Peritubular capillaries are derived from efferent arteriole and therefore receive blood from the glomerulus.

- As the blood draining from glomerulus has already been filtered in the glomerular capillary and **protein has not been filtered** through the filtration barrier in the renal corpuscle, **blood in peritubular capillary has high oncotic pressure**.
- Moreover, the **hydrostatic pressure is also less in peritubular capillaries** as blood has passed through the upstream resistance vessels before entering these capillaries.
  - Thus, **high oncotic and low hydrostatic pressures** favor ***uptake of water*** from the interstitial tissue space surrounding tubules.
- This transfer of water **from peritubular space into peritubular capillaries** maintains the ***gradient for water reabsorption*** from tubular lumen.

Glucose Reabsorption

Glucose is **reabsorbed completely from tubular fluid in the proximal tubule.**

- It is reabsorbed **along with Na^+** in the tubule. Na^+ is pumped out of the tubular cells by Na^+-K^+ pump located on the basolateral membrane. This decreases intracellular Na^+ concentration and creates gradient for Na^+ entry into the cell from the tubular fluid.
- The carrier protein that transports Na^+ also reabsorbs glucose (**sodium-glucose cotransporter**).
- Thus, reabsorption of glucose from the luminal membrane is **secondary transport to the active process** located on the basolateral membrane of the cells and therefore, is a typical example of **secondary active transport** (Fig. 88.5).
  - Glucose transport mechanism in the kidney is similar to the transport of glucose in the intestine. Glucose and Na^+ bind to the **SGLT 1 and 2** (***sodium-glucose cotransporter***, the common carrier protein that transports Na^+, glucose and many other solutes like amino acids, lactate, phosphates, etc.).
  - This helps in reabsorption of glucose along with Na^+, when Na^+ is reabsorbed into the tubular cell from the tubular fluid.
  - From the cell, **glucose is transported into the interstitial fluid by GLUT 2**.
- Thus, glucose reabsorption is closely associated with Na^+ reabsorption.

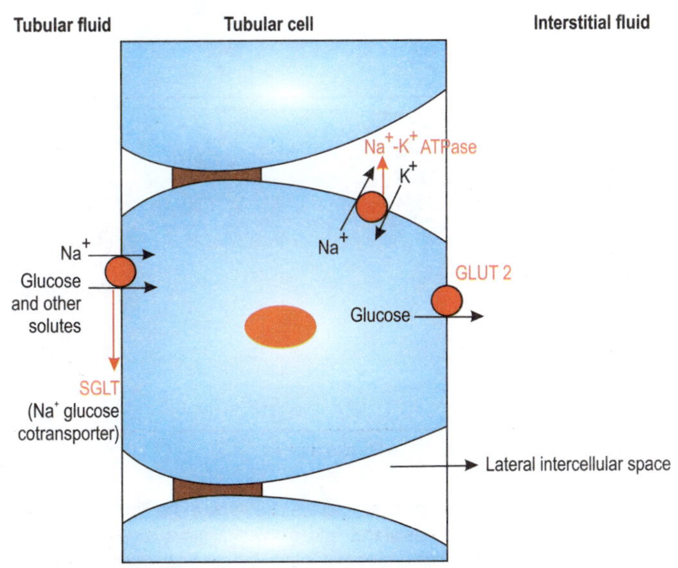

Fig. 88.5: Mechanism of glucose reabsorption in proximal tubule. From tubular fluid, glucose is reabsorbed into tubular cell along with Na^+ by SGLT (sodium-glucose cotransporter). Na^+-K^+ ATPase located on the basolateral membrane actively pumps Na^+ (primary active transport) out of the cell and creates the gradient for Na^+ transport from tubular fluid into the tubular cells. Glucose is cotransported into tubular cell by the same carrier protein (secondary active transport), and then from cell into interstitial fluid by GLUT 2.

Tm_G and Renal Splay

Glucose is **filtered at a rate of 100 mg/min.** This is because the normal plasma glucose concentration is about 80 mg/dL and GFR is 125mL/min (80 × 125). However, almost all the filtered glucose is reabsorbed in the proximal tubule, so that in normal condition, **urine is essentially glucose free**.

- The **rate of reabsorption of glucose is proportional to the amount of glucose filtered**.
  - Therefore, plasma glucose level determines the **transport maximum for glucose** (Tm_G).
- The normal Tm_G is 375 mg/min. in males and 300 mg/min in females. When Tm_G is exceeded, the glucose appears in urine.
  - As the **renal threshold** is the Tm_G divided by GFR, the predicted value for renal threshold will be about 300 mg/dL, when Tm_G is 375 mg/min and the GFR is 125mL/min (Tm_G divided by GFR should have been about 300 mg/dL).
- However, the **actual renal threshold is much below** the predicted value, i.e. about 200 mg/dL in arterial plasma and 180 mg/dL in venous plasma.
- Therefore, when the graph of Tm_G is plotted, the **actual curve deviates** from the ideal curve. This deviation is called **renal splay** (Fig. 88.6). The splay is due to *two reasons*:
  - Tm_G is **not same in all the tubules**, and
  - Amount of glucose removed from each tubule **is not complete** even when the amount filtered is below the Tm_G.

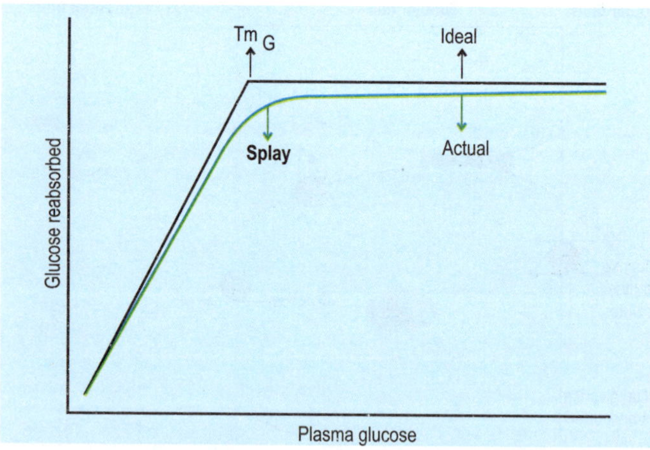

Fig. 88.6: Mechanism of renal splay for glucose. Note, once the Tm_G for glucose is reached, glucose reabsorption saturates and glucose appears in urine. However, saturation of glucose reabsorption occurs earlier than the expected plasma level, which is called renal splay. Therefore, the actual curve for glucose transport deviates from the ideal curve.

Protein Reabsorption

Normally proteins do not appear in the urine as they are almost **totally reabsorbed in the proximal tubule**. The glomerulus filters only a small quantity of proteins, which is about 7 g/day.

1. Amino acids from the tubular fluid are also *reabsorbed by means of the carrier proteins that reabsorb Na^+ and glucose* (**secondary active transport**).
1. Also, enzymes present on the apical membrane of the epithelial cells of PCT partially degrade the proteins and endocytose them.
2. The proteins in the cell are **degraded by the cellular enzymes** into their **respective amino acids**.
3. Amino acids are then transported from the cell across the basolateral membrane into the interstitial tissue space and from there into the blood.
4. By these mechanisms almost all the filtered proteins and amino acids are reabsorbed in proximal tubule. Therefore, urine is practically **protein free**.
5. But, when amount of protein filtered is more or protein reabsorption is less, **proteinuria occurs** (Clinical Note 88.1). Usually proteinuria occurs due to the disruption of the glomerular filtering membrane as occurs in **glomerulonephritis** that increases the tubular load of proteins.

Clinical Note 88.1

Proteinuria: The protein that appears in urine comes from two sources. The primary source of protein in the urine is the **excess filtration** by the glomerular membrane or **less reabsorption** in the proximal tubule. The other source may be the **protein synthesized** by the cells of thick ascending limb of loop of Henle, which is called **Tamm-Horsfall protein**. This protein is usually excreted in urine as the mechanism for protein reabsorption is primarily located in the proximal tubule.

Transport of Organic Solutes

The proximal tubule **secretes various organic cations and anions**. Many of these ions are produced by metabolism such as uric acid.

- Many exogenous organic substances like PAH, drugs, etc. are also secreted by the proximal tubule.
  - Usually these organic compounds are bound to plasma proteins that prevent filtration of the substances via the glomerular membrane.
  - However, the substances are **transported from the peritubular capillaries into the tubular cells** from where they are secreted into the tubular fluid.
- Therefore, the excretion of this organic compound in urine via their secretion by the tubular cells (rather than through filtration), constitutes an *important mechanism for their elimination* from the body.

Physiological Significance: Interference in renal transport of organic compounds help in treatment of many metabolic diseases. For example, **gout** occurs due to accumulation of uric acid in plasma. Therefore, aim of treatment of gout is **to decrease the plasma uric acid level**.

- Uric acid is both secreted and reabsorbed in proximal tubule.
- Thus, one mechanism to decrease uric acid level in gout is to promote its excretion by decreasing absorption in PCT.

PAH Transport

PAH is an **organic anion secreted across the proximal tubular cells.** The pathway for this secretion **has low specificity,** which means many other organic anions like bile salts, oxalates, urates, etc. are also secreted by this mechanism.

- PAH enters the proximal tubular cells via basolateral membrane in exchange for α-ketoglutarate (αKG), i.e. via PAH-αKG antiport mechanism.
  - Normally, αKG is produced in the cell by glutamate metabolism (Fig. 88.7).
- The αKG that comes out of the cell into the interstitial tissue space is taken back into the cells by **Na^+-α KG symport.**
- PAH is then taken into the tubular fluid along its concentration gradient.
  - The mechanism that transports PAH into the tubular cell is **non-specific.**
- Therefore, increased plasma concentration of one anion decreases the secretion of the other. For example, urinary excretion of PAH decreases in individual receiving penicillin, and, similarly, excretion of penicillin decreases in individual receiving PAH.

Defects in proximal tubular reabsorption causes Fanconi syndrome (Clinical Note 88.2).

Clinical Note 88.2

Fanconi syndrome: This is a **generalized defect in proximal tubular reabsorption** involving amino acids, glucose, phosphate, uric acid, sodium, potassium, bicarbonate and proteins. This renal disease occurs due to **mutation of the carrier or transporter proteins** or acquired secondary to diseases or drugs. Manifests as glucosuria, aminoaciduria, low molecular weight proteinuria and proximal renal tubular acidosis. **Rickets and osteomalacia** commonly occurs. **Salt wasting and polyuria** are also common.

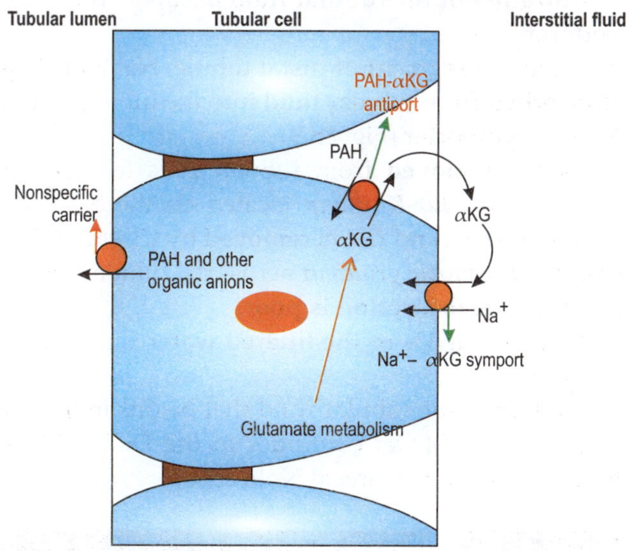

Fig. 88.7: Mechanism of PAH secretion. Note, PAH-αKG antiport located on the basolateral membrane exchanges PAH from interstitial fluid with αKG produced in the cell. PAH is then secreted into the tubular lumen by a less specific carrier protein that also transfers other organic anions. Therefore, presence of other organic anions impairs PAH secretion and vice versa.

Chloride Reabsorption

Chloride is mainly **reabsorbed secondary to Na^+ reabsorption** in the proximal tubule to maintain electroneutrality. Recently, ***separate chloride channels*** have been identified in the kidney tubules.

- It has been observed that these Cl^- channels are **linked with Ca^{++} channels.**
- Defect in Cl^- channels causes Dent's disease (Clinical Note 88.3).

Clinical Note 88.3

Dent's Disease: This is a disease of childhood that results from **mutation of gene for chloride channels.** Number of Cl^- channels decreases in kidney tubules in this dysfunction. As Cl^- channels are linked with Ca^{++} channels, abnormality also occurs in calcium excretion. Therefore, hypercalciuria and kidney stones occur in this disease.

Functions of Loop of Henle

The loop of Henle (LOH) has descending and ascending limbs. **LOH of juxtamedullary nephrons** are longer than cortical nephrons and dip deep into the medullary pyramid.

- Fluid from proximal tubule that enters LOH **is almost isotonic,** whereas **fluid leaving LOH is considerably hypotonic** having osmolality of 100 msom/kg of H_2O (in comparison to 285 msom/kg of H_2O of plasma and proximal tubular fluid).
  - This is because solutes are reabsorbed in ascending limb of LOH without reabsorption of water that makes the fluid more dilute.

Transport of Solutes

LOH reabsorbs about 25% of the filtered NaCl and K^+, 30% of filtered Ca^{++}, and 65% of filtered Mg^{++}.

In Descending Limb: Descending limb **is permeable to water,** but **not to solutes.** Therefore, fluid in terminal part of descending limb becomes **hypertonic as water moves out** of the tubule to enter the interstitial space.

In Thin Ascending Limb: In the thin part of ascending limb of LOH, transport mechanism is predominantly a **passive phenomenon,** and **permeability to water is less.** Though passive transport of NaCl occurs to some extent, **active transport of Na^+ is almost nil.**

In Thick Ascending Limb: In the thick ascending limb of LOH, the **fluid becomes more dilute** (hypotonic) as **Na^+ and Cl^- are taken out** of the tubular fluid.

- The **active transport** system for Na^+ is *well developed* in this segment of LOH.
  - Reabsorption of Na^+ from tubular fluid is dependent on a carrier protein on the apical membrane that transports **1 Na^+, 1 K^+, and 2Cl^-** from the lumen into the cell. $1Na^+$-$1K^+$-$2Cl^-$ cotransporter membrane protein is also present in airways, epithelial cells of *GI tract and salivary gland.*

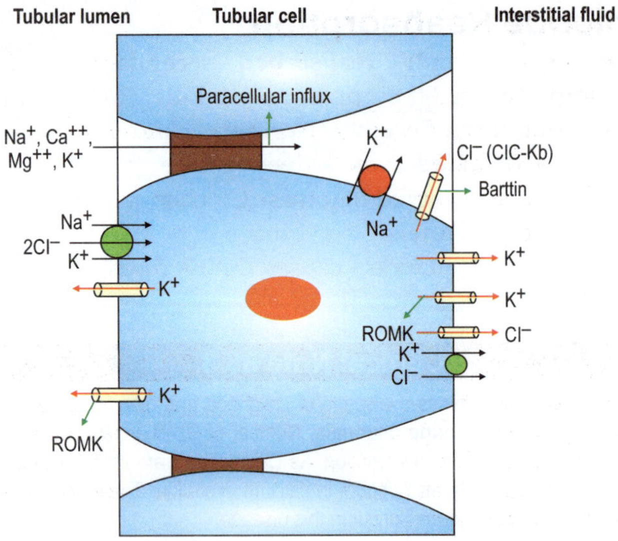

Fig. 88.8: Mechanism of solute transport in thick portion of ascending limb of LOH. Na^+–K^+ ATPase located on the basolateral membrane actively pumps Na^+ out of the cell and creates the gradient for Na^+ transport from tubular fluid into the tubular cells. However, in this part of nephron, Na^+ transport is coupled with K^+ and Cl^- via Na^+–K^+–$2Cl^-$ channel (1 Na^+–K^+–$2Cl^-$ cotransporter, which is blocked by furosemide group of diuretics). K^+ from the cell is taken out by K^+ and ROMK channels located on both basal and apical membranes. Cl^- from the cell is taken out by Cl^- channel and ClC-Kb channel formed by Barttin, a membrane protein located on basolateral membrane. K^+–Cl^- symport on basal membrane also transfers Na+ and Cl^- from the cell.

- From tubular cells, Na^+ is transported into the interstitial fluid by **Na^+–K^+ pump**, which is quite efficient in thick ascending limb of LOH (Fig. 88.8).

- K^+ from cells diffuses back into the tubular fluid and also into the interstitium passively through **ROMK and other membrane K^+ channels**.
- Cl^- that enters the cell is **co-transported with K^+** into the interstitial fluid.
  - Transepithelial transfer of these solutes creates a *potential difference* between tubular and interstitial fluid space, which drives transfer of solutes, especially **transport of Na^+, K^+, Mg^{++} and Ca^{++} via paracellular pathway**.
- Thus, **transport of solute**s occurs by both ***transcellular and paracellular routes***.
- However, the tubular epithelium of thick ascending limb of LOH **is almost impermeable to water**; therefore, solute transfer in this part of the tubule is **not associated with transfer of water**.

Defect in thick ascending limb transport process causes *Batter syndrome* (Clinical Note 88.4)

Clinical Note 88.4

Bartter syndrome: This is a rare syndrome that occurs due to defective transport of solutes in thick ascending limb of LOH. It occurs due to mutation of gene for barttin, an integral membrane protein essential for function of Cl^- channels (ClC-Kb Cl^- channels). Also, mutation of gene that causes synthesis of transporter proteins such as 1Na^+-1K^+-2Cl^- cotransporter and ROMK K^+ channel occurs in this syndrome.

- The disease is characterized by chronic hyponatremia and hypovolemia that causes activation of renin-angiotensin system.
- The resultant increase in aldosterone secretion causes hypokalemia and alkalosis.
- **Hypertension does not occur.**
- Patients of Bartter syndrome with mutated barttin are **deaf** because the defect in stria vascularis in inner ear, which maintains high concentration of K^+ in scala media contains ClC-Kb Cl^- channels.

Reabsorption of Water

The loop of Henle reabsorbs approximately **15% of the filtered water, which occurs exclusively in the descending limb**, the ascending limb being impermeable to it.

- The **descending limb** except at its terminal portion is ***highly permeable*** to water.
- Inspite of active transport of solutes **in thick ascending limb** of LOH, **water is not reabsorbed**.
- Both thin and thick portions of ascending limb of LOH are **almost impermeable to water**.
- Furosemide is a loop diuretic (Clinical Note 88.5)

Clinical Note 88.5

Loop Diuretics: The loop diuretics like furosemide inhibit the 1Na^+-1K^+-2Cl– symporter. This inhibits NaCl reabsorption from the thick ascending limb of loop of Henle. Thus, loop diuretics cause **natriuresis and kaliuresis and increase osmolality of tubular fluid** that lead to increase water excretion. However, K^+ depletion may result from long use of loop diuretics. Hence, K^+ supplement is usually given to patients under chronic furosemide therapy

Functions of Distal Convoluted Tubule

Reabsorption of Solutes and Water

DCT is **relatively impermeable to water** whereas solutes are transported. As solute is removed in excess of solvent, **further dilution of the tubular fluid occurs** in this part of the nephron.

- In the initial segment of distal tubule, **Na^+ and Cl^- are reabsorbed** from tubular fluid into the tubular cells by **Na^+-Cl^- symporter** (Fig. 88.9).
  - **Na^+ is removed** from tubular cells to interstitial space by ***Na^+-K^+ pump*** located on the basolateral membrane, and **Cl^- is removed** by Cl^- channels.
- ***Inspite of osmotic gradient*** across the tubular epithelium, **water reabsorption is poor**.
  - Only about **5% of the filtered water** is removed in DCT.

Thus, dilution of the tubular fluid that begins in the thick ascending limb of LOH continues in the DCT. Thiazide diuretics act on DCT (Clinical Note 88. 6).

Clinical Note 88.6

Thiazide Diuretics: Thiazide diuretics such as chlorthiazide, and metolazone diuretics act by inhibiting Na^+-Cl^- cotransporter in the early part of DCT. This causes natriuresis and diuresis.

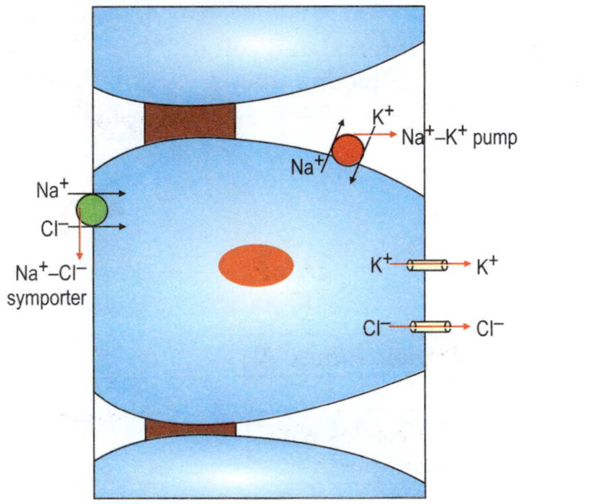

Fig. 88.9: Mechanism of solute reabsorption in distal convoluted tubule. Na^+–K^+ ATPase located on the basolateral membrane actively pumps Na^+ out of the cell and creates the gradient for Na^+ transport from tubular fluid into the tubular cells. However, in this part of nephron, Na^+ transport is coupled with Cl^- via Na^+–Cl^- cotransporter, which is blocked by thiazide group of diuretics. K^+ and Cl^- from cell are taken out by K^+ and Cl^- channels located on basal membrane.

Functions of Collecting Duct

Reabsorption of Solutes

Epithelium of collecting duct contains **two types of cells:** principal cells and intercalated cells.

Principal Cells

Principal cells are present abundantly in the epithelium of collecting duct.

- The **reabsorption of Na^+ and secretion of K^+** in the principal cells depends on Na^+-K^+ pump in the basolateral membrane (Fig. 88.10).
  - This pump provides chemical gradient for the movement of Na^+ from the distal tubular fluid into the cells.
  - K^+ is secreted from blood via principal cells into the tubular fluid.
- K^+ secretion in the collecting duct mainly occurs **in the cortical part.**
- In physiological conditions, most of K^+ in urine comes from collecting duct secretion.
- Though, in conditions of K^+ excess like high K^+ diet, collecting duct secretes more K^+, in **K^+ depletion it reabsorbs K^+.**
- K^+ secretion is **facilitated by aldosterone**.

Role of Aldosterone: Na^+ is reabsorbed from tubular fluid by principal cells by diffusion through Na^+ channels in the apical membrane of epithelial cells. These Na^+ channels are known as **epithelial sodium (Na) channels** or **ENaC**.

1. **Aldosterone facilitates genomic activity** to produce **sgk and other proteins** that form ENaC in the cells and their insertion into the luminal membrane (Fig. 88.10).
   - Aldosterone increases the activity of ENaC and increases reabsorption of Na^+. Na^+ that enters cell is pumped out into interstitial space by **Na^+-K^+ pump**, the activity of which is **also promoted by aldosterone**.
2. Thus, aldosterone, acting on collecting duct (mainly cortical part) increases Na^+ absorption and facilitates K^+ excretion.

Therefore, **hypernatremia** (and expansion of ECF) and **hypokalemia are features of hyperaldosteronism.**

K^+-sparing diuretics inhibit Na^+ reabsorption in collecting duct (Clinical Note 88.7)

Clinical Note 88.7

K^+-sparing diuretics: K^+-sparing diuretics like amiloride and spironolactone inhibit **Na^+ reabsorption from collecting** duct by antagonizing the effect of aldosterone. **Amiloride** directly inhibits the Na^+ channels (ENaC) on the luminal membrane and spironolactone inhibits Na^+-K^+ pump on the basolateral membrane.

- The disease is characterized by chronic hyponatremia and hypovolemia that causes activation of renin-angiotensin system.
- K^+ sparing diuretics: K^+ sparing diuretics like amiloride and spironolactone inhibit Na^+ reabsorption from collecting duct by antagonizing the effect of aldosterone. Amiloride directly inhibits the Na^+ channels (ENaC) on the luminal membrane and spironolactone inhibits Na^+-K^+ pump on the basolateral membrane.

Intercalated Cells

These cells are scattered among the major cells in the collecting duct.

- On the luminal side, the membrane contains **H^+-K^+ ATPase that pumps K^+ into the cell and H^+ into the tubular fluid** (Fig. 88.11).
- In the cell, H^+ and HCO_3^- are formed from dissociation of H_2CO_3. H^+ is secreted into the tubular lumen and HCO_3^- is reabsorbed into the interstitial space.
  - Thus, intercalated cells contribute **to acidification of urine** and conservation of K^+.

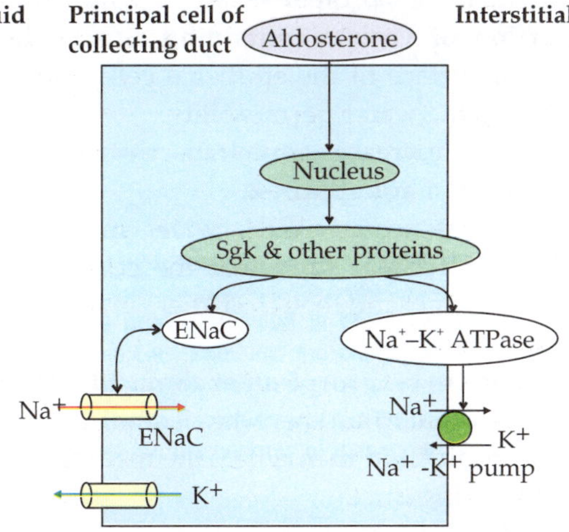

Fig. 88.10: Mechanism of Na^+ reabsorption and K^+ secretion in principal cells of collecting duct. Note, aldosterone increases activity of epithelial Na^+ channels (ENaC) that increase Na+ reabsorption, and also stimulates activity of Na^+–K^+ ATPase that helps in generating gradient for Na^+ absorption and K^+ secretion.

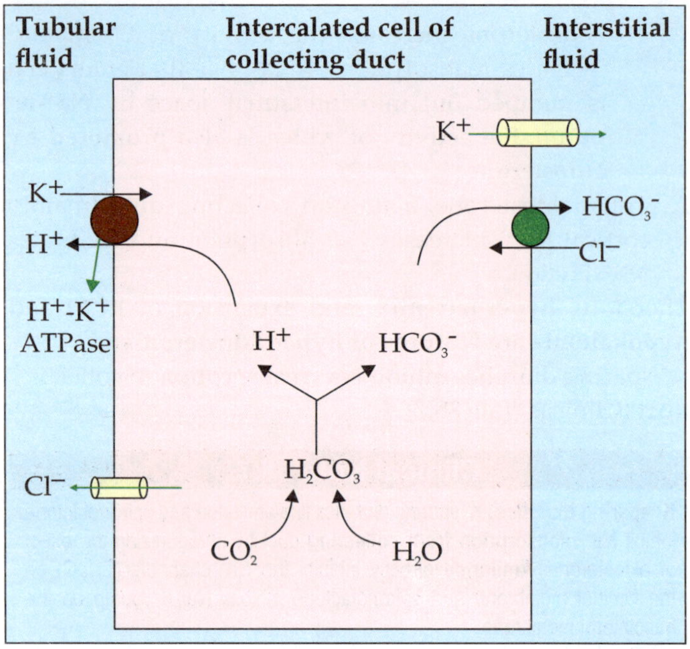

Fig. 88.11: Mechanism of H^+ secretion by intercalated cells of collecting duct. Note, H^+ is secreted by activation of K^+-H^+ pump activity.

Reabsorption of Water

Collecting duct has two parts: the cortical part and the medullary part. The reabsorption of solute and water from the collecting duct mainly **depends on the efficacy of ADH acting on it**.

In Cortical Part

In the cortical part, ADH increases the permeability of collecting duct to water by inserting aquaporin-2 water channels, especially on the luminal membrane of the principal cells.

- **ADH binds with V_2 receptor** on the basolateral cell membrane, where it activates adenylate cyclase to **increase the production of cAMP**.
- cAMP activates protein-kinase A, which promotes the **insertion of vesicle containing aquaporin-2** on the luminal surface of the epithelial cells (Fig. 88.12) that increases the water permeability.
- cAMP also **increases gene transcription** that increases **formation of aquaporin-2**.
- In the presence of ADH, water moves out of the hypotonic tubular fluid into the cells of the cortical collecting duct and then from there into the interstitium of the cortex.
- This helps in **reabsorption of about 10% filtered water** and the tubular fluid becomes isotonic.
- The isotonic fluid then enters the medullary portion of the collecting duct.

In Medullary Part

In this portion of the collecting duct **osmolality of interstitium is very high**.

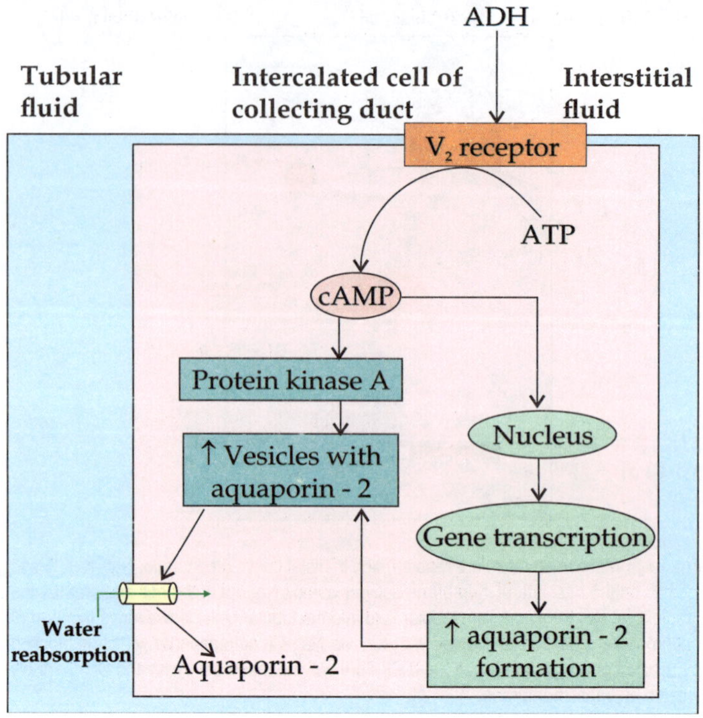

Fig. 88.12: Mechanism of water reabsorption by epithelial cells of collecting duct. ADH increases cAMP formation in the cell by acting on V_2 receptors. cAMP stimulates protein kinase A activity that promotes insertion of vesicles containing aquaporin-2 on cell membrane. cAMP also stimulates gene transcription that promotes formation of new aquaporin-2 in the cell.

1. Water is reabsorbed from the tubular fluid into the hypertonic medullary interstitium by osmotic effect, which **accounts for about 5% of water reabsorption**.
2. This plays an important role in **counter-current mechanism** and makes the urine concentrated.

Role of ADH: In human beings, **in the presence of adequate ADH**, osmolality of urine may reach 1400 mosm/kg of H_2O (99.7% of filtered water is reabsorbed).

- **In the absence of ADH**, the cells of collecting duct are relatively impermeable to water.
- Therefore, **urine becomes hypotonic** (osmolality as low as 30 mosm/kg. of H_2O) in the absence of ADH (Clinical Note 88.8).
- However, collecting duct is **not totally impermeable to water** and therefore, even in complete absence of ADH, about 2% filtered water is reabsorbed.

Clinical Note 88.8

Diabetes Insipidus: This is a condition of excess urine formation (polyuria) that occurs due to ADH deficiency **(neurogenic DI)** or failure of collecting duct to respond to the hormone **(nephrogenic DI)**. The nephrogenic form, which is an X-linked recessive type, occurs due to **mutation of the gene for V_2 receptors.**

Other Tubular Dysfunctions

Liddle's Syndrome

This is a rare **autosomal dominant disorder** characterized by clinical **features similar to hyperaldosteronism** consisting of increase in ECF volume, hypertension, hypokalemia, and metabolic alkalosis. However, **aldosterone and renin level in plasma are less**.

- In this disease, the **amiloride-sensitive Na^+ channels become hyperactive**, which results in reabsorption of inappropriately large quantity of Na^+ and increased K^+ excretion from the tubular fluid.
- This is accompanied by reabsorption of large quantity of water. Thus, ECF expansion occurs that causes hypertension.

Pseudohypoaldosteronism

There are **two forms** of pseudohypoaldosterinism: **type I and type II**.

Pseudohypoaldosteronism Type 1: This is a rare autosomal disease, which is just opposite to that of Liddle's syndrome. The **dominant form** is due to the *mutation of mineralocorticoid receptor gene* and the **recessive form** is due to the *mutation of amiloride-sensitive epithelial Na^+ channels*.

- The disease is characterized by significant **reduction in ECF volume** and therefore, the condition is **associated with hypotension**.
- The decreased Na^+ channels and decreased aldosterone activity in the tubule ***impair Na^+ reabsorption.*** Consequently, **increased Na^+ excretion** is accompanied by **excretion of large amount of water**.
- This causes contraction of ECF compartment and **hypotension**.

Pseudohypoaldosteronism Type II: In type II pseudohypoaldosteronism, (also called as **Gordon syndrome**), an autosomal dominant disease, hyperkalemia, hypertension and metabolic acidosis occur secondary to **overactivity of thiazide-sensitive Na^+-Cl^- cotransporter** in DCT.

Gitelman's Syndrome

This is an **autosomal recessive** disorder that has similarity with features of Bartter syndrome like hypokalemia, metabolic alkalosis, salt wasting, elevated renin and aldosterone level, and normal BP. However, hypomagnesemia and hypocalciuria differentiates it from Bartter syndrome.

- The disease occurs due to **mutation of thiazide-sensitive Na^+-Cl^- transporter**.
- **Decreased Na^+ reabsorption in DCT** leads to volume depletion and hypokalemia.
- Loss of activity of thiazide-sensitive transporter **increases calcium reabsorption** causing hypocalciuria.

Summary of Tubular Functions

From the above discussion on tubular functions, we learn that nephron is **functionally divided into three parts**: proximal segment, middle segment and distal segment.

Proximal Nephron

The proximal nephron **is the proximal tubule** that absorbs about **67% of the solutes and water** (Fig. 88.13). Proximal nephron is nonselective and reabsorbs solute and solvent maximally. Thus, it greatly **contributes to electrolyte and volume homeostasis**.

- In proximal nephron, Na^+ and water reabsorption are closely coupled as the epithelial water permeability is very high and **paracellular pathway** of absorption of solute and water **is well developed** (as the *tight junctions between the cells are leaky*).
- Inspite of a small osmotic gradient across tubular epithelium, the **quantity of water reabsorbed is large** due to greater permeability of PCT to water.
- However, the **tubular fluid is isosmotic.**

Middle Nephron

Loop of Henle constitutes the middle segment of the nephron.

- In this segment, **reabsorption of solute in excess of water** contributes to hyperosmolality of medullary interstitium and makes the **tubular fluid hypotonic**.
- Thus, LOH plays an important role in **generating hyperosmolar interstitium** that is essential for counter current mechanism of **urine concentration**.

Distal Nephron

DCT and collecting duct form the distal nephron. Distal nephron **is selective in reabsorption** and absorbs smaller quantity of water and solutes. About **8% of Na^+ and 18–20% of water is reabsorbed** in this part of the tubule (Fig. 88.14).

- **Na^+ and water reabsorption are not coupled as water permeability is very poor** in distal nephron.
- The tubular fluid is hypotonic.
- Inspite of a steep osmotic gradient across the epithelium, **reabsorption of water is extremely poor** in the absence of aldosterone and ADH.

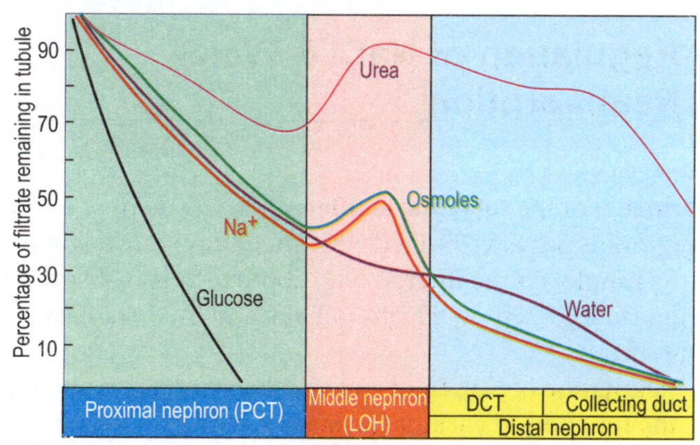

Fig. 88.13: Magnitude of reabsorption of water and various solutes (expressed as percentage of the filtrate remaining in tubular fluid) in different parts of nephron. PCT: proximal convoluted tubule; LOH: loop of Henle; DCT: distal convoluted tubule.

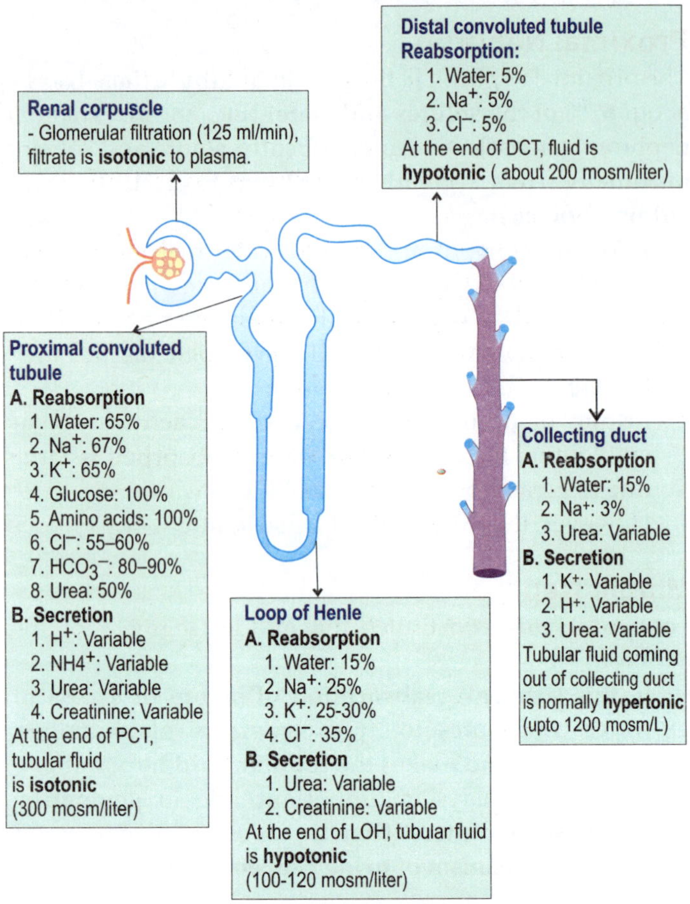

Fig. 88.14: Summary of functions of nephron. Note, the change in composition and osmolality of the filtrate as it passes through different parts of nephron, starting from the glomerular filtration to urine (fluid coming out of collecting duct) formation.

- The **paracellular route of transport is not well developed** as the junctions between epithelial cells are really very tight.
- Distal nephron **contributes to concentration and acidification of urine**.

PY7.5

REGULA TION OF IONS & WATER REABSORPTION IN KIDNEY

Regulation of NaCl & Water Reabsorption

Normally, of the **total Na^+ is filtered** (26,000 meq) of in the glomerulus per day, 99.4% (25,850 meq/day) is reabsorbed in the tubule. Of the filtered Na^+, about 67% is reabsorbed in the PCT, 25% in LOH, 5% in DCT and 3% in collecting duct (Fig. 88.15).

1. Regulation of NaCl and water reabsorption is primarily the function of various **hormones acting on kidneys**.
2. **Neural factors, starling forces, tubuloglomerular feedback and glomerulotubular balance** also play role in Na^+ regulatory mechanisms.

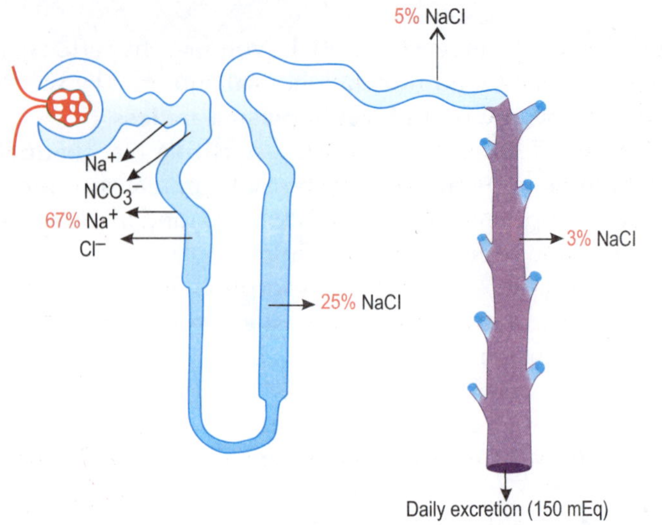

Fig. 88.15: The percentage of Na^+ reabsorption in different parts of nephron and the major accompanying anions reabsorbed with Na^+.

Hormonal Factors

The major hormones that influence NaCl and water reabsorption form kidney are angiotensin II, aldosterone, ADH, dopamine, glucocorticoid, urodilatin and ANP.

Angiotensin II: Angiotensin II acts mainly on proximal tubule of the kidney. It increases **NaCl and water reabsorption** and causes expansion of ECF volume. It is secreted in conditions of hypovolemia and hypotension.

Aldosterone: Aldosterone stimulates reabsorption of NaCl and water from collecting duct. It **acts on Na^+-K^+ pump and ENaC**. It facilitates K^+ excretion in tubular fluid. Thus, it increases Na^+ concentration in the plasma and decreases K^+ concentration. Among the important regulator of aldosterone secretion are hyperkalemia and angiotensin II.

ADH: This is an **important hormone for volume homeostasis**. It is secreted from posterior pituitary in response to hyperosmolality of plasma and hypovolemia. It **increases the permeability of collecting duct to water** by incorporating water channels (aquaporins).

Dopamine: Dopamine **inhibits NaCl and water reabsorption** in the proximal tubule. Thus, it causes **natriuresis and diuresis**. Dopamine secretion increases in expansion of ECF volume.

Glucocorticoids: Glucocorticoids have **mild mineralocorticoid (aldosterone) activity**. They increase water and NaCl reabsorption.

Urodilatin: This is a polypeptide hormone containing 32 amino acids **secreted by the distal tubule and collecting duct**. It acts on the kidney tubule locally. It acts exclusively on collecting duct to **inhibit NaCl and water reabsorption** from the medullary part of the collecting duct. It is a potent natriuretic and diuretic hormone like that of ANP. However, recently the validity of this hormone has been questioned.

ANP: This is a polypeptide hormone containing 28 amino acids, secreted from myocytes of atria of the heart. It acts on distal tubule and collecting duct to **inhibit NaCl and water reabsorption**. Thus, it produces **natriuresis and diuresis**. It is secreted in response to ECF expansion and hypertension.

Neural Factors

Neural regulation is mainly through **sympathetic innervation** of kidney that controls water and NaCl reabsorption.

- Activation of sympathetic fiber results in **increased NaCl and water reabsorption** from the proximal tubule, thick ascending limb of LOH, distal tubule, and collecting duct.
- Actions are mediated via release of norepinephrine, and epinephrine from the sympathetic nerve endings locally.

Starling Forces

Starling forces regulate NaCl and water reabsorption across the proximal tubule.

- The peritubular capillary oncotic pressure and the hydrostatic pressure in the interstitial space favor this process.
- The interstitial space oncotic pressure and peritubular capillary hydrostatic pressure oppose this process.
- When solutes are reabsorbed from the tubular cells into the interstitial space, **osmolality of the interstitium** increases, this favors movement of water from tubular fluid into the interstitium via **transcellular and paracellular pathways**.

Tubuloglomerular Feedback

Signals originating **from renal tubules provide feedback for control of glomerular filtration**, which is called as tubuloglomerular feedback.

- In this process, the **rate of flow of and the concentration of NaCl** in the tubular fluid of thick ascending limb of LOH and initial part of distal tubule provide **feedback information to the glomerulus** to control the rate of filtration.
- When the rate of flow through the tubule increases, rate of filtration decreases and when the rate of tubular flow decreases, rate of filtration increases in the same nephron.
- Thus, the change in glomerular filtration maintains a **constancy of tubular load**, i. e. a constant volume of fluid delivered to the tubule.

Role of Macula Densa: The **macula densa** in the terminal part of thick ascending limb of LOH act as **sensor** that detects the rate of flow of fluid through it.

- Macula densa cells provide **signal to the afferent arteriole**. When tubular flow is high, concentration of Na^+ and Cl^- in tubular fluid becomes high.
- More quantity of **Na^+ and Cl^- enters the macula densa cells** via $1Na^+$-$1K^+$-$2Cl^-$ cotransporter located in their apical membrane.
  - Increased Na^+ in the cell **increases Na^+-K^+ ATPase activity**.
- Increased ATP hydrolysis results in formation of more **adenosine**.
  - Adenosine acts on the A_1 adenosine receptors to increase the **release of Ca^{++}** from macula densa cells that causes **constriction of afferent arteriole** (Flowchart 88.1).
- Thus, **glomerular filtration is decreased**. Opposite mechanism operates when tubular flow decreases.

Other Factors: It is also believed that a similar mechanism operates to **control renin secretion** from JG cells that influence glomerular function through angiotensin II.

1. Also, **change in diameter of the afferent arteriole** is mediated by secretion of chemicals like **thromboxane A_2 and prostaglandins** locally.
2. Alteration in glomerular filtration is also achieved by **changing the surface area for filtration**, which is brought about by constriction or relaxation of the **mesangial cells**.

Glomerulotubular Balance

Increase in GFR increases the load of solutes, especially of Na^+ in the tubular fluid. This increases reabsorption of Na^+ from the proximal tubule.

- Normally, a **constant fraction of filtered solute is reabsorbed**.
- That means, a **constant percentage of the tubular load** is reabsorbed by the proximal tubule. This is called **glomerulotubular balance**.

Mechanisms: There are **two possible mechanisms** for glomerulotubular balance:

1. **Change in oncotic & hydrostatic pressures between peritubular capillaries & lateral intercellular space:** This mechanism is more effective for Na^+.
   - Increase in GFR **increases protein concentration** in the blood that leaves glomerular capillary, i.e. protein content becomes more **in efferent arteriole**.
   - Efferent arteriolar blood enters the peritubular capillaries. Therefore, **oncotic pressure in the peritubular capillaries increases**, which causes increased **Na^+ reabsorption** from tubular fluid.
   - This is also accompanied by **increased fluid movement** into the interstitial space (lateral intercellular space) and then from there into the blood.
2. **Increased load on the tubule:** With increased GFR, filtered load of Na^+, glucose and amino acids on the tubule increases.

- Increased Na^+ reabsorption is associated with increase in glucose and amino acid reabsorption through the same carrier proteins.
- Thus, more solutes are reabsorbed.

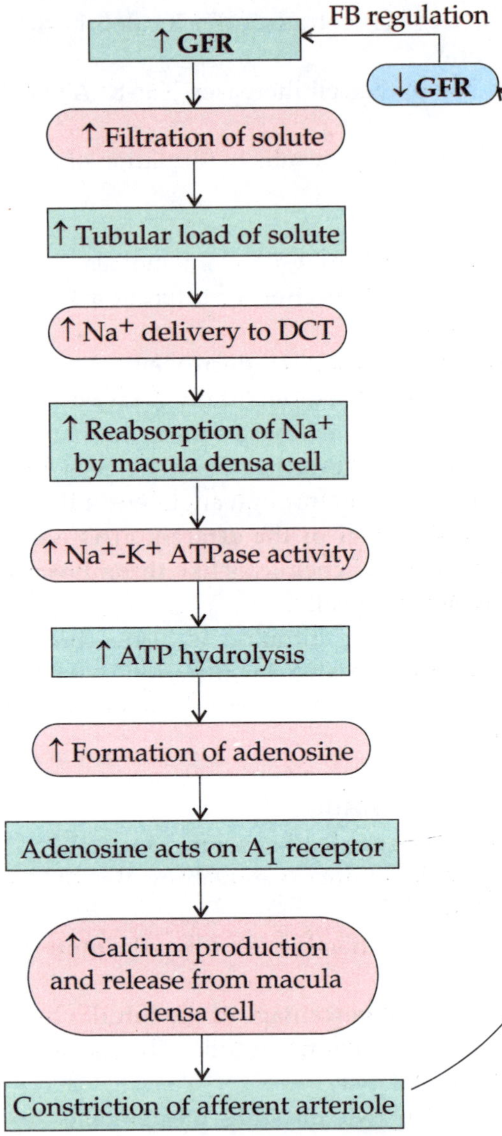

Flowchart 88.1: Mechanism of tubuloglomerular feedback (FB).

REGULATION OF K+ EXCRETION

K^+ is the primary intracellular cation. Its gradient across the cell membrane is mainly determined by the electrical potential across the membrane. As excitability of nerves and muscles depends on this electrical potential, precise control of K^+ level in plasma is very essential, in which kidneys play an important role.

1. Normally **600 meq of K^+ is filtered in 24 hours** of which **99.3% (560 meq) is reabsorbed**.
   - The major reabsorption of K^+ takes place in the **proximal tubule**, which removes about **65% of its filtered load.**
   - In thick ascending portion of **LOH**, about **25–30% of K^+ reabsorption** takes place.
   - However, about **50 meq of K^+ is secreted** from the **distal tubule**.
   - Thus, the net excretion of K^+ in urine is about **90 meq/day**.
   - Minor **reabsorption and secretion** of K^+ also take place in **collecting duct**, especially by the intercalated cell (Fig. 88.16).
2. The rate of **secretion of K^+ by distal tubular cells** is *proportionate to the rate of flow* of fluid through it.
   - When the flow of fluid in the distal tubule **is rapid**, the **secretion is more**. This is because with rapid flow, the K^+ in the tubular fluid gets less opportunity to oppose or prevent K^+ secretion.
   - In the distal tubule, usually Na^+ is reabsorbed and K^+ is secreted. Though, the transport of K^+ is mainly passive, **movement of Na^+** from the tubular fluid **decreases the potential difference** across the tubular cells; thus, **K^+ movement into the tubular lumen is favored.**

Linked to H^+ Secretion: Na^+ is reabsorbed along with secretion of H^+ into the lumen. Therefore, a competition between **H^+ and K^+ exists for exchange with Na^+.**

- When K^+ in the body increases H^+ secretion decreases and when **H^+ secretion increases K^+ secretion is inhibited.**
- K^+ secretion is mainly **regulated by aldosterone**.

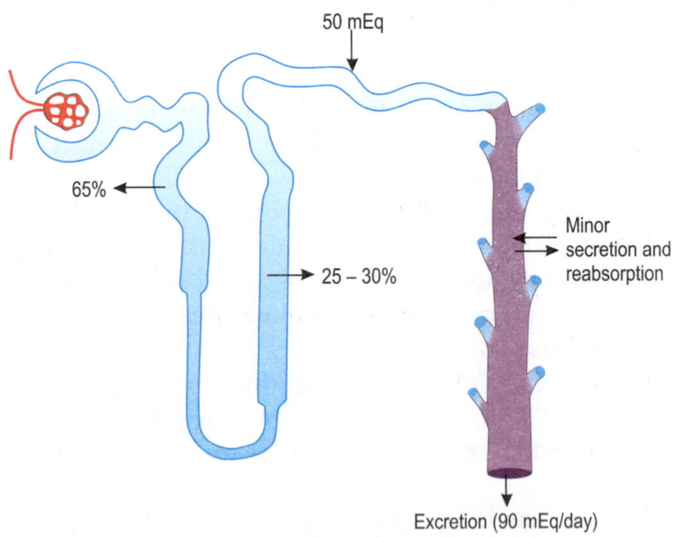

Fig. 88.16: Transport of K^+ in different parts of the nephron.

Exam Questions

1. Describe the mechanism of Na^+ and glucose reabsorption in proximal renal tubule. Add a note on renal splay.
2. Describe the mechanism and importance of tubuloglomerular feedback and tubulomerulotubular balance.
3. Describe the mechanism of solute and water reabsorption in collecting duct. Add anote on renal transport maximum.
4. Describe the regulation of ions and water reabsorption in kidney tubule.

Multiple Choice Questions

1. **All of the following statements are true, EXCEPT:**
   A. Bicarbonate is 100% reabsorbed from kideny
   B. The transport maximum (Tm) value of urea is equal to that of glucose
   C. H^+ is not absorbed from PCT
   D. Active reabsorption of glucose occurs in the proximal tubule
2. **ANP acts at which site?**
   A. Glomerulus B. Loop of Henle
   C. PCT D. Collection duct
3. **Transport maximum (Tm) means:**
   A. Maximum reabsorption & secretion
   B. Maximum amount of glomerular filtration/min
   C. Substance cleared from plasma/min
   D. Amount of toxic substances excreted/min
4. **In the presence of vasopressin, the greatest fraction of filtered water is re-absorbed which part of the nephron?**
   A. Proximal tubule B. Distal tubule
   C. Loop of Henle D. Collecting duct
5. **The main site of bicarbonate reabsorption is**
   A. Proximal convoluted tubule
   B. Distal convoluted tubule
   C. Cortical collecting duct
   D. Medullary collecting duct
6. **The most sensitive index for renal tubular function is**
   A. Specific gravity of urine B. Blood urea
   C. GFR D. Creatinine clearance
7. **All are absorbed in the DCT, except:**
   A. Water B. Potassium
   C. Chlorine D. Sodium
8. **Major portion of glomerular filtrate is absorbed in**
   A. Loop of Henle B. Distal convoluted tubule
   C. Collecting duct D. Proximal segment
9. **Loop of Henle handles the following ions except**
   A. Na^+ B. K^+
   C. Cl^- D. Urea
10. **Where in the kidney does active reabsorption of sodium ions occur?**
    A. Collecting duct
    B. Distal tubule
    C. Ascending limb of Henle
    D. All of the above
11. **K^+ secretion from loop of Henle is decreased by:**
    A. Furosemide B. Thiazide
    C. Spironolactone D. Acetazolamide
12. **Aldosterone mainly acts upon:**
    A. PCT B. Loop of Henle
    C. Glomerulus D. Collecting duct
13. **Functions of vasopressin is:**
    A. Absorption of water in PCT
    B. Absorption of water in loop of Henle
    C. Absorption of water in collecting duct
    D. Absorption of Na^+ in PCT
14. **Hypertonic urine is excreted due to absorption of water in:**
    A. Collecting duct
    B. DCT
    C. Ascending part of loop of Henley
    D. Descending part of loop of Henley
15. **Substance that is completely reabsorbed from the kidney tubule is:**
    A. Na^+ B. K^+
    C. Urea D. Glucose
16. **Which substance is least reabsorbed in tubule?**
    A. Glucose B. Urea
    C. Na^+ D. HCO_3
17. **How much sodium is normally reabsorbed in PCT?**
    A. 67% B. 75%
    C. 98% D. 50%
18. **How much of filtered sodium is reabsorbed in the tubule?**
    A. 67.8% B. 95.6%
    C. 99.4% D. 100%
19. **Which of the following hormone inhibits sodium and water reabsorption in kidney?**
    A. Aldosterone B. Angiotensin II
    C. Glucocorticoid D. ANP
20. **The tubuloglomerular feedback is mediated by**
    A. Sensing of Na^+ concentration in the macula densa
    B. Sensing of Cl^- concentration of macula densa
    C. Sensing NaCl concentration in the macula densa
    D. Opening up of voltage gated Na^+ channels in afferent arteriole
21. **The sensor for the rate of flow of tubular fluid in tubuloglomerular feedback is located in:**
    A. JG cells B. Macula densa cells
    C. Lacis cells D. Interstitial cells
22. **Which of the following factor does not contribute to glomerulotubular balance?**
    A. Oncotic pressure in peritubular capillaries
    B. Hydrostatic pressure in peritubular capillaries
    C. Load of concerned solute on the tubule
    D. Molecular weight of the substance
23. **How much of filtered K^+ is reabsorbed in LoH?**
    A. 65% B. 27%
    C. 50% D. 15%
24. **Which of the following hormones is the physiological regulator of K^+ reabsorption in kidney tubule?**
    A. ADH B. ANP
    C. Aldosterone D. Angiotensin II

Answers

1. B	2. D	3. A	4. A	5. A	6. A	7. B	8. D	9. D	10. D
11. C	12. D	13. C	14. A	15. D	16. B	17. A	18. C	19. D	20. C
21. B	22. D	23. B	24. C						

Chapter 89

PY7.3

Concentration and Dilution of Urine

Learning Objectives

On completion of study of this chapter:

The student will be able to (must know):

1. Understand the concept and importance of a counter current system.
2. Describe the countercurrent mechanism of urine concentration.
3. Justify LoH as counter-current multiplier and vasa recta as counter-current exchanger.
4. Appreciate the role of collecting duct in urine concentration.

The student may also be able to (desirable to know):

1. Explain the application of counter current mechanism in different situations. .

GENERAL CONCEPT

In human beings, urine can be formed with an osmolality of as high as 1400 mosm/kg of H_2O and as low as 30 mosm/kg of H_2O. Such a capability of kidneys to pass urine with extremes of osmolality is a fundamental necessity for volume and electrolyte homeostasis. The **osmolality of urine is an index of its concentrating and diluting capacity**.

1. **In physiological conditions**, urine osmolality is a **function of solvent (water) excretion**. When kidney excretes osmotically concentrated urine, water output is reduced considerably, and when kidney excretes osmotically dilute urine, water excretion is increased significantly.
   - For example, when the individual is exposed to a desert like condition **kidney maintains effective blood volume by reducing the urine output**, and in the process it excretes concentrated urine. For excreting **urine with osmolality of 1400 mosm/kg** of H_2O, kidney excretes about *0.5 L of urine in a day*. Thus, kidney prevents dehydration in such conditions.
   - Conversely, kidney has the **task of excreting a water load** from the body by forming a large quantity of dilute urine.
2. **In pathological conditions**, increased urine osmolality is due to **change in solute output**, and *excretion of water is secondary to the* **change in osmolality** of tubular fluid.
   - For example, **in diabetes mellitus, glycosuria results in osmotic diuresis**. Increased excretion of solute in urine is accompanied by **increased volume output** that results in dehydration.

Thus, mechanisms and the consequences of increased urine osmolality in physiological and pathological situations are different.

Diluting and Concentrating Ability of Kidney: Normally, the change in urine osmolality is brought about **mainly by the action of ADH** on collecting duct of kidney.

- **In the presence of ADH,** urine osmolality may be as high as 1400 mosm/kg of H_2O with volume of urine at about *0.5 liter per day* (0.27% of glomerular filtrate) and **in the absence of ADH**, urine osmolality may fall to as low as 30 mosm/kg of H_2O with urine volume at about *23 liters per day* (more than 12.7% of glomerular filtrate).
- **In ADH deficiency like diabetes insipidus**, urine output is **more than 20 liters per day**.

Thus, **ADH,** which is an external factor for kidney plays an important role in urine concentration and dilution. Nevertheless, kidney has its own **intrinsic mechanism** to concentrate and dilute urine. As such, kidneys normally excrete concentrated urine, which is less than 1% of glomerular filtrate. Kidneys **further concentrate urine** in the presence of volume contraction. The mechanism is known as **countercurrent mechanism** of urine concentration.

Requirements of a Countercurrent System

Countercurrent means **flow of fluid in opposite direction in the adjacent structures**. Countercurrent system has **three requirements**:

1. There should be **two tubes** (inflow and outflow tubes) that should **run parallel to each other**.
2. The movement of fluid in one tube should be **in opposite direction** to the other.
3. The tubes should be **in close proximity** to each other and should be selectively permeable.

Furnace is a Prototype: The best example is the **maintenance of air temperature in a furnace**, in which the input duct carries cool air from outside into the furnace and output duct carries hot air from the inner furnace to outside.

- The temperature of the hot air in the output duct is exchanged with the cool air of the input duct as both are in close thermal contact with each other (Fig. 89.1).
- Thus, temperature of fresh air of the input pathway increases as it passes deep into the furnace and becomes maximum at the tip (deepest part) and the temperature in the output pathway decreases as air comes out of the furnace.
  - As a result, *inner temperature of the furnace circulates in the furnace without much loss to the environment*.
  - Consequently, **a high temperature is maintained** inside the furnace.

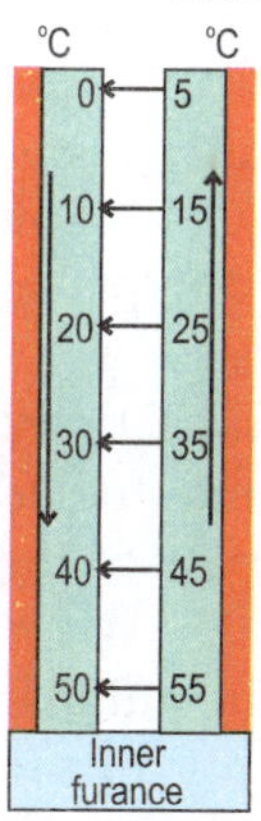

Fig. 89.1: Mechanism of counter-current heat exchange between inflow (downward arrow) and outflow (upward arrow) tubes of a furnace. Note, cooler air of inflow tube exchanges heat with hot air of outflow tube, so that the heat is maintained in the inner furnace. Thick outer wall of inflow and outflow tubes are meant to insulate the tubes.

In Kidney: **Two countercurrent processes** work in the medulla of the kidney: countercurrent multiplication system and countercurrent exchange system. Loop of Henle (LOH) acts as **countercurrent multiplier** and vasa recta as **countercurrent exchanger**.

1. **In LOH,** fluid flows deep into the medulla along the descending limb and from medulla into the cortex along the ascending limb.
   - The descending and ascending limbs for their selective permeabilities for water and solutes, **establish an osmotic gradient** in the medulla.
2. **In vasa recta,** blood flows in opposite direction in descending and ascending vessels during which **water and solutes are exchanged passively** between capillary blood vessels.
   - This passive exchange in vasa recta **maintains the osmotic gradient**.
3. Collecting duct is juxtaposed to LOH and vasa recta and acts as an **osmotic equilibrating device** (Fig. 89.2).

Countercurrent mechanism also operates in other vascular beds (Application Box 89.1).

IMPORTANT NOTE

Countercurrent mechanism in scrotal vessels: Countercurrent mechanism in pampiniform plexus in scrotum contributes to less temperature in the scrotum compared to core body temperature, and less scrotal temperature promotes spermatogenesis.

Application Box 89.1

Countercurrent mechanism helps penguin to stand on ice for a long: Countercurrent mechanisms operate in many vascular beds where the blood vessels lie close to each other and allow exchange of solute, solvent and temperature between them. For example, exchange of heat between the inflowing and outflowing vessels of the feet of penguin helps penguin maintain body temperature when it stands on ice for a long.

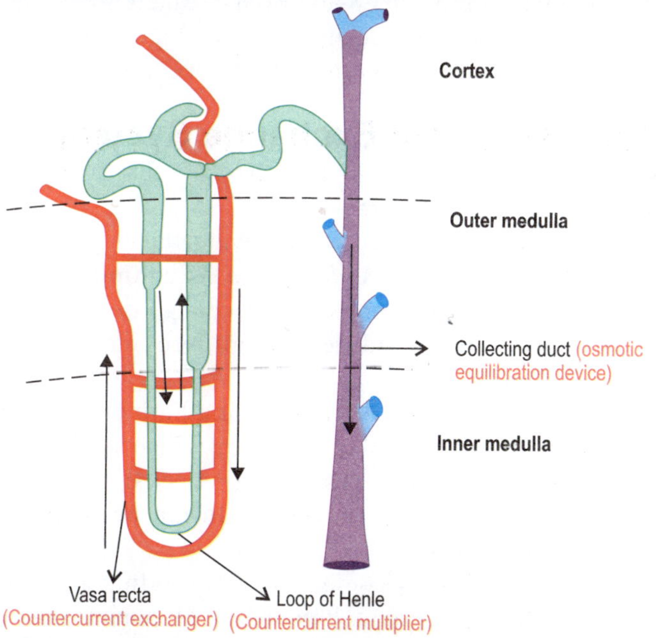

Fig. 89.2: Components of countercurrent mechanism in kidney for concentration of urine. Note that the flow is in opposite direction in descending and ascending limbs of loop of Henle (as indicated by arrows inside) and vasa recta (as indicated by arrows outside vasa recta). This close proximity of descending and ascending limbs in a parallel arrangement and the opposite direction of flow in limbs are essential components of a countercurrent mechanism to be effectively operative. Also, note the direction of flow in collecting duct (as indicated by arrow within the collecting duct).

Countercurrent Multiplication System

This is the process in which a **small osmotic gradient** established at any level of LOH is **multiplied into a larger gradient**.

- The osmotic gradient created at any level of LOH is called **single effect**, which is due to *movement of solute out of the water impermeable ascending limb of LOH*.
- **Solute deposition** in medulla is accompanied by **removal of water** from the descending limb.
- As tubular fluid in the loop enters the deeper layers of medulla, it is more concentrated that creates increasing gradient of osmolality along the axis of the loop, called **axial gradient**.

Magnitude of the Axial Gradient: Magnitude of gradient depends on **three factors:**

1. The rate of fluid flow
2. Strength of single effect
3. The length of LOH

More axial gradient: Slower the fluid flow, larger the single effect and greater the loop length, the bigger is the axial gradient.

Less axial gradient: Conversely, faster the fluid flow, smaller the single effect and shorter LOH reduces the axial gradient.

Rate of Flow is Important: When the **rate of flow is slower**, time taken for transport of solutes in the ascending limb of LOH is more, and therefore, the **strength of single effect** and consequently the magnitude of axial gradient is enhanced.

When LOH is longer, a greater axial gradient is generated as the chance for multiplication becomes higher. However, the length of LoH of a nephron does not change.

Countercurrent Exchange System

The solute gradient created in the medulla by LOH is **maintained by vasa recta.**

- The **exchange of solutes and water** takes place **passively** between descending and ascending limbs of vasa recta and this process of exchange **decreases the dissipation of the solute gradient** from medullary interstitium.
- Water is removed from descending limb of vasa recta into the hyperosmolal interstitium, which is taken back by ascending limb of vasa recta (Fig. 99.3).
  - Thus, vasa recta **prevents dilution of osmolality of interstitium.**
- Moreover, solutes come out of ascending limb and enter the descending limb of LOH, which ensures **trapping of solutes** in the medulla.
  - Thus, the process of exchange of water and solutes between descending and ascending limbs of vasa recta **maintains the gradient of osmolality established by LOH.**

COUNTERCURRENT MECHANISM

The countercurrent mechanism for urine concentration depends on **generation and maintenance of an increasing osmolality gradient** along the medullary pyramid from its outer layer to its deepest part.

1. The osmolality gradient is **generated by the loop of Henle**, which acts as countercurrent multiplier, and **maintained by vasa recta**, which acts as countercurrent exchanger.
2. The **collecting duct** contributes to this process **by equilibrating the gradient** (acts as *equilibrating device*).

Thus, renal countercurrent mechanism depends on integrated functioning of loop of Henle, vasa recta and collecting duct.

Role of Loop of Henle: The Counter Current Multiplier

The loop of Henle acts as counter current multiplier. About 30% of the volume originally filtered by the renal corpuscle enters LOH, which is **isosmotic**. In LOH, **selective reabsorption of solutes and water** occurs in its different segments that contribute to generate higher osmolality in medullary interstitium.

1. **Descending limb of LOH is highly permeable to water**, but **impermeable to solutes.**
   - Therefore, fluid that flows down in the descending limb **becomes increasingly hypertonic** as water is selectively removed.
   - Thus, **fluid in the tip** of the loop **is highly concentrated** and its osmolality is more than the interstitial osmolality.
2. **Thin ascending limb of LOH** is passively permeable to solutes and relatively impermeable to water.
   - Due to high osmolality of fluid at the tip of the hairpin loop and in thin ascending limb of LOH, and the permeability of thin ascending limb to solutes, **solutes are passively transported from the hypertonic tubular fluid in to the interstitium.**
   - However, the thin ascending limb of LOH is **relatively impermeable to water.**
   - Therefore, every time the tubular fluid passes through the thin ascending limb of LOH, **extra solutes enter the interstitium**. This helps in **multiplication** of the interstitial osmolality.
3. **In thick ascending limb of LOH**, Na^+ and Cl^- are **actively transported** from the tubular fluid due to vigorous *activity of Na^+-K^+ ATPase* in this part of the loop (Fig. 89.3).
   - This **actively removes solutes** from the tubular fluid into the interstitium and **considerably aids in building up of a higher interstitial osmolality.**
   - This makes the tubular fluid entering the distal tubule hypotonic.

Length of LoH Contributes: The countercurrent multiplier role of LOH **depends on its length.**

- LOH of medullary nephrons are much longer than that of cortical nephrons. Therefore, higher osmolality is built only in the medullary interstitium.
- This is due to **more Na^+ and Cl^- move down their concentration gradient along a longer thin ascending limb** into the interstitium and **more solutes are actively transported** along a greater length of thick ascending limb of LOH

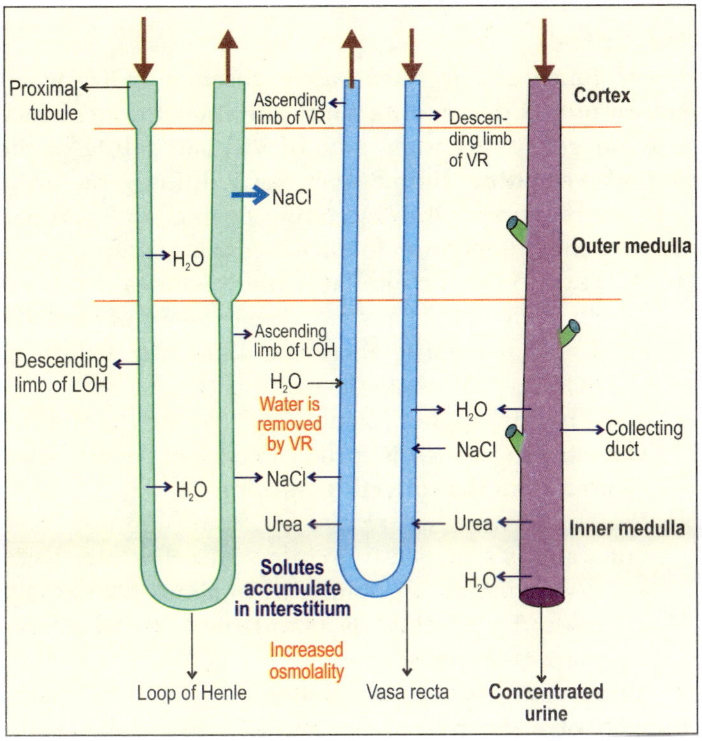

Fig. 89.3: Mechanism of urine concentration. Note, the descending limb of LOH is permeable to water that makes the tubular fluid hyperosmolal and therefore, NaCl comes out of thin ascending limb into medullary interstitium passively. NaCl is transferred actively (as indicated by thick arrow) out of thick ascending limb of LOH into medullary interstitium, which contributes considerably to increase the osmolality of interstitium. In collecting duct, urea diffuses out of the tubular fluid that aids to increase the interstitial osmolality. Water that comes out of collecting duct (and also from descending limb of LOH) is removed from medullary interstitium by vasa recta, which helps to maintain higher osmolality in the interstitium. This higher interstitial osmolality transfers water from tubular fluid leaving collecting duct and makes the urine concentrated. Arrows indicate direction of flow.

Role of Collecting Duct

Collecting duct acts as **osmotic equilibrating device**. It contributes to urinary concentration by *two ways*: first by its permeability to water and second for its permeability to urea.

1. Collecting duct is **permeable to water**.
   - Therefore, **water moves out of tubular fluid** in the collecting duct into the hyperosmolal interstitium both in the cortical and medullary part.
   - This **makes the tubular urine hypertonic**.
2. **Urea transported in collecting duct** greatly helps in *generating osmotic gradient* in the medullary pyramid.

- Except in the inner medullary portion of collecting duct, *the rest of tubular epithelium is relatively impermeable to urea*.
- Some amount of **urea is secreted** into tubular fluid in the *descending limb of LOH*.
  - Therefore, by the time tubular fluid reaches the medullary part of collecting duct, its urea **concentration is high**.
- In the collecting duct in inner medulla, **urea moves from the tubular fluid into the interstitium passively**.
  - When urea is removed from tubular fluid into the interstitium, *water moves out* of tubular lumen along with urea to maintain osmotic balance.
  - Thus, **urine is more concentrated**.
- Water that enters the interstitium is **taken up by vasa recta** and consequently **osmolal dilution of interstitium is prevented.**

Urea Transporters

The movement of urea in collecting duct of kidney is facilitated by **urea transport protein A1** (UT-A1). There are **two types of urea transporters** that help urea transport by facilitated diffusion: urea transporter A (UT-A) and urea transporter B (UT-B).

- **UT-A** is found in kidney and **UT-B** in red cells.
- In kidney, **UT-A has four subtypes**: UT-A1 to UT-A1-4.
- The **UT-A1 is influenced by ADH**. Therefore, ADH facilitates urea reabsorption in kidney.

The transport of urea and water in the collecting duct further helps in building up of hyperosmolality of the interstitium. Diet affects urine concentration (Application Box 89.2).

Application Box 89.2

Protein content of diet controls concentration of urine: Urea content of tubular fluid depends mainly on the urea filtered in the glomerular filtering membrane, which depends on the **protein content of the diet**.

- **Low-protein diet** impairs the ability of kidney to maximally concentrate urine as this decreases the urea content in the medullary interstitium.
- **High protein diet** makes the urine concentrated.

Role of Vasa Recta: The Counter Current Exchanger

The concentration gradient generated by loop of Henle will not continue for a long time if NaCl and urea accumulated in the interstitium are removed by circulation. However, the **osmolal gradient is maintained by the vasa recta**, which acts as counter current exchanger.

1. **In the descending limb** of vasa recta, **solutes diffuse into the vessels** (that carries blood into the medullary pyramid), and in the ascending limb **solutes diffuse out of the vessel** that carries blood towards the cortex.
   - Thus, **solutes keep circulating in the interstitium**.
2. The **movement of water is opposite** to the movement of solutes. **Water diffuses out of the descending limb and enters into the ascending limb** of the vasa recta (Fig. 89.3).
   - Thus, while solutes recirculate in the medulla, **water is removed** from it. Therefore, hypertonicity of the interstitium is maintained.

Water in the vasa recta enters general circulation and helps in maintaining ECF volume.

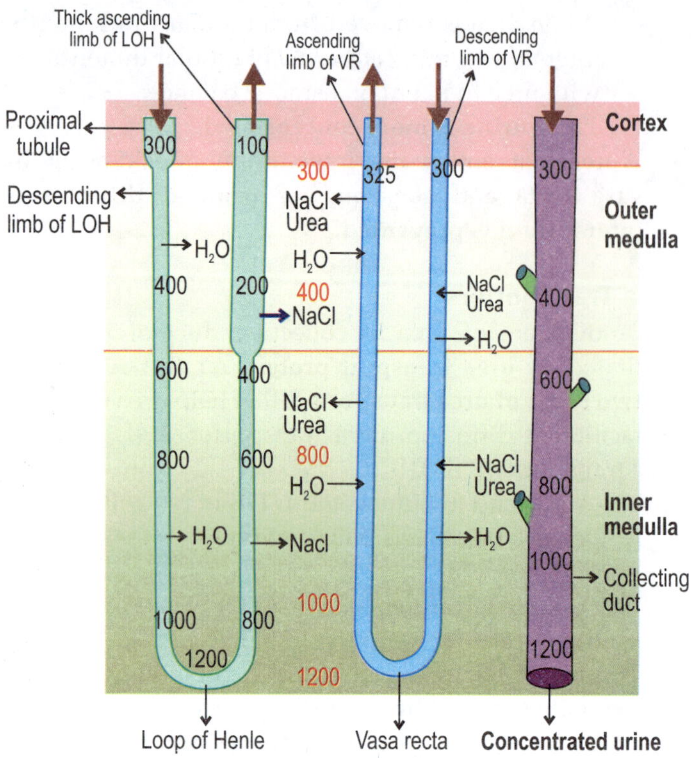

Fig. 89.4: Osmotic gradient across the medulla of kidney from its outer regions to the inner regions. Note, the tubular fluid and blood in vasa recta entering into medulla becomes gradually hyperosmolal and fluid and blood leaving medulla becomes gradually hypoosmolal. This occurs due to mechanisms as described in Fig. 89.3. Thus, interstitial osmolality (mosm/kg of water) increases gradually from outer layers to inner layers of medulla reaching about 1200 mosm/kg of water in innermost part (increased osmolality from cortex to inner medulla it shown by increased in the darkness of the colour). This osmolal gradient transfers water from tubular fluid of collecting duct leaving the medulla that makes urine concentrated. Arrows indicate direction of movement. VR: Vasa recta.

Net Effect

Every time tubular fluid passes through LOH, **water comes out of descending limb** into interstitium (which is removed by ascending limb of VR) and **solutes come out of ascending limb** (*Note:* NaCl diffuses passively into interstitium in thin ascending portion and pumped actively into interstitium in thick ascending limb).

- A **longer LOH accumulates more solutes** across its length from outer layers into deeper layers of medulla.
  - Thus, **osmolality increases along the length of LOH** as it dips into the medulla (Fig. 89.4).
- This builds **higher osmolality in the medullary interstitium**, which is further enhanced by **diffusion of urea from the collecting duct** into it.
- Water also moves out passively from collecting duct, but **water is removed from interstitium by vasa recta**.
  - Consequently, an **osmolality of about 1200 to 1400 mosm/kg of H2O is maintained** in the deeper portion of medulla.

A **preserved higher osmolality** in medulla causes **transfer of water** from collecting duct and **makes urine concentrated.**

Exam Questions

1. Describe the countercurrent mechanism of urine concentration.
2. With the help of suitable diagrams, explain the role of the loop of Henle and vasa recta in the countercurrent mechanism of urine concentration.

Multiple Choice Questions

1. **For counter current mechanism, all are true, EXCEPT:**
   A. Occurs due to opposite flow in vasa recta and loop of Henle
   B. Seen in medullary nephron
   C. Helps in creating osmolarity gradient
   D. Urea has no role
2. **Counter current mechanism in the kidney is responsible for:**
   A. Absorption of glucose
   B. Maintenance of blood flow
   C. Osmotic gradient in medulla
   D. Secretion of uric acid
3. **Substance (s) involved in countercurrent mechanism for maintaining medullary osmotic gradient are:**
   A. NaCl but not urea B. Urea
   C. NaCl, but not water D. NaCl, urea, water
4. **The high sodium content of the filtrate in renal medulla is because:**
   A. At the loop of Henle, there is counter current mechanism
   B. Increased blood flow to vasa recta
   C. Increased excretion of Na^+ from PCT
   D. Increased absorption of Na from PCT
5. **Renal medullary hyperosmolarity is due to all, EXCEPT:**
   A. Increased Na^+ B. Increased Glucose
   C. Increased urea D. Increased Potassium
6. **The prime driving force for counter current multiplier system is:**
   A. Medullary hyperosmolarity
   B. Reabsorption of Na^+ in thick ascending limb
   C. Action of ADH via aquaporin channels
   D. Urea recycling
7. **Countercurrent mechanism is not is not seen in:**
   A. Kidney B. Testes
   C. Eye D. Intestine
8. **Which of the followings is not a component of counter current multiplier mechanism?**
   A. Vasa-recta
   B. Thick ascending limb of loop of Henle
   C. Thin descending limb of loop of Henle
   D. Collecting duct
9. **Urinary concentrating ability of the kidney is increased by:**
   A. ECF volume contraction
   B. Increase in RBF
   C. Reduction of medullary hyperosmolarity
   D. Increase in GFR
10. **In counter-current process, the collecting duct works as:**
    A. Multiplier B. Exchanger
    C. Osmotic equilibrating device D. Osmotic enforcer

Answers: 1. D 2. C 3. D 4. A 5. B 6. B 7. C 8. A 9. A 10. C

Chapter 90

Water Excretion, Diuresis and Diuretics

Learning Objectives

<u>On completion of study of this chapter:</u>

The student will be able to (must know):

1. Outline the process of obligatory and facultative reabsorption of water.
2. List the difference between water diuresis and osmotic diuresis.
3. Describe the mechanism of water reabsorption in kidney tubules.
4. Name common diuretics and give their mechanism of action.

The student may also be able to (desirable to know):

1. Describe the functions of aquaporins
2. Describe the physiological basis of use of diuretics.

WATER EXCRETION

Normally, kidney **reabsorbs more than 99% of the filtered water**. Therefore, though the GFR is about 180 liters per day, only 1 to 1.5 liters of urine is formed in 24 hours.

Types of Water Reabsorption

Water reabsorption in renal tubules is of **two types**: obligatory and facultative.

Obligatory Reabsorption: Obligatory reabsorption of water is the water reabsorption that occurs secondary to reabsorption of solutes.

- This accounts for about 85% of the total water reabsorption in tubules and most part of it occurs in proximal tubule.

Facultative Reabsorption: Facultative reabsorption of water is the water reabsorption that occurs secondary to the effects of hormone, especially **ADH and aldosterone**.

- This accounts for about 15% of total water reabsorption from kidney and occurs mostly in distal parts of nephron (in collecting duct and DCT).

Aquaporins

Transport of water across the membrane of epithelial cells depends on the presence of **aquaporins**, the water channels made up of proteins.

Types of Aquaporins

13 aquaporins have been identified till date. **Aquaporins-1 and 2** are mainly involved in water reabsorption from kidney (Table 90.1).

Aquaporins in Kidney: Most of the aquaporins are found in kidney. **Aquaporin-1** is found mainly in proximal tubule and loop of Henle, and **aquaporin-2** in the collecting duct.

- These aquaporins (**aquaporins-1 and 2**) control water reabsorption in renal tubules.
- **Knock out of aquaporin 1 in PCT** in experimental animals ***decreases water reabsorption by about 70%.*** These animals fail to maintain water balance in dehydration.

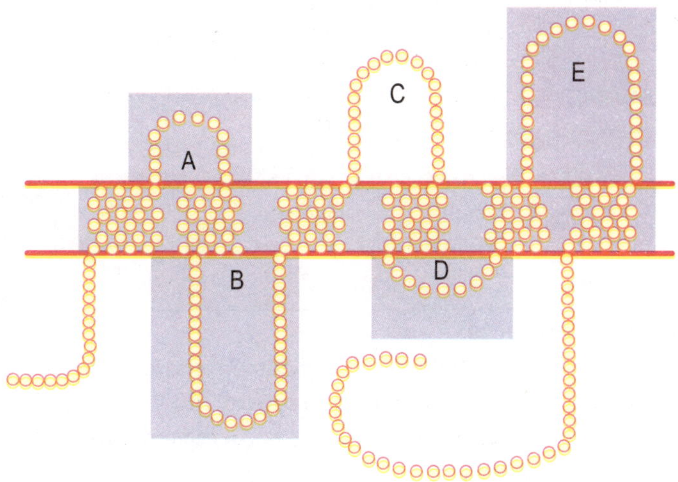

Fig. 90.1: Structure of aquaporin 1.

- This signifies the importance of aquaporin 1 in proximal tubule in water reabsorption.

Aquaporins in Extrarenal Tissues: In addition, **aquaporin-5** is found in lacrimal gland and **aquaporin-9** is present in liver, spleen, lungs and leucocytes. The role of aquaporins in extrarenal tissues is not clearly known.

Structure & Functions of Aquaporins

Aquaporins have **six membrane spanning regions**, with intracellular membrane spanning both amino and carboxy terminals (Fig. 90.1). They form tetramers in the cell membrane, with **each monomer acting as a water channel**. The distribution and function of main 9 types of aquaporins are listed in Table 90.1

Table 90.1 | Distribution and function of main types of aquaporins.

Types	Distribution	Functions	Expression in other tissues
A. Renal aquaporins Aquaporin 1	Apical and basolateral membrane of PCT & thin descending limb of LOH	67% of water reabsorption in PCT is due to AQP-1 Imparts free water permeability in thin descending limb of LOH	Multiple organs
Aquaporin 2	Apical membrane of late DCT & vesicles of principal cells of cortical part of CD	Mediate ADH effects	Testis
Aquaporin 3	Basolateral membrane of late DCT & cortical CD	Mediate ADH effects	Multiple organs
Aquaporin 4	Basolateral membrane of late DCT & cortical CD	Mediate ADH effects	Brain, other organs
Aquaporin 6	Vesicles of intercalated cells of CD	Acts as an internal ion channel of I cells	
Aquaporin 7	Apical membrane of PCT	Water absorption in PCT	Testis & adipocytes
Aquaporin 8	Intracellular vesicles in cortex & medulla; in PCT	Exact function not known	Testis, epididymis pancreas, liver,

Applied Aspects

1. Nephrogenic diabetes insipidus is characterized by **decreased expression of aquaporin 2** in CD & DCT.
2. In chronic **heart failure**, there is **increased expression** of aquaporin 2.

Mechanism of Water Reabsorption

Details of water reabsorption in kidney tubules have been described in Chapter 88.

In Proximal Tubule: Normally, **65% of the filtered water** is reabsorbed in the proximal tubule.

- The driving force for water reabsorption is the **transcellular osmotic gradient**, which is established by absorption of Na^+ and accompanying solutes.
- Permeability of epithelium of **proximal tubule to water is extremely high**, due to the presence of **aquaporin 1** in the cell membranes.

In LOH: The loop of Henle reabsorbs approximately **15% of the filtered water**.

- The ascending limb of LOH is impermeable to water and water reabsorption **occurs mainly in the descending limb**.
- The water reabsorption in descending limb of LOH **is a passive process** that occurs secondary to higher osmolality of medullary interstitium.

In DCT: Only about 5% of the filtered water is removed in DCT, which is influenced by **aldosterone** and ADH.

In Collecting Duct: Reabsorption of solute and water from the collecting duct mainly depends on ADH (details of ADH effects are described in Chapter 72). About **12–15% of water is reabsorbed** in collecting duct.

DIURESIS AND DIURETICS

Diuresis

Diuresis is the **excess excretion of water** in the urine. Diuresis is of **two categories**: water diuresis and osmotic diuresis.

Water Diuresis: Water diuresis is the **excretion of large volume of water without loss of excess of solute.** This occurs when the capacity of the kidney tubule to reabsorb water is impaired.

1. **ADH deficiency, results in water diuresis.** For example, in **diabetes insipidus**, urine is dilute and more in volume.
2. Water diuresis can be physiologically demonstrated by **drinking a large amount of hypotonic fluid** like water, in which polyuria occurs in 15 to 40 minutes of water ingestion.

Osmotic Diuresis: Increased concentration of **osmotically active particles in the tubular fluid** increases the excretion of water. This is called as osmotic diuresis.

1. This is typically seen in **diabetes mellitus** in which increased filtration of glucose (increased tubular glucose load) causes **glycosuria**, this causes osmotic diuresis.
2. Osmotic diuresis is also produced by **administration of mannitol.**
    - **Mannitol** is filtered in kidney but not reabsorbed and therefore, produces diuresis by its osmotic effect.

- Mannitol is usually used in the treatment of cerebral edema, acute kidney failure.

3. Osmotic diuresis can also be produced by infusion of large amount of NaCl or urea.

Diuretics

Diuretics are substances that promote diuresis (increased excretion of water in urine). Frequently, administered diuretics are loop diuretics, aldosterone antagonists, thiazide diuretics, carbonic anhydrase inhibitors, xanthines, large quantities of osmotically active substances, ethanol, acidifying salts, vasopressin antagonists, and water.

Loop Diuretics: **Furosemide** (Lasix) and ethacrynic acid are loop diuretics.

- They act by ***inhibiting*** Na^+-K^+-$2Cl^-$ ***cotransporter in the thick ascending limb*** of loop of Henle.
- This inhibits Na^+, K^+ and Cl^- reabsorption causing diuresis with loss of these electrolytes.

Aldosterone Antagonists: **Spironolactone** is the commonly administered aldosterone antagonist.

- It **inhibits the action of aldosterone** on the kidney tubule.
  - Thus, it ***inhibits*** Na^+-K^+ ***exchange*** that leads to natriuresis and diuresis with retention of K^+ in the body.
  - Hence, it is called K^+ ***sparing diuretic***.

Amiloride and triamterene, other K^+ sparring diuretics compete with sodium for a site in the ENaC (epithelial Na channel) and block sodium reabsorption and potassium secretion.

- Thus, they produce diuresis with retention of K^+.

Thiazide Diuretics: Usually administered thiazide diuretic is **chlorothiazide**.

- It **inhibits** Na^+-Cl^- **cotransporter in the early part of distal tubule**.
- Thus, increased excretion of NaCl produces diuresis.

Carbonic Anhydrase Inhibitors: The usually administered diuretic is **acetazolamide** (Diamox). As the name suggests, it inhibits carbonic anhydrase activity in renal tubular cells.

- It **decreases** H^+ **secretion** into tubular fluid.
  - Normally, H^+ is exchanged with Na^+ in luminal membrane of tubular epithelial cells by Na^+-H^+ **antiport**.
- Therefore, decreased H^+ secretion results in **increase in** Na^+ **(and also** K^+**) excretion** that leads to diuresis.

Xanthines: Xanthines such as caffeine and theophylline act as diuretics.

They inhibit tubular reabsorption of Na^+. They also increase GFR.

Osmotically Active Substances: Administration of large quantities of osmotically active substances like mannitol and glucose produce osmotic diuresis by increasing their concentration in tubular fluid.

Ethanol: Ethyl alcohol produces diuresis by **inhibiting ADH secretion.**

Acidifying Salts: Acidifying salts like calcium and ammonium chloride act as diuretic by **increasing the tubular acid load.**

- The H^+ is buffered, but an anion is excreted with Na^+ when the ability of kidney to replace Na^+ with H^+ is exceeded.

Vasopressin Antagonists: ADH antagonists inhibit the action of ADH on kidney tubules.

Water: Increased water consumption (hypervolemia) *inhibits ADH secretion*

Exam Questions

1. Describe the mechanism of water reabsorption in kidney. Give a note on Aquaporins
2. Name the types of diuresis. Briefly describe the physiological actions of 4 important types of diuretics.

Multiple Choice Questions

1. In nephrogenic DI, which aquaporin is deficient in DCT?
A. Aquaporin 9 B. Aquaporin 1
C. Aquaporin 2 D. Aquaporin 4

2. Water reabsorption that occurs secondary to solute reabsorption is called:
A. Obligatory reabsorption B. Facultative reabsorption
C. Complementary reabsorption D. Compulsive reabsorption

3. Which of the following does not produce osmotic diuresis?
A. Mannitol B. Glucose
C. NaCl D. Water

4. Which of the following diuretic causes retention of K+ in the body?
A. Spironolactone B. Furosemide
C. Xanthines D. Acetazolamide

5. Which of the following diuretic decreases H+ in the tubule?
A. Spironolactone B. Furosemide
C. Xanthines D. Acetazolamide

6. Ethanol produces diuresis mainly by:
A. Opposing aldosterone secretion
B. Inhibiting ADH secretion
C. Inhibiting sodium reabsorption
D. Decreasing osmole reabsorption

Answers

1. C 2. A 3. D 4. A 5. D 6. B

Chapter 91

Acidification of Urine

Learning Objectives

On completion of study of this chapter:

The student will be able to (must know):

1. Understand the purpose of acidification of urine.
2. List the factors that contribute to acidification of urine.
3. Elucidate the mechanism of renal acid excretion and bicarbonate reabsorption.
4. Outline the mechanisms of acidification of urine.

The student may also be able to (desirable to know):

1. Describe the renal handling of acids and bicarbonate in tubular fluid.

PHYSIOLOGICAL ASPECTS

Kidneys play important role in the control of pH of blood as most of the acid load from plasma is removed through renal system. Kidneys are vital for **acid-base balance** of body

Factors Influencing Acidification of Urine

Four important factors contribute to acidification of urine:

1. Renal acid excretion
2. Renal bicarbonate reabsorption
3. Acid-base status of the body
4. Other factors (mainly hormonal).

Renal Acid Excretion

Kidney contributes to acid-base balance **by excreting acid**, which is proportionate to the production of non-volatile acids in the body. Kidney also **prevents bicarbonate loss** to achieve this purpose.

1. The major contribution to acid-base balance is by **renal bicarbonate loss or gain** as filtered *load of* HCO_3^- (about 4300 meq/day) is much higher than the filtered ***load of non-volatile acid***, which is about 80 meq/day.
   - **Most of the filtered HCO_3^- is reabsorbed.**
   - The reabsorption of filtered HCO_3^- and excretion of acid are achieved through the **process of H^+ secretion**.
2. Most of the **H^+ secreted into the tubular fluid**, which is about 4400 meq/day, *serves to reabsorb the filtered* HCO_3^-, and **only about 100 meq/day is excreted** in urine.
   - Therefore, normally urine is mildly acidic.

Role of Ammonium: Ammonium (NH_4^+) **synthesis and excretion** by kidney plays an important role in maintenance of acid base balance.

- For each NH_4^+ excreted in urine, one HCO_3^- is added to the systemic circulation.
  - This replenishes the HCO_3^- lost during titration of non-volatile acid (Application Box 91.1).

For acid-base balance, the net acid excretion should be equal to the net non-volatile acid production. In general, the process is designated as **net acid excretion**.

Application Box 91.1

Titrable Acids: Kidney excretes non-volatile acids and replenishes HCO_3^- lost, during titration. However, kidney cannot excrete the free acids; instead excretes the salts of free acids while excreting H^+ with other anions, the **urinary buffers**.

- The main buffer in the urine is phosphate buffer. Other buffers are bicarbonate and ammonia buffers. **The different urinary buffers are collectively known as titrable acids.**
- The term titrable acid refers to the method of estimation of an acid.
- In a laboratory, to estimate urine acids, alkali is added to urine sample to titrate its pH to that of plasma. The quantity of alkali added is equal to the H^+ titrated by these urine buffers. Therefore, this is called the titrable acid.

Renal Bicarbonate Reabsorption

Normally, the amount of bicarbonate reabsorbed from tubular fluid equals the amount filtered. Thus, **bicarbonate reabsorption in the tubule is 100%**. Therefore, under normal conditions, **HCO_3^- is not excreted in urine**.

1. About 80% of the total filtered bicarbonate is reabsorbed in PCT and 15% in thick ascending limb of LOH and 5% in the collecting duct (Fig. 91.1).
   - The mechanism of **bicarbonate reabsorption in PCT** involves **Na^+-H^+ antiporter** in the apical surface of the epithelial cells.
2. In the thick part of ascending limb of LOH, mechanism is similar to that in the PCT.
3. **In DCT and collecting duct**, reabsorption does not require Na^+-H^+ antiporter.
   - In **intercalated cells (I cells)** in these parts of nephron, H^+ and HCO_3^- are produced by hydration of CO_2, which is catalyzed by carbonic anhydrase.
   - From the cell, H^+ is secreted into the tubular fluid **by H^+-ATPase or K^+-H^+ ATPase** and HCO_3^- is added to interstitium by **Cl^--HCO_3^- antiporter** present in the basolateral membrane.

pH of Tubular Fluid in PCT and DC: In PCT, permeability to H^+ and HCO_3^- is more. Therefore, the pH of tubular fluid in the PCT ***is about 6.5***. **In collecting duct**, permeability to H^+ is low. Therefore, tubular fluid in this part of the tubule is ***more acidic***, having pH about 4.5. This ability of the collecting duct to reduce the tubular fluid pH is **physiologically important for excretion of urinary buffers**.

Formation of New Bicarbonate (Role of Ammonia):

Urinary ammonium excretion is intimately associated with acid-base balance.

1. Ammonium is **important in HCO_3^- formation**.
   - In the kidney, ammonium is produced by **metabolism of glutamine**.
2. Glutamine and Na^+ salts are the non-volatile acids (fixed or metabolic acids)

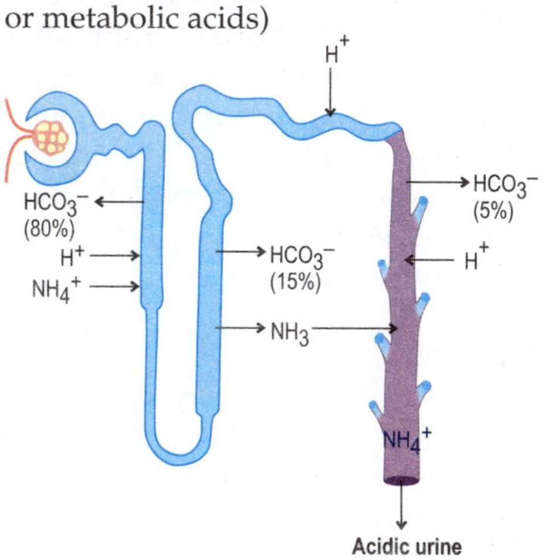

Fig. 91.1: Renal tubular handling of HCO_3^-, H^+ and NH_4^+. Arrows indicate the direction of movement.

   - Kidney metabolizes glutamine, excrete NH_4^+ with acid-salts and add $NaHCO_3$ to the body.
3. In this process, **new HCO_3^- is formed** which is dependent on the ability of the kidney to excrete the NH_4^+ in the urine (details given below).

Acid-Base Status of the Body

Systemic acid-base balance affects acid secretion and HCO_3^- reabsorption and hence, acidification of urine. Therefore, acidification of urine is part of acid base balance of the body, which is discussed in Chapter 134.

Other Factors

Aldosterone, parathormone, angiotensin II and plasma K^+ contribute to acidification of urine.

1. **Aldosterone** increases H^+ secretion from the tubular cells into the tubular fluid. Therefore, it contributes to urine acidification and alkali reabsorption in the kidney.
2. **Angiotensin II** secondarily affects Na^+ concentration and Na^+-H^+ exchange, hence affects urine acidification.

PY7.5

MECHANISM OF URINE ACIDIFICATION

Acidification of urine is due to various mechanisms operating in different parts of the nephron, especially in PCT, DCT and collecting duct.

Acidification in Proximal Tubule

Increased CO_2 in the body represents ***increased acidity*** in systemic circulation.

1. In proximal tubular cells, CO_2 binds with H_2O to form carbonic acid. Dissociation of carbonic acid produces H^+ and HCO_3. Both the formation and dissociation of carbonic acid is catalyzed by the enzyme **carbonic anhydrase** at the brush border. This **serves two purposes**.
   - First, it helps to ***trap the acid*** in the form of CO_2 which can't be removed from kidney fully even after diffusion through tubular walls.
   - Second, it ***cleaves and extracts the acid*** and helps in its active secretion into the lumen while retaining the alkaline bicarbonate inside the cell.
2. **Secretion of H^+ into tubular fluid** occurs via Na^+-H^+ antiporter (Fig. 91.2).
3. The **bicarbonate ion diffuses into the interstitium** as K^+ ion does.
4. The Na^+ ion from tubular cells enters interstitium in exchange of a K^+ by Na^+-K^+ ATPase.
   - Thus, cellular K^+ concentration remains unaffected, while **Na^+ concentration decreases**. The decreased Na^+ concentration initiates entry of Na^+ ions from

luminal side into cell, which is coupled with **secretion of H^+** (Na^+-H^+ exchanger).

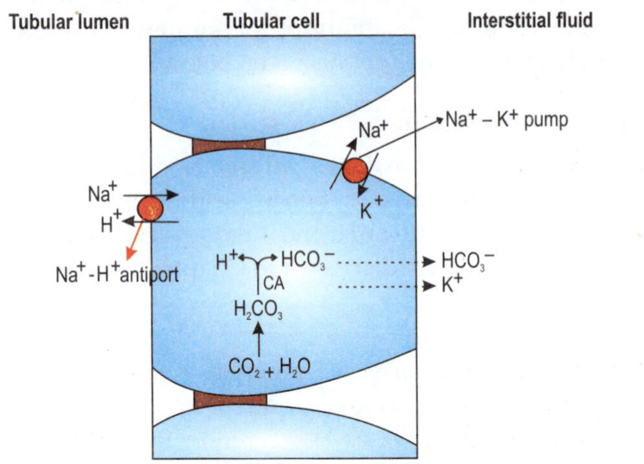

Fig. 91.2: Mechanism of acid secretion in PCT. H^+ formed from dissociation of $H2CO_3^-$ is transferred into tubular fluid by Na^+–H^+ antiport located on apical membrane of tubular epithelial cell and HCO_3^- diffuses into interstitial fluid. Thus, H^+ secretion in PCT is Na^+ dependant. CA: Carbonic anhydrase.

Thus, urine **acidification at PCT is dependent on Na^+ concentration**.

Effects of Parathormone & CAI:

i. **Parathormone** inhibits Na^+-H^+ exchanger in apical cell membrane of PCT and therefore, affects urine pH.

ii. As carbonic anhydrase plays a vital role in PCT, drugs that inhibit its action (**carbonic anhydrase inhibitors**) decrease the process of acidification of urine.

Acidification in Distal Tubules and Collecting Duct

Unlike in PCT, the distal tubular cells acidify urine independent of their Na^+ concentration. In DCT, secretion of H^+ occurs by **active (ATP-driven) proton pumps**.

- Aldosterone increases distal tubular acid secretion by acting on these pumps directly.
- The **I cells of DCT** are equivalent to the parietal cells of stomach as they actively secrete acid.
  - These cells are rich in carbonic anhydrase. The number of H^+ pumps employed at the membrane increases for increased acid secretion.
- **Band 3 protein**, an anion exchanger protein located at the basolateral membrane acts as **chloride-bicarbonate exchanger** (Fig. 91.3).
  - It transports bicarbonate ion into interstitium, thereby it retains bicarbonate ion and acidifies urine.
- Apart from this, **H^+-K^+ ATPase** to some extent secretes H^+ and absorbs K^+ in the collecting tubules. pH changes of tubular fluid in DCT may be acute (Application Box 91.2)

Application Box 91.2

Maximum acidification: The minimum urinary pH at which maximal acidification can be achieved is 4.5. At this pH, H^+ concentration of urine is 1000 times more than that in plasma. This pH of tubular fluid is usually attained in the collecting ducts. Though acid secretion is more in PCT, it contributes to moderate change in urinary pH as the carbonic acid breaks down into carbon dioxide and water. On the other hand, urinary pH changes are acute in DCT though its acid secreting capacity is less.

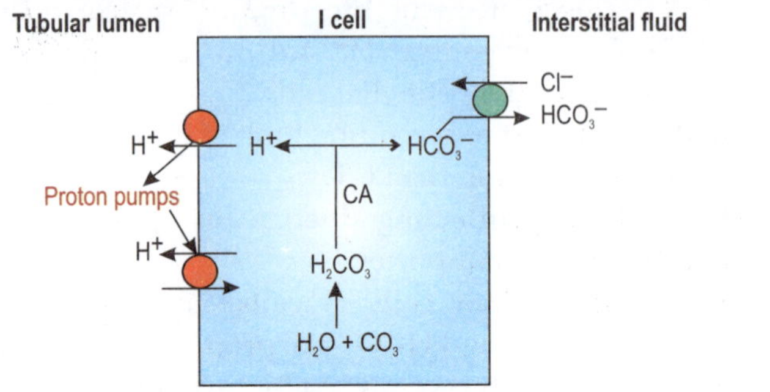

Fig. 91.3: Mechanism of acid secretion in distal tubular cells (by intercalated (I) cells in DCT and CD). H^+ formed from dissociation of $H_2CO_3^-$ is transferred into tubular fluid by proton pumps (H^+ ATPase or K^+-H^+ ATPase) located on apical membrane of tubular epithelial cell and HCO_3^- diffuses into interstitial fluid by HCO_3^-– Cl^- antiport located on basolateral membrane. Thus, H^+ secretion in DCT and CD is mostly Na^+ independent. CA: Carbonic anhydrase.

Further Modifications in Acidification

After saturation of acid secreting mechanisms, there would be no further urine acidification. However, constant removal of H^+ by the action of urinary buffers from the tubules makes it possible for further acid secretion. It occurs via three different **buffering mechanisms** at different regions of tubules (Fig. 91.4)

In PCT

Reaction with **bicarbonate buffers** occurs in the tubular fluid in PCT.

- Bicarbonate ion after filtration into tubular fluid reaches a concentration of about **24 millimoles**. At this concentration, it is an **effective buffer for the tubular acids**.
- It forms carbonic acid that breaks down into carbon dioxide and water at the brush border of PCT by the action of carbonic anhydrase. The carbon dioxide diffuses into tubule cell and reacts with water molecule to resecrete acid into tubule and reclaim bicarbonate ion into interstitium (Fig. 94.4A).

In DCT and Collecting Duct

Secreted acid reacts with dibasic **phosphate buffer** whose pK value is closer to urinary pH (Fig. 94.4B). The relative concentration of **phosphate buffer here is more and effective**, as it is not reabsorbed in PCT. The reaction is:

$Na_2HPO_4 + H^+ \rightarrow Na^+ + NaH_2PO_4$

The monobasic phosphate gets excreted while sodium gets reabsorbed.

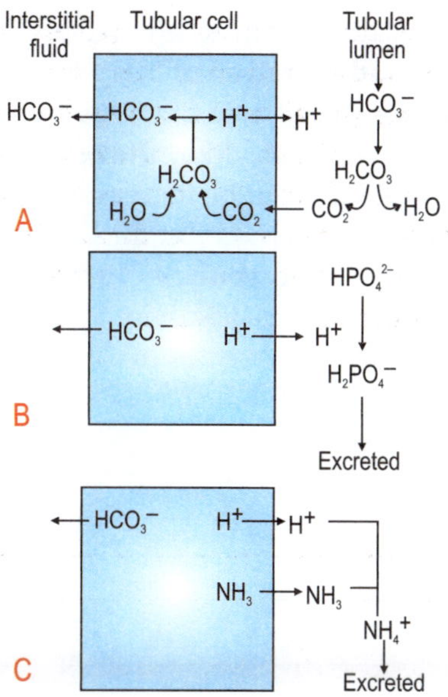

Fig. 91.4: Fate of H^+ secreted by tubular cells in different segments of renal tubule. H^+ is buffered by bicarbonate buffer mostly in proximal tubule (A); by phosphate buffer mostly in distal part of the tubule (B); and by ammonia buffer in PCT and DCT (C).

- In DCT and collecting tubules, **phosphate gets concentrated** due to increased absorption of water.
- Hence, **phosphate buffer** is more active in these parts of nephron.

In PCT and DCT

In PCT and DCT, **ammonia buffer** also works. Soluble **ammonia diffuses** through cell membrane down its concentration gradient into tubular fluid. Here it reacts with acid to form ammonium ion, which subsequently gets excreted. Hence, it maintains the ammonia gradient for further ammonia diffusion. This is called **nonionic diffusion**.

- In case of acidosis, amount of ammonia diffusion into urine increases and hence the excretion of ammonium ion increases (Fig. 94.4C).
- The mechanism that increases ammonia diffusion into urine in acidosis is still not clear. However, the probable mechanism may be as follows.

In PCT

In proximal tubular cells, ammonium is produced from glutamine. Each **glutamine molecule produces two molecules of NH_4^+** and a **divalent anion**.

- Each anion is metabolized to produce two molecules of HCO_3^- that enter the blood as new HCO_3^- and NH_4^+ enters the tubular fluid.
- **Glutamine becomes glutamate** by glutaminase, which in turn forms **α-ketoglutarate** (α-KG) by glutamic dehydrogenase.
  - **α-KG is converted to glucose** by gluconeogenesis that enters interstitial fluid and from there into blood. NH_4^+ formed during this process is secreted into tubular fluid.

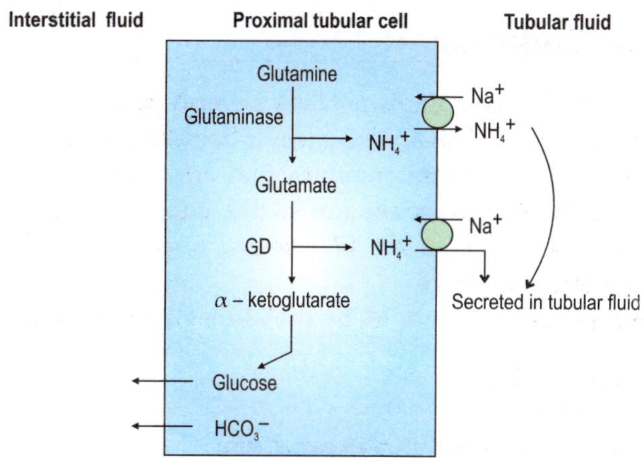

Fig. 91.5: Mechanism of NH_4^+ secretion that occurs mostly in proximal tubule. Note, NH_4^+ is formed during glutamine metabolism and its secretion involves Na^+– H^+ antiporter that substitutes NH_4^+ for H^+. GD: glutamic dehydrogenase.

- The mechanism of **NH_4^+ secretion** involves **Na^+-H^+ antiporter** that substitutes NH_4^+ for H^+ (Fig. 91.5).

A substantial amount of this NH_4^+ is reabsorbed in thick ascending limb of loop of Henle, which accumulates in the medullary interstitium.

In Collecting Duct

In the collecting duct, the tubular cells are **not permeable to NH_4^+** but permeable to NH_3.

1. NH_3 diffuses from the interstitium into the tubular fluid.
2. **H^+ is also secreted** by the intercalated cells into the tubular fluid, and **combines with NH_3 to form NH_4^+**, which is excreted in the urine.
3. Thus, ***H^+ secreted*** in the collecting duct **is essential for the excretion of NH_4^+.**
4. Therefore, when H^+ secretion in collecting duct is decreased, **net acid excretion is decreased** (Clinical Note 91.1). This in turn **decreases the transfer of new HCO_3^- to the blood** to replenish the amount utilized by buffering of non-volatile acid.

Clinical Note 91.1

Fanconi Syndrome: Renal tubular acidosis (RTA) is the condition in which acidification of urine is decreased. In such a situation, kidneys are incapable of excreting a large amount of acid to balance the production of non-volatile acid. This results in **metabolic acidosis**. An example of RTA is Fanconi syndrome.

- When the defect is in the proximal tubule, the condition is called **proximal RTA** and when the defect is in distal part of the tubule, the condition is called **distal RTA**.
- Failure to produce and excrete NH_4^+ decreases the amount of net acid excreted by kidneys that results in metabolic acidosis.

RENAL DEFENSE IN ACID-BASE DISORDER

Body's responses to metabolic acidosis or alkalosis, and respiratory acidosis or alkalosis are discussed in Chapter 134.

Renal Defense

The renal defense mechanism **takes several days** to be effectively operative. This is because kidney takes hours to **days to synthesize the enzymes** that are involved in NH_4^+ synthesis. **Ammonium ion is the major urinary acid**. When the pH of urine falls below 6, excretion of ammonium ions increases.

1. **In acidosis**, secretion of H^+ by the kidney is increased, and filtered bicarbonate is totally reabsorbed.
   - **Synthesis and excretion of NH_4^+** are also increased.
   - This **increases total acid excreted by the kidney**.
   - In chronic acidosis like **diabetic ketoacidosis**, excretion of NH_4^+ can be increased **10 folds**.
2. **In alkalosis,** secretion of H^+ by the kidney is inhibited. This **decreases bicarbonate reabsorption** and therefore, urine becomes alkaline.

Exam Questions

1. Describe the mechanism of acidification of urine.
2. Describe the renal handling of acid-base imbalance.

Multiple Choice Questions

1. **Principal site of acidification of urine:**
   A. Distal convoluted tubule
   B. Proximal convoluted tubule
   C. Loop of Henle
   D. Collecting duct
2. **Which part of kidney tubule plays less role in acidification of urine?**
   A. PCT
   B. Loop of Henle
   C. DCT
   D. Collecting duct
3. **In metabolic acidosis, which of the following changes are seen:**
   A. Increased K^+ excretion
   B. Decreased K^+ excretion
   C. Increased Na^+ excretion
   D. Increased Na^+ reabsorption
4. **All of the following statements are correct about potassium balance, EXCEPT:**
   A. Most of potassium is intracellular
   B. Three quarter of the total body potassium is found in skeletal muscle
   C. Intracellular potassium is released into extracellular space in response to severe injury
   D. Acidosis leads to movements of potassium from extracellular to intracellular fluid compartment
5. **Anion gap is mostly due to:**
   A. Proteins
   B. Sulphates
   C. Phosphates
   D. Nitrates
6. **Metabolic alkalosis is seen in all except:**
   A. Thiazide diuretics
   B. Ureter-sigmoidostomy
   C. Prolonged vomiting
   D. Systemic antacid therapy
7. **Increased anion gap is seen in**
   A. Enterocutaneous fistula
   B. Ileostomy fistula
   C. Lactic acidosis
   D. Diabetic ketoacidosis
8. **Normal anion gap metabolic acidosis is seen in:**
   A. Diarrhea
   B. Renal failure
   C. Lactic acidosis
   D. Diabetic ketoacidosis
9. **In severe exercise, decrease in pH is due to**
   A. Respiratory acidosis
   B. Lactic acidosis
   C. H^+ retention
   D. HCO_3^- excretion
10. **Which of the following is not a buffer in kidney?**
    A. Bicarbonate buffer
    B. Ammonia buffer
    C. Phosphate buffer
    D. Hemoglobin buffer

Answers

1\. D 2. B 3. B 4. D 5. A 6. B 7. C 8. A 9. B 10. D

Chapter 92

Kidney Function Tests and Renal Failure

Learning Objectives

On completion of study of this chapter:

The student will be able to (must know):

1. Classify kidney function tests (KFTs) and outline their principle and give normal values.
2. Define the concept of clearance tests.
3. Name the tubular function tests and give their physiological significance.
4. Understand the concept of acute kidney injury (AKI) and chronic renal failure (CRF).

The student may also be able to (desirable to know):

1. Describe the procedure, application, merits and demerits of KFTs.
2. Learn the physiological basis of dialysis.

PY7.8

KIDNEY FUNCTION TESTS

Kidney function tests (KFTs) are classified physiologically and clinically.

Physiological Classification

KFTs are physiologically grouped into *two categories*: glomerular function tests and tubular function tests.

A. Glomerular function tests:

1. Blood urea determination
2. Blood creatinine estimation
3. Inulin clearance test
4. Creatinine clearance test
5. Urea clearance test
6. PAH clearance test
7. Estimation of proteins in the urine

B. Tubular function test

1. Urine concentration test
2. Urine dilution test
3. Detection of uric acid excretion
4. Test for acidification of urine
5. Test for alkalinization of urine
6. Test for amino acids in urine

Clinical Classification

Clinically, KFTs are grouped into *four categories:*

1. **Routine tests:** Complete *urine analysis*, measurement of *BUN in blood*, and measurement of *serum electrolytes*.
2. **Tests for further assessments:** Clearance test, determination of urine and plasma osmolality, and concentration and dilution tests.
3. **Specific tests:** Tests to assess renal acidification, tests to assess renal handling of sodium, measurement of renal plasma flow, and excretion of exogenous compound like PSP.
4. **Special tests:** Ultrasonography, CT scan, MRI, etc.

Routine Urine Analysis

Routine urine analysis includes assessment of **physical and biochemical characteristics** of urine.

Physical Characteristics

Volume

The normal volume of urine excreted is about **1–1.5 liters** per day.

Oliguria and Anuria: A person on normal diet can excrete the solute load at maximum concentration when the urine volume is between 300 to 500 ml/day. Volume below this is termed as **oliguria**.

1. When urine flow is less than 50 ml/day, is called as **anuria**.
2. Oliguria and anuria could be due to **decreased urine production** (as seen in renal failure, renal infarction, rapidly progressive glomerulonephritis etc.) or **due to**

obstruction to urine flow (as seen in urinary calculi, prostatic enlargement, atonic bladder, pelvic or retroperitoneal tumors, urethral strictures, urethral infection, urethral valves etc.).

Polyuria: When urine volume is inappropriately high (> **3 liters per day**), is called polyuria. Polyuria could be due to **osmotic diuresis** (increased urinary solute excretion) or due to **water diuresis**.

Common causes of polyuria are:

1. Excessive fluid intake
2. ***Osmotic diuresis*** (due to hyperglycemia as in DM and hypercalcemia)
3. Diabetes insipidus
5. Diuretics
6. Increased frequency of micturition as occurs in urethritis, cystitits, prostitis etc.

Nocturia: Waking up in the night to void urine is called nocturia.

- It may occur due to **polyuria** of any cause.
- Seen in **chronic kidney diseases** and **prostatic enlargement**.

Appearance

Normally, urine is clear.

- Urine may be turbid if it contains more **phosphates** (as in alkaline urine) or **pus** (infection of urinary tract) or **chyle** (obstruction of urinary tract lymphatics as occurs in filariasis).

Odor

Normally, the odor of urine is **mildly aromatic** due to presence of volatile organic acids.

- **Diabetic urine** gives acidotic-fruity odor due to the presence acetone in the urine.
- Excretion of different drugs in the urine also changes the smell of urine.

Color

Normal urine is **straw colored** or amber-yellow in color, which is due to the presence of the pigment **urochrome** in it.

1. Urine becomes **yellow in hyperbilirubinuria**.
2. Urine becomes **dark** in alkaptonuria, melanuria (seen in malignant melanoma), and,
3. **Red** in hematuria, hemoglobinuria, myoglobinuria, etc.

Biochemical Characteristics

Reaction of Urine

Normally, urine is ***mildly acidic***; the average pH being 6 (ranging between **4.5–7.5**).

1. **After a normal meal**, urine becomes alkaline due to ***alkaline tide***.
2. If the meal is **rich in protein**, urine becomes acidic.
3. If the meal is **rich in vegetables**, urine becomes alkaline.
    - **Alkaline urine** is also a feature of type II distal renal tubular acidosis, urinary tract infection by urease producing organisms, acetazolamide therapy and following ingestion of alkali.

Proteins in Urine

Normally, glomerulus is not permeable to substances with molecular weight more than 69000. Therefore, **normally proteins are absent in urine**. The normal protein content of 24-hour urine is < 0.03 g.

Protein-Creatinine Ratio: The normal protein-creatinine ratio in a random urine sample is < 2.5 mg/mM in males and < 3.5 mg/mM in females (Table 92.1).

- Ratio > 3.5 mg/mM indicates microalbuminuria and > 15 mg/mM indicates proteinuria.

Proteinuria

Proteinuria is seen in nephritis, nephrosis, urinary tract infections (UTIs), eclampsia, heart failure and later part of pregnancy.

Bence-Jones Proteinuria: occurs in **multiple myeloma, amyloidosis and plasma cell dyscrasias**.

- This is used as a marker in myeloma in which **myeloma protein** (*Bence-Jones proteins*) increases in plasma.

Microalbuminuria: Excretion of 24 hr urinary protein > **300 mg** (0.03 to 0.3 g) is described as microalbuminuria.

1. This is an **early sign** of glomerular dysfunction.
2. Patients with **diabetic nephropathy**.
3. A persistent microalbuminuria is risk of atherosclerosis and cardiovascular mortality.

Table 92.1 | 24 hr urinary protein and protein-creatinine ratio in different conditions.

24 h urinary protein (g)	Protein/Creatinine ratio mg/mM	Significance
< 0.03	<2.5 in males <3.5 in females	Normal
0.03 – 0.3	3.5 – 15	Microalbuminuria
0.3 – 0.5	15 – 50	Dipstick positive
> 2.5	100-300	Glomerular disease likely
> 4.0	> 300	Glomerular disease

Blood in Urine

Blood in urine is called **hematuria**. Occurs in infection or injury in any part of urinary tract.

Hemoglobinuria & Myoglobinuria: Presence of hemoglobin in urine (hemoglobinuria) indicates **intravascular hemolysis** and presence of myoglobin in urine (myoglobinuria) indicates **rhabdomyolysis**.

Reducing Sugars in Urine

The presence of sugar in urine is called glycosuria (or more accurately, glucosuria). Normally, glucose does not appear in urine.

Glycosuria occurs due to:

1. **Diabetes mellitus**
2. Kidney diseases (**renal glycosuria**) due to decreased renal threshold
3. Alimentary glycosuria (lag storage glycosuria) following meals.
4. Gestational glycosuria.

Other Biochemical Tests

Ketone Bodies in Urine: Excretion of ketone bodies in urine is called **ketonuria**. Normally, **ketone bodies are not present** in urine.

- Ketonuria occurs in severe diabetes mellitus, starvation, chronic vomiting, etc.

Bile salts in Urine: Bile salts appear in urine in the **early phase of obstructive jaundice**.

Bile-Pigments in Urine: Bile pigments (bilirubin and biliverdin) appear in urine in obstructive jaundice.

Urobilinogen in Urine: Normally, the main pigment in the urine is **urochrome**.

- Urobilinogen excretion increases in persistent fevers, liver diseases, diseases of biliary tract and hemolysis.

Measurement of NPN in Urine: The non-protein nitrogen (NPN) in urine includes **urea, creatinine and uric acid.** These compounds are excreted from the body mainly through urine. Their concentration in urine increases in different physiological and pathological conditions.

1. Determination of **creatinine** is an important test for renal function.
2. **Urea** level is altered in many conditions. Blood urea concentration is a good index of renal functions.
3. **Uric acid** is increased in urine in conditions that are associated with increased purine catabolism.

Clearance Tests

Clearance tests mainly determine the glomerular function. **GFR provides the most useful index** for assessment of severity of the renal disease.

Clearance is defined as the **quantity of blood or plasma cleared of a substance for unit time.** This is expressed as ml per minute.

Details of clearance and clearance tests are described in Chapter 87, in glomerular filtration rate (GFR). The relation between clearance value and GFR is depicted in Table 92.2.

Table 92.2 | Relationship between GFR and clearance value.

Mechanism	Result	Example
Substances filtered but neither reabsorbed nor excreted.	GFR = clearance	Inulin
Substances filtered, reabsorbed & excreted	GFR = clearance	Uric acid
Substances filtered & partially reabsorbed	Clearance < GFR	Urea, & creatinine
Substances filtered & secreted, but not reabsorbed	Clearance > GFR	Diodrast & PAH

Blood Investigations

Blood tests for assessing kidney functions are serum urea, creatinine, uric acid and electrolytes.

Serum Urea: Normal serum urea level is **15 – 40 mg%.** Increased serum urea is seen in:

1. High intake (high protein diet, GI hemorrhage)
2. High production (trauma, burn, infections)
3. Reduced urinary excretion (renal failure, hypovolemia)

Serum Creatinine: Normal serum creatinine level **0.7 – 1.5 mg% in males and 0.5 to 1.2 mg% in females.**

Increased serum creatinine is seen in:

1. High production (increased muscle mass, rhabdomyolysis)
2. Reduced excretion in urine (renal failure, drugs like trimethoprim, cimetidine)

Serum Electrolytes: Hyperkalemia is an important feature of renal dysfunctions.

Tubular Function Tests

The primary function of tubule is to reabsorb solutes and water from the tubular fluid. Therefore, **detecting concentration of solutes in urine** gives the knowledge of tubular functions. The simplest tubular function test is the **measurement of specific gravity** of the urine.

Tubular functions are determined by **concentration** and **dilution tests.**

Concentration Test: The patient is advised to eat normal food at 6 PM but fluid intake is restricted to 200 ml. He is further advised not to take anything throughout night. Next morning, at 7AM, the bladder is emptied and this first specimen is discarded. At 8 AM, urine collected and this second specimen is obtained for measuring specific gravity.

1. **If specific gravity is more than 1.022**, the renal function is normal.
2. **If specific gravity is below this value**, a third sample is collected at 9AM.
3. If this sample gives **specific gravity less than 1.022**, then the concentrating ability of the kidney is considered to be impaired.

Dilution Test: The patient is not allowed to drink water or fluid after 10 PM. The bladder is emptied at 7AM in the next morning and patient is allowed to take a water load of 1.2 liter in half an-hour.

- Hourly urine samples are collected for four hours for determination of volume, specific gravity, and osmolality of each sample.
- Normally, a person **excretes the total water load in four hours** and the specific gravity of at least one sample should fall to 1.003 and osmolality to 50 mosm/kg.

Specific Tests

Tests for Urine Acidification: Usually, acid loading test is performed to detect the ability of the kidney to acidify urine. Ammonium chloride is given to the subject as an enteric coated tablet (0.1 g/kg b.w.).

1. Urine is collected every hour for 4–8 hours for determination of pH of urine and ammonia excretion of each sample.
2. At least, **one sample should have pH of 5.3** or less and **ammonia excretion should be 30–90 mmole per hour.**

Test for Renal Handling of Na^+: The patient is given **sodium free diet for 7 days** (daily intake less than 10 mmole). After a week, urinary sodium output is estimated.

1. A normal person **decreases Na^+ excretion to 10 mmole** per day after 7 days. When tubular function is impaired, ability to reabsorb sodium is lower.
2. In such conditions, natriuresis continues regardless of Na^+ intake.

PSP Test: The PSP or phenol-sulphonphthalein (phenol red) test is used for determining the secretory capacity of the tubule.

- The subject is allowed to drink 600 ml of water following which PSP is given intravenously (6 mg in 1 ml solution). Bladder is emptied after 15 minutes, 30 minutes, 60 minutes and 120 minutes, and excretion of the phenol red is noted in each sample.
- Normally, the **phenol content is 35% in the first sample** and **70% of the dye should be eliminated in two hours**.
- **In tubular dysfunctions**, the dye excreted in first sample is less and also the total amount excreted in two hours will be less.
- This is a useful test for detection of **early stage of kidney disease**.

Special Tests

Special tests to assess kidney functions include **utrasonography, intravenous pyelogrphy, computed tomography** and **magnetic resonance imaging. Renal biopsy** is useful in some selective diseases.

PY7.7

RENAL FAILURE

Renal failure is the condition of decreased urine output due to loss of renal function that develops over a period of days to years. This is of two types: acute kidney injury (acute renal failure) and chronic renal failure.

Acute Kidney Injury

Definition and Causes: Acute kidney injury (AKI) was previously known as acute renal failure (ARF). The other term used is Azotemia.

- AKI refers to a sudden, but usually reversible deterioration in renal function that develops over a period of hours or few days and is usually accompanied by a reduction in urine volume.
- AKI includes an increase in serum creatinine >0.3gm/dL within 48 hours, or an increase to >1.5 times the presumed baseline value or presumed to have occurred within prior seven days or a decrease in urine volume <3ml/kg over six hours.

The causes of AKI (ARF) are listed in Table 92. 3. The commonest pre-renal cause of ARF is hypovolemic shock and commonest renal cause is acute tubular necrosis (ATN).

Table 92.3 | Causes of renal failure
I. Causes of AKI or acute renal failure
A. Pre-renal causes
1. Systemic causes
- Heart failure
- Blood or fluid loss
2. Local causes
- Renal artery stenosis
3. Under-perfusion of kidney
B. Renal causes
1. Acute tubular necrosis/toxic/septic renal failure
2. Glomerular diseases
3. Interstitial kidney diseases
C. Post-renal causes
1. Obstruction to urine outflow
- Kidney stones
- Kidney tumors
- Prostatic enlargement
II. Causes of chronic renal failure.
1. Diabetes mellitus
2. Hypertension
3. Glomerular diseases (e. g. IgA nephropathy)
4. Renal interstitial diseases
5. Renal artery stenosis
6. Congenital and inherited (e.g. polycystic kidney disease, Alport syndrome)
7. Systemic inflammatory diseases (e.g. SLE, vasculitis)

Features: Patient is usually oliguric (24 hr urine volume < 500 ml).

1. Hyperkalemia is common. Dilutional hyponatremia

and metabolic acidosis may be present. Hypocalcemia is common due to decreased production of 1,25 dihydroxycholecalciferol.

2. Uremic features include anorexia, nausea, vomiting, apathy, confusion, muscle twitching, hiccoughs, fits and coma.
3. Pulmonary edema may be present due to increased pulmonary capillary permeability.
4. Anemia is common.
5. Bleeding may occur due to platelet dysfunctions or disturbances in coagulation cascade. Spontaneous GI hemorrhage is not uncommon.

Treatment: Emergency resuscitation and follow up treatment include:

1. **Hyperkalemia is treated immediately** to prevent development of life threatening cardiac arrhythmias.
   - ***Calcium gluconate*** (10 ml of 10% solution) is given i.v. to stabilize membrane potential.
   - ***Insulin and glucose solution*** (5 units of insulin + 50 ml of 50% glucose) is injected i.v. along with sodium bicarbonate. **Insulin** facilitates entry of K^+ into the cell and immediately decreases plasma K^+ level. **Glucose** is given to combat insulin-induced hypoglycemia.
   - **Sodibicarb** prevents acidosis. Dialysis may be needed in extreme cases.
2. Circulating blood volume should be optimized.
3. **Metabolic acidosis is corrected** by isotonic sodium bicarbonate infusion.
4. **Fluid intake** should equal the urine output.
5. **Treatment of underlying cause**

Exam Questions

1. Classify KFTs. Briefly describe their basic principle and clinical application.
2. Briefly describe glomerular function tests and tubular function tests. Add a note on acute kidney injury.

Multiple Choice Questions

1. ADH does not act on:
A. PCT B. Collecting duct
C. Collecting tubules D. DCT

2. Which of the following is true about Nephron function?
A. Ascending thick limb is permeable to water
B. Descending thin limb is impermeable to water
C. Osmolality of intra-tubular content in DCT is more than surrounding interstitium
D. Osmolality of intratubular content in PCT is isotonic to surrounding interstitium

3. Which of the following occurs along with glucose transport into renal tubular cells?
A. Sodium symport/cotransport B. Sodium antiport
C. Potassium transport D. Amino acid transport

4. As fluid comes down the PCT, what is true?
A. Concentration of urea falls
B. Concentration of HCO_3 falls
C. Concentration of Na^+ increases
D. Concentration of inulin decreases

5. Which one of the following is not responsible for concentration of urine in the kidney?
A. Aldosterone B. Angiotensin II
C. Vasopressin D. Epinephrine

6. Which of the following estimation is a better tubular function test?
A. Serum creatinine B. Serum urea
C. Protein in urine D. Urine dilution test

7. Urine volume decreases in all of the following, EXCEPT;
A. Hypovolemia B. High protein diet
C. Dehydration D. Hypotension

8. Elimination of waste product from a normal person required minimal amount of urine formation is:
A. 200 ml B. 500 ml
C. 800 ml D. 2000 ml

9. Normal excretion of protein in urine per day is:
A. 100 mg B. 150 mg
C. 400 mg D. 600 mg

10. Determination of specific gravity of urine indicates more of:
A. Tubular function B. Glomerular function
C. Function of JG apparatus D. Function of mesangial cells

11. Normal urinary protein-creatinine ratio in male is:
A. <3.5 B. <4.7
C. <5.8 D. <7.2

12. Increase in serum urea seen in all, EXCEPT:
A. High protein diet B. Burn
C. Renal failure D. Increased blood volume

13. Serum creatinine more than 1.5mg% is seen in all, EXCEPT:
A. Increased skeletal muscle mass
B. Trimethoprim therapy
C. Rhabdomyolysis
D. Excess day time sleep

14. Which one of the following statements regarding water reabsorption in the tubules is correct?
A. The bulk of water reabsorption occurs secondary to Na^+ reabsorption
B. Majority of facultative reabsorption occurs in proximal tubules
C. Obligatory reabsorption is ADH dependent
D. 20% of water is always reabsorbed irrespective of water balance

Answers

1. A	2. D	3. A	4. B	5. D	6. D	7. B	8. B	9. A	10. A
11. A	12. D	13. D	14. A						

Chapter 93

Physiology of Micturition and Bladder Dysfunctions

Learning Objectives

On completion of study of this chapter:

The student will be able to (must know):

1. Remember the innervation and arrangement of sphincters of urinary bladder
2. Draw a labelled diagram of micturition reflex and describe its mechanism and control.
3. Draw the graph of cystometrogram.
4. Name the common bladder dysfunctions.

The student may also be able to (desirable to know):

1. Describe the abnormalities of bladder dysfunctions

PY7.6

URINARY BLADDER

Functional Aspects

Bladder Wall

Urinary bladder is a **distensible organ** made up of smooth muscle, called **detrusor muscle** (Fig. 93.1), depicting the Latin word 'pushes down'.

- Contraction of the detrusor causes emptying of the bladder.
- The **epithelium of the bladder** is formed by a superficial layer of flat cells and a deep layer of cuboidal cells.

Innervation

Bladder is innervated by sympathetic, parasympathetic and somatic fibers (Fig. 93.1).

1. **Parasympathetic fibers** originate from the **sacral 2, 3 and 4 segments** of the spinal cord and reach the bladder via pelvic nerves,
2. The **sympathetic fibers** originate from **lumbar 1, 2 and 3 segments** of the spinal cord and reach the bladder via hypogastric nerve.

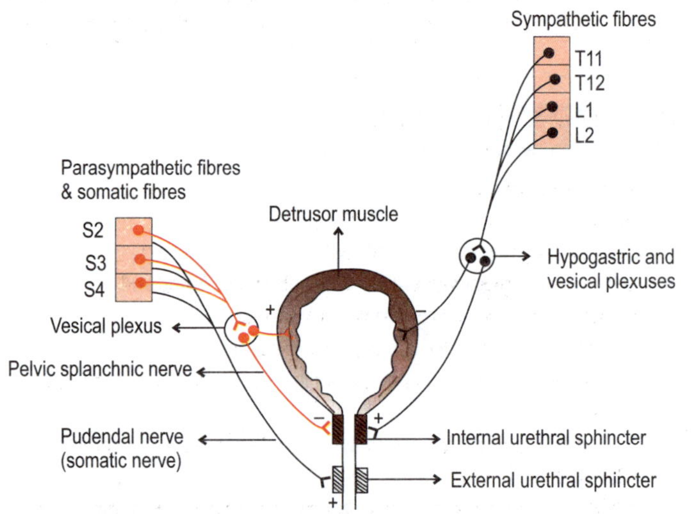

Fig. 93.1: Structure and innervation of urinary bladder. Plus sign indicates stimulatory and minus sign indicates inhibitory.

3. The **somatic fibers** originate from **S_2, S_3 and S_4** and innervate bladder and external sphincter via pudendal nerve.

Filling of bladder, desire to pass urine and painful distension, all these sensations of bladder are mediated by **afferents in the pelvic nerve.**

Urethral Sphincters

There are **two sphincters**: internal and external (Fig. 93.2).

1. The **internal sphincter**, which is located at the neck of the bladder, is made up of a bundle of smooth muscle (*sphincter vesicae*) and innervated by **sympathetic (hypogastric) and parasympathetic (pelvic) nerves**.
   - Therefore, the internal sphincter is **under autonomic control**.
2. The **external sphincter** is made up of a flap of skeletal muscle, which is present around the urethra in its proximal part (*sphincter urethrae*).

- The external sphincter is **innervated by somatic (pudendal) nerve** and therefore **under voluntary control**.

Functions of Urinary Bladder

Urinary bladder serves **two functions**:

1. **Storage of urine** upto a critical volume.
2. **Emptying urine** into urethra when the critical volume is attained.

The external sphincter is kept closed most of the time.

- The sensation of bladder filling is experienced at the bladder volume of about 150 ml and the **sensation to pass urine** is experienced at bladder volume of **150–250 ml.**
- **At volume of about 400 ml**, the sensation to pass urine becomes **uncomfortable** and at about 700 ml, it becomes very painful leading to loss of control.

MICTURITION REFLEX

Micturition is the process of passing urine. This is primarily a **reflex phenomenon**, which is mostly **integrated in the spinal cord**. This spinal reflex is **influenced by activities of the higher centers**.

- Unless the bladder is filled, urine accumulates in urinary bladder without much increase in the intravesical pressure, as bladder wall is made up of smooth muscles that exhibit the property of **plasticity**.
- Due to plasticity, tension produced by stretching is not maintained. This relationship between the bladder volume and pressure is best studied by **cystometry.**

Cystometry **PY7.9**

Cystometry is the procedure to study the **relationship between the bladder volume and pressure**. For this purpose, a catheter is inserted into the bladder and bladder is completely emptied. Then, as bladder volume is gradually increased by slowly pushing water to fill bladder, intravesical pressure is recorded at different bladder volumes. This recording of pressure-volume relationship is called **cystometrogram** (Fig. 93.2).

1. The **initial rise in intravesical pressure** occurs when bladder is filled with 50 ml of water (at point A, Fig. 93.2) and thereafter no significant increase in pressure occurs with increase in volume to about 400 ml (between the points B and C, Fig. 93.2).
2. The intravesical pressure increases steeply when the intravesical volume exceeds 400 ml (between the points C and D, Fig. 93.2).
   - This **sharp rise in pressure initiates the reflex** triggering of micturition.
3. The limb B-C of cystometrogram is flat due to the application of **Laplace law,** which states that the pressure in a spherical viscus is equal to twice the wall tension divided by radius.

- Urinary bladder being a spherical viscus, the tension increases as the organ fills.
- However, at the same time also the radius increases.

Therefore, increase in intravesical pressure is minimal unless the viscus is relatively full. However, **above the volume of about 400 ml, pressure increases sharply** as wall tension increases abruptly.

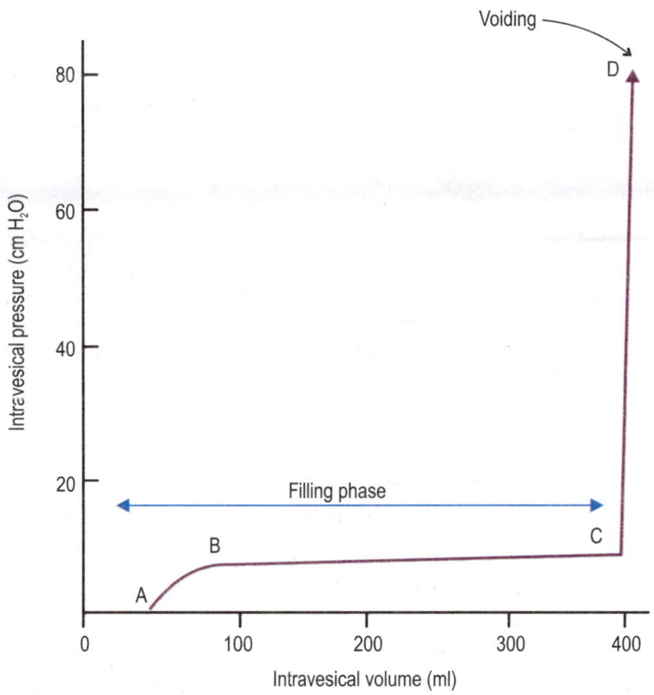

Fig. 93.2: Cystometrogram.

Mechanism of Micturition

Stimulus and Reflex Arc

Filling of the bladder, cussing stretch of bladder wall is the stimulus.

1. The **stretch receptors** that are present in the wall of the bladder send impulses in the afferent nerve that initiate reflex contraction.
2. The **fibers in the pelvic nerve** form the **afferent limb** for the micturition reflex (Fig. 93.3).
   - The **center** for this spinal reflex is the **sacral 2, 3, and 4 segments** of the spinal cord.
3. The **parasympathetic fibers** to bladder constitute **efferent limb**, which also travel in the pelvic nerve.
   - The reflex is initiated at about 300–400 ml of intravesical volume.
4. Normally, the **sympathetic fibers do not play role** in micturition.
   - However, the sympathetic activation causes **contraction of bladder muscle** that prevents semen from entering the bladder during ejaculation.

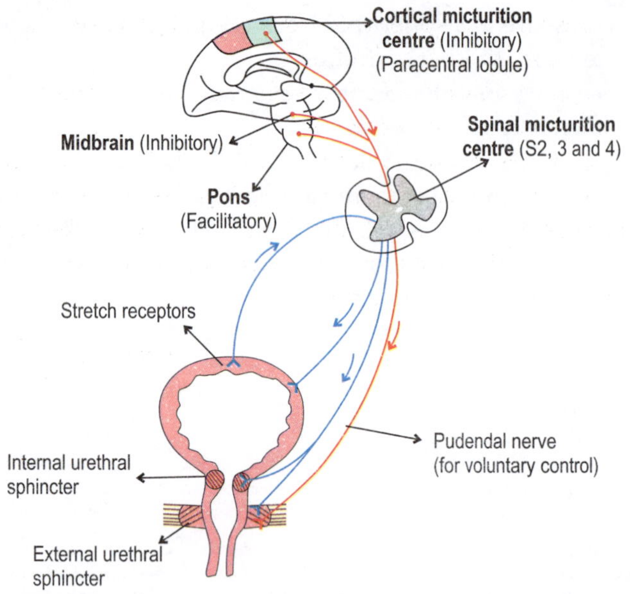

Fig. 93.3: Control of micturition reflex. Fullness of bladder is sensed by afferents in pelvic nerve and parasympathetic efferents also travel in pelvic nerve. Note, midbrain and cortex inhibit and pons facilitates reflex activity. Voluntary prevention of micturition is achieved by contracting external urethral sphincter, which is mediated through somatic efferents in pudendal nerve.

Mechanism

Micturition is a **parasympathetic activity**.

1. Parasympathetic stimulation causes **contraction of detrusor and relaxation of internal sphincter**, so that the urine passes forcefully into the urethra.
   - Contraction of abdominal muscle and descent of diaphragm ***increases intra-abdominal pressure***.
2. During micturition, the **pelvic, perineal and levator ani muscles relax**.
   - This causes **downward pull of detrusor muscle** and aids to initiation of its contraction.
   - At this stage, *perineal muscles and external sphincter can be made to contract voluntarily* to prevent micturition to occur.
3. The **voluntary control** of micturition is influenced by **cortical activities** and by *learning to contract the external urethral sphincter*.
   - Once in the urethra, the urine is emptied **in females** by the effect of gravity and pressure from the pelvic floor, whereas **in males**, urine is emptied by *contractions of bulbocavernosus muscle*.
4. The voluntary contraction of abdominal muscles helps in expulsion of urine.

Control of Micturition

The micturition reflex is controlled by **centers in the brainstem**.

1. The **facilitatory area** is present in pons and the **inhibitory area** is present in midbrain (Fig. 93.3).
   - Therefore, **section of neuraxis above pons** promotes activity of micturition reflex in which less filling of bladder triggers its reflex evacuation, and **section above midbrain** does not affect it.
2. **Posterior hypothalamus** also contains a **facilitatory area for micturition**.
3. **Cortex** has ***voluntary inhibitory control*** on micturition.
   - In children, below three years of age, cortical inhibition is not well developed; hence they often pass urine without their knowledge.
4. Control on urination starts to **develop at about two years** of age and completes by three years.

BLADDER DYSFUNCTIONS

Abnormalities of Micturition

The **lesions at different segments of neuraxis** result in bladder dysfunctions. There are ***three major neural defects*** that produce bladder dysfunctions:

1. Interruption of afferent fibers (**deafferentation**)
2. Interruption of both afferent and efferent fibers (**denervation**)
3. Interruption of influences from the facilitatory and inhibitory areas in the brain (**spinal cord transection**).

In these lesions, bladder may contact, but the contraction is not enough to empty the viscus. Therefore, **residual urine** is always left in the bladder.

Deafferentation

When, fibers originating from **the sacral roots** of the spinal cord are experimentally destroyed, **reflex contraction of bladder is abolished**.

- The bladder is **distended, thin-walled and hypotonic**.
  - However, some contractions occur (due to intrinsic response of the smooth muscles to stretch).
- Such type of bladder is seen in ***tabes dorsalis.***

Denervation

When both the **afferent and efferent fibers are cut**, bladder becomes **flaccid and distended** at the beginning.

- Gradually the muscle of the bladder becomes active and the contraction of the bladder muscle removes urine in the form of dribbles.
- Later, the bladder is **shrunken and bladder wall becomes hypertrophied**.
  - This is typically seen in the **tumors of cauda equina or filum terminale**.
- The hyperactive bladder suggests **denervation hypersensitivity** of bladder muscles.

Spinal Cord Transection

When the spinal cord is transected, typically **three phases** are observed: phase of shock, phase of recovery (increased reflex activity), and phase of failure.

1. During **the phase of spinal shock**, the bladder becomes **flaccid and unresponsive**.

- The **overflow incontinence** (urine dribbles through the sphincter when the bladder is overfilled) occurs.

2. In the **phase of recovery**, micturition reflex is the **first reflex activity to return**. However, voluntary control or control by the higher centers is abolished after transection.
   - The spinal man (the human being following transection of the spinal cord) can train himself to initiate the micturition reflex by voluntarily **activating the mass reflex** (for details, refer to 'Spinal Regulation of Motor Control', Chapter 107).
3. The **bladder capacity is decreased,** and the muscle of bladder **is hypertrophied**.
   - This type of bladder is known as **spastic neurogenic bladder**.
4. In the **phase of failure,** the infection of bladder makes the reflex activity worse.

Exam Questions

1. With the help of a schematic diagram, describe the mechanism of micturition reflex. Add a note on cystometrogram.
2. With the help of a diagram of cystometrogram, explain the intravesical volume-pressure pressure relationship. Add a note on effects of spinal cord transection on bladder function.

Multiple Choice Questions

1. **All of the following statements are true about external urethral sphincter, EXCEPT:**
   A. Present around the urethra in its proximal part
   B. Made up of a bundle of smooth muscle
   C. Innervated by somatic pudendal nerve
   D. Is known as sphincter urethrae
2. **All of the following statements are true about internal urethral sphincter, EXCEPT:**
   A. Located at the neck of the bladder
   B. Made up of a flap of skeletal muscle
   C. Innervated by sympathetic hypogastric nerve
   D. Innervated by parasympathetic pelvic nerve
3. **Peristaltic waves in ureters originate by a pacemaker tissue at a frequency of:**
   A. One every 5 sec B. One every 10 sec
   C. One every 20 sec D. One every 60 sec
4. **Which of the following is not true about innervation of bladder?**
   A. Parasympathetic fibers to bladder originate from sacral 2, 3 and 4 segments.
   B. Sympathetic fibers to bladder originate from lumbar 1, 2 and 3 segments.
   C. Somatic fibers originate from sacral 2, 3 and 4 segments.
   D. Parasympathetic fibers reach bladder in hypogastric nerve.
5. **The urge for micturition is felt when the bladder is filled with**
   A. 150-200 cc of urine B. 200-300 cc of urine
   C. 500-700 cc of urine D. 700-800 cc of urine
6. **In a normal adult, the marked desire for micturition is felt:**
   A. When about 100-200 cc of urine has collected in the bladder
   B. When about 300-400 cc of urine has collected in the bladder
   C. When about 600-800 cc of urine has collected in the bladder
   D. When about 1000 cc of urine has collected in the bladder
7. **True statement among the following is:**
   A. Bladder emptying cannot occur if volume less than 100ml
   B. Bladder muscle contains intrafusal fibers
   C. Pressure increase in bladder very linearly with time
   D. One liter of fluid intake results in complete excretion in one hour
8. **In cystometrogram, the intravesical pressure rises steeply at what intravesical volume:**
   A. 100 ml B. 250 ml
   C. 400 ml D. 600 ml
9. **Spastic neurogenic bladder is seen in:**
   A. Spinal cord transaction
   B. Deafferentation
   C. Denervation
   D. Bladder tumor
10. **The flat limb of cystometrogram is due to application of:**
    A. Laplace law
    B. Poiseuille's law
    C. Ohm's law
    D. Bernoulli's principle
11. **In deafferentation, the bladder is:**
    A. Spastic B. Distended, thin walled
    C. Shrunken D. Hypertrophied
12. **For micturition, parasympathetic stimulation causes:**
    A. Contraction of detrusor and contraction of internal sphincter
    B. Relaxation of detrusor and contraction of internal sphincter
    C. Contraction of detrusor and relaxation of internal sphincter
    D. Relaxation of detrusor and relaxation of internal sphincter
13. **During micturition, all of the following muscles relax, EXCEPT:**
    A. Pelvic B. Perineal
    C. Levator ani D. Detrusor
14. **All of the following statements are true regarding control of micturition, EXCEPT:**
    A. Facilitatory area is present in the midbrain
    B. Inhibitoy area is present in the cortex
    C. Facilitatory area is present in the pons
    D. Facilitatory area is present in the posterior hypothalamus

Answers

1. B	2. B	3. D	4. D	5. A	6. B	7. A	8. C	9. A	10. A
11. B	12. C	13. D	14. A						

Section XI

Neurophysiology

To receive the divine grace, not only one must have a great aspiration, but also a sincere humility and an absolute trust.

The Mother
(of Sri Aurobindo Ashram, Pondicherry, INDIA)

Chapter 94

PY10.1

Functional Organization of Nervous System

Learning Objectives

On completion of study of this chapter:

The student will be able to (must know):

1. Name the divisions of nervous system and outline functions of each division.
2. Name the different parts of brain and briefly mention functions of each part.
3. Outline the integrated functions of CNS.
4. Name the cell types of CNS and give their functions.
5. Classify neurons and give example of each category of neurons.

The student may also be able to (desirable to know):

1. Describe the structure and functions of neurons and glial cells.

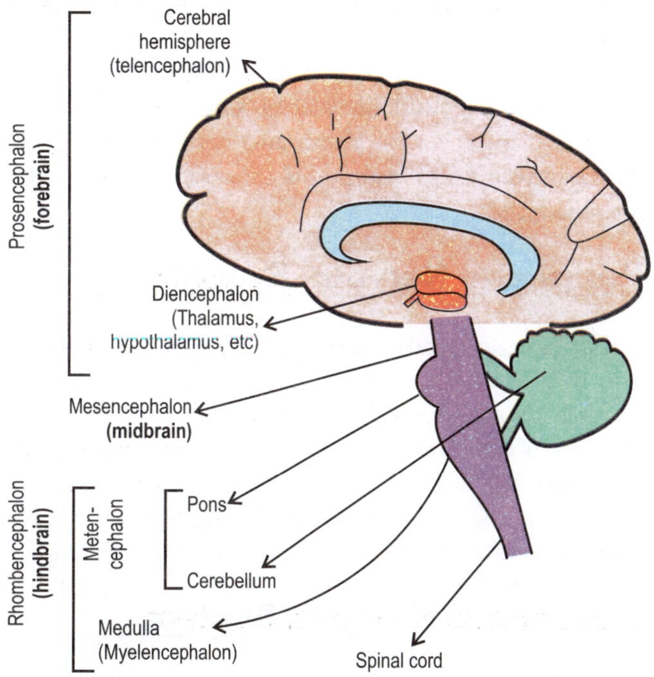

Fig. 94.1: Parts of CNS. Note the structures included in forebrain, midbrain, and hindbrain. Midbrain, pons and medulla are combinely designated as brainstem.

DIVISIONS OF NERVOUS SYSTEM

The nervous system consists of **three divisions**: central nervous system, peripheral nervous system, and autonomic nervous system.

Central Nervous System

The central nervous system (CNS) includes **brain and spinal cord**.

Brain

Brain is divided into three parts (Fig. 94.1): prosencephalon, mesencephalon and rhombencephalon

Prosencephalon: This is **the forebrain**, which consists of the ***telencephalon*** (the two cerebral hemispheres) and the ***diencephalon*** (thalamus, hypothalamus, metathalamus, and subthalamus).

1. The **telencephalon** is meant for perception of sensations, cognition, learning and memory, and planning and programming of responses.
2. The **diencephalon** is primarily meant for relay of information to cortex, and control of autonomic and endocrine functions.

Mesencephalon: This consists of **the midbrain** structures, which includes corpora quadrigemina, cerebral peduncles, substantia nigra, tegmentum and many midbrain nuclei.

- Midbrain contains central pattern generator for locomotion and nuclei for righting reflexes.
- It also contains a part of reticular formation.

Rhombencephalon: This is **the hindbrain**, which consists of ***metencephalon*** (the pons and the cerebellum) and ***myelencephalon*** (the medulla oblongata).

- The midbrain, pons, and medulla are combinely known as **brainstem**.
- The *main functions of brainstem* are control of cardiovascular and respiratory functions, motor activities, sleep-wakefulness and visceral functions.

Spinal Cord

Spinal cord starts from the base of the skull as the extension of medulla and continues till the body of first lumbar vertebra. Thus, spinal cord does not run the full length of the vertebral column in adults.

- The space at the end of spinal cord, especially between L_3 and L_4 vertebral segments is used in *tapping cerebrospinal fluid* during **lumbar puncture**.
- Spinal cord has 31 segments, each having a motor and a sensory nerve root.
  - The nerve roots combine to form the **31 bilaterally symmetrical pairs of spinal nerves**.
- Spinal cord contains all the **ascending and descending tracts**.

The main **function of spinal cord** is to receive sensory inputs from peripheral structures via somatic nerves and transmit them to the brain, and convey the signals originating from brain motor and autonomic areas to the target structures.

Peripheral Nervous System

The peripheral nervous system (PNS) includes **somatic nerves** that come out of the spinal cord to innervate different body structures like skin, muscles, bones etc.

- The main function of PNS is to **collect and convey information** from peripheral structures to CNS via sensory axons and **convey motor signals** from CNS to muscles and related structures via motor neurons.

Autonomic Nervous System

The autonomic nervous system consists ***sympathetic*** and ***parasympathetic divisions*** that work reciprocally to regulate visceral functions (for details, refer chapter 24).

FUNCTIONS OF NERVOUS SYSTEM

The **major functions** of the nervous system are:

1. Communication between body parts and integration of systemic functions.
2. Appropriate regulation of body functions.
3. Coordinated interaction of the body with the environment.

The neural regulation is the major controlling mechanism of many functions and processes of the body. Nervous system achieves its objectives through neurons that are designed for rapid transmission of information from one body part to the other.

Execution of Functions

CNS accomplishes its functions through **three major processes** (Fig. 94.2):

1. Recognition of stimulus and transmission of information in the form of nerve impulse to CNS.
2. Processing of information in CNS and generation of appropriate command signal in CNS.
3. Specific responses in accordance with the command signal conveyed by CNS.

Stimulus Recognition and Transmission of Information to CNS: This is the process by which we become aware of our environment through various sensations.

- **Sensation** is the basic recognition of the stimulus.
- The **receptors** transduce stimulus into the action potentials in the sensory neurons.
- **Sensory neurons** transmit information in the form of nerve action potentials from receptors to the CNS via ***sensory pathways***.

Details of sensory mechanisms are discussed in **physiology of sensory system**.

Information Processing and Generation of Command Signal: The general outline of central processing is as follows:

- The action potential (***sensory signal***) transmitted is first **relayed in the thalamus and then processed in sensory cortex**.

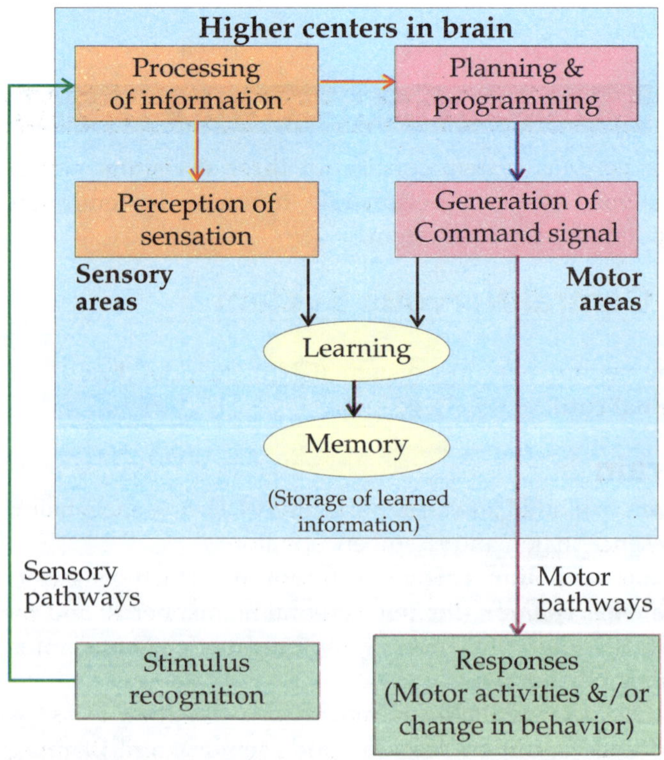

Fig. 94.2: Integration of functions of central nervous system.

- The processed signal is then *transformed into other signals* in sensory networks in the brain.

- Integration of the processed signals into **appropriate command signals** through detailed **planning and programming mechanisms**.
- Transmission of the command signal to the effector organs for implementation of the plan.
- **Learning** based on sensory inputs and then ***storage of learned information*** in memory for future utilization of the knowledge (described in detail in **the higher functions**).

Responses: Responses consist of movement of body parts (**motor activities**), change in visceral functions (**autonomic responses**) or even the **change in behavior** of the individual.

- Thus, the responses may be an internal change such as alteration in cognition, behaviour etc. or an external change such as motor activities.

Details of responses are discussed in **physiology of motor system.**

CELLULAR COMPONENTS OF CNS

CNS consists of only **two principal cell types**: Glial cells and neurons. **Glial cells** of nervous system are called **neuroglia**. Neuroglias are 10 – 30 times plentiful than neurons.

Glial Cells PY3.1

Glial cells **neither conduct action potential** *nor form functional synapse* with other cells. Though glial cells generally **provide support for neurons**, their functions are complex and not completely understood. Glial cells can multiply (Application Box 94.1)

Application Box 94.1

Gliomas: Neurons cannot multiply, whereas neuroglia can. Following brain injury, neuralgia multiply to fill the space formerly occupied by neurons. Excessive multiplication of glial cells results in **gliomas**. Gliomas are common malignant tumors of brain.

Functions of Glial Cells

1. They **form the mechanical matrix** in which neurons are embedded.
2. They play **metabolic and nutritive** roles for neurons.
3. They may help to *regulate blood flow* through the brain.
4. They may act as a *sink or source of ions*.
5. They **insulate axons and synapses** and electrically isolate them from one another.
6. They phagocytose neural debris.

Types of Glial Cells

Four types of glial cells have been described in CNS: *astrocytes* (astroglia), *oligodendrocytes* (oligodendroglia), *ependymal cells* and *microglia*. Schwann cells are glial cells in PNS.

Astrocytes: Astrocytes are so named because of their **star shape** (Fig. 94.3A).

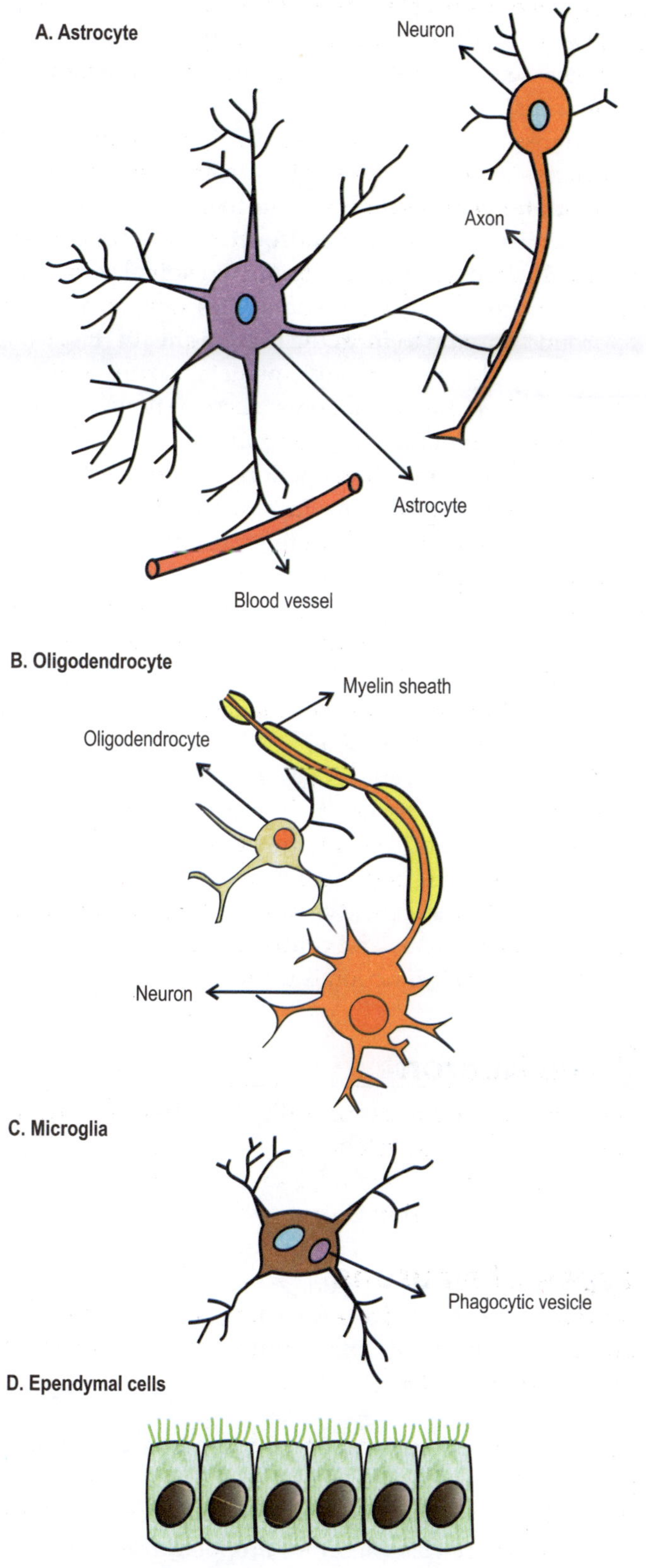

Fig. 94.3: Glial cells in CNS. Note, processes of astrocyte terminate on blood vessel and axon, processes of oligodendrocyte form myelin sheath of myelinated axon, and microglia contains phagocytic vesicle.

- They are found abundantly throughout the brain and spinal cord.
- Processes of astrocytes surround the neurons and their axons, and often terminate on the wall of blood vessels.

Functions of astrocytes are as follows:

1. They provide the mechanical matrix.
2. They serve metabolic and nutritive functions for neurons.
3. Synapses in CNS are usually surrounded by the processes of astrocytes. Thus, astrocytes **electrically insulate synapses** and separate them from one another.

Oligodendrocytes: Oligodendrocytes are found **close to the myelinated axons** in the brain and spinal cord.

- The processes of oligodendrocytes wrap many times around an axon to **form the myelin sheath** (Fig. 94.3B).
  - This sheath not only insulates axons from one another, but also limits current flow across the axon membrane (axolemma).
- Because of this myelination, action potential is conducted in a saltatory fashion in myelinated fibers, which is much faster than the transmission of impulse in unmyelinated fibers.
- Oligodendrocytes provide myelin sheath for neurons in CNS in a much similar way the *Schwann cells do for peripheral nerves*.

Microglia: Microglia are the smallest cells in the central nervous system (Fig. 94.3C).

- They are the scavenger cells in brain.
- If the nervous tissue is damaged or infected, these cells enlarge and become mononuclear phagocytes to eliminate debris and organisms.

Ependymal Cells: Ependymal cells **line the surfaces of the brain's ventricles and central canal** of the spinal cord (Fig. 94.3D). Their function is unclear.

The Neuron

The nerve cell or the neuron is the structural and functional unit of the nervous system.

Details of the structure and function of the neuron have been discussed in Chapter 18.

Types of Neurons

Neurons are classified according to the number of processes, length of axon, functions of neurons and patterns of dendrites.

A. According to the arrangement of axon or processes

According to the arrangement and number of processes, the neurons are classified into unipolar, pseudounipolar, bipolar, and multipolar neurons (Fig. 94.4).

Unipolar Neurons: They have a **single process** (Fig. 94.4A).

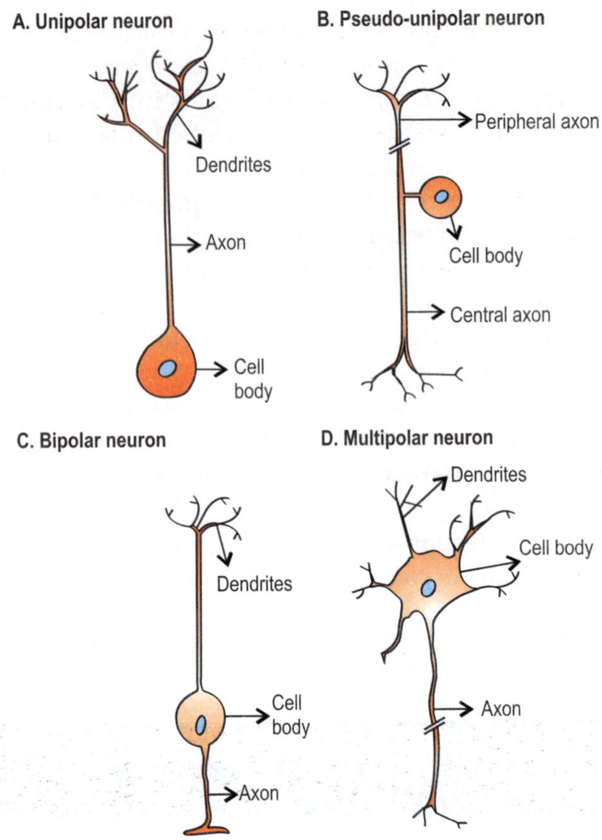

Fig. 94.4: Types of neurons based on the arrangement of processes.

- They are usually found in invertebrate. In vertebrates, they are found in ANS.

Pseudounipolar Neurons: In pseudounipolar neurons, axon after originating from soma **splits into central and peripheral processes** (Fig. 94.4B).

- The example is dorsal root ganglion cell (primary sensory neurons with cell bodies in dorsal root ganglion).

Bipolar Neurons: In these neurons, **two processes arise from the cell body** (Fig. 94.4C).

- The example is the bipolar cell of retina.

Multipolar Neurons: In multipolar neurons, **many processes arise from the soma** (Fig. 94.4D).

- The example is a spinal motor neuron.

B. According to the length of axon

According to the length of the axon, neurons are classified into two categories: Golgi type 1 and type 2.

Golgi Type 1: These are the neurons ***with short axons***. Dendrites of these neurons terminate near the soma. The example is cortical inhibitory neurons.

Golgi Type 2: Axons of Golgi type 2 neurons ***are long***. Cortical motor neurons (neurons that give rise to corticospinal tract) are the examples.

C. According to function

According to functions, neurons can be divided into sensory and motor neurons.

Sensory Neurons: These are the neurons that carry impulses from the receptors to the central nervous systems. These are called **afferent neurons** *(afferent fibers)*.

Motor Neurons: These are the neurons that carry impulses from the central nervous system to the target organs. These are called **efferent neurons** *(efferent fibers)*.

D. According to dendritic pattern

According to dendritic pattern, two types of neurons are present: pyramidal cells and stellate cells.

Pyramidal Cells: Dendrites of these cells spread like pyramids. The example is hippocampal pyramidal neurons.

Stellate Cells: Radial shaped spread of dendrites occurs in these cells. The examples are cortical stellate cells.

Exam Questions

1. Describe the structure and functions of glial cells in the brain.
2. Briefly describe the functional organization of CNS. Add a note on types of neurons.

Multiple Choice Questions

1. The Nobel prize for the work on structure of nervous system was awarded to
   A. Filippo Pacini
   B. Camillo Golgi
   C. Friedrich Goll
   D. Henry Head

2. Which of the following is not a part of hind brain (rhombencephalon)?
   A. Pons
   B. Cerebellum
   C. Substantia nigra
   D. Medulla oblongata

3. Which of the following is a type of glial cell in brain?
   A. Ependymal cells
   B. Basket cells
   C. Stellate cells
   D. Purkinje cells

4. Which of the following is NOT the function of astrocytes?
   A. Provide the mechanical matrix
   B. Form the myelin sheath
   C. Electrically insulate the synapses
   D. Nutritive function for neurons

5. Which cell in CNS lay myelin sheath?
   A. Basket cells
   B. Oligodendrocytes
   C. Stellate cells
   D. Astrocytes

6. Action potential is generated in which part of the neurons in CNS?
   A. Axon
   B. Soma
   C. Dendrite
   D. Initial segment

7. Dorsal root ganglion cells (DRG) that carry sensation from peripheral receptors to spinal cord are examples of:
   A. Bipolar cells
   B. Unipolar cells
   C. Pseudounipolar cells
   D. Multipolar cells

8. Which of the following is not a part of diencephalon?
   A. Hypothalamus
   B. Metathalamus
   C. Epithalamus
   D. Substantia nigra

9. Which of the following is not a function of glial cells in the brain?
   A. Form mechanical matrix
   B. Transmit electrical impulses
   C. Phagocytosis of organisms and debris
   D. Provide metabolic and nutritive support to neurons

10. Which of the following is not a type of glial cell in brain?
   A. Astrocyte
   B. Oligodendrocyte
   C. Golgi cells
   D. Microglia cells

11. Which of the following is the component of MPS in the brain?
   A. Ependymal cells
   B. Oligodendrocytes
   C. Microglia
   D. Granule cells

12. All of the following are true about Nissl bodies, EXCEPT:
   A. Present in axon hillock area
   B. Are modified rough endoplasmic reticulum
   C. Synthesize proteins
   D. Special granules present in the cytoplasm

13. The cells lining the surface of brain's ventricles are
   A. Ependymal cells
   B. Stellate cells
   C. Astrocytes
   D. Basket cells

14. Bipolar neurons are present in:
   A. Anterior horn of spinal cord
   B. Cerebellum
   C. Retina
   D. Dorsal root ganglion

Answers

1. B	2. C	3. A	4. B	5. B
6. D	7. C	8. D	9. B	10. C
11. C	12. A	13. A	14. C	

Chapter 95

Synaptic Transmission in Central Nervous System

Learning Objectives

On completion of study of this chapter:

The student will be able to (must know):

1. Classify synapses and give example of each category of synapse.
2. Draw a labelled diagram of a synapse.
3. Describe the mechanism of synaptic transmission.
4. Understand the genesis of synaptic potentials (EPSP and IPSP).
5. List the properties of synapses and briefly describe each of them.
6. Name types of synaptic inhibitions, give example of each with their mechanisms.
7. Classify neurotransmitters (NTs) in CNS and list the functions of common NTs.

The student may also be able to (desirable to know):

1. Explain the properties of synapses.
2. Describe the receptors, functions and dysfunctions of neurotransmitters.

SYNAPSES IN CNS

Types of Synapses

There are innumerable synapses in the nervous system. On average, **each neuron forms about 2000 synapses**. As there are about 10^{11} neurons in CNS, the total number of synapses may be about 2×10^{14}.

Synapses are usually classified, as follows:

According to Part of the Neurons Involved in the Formation of Synapse

Based on the parts of the neurons involved in the formation of synapse, **four types of synapses** are found in CNS: axodendritic, axosomatic, axoaxonic and dendrodendritic (Fig. 95.1).

Axodendritic Synapse: In this type of synapse, axon of presynaptic neuron connects with dendrite of postsynaptic neuron.

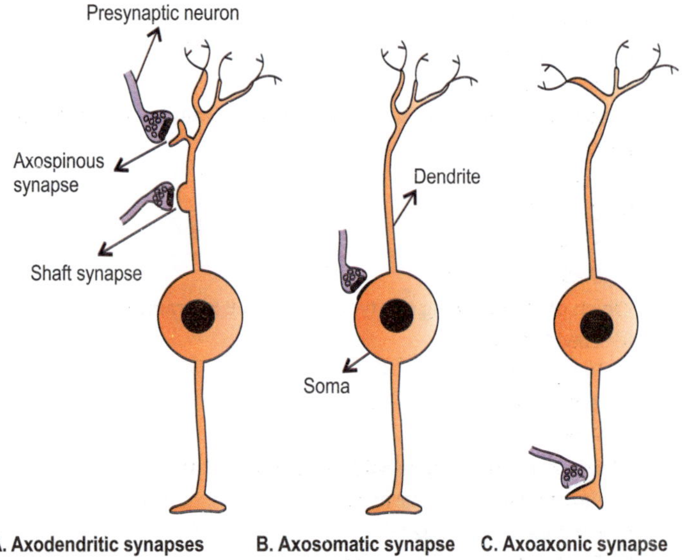

Fig. 95.1: Types of synapses. A: Axodendritic synapse; B: Axosomatic synapse; C: Axoaxonic synapse.

- This is the **commonest synapse** in CNS.
- The axon terminal may synapse with the spinous process of the dendrite (**axospinous synapse**) or with the shaft of the dendrite (**shaft synapse**) (Fig. 95.1A).

Axosomatic Synapse: In this variety, axon of presynaptic neuron **synapses with cell body** of postsynaptic neuron (Fig. 95.1B).

- This is also a **common form of synapse** in CNS.

Axoaxonic Synapse: In axoaxonic type, axon of presynaptic neuron synapses with axon of postsynaptic neuron (Fig. 95.1C).

Dendrodendritic Synapse: In this type, dendrite of presynaptic neuron connects to the dendrite of postsynaptic neuron.

According to the Nature of Transmission

Synapses are of three types according to the mode of transmission of the impulse.

Chemical Synapse: Transmission of the impulse occurs through release of neurotransmitters.
Electrical Synapse: Transmission of the impulse occurs through gap junctions.
Conjoint Synapse: Partly electrical and partly chemical.

According to the Number of Neurons Involved

1. One neuron ends on another (**one to one**).
2. Multiple neurons terminate on a single neuron (**many to one**).
3. One neuron contacts many neurons (**one to many**).

Example of 'one to one' synapse is the neuromuscular junction, 'many to one' is the usual type found in CNS and 'one to many' is less frequent. In ANS, usually 'one to one' synapse is found in parasympathetic and 'one to many' type is found in sympathetic system.

PY10.2

MECHANISM OF SYNAPTIC TRANSMISSION

Functional Anatomy of a Synapse

The neuron from which the information passes through the synapse is the **presynaptic neuron** and the neuron, which receives the information, is the **postsynaptic neuron**.

- The part of the presynaptic axon terminal forming the synapse is called **presynaptic membrane** and that of the postsynaptic neuron is called the *postsynaptic membrane*.
- The space between presynaptic and postsynaptic membrane is called the **synaptic cleft**.

The presynaptic axon terminal, postsynaptic membrane and the synaptic cleft form the synapse (Fig. 95.2).

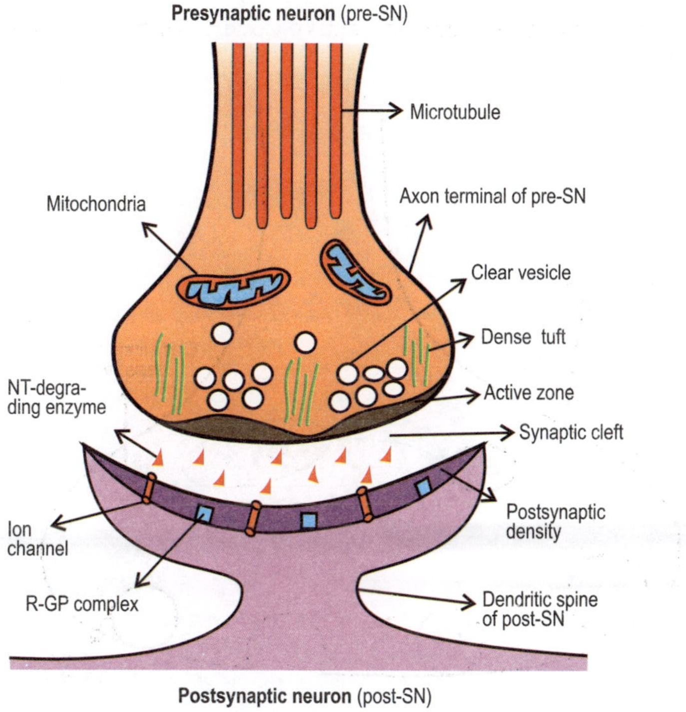

Fig. 95.2: Functional anatomy of an axodendritic synapse. Note the components of presynaptic (pre-SN) and postsynaptic (post-SN) neurons. NT: Neurotransmitter; R-GP: Receptor-G protein.

Presynaptic Axon Terminal

The **presynaptic membrane** is the part of an axon terminal of the presynaptic neuron. The terminal of presynaptic neuron typically ends in small bulbous enlargement called **terminal bouton** or **synaptic knob**, which is about 1 mm in diameter.

Synaptic bouton contains **two specialized structures**:

i) Numerous *synaptic vesicles* that contain neurotransmitters.
ii) *Dense tufts* or projections that are made up of filamentous proteins, which contact larger filaments in the axoplasm.

Synaptic Vesicles

There are **three types of synaptic vesicles**: i) small vesicles with clear-core, ii) small vesicle with dense-core, and iii) large vesicle with dense-core.

- **Small-clear vesicles** contain acetylcholine, GABA, glycine or glutamate.
- **Small-dense vesicles** contain catecholamines and **large-dense vesicles** contain neuropeptide.

1. **Large vesicles** are present throughout the presynaptic terminals and are released by exocytosis from all parts of the presynaptic membrane.
2. **The small vesicles** are located close to the presynaptic membrane and are released to the synaptic cleft through the active zone by exocytosis.
   - The small vesicles after discharging their content are recycled back into the terminal. The vesicles are endocytosed and then fused with the endosomes.
   - New vesicles that are formed from endosomes by budding are refilled with the transmitter chemicals.
   - Vesicles then move close to the active zone and undergo **docking and priming** (Fig. 95.3) before discharging their content into the synaptic cleft.

Dense Tufts

These are **filamentous projections** present in close contact with vesicles and play an important role in **exocytosis of vesicles**. Dense tufts are present mainly in active zone (see below).

Active Zone

Presynaptic terminal also contains few large mitochondria. A region of presynaptic membrane is modified to form active zone, which contains many **proteins and calcium channels**. Release of vesicles containing neurotransmitters occurs mainly through the active zone (Application Box 95.1).

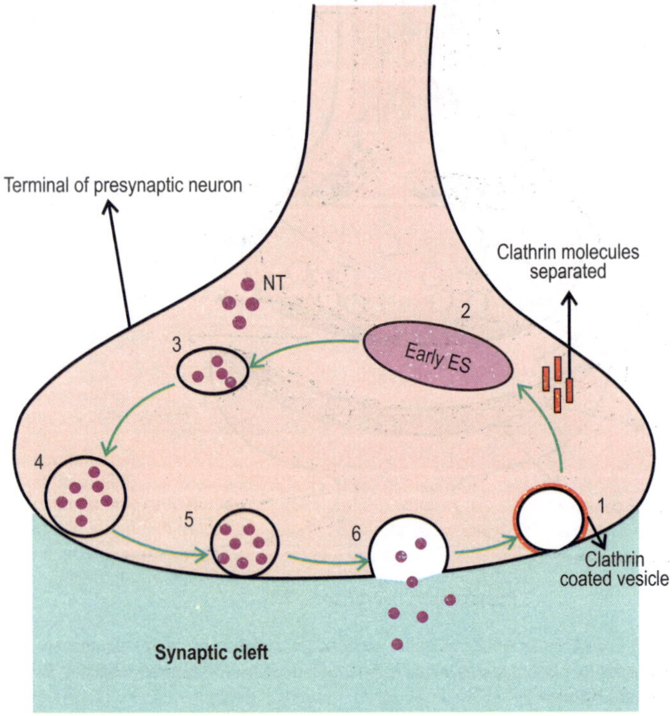

Fig. 95.3: Recycling of neurotransmitter (NT) vesicle in presynaptic neuron terminal. This occurs in six steps. **1.** The vesicle that has discharged its content into the synaptic cleft is coated with clathrin and gets detached from the membrane; **2.** Clathrin is separated from the vesicle and vesicle fuses with early endosomes (early ES); **3.** New vesicle is formed from early ES, which picks up NT from nerve terminal; **4.** Docking of vesicle-containing NT with the membrane of presynaptic neuron terminal; **5.** Priming of the vesicle; **6.** Discharge of NT into synaptic cleft from vesicle by calcium-mediated exocytosis.

Application Box 95.1

Presynaptic receptors are autoreceptors: The receptors in the presynaptic membrane sense the release of neurotransmitters from presynaptic nerve terminal and control their rate of secretion. Therefore, they are called autoreceptors. Usually, they inhibit the secretion of neurotransmitters when the rate of secretion is more. For example, noradrenaline secretion is inhibited from noradrenergic nerve terminal by α2 receptors. Sometimes, they also stimulate the secretion of neurotransmitters.

Synaptic Cleft

The synaptic cleft is the gap between pre- and postsynaptic membranes, which is about **20 to 50 nm wide**.

- This space is filled with extracellular fluid.
- Transmitter molecules released from the presynaptic terminal diffuse across the cleft to reach the postsynaptic receptors.

Postsynaptic Membrane

The postsynaptic membrane usually is a part of a dendritic spine, but may be a part of a cell body (soma) or part of an axon, which contains receptors for the neurotransmitters.

- The area of the postsynaptic membrane modified for synaptic transmission is called **postsynaptic density**.
- Postsynaptic density is the **cluster of receptors** for transmitter embedded within the postsynaptic membrane.

Neurotransmitter is the chemical substance used for transfer of information through the synapse. The neurotransmitter **amplifies the effect of the action potential** arriving at the synapse.

- Due to this amplification, presynaptic action potential after passing through the synaptic cleft **stimulates the postsynaptic neuron**.
- The arrangement in the synapse is such that the neurotransmitter released from presynaptic nerve ending acts on a wide area of the postsynaptic membrane and activates a large number of receptors (ion channels) to activate postsynaptic potential (Application Box 95.2).

Role of Neurexins

Neurexins are proteins attached to the presynaptic membrane.

1. There are **neurexin receptors** in the postsynaptic membrane to which neurexins bind.
2. Thus, neurexins that link presynaptic and postsynaptic membranes provide **structural stability to the synaptic architecture**.
   - In fact, the systematic organization of the synapse depends partly on neurexins.
   - In many vertebrates, neurexins are produced by a single gene that codes for the α isoform.
3. Neurexins are coded by three genes and there are both **α and β isoforms**.
   - As each of the genes has two regulatory regions and extensive alternative splicing of their mRNAs occurs, there are more than 1000 different neurexins.
4. It is proposed that neurexins not only bind the synapses together, but also provide **basis for synaptic specificity**.

Application Box 95.2

Specific binding proteins for postsynaptic receptors: Postsynaptic receptors are present in clusters close to the presynaptic nerve terminal that secretes the neurotransmitters. This occurs due to presence of specific binding proteins for the receptors on the postsynaptic membrane.

- For example, for glutaminergic receptors, the binding protein is **PB2-binding protein**, for GABA receptors binding protein is **gephyrin**, for nicotinic acetylcholine receptors binding protein is **rapsyn**.

PY10.10

Steps of Synaptic Transmission

The mechanism of synaptic transmission can be divided into presynaptic and postsynaptic mechanisms.

Presynaptic Mechanisms

Five major steps are involved in the presynaptic mechanism of synaptic transmission.

1. Vesicles containing neurotransmitter molecules that are concentrated at active zone of the presynaptic axon terminal undergo docking and priming.
    - **Docking** is the process by which vesicles attach with the membrane and **priming** is the process by which the vesicles become ready to discharge their content in response to a stimulus.
2. The action potential that arrives at presynaptic axon terminal **depolarizes the presynaptic membrane**.
3. Depolarization of membrane causes **opening of voltage-gated calcium channels** that allows calcium to enter the axon terminal through the active zone.
4. Increase in calcium concentration in the presynaptic terminal increases **calcium-mediated exocytosis** of the vesicles.
    - Calcium causes fusion of vesicles to the presynaptic membrane by causing contraction of microfilaments in the dense tuft that facilitates their movement, and then help to discharge their content into the cleft.

Kiss and Run Discharge: Discharge of synaptic vesicular contents takes place through a small hole in the cell membrane, which immediately closes rapidly.

- In this process, the main vesicle remains inside the cell. This is called kiss-and-run discharge.
- Following discharge, some vesicles are quickly recovered by endocytosis and refilled locally, in which the endocytic process is short- circuited.

5. Transmitter is released into the synaptic cleft in a quantized amount that diffuses passively across the cleft to the postsynaptic membrane.
    - Quantal release of neurotransmitter is sometimes called **Dale's phenomenon**.
    - From the **calcium influx to the transmitter release takes about 200** μs.

Role of Membrane Proteins

Normally, small synaptic vesicles recycle in the presynaptic nerve terminal. The mature vesicles move to the active zone, dock and get primed. When action potential arrives, calcium influx facilitates fusion of vesicles with presynaptic membrane that causes discharge of granular content into the synaptic cleft.

1. Vesicle membrane then gets **coated with clathrin** and taken up by endocytosis into the presynaptic terminal where it is reutilized for neurotransmitter packaging (Fig. 95.3).
2. Fusion of synaptic vesicle with cell membrane is facilitated by **synaptobrevin**, a ***v-snare protein*** present in vesicular membrane, and **syntaxin**, a ***t-snare protein*** present in the cell membrane.
    - In fact, synaptobrevin attaches and interacts with syntaxin for docking and priming of vesicles.

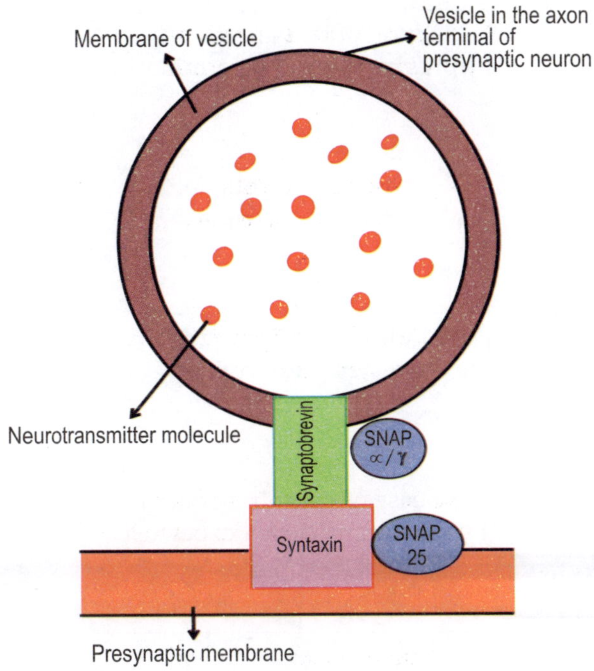

Fig. 95.4: Priming and docking. Note the role of syntaxin and synaptobrevin.

3. Various other synaptic proteins (**SNAP 25** connected with syntaxin, and **α/γ SNAPs** connected with synaptobrevin) facilitate the interaction between synaptobrevin and syntaxin (Fig. 95.4).
    1. A **multi-protein complex** regulated by small GTPase like **rab3** also participates in the process.

Clinical Significance

Many **neurotoxins inhibit release of neurotransmitters** by preventing attachment of synaptobrevin and syntaxin.

1. For example, **tetanus and botulinum toxins** act on synaptobrevin and syntaxin that in turn prevents fusion of vesicles with membrane that blocks release of neurotransmitters from presynaptic terminals.
2. **Botulinum toxins** are of seven types (A to G).
    - **A and B botulinum toxins** act on SNAP 25 and prevent the interaction between synaptobrevin and syntaxin that in turn prevents docking and priming of vesicles.
    - **Botulinum toxin C** acts on syntaxin and prevents its attachment with synaptobrevin.
    - **Botulinum toxin B, D, F and G** act on synaptobrevin and prevents its attachment with syntaxin. Thus, botulinum toxins produce flaccid paralysis by inhibiting release of acetylcholine at neuromuscular junction.
3. **Tetanus toxin** act on synaptobrevin and prevents its attachment with syntaxin. Tetanus toxin prevents release of other neurotransmitters from vesicles at different synapses in CNS, and therefore produces spastic paralysis (Clinical Note 95.1).

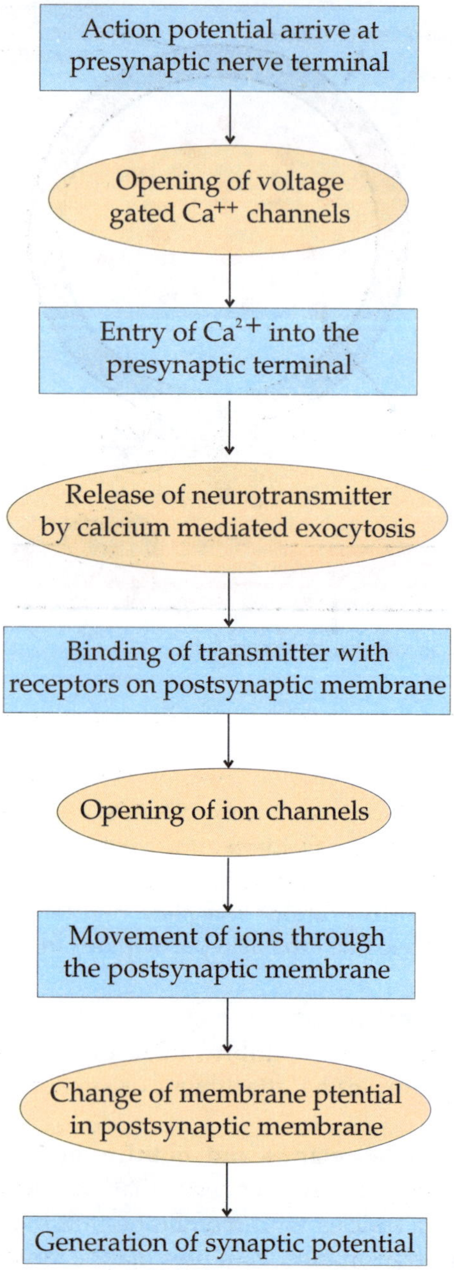

Flowchart 95.1: Steps of synaptic transmission.

> **Clinical Note 95.1**
>
> **Clinical uses of botulinum toxin:** For its muscle relaxation effect, botulinum toxin in small doses is used for the treatment of conditions that produce muscle hyperactivity, for example, injection of the toxin into lower esophageal sphincter in **achalasia cardia** produces relaxation of the sphincter. In low doses, it is also used to **decrease the facial wrinkles** by causing relaxation of facial muscles.

Postsynaptic Mechanisms

The **following events** take place in postsynaptic cell.

1. Neurotransmitter binds with the receptors in the postsynaptic membrane and brings about **conformational change** in the receptor that either **opens an ion channel** or triggers a cascade of biochemical reactions that **generate a second messenger**, which in turn generates **change in ionic permeability** of the cell.
2. Some of the transmitter molecules diffuse away from the postsynaptic receptor that are cleared either by **enzymatic degradation** or **taken back** into the presynaptic cell by endocytosis (Application Box 95.3).

After the binding of the neurotransmitter with receptors, the **ion channels** in the postsynaptic membrane open up and **movement of ions occurs**. Depending on the ion (cation or anion) and the direction of their movement, the membrane potential of the postsynaptic membrane changes either towards **depolarization or hyperpolarization**. This change in membrane potential, also called **synaptic potential**, creates signal in the postsynaptic neuron. **Summary of synaptic transmission** is depicted in Flowchart 95.1.

> **Application Box 95.3**
>
> **Desensitization of receptors:** When postsynaptic receptors are exposed chronically (for a prolonged period), they gradually become hyporesponsive to the ligand. This is called desensitization. When the responsiveness decreases to that particular ligand, the process is called **homologous desensitization**.
>
> - For example, continuous secretion of catecholamines in excess causes desensitization of β receptors to catecholamines. The carboxy terminal region of β receptors undergoes phosphorylation by β adrenergic receptor kinase (β-ARK) that decreases β receptor responsiveness. Also, β receptors bind with β-arrestin, which inhibits responsiveness of the receptors.
> - There are four types of β-arrestins that desensitize adrenergic receptors and also promote endocytosis of ligands.
> - Chronic exposure to a ligand also decreases responsiveness of receptors to other ligands, the process is called **heterologous desensitization**.

Synaptic Potentials

Synaptic potential is of longer duration than an action potential. When it is excitatory, it can cause repeated firing of initial segment of the postsynaptic neuron. Postsynaptic potentials are of **two types**: excitatory and inhibitory.

Excitatory Postsynaptic Potential

If the potential change in the postsynaptic membrane during synaptic transmission is **towards depolarization**, the potential is called EPSP. For example, if initially the RMP was –70 mV, which becomes –60 mV during synaptic transmission, then it is EPSP (Fig. 95.5).

- The **latency** of EPSP is about 0.5 ms. EPSP reaches its peak at 11.5 ms after the entry of afferent impulses into the spinal cord, which then declines exponentially.
  - A single EPSP leads to a change of 0.5–2 mV only.
  - Though the EPSP produced at one synaptic knob is small, EPSP at many synaptic knobs summate.

- EPSP of optimum magnitude leads to excitation of the postsynaptic neuron.
- During this potential, **excitability of postsynaptic neuron increases to other stimuli**, and therefore, the potential is called excitatory postsynaptic potential.
- EPSPs are produced by transmitters like **acetylcholine, nor-adrenaline** etc.

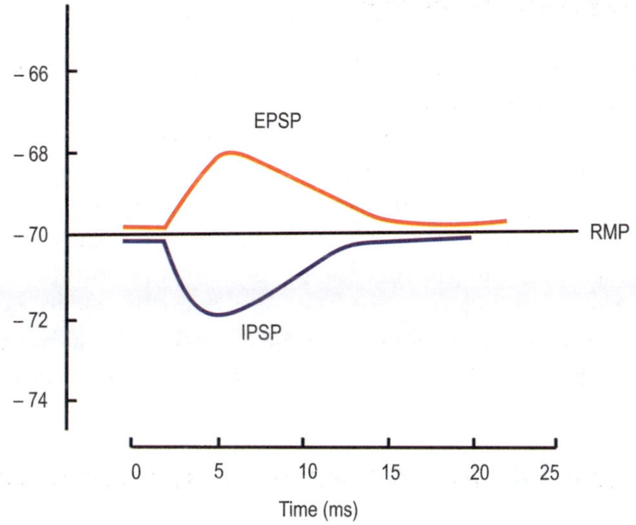

Fig. 95.5: Excitatory (EPSP) and inhibitory (IPSP) postsynaptic potentials.

Ionic Basis: EPSP is caused by **opening of Na^+ or Ca^{++} ion channels** in the postsynaptic membrane that results in influx of Na^+ or Ca^{++} and causes depolarization.

- EPSP is also caused by **closure of K^+ ion channels**.

Slow EPSP

Slow EPSP has been observed in autonomic ganglia and cortical neurons.

- They have the latency of 100–500 ms, and they persist for several seconds.
- They are usually due to **decreased K^+ conductance**.

Inhibitory Postsynaptic Potential

During synaptic transmission, if the **potential of postsynaptic membrane is carried towards hyperpolarization**, then the potential is called IPSP (Fig. 95.5).

- This is because the hyperpolarization leads to **inhibition of the postsynaptic neuron**. For example, if the RMP was –70 mV, and after transmission it becomes –80 mV, then the potential is IPSP, which is of –10 mV.
- Actually, a very small change occurs due to an IPSP, i.e. about 0.5 mV. During this potential, **excitability of postsynaptic neuron decreases to other stimuli**, and therefore, the potential is called inhibitory postsynaptic potential.
- IPSP, like EPSP is a **local response** and can be summated. IPSPs are caused by transmitters like GABA (gamma amino butyric acid), glycine, etc. IPSP reaches its peak at 11.5 ms after the application of stimulus, which then decreases exponentially

Ionic Basis: IPSP is produced by **opening of Cl^- channels** (Cl^- enters into the cells along the concentration gradient). **Opening of K^+ cannels** that result in K^+ efflux can produce IPSP. **Closure of Na^+ or Ca^{++} channels** also produce IPSP.

Slow IPSP

Slow IPSP are also observed in autonomic ganglia and cortical neurons. They usually occur due to **increased K^+ conductance**.

Reversal Potential

As it is known, the IPSP is mediated by Cl^- influx. However, in an experimental set up, Cl^- influx occurs only when the membrane potential is less than –70mV, for example the RMP at –50mV.

- At the membrane potential of –70mV, influx or efflux of Cl^- across the membrane disappears, as the E_{Cl} is –70mV.
- If the membrane potential becomes more negative, such as at RMP of –90 mV, Cl^- efflux takes place that makes the interior of the cell positive. This is called the **reversal potential**.

Genesis of Action Potential

The message arriving at postsynaptic neuron usually comes from a large number of presynaptic neurons. These neurons can end on any part of the soma and dendrites of the postsynaptic neuron.

1. In CNS, many excitatory and inhibitory inputs **continuously and simultaneously arrive** at the postsynaptic membrane.
   - **All the EPSPs or IPSPs** produced at various postsynaptic membranes **act together to summate electronically**.
   - The **soma of the neuron integrates** these potentials and the ***algebraic sum*** of these depolarizing and hyperpolarizing potentials finally produce the **change in resultant potential**.
2. **If the resultant potential is depolarizing** and the change is about +15 mV, the ***firing level is reached*** that leads to genesis of a **propagated spike potential.**
   - However, a full phased action potential is generated **only at initial segment**, as this part of the neuron **has the lowest threshold**.
3. The action potential propagates **in two directions**, towards axon terminal down the axon (**orthograde propagation**) and towards the cell body (**retrograde propagation**).
   - The propagation of action potential into the soma ***cleans the soma for subsequent renewal*** of postsynaptic activities.

Role of Dendrites

Dendrites are the extensions of soma.

1. They **increase the surface area** for presynaptic knobs to end on them.
    - Thus, more the number of dendrites, better the integration of excitatory and inhibitory activities.
2. Number and pattern of dendritic spine change during development.
    - A special type of neural protein called **neuroligin** controls synapse formation.
3. **Alteration in dendritic spine** occurs in learning and long-term potentiation (Application Box 95.4). It has been recently observed that the *propagated action potentials are also initiated* in few dendrites.
4. It has also been noted that **protein synthesis**, which usually occurs in soma, also occurs in ribosome in dendritic spine that can alter inputs from glutaminergic neurons.

Application Box 95.4

Change in dendritic spine occurs in motivation, learning and long-term memory: Pattern and arbor of dendritic spines can change in different conditions. New dendrites can appear and grow or they can also disappear even in minutes and hours. Changes in dendritic spines have been observed to provide the physiological basis in motivation, learning and long-term memory.

Transmission Through an Electrical Synapse

Gap junctions are electrical synapses. The pre- and post-synaptic membranes come close together to form **gap junctions**.

- Gap junctions are *low resistance channels* through which ions pass easily.
- Electrical activities of one neuron can pass to the other directly through gap junctions.
- There are sparse electrical synapses in CNS.

Difference From Chemical Synapse: Transmission through electrical synapse **differs from that of a chemical synapse** by following ways:

1. EPSP generated in the postsynaptic neuron by electrical transmission has **short latency** than the EPSP generated in the chemical transmission.
2. In chemical synapse, the transmission is usually unidirectional, whereas in electrical synapse the **transmission is bidirectional**.
3. The **signal is not magnified** in electrical transmission.
4. The **time taken for impulse to travel** an electrical synapse **is much less** than the chemical synapse.

PROPERTIES OF SYNAPSES

The synapses or rather the synaptic transmissions exhibit the following properties:

Law of Forward Conduction

Through a synapse, impulse travels in one direction only i.e. from presynaptic to postsynaptic neuron. This is called **law of forward conduction**. However, transmission of impulse is bidirectional in electrical synapses.

Synaptic Delay

The **time required for the impulse to be transmitted through the synapse** is called synaptic delay.

1. Synaptic delay is **about 0.5 ms**. It occurs due to the time spent in entry of Ca^{++} into the presynaptic knob, release of neurotransmitter into the synaptic cleft and for the action of neurotransmitter on the postsynaptic membrane to produce the postsynaptic potential.
2. The knowledge about synaptic delay helps to **find out the number of synapses present in a neural pathway** (monosynaptic, disynaptic or polysynaptic reflex arc).

Law of Convergence and Divergence

Convergence means **many to one projection**, in which many presynaptic neurons project to a single postsynaptic neuron (Fig. 95.6A).

- **Divergence** means **one to many projections** (Fig. 95.6B). This means information from one presynaptic neuron passes to many postsynaptic neurons.
- Divergence and convergence are very common in CNS and form the **physiological basis for summation and facilitation** at synapses.

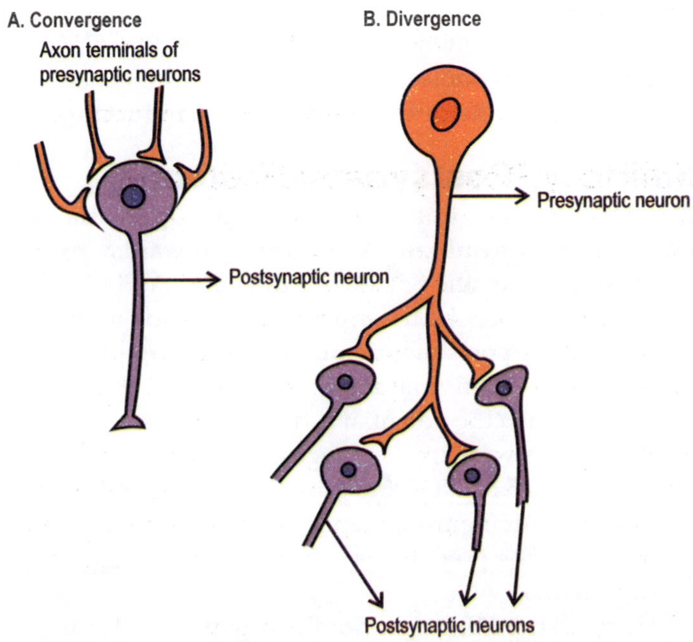

Figs. 95.6: Convergence (A) and divergence (B). In convergence, many presynaptic neurons project to one postsynaptic neuron, and in divergence, one presynaptic neuron projects to many postsynaptic neurons.

Postsynaptic Potentials

During synaptic transmission, if the potential of the postsynaptic membrane is carried towards depolarization, is called **excitatory postsynaptic potential** (EPSP) or, if the potential of the postsynaptic membrane is carried towards hyperpolarization, then it is called **inhibitory postsynaptic potential** (IPSP).

Synaptic Inhibitions

In CNS, neurons are highly interconnected, and therefore, any trivial stimulus would lead to an widespread activation of many neurons. **Synaptic inhibition prevents this explosive situation** by stabilizing the neurons and by preventing unnecessary spread of impulse.

Types: There are **two different types of synaptic inhibitions**: direct inhibition vs. indirect inhibition, and feedback inhibition vs. feedforward inhibition.

Direct and Indirect Inhibitions

(Postsynaptic and Presynaptic Inhibitions)

Direct Inhibition

When synaptic inhibition occurs through formation of **IPSP on the postsynaptic neuron**, is called **direct inhibition** as the postsynaptic neuron is directly inhibited (**postsynaptic inhibition**).

- Example of direct inhibition is inhibition of anterior horn cells (AHC) by the descending inhibitory fibers in the spinal cord or by the afferent inputs originating from the Golgi tendon organs that influences AHC via an inhibitory interneuron.

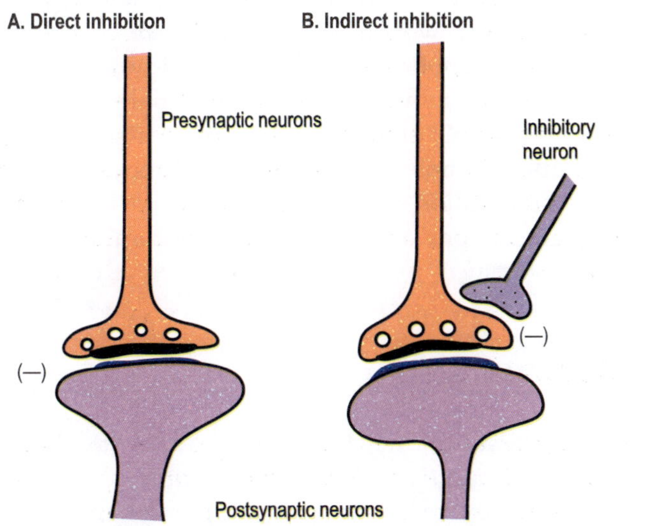

Figs. 95.7: Direct (A) and indirect (B) inhibitions at synapses. In direct inhibition, an inhibitory presynaptic neuron directly inhibits postsynaptic neuron by releasing inhibitory neurotransmitter. In indirect inhibition, presynaptic neuron is not inhibitory, but another inhibitory neuron projects to the axon terminal of presynaptic neuron that inhibits the release of neurotransmitter from it (therefore, the transmission is inhibited). Minus sign depicts inhibition.

- In both these situations, there is ***release of inhibitory transmitter*** from presynaptic neurons (Fig. 95.7A).

Indirect inhibition

Indirect inhibition occurs when the passage of impulse through a synapse is inhibited by another earlier impulse originating from a separate neuron terminating on presynaptic ending (Fig. 95.7B).

- This inhibition occurs due to **decreased release of neurotransmitter** from the presynaptic nerve terminal (**presynaptic inhibition**).
- Indirect inhibition could also be due to the effects of previous postsynaptic neuron discharge. For example, the neuron can be refractory to excitation because it is in its refractory period as it has just fired.
- During after-hyperpolarization cells are less excitable.
- In spinal neurons, after-hyperpolarization may be prolonged, especially after repeated firing.

Mechanisms of Presynaptic Inhibition: For presynaptic inhibition, **three mechanisms** of have been proposed.

1. Activation of the presynaptic receptors **facilitate Cl^- conductance**, which ***decreases the magnitude of action potential*** reaching the excitatory ending.
   - Thus **Ca^{++} entry is decreased** and consequently the quantity of ***neurotransmitters released is reduced***.
2. Activation of the presynaptic receptors also causes **voltage-gated K^+ channels to open**.
   - The resulting ***K^+ efflux decreases Ca^{++} influx***.
3. Direct **inhibition of transmitter release** can occur, independent of Ca^{++} influx into the excitatory ending.

GABA: GABA was the first neurotransmitter shown to produce presynaptic inhibition. There are **two GABA receptors**: $GABA_A$ and $GABA_B$.

- GABA acting through its **$GABA_A$ receptors** produces presynaptic inhibition by ***increasing Cl^- conductance***.
- Through **$GABA_B$ receptors**, it produces presynaptic inhibition via a G protein that produces an ***increase in K^+ conductance*** (Application Box 95.5).
- Other neurotransmitters also produce presynaptic inhibition by G protein-mediated effects on Ca^{++} channels and K^+ channels.

Application Box 95.5

Baclofen causes presynaptic inhibition: Baclofen, a $GABA_B$ receptor agonist, is useful in the treatment of the spasticity of spinal cord injury and multiple sclerosis. It is administered intrathecally via an implanted pump. It inhibits neuronal transmission by causing presynaptic inhibition.

Feedback and Feedforward Inhibitions

Feedback Inhibition

Renshaw cell inhibition in the spinal cord is an example of feedback inhibition.

- This is a ***negative feedback inhibition*** in which collateral from spinal motor neurons ends on an

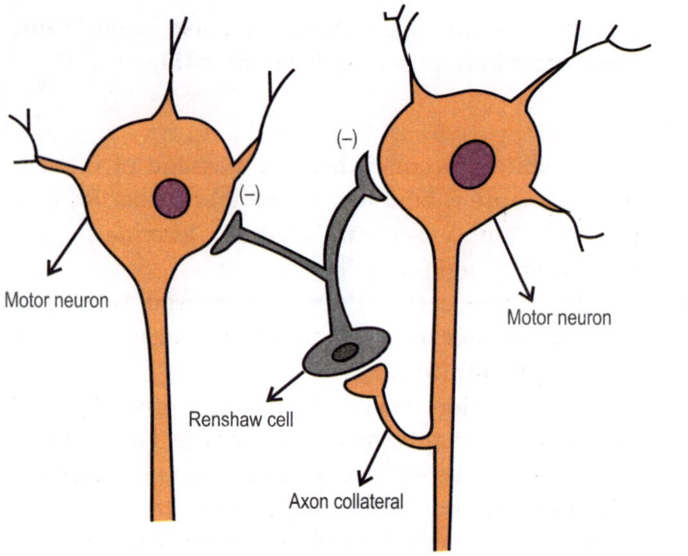

Fig. 95.8: Negative feedback inhibition by Renshaw cell. Collateral from spinal motor neuron ends on an inhibitory interneuron (Renshaw cell) that in turn inhibits (minus sign) the discharge of the same motor neuron. Collateral from Renshaw cell also inhibits neighbouring motor neuron, which is called lateral inhibition.

inhibitory interneuron, known as **the Renshaw cell**, which in turn inhibits the discharge of the same motor neuron (Fig. 95.8).

- A collateral from Renshaw cell also inhibits neighboring motor neuron, which is called **lateral inhibition**.

Feedforward Inhibition

The example of feedforward inhibition is the **inhibition of Purkinje cell output** by parallel fibers originating from granule cells in the cerebellum.

- Mossy fiber inputs stimulate granule cell, which through its parallel fibers activates Purkinje cells. Output of Purkinje cell is inhibitory as neurotransmitter secreted by Purkinje cells is GABA.
- Thus, stimulation of **mossy fiber-parallel fiber pathway** finally activates the inhibitory output of Purkinje cells. This is called **feedforward inhibition**.

Synaptic Facilitation

This is the process by which **transmission through a synapse is increased**.

- It is usually caused by increase in the transmitter release from the presynaptic terminal. Therefore, this is also called **presynaptic facilitation**.
- Prolongation of action potential at presynaptic ending helps **voltage gated Ca^{++} channel to remain open** for a longer duration.
- This ensures more Ca^{++} influx that in turn **increases transmitter release** from the presynaptic ending. Thus, transmission through the synapse is facilitated.

Action of Serotonin: Serotonin released at an axoaxonal ending causes synaptic facilitation by **increasing intraneuronal cAMP** levels.

- This induces phosphorylation of one group of K^+ channels that closes the K^+ channels.
- This **slows the process of repolarization** and prolongs the duration of action potential.

Summation

Summation literally means **to add up**. Since synaptic potentials are graded, individual potential changes can summate. The phenomenon of summation is seen in neuronal networks involving multiple synapses in which synapses are shared by many neurons.

There are **two types of summations**: temporal summation and spatial summation.

Temporal Summation: In temporal summation, the same input **stimulates the postsynaptic neuron repetitively** in such a way that the second synaptic potential arrives before the postsynaptic cell recovers from the first synaptic potential.

- This happens because **action potentials arrive in rapid succession** at the presynaptic terminal, which in turn stimulates the postsynaptic membrane in quick succession so that resultant **postsynaptic potential overlap in time**.
- Thus, postsynaptic potential is elevated to the firing level.

Spatial Summation: In spatial summation, instead of repeated stimulation by the same input, **two or more separate inputs arrive simultaneously** at the postsynaptic membrane.

- In this situation, if the **inputs have the same sign** (either all are excitatory or all are inhibitory), the postsynaptic response evoked by all inputs becomes larger than response that would have occurred in response to their individual application.
- This type of summation is called spatial summation.

Thus, temporal summation occurs when a single presynaptic knob is stimulated repeatedly and spatial summation occurs when many synaptic knobs converging on one postsynaptic membrane are stimulated simultaneously.

Occlusion

When a presynaptic neuron (say A) fires, five postsynaptic neurons discharge and when another presynaptic neuron (say B) fires separately, another five postsynaptic neurons discharge. However, as **two presynaptic neurons share their discharge zone** (common discharge zone of A and B), simultaneous firing of A and B results in activation of eight postsynaptic neurons instead of ten (Fig. 95.9). This is called occlusion.

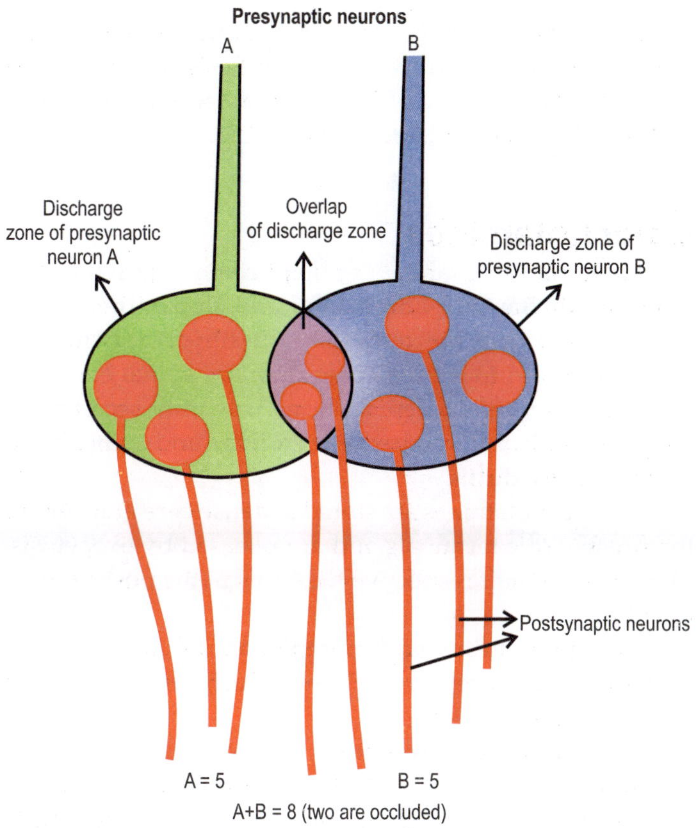

Fig. 95.9: Mechanism of occlusion. Activation of presynaptic neuron A stimulates a set of five postsynaptic neurons and activation of presynaptic neuron B stimulates another set of five postsynaptic neurons, when A and B are activated separately. But, as two presynaptic neurons share their discharge zone (common area of A and B), simultaneous activation of A and B results in activation of eight postsynaptic neurons instead of ten. This is called occlusion.

Habituation, Sensitization & Potentiation

Habituation

Habituation is the **gradual decrease of transmitter release** in response to repeated transmission of impulses.

- This is probably caused by prolonged inactivation of the Ca^{++} channels in the synaptic knob or due to decreased number of vesicles in the presynaptic terminal.

Sensitization

Sensitization occurs when a transmission is accompanied by a **painful or unpleasant sensation**.

- The response increases more and more by the mechanism of **presynaptic facilitation**.
- Sensitization is short lived and is explained on the basis of *increased Ca^{++} entry into the presynaptic terminal.*

Potentiation

Potentiation is **enhanced synaptic transmission** for a prolonged duration.

1. In **post-tetanic potentiation,** the duration is shorter in comparison to other potentiation called long-term potentiation.
   - Post-tetanic potentiation is due to increased Ca^{++} in the presynaptic knob in response to the arrival of a series of stimuli that causes increased transmitter release.
2. **Long-term potentiation** occurs due to increased Ca^{++} in the postsynaptic neuron due to opening of NMDA (N-methyl-D-aspartate) channels (e.g. by glutamate) along with increase of intracellular proteins.

Synaptic Plasticity

There are several ways by which synaptic transmission is **modified to suit the need of the body**, and to learn to react against a particular stimulus in an appropriate manner. These changes are memorized for a variable period by the concerned cells that are involved in the process of learning and memory. This involves a **long-term change in the synapses**, which is also called synaptic plasticity.

PY10.10

NEUROTRANSMITTERS

Classification

Neurotransmitters may be classified based on their chemical structure:

1. Acetylcholine

2. Amines

Norepinephrine, Epinephrine, Dopamine
Serotonin, Histamine

3. Amino acids

A. Excitatory amino acids
Glutamate, Aspartate
B. Inhibitory amino acids
Glycine, GABA

4. Polypeptides

ADH, Oxytocin
Tachykinins like Substance P
CRH, TRH, GnRH
Somatostatin
Endorphins, Enkephalins
CGRP, Neuropeptide-Y
Angiotensins
Activins, Inhibins

5. Purines

Adenosine, ATP

6. Gases

Nitric oxide (NO), CO

Acetylcholine

Distribution

Acetylcholine (Ach) is found as neurotransmitter in many parts of the nervous system, as given below.

1. All autonomic preganglionic neurons,

2. Postganglionic parasympathetic neurons,
3. Postganglionic sympathetic neurons supplying sweat glands and blood vessels of skeletal muscles,
4. Axons of motor neurons arising from spinal cord (neuromuscular junctions),
5. Many parts of the brain including Betz cells of the motor cortex and basal ganglia and
6. Amacrine cells in retina.

Receptors

The cholinergic receptors are of **two types**: nicotinic and muscarinic.

Nicotinic Receptors

These receptors behave like ligand gated ion channels but with some differences. The receptors at **motor end plate** but not at **ganglia** can be blocked by α bungarotoxin, whereas mecamylamine blocks receptors at the ganglia but not at the neuromuscular junction.

- The nicotinic receptors are members of a **superfamily of ligand gated ion channels** that includes $GABA_A$, glycine and few glutamate receptors.
- Each nicotinic receptor is made up of **five subunits** (**α**, β, γ, δ and ε) that form a central channel, which permits Na^+ and other ions to pass through when the receptor is activated. There are ***16 known subunits*** for these 5 subunits of nicotinic receptors.
  - These are: **α_1- α_9, β_2-β_5, γ, δ and** ε. In fetus, nicotinic receptor is made up of two **α_1**, one β_2, one γ and one δ subunits.
  - In adults, the γ subunit is replaced by δ subunit, which decreases the time duration of channel opening, but increases the rate of conductance of ions through the channel.
- The receptors in the **autonomic ganglia** usually contain **α_3** subunits in addition to other subunits. Nicotinic receptors **in the brain** are located in the postsynaptic membrane, especially in glutaminergic axon terminals.
- A special characteristic of neuronal nicotinic receptors is that they are **highly permeable to Ca^{++}.**

Muscarinic Receptors

These receptors are found in **brain, involuntary muscles, glands**, etc.

- **Five subtypes** of muscarinic receptors such as **M_1, M_2, M_3, M_4 and M_5** have been described.
- Though specific blockers are available for each receptor subtypes, **atropine blocks all.**
- These receptors are serpentine membrane proteins **coupled to G proteins, K^+ channel**, etc., for their intracellular activities.

In the synaptic cleft, Ach is **rapidly hydrolyzed to choline and acetate** by specific enzyme, the **cholinesterase**. The choline is taken up by the presynaptic nerve ending (reuptake) and reutilized for synthesis of new Ach molecule. For details of distribution and functions of acetylcholine in brain, refer Chapter 156.

Catecholamines

Catecholamines are **epinephrine** (adrenaline), **norepinephrine** (nor-adrenaline) and **dopamine**. All of them have a catechol nucleus (1, 2-dihydroxybenzene). They are found in the synapses in brain, spinal cord and peripheral nerves. Norepinephrine is mainly secreted by the **postganglionic sympathetic endings** and epinephrine by **adrenal medulla**.

The catecholamines are stored in **dense core granules** in the presynaptic terminals and are released by exocytosis. They bind to their respective receptors in the postsynaptic membrane.

- The epinephrine and norepinephrine bind to the adrenergic receptors, all of which are serpentine membrane proteins.
- **The adrenergic receptors** are divided into **two main types**: α and β. The **α adrenergic receptors** are of two subtypes: α_1 and α_2, and **β adrenergic receptors** are of three subtypes: β_1, β_2, and β_3. These receptors are found not only on the postsynaptic membrane but also on presynaptic membrane (especially the α_2 receptors).
- The catecholaminergic receptors are present in almost all tissues of the body. The receptors bind with circulating transmitters or the transmitters secreted from the nerve endings.
- The enzymes **monoamine oxidase** (MAO) and **catechol-o-methyl transferase** (COMT) metabolize epinephrine and norepinephrine respectively. Norepinephrine is also taken up by the presynaptic nerve endings (reuptake).

Dopamine

Dopamine is secreted by dopaminergic neurons and bind to dopaminergic receptors on the postsynaptic membrane, mostly in the synapses in brain. **Nigrostriatal dopaminergic neurons** in the basal ganglia are important in normal motor functions.

1. **Five types of dopamine receptors** have been described such as **D_1, D_2, D_3, D_4 and D_5**. All dopaminergic receptors are membrane proteins and many of them have subtypes.
2. It is observed that the number of **D_2 and D_4 receptors increases in schizophrenia** as the use of D_2 receptor blocker is very helpful in the treatment of schizophrenia, and D_2 receptor blockers also bind to D_4 receptors.

Gamma Aminobutyric Acid

Gamma aminobutyric acid (GABA) is a major inhibitory neurotransmitter in brain and retina.

Synthesis and Metabolism: It is formed **from glutamate by decarboxylation** by the action of enzyme **glutamate decarboxylase**. GABA is present in body fluids as β-aminobutyrate.

- It is metabolized mainly by transamination reaction by the enzyme GABA transaminase to succinate in the Kreb cycle.

Receptors: GABA has **three receptors** called **$GABA_A$, $GABA_B$ and $GABA_C$**. $GABA_A$ and $GABA_B$ receptors are present in the brain and $GABA_C$ is present in retina.

1. $GABA_A$ and $GABA_C$ receptors are ion channels and have five subunits surrounding a pore similar to that of nicotinic receptor. These are membrane proteins that on activation lead to increased Cl^- conductance. Different tranquillizer drugs like benzodiazepins act on these receptors.
2. $GABA_B$ receptors are metabotropic receptors coupled to G proteins that on activation produce increased K^+ conductance, decreased Ca^{++} influx and decreased adenylyl cyclase activity.

Functions: GABA is a **major inhibitory neurotransmitter** in brain.

1. The actions of GABA such as increased Cl^- conductance, increased K^+ conductance and decreased Ca^{++} influx all lead to hyperpolarization of neuron, causing **generation of IPSP**.
2. Recently it has been observed that chronic low level stimulation of GABA receptor in brain is aided by GABA present in intestinal fluid, which **controls neuronal discharge** of billions of neurons in the brain by decreasing the signal to noise ratio.
   - Also it is observed that **GABA activity declines with age**, which decreases the specificity retinal neuronal responses.
3. **Benzodiazepin drugs** that are used as ***sedatives, muscle relaxants, anticonvulsants and anti-anxiety medicine*** act by increasing Cl^- conductance via $GABA_A$ receptors. They bind to α subunit of GABA receptors.
   - A second set of benzodiazepin receptors has been found in peripheral tissues and steroid secreting endocrine cells.
   - These are called **peripheral benzodiazepin receptors (PBR)**.
   - PBR may be involved in steroid synthesis.
4. **Alcohol and barbiturates** also act partly by increasing Cl^- conductance through Cl^- channels (Clinical Note 95.2).
5. **Progesterone and deoxycorticosterone** in high doses ***induce sleep and act as anesthetics*** by acting through $GABA_A$ receptors.

Clinical Note 95.2

Anesthetics act via GABA receptor: Alcohol, barbiturates and many volatile inhaled anesthetics increase Cl− conductance by acting on GABA and glycine receptors. Some anesthetics act by inhibiting NMDA and AMPA receptors instead of acting on GABA receptors. Local anesthetics produce anesthesia by blocking Na+ channels in peripheral nerves.

Glycine

Glycine is both inhibitory and excitatory neurotransmitter. Glycine receptor is a pentamer having two subunits: the α subunit that binds with the ligand and the β subunit.

1. Glycine receptor is a **Cl^- channel** that **increases chloride conductance and produces IPSP**. Hence, glycine is mainly an inhibitory transmitter. It causes direct post-synaptic inhibition in brainstem and spinal cord.
2. However, it also acts as an **excitatory transmitter** in some parts of the brain where it influences the activity of NMDA (N-methyl-D-aspartate) receptors, which is bound to glutamate.
3. For example, in dorsal horn of spinal cord, glycine binds with NMDA receptor and facilitates pain transmission.

Neurons causing direct inhibition: Recently neurons causing direct inhibition have been categorized into 3 categories: neurons that secrete glycine, neurons that secrete GABA and neurons that secrete both glycine and GABA. **GLYT2**, the glycine transporter is present in neurons secreting glycine, and **GAD**, the GABA transporter is present in neurons secreting GABA.

Glutamate

Glutamate is the common **excitatory neurotransmitter** in CNS that causes about *75% of excitatory transmission* in brain.

- It is formed from α-ketoglutarate in the Kreb's cycle.
- It accumulates in synaptic vesicle by the **transporter BNP_1.**
- Glutamate released from nerve terminal is taken up by astrocytes that convert it first to glutamine and then transfer glutamine to nerve ending where it is converted to glutamate.
- Glutamate is used for **making lesion** (Clinical Note 95.3).

Clinical Note 95.3

Glutamate in excess produces lesion in brain: Glutamate in higher concentration increases Ca^{++} influx into the cell that causes cell death. Thus, glutamate in higher concentration acts as an excitotoxin. Therefore, glutamate is used to produce excitotoxic lesion in the brain in experimental animals. This is one of the mechanisms of damage to brain tissue that occurs in stroke.

Serotonin

Serotonin or 5-hydroxytryptamine (5HT) is a transmitter in **CNS, enteric nervous system and retina**.

Most of the receptors act by activating **adenylyl cyclase**

and phospholipase C (Serotonin receptor types and functions are described in Chapter 78, Local Hormones).

1. Serotonergic transmission in the ***raphespinal pathway*** (nucleus raphe magnus to spinal cord neurons) is an important component of **endogenous analgesia system**.
2. Serotonin is a **mood elevator** and lysergic acid diethylamide (LSD), the **hallucinogenic agent** is a serotonin agonist, which acts through $5HT_2$ receptors.
3. Serotonin is also a circulating chemical secreted by many cells (**enterochromaffin cells, platelets, basophils**, etc.) and takes part in physiological processes like contraction of smooth muscles, formation of platelet plug etc.

Histamine

Histamine acts as neurotransmitter as well as a circulating hormone. Histaminergic neurons are present mainly in hypothalamus and limbic system.

1. There are **three receptor types**: H_1, H_2 and H_3.
2. Histamine controls behavioral functions and also has important peripheral actions like smooth muscle contraction (leading to bronchospasm etc.), secretion of HCl in stomach, increased capillary permeability, arteriolar dilatation etc.

Substance P and Other Tachykinins

Substance P is a major tachykinin. It is a polypeptide containing 11 amino acids. It is found in many parts of CNS, intestine and peripheral nerves.

- There are other tachykinins such as **neurokinin A** (3-10), **neurokinin B**, neuropeptide K and neuropeptide α.
- There are **3 types of neurokinin receptors**: NK-1, NK-2 and NK-3. NK-1 and NK-2 receptors are G protein coupled receptors.
    - **NK-1** is the receptor for substance P, **NK-2** is the receptor for neurokinin K and **NK-3** is the receptor for neurokinin B.
- Substance P activates phospholipase C and increases intracellular concentration of IP_3 and DAG.

Functions of Substance P:

1. Substance P causes **transmission of pain** in the dorsal horn of spinal cord.
2. In nigrostriatal pathway in basal ganglia, it is a **cotransmitter** with dopamine and its concentration is proportionate to the concentration of dopamine.
3. In hypothalamus, it causes **neuroendocrine modulation**.
4. It mediates **axon reflex** in skin.
5. It mediates **peristalsis** in intestine.
6. It suppresses mood.
    - Recently, NK-1 receptor antagonist has been used as **antidepressant**.

Calcitonin-Gene Related Peptide

Calcitonin-gene related polypeptide (CGRP) is a polypeptide, which has two forms: **CGRP α and CGRP β**.

1. **CGRP β** is mainly present in GI tract.
2. **CGRP α** is present along with substance P in ***primary sensory afferent neurons*** in spinal cord and in the neurons of blood vessel.
    - It is also present in thalamus and median forebrain bundle.
    - **In spinal cord** it modulates transmission of pain.
    - It is **potent vasodilator**.

Though the same gene produces CGRP and calcitonin, CGRP has little calcium lowering effect and calcitonin has little vasodilation effect.

Neuropeptide Y

Neuropeptide Y (NP-Y) is a polypeptide containing 36 amino acids distributed widely in brain and ANS.

1. Cell bodies of NP-Y secreting neurons are highly concentrated in **arcuate nucleus of hypothalamus** that project to paraventricular nuclei.
2. NP-Y is potent **orexigenic neurotransmitter** that profoundly increases food intake.
    - **NP-Y antagonists** are used to ***decrease food intake***.
3. NP-Y acts through **Y receptors** that are G protein coupled. There are known **4 Y receptors** for NP-Y: Y_1, Y_2, Y_4 and Y_5.

Purines and Pyrimidines

Known transmitters in this group are **adenosine, ATP, uridine, and adenosine metabolites**.

Adenosine

Adenosine is a general **depressant in CNS** and **potent vasodilator** in many regional circulations.

- It has **four receptor subtypes**: A_1, A_{2A}, A_{2B} and A_3.
- All the receptors are G protein coupled. Adenosine acting through A_{2A} and A_{2B} receptors **increase cAMP** formation and acting through A_1, and A_3 receptors decrease cAMP formation.
- **Theophylline and caffeine** in tea and coffee exert stimulatory effect by blocking adenosine receptors.
- **A_1 receptor antagonists** are used in the treatment of stroke ***to decrease glutamate release*** and prevent excitotoxin effects of glutamate.

ATP

ATP has recently been emerged as a neurotransmitter in CNS. In ANS it causes rapid synaptic responses and in habenula it causes fast neurophysiological responses.

- ATP acts through **P2X and P2Y receptors** that are widely distributed in the body.

- **P2X receptors** are ligand-gated ion channel receptors that have ***seven subtypes***: $P2X_1$ to $P2X_7$.
- There are **eight P2Y receptor subtypes**: $P2Y_1$, $P2Y_2$, $P2Y_4$, $P2Y_6$, $P2Y_{11}$, $P2Y_{12}$, $P2Y_{13}$ and $P2Y_{14}$.
- Presence of P2X receptors in dorsal horn of spinal cord indicates the role of ATP in **transmission of sensory information** in the spinal cord.

Nitric Oxide

Nitric oxide (NO), also called **endothelium-derived relaxing factor** (EDRF) is released from endothelial cell of blood vessels. It is also found as a transmitter in brain.

- NO is formed from **arginine by NO synthase**. NO synthase requires NADPH, which is also called as NADPH diaphorase (NAD).
- In brain it acts as a signal for postsynaptic neurons to communicate with presynaptic neurons in mediating **long-term potentiation and long-term depressions.**

Co-transmitters

The chemicals that are **secreted along with the neurotransmitters** are called co-transmitters. Examples are release of VIP with Ach or neuropeptide-Y with norepinephrine, etc.

- Sometimes, cotransmitters facilitate the actions of regular transmitters in synapses.
- Aspartate, enkephalins, prostaglandins, etc. are also described as transmitters in the CNS.

Exam Questions

1. With the help of a suitable diagram of structure of a synapse, describe the mechanism of synaptic transmission in CNS.
2. Describe the properties of synapses.
3. Describe the synaptic potentials. Write a note on synaptic inhibitions
4. Describe distribution and functions of important neurotransmitters in the brain.

Multiple Choice Questions

1. Botulinum toxins type A and B act by which mechanism?
A. Prevent calcium influx
B. Prevents priming mechanism
C. Prevent release of neurotransmitter by acting on SNAP 25
D. Prevent binding of neurotransmitter to postsynaptic receptors

2. EPSP can be caused by all EXCEPT:
A. Opening of sodium channels
B. Opening of calcium channels
C. Opening of chloride channels
D. Closure of potassium channels

3. IPSP can be produced by:
A. Opening of potassium channel
B. Closure of chloride channel
C. Opening of sodium channel
D. Opening of calcium channel

4. Which of the flowing is not true about slow IPSP?
A. Seen in autonomic ganglia
B. Seen in cortical neurons
C. Due to increased potassium conductance
D. Due to decreased potassium conductance

5. All are true about synaptic delay, EXCEPT:
A. Usual duration is 0.5 ms
B. Is due to time taken in calcium influx, exocytosis and release of NT and generation of synaptic potential
C. Is due to time taken in degradation of the NT in the synaptic cleft
D. Can help in identifying the number of synapses in the conduction pathway

6. Renshaw cell inhibition is an example of:
A. Negative feedback inhibition
B. Positive FB inhibition
C. Postsynaptic inhibition
D. Feedforward inhibition

7. Which of the following is an example of feed forward inhibition?
A. Inhibition of AHC in spinal cord by descending pathways
B. Inhibition of Purkinje cell in cerebellum by mossy fiber-parallel fiber pathway
C. Inhibition of AHC by Golgi bottle neuron
D. Inhibition of granule cell by Golgi cell in cerebellum

8. Which is not a peptide neurotransmitter?
A. Enkephalin B. Substance P
C. Endorphin D. Serotonin

9. Which of the following is the commonest type synapse in CNS?
A. Axodendritic B. Axosomatic
C. Axoaxonic D. Dendrodendritic

10. Substance P is increased in response to pain in periphery by which of the following?
A. Mast cells B. Endothelium
C. Plasma D. Nerve terminals

11. The main excitatory neurotransmitter in the CNS is:
A. Glycine B. Acetylcholine
C. Aspartate D. Glutamate

12. The inhibitory neurotransmitter in CNS neurons is:
A. Glutamate
B. Aspartate
C. Gamma-amino butyric acid
D. Taurine

Answers

1. C 2. C 3. A 4. D 5. C 6. A 7. B 8. D 9. A 10. D
11. D 12. C

Chapter 96

Introduction to Sensory System and Physiology of Receptors

Learning Objectives

On completion of study of this chapter:

The student will be able to (must know):

1. Define sensation, receptor and classify receptors.
2. Illustrate structure and functions of Pacinian corpuscle.
3. Mention the functions of other receptors.
4. Draw the diagram of a receptor potential and describe its mechanism of genesis.
5. List the properties of receptors and explain their significance.
6. Define sensory unit, receptive field, receptor recruitment and sensory unit recruitment.

The student may also be able to (desirable to know):

1. Describe the structure and functions of each receptor.
2. Describe the properties of receptors.

INTRODUCTION

The sensory system consists of the **receptors** that receive and transduce the stimulus into action potential in sensory neurons, the **afferent pathways** (sensory neurons) that transmit the stimulus in the form of action potential to the CNS, the **neurons in the CNS** that modulate sensory information and the **areas in the brain** that recognize the stimulus.

Sensation

Definition: The **basic recognition of a stimulus** is defined as sensation.

Clinically, sensation is called **aesthesia**, a Greek word, which means 'feeling'. Accordingly, absence of sensation is called **anesthesia**, abnormal sensation is called **paresthesia**, sensation of movement is called **kinesthesia** etc.

Types of Sensations

Sensation is broadly classified into **three categories**: somatic sensation, visceral sensation, and special sensation.

Somatic Sensations: The somatic sensations (somesthesia) arise from receptors present on the body surface, in the body wall, muscles, tendons, bones, joints, and connective tissues.

- These include sensation of touch, pain, temperature, vibration, joint movement (proprioception) etc.

Visceral Sensations: Visceral sensations originate from stimulation of receptors in the viscera.

- Usually, receptors are located in the wall of the viscera (if the viscera have a wall) or *in the connective tissue* of the viscera. The visceral organs are present in the skull, thorax, abdomen and pelvis.

Special Sensations: The special sensations originate in the special sense organs and include vision, audition, olfaction, gustation (taste), and the vestibular senses.

- These are sensed by special sensory receptors present in eye, ear, nose and tongue.

Perception

Appreciation and interpretation of sensation is called perception. It involves first the recognition and then the comparison, discrimination and integration of the sensations.

Sensory Modulation

Sensation elicited by a stimulus differs in quality and intensity depending on the afferent pathways carrying the sensation, CNS areas activated by it and the nature of processing of information in the CNS areas.

- This may result in either accentuation or inhibition of the sensations.
- This type of control of sensation is known as sensory modulation.

Dimensions of Sensation

Sensation has several aspects like **modality, intensity, affect and acuity.**

Modality: The quality or type of sensation is known as its modality.

- For example, modality of tactile sensation is touch.

Intensity: This is the **degree of perception** of a stimulus.

- The sensation that spontaneously decreases in intensity quickly when the stimulus is applied for a little longer duration is said to be **rapidly adapting**, the sensation that decreases in intensity slowly is **slowly adapting**, and the sensation that does not change its intensity is said to be **non-adapting.**
- For example, pain is non-adapting whereas touch is rapidly adapting.

Affect: The **emotional component** of a sensation is called affect.

- The sensation that do not have emotional component is said to be neutral.
- The affect may be **positive** (when it evokes pleasant emotional response), or **negative** (when it evokes unpleasant emotional response).
- For example, pain which is associated with unpleasant sensation has negative affect.

Acuity: The **precision of stimulus localization** is called acuity.

- It varies with the concentration of receptors (**innervation density**) and the **receptive field size** of the area where the stimulus is applied and the size of the cortical area representing that somatic body part.

PY10.2

RECEPTORS

Definition

Receptors are **transducers that convert various forms of energy** in the environment **into action potentials** in sensory neurons.

- The receptors are the **endings of afferent nerve fibers.** The sensory receptor may be a part of the neuron or a specialized cell that generates action potentials in the neuron.
- The receptor is usually associated with non-neural cells that surround it. The receptor and non-neural structure are together known as a **sense organ.**
- The receptors are specific for a particular stimulus (i. e. a particular form of energy).
  - The form of energy to which the receptor is *most sensitive* is called its **adequate stimulus.** For example, adequate stimulus for rods and cones in the retina is the light.

Classification

Receptors are classified in various ways such as by function, by adequate stimulus or by location.

A. Based on Function

Receptors are classified into **four categories**: exteroceptors, interoceptors, proprioceptors and teleceptors.

Exteroceptors: These receptors are present in the skin and subcutaneous tissue and are concerned with a change in the external environment close to the body.

- These are present in the *cutaneous sense organs.*

Interoceptors: These are the receptors that detect change in the internal environment of the body.

- For example, the baroreceptors detecting change in blood pressure, the osmoreceptors detecting change in osmolality of the body fluids, etc.

Proprioceptors: These receptors provide information about the **position of the body in space** at any given time.

- Proprioceptors are mechanoreceptors present in the muscles, tendon and joints.
- Sense of position also depends on **kinesthesia**, which is the sensation of movements of body parts, i. e. dynamic movements and static position of the body.

Teleceptors: These are the receptors that receive stimuli or the sensation that are present **far away from the body.**

- For example, the auditory receptors that detects sound coming from a distance.

B. Based on Adequate Stimulus

There are different types of **adequate stimuli** (forms of energy). These are touch-pressure, cold- warmth, pain, chemical and photons.

- They are detected by the presence of various sense organs in the skin and the subcutaneous tissues, and in epithelia.
- The major receptors are mechanoreceptors, thermoreceptors, nociceptors, chemoreceptors and photoreceptors.

Mechanoreceptors: Mechanoreceptors respond to **application of a mechanical stimulus**; for example, touching or stroking the skin.

- The mechanoreceptors are broadly divided into **three categories**: expanded endings, encapsulated endings and naked nerve endings.

Expanded Endings: These are Merkel's disks and Ruffini endings.

Encapsulated Endings: These are Pacinian corpuscles, Meissner's corpuscles, and Krause's end-bulbs.

Naked Nerve Endings: The expanded and encapsulated endings are not very much essential for elicitation of the cutaneous sensations.

All the four cutaneous sensory modalities can be elicited from the areas that contain only naked nerve endings.

Thermoreceptors: These receptors are sensitive to **changes in the temperature** of the skin. Accordingly, there are *two types* of thermoreceptors: the **warmth receptor and the cold receptor.**

These receptors are active over a broad range of change in temperature.

Nociceptors: They **respond to painful stimuli**, the stimuli that are harmful (damages the tissue or threaten to produce damage) to the organism.

There are ***two types of nociceptors***: Aδ-mechanical nociceptors and C-polymodal nociceptors.

- **Aδ-mechanical nociceptors** respond to fast pain, for example, sharp pain due to pricking. They do not respond to pain activated by thermal or chemical stimuli.
- On the other hand, **C-polymodal nociceptors** respond to several types noxious stimuli including thermal and chemical ones.

Chemoreceptors: Receptors that respond to chemical stimuli are chemoreceptors. Examples are taste receptors, olfactory receptors etc.

Photoreceptors: Stimulus for photoreceptors is the light (photons). Example is rods and cones of retina.

C. Based on Location

Superficial: Receptors are located in the skin. Examples are touch and pressure receptors.

Deep: Receptors are present in muscles, bone, tendons etc.

Visceral: Receptors are located in the viscera. Example is visceral pain receptors.

Important Mechanoreceptors

Pacinian Corpuscles

These are mechanoreceptors located in the skin and deep tissues. They mediate the **sensation of vibration, touch and pressure.**

Structure: Pacinian corpuscle consists of a body composed of **concentric layers (lamellae)** much like an onion.

- There are 20 - 70 lamellae in each corpuscle arranged concentrically (Fig. 96.1).

Dimensions: 0.5 to 2 mm long (it is the **largest mechanoreceptor**) and 0.7 mm in diameter

The distal end of a primary afferent fiber penetrates into the **concentric lamellae** of Pacinian corpuscle.

- The cell body of this **Aβ fiber** lies in the dorsal root ganglion and the axon enters the spinal cord through dorsal root.
- The fiber is myelinated but the ending which lies in the concentric lamellae of the Pacinian corpuscle is unmyelinated.

Function: This is a **rapidly adapting mechanoreceptor** capable of receiving **high frequency vibration**. Therefore, it senses **vibration and fine touch**. It also senses **pressure sensation**.

- The distal ***end of the axon***, not the lamellae of the Pacinian corpuscle is the **actual transducer**.
- Thus, when the concentric lamellae are stripped away, the force applied to the nerve ending continues to result in the genesis of receptor potential.

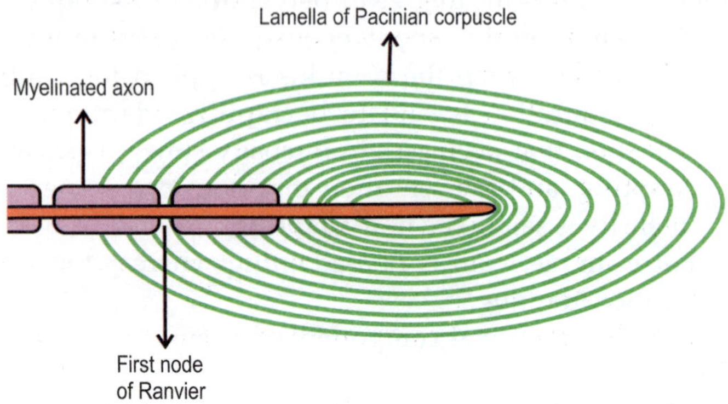

Fig. 96.1: Pacinian corpuscle. Usually, first node of Ranvier remains within the lamella of the corpuscle.

Meissner's Corpuscle

This is a relatively large receptor located in the dermal ridges of the glabrous (hairless) skin.

Structure: The dimensions are:

Length : 150 µm

Diameter : 50 µm

This is an **encapsulated ending** having a *single layered capsule* (Fig. 96.2) into which the ending of the afferent nerve penetrates.

- The afferent fiber is myelinated but ending is unmyelinated.
- The characteristic of the ending is that it is **branched to form a complex structure** inside the corpuscle.

Function: This is a **rapidly adapting receptor that senses vibration sensation**. It also senses the sensation of **contact (touch).**

Merkel's Disks

These are the most superficial mechanoreceptor present in the epidermis of glabrous and hairy skin.

Structure: They are formed by **flattened terminations** of primary afferent axons (Fig. 96.3). The fibers are myelinated but lose their myelin sheath before entering the epidermis.

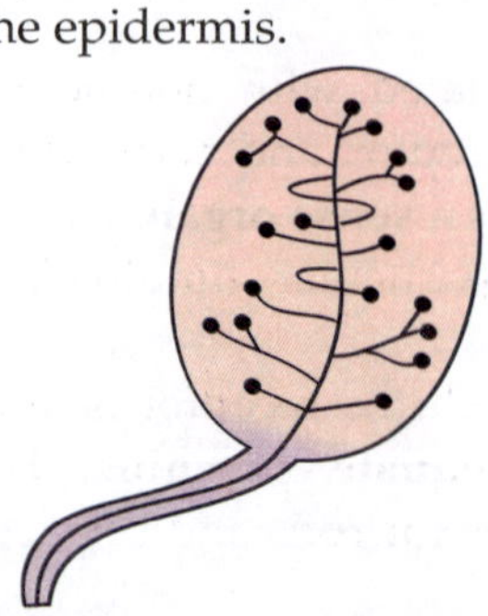

Fig. 96.2: Meissner corpuscle.

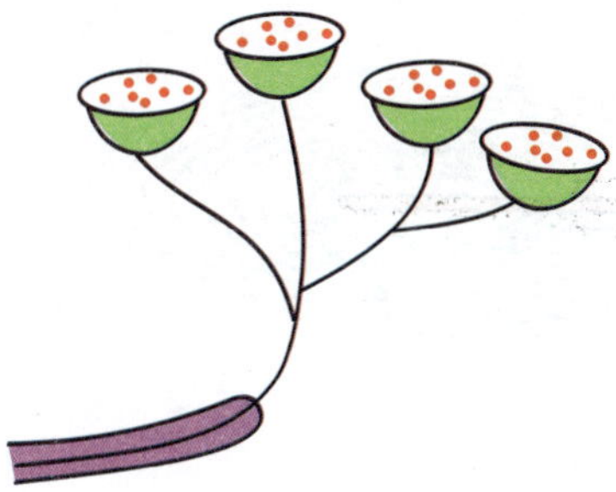

Fig. 96.3: Merkel disk.

- The afferent ending branches to form cup like flattened structures called *Merkel disks* which synapses with the special modified cells, **the Merkel cells**.
- The Merkel cells along with the Merkel disk are combinely called as **Merkel apparatus** or **Iggo-dome receptor** (because they elevate the epithelium of the skin).

Function: Merkel disks are **slowly adapting mechanoreceptor that senses touch-pressure**. The functions of the associated Merkel cells are not clearly known.

- Because the Merkel cells form a synaptic junction like structure with the Merkel disks, they are assigned the role of primary electromechanical transduction.

Ruffini Endings

These are **smallest mechanoreceptors** present in both glabrous and hairy skin.

Structure: These are **expanded endings** of the afferent Aβ nerve fibers. The myelinated nerve fiber and its unmyelinated endings branch out to form a complex expanded structure (Fig. 96.4).

Function: These are **slowly adapting** receptors that usually receive the sensation of crude touch.

Krause's End-Bulb

These are rapidly adapting mechanoreceptors present in the dermis and are widely distributed in the skin.

Structure: These are **encapsulated receptors** into which the primary afferent nerve penetrates.

- The capsule is made up of modified cells that encircle the branched unmyelinated endings of Aβ myelinated nerve fiber (Fig. 96.5).

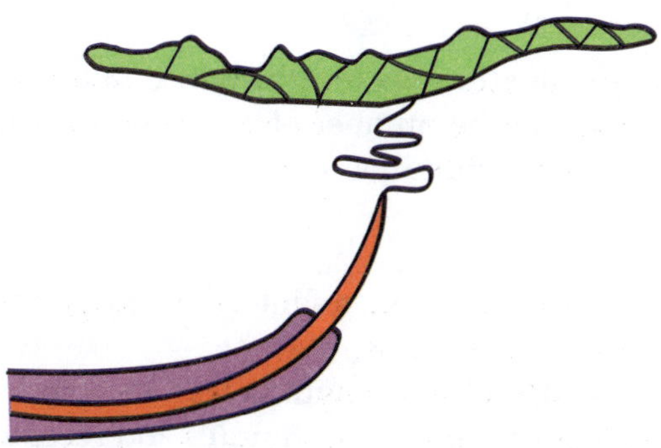

Fig. 96.4: Ruffini ending.

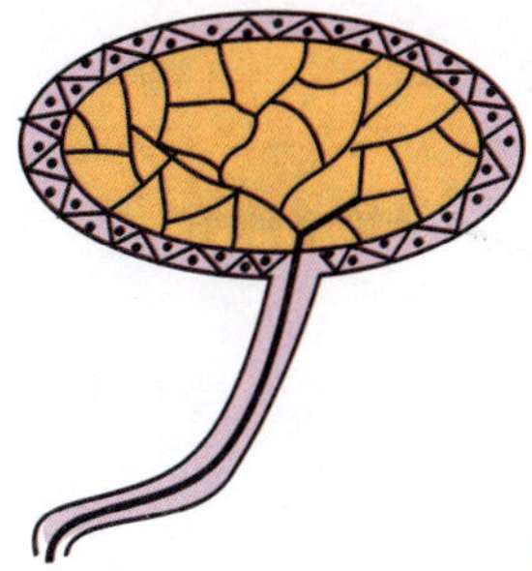

Fig. 96.5: Krause end-bulb.

Function: These are **rapidly adapting mechanoreceptors** that mediate the sensation of touch and pressure.

Golgi-Mazoni Corpuscle

These are first identified in the tendons and muscles, but afterward also found in skin.

Structure: These are **encapsulated receptors** consisting of ***10–15 lamellae***. They are 150–250 μm in diameter.

Function: These are **rapidly adapting mechanoreceptors**. The function is not exactly known but probably they are involved in the elicitation of the sensation of touch-pressure.

Hair Follicle Endings

The endings of the afferent fibers are often present adjacent to the hair follicles. The pressure on the hair distorts and stimulates the associated afferent endings in the hair follicle. Just by bending a hair (without touching skin) therefore touch sensation can be well elicited.

There are **three types of hair follicles** innervated by three morphologically distinct afferent endings: simple hair-follicle, nonsinus facial hair follicle and sinus hair follicle.

Simple Hair Follicle: These are hair follicles **without erectile tissue**. They are innervated by unmyelinated nerve terminals of many myelinated axons.

- The receptors are functionally **rapidly adapting mechanoreceptors**.

Sinus Hair Follicle: These are associated with hairs having large diameter and **erectile tissue at the base** surrounding the follicle. These follicles are rich in nerve supply.

- Slowly and rapidly adapting endings are present in these follicles.
- Thus, they have the properties of **both slow and rapid adaptation**. The hairs with these follicles are called *vibrissae or tactile hairs*.

Nonsinus Hair Follicle: These are associated with spray like terminals resembling Ruffini endings.

- They are present mainly in the skin of the face. They behave like *slowly adapting mechanoreceptors*.

Receptor Potential

Receptors convert environmental energy into action potential in the sensory nerves. On application of stimulus

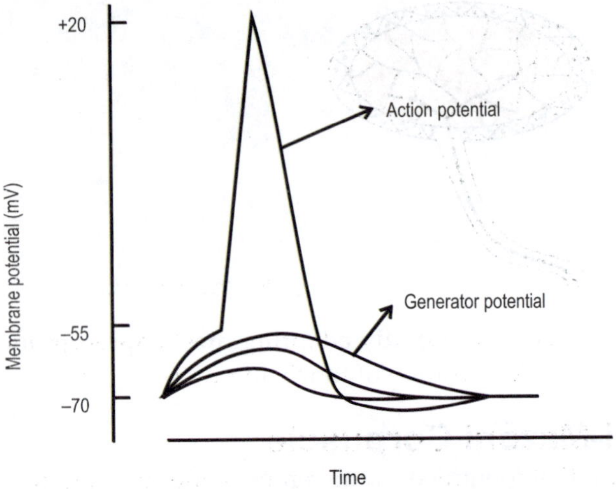

Fig. 96.6: Receptor (generator) potential and action potential formed in receptors.

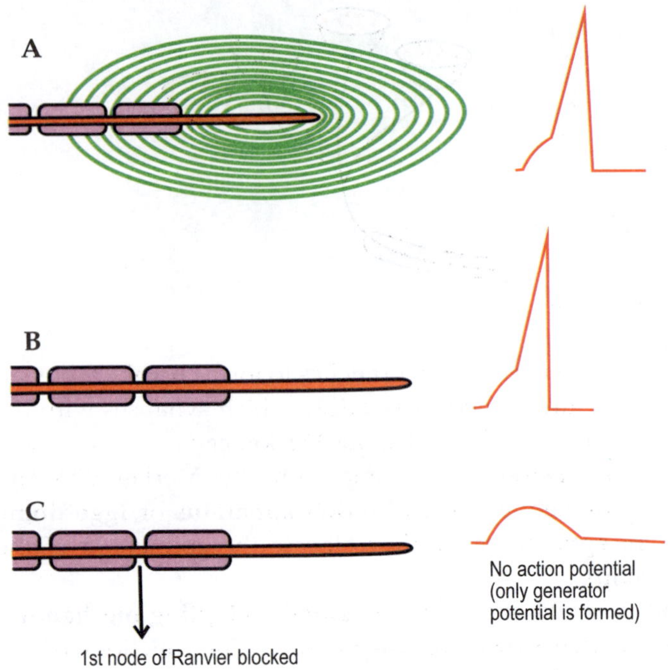

Figs. 96.7: Demonstration of site of action potential genesis in Pacinian corpuscle. Note, action potential is formed following removal of lamella of Pacinian corpuscle (B); but, action potential is not formed following blockade of first node of Ranvier (C).

(change in energy), a potential change is observed in the receptor. This is usually a nonpropagated depolarizing potential that resembles an EPSP. This is called *receptor potential* or **generator potential**.

- When the stimulus intensity is increased, the magnitude of the potential is proportionately increased.
  - When it reaches about 10-15 mV, the action potential is generated in the sensory nerve (Fig. 96.6).
- Pacinian corpuscles, due to their large size are the best-studied receptors for studying the genesis of receptor potential.
- It has been experimentally observed that for the generation of receptor potential, the lamellae of the Pacinian corpuscles are not required.
  - It is the **unmyelinated nerve terminal that generates the receptor potential** (Fig. 96.7).
- It is further observed that the receptor potential forms action potential in the sensory nerve **at the first node of Ranvier**, which is located in the lamellae of the Pacinian corpuscle.

Mechanism of Genesis of Receptor Potential

The pressure on the Pacinian corpuscle causes mechanical **distortion of the lamellas** which in turn **opens stretch sensitive sodium channels** in the nerve terminal, the actual receptors. This increases **influx of sodium ions** that results in the production of receptor potential.

- At the **first node of Ranvier**, the action potential is generated.
- The magnitude and frequency of action potential is proportionate to the intensity of the stimulus.

Properties of Receptors

Specificity

Receptors are **specific to a particular type of stimulus**. For example, pain receptors are stimulated by application of a painful stimulus and touch receptors by tactile stimulation.

Adequate stimulus

The particular **form of energy to which the receptor is most sensitive** is called adequate stimulus. For example, adequate stimulus for rods and cones is the light.

Adaptation

When a stimulus of constant strength is applied continuously to a receptor, frequency of action potential in the sensory nerve decreases.

- This is called adaptation (**desensitization**). Based on this property, receptors are classified to **two types**: phasic and tonic receptors.

Phasic Receptors: The receptors that **adapt rapidly** are called phasic receptors. For example, touch and pressure receptors.

Tonic Receptors: The receptors that **adapt slowly** (or do not adapt at all) are called tonic receptors; for example, the baroreceptors present in the carotid sinus and aortic arch or the pain receptors.

Acuity

The **precision of stimulus localization** is called acuity.

- It depends on the number of receptors present in the area where the stimulus is applied.

Intensity

When a stimulus is applied, receptors discharge depending on the strength of stimulus.

- When the **stimulus strength is less,** receptors that are present close to the site of stimulus and receptors with low threshold, discharge.

- When the **stimulus strength is more**, the activated neurons fire at more rate, and receptors that are present some distance away from the stimulus, also discharge. This is called **receptor recruitment**.

Weber-Fechner Law

The **magnitude of sensation** felt is proportionate to the **log of the intensity of the stimulus**. This is called Weber-Fechner law.

Law of Projection

No matter where a specific sensory pathway is stimulated along its course to the cortex, the **sensation formed is referred to the location of the receptors**. This is called the law of projection.

- This means, irrespective of the site of application of the stimulus in the sensory pathway, the **sensation evoked is felt at the nerve endings** (the receptors).
- This forms the basis of **phantom limb**. In phantom limb phenomenon, the limb actually does not exist (as the limb has been amputated), but the patient complains that he feels pain or itch in the limb.

Doctrine of Specific Nerve Energy

The sensation evoked by a stimulus that generates impulse in the specific sensory pathway depends on the **precise area of the brain that is eventually activated by the stimulus**. This was first described by Muller; therefore, it is called **Muller's doctrine of specific nerve energy**.

- For example, when the sensory fiber for touch is stimulated anywhere along its course to the cortex, the sensation evoked is touch.
- It becomes possible because the **pathways are specific and discrete** from the sense organ to the cortex.
- Therefore, when a nerve pathway from a particular sense organ is stimulated, the **sensation evoked is that for which the receptor is specialized**, no matter how or where along the pathway the activity is initiated.

Sensory Unit and Receptive Field

1. **Sensory unit** is defined as a single sensory axon and all its peripheral branches.
2. **Receptive field** of a sensory unit is the area from which a stimulus produces a response in that unit. Usually, there is some degree of overlap of sensory units of the nearby regions.

Recruitment of Sensory Unit

Receptors spread over a large area are activated when the **strength of stimulus is increased.** This, not only activates the sense organs that are in direct contact with receptor but also the sensory units present in the surrounding areas. This is called recruitment of sensory units or receptor recruitment.

Exam Questions

1. Classify receptors and give the structure and functions of each and describe the mechanism of genesis of receptor potential.
2. Describe the properties of receptors. Add a note on Pacinian corpuscle.

Multiple Choice Questions

1. **Which of the following receptor organ is largest in size?**
   A. Pacinian corpuscle
   B. Merkel disc
   C. Ruffini ending
   D. Krause end-bulb
2. **Which of the following receptor organ is smallest in size?**
   A. Golgi-Mazzoni Corpuscle
   B. Hair follicle ending
   C. Ruffini ending
   D. Krause end-bulb
3. **Which of the following phrase adequately describes Pacinian corpuscles:**
   A. A type of pain receptors
   B. Slowly adapting touch receptors
   C. Rapidly adapting touch receptors
   D. Located in the joints
4. **Meissener's corpuscle are for:**
   A. Touch
   B. Temperature
   C. Pressure
   D. Proprioception
5. **The mechano-stretch receptors in joints and ligaments are:**
   A. Fast adapting
   B. Slow adapting
   C. Non adapting
   D. Adapt differentially for different stresses
6. **The increase in threshold of a receptor when a series of stimuli of sub-threshold intensity are applied in succession is called:**
   A. Adaptation
   B. Accommodation
   C. Initiation
   D. Resistance

Answers

1. A **2.** C **3.** C **4.** A **5.** B **6.** B

Chapter 97

Sensory Communication to Spinal Cord

Learning Objectives

On completion of study of this chapter:

The student will be able to (must know):

1. Name the afferent fibers in peripheral nerves and give their functions.
2. Define sensory map of the body and the segmental distribution in the map.
3. Learns involvement of nerve in axotomy, demyelination, ischemia and compression.
4. Define Bell-Magendie law and gives its application.
5. Outline the spinal cord laminae and the fiber groups terminating in them.

The student may also be able to (desirable to know):

1. Describe the physiological basis of dysfunctions in peripheral nerves in various clinical conditions.
2. Draw the sensory map of the body.

Somatic sensations are carried from the receptors via **sensory fibers in the peripheral nerves** to the spinal cord. They enter spinal cord **via dorsal root** (Fig. 97.1). From spinal cord, they are carried to the different centers in the brain in various ascending pathways.

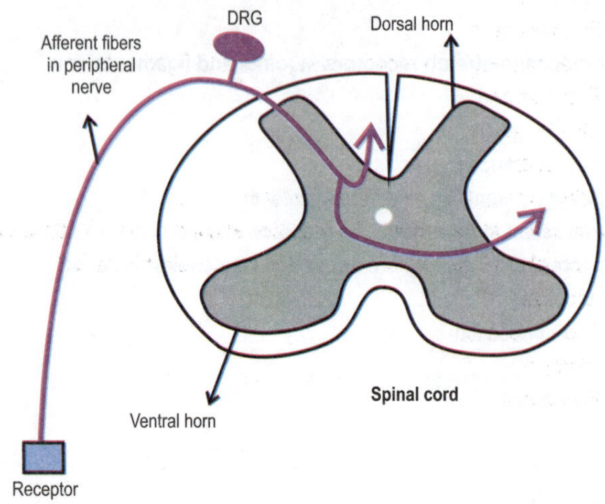

Fig. 97.1: Transmission of sensations from receptors to spinal cord. (DRG: Dorsal root ganglia)

PERIPHERAL NERVE

The somatosensory signals travel to the CNS via the peripheral nerves.

- The peripheral nerves contain **axons of the pseudounipolar sensory neurons**. The cell bodies of these neurons are located in the **dorsal root ganglia** (DRG).
  - The sensory fibers have different diameter and conduction velocity depending on the receptors they innervate and the sensation carried by them.
- Sensory nerve originating from a **particular segment of a spinal cord** innervates a specific **dermatome** (Fig. 97.2).

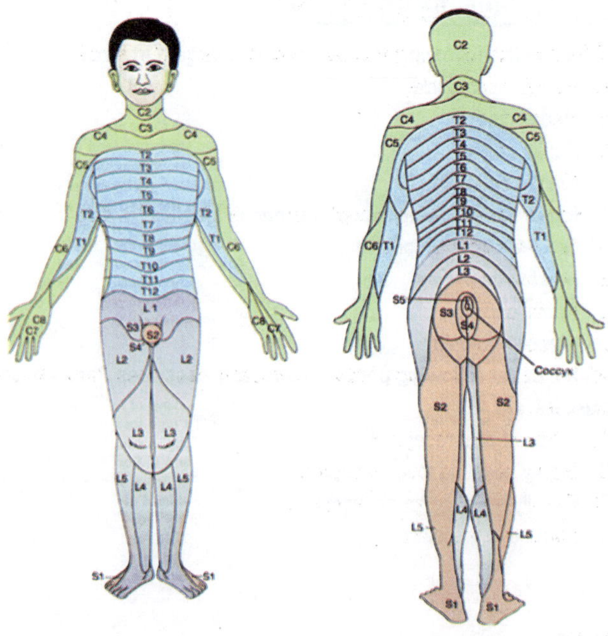

Fig. 97.2: Dermatomal distribution of spinal nerve innervations.

- That means, an area of the skin is supplied by a particular sensory nerve.
- This is called as the **somatosensory map** of the body.

- Therefore, lesion of a particular segment of the spinal cord, or a particular dorsal root or a particular nerve results in loss of sensation from the corresponding skin area supplied by the nerve.
  - This helps in **localizing the nerve or the spinal cord segment** involved in the disease process.

Afferent Fibers in Peripheral Nerves

The afferent fibers that transmit cutaneous sensations are broadly divided into **three categories**:

Large Myelinated Aα and Aβ Fibers: These fibers transmit impulses generated in **mechanoreceptors**.

Small Myelinated Aδ Fibers: These fibers transmit **impulses from nociceptors** (fast pain) and **cold receptors**. Some fibers also transmit impulses generated in mechanoreceptors.

Small Unmyelinated C Fibers: These fibers primarily transmit **slow pain**, and **temperature**. Few fibers also transmit impulses generated in mechanoreceptors.

Clinical Importance

Peripheral nerves are affected by **four major types of disease processes**: axotomy, demyelination, ischemia and compression.

Axotomy: Axotomy is the **transection of nerve fiber**. This usually happens in cut injuries.

1. The part of the axon distal to axotomy degenerates, which is called **Wallerian degeneration** (for details, refer Chapter 19).
   - Degeneration also occurs in the proximal part of the neuron, which includes *swelling of cell body*, *chromatolysis* in soma, and *retraction of axon* from the point of injury.
2. During the ***process of regeneration***, *sprouting of new fibers* starts from the proximal axon.
3. The peripheral axons regenerate faster than the central axons. Sensory fibers regenerate faster than the motor fibers.

Demyelination: **Demyelination occurs in many neuropathies.**

- **Distal axonopathy** (degeneration of distal part of peripheral neurons) occurs commonly in ***diabetes and chronic alcoholism***.
- Usually, these diseases manifest in the form of sensory loss in the distal parts of the limbs (**distal sensory neuropathy**).

Ischemia: Ischemia for more than 15 minutes **results in loss of touch, temperature and fast pain.** *Slow pain is usually not affected*, as unmyelinated ***C fibers are less sensitive to hypoxia*** than myelinated fibers.

1. **Acute ischemia** inhibits axoplasmic transport and impulse propagation, known as ***conduction block***.
2. **Chronic ischemia** results in *degeneration of nerve fibers*.

Compression: Compression of nerve fiber is called compressive neuropathy.

- In compressive neuropathy, large diameter fibers (fibers>5 μm in diameter) are affected early and more severely than the small unmyelinated fibers.
- Therefore, usually **slow pain is not affected** initially.
  - Example of compressive neuropathy is entrapment of median nerve in carpal tunnel (**carpal tunnel syndrome**).

IMPORTANT NOTE

In ischemia and compression, **elimination of touch sensation** occurs first and then the pain sensation, whereas **local anesthetics first eliminate the pain sensation** and then the touch.

- Small unmyelinated fibers are more sensitive to local anesthetics but less sensitive to hypoxia and mechanical compression than the large diameter fibers.

Dorsal Root

The afferent fibers that travel in the peripheral nerve enter the spinal cord via the dorsal root.

1. The cell bodies of the afferent neurons are present in the DRG. The distal axons are the peripheral nerve fibers. The proximal axons are the dorsal root fibers that enter the spinal cord.
2. The ***region of the skin innervated by a single dorsal root ganglion*** is called a **dermatome** (Fig. 97.2).
   - Usually, there is no significant overlapping of the dermatomes of the adjacent ganglia.
   - This helps in **mapping** (detecting the defect according to dermatomal innervation) the sensory loss of a particular segment of the spinal cord and thereby **locating the disease process**.
3. However, the distribution of *innervations of muscles* (**myotomes**) or bones (**sclerotomes**) by individual dorsal root ganglia is loose, as there is greater degree of overlapping.

Clinical Significance

The dorsal roots may be affected by compression, transection or various other disease processes. The features of dorsal root involvement depend on severity and distribution of the fibers. For example, mild compression causes irritation whereas more compression causes damage to the dorsal root fibers.

Compression of Dorsal Root

Compression of dorsal root is not uncommon. This occurs usually from the **herniation of an intervertebral disk**.

- The injury produced by compression results in **pain** in all the affected dermatomes.
- Irritation of the dorsal root can produce **paresthesia or hyperesthesia** in the corresponding dermatome, whereas damage to the dorsal root can cause **frank segmental anesthesia**.

Other Diseases Affecting Dorsal Root

Dorsal root damage can also occur in following pathological processes.

- Traction
- Inflammation
- Ischemia
- Infection (Tabes dorsalis)
- Degeneration

PY10.6

SPINAL CORD

Afferent fibers enter spinal cord through the dorsal root and efferent fibers leave the spinal cord through the ventral root.

- Thus, ***dorsal root is sensory*** **and** ***ventral root is motor***.
  - This is called **Bell-Magendie Law.**
- The ventral root afferents are usually small unmyelinated nociceptors arising from visceral structures.

Spinal Connections

Afferent fibers (the first order of neurons of sensory pathway), after entering the spinal cord may have the following **three major destinations** (Fig 97.3):

1. They **ascend directly in the dorsal column** of the spinal cord (without relay on second order neuron) as a major ascending tract (***dorsal column pathway***) to reach the second order of neuron in the medulla.
2. They **terminate in the dorsal horn** and relay on the second order of neuron in the same segment and the same side of the spinal cord. The second order neuron then crosses to the opposite side and ascend in the ***anterolateral system***.
   - They **may ascend or descend few segments in the spinal cord** before contacting the second order of neurons.
   - They may also contact commissural neurons.
3. Many afferent neurons originating from muscle spindle, Golgi tendon organs or joint receptors **mostly directly** or sometimes indirectly contact the corresponding **motor neurons in the anterior horn cells.**
   - Some afferent fibers also **make connections with the interneurons** present in the spinal cord segment or with the terminals of the fibers in the descending pathways originating from different areas of the brain.

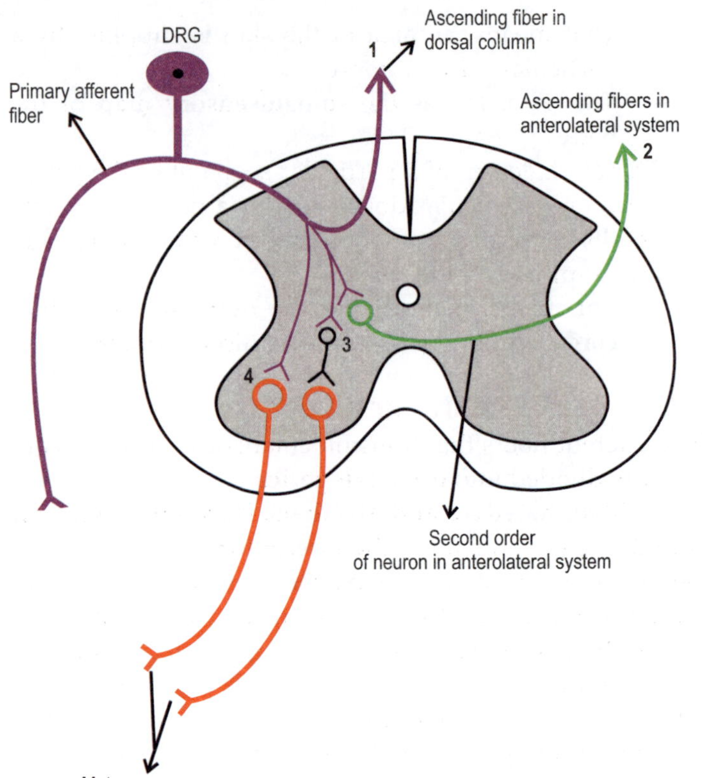

Fig. 97.3: Destinations of primary afferent fibers after entering spinal cord. **1.** They may ascend up in the dorsal column pathway; **2.** They may terminate on second order neuron of anterolateral system; **3.** They may contact interneuron that in turn terminates on motor neuron; **4.** They may directly terminate on motor neurons of anterior horn. They may also ascend or descend few spinal cord segments (not shown in picture). DRG: Dorsal root ganglia.

Somatotopic Organization

Fibers are somatotopically (somatotopic means representing a body part) arranged in the spinal cord.

- The afferent fibers arising from **distal part of the extremities and the ventral surface of the trunk** terminate in or occupy the ***medial part*** of the spinal cord.
- The fibers coming from the **proximal part of the extremities and the dorsal body surface** terminate ***laterally*** in the spinal cord.

Spinal Cord Laminae

There are different laminae in the dorsal and ventral horns of the spinal cord. The laminae in the dorsal horn are called **sensory laminae** as they accommodate the afferent fibers.

1. **Sensory laminae** are lamina I to VI. The laminae in the ventral horn are called **motor laminae** as they accommodate efferent fibers.
2. The **motor lamina** is mainly lamina IX. However laminae VII and VIII also contribute to motor laminae, but contain mainly interneurons.
3. Lamina X is the **intercomissural lamina.**

As spinal laminae were first described by **Rexed in 1954,** they are known as **Rexed laminae**. The nerve fibers with different diameters terminate preferentially in the different sensory laminae in the dorsal horn of the spinal cord (Fig 97.4).

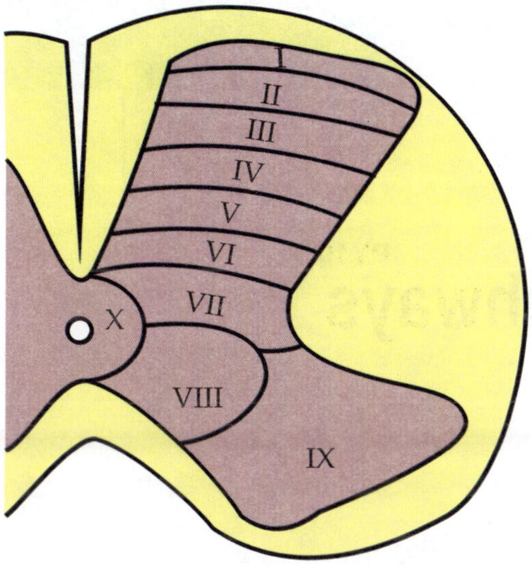

Fig. 97.4: Spinal cord laminae. Note, laminae I to VI are dorsal horn laminae.

Lamina I: Lamina I receives **small nociceptive A and C fiber inputs**. Therefore, this lamina responds primarily to the noxious stimuli.

- The cells of lamina I project their axons to a variety of spinal and supraspinal nuclei.
- They send axons to lateral cervical nucleus, dorsal column nuclei, thalamus, etc.

Lamina II: Laminae II is known as **substantia gelatinosa**. It receives primarily **C fiber inputs**.

- Thus, most of the lamina II cells respond to nociceptive or strong mechanical stimuli.
- The axons of laminae II terminates locally, a few neurons project to the other segments of the spinal cord.

Laminae III–VI: These laminas mainly receive myelinated A fiber inputs. These neurons respond to **fine touch, vibration and proprioception**.

- The axons of these cells ascend up in the somatosensory pathway in the dorsal column.
- In addition, lamina V receives inputs from nociceptors.

Descending Influences on the Spinal Cord Laminae

The descending influences come primarily **from the cortex** via corticospinal tract and **from the brainstem** via extrapyramidal tracts.

1. These descending tracts primarily terminate **(directly or indirectly) on the motor neurons** located in the ventral horn (anterior horn cells). However, a significant number of descending fibers **also terminate on the cells of the dorsal horn laminae** (the sensory laminae).
2. The main purpose of this termination of the descending tract is to bring about **sensory-motor coordination** or to modify the sensory input entering into the central nervous system according to the motor need of the body. This provides a feedback for sensory motor regulations.
3. The following are the **sites of termination of the descending tracts** in the sensory laminae, in addition to their terminations on motor neurons and other spinal neurons:

Tracts	Terminations
1. Corticospinal	III, IV, V, VI
2. Raphespinal	I, II, V, VI, VII
3. Medullary reticulospinal	I, II, V, VI, VII
4. Pontine reticulospinal	V, VII, VIII

Exam Questions

1. With the help of a suitable diagram, describe how afferent fibers are organized at the spinal cord level. Add a note on Rexed laminae in the spinal cord.

Multiple Choice Questions

1. All of the following are sensory lamina, EXCEPT:
A. Lamina VI B. Lamina IV C. Lamina V D. Lamina IX

2. Sensory nerve originating from a particular segment of spinal cord innervate a defined area of the body. This is called:
A. Myotome B. Sclerotome
C. Dermatome D. Viscerotome

3. Sensory fibers from peripheral structures after entering spinal cord have the following destinations EXCEPT:
A. Ascend in dorsal column
B. Ascend in anterolateral system
C. Terminate on gamma motor neurons directly
D. Contact motor neurons directly or indirectly

4. The dorsal root of spinal cord is sensory and ventral root is motor. This is called:
A. Weber-Fechner law B. Muller's doctrine of nerve energy
C. Bell-Magendie law D. Rexed laminar principle

5. Laminae in spinal cord were described by:
A. Cajal B. Rexed
C. Magendie D. Muller

6. Lamina II of spinal cord mainly receives:
A. C fiber inputs B. Aδ fiber inputs
C. Aα fiber inputs D. Aβ fiber inputs

Answers
1. D 2. C 3. C 4. C 5. B 6. A

Chapter 98

PY10.3

Ascending Pathways

Learning Objectives

On completion of study of this chapter:

The student will be able to (must know):

1. List the sensations carried in dorsal column pathway and anterolateral system.
3. Draw a labeled schematic diagram to trace the pathway for dorsal column.
4. Draw a labeled schematic diagram to trace the pathway for anterolateral system
5. Trace the pathway for each sensation such as touch, vibration, proprioception etc.
6. Define various abnormalities of sensations and name common causes for these sensory deficits.

The student may also be able to (desirable to know):

1. Describe the pathway for each sensation.
2. Explain the physiological basis of abnormalities of dorsal column sensations.

Neurons in Ascending Pathways

Usually, there are three sets of neurons: first order, second order, and third order of neurons.

- These neurons are arranged sequentially in the central nervous system.
- Some of the pathways also have the higher order of neurons (fourth order neurons) for further processing of information in other parts of the cerebral cortex.

First Order of Neurons: These are **primary afferent neurons.**

1. They start from the receptor and travel in the peripheral nerves to **reach the spinal cord via the dorsal root**.
2. **Cell bodies** are located **in the DRG**.
3. After entering the spinal cord, they **terminate on the second order of neurons** in the spinal cord laminae itself or **ascend up** in dorsal column to terminate on the second order of neurons in the medulla.

Second Order of Neurons: They are either located **in the spinal cord or in the brainstem.**

- The primary function of these neurons is to *transmit impulse from the first order of neurons to the thalamus.*
- As a general rule, the **second order of neurons typically cross the midline** (either in the spinal cord or in the medulla).
- Thus, these neurons transmit the impulses originating in one side of the body ***to the opposite side of the thalamus***.

Third Order of Neurons: These neurons originate from the **specific nuclei in the thalamus** and terminate in the **specific areas in the sensory cortex.**

- Sensations transmitted from different parts of body are relayed in the thalamus before being projected into the cortex.
- Therefore, thalamus is considered as the **main sensory relay center** in the brain.

Higher (Fourth) Order of Neurons: These neurons are usually not included in the sensory pathways. However, sometimes a higher order of neuron originates from the terminals of third order of neurons in the sensory cortex and **project to other areas of the brain,** especially to the cortical sensory association area, for further processing of the sensory information.

Classification

The ascending pathways are typically **divided into three categories**: dorsal column pathways, anterolateral systems and other ascending pathways.

Dorsal Column Pathways: Fibers ascending in the **dorsal column of the spinal cord** are included in this pathway.

- This is also called **lemniscal system** as fibers occupy medial lemniscus in the brainstem.

Dorsal column pathways transmit **following six sensations**:

1. Fine touch
2. Vibration
3. Proprioception
4. Tactile localization
5. Tactile discrimination
6. Stereognosis

Anterolateral Systems: It is divided into **two parts: anterior** spinothalamic tract and lateral spinothalamic tract.

1. The **anterior spinothalamic tract** carries the ***sensation of crude touch***.
2. The **lateral spinothalamic tract** carries the ***sensation of pain and temperature***.

Other Ascending Pathways: These include many other ascending pathways such as:

1. Spinocerebellar tract (dorsal and ventral)
2. Spinoreticulothalamic tract
3. Spinocervicothalamic tract

DORSAL COLUMN PATHWAYS

The large myelinated afferent fibers that enter the dorsal column of the spinal cord to reach the medulla constitute dorsal column pathways.

- They carry the sensations of **fine touch, vibration, proprioception, tactile localization, tactile discrimination and stereognosis.**
- In the spinal cord, they ascend up in two fasciculi: the gracile fasciculus and the cuneate fasciculus (Fig. 98.1).
- These ascending tracts in spinal cord are also called **tract of Goll and Burdach**.

First Order of Neuron

Neurons arriving from lower extremity and lower part of the trunk ascend up in the gracile fasciculus, whereas the neurons arriving from upper extremity and upper part of the trunk ascend in the cuneate fasciculus.

1. The **gracile fasciculus is located medially** in the spinal cord and carries sensations from hindlimb and trunk.
2. The **cuneate fasciculus is situated laterally** that transmits impulses from upper limb and upper part of the trunk.
3. The first order of neurons terminates in the **nucleus gracilis and nucleus cuneatus** in the medulla.

Second Order of Neuron

The cell bodies of these neurons are present in the **nucleus gracilis and cuneatus** in the medulla.

- These two nuclei are known as the ***dorsal column nuclei***.
- The fibers originating from these nuclei cross the midline and pass on to the opposite side in the medulla and ascend up in the ***medial lemniscus*** to reach thalamus.
- The second order of neurons, thus transmit impulses ***to the contralateral thalamus***.

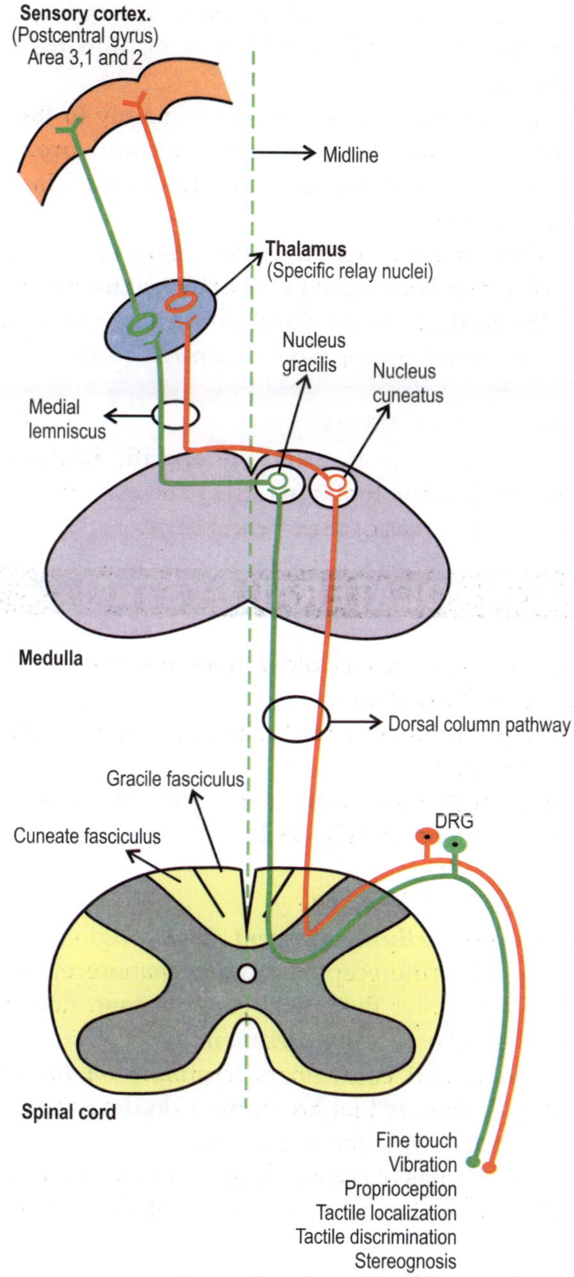

Fig. 98.1: Dorsal column pathways.

Dorsal Column Nuclei

There is a **somatotopic organization** in the dorsal column nuclei with face placed laterally and trunk and hind limb medially. Dorsal column nuclei are divided into two different zones: cluster and non-cluster zones.

Cluster Region: This is the main part of the dorsal column nuclei in which *cells are arranged in clusters*.

1. This region *receives direct input from the fibers* ***in the dorsal column pathways***.
2. The second order of neurons from this region cross over to the opposite side to reach thalamus.

- This region informs the thalamus and cortex about the sensory stimulation.

Non-Cluster Region: The noncluster region is present more rostrally in the dorsal column nuclei.

1. This region receives inputs ***from descending fibers*** from the cortex and *from fibers in the* ***dorsal column pathways***.
2. The projection from this region is mainly **to the non-thalamic areas** like cerebellum, tectum, pretectum, inferior olive, red nucleus and areas that are involved in motor control.
   - Thus, **main function of this region** is to provide direct sensory input **to the different motor areas of the brain** to bring about immediate regulation of movement by appropriate sensory feedback.

Third Order of Neuron

These neurons originate from the **specific nucleus (the VPL nucleus) in the thalamus**. The neurons project to the somatosensory areas of the cerebral cortex.

ANTEROLATERAL SYSTEM

Phylogenetically, this is older than the dorsal column system. It is divided into:

Anterior spinothalamic tract that carries the sensation of *crude touch*, and,

Lateral spinothalamic tract that carries the sensation of *pain and temperature* (Fig. 98.2).

First Order of Neuron

These are ***primarily the afferent fibers*** originating from nociceptors, thermoreceptors, and mechanoreceptors.

- The fibers enter the spinal cord through dorsal root and the cell bodies are present in the DRG.
- **In the spinal cord**, fibers ***terminate on the second order of neurons*** that are present on the same side of the dorsal horn of the spinal cord.
- The cell bodies of second order of neurons are located mainly in the laminae I, II and V in the dorsal horn.

Second Order of Neuron

The cell bodies of these neurons are present ***in the dorsal horn of the spinal cord***.

- The axons **cross the midline** in the same spinal segment and ascend up in the opposite side of the anterolateral funiculus to reach the thalamus.
  - The fibers carrying the **sensation of crude touch** are placed anteriorly and therefore called ***anterior or ventral spinothalamic tract***.
  - The fibers carrying the **sensations of pain and temperature** are placed laterally and therefore called ***lateral spinothalamic tract***.

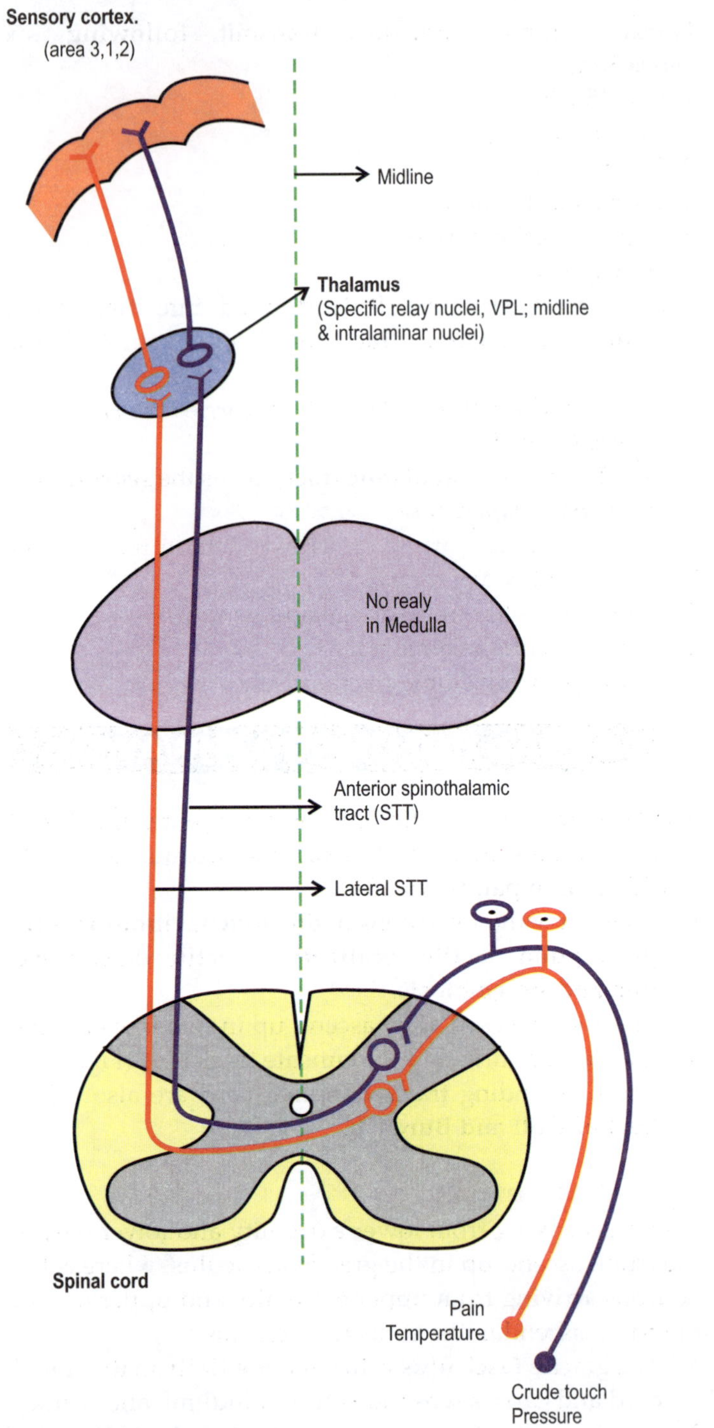

Fig. 98.2: Anterolateral system.

Third Order of Neuron

The neurons originate from the VPL, midline and intralaminar nuclei of the thalamus and **project to the specific areas in the sensory cortex**.

PATHWAYS FOR SPECIFIC SENSATIONS

Touch

Receptors: Touch can be elicited from the skin areas containing no specialized receptors. Thus, it is observed that the free nerve endings mediate touch sensation.

- However, it has been known that **Meissner's corpuscle and Pacinian** corpuscles are ***rapidly adapting touch receptors***, whereas **Merkel disk and Ruffini endings** are slowly adapting touch receptors.
- The **Na^+ channel BNC1** is closely linked with touch receptors.
  - This ion channel belongs to a group of proteins called **degenerins** that if hyper-expressed cause degeneration of the neurons.
- The receptors are activated by mechanical pressure.

Distribution of Receptors: Touch receptors are abundantly present in hands especially in fingertips, and lips, and are less in number in the proximal part of the limbs and trunk of the body.

1. Receptors are *very less on back of the trunk*. Usually, the receptors are present **in more numbers around the hair follicles**. Therefore, *movement of hair is a potent stimulus* to elicit touch sensation.
2. They are also present in skin and subcutaneous tissues of the hairless areas.

Pathway: The fibers carry the touch sensations are **Aβ fibers.**

1. The fibers ascend in ***two pathways***: the **dorsal column pathway** for the *fine touch* and the **anterior spinothalamic tract** for the *crude touch* (for details, see above).
2. The touch sensation carried in the dorsal column is well localized and have better discriminative aspects, whereas, the touch sensation carried in the anterolateral system is poorly localized and has less discriminative aspects.

Proprioception and Kinesthesia

Definitions:

1. **Proprioception** is defined as the afferent input arising from stimulation of muscle, tendon, and joint mechanoreceptors that inform about the ***movement of joints and body parts*** in space.
2. **Kinesthesia** is defined as the sensation arising from ***movement of the body parts in relation to one another***.

These two terms are used to describe the sense of position and movement of the parts of the body. This excludes the sense of position and orientation of the body obtained by the stimulation of visual and vestibular receptors.

Receptors: The receptors are slowly adapting spray endings in the joints and muscles that resemble the Golgi tendon organs.

- The **Pacinian corpuscles** in the synovia and ligaments are also included in the proprioceptors.
- The touch receptors in the skin overlaying the joint may also be the part of the receptors.

Pathway: Proprioception (sensation of movement of body parts due to joint movements) is transmitted in the dorsal column of the spinal cord.

- From medulla (nucleus gracilis and cuneatus) a significant proprioceptive projection goes to the cerebellum.
- Therefore, diseases affecting dorsal column produce ataxia, as they interrupt the fibers to cerebellum.

Vibration

Application of mechanical stimuli oscillating rapidly from 2 to 400 Hz elicits this sensation, which is described as trembling or vibrating.

- Ability to feel mechanical vibration is also called **pallesthesia**.
- The sensation elicited in the **lower range of this frequency is flutter** and **at higher frequency range is sense of vibration.**
- Vibratory sense is a composite sensation comprising of touch and rapid alterations of deep-pressure sense.

Receptors: The receptors are touch receptors that are rapidly adapting, especially **Pacinian corpuscles**.

Pathway: Sense of vibration is carried in the **dorsal columns.**

Clinical Importance:

1. Vibratory sensibility and proprioception are closely related. The diseases that decrease proprioception also decrease vibratory sensibility and vice-versa.
2. **In cortical lesions**, proprioception and sense of vibration ***are affected early and impaired severely***.
3. Depression of the threshold for vibratory sensibility is an **early symptom of degeneration of the spinal cord** involving the dorsal column. Such degenerations are seen in chronic diabetes mellitus, vitamin deficiencies, especially deficiency of vitamin B_{12} (pernicious anemia) and early part of tebes dorsalis. .

Two-Point Discrimination

The minimal distance that permits two-touch stimulus to be perceived as two separate points, when applied simultaneously on the skin, is called as two-point discrimination. Two-point discrimination threshold is a **measure of tactile acuity**.

Receptors: The receptors are **fine touch receptors**. However, identifying two points depends on the intactness of the cortex.

- The magnitude of two-point threshold is different in different body parts.
- The body parts **with abundant touch receptors have the smallest magnitude**. For example, on the back the two points must be separated 65 mm or more to be distinguished as separate points, whereas on the finger tips this distance is reduced to as low as 3 mm.
- This also depends on the **degree of representation of body parts** in the sensory cortex.

Pathway: The sense of two-point discrimination is carried by **dorsal column pathway.**

Clinical significance: This sensation is abolished when cortex is damaged.

- Two-point discrimination, tactile localization and stereognosis are severely impaired in cortical lesions as they are integrated in cortex.
- Therefore, they are called cortical sensations.

Stereognosis

The ability to **identify known objects** by handling them with eyes closed is called stereognosis.

Receptors: Receptors are **touch and pressure receptors.**

Pathway: This sensation is transmitted by **dorsal column pathway** to the brain.

Clinical significance: Inability to identify the object by touch is called astereognosis or tactile agnosia. Inability to identify an object by sight is called **visual agnosia**, inability to identify sounds or words is called auditory agnosia and inability to identify position of limb is called **positional agnosia**.

1. Stereognosis is one of the important cortical sensations. Therefore, impaired stereognosis is an **early sign of cortical pathology**, which may occur with intact touch and pressure sensations.
2. This is also compromised in diseases that affect dorsal column of the spinal cord.

ABNORMALITIES OF DORSAL COLUMN SENSATIONS

Abnormalities of Tactile Sensations

Anesthesia

Definition: Anesthesia means complete loss of all forms of sensations.

- **Hypesthesia** refers to partial loss of sensations.
- Loss of a particular sensation is depicted specifically with a prefix; for example, **thermoanesthesia** indicates loss of temperature sensation or **pallanesthesia** means loss of vibratory sense.

Causes:

A. Hypesthesia: This is usually seen in **central lesions** like lesions at thalamus, internal capsule and cortex. It affects the distal parts of the limbs more than the peripheral parts.

B. Complete anesthesia: Usually occurs in **peripheral nerve lesions**. The commonest cause is leprosy.

- Lesion of peripheral nerve results in anesthesia corresponding to the distribution of sensory fibers.
- Complete anesthesia also occurs in complete transaction of the spinal cord where anesthesia is seen in the limbs and trunk below the level of the lesion.

Dissociated Anesthesia

Definition: When the sensation of pain and temperature is lost with the preservation of touch, the condition is known as dissociated anesthesia.

Causes:

1. Syringomyelia
2. Intramedullary tumors
3. Brainstem lesions (syringobulbia)
4. Thrombosis of the posterior inferior cerebellar artery.

Physiological Basis: Dissociated anesthesia occurs in diseases when **spinal cord grey matter surrounding the central canal is damaged.**

- The fibers of dorsal column pathway are spared in the disease process as they are placed in the periphery of the spinal cord. Therefore, tactile sensibility is preserved.
- The **fibers of spinothalamic tract** (that carry the sensation of pain and temperature) while crossing over to the opposite side in the spinal cord are **placed close to the central canal**.
- These fibers are damaged in the disease process that results in loss of pain and temperature.

Hemianesthesia

Definition: Loss of sensations that affect face, arm, trunk and leg of one side of the body is called hemianesthesia.

Causes: Usually seen in lesions of the thalamus, internal capsule or cortex of contralateral side.

Hyperesthesia

When the **response to the sensory stimulation is exaggerated**, the condition is called hyperesthesia. The increased sensitivity to various stimuli indicates heightened activity of sensory apparatus like *increased receptor sensitivity*. It is seen in thalamic lesions.

Hyperpathia: Exaggerated perception of sensations is called hyperpathia. It is interchangeably used for hyperesthesia.

Alloesthesia

Definition: When a tactile or a painful stimulus delivered on the side of hemisensory loss is experienced on the corresponding area of the opposite side, is called alloesthesia or allesthesia.

Causes:

1. Lesion of right side putamen (usually that occurs due to putamen hemorrhage)
2. Anterolateral lesion of the cervical spinal cord (this may be due to existence of few uncrossed spinothalamic fibers).

Paresthesia

Definition: When the sensations are abnormal and distressing (touch may produce an unpleasant sensation almost amounting to pain) the condition is called **paresthesia or dysesthesia**. This may occur in the form of pricking, numbness, or band like sensations around the trunk.

Causes:

1. Nerve compression
   - This is the commonest cause of paresthesia. It occurs when peripheral nerves are stretched or subjected to pressure. The commonest example is the experience of paresthesia (numbness and pricking) when sitting posture is maintained for a longer time with legs crossed.
2. Spinal tumors
3. Subacute combined degeneration of spinal cord
4. Disseminated sclerosis
5. Thalamic lesions

Agraphesthesia

Definition: Loss of graphesthesia, i. e. the **loss of sense of cutaneous localization and figure writing** (sense of writing figures on the body). Graphesthesia is the function of posterior column.

Cause: This is commonly seen in lesion of the sensory cortex.

Astereognosis

Definition: Inability to identify a known object by palpation with eyes closed even though the primary tactile sensibility is intact.

Cause: It is seen in cortical disease. However, it should be differentiated from *stereoanesthesia*, in which lesions of the spinal cord or brainstem interrupt proprioceptive and tactile sensations.

Abnormalities of Proprioceptive Sensations

Proprioceptive sensation means the sensation of joint movement, or the sense of position of different parts of the body in space. The sense of vibration is closely linked to proprioceptive sensation.

The loss of proprioceptive sensation can occur without loss of other sensations. It occurs in lesions of the posterior column.

It is typically seen in:

1. Tabes dorsalis
2. Subacute combined degeneration of spinal cord
3. Proprioception and vibration sense are severely affected in lesion of the sensory cortex

Romberg Sign

Inability to maintain a balanced standing position **with feet together and eyes closed** is called Romberg sign. This displays the lack of sense of position in both the legs. The patient should be tested in bare-foot. This is called **sensory ataxia**. However, ataxia also occurs in cerebellar disease and vestibulopathy, and should be differentiated from posterior column lesion.

Exam Questions

1. With the help of a labeled schematic diagram, describe the pathway for dorsal column sensations. Add a note on Romberg sign.
2. With the help of a labeled schematic diagram, describe the pathway for crude touch and pressure. Add a note on dissociated anesthesia.

Multiple Choice Questions (of Chapter 98 and 99)

1. **Which of the following area has least concentration of fine touch receptors?**
   A. Finger tips B. Buttock
   C. Lips D. Around hair follicles
2. **Third order neurons of dorsal column pathway arise from:**
   A. Anterior nucleus of thalamus
   B. Gracile nucleus of medulla
   C. Cell bodies in the spinal cord lamina II
   D. VPL nucleus of thalamus
3. **All of the following sensations are called cortical sensations, EXCEPT:**
   A. Stereognosis B. Crude touch
   C. Tactile discrimination D. Tactile localization
4. **All of the following sensations are true for vibration sensations, EXCEPT:**
   A. Receptors are Pacinian corpuscles
   B. A composite sensation comprising of touch and rapid alteration of deep pressure
   C. Impaired in degeneration of spinal cord
   D. Not affected in cortical lesions
5. **All of the following statements are true for dorsal column nuclei, EXCEPT:**
   A. Cluster region receives direct input from fibers in the dorsal column pathways
   B. Noncluster region is located more rostrally
   C. Noncluster region projects mainly to thalamic areas
   D. Noncluster region receives inputs from descending fibers from cortex

Answers

1. B 2. D 3. B 4. D 5. C

MCQs continue in Page No. 815

Chapter 99

Physiology of Pain, Itch, Temperature and Trigeminal System

Learning Objectives

On completion of study of this chapter:

The student will be able to (must know):

1. Define pain, classify pain, name the nociceptors, and trace afferent projections to spinal cord.
2. Draw labeled diagrams of pain pathways and describe the pathways.
3. List the differences between somatic pain and visceral pain.
4. Define referred pain, give examples and explain the theories of referred pain.
5. Understand the mechanism of pain recognition & perception.
6. Draw the schematic diagram of endogenous neural analgesia systems.
7. Outline the mechanisms of endogenous analgesia systems.

The student may also be able to (desirable to know):

1. Describe the pathway for each sensation.
2. Explain the physiological basis of abnormalities of dorsal column sensations.

PAIN

Definition: Pain (as defined by International Association for the Study of Pain, IASP) is an unpleasant sensory and emotional experience associated with actual or potential tissue damage or described in terms of such damage.

Nociceptive Stimuli

Stimulus that elicits pain is called **noxious** or **nociceptive stimulus**.

- Nociceptive means the one, which is ***potentially damaging***.
- Thus, a stimulus that is capable of damaging or causing harm to the tissue is a nociceptive stimulus and the sensation elicited is called **nociception** (pain sensation).

Nociceptive stimuli are different for different tissues, such as pricking or cutting in skin, distension of intestine, ischemia of cardiac muscle, traction on cerebral arteries or meningeal structures in brain, etc.

Types of Pain

Fast Pain vs. Slow Pain: A painful stimulus first elicits a **sharp-localized pain**, which is followed by ***diffuse-dull pain***.

- The **first component** is called *fast pain* or first pain and the **second component** is called the *slow pain* or second pain.
- The fast pain is transmitted by **Aδ fibers** and the slow pain is transmitted by **C fibers**.

Superficial Pain vs. Deep Pain: The pain elicited in the **superficial structures** like skin and subcutaneous tissues is the superficial pain, which is usually the fast pain.

- The pain felt in the **deeper structures** like bones, muscles, connective tissues etc. is the deep pain.
- **Deep pain is usually the slow pain** that occurs due to stimulation of C fibers in the deeper structures of the body.

Somatic Pain vs. Visceral Pain: Pain originating in the **somatic structures** is the somatic pain and pain originating in the **visceral structures** is the visceral pain (details of visceral pain are described below).

Peripheral Pain vs. Central Pain: Pain occurring due to **direct stimulation of receptors or nerves** is the peripheral pain. Example is the *neuropathic or neurogenic pain* (as seen in neuralgias).

- Stimulation of **central pain fibers** resulting in pain is called central pain.
- Example of central pain is the *pain below the level of lesion* in spinal transection.

Physiologic Pain vs. Pathologic Pain: **Acute pain** is sometimes referred to as ***physiologic pain***. Acute pain has sudden onset and subsides faster with the natural healing process or due to treatment. It is called physiologic pain or 'good pain' as it serves an important protective mechanism.

- **Chronic pain** is often referred to as ***pathologic pain*** or 'bad pain' as it persists even after the healing from the injury or following treatment as usually, they do not respond to usual anti-inflammatory analgesics.

Types of Pathologic Pain: There are two categories of pathologic pain: neuropathic and inflammatory.

  i. **Neuropathic pain** is due to nerve damage as occurs in chronic diabetes, ischemia or toxins.
  ii. **Inflammatory pain** is due to inflammatory diseases such as rheumatoid arthritis.

- Usually, inflammatory pain is accompanied by ***hyperalgesia and allodynia*** (details given at the end of this chapter).

Receptors and Peripheral Fibers

Types of Nociceptors

Receptors for pain are called **nociceptors**. Nociceptors are the **free nerve endings**. They are distributed widely throughout most parts of the body. However, there are few tissues like brain (only the neural tissue of the brain) that are devoid of nociceptors. Though the brain tissue does not contain nociceptors, the coverings of the brain are rich in these receptors.

TYPES: The nociceptors are broadly divided into **three categories**: Aδ mechanical nociceptors, multimodal C fiber nociceptors and other nociceptors.

Aδ Mechanical Nociceptors

These are the **terminals of Aδ fibers**. The Aδ fibers are small, myelinated axons that discharge only in response to intense mechanical stimuli (but, not to thermal or chemical stimuli).

- The fibers are usually 1–5 mm in diameter with **conduction velocity of 10–30 m/s.**
- Aδ fibers conduct the **fast pain**.

Polymodal C Fiber Nociceptors

The polymodal nociceptors are activated by high-intensity mechanical, chemical and thermal (both hot and cold) stimuli. As they respond to varieties of stimuli, they are polymodal in nature.

- These are **terminals of C fibers**, which are fine-unmyelinated fibers having diameters of about 0.3–1.2 mm and **conduction velocity of 0.5–2 m/s.**
- The C fiber nociceptors usually respond to thermal and chemical stimuli.
- They respond to high skin temperature (at least 45° C) and locally applied chemicals.
- The C fibers carry the **slow pain**.

Other Nociceptors

These include **thermal nociceptors** (Aδ and C fiber terminals that respond to very low and high temperature, i. e. < 5° C and > 45° C respectively), Aδ fibers responding to heat and non-multimodal C fibers responding to strong mechanical stimuli.

Three types of receptors for thermal pain have been cloned:

- Cold and methanol-sensitive receptor 1 (**CMR 1**), 2. **VR-1**, and 3. **VRL-1**.
- No. 2 and 3 are vanilloid receptors for nociceptive heat that are sensitive to vanillins, a group of chemical substances including capsaicin that induce pain.

Vanilloid Receptors: Vanilloid receptor–1 (**VR–1**) at **C fiber terminals** have been described recently.

1. These receptors are so named as they **respond to vanillin**, a group of pain producing compounds that include capsaicin.
2. **VR–1** responds not only to nociceptive stimuli such as capsaicin, but also to increase in temperature > 43C, and change in pH.
3. Another type, celled **VRL–1 receptor** isolated from C fibers respond to temperature above 50°C, but not to capsaicin.

Thus, it appears that there are **multiple receptors in C fiber endings** responding to various stimuli or possibly, there may be different C fiber systems.

TRP Family of Ion Channels: CMR 1, VR-1 and VRL-1 receptors belong to **transient receptor potential family (TRP family) of ion channels**. These are *excitatory ion channels*.

1. Especially, **VR-1 has a PIP_2 binding site**.
   - When the quantity of PIP_2 bound to VR-1 is decreased, the sensitivity of this thermal nociceptor is increased.
2. The **mechanism of action** of these receptors is fully understood.
   - In general, **depolarization** in the cutaneous receptors could be due to **inhibition of K^+ channels** that decreases K^+ efflux or **activation of Na^+ channels** that causes Na^+ influx or inhibition of Na^+- K^+ pump.
3. **Depolarization of cool receptors** is observed to be due to **Ca^{++} influx**.

Spinal Cord Termination of Pain fibers

The cell bodies of pain fibers are located in DRG. Fibers **enter spinal cord** via dorsal horn. In case of **cranial pain fibers**, the afferents project to the ***nucleus of trigeminal nerve*** (the medullary analogue of dorsal horn).

1. **In the dorsal root**, pain fibers occupy the most lateral part of the root.
2. In the dorsal horn, **Aδ fibers terminate in laminae I and V** and **C fibers terminate in lamina II** (Fig. 99.1).

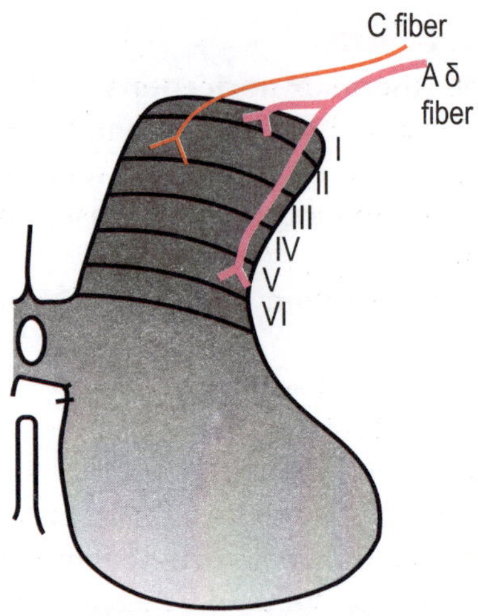

Fig. 99.1: Termination of pain fibers in the dorsal horn of spinal cord.

3. In the spinal cord, the ascending pain fibers **occupy the lateral fasciculus**.
4. However, the thinnest pain fibers (C fibers) form a discrete bundle in the spinal cord, the **tract of Lissauer**.
   - The Lissauer's tract also contains few **deep sensory and propiospinal fibers**.

Specificity of Nociceptors

Many theories have been forwarded to explain the specificity of nociceptors and nociceptive pathways. These are:

Specificity Theory: This theory states that the pain sensation has a **specific sensory modality, specific receptors, and a specific pathway** in the CNS. Stimulation of these receptors and pathway produces the sensation of pain.

Overstimulation Theory: This theory explains that the pain results from **over-stimulation of various types of afferent ending**. Therefore, according to over-stimulation theory, pain can be transmitted via different afferent pathways.

Pattern Theory: This theory states that the pain sensation can be elicited by **stimulation of receptors by a particular pattern**.

However, finally it has been agreed that **specificity theory explains all the aspects of pain**. Thus, the receptors for pain are specific and the pathways.

Dermatomal Distribution of Pain Fibers

Pain fibers are distributed in the somatic structures as per the **sensory map** of the body, which is useful to the physician to locate the site of lesion.

- The distribution of **pain fibers from deep structures** however does not fully correspond to the cutaneous pattern, though they also follow a segmental pattern.
- For example, **T_1 to T_4 nerve roots** mainly innervate thoracic organs like heart and lungs, **T_6 to T_8 nerve roots** are for upper abdominal organs and **T_{10} to L_2** nerve roots are for lower abdominal viscera.

Localization

Pain is localized like other sensory *modalities.*

1. **Sharp pain is better localized than the dull pain,** because it preserves ***its specific dermatomal representation*** and also ***its somatotopic organization in the CNS.***
   - However, in general, **pain is relatively poorly localized**, because pain endings have **low innervation density** and pain pathways exhibit *extensive branching* than any other sensory pathways.
2. **Visceral pain is very poorly localized** than the somatic pain due to **less number of receptors** present in visceral structures and also due to their **poor cortical representation.**

Pain Pathways

Pain is transmitted to the higher centers in the brain in the *lateral spinothalamic tract* of the anterolateral system. The pain pathways are divided into ***two types***: the **paleospinothalamic pathway** and **neospinothalamic pathway**.

Paleospinothalamic Pathway

Phylogenetically, paleospinothalamic is the **oldest pathway**.

- This pathway ***mainly carries the sensation of slow pain.***
- This is the slow conducting multineuron system that mediates the poorly localized pain **from deep somatic and visceral structures.**
- The fibers are mostly *C fibers* (Fig. 99.2).

First Order Neurons: First order neurons enter the spinal cord and terminate mainly in the **laminae II** of the dorsal horn.

Second Order Neurons: Second order neurons decussate and ascend up in the ***contralateral spinothalamic pathway***. The fibers are more medially placed in the spinothalamic tract. In the brainstem on their way to thalamus, fibers project to **three major nuclear groups** forming ***three subsystems***.

1. At the level of medulla, the collaterals from the second order of neurons heavily **project to the reticular formation**; therefore, this pathway is also called as ***spinoreticulothalamic pathway***.
2. Fibers also **project heavily to the midbrain nuclei** (***spinomesencephalic fibers***) like midbrain reticular formation, parabrachial nuclei and periaqueductal gray.
3. Fibers also **project to hypothalamus** forming ***spinohypothalamic fiber system***.

Third Order Neurons: In the thalamus, the fibers terminate mainly in the **medial nuclear group** (the midline and intralaminar nuclei; also called as ***non-specific nuclei***) from where the third order of neurons arise and project to different areas of the cortex **including limbic cortical areas.**

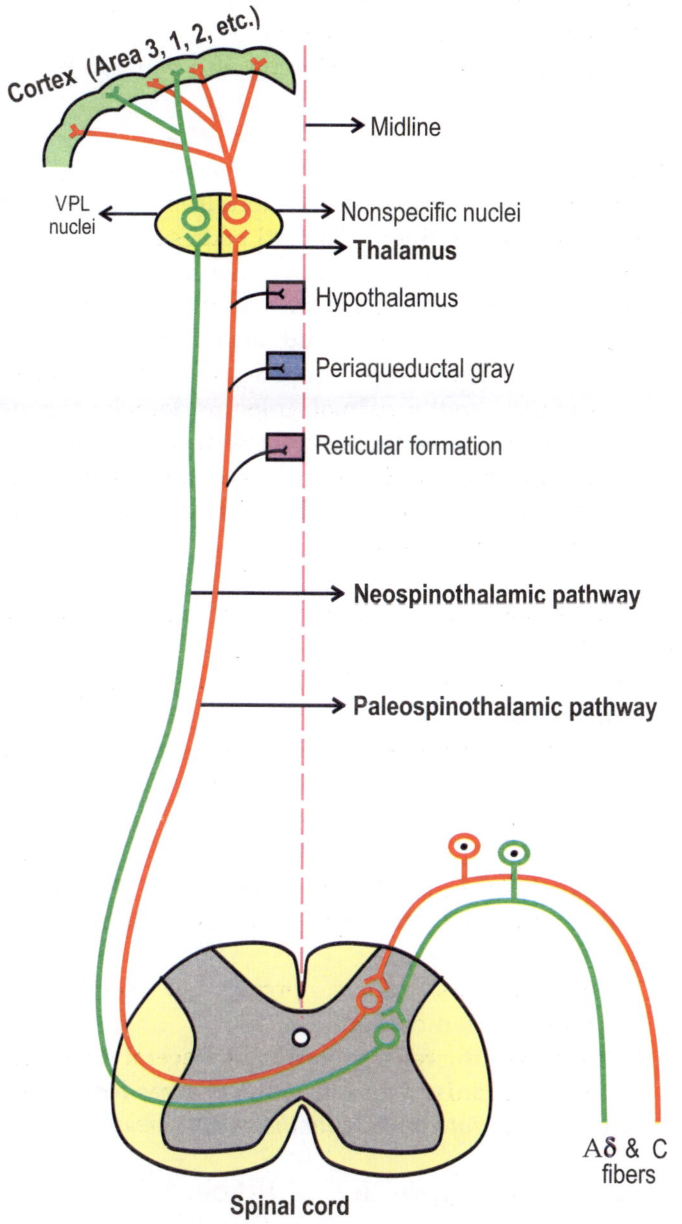

Fig. 99.2: Paleospinothalamic and neospinothalamic pain pathways. Note the collaterals in the brainstem from the paleospinothalamic pathway terminating in different brainstem nuclei.

Special Features

1. Because of **non-specific projection** of paleospinothalamic fibers that mainly transmits slow pain; the slow pain **is poorly localized.**
2. Through its substantial projection to the reticular formation, the **slow pain keeps a person awake.**
3. Also, through its connection with limbic system, paleospinothalamic pathway **evokes the emotional experience** of pain and through hypothalamic connections it **mediates autonomic responses.**
4. This pathway mediates **motivational-affect component** of pain.

Thus, the paleospinothalamic pathway mediates **arousal, affective aspects and autonomic responses of pain.**

Neospinothalamic Pathway

The neospinothalamic tract is most developed in primates. This pathway **carries mainly the fast pain.** The fibers are mostly **Aδ fibers.**

First Order Neurons: First order of neurons terminates mainly in the **lamina I and V** in the dorsal horn of the spinal cord (Fig. 99.1). The neurotransmitters released at the terminals of primary nociceptive afferents (1st order of neurons) are glutamate and neuropeptides (of which most important is **substance P**).

Second Order Neurons: Second order neurons cross over to the opposite side in the same segment of the spinal cord and ascend in the lateral spinothalamic tract. In the spinal cord, there is a **topographic organization** of fibers.

1. The fibers from **lower body parts** are ***placed laterally*** and fibers **from upper body parts** are located more ***medially*** in the lateral fasciculus.
2. The fibers from **sacral spinal segments** occupy the ***most lateral part*** and the fibers **from cervical region** are present in ***most inner part*** in the spinothalamic tract (Fig. 99.3).
3. Second order neurons terminate in **lateral nuclear group** (the ventrobasal and posterior nuclear complexes; or also called VPL nuclei or **specific nuclei**) of the thalamus.
4. On their way to thalamus, the neospinothalamic tract project sparsely to the midbrain reticular formation, periaqueductal gray, and hypothalamus.

Third Order Neurons: The third order of neurons originate from **specific thalamic nuclei** and project to the ***postcentral gyrus*** (the sensory cortex).

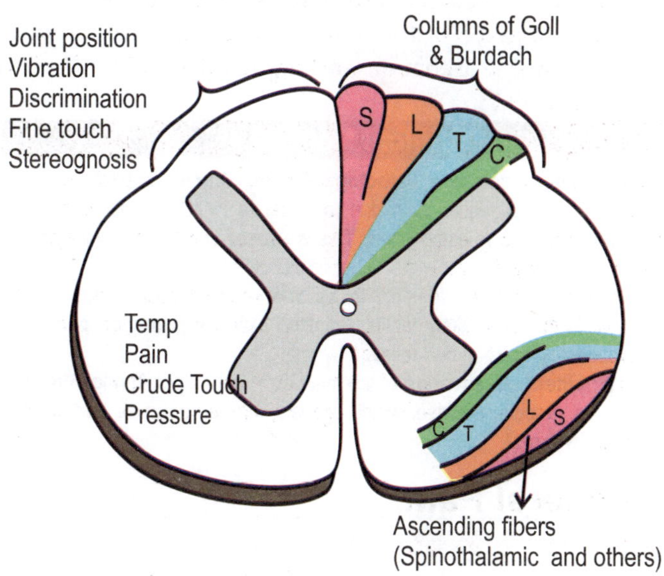

Fig. 99.3: Topographic organization of pain and other sensory fibers in the spinal cord. S: Sacral; L: Lumbar; T: Thoracic; C: Cervical.

- The **topographic organization** of these fibers in the thalamus and cortex **is very concrete**, and in the sensory cortex, the neurons are organized in modality specific columns.
- Therefore, the **fast pain is better localized**.

Special Features

1. The **topographic organization** of neospinothalamic fibers in the thalamus and cortex **is more precise.**
2. In sensory cortex, the neurons are organized in **modality specific columns**. Therefore, the fast pain is better localized.
3. The neospinothalamic pathway for its termination in the specific and discrete areas in thalamus and cortex, sub-serves the **sensory-discriminative aspects of pain** such as the ***localization of pain*** and detection of ***quality and intensity*** of the noxious stimuli.

Deep Pain

Pain originating from nociceptors in the deeper somatic structures such as muscles, tendons, bones, periosteum, internal ligaments etc. is the deep pain.

- It differs from superficial pain by the nature of pain evoked by the stimuli, which is usually dull aching with poor localization.
  - This is mainly due to deficiency of Aδ fibers in the deeper structures and the relatively less no of receptors in the deep structures.
- Like visceral pain (see below), often deep pain is associated with autonomic symptoms as autonomic fibers accompany the neurons originating these deeper body structures.
- Pain from a deeper body part is usually accompanied by contraction of surrounding skeletal muscles.
  - Prolonged contraction of these muscles induces muscle ischemia and aggravates pain (Clinical Note 99.1).

Clinical Note 99.1

Muscle pain is common pathological pain: Muscle contraction for a longer duration produces pain due to ischemia, which usually subsides once blood flow is re-established. This is usually due to accumulation of **Lewis factor or P factor** in the ischemic muscles.

- The exact chemical nature of P factor is not known, though accumulation of K^+ is the most likely factor. Common example is **angina pectoris** induced by exertion and relieved by rest.
- **Intermittent claudication** of leg muscles in persons suffering from occlusive vascular disease, which appears with leg exercise and disappears with rest.

Visceral Pain

Receptors and Stimulus

The receptors for pain are similar to the nociceptors in the somatic structures, but the receptors are much **less in number**.

- Due to the ***paucity of nerve endings*** in viscera, the ***margins of the painful zone*** *are not well delineated* and the pain is **poorly localized**.
- **Stimulus** for visceral pain is usually the **distension of the organ**, if it is a hollow viscus.
- **Chemical irritation** or **ischemia** also causes visceral pain.

Afferent Fibers

Afferent fibers carrying pain sensations from viscera reach CNS **via autonomic fibers**. The cell bodies are located in the DRG and homologous cranial nerve ganglia.

- The **cranial nerves** that carry visceral pain fibers are **vagus, glossopharyngeal, and facial** nerves.
  - Visceral pain from esophagus, stomach, small intestine and proximal colon is largely carried in **vagus nerve** and terminate in the nucleus of solitary tract (NTS) before projecting to thalamus.
- Pain fibers from abdominal viscera also accompany the **sympathetic fibers**.
  - Therefore, visceral pain is associated with **autonomic features** like sweating, alteration in blood pressure etc.
- Pain fibers from pelvic structures accompany **lumbosacral roots**.
- The **trigeminal nerve** carries the sensation from face and eye.

Ascending Pathway

From spinal cord, the fibers travel along the **lateral spinothalamic tract**, the same pathway as that for the somatic sensation.

1. From thalamus, fibers project to cortex via thalamocortical radiation.
2. In the cortex, the **representation of visceral structures is poorly organized** and the cortical areas for visceral sensation are *intermixed with the somatic areas*.

Special Characteristics of Visceral Pain

1. As the pain receptors are less in number in the viscera, the visceral pain is **poorly localized**.
2. The important stimulus for elicitation of visceral pain is the **distention of viscera**. Inflammation of viscera also increases the sensitivity to pain.
3. Visceral pain is usually **unpleasant**, because, it has an affective component, and the afferent fibers stimulate the vomiting center in the brain.
4. Visceral pain is usually **associated with autonomic symptoms** like change in blood pressure, sweating, etc. because the afferent fibers travel in sympathetic and parasympathetic pathways. Thus, visceral pain causes autonomic changes.
5. Visceral pain (especially abdominal pain) causes **muscle spasm and rigidity**. It is especially observed

if the inflammatory process that produces pain also involves the peritoneum. Muscle guarding (abdominal wall rigidity) as seen in **acute abdomen** is a protective mechanism that prevents further injury to the viscera.

6. Visceral pain often radiates to other structures (**referred pain**).

Referred Pain

Visceral pain may be referred to the somatic structures that are located away from the viscera.

1. The pain **perceived in the somatic structure due to visceral irritation or injury** is called the referred pain.
2. Usually, the visceral pain is not referred to the skin overlying the viscera, but to the other areas of the skin innervated by the same embryonic spinal segment. For example, the referred pain is typically seen in acute myocardial infarction or in acute cholecystitis.
3. In **acute myocardial infarction**, the pain is referred to the ***inner aspect of the left arm***, and in **acute cholecystitis** to the tip of the right shoulder.
4. In cholecystitis, the inflamed gall bladder irritates the diaphragm, which stimulates the phrenic nerve. Therefore, ***cholecystitis pain radiates to the tip of the shoulder***, as the shoulder and diaphragm develop from the same dermatomal segments.

Theories of Referred Pain

The referred pain is explained by the following theories:

1. Dermatomal theory
2. Convergence theory
3. Facilitation theory
4. Experience theory

Dermatomal Theory

Visceral pain is referred usually to a structure that **develops from the same embryonic segment** (dermatome). This is called dermatomal theory.

- For example, the heart and the inner aspect of the arm develop from the same embryonic segment.
- Therefore, the **pain of acute myocardial infarction** radiates to ***ulnar border of the left arm***.

Convergence Theory

The **visceral and somatic afferent fibers converge on the second order of neuron** in the spinothalamic tract, as the number of second order neurons is less than the afferent fibers (the first order neurons).

- Therefore, the fibers carrying the pain sensation from the somatic structures also carry the pain sensation arising from the visceral structures (Fig. 99.4).
- The **cortex sometimes cannot differentiate** the site of origin of the pain sensation because the ascending fibers projecting to cortex from both structures are the same.

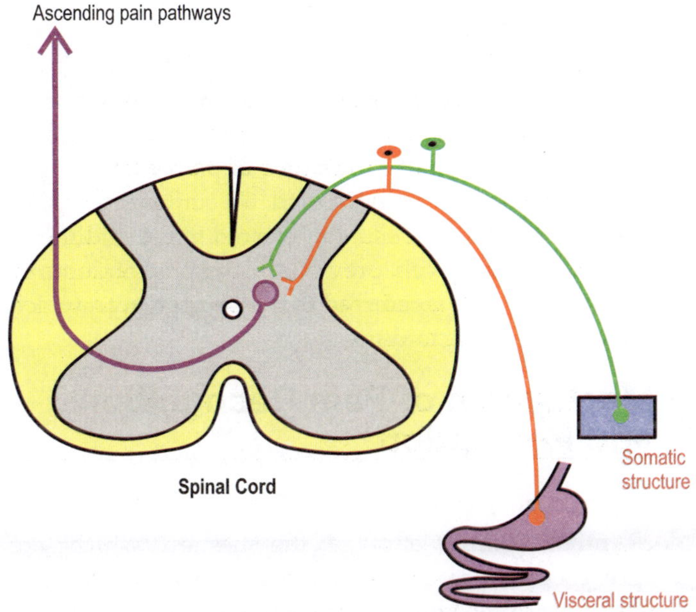

Fig. 99.4: Convergence theory of referred pain. Note that, due to the convergence of fibers from the somatic and visceral structures on a single second-order neuron, fibers transmitting pain sensation from the somatic structure also carry the pain sensation arising from the visceral structures.

- Therefore, signal conveyed by brain for perception is also referred to the somatic area in addition to the projection to the viscera.

Facilitation Theory

The collaterals arising from the visceral afferent fibers **project to the spinothalamic neurons** that receive afferents ***from the somatic structures*** (Fig. 99.5).

- Therefore, the pain sensation arising from somatic structure is **facilitated (strengthened) by activity in the visceral afferents**.
- Thus, minor activity in the somatic afferent can cause pain.

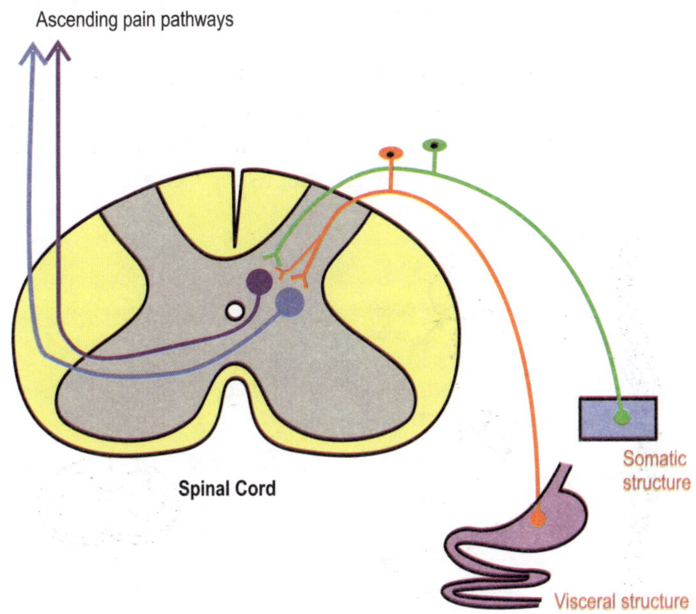

Fig. 99.5: Facilitation theory of referred pain.

Experience Theory

Experience plays a role in the genesis of referred pain. According to this theory, pain instead of being felt at its usual site, may be referred to some other structure or area in which the **patient had experience of pain earlier**.

- For example, the pain due to the inflammation of abdominal viscera is usually referred to the midline.
- But, in patients with previous history of abdominal surgery, the pain is **referred to the surgical scar**, which may not be in the midline.

Mechanism of Pain Recognition and Perception

Pain Recognition

Nociceptive stimuli damage the tissues, which are recognized by the body as sensation of pain. **Proteolytic enzymes** are released from damaged tissues.

1. These enzymes act on tissue proteins and cells locally to release many substances that activate nociceptors.
2. The ***chemical substances that mediate pain*** are histamine, prostaglandins, serotonin, kinins and other polypeptides like leukotrienes (Fig. 99.6). Locally released potassium ions from the damaged cells also activate nociceptors.
3. Activation of nociceptors directly releases polypeptide mediator by the primary afferent fibers that sensitizes nociceptors.
4. The mediator is the **substance P** released from C-fiber endings in skin. Substance P enhances pain perception. Substance P also mediates other features of inflammation as well.

Modulation of Pain Perception

The **threshold for pain perception** may be same in all, but *is lowered in inflammation*.

1. **Local anesthetics** and many centrally acting **analgesics** (and also placebos) act by raising the pain threshold.
2. **Distraction** that turns the attention away from the painful part of the body decreases awareness to pain.
3. **Strong emotion** also decreases pain perception probably by acting on descending adrenergic system (for details see below). However, the degree of emotional reaction varies in individual.

The conscious awareness of pain occurs when the impulse reaches thalamocortical level.

- **Recognition** of noxious stimulus is the *function of thalamus*, and appreciation of **intensity, localization and discrimination** are the *functions of sensory cortex*.

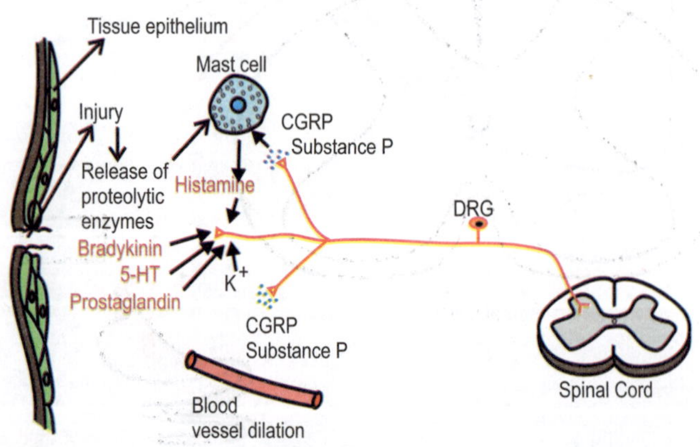

Fig. 99.6: Mechanism of pain recognition. CGRP: calcitonin gene-related peptide; DRG: dorsal root ganglion; 5-HT: 5-hydroxytryptamine.

ANALGESIA SYSTEMS

Endogenous Pain Control Mechanisms

Prominent among the analgesia systems are **neuronal analgesia** (descending pain-inhibiting) systems and **opioid systems**.

Descending Pain Modulating Systems

Neuronal analgesia systems were described following discovery by V. Raynold in 1969 that stimulation of ventrolateral **periaqueductal gray** (PAG) in rats produces profound analgesia. Subsequently other areas were found to have analgesic properties.

- Important among them are **nucleus raphe magnus** and **nucleus paragigantocellularis** in medulla.
- **Two descending analgesia systems** have been described: raphespinal serotonergic pathway and ceruleospinal norepinephrinergic pathway.

Descending Raphespinal Serotonergic Pathway

This pathway originates from the frontal cortex and hypothalamus and projects to the cells in the **periaqueductal region** of the midbrain.

- Fibers from PAG project to the **nucleus raphe magnus** and reticularis magnocellularis in the medulla.
- From raphe nucleus, fibers descend down to the spinal cord via **raphespinal pathway** (Fig. 99.7).
    - Fibers of raphespinal pathway are **serotonergic** and they terminate in laminae I, II, and V of dorsal horn.
- In the spinal cord, raphespinal fibers mainly *terminate on the interneurons* that by **presynaptic mechanisms** inhibit the transmission of impulses from primary afferent fibers to second order of neurons.
    - These interneurons release **enkephalins** as their neurotransmitters that inhibit the release of substance P from the presynaptic ending.
    - Thus, transmission of impulse in the pain pathway in the dorsal horn is inhibited.

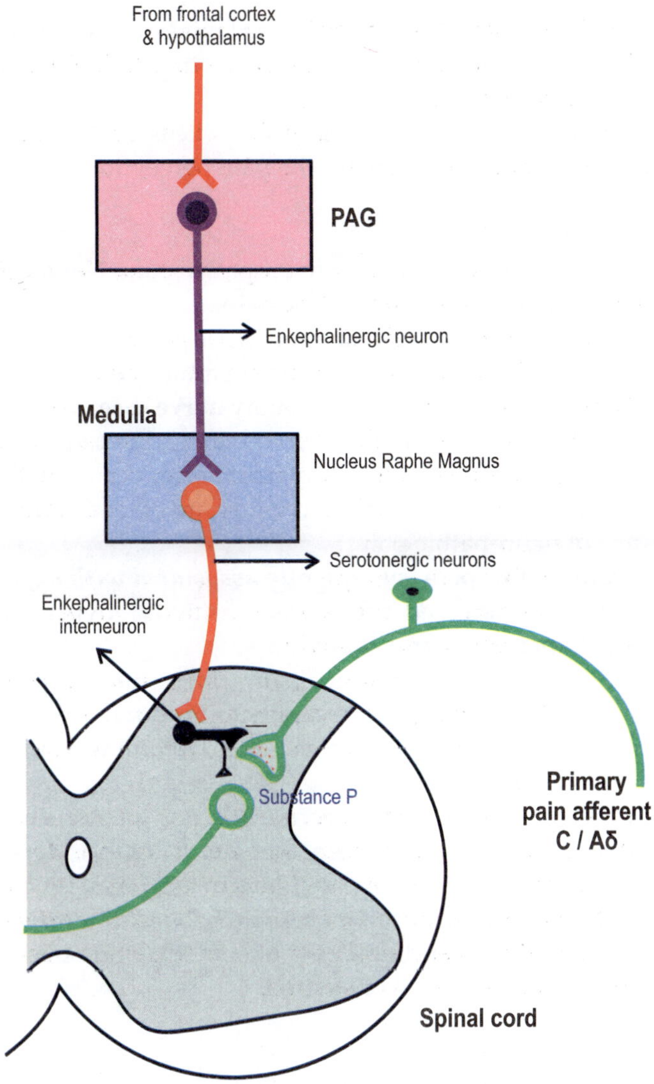

Fig. 99.7: Endogenous neural analgesia system. PAG:Periaqueductal gray; Minus sign is inhibition.

In Chronic Pain: This endogenous pain-inhibiting pathway is activated by prolonged pain that chronically **activates the ascending pain pathways.**

- Fibers from ascending pain pathway **terminate on PAG and raphe nucleus** that in turn activates descending endogenous analgesia system.
- Therefore, in chronic pain, intensity of pain automatically decreases (**auto-inhibition of pain**).

Descending Ceruleospinal Norepinephrinergic Pathway

Cell bodies of descending noradrenergic fibers are located in the **locus ceruleus** of dorsolateral pons. These neurons do not receive inputs from PAG. The fibers **project to dorsal horn** of spinal cord **to inhibit the transmission of nociceptive impulses** from primary afferents.

Endogenous Opioid Systems

Morphine is a potent endogenous **analgesic peptide.** It acts at synapses of the nociceptive pathways by binding to specific sites, the **opiate receptors**. The binding of morphine molecules to an opiate receptor decreases nociceptive synaptic excitability.

There are **three major classes of opiate receptors**: μ, δ and κ. Genes encoding these receptors are found to be members of G protein-coupled class of receptors. Morphine is a **potent agonist at the μ receptor.**

- Opiates such as morphine act **presynaptically and postsynaptically** to inhibit the transmission of impulses from Aδ and C fibers.
- **Increased potassium conductance** of postsynaptic membrane produces postsynaptic inhibition and **inhibition of release of substance P** *from terminals of sensory neurons* results in ***presynaptic inhibition.***
  - These effects are **reversed by** naloxone, the narcotic antagonist that binds to μ receptor.
- **Acupuncture and acupressure** produce analgesia by facilitating the release of ***endogenous opioids.***
  - There are many opioid peptides synthesized endogenously in our body.
  - These are collectively known as **endorphins** (endogenous morphine like substances).
- The important endorphins are **enkephalins** (leu-enkephalin and met-enkephalin), **β-endorphin, γ-endorphin, dynorphin, α-neoendorphins**, etc.
- The ***endorphin receptors*** are particularly present in the spinal cord, PAG of midbrain and raphe nucleus in the medulla.
  - The endorphins produce **profound analgesia** when they are secreted from different parts of the brain in response to different stimuli.

However, the major disadvantage of opioid is that on chronic use they produce **addiction and tolerance** (Clinical Note 99.2)

Clinical Note 99.2

Chronic opioid use produces addiction & tolerance: Repeated use of opioid analgesics results in **addiction and tolerance**, mechanisms of which are not clearly known. It has been proposed that tolerance results from an uncoupling of opioid receptor from its associated G proteins. A protein called **β-arrestin-2** that phosphorylates G protein is responsible for development of addiction, but not tolerance.

Gate Control Theory of Pain

According to this theory, pain can be modulated by the peripheral mechanisms, especially by **gating the impulses** in the spinal cord.

- This theory postulates that the **collaterals from large myelinated afferent fibers** associated with tactile sensibility produce **presynaptic inhibition of Aδ and C fibers** in the dorsal horn of spinal cord.
- Thus, activity in the large afferent fibers regulates (as a gate in the spinal cord) the transmission of impulses originating in the pain receptors.

- **Acupuncture analgesia** acts by gate control mechanism and **release of endorphins** (Clinical Note 99.3).

Clinical Note 99.3

Acupuncture-Induced Analgesia: In acupuncture, needle-puncture is made at a distant but specific location from the site of pain. The exact anatomical link between the site of pain and the site of acupuncture is not known. It is proposed that analgesia in this method occurs by two important mechanisms: **release of endorphins** and the **gate control mechanism** as described above.

Stress-induced Analgesia

During stress, reaction of the individual to pain is suppressed. This results in analgesia. Stress induced analgesia occurs by **both opioid and nonopioid mechanisms**. Stress **activates descending analgesia systems**.

Specific Pain Syndromes

Terminologies

Hyperalgesia: Hyperalgesia refers to increased sensitivity and lowered threshold to painful stimuli. Inflammation of skin is among the common causes of hyperalgesia.

Hypoalgesia: Hypalgesia or hypoalgesia refers to decreased sensitivity and raised threshold to painful stimuli.

Analgesia: Complete loss of pain sensation. Analgesia may not be associated with loss of other sensations.

Hyperpathia: This is a **defect in pain perception**, which is associated with an increased reaction to the pain stimulus once it is perceived. In general term, it is the exaggerated response to pain. However, in this condition there is also an increased reaction to other stimuli.

Allodynia: This is a state in which there is **excessive response to even mild stimuli**. For example, a stimulus like light touch which is never painful, elicits pain in allodynia.

Causalgia

Causalgia is a burning pain that usually develops following a **traumatic peripheral nerve injury**. The pain is continuous and often accompanied by hyperalgesia and allodynia. It is interesting to note that causalgia *persists even after the complete recovery from the nerve damage.*

- The sympathetic fibers are proposed to be responsible for maintaining causalgia, as it is **relieved by sympathectomy** or by using **adrenergics blockers**.
- The noradrenergic sympathetic fibers overgrow into the dorsal root ganglia of sensory nerves from the injured area. Therefore, sympathetic discharge results in pain in the injured area.

Inflammatory Pain

Commonest cause of pain is inflammation. Inflammation occurs following injury.

- Mediators of inflammation like cytokines and substance P increase sensitivity and lower the threshold for pain in the injured area.
- Thus, a minor painful stimulus elicits severe pain. These substances increase the pain perception.

Neuropathic Pain

Injury to the nerve results in neuropathic pain. **Neuralgia** is a general term for neuropathic pain.

- **Trigeminal neuralgia** due to herpes zoster (including causalgia) is an example of neuropathic pain.
- Neuropathic pain occurs in **many nerve diseases**.
  - Diabetic neuropathy, nerve injury, different types of polyneuropathies, root irritation as occurs in disc prolapse and spinal cord injury are other examples of neuropathic pain.
- Neuropathic pain is frequently ***associated with hyperesthesia*** (increased cutaneous sensitivity), hyperalgesia, hyperpathia and allodynia.
  - Usually, neuropathic pain **does not respond well to analgesic** treatment. Epidural injection of mixture of ***analgesic and steroid*** is usually helpful.
- In severe cases, ***nerve section*** (section of the nerve that caries sensation from the site of injury), ***dorsal rhizotomy*** (cutting the pain fibers in the dorsal root) or ***anterolateral cordotomy*** or ***spinothalamic tractotomy*** (cutting the ascending fibers of spinothalamic tract in the spinal cord) are considered.

Tic Douloureux

This is also known as **trigeminal neuralgia**. This is severe and stabbing type of acute facial pain that persists briefly. Most patients develop this syndrome following **compression of the trigeminal nerve roots**.

Thalamic Syndrome

The patients with thalamic syndrome experience chronic, severe and extremely unpleasant pain that occurs either spontaneously or in response to a trivial stimulus.

- The pain is felt in the brain, in the absence of any peripheral pathology.
- It occurs due to **ischemic or hemorrhagic lesions of posterior thalamic nuclei** following obstruction of the ***thalamogeniculate branch of posterior cerebral artery.***
- Pain is cured by surgical destruction of the posterior thalamic nucleus by stereotaxic surgery.

Toothache

Teeth have plenty nociceptors. Teeth are innervated by axons of maxillary and mandibular divisions of trigeminal nerve. The fibers include **unmyelinated C fibers**, and myelinated Aδ and Aβ fibers.

- The fibers enter the tooth through the root apex,

branched within the pulp and then terminate in the plexus of the pulp.
- Enamel and cementum contain no nerve fibers. The pulp is protected and covered by enamel.

- Thus, **exposure of pulp or pulp inflammation** is painful.
- Toothache is caused by heat, cold, inflammation, and mechanical probing of the dental pulp.

ITCH

Receptors and Pathway

Definition

It is defined as an **unpleasant sensation that evokes the desire to scratch**. This is a distinct sensory modality. It can be evoked by mechanical or chemical stimuli. In contrast, **tickle** is a pleasurable sensation.

Receptors

Itch is produced by stimulation of **itch receptors** that are the **endings of unmyelinated C fibers** (these are not the same C fibers that are responsible for pain).

- Itching can be produced by mechanical stimulation of the skin and by application of various chemical agents. Itching invariably occurs when *plasma concentration* **bile salt is high.**
- **Histamine** is the most important chemical agent that produces itching (**antihistaminics** are prescribed to stop itching), though itching can occur without histamine.
- Kinins also produce severe itching.

Pathway

The pathway for transmission of sensation of itch and tickle is **lateral spinothalamic tract**.

TEMPERATURE

Receptors and Pathway

Receptors

There are two types of temperature receptors:

1. The **warmth receptors**, the receptors that respond maximally to the temperature above the body temperature, and,
2. The **cold receptors**, the receptors that respond maximally to temperature below body temperature. Cold receptors respond to the temperature ranging from 10 to 40°C and warm receptors respond from 30–50°C (Fig. 99.8).
3. The sense organs are **naked nerve endings**.

Three special sets of temperature receptors have been recently described.

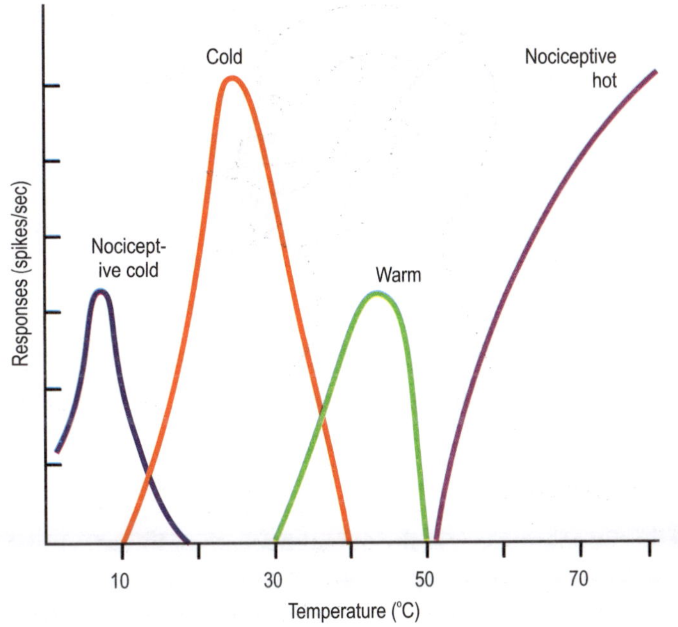

Fig. 99.8: Temperature range for the activation of warm and cold receptors and hot and cold nociceptors.

1. **Cold and methanol sensitive** receptors 1 (**CMR 1**): these are the receptors for moderate cold.
2. **VR 1:** respond to ***very high temperature*** (nociceptive thermoceptors).
3. **VRL 1:** respond to ***moderate to high temperature***.

All these three set of receptors (CMR 1,VR 1 and VRL 1) are ion channels and they belong to **transient receptor potential** (TRP) subfamily.

Pathway

The afferents for cold are **Aδ and C fibers**, and afferents for heat are **C fibers**. The temperature sensation is transmitted by **lateral spinothalamic tract**.

TRIGEMINAL SYSTEM

Trigeminal Pathway

A complete somatosensory representation of the body includes inputs from the trigeminal nerve.

- Trigeminal nerves supply **face, oral cavity, and head.** Trigeminal pathway is different from the pain sensory pathway from other body parts.
  - Trigeminal nerve has **three branches** that supply three different parts of the face (Fig. 99.9).
- The neurons of trigeminal nerve are **pseudobipolar neurons.** They have their cell bodies in the semilunar or gasserian ganglion (trigeminal ganglion).
  - The proximal axons divide into ascending and descending branches to reach two brainstem nuclei.
- These brainstem nuclei are: **spinal nucleus** (spinal V), and the **main sensory nucleus** (main sensory V) of the trigeminal nerve (Fig. 99.10).

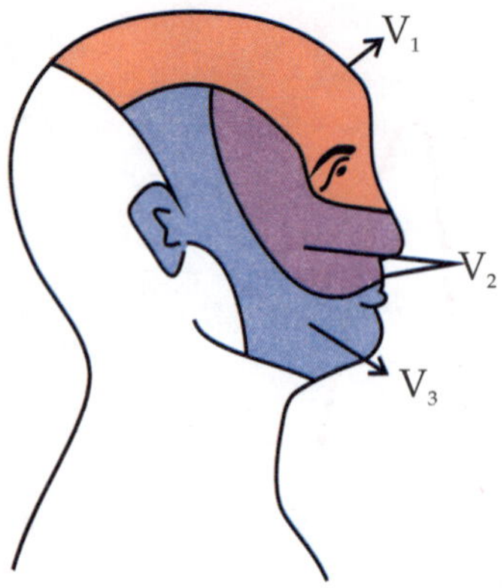

Fig. 99.9: Innervation of face ophthalmic (V_1), maxillary (V_2), and mandibular (V3) divisions of the trigeminal nerve.

Spinal V

The caudal nucleus is the spinal nucleus of the trigeminal nerve, which has **three sub-divisions**:

1. The lower most is the **caudal sub-division** of spinal V that receives *many nociceptive afferent fibers* from the face.
   - Therefore, to relieve untreatable chronic facial pain as occurs in trigeminal neuralgia, surgical lesion of the caudal sub-division spinal nucleus of trigeminal nerve is performed.
2. The middle sub-division is the **interpolar sub-division**, which receives mechanosensitive and nociceptive inputs from teeth and gums, and the mucous membrane of the mouth.
3. The upper most is the **oral sub-division** that receives nociceptive inputs mainly from the oral cavity.

The spinal nucleus receives mainly the nociceptive inputs via **small diameter fibers**. Therefore, this is considered as the **spinothalamic pathway** of the trigeminal system.

Main Sensory V

This nucleus is situated rostrally. It receives ipsilateral projections from the *low threshold mechanoreceptors* from face and teeth. The fibers are large diameter fibers. Therefore, the main sensory V is considered to be the **trigeminal homologue of dorsal column nuclei**.

1. The input from trigeminal nuclei reaches thalamus via **trigeminal lemniscus** (Fig. 99.10), which runs along the medial lemniscus.
2. The projections are primarily contralateral thalamus. In thalamus fibers terminate in the specific nuclei i. e. ventral posterior and lateral (VPL) and posterior (PO) nuclei of thalamus. The VPL receives inputs from the rostral sub-divisions of spinal V and from main sensory V, whereas the PO receives inputs from the caudal sub-divisions of spinal V (Fig. 140.2).

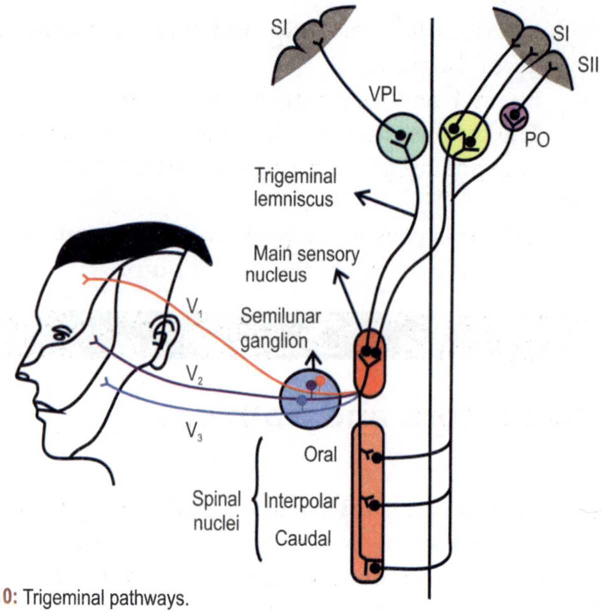

Fig. 99.10: Trigeminal pathways.

The VPL nucleus of the thalamus projects to the **ventrolateral portion of the somatosensory cortex** (SI). The cortical representation of the face is relatively enormous, due to its high innervation density. The representation of mouth and tongue is also larger. Both SI and SII receive trigeminal inputs from the thalamus.

Applied Physiology

Trigeminal Neuralgia

This is a condition of severe and stabbing type of ***acute facial pain*** that persists briefly.

- The pain is initiated by application of an innocuous stimulus to the **trigger zone**, which is a very specific and restricted area on the face.
  - The trigger zone may be located on the cheek, nose, lip, oral mucosa, teeth, or scalp.
  - The trigger zone may not have a particular relation to the area from which the pain is perceived.
- Most patients develop this syndrome following **compression of the trigeminal nerve roots.**
  - The root compression causes nerve irritation or degeneration that results in episodic bursts of severe pain.
- If adequate control is not achieved with analgesic, **surgical release of trigeminal compression or lesions of trigeminal ganglion** may be considered.

Exam Questions

1. With the help of a labeled schematic diagram, trace the pathway for pain. Describe the physiology of pain recognition and perception.
2. With the help of a labeled schematic diagram, trace the pathway for endogenous analgesia system, and give a note on opiate receptors.
3. Define referred pain and give two examples. Describe the theories of refereed pain.
4. With the help of a labeled schematic diagram, describe the pain pathway in trigeminal system

Multiple Choice Questions (of Chapter 98 and 99)

6. All of the following statements are true for dorsal column nuclei, EXCEPT:
   A. Present in the medulla
   B. Nucleus gracilis is located medially
   C. Nucleus cuneatus is located laterally
   D. Nucleus gracilis receives sensation from upper limb

7. Sensation of tactile discrimination is transmitted in:
   A. Dorsal column pathway
   B. Anterior spinothalamic tract
   C. Lateral spinothalamic tract
   D. Dorsal spinocerebellar tract

8. Sensation of fast pain is transmitted in:
   A. Dorsal column pathway
   B. Anterior spinothalamic tract
   C. Paleospinothalmaic tract
   D. Neospinothalamic tract

9. Sensation of slow pain is transmitted in:
   A. Dorsal column pathway
   B. Anterior spinothalamic tract
   C. Paleospinothalmaic tract
   D. Dorsal spinocerebellar tract

10. Sensation of temperature is transmitted in:
   A. Dorsal column pathway
   B. Anterior spinothalamic tract
   C. Lateral spinothalamic tract
   D. Dorsal spinocerebellar tract

11. All of the following are true for the second order neurons of sensory system, EXCEPT:
   A. Transmit the sensation to ipsilateral thalamus
   B. Always cross the midline
   C. Cell bodies are present in spinal cord or in the brainstem
   D. Known as medial lemniscus in dorsal column pathway

12. Sensation of itch is transmitted in:
   A. Dorsal column pathway
   B. Anterior spinothalamic tract
   C. Lateral spinothalamic tract
   D. Dorsal spinocerebellar tract

13. Usually how many order of neurons are present in a sensory pathway from receptor to cortex?
   A. Two B. Three
   C. Four D. Five

14. Which of the following sensation is not carried in dorsal column pathway?
   A. Vibration B. Stereognosis
   C. Crude touch D. Proprioception

15. Anterior spinothalamic tract carries the sensation of:
   A. Pain B. Temperature
   C. Vibration D. Crude touch

16. Tract of Goll and Burdach belong to:
   A. Dorsal column pathway
   B. Dorsal spinocerebellar pathway
   C. Anterior spinothalamic tract
   D. Lateral spinothalamic tract

17. Maximum distance for tactile localization is observed at:
   A. Tip of fingers B. Lips
   C. Palm and hand D. Back of scapula

18. Vibration sensation is impaired in all of the following, EXCEPT:
A. Vitamin B12 deficiency
   B. Early part of tabes dorsalis
   C. Chronic diabetes mellitus
   D. Tuberculosis

19. All of the following are true for proprioception and kinesthesia, EXCEPT:
   A. Receptors are slowly adapting spray endings
   B. Receptors are Pacinian corpuscles in the synovia and ligaments
   C. Fibers project to midbrain
   D. Describe the sense of position and movement of body parts

20. Inability to maintain a balanced standing position with feet together and eyes closed, is:
   A. Romberg sign B. Sign of cerebellar dysfunction
   C. Sign of vestibular dysfunction D. Sign of thalamic lesion

21. Nerve ending sensitive to noxious stimuli are present in all, EXCEPT:
   A. Stomach B. Intestine
   C. Mesentery D. Brain

22. Pain-sensitive intracranial structure is:
   A. Piamater B. Pial vessels
   C. Duramater D. Brain matter

23. Vanilloid receptors are activated by:
   A. Pain B. Vibration
   C. Touch D. Pressure

24. Which of the following is 'True' about visceral pain:
   A. It is poorly localized
   B. Resembles 'fast pain' produced by noxious stimulation of the skin
   C. Mediated by B fibers in the dorsal roots of the spinal nerves
   D. Causes relaxation of nearby skeletal muscles

25. Endogenous analgesia neurons from PAG to raphe nucleus mainly release:
   A. Serotonin B. Enkephalin
   C. Glutamate D. Substance P

26. Primary sensory afferent carrying pain sensation release which of the following neurotransmitter in dorsal horn at its ending on second order neuron?
   A. Substance P B. GABA
   C. Enkephalin D. Serotonin

27. Transcutaneous Electrical Nerve Stimulation (TENS) is based on
   A. Central pain B. Referred pain
   C. Gate controlled theory of pain D. Allodynia

28. Which of the following is not a theory of referred pain:
   A. Gate control theory B. Facilitation theory
   C. Convergence theory D. Dermatomal theory

29. The ascending pain fibers in paleospinothalamic pathway while ascending to cortex, provide collaterals to all the following structures, EXCEPT:
   A. PAG B. Reticular formation
   C. Hypothalamus D. Nucleus tractus solitarius

Answers:

6. D	7. A	8. D	9. C	10. C
11. A	12. C	13. B	14. C	15. D
16. A	17. D	18. D	19. C	20. A
21. D	22. C	23. A	24. A	25. B
26. A	27. C	28. A	29. D	

Chapter 100

Thalamus

Learning Objectives

On completion of study of this chapter:

The student will be able to (must know):

1. Name the major nuclear groups in the thalamus and give their functions.
2. Describe the connections and functions of thalamus.
3. Correlate the functions of thalamus with thalamic dysfunctions.
4. Outline the functions of epithalamus and subthalamus.

The student may also be able to (desirable to know):

1. Describe the physiological basis of thalamic syndrome.

FUNCTIONAL ORGANIZATION

Thalamus is an egg-shaped nuclear structure present obliquely atop the brain stem. There are two thalami on both sides. Anteriorly they are separated by the third ventricle and the corpora quadrigemina is present between their posterior parts.

Thalamic Nuclei

The thalamus is composed of a number of discrete nuclei. Anatomically, a **Y shaped internal medullary lamina** splits thalamus into **three parts**: anterior, medial and lateral group of nuclei (Fig. 100.1).

1. **The anterior group** of nuclei is enclosed by the bifurcation of the internal medullary lamina.
2. **The medial group** of nuclei consists of the medial nucleus, the midline nucleus, centromedian and the intralaminar nucleus.
3. **The lateral group** of nuclei is further divided into dorsal and ventral nuclear groups of nuclei.

- The ***dorsal nuclear group*** contains lateral posterior nucleus, lateral dorsal nucleus and pulvinar.
- The ***ventral nuclear group*** is comprised of ventral anterior, ventral lateral and ventral posterior nuclei, and medial and lateral geniculate bodies.

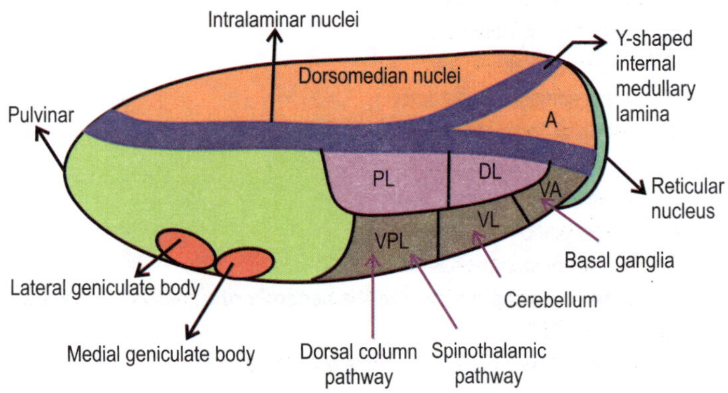

Fig. 100.1: Nuclei of thalamus (A: Anterior; VA: Ventral anterior; VL: Ventral Lateral; VPL: Ventral posterolateral; DL: Lateral dorsal; PL: Lateral posterior). Purple arrows indicate afferent fibers.

The ventral posterior group, also known as **ventrobasal complex**, consists of venteroposterolateral and ventroposteromedian groups of nuclei.

Physiological Nuclear Groups and their Connections

Physiologically, thalamic nuclei are divided into **four groups**:

1. **Specific relay nuclei:** Ascending afferent inputs synapse on these nuclei. The axons arising from them transmit the afferent impulse to cortex. This nuclear group consists of **ventrobasal complex** (VBC), **lateral geniculate body** (LGB), **medial geniculate body** (MGB), and anterior nucleus.
   - **Ventrobasal complex** receives inputs from dorsal column pathway, anterolateral system and corticothalamic fibers, and projects to somatosensory cortex.
   - The trigeminal lemniscus carries the general sensations from face along with the gustatory afferents and project to the **ventral posterior (VP)**

nucleus that transmits the afferent inputs to the postcentral gyrus (Fig. 100.2).

- **LGB** receives input from optic tract and projects to visual cortex.
- **MGB** receives input from auditory pathway and projects to auditory cortex.
- The **anterior nucleus** receives inputs from the hypothalamus through the mamillothalamic tract and relays the information to the cingulate gyrus.

2. **Association nuclei:** This nuclear group consists of **pulvinar, dorsal nuclei** and **lateral posterior nucleus**.
   - These nuclei receive inputs from sensory cortex and limbic system and project diffusely to the association cortex or to sub-cortical structures.

- The pulvinar projects to the inferior parietal lobe.
- The dosolateral nucleus is reciprocally connected to the precuneate gyrus.

3. **Non-specific nuclei:** These include **intralaminar** (IM), **midline**, **centromedian** (CM) nuclei, and reticular nuclei (RET).

- They receive inputs mainly from reticular formation and paleospinothalamic tract, and also inputs from striatum, hypothalamus and other thalamic nuclei.
- They project diffusely to wide areas of cerebral cortex, to thalamus and limbic system.

4. **Motor nuclei:** These include **lateral, ventral anterior** and **ventral lateral nuclei**.

- The ventral lateral nucleus receives input from the cerebellum through the dentato-rubro-thalamic tract and projects to the motor cortex area 4 and 6. The ventral anterior nucleus receives inputs from basal ganglia (globus pallidus) and projects to the premotor cortex (Fig. 100.2).

The thalamic nuclei are also divided into **extrinsic and intrinsic nuclei**. The specific relay nuclei are known as extrinsic nuclei and rest others as intrinsic nuclei. It should be noted that all somatosensory information reaches all of these different types of thalamic nuclei.

CONNECTIONS AND FUNCTIONS

The ascending somatosensory pathways terminate in certain thalamic nuclei. The sensory signals mostly arise form contralateral receptors of the body (Fig. 100.3).

1. Axons from cells in the **dorsal column nuclei** cross the brain stem immediately at the level of the medulla and travel in the contralateral medial lemniscus to terminate primarily in the **ventral-posterolateral nucleus** (VPL) of the thalamus.

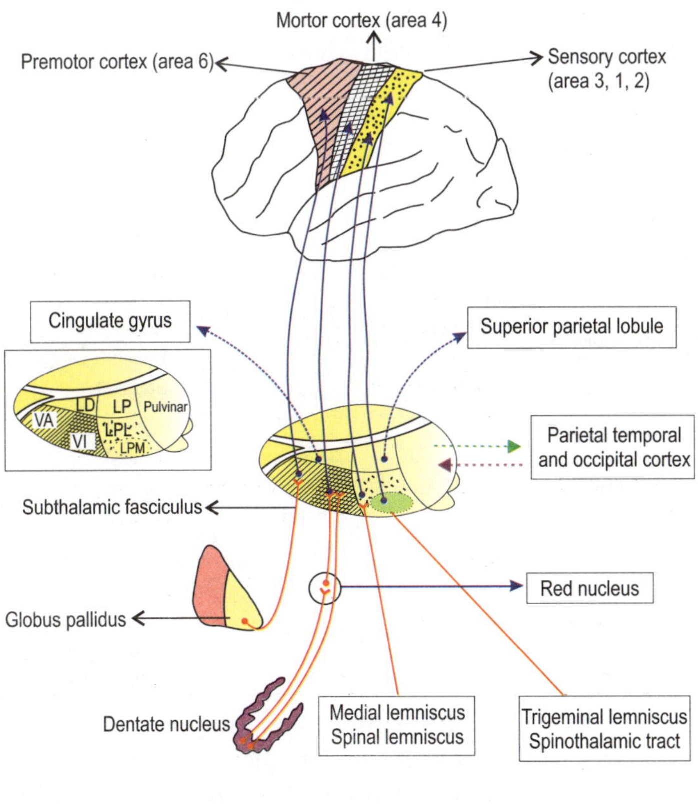

Fig. 100.2: Affarent and efferent connections of specific nuclear groups of thalamus. Note that sensory lemniscal inputs (medial lemniscus, spinal lemniscus and trigeminal lemniscus) project to VPL and VPM nuclei, which in turn project to Area 3, 1, 2 of sensory cortex. Basal ganglia (globus pallidus) project to ventral anterior (VA) nucleus, which in turn projects to premotor cortex and cerebellum (dentate nucleus) projects to ventral intermediate (VI) nucleus, which in turn projects to motor cortex (area 4).

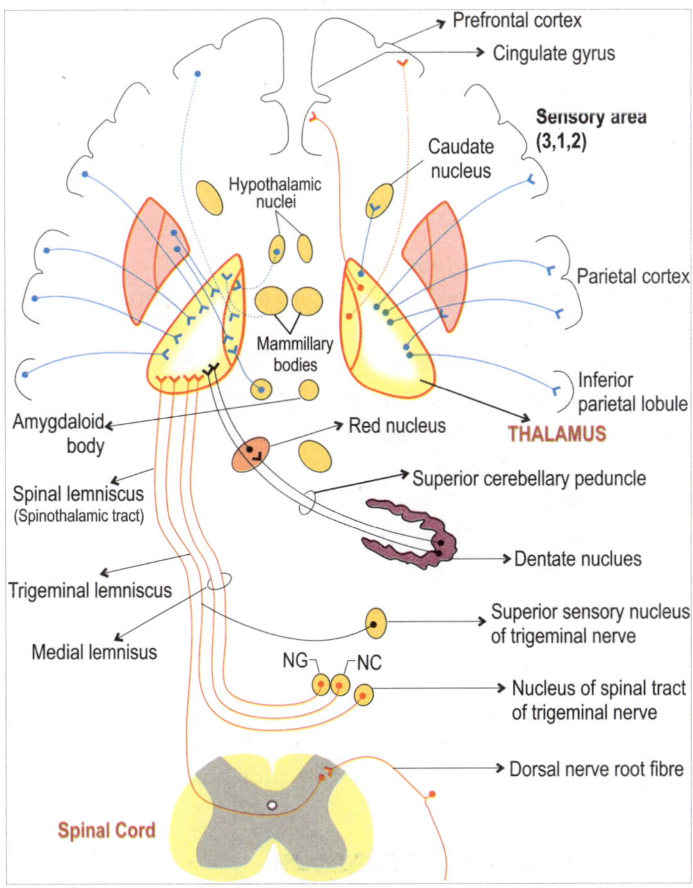

Fig. 100.3: Main afferent and efferent connections of thalamus. NG: Nucleus gracilis; NC: Nucleus cuneatus.

2. The fibers of the **anterolateral system** (lateral and anterior spinothalamic tracts) travel in the contralateral anterolateral funiculus of the spinal cord to terminate in the VPL, posterior (PO) and intralaminar (IM) nuclei.
3. **Reticulothalamic fibers** of the spinoreticulothalamic pathway remain *largely uncrossed* and terminate in IM, midline or centromedian (CM) nuclei, and in the thalamic reticular nuclei (RET).

The VPL and PO project to cortical regions. IM diffusely projects to cortex and RET is reciprocally connected with other thalamic nuclei.

Ventral Posterolateral Nucleus (VPL)

The VPL receives input from **many of ascending sensory pathways.** Each pathway has a typical pattern of termination in VPL nucleus.

- The central core of VPL nucleus receives largely cutaneous inputs.
- The dorsal aspect of VPL receives mostly deep inputs, whereas anterior surface receives muscle inputs.

Thus, the VPL consists of a **core of cutaneous inputs** and a **shell of deep inputs**.

- The afferent fibers from the face, arm and leg are represented in a medial to lateral manner in the VPL nucleus.

Posterior Nuclei (PO)

PO receives nociceptive inputs. Cells in PO respond to a variety of somatic and non-somatic modalities.

- PO is mainly involved in the **transmission of nociceptive impulses**.
- Large lesion in PO produces analgesia and stimulation of PO produces pain sensations.

However, there is no somatotopic organization in PO.

Intralaminar Nuclei and Reticular Nuclei

Cells in intralaminar nuclei (IM) have large, somatic receptive fields. They are activated by nociceptive and other sensory stimuli.

- Responses in IM are strongly affected by the level of **arousal, attention and affect.**
    - IM has diffuse but **strong projection to the cortex, striatum and limbic system.**
- Cells in reticular nuclei (RET) respond to a variety of somatosensory modalities.
- RET does not project to cortex but is reciprocally connected to other thalamic nuclei.
- Thus, RET is involved in the modulation of thalamic activity.

Functions of Thalamus PY10.7

All afferent impulses on their way to the sensory cortex terminate in the thalamus.

1. **Relay station for all somatic sensations:** Thalamus conveys the sensory information to the cortex through thalamocortical projections (Table 100.1).

Table 100.1 | **Table 100.1: Connections and functions of major thalamic nuclei.**

Nuclear Group	Major Afferents	Major Efferents	Functions
A. Specific Nuclei			
Lateral-ventral cortex, movement.	Dentatothalamic tract, & pallidothalamic tract	Thalamocortical tract (to motor area 4 and 6)	Proprioceptive input to control of voluntary
Postero-ventral	Spinothalamic fibers, trigeminothalamic fiber, & medial lemniscus.	To sensory cortex (area 3, 1 and 2)	Relay of all somatosensory inputs including face.
Dorsal-lateral	From parietal lobe	To parietal lobe	Language and speech.
Pulvinar	From parietal, temporal and occipital lobes	To parietal, temporal and occipital lobes	Integrates somatic, auditory and visual information.
LGB	From optic tract	To visual cortex	Vision
MGB	From cochlea and inferior colliculi	To auditory cortex	Audition
A. Nonspecific Nuclei			
Anterior group	Mammillothalamic tract	To cingulated gyrus	Memory and emotion
Midline group	All ascending fibers, & from hypothalamus and reticular formation	To neocortex, BG & hypothalamus	Integration of somatic and visceral sensations, & arousal.
Intralaminar	From RAS & BG	To neocortex and prefrontal cortex	Arousal and motor functions.
Dorso-medial	From hypothalamus & prefrontal cortex	To prefrontal cortex	Association center for synthesis of crude somatic sensations.

- Thus, it is the **major relay station** for sensory inputs in humans and higher order of animals, whereas in lower order of animals, it acts as the center for **sensory integration**.

2. **Relay of special sensations:** Thalamus is the relay center for all special sensations **except olfaction**.

- The lateral and medial geniculate bodies receive the visual and auditory afferents respectively.

- The VPL nucleus receives the taste afferents.

3. **Arousal mechanisms:** Thalamocortical projects from nonspecific nuclei to cortex contributes to reticular activating system that activates arousal mechanisms and keeps the individual awake.
4. **Subcortical Perception of Sensations:** Subcortical perception of **pain, temperature, pressure (crude touch)** occurs to some extent in thalamus.
   - Thalamus is not only the relay station, but also the integration center for these sensations. Therefore, these sensations remain intact considerably in cortical lesion.
5. **Motor Functions:** Thalamus is an integral part of motor loop of the brain in which globs pallidus of basal ganglia projects mainly to VPL nucleus of thalamus (via pallidothalamic tract) and thalamus projects to the motor cortex (via thalamocortical fibers), which projects back to the basal ganglia.
   - Through motor loop thalamus influences postural movements.
   - Thalamus also links cerebellum and motor cortex via dentato-rubro-thalamo-cortical tract.
   - Thorough this connection, thalamus influences planning and programming of movements.
6. **Memory and Emotion:** Anterior thalamus is a constituent of **Papez circuit**.
   - It receives input from mamillary body of limbic system via mamillothalamic tract.
   - Through this connection, thalamus is concerned with recent memory and emotion.
7. **Synchronization of EEG:** Stimulation of intralaminar thalamic nuclei at low frequency causes synchronization of EEG waves recorded from ipsilateral cortex.
   - This is called recruiting response.
   - However, high frequency stimulation causes arousal and desynchronization.
8. **Role in Sleep:** A circuit linking the thalamus and cortex **(thalamocortical loop)** is important in generating the pattern of brain activity in sleep-wake cycle.
   - Inhibitory thalamic reticular neurons are proposed to be the part of this neuronal network that causes induction of sleep.
9. **Sensory Motor Coordination:** Thalamus receives all sensory inputs from the body and closely interacts with basal ganglia, cerebellum and motor cortex.
   - Therefore, thalamus is one of the major structures in the brain for coordination between sensory and motor functions, especially in the **sensory feedback for correction and improvement in motor output.**
10. **Language and Speech:** Dorsal lateral nucleus of thalamus is reciprocally connected with parietal lobe of the brain, and therefore is concerned with language and speech and complex integrated functions.

APPLIED ASPECTS

Thalamic Syndrome

Lesion of the VPL occurs due to thrombosis of **posterolateral branch of the posterior cerebral artery**.

1. This results in **severe impairment of the discriminative touch and pressure** sensations of **contralateral side**, whereas diffuse touch, temperature, and pain sensations are often less impaired.
2. Also, there will be decreased muscle tone, profound weakness of the muscles and ataxia as VPL nucleus receives afferent impulses from cerebellum and relays them to the motor cortex, area 4 and 6.
3. The emotion may be affected.

Vascular lesions **usually spare the medial thalamus** including VPM nuclear group. Therefore, sensations in the face and head often remain intact.

Other Deficits: When the thalamus is damaged, not only thalamic functions are lost, but also many cortical functions are affected, as cortex is intimately connected with thalamus.

Electrical lesion of intralaminar nuclei relieves chronic suffering type of pain, though the acute perception of pain remains intact.

EPITHALAMUS

The epithalamus consists of the structures that **form the roof of the third ventricle**.

- These include the **pineal gland, the habenular nuclei and the striae medullaris**.
- Externally, it is seen above the superior colliculi.

SUBTHALAMUS

The subthalamus is located **between the upper end of substantia nigra and the thalamus**.

- Subthalamus contains sensory fasciculi, rostral extensions of midbrain nuclei, fiber bundle from cerebellum and globus pallidus, and subthalamic nuclei.
- Fibers in the supramamillary commissure interconnect subthalamic structures.
- The subthalamic nucleus (body of Luys) has reciprocal connection with the globus pallidus

Lesion of subthalamic nucleus results in **hemiballismus** (for detail, see Basal Ganglia).

Exam Questions

1. With the help of a labeled schematic diagrams, describe the connections and functions of thalamus.
2. Classify thalamic nuclei. Briefly describe connections and functions of specific nuclei of thalamus. Add a note on thalamic syndrome.

Multiple Choice Questions

1. Which of the following is the specific nucleus of thalamus?
A. VPL
B. Midline
C. Intralaminar
D. Centromedian

2. Which of the following nucleus of thalamus is not directly involved in regulation of motor functions?
A. Lateral
B. Ventral anterior
C. Ventral lateral
D. Centromedian

3. Which nucleus of thalamus controls visual functions?
A. MGB
B. LGB
C. Pulvinar
D. Anterior

4. Which of the following nucleus is not association nucleus of thalamus?
A. Pulvinar
B. Dorsal
C. Lateral posterior
D. Intralaminar

5. Which of the following is not the direct function of the thalamus?
A. Relay center of all sensations
B. Perception of pain temperature and pressure
C. Sensory motor coordination
D. Secretion of hormones

6. Which of the following statement is not correct about thalamic syndrome?
A. Usually occurs due to thrombosis of posterolateral branch of posterior cerebral artery
B. There will be severe impairment of discriminative touch and pressure sensations of opposite side
C. Emotion is never affected
D. Vascular lesion usually spares medial nuclear group, hence sensation of head and face often remain intact.

Answers

1. A **2. D** **3. B** **4. D** **5. D** **6. C**

Chapter 101

Sensory Cortex

Learning Objectives

On completion of study of this chapter:

The student will be able to (must know):

1. Name cortical sensory areas and give their connections and functions.
2. Mention the effects of lesion of each sensory area.
3. Illustrate the organization of sensory homunculus and its physiological significance.

The student may also be able to (desirable to know):

1. Describe the connections and functions of sensory cortex.

CORTICAL SENSORY AREAS

The cortical areas associated with processing of somatic sensory information collectively form **somatosensory cortex**. These are:

Primary Somatosensory Area I (SI): SI is present **in the post-central gyrus**, especially on the posterior bank and floor of the central sulcus.

- SI includes the **Brodmann's area 3, 1, and 2** (Fig. 101.1).
- Area 3 has two sub-areas: 3a and 3b.

Primary Somatosensory Area II (SII): SII is located in the **wall of the Sylvian fissure** (superior bank of the lateral sulcus).

Somatosensory Association Cortex (Brodmann's area 5): This is present in the **posterior parietal lobe**.

- This is also called **higher somatosensory cortex**, as it largely receives inputs from SI and SII.
- Lesion of this area produces more subtle deficits of sensations.

Supplementary Sensory Area: This is part of the posterior parietal association area located on the **medial wall of the parietal lobe.**

Other Somatosensory Areas: Other areas include:

1. ***Pre-central gyrus (area 4):*** Though this is the primary motor cortex, it also receives somatosensory signals.

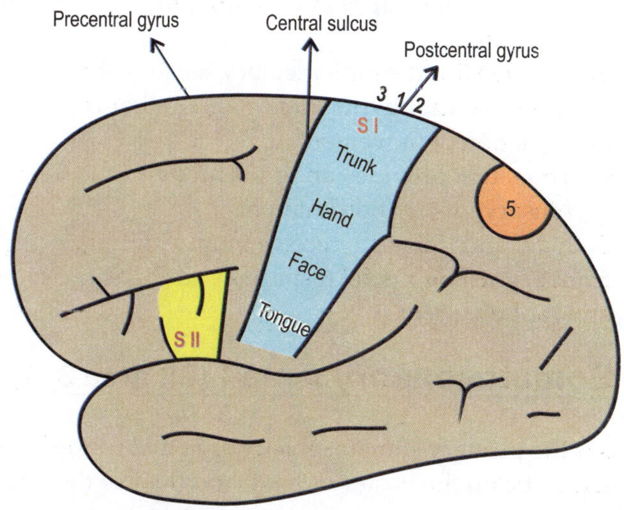

Fig. 101.1: Cortical sensory areas.

2. ***Cortical areas surrounding SII (area 7b):*** The cells in this area also respond to somatosensory stimuli.

Connections of Somatosensory Areas

Somatosensory areas are interconnected to each other (Fig. 101.2) as follows:

1. All sub-areas of **SI** make reciprocal and specific point-to-point connection with the **VPL nuclear group in the thalamus.**
   - The main projection to the thalamus is from the **area 3a.**
2. **SII** receives inputs from **ventrobasal nucleus** of the thalamus.
   - There is a serial flow of information from area 3b to area 5.
   - **Area 3a** is reciprocally connected with area 1 and 2.
4. **SI and SII** have extensive **reciprocal connections**.

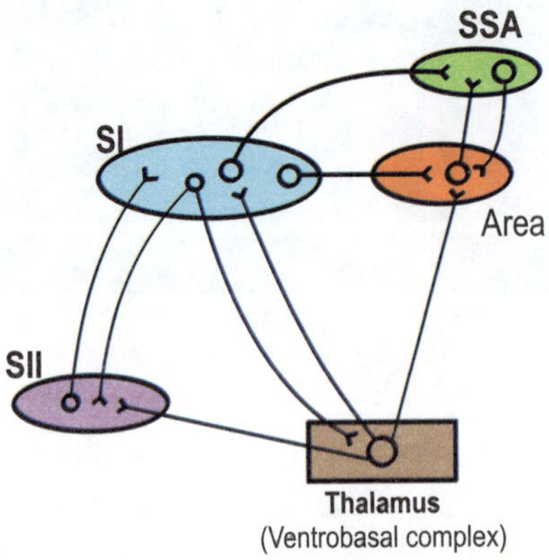

Fig. 101.2: Interconnections between cortical sensory areas. SSA: Supplementary sensory area

5. **Area 5** receives input only from the lateral posterior nucleus of the thalamus, which does not receive direct somatosensory inputs.
   - SI and SII are connected with their homologous areas in the **opposite hemisphere** via corpus callosum.
7. **SI, SII, area 5** and supplementary sensory areas project to the **pre-central gyrus** (area 4 and 6) that is involved in regulation of movement.
   - Thus, this provides an opportunity in the CNS for sensory motor coordination.
8. Both SI and SII also receive **monoaminergic input from brainstem nuclei** (especially from locus ceruleus and raphe nuclei).

Somatosensory Area I (SI: area 3, 1, 2)

This is the **primary somatosensory area** that resides in the parietal lobe on the posterior bank and floor of the central sulcus.

Inputs

SI receives inputs mainly from following **thalamic and cortical areas**.

1. VPL nucleus of the thalamus,
2. SII area, and
3. Brainstem nuclei (locus ceruleus and raphe nucleus)

Outputs

SI projects mainly to the following thalamic and cortical areas

1. VPL nucleus of the thalamus
2. Supplementary sensory area
3. SII
4. Area 5
5. Area 4 and 6 (motor cortex)

Sub-Regions (based on modality specificity)

SI is the **area 3, 1, and 2**. Area 3 is subdivided into area **3a and 3b**.

- This division of SI is ***based on their modality specificity***.
- That means whether they respond to cutaneous (from the skin) or deep (from muscles and joints) stimuli.

Area 3a and 2: Respond mainly to deep stimulation (i. e. from the muscles and joints).
They respond poorly to cutaneous stimulation.
Area 1: Responds to both cutaneous and deep stimulation.
Area 3b: Responds mainly to cutaneous stimulation.

Topographic Organization

Entire body is **represented twice** in SI (once in area 3b, and again in area 1). The topographic representation is called the **sensory homunculus** (Fig. 101.3).

- In this sensory map in brain, face is represented in the lateral part, hand and upper extremity are represented in the dorsolateral part of the post central gyrus, and lower extremity on the medial surface of the hemisphere.
- The **greatest area of the map is devoted for face, especially lips** (area devoted for speech), **and hand, especially the digits** (cutaneous sensations from areas involved in skilled activities).
- The cortical receiving areas **for trunk and back are small.**

Columnar Organization

Especially in SI, the neurons are arranged along a line **perpendicular to the cortical surface**, which is known the *columnar organization*.

- Cortical columns that are located adjacently **process different sensory modalities.**
-

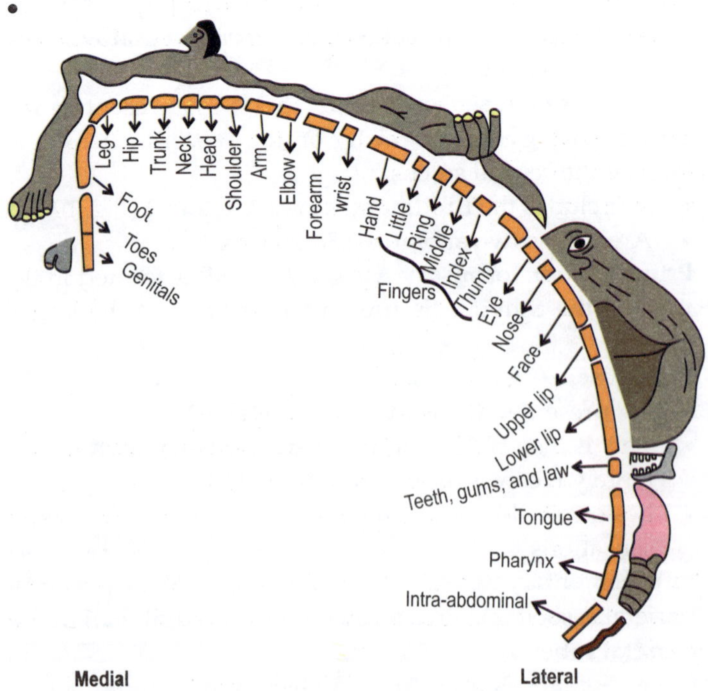

Fig. 101.3: Sensory homunculus. Note that larger cortical representations are from face and hands.

- For example, the column in the area 3b responds to cutaneous stimulation (that come from rapidly adapting mechanoreceptors), whereas the column in the area 3a responds to deep stimulation (mainly from slowly adapting mechanoreceptors).

Functions

SI is involved in the **initial processing of the somatosensory input**. It also processes higher sensory orders like perception of the direction of an applied stimulus. The functions of SI are best studied by producing lesions.

Effects of Lesions: Cortical lesions do not completely abolish somatic sensation.

- **Proprioception and fine touch are most affected** by cortical lesions.
- **Temperature and pain** sensibility are *least affected*.
- **Cortical sensations** (tactile localization, tactile discrimination, and stereognosis) are ***almost abolished***.

However, damage to different parts of SI produces different sensory deficits.

1. **Lesion of SI** of one side results in clear deficit in all aspects of somesthesis in the *contralateral body parts*.
2. With selective **lesions of area 3**, there is *failure to learn the discriminative task* even after repeated trials.
3. **Lesion of area 1** causes significant *impairment of hard-soft, or smooth-rough discrimination*, but no deficit in other aspects of sensory learning.
4. Damage to **postcentral gyrus** also causes *impairment of kinesthesia* (inability to appreciate passive position and movements of different body parts).
5. Damage to **area 5** specifically *affects stereognosis*, with other tactile sensation remaining intact.

There is least impairment of pain and temperature sensation in cortical lesion.

Somatosensory area II (SII)

SII is **located in the superior wall of the Sylvian fissure** (the fissure that separates temporal lobe from frontal and parietal lobe).

- The topographic organization is such that head is represented at the inferior end of the post central gyrus and the feet at the bottom of the sylvian fissure.

Functions: Most of the neurons of SII **respond to light mechanical stimulation** of the hair or skin (rapidly adapting mechanoreceptors).

- They *poorly respond to deep stimuli.*

Effects of Lesion: Lesion of SII results **deficit in learning based on tactile discrimination**.

Association Cortex

Association sensory cortex is present in the parietal lobe (**parietal association cortex**).

- It receives inputs mainly from SI, but also from SII and visual cortex.

Functions: The major function of the parietal association cortex is to **coordinate the relationship of the body to extrapersonal space**, for example, *hand-eye coordination*.

- In the **non-dominant hemisphere**, the association cortex is involved in ***spatial relations***, whereas in the **dominant hemisphere** it is concerned with ***language***.

Effects of Lesion: A lesion of parietal association cortex of the non-dominant hemisphere produces **impairments in the ability to relate to extrapersonal space**.

- For example, if the subject is asked to copy a geometry, the figures are distorted.
  - The person develops **constructional apraxia** (defect in constructing a picture) and **hemineglect syndrome** (he denies existence of the opposite side of the body).

Exam Questions

1. Describe the connections and functions of sensory cortex. Add a note on sensory homunculus.
2. List the cortical sensory areas and give their functions. Briefly describe the connections, functions and effects of lesion of S-I

Multiple Choice Questions

1. All of the following areas are classified under sensory cortical areas, EXCEPT:

A. Area 3 B. Area 4
C. Area 8 D. Area 5

2. What is the correct arrangement for areas of primary sensory cortex (S-I)?

A. Area 3,1,2 B. Area 1,2,3
C. Area 3,5,7 D. Area 5,7

3. Which of the following sensation (s) is/are affected most in lesion of S-I?

A. Pain and temperature B. Crude touch
C. Pressure D. Stereognosis

4. Which of the following sensation (s) is/are affected least in lesion of S-I?

A. Fine touch B. Pain and temperature
C. Vibration D. Tactile localization

5. In sensory homunculus, which body part is most represented?

A. Face B. Neck
C. Trunk D. Legs

Answers: 1. C 2. A 3. D 4. B 5. A

Chapter 102

Applied Sensory Physiology

Learning Objectives

<u>On completion of study of this chapter:</u>

The student will be able to (must know):

1. Name the common causes of lesion and list the sensory defects produced by lesions at various levels of sensory pathways.
2. Understand the physiological basis of sensory deficits produced by the lesions.
3. Outline the physiological basis of sensory deficit in Brown-Sequard syndrome.

The student may also be able to (desirable to know):

1. Describe the physiological basis of sensory abnormalities.

LESIONS AT DIFFERENT LEVELS

Nerve Lesion

Single Peripheral Nerve Lesion

Features of lesion of a peripheral nerve depend on whether the nerve is predominantly cutaneous, muscular or mixed.

1. Lesion of a cutaneous nerve results in **sensory loss in the corresponding areas of distribution** of that particular nerve.
    - However, **deficit is always less** than the anatomic distribution because of ***overlap from the adjacent nerve***.
2. Perception of **deep pressure and passive movements is usually not affected**, as these modalities are mediated by nerve fibers from subcutaneous structures and joints.
3. **If the nerve is affected by compression**, large fibers carrying ***touch and pressure are affected*** whereas small fibers carrying ***pain and temperature remain intact.***

Multiple Nerve Lesions (Polyneuropathy)

Diabetic, inflammatory and vasculitic neuropathies are common form of polyneuropathies. Usually, the sensory **impairment is bilateral.**

1. As the long and large fibers are most affected, sensory deficits are *more marked in legs and feet in lower limb and hands in upper limb*.
2. Sensory loss **involves all modalities of sensation**. If the loss is distal and symmetrical, **glove and stocking anesthesia** (anesthesia of hands and feet of both sides) occurs.

- However, if the degeneration is **more demyelinating** than the axonal type, ***paresthesia is an early feature***.
- As large fibers (kinesthetic fibers that carry sense of position and vibration) are more affected, sensory ataxia may occur.
- In chronic cases, due to prolonged analgesia, **trophic ulcers** develop.

Nerve Root Lesion (Radiculopathy)

Segmental anesthesia occurs in root lesions corresponding to the involvement of the segment of the spinal cord from where the nerve root arises.

- This usually occurs in **compression of a single sensory nerve root** as occurs in herniation of intervertebral discs.
    - However, considerable overlap from adjacent root usually occurs.
- Therefore, lesion of a single sensory root **does not produce complete loss of sensation** in area of the skin.

Lesion of Sensory Ganglia

Dorsal root ganglia are affected in many **inflammatory, toxic and neoplastic** diseases. This produces same sensory loss as that of root lesion, but loss of sensation in **proximal parts of the body is more pronounced**.

Spinal Cord Lesions PY10.6

Features of spinal cord lesion depend on the part of the spinal cord involved in the disease process. Accordingly following sensory **spinal cord syndromes** are observed:

Tabetic Syndrome

In tabes dorsalis, destruction of large proprioceptive and other posterior column fibers of one side (Fig. 102.1A) results in loss of sense of position and vibration.

- Numbness and paresthesia may occur.
- ***Romberg sign** may be positive.*

This is typically seen in **neurosyphilis.** Tabetic syndrome also occurs in **diabetes.**

Posterior Column Syndrome

Destruction fibers in the posterior column (Fig. 102.1B) results in loss of vibratory and position sense, without affecting pain and temperature.

- **Stereoanesthesia**, impairment of **graphesthesia** and tactile sensibility also occur.
- This resembles the cortical lesion, but *loss of vibration differentiates it*.

Brown Sequard Syndrome:

Cause: Brown-Sequard Syndrome occurs in **hemisection of the spinal cord** (Fig. 102.1C). It is usually seen in **injury to the spinal cord or in tumors** of the spinal cord that affects *only half of the cord*.

Sensory Deficit:

1. **On the side of lesion**, the fine-touch sensation, proprioceptive sensations (sensations from tendons, muscles, joints and vibration sense) and tactile discrimination are lost.
2. **On the opposite side,** pain and thermal sensations are lost.
    - This occurs because sensation for fine-touch, proprioception, and two-point discrimination ascend up in the dorsal column of the same side, whereas the sensation for **pain and temperature ascend up in the anterolateral system in the opposite side** of the spinal cord.

Motor Deficit: There is also ***damage to corticospinal tract*** on the side of hemisection of spinal cord. This causes paresis (muscle weakness) and spasticity of muscles of the same side of the body.

Complete Spinal Sensory Syndrome

In complete section of spinal cord (Fig. 102.1D), all forms of sensation are abolished below the level of lesion. Usually, **a narrow zone of hyperesthesia** occurs at the upper margin of anesthetic zone.

Syringomyelic Syndrome

Syringomyelia is a disease in which there is lesion **around the central canal** of the spinal cord (Fig. 102.1E).

- The lesion interrupts the **lateral spinothalamic fibers** (for pain and temperature) without affecting fibers of dorsal column.
- Thus, pain and temperature are lost without affecting touch and postural sensibility (**dissociated sensory loss**).

Anterior Spinal Artery Syndrome

Anterior spinal artery supplies **ventral part of the spinal cord**. Thus, obstruction or hemorrhage of this artery causes infarction of anterior half of the cord (Fig. 102.1F). This results in **anterior myelopathy**.

- Usually, ***pain and temperature sensation are lost*** *without affecting proprioceptive sensations* below the level of lesion.
- Spastic paralysis occurs due to involvement of corticospinal tract.

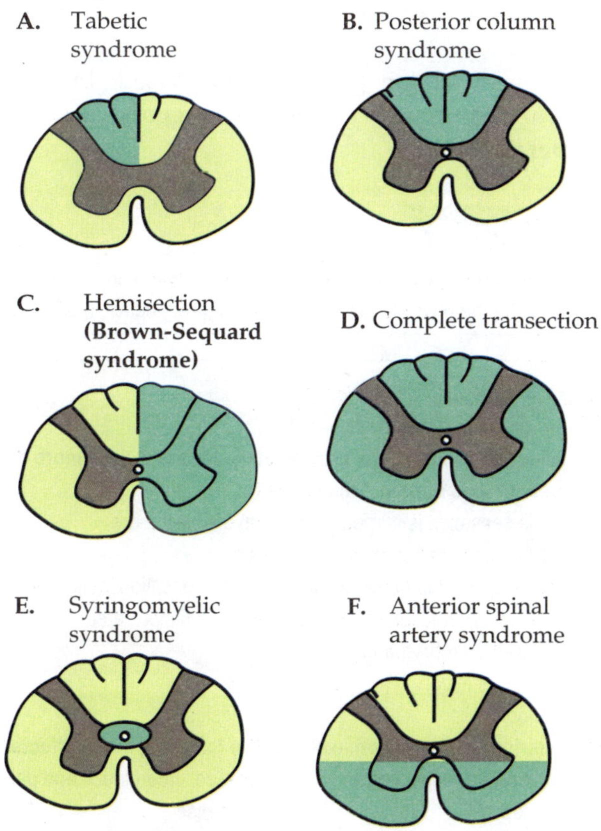

Figs. 102.1: Effects of different pattern of lesions in spinal cord that produces various sensory deficits (lesioned area represented by green color). **A:** Tabetic syndrome that occurs due to lesion of the posterior column of one side; **B:** Posterior column syndrome that occurs due to bilateral lesion of the posterior columns; **C:** Brown-Sequard syndrome that occurs due to hemisection of the spinal cord; **D:** Complete spinal sensory syndrome that occurs due to total transection of spinal cord; **E:** Syringomyelic syndrome that occurs due to lesion around the central canal of spinal cord; **F:** Anterior spinal artery syndrome that affects ventral half of both sides of spinal cord.

Brainstem Lesion

Lesion at the medulla affects **descending trigeminal tract** and the **crossed lateral spinothalamic tract** on one side of the brain stem. This results in **crossed sensory loss**, i. e., loss of pain and temperature on one side of the face and on the opposite side of the body.

1. **In the upper medulla, pons and lower midbrain**, the crossed spinothalamic and trigeminothalamic tracts run together.
   - Thus, lesion at these levels causes **loss of pain and temperature on the opposite half of the face and body** without affecting other sensations (as the medial lemniscus is spared).
2. **In the upper brainstem**, spinothalamic tract and medial lemniscus become confluent.
   - Thus, lesion at this level results in **contralateral loss of all superficial and deep sensations** (posterior column sensations and pain and temperature).

Thalamic Lesion

Severe and extensive lesion of the thalamus results in ***gross impairment of sensory modalities on the opposite side*** of the body.

- The threshold for pain may be raised, but a less painful stimulus may cause an exaggerated response (**hyperalgesia**).
- The touch sensation may induce ***unpleasant sensation (paresthesia).***

This is called **thalamic syndrome**, which occurs in the lesion of lateral and ventral nuclei.

Cortical Lesion

The cortex is mainly involved in integration of finer aspect of sensations, especially the **spatial and discriminatory sensibility.**

- **Tactile localization, two-point discrimination and stereognosis** are therefore called as **cortical sensations.**
  - The cortical lesion results in **topagnosia** (inability to localize touch and pain stimuli), **astereognosis** and widening of two-point discrimination.

1. **Proprioception and sense of vibration** are also impaired.
2. Sensory inattention, extinction or neglect is characteristic manifestation of **parietal lobe lesion.**

SENSORY FUNCTION TESTS

PY10.11

Functions of sensory system can be assessed by performing clinical examination of sensory system, sensory nerve conduction studies and by studying somatosensory evoked potentials. All these tests are described in 'Textbook of Practical Physiology' 5th Edition, 2020, by GK Pal and Pravati Pal)

Exam Questions

1. Describe the physiological basis of sensory deficits in different levels of lesion in the sensory pathway.
2. Describe the physiological basis of the sensory deficit in different kinds of nerve lesions. Add a note on Brown-Séquard syndrome.

Multiple Choice Questions

1. **If a spinal nerve is cut, the area of tactile loss is always more than the area for loss of pain. This is due to:**
   A. Tactile sensation is carried by more myelinated fibers
   B. Tactile receptors have quick adaptation
   C. Degree of overlap of fibers carrying tactile sensation is much less
   D. In S-I, representation of tactile sensation is in more area
2. **Dissociated anesthesia is seen in:**
   A. Dorsal root lesion B. Nerve lesion
   C. Syringomyelia D. Thalamic lesion
3. **In posterior column lesion, which of the following is not affected?**
   A. Vibration & proprioception B. Temperature, crude touch and pain
   C. Fine touch D. Position sense
4. **A lesion of ventrolateral part of spinal cord will lead to loss (below the level of lesion) of:**
   A. Pain sensation on the ipsilateral side
   B. Proprioception of the contralateral side
   C. Pain sensation on the contralateral side
   D. Proprioception on the ipsilateral side
5. **An anterolateral (ventrolateral) cordotomy to relieve pain in right leg is effective because it interrupts the:**
   A. Left dorsal column
   B. Left ventral spinothalamic tract
   C. Left lateral spinothalamic tract
   D. Right lateral spinothalamic tract
6. **Which of the following is true about Brown-Sequard syndrome?**
   A. Ipsilateral loss of joint sensation
   B. Contralateral loss of joint sensation
   C. Ipsilateral loss of pain and temperature
   D. Contralateral loss of vibration
7. **Unlikely to be involved in lesion of anterior spinal artery is:**
   A. Pain and temp B. Vibration and proprioception
   C. Pyramidal tract D. Sphincters

Answers

1. C 2. C 3. B 4. C 5. C
6. A 7. B

Chapter 103

Introduction to Motor Physiology and Organization of Motor System

Learning Objectives

On completion of study of this chapter:

The student will be able to (must know):

1. Name the types of movements and list their characteristic features.
2. Name the feedback control systems and outline their role in improvement of motor functions.
3. Appreciate the general organization of motor system.
4. Understand the segmental organization of motor system at the level of spinal cord.
5. Define upper & lower motor neurons and give their functions.
6. Understand the importance of motor unit recruitment.
7. Comprehend the topographical organization of motoneuron pool and spinal interneurons.

The student may also be able to (desirable to know):

1. Describe the feedback control systems of motor functions.
2. Describe the importance of spinal cord organization of motor control.

INTRODUCTION TO MOTOR PHYSIOLOGY

Motor system deals with the **study of physiology of movement**. Motor physiology involves **initiation, execution, and control of movements.**

- With the help of **stable postural background** and with **appropriate postural adjustments**, coordinated movement becomes possible.
- Therefore, motor physiology deals with the study of **control of movement and posture together**.

Types of Movements

Movements can broadly be divided into **two categories**: automatic movements and volitional movements.

Automatic Movements

The automatic movements are **reflexive in nature**. An example of an automatic movement is a *rapid response* to a nociceptive stimulus.

The **following are the characteristics** of reflexive movements:

1. They have short latency
2. They are stereotyped in nature
3. They are executed rapidly
4. Usually, they cannot be modified
5. They are not under voluntary control
6. They are triggered by a specific sensory stimulus

Volitional Movements

The movements that are **under voluntary control** are the volitional or intentional movements. They can **easily be modified**. An example of a volitional movement is painting, or threading a needle.

The **characteristics** of such movements are that they:

1. Have long latency
2. Are slow in execution
3. Can be modified easily
4. Are under voluntary control
5. Are rarely triggered by a specific sensory stimulus
6. May be affected by factors like attention, emotion and motivation.

What is Movement?

Movement is defined as **displacement of the body parts that results in change in position of the body** as a whole or a part of the body. Movement is produced by the contraction and relaxation of the muscles.

- The muscles that facilitate a particular movement (**decrease angle at the joint**) are called as **agonists**.
- The muscles that oppose the movement (*increase angle at the joint*) are called as **antagonists**. In fact, movement is facilitated by **relaxation of the antagonist** muscle.

How Does the Movement Occur?

Movement occurs due to the **motor signals** generated in the motor neurons in the spinal cord. This is accomplished by the activities initiated in the central nervous system.

- For a basic or reflexive movement to be executed, the motor signal generated in the spinal cord is **conveyed to the appropriate muscles via motor neurons**.
- However, for complex or volitional movements to be appropriately executed, first, the **signals are generated in the forebrain** (mainly in motor cortex) **and brainstem**, and then, the signals are **relayed to the spinal cord**.
- Spinal cord interacts with supraspinal influences for the integration and refining of the final output signal (Fig. 103.1).

Thus, the precision and stability of movements are achieved by various **feedback control mechanisms**.

Feedback Control Systems

The feedback systems are meant to improve quality of movement. The feedback mechanisms are divided into **three types**: local feedback, central feedback, special sensory feedback.

Local Feedback

The local feedback is the **lowest level of feedback systems**. It is exclusively integrated in spinal cord (Fig. 103.2).

- The afferent signal does not interact with supraspinal signals originating from various parts of CNS. Thus, it acts fast and **controls gross reflexive movement**.
- The local feedback operates for movements in which the **speed is more important than the accuracy** of the movement.

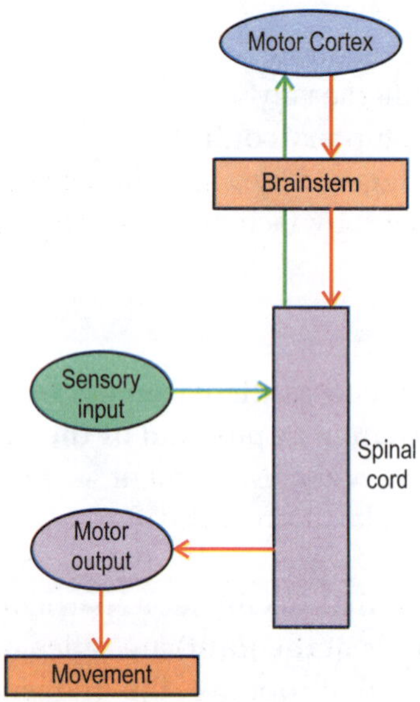

Fig. 103.1: General schematic representation of control of movement. Note, efferent signals originating in cortical and brainstem areas determine the motor output signal from spinal cord that finally produces movement.

  - For example, during withdrawal of body parts in response to a noxious stimulus, the body part must be withdrawn faster no matter how precisely it is done.
- However, the pattern of movement depends on the strength and nature of afferent inputs.

Central Feedback

This is the second level of feedback control system. It is integrated in spinal cord, brain stem and cortex (Fig. 103.2).

- In this feedback mechanism, the afferent signal satisfactorily **interacts with the other signals arising from different parts of the supraspinal segments**.
- For processing and integration of signals at various levels, the speed of execution is considerably delayed.
  - However, with slowness, the **precision of movement is achieved**.
  - Thus, central feedback mechanism operates when ***accuracy of movement is of paramount importance*** than the speed of execution.
- For example, for threading a needle, the movement needs proper balance and coordination to achieve its precision.

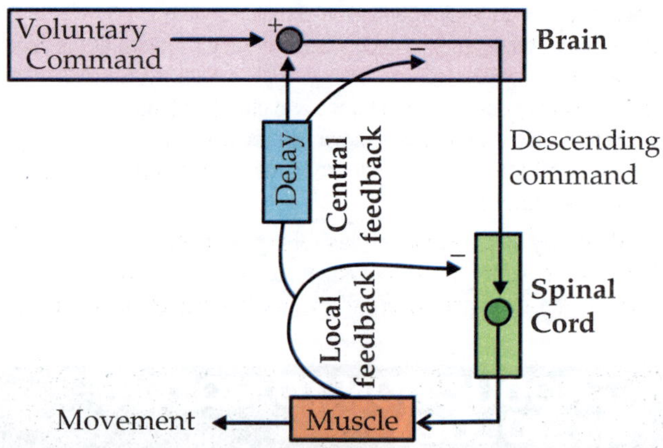

Fig. 103.2: Local and central feedback mechanisms in motor control.

Special Sensory Feedback

This feedback mechanism involves special sensory information like visual and auditory inputs.

- The movement **becomes most accurate** with control by this feedback system. For example, to hit a nail with a hammer becomes easier and accurate with eyes open.
- In this system, the **inputs from special sensory structures** interact with different parts of the central nervous system to improve the accuracy of the movement.

ORGANIZATION OF MOTOR SYSTEM

The components of motor systems are: muscle and its efferent connections, the segmental circuit (in the spinal cord), the brainstem controlling centers, the basal ganglia, cerebellum, and cerebral cortex (Fig. 103.3).

Muscle and its Efferent Connections: The important components of the motor system are the muscles and their efferent connections (the motor neurons). Tone of muscle depends on its ***intact innervation***.

- Without muscle tone, the adequate force cannot be generated for execution of movements.
  - Therefore, lesion of the motor neurons that abolishes muscle tone and function results in **complete paralysis**.
- Thus, muscle and the motor neurons are fundamental parts of the motor system.

Spinal Segmental Circuit: Sensory inputs from muscle influence the motor neurons that in turn innervate the same muscle.

- This circuit of neural connection constitutes the **local or segmental spinal circuit,** which is *essential for all reflexive movements*.
- Also, spinal cord generates and controls **basic neural patterns** required for genesis and coordination of limb movements.

Brainstem Controlling Centers: The activities of motor neurons and interneurons in the spinal cord are largely influenced by the descending inputs arising from the brainstem motor nuclei.

- The descending pathways from the brainstem especially **reticulospinal tract** and **vestibulospinal tract profoundly influence the activities** of the motor neurons in the spinal cord.

Cortex: The motor cortex directly controls the spinal cord motor neurons through the corticospinal tracts and controls brainstem motor nuclei via ***corticobulbar projections*** from where the **extrapyramidal tracts originate**.

- Thus, motor cortex regulates all peripheral motor activities.
- Sensory cortex projects to the motor cortex for **sensory-motor coordination.**

Basal Ganglia: Basal ganglia project to motor cortex via the thalamus and **strongly influence the motor output to spinal cord.**

- Basal ganglia are involved in **initiation, smoothening and coordination of the movement**.

Cerebellum: Cerebellum influences all parts of motor neuraxis.

1. It **receives inputs from almost all sensory modalities** and projects heavily **to the brainstem motor nuclei, and motor cortex.**
   - Therefore, cerebellum plays a crucial role in the regulation of posture and movement.
2. It controls almost **all the aspects of movement,** starting from *planning, programming, and initiation to the smoothening and coordination, and termination of movement*.

Thalamus: Thalamus is the major sensory relay station in the brain.

1. Thalamus also receives **inputs from cerebellum and basal ganglia**.
2. Thus, thalamus plays an important role in **sensory-motor coordination**.

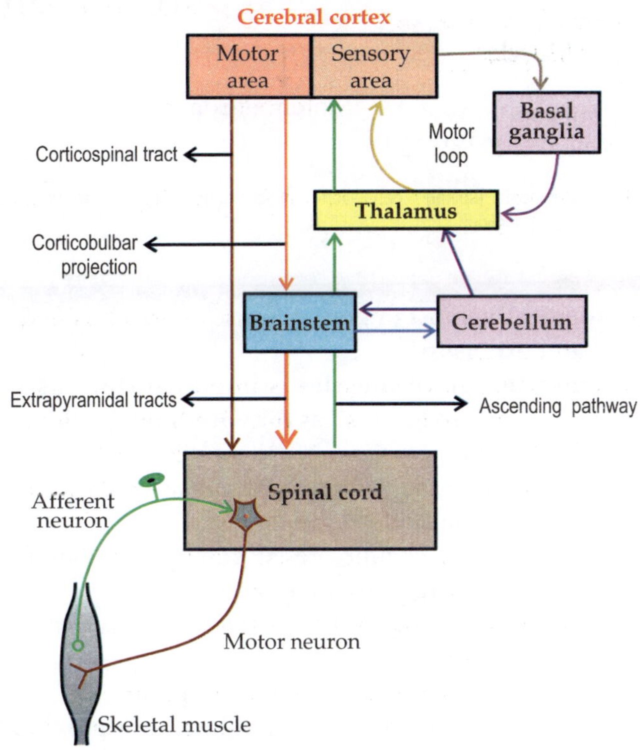

Fig. 103.3: General organization of motor system.

Segmental Organization

Organization of motor control at spinal cord level is called **segmental organization**. Organization ***above the spinal cord segment*** (mainly by brainstem and forebrain areas) is called **suprasegmental organization.**

Components of Organization

Each spinal cord segment has its **input and output connections** with various muscles.

1. From muscles, input reaches spinal cord via muscle **afferents** (Ia, Ib and other afferents).
2. From spinal cord, output reaches muscles via **motoneurons**.
3. In the spinal cord, between afferent neurons and motoneurons are many **interneurons**.
   - In addition to the inputs from afferents, the interneurons and motoneurons are the **targets of descending fibers** from various suprasegmental centers.

Segmental organization includes **muscles, afferent neurons, motoneurons, motoneuron pool,** and **spinal interneurons** (Fig. 103.4).

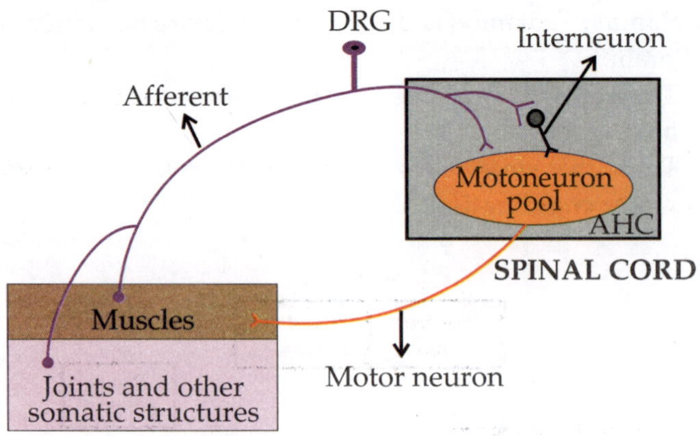

Fig. 103.4: Segmental (spinal) organization of motor control. AHC: anterior horn cell; DRG: dorsal root ganglion.

Muscles

Physiologically, most important muscles are classified as **flexors and extensors**.

- **Extensor group of muscles is important for posture** *and* **flexor group of muscles for withdrawal reflexes.**
  - By definition, **extensors** are muscles that increase the angle at the joint, and **flexors** are muscles that decrease the angle at the joint.
- Extensors of lower limbs resist gravity and therefore are the main **antigravity muscles**.
- The **tone of antigravity muscles** *is important for maintaining posture*.

However, from **neurophysiological point** of view, muscles are best classified as **medial-lateral or proximal-distal groups**.

Medial or Proximal Group of Muscles: The medial or proximal groups of muscles include the *axial and girdle muscles, and proximal limb muscles*.

- Axial muscles are muscles attached to axial skeletons and girdles of the body.
- These muscles are **involved in postural adjustments** as they produce body and whole limb movements.
- The medial extensors perform **antigravity function**, and therefore are important for **control of posture**.

Lateral or Distal Group of Muscles: The lateral or distal muscles include the intrinsic **muscles of digits and distal muscles** of the extremities. These muscles subserve the manipulatory activities, i. e., the **skilled voluntary movements**.

Thus, to summarize, the **proximal group of muscles control posture** and **distal group of muscles control skilled voluntary activities**.

Afferents

The main afferent fibers for motor activities are **Ia afferents** that arise from muscle spindles.

- **Type II and Ib afferents** also play role in motor control.
- **Flexor reflex afferents** mediate withdrawal reflexes.

Motor Neurons

The motor neurons (also called, motoneurons) are neurons that are involved in control of motor functions. They are broadly divided into **two categories**: Upper motor neurons and lower motor neurons.

Upper Motor Neurons (UMNs)

UMNs are motor neurons that are derived from various motor areas of brain like motor cortex, brainstem motor nuclei etc. and **terminate directly or indirectly (via interneurons) on lower motor neurons** in the spinal cord (Fig. 103.5).

- Axons of these neurons **form the descending pathways**.
- Some important examples of these pathways are corticospinal, rubrospinal, vestibulospinal, and reticulospinal tracts.

Lower Motor Neurons (LMNs)

LMNs originate in the anterior horn of the spinal cord or in cranial nerve motor nuclei, and **innervate various skeletal muscles** (Fig. 103.5).

- The **cell bodies** of motor neurons are located in the ventral horns of the spinal gray matter (**anterior horn cells**) and *brainstem nuclei*.
- Though some of the fibers in the descending pathways terminate directly on motor neurons, most of the fibers terminate on interneurons, which in turn project to motor neuron.

There are **two types of lower motoneurons:** α motoneurons and γ motoneurons.

The α Motoneurons: The **α** motoneurons constitute the **final common path of motor output signals** from the CNS, the route by which central neural activity influences the skeletal muscles.

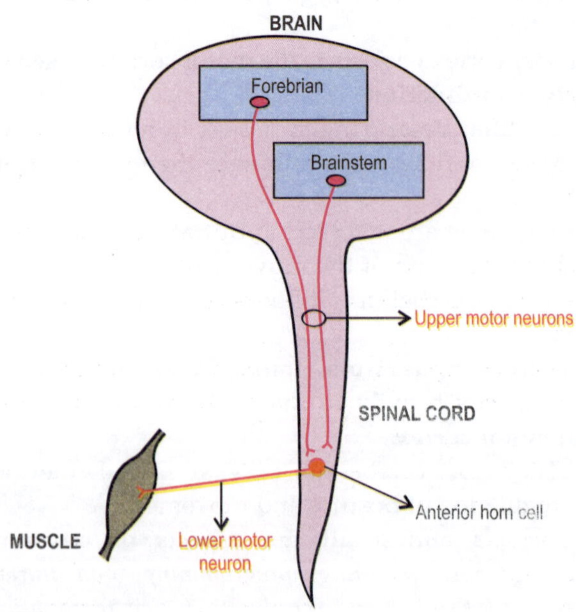

Fig. 103.5: Upper and lower motor neurons.

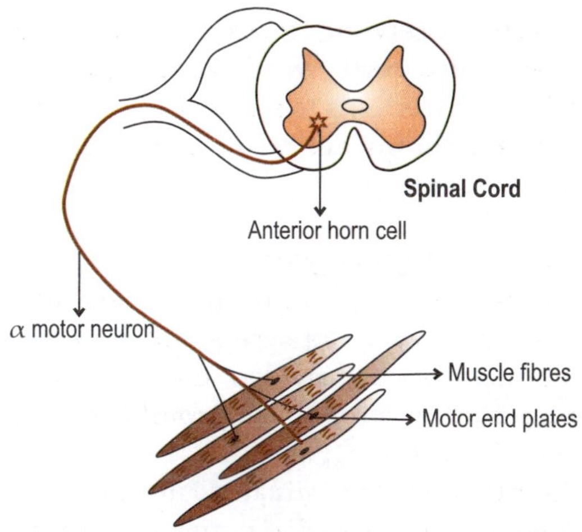

Fig. 103.6: A motor unit. Note it consists of an alpha motor neuron and the muscle fibers innervated by it.

1. The α motor neurons **innervate extrafusal muscle fibers**, which are responsible for force generation. One alpha motor neuron innervates 10 to 1,000 muscle fibers, depending on the muscle.
   - A **Motor unit** constitutes a motor neuron, its axon, the branches of the axon, the neuromuscular junctions at the distal end of each axon branch, and all of the extrafusal muscle fibers innervated by that motor neuron (Fig. 103.6).

1. When a motor neuron generates an action potential, all its muscle fibers are activated (Application Box 103.1).

Physiologic Significance: According to their cell body size and axon diameter, α motor neurons are divided into **two types**; the larger and smaller motoneurons.

1. **The larger motoneurons** have fast conduction velocities and are active in high-effort force generation.
   - They **innervate fast-twitch**, high-force but fatigable muscle fibers.
2. **The smaller motor neurons** have lower thresholds to synaptic stimulation, have slower conduction velocity, and **innervate slow-twitch**, low-force and fatigue resistant muscle fibers.
   - Thus, all muscle fibers of a motor unit belong to one category, i. e., either **fast-twitch or slow-twitch type**.

Application Box 103.1

Motor unit recruitment follows size principle: The smaller motor neuron with small motor unit size has the low threshold. Therefore, when synaptic activity is low, they are activated first. When drive increases the larger motor neurons (with large motor unit size) are recruited. This phenomenon of orderly recruitment of motor unit follows the **size principle**, i.e., the smaller motor units are activated first and then the larger motor units.

The γ Motor Neurons: The γ motor neurons **innervate the intrafusal fibers** that are fibers of the muscle spindle.

- They constitute **30% of fibers** arising from anterior horn cells.

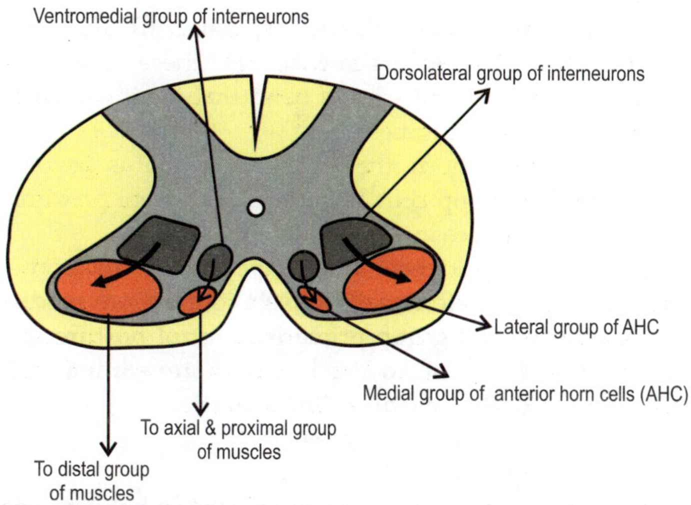

Fig. 103.7: Topographic organization of interneurons and motoneuronal pool. Arrows indicate the projection of interneuronal group to motoneuronal pool.

  - They do not contribute to the total force generated in the muscle.
  - Rather, they **modulate the sensitivity of muscle spindle** and thereby regulate muscle length and muscle tone.
- The γ motor neurons with intrafusal fibers constitute the **fusimotor system**.
- The γ motor neurons **do not receive inputs from sensory afferents**.
  - They receive inputs from ***descending pathways*** that influence them.
  - Thus, **supraspinal motor centers** regulate muscle tone mainly by altering the discharge of motor neurons.

Spinal motoneurons are final common path for central motor outputs.

Motoneuron Pools

The cell bodies of motoneurons are located in the ventral horn of the spinal cord, which are known as **anterior horn cells**. The anterior horn cells constitute the motoneuron pools.

Topographical Organization

There is a topographical organization of motoneurons in the spinal cord with regard to the target muscles they innervate. Accordingly, motoneuron pool is divided into **two parts**: the ***medial group and the lateral group***.

- **The medial group** of anterior horn cells innervates the axial and proximal muscles, and **the lateral group** of anterior horn cells innervates the distal muscles (Fig. 103.7).
  - Thus, **medial group of anterior horn cells control posture** whereas **lateral group of anterior horn cells control skilled voluntary activities**.
- Consequently, **lateral motoneuron pool** is enlarged to occupy about ***70% of the ventral horn*** in the lower

cervical and upper thoracic spinal cord segments (**the brachial enlargement**), as these segments supply intrinsic muscles of hand that are involved in manipulatory activities.

- In the ventral horn, the motoneuron pool is devoted for medial group cells as successively more proximal limb muscles are innervated by them.

Physiologic Importance: It is important to remember the inputs that preferentially project to the more **medial motoneuronal cell group primarily control posture** and inputs that distribute to the **lateral motoneuronal cell group principally control skilled activities**.

Spinal Interneurons

Interneurons in the spinal cord are **placed in between the dorsal and ventral horns**.

- Interneurons that are **concerned mainly in motor functions** are placed more ***towards the ventral horn*** and interneurons **concerned with sensory functions** are placed more ***towards the dorsal horn***.
- Most of the descending influences on the motoneurons are **exerted indirectly via interneurons**, rather than their direct projections to the spinal motoneurons.
- Thus, **interneurons are major targets of descending tracts**.

Topographical Organization

Like motoneuronal cell groups, interneuronal cell groups are arranged topographically in the spinal cord. Interneurons are divided into **two cell groups**: *ventromedial interneuronal cell group* and *dorsolateral interneuronal cell group* (Fig. 103.7).

- The **ventromedially situated** interneurons project preferentially ***to the medial group*** of motoneurons and **dorsolaterally placed** interneurons project ***to lateral group*** of motoneurons.
  - Consequently, **ventromedial interneuronal cell group** is primarily involved in ***controlling posture*** and **dorsolateral interneuronal cell group** in regulating ***skilled voluntary activities***.

Exam Questions

1. Describe the role of feedback control systems for improvement of motor functions.
2. Describe the segmental organization of motor control. Add a note on size principle.
3. Describe the general organization of upper and lower motor neurons in motor control. Give a note on topographical organization of motoneurons and interneurons in spinal cord.

Multiple Choice Questions

1. All of the following are true for local feedback systems, EXCEPT:
A. It is the lowest level of feedback system
B. Controls fine, precise movements
C. Integrated at the level of spinal cord
D. Speed of movement is of paramount importance

2. Which of the following is true for central feedback system?
A. It is the first level of feedback system
B. Controls gross, reflexive movements
C. Integrated at the level of cortex only
D. Accuracy of movement is of paramount importance

3. Which of the following is not a feature of automatic or reflexive movements?
A. Modified by feedback inputs
B. Short latency
C. Stereotype in nature
D. Rapid execution

4. All the following are features of volitional movements, EXCEPT:
A. Long latency
B. Slow execution
C. Can't be modified
D. Affected by attention and motivation

5. Which of the following is not a feedback system for regulation of motor activities?
A. Local feedback
B. Central feedback
C. Humoral feedback
D. Special sensory feedback

6. Which of the following structure is anatomically located outside the central neuraxis of the motor control?
A. Spinal cord
B. Brainstem
C. Cerebellum
D. Motor cortex

7. Medial group of motoneurons contain cell bodies of neurons that supply:
A. Distal group of muscles
B. Proximal and axial group of muscle
C. Muscles of limb
D. Muscles of Head and neck

8. Dorsolateral group of interneurons project to the motoneurons that contain cell bodies of neurons that supply:
A. Distal group of muscles
B. Proximal and axial group of muscle
C. Muscles of limb
D. Muscles of Head and neck

9. The motoneurons are mainly influenced by:
A. Afferent neurons
B. Interneurons
C. Neurons of descending tracts
D. Commissural neurons

Answers

1. B 2. D 3. A 4. C 5. C 6. C 7. B 8. A 9. C

Chapter 104

Muscle Spindle and Golgi Tendon Organ

Learning Objectives

On completion of study of this chapter:

The student will be able to (must know):

1. Draw a labeled diagram of muscle spindle and describe the functions of muscle spindle.
2. Outline the innervations and functions of nuclear bag fibers and nuclear chain fibers
3. Define the role of γ motor neuron in the control of muscle tone.
4. Briefly describe the structure and function of Golgi tendon organ.
5. Illustrate the length feedback and force feedback for regulation of muscle tone and function.
6. Give the significance of α–γ coactivation.

The student may also be able to (desirable to know):

1. Explain the role of [illegible] motor neuron in motor control.
2. Describe the role of Golgi tendon organ in motor functions.

MUSCLE SPINDLE

Muscle spindles are specialized **sense organs present in all skeletal muscles.** They are **long spindle (fusiform) shaped,** present inside the fusiform capsules. Therefore, they are known as **intrafusal fibers**.

- This differentiates spindle fibers from the **extrafusal fibers**, the regular muscle fibers.
- Muscle spindles are the **receptors that respond to change in muscle length and the velocity of lengthening**.

Structure

About **2 to 12 fibers** are present in a muscle spindle. Each muscle spindle is enclosed in a connective tissue capsule. The muscle spindle is about **100 µm in diameter and 5 to 10 mm** in length.

- The muscle spindle lies in parallel to the regular muscle fibers and their distal ends are attached to the tendon of the muscle or to the sides of extrafusal fibers (Fig. 104.1).

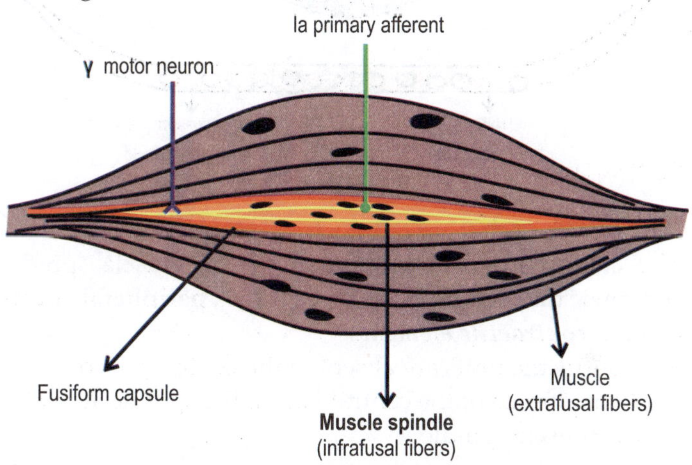

Fig. 104.1: Location of muscle spindle. Note that, in the muscle, spindle is surrounded by a fusiform capsule. The peripheral part of the muscle spindle is innervated by γ motor neuron and central part receives Ia afferent fiber.

- This parallel arrangement and special attachment help the spindle to respond to muscle stretch.

Intrafusal fibers are of **two types**: the nuclear bag fibers, and the nuclear chain fibers.

Nuclear Bag Fibers

Nuclear bag fibers are longer than the nuclear chain fibers (Fig. 104.2).

- These fibers are called nuclear bag fibers as they are **dilated at their center to form a bag** like structure that contains multiple nuclei.
- Usually, ***two nuclear bag fibers*** are present in a spindle: the nuclear bag fiber 1, and the nuclear bag fiber 2.

1. The **bag fiber 1** has *low myosin ATPase activity* and responds best in the dynamic phase of muscle stretch.

2. The **bag fiber 2** has ***high myosin ATPase activity*** and responds best in the static phase of muscle stretch.

Nuclear Chain Fibers

These are thinner and shorter fibers.

- They are present by the side of the nuclear bag fiber and **do not have a definitive bag**.
- The **nuclei in these fibers are arranged in a row** in the form of a chain, for which they are called nuclear chain fibers.
- Usually, four or more nuclear chain fibers are present in a spindle.

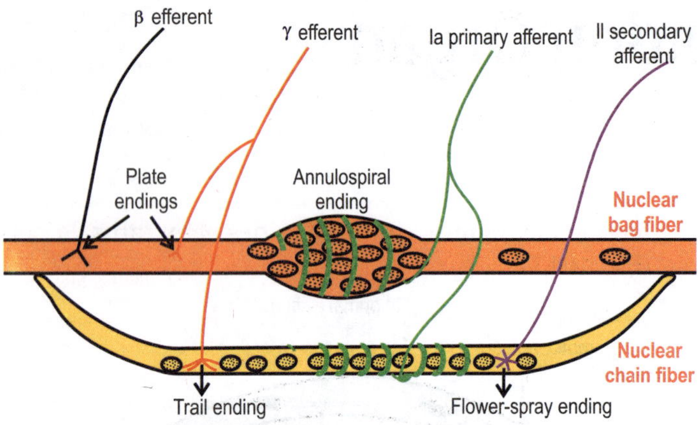

Fig. 104.2: Structure of muscle spindle.

Location of Receptors

The **central noncontractile part** of the muscle spindle contains the receptors whereas the **peripheral parts** contain ***contractile elements***.

- Contractile units are absent in the central portion.
- Thus, stretch of the central part of the spindle activates the muscle spindle.

Innervation of Muscle Spindle

The muscle spindles have both **afferent (sensory) and efferent (motor) innervations**.

Afferent Innervation (Sensory Fibers)

Afferent fibers for muscle spindle are Ia and II fibers. Ia fibers have larger diameter (12 to 20 µm) than type II fibers (6 to 12 µm) and have faster conduction velocity.

There are **two types of sensory endings** in each muscle spindle: the primary endings, and the secondary endings.

Primary Endings: The primary endings are the terminals of **type Ia afferent fiber.**

These are also called **annulospiral endings** as they are coiled spirally around the center of the intrafusal fibers.

- Type Ia afferent fiber has two branches.
- One branch of Ia fiber terminates on nuclear bag fiber 1, and the other branch terminates on the nuclear bag fiber 2 and the nuclear chain fibers.

Secondary Endings: The secondary endings are the terminals of **type II afferent fiber.**

- They are also called **flower-spray endings**, as they appear like flowers.
- They are usually present on the nuclear chain fibers.
- The secondary endings are located in paracentral part of the spindle.

Efferent Innervation (Motor Fibers)

The spindles are innervated by a separate set of motor neurons, the **γ motor neurons**. They are also called **fusimotor fibers**.

- These are small nerves arising from the anterior horn cells and are having the diameter of 3 - 6 µm.
  - They constitute only about 30% of the fibers in the ventral root (70% of fibers are **α** motor neurons).
  - Because of their size and number, they comprise the **small motor nerve system**.
- The γ motor neurons supply the peripheral parts of intrafusal fibers.
- The terminals of the γ efferent fibers on the nuclear bag fiber 1 form the **plate ending** (as they end on the motor endplates), and on the nuclear bag fiber 2 and chain fiber form the **trail ending**.

Types of γ Motor Neurons: The γ motor neurons are of ***two types***: the **dynamic γ motor neurons** that terminate on the nuclear bag fiber 1, and the **static γ motor neurons** that innervate the nuclear bag fiber 2 and nuclear chain fiber.

1. **Stimulation of dynamic γ motor neurons** increases response in ***type Ia afferent fibers*** (only during the dynamic phase of muscle stretch; i. e. during change in muscle length).
2. **Stimulation of static γ motor neurons** increases response in ***type II afferent fibers*** (only during the static phase of muscle stretch; i. e. the maintained stretch).

Thus, **γ motor neurons monitor the muscle length and the speed of change in length**.

The muscle spindle is also innervated by **β efferent fibers** and there are both ***dynamic and static β efferents***.

Afferent Discharge Patterns

Two patterns of afferent discharge are obtained following stimulation of motor neurons: the **dynamic pattern**, and the **static patterns**. Both γ and β motor neurons produce these two types of responses.

- Stimulation of dynamic fusimotor fibers results in **dynamic response** and stimulation of the static fusimotor fibers produces **static response**.
- Fibers **from nuclear bag fibers** show ***dynamic response*** and fibers **from the nuclear chain fibers** show ***static response***.

Functions of Muscle Spindle

Muscle spindles are **receptors that are sensitive to stretch**. When the muscle spindle is stretched, the **sensory endings are distorted,** and action potential is generated in the afferent fibers.

- The **frequency** of afferent signal is **proportional to the degree of stretching.**
    - Spindle is **stretched by the stretch of the muscle,** as the spindle is present in parallel with the extrafusal fibers.
    - Therefore, **stretch of the muscle initiates the activities** in the spindle afferents.
- The **spindle afferents** directly terminate on the ***cell bodies of α motor neurons*** in the spinal cord.
    - Therefore, spindle afferent activity stimulates α motor neurons that in turn results in muscle contraction (Flowchart 104.1).
- On the contrary, **when muscle contracts,** the spindle activity (firing in the spindle afferents) is less, as the muscle spindle is no more stretched.
    - Thus, **stretch of the muscle causes muscle contraction** *by stretching the muscle spindle* whereas **contraction of the muscle causes muscle relaxation** by inhibiting the spindle.
- Therefore, muscle spindle and its reflex connection with the motor neurons constitute a **feedback device that controls muscle length.**

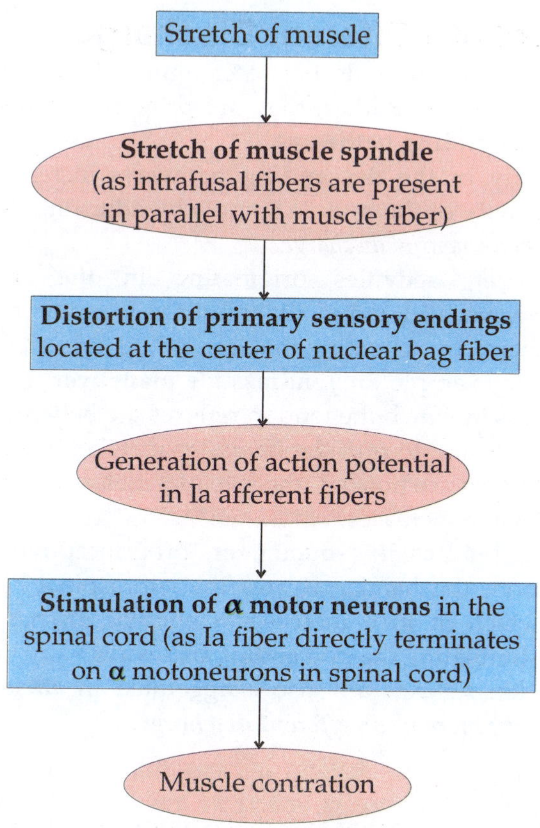

Flowchart 104.1: Mechanism of muscle contraction in response to muscle stretch.

Effects of Stimulation of γ Motor Neurons

Muscle also contracts in response to **stimulation of γ motor neurons**. But, in this situation, muscle contraction is not a direct response to the γ motor neuron discharge.

1. The stimulation of γ motor neuron causes **contraction of the peripheral portions** (that contains the contractile elements) of the muscle spindle.
2. This in turn **stretches the central portions** of the muscle spindle, which contains primary endings.
    - This **distorts the primary endings** in the muscle spindle, which in turn increases the discharge of the afferent fibers.
3. Afferent fibers stimulate α motor neurons and cause muscle contraction (Flowchart 104.2).
4. **Thus, γ motor neurons increase the sensitivity of the spindle to stretch.**

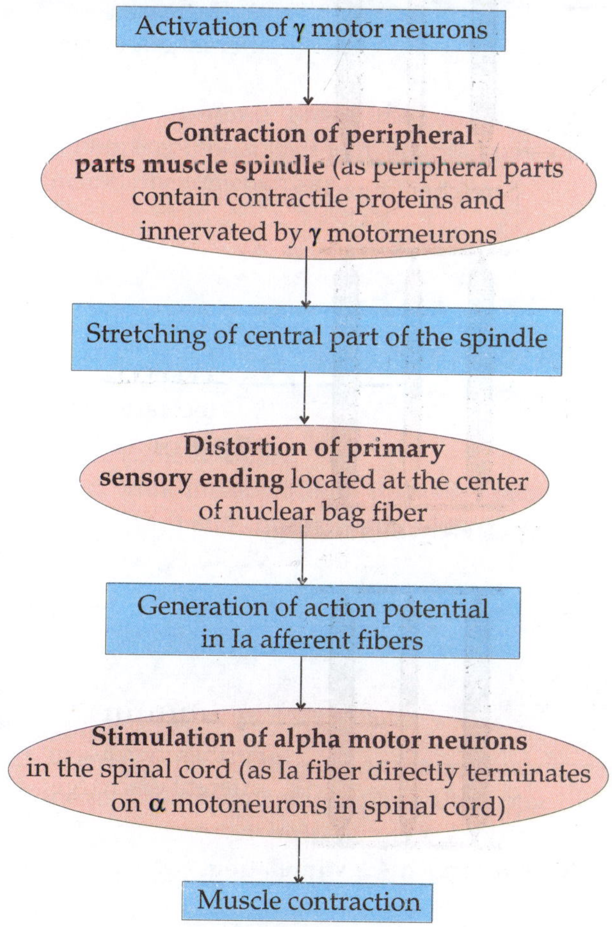

Flowchart 104.2: Mechanism of muscle contraction in response to stimulation of γ motor neuron.

It should thus be noted that the muscle contracts by stimulation of α motor neurons directly or by stimulation of γ motor neurons indirectly.

- In fact, the ***sensitivity of the muscle spindle to stretch varies with the state of γ efferent discharge.***
    - Therefore, stimulation of γ motor neuron in a stretched muscle leads to maximum spindle response (Fig. 104.3).

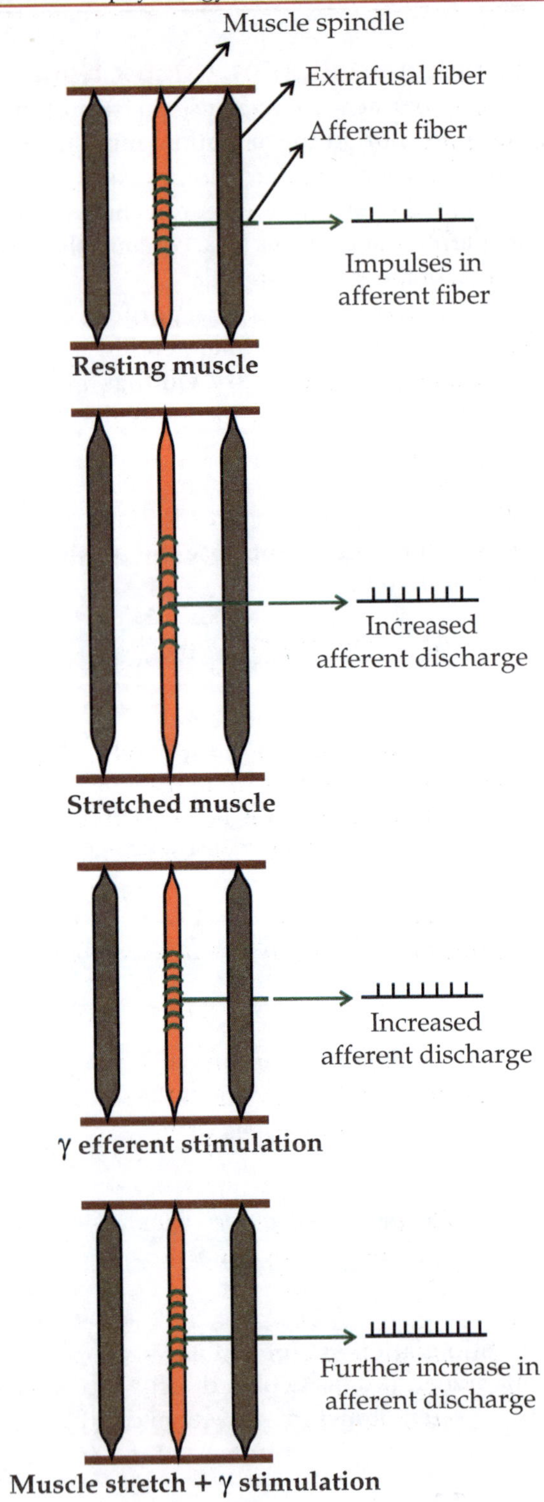

Fig. 104.3: Effects of stretch and stimulation of γ motor neuron on spindle activity.

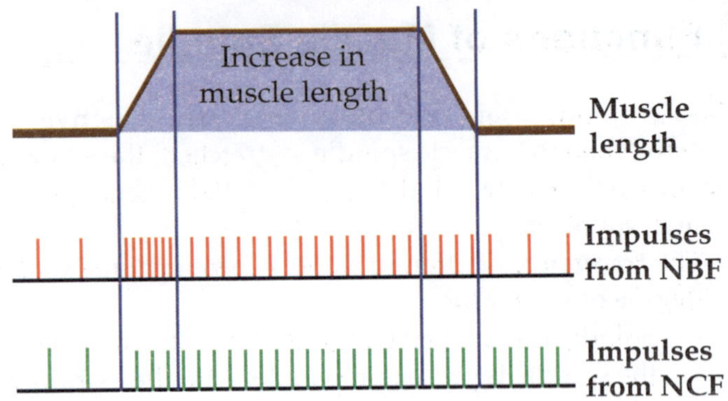

Fig. 104.4: Dynamic and static spindle responses. Nuclear bag fiber (NBF) exhibits dynamic responses (increased rate of impulse) during the act of stretch, whereas nuclear chain fiber (NCF) shows static responses (same impulse rate) throughout the stretch.

Spindle Responses

The primary endings on the nuclear bag fibers and nuclear chain fibers are stimulated in response to stretch, but the patterns of responses are different.

Dynamic Response: The **endings on the nuclear bag regions show a dynamic response,** that is, they discharge more rapidly when the ***muscle is being stretched*** and less in response to sustained stretch.

Static Response: The primary **endings on the nuclear chain fibers show a static response,** that is, they discharge at an increased rate throughout the period of stretch of the muscle (Fig. 104.4).

Thus, the primary endings are capable of exhibiting both dynamic and static responses, which means they respond to both change in length and the velocity of lengthening of the muscle.

- The **static response is the response to muscle stretch,** i. e., change in muscle length at a maintained stretch, whereas,
- the **dynamic response is the response to the rate at which the muscle is being stretched,** i. e., the velocity of lengthening of the muscle.

Control of γ Efferent Discharge

The γ motor neurons do not receive input from primary sensory afferents. Rather, they are **primarily influenced by the descending pathways.**

1. Activity **in the descending pathways** increases the sensitivity of the muscle spindle by adjusting the *rate of γ motor neuron discharge.*
2. However, activities originating **in the sensory pathways** also indirectly influence γ motor neuron discharge by activating the descending influences.
   - For example, in **Jendrassik's maneuver,** the process in which the tendon reflexes are better elicited by trying to pull the hands apart when the flexed fingers are hooked, the rate of γ motor neuron discharge increases.
   - In **Jendrassik's maneuver,** proprioceptive input from the hand activates the supraspinal centers, which in turn increases γ efferent discharge by stimulating the descending pathways.
3. Tendon reflexes are also exaggerated in anxiety, as ***anxiety increases γ efferent discharge.***

α-γ Colinkage

The descending pathways that stimulate the γ motor neurons also stimulate the **α** motor neurons.

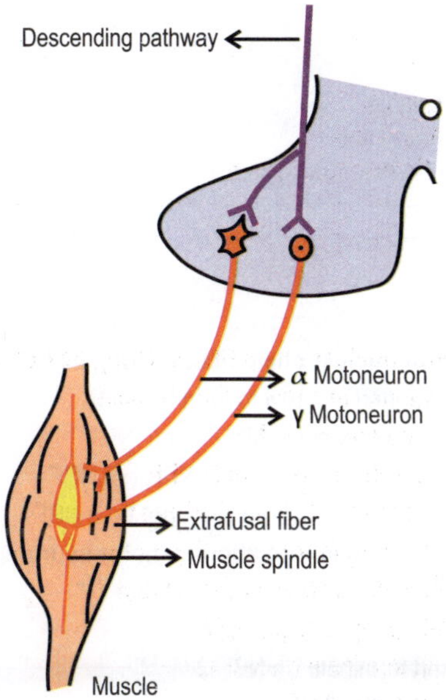

Fig. 104.5: Mechanism of α–γ coactivation.

- Therefore, γ efferent discharge increases along with the increased discharge of α motor neurons. This is called α-γ **colinkage** (α-γ **coactivation;** Fig. 104.5).
  - Because of this α–γ co-interaction, muscle spindle continues to discharge even when the muscle is in contracted state.
- Thus, **spindle adjusts motor neurons discharge throughout the period of muscle contraction.**

GOLGI TENDON ORGAN

Location

Golgi tendon organs (GTO) are found in the **tendon of the muscles.**

Structure

The GTOs are formed by the terminals of the **group Ib afferent fibers** (Fig. 104.6).

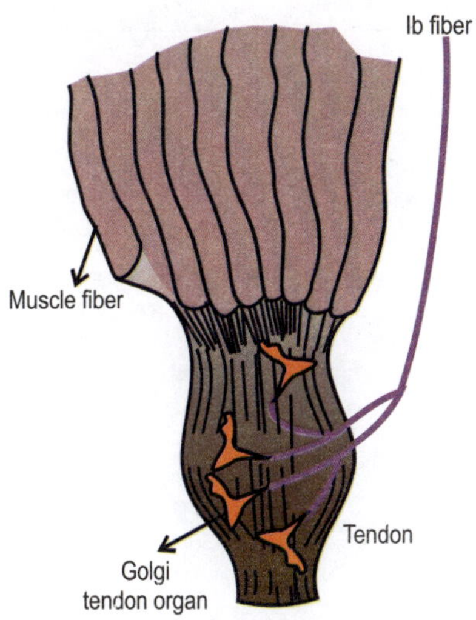

Fig. 104.6: Structure of Golgi tendon organ (GTO).

- The diameter of GTO is about 100 um and the length is about 1 mm. These sensory endings are **arranged in series** with that of the muscle fibers.
- The Ib fibers originating from GTO ***terminate indirectly on α motor neurons*** *via interneurons.*
- As the interneurons are inhibitory, stimulation of Ib fibers **inhibit the motor neuron activity.**

Function

Because of their arrangement (in series) with the muscle, GTO can be activated either by muscle stretch or by contraction of the muscle.

1. However, a **strong muscle contraction is a stronger stimulus** than the passive stretch of the muscle (Fig104.7).
   - The passive stretch does not effectively stimulate GTO because the elastic muscle fibers take up much impact of the stretch.
   - But, the afferents from **GTO discharge actively in response to muscle contraction** as muscle contraction stretches the tendon to a greater extent.
2. The actual stimulus for activation of GTO is **the force that develops in the tendon** (by muscle contraction or muscle stretch).

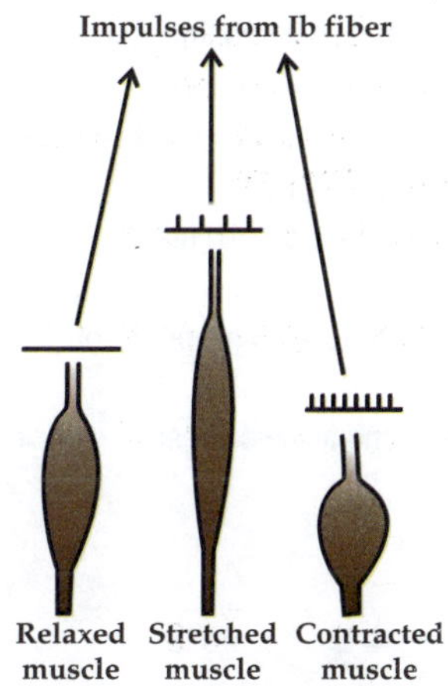

Fig. 104.7: Comparison of muscle stretch and strong active contraction on GTO activity. Note that there is no impulse from relaxed muscle and maximum impulse from contracted muscle.

Thus, GTO **signals the force of muscle contraction,** whereas the muscle spindle signals the muscle length.

- Therefore, **GTO provides the force feedback whereas muscle spindle provides the length feedback** (Fig. 104.8).

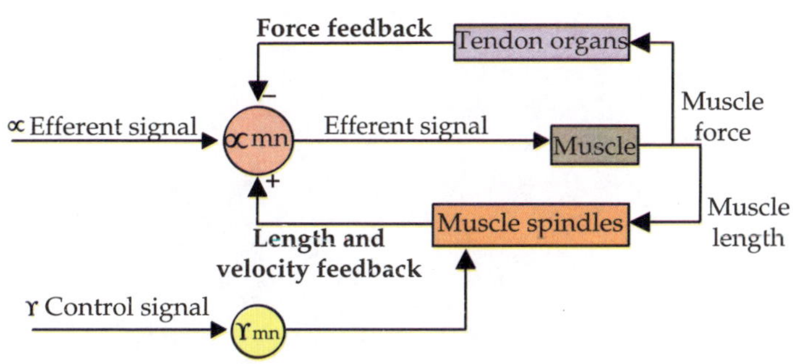

Fig. 104.8: Force and length feedbacks in motor control. mn: motor neuron.

Exam Questions

1. With the help of labeled schematic diagrams, describe the structure and functions of muscle spindle.
2. Briefly describe the role of γ motor neuron discharge on muscle tone. Add a note on spindle responses.
3. Describe the influence of length feedback and force feedback in motor control. Add a note on Golgi tendon organ.

Multiple Choice Questions

1. **The afferent from muscle to spinal cord is:**
   A. Ia fiber
   B. Ib fibers
   C. III fibers
   D. IV fibers
2. **In the motoneuron pool of anterior horn of spinal cord, γ-motor neurons constitute about:**
   A. 10%
   B. 30%
   C. 50%
   D. 70%
3. **During Jendrassik's maneuver, there is increased discharge of:**
   A. α-motor neurons
   B. β-motor neurons
   C. γ-motor neurons
   D. Ia afferent fiber
4. **Which of the following is not correct about muscle spindle (MS)?**
   A. Abut 2 to 12 fibers are present in a muscle spindle
   B. length of MS is about 5 to 10 mm and width about 100μm.
   C. Fibers of MS are present in parallel to regular muscle fibers
   D. They are the receptors for muscle force, not for lengthening of muscle
5. **All are true about nuclear bag fibers (NBF), EXCEPT:**
   A. The central portion is dilated to form a bag that contain nuclei
   B. About 10 NBF are present in a MS.
   C. NBF-1 has low myosin activity and respond to dynamic phase of muscle contraction
   D. NBF-2 has high myosin activity and respond to staic phase of muscle contraction
6. **All are true about nuclear chain fibers (NCF), EXCEPT:**
   A. Nuclei are arranged in a raw to form a chain
   B. About 5 NCF are present in MS
   C. Ia primary afferents innervate only NBF, not NCF
   D. Type II afferent arise only from NCF, not from NBF
7. **Which of the following is true about γ-motor neurons?**
   A. They constitute >50% fibers in ventral root
   B. They innervate peripheral part of MS
   C. Dynamic γ-mn terminate on NBF-2
   D. Static γ-mn innervate NBF-2
8. **Which of the following is not correct about functions of MS**
   A. MS is sensitive to muscle stretch, but not the speed of stretch
   B. γ-motor neuron increases sensitivity of spindle to stretch
   C. Endings on NBF show dynamic response
   D. Endings on NCF show static response
9. **True about Golgi tendon organs (GTO), EXCEPT:**
   A. Afferents are Ib fibers
   B. Muscle contraction is a stronger stimulus than muscle stretch for GTO
   C. Arranged in parallel with muscle fibers
   D. Stimulation of GTO inhibits motor neuron activity
10. **The muscle spindle continues to discharge even when the muscle is contracted due to:**
    A. Increased spindle sensitivity by increased muscle contraction
    B. Increased α-motor neuron discharge
    C. Stimulation of GTO
    D. α-γ coactivation

Answers

1. A 2. B 3. C 4. D 5. B 6. C 7. B 8. A 9. C 10. D

Chapter 105

PY10.2

Spinal Reflexes

Learning Objectives

On completion of study of this chapter:

The student will be able to (must know):

1. Name the spinal reflexes.
2. Draw diagrams of stretch reflex, inverse reflex and withdrawal reflex and briefly explain their physiological and clinical significance.
3. List the differences between stretch and withdrawal reflexes.
4. Explain the significance and mechanism of after-discharge of withdrawal reflex.
5. List the properties of spinal reflexes.
6. Illustrate the mechanism of inhibitions in the spinal cord.

The student may also be able to (desirable to know):

1. Describe the properties of spinal reflexes.
2. Describe the role of spinal reflexes in motor control.

A spinal reflex is defined as a **stereotyped motor response** to a *specific stimulus like stretch of the muscle*.

Components: Typically, the spinal reflexes include receptors, afferents, interneurons, motor neurons, and the muscle (Fig. 105.1).

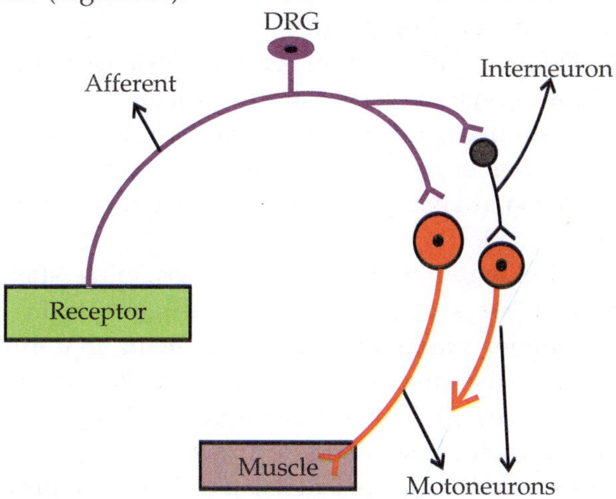

Fig. 105.1: Components of a spinal reflex. DRG: dorsal root ganglion.

The reflexes integrated in the spinal cord are:

1. Stretch reflex (Myotatic reflex)
2. Inverse stretch reflex (Inverse myotatic reflex)
3. Withdrawal reflex (Flexion reflex)
4. Positive supporting reaction
5. Negative supporting reaction

The last two reflexes are not observed in normal subjects, rather elicited in spinal human/animal.

STRETCH REFLEX (Myotatic Reflex)

Definition: The reflex contraction of the muscle to stretch when a skeletal muscle with its intact nerve supply is stretched is called the stretch reflex.

- The **stimulus is the stretch of the muscle,** and the **response is the contraction of the stretched muscle.**
- Stretch reflex is a **monosynaptic reflex** (a single synapse between the afferent and efferent limbs).

Types: There are **two types of stretch reflexes**: the phasic stretch reflex and the tonic stretch reflex.

Phasic Stretch Reflex

The phasic stretch reflex is elicited by stimulating the **primary endings of the muscle spindle**.

Stimulus

The stimulus for phasic stretch reflex is the **sudden stretch** of the muscle.

Reflex Arc

The receptor is the **muscle spindle** and afferent is the group **Ia afferent** fiber (Fig. 105.2).

1. In the spinal cord, afferent fiber divides into **two main branches.**

- The one of the branches of **Ia fiber directly terminates monosynaptically on the homonymous motor neurons** (i.e. the motor neuron that supplies the protagonist muscle).
- The other branch **terminates disynaptically via an inhibitory interneuron** (**Golgi bottle neuron**) on the heteronymous motor neuron (i.e. the motor neuron supplying the antagonist muscle).

2. Activity in the Ia afferent fiber **stimulates the homonymous motor neuron** that causes contraction of the protagonist muscle, and **inhibits the heteronymous motor neuron** that causes relaxation of the antagonist muscle.
   - Therefore, when the **agonist muscle contracts**, simultaneously the ***antagonist muscle relaxes***.
3. **Relaxation of antagonist muscle facilitates movement** caused by contraction of agonist muscle.
   - Such an innervation that ensures activation of a set of motor neuron and inhibition of another set of motor neuron is called **reciprocal innervation**, and the inhibition of antagonist muscle is called ***reciprocal inhibition***.

Function

Reflex contraction of muscle in response to a **sudden stretch** is the phasic stretch reflex.

1. The phasic reflex contraction results in **rapid limb movement**.
   - The examples are **tendon reflexes.**
   - The tendon reflex is elicited by tapping the tendon, which provides a quick stretch of the muscle.
2. By making rapid and transient movements, phasic stretch reflex ensures **immediate corrections of spinal motor output** in the moment-to-moment motor control.

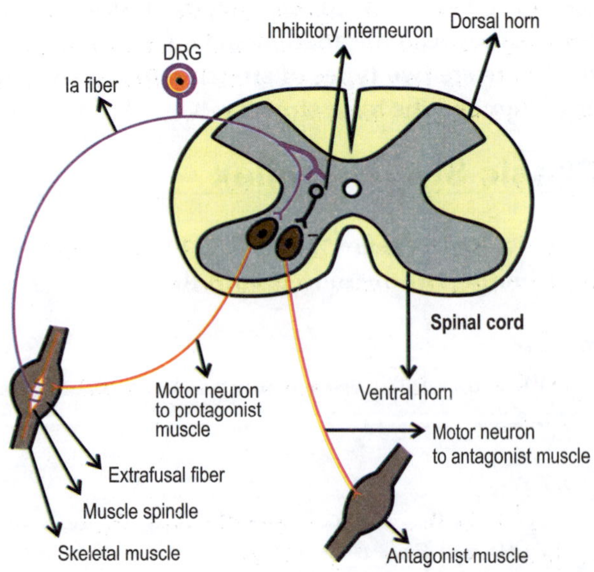

Fig. 105.2: Schematic representation of a stretch reflex. DRG: dorsal root ganglion

Clinical Significance

Tendon reflex reflects the **general excitability of motor neurons**.

1. When **excitability of the motor neurons is altered** in different clinical or pathological conditions the tendon reflexes are **depressed or exaggerated.**
   - This helps the physician to diagnose the nature of the **neurological deficit based on the response of the tendon reflexes**. Especially, the excitability of γ motor neurons is more important as it controls spindle sensitivity.
2. **Exaggeration of tendon reflex** is an index of ***increased γ motor neuron*** discharge and **depression of reflex** indicates ***decreased γ motor neuron*** activity.

Tonic Stretch Reflex

Stimulus

The tonic stretch reflex is elicited by a **sustained stretch** of the muscle.

Reflex Arc

It is same as that of the phasic stretch reflex except that the **receptors are both primary and secondary endings**.

1. Therefore, the **afferents are both Ia and II afferent fibers** from the muscle spindle.
2. Group II afferents make ***direct connections*** with the α motor neurons. Thus, this is also a **monosynaptic reflex**.

Function

Tonic stretch reflex **contributes to the muscle tone.**

1. **Muscle tone** is the resistance of muscle to stretch.
2. Tonic stretch reflex is also important for **regulation of posture**.
3. To maintain standing position after assuming the position, the extensors of knees should contract so that knees remain extended and legs do not bend.
   - This is achieved by the **action of gravity on medial extensors of the thigh**.
   - Due to the effect of gravity, extensor muscles (**antigravity muscles**) are stretched.
4. The **sustained stretch of extensors** results in sustained contraction of these antigravity muscles that maintains extension at knee joint. Thus, the standing position is maintained.
5. **On Prolonged Standing:** After assuming standing posture for a longer duration, **fatigue sets in**. Due to fatigue, gradually the **knees bend** that further stretches the quadriceps muscles. The flexion at knee joints **elicits additional tonic stretch reflex** that in turn causes **added sustained contraction** of quadriceps. This maintains further extension of knees and prevents the person from falling. Thus, stretch reflex helps **to**

restore and maintain the posture for a very long period.

- For example, a **traffic police** who is standing for a longer duration flexes his knees due to physical fatigue. This stretches his quadriceps and elicits tonic stretch reflex.
- **Contraction of quadriceps** opposes the flexion at the knee and restores his posture. Thus, tonic stretch reflex **maintains posture**.

In summary, the phasic stretch reflex mediates tendon jerk and controls rapid corrections in motor output, whereas the tonic stretch reflex maintains body position despite alteration in load on the body.

INVERSE STRETCH REFLEX (Inverse Myotatic Reflex)

Definition: Relaxation of the muscle in response to a strong stretch is called inverse stretch reflex. This is also known as **autogenic inhibition**.

Reflex Arc

Receptors: Receptors are Golgi tendon organs (GTO).

- These are netlike collection of knobby nerve endings located in the fascicles of a tendon.
- There are 3 - 25 muscle fibers per tendon organs.

Stimulus: The stimulus for inverse stretch reflex is **a stronger stretch.**

An active muscle contraction also elicits this reflex.

Reflex Circuit: Afferent fibers from GTO are **Ib fibers (Fig. 105.3).**

1. Ib fibers terminate on the **inhibitory interneurons** that in turn project to the homonymous α motor neurons.
2. This results in *inhibition of the agonist muscle*. This is a **disynaptic reflex**.

Functions

Golgi tendon organ **monitors force developed in the muscle**.

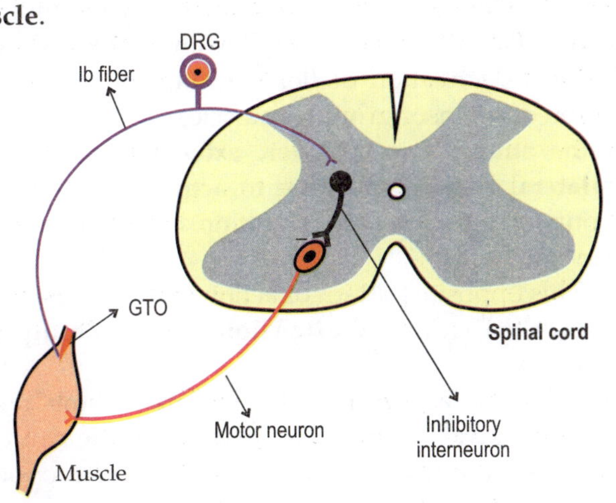

Fig. 105.3: Schematic representation of an inverse stretch reflex. DRG: dorsal root ganglion; GTO: Golgi tendon organ.

1. The force is detected either by strong stretch or by an active contraction. Stimulation of the GTO **inhibits the agonist muscle** through its reflex connections.
2. The agonist muscle relaxes in response to activation of GTO.
3. Thus, a **stronger stretch** imparted on the muscle automatically **inhibits the muscle**.
   - Therefore, the reflex is also called **autogenic inhibition**.

Physiologic Significance

Muscle spindle (stretch reflex) monitors muscle length and GTO (inverse stretch reflex) monitors muscle tension, i.e. the force of contraction.

1. Thus, muscle spindle provides **length feedback** and GTO provides **force feedback** (refer Fig. 104.8, Chapter 104).
2. Stretch reflex and inverse stretch reflex by acting together maintain **optimal motor responses** (of muscle tension and muscle length) for postural adjustments.
3. Inverse stretch reflex, by allowing the muscle to relax, **prevents rupture of muscle** when the muscle is stretched to greater extents.

Effect of γ Motor Neuron on Stretch Reflexes & Muscle Tone

The γ motor neurons control the activity of stretch reflexes by **altering the sensitivity of muscle spindle to stretch.**

1. Spindle afferents **do not influence** the activities of γ motor neurons, as they **have no direct contact** with them.
   - However, ***descending influence from supraspinal segments*** increases the discharge of γ motor neurons, which in turn ***increases the sensitivity*** of the spindle to stretch.
2. **In upper motor neurons paralysis**, for example following spinal transection (in the recovery phase), the increased γ motor neuron discharge (due to loss of inhibitory suprasegmental inputs on the motor neurons) increases the reflex activity.
   - The muscle becomes **hyper-reactive due to increased phasic stretch reflex activity** and becomes **hypertonic due to increased tonic stretch reflex activity**.

Muscle Tone

Resistance of the muscle to stretch is called tone.

1. Muscle becomes **hypertonic or spastic** when the resistance to stretch is more due to hyperactive stretch reflexes (**increased γ motoneuron discharge**).
2. Muscle becomes hypotonic (flaccid) when the motor neurons supplying the muscle are damaged or when the discharge of γ motor neurons is decreased.

Clasp-Knife Phenomenon

When a hypertonic muscle as seen in upper motor neuron paralysis is stretched, muscle contracts, but **if the stretch is continued then muscle relaxes**.

- For example, flexing the elbow of such a patient first meets with greater resistance, but if the flexion continues then the muscle relaxes and ***suddenly the resistance force disappears*** (flexion occurs easily).
- This type of **high resistance followed by sudden collapse** is known as clasp-knife phenomenon as it resembles the **closing a clasp-knife**.
- Physiologically, this is called **lengthening reaction** as the response occurs due to lengthening of spastic muscle.

Physiological Basis: As the muscle tone is more, resistance against flexion of the limb is more. However, when flexion is continued, further stretch of the triceps muscle **activates inverse stretch reflex** that relaxes the muscle due to ***autogenic inhibition***. Thus, the resistance force against flexion suddenly disappears.

Clonus

This is defined as a **regular rhythmic contraction of a muscle *subjected to a sudden and maintained stretch***. The best example is the **ankle clonus**. This is elicited by dorsiflexing the foot and trying to maintain the dorsiflexion, which results in rhythmic planter flexion at the ankle.

1. It is typically seen in ***upper motor neuron paralysis*** in which the **spindles are hyperactive**.
2. When the muscle is suddenly stretched the spindle discharges and muscle contracts. Muscle contraction stops the spindle discharge and muscle relaxes. But, **maintained stretch stimulates the spindle again** and the process is repeated.

WITHDRAWAL REFLEX

Withdrawal reflex is an example of **polysynaptic spinal reflex**. This is also called **flexor withdrawal reflex** because activation of it causes withdrawal of the body parts by flexing the limbs.

Receptors and Stimuli

The receptors are **nociceptors** that are present in the skin, muscle, tendon, or joints. Noxious or painful stimulation of skin, subcutaneous tissue or muscle elicits this reflex.

Reflex Circuit

The afferents are called **flexor reflex afferents** (FRA).

1. This includes **type III and IV somatic afferents**. The afferents, after entering the spinal cord divides into **two branches** to terminate on two separate sets of interneurons (Fig. 105.4).
    - One branch activates a set of interneurons that in turn **excites α motor neurons supplying flexor muscles** of the same side.
    - Another branch activates a separate set of interneurons that in turn **inhibits α motor neurons supplying the same side extensor muscles.**

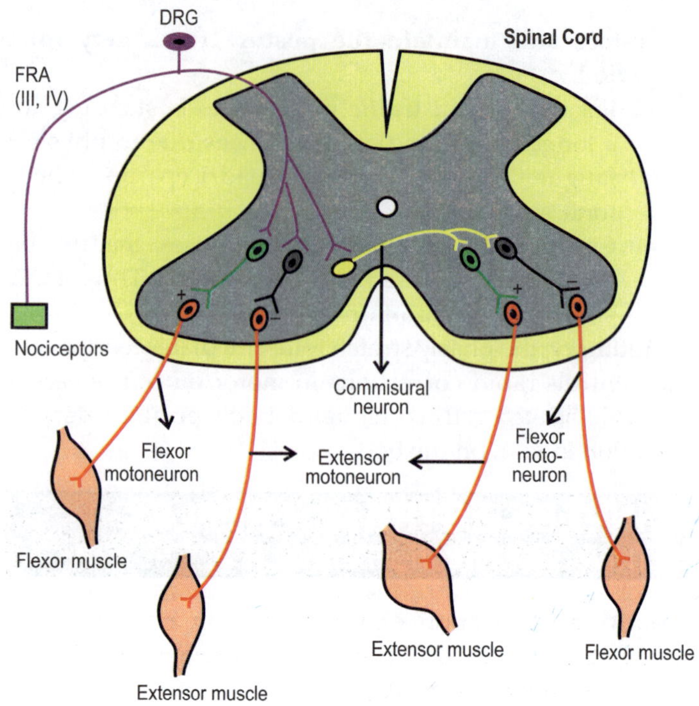

Fig. 105.4: Schematic representation of a withdrawal reflex. DRG: dorsal root ganglion; FRA: flexion reflex afferents.

2. A branch of the interneuron (**commissural interneurons**) excited by FRA crosses the midline to enter the opposite side of the ventral horn and **terminate on opposite set of interneurons**.
    - That means, the commissural interneurons activate the interneurons that in turn ***stimulate motoneurons supplying contralateral extensor muscles*** and activate interneurons that in turn ***inhibit motor neurons supplying contralateral flexor muscles.***

Responses

As per the reflex connections described above, stimulation of flexor reflex afferents causes **flexion of the ipsilateral limb** due to activation of flexor group of muscles and inhibition of extensor group of muscles.

1. If the stimulus is stronger, **extension of the contralateral limb** occurs due to activation of extensor group of muscles and inhibition of flexor group of muscles.
    - This opposite pattern of action in the opposite limb is called as **crossed extension reflex** or **Phillipson's reflex.**
2. The flexion response of the ipsilateral limb results in **withdrawal of the body parts** from the source of noxious stimulus and the extension of the opposite limb **maintains balance during the act**.

Widespread Response

If the stimulus is still stronger, **impulses irradiate upward and downward** in the spinal cord and activate motor neurons that supply muscle of other limbs to produce **widespread response**.

1. This results in **extension of the other limb of the same side and flexion of other limb of the opposite side**.
   - This is one of the examples of ***irradiation of impulse*** in the spinal cord generated by the stimulus and also of the **recruitment of motor neurons or motor units**.
2. This is also an example of **divergence of impulses** in the spinal cord. That is, impulses in FRA project to **many interneurons** and motor neurons in the spinal cord that finally results in:
   i) **flexion of the same limb** and with ***extension of the opposite limb***, and
   ii) **extension of the other limb** of the same side and ***flexion of the other limb*** of the opposite side.
3. Various patterns of these limb movements **provide postural support and balance** for immediate and appropriate withdrawal of body parts.

Special Features of Withdrawal Reflex

1. **Protective Reflex:** Withdrawal reflex is a protective reflex ***protects body parts*** from damage caused by noxious (potentially harmful) stimuli.
   - Flexion of the stimulated limb withdraws the limb and extension of the opposite limb supports or balances the body.
2. **Pre-Potent:** Withdrawal reflex is pre-potent. This means when this reflex is activated, temporarily other reflex activities in the spinal cord almost stop at that moment, so that the spinal cord carries out the reflex responses precisely and without delay (Table 105.1).
3. **Local Sign:** The pattern of response of flexor withdrawal reflex depends on the **nature and the location of the stimulus**.
   - For example, abduction occurs when the medial surface of the limb is stimulated, and adduction occurs when lateral surface is stimulated. This is called **local sign.**
4. **After-Discharge:** A stronger stimulus not only causes **widespread response** but also **prolongs the response**. The prolongation of response is due to ***prolonged and repeated firing*** of the target motor neurons. This process is called **after-discharge**. After-discharge occurs due to ***two mechanisms*** (Fig. 105.5):

i) Involvement of **many interneuronal pathways** of different length between afferent and efferent neurons. The pathways containing less number of interneurons ***stimulate the motor neuron early*** (as the impulses arrives at motor neuron early), and the pathways containing more interneurons ***stimulate the motor neurons later*** (as the impulses arrive at motor neuron later through these pathway) (Fig. 105.5). Thus, motor neurons are **stimulated repeatedly.**

ii) Presence of **reverberating circuits** in the interneuronal pathways in the spinal cord. The branches of the interneurons project onto the other interneurons that ***project back to the same interneurons***. Thus, stimulation of interneurons reverberates the impulses circuitously. Therefore, motor neurons are stimulated repeatedly.

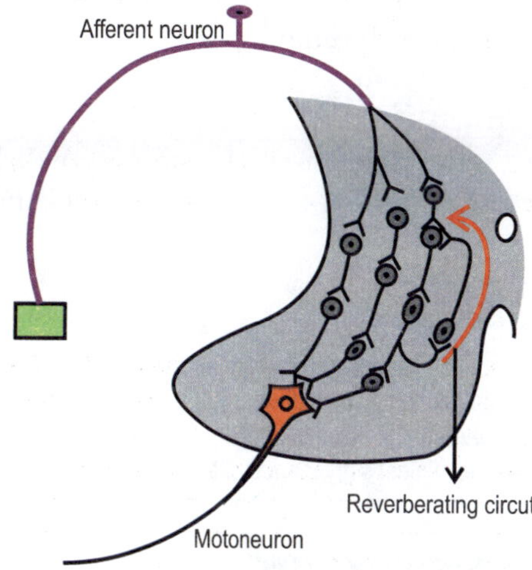

Fig. 105.5: Mechanism of after-discharge in withdrawal reflex. Note the presence of many interneuronal pathways and reverberating circuits between afferent and efferent neurons.

Table 105.1 | Differences between Stretch and Flexion (withdrawal) reflex.

	Stretch reflex	Flexion reflex
1. Receptors	Muscle spindle	Nociceptors
2. Afferents	Ia afferents	Flexor reflex afferents (FRA)
3. Divergence	Less	Widespread
4. Latency	Short (as it is monosynaptic)	Long (as polysynaptic)
5. Target muscle	The same muscle	Flexor muscles of the same side and extensor muscles of the opposite side.
6. Reciprocal Innervation	Single reciprocal innervation	Double reciprocal innervation
7. Response	Linear or stereotyped	Non-linear and may be widespread
8. Duration	Reflex stops as the stimulus is withdrawn	Reflex activity continues even after the withdrawal of the stimulus. This occurs to after discharge.
9. Specificity	Specific to a set of muscles	Less specific (involves many muscle groups).
10. Local sign	Absent	Present
11. Importance	Not pre-potent	Pre-potent

PROPERTIES OF SPINAL REFLEXES

Convergence, divergence, facilitation, inhibition, summations, occlusion have been discussed in Chapter 95.

Adequate stimulus

The **quality of a stimulus** that evokes a reflex response is a very precise one.

- This is called the adequate stimulus for that particular reflex.
- For example, stretch of the muscle is the adequate stimulus for stretch reflex.

Habituation and Sensitization

Usually, the reflex responses are stereotyped. However, with experiences, reflexes can also be modified. These are called habituation and sensitization. Habituation and sensitization forms the physiological basis of learning and memory in the CNS.

Habituation: Decreased response of the target neuron to a afferent stimulations, when the stimulus is applied repeatedly is called habituation.

Sensitization: Increased response of the target neuron to afferent stimulations, when the stimulus is applied repeatedly is called sensitization.

Final Common Pathway

The motor neurons that supply the skeletal muscle especially the α motor neurons are considered to be the *final common path* for the motor output. This is because all the neural influences arriving from different parts of the CNS, regulate muscle activity through these motor neurons.

Exam Questions

1. Draw a labelled schematic diagram of stretch reflex. Describe the role of stretch reflex in motor function. Add a note on reciprocal inhibition.
2. Draw a labelled schematic diagram of withdrawal reflex. List the differences between stretch reflex & withdrawal reflex. Describe the mechanism of after-discharge.
3. Describe the clinical significance of lengthening reaction and clasp knife phenomenon. Add a note on types of inhibition in spinal cord.

Multiple Choice Questions

1. All of the following reflexes are integrated at the level of spinal cord, EXCEPT:
A. Inverse stretch reflex
B. Withdrawal reflex
C. Tonic neck reflex
D. Positive supporting reaction

2. All of the following are true about tonic stretch reflex, EXCEPT:
A. Contributes to muscle tone
B. Important for regulation of posture
C. Elicited by sudden stretch of the muscle
D. Afferents are both Ia and II afferent fibers

3. Which of the following is not true about stretch reflex?
A. Also called myotatic reflex
B. Afferent is Ib fiber
C. Monosynaptic reflex
D. A branch of afferent terminates on inhibitory interneuron

4. All are true about inverse stretch reflex, EXCEPT:
A. Receptor is GTO
B. Afferent is Ib fiber
C. Afferent terminates on interneuron that contacts homonymous motoneuron
D. Monosynaptic reflex

5. Salivation by dog seen when food is given along with ringing of bell is:
A. Conditional reflex
B. Reinforcement
C. Habituation
D. Innate reflex

6. Decreased reflex response after repetitive stimulation:
A. Summation
B. Fatigue
C. Irradiation
D. Occlusion

7. All are true properties of spinal cord reflex, EXCEPT:
A. Memory
B. Summation
C. Delay
D. Fatigue

8. All of the following are true for withdrawal reflex, EXCEPT:
A. Afferents are FRA (III and IV fibers)
B. Polysynaptic reflex
C. Prolongation of response due to after-discharge is an important property
D. Local sign is absent

Answers

1. C 2. C 3. B 4. D 5. D 6. B 7. B 8. D

Chapter 106

Descending Pathways

Learning Objectives

On completion of study of this chapter:

The student will be able to (must know):

1. Classify the descending pathways and justify the basis of physiological classification.
2. Name the descending tracts in lateral system and medial system pathways
3. Draw a diagram of corticospinal tracts (CSTs) and explain the effects of lesion of CSTs at internal capsule.
4. List the differences between UMN & LMN paralysis and explain the physiological basis of these differences.
5. Give the course and functions of other descending pathways.
6. Define monoplegia, hemiplegia, paraplegia & quadriplegia and give the common causes for each.
7. Outline the importance of examination of cranial nerves in hemiplegia and justify why 7th cranial nerve examination is very helpful in a hemiplegic patient.
8. Name the brainstem syndromes associated with hemiplegia.

The student may also be able to (desirable to know):

1. Describe the extrapyramidal system pathways.
2. Describe the physiological basis of features of a patient of stroke with hemiplegia and explain the brainstem syndromes associated with hemiplegia.

PY10.4

CLASSIFICATION

Clinical Classification: Descending motor pathways have been traditionally classified into **pyramidal and extrapyramidal tracts.**

1. **The pyramidal tracts** are the descending tracts that pass through the pyramid in the medulla.
   - **Pyramidal tract diseases** clinically refer to dysfunctions that ***interrupt fibers of the corticospinal tracts,*** as these fibers pass through the medullary pyramid.
2. **Extrapyramidal tracts** are the descending pathways that **do not pass through the pyramid** in the medulla.
   - Extrapyramidal tracts include **reticulospinal, vestibulospinal, rubrospinal, and tectospinal tracts.**

Confusion in clinical classification: Pyramidal-extrapyramidal classification is not appropriate physiologically for the following reasons.

1. All the fibers of corticospinal tracts do not pass through pyramid, and especially most of the **fibers in the anterior corticospinal tract bypass the pyramid.**
2. **Pyramidal tract signs** seen in patients suffering from pyramidal tract disease are ***not similar with the features of the isolated lesion of corticospinal tract*** produced in experimental animals.
3. Clinically, extrapyramidal diseases refer to the **diseases of basal ganglia and cerebellum.**
   - But major descending pathway **involved in basal ganglia function is the corticospinal tract** rather than the extrapyramidal tracts.

Thus, classification of pyramidal versus extrapyramidal pathways is **physiologically inappropriate.**

Physiological Classification: Physiologically, descending pathways are divided into two: **lateral system and medial system pathways.**

- This classification is based on the **termination of the descending pathways on the motor neurons** in the spinal cord, **and the function** of the pathways.

Lateral System Pathways

Lateral system pathways **descend down in the lateral column** of the spinal cord.

1. These include **lateral corticospinal tract** and **rubrospinal tract.**
2. The fibers of these tracts are placed in the lateral funiculus in the spinal cord and fibers **terminate on the**

motor neurons that are placed laterally in the ventral horn of the spinal cord, i. e., on the lateral group of motor neurons (Fig. 106.1).

3. These tracts are involved in the **regulation of skilled voluntary movements** as lateral group of motor neurons innervate the distal limb muscles.

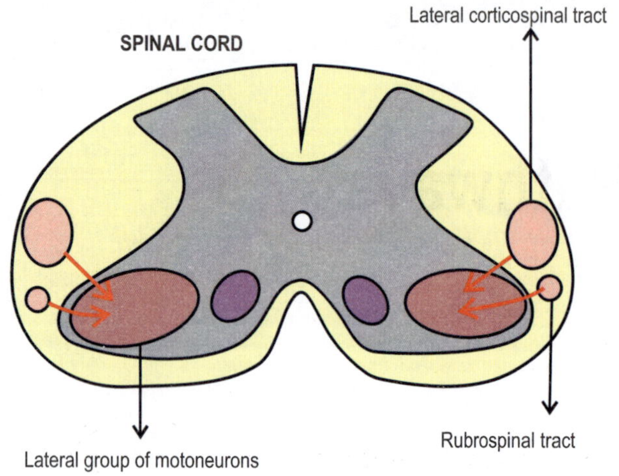

Fig. 106.1: Placement of lateral descending pathways in spinal cord.

Medial System Pathways

Medial system pathways **descend down in the medial and anterior columns** of the spinal cord.

These pathways include:

1. Reticulospinal tract
2. Vestibulospinal tract
3. Tectospinal tract
4. Anterior corticospinal tract

The fibers of these tracts are placed in the ***medial and anterior funiculi*** in the spinal cord and they **terminate on the motor neurons that are placed medially** in the ventral horn, i. e., on the **medial group of motor neurons** (Fig. 106.2). Therefore, these tracts are involved in **regulation of posture** as the motor neurons of medial group innervate the ***proximal limb muscles and the muscles of the axial skeleton*** of the body.

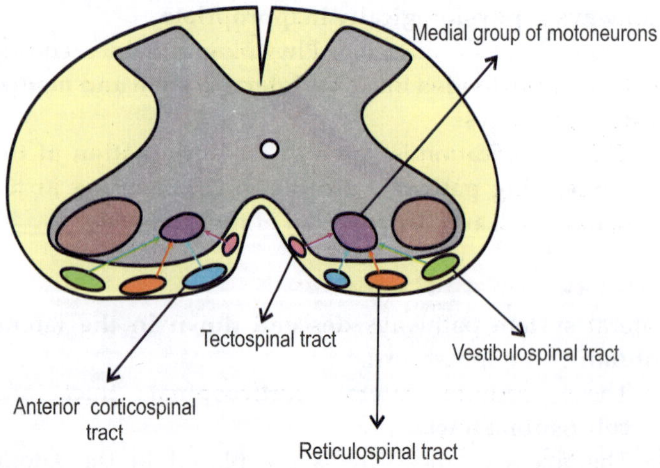

Fig. 106.2: Placement of medial descending pathways in spinal cord.

Corticospinal Tracts

Traditionally, corticospinal tract, pyramidal tract and upper motor neurons are used interchangeably.

There are **two groups** of corticospinal tracts (CST): the lateral CST and anterior CST.

1. The **lateral corticospinal tract** constitutes about 80% of the fibers in the corticospinal pathway.
   - This is the most important descending pathway for the control of skilled voluntary activities.
2. The **anterior or ventral corticospinal tract** constitutes only 20% of the fibers in the corticospinal pathway and is involved in control of posture.

Origin

The fibers of corticospinal tract **originate from the primary motor cortex (area 4)**, especially from the large motor cells of Betz in the fifth layer of the precentral gyrus.

- There are about 30, 000 Betz cells in the cortex, whereas about one million axons are present in corticospinal tract, which clearly indicate that the corticospinal fibers also originate from other areas in the cortex.
- The **other cortical motor areas** include **premotor cortex** (lateral part of area 6), **supplementary motor area** (medial part of area 6), **primary somatosensory cortex** (area 3, 1, and 2) and **parietal cortex** (area 5 and 7).
- Motor cortex contributes to **60% of fibers** (30% from area 4 and 30% from area 6) and **sensory cortex contributes to 40%** of fibers in the corticospinal tract.

Course

Fibers arising from different parts of the cortical areas converge **through the posterior limb of the internal capsule** (Fig. 106.3).

1. As the fibers in the subcortical areas appear in a ***radiating pattern***, they are collectively known as **corona radiata.**
2. After passing through internal capsule, fibers descend down in the ventral brainstem as the cerebral peduncles.
   - In the medulla, fibers **pass through the pyramid** (medullary pyramid).
3. About **80% of the fibers** after passing through the pyramid, **immediately decussate** (cross over to the opposite side) and descend down in the lateral funiculus of the spinal cord.
   - This forms the **lateral corticospinal tract.**
   - The lateral corticospinal fibers have **monosynaptic connections with anterior horn cells.**
4. The remaining **20% of the fibers** descend down ipsilaterally (do not decussate) in the anterior funiculus of the spinal cord.
   - This constitutes the ventral or **anterior corticospinal tract.**

- The fibers cross over to the opposite side ***only at the spinal cord segments*** through their termination **on the interneurons**.

Termination

1. Fibers of **lateral corticospinal tract terminate on lateral group of motor neurons** in the ventral horn of spinal cord.
   - About 30% of Lateral CST fibers **terminate directly on motor neurons** and 70% fibers terminate **through interneurons**.
   - These motor neurons **innervate the distal limb muscles**.
2. The fibers of **ventral corticospinal tract** do not directly terminate on the motor neurons, rather they **end on the interneurons** in the same side of the spinal cord.
   - These interneurons in turn **cross over to the opposite side** and terminate on the **medial group of motor neurons**. Few fibers from the interneurons terminate on the same side of medial group of motor neurons.
   - These motor neurons supply the **proximal limb muscles and axial muscles** of the body.

Functions

The motor cortex is mainly involved in **initiation, planning and control of movement** (for details of functions of motor cortex, refer Chapter 107). Corticospinal tracts **transmit central command signal** from motor cortex to the spinal cord interneurons and motor neurons.

1. **Lateral corticospinal tract** controls the ***skilled voluntary movements*** of the body.
2. **Anterior corticospinal tract** controls ***posture.***

Functions of corticospinal tracts are better appreciated by making lesions of these tracts.

Effects of Lesions:

1. **Lesion of lateral corticospinal tract** results in **impairment of skilled voluntary activities** like writing, painting, etc. But, as the rubrospinal tract is intact, the subject recovers after few days or weeks.
   - However, isolated lesion of lateral corticospinal tract is very uncommon in humans.
   - In addition, diseases that affect corticospinal tract **also affect the corticobulbar tracts** that influence activities of extrapyramidal systems.
   - Thus, a pure corticospinal tract disease is not seen in humans.
2. **Lesion of anterior corticospinal tract** in animals results in **inability to maintain posture** while walking, climbing etc.
   - But in human beings, postural deficit following lesion of anterior corticospinal tract is not prominent because of two reasons:

   i) First, this tract is ***not well developed*** in humans and,

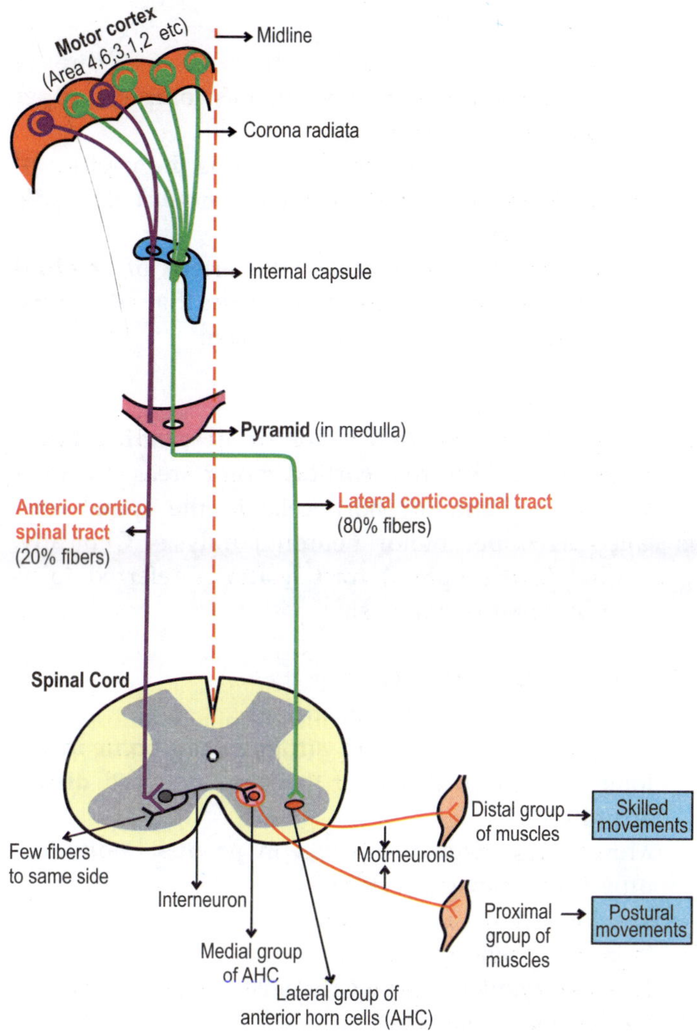

Fig. 106.3: Course of corticospinal tracts. Note, 80% of fibers after passing through medullary pyramid decussate (cross over to opposite side) and descend down as lateral corticospinal tract to contact lateral group of motoneurons in the spinal cord. Remaining 20% fibers descend down ipsilaterally on the same side as anterior corticospinal tract to terminate mostly indirectly (through interneurons) on medial group of motoneurons.

   ii) Second, ***other major posture regulating pathways*** especially the reticulospinal tract and vestibulospinal tracts **are still intact**.

Clinical Importance

Corticospinal pathway may be interrupted anywhere along its course from cortex to spinal cord. However, the lesion of corticospinal tract at the internal capsule (**capsular lesion**) is the commonest pyramidal tract lesion.

Capsular Lesion: As the fibers coming from different parts of the cortex pass through a narrow tunnel in the **posterior limb of the internal capsule,** disease of the internal capsule results in **complete interruption of corticospinal fibers**.

1. This leads to complete paralysis of opposite half of the body (**contralateral hemiplegia)**.
2. The ascending fiber systems from basal ganglia and cerebellum pass close to the internal capsule.
   - Therefore, **extrapyramidal systems are also affected** in addition to involvement of corticospinal

fibers.
- Consequently, pyramidal tract disease due to capsular lesion is often termed as **complete upper motor neuron paralysis**.

3. The usual ***cause of capsular lesion*** is the rupture of **Charcot's artery,** the ***lenticulostriate branch*** of middle cerebral artery.
   - This artery is also called the **artery of cerebral hemorrhage** as it accounts for more than 60% of the causes of intracerebral hemorrhage.

UMN Paralysis

Paralysis that results from **lesion of descending fibers** between their origin from cortical motor areas and their termination on anterior horn cells in the spinal cord is called as upper motor neuron paralysis. Clinically, **pyramidal (corticospinal) tract lesion** is referred to as upper motor neuron paralysis.

Features of UMN Paralysis

1. Increased muscle tone (**spasticity**).
2. No muscle atrophy (mild atrophy may occur in the long run due to disuse of the muscle, called **disuse atrophy**).
3. Muscles are usually affected in groups (individual muscles are never affected).
4. Tendon reflexes are exaggerated.
5. Superficial reflexes are lost
6. Extensor planter response (Babinski's sign positive)
7. No fascicular twitches
8. No denervation potential in EMG
9. Normal nerve conduction studies

However, if **only the corticospinal fibers are interrupted** by the disease process that affects medullary pyramid (or, experimentally produced lesion of medullary pyramid), most of the *above-mentioned features are not observed.*

- The most prominent features of such a isolated lesion of CST are paralysis or weakness of the distal muscles of the limbs and positive Babinski's sign. **Spasticity is not seen**; muscle tone even may be decreased. This indicates that descending fibers passing through pyramid are **mostly the fibers of lateral corticospinal tract**.
- The features described for pyramidal tract disease indicate the **involvement of corticobulbar fibers** that influence brainstem motor nuclei in **addition to the interruption of corticospinal fibers**.

Physiological Basis of Features of UMN Paralysis

Spasticity: Spasticity occurs due to **increased discharge of motor neurons** and ***increased excitability of the motor neuron pool.***

- In upper motor neuron lesions, not only the corticospinal fibers are interrupted, but also the **corticoreticular fibers** are damaged.
- Normally, corticoreticular fibers (fibers from motor cortex to the brainstem reticular formation, especially to the pontine reticular nuclei that forms pontine reticulospinal tract) **inhibit reticulospinal pathway**.
  - Therefore, interruption of corticoreticular pathway **facilitates reticulospinal activity**.
  - Normally, pontine reticulospinal tract excites the proximal extensor muscles.
- Loss of inhibitory corticoreticular influence **makes the reticulospinal tract more facilitatory**, and therefore, muscle tone increases.
  - Hence, spasticity and hypertonia are important features of UMN paralysis.

Absence of Muscle Atrophy: Muscle atrophy occurs when either the blood supply or the nerve supply to a muscle is disrupted.

- In UMN paralysis, the nerve supply is not interrupted (the **lower motor neurons remain intact**).
  - Therefore, atrophy is not a feature of UMN paralysis.
- However, in long standing cases, mild atrophy occurs due to disuse of the muscle. This is called **disuse atrophy**.

Exaggeration of Deep Tendon Reflexes: Usually, the upper motor neurons are inhibitory to the lower motor neurons.

- In UMN paralysis, **loss of these inhibitory influences** increases the motor neuron discharge.
- Especially, the **increased γ motor neuron discharge** increases the sensitivity of the muscle spindle to stretch. This results in increased deep tendon reflex.

Loss of Superficial Reflexes: Superficial reflexes are **long polysynaptic reflexes** that involve different parts of CNS (unlike stretch reflexes that are monosynaptic and integrated at the level of spinal cord).

- The **afferent pathways** of superficial reflexes ascend up in the ascending sensory systems.
- The **efferent pathways** are the descending motor pathways that finally terminate in skeletal muscles.
- As **efferent pathway is disrupted** in UMN paralysis, the superficial reflexes are abolished.

Extensor Planter Response: Corticospinal tract **excites the flexor motor neurons and inhibits the extensor motor neurons** supplying the muscles of the digits of the limbs.

- Therefore, normally stroking the sole of the foot elicits planter flexion.
- In UMN paralysis, **disruption of corticospinal influence** on the lumbosacral motor neurons causes dorsiflexion of big toe and fanning of other toes (extensor planter response; **Babinski's sign positive**).

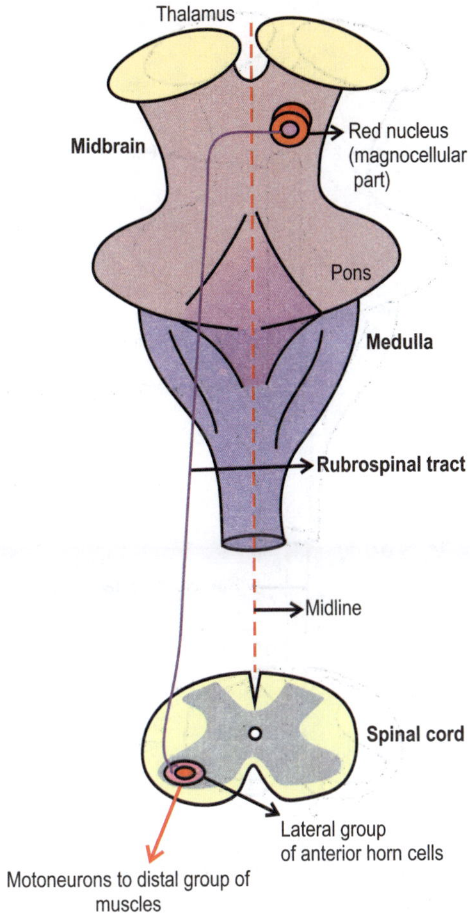

Fig. 106.4: Course of the rubrospinal tract.

Rubrospinal Tract

Origin: Rubrospinal tract **originates from red nucleus,** located in the midbrain.

- Red nucleus receives **strong excitatory input from motor cortex and cerebellum.**

Course: Immediately after originating from red nucleus, fibers **cross over to the opposite side** at the same level (Fig. 106.4).

IMPORTANT NOTE

Both lateral descending systems, viz, **lateral corticospinal and rubrospinal tracts, cross over to opposite side.**

After descending down through contralateral brain stem, fibers ***occupy the lateral column*** of the spinal cord.

- The fibers **terminate on lateral group of motor neurons** that innervate distal limb muscles.
- Rubrospinal tract **excites flexor group of muscles** and inhibits extensor muscles.

Functions: Rubrospinal tract controls **skilled voluntary movements.**

Applied Physiology: In experimental animal, lesion of rubrospinal tract produces deficit in the distal limb muscles, especially in the flexor group of muscles. However, if the lateral corticospinal tract is intact, the deficit persists temporarily.

MEDIAL SYSTEM PATHWYAS

Vestibulospinal Tracts

Vestibulospinal tracts (VST) originate from vestibular nuclei. There are **two vestibulospinal tracts:** lateral VST and medial VST.

Lateral Vestibulospinal Tract

Origin: Lateral VST originates from **lateral vestibular nucleus** (*Deiter's nucleus*) in the brainstem.

Course: This tract descends down **ipsilaterally through the brainstem and spinal cord.**

The fibers occupy the ventral funiculus of the spinal cord and **terminate on the medial group of interneurons and motor neurons** in the ventral horn of spinal cord (Fig.106.5).

This tract extends throughout the rostrocaudal extent of the spinal cord.

Functions: It excites motor neurons that supply the proximal group of muscles (especially the extensor muscles of the limb).

- Thus, LVST **controls posture**.
- The input to lateral vestibular nucleus comes **mainly from semi circular canals and otolith organs** of the inner ear.
- Therefore, LVST controls body posture *in relation to angular and linear accelerations* of the head.

Clinical Importance: In decerebrate animals (following mid-collicular section), LVST becomes hyperactive due to loss of inhibitory controls from the cortical areas on it.

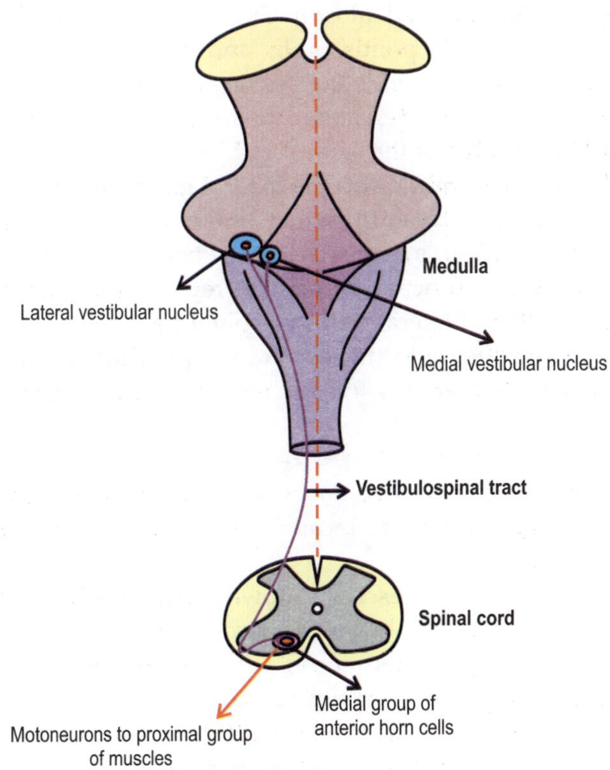

Fig. 106.5: Course of the vestibulospinal tract.

- Therefore, **extensor rigidity** is the hallmark of **decerebrate animals**.
- In humans, brainstem lesion due to stroke or injury facilitates vestibulospinal tract activity that manifests in the form of neck, arms and leg rigidity.

Medial Vestibulospinal Tract

Origin: Medial vestibulospinal tract (MVST) originates from **medial vestibular nucleus.**

Course: MVST **descends down ipsilaterally** in the brainstem and ventral funiculus of the spinal cord. It extends upto the midthoracic spinal cord segments.

The fibers of MVST terminate on the **medial group of interneurons and motor neurons** (Fig. 106.5).

Functions: MVST controls body posture.

The input to medial vestibular nucleus comes mainly from the semicircular canals. Therefore, MVST adjusts body posture especially the **head position in response to angular acceleration**.

Reticulospinal Tracts

Reticular formation **receives inputs** from spinal cord, vestibular nuclei, cerebellum, hypothalamus, tectum and cortex, and projects mainly to cortex, thalamus, and spinal cord. Reticulospinal tracts **profoundly affect motoneuronal excitability**, especially of the γ **motor neurons**. There are two reticulospinal tracts: pontine and medullary.

Pontine Reticulospinal Tract

Origin: Pontine reticulospinal tract originates from nucleus reticularis pontis oralis and nucleus reticularis pontis caudalis located in the pontine reticular formation.

Course: This tract descends down **ipsilaterally in the medial funiculus** of the spinal cord.

- The fibers **terminate on the medial group of interneurons and motoneurons** that innervate the proximal and axial groups of muscles of the body (Fig. 106.6).

Functions: The function of pontine reticulospinal tract is similar to that of lateral vestibulospinal tract.

- It excites the motor neurons of the **proximal extensor muscles** that are involved in **regulation of posture**.

Medullary Reticulospinal Tract

Origin: Medullary reticulospinal tract originates from nucleus gigantocellularis located in the reticular formation of the medulla.

Course: The tract **descends down ipsilaterally** in the ventral funiculus of the spinal cord to terminate on the medial group of interneurons and motoneurons that innervate the proximal group of muscles.

Functions: This tract is mainly inhibitory. It **inhibits the activities of the motor neurons** that innervate extensor neurons.

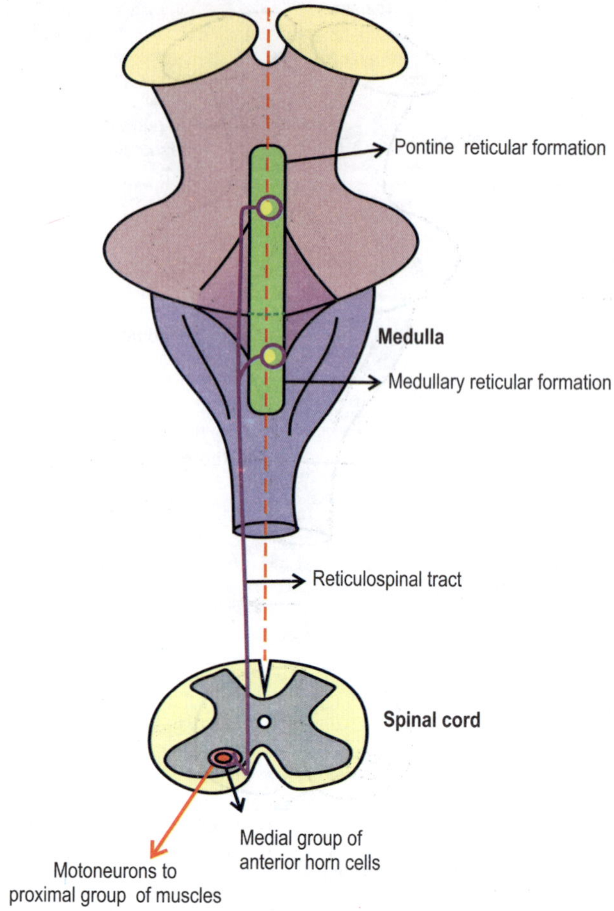

Fig. 106.6: Course of the reticulospinal tract.

Tectospinal Tract

Origin: Tectospinal tract originates from the tectum or **superior colliculus** (from deep layers).

Course: Immediately after originating from superior colliculus, fibers **cross-over to the opposite** side below the periaqueductal gray.

- The fibers then descend down in the ventral funiculus of the spinal cord to **terminate on the medial group of interneurons and motor neurons**.
- This is the **smallest** of all descending tracts as it ***extends upto the midcervical region*** of the spinal cord.

IMPORTANT NOTE

All medial descending pathways **descend down ipsilaterally** in brain and spinal cord except, tectospinal tract that crosses over to opposite side.

Functions: Superior colliculus mainly receives **visual inputs.**

Therefore, tectospinal tract regulates **contralateral movement of the head in response to visual stimuli**.

OTHER DESCENDING PATHWAYS

Monoaminergic Pathways

This includes monoaminergic (raphespinal and ceruleospinal tracts) pathways.

Raphespinal Tract

Origin: This tract originates from **nucleus raphe magnus in the medulla.**

Course: The fibers descend down ipsilaterally and **terminate on the interneurons in the dorsal horn** (refer Fig. 99.7; Chapter 99) that *inhibit the transmission of impulses in the nociceptive pathway*.

Functions: The fibers of the raphe spinal pathway are serotonergic.

They inhibit the nociceptive transmission in the spinal cord (*endogenous pain inhibiting system*). Through their termination on the motor neurons, they are involved in **sensory-motor coordination** at the level of spinal cord.

Ceruleospinal Tract

Origin: Fibers originate from the **nucleus locus ceruleus and nucleus subceruleus.**

Course: Fibers mainly descend down **ipsilaterally in the spinal cord** to terminate on the interneurons and motor neurons.

Functions: The fiber of this pathway contains norepinephrine.

- The pathway is inhibitory to the nociceptive afferents, and also to the motor neurons.
- It **alters the excitability of the motor neurons** to different stimuli and brings **sensory-motor coordination** in the spinal cord.

DIFFERENCES BETWEEN UMN & LMN PARALYSIS

Lower Motor Neuron Paralysis

Lower motor neurons (LMN) paralysis occurs in diseases that cause destruction of anterior horn cells or their axons in dorsal root, nerve plexuses, or the peripheral nerves.

- The examples of LMN disease are **nerve lesion** as occurs in nerve injury or **diseases of the nerve, poliomyelitis, motor neuron disease, and lesion of nerve roots.**

Features of LMN Paralysis

1. Flaccid paralysis (**muscles are hypotonic**).
2. Pronounced **muscle atrophy.**
3. Individual muscles are affected depending on the muscles supplied by that particular nerve.
4. Tendon reflexes are **diminished or absent.**
5. **Superficial reflexes are lost.**
6. Flexor planter response (**Babinski's sign is not elicited**).
7. Involuntary movements like fascicular twitches are observed.
8. Denervation potentials (fibrillation, fasciculation, and sharp waves) are seen in EMG.
9. Nerve conduction is decreased or absent.

Physiological Basis

1. As the lower motor neurons are interrupted, the **innervation to the muscle is lost**. Therefore, ***pronounced muscle atrophy*** occurs as secretion of nerve growth factors is abolished and muscle function is lost.
2. The *muscles that are innervated by the nerve are only affected*, not the muscles of one limb or side of the body as seen in UMN paralysis (Table 106.1).
3. Loss of motor neurons **disrupts the reflex arc** of the stretch reflexes, as well as superficial reflexes.
4. Therefore, both the **tendon and superficial reflexes are diminished or lost** in LMN paralysis. The denervation abolishes influence of γ motoneurons that results in *hypotonia* (**flaccidity of muscles**), an important feature of LMN paralysis.
5. Usually, muscular paralysis is associated with *sensory changes*, because the nerve that carries the motor impulses from the spinal cord also transmits sensory information to the spinal cord.
6. *Nerve conduction is decreased* because of damage to the nerve fibers.
7. **Babinski's sign** *is not elicited* due to loss of motor neuron activity, but if at all present, is of normal flexor type.
8. As the muscle is denervated the **denervation potentials (fibrillation or fascicular twitches)** are observed in EMG recordings.

Differences between the UMN and LMN paralysis are listed in Table 106.1.

Table 106.1 | TDifferences between the UMN and LMN paralysis.

	UMN Paralysis	LMN Paralysis
1. Muscles affected	In groups (not individual muscles)	Individual muscles are affected
2. Size of the muscles	No atrophy	Atrophy is a pronounced feature
3. Type of paralysis	Spastic paralysis (hypertonia)	Flaccid paralysis (hypotonia)
4. Tendon reflexes	Exaggerated	Diminished or absent
5. Superficial reflexes	Absent	Absent
6. Babinski's sign	Extensor planter response	Flexor planter response
7. Involuntary movements	Absent	Present (in the form of fascicular twitches)
8. EMG changes	No denervation potential	Denervation potential seen in EMG
9. Nerve conduction study	No abnormalities	Decreased nerve conduction

CLINICAL ASPECTS

Patterns of Paralysis

Paralysis or plegia means complete loss of voluntary movement, whereas **paresis** refers to the weakness of muscles (incomplete paralysis).

Monoplegia: Monoplegia refers to weakness or paralysis of all the muscles **of one limb** (leg or arm).

Hemiplegia: Hemiplegia means paralysis of **one half of the body**.

- Usually, it occurs due to **lesion of the corticospinal pathway** at the internal capsule that results in **contralateral hemiplegia** (detailed discussed below).

Paraplegia: Paraplegia refers to **paralysis of both lower limbs**.

It usually occurs due to spinal cord injury or diseases that cause **transection of the cord.**

Quadriplegia: Quadriplegia or tetraplegia indicates **paralysis of all four extremities.**

- It usually occurs due to transection of spinal cord in the upper cervical segments.
- **Triplegia** occurs most often as a transitional condition in the development of or partial recovery from tetraplegia.

Isolated Paralysis: Isolated paralysis of one or more muscle groups occurs due to disease of a particular nerve or the branch of the nerve.

Stroke and Hemiplegia

The term '**Stroke**' is used to identify all forms of **cerebrovascular accidents** (CVA). The details of stroke have been discussed in Chapter 39, in 'Cerebral Circulation'. The commonest manifestation of stroke is hemiplegia.

Hemiplegia

Hemiplegia is **paralysis of one half of the body**. This manifests as paralysis of face, arm and leg. Paralysis in trunk is not well marked for its bilateral innervation. The paralysis is of **UMN type.**

- This occurs due to **lesion of corticospinal tract** (pyramidal tract) and the usual site of lesion is **internal capsule**. However, lesion can be in brainstem or at any other site of CST starting from cortex to AHC.
- Hemiplegia due to lesion at internal capsule is called **classical hemiplegia**.
- The paralysis occurs on the opposite side of the body (opposite side of the lesion), hence called **contralateral hemiplegia**.
- However, **crossed hemiplegia** (ipsilateral LMN type of cranial nerve palsy and contralateral hemiplegia) and **bilateral hemiplegia** (paralysis of all four limbs, trunk and total face) are not uncommon.

Features

Features depends on the stage of the disease.

In the stage of Shock: All reflexes are depressed, aphasia, hypotonia, absent jerks, planter no response or equivocal.

Stage of Recovery: Occurs in the following order.

1. Face earliest to recover
2. Lower limbs (first extensors recover)
3. Upper limbs (first flexors recover)
4. Dorsiflexion of foot (minimally recovers)
5. Finer movements of fingers (usually do not recover, or very late recovery)

Deep tendon **reflexes are exaggerated** and **hypertonia (clasp-knife spasticity) of the muscles** are prominent features. Planter response is **extensor type**. Other features of **UMN paralysis** are seen (as discussed above in this chapter)

Stage of Residual Paralysis: Patient recovers, but lives with residual paralysis. He walks with classical hemiplegic gait. Planter response may remain extensor throughout life.

Why 7th nerve Palsy in Hemiplegia?

The 7th **cranial neve nuclear group** is strategically close to internal capsule. The 7th cranial neve nucleus is divided into **upper and lower part** by an arbitrary horizontal line. Upper part supplies muscles of upper face while the lower part supplies muscles of lower face.

- All cranial nerve nuclei are bilaterally supplied by pyramidal fibers (corticonuclear fibers), **except the lower part of the 7th cranial nerve** which receives pyramidal fibers ***only from the opposite side***.
- Therefore, lower face is easily affected (i.e., UMN of 7th nerve palsy) in a patient of hemiplegia.

Importance of Examination of Cranial Nerves in Hemiplegia: Examination of cranial helps in **localization of site of lesion** in hemiplegia.

- Though classical hemiplegia is due to lesion at internal capsule, **lesions of brainstem** (midbrain, pons and medulla) are not uncommon.
- Even the lesion at internal capsule may extend to brainstem.
- As there are **specific cranial nerve nuclei** in three different parts of brainstem, their involvement helps in localizing the site of lesion.
- **Midbrain:** 3rd and 4th cranial nerves
- **Pons:** 5th, 6th, 7th and 8th cranial nerves
- **Medulla:** 9th, 10th, 11th and 12th nerve.

Importance of 7th CN Examination in Hemiplegia: 7th CN examination is more helpful in detecting the site of lesion, as it is the common CN to be affected and it has a wider distribution and differential innervation.

1. **UMN paralysis with 7th CN** palsy in the side of hemiplegia (side of paralysis): ***Lesion is above the Pons*** (opposite side)

2. **LMN type of 7th CN palsy** with contralateral hemiplegia, i.e., crossed hemiplegia (lesion at 7th CN nerve nucleus): ***Lesion is at Pons*** on the side of 7th nerve palsy.
3. **No facial nerve involvement** (incomplete hemiplegia): ***Lesion is below the level of Pons.***

IMPORTANT NOTE

7th nerve palsy and hemiplegia: UMN type of 7th CN palsy is always associated with same sided hemiplegia. When hemiplegia, if at all present with LMN type of 7th CN palsy, it is always crossed hemiplegia.

Common Brainstem Syndromes

Weber Syndrome: Paralysis of 3rd cranial nerve of one side (LMN type) with contralateral hemiplegia (crossed hemiplegia). The ***lesion is at midbrain.***

Millard-Gubler Syndrome: Paralysis of 6th cranial nerve (LMN type) + 7th cranial nerve (LMN type) with contralateral hemiplegia. The ***lesion is at pons.***

Avellis Syndrome: Paralysis of 10th cranial nerve of one side (LMN type) with contralateral hemiplegia (crossed hemiplegia). The ***lesion is at medulla.***

Exam Questions

1. With the help of a suitable diagram, trace the pathway of corticospinal tract (CST), and describe the physiological basis of features of lesion of CST at internal capsule.
2. List the differences between UMN paralysis and LMN Paralysis. Briefly describe the physiological basis of these differences.

Multiple Choice Questions

1. **Which of the following descending tract is not a component of medial system pathways?**
   A. Anterior corticospinal tract
   B. Rubrospinal tract
   C. Vestibulospinal tract
   D. Reticulospinal tract
2. **Which of the following tract controls skilled voluntary movements?**
   A. Corticospinal tract
   B. Tectospinal tract
   C. Vestibulospinal tract
   D. Reticulospinal tract
3. **All the following tracts are mainly involved in regulation of posture, EXCEPT:**
   A. Reticulospinal tract
   B. Vestibulospinal tract
   C. Rubrospinal tract
   D. Tectospinal tract
4. **Pyramids are formed by:**
   A. Arcuate nucleus
   B. Vestibular nuclei
   C. Interstitial cells of Cajal
   D. Lateral corticospinal tract
5. **Cell bodies of UMN includes:**
   A. Pyramidal cells
   B. Anterior horn cells
   C. Glial cells
   D. Schwann cells
6. **Which of the following is true about lateral corticospinal tract?**
   A. Crossed tract
   B. Uncrossed tract
   C. Stops in midthoracic region
   D. Crossed at midspinal level
   E. Only 20% fibers cross to opposite side
7. **Corticospinal tract lesion leads to all, EXCEPT:**
   A. Spasticity
   B. Extensor plantar response
   C. Cogwheel rigidity
   D. Exaggerated reflexes & increased tone
8. **Following are the features of corticospinal involvement EXCEPT**
   A. Cog-wheel rigidity
   B. Spasticity
   C. Planter extensor response
   D. Exaggerated deep tendon reflexes
9. **LMN paralysis will not manifest as:**
   A. Muscle hypertonia
   B. Muscle atrophy
   C. Depressed tendon reflexes
   D. Babinski no response or negetive
10. **Amyotrophic lateral sclerosis involves:**
    A. Upper motor neuron and lower motor neuron both
    B. Posterior column only
    C. Lower motor neuron only
    D. Raphae nucleus
11. **If UMN type of 7th nerve palsy in the side of hemiplegia, the lesion is at:**
    A. Pons
    B. Above pons
    C. Below pons
    D. Spinal cord
12. **LMN type of 7th CN palsy with contralateral hemiplegia, the lesion is likely in:**
    A. Pons
    B. Below pons
    C. Above pons
    D. Spinal cord

Answers: 1. B 2. A 3. C 4. D 5. A 6. A 7. C 8. A 9. A 10. A 11. B 12. A

Chapter 107

PY10.4

Regulation of Posture and Movement

Learning Objectives

On completion of study of this chapter:

The student will be able to (must know):

1. List the postural reflexes integrated at different levels of neuraxis.
2. Describe the features in spinal, decerebrate, midbrain and decorticate preparations.
3. Explain the mechanism of decerebrate rigidity.
4. Name the cortical motor areas and give their functions.
5. Appreciate organization of body parts in motor homunculus.

The student may also be able to (desirable to know):

1. Describe the mechanisms of regulation of posture and movement.
2. Explain the dysfunctions of regulation of posture and movement.

GENERAL ORGANIZATION

The movements are planned in the cortex, basal ganglia, and cerebellum. The supraspinal inputs controlling the spinal motor neurons carry out **three important functions**:

1. Initiation and execution of voluntary activities.
2. Coordination and smoothening of movements.
3. Postural adjustments to provide a stable background for movement.

Major Steps of Motor Control: The execution and control of motor activities are carried out in **six broad steps.**

- *Motor planning:* The plan for motor function is initiated in motor cortex.
- *Generation of command pattern:* A copy of the plan is conveyed to brainstem areas that interact with basal ganglia and cerebellum for generation of appropriate command pattern (Fig. 107.1).
- *Transmission of command to the effector organs:* The pattern of command is conveyed to spinal motor neurons as motor ***command signal*** by descending motor pathways for initiation of motor activities.
- *Sensory feedback:* Once movement is initiated, activities in the muscle, tendon, ligaments, joints and skin ***provide sensory feedback*** to the CNS.
- *Smoothening and coordination of movement:* Smoothening and coordination and postural adjustments during movement are regulated mainly by the **extrapyramidal systems** that originate from the brainstem.

The **major extrapyramidal pathways** are vestibulospinal, reticulospinal, and tectospinal tracts. As the activities in these tracts are profoundly influenced by **cerebellum and basal ganglia**, these structures are largely considered as **extrapyramidal structures.**

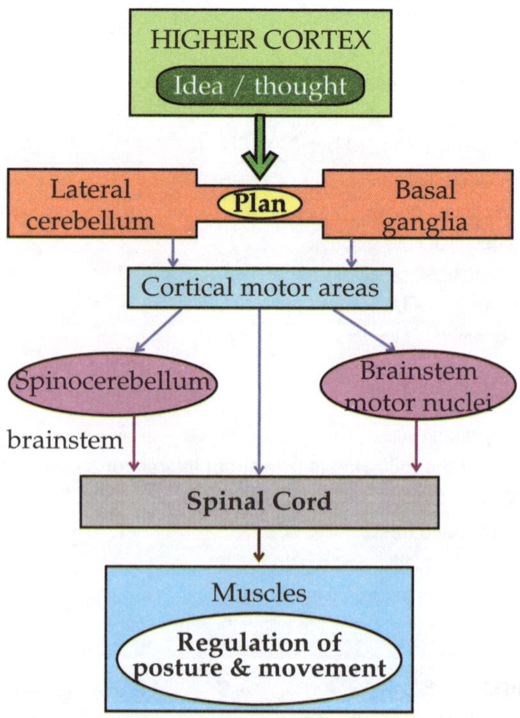

Fig. 107.1: Overall organization of motor control.

GENERAL ORGANIZATION

Levels of Integration

The mechanisms involved in regulation of posture and movement are **integrated at six levels** of the CNS: **spinal cord, medulla, midbrain, cortex, basal ganglia and cerebellum.**

Release Phenomenon: When the neuraxis is transected at a particular level, motor activities carried out by the centers below the section are **usually accentuated**. This is called *release phenomenon*, which **facilitates the final motor output**.

The **facilitation** of motor activity is due to **two main reasons**:

i) **Release of the center** from the inhibitory control of higher centers.
ii) **Denervation hypersensitivity** of the center below the transection.

Postural Reflexes

Postural reflexes **maintain a balanced posture** of the body, **provide a stable background** for movement and **adjust body posture** constantly during the movement.

The postural reflexes are broadly classified into **two broad categories**: phasic and static reflexes.

Phasic or Dynamic Reflexes: These are the reflexes that are short-term in nature and produce transient movements for immediate change in posture and rapid postural adjustments. The examples are:

- Phasic stretch reflex,
- Righting reflexes,
- Vestibular placing reactions, etc.

Tonic or Static Reflexes: These reflexes produce sustained contraction of the muscle and mainly provide a stable background for maintaining a posture. They also adjust posture during movement. The examples are:

- Tonic stretch reflex,
- Tonic neck reflexes,
- Tonic labyrinthine reflexes, etc.

SPINAL INTEGRATION

The spinal cord plays a crucial role in the regulation of posture and movement. It helps in execution of **four important motor functions**:

1. Spinal cord contains neural circuitry that generates basic postural reflexes, called **spinal reflexes.** Spinal reflexes produce **immediate change in motor output** that leads to rapid responses.
   - For example, withdrawal of body parts in response to a noxious stimulus.
2. Spinal cord contains **neural circuitry that can alter motor neuron output** to maintain the tone of the muscle. Especially, the change in γ motor neuron activity alters the muscle spindle sensitivity to stretch that in turn greatly influences muscle tone.
   - However, the γ motor neuron activity is primarily influenced by activities in the descending fibers.
3. Spinal cord contains neural circuitry (**pattern generator for locomotion**) that on appropriate stimulation produces **basic movements** like walking.
4. **Tonic stretch reflex executed** in spinal cord is essential for maintaining posture.

The role of spinal cord in regulation of movement and posture is best studied in a spinal preparation (Spinal Animal).

Spinal Preparation

A **spinal animal** is the animal (usually performed in a cat) in which influence of brain on spinal cord is removed by **making a section below the medulla**.

- Ideally, in the spinal preparation, the section is **made below the C_5** so that the respiration (diaphragm activity) remains intact.
- However, usually, section is made **below the mid-thoracic level** so that cardiovascular activity also remains intact and it becomes easy to maintain the preparation.

Phases: Following transection**, three phases** (stages) are distinctly marked in spinal preparation.

1. The stage of shock (stage of flaccidity)
2. The stage of recovery (stage of reflex activity)
3. The stage of failure

Stage of Shock

As soon as the section is made, animal enters into the stage of shock (**spinal shock**). This is also called as the **stage of flaccidity**.

- Spinal transection causes immediate loss of sensations and voluntary movements below the level of lesion.
- In all vertebrates, transection of the spinal cord is followed by a period of spinal shock during which all **spinal reflex responses are profoundly depressed.**

Duration of Shock: The duration of spinal shock is proportionate to the **degree of encephalization** of motor function. Accordingly, the duration of shock is different in different species.

In frogs : few minutes (2 - 4 minutes)
In dogs and cats : few hours (2 - 4 hrs)
In monkeys : few days (2 - 4 days)
In humans : few weeks (1 - 4 weeks)

Mechanism of Shock: The spinal shock results from **immediate abolition of tonic bombardment** of motor neurons by descending fibers.

- Neurophysiological evidence indicates that **motor neuron excitability is profoundly depressed** after spinal transection.

Features of Shock:

Below the level of the lesion: 1. The muscles are completely paralyzed (**flaccidity**).

1. All the reflexes are abolished (**areflexia**).
2. Complete loss of all sensation (**anesthesia**)

At the level of lesion: Cramp like pain is present.

Other Features: The **bladder and rectum are generally paralyzed**. The sphincter vesicae, however, frequently retains its function or recovers rapidly.

- The **penis remains flaccid** and erection becomes impossible.
- Section below T_1 leads to **gross fall in BP** which resembles to the degree of hypotension observed following destruction of vasomotor center.
- Absence of muscle pump activity due to muscle paralysis significantly decreases blood flow and venous return.
  - **Cardiac output decreases grossly**. Therefore, legs become blue and cold.
- If the lesion is at T_6, impulses coming from abdominal viscera are interrupted. Therefore, griping sensation or distension of the viscera cannot be appreciated.

Stage of Recovery (Reflex Activity)

Smooth Muscle Function

As the stage of shock passes off, **activity returns first in smooth muscle**.

- The **sphincter vesicae recovers very soon**, but detrusor muscle regains slowly.
- The paralyzed **blood vessels regain tone** and BP slowly returns to normal.

Reflex Responses

The first reflex response to appear is **slight contraction of leg flexors** in response to a noxious stimulus. **Adductors** also respond to painful stimulus. In some patients, knee jerk recovers first.

Mechanism of Recovery: Mechanism of reflex recovery from spinal shock is not clearly known.

- It may possibly be due to the segmental influences that become more effective during the recovery. This occurs due to the **axonal sprouting**.
- The sensory fibers that enter the cord give **more collaterals** and **spinal interneurons sprout additional terminals**.
- These nerve terminals occupy the synaptic space vacated by degeneration of sectioned descending fibers.

Muscle Tone and Size

Tone in skeletal muscle returns after 2 to 3 weeks in humans.

1. Tone reappears first in **the flexor muscles** of lower limbs, then in the flexors of upper limbs and trunk. Extensor muscles remain flabby for a longer period.
2. Due to **increased flexor tone**, the body adopts a **position of flexion**. Thus, the paralysis in this stage is referred to as **paraplegia in flexion**.
3. Though paralyzed, muscles **usually do not undergo wasting** due to constant reflex activity.

Reflex Movements

Spontaneous involuntary **flexor movements** of the limb occur. The small toes are separated and raised. Contraction of flexor group of muscles occurs, which is accompanied by the reciprocal inhibition of the extensor muscles.

Flexor Reflex: **The reflex response that returns first is the flexor reflex to a noxious stimulus.**

- Stimulation of the lateral aspect of the sole of the foot leads to **Babinski sign** with dorsiflexion of big toe, abduction of other toes, flexion of knee and hip and abduction of the thigh.
- The antagonistic muscles are inhibited.
- Flexor reflex is a ***protective withdrawal reflex***, which removes the limb from the site of injury.

Mass Reflex: By scratching any point on the inner aspect of the thigh or lower anterior abdominal wall, a very widespread response is readily elicited. This is called mass response, which consists of:

i) **Flexor spasm** of lower extremities and contraction of the anterior abdominal wall.

ii) **Evacuation of bladder and bowel**, those occur partly due to increased abdominal pressure.

iii) **Profuse sweating** below the level of lesion. Sweat fibers to head and neck arise from $T_{1,2}$ and to arm from $T_{5–9}$. Thus, with a lesion at T_1 or above, the whole-body sweats when mass reflex is activated.

Mass reflex appears late, may be after several months of transection.

Coitus Reflex: This is elicited by stimulation of glans penis, or the skin around the genitals.

- The response consists of **swelling and stiffening of penis**, withdrawal of testis (because of contraction of cremasteric muscle) and curling up of the scrotal skin by the action of the dartus.
- Flexors of hip and abductors of thigh also contract.
- Seminal emission may occur. However, **full intercourse never becomes possible**.

Deep Reflexes: Knee jerk returns in 1 to 5 weeks after the recovery of flexor response.

- Quadriceps muscle, though contracts adequately, relaxes immediately and therefore, limb drops soon. **Ankle jerk** returns later. Ankle clonus may be present in the mild form.

Extensor Responses: Increase in extensor activity occurs later.

Generally, **in six months tone appears** and slowly becomes **marked in extensors**.

- This leads to appearance of extensor spasm. The body assumes an **attitude in extension**.
- In this stage, the condition is called **paraplegia in extension**.

The following **findings** are observed in this stage:

- **Ankle and knee jerks become exaggerated**.
- If limb muscles are stretched passively and abruptly (e.g. if the flexed thigh is suddenly extended), a **reflex extension** of it or both limbs occurs. Contraction involves both extensor and flexor muscles that convert the limbs into **"solid pillars"**.
- Mass reflex as described above may not be obtained any more.
- Stimulation of glans penis produces the genital response as seen in the recovery of flexor group of muscles, but occurs without seminal emission.

Autonomic Reflexes

1. **Micturition reflex** becomes hyperactive. Though reflex evacuation of bladder occurs, bladder is not emptied completely.
   - Hyperactive bladder reflex for a long duration keeps the bladder in a **shrunken state that results in hypertrophy and fibrosis** of the bladder wall and decreases bladder capacity.
   - This type of bladder is called **spastic neurogenic bladder**.
2. **Defecation reflex** also regains, but reflex contraction of rectum does not empty it completely.
3. **Blood pressure** remains normal at rest. However, due to lack of feedback regulation by the baroreceptor reflex, **wide swing in pressure** occurs in various conditions.
4. Sweating occurs and skin becomes healthy.

Supporting Reactions

Once the **spinal reflexes** reappear, their **threshold steadily drops**. A minor noxious stimulus may cause prolonged withdrawal response.

- Repeated flexion movement may occur for a prolonged period.
- **Stretch reflexes become hyperactive**. An example of this is **supporting reactions**.

There are **two supporting reactions**:

1. **Positive supporting reaction (PSR):** When a finger is placed on the sole of the foot of a spinal animal and then withdrawn, the limb of the animal extends following the examining finger. This is called PSR or **magnet reaction** (as the limb is withdrawn like a magnet).
   - The **receptors** are tactile receptors and afferent pathways involve both tactile and proprioceptive afferents.
   - The motor responses **transform the limb into a rigid pillar that resist gravity.**
   - Other limbs also become rigid like pillars **to support the animal**. Therefore, this is called supporting reaction.
2. **Negative supporting reaction:** The disappearance of positive supporting reaction is an active phenomenon, and called as **negative supporting reaction**. This is initiated by stretch of the extensor muscles.

On the basis of positive supporting reaction, spinal cats and dogs can be **made to stand and walk** though ineptly, for about 2 minutes.

Locomotion Generator

As spinal animals can stand and walk with appropriate stimulation, it indicates that a **circuit intrinsic to the spinal cord** produces locomotion. This is called **central pattern generator** (CPG) for locomotion.

- There are **two spinal cord CPGs**, one is located in the ***cervical region*** for upper limbs and another in the ***lumbar region*** for lower limbs.
- The CPGs are **group of interneurons** that activate the motor neurons.
- CPGs **on stimulation** produce alternate contractions of flexors and extensors of limbs, which is needed for locomotion. Experimentally, it is also observed that **injection of glutamate or L-dopa** into the spinal cord produces rhythmic action potentials for locomotion in motoneurons.
- CPGs in spinal cord are activated by discharge of a locomotor center present in the midbrain, called **mesencephalic locomotion generator** (MLG) (discussed later in this chapter in 'Midbrain Integration').
- In spinal animal, as the **influence of MLG on CPG is interrupted**, CPG requires appropriate stimulation to be activated.

Stage of Failure of Reflex Activity

In chronic spinal patients, due to lack of proper nutrition and hygiene, and repeated general infections or toxemia, failure of reflex activity develops.

1. It becomes difficult to elicit reflexes as **threshold for all reflexes is raised**. The **mass reflex disappears**.
2. Muscle wasting occurs and **muscles become flaccid**.
3. Bedsores develop at pressure points, which results in **decubitus ulcers**. Immunity is suppressed due to protein depletion. Poor healing of ulcers leads to septicemia.
4. **Prolonged immobilization and lysis of protein matrix** of bones cause *hypercalcemia and hypercalciuria*. This results in formation of **stone in the urinary tract** that causes repeated urinary infection.

Frequent **septicemia and uremia** cause death of most of the patients. However, early and appropriate use of modern

antibiotics and glucocorticoids, and **proper nutrition and nursing care** prolong the life of such patients.

MEDULLARY INTEGRATION

Medulla mainly integrates the **tonic reflexes** that maintain posture.

- The role of medulla in regulation of posture and movement is best studied by producing a **mid-collicular lesion** (section between superior and inferior colliculi) in an experimental animal.
- The preparation is known as **decerebrate preparation** and the procedure is called **decerebration**.

Features of Decerebrate Preparation

1. No phenomenon similar to spinal shock occurs in decerebrate preparation.
2. Following the mid-collicular section, **severe spasticity** is immediately observed in the extensor group of muscles of the body.
   - This is called **decerebrate rigidity**.
   - Rigidity is so prominent that the **limbs are fully extended and the spine is hyperextended**.
3. **Righting reflexes are absent**. Therefore, animal lies on the ground.
4. **Tonic reflexes** are prominently marked.

Mechanism of Decerebrate Rigidity

Rigidity occurs due to **increased activity of motoneurons** that facilitate stretch reflexes. Facilitation of stretch reflexes occurs due to **two mechanisms**:

1. Increased excitability of the motor neuron pool in general.
2. Increased rate of γ **motor neuron discharge**.

Increased general excitability of motor neurons occurs due to **facilitation of descending neural inputs** converging on the anterior horn cells. In the brainstem, the reticular nuclei for motor control are largely divided into **two areas**: the large **facilitatory area**, which is mainly located in pons (that gives rise to pontine reticulospinal tract) and the small **inhibitory area** (Fig. 107.2), which is located in medulla (that gives rise to medullary reticulospinal tract).

1. The **facilitatory area discharges spontaneously** whereas the inhibitory area does not.
   - Discharge of inhibitory area requires inputs from the cortex, basal ganglia and cerebellum. Basal ganglia do not directly influence the brainstem reticular activity.
   - Basal ganglia projects to the motor cortex and via cortical projection to brainstem, it controls the medullary reticular activity.
2. Normally, **medullary reticulospinal fibers inhibit motor neurons** in the spinal cord.

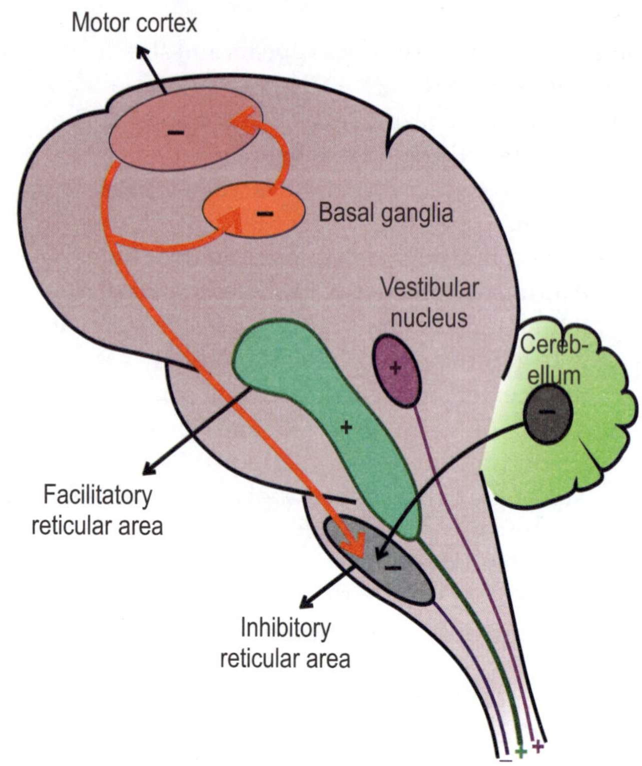

Fig. 107.2: Control of output of reticulospinal tract activity. The facilitatory reticular area discharges spontaneously, whereas the inhibitory reticular area to discharge effectively requires input from cortex, basal ganglia and cerebellum. Basal ganglia influences reticulospinal activity via its projection to the motor cortex. As cortex, basal ganglia and cerebellum drive the inhibitory medullary reticular activity, they are classified under inhibitory brain areas (as indicated by 'minus' sign). Output of vestibulospinal tract is facilitatory.

   - As the cortex drives the inhibitory (the medullary) reticular area, the **cortex and basal ganglia** are classified under **inhibitory brain areas**.
3. Likewise, **cerebellum** is also classified under **inhibitory brain areas** as it also drives the inhibitory reticular area.
4. Thus, three areas (**cortex, basal ganglia and cerebellum**) drive the inhibitory center in medulla.

In mid-collicular lesion, the ***influence of two (cortex and basal ganglia)*** out of the three inhibitory centers ***on medullary reticular formation is removed*** (Fig. 107.3).

- Thus, **inhibitory output** of the medullary reticulospinal tract becomes **less inhibitory**, whereas the discharge of *facilitatory pontine reticulospinal tract continues* (as it discharges spontaneously).
- Consequently, the **net discharge of reticulospinal tract shifts more towards facilitation**.
- The output of γ motor neurons is mainly influenced by reticulospinal tract.
- Therefore, γ **motor neuron discharge increases** following decerebration. This causes decerebrate rigidity.

Importance of Decerebrate Rigidity

Rigidity observed in decerebrate animal is **more marked in the extensor muscles**.

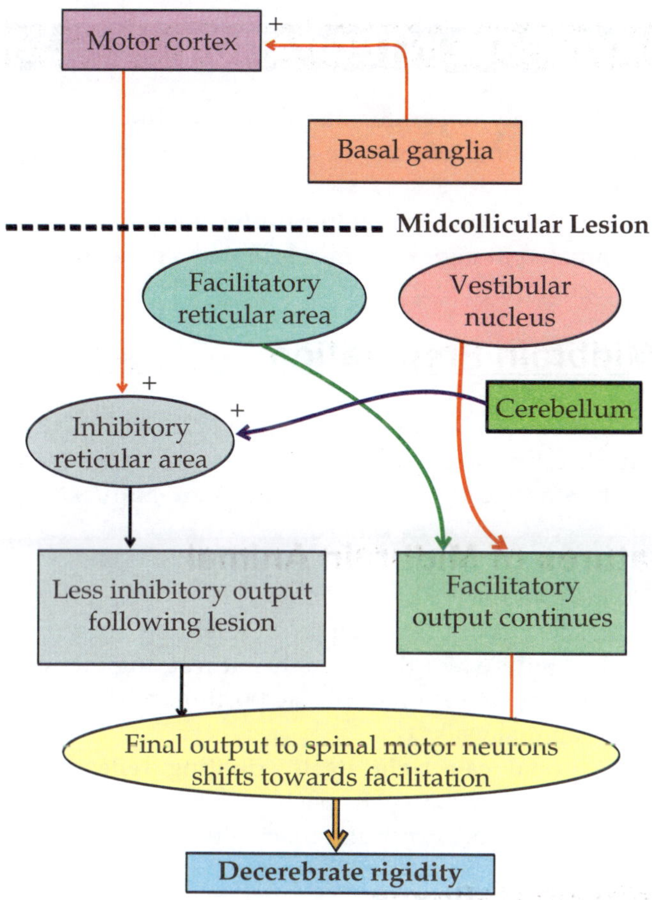

Fig. 107.3: Mechanism of decerebrate rigidity. In mid-collicular lesion, the influence of cortex and basal ganglia on inhibitory reticular area is abolished (only cerebellar drive remains). Therefore, inhibitory output of the medullary reticulospinal tract becomes less inhibitory, whereas facilitatory area continues to discharge spontaneously. Consequently, the net output of reticulospinal tract becomes more facilitatory. As, motor neurons are primarily driven by reticulospinal tract influence, decerebration causes severe rigidity.

1. **Extensor muscles** are the most important components of posture regulating system as they maintain erect posture of the body by keeping the limbs extended.
   - The **tone of these muscles**, which is a **static postural reflex**, is highly essential to **support the animal against gravity**. Therefore, these muscles are called **antigravity muscles**.
2. In humans, the major antigravity muscles are the **extensors of the lower limbs**.
3. The **increased extensor rigidity** in decerebrate preparation indicates that **medulla controls the tone of the antigravity muscles** that are involved in maintaining posture.

Medullary Reflexes

Reflexes integrated in medulla for control of motor activities are mainly **static postural reflexes**. Activities of these reflexes are accentuated following mid-collicular lesion. These reflexes are:

1. Extensor rigidity
2. Tonic labyrinthine reflexes
3. Tonic neck reflexes

Extensor Rigidity

The tone in the extensor muscles (antigravity muscles) is a prominent static postural reflex, which is essential for ***maintaining posture against gravity***.

1. This extensor muscle tone is mainly due to the **discharge of motor nuclei located** in pons and medulla.
   - Reticulospinal and vestibulospinal tracts primarily contribute to muscle tone.
2. **Reticulospinal tract** controls tone of antigravity muscles via its **influence on γ motor neurons** and **vestibulospinal tract via α motor neurons** in the spinal cord (Application Box 107.1).
   - The **γ motor neurons control muscle tone** by regulating muscle spindle sensitivity.
3. Hence, γ motor neuron discharge, and therefore the **reticulospinal tract activity** is the principal regulator of muscle tone.

Application Box 107.1

Experimental Deafferentation: The vestibulospinal tract mainly influences α motor neurons and reticulospinal tract influences γ motor neurons in the spinal cord. This can be experimentally proved by making **dorsal rhizotomy that causes deafferentation.**

- When afferent fibers (Ia) are interrupted by deafferentation, the input from muscle spindle to spinal cord is abolished. As γ motor neurons control muscle tone via spindle sensitivity, deafferentation removes the influences through γ motor neurons.
- Therefore, following dorsal rhizotomy, influence of reticulospinal tract on muscle tone is abolished, which indicates that this tracts acts through γ motor neurons.
- However, influence of vestibulospinal tract on muscle tone is not affected (as it terminates mainly on α motor neurons that contact extrafusal fibers) indicating that this tract acts through α motor neurons (Fig. 107.4).

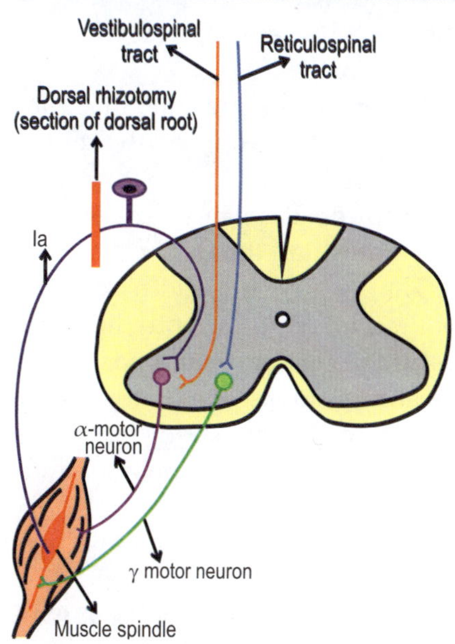

Fig. 107.4: Effects of dorsal rhizotomy (deafferentation). Section of Ia fibers that carry sensation from muscle spindle abolishes influence of reticulospinal tract on muscle that mediates effects mostly through γ motor neurons. The influence of vestibulospinal tract on muscle remains unaffected as it mediates its effects mostly through α motor neurons that directly contact extrafusal fibers.

Tonic Labyrinthine Reflexes

The decerebrate animal cannot right itself, and therefore remains static in the position in which it is placed.

- If the **position of the animal is changed** passively, the **pattern of rigidity in the limbs alters**. This is called tonic labyrinthine reflexes.
- The rigidity is maximum in supine position and minimum in prone position.

Receptors: **Otolith organs** of the vestibular apparatus are receptors for tonic labyrinthine reflexes.

Stimulus: **Action of gravity on the otolith organs**, as altered by change in body position is the potent stimulus for this reflex.

Reflex Pathway: The effects are mediated by **vestibulo-spinal tracts.**

Response: When the animal is **placed on its back**, the ***rigidity is maximum*** in the extensor muscles (all four limbs are maximally extended).

If the **animal is turned to either side**, the rigidity decreases and rigidity becomes minimum **in prone position**.

Importance: These reflexes help animal to **maintain the tone of muscle, especially in erect posture.**

Tonic Neck Reflexes

This is the change in pattern of rigidity when position of the head is changed in relation to the body.

Receptors: **Proprioceptors** in the upper part of the neck are receptors for tonic neck reflexes.

Stimulus: **Change in head position** that stimulates proprioceptors in the neck.

Reflex Pathway: The reflex is mediated via reticulospinal and tectospinal pathways.

Response: If the head is ventroflexed, the upper limbs flex and the hind limbs extend.

- If the **head is turned to one side,** the limb of that side (the jaw limb) is extended while the contralateral limb (occipital limb) is flexed.
- **Extension of the head** causes extension of the forelimbs and flexion of the hind limbs.

Importance: The change in rigidity due to change in head position in relation to the body helps the **animal to maintain posture in that particular position.**

- When the **animal looks above**, for example, looking for an object in the tree, during which extension of the head extends the forelimb and flexes the hindlimb.
  - This helps the animal to maintain posture in that position.
- Similarly, when the **animal looks downward** for an object on the ground or below the ground level, flexion of head causes extension of hind limb and flexion of the forelimbs.
  - This helps the animal to maintain posture in that position.

MIDBRAIN INTEGRATION

Midbrain mainly integrates the **phasic postural reflexes**. These are righting reflexes, vestibular placing reflex and grasp reflex.

- **Central pattern generator for locomotion** (CPG) is situated in midbrain (**mesencephalic generator for locomotion**) that drives the spinal CPG.

Midbrain Preparation

The influence of midbrain on posture and movement is best studied by making a section at the superior border of the midbrain. The animal is called **midbrain animal**.

Features of Midbrain Animal

1. No features of shock.
2. Extensor rigidity (as seen in decerebrate animal) is present **only when the animal is at rest**. Rigidity disappears on activation of phasic postural reflexes, e.g., when animal walks.
3. The **animal can right itself** (**righting reflexes are preserved**) and change its posture.
4. **Grasp reflex** and **vestibular placing reaction** are intact.

Midbrain Reflexes

Righting Reflexes

These are a series of reflexes that operate **to correct the body position and maintain it by keeping the animals head upright**.

- Maintaining ***stable head position*** is an integral part of the posture regulating mechanisms. **Righting reflexes keep the head in a stable position** and the eyes fixed at visual targets despite movement of the body.
- They tend to restore the position of the body when it is altered, by stimulating proprioceptors, tactile receptors and vestibular receptors.
- The responses are initiated by vestibular stimulation, stretching of neck muscle, pressure on the side of the body or on the limbs, and stimulation of visual receptors.
- Righting reflexes are **series of responses integrated in midbrain** (Table 107.1). Following are the righting reflexes:

Table 107.1 | Righting reflexes (RR).

Reflexes	Stimulus	Receptors	Center	Responses
1. Labyrinthine RR	Tilting of head (effect of gravity)	Otolith organ	Midbrain	Head kept level
2. Neck RR	Stretch of neck muscle	Muscle spindle	Midbrain	Righting of shoulders, thorax& then pelvis

Table 107:1 contd...				
3. Body RR				
i. Body on head RR	Pressure on the side of the body	Exterocep-tors	Midbrain	Righting of head
ii. Body on body RR	Pressure on the side of the body	Exterocep-tors	Midbrain	Righting of body even head held sideways
4. Limb RR	Stretch of the limb muscles	Muscle spin-dle	Midbrain (red nucleus)	Righting of the body
5. Optical RR	Visual cues	Visual recep-tors	Visual cortex	Righting of head

Labyrinthine Righting Reflex

When the animal is held by its body and tipped from side to side, the head stays level due to activation of labyrinthine righting reflexes.

Receptors: Receptors are present in the **otolith organs**.

Stimulus: Tilting of the head that stimulates otolith organs.

Response: Contraction of neck muscles that keep the head level.

Body on Head Righting Reflex

When the animal is **laid on its side**, the pressure on that side of the body initiates reflex righting of the head. This reflex is operated even after labyrinthectomy. This is called body on head righting reflex.

Neck Righting Reflex

If above-mentioned two reflexes right the head but the body remains tilted, the neck muscles are stretched. Contraction of neck muscles rights the thorax and abdomen. This is called neck righting reflex.

Body on Body Righting Reflex

Pressure on the side of the body rights the body even if the head is prevented to right. This is called body on body righting reflex.

Limb Righting Reflex

Pressure on the limbs rights the body.

Optical Righting Reflex

The righting reflexes are best operated with eyes open (even in the absence of labyrinthine or body stimulation). This is the optical righting reflex. The center for this reflex is ***not the midbrain***, but **the cortex**. Therefore, this reflex depends on the intact cortical functions.

Grasp Reflex

When a stick or an object is brought close to the limbs of a midbrain animal, the animal grasps the object and the limbs are extended. This is the grasp reflex.

- This reflex is a **primitive reflex** that helps the animal to stand up and **support the posture**.
- In humans, it is better observed *during infancy and early childhood*.

Vestibular Placing Reaction

When a blind folded animal is brought down from a height rapidly, the forelimbs of the animal extend and the toes spread, which assist the animal to steadily land on the ground.

Receptors: Vestibular receptors.

Stimulus: Linear acceleration of the body.

Pathway: Vestibulospinal tract.

Response: Extension of forelimbs and spreading of the toes. This helps the animal **to land steadily on the ground**.

Mesencephalic Locomotion Generator

The generator for locomotion is located in the midbrain. This is called **mesencephalic locomotion generator** (*midbrain locomotion center*). This midbrain center drives the spinal locomotion generator.

- It organizes the **command signals that arrives from the motor cortices** via corticobulbar fibers and accordingly **influences spinal motor neurons** mainly via reticulospinal tract (Fig. 107.5).
- Locomotion is not only activated and initiated but also **altered rapidly during swift motor activities** like running, swimming etc., by adjustment of activities of phasic postural reflexes.
- All these postural mechanisms are integrated in midbrain.

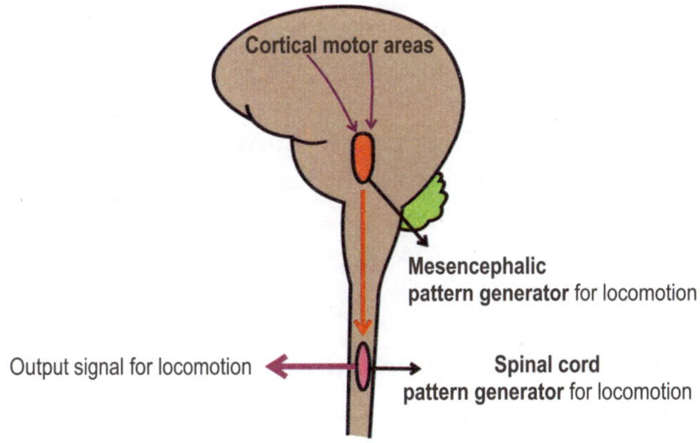

Fig. 107.5: Central pattern generators for locomotion. Note that mesencephalic pattern generator drives the spinal cord pattern generator that produces final motor signal for locomotion.

CORTICAL I NTEGRATION

For the command signal for movement to be conveyed to spinal motor neurons, first, the **motor plan** is generated in the cortex.

- Motor cortex **interacts with basal ganglia and cerebellum** for finalizing the plan and programme of the movement, and later, **interacts with the sensory cortex and association cortex** to fine-tune and modify the command signal for implementation of the initial plan.

- Information is also transmitted partly to the **premotor cortex and supplementary motor area**, for generating further motor signal for initiating appropriate movement.
- Motor signal is then conveyed to spinal motor neurons via descending motor pathways.

Decortication

The role of motor cortex in regulation of posture and movement is best studied by removing the cerebral cortex in experimental animals. The surgical procedure is called **decortication** and the animal is called **decorticate animal.**

Features of Decorticate Animal

1. No features of shock.
2. All the reflex activities of midbrain animal are intact.
3. Rigidity (**decorticate rigidity**) is very minimal and present only at rest.
4. **Hopping and placing reactions** are severely impaired.
5. Striking defect is the **inability to react in terms of past experience.**
6. Conditioned reflexes are absent but can be reestablished with special training.
7. Temperature regulation is intact.
8. Visceral homeostatic mechanisms are intact.

As the hypothalamus is intact in decorticate animal, it is easier to maintain such an animal due to intact visceral homeostatic mechanisms including the process of temperature regulation.

Decorticate Rigidity

Cortex **drives medullary reticulospinal tract** (Fig. 107.3).

- Therefore, removal of cortex results in **facilitation of γ motor neuron discharge**.
- Rigidity is seen only at rest and disappears when phasic postural reflexes are activated.

Hopping and Placing Reactions

When a normal animal (or a human being) is pushed laterally, the animal takes short steps to balance the body (**hopping reaction**) and then places its feet firmly on the ground (**placing reaction**) to attain and maintain the new stable position.

- These reflexes are **seriously impaired following decortication**.
- This indicates that center for integration of hopping and placing reactions is the motor cortex.

Summary of Spinal Reflexes

Thus, in summary, spinal reflexes including supporting reactions are integrated in spinal cord, antigravity (static postural) reflexes are integrated in medulla, righting reflexes are integrated in midbrain, and hopping and placing reactions in cortex as studied in above-mentioned preparations (Table 107.2).

Table 107.2 | Integration of postural reflexes at various levels of CNS as studied in different preparations.

Reflexes	Spinal preparation	Decerebrate Preparation	Midbrain preparation	Decorticate preparation
1. Spinal reflexes	++	+	+	+
2. Antigravity reflexes	Absent	++	+	+
3. Righting reflexes	Absent	Absent	++	+
4. Conditioned reflexes	Absent	Absent	Absent	±
5. Hopping and placing reactions	Absent	Absent	Absent	Grossly impaired

Cortical Motor Areas

Cortical motor areas include a large number of areas in the brain that are involved in or associated with movement (Fig. 107.6). These include:

1. Primary motor cortex (precentral gyrus)
2. Pre-motor cortex
3. Supplementary motor area
4. Somatosensory cortex
5. Frontal eye field

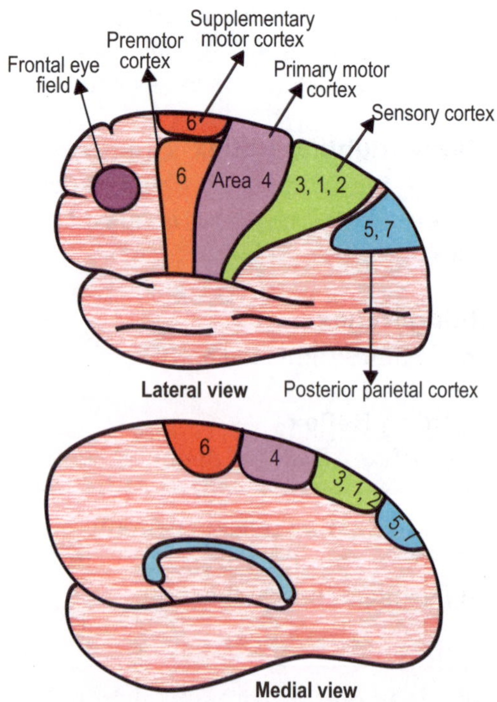

Fig. 107.6: Motor areas in the cortex.

Primary Motor Cortex

Primary motor cortex (**area 4**) is present in the precentral gyrus. Corticospinal and corticobulbar tracts mainly originate from this area of the cortex. This area is involved in **planning and initiation of voluntary movements**.

Connections: Motor neurons originating from area 4 project to premotor cortex, brain-stem and spinal cord. It is reciprocally connected with thalamus, sensory cortex and supplementary motor area (Fig. 107.7).

- The connections are such that the cortical motor areas **control the muscle activity of the opposite side of the body**.

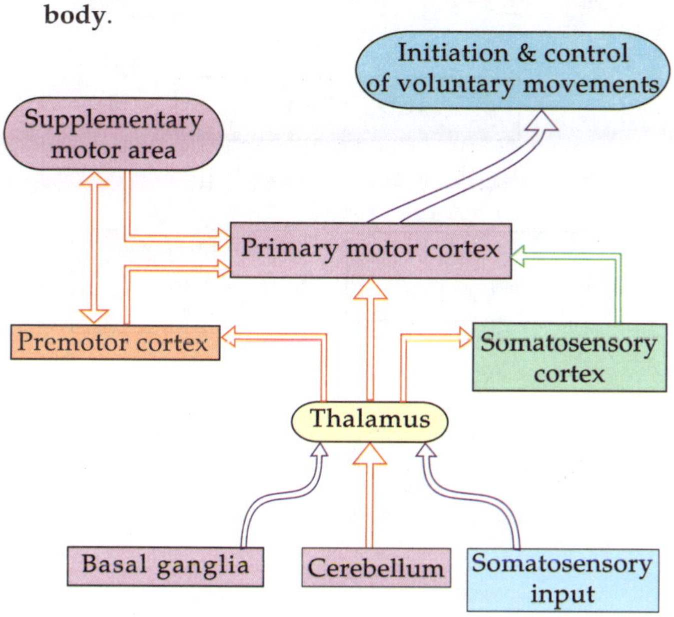

Fig. 107.7: Connections and functions of primary motor cortex.

Motor Homunculus: The motor areas of various parts of the body are **represented in the pre-central gyrus.**

- The areas for face are represented bilaterally, whereas representation of rest of the body is unilateral. The representation is such that the **feet remain at the top of the gyrus and the face at the bottom** (Fig. 107.8).
  - The cortical representation is *proportionate to the skill with which the body part is involved in voluntary activities*. Therefore, **hand and digits occupy a large area** in the cortex since they are involved in execution of skilled activities.
- As human beings are specialized in speech, the **lips, jaw, and tongue also occupy a significantly large area** in the cortex.
- This is called the **vocalization of the cortex**.

Pre-motor Cortex

Pre-motor cortex (**lateral area 6**) receives information from supplementary motor area and primary motor cortex and projects to brainstem areas that are concerned with postural control (Fig. 107.9).

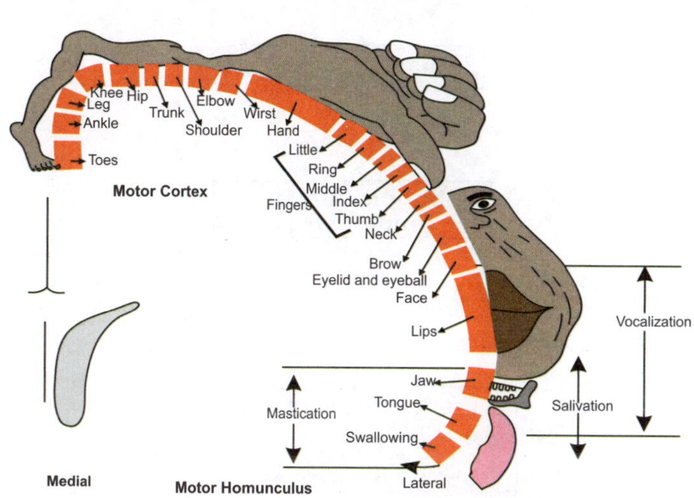

Fig. 107.8: Motor homunculus. Note that hands (including digits) and face have maximum representation in the motor cortex.

Pre-motor Cortex

Pre-motor cortex (**lateral area 6**) receives information from supplementary motor area and primary motor cortex and projects to brainstem areas that are concerned with postural control (Fig. 107.9).

- It **sets posture at the beginning of a planned movement**.

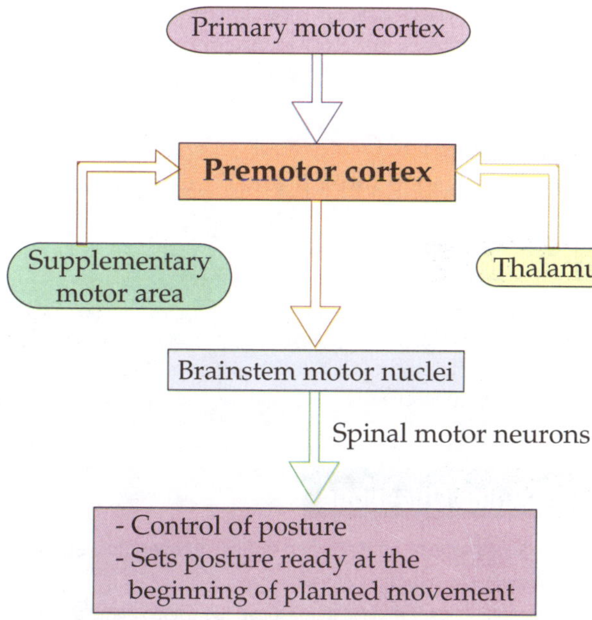

Fig. 107.9: Connections and functions of premotor cortex.

- Thus, it helps the individual to ***prepare for execution of movement.***

Supplementary Motor Area

This is the **medial portion of area 6**. It receives input from somatosensory cortex.

- It is involved in higher motor functions like **planning and programming the motor sequences** and it **controls bimanual tasks** (Fig. 107.10).
- **Lesion of this area** produces difficulty in performing complex motor activities, and the activities that involve bimanual coordination.

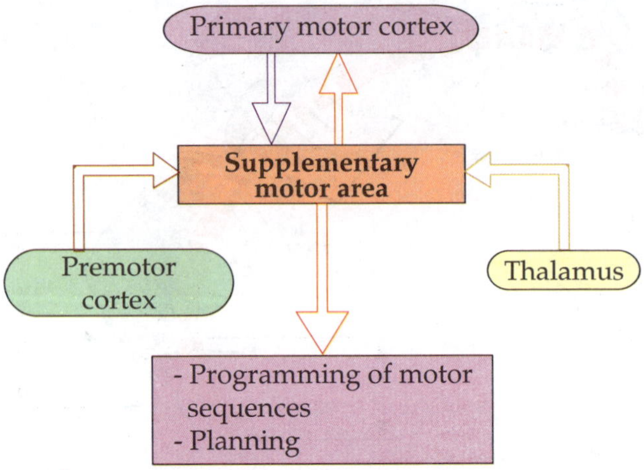

Fig. 107.10: Connections and functions of supplementary motor area.

Primary Somatosensory Cortex

The somatosensory cortex (**area 3 1, and 2**) projects to the supplementary motor area and pre-motor cortex.

- Lesion of this area produces *defect in motor performance* that involves **execution with learned sequences of events**. For example, eating with knife and fork is severely affected.
- Fibers in the corticospinal tract that originate from somatosensory cortex terminate more in the dorsal horn. These fibers modulate afferent inputs into the CNS.

Posterior Parietal Cortex

Posterior parietal lobe (**area 5 and 7**) contributes to the corticospinal tract and is also connected with motor cortex. This area utilizes complex sensory information for producing movements.

Frontal Eye Field

This is the **area 8**. It receives input from primary and pre motor cortices and projects to pontine nuclei that **control eye movements** and superior colliculus that integrates **saccadic movements** (Fig. 107.11).

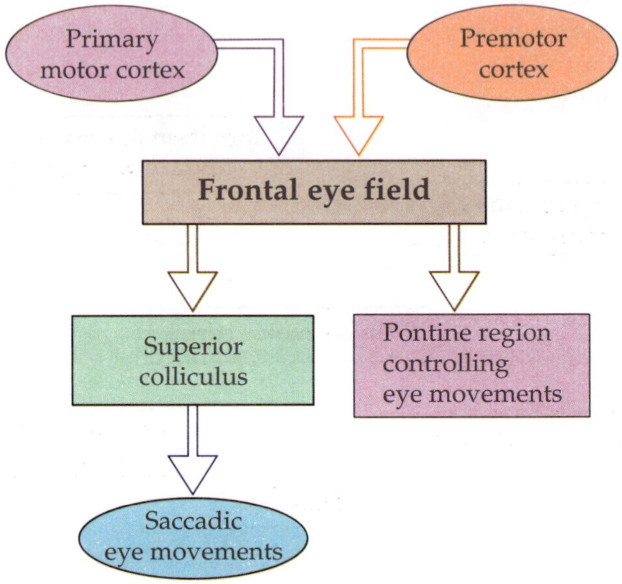

Fig. 107.11: Connections and functions of frontal eye field.

Exam Questions

1. Describe the mechanisms of regulation of posture and movement.
2. Describe the spinal and medullary integration of regulation of posture and movement. Add a note on pattern generator (CPG) of locomotion
3. Describe the midbrain and cortical integration of regulation of posture and movement. Add a note on central pattern generator (CPG) of locomotion
4. Describe the connections and functions of different cortical motor areas. A dd a note on motor homunculus.

Multiple Choice Questions

1. Which reflex response appears first during recovery in a spinal being following transection of spinal cord.
A. Contraction of flexor muscle in response to noxious stimulus
B. Triceps jerk
C. Mass reflex
D. Babinski sign

2. Which of the following is not a feature of decerebrate preparation?
A. Intense rigidity in extensor group of muscle
B. Tonic reflexes are prominent
C. Righting reflexes are present
D. No phase of shock

3. Which of the following is not seen in midbrain animal?
A. No features of shock
B. Minimal extensor rigidity
C. Righting reflexes present
D. Grasp reflex absent

4. Setting posture before planned movements, is the function of:
A. Premotor cortex
B. Motor cortex
C. Frontal
D. Supplementary motor cortex

5. In decorticate animal, which reflex is lost:
A. Hoping and placing reflex
B. Tonic neck reflex
C. Tonic labyrinthine reflex
D. Stretch reflex

Answers

1. D 2. C 3. D 4. A 5. A

Chapter 108

Basal Ganglia

Learning Objectives

On completion of study of this chapter:

The student will be able to (must know):

1. Name the parts of basal ganglia.
2. Outline the inputs, outputs and internal connections of basal ganglia.
3. Draw a schematic diagram of direct and indirect pathways through basal ganglia and briefly describe their role in motor functions.
4. List the functions of basal ganglia.
5. Learn the physiological basis of etiology, features and management of Parkinsonism.
6. Define chorea, athetosis and ballism.

The student may also be able to (desirable to know):

1. Describe the role of basal ganglia in motor function.
2. Mention the abnormality of Huntington's disease.

Basal ganglia are a group of **deep subcortical nuclei** located at the base of forebrain. Unlike cerebellum, basal ganglia **do not receive inputs directly** from the spinal cord.

1. They **do not directly project to the brainstem areas** that control motor activities.
2. They receive **inputs mainly from cortex** and **project to the cortex** via thalamus.

- Basal ganglia via their cortical connections project principally **to brainstem areas** that give rise to all ***extrapyramidal tracts***.
- Therefore, basal ganglia **mainly influence extrapyramidal functions**.

Consequently, they are classified as important **extrapyramidal structures**.

FUNCTIONAL ORGANIZATION

Basal ganglia mainly include **caudate nucleus, the putamen and the globus pallidus** (Fig. 108.1).

- Subthalamic nucleus, and substantia nigra are also included in basal ganglia.
  - The caudate nucleus and putamen are together known as **striatum** (**neostriatum**), and putamen and globus pallidus are combinely known as **lenticular nucleus**.
- **Globus pallidus** is divided into an **external part** (globus pallidus externus) and an **internal part** (globus pallidus internus).
- Substantia nigra is divided into **two parts**: pars compacta and pars reticulata.

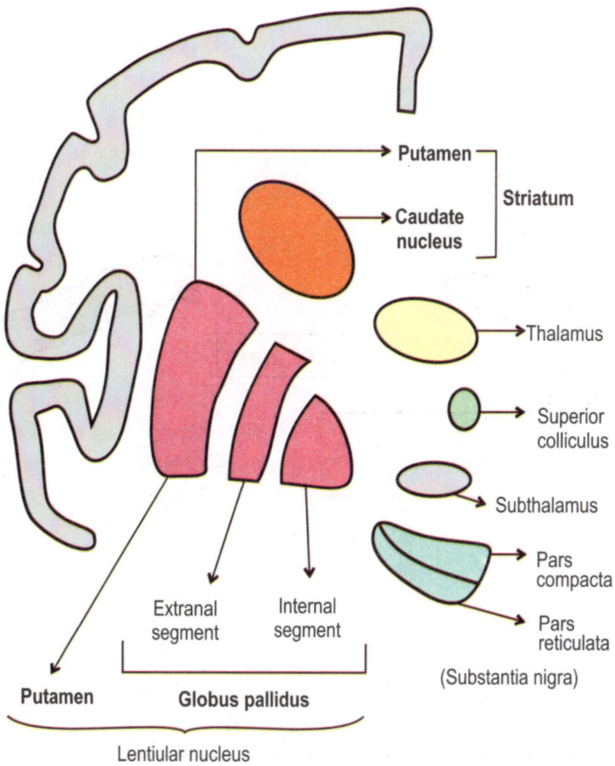

Fig. 108.1: Parts of basal ganglia.

Inputs

In contrast to cerebellum, basal ganglia **do not receive direct sensory input** from the peripheral structures, spinal cord or sensory nuclei in the brainstem.

- The main inputs to basal ganglia come **from cerebral cortex** (Fig. 108.2).
- Basal ganglia also receive inputs **from thalamus**, dorsal raphe nucleus and pedunculopontine region of the brainstem.
- Most *afferent information* enters basal ganglia ***via striatum*** (caudate nucleus and putamen).

The afferent fibers are:

1. **Corticostriate projection:** Basal ganglia receive afferents from all parts of cerebral cortex via corticostriate projection.
   - **Putamen** receives input mainly from the ***sensorymotor cortex*** and caudate nucleus receives inputs from remainder of the cortex.
2. **Thalamostriate projection:** The centromedian nucleus of thalamus projects to the striatum via thalamostriate projections.
3. **Raphestriate projection:** Striatum also receives input from dorsal raphe nucleus.
4. **Pedunculostriate projection:** Pedunculopontine nucleus of brainstem projects to basal ganglia.

Outputs

The **principal output nucleus** of basal ganglia is the *internal segment of globus pallidus* (Fig. 108.3).

- The fibers project mainly to the ventral-lateral, ventral-anterior, and centromedian **nuclei of thalamus** from where fibers project **to prefrontal and premotor cortices** (extrapyramidal pathways mainly originate from these cortical areas).

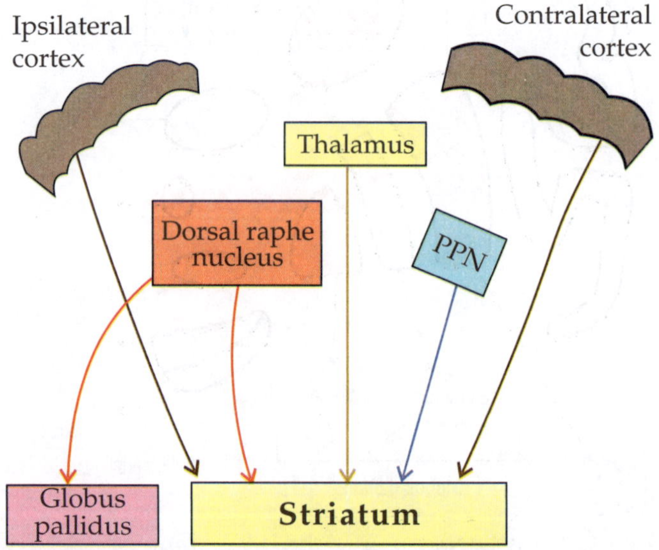

Fig. 108.2: Inputs to basal ganglia. The major input arrives from the cortex. PPN: pedunculopontine nucleus.

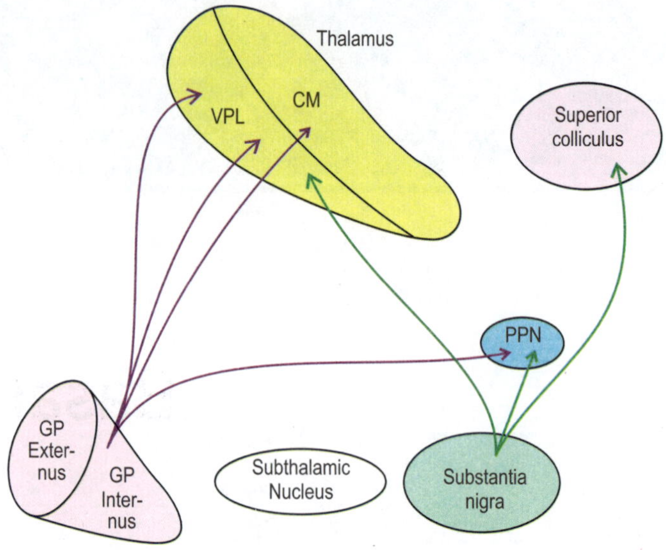

Fig. 108.3: Outputs from basal ganglia. The major outputs are to ventral-posterolateral (VPL) and centromedian (CM) nuclei of the thalamus. PPN: pedunculopontine nucleus.

- The output from the internal segment of the globus pallidus to the thalamus is **inhibitory**, whereas the output from the thalamus to the cerebral cortex is **excitatory**.

- Pars reticulata portion of substantia nigra projects to thalamus.
- Basal ganglia also project to pedunculopontine nucleus, habenula and superior colliculus.

Motor Loop

The main feature of input and output of basal ganglia is that ***cerebral cortex projects to striatum***, striatum projects to internal segment of globus pallidus, globus pallidus projects to thalamus, which projects ***back to the cortex***, completing the **motor loop** (Fig. 108.4).

Motor loop forms two major neuronal circuits through basal ganglia: putamen circuit and caudate circuit

Putamen Circuit: Fibers from premotor cortex, primary motor cortex and prefrontal cortex project to putamen and from there via interneurons to globus pallidus (GP).

- From GPi either directly or via subthalamic nuclei and substantia nigra fibers project to ventroanterior and ventrolateral nuclei of thalamus.
- From thalamus fibers project to the cortex, completing the circuit. This is called putamen circuit.
- Putamen circuit is for subconscious execution of learned patterns of movement.

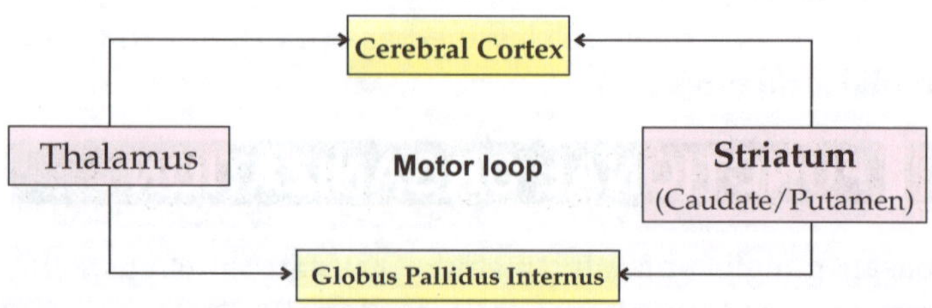

Fig. 108.4: The motor loop in the brain.

Cudate Circuit: Fibers from various part of the cortex project to caudate nucleus and from there to globus pallidus internus.

- From GPi fibers project to ventroanterior and ventrolateral nuclei of thalamus.
- From thalamus fibers project to the prefrontal cortex, completing the circuit. This is called caudate circuit.
- Caudate circuit is **for cognitive planning of sequential and parallel motor patterns** to achieve specific conscious goal on a movement.

Connections within Basal Ganglia

Major connections within the basal ganglia are as follows (Fig. 108.5):

1. **Nigrostriatal projection:** The pars compacta portion of substantia nigra projects to striatum. The nigrostriatal projection is dopaminergic.
   - Degeneration of this system produces **Parkinsonism**.
2. **Striatonigral projection:** Striatum also projects to substantia nigra. The striatonigral projection is inhibitory and neurotransmitter secreted in this pathway is GABA.
   - Degeneration of this pathway produces **Huntington's disease**.
3. **Projection from subthalamic nucleus** to globus pallidus internus: Subthalamic nucleus projects to internal segment of globus pallidus. **This projection is excitatory.**

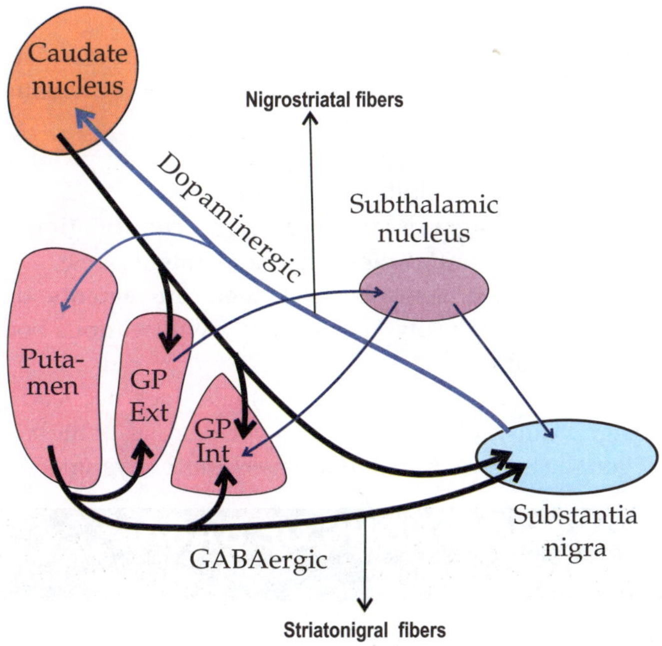

Fig. 108.5: Connections within the nuclei of basal ganglia. Note the dopaminergic nigrostriatal projections and GABAergic striatonigral projections.

Neural Pathways through Basal Ganglia

The inputs, interconnections, and outputs constitute **two important neural pathways** through the basal ganglia that are involved in control of motor activities: the direct pathway, and the indirect pathway.

Direct Pathway

Cortex projects to striatum. Striatum projects to globus pallidus internus, which projects to thalamus and thalamus in turn projects to motor cortex. This is the direct pathway (Fig. 108.6).

- The projection of cortex to striatum is excitatory (glutaminergic).
- ***Projection of striatum to globus pallidus internus is inhibitory*** (GABAergic), and projection ***from globus pallidus internus to the thalamus is inhibitory*** (GABAergic).
- Thus, stimulation of striatum results in stimulation of thalamus by **disinhibition.**

The direct pathway is stimulated during movement. Usually, neurons in the striatum have less resting background activity.

- During movement, they are activated by inputs from cortex and thalamus.
- Activation of striatum inhibits globus pallidus internus.
  - However, pallidal neurons themselves are inhibitory to thalamus.
  - Therefore, ***activation of striatum finally*** **excites the thalamic neurons.**
- Consequently, the **target neurons in the motor cortex are stimulated** via thalamocortical projection.

Indirect Pathway

This involves connection from striatum to the external segment of globus pallidus, which projects to subthalamic nucleus. Subthalamic nucleus projects to internal segment of the globus pallidus, which in turn projects to thalamus (Fig. 108.6).

- In this pathway, **striatum inhibits globus pallidus externus**, which ***inhibits subthalamic nucleus.***
- Subthalamic nucleus **activates globus pallidus internus**.
  - Therefore, **stimulation of striatum activates globus pallidus internus** through this indirect pathway.
- The final output of striatum through this **indirect pathway is inhibitory** (as globus pallidus internus activation inhibits thalamocortical projections).

Modulation by Nigrostriatal Projections

The direct and indirect pathways have opposite effects. Normally, there is a balance between these two pathways.

Alteration of activity in either of the pathways leads to imbalance in motor output from basal ganglia. Therefore, in basal ganglia disorders both **hypokinetic and hyperkinetic features** are observed.

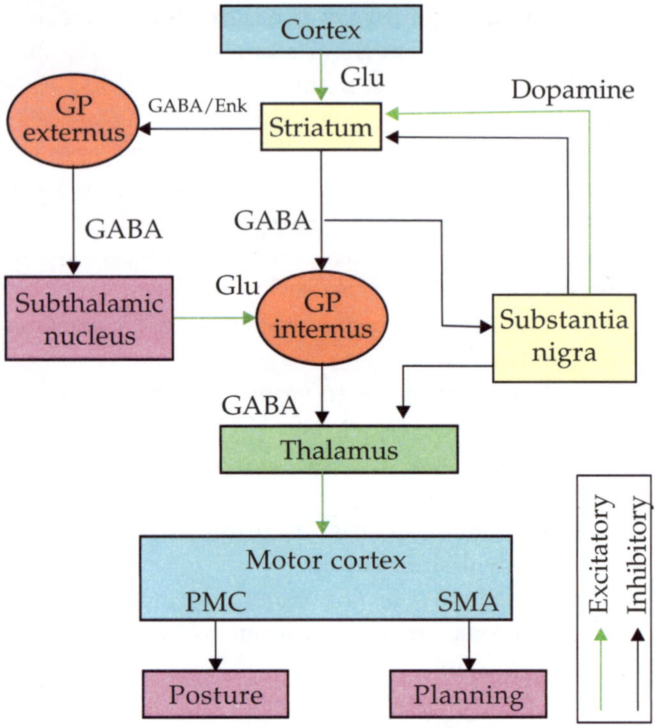

Fig. 108.6: Direct and indirect pathways through basal ganglia. In direct pathway, projection of striatum to globus pallidus internus is inhibitory (GABAergic), and from there to the thalamus is inhibitory (GABAergic). Therefore, stimulation of striatum results in stimulation of thalamus by disinhibition that leads to stimulation of cortical neurons. In indirect pathway, striatum inhibits globus pallidus externus, which in turn inhibits subthalamic nucleus and subthalamic nucleus activates globus pallidus internus. Therefore, stimulation of striatum activates globus pallidus internus. The final output of striatum through indirect pathway is inhibitory (as globus pallidus internus activation inhibits thalamocortical projections). Thus, direct and indirect pathways have opposite nature of projections to cortex. Enk: enkephalin; Glu: glutamate; GP: globus pallidus; PMC: premotor cortex: SMA: supplementary motor area.

- Another important connection of these pathways is the **nigrostriatal projections**.
  - The **dopaminergic projections** from pars compacta of substantia nigra to the striatum appear to have an **excitatory influence** *on the direct pathway and* ***inhibitory influence*** *on the indirect pathway.*
  - It also modulates the input from cortex to the striatum.
  - Therefore, projection from substantia nigra to striatum is important physiologically.
- The **neurons in the striatum** are cholinergic.
- In striatum, the **ratio of acetylcholine and dopamine** keeps the striatal neurons active.
  - **Alteration in this Ach-DA ratio** results in abnormalities in motor activities.

Subdivisions of Striatum

Striatum is subdivided into two zones: striosomes, and matrix.

Striosomes: Limbic system mainly projects to the striosomes of striatum. Therefore, striosomal part of basal ganglia is concerned with **limbic functions**.

Matrix: This zone receives projection from motor cortex. Thus, matrix zone of basal ganglia is connected with **motor functions**.

PY10.7

FUNCTIONS OF BASAL GANGLIA

1. The neurons of basal ganglia are observed to **discharge before the movement begins**. This indicates that basal ganglia is involved in **planning and programming** of motor activities.
2. Basal ganglia **controls posture**.
   - Basal ganglia-thalamic-cortical projection to brainstem **influences descending pathways** that control posture.
   - Diseases of basal ganglia result in profound postural abnormalities.
3. Basal ganglia **inhibits stretch reflexes** by stimulation of caudate nucleus.
   - This is achieved by **stimulation of inhibitory motor cortex** through thalamocortical feedback pathway and by **stimulation of inhibitory reticular formation.**
4. Neostriatum regulates **subconscious gross movements**.
5. Basal ganglia also play a role in **cognitive functions**.
   - This is especially performed by the caudate nucleus through its connections with the frontal portion of the neocortex.
   - Lesion of caudate nucleus results in deficit in performance based on learning.
6. Lesion of head of the left caudate nucleus is associated with **dysarthric aphasia** (difficulty in articulating words).
7. Globus pallidus provides inputs for appropriate **muscle tone** for skilled movements.
8. Substantia nigra is the center for **coordination of impulses essential for skilled movements**.
9. Basal ganglia controls **associated movements** that occur automatically and normally with various body movements.
10. Lesion of basal ganglia in animals does not lead to significant motor deficit. However, diseases of the basal ganglia in humans result in severe motor dysfunctions.

DYSFUNCTIONS OF BASAL GANGLIA

Parkinson's Disease

Parkinson's disease (as described by James Parkinson) results from degeneration of nigrostriatal dopaminergic neurons. With age, there is progressive loss of dopamine and dopamine receptors in the basal ganglia. When this processes is accentuated, Parkinsonism results.

Causes

1. **Idiopathic:** The cause of degeneration of dopaminergic neurons is not exactly known.
2. **Drugs:** It occurs secondary to chronic use of many drugs like phenothiazine, D2 receptor blockers, etc.
3. **MPP:** It has been recently described that **methyl-phenyl-pyridinium** (MPP) concentration in the brain of Parkinsonism is high.
    - MPP is formed from methyl-phenyl-tertahydropyridinum (MPTP) by the action of ***monoamine oxidase B*** (MAO-B) enzyme.
    - MPP rapidly **accumulates in the neurons of basal ganglia** and destroys them.

Features

Both **hypokinetic and hyperkinetic** movements are observed in Parkinsonism.

Hypokinetic Movements

1. **Akinesia:** Akinesia is defined as **difficulty in initiating movements** and **decreased spontaneous movements.**
2. **Bradykinesia:** Bradykinesia is defined as **slowness of movement.**
    - All activities are grossly reduced and slowed. Difficulty in tying shoelaces and buttoning is frequently observed.
3. **Decreased associated movements:** Examples of associated movements are swinging of the arms during walking or the facial expressions during speaking.
    - These associated movements are grossly diminished in Parkinsonism.
    - The patient suffering from Parkinsonism speaks without any emotional expression, which is called as **expressionless face** or **mask face** (facial immobility).
4. **Serpentine Stare:** Frequency of spontaneous blinking of eyes decreases producing a serpentine stare.
    - *Myerson's sign:* Repetitive tapping (about 2 Hz) over the glabella (Glabellar tap) produces a sustained blink response.

Hyperkinetic Movements

1. **Rigidity:** Rigidity of Parkinsonism is different from spasticity that occurs in UMN paralysis.
    - In rigidity, the ***motor neuron discharge is increased in both agonists and antagonists***.
    - Therefore, the limbs offer resistance to passive bending throughout the movement (**lead pipe rigidity**).
    - Sometimes, **cogwheel rigidity** (series of catches during passive movement) is also seen.
    - However, the clasp-knife spasticity (sudden loss of resistance while moving a rigid limb) of UMN paralysis is never seen.
2. **Tremor:** Tremor occurs due to *regular alternating contractions of antagonist muscles*, at a frequency of about 8 per second.
    - Typically, **tremor is observed only at rest.**
    - Once patient initiates the movement, tremor disappears. This is described as **resting tremor.**
3. **Festinant gait:** Patient walks in an attitude that as if he is **trying to catch the center of gravity**. Usually, he bends forward but does not fall, instead takes short and shuffling steps (Fig. 108.7).
4. **Micrographia:** Combination of tremor rigidity and bradykinesia results in small, tremulous and often illegible or difficult handwriting, called micrographia.

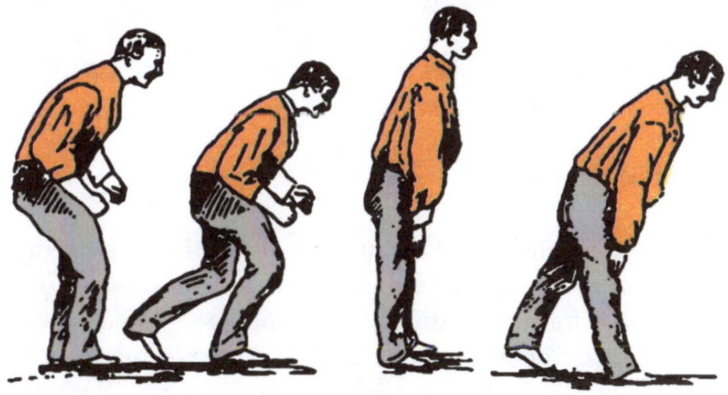

Fig. 108.7: Pictorial demonstration of festinant gait. Note, tries to catch the center of gravity, bends forward and takes short and shuffling steps.

Management

Diagnosis: Disease is diagnosed by **functional dopaminergic imaging by SPECT**, in which uptake of striatal dopaminergic marker, particularly in posterior putamen is reduced.

- **Dopamine transporter (DaT) imaging** by using radiolabeled ligand binding to dopaminergic terminals, is done to assess the nigrostriatal cell loss.

Treatment

1. **Replacement of dopamine:** Dopamine cannot cross the blood brain barrier. Therefore, ***Levodopa (L-dopa),*** a precursor of dopamine that easily crosses blood brain barrier, is the drug of choice for Parkinsonism. It also helps repair dopamine deficiency.
    - **Dopamine receptor agonists:** Dopamine agonists like **bromocriptine, pergolide** are also used.
2. **Anticholinergics:** Though Parkinson's disease occurs due to dopamine deficiency in the striatum, the alteration in the **ratio of dopamine to acetylcholine plays an important role.**

- Therefore, injection of anticholinergics that decreases acetylcholine concentration in the basal ganglia and ***reestablishes acetylcholine dopamine ratio***, improves the symptoms.

3. **MAO-B Inhibitors: Deprenyl** is the drug of choice. Deprenyl **inhibits monoamine oxidase B**, therefore, prevents formation of MPP from MPTP.
   - **Selegiline,** a MAO-B inhibitor reduces metabolic breakdown of dopamine and also slowdown degeneration of neurons in substantia nigra.
4. **Transplantation of adrenal:** Transplantation of adrenal medulla from one of the adrenal gland of the patient into his basal ganglia helps in regenerating the dopaminergic neurons.
5. **Implantation of fetal basal ganglia:** Implantation of tissue from the basal ganglia of fetuses into the basal ganglia of the patient improves the condition.
6. **Transplantation of glomus cells:** Recently, for treatment of Parkinsonism, glomus cells from carotid body are isolated and transplanted into basal ganglia. Glomus cell **releases dopamine locally**. This has been found to be encouraging.

Huntington's Disease

This is a genetic defect of **autosomal dominant** type that occurs due to a defective gene ***on the chromosome 4***. The gene codes for **huntingtin,** an abnormal protein that causes the disease. The abnormal gene has a many-times-repeating codon, CAG, that codes for multiple extra glutamine amino acids in the molecular structure of huntingtin, the abnormal neuronal cell protein that causes the symptoms.

Cause

The disease occurs due to **degeneration of GABAergic striatonigral pathway**.

- **GABAergic and cholinergic neurons** are lost in the striatum.

Features

Age: Disease usually starts between the age of 30–40 years and progresses uniformly till death that usually occurs within 10–15 years. Disease has three important features: chorea, dementia and slurred speech.

Chorea: Chorea is defined as **rapid involuntary and dancing movements**.

- The chorea is called as **Huntington's chorea**.
- The loss of GABA-ergic neurons in the striatum removes its inhibitory influence on the globus pallidus, which reduces the activities in the thalamic nucleus that results in chorea.

Dementia: Dementia occurs due to simultaneous and progressive loss of cholinergic neurons in the cerebral cortex.

Slurring speech: Gradually, speech is slurred in Huntington disease.

Treatment

There is no definite treatment of Huntington's chorea. The disease is ***progressively fatal***. Drugs are used to reduce the symptoms.

- **Tetrabenazine** has been used recently to reduce the choreiform movements. It reversibly binds with vesicular monoamine transporter (VMAT) and ***inhibits the uptake of monoamine*** into synaptic vesicles.
- It also acts as ***dopamine receptor antagonist***. Tetrabenazine is used in other movement disorders such as tardive dyskinesia.

Other Dysfunctions

Ballism

Ballism is defined as **involuntary movements that are flailing, intense, and violent in nature**. Usually it occurs suddenly.

- Ballism occurs when the **subthalamic nucleus is damaged**.
- **Hemiballism** is common than ballism and occurs due to hemorrhage in the subthalamic nucleus of the opposite side of the brain.

Athetosis

Athetosis is defined as **continuous but slow writhing movements**.

- It occurs due to **damage to striatum.**

Chorea

Chorea is defined as **rapid involuntary dancing movements**.

- It occurs due to **damage to caudate nucleus**.

Exam Questions

1. Describe the connections, functions and dysfunctions of basal ganglia.
2. With the help of a suitable diagram, describe the functions of direct and indirect pathways passing through basal ganglia, in the regulation of motor functions. Add a note on features and treatment of Parkinsonism.

Multiple Choice Questions

1. **All the following statements are true about basal ganglia, EXCEPT:**
   A. Receives inputs directly from the spinal cord
   B. Receives inputs mainly from the cortex
   C. Gives outputs to cortex through thalamus
   D. Mainly influences extrapyramidal tracts
2. **Striatum is:**
   A. Caudate and putamen
   B. Putamen and globus pallidus
   C. Subthalamus and substantia nigra
   D. Putamen and thalamus
3. **All the following are afferent (input) fibers to basal ganglia, EXCEPT:**
   A. Corticostriate B. Pedunculostriate
   C. Niagrostriate D. Thalamostriate
4. **The motor loop of basal ganglia is:**
   A. Cortex to globus pallidus to thalamus to cortex
   B. Cortex to striatum to thalamus to cortex
   C. Cortex to thalamus to striatum to cortex
   D. Cortex to striatum to globus pallidus to thalamus to cortex
5. **Cognitive planning of sequential and parallel motor patterns to achieve specific conscious goal on a movement is done by basal ganglia's:**
   A. Motor loop B. Putamen circuit
   C. Caudate circuit D. Striatonigral projections
6. **All the following are nuclear group of basal ganglia, EXCEPT:**
   A. Putamen
   B. Globus pallidus
   C. Caudate nucleus
   D. Red nucleus
7. **Striatum does not receive input from which of the following structure?**
   A. Thalamus
   B. Cortex
   C. Raphe nucleus
   D. PAG
8. **Basal ganglia project to all structures, EXCEPT:**
   A. Thalamus
   B. Hippocampus
   C. Pedunculopontine nucleus
   D. Superior colliculus
9. **The efferent fiber bundle from substantia nigra transmits dopamine to which of following area?**
   A. Thalamus
   B. Corpus striatum
   C. Tegmentum of pons
   D. Tectum of midbrain
10. **The highest density of glutamate receptors in basal ganglia are found in:**
    A. Substantia nigra
    B. Globus pallidus interna
    C. Globus pallidus externa
    D. Putamen
11. **Which of the following basal ganglia nucleus is primarily glutaminergic?**
    A. Putamen
    B. Subthalamic nucleus
    C. Globus pallidus
    D. Substantial nigra
12. **Which of the following is the major neurotransmitter in nigrostriatal pathway?**
    A. Dopamine
    B. Noradrenaline
    C. Acetylcholine
    D. Serotonin
13. **Functions of basal ganglia include:**
    A. Righting reflex
    B. Skilled movements
    C. Memory
    D. Maintenance of equilibrium
14. **Which of the following is the main function of basal ganglia in motor control?**
    A. Planning & programming of movement
    B. Skilled functions
    C. Coordinate the motor functions
    D. Balance & coarse movements
15. **Continuous but slow writhing movement is known as:**
    A. Chorea
    B. Ballismus
    C. Athetosis
    D. Akinesia
16. **Diseases of basal ganglia dysfunction are all, EXCEPT:**
    A. Alzheimer's disease
    B. Parkinsonism
    C. Chorea
    D. Athetosis
17. **Striatonigral projection is mainly:**
    A. GABAergic
    B. Cholinergic
    C. Dopaminergic
    D. Histaminergic
18. **Ballism is due to damage to:**
    A. Substantia nigra
    B. Globus pallidus interna
    C. Subthalamic nucleus
    D. Putamen
19. **Huntington's disease is due to degeneration of:**
    A. Corticostriate fibers
    B. Thalamostriate fibers
    C. Niagrostriatal fibers
    D. Striatoniagral fibers
20. **Treatment of Parkinson's disease include all of t:e following, EXCEPT:**
    A. Transplantation of glomus cells
    B. Implantation of fetal basal ganglia
    C. Transplantation of adrenal medulla
    D. Transplantation of adrenal cortex

Answers

1. A	2. A	3. C	4. D	5. C	6. D	7. D	8. B	9. B	10. D
11. B	12. A	13. B	14. A	15. C	16. A	17. A	18. C	19. D	20. D

Chapter 109

Cerebellum

Learning Objectives

On completion of study of this chapter:

The student will be able to (must know):

1. Draw a schematic diagram of functional divisions of cerebellum, depicting functions of each division.
2. Name deep cerebellar nuclei and give their functions.
3. Outline the internal connections of cerebellum, describe the projection of deep cerebellar nuclei to the descending pathways.
4. List functions of cerebellum and briefly describe each of them.
5. Describe the connections and functions of cerebellum.
6. List the features of cerebellar disorder.
7. List the cerebellar function tests.

The student may also be able to (desirable to know):

1. Explain the physiological basis of cerebellar disorder.
2. Describe connections of Purkinje cells.

Cerebellum literally means the '**little brain**'. Cerebellum receives inputs of almost **all sensory modalities** and projects to almost **all areas of brain that are involved in control of motor activities**.

- Cerebellum strongly influences **all aspects of movement**, starting from the **rate, range, force, and direction to the termination of movement**.
- Hence, damage to cerebellum results in severe **incoordination of movement and postural abnormalities**.

FUNCTIONAL ORGANIZATION

Cerebellum is located in the posterior cranial fossa, behind the brainstem.

1. It is connected to midbrain through **superior cerebellar peduncle**, to pons through **middle cerebellar peduncle** and to the medulla through **inferior cerebellar peduncle** (Fig. 109.1).
2. The surface area of cerebellum is **about 75% of the cerebral cortex**, but in weight it is only 10% of the cortex. Thus, ***cerebellar cortical tissue is much folded***.
3. There are **two main fissures** in the cerebellum that divides it into **two major parts**:
   - ***the posterolateral fissure*** that separates flocculonodular lobe from rest of the cerebellum and,
   - ***the primary fissure*** that separates the anterior lobe from the posterior lobe.

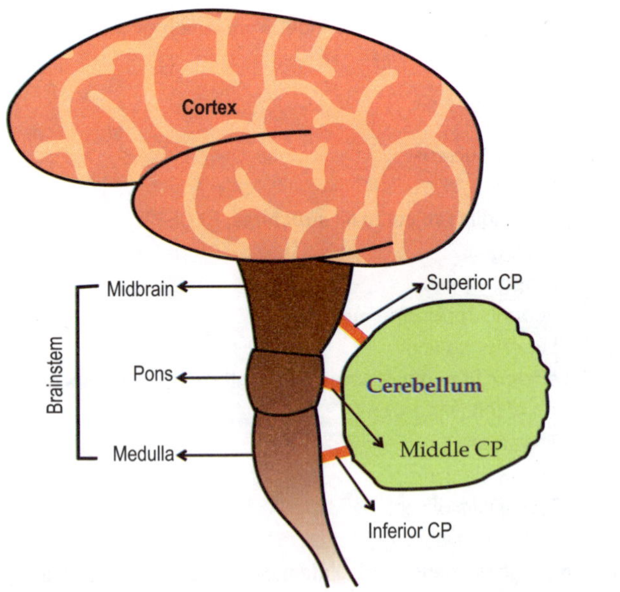

Fig. 109.1: Location of cerebellum and connection of cerebellum with brainstem via cerebellar peduncles.

Functional Divisions and Functions of each Division

Functionally, cerebellum is divided into **three major subdivisions**: vestibulocerebellum, spinocerebellum and cerebrocerebellum (Fig.109.2).

Vestibulocerebellum

This is also called **archicerebellum**, as phylogenetically it is the oldest part.

- It consists of **flocculonodular lobe**.
  - This part of cerebellum is called vestibulocerebellum for its extensive and reciprocal **connection with the vestibular nuclei**.
- It is concerned with **equilibrium and learning induced changes in vestibulo-ocular reflex**.

Spinocerebellum

This is also called **paleocerebellum**, as it is intermediate in development.

- It consists of the **vermis and the paravermal regions** of cerebellum.
  - It is called spinocerebellum, as it receives **proprioceptive and other sensory inputs** from all the body parts **through spinal cord.**
- It also receives **inputs from the motor cortex**, where motor planning is carried out.
  - By comparing plan with performance, it **smoothens and coordinates movement**.
- The **vermal portion** of spinocerebellum projects to the brainstem areas that control axial and proximal limb muscles.
  - Therefore, vermal spinocerebellum **controls posture**.

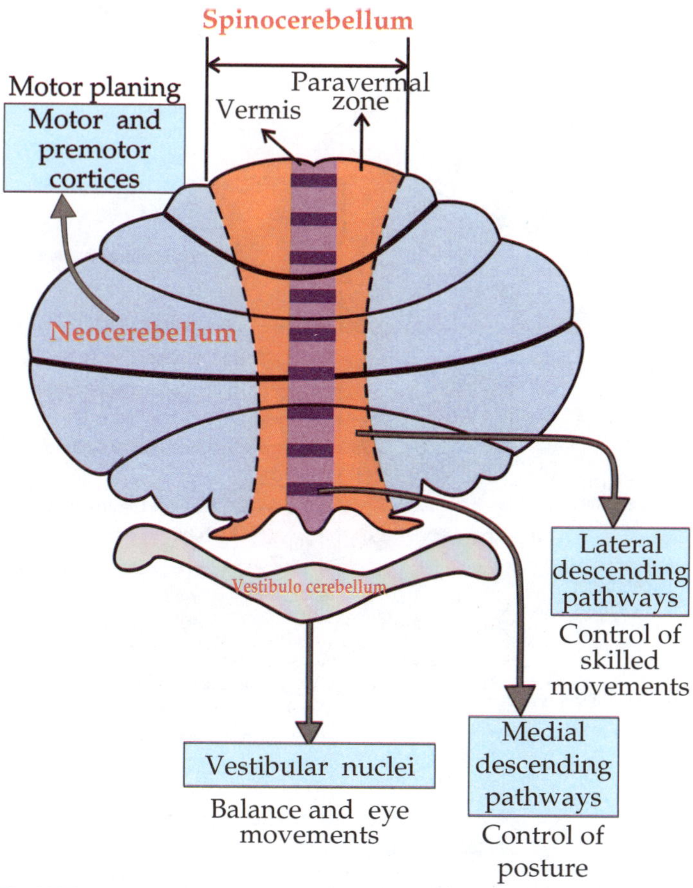

Fig. 109.2: Functional divisions and functions of cerebellum.

- The **paravermal region** of spinocerebellum projects to the brainstem nuclei that influence distal limb muscles.
  - Therefore, paravermal spinocerebellum **controls skilled voluntary movements**.

Cerebrocerebellum

This is also called **neocerebellum**, as it is newest phylogenetically.

- It consists of the two main **cerebellar hemispheres**.
  - This is called cerebrocerebellum for its connections with the cortex.
- Cortex projects to neocerebellum via the pontine nuclei; hence, this is also called **corticopontocerebellum**.
- As it interacts with the cortex, it is involved in **planning and programming of the movements**.

Functional Histology

Cerebellum is divided into the **outer cortex** and the inner part containing **deep cerebellar nuclei**.

Cerebellar Cortex

The cerebellar cortex has **three layers**: outer molecular layer, middle Purkinje cell layer, and inner granular layer (Fig. 109.3).

Molecular Layer: This layer contains interneurons that are basket cells and stellate cells.

Purkinje Cell Layer: This layer contains **Purkinje cell**.

- Purkinje cells are the largest neurons with extensive dendritic branches.
  - Dendrites of Purkinje cells enter into the molecular layer.
- The axons of the interneurons of the molecular layer project to the dendrites of the Purkinje cells.
- Purkinje cells also *receive inputs directly from the climbing fibers*.

Purkinje cells are the only cells that **project form the cortex of cerebellum to the deep cerebellar nuclei**. Thus, Purkinje cells are **connecting links** between cerebellar cortex and deep cerebellar nuclei.

Granular Cell Layer: This layer contains **granule cells and Golgi cells (interneurons).**

- The Golgi cells project to the granule cells and modify granular cell output.
- The **granule cells receive inputs from the mossy fibers** and project to the Purkinje cells, basket cells, stellate cells and Golgi cells via parallel fibers.

Significant contribution of Scientist

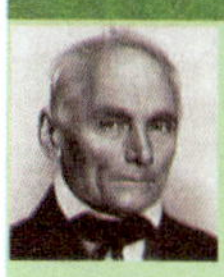

Johan Evangelista Purkinje (1787–1869), a Czech Physiologist, created the world's first Department of Physiology at the University of Breslau in Prussia (Poland) in 1839 and the world's first official physiology laboratory in 1842. He is best known for his 1837 discovery of **Purkinje cells**, large neurons with many branching dendrites found in e cerebellum. Purkinje also pioneered in subjective visual phenomena. He is also popular for describing the **Purkinje fibers** in in the ventricle of heart and **Purkinje images** in the eyes.

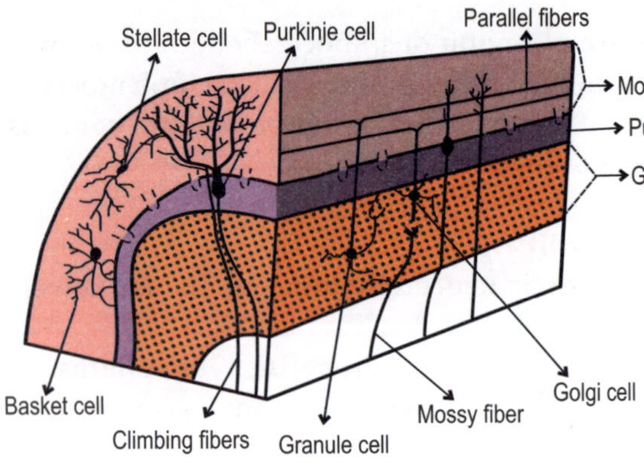

Fig. 109.3: Layers of cerebellar cortex. Note the outer molecular layer, middle Purkinje cell layer and inner granular layer.

Deep Cerebellar Nuclei

There are **four deep cerebellar nuclei** (Fig. 109.4).

Nucleus Fastigius: The nucleus fastigius is present in the **deep vermal portion of the cerebellum.**

- The vermal cortical portion of spinocerebellum projects to the fastigial nucleus.

Nucleus Globosus & Nucleus Emboliformis: The globos and emboliform nuclei are combinely known **as nucleus interpositus.**

- The **paravermal portion** of spinocerebellum projects to nucleus interpositus.

Nucleus Dentatus: This is present in the **hemispheric portion of the cerebellum.** It receives inputs from neocerebellum.

- The name of the nucleus is '**dentate**' for its appearance, which has teeth like serrated morphology.
- The deep cerebellar nuclei project to the different parts of the brainstem and thalamus (discussed in cerebellar output).

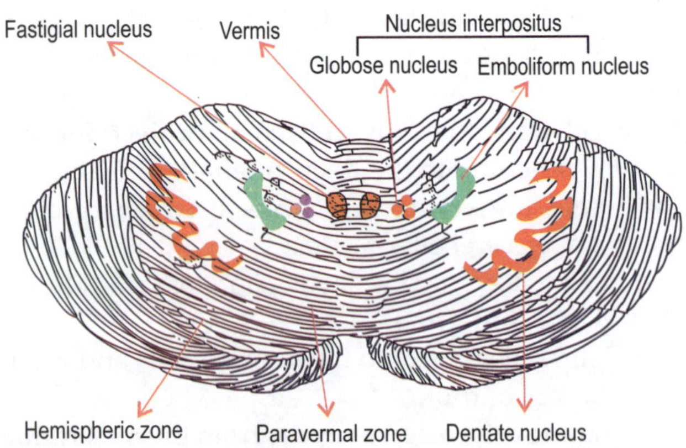

Fig. 109.4: Location of deep cerebellar nuclei.

CEREBELLAR CONNECTIONS

Cerebellar Inputs

Cerebellum receives **somatosensory inputs from almost all parts of the body** and inputs of all sensory modalities including special sensory inputs (Fig. 109.5). The cerebellar afferents are:

1. **Vestibulocerebellar tract:** Through this tract cerebellum receives impulses directly from ***the vestibular apparatus*** and also from the vestibular nuclei.
2. **Dorsal spinocerebellar tract:** This tract conveys ***proprioceptive and exteroceptive*** impulses from different parts of the body to cerebellum
3. **Ventral spinocerebellar tract:** This pathway also conveys ***proprioceptive and exteroceptive*** impulses from different parts of the body.
4. **Cuneocerebellar tract:** This tract originates from **lateral cuneate nucleus** in the caudal medulla and conveys proprioceptive inputs from head and neck.
5. **Tectocerebellar tract:** This tract conveys **visual information** from superior colliculus and **auditory information** from inferior colliculus to the cerebellum.
6. **Pontocerebellar tract:** Impulses ***from motor cortex*** reach cerebellum via pontine nuclei.
7. **Olivocerebellar tract:** *Proprioceptive inputs from the whole body* reaches cerebellum via **inferior olive**.
   - Inferior olivary nucleus is located in the rostral medulla that receives input from the *vestibular system, spinal cord and cerebral cortex*.
   - It projects to cerebellum via climbing fibers.

Mode of Inputs

Inputs to cerebellum reach via **three routes**: mossy fibers, climbing fibers and other inputs (Table 109.1).

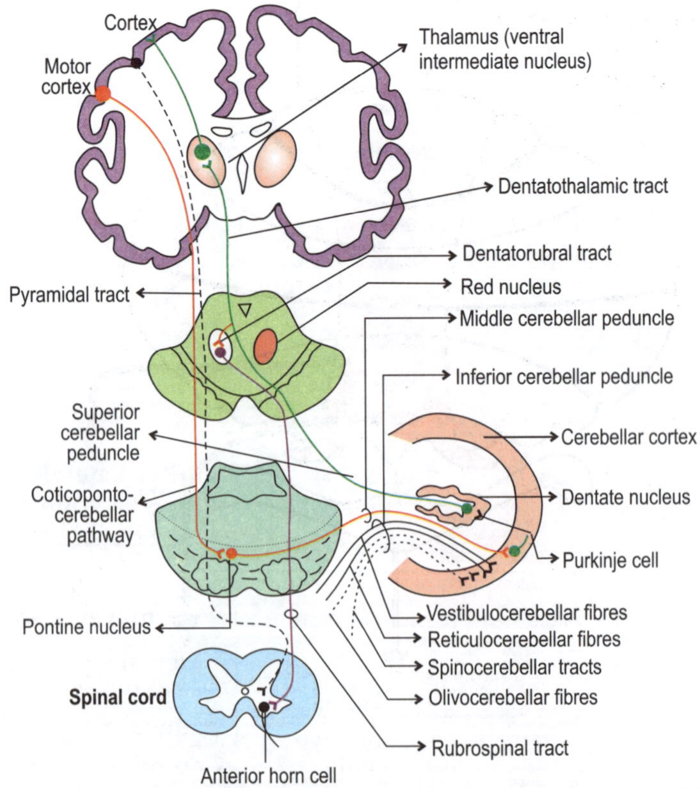

Fig. 109.5: Major afferent and efferent connections of cerebellum.

Table 109.1 | Cerebellar inputs via different fiber systems.

Fiber systems	Tracts	Nature of input
I. Through climbing fibers	Olivocerebellar tract	Proprioceptive inputs from whole body via relay in inferior olivary nucleus.
II. Through mossy fibers	1. Dorsal spinocerebellar tract	Proprioceptive and exteroceptive inputs
	2. Ventral spinocerebellar tract	Proprioceptive and exteroceptive inputs
	3. Vestibulocerebellar tract	Inputs from vestibular nuclei
	4. Tectocerebellar tract	Visual information from superior colliculus & auditory inputs from inferior colliculus
	5. Cuneocerebellar tract	Proprioceptive inputs from head and neck
	6. Corticopontocerebellar tract	Inputs from cortex via pontine nuclei
III. Other fiber systems	1. Monoaminergic inputs	
	a. Serotonergic inputs	From nucleus raphe magnus
	b. Noradrenergic input	From nucleus locus ceruleus
	2. Thalamic and other inputs	From thalamus and other brain areas

Mossy Fiber Inputs: Mossy fibers are major source of inputs to cerebellum. These fibers carry **direct proprioceptive inputs** from all parts of the body and also convey input **from cerebral cortex**. Mossy fibers project mainly to the granule cells.

Climbing Fiber Inputs: Climbing fibers convey inputs from **inferior olivary nucleus** to cerebellum. Inferior olive receives proprioceptive input from all parts of the body. Climbing fibers project to Purkinje cells of cerebellum.

Other Inputs: Cerebellum receives **monoaminergic inputs**, and inputs *from thalamus* and other parts of the brain. These fibers project to the deep cerebellar nuclei.

Cerebellar Outputs

Different parts of cerebellum project to various descending pathways via deep cerebellar nuclei (Fig. 109.6). Deep cerebellar nuclei are the output pathway of cerebellum.

Output from Vestibulocerebellum: Vestibulocerebellum **directly projects to the vestibular nuclei** without any relay in the deep cerebellar nuclei.

- Thus, vestibulocerebellum directly controls **vestibulospinal tract** activity

Output from Spinocerebellum

- The **vermal portion** of the spinocerebellum projects to fastigial nucleus, which in turn projects to pontine reticular formation and vestibular nuclei in the brainstem.
- Thus, vermal part of spinocerebellum controls the activity of pontine **reticulospinal tract and vestibulospinal tract**.

1. The **paravermal portion** of the spinocerebellum projects to the nucleus interpositus, which in turn projects to the red nucleus.
   - Thus, paravermal part of the spinocerebellum controls the activity of **rubrospinal tract**.

Output from Cerebrocerebellum: The cerebellar hemisphere **projects to the dentate nucleus**, which in turn project to the motor cortex via thalamus.

- Thus, cerebrocerebellum controls the activity of the **corticospinal tract**.

IMPORTANT NOTE

Cerebellum controls all motor functions: As different parts of the cerebellum project to all the motor nuclei in the brainstem and to the motor cortex, cerebellum controls activities of a**ll the descending pathways** (corticospinal and extrapyramidal systems). Therefore, diseases of the cerebellum affect both regulation of posture and skilled voluntary movements.

Internal Connections of Cerebellum

Cerebellum receives inputs from **two sources**: the **climbing fibers** (from olivary nucleus), and the **mossy fibers**.

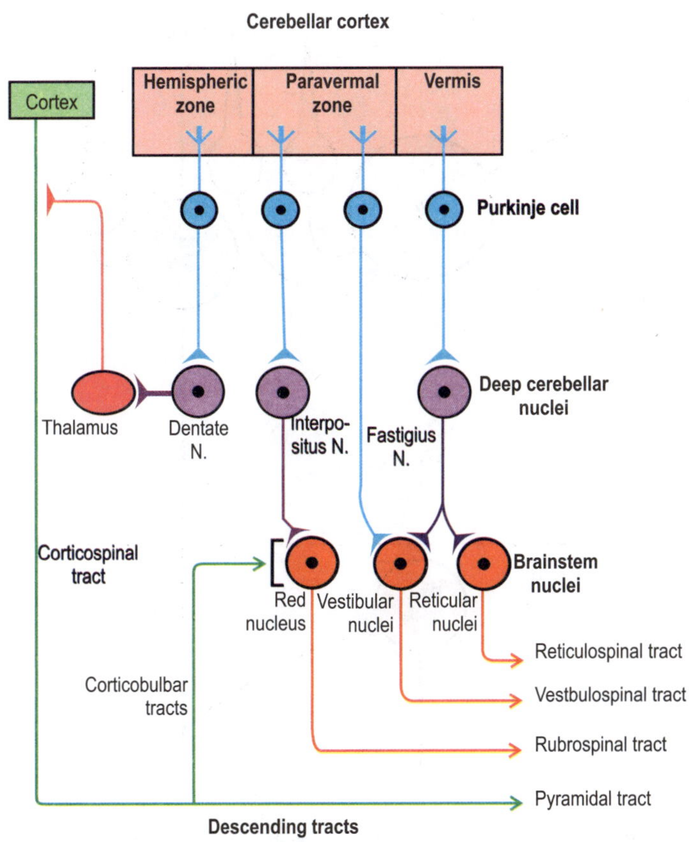

Fig. 109.6: Major output pathways from cerebellum. Note, cerebellum projects the all descending pathways.

1 .The Purkinje cells are stimulated **directly by climbing fiber** input, whereas **mossy fibers** stimulate Purkinje cells **indirectly via granule cell-parallel fiber** pathways (Fig. 109.7).
   - Mossy fibers project to granule cell.
   - Granule cells via its parallel fibers provide excitatory input to the basket and stellate cells, and Purkinje cell.
2. Basket and stellate cells that are activated by mossy fiber-parallel fiber pathway finally **inhibit Purkinje cell**.
   - This is an example of **feed-forward inhibition**.
3. Granule cell also stimulates the Golgi cells (the interneurons in granular cell layer), which in turn inhibit the activity of granule cells.
   - This is an example of **local feedback inhibition** and is meant to regulate the granule cell output.

Excitatory Output from Cerebellum: The **Purkinje cell output** to the deep cerebellar nuclei **is inhibitory** because the neurotransmitter secreted by Purkinje cells is GABA.

But deep cerebellar nuclei receive **excitatory inputs** from mossy fibers and climbing fibers, and from other sources.
   - Therefore, inspite of inhibition by the Purkinje cells, the **output of deep cerebellar nuclei to the brainstem is always excitatory**.

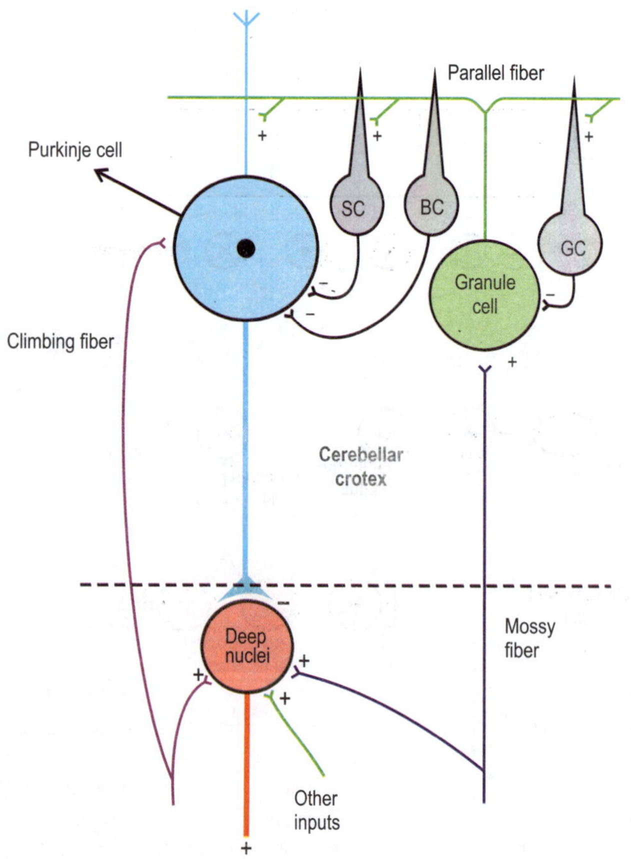

Fig. 109.7: Inputs and internal connections of cerebellum. Note, inspite of inhibitory inputs from Purkinje cells, the output of deep cerebellar nuclei is always excitatory. BC: basket cell; SC: stellate cell; GC: Golgi cell.

2. The internal circuitry of cerebellar neurons is designed mainly to **modulate the excitatory output** of the deep cerebellar nuclei.
   - Therefore, lesion of the cerebellum in human beings results in **hypotonia**.

Purkinje Cell Activity

Purkinje cells exhibit two types of action potentials: the simple spikes, and the complex spikes.

Simple Spikes: Simple spike action potential is generated in response to **stimulation of mossy fiber-parallel fiber input**.

Complex Spikes: Complex (multi-peaked) spike action potential is generated in response to **stimulation of climbing fiber input** that comes from olivary nucleus.
- These complex spike action potentials are involved ***in motor learning*** as climbing fiber activity is observed to be increased when a new motor task is learned.
- They also produce **long-term adjustment in motor responses.**

PY10.7

FUNCTIONS OF CEREBELLUM

1. **Control of postural balance and equilibrium:** This is the function of vestibulocerebellum, which has extensive and reciprocal **connection with the vestibular nuclei**.
   - Afferents from vestibular apparatus in the inner ear project to vestibulocerebellum via vestibular nuclei.
2. **Vestibulo-ocular reflex:** Vestibulocerebellum is concerned with **learning induced changes** in vestibulo-ocular reflex.
3. **Smoothening and coordination of movement:** This is the function of **spinocerebellum** that receives proprioceptive and other sensory inputs from all the body parts through the spinal cord.
   - It also receives inputs from the motor cortex, where **motor planning** is carried out.
   - By comparing plan with performance, it **smoothens and coordinates movement**.
4. **Control of posture:** The **vermal portion** of spinocerebellum projects to the brainstem areas that control axial and proximal limb muscles. Therefore, vermal spinocerebellum has **profound influence on posture**.
5. **Control of skilled voluntary movements:** The **paravermal region** of spinocerebellum projects to the brainstem nuclei that influence distal limb muscles. Therefore, paravermal spinocerebellum **controls skilled voluntary movements**.
   - Cerebellum controls all aspects of movement starting from ***rate, range, force and direction to termination*** of movement. Although, functionally cerebellum has three lobes (vestibulocerebellum, spinocerebellum and neocerebellum), they

work in a coordinated and integrated manner, that means it acts as "**Comparator of a servo mechanism**".

i) Cerebellum receives **information from corticospinal output** transmitted to the muscles, **receives proprioceptive inputs** from muscles (via spinocerebellar tracts) that informs about ongoing movements and position of the limbs, and also **receives all special sensory inputs** (visual, auditory and vestibular inputs).
ii) Cerebellum **projects to cortex** via red nucleus and pontine nuclei (Fig. 109.8).
iii) Cerebellum coordinates all the **cortical and spinal information** and appropriately modifies the ongoing movements via its influence on all descending pathways.
iv) It sends **error signal to the cortex** for alteration in programming of the movement for any ***desirable change in motor outputs*** to be achieved.

6. **Planning and programming of the movements:** This is the function of **neocerebellum** that interacts with the cortex.
   - Hence, neocerebellum controls planning and programming of the movements.
   - Especially, **planning of sequential movements** is carried out by hemispheric part of cerebellum that communicates with premotor cortex and sensory cortex.
   - Also, **timing of the sequential movements** is done by cerebellar hemisphere. It controls and provides ***appropriate timing for each succeeding movement.***
7. **Control of muscle tone and stretch reflexes:** Cerebellum influences the activity of the major descending medial system pathways through its output from fastigial nucleus, especially the vestibulospinal and reticulospinal tracts.
   - As vestibulospinal tract mainly controls α neuron activity and reticulospinal tract controls γ neuron activity in the spinal cord, cerebellum is one of the **major sites of α-γ co-linkage**.
   - In human beings, the output of deep cerebellar nuclei to the brainstem motor nuclei is excitatory that facilitates muscle tone. Therefore, **cerebellar disorder produces hypotonia**.
   - Though cerebellum has profound influence on all descending brainstem pathways, its influence on stretch reflexes is minimal, except in some patient **pendular knee jerk** is elicited. Therefore, **stretch reflexes remain usually normal** in cerebellar disorder.
   - However, **in animals** the connection of cerebellum with brainstem nuclei is complex, which inhibits the output of inhibitory reticular area. Therefore, **cerebellectomy** in decerebrate animals ***increases spasticity*** of extensor group of muscles (facilitates decerebrate rigidity).
8. **Control of movements of same side of the body:** Motor cortex of one side is connected to the cerebellar hemisphere of opposite side through a closed feedback circuit, known as **cerebral-cerebellar-cerebral circuit** via cortico-ponto-dentato-thalamo-cortical connections.
   - Thus, each cerebellar hemisphere influences the output of **opposite cerebral cortex**.
   - However, **cerebral cortex** via corticospinal tract that ***decussates to opposite site*** just after passing through pyramid controls the motor functions of contralateral half of the body.
   - Therefore, **due to double decussation**, each cerebellar hemisphere controls movements of its **own side of the body**.
9. **Learning and improvement of motor skill:** Cerebellum plays a critical role of comparing information of the ongoing movements and the changes required to improve performance.
   - Hence, for every activity, cerebellum **improves the learning and performance**.
   - Cerebellum also controls **long-term adjustment of motor skills**.
   - Especially, climbing fiber inputs that produce **complex spikes** in Purkinje cells is involved in motor learning.
   - **Climbing fiber activity** is increased every time a new activity is learned.
10. **Prevents overshoot and damp movements:** There is tendency to overshoot, especially when a movement (act) is done faster. But, intact cerebellum generates appropriate signals to prevent the overshoot and tremor. This is the basic feature of a damping system.
11. **Eyeball movement:** The *paraflocculus and pyramis* of cerebellum are concerned with movement of eye ball especially in upward direction.
    - Stimulation of these parts of cerebellum causes **upward eye movement** of the ipsilateral side.
    - Especially visual judgment of distance is the function of cerebellum, which is more developed in monkeys.
12. **Vestibular functions:** For its dense and reciprocal connection with vestibular apparatus, **vestibulocerebellum** is involved in control of all vestibular functions such as **balance during movement**, execution of **vestibule-ocular reflex**, **vestibular postural reflexes**, and change in body posture and movement in response to head movement and acceleration.

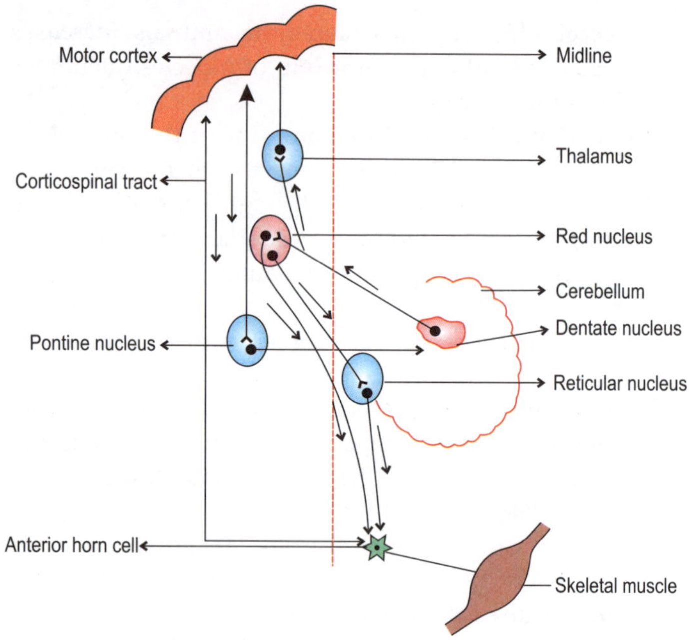

Fig. 109.8: The cerebellar connection to explain its comparator of a servo mechanism.

CEREBELLAR DISORDERS

Diseases affecting flocculonodular lobe: Diseases affecting flocculonodular lobe result in **abnormalities in maintaining equilibrium**.

- For example, stimulation of vestibulocerebellum or vestibular nuclei leads to the **motion sickness**.
- Intractable motion sickness, in fact, is cured by selective removal of flocculonodular lobe.

Diseases affecting main lobe: Features of cerebellar disorder depend on the part of cerebellum affected and whether the **cortex or the deep cerebellar nuclei** are involved in the disease process.

- Effects of lesion of *one side cerebellar hemisphere* ***manifest on the ipsilateral side of the body***.

In general, cerebellar disorders have the **following features**:

1. **No paralysis** (voluntary movements are intact, though defective)
2. Usually, *reflexes are normal*, except that sometimes, **pendular knee jerk** is elicited.
3. No sensory deficit.
4. **Hypotonia** is a usual feature.
5. **Ataxia**: Motor deficit in cerebellar disorder manifests mainly in the form of ataxia, which is defined as a ***defect in coordination*** *due to errors in the rate, range, force, and direction of movement*. If only cerebellar cortex is involved in the disease process, ataxia is temporary. But, if the lesion involves deep cerebellar nuclei, the ataxia almost becomes permanent.

Ataxia manifests in the following forms:

i) **Drunken gait:** Unsteady and wide-base gait.

ii) **Scanning speech:** Ataxia involving muscles of speech manifests in the form of scanning speech. Patient scans the syllables while speaking.

iii) **Dysmetria:** When patient attempts to touch an object, usually the hand overshoots instead of reaching the target. This is called **dysmetria (inability to measure the length or distance)**. This is also called **past pointing.**

iv) **Intention tremor:** Due to dysmetria, the corrective measures are immediately initiated, but this time hand overshoots in the opposite direction. Repeated overshoot and re-correction results in **intention tremor** (hand oscillating back and forth). Tremor is not seen at rest.

v) **Rebound phenomenon:** This results due to **inability to put on brake** (suddenly stop) of the ongoing movement. For example, if the patient is asked to flex his limb against resistance and then asked to stop immediately by withdrawing the resistance, he cannot stop, rather his arm moves with a wide arc. This is called rebound phenomenon.

vi) **Adiadochokinesia:** The ***inability to perform alternate movements rapidly*** is called adiadochokinesia. For example, patient cannot perform supination and pronation rapidly.

vii) **Decomposition of movement:** Inability to perform movement that *involves more than one joint simultaneously*. Therefore, cerebellar patient dissects such complex movement and performs movement at each joint slowly and separately.

6. **Inability to carry out long-term adjustment** in motor response.
7. Defect in vestibulo-occular reflex leads to pathological **nystagmus**.
8. **Charcot's triad:** Presence of ***nystagmus, intention tremor and scanning speech*** (or lalling speech like a baby) together is called Charcot's triad. This is seen in cerebellar disorder and disseminated sclerosis that affects cerebellar functions.
9. **Friedreich's Ataxia:** This is a form of hereditary ataxia in which **spinocerebellar tract degenerates** producing the ataxia as described above.

Cerebellar Function Tests

Many **clinical tests** detect cerebellar functions. These are:

1. **Test for coordination**
   In upper limbs: Finger-nose test, making circle in the air etc.
   In lower limbs: Knee-heel test, walking on a straight line etc.
2. **Tests for postural stability**
   To stand erect with feet closed but eyes open.
3. **Assessment of various aspects of ataxia** by eliciting different movements as described above.
4. **Assessment of gait and speech.**

Exam Questions

1. Describe the connections and functions of cerebellum.
2. Draw a schematic diagram to depict functional divisions and functions of each division of cerebellum. Add a note on Purkinje cells.
3. With the help of a schematic diagram, describe how Purkinje cells in cerebellar cortex control the functions of descending tracts through corresponding deep cerebellar nuclei. Add a note on features of cerebellar dysfunctions.

Multiple Choice Questions

1. Which of the following is NOT a functional division of cerebellum?
A. Vestibulocerebellum
B. Tectocerebellum
C. Spinocerebellum
D. Neocerebellum

2. Flocculonodular lobe has direct connection with:
A. Red nucleus
B. Inferior olivary nucleus
C. Vestibular nucleus
D. Dentate nucleus

3. Vestibulocerebellar tract terminates in which part of cerebellum?
A. Flocculus and nodules
B. Vermis
C. Paravermis
D. Cerebellar cortex

4. Cerebellar connection to the other parts of the brain is projected through which cell?
A. Golgi cells
B. Basket cells
C. Purkinje cells
D. Stellate cells

5. Purkinje cells from the cerebellum end on?
A. Extrapyramidal system
B. Cranial nerve nuclei
C. Deep Cerebellar nuclei
D. Cerebral cortex

6. All are true about cerebellum, EXCEPT:
A. It has 3 cortical layers, 4 deep cerebellar nuclei & 5 cells in cortex
B. Climbing fibers are afferent inputs
C. Mossy fibers inhibit Purkinje cells
D. Climbing fibers excite Purkinje cells

7. Which is a cerebellar nucleus?
A. Caudate nucleus
B. Subthalamic nucleus
C. Red nucleus
D. Dentate nucleus

8. Cells present in cerebellar cortex are all, EXCEPT:
A. Purkinje cell
B. Renshaw cell
C. Granule cell
D. Golgi cell

9. All are true about cerebellum, EXCEPT:
A. Cerebral cortex has mostly inhibitory effects on deep nuclei
B. Smoothening and co-ordination is a major function
C. Decreased muscle tone in cerebellar disorder
D. Inhibitory effect from deep nuclei to descending tracts

10. Which one of the following is the most important role of cerebellum in motor performance?
A. Planning and programming of movement
B. Convert abstract thought into voluntary action
C. Initiation of skilled voluntary action
D. Smoothens and coordinates ongoing movements

11. Lesions of the lateral cerebellum cause all of the following, EXCEPT:
A. Incoordination of movement
B. Dysmetria
C. Resting tremor
D. Ataxia

12. Which of the following does NOT carry proprioceptive impulses?
A. Olivocerebellar tract
B. Tectocerebellar tract
C. Spinocerebellar tract
D. Cuneocerebellar tract

13. Destruction of anterior cerebellum in a decerebrate animal leads to:
A. No effect on rigidity
B. Increased flexor muscle tone
C. Increased rigidity via alpha motor neurons
D. Decreased rigidity

14. Which of the following Is 'True' about functions of spinocerebellar tract?
A. Equilibrium
B. Smoothening and coordination of movement
C. Learning induced by change in vestibulo-ocular reflex
D. Planning and programming

15. Vestibulo ocular reflex is concerned with
A. Spinocerebellum
B. Flocculonodular lobe
C. Neocerebellum
D. Pontocerebellum

16. Setting posture before planned movements is function of:
A. Premotor cortex
B. Motor cortex
C. Cerebellar cortex
D. Supplementary motor cortex

17. Which of the following is NOT a usual feature of cerebellar disorder?
A. Hypotonia
B. Drunken gait
C. Exaggerated DTR
D. Intention tremor

Answers: 1. B 2. C 3. A 4. C 5. C 6. C 7. D 8. B 9. D 10. D
11. C 12. B 13. C 14. B 15. B 16. A 17. C

Chapter 110

PY10.4

Vestibular Apparatus

Learning Objectives

On completion of study of this chapter:

The student will be able to (must know):

1. Name the components of vestibular apparatus and mention function of each component.
2. Understand the mechanism of action potential generation in vestibular hair cells.
3. Outline the mechanism of activation of hair cells due to acceleration or during head rotation.
4. Trace the vestibular pathways.
5. Name vestibular reflexes and describe vestibulo-ocular reflex.
6. Get a concept of vestibular dysfunctions.
7. List the vestibular function tests.

The student may also be able to (desirable to know):

1. Describe the connections and functions of vestibular apparatus
2. Describe the vestibular function tests

FUNCTIONAL ANATOMY

Vestibular apparatus is enclosed in the bony labyrinth of temporal bone. Vestibular apparatus is also known as **membranous labyrinth**. The vestibular apparatus consists of the **otolith organs** and three **semicircular canals** (Fig. 110.1).

1. **Otolith organs** are two sacs like structures called **saccule and utricle**.
   - Saccule and utricle contain calcium carbonate crystals (crystals of the ear or **otoliths**), for which they are called the otolith organs.
   - The saccule communicates with the cochlea via the ductus reuniens.
2. **Three semicircular canals** on each side are arranged in three **mutually perpendicular planes**.
   - Accordingly, they are named as the **horizontal, anterior and posterior canals** respectively. Their arrangement ensures that at least any one of them of either ear can detect change in rotational acceleration in any plane.

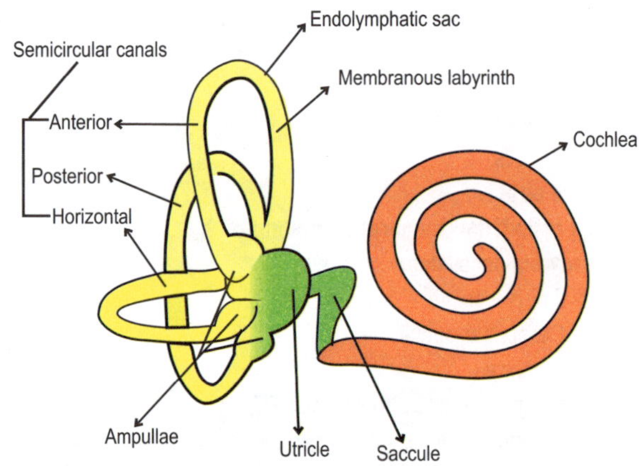

Fig. 110.1: Components of vestibular apparatus.

Hair Cells

The hair cells are **receptors in vestibular apparatus**.

1. Hair cells have a large number of cilia **arranged according to their length** (Fig. 110.2).
   - The longest cilium is the **kinocilium**, which is located to one extreme end.
   - Other cilia are called **stereocilia**, which are arranged in a graded length with longest stereocilium remaining next to kinocilium.
2. Hair cells have **directional sensitivity**.
   - When **cilia bend towards the kinocilium hair cells are depolarized** or stimulated and when cilia **bend away from the kinocilium hair cells are hyperpolarized** or inhibited (Fig. 110.3).
3. Hair cell activity is conveyed to the higher centers through **eighth cranial nerve**.

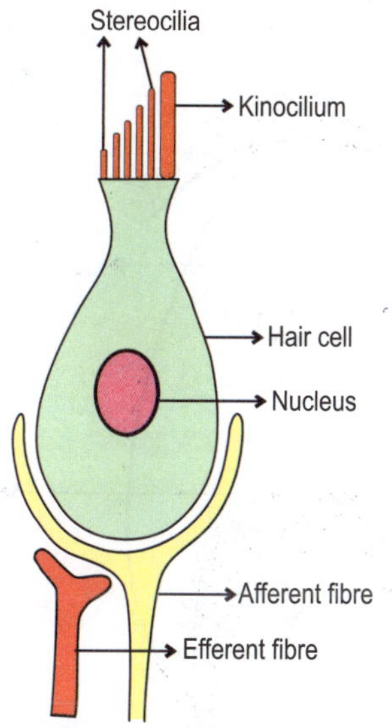

Fig. 110.2: Structure of a hair cell.

4. **Bending of cilia towards kinocilium** opens K^+ channels, through which Ca^{++} enters hair cells and produce **depolarization**.
   - **Bending of cilia away from kinocilium** closes K^+ channels, and prevents entry of Ca^{++} that produce **hyperpolarization.**

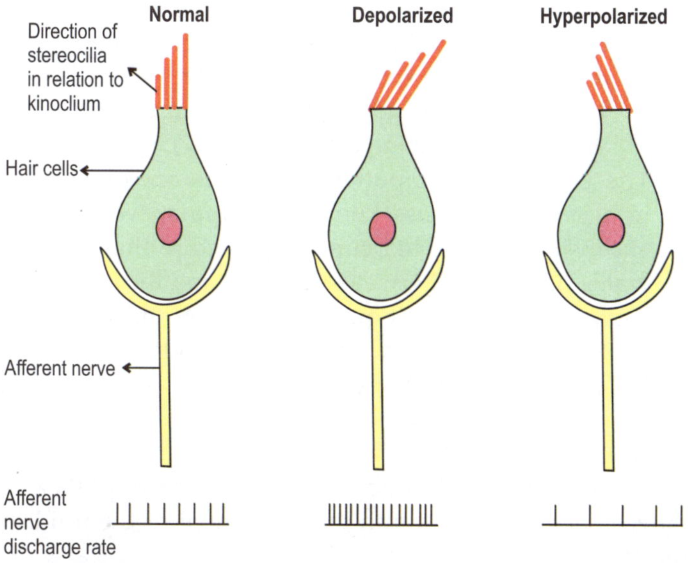

Fig. 110.3: Stimulation and inhibition of hair cell. Note that bending of cilia toward kinocilium produces depolarization and bending of cilia away from kinocilium produces hyperpolarization.

Otolith Organs

The receptors in otolith organs are hair cells. Hair cells in saccule and utricle are located in the **macula**, the sensory epithelium.

1. The **macular hair cells** are covered with an **otolith membrane**, which is a gelatinous mass containing crystals of calcium carbonate, known as **otoliths** or **otoconia** (Fig. 110.4).
   - **The cilia** of the hair cells project into the gelatinous mass and are **embedded in the otolith membrane**.

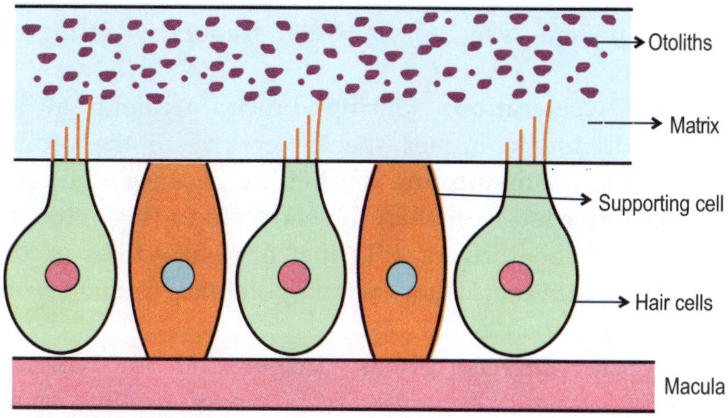

Fig. 110.4: Structure of otolith organs.

2. The **macula** of the saccule is oriented ***vertically*** and macula of the utricle is oriented ***horizontally*** (Fig. 110.5).
3. Hair cells of otolith organs are stimulated by **linear acceleration.**
   - Thus, **saccule detects linear acceleration in vertical direction** and **utricle detects linear acceleration in horizontal direction.**
4. They also detect **change in head position**, like tilting or bending of head.

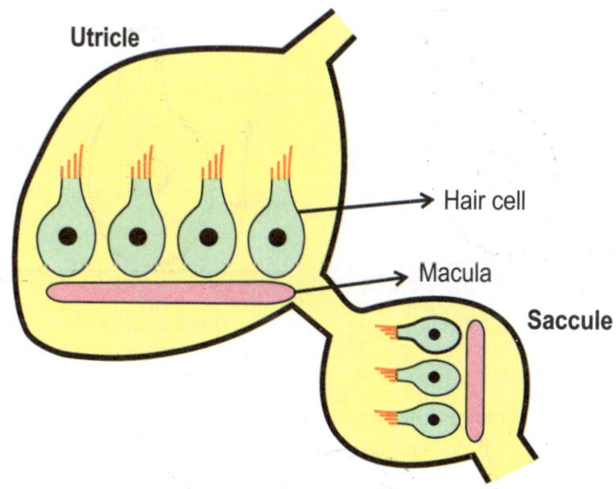

Fig. 110.5: Position of macula and arrangement of hair cells in utricle and saccule.

Mechanism of Action

The cilia of hair cells are embedded in otolith membrane that contains otoliths.

- **Otoliths are heavier than endolymph.**
  - Thus, **specific gravity** of the otolith membrane is more than that of the endolymph.
- Therefore, **a change in the direction of the gravitational pull** exerted on the otolith membrane bends the cilia of hair cells.
- Otolith organs detect change in head position and linear acceleration.

Change in Head Position: With change in head position like tilting of head, **change occurs in the direction of the gravitational pull** exerted on its otolith membrane. This results in **gravitational movement of otolith membrane** (Fig. 110.6A).

- As cilia are entrenched in otolith membrane, head-tilt **bends the cilia of some of hair cells** towards the kinocilium.

- This increases action potential frequency in eighth nerve.

Linear Acceleration: During linear acceleration of the head, due to higher specific gravity of the otolith membrane, the **membrane lags behind because of greater inertia imparted to it** than the endolymph (Fig. 110.6B). This causes bending of cilia that are embedded in the otolith membrane. Thus, action potential frequency in eighth nerve increases.

- **Saccule detects linear acceleration in vertical direction**; e. g. experiencing acceleration while using the lift.
- **Utricle detects linear acceleration in horizontal direction**; e. g., experiencing acceleration in a car when the car starts moving.

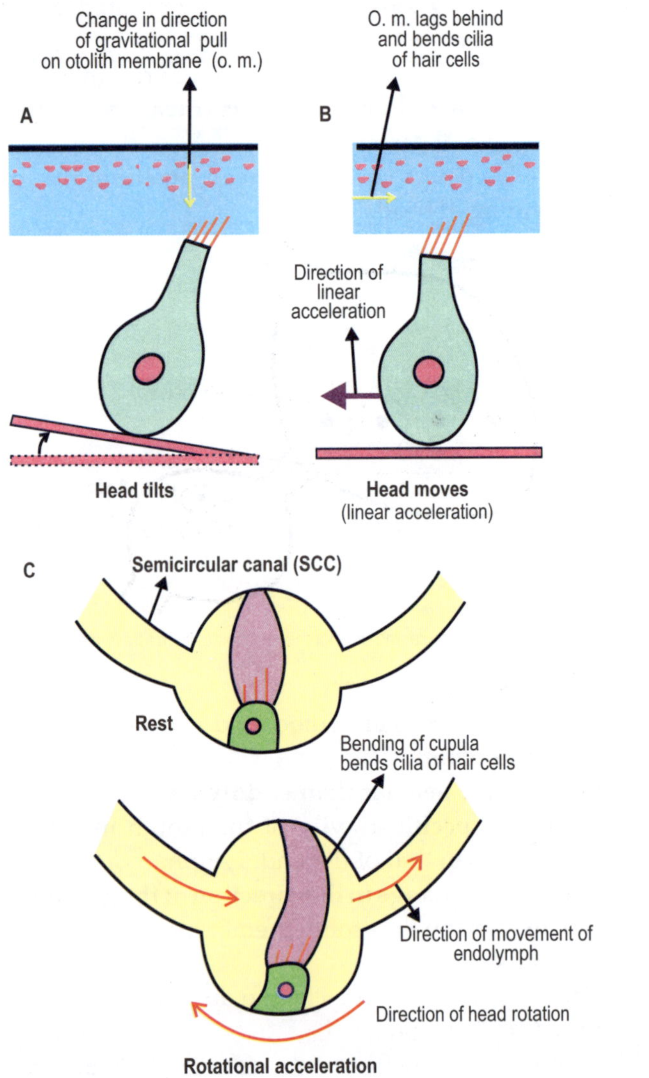

Figs. 110.6: Mechanism of stimulation of hair cells of otolith organs during change in head position (A) and linear acceleration (B); and of hair cell of SCC during head rotation (C).

Semicircular Canals

In semicircular canals, hair cells are located in **ampulla**, the dilated end of each canal.

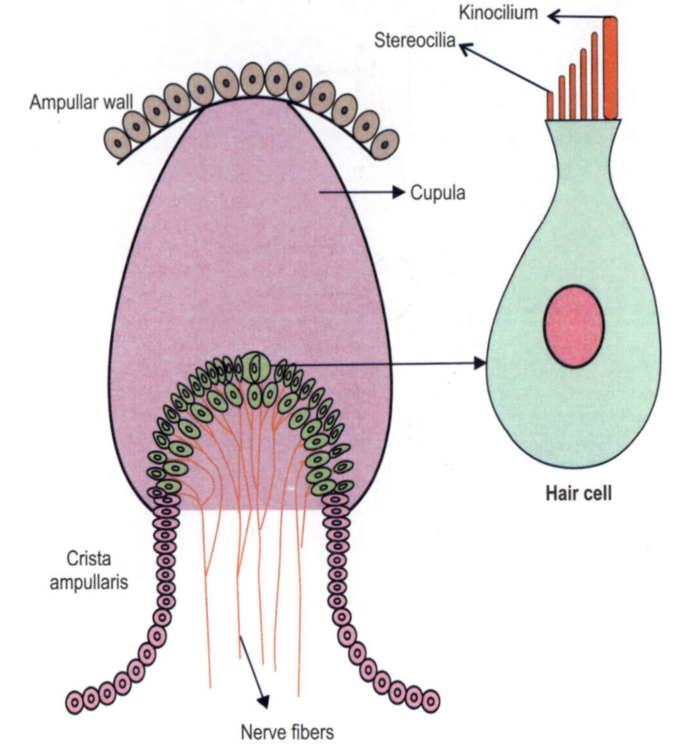

Fig. 110.7: Structure of ampulla of semicircular canal.

- The ampullae open into the utricle. Each ampulla contains **crista terminalis** located on a pendular hillock (as it appears like a small hill).
  - Hair cells are present in the crista ampullaris along with the supporting cells (Fig. 110.7).
- The cilia of the ampullary hair cells are embedded in a gelatinous mass known as **cupula**, which is an encapsulated-inverted cup like structure that forms a water-tight space between the canal and the utricle.
- However, the gelatinous mass of cupula does not contain otoliths. Thus, the **specific gravity of cupular fluid is same as that of endolymph**.

Mechanism of Action

The cupula extends from crista to the top of ampulla and moves back and forth with the movement of the fluid in the canal.

1. **When head rotates to one side**, canals being part of the head automatically rotate to that side.
   - However, the endolymph in the canals due to its **natural inertia of a gelatinous fluid** does not move immediately for about 20 seconds.
   - Therefore, ***initially endolymph lags behind***, as if the endolymph moves in an opposite direction to that of the direction of canal movement (Fig. 110.6C).
2. Thus, if head rotates to the right, for initial 20 seconds endolymph practically rotates to the left.
   - Cupular fluid having the same specific gravity as that of endolymph moves along the direction of endolymph.
   - The cupular deflection bends the cilia of the hair

cells.

3. In the ampulla, the **kinocilia are located towards the utricle**. Therefore, **displacement of cupula towards the utricle** bends cilia towards the kinocilium and stimulates hair cells (Fig. 110.8).
4. Thus, head rotation is **detected in the first 20 seconds**.
   - After the initial lag period, the movement of endolymph equalizes with the movement of the canal.
   - Therefore, rotation is not detected after the initial phase.
5. **When head rotation stops**, endolymph in the canal continues to move in the same direction for about 20 seconds, which causes deflection of cupula away from the utricle and the hair cells are inhibited.
   - However, arrangement of hair cells in the canals of both the ears is such that the **beginning of rotation is detected** by the hair cells in the ear towards which rotation takes place, and **termination of rotation is detected** by the hair cells in the opposite ear.

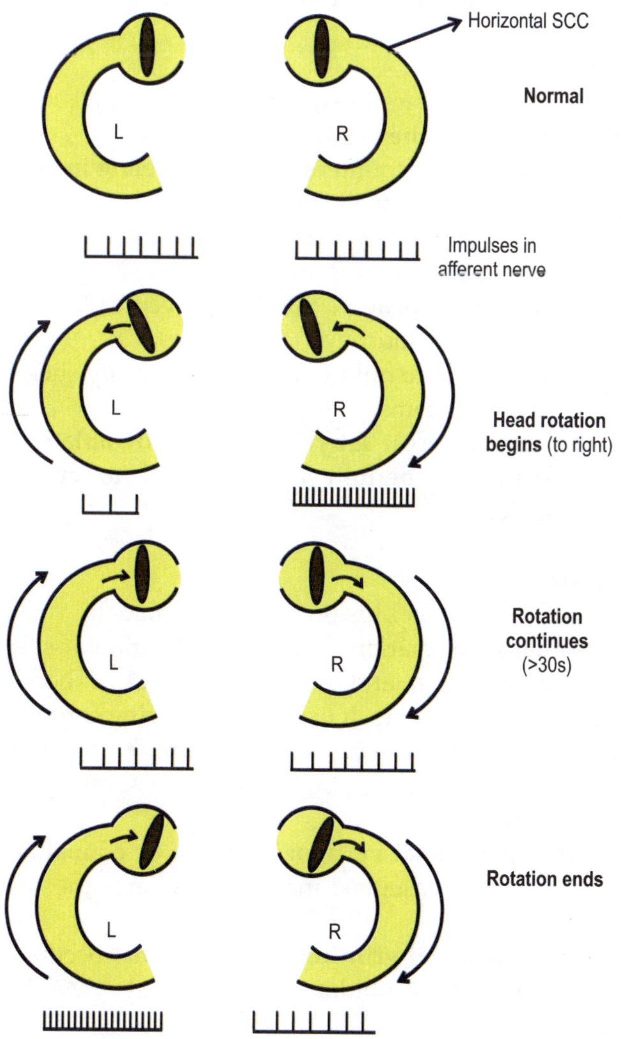

Fig. 110.8: Mechanism of activation of hair cells of semicircular canal during rotation of head. SCC: Semicircular canal.

Vestibular Pathways

Vestibular information is conveyed to CNS via vestibular division of the 8th **cranial nerve**.

- The cell bodies of afferent fibers are located in the **Scarpa's ganglion** (vestibular ganglion).
- These neurons are bipolar neurons. The central axons travel in 8th cranial nerve, which enter the brain at the level of the pons and **terminate in vestibular nuclei** in the brainstem (Fig. 110.9).

There are **four vestibular nuclei**: lateral, medial, superior and inferior.

1. **Lateral vestibular nucleus:** This receives fibers mainly from the utricle, cerebellum and spinal cord. Efferent fibers form the lateral vestibulospinal tract that facilitates the extensor group of motor neurons supplying antigravity muscles.
2. **Medial and superior vestibular nuclei:** These two nuclei receive fibers from the otolith organs, semicircular canals and cerebellum. Efferent fibers from medial nucleus form medial vestibulospinal tract. Fibers from superior nucleus project to the vestibulocerebellum and occulomotor nerve nucleus.
3. **Inferior vestibular nucleus:** It receives fibers from cerebellum and project to cervical spinal cord.

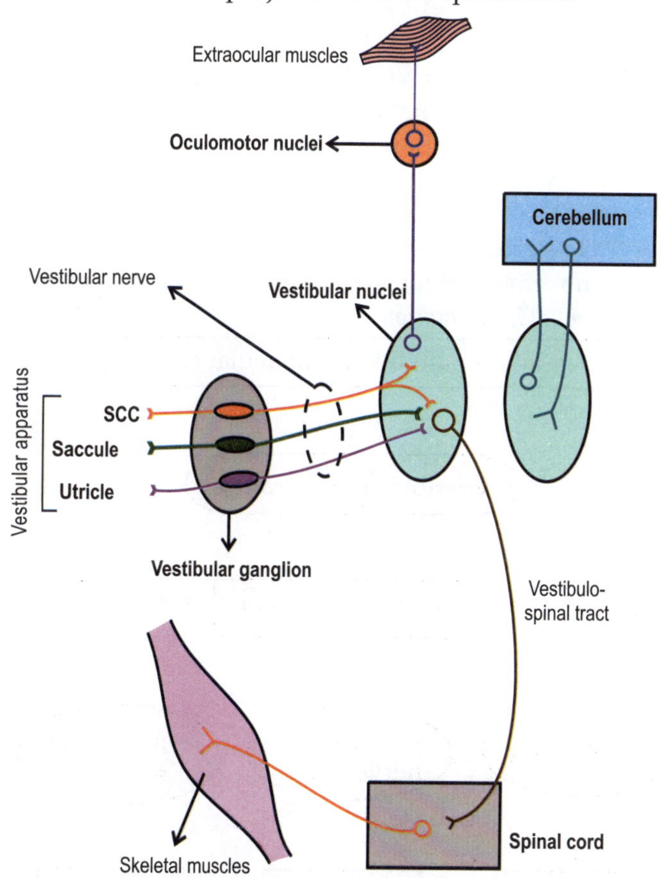

Fig. 110.9: Vestibular pathways. SCC: Semicircular canals.

Thus, vestibular apparatus through vestibular nerve and nuclei conveys information to **three major structures**:

cerebellum, oculomotor nuclei and spinal cord motor neurons.

1. Through **cerebellar connections**, it maintains equilibrium and coordinates postural movements.
2. Through **oculomotor nucleus**, it regulates eye movements coordinated with bodily movements.
3. Through **spinal motor neurons**, it controls postural reflexes. Especially by controlling postural muscles of head and neck, vestibular apparatus maintains postural stability during movement (Fig. 110.10).

VESTIBULAR REFLEXES

Vestibular reflexes are broadly divided into **two categories**: Postural and visual reflexes.

Postural Reflexes

Postural reflexes activated by vestibular apparatus are:

1. **Tonic labyrinthine reflex**
2. **Labyrinthine righting reflex**
3. **Vestbulocollic reflex:** Contraction of head and neck muscle in response to vestibular stimulation provides stability of head position during movement.

Postural reflexes are described in detail in Chapter 107.

Vestibuloocular Reflex

The visual reflex is the **vestibuloocular reflex** (VOR).

- When head rotates, VOR helps to **fix vision on the same object** inspite of rotation of head. The visual fixation is an important component of postural regulation.
- When head rotates, **eyes move in opposite direction** so that the visual image remains constant.
    - However, when rotation ***exceeds 60°***, rapid movement of the eyes *occurs in the same direction of that of head rotation*.

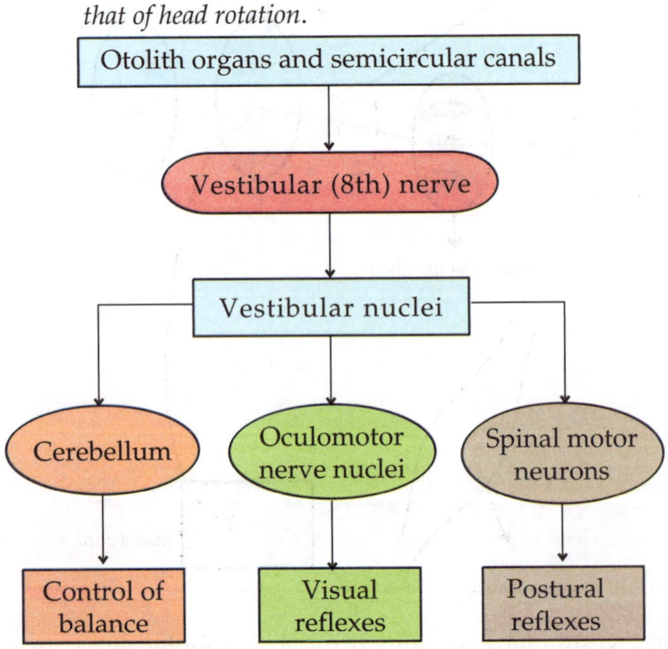

Fig. 110.10: Components of vestibular pathways and their functions.

    - This rapid movement leads to visual fixation on a new object.
- Then, again **eyes move slowly in the opposite direction**. This slow movement of the eyeballs alternating with a rapid movement in the opposite direction gives rise to **nystagmus**.
- The **slow component** *of this reflex is vestibular component*, whereas **rapid component** is integrated in ***superior colliculi*** and ***prepontine reticular formation***.

Pathway for VOR: The **first order** neurons start from vestibular apparatus (afferent in vestibular nerve) and terminate in the vestibular nuclei in brainstem. The **second order** neurons project from vestibular nuclei to oculomotor nerve nucleus. The **third order** neurons originate from oculomotor nucleus to innervate extraocular muscles. The latency of the reflex is about 10 ms.

APPLIED PHYSIOLOGY

Importance of vestibular function is not realized unless there is vestibular dysfunction.

Motion Sickness

Motion sickness occurs in susceptible individuals due to **overstimulation of the vestibular apparatus**.

- Very often it is encountered while traveling in ship or a fast moving vehicle like bus.
- It heralds with nausea and palpitation, and culminates with sweating, dizziness and vomiting.
    - However, repeated vomiting occurs if person continues the journey.

Antiemetics may give mild relief. Closing the eye helps in reducing the symptoms.

- In severe cases, **labyrinthectomy or ablation of vestibulocerebellum** is performed to cure the disease.

Vertigo

Vertigo is defined as illusion of motion, usually rotation when actually no rotation is occurring. Vestibular system that senses position and rotation of head, if becomes abnormal vertigo occurs. It occurs in following conditions:

1. **Physiological vertigo:** Usual example is motion sickness. However, motion sickness in severe form is pathological.
2. **Central positional vertigo:** Lesion of 8th cranial nerve and vertebro-vascular insufficiency are the usual cause.
3. **Peripheral or labyrinthine vertigo:** This occurs due to disease of vestibular apparatus, e.g., **Ménière's disease.**
4. **Benign positional vertigo:** It happens by assuming a particular position of the head. Usually it occurs in elderly.

Vestibular Function Tests

1. **Clinical tests:** Assessment of postural balance tests vestibular functions. For example, ask the subject to walk on a straight line, or stand erect with feet together but **with eyes open**. (with eyes closed, the test is **Romberg sign** that assesses postural imbalance other than cerebellar and vestibular origin).
2. **Rotational stimulation (Postrotatory Nystagmus):** Vestibular stimulation can be produced by rotating the patient in a **Bàrány chair**.
   - The subject seats on the chair with his head bent 30° forward as the horizontal semicircular canals remains horizontal in this position and can be stimulated most effectively by rotation around a vertical axis.
   - Subject's eyes are closed or he uses Frenzel lenses to avoid the effect of optokinetic nystagmus.
   - The chair is revolved at the rate of one revolution per two seconds for 10 revolutions, and then suddenly stopped.
   - If vestibular function is normal, nystagmus will be observed for 20-30s.
3. **Caloric stimulation (Caloric nystagmus):** Vestibular stimulation can be produced by irrigating ear canal alternatively with **warm and cold saline**.
   - The test is based on **Bàrány's theory** that warming the endolymph decreases its specific gravity, which sets up convection currents that produce movement of endolymph as occurs during angular acceleration.
   - Patient is kept in supine position with his head bent forward by 30°. In this position the horizontal SCC remains in vertical position. External auditory canal is syringed gently first with cold (30° C) water for 30 seconds and then with warm water (44° C) with a gap of 5 seconds between them.
   - The procedure leads to nystagmus if semicircular canal function is normal. With warm water, nystagmus occurs to the irrigated side for about 90 seconds.
4. **Electronystagmography:** This provides more accurate assessment of labyrinth functions.

Exam Questions

1. Describe the connections and functions of vestibular apparatus. Add a note on vestibular function tests.
2. Describe the mechanism of action of hair cells. Briefly describe how hair cells respond to change in head position and change in acceleration.
3. With the help of suitable diagram, trace the vestibular pathway. Add a note on vestibuloocular reflex.

Multiple Choice Questions

1. Linear acceleration in horizontal direction is detected by:
A. Utricle B. Saccule
C. Cochlea D. Semicircular canals

2. Linear acceleration in vertical direction is detected by:
A. Utricle B. Saccule
C. Cochlea D. Semicircular canals

3. Angular rotation of head is detected by:
A. Utricle B. Saccule
C. Cochlea D. Semicircular canals

4. Which of the following is not a component of vestibular apparatus?
A. Utricle B. Saccule
C. Cochlea D. Semicircular canals

5. Which of the following is not correct about vestibular hair cells?
A. They are the receptors that initiate the action potential in 8th nerve
B. Bending of cilia towards kinocilium causes depolarization
C. Bending of cilia away from kinocilium causes hyperpolarization
D. Sodium influx into the cell causes depolarization

6. All of the following are target nuclei of afferents from vestibular organs EXCEPT:
A. Oculomotor nerve nuclei B. Midbrain motor nuclei
C. Spinal motor nuclei D. Flocculonodular lobe

7. Which of the following is not a vestibular reflex?
A. Tonic labyrinthine reflex
B. Labyrinthine righting reflex
C. Optical righting reflex
D. Vestibulocollic reflex

8. Which of the following is not a vestibular function test?
A. Romberg sign
B. Rotational stimulation by Barany's chair
C. Caloric stimulation by irrigating ear canal with cold and warm solutions
D. Asking the subject to walk on a straight line or stand erect with eyes open

9. All of the following are true about vestibuloocular reflex (VOR), EXCEPT:
A. When rotation of head exceeds 60-degree, rapid movement of the eye occurs in same direction and then again move slowly in opposite direction.
B. Slow component is the vestibular component and part of VOR
C. Fast component is integrated in superior colliculi
D. The second order neuron in VOR projects from vestibular nuclei to optic nerve nuclei

Answers

1. A 2. B 3. D 4. C 5. D 6. B 7. C 8. A 9. D

Chapter 111

Functions of Hypothalamus

Learning Objectives

On completion of study of this chapter:

The student will be able to (must know):

1. Name the major nuclear groups of hypothalamus and give their functions.
2. Briefly describe hypothalamic regulation of temperature, circadian rhythm and sleep.
3. Describe the regulation of food intake and water intake.
4. Outline the physiological basis of hypothalamic dysfunctions.

The student may also be able to (desirable to know):

1. Describe the connections and functions of hypothalamus.
2. Explain the physiological basis of hypothalamic disorders.

FUNCTIONAL ANATOMY

Hypothalamus is a small structure in the brain lies on each side of the third ventricle. It weighs about 10 g.

1. It is located below the thalamus, hence called hypothalamus.
2. Along with thalamus and subthalamus it forms the **diencephalon**. The hypothalamus consists of a **large number of nuclei and nuclear groups** (Fig. 111.1).

Hypothalamic nuclei are divided into **four main groups**:

Anterior group : Includes the preoptic, supraoptic and paraventricular nuclei.

Middle group : Consists of the tuberal, arcuate, ventromedial and dorsomedial nuclei.

Posterior group: Contains supramamillary, mammillary and posterior hypothalamic nuclei.

Lateral group : Comprises of lateral preoptic area and lateral hypothalamic nuclei.

Connections of Hypothalamus

Hypothalamus through its afferents and efferents is connected with almost all parts of the brain (Fig. 111.2). Following are the major connections of hypothalamus:

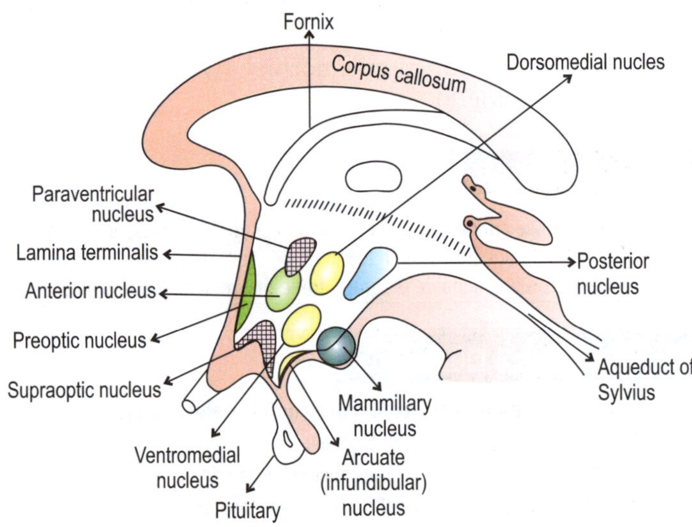

Fig. 111.1: Hypothalamic nuclei in sagital section.

1. **Fornix:** Through fornix hypothalamus is reciprocally connected with limbic system.
2. **Medial forebrain bundle:** Hypothalamus is extensively and reciprocally connected with brainstem including reticular formation and limbic system especially the septum via median forebrain bundle. Median forebrain bundle also connects brainstem with the cerebral cortex.
3. **Periventricular system:** Reciprocally connects midbrain and sensory pathways to hypothalamus.
4. **Mammillothalamic tract:** This tract conveys information from mammillary body of hypothalamus to the anterior nucleus of thalamus.
5. **Retinohypothalamic fibers** (Optic nerve): It carries visual information from retina to suprachiasmatic nucleus of hypothalamus.
6. **Mamillotegmental tract:** Connects mammillary body to tegmental reticular nuclei of midbrain.

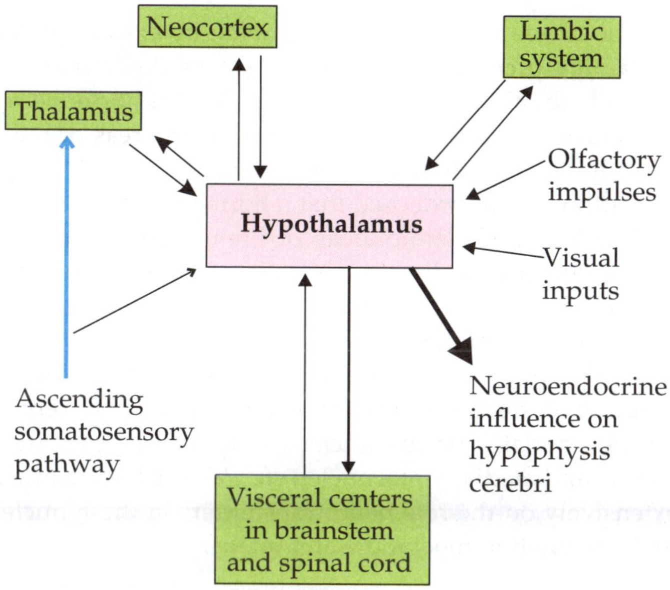

Fig. 111.2: Major connections of hypothalamus.

7. **Hypothalamohypophyseal tract:** Connect supraoptic and paraventricular nuclei of hypothalamus to posterior pituitary.
8. **Tuberoinfundibular tract:** Connects accurate and ventromedial nuclei of hypothalamus to infundibulum.
9. **Dorsal noradrenergic bundle:** Connects locus ceruleus to dorsal hypothalamus
10. **Serotonergic neurons:** Connect raphe nuclei to hypothalamus
11. **Mesolimbic dopaminergic system:** Connects third ventricle to medial hypothalamic nuclei and within hypothalamic nuclei
12. **Corticohypothalamic fibers:** Connect cerebral cortex to hypothalamus directly.

Hypothalamic Areas outside Blood-Brain Barrier

The hypothalamic areas present outside the blood-brain barrier (BBB) are:

1. Organum vasculosum of lamina terminalis (OVLT)
2. Sub-fornical organ (SFO)
3. Area postrema

These hypothalamic areas are present in the **ventral part of median eminence.** Since portal vessels arise in the median eminence, the regions in median eminence of the hypothalamus are present outside the blood-brain barrier.

IMPORTANT NOTE

Hypothalamic areas outside BBB control water intake: These regions of the hypothalamus (OVLT, SFO, are postrema) as they are present outside BBB easily **detect change in osmolality of blood** and are involved in **regulation of blood volume and water intake.**

PY10.7

FUNCTIONS OF HYPOTHALAMUS

The hypothalamus controls many homeostatic and visceral functions as listed below.

1. Endocrine functions
2. Autonomic functions
3. Circadian rhythm
4. Temperature regulation
5. Regulation of food intake
6. Regulation of water intake
7. Reproductive functions
8. Influence on emotion and other limbic functions
9. Role in sleep
10. Immunological functions

Endocrine Functions

Hypothalamus controls endocrine functions via its connections with pituitary gland. It controls both anterior and posterior pituitary functions (Application Box 111.1).. Details of endocrine functions of hypothalamus have been described in Chapter 70.

Autonomic Functions

Sympathetic Control

Stimulation of lateral and posterior hypothalamic areas results in sympathetic responses.

1. **Stimulation of lateral area** results in general sympathetic activation in the form of piloerection, rise in BP, increase in heart rate, sweating, papillary dilation, and increase in secretion of catecholamines.
2. **Stimulation of posterior hypothalamus** results in activation of emotional behavior pattern such as aggression, fear or rage, which may be due to its connection through limbic system.

Parasympathetic Control

Stimulation of **anterior hypothalamus** results in parasympathetic activation and vagal responses.

Application Box 111.1

Head ganglion of ANS: Hypothalamus has strong influence on ANS. For its close link with autonomic functions, Sherrington had described hypothalamus as the "head ganglion of ANS".

Circadian Rhythms

Circadian rhythm means 24 hours fluctuation in body functions, i.e., **day-night variation** or variation during light-dark cycle. Many body functions such as sleep habit, corticosteroid secretion, variation in body temperature, melatonin secretion, show a circadian pattern. Some of these important functions include. Hypothalamic nucleus regulating and maintaining the circadian rhythmicity is the **suprachiasmatic nucleus**, which is known as **biological clock.** Details of circadian rhythm is describe in Chapter 112, in 'Theories of Sleep'.

Temperature Regulation

Hypothalamus plays the key role in temperature regulation.

- Anterior hypothalamus **activates mechanisms that promote heat loss**, especially by causing cutaneous vasodilation and sweating.
- The posterior hypothalamus **activates mechanisms that increase heat production and promote heat gain.**

Details of temperature regulation by hypothalamus have been described in Chapter 132.

IMPORTANT NOTE

Hypothalamus acts as Thermostat: Thermosensor cells in hypothalamus detect changes in temperature of blood and receive inputs from thermosensitive receptors in the skin. The information received is matched with the set point for body temperature and accordingly hypothalamus initiates appropriate temperature regulating mechanisms.

Regulation of Food Intake

Factors regulating food intake are of **three major categories**: neural factors, hormonal factors and metabolic factors. Hypothalamus plays the key role in integrating all these factors.

Neural Factors

Role of Hypothalamus

Two areas in hypothalamus control food intake: the **feeding center and the satiety center.**

Feeding Center: Feeding center is the **lateral hypothalamus** (LH).

- LH is called feeding center as its **stimulation greatly increases food intake**.
- On the contrary, experimental lesion of LH results in fatal anorexia in otherwise healthy animals.

Satiety Center: The **ventromedial hypothalamus** (VMH) is called satiety center, because stimulation of it causes cessation of eating.

- **Lesion of VMH** causes severe hyperphagia that results in ***morbid obesity***, which is called **hypothalamic obesity**.

Interaction between Feeding & Satiety Center: Normally, **satiety center decreases food intake by inhibiting feeding center**. Feeding center is chronically active. Following feeding, activity of satiety center increases that in turn inhibits feeding center and finally stops eating.

Extrahypothalamic Factors

In human beings, the appetite for food is greatly controlled by **the preference and the desire for food. Uncontrolled desire for eating** results in excess calorie intake that leads to obesity.

1. The desire to eat food is controlled by **extrahypothalamic structures** such as limbic system. Preliminary reports (by Dr. G. K. Pal et al) suggest that hormones or neurotransmitters secreted from limbic areas of brain influence hypothalamic feeding areas.
2. Authors have proposed that a hormone secreted from limbic-hypothalamic areas of brain **influences body weight gain** by directly controlling deposition of fat in the fat cells (adiposity) and they have designated it as "**Greed Hormone**".

Role of other Centers: Extrahypothalamic areas in the brain suggested are amygdala (basolateral and central nuclei), caudate nucleus, nucleus accumbens, septal areas (lateral and medial septal nuclei) etc. Pal et al have worked extensively on the role neurotransmitters in these nuclei, in the regulation food and water intake.

Role of Vagus Nerve

Vagus nerve provides **sensory signals** regarding the filling of the stomach to the hypothalamic regulatory centers.

- Therefore, **stretching of stomach wall** by accumulation of food is the immediate factor to **inhibit feeding**.

Hormonal Factors PY8.5

Many hormones are either secreted from hypothalamus or act on hypothalamus to influence food intake. **In obesity, many of these hormones are altered** in the body and contribute to obesity dysfunctions.

A. **Hormones that increase food intake:** Neuropeptide Y, orexins, grehlin, MCH (melanin concentrating hormone), AGRP (Agouti related peptide), galanin and GHRH.

B. **Hormones that decrease food intake:** Estrogen, dopamine, α – MSH, CART (cocaine and amphetamine regulated transcript), CRH, gut hormones, oxytocin, CCK, peptide YY, and leptin.

Leptin

Leptin is the key hormone for regulation of food intake and body weight.

- Leptin is secreted from white fat cells (adipocytes).
- The receptors for leptin are located in hypothalamus.
- Leptin, by acting oh hypothalamus **decreases food intake** and increases energy consumption.
- The **arcuate nucleus of hypothalamus** is the sensor to detect plasma leptin concentration.

Physiological Responses to High Leptin Level: High leptin level as occurs in obesity decreases food intake, increases energy expenditure and increases sympathetic activity.

Physiological Responses to Low Leptin Level: Low leptin level as occurs in starvation increases food intake, decreases energy expenditure and increases parasympathetic activity.

Lipostatic Hypothesis

Hypothalamus controls food intake according to the **adipose tissue mass** (degree of obesity) in the body. Hypothalamus **senses adiposity via leptin** and accordingly controls food intake and energy expenditure of the body. This is called **lipostatic hypothesis** of food intake.

IMPORTANT NOTE

Other actions of leptin: In addition to inhibition of food intake, leptin has following functions.
1. Regulates the onset of puberty.
2. Stimulates thyroid function.
3. Controls glucocorticoids secretion.
4. Increases sympathetic activity.
5. Increases the activity of uncoupling of protein in the brown adipose tissue cells.

The last four actions increase peripheral energy expenditure.

Other hypothalamic hormones controlling food intake (NPY, orexin, MCH and CART) have been described in Chapter 70.

Metabolic Factors

Plasma Glucose

Plasma glucose concentration is the important metabolic factor for regulation of feeding. Discharge of ventromedian hypothalamus (**satiety center**) partly **depends on its glucose utilization**.

- Following feeding, plasma **glucose concentration** rises that in turn increases the **activity of neurons of satiety center**. Increased discharge of satiety center **inhibits the feeding center** that finally inhibits food intake. Thus, the person feels sated.

Glucostatic Hypothesis: Food intake **remains inhibited** till the blood glucose concentration remains high. This is called **glucostatic hypothesis** of regulation of food intake.

- Hypothalamus by sensing plasma glucose concentration not only **regulates food intake**, but also indirectly **regulates plasma glucose concentration**.
  - Therefore, hypothalamus is called "**Glucostat**".
- Hypoglycemia is a potent stimulus for food intake.

Body Temperature

Decrease in body temperature increases food intake and increase in body temperature inhibits food intake.

- This is called "**Thermostatic Hypothesis**" of food intake.

Therefore, ***anorexia is a common feature*** of fever due to any cause.

In fact, change in food intake changes body temperature (by changing body metabolism) and vice versa.

Regulation of Water Intake

Hypothalamus plays an important role in water intake. Two major factors that affect water intake are **plasma osmolality and extracellular fluid volume** (mainly blood volume).

Change in Osmolality: Osmoreceptors are located in the anterior hypothalamus. Osmoreceptors detect the change in the osmolality of plasma.

- Hyperosmolality of plasma **stimulates hypothalamic thirst center** that increases water intake.
- Hyperosmolality also **increases ADH secretion** that decreases loss of water in urine by increasing water reabsorption from kidney tubule.

Change in Fluid Volume: Volume change is detected by volume receptors in the right and left atria and pulmonary vessels.

- **Hypovolemia** (decrease in blood volume) increases **secretion of rennin** from JG cells of kidney that in turn forms angiotensin II (A II).
- A II is a strong **dipsogen** (dipsogen is a substance that stimulates thirst).
- A II ***stimulates OVLT and SFO*** to increase water intake.

Control of Reproductive Functions

Hypothalamus **secretes gonadotropin-releasing hormone** (GnRH).

1. GnRH secreting neurons are located in **preoptic area** and these neurons contain receptors for gonadal hormones that **regulate GnRH secretion**.
   - GnRH is essential for attainment of reproductive functions **in both males and females**.
2. Hypothalamus also **controls sexual behavior**. Stimulation of medial forebrain bundle in experimental animals induces penile erection and sexual drive, whereas **lesion of anterior hypothalamus abolishes this sexual behavior**.

Other Functions

Influence on Emotion

Limbic system is the principal seat of emotion. Hypothalamus forms one of the output pathways of limbic system for emotional responses.

- Suitable stimulation of **lateral hypothalamus activates rage reactions** in animals.
- Self-stimulation experiments have established that the **reward system** in hypothalamus is **located in lateral preoptic area.**

Role in Sleep

There are three subcortical regions that on appropriate stimulation induce **slow wave sleep**.

- **Diencephalic sleep zone** is mainly the **posterior hypothalamus**.
- Stimulation of **pre-optic area** of the hypothalamus also induces sleep.

Role of Hypothalamus in Immunity

Hypothalamus influences immunity by controlling the secretion of **ACTH and cortisol** vis hypothalamo-pituitary-adrenal (cortex) axis.

Table 111.1 | **Major hypothalamic nuclei and their functions.**

Nucleus/nuclei	Functions
Preoptic nucleus	Regulates release of gonadotrophic hormones
Supraoptic and paraventricular nuclei	Produce antidiuretic hormone (ADH) and oxytocin. Regulate water balance
Anterior nucleus	Regulates body temperature by dissipation of heat. Stimulates parasympathetic nervous system
Arcuate (infundibular nucleus)	Produces hypothalamic releasing factors
Venteromedial nucleus	Its stimulation inhibits the urge to eat (Satiety center)
Dorsomedial nucleus	Its stimulation causes obesity and results in savage behavior
Posterior nuclei	Regulates body temperature by conservation of heat. Stimulates sympathetic nervous system
Mammillary nuclei	Receives input from hippocampal formation through fornix
Lateral nucleus	Its stimulation induces eating (Feeding Center)

APPLIED PHYSIOLOGY

Hypothalamic dysfunctions are usually known as **hypothalamic syndromes**. Hypothalamic syndromes are of two types: Global hypothalamic syndrome and partial hypothalamic syndromes.

Global Hypothalamic Syndrome

In global hypothalamic syndromes, the disease process **involves either all parts or a large part** of hypothalamus.

- Primary tumors or metastatic carcinoma, lymphoma, or granulomatous diseases like sarcoidosis affecting hypothalamus result in such syndromes.
- Usually, patient **dies due to failure of visceral homeostatic mechanisms** and failure to regulate **body temperature**.

Partial Hypothalamic Syndromes

Partial hypothalamic syndromes occur due to **selective lesion** of a specific part of hypothalamus, resulting in deficiency or overproduction of a single hormone.

Examples of few such syndromes are given below.

Neurogenic Diabetes Insipidus (DI): Neurogenic DI occurs in hypothalamic or pituitary tumors affecting secretion of ADH.

Neurogenic Salt Wasting: It occurs as part of **SIADH** (syndrome of inappropriate ADH secretion).

Precocious Puberty: Hypothalamic tumor resulting in premature and **excess secretion of GnRH** is one of the causes of precocious puberty.

Neurogenic Pulmonary Edema: The **lesion of caudal hypothalamus** causes pulmonary edema. There is ***rapid rise in pulmonary vascular resistance***, which may be fatal unless treated immediately.

Exam Questions

1. Describe the nuclear groups, connections and functions of hypothalamus.
2. Describe role of hypothalamus on food intake and water intake.

Multiple Choice Questions

1. Which of the following is not a function of hypothalamus?
A. Regulation of water intake
B. Control of sleep
C. Sexual behaviour
D. Motor activity

2. The principal polypeptide that increase food intake are all, EXCEPT:
A. Neuropeptide Y
B. Leptin
C. Orexin A
D. Ghrelin

3. Location of osmoreceptors in hypothalamus is:
A. Posterior region
B. Paraventricular
C. Preoptic nucleus of anterior hypothalamus
D. Supraoptic

4. Vasopressin induces thirst by acting through:
A. Subfornical organ
B. Posterior hypothalamic osmoreceptors
C. Pretectal nucleus
D. Lamina vasculosum

5. Function of preoptic nucleus of hypothalamus
A. Temperature regulation
B. Thirst
C. GI stimulation
D. Satiety centre

Answers

1. D 2. B 3. C 4. A 5. A

Chapter 112

Reticular Activating System, EEG, Physiology of Sleep and Brain Death

Learning Objectives

On completion of study of this chapter:

The student will be able to (must know):

1. Outline the connections and functions of reticular formation and reticular activating system.
2. Name the EEG waves and their mechanism of genesis.
3. Name the stages of sleep and draw the EEG waves in different stages.
4. Understand the mechanisms of NREM & REM sleep.
5. List the differences between NREM and REM sleep.
6. Outline the theories of sleep.
7. Define common sleep disorders.

The student may also be able to (desirable to know):

1. Explain the electrophysiological basis of EEG
2. Describe the theories of sleep.

PY10.5

RETICULAR ACTIVATING SYSTEM

Organization of Reticular Formation

There are groups of cells in the core of the brainstem that constitute **brainstem reticular formation**.

- This is formed by a **diffuse system of neurons** having widely branching axons.
- According to their location, they are named as **midbrain, pontine and medullary reticular formation** (Fig. 112.1).
    - Characteristically, these neurons have **very long dendrites and axons**.
- They have **long ascending branches** projecting to the thalamus, hypothalamus and cortex and **long descending branches** projecting to the spinal cord.

The neurons are organized into **two columns**: medial and lateral columns.

Medial Column: Medial group of cells constitute gigantocellular part (large cell group) that contains the raphe nuclei and central group of nuclei.

1. They **receive afferents** from all sensory pathways, especially from **spinoreticular tracts**.

- Fibers from this part ***project upwards*** as the **reticular activating system** (RAS).
- The fibers ***project downward*** as the medial and lateral **reticulospinal tracts**.

Lateral Column: Laterally placed is the **parvocellular part** containing small-celled nuclei.

- This part contributes to seep-wakefulness.

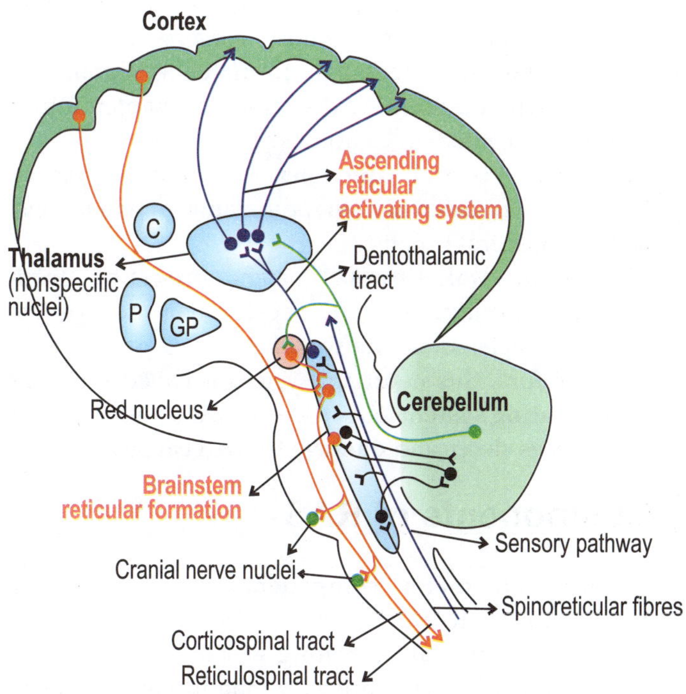

Fig. 112.1: Afferent and efferent connections of reticular formation. Ascending reticular activating system is also shown in the picture. C: Caudate nucleus; P: Putamen; GP: Globus pallidus.

ok

Connections of Reticular Formation

Afferents: Reticular formation receives input from all sensory pathways, cerebellum (mainly from fastigial nucleus), basal ganglia (mainly from striatum), thalamus, hypothalamus, limbic system, cortex (motor and sensory areas), red nucleus and substantia nigra.

Efferents: Reticular formation projects to motor and autonomic centers in brainstem and spinal cord, cranial nerve nuclei (e.g., dorsal nucleus of vagus), thalamus, cortex (mainly via nonspecific nuclei of thalamus), red nucleus, tectum, hypothalamus and limbic system.

Functions of Reticular Formation

1. **Control of motor activities:** Reticular formation gives rise to **reticulospinal tracts (RST).**
   - RST are important components of medial system pathways that are involved in **regulation of posture** (discussed in detail in Chapter 106).
2. **Control of sensory activities:** Many of the **ascending sensory pathways** provide their collaterals to reticular formation.
   - Especially for **pain sensation**, along with alertness for the sensation, there is simultaneous activation of **endogenous analgesia system**.
     - The neurons of raphe nucleus in reticular formation are activated by paleospinothalamic and spinoreticulothalamic fibers.
     - Consequently, **activation of raphespinal pathway** inhibits transmission of pain in the dorsal horn of spinal cord.
3. **Control of cardiovascular and respiratory functions:** Cardiovascular and respiratory centers are located in the brainstem reticular formations. Details of cardiovascular centers are discussed in Chapter 37 and respiratory centers in Chapter 49.
4. **Control of visceral functions:** Reticular formation, through its extensive hypothalamic connections, controls visceral functions.
5. **Sleep and wakefulness:** Fibers projecting from reticular formation to the cortex via nonspecific thalamic nuclei, maintain wakefulness.
   - Therefore, this neuronal system is called **reticular activating system** (RAS). Decreased activity of RAS induces sleep, and **damage to RAS causes coma**.

Components of RAS

There are **four major components** of the reticular activating system (RAS):

1. **Ascending reticular activating system:** From central group of reticular nuclei (magnocellular part), ascending neurons **project to the intra-laminar and midline nuclei of the thalamus (nonspecific nuclei)**.
   - From these nonspecific thalamic nuclei, fibers project to all parts of the cerebral cortex and limbic system.
     - Few fibers from reticular formation bypass thalamus and project directly to the cortex.
   - These neuronal projections form a major part of brainstem **ascending reticular activating system**, which maintains arousal of the being.
   - Increased activity in these projecting neurons causes excitation of cortical neurons and **creates alertness and wakeful state.**
   - Diminished activity in these systems induces sleep.
2. **Monoaminergic and cholinergic fibers:** **Locus ceruleus** is located in the reticular formation at the junction between pons and medulla.
   - The **noradrenaline-secreting neurons** originate from locus ceruleus.
   - Major monoaminergic and cholinergic systems of the brain are located in the reticular activating system.
   - These fibers are involved in integration of various sensory and behavioral activities.
3. **Fibers from parvocellular part:** Fibers originating from small-celled neurons located in lateral part of the brainstem reticular formation (**parvocellular part**) are **active only during the awaken state** and silent during sleep.
   - This indicates that they control **sleep-wakefulness.**
4. **Serotonergic neurons:** The serotonergic neurons **originating from raphe nuclei** project to all part of CNS.
   - These neurons are **active during deep sleep**.
     - This indicates that these neurons are involved in genesis of sleep.
   - **Histaminergic neurons** projecting from hypothalamus to all parts of CNS play a major role in arousal.

ELECTROENCEPHALOGRAM

Electroencephalogram (EEG) is the *record of spontaneous electrical activities generated in the cerebral cortex* that are picked up from brain's surface through electrodes placed on designated site in the scalp.

- These electrical currents reflect the **summated effects of innumerable excitatory and inhibitory synaptic potentials** upon the cortical neurons.

Procedure of Recording

Hans Berger, a German psychiatrist in 1929 for the first time demonstrated that electrical activities of the human brain could be recorded using external electrodes on the scalp, which he termed as electroencephalogram (EEG). As the EEG waves are of very low voltage, they require more amplification before recording.

1. **EEG leads** may be bipolar (comparing the potentials between two active leads) or unipolar (measuring the potential changes at a single lead against a reference lead placed on the ear or nose or chin).
2. EEG electrodes are solder or **silver-silver chloride disc** of 0.5 cm diameter.
3. Recording is done with subject preferably in recumbent position with his head and neck supported to ensure that the posterior electrodes are secure.
4. Usually, four leads are attached to the scalp by means of adhesive material on standard skull locations on each side.
5. A **multi-channel pen recorder** is used to record the activities from the **eight leads simultaneously**.

The EEG waves are analyzed manually or by using a computer.

EEG Waves PY10.12

EEG waves are described in terms of their frequency, which usually ranges from **1 to 30 Hz**, and amplitude, which ranges from **20 to 100 μV**. Characteristics of EEG wave vary according the state of consciousness.

- When the **individual is fully alert** (sensory inputs are maximum), the waves are mostly of ***high frequency and low amplitude*** with as many units ***asynchronized***.
- When the person is **minimally alert** as in deep sleep (least sensory input), the waves are of ***low frequency and high amplitude, and synchronized***.
- Absence of EEG waves indicates brain death.

Wave Patterns and Rhythms

EEG wave patterns are classified into **four types**: α, β, θ and δ according to their frequency. The characteristic features of the various EEG rhythms are as follows:

Alpha Rhythm

Frequency ranges from **8 to 13 Hz** and amplitude from **50 to 100 μV** (Fig. 112.2).

- This is the most prominent EEG rhythm seen in a **normal adult at rest** (awake but relaxed) with eyes closed.
- It is found in the posterior half of the brain, especially **in the parieto-occipital regions**.

Alpha Block

The alpha rhythm **disappears upon opening of the eyes** or the subject engaging in mental effort such as mental arithmetic. The regular alpha rhythm is replaced by irregular low voltage activity. This phenomenon is known as alpha block or **desynchronization**. This is also called **arousal or alerting response**.

Factors affecting α Wave Frequency:

1. Frequency of alpha rhythm **is decreased by** hypoglycemia, hypothermia, high arterial pressure and low levels of glucocorticoids.
2. High blood glucose, increased body temperature, low arterial pressure and high levels of glucocorticoids **increase frequency of alpha rhythm**.

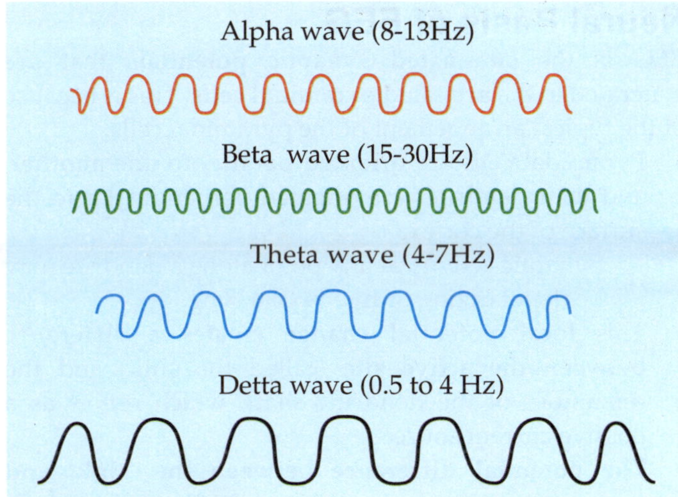

Fig. 112.2: Various EEG waves.

Beta Rhythm

Frequency of beta waves ranges from **13 to 30 Hz** with low amplitude ranging from **5-10 μV**.

- This is seen in adults, when the **eyes are open**.
- These waves appear **in posterior regions**. Beta rhythms are sometimes seen in the frontal regions regardless of whether the eyes are closed or open.

Theta Rhythm

Frequency of theta waves ranges from **4 to 8 Hz** with large amplitude.

- Usually, theta rhythm is **seen in normal children**.
- It also occurs **during moderate sleep**.
- It may sometimes appear in adults when they are severely disappointed or depressed.

Delta Rhythm

Frequency of delta waves ranges from **0.5 to 4 Hz** and amplitude from **20 to 200 μV**.

- Delta rhythm occurs normally **during deep sleep**.
- Its appearance in an alert state in adult, suggests a serious organic brain damage.

EEG Rhythms in Infants and Children

The EEG recordings in children show wide range of patterns.

- Usually, **in awakened infants**, there is **fast beta rhythm**.
- The rhythm speeds up **during childhood** and **theta rhythm appears**.

- As the child matures, the theta rhythm is replaced by **faster alpha rhythms**.
- The **alpha rhythm of adults** gradually appears **during adolescence**.
- The theta rhythm is prominent in the temporal or parietal region, while alpha rhythms are in the occipital region.

Neural Basis of EEG

EEG is the **summated synaptic potentials** that are generated in the activated **pyramidal cells**. This is because of the typical arrangement of the pyramidal cells.

- Pyramidal cells are **oriented parallel to one another**, and their dendrites are oriented perpendicular to the surface of the cortex.
    - Synaptic activity at any point along a dendrite may be depolarizing or hyperpolarizing.
- This **local potential change creates a difference between the active site** (called the **sink**) and the remainder of the dendritic shaft, which serves as a passive current source.
- The **potential difference between the 'sink' and 'source'** is similar to an electrical dipole, and the **flow of current between them** is responsible for the EEG wave.

PY10.8

PHYSIOLOGY OF SLEEP

Sleep is defined as temporary state of unconsciousness (more accurately, withdrawal of conscious from the physical world) from which the subject can be aroused with appropriate sensory stimuli. Though, about **one-third of our life is spent in sleep**, the time spent in sleep is not wasted as ***sleep is essential for normal growth and development*** of mind and body (Application Box 112.1).

- An individual is kept awake by activation of RAS.
    - Sleep occurs due to **periodic shutdown of RAS** by influences from brainstem and other regions of brain.
- **Aserinsky, Dement and Kleitman in 1953** through EEG and polygraphic analysis, described that normal sleep consists of **recurring cycles of different stages**, each of which is characterized by specific EEG changes associated with autonomic and endocrine changes.

Application Box 112.1

Sleep potentiates growth: Growth hormone secretion is more in sleep though the secretion is less in REM period. As infants and children spend more time in sleep, this helps them to attain adequate growth. Sleep deprivation invariably leads to growth deficiency.

-
    - They discovered that some particular stages of sleep are accompanied by **rapid eye movements** (REMs), which do not occur in the other stages.
- Accordingly, the sleep was divided **into two phases**: REM sleep and non-REM sleep.
    - The non-REM sleep is known as **slow wave sleep**, whereas REM sleep is known as **paradoxical sleep**.

Sleep Cycles

The EEG pattern recorded during sleep varies in a cyclic fashion, which **repeats in about every 90 minutes**. Thus, there are about **four cycles** in normal 6 to 7 hours of sleep.

1. In normal individuals, sleep cycle begins with slow-wave sleep or **Non-REM sleep**.
    - There are **four stages** of slow-wave sleep: **stages 1 to 4**.
    - A person when falls asleep, passes sequentially through these four stages of increasingly deep sleep.
2. After that the sleep lightens and enters into **REM period**.
    - With completion of REM phase, sleep cycle completes.
3. The REM phase is followed by the **next new cycle**, i.e., with stage 1 of non-REM sleep.
    - Thus, the **cycle repeats in every 70 to 90 minutes**.

There are differences in the proportion of time spent in the various sleep stages in different age groups. Moreover, each individual has his or her own characteristic pattern.

- Usually, there is a predominance of **deep slow wave sleep during the early part of the night**, and the first REM sleep may occur after an hour.
- **REM stage** becomes prevalent during the **later part of the night**.
- In general, **REM sleep occupies about 25 per cent** of total sleep period.

Slow Wave Sleep (Non-REM sleep)

Stages

As the individual goes to sleep, he advances from **stage 1 to stage 4** of slow wave sleep. These are ***four stages of progressively deepening sleep*** (it is difficult to wake up the subject in slow wave sleep) during which EEG pattern becomes progressively slower in frequency and higher in amplitude (Fig. 112.3).

Stage 1

First, subject becomes drowsy; the EEG shows a change from beta to **alpha rhythm**. Immediately, light sleep begins during which the alpha rhythm is replaced by **high frequency and low amplitude** EEG waves.

Stage 2

The subject then enters into stage 2 sleep. The amplitude of EEG waves slightly increases in this sage. The hallmarks of EEG pattern in stage 2 are **sleep spindles and K-complexes.**

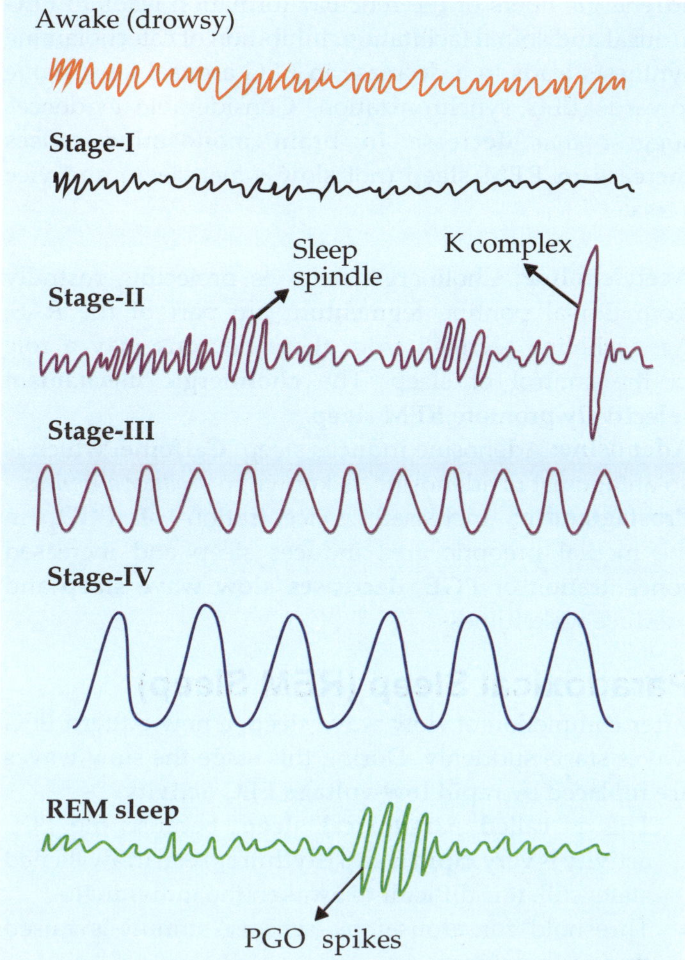

Fig. 112.3: EEG waves in different stages of sleep. Note the presence of sleep spindles and K complexes in stage 2 NREM sleep and PGO spikes in REM sleep.

Sleep Spindles: Sleep spindles are **bursts of alpha like waves** having frequency of 12-14 Hz and amplitude of about 50 μV, each lasting for about two seconds. They are called sleep spindles because of their characteristic **waxing and waning amplitude**.

K-Complexes: K-complexes are high amplitude-sharp waves appearing irregularly in EEG.

Stage 3

This is the stage of moderately deep sleep. The rhythm of the EEG waves shows **lower frequency and higher amplitude**.

Stage 4

This is the **stage of deep sleep**, with **delta rhythm predominant** over the whole scalp.

- Maximum slowing (lowest frequency) with large amplitude waves is seen in this phase.
- It is **very difficult to wake up the subject** in this stage. In young adults, maximum time of sleep is spent in stage 4 (Fig. 112.4).

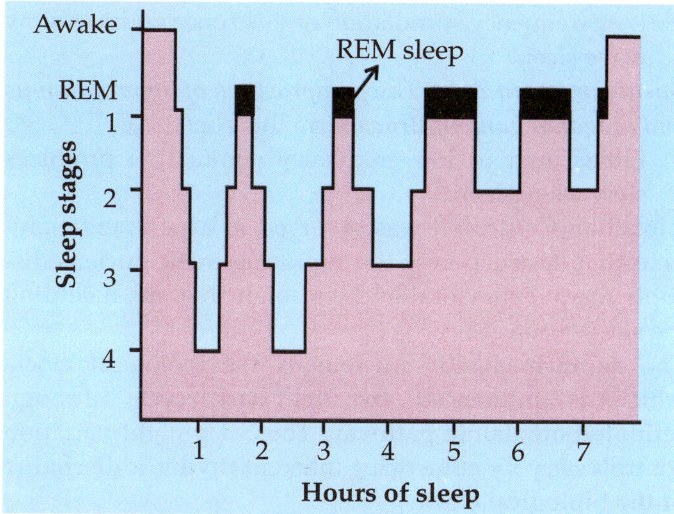

Fig. 112.4: Distribution of different stages of NREM and REM sleep in a normal night sleep in young adults.

Physiological Changes during Slow Wave Sleep

1. Decrease in heart rate and blood pressure
2. Fall in body temperature
3. Slow and regular respiration
4. Increase in gastrointestinal activity, which indicates increased parasympathetic activity.
5. Decreased muscle tone
6. No rapid-eye movements (**NREM stage**)
7. Sleep is deep in stage III and IV.

Control Mechanisms of Slow Wave Sleep

Mechanisms controlling slow wave sleep may be broadly divided into ***neural and chemical mechanisms***.

Neural Control Mechanisms

Neural control mechanisms of slow wave sleep may be subdivided into ***three categories***: afferent control, central control and circadian control.

Afferent Control: It is known that repeated and monotonous **stimulation of mechanoreceptors or afferents** from these receptors at a frequency less than 10 Hz produces sleep.

This is mediated by **low frequency stimulation** of brainstem and other areas (see below) that activates the sleep producing areas in the brain.

Central Control: There are **three brain areas** that on appropriate stimulation produce slow wave sleep. These sleep zones are diencephalic zone, medullary zone and basal forebrain zone.

Diencephalic Zone: This zone is formed by ***posterior hypothalamus and intralaminar & anterior thalamic nuclei*** close to hypothalamus.

- Low frequency stimulation of this zone produces an EEG pattern that resembles slow wave sleep.

Medullary Zone: The **reticular formation at the level of NTS** in medulla constitutes the medullary sleep zone.

- Low frequency stimulation of this zone produces slow wave sleep.

Basal Forebrain Zone: The ***preoptic area of hypothalamus and diagonal band of Broca*** form this zone.

- Either high or low frequency stimulation produces slow wave sleep.

Circadian Control: It was observed in experimental animals that destruction of the suprachiasmatic nucleus disrupts many behavioral and circadian rhythms including the sleep-wake cycle.

The **suprachiasmatic nucleus** is the biological clock, which is influenced by light-dark cycle through **retinohypothalamic pathway**. Thus, day-night variation controls sleep by influencing inherent **rhythmic discharge of the biological clock**.

- The physiological basis of suprachiasmatic nucleus (SCN) seems to be the **rhythmic discharge** exhibited by this nucleus.
  - It has been observed that neurons of SCN continue to discharge rhythmically in vitro even after its removal from the brain.
- It has been recently observed that, there are **specific genes in neurons of SCN** that regulate the rhythmic discharge pattern. **Four such genes** have been identified in mammals.
- In the neurons of SCN, **genes are activated diurnally** that synthesize **new proteins**.
  - The proteins that are formed enter cytoplasm and modify cell functions. Change in cytoplasmic activity alters their discharge patterns.
- Later, these **proteins return back** to nucleus and **inhibit the genes** that produce them.
  - Thus, genes that control rhythmic discharge of SCN are also **regulated by negative feedback mechanism** so that the biological clock acts within the physiological range.
- It has been evidenced that the rhythmic discharge of biological clock (SCN) and alteration of cellular protein are the primary regulator of sleep-wake cycle.

Chemical Control Mechanisms

Centers for mechanisms governing NREM and REM sleep lie in pons, which is influenced by serotonin, norepinephrine, acetylcholine, adenosine and prostaglandins.

Serotonin: It is clearly known that **serotonin agonists suppress sleep** and **serotonin antagonists induce slow wave sleep**. Serotonergic projection from raphe nucleus to thalamus and cortex plays role in the control of sleep.

Norepinephrine: Cells in the **locus ceruleus release norepinephrine**. Fibers from locus ceruleus project to spinal cord and also to the cortex. The **ascending fibers on stimulation prevent sleep** and descending fibers inhibit motor neurons that produce hypotonia during slow wave sleep.

Administration of L-DOPA (catecholamine precursor) causes an increase in wakefulness. Stimulation of the adrenergic fibers of the reticular formation leads to EEG arousal and spinal facilitation. Inhibition of catecholamine synthesis leads to a decrease in EEG arousal i.e. a move towards EEG synchronization. Considerable evidences suggest that **decrease in brain monoamine causes increase in REM sleep** (not slow wave sleep) and vice versa.

Acetylcholine: Cholinergic neurons projecting rostrally from dorsal pontine tegmentum are part of the RAS. Acetylcholine secreted from these neurons play a role in the control of sleep. The **cholinergic mechanism selectively promote REM sleep**.

Adenosine: Adenosine induces sleep. **Caffeine**, which is an antagonist of adenosine, is known to *produce alertness*.

Prostaglandin: Increased concentration of PGD_2 in the medial preoptic area induces sleep and increased concentration of **PGE_2 decreases slow wave sleep** and produce wakefulness.

Paradoxical Sleep (REM Sleep)

After completion of slow wave sleep, a new pattern EEG waves starts suddenly. During this stage the slow waves are replaced by **rapid low-voltage EEG activity**.

- This is called **paradoxical sleep**, because the EEG activity is **very rapid like β rhythm** as seen in awakened state; still, it is difficult to awaken the individual.
- Threshold for arousal by sensory stimuli is raised during this stage.
- This phase lasts for about **10 to 15 minutes**.

Features of Paradoxical Sleep

1. Paradoxical sleep is characterized by rapid and roving eye movements, even visible under the closed eyelids. Therefore, paradoxical sleep is also called **rapid eye movement (REM) sleep**.
2. The **EEG pattern** shows a desynchronized *high frequency and low-voltage* like **fast β rhythm**.

- Yet it is difficult to arouse the individual from sleep as the threshold for sensory stimuli is raised.
- However, the **subject is likely to wake up spontaneously** from REM sleep than at any other stage.

3. Another characteristic feature of REM sleep is the appearance of **PGO spikes** in EEG (Fig. 112.3).
   - PGO spikes are phasic potentials that occur in groups of three to five.
   - They originate in pons and through ***lateral geniculate body travel to occipital cortex***. Therefore, they are called *ponto-geniculo-occipital spikes* or PGO spikes.
4. If the subject is awakened from REM sleep, he commonly reports that he was dreaming.

- The **dream is easily remembered** in this stage, but usually it is not of frightful type, which occurs in slow wave sleep.
- The REM sleep is customarily considered as **dream sleep**.

5. **Sympathetic system is stimulated**: Heart rate and blood pressure are increased, and respiration is rapid and sometimes may be irregular (Table 112.1).
6. In males, **penile erection** occurs.
   - This is **used in diagnosing impotence**, in which *erection does not occur in REM sleep*.
7. **Muscle tone is profoundly depressed**. Hypotonia is widespread. However, there are **two exceptions**.
   - The two groups of skeletal muscles not involved in hypotonia are the **extraocular muscles** (that cause rapid eye movements), and **muscles of the middle ear ossicles** (that protect the inner ear).
   - Hypotonia occurs due to ***active inhibition of motor neurons*** by a group of neurons located close to the locus ceruleus in brain stem. The stretch reflexes are inhibited.

Table 112.1 | Differences between NREM and REM sleep.

	NREM sleep	REM sleep
1. Timing in sleep-cycle	Occurs first	Occurs after NREM sleep
2. Duration in normal adults	75% of total sleep	25% of sleep
3. Autonomic symptoms	Sympathetic inhibition (low HR, BP, respiration)	Sympathetic excitation (high HR, BP, respiration)
4. Eyeball movement	No eye movement	Rapid eye movement occurs
5. Dreams	Dreams are not memorized	Dreams well memorized
6. Muscle tone	Is inhibited	Is profoundly depressed
7. Type of sleep	Enters into deep sleep	Sleep lightens
8. EEG waves	Slow wave-high amplitude (in stage 3 and 4)	High frequency-low voltage
9. Mechanism	Inhibition of RAS	Activation of pontine reticular formation

Mechanisms for Paradoxical Sleep

Neural mechanisms

The EEG pattern of REM sleep resembles EEG recording **during alerting response.** Form PET scanning in humans, it is observed that neuronal activity increases in **pons, amygdala and cingulate gyrus** during REM sleep.

- The mechanisms that generate REM sleep are **located in the pontine reticular formation.**
- Rapid eye movement, the hallmark of REM sleep is triggered by potentials originating from pons in the form of **PGO spikes**.

Chemical mechanisms

Acetylcholine seems to mediate REM sleep. In cat, administration of atropine suppresses paradoxical sleep, whereas injection of physostigmine (which promotes acetylcholine activity) increases the duration of REM sleep.

- It is also seen that **decrease in brain monoamine** causes increase in REM sleep.
- **Reserpine,** a drug that depletes monoamine stores, blocks slow wave sleep, and hypotonia and EEG desynchronization seen in REM sleep. However, reserpine enhances the rapid eye movements by facilitating PGO activity. Thus, the role of monoamines in paradoxical sleep appears to be complex one.
- **Barbiturates** decrease the duration of REM sleep.

Effect of Age on Sleep

The duration of REM sleep and stage 4 sleep **decreases gradually with advancing age**.

- **Newborns and infants** sleep 18 – 20 hours a day of which 50% is spent in REM sleep (Fig. 112.5).

Functions of Sleep

Sleep is essential for normal functioning of the body.

1. Sleep restores strength, both physical and mental.
2. Ability to think and concentrate is enhanced with adequate sleep.
3. Sleep consolidates learning and memory.
4. Adequate sleep promotes and maintains growth, as during sleep growth hormone secretion is more.
5. Dreams are produced during sleep. However, utility of dreams depends on the ability to remember and interprete them.

Theories of Sleep

Sleep-Wake Cycle

The exact mechanism of induction of sleep or to arouse from sleep is not known. Sleep-wake cycle is entrained

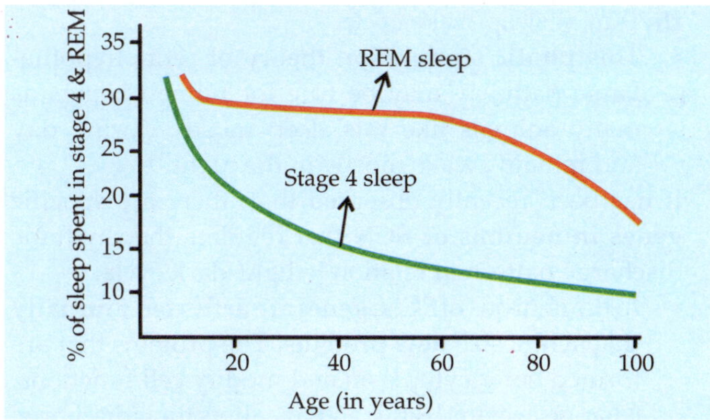

Fig. 112.5: Percentage distribution of stage 4 and REM sleep at different age.

with the diurnal rhythm, which means sleep-wakefulness is synchronized to the day-night variation in the environment. Circadian rhythm plays an important role in shift between sleep-wake cycles, at least in human beings. **Following theories** have been proposed to explain the sleep-wake cycle:

1. Role of circadian rhythm
2. Role of pineal gland
3. Thalamocortical loop
4. Role of neurochemicals

Circadian Rhythm

Many mammalian functions and behaviors are linked to the circadian rhythm. The center of circadian rhythm is the **suprachiasmatic nucleus** (SCN) of hypothalamus. SCN is so named for its location bilaterally above the optic chiasm. For its major influence on physiological alterations in diurnal rhythm, SCN is designated as the **biological clock.**

1. Experimental findings suggest that the peaks of circadian activity of SCN **correlate with the light-dark cycle.**
   - It has been observed that sleep-wake cycle depends on the time of exposure to the bright light.
2. If the individual is exposed to bright light during the day, sleep-wake cycle is usually not affected; if exposed to bright light after the evening, onset of sleep is delayed; if exposed in the early morning (before dawn), onset of next sleep period is accelerated.
   - Therefore, it was suggested that the exposure to light **(photic stimulation retina)** is an important determinant of sleep-wake cycle.
   - The retinal stimulation during day stimulates **retinohypothalamic pathway** that activates SCN, which keeps the individual awake by activation of reticular activating system.
3. **Cessation of retinohypothalamic activation** with the onset of night (loss of photic stimulation of retina) **induces the onset of sleep.**
4. It has been proposed that SCN initiates the neurohumoral signals that **entrain the circadian rhythm** of sleep-wake cycle.
   - This **photic stimulation theory** of retinohypothalamic pathway may be true for human beings as many animals like rats sleep mostly during day and remain awake mostly in the night.
5. It has been recently observed that, there are **specific genes in neurons of SCN** that regulate the rhythmic discharge pattern in relation to light-dark cycle.
   - In the neurons of SCN, **genes are activated diurnally** that synthesize **new proteins**. The proteins that are formed enter cytoplasm and modify cell functions. Change in cytoplasmic activity alters their discharge patterns.
   - It has been evidenced that the **rhythmic discharge of biological clock** (SCN) and **alteration of cellular protein** are the primary regulator of sleep-wake cycle.

Role of Pineal Gland

Earlier it was thought that pineal gland is a small vestigial organ in the brain like that of vermiform appendix in GI tract. Recent evidences suggest that pineal plays important roles in hypothalamic control of hormonal secretion and regulation of circadian rhythm.

1. It has been observed that activity of sympathetic fibers to pineal gland is entrained with the light-dark cycle of the environment via ***retinohypothalamic connections*** of SCN and ***melatonin secretion*** from pineal gland.
2. The alteration in melatonin secretion varies with the **light-dark cycle.**
   - The secretion is more in the evening and first half of night and less in the second half of the night and first half of the day.
3. It is substantiated that the melatonin secretion from pineal is controlled by ***post-ganglionic sympathetic fibers*** innervating pineal gland that secrete norepinephrine, which increases cAMP by acting on β receptors on the pinealocytes.
4. Melatonin released into circulation from the fenestrated capillaries of pineal gland is suggested to act on brain **reticular activating neurons** to mediate sleep-wake cycle (Flowchart 112.1).

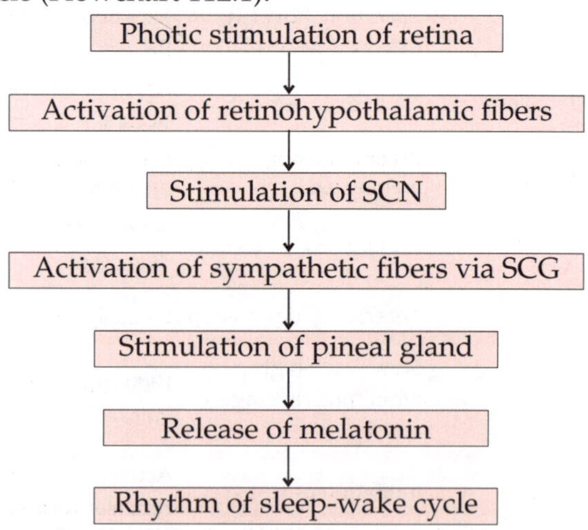

Flowchart 112.1: Circadian control of sleep-wake cycle. Note, photic stimulation of retina through retinohypothalamic pathway causes sympathetic activation of pineal gland and releases melatonin that controls sleep-wake cycle rhythm. SCN: suprachiasmatic nucleus; SCG: Superior cervical ganglion.

5. Melatonin acting on **ML_1** receptors inhibits cAMP formation and acting on **ML_2** receptors stimulates formation IP_3 and DAG.

Role of Thalamocortical Loop

The **neural circuit between thalamus and cortex** has been proposed to be an important component of pattern generator of sleep-wake cycle.

- The thalamocortical circuitry **generates this rhythmic activity**, and the inhibitory reticular neurons are believed to be the main elements in the network.
- The recordings from thalamic and cortical neurons show typical **patterns of rhythmic activity** in different phases of sleep-wake cycle.
    - **In the waking state**, thalamocortical neurons exhibits high frequency rhythmic activity and **in sleep** the activity is of low frequency rhythm.
- The **gamma rhythm** has been suggested to link the various sensory inputs that generate induction of sleep.

Role of Neurochemicals in Brainstem

The neurons in brainstem RAS projecting to various areas in the cortex secrete norepinephrine (NE), serotonin and acetylcholine.

1. It has been observed that concentration of **NE and serotonin** secreted from these neurons modulate the **release of acetylcholine** and this controls the rhythm of sleep-wake cycle.
2. **Decreased acetylcholine** keeps the individual **awake** and **increased acetylcholine induces sleep** (Flowchart 112.2).
3. The **serotonergic neurons** originating from raphe nucleus and **NE secreting neurons** from locus ceruleus in the brainstem ***inhibit cholinergic neurons*** in pontine RAS and decrease the content of acetylcholine that **keeps the individual awake**.

Role of Hypothalamic Neurochemicals: Secretion of **histamine from posterior hypothalamic neurons** and **GABA from preoptic neurons** of hypothalamus play a crucial role in **activation of thalamocortical neurons** mediating sleep-wake cycle.

In this mechanism:

- **decreased GABA** concentration increases histamine release that activates thalamocortical neurons and ***keeps the individual awake***, and,

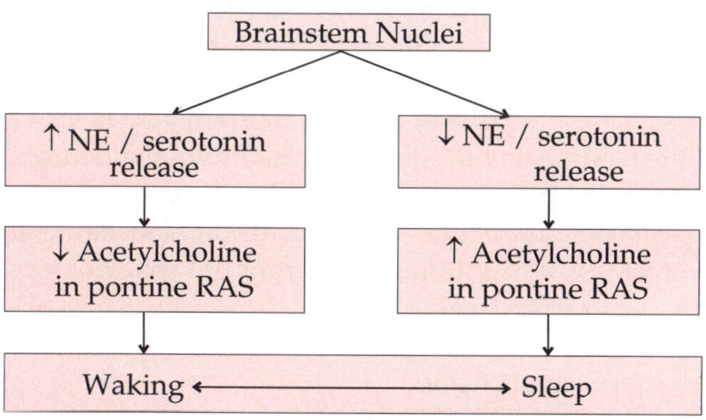

Flowchart 112.2: Modulation of acetylcholine content of pontine reticular activating system (RAS) by serotonin secreted from neurons projecting from raphe nucleus and norepinephrine (NE) secreted from neurons projecting from locus ceruleus in the brain stem control the sleep-wake cycle.

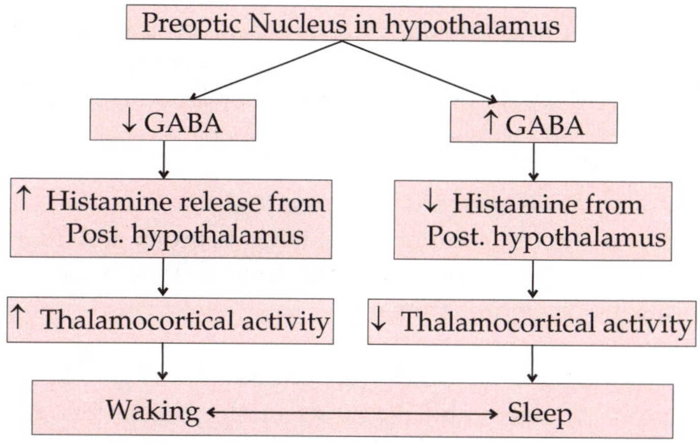

Flowchart 112.3: GABA secreted from preoptic nucleus of hypothalamus modulates histamine release from posterior hypothalamus that influences thalamocortical activity, which controls the sleep-wake cycle.

- **increased GABA** level inhibits histamine secretion that suppresses thalamocortical neurons and ***induces sleep*** (Flowchart 112.3).

Clinical Aspects of EEG and Sleep

Usage of EEG

Epilepsies

1. Diagnosis of various types of epilepsies

Epilepsy is defined as the intermittent disorder of cerebral function associated with a sudden uncontrolled discharge of cerebral neurons, which may or may not be accompanied by loss of consciousness. The epileptogenic focus in the cerebral cortex discharges **irregular slow waves** or sometimes, high voltage waves that can be recorded in EEG.

There are two main groups of epilepsies depending on type of seizures:

Generalized Seizures: Generalized seizures with loss of consciousness associated with generalized synchronous EEG discharge from both hemispheres; e.g., grand mal and petit mal epilepsies.

1. ***Grand mal epilepsy*** is characterized by immediate loss of consciousness followed by sustained contraction of limb muscles (*tonic phase*) and then jerky movements due to rhythmic contraction-relaxation of limb muscles (*clonic phase*). In EEG, **fast activities** are recorded in tonic and slow activities in clonic phase.
2. ***Petit mal epilepsy (absence seizure)*** manifests in the form of short-lived loss of consciousness with mild or no motor activity. EEG recording shows **doublets consisting of a spike and a dome**. Three such doublets occur typically per second.

Focal Epilepsy: Focal epilepsy, the manifestations of which depend on the site of the cortex from which the discharge occurs e.g. temporal lobe epilepsy and Jacksonian (motor cortex) epilepsy.

The value of EEG is to diagnose epilepsy, confirm the type of epilepsy, and to identify the cortical site that may be the focus of the abnormal discharge of epilepsy. However, EEG recording between the attacks may be normal.

2. Intracranial space occupying lesion

Cerebral tumors compress adjoining neurons and may manifests as **irregular or slow waves**. This helps in localizing cerebral tumors.

3. Diagnosis of sleep disturbances

Analysis of sleep, and diagnosis of sleep disorders are accomplished with the help of EEG.

Sleep Disorders

Insomnia: The chronic inability to sleep inspite of adequate opportunity to do so is called insomnia.

There are **two types** of insomnia: ***primary insomnia***, in which there is abnormality in normal sleep mechanism (normal nocturnal sleep is disturbed chronically), and ***secondary insomnia*** in which the sleep disturbance is secondary to medical or psychological disorders.

Narcolepsy: Narcolepsy is a condition in which there is **episodic sudden loss of muscle tone accompanied with irresistible urge to sleep.**

- Sleep may start with REM phase of sleep, which never occurs in normal individuals in whom slow wave sleep always precedes REM sleep.

Cataplexy: Cataplexy is a condition in which there is a **sudden loss of power of movement and posture** while the subject is awake, followed by irresistible desire to sleep. Even, there may be brief period of paralysis at the beginning or end of the sleep.

- Catalepsy is usually triggered by strong emotional excitement, which persists for few seconds or minutes.
- Three-fourth of narcoleptic patients present first with catalepsy.

Bruxism: This is **nocturnal grinding of teeth** that is usually is associated **with dreams in REM sleep.**

- Sometimes it occurs during daytime sleep.
- It can occur in all ages.
- EMG studies have revealed that masseter and temporalis muscles contract excessively during bruxism.

Nocturnal Enuresis: Bed-wetting in the night with daytime continence is a frequent disorder in childhood. It may persist into adult life.

- Boys are affected more than girls in a ratio 4:3.
- It occurs usually after 3 to 4 hours of sleep **in the stage 3 or stage 4 of slow wave sleep**.
- It could be due to **failure of neural regulation of micturition** in sleep.
- It is preceded by a burst of **rhythmic delta waves in EEG**, associated with general body movements.

Parasomnic Disturbances: These include several disorders that occur only during sleep.

- These are somnolescent starts, sensory paroxysms, nocturnal paroxysmal dystonia, sleep paralysis, night terrors and nightmares, somnambulism, and REM sleep behaviour disorder.

Night terrors and nightmares: Night terror (***pavor nocturnus***) and nightmares are usually the **problems of childhood.**

- Usually, this occurs after falling asleep, in the **stage 3 or 4** of NREM sleep. Child awakens abruptly in a state of **intense fright** with marked tachycardia (150-170/min) and tachypnea and then he sleeps automatically.
- The episode occurs only for 1 to 2 minutes, and child **does not remember** anything in the morning.

Somnambulism: Somnambulism is the condition in which the sleeping individual is ***able to stand and walk about***. This is called **sleep walk**, which is just opposite of cataplexy.

- Usually patient sits up at the edge of the bed, but sometimes he gets down from the bed and really **walks with eyes open**. He may even perform some familial act without outward show of emotion.
  - Usually, it is seen in children and is benign; but in adults it may be an aggressive motor act.
- During the act they ***do not respond to external stimuli***.
- It occurs in **stage 4 of slow wave sleep** in the first third part of sleep when usually dream does not occur.
  - Next morning, patient ***does not recall anything***.

REM sleep behaviour disorder: This parasomnic disorder occurs more commonly in adults or older men, characterized by vigorous and often **dangerous motor activity** that accompanies vivid dreams.

- They do not have history of childhood sleepwalking.
- Characteristically, they become aggressive, angry and shout loudly or even become **violent and cause injury** to themselves or to the bedmate.
- The violent episodes occur during the **REM phase**, during which ***hypotonia fails to occur***.

Hypersomnia (Excessive Sleep): Patient sleeps for days to weeks continuously.

- It usually occurs due to **damage to brainstem RAS**, or to the neurons in the subthalamus or hypothalamus.
- Recently, it has been suggested that *destruction of dopaminergic neurons* in the substantia nigra resulting in **overactivity of serotonergic neurons of raphe nucleus** causes hypersomnia.

Obstructive Sleep Apnea

Obstructive sleep apnea (OSA) is a common sleep disorder of middle-aged people in which **time spent in stage 1 is more**. Normally, the duration of stage 1 of **NREM** sleep is about 10% of total duration of night sleep. In OSA, this duration increases to **30 – 50%** and there is marked reduction in stage 3 and 4 of NREM sleep (slow wave sleep).

- There is **reduction in muscular tone and respiratory** drive at the ***onset of sleep*** that causes obstruction of upper airway, especially of the pharynx (decreased tone of pharyngeal muscles).
- **Apnea** (cessation of breathing) occurs for more than 10 seconds during frequent episodes of obstruction.
  - Apnea causes **brief arousal** from sleep that reestablishes the airway tone.
- But **airway obstruction is repeated** often throughout the night that decreases the duration of sleep and **sleep is usually disturbed**.
  - Therefore, the subject **feels often sleepy during day time.**

PY11.11

BRAIN DEATH

EEG can confirm brain death when it shows no electrical activity more than 2 microvolts, at a sensitivity of 2 microvolts/mm for at least 30 seconds. Also, it should show no reactivity to intense somatosensory stimuli.

Definition and Meaning

According to the American Academy of Neurology guidelines, brain death is clinically equivalent to the **irreversible loss of all brain stem functions**, which refers to the impossibility of recovery, regardless of any medical intervention.

- However, patients with brain death could be maintained physiologically for prolonged periods in the intensive care units.

Criteria for Diagnosis of Brain Death

Brain death **can be assessed** by doing physical examination, apnea test, and ancillary tests.

Physical Examination

This includes the **response to pain and assessment of brain stem reflexes**.

- Loss of eye response and motor reflexes in response to deep pain stimuli occur in brain death.
- Brain death can be confirmed if **brain stem reflexes are lost**, including:

CN II: Loss of light reflex, pupils should be mid-dilated 4 to 9 mm, and not reactive to light.

CN III, IV, VI: Eye motion is lost in reaction to head movement (Doll's eyes).

CN V, VII: Loss of corneal reflex.

CN VIII: Loss of oculovestibular reflex (caloric test)—with irrigation of each by 60 ml of ice water, the eye will not move towards the irrigated ear.

CN IX: Loss of gag reflex.

CN X: Loss of cough reflex

Apnea Test

The apnea test is used to assess the brain's ability to drive pulmonary function **in response to the rise of CO_2**.

- During the test, oxygen should be supplemented using a cannula connected to the endotracheal tube at 6 l/min.
- In the case of loss of respiratory drive, CO_2 is expected to rise 5 mmHg every minute in the first 2 minutes, then by 2 mmHg every minute.
- The rise of CO_2 more than 20 mmHg above baseline is consistent with brain death.

Ancillary tests

Two types of ancillary tests are considered if there is uncertainty of diagnosis or if apnea test cannot be performed.

A. For Detection of Cessation of Cerebral Blood Flow

Cerebral angiography: Four vessel angiography is considered the gold standard.

Transcranial ultrasound: This is used to assess pulsations of middle cerebral arteries, vertebral and basilar arteries bilaterally.

Computed tomogram (CT) brain angiography and MR angiography: This shows cessation of cerebral blood flow.

Radionuclide brain imaging: This can be done using a 99mTc-isotope tracer, then imaging by SPECT brain scintigraphy. The absence of a tracer in the brain circulation (the hollow skull phenomenon) is consistent with brain death.

B. For Detection of Loss of Bioelectrical Activity of the Brain

Electroencephalogram (EEG): This can confirm brain death when it shows no electrical activity more than 2 microvolts, at a sensitivity of 2 microvolts/ mm for at least 30 seconds.

Somatosensory evoked potentials: Patients with brain death show no SEP in response to bilateral median nerve stimulation, and no BAEP in response to auditory stimuli.

Implications

It is crucial to differentiate brain death from other forms of severe brain damage, which can cause vegetative states when some of the brain functions are maintained, and recovery can occur even after prolonged periods, especially in patients with traumatic brain injuries.

Dead Donor Rule: Another essential topic that evolved in parallel with brain death is the need of obtaining organs for transplantation. According to the "dead donor rule," organ procurement can occur only after death. So, for patients who are brain dead, the procurement of viable organs is allowed, even if they still have some circulatory and pulmonary functions.

Exam Questions

1. Describe the connections and functions of reticular formation. Add a note on reticular activating system.
2. Draw EEG waves in different phases of sleep and list the differences between NREM and REM sleep. Briefly describe the theories of sleep.

Multiple Choice Questions

1. Which of the following is NOT true about medial column of brainstem reticular formation?
A. Constitute the gigantocellular part
B. Mainly contribute to sleep-wakefulness
C. Contain the raphe nuclei and central group of nuclei
D. Project downward as reticulospinal tracts

2. Which of the following is NOT true about brainstem reticular formation?
A. They are diffuse system of neurons having widely branching axons
B. Very long dendrites
C. Long ascending axons that project to thalamus, hypothalamus and cortex
D. Descending branches of axons are small

3. Which of the following structure does not project to reticular formation?
A. Cerebellum B. Corpus striatum
C. Corpus callosum D. Amygdaloid complex

4. Reticular formation has direct projection to all the following structures, EXCEPT:
A. Olivary nucleus B. Tectum
C. Substantia nigra D. Posterior pituitary

5. Which of the following is not a major function of RAS?
A. Arousal and sleep
B. Sensory behavior
C. Heart rate, BP and respiration
D. GI motility

6. What are the EEG waves recorded from parieto-occipital region with subject awake & eye closed?
A. Alpha waves B. Beta waves
C. Delta waves D. Theta waves

7. Which of the following is not true about α wave of EEG?
A. Frequency is 8-13/sec
B. Voltage is 50 microvolts usually
C. Seen in awake patients at rest with eyes closed and mind wandering
D. Seen in hippocampus

8. Which of the following is true about β wave of EEG?
A. Frequency is 8-13 per second
B. Seen in emotional states
C. Predominant activity in REM sleep
D. Predominant activity in transition phase

9. Beta waveforms in electroencephalogram indicate which of the following states of the patient
A. Deep anaesthesia
B. Surgical anaesthesia
C. Light anaesthesia, eyes closed, relaxed
D. Awake or alert state

10. Delta waves are seen in:
A. Deep sleep B. REM sleep
C. Awake sleep D. Stage I NREM sleep

11. EEG rhythm having lowest frequency is:
A. Alpha B. Beta
C. Delta D. Theta

12. Slow wave sleep associated with:
A. Dreams B. Cardiac arrhythmia
C. Penile intumescence D. Delta activity

13. About paradoxical sleep, which of the following statement is true?
A. Prominent beta waves
B. Prominent alpha waves
C. Also known as NREM sleep
D. Low amplitude, mixed frequency waves

14. Nightmare is seen in:
A. REM sleep B. Stage II NREM sleep
C. Stage IV NREM sleep D. Stage I NREM sleep

15. Which one of the following phenomena is closely associated with slow wave sleep?
A. Dreaming B. Atonia
C. Sleep walking D. Irregular heart rate

16. The normal adult human electroencephalogram (EEG):
A. Will show high frequency waves during state 3 sleep
B. Shows alpha rhythm when a person is awake but inattentive
C. Has lower frequency waves during mental activity
D. Is predominated by large amplitude waves during REM sleep

17. Polysomnography contains all of the following tests EXCEPT:
A. Electroencephalography
B. Pulse oximetry
C. Electrooculography
D. Arterial pCO_2 measurement

18. Sleep spindles and K-complexes are seen in:
A. REM sleep B. Stage II NREM sleep
C. Stage IV NREM sleep D. Stage I NREM sleep

19. All of the following induce sleep, EXCEPT:
A. Serotonin B. Acetylcholine
C. Adenosine D. PGD_2

20. All of the following are true for narcolepsy, EXCEPT:
A. Episodic sudden loss of muscle tone
B. Has a strong genetic susceptibility
C. Irresistible urge to sleep
D. Hypothalamus shows more hypocretin producing neurons

Answers

1. B 2. D 3. C 4. D 5. D 6. A 7. D 8. C 9. D 10. A 11. C
12. D 13. D 14. A 15. C 16. B 17. D 18. B 19. A 20. D

Chapter 113

Limbic System

Learning Objectives

On completion of study of this chapter:

The student will be able to (must know):

1. List the components of limbic system and Papez circuit and give their functions.
2. Outline the pathway and functions of different mesocortical neurotransmitters systems
3. Describe the functions of limbic system.
4. Name the structures and neurotransmitters of reward system and avoidance system.
5. Elucidate the role of limbic system in motivation, addiction, and emotional responses.
6. Define abnormalities of limbic functions, especially the Kluver Bucy syndrome.

The student may also be able to (desirable to know):

1. Describe the connections and functions of limbic system.
2. Describe various neurotransmitter systems of limbic cortex.
3. Explain the physiological basis of limbic dysfunctions.

Phylogenetically, limbic system is the **oldest part** of cortical and subcortical areas of the brain that mainly controls emotional responses and visceral functions.

Functional Anatomy

The limbic system comprises **limbic lobe** of the cortex and **subcortical structures** associated with it

Limbic Lobe

The structures of limbic lobe include **cingulate gyrus, subcallosal and parahippocampal gyri** including subiculum, and hippocampal formation that includes dentate gyrus and hippocampus (Fig. 113.1).

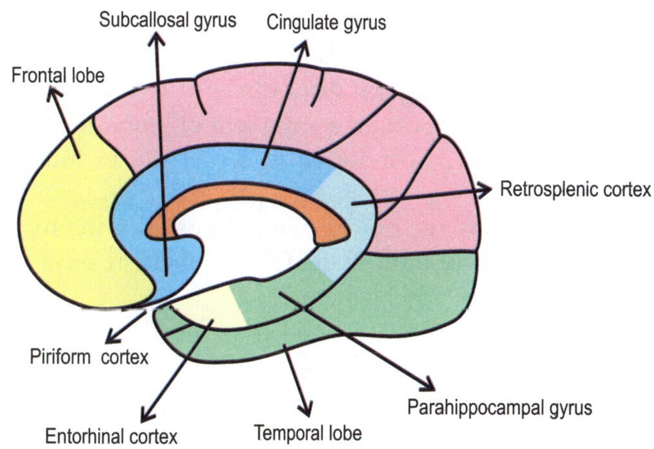

Fig. 113.1: Components of limbic lobe.

Subcortical Structures

The subcortical structures associated with limbic functions are categorized into **two parts**: diencephalic components and other components (Fig. 113.2).

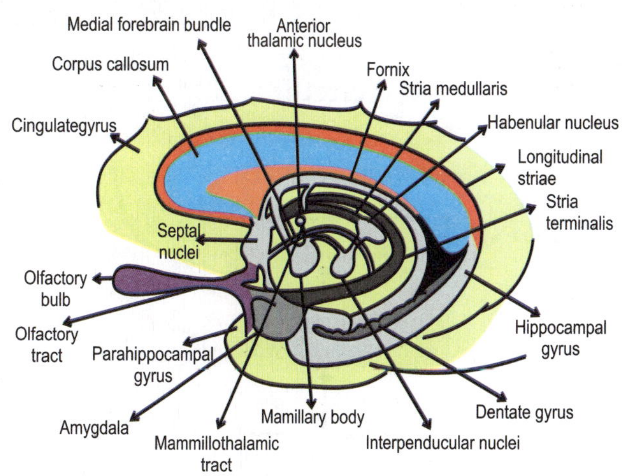

Fig. 113.2: The limbic system and its associated subcortical structures.

Diencephalic Components: Diencephalic components of the limbic system are the hypothalamus (including mamillary body), epithalamus and anterior thalamus.

Other Components: Other components include the amygdala, nucleus accumbens, septal nuclei, the prefrontal cortex (anterior and inferior components of the frontal lobe) and the habenula.

Papez Circuit: The limbic structures are interconnected by **circuitous tracts**, which were initially described by Papez, hence called **Papez circuit** (Fig. 113.3).

- The major circuitous tract of limbic system connects **hippocampus to the mamillary body** of the hypothalamus, the hypothalamus to the **anterior thalamic nuclei** via the mamillothalamic tract, and the anterior thalamus **to the cingulate gyrus** by thalamic projections.
- The circuit is completed by **cingulate gyrus projecting to hippocampus**.
- The minor circuitous tracts of limbic system connect other structures within the major circuit.

Important Physiological Aspects:

1. **Septum** is an important component of limbic system.
2. **Hippocampus** is connected to septal nuclei through fornix.
3. **Brainstem has reciprocal connections** with the hypothalamus. Ascending fibers from brainstem send collaterals to the limbic system.

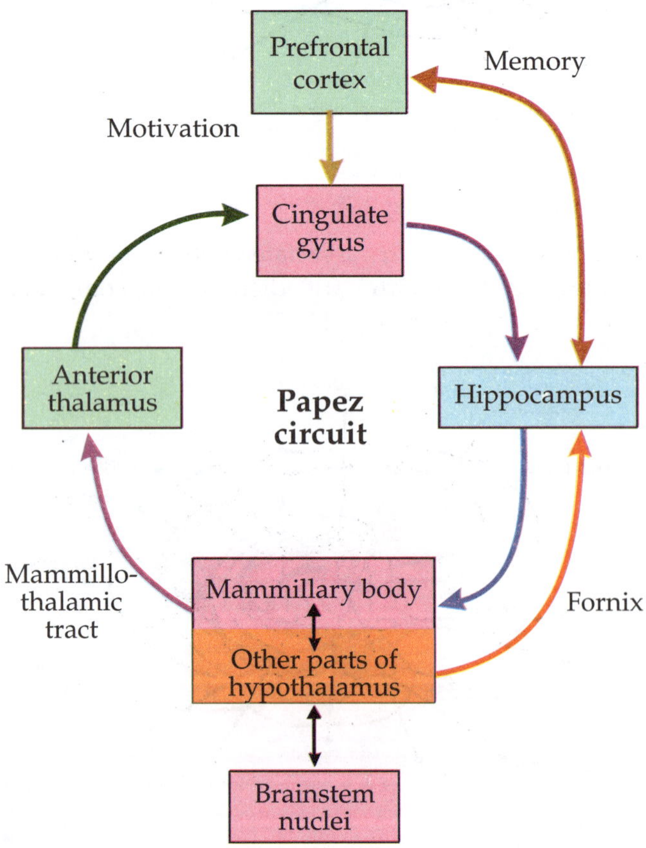

Fig. 113.3: Papez circuit.

4. Brainstem projections provide **visceral and somatic sensory signals** including pain and temperature and sensory information from sexual organs to the limbic system.
5. Information about **learning and memory** from cortex, especially from prefrontal cortex is referred to the limbic system mainly through cortico-hippocampal connections.

MAJOR AMINERGIC & CHOLINERGIC SYSTEMS

The limbic system is richly distributed by the neurons of monoaminergic and cholinergic systems that play major role in emotional and other behavioral responses.

Dopaminergic Systems

The major dopaminergic systems are: **mesocortical, tuberoinfundibular, nigrostriatal, and incertohypothalamic** systems.

Mesolimbic or Mesocortical System

The mesocortical system of dopaminergic neurons originate in the ventral tegmental area of the midbrain region of the brainstem and project to the limbic system (olfactory tubercles, septal nuclei, amygdala, nucleus accumbens) and limbic cortex (frontal and cingulate cortices) (Fig. 113.4).

- This dopaminergic system **plays an important role in motivation and drive** (Application Box 113.1).
- Especially, dopaminergic neurons in the more ventral structures such as the septal and accumbens are associated with the **brain's reward system**.

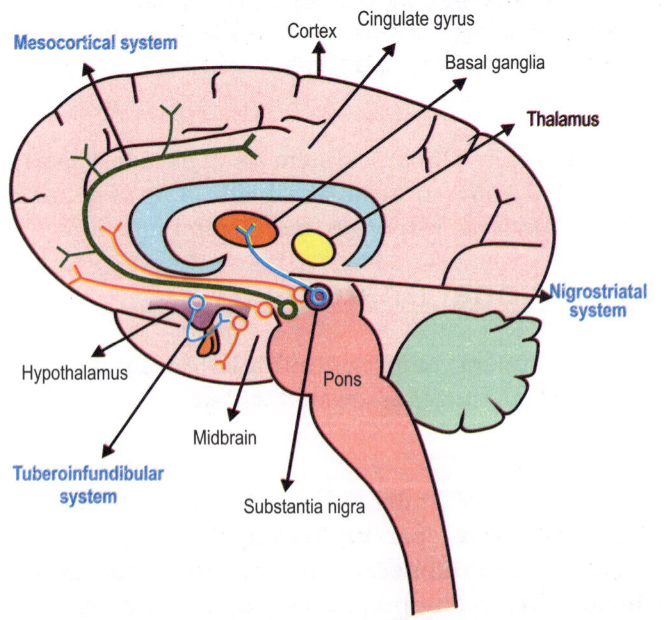

Fig. 113.4: Dopaminergic systems in the brain. Note, most prominent among them are mesocortical system, nigrostriatal system, tuberoinfundibular system, etc.

Application Box 113.1

Drug abuse and use: Due to its importance, dopamine is significant for drug use and drug abuse.

- **Drug abuse:** Drugs such as cocaine increase dopaminergic transmission that stimulate the brain's reward system and motivation. Therefore, these drugs are potential candidate for drug addiction (drug abuse).
- **Drug use:** The mesolimbic dopaminergic system is major site of action of neuroleptic drugs that are used to treat schizophrenia and other psychotic conditions. Amphetamine that promotes dopamine release causes schizophrenia and antischizophrenic drugs act by blocking D_2 and D_4 receptors.

Tuberoinfundibular System

The tuberoinfundibular system of dopaminergic neurons is located within the hypothalamus.

- The cell bodies are in the arcuate nucleus and periventricular nuclei fibers terminate in the median eminence.
- The tuberoinfundibular system **controls secretion of hypothalamic releasing factors** into a portal system.
- Especially, it **inhibits prolactin** secretion.

Nigrostriatal System

Cell bodies are located in the pars compacta of substantia nigra and fibers project to neostriatum (caudate and putamen) (Fig. 113.4). This dopaminergic pathway is essential for maintaining normal ***muscle tone*, posture and voluntary movements** (For details, refer 'Basal Ganglia').

Incertohypothalamic System

This system connects zona incerta of lateral septum with hypothalamus. It is involved in **motivation and ingestive behaviour**.

Noradrenergic System

Noradrenergic neurons secrete norepinephrine. **Two major noradrenergic systems** have been described: **locus ceruleus system, and tegmental system**.

Locus Ceruleus System

Cell bodies of noradrenergic neurons are located mainly in the locus ceruleus from where fibers project to all parts of the CNS (Fig. 113.5).

- Fibers project to spinal cord, cerebellum, hypothalamus (paraventricular, supraoptic and periventricular nuclei), thalamus, basal forebrain and the whole of neocortex.
- The fibers ascending from locus ceruleus form **dorsal noradrenergic bundle**.
- This system is involved in **modulation of sensory and motor functions**, and influences cardiovascular regulation and other autonomic functions.
- The ceruleospinal noradrenergic pathway is a component of **endogenous analgesia system**.

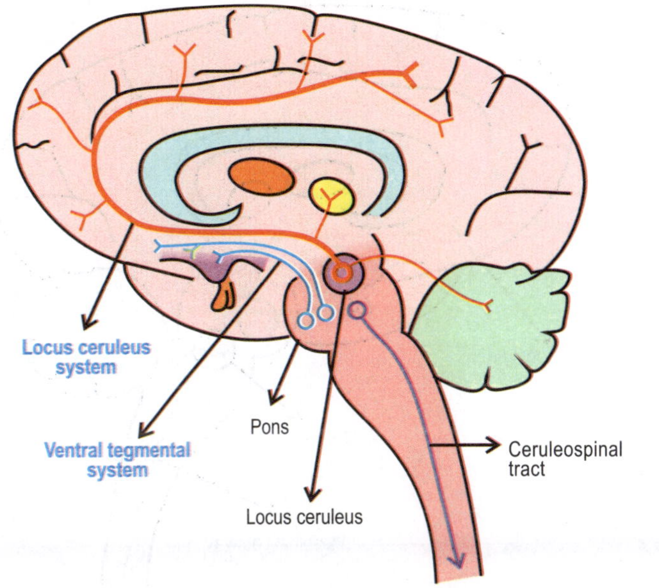

Fig. 113.5: Noradrenergic systems in the brain. Note, locus ceruleus and ventral tegmentum are the primary areas that contain cell bodies of noradrenergic neurons.

Tegmental System

This system includes neurons that are located in dorsal and ventral tegmentum, dorsal motor nucleus of vagus, and nucleus tractus solitarius (NTS).

- Fibers originating from ventral tegmentum form **ventral tegmental system** and fibers originating from lateral tegmentum forms **lateral tegmental system**.
- The fibers of tegmental systems project to spinal cord, brainstem, all parts of hypothalamus and basal forebrain.
- The fibers ascending from tegmental systems form **ventral noradrenergic bundle**.
  - Ventral tegmental system is involved in regulation of **secretion of ADH and oxytocin**.
  - It also controls **hypothalamic secretion** that in turn regulates hypophysiotropic secretion.
- Fibers of dorsal motor nucleus of vagus, and NTS **control cardiovascular and respiratory functions**.

Noradrenergic transmission controls mode and behavioral functions (Application Box 113.2).

Application Box 113.2

Drug abuse: Drugs that interfere with noradrenergic transmission significantly influence the mood and affect (the emotional state like euphoria, depression, anxiety etc.). Drugs like **reserpine** that decreases brain norepinephrine produce depression and drugs that increase norepinephrine availability like **MAO inhibitors** produce elevation of mood. Therefore, such drugs are candidates for drug abuse.

Adrenergic System

Cell bodies of neurons secreting **epinephrine** are located in the **medulla** and project to spinal cord, hypothalamus, thalamus and periaqueductal gray. Exact role of these neurons are not known.

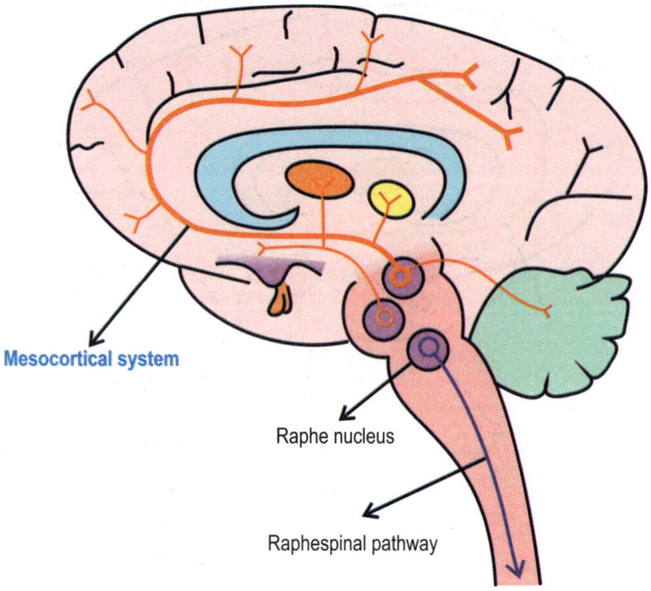

Fig. 113.6: Serotonergic systems in the brain. Cell bodies of serotonergic neurons are located in brainstem raphe nucleus and other nuclei from where fibers mainly project to spinal cord and cortex.

Serotonergic Systems

Cell bodies of serotonergic neurons are located in the midline raphe nucleus of the brainstem (Fig. 113.6).

- The fibers project to spinal cord, hypothalamus, limbic system, neocortex and cerebellum.
  - Serotonin is an important **mood elevator** (Clinical Note 113.1).
- Serotonin **suppresses sleep**. Serotonin neurons are most active during awake state and least active during slow wave sleep (not during REM sleep).
- Serotonin also stimulates **prolactin secretion**, **inhibits pain transmission** in the dorsal horn of the spinal cord and controls **circadian rhythm** by influencing function of suprachiasmatic nucleus.

Clinical Note 113.1

Antidepressant and ecstasy drugs: Drugs that increase serotonin transmission are effective antidepressant agents. For example, the serotonin agonist LSD (lysergic acid diethylamide), a popularly known hallucinogen acts by activating 5-HT_2 receptors.

- The ecstasy drug, MDMA (3,4-methylene dioxy-methamphitamine) produces euphoria by releasing serotonin.
- Drugs that inhibit norepinephrine reuptake also inhibit serotonin reuptake.

Histaminergic System

Cell bodies of histaminergic neurons are located in **tuberomamillary nucleus** of posterior hypothalamus. The fibers project to **olfactory bulb and all part of cortex**.

- Histamine is proposed to be involved in **regulation of limbic functions**, especially in arousal and sexual behavior, regulation of blood pressure, water intake, pain and anterior pituitary secretion.
- Recently, it has been observed that histamine release from posterior hypothalamus ***inhibits thalamocortical projection*** neurons that induce sleep.

Cholinergic Neurons

Cholinergic neurons are plentily available in basal telencephalon, thalamus and cortex. Distribution of these neuron closely resemble to that of monoaminergic neurons.

1. A major cholinergic system of neurons projects from **nucleus basalis of Meynert** to amygdala and neocortex (Fig. 113.7).
2. Both nicotinic and muscarinic receptors are present in brain. Cholinergic neurons are involved in many physiological functions such as **learning, memory** (Clinical Note 113.2), **motivation, perception, cognition and REM-sleep**.
3. Muscarinic blockers produce hallucination.

Clinical Note 113.2

Alzheimer's disease: In old age, degeneration of cortical cholinergic neurons produces senile dementia. Degeneration of cholinergic neurons projecting from nucleus basalis of Meynert produces Alzheimer's disease (for details, refer next chapter).

PY10.7

FUNCTIONS OF LIMBIC SYSTEM

Limbic system is called as **'the visceral brain'** for its close association with hypothalamus and visceral autonomic functions. Limbic system is primarily involved in **motivation, addiction, emotions** of rage and fear, **sexual behavior and autonomic responses**.

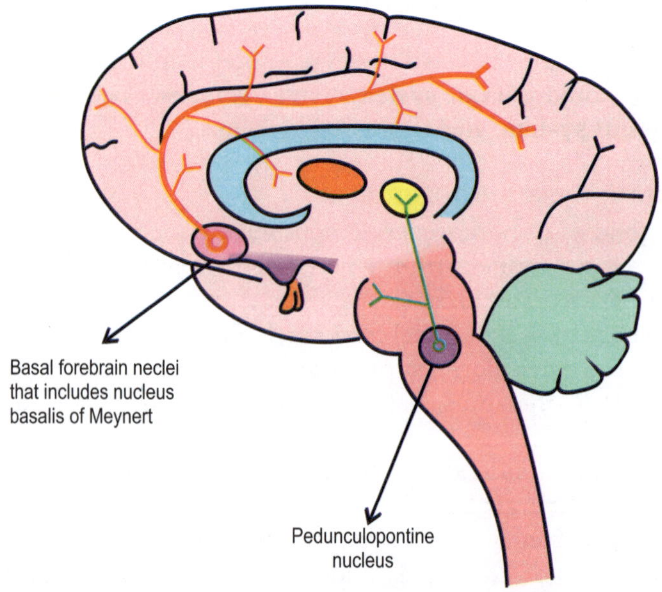

Fig. 113.7: Cholinergic systems in the brain. Cell bodies of cholinergic neurons are located in and around nucleus basalis of Meynert in the forebrain basal nuclear group from where fibers mainly project to cortex.

Motivation

There are different areas in the brain that on stimulation produce either pleasurable feeling (reward system) or unpleasant (averse or avoidance system) feelings. About, 35% of brain areas are rewarding, 5% aversive and 60% neutral.

Reward System

The reward system is also called **approach system.**

- It consists mainly of **dopaminergic pathways starting from ventral tegmental area to the nucleus accumbens.**
- **Frontal cortex and hypothalamic nuclei** also belong to this system.
    - **Nucleus accumbens** is found to be the main reward center in which **dopamine** is the major neurotransmitter for it (Fig. 113.8).

Avoidance System

Structures of avoidance system includes lateral portion of **posterior hypothalamus, dorsal midbrain and entorhinal cortex.**

- In humans, the feeling on stimulation of these areas ranges from **fear to terror**. Therefore, this system is also called **punishment system.**

Addiction

Addiction is defined as the **compulsion to repeatedly use a substance** in spite of knowing the negative impact of the substance on health.

- Addiction commonly occurs to opiates such as **morphine and heroin**. Other usually addictive drugs are **cocaine, amphetamine, ethyl alcohol and nicotine.**
    - Irrespective of the chemical nature of the substance, the major mechanism for addiction is the **increase in dopamine concentration** in the reward system of the brain.
- The primary center for the neural mechanism of addiction is the **nucleus accumbens.**

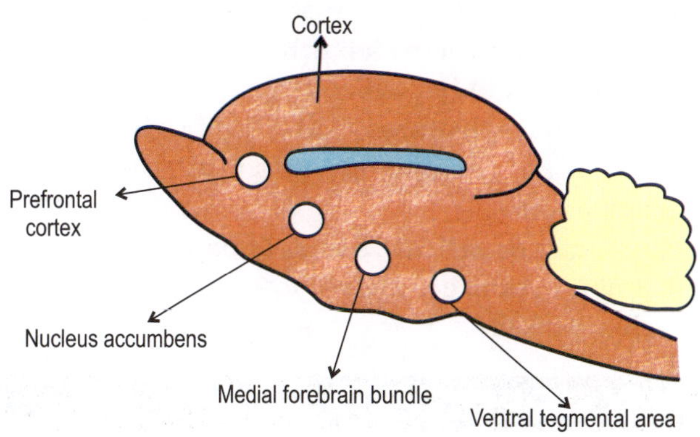

Fig. 113.8: Components of brain reward system in rat brain.

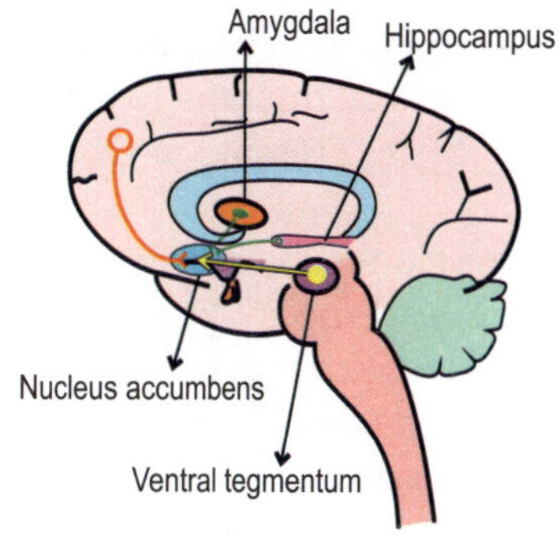

Fig. 113.9: Brain systems involved in addiction.

- Ventral tegmental area projecting to nucleus accumbens through mesocortical dopaminergic fibers is the major afferent pathway for addiction (Fig. 113.9).
- Projection from frontal cortex, amygdala and hippocampus also form part of this system.
    - Dopamine released at the nerve terminals act on the D_3 **dopaminergic receptors** in the nucleus accumbens.

Emotions of Fear, Anxiety, Rage and Aggression

Fear: Centers for fear reaction are located in hypothalamus and amygdala.

- Following experimental destruction of amygdala, animals become fearless and autonomic reactions associated with fear are not elicited.
- In humans, **left amygdala is activated** by looking at the ugly faces that evoke fear.

Anxiety: Anxiety is the normal emotional reaction to a stimulus in which there **is uncertainty or doubt about future** and apprehension for the unknown.

- Anxiety is part of routine normal life.
    - However, *inappropriate or excessive anxiety* in any condition is abnormal.
    - *The seat of anxiety is the* **frontal part of temporal lobes.**
- The α_2**-GABA$_A$ receptors** have been identified to mediate anxiety.
- **Benzodiazepins**, the known anxiolytics, act by **increasing chloride conductance** in these receptors.

Rage and Placidity: Rage is the anger reaction in which a person loses his temper in response to a minor stimulus.

- **Placidity** is the emotional state in which the individual is not disturbed even in response to a major irritating stimulus.
    - *Destruction of* **neocortex, ventromedian hypothalamus and septal nuclei** results in rage in response to a minute stimulus, whereas **bilateral lesions of amygdaloid nuclei** lead to greater placidity.
- **Sham Rage** is the rage or aggression without emotional expression, demonstrated in cat by removing

cerebral hemisphere and keeping the hypothalamus and brainstem intact, in which the animal reacted to all stimuli by expressing anger and autonomic overactivity.

Aggression: Aggression is the violent form of rage.

- Gonadal hormones, especially **testosterone**, are known to produce aggressive behaviors.
  - Aggression decreases following castration.
- Fight-or-flight response, rage and aggression are fighting behaviors that can be elicited by **stimulation of hypothalamic and amygdalar nuclei**.
- If the connections of frontal cortex to the limbic system are removed, aggressiveness becomes more intense and permanent.
- In contrast, **bilateral amygdalectomy results in permanent placidity**.

Sexual Activity

The sexual activities include sexual reflexes and behavior.

- Though **sexual behavior** is controlled primarily by the limbic system, in human beings the higher cortical centers override limbic influences and refine the behavior.

In Males

In males, **lesion of neocortex inhibits sexual behavior**, which shows that connection of the limbic system with the cortex is required for integration of the same.

- Bilateral lesion of limbic system confined to pyriform cortex overlying amygdala and **destruction of amygdala** result in intense sexual activity (**hypersexuality**).

In Females

Female animals usually do not seek for mating always throughout their estrous cycle. Suddenly in the **heat phase**, sexual activity increases in females and they deeply seek for mating.

- **Lesion of anterior hypothalamus abolishes** sexual activity in female animals.
- In human also, sexual passion increases in females in periovulatory phase, though the basal desire for mating remains throughout the menstrual cycle.

Role of Pheromones: Olfactory stimuli are important in initiating sexual activity.

- **Pheromones** in female animals signal the onset of estrus cycle. Pheromones increase sexual receptivity to the male.
- The **olfactory system**, through its direct connections with the limbic system integrates the behavioral, endocrine, and autonomic responses of sexual behavior.

Autonomic Responses

Hypothalamus, for its major role in autonomic functions, is called the **head ganglion of ANS**.

- **Insular and prefrontal areas** of cortex are involved in the regulation of autonomic functions.
- Autonomic component of **emotional responses** is controlled by **amygdala**.
- Parts of limbic system that *project to brainstem and spinal cord centers* have major influence on autonomic functions.

DISORDERS AFFECTING LIMBIC SYSTEM

Types of Limbic Dysfunctions

Affective Disorders

The affective disorders include *depression*, **mania or manic-depressive psychoses** (MDP).

- **In MDP**, periods of depression follow the periods of mania in a cyclic pattern.
  - **During depression periods** brain *NE concentration is decreased* and **in maniac periods**, *NE transmission is increased*.
  - Both in depression and mania, there is **decreased brain serotonergic transmission**.
- The **antidepressant drugs** like MAO inhibitors or serotonin reuptake inhibitors stimulate both noradrenergic and serotonergic neurons of limbic system.
- **Acute treatment of mania** involves use of drugs that block dopamine receptors and **long-term treatment for mania** is lithium.
  - **Lithium** inhibits regeneration of the second messenger phosphatidylinositol in neuronal membranes by blocking the hydrolysis of inositol-1-phosphate.

Schizophrenia

Schizophrenia refers to a group of closely related psychotic disorders characterized by a **particular type of disordered thinking, affect and behavior**.

- The **usual features** are thought disorder, inappropriate emotional response, and auditory hallucinations.
- Neuroleptic drugs that **block dopamine receptors** in the limbic system are known to ameliorate the features of schizophrenia.

PHYSIOLOGY OF EMOTIONS

Emotion is a state of feeling that manifests mentally and

physically through cardiovascular and other autonomic changes.

Phases of Emotion

Emotional activation and responses occur in three phases: stimulus recognition and evaluation, emotional responses and emotional experience.

Stimulus Recognition and Evaluation

First, the stimulus should be perceived, which is called **recognition** or the awareness of sensation. Then, the next step is the **stimulus evaluation**, the process by which the output is compared with stored information.

- The stored information is available either by experience or by inheritance. The knowledge and experience that are acquired are used for emotional expression.
- The inherited information also helps in emotional integration, for example inherent fear in monkeys for snakes.

Emotional Responses

Emotional response has three components: affect, conation and physical changes.

- **Affect** is the feeling of emotion itself, conation is the urge to take immediate action and the **physical changes** are the sympathetic effects like rise in heart rate, BP and respiration, and sweating.
- However, emotional manifestations mainly depend on the type of emotional response.
- There are three types of emotional response may be a **natural response, defense response and conditional response**.

Natural Response: Natural emotional response is the normal response of fear, anxiety or pleasure encountered in daily life.

- In humans, **cingulate gyrus** is believed to play an important role in emotion as it interacts with neocortex.
- Stimulation of cingulate cortex during neurosurgery has been reported to evoke normal pleasure or fear responses and cingulectomy produced for psychotic or neurotic patients is reported to produce diminished emotional responses.

Defense Response: Defense response is **the response for a natural attack or responses to prevent from an attack.**

- In experimental animals, the defense response is elicited by **stimulation of hypothalamic areas** that in cat elicits hissing, arching of the back, piloerection and dilation of the pupil.
- This is associated with **autonomic cardiovascular responses** consisting of an increased heart rate and blood pressure, and a large increase in skeletal muscle blood flow.
- **Respiratory rate and depth** also increase.

Conditioned Response: This is the emotional response attached to a **conditioned stimulus.**

- Most of our emotional responses are **conditioned emotional responses** as they are usually evoked by a conditioned stimulus.

Emotional Experience

Emotional experiences are stored effectively in the memory. The subsequent emotional reactions to the similar stimuli mostly depend on the knowledge of the previous experiences.

Control of Emotional Responses

Though the emotional responses are profoundly influenced by external factors like social and cultural influences, they are mainly mediated by neural and hormonal mechanisms. The **neural control mechanisms** for emotion are divided into **peripheral and central** mechanisms.

Peripheral Control of Emotion

The main output pathway for emotional responses is the autonomic nervous system. The pattern of ***autonomic activation*** depends on the type of emotion.

- The emotion of fear and rage closely resembles the effects of injection of norepinephrine. Thus, it is clear that emotional responses of fear and anger are mediated by **sympathetic activation**.

Central Control of Emotion

Emotional responses have been experimentally seen to occur in the absence of cortex. **Hypothalamus and other limbic structures** are important for expression of emotion.

- As suggested by Papez, for emotional expression and experience, the sensory information from environment passes through the **thalamus to the hypothalamus**.
- From hypothalamus, projections are divided into **ascending and descending outputs**.

Ascending Output: The ascending output reaches anterior thalamus via mamillothalamic tract and from there it projects **to cingulate cortex**. The cingulate cortex interacts with the cortical signals. The cingulate gyrus projects to hippocampus. The circuit is completed by the hippocampus projecting back to the hypothalamus.

Descending Output: The descending output of the hypothalamus is directed **to the brainstem and spinal cord centers** from where autonomic fibers originate. The autonomic output is primary basis for manifestations of emotional expression.

Role of Limbic System

Limbic system receives both exteroceptive and interoceptive sensory inputs.

1. **Exteroceptive inputs** reach limbic system via **two ways**; first, through collaterals arising from ascending sensory projections before the fibers reach cortical

areas, and second, form sensory cortex.

2. **Interoceptive inputs** reach hypothalamic and amygdalar nuclei of limbic system from brainstem especially from the nucleus tractus solitarius.

The major output of limbic system to autonomic control areas is via its connections with brainstem and spinal cord.

- Amygdala has direct connections with hypothalamus and brainstem autonomic areas.
- The Papez circuit forms the limbic-hypothalamic connections for emotional expression through autonomic pathways.

APPLIED PHYSIOLOGY

Psychosurgery

In 1935, John Fulton observed that frontal lobotomy in monkeys cures experimentally induced neurosis.

- Since then, **selected lesions of the brain, especially of the limbic areas** have been performed for the treatment of psychiatric disorders, which are popularly known as psychosurgery.
- Psychosurgery is usually used for the treatment of psychiatric illness in which extremes of aggression is the main symptom.

Types of Emotional Disturbances

1. Disturbances of emotionality due to perceptual or cognitive abnormalities
   a. Perceptual dysfunction: illusion and hallucination
   b. Cognitive disorder: delusion
2. Disinhibition of emotional expressions
   a. Emotional lability
   b. Pathological laughing and crying
3. Rage reaction and aggressiveness
4. Apathy and placidity: Klüver-Bucy syndrome & others
5. Altered sexuality
6. Endogenous fear, anxiety, depression and euphoria

Klüver-Bucy Syndrome

Klüver-Bucy syndrome (was first described by **H. Klüver and P. C. Bucy**) is experimentally induced in rhesus monkey by **bilateral temporal lobectomy, particularly involving the amygdala**.

- Animal exhibits placidity and inability to recognize object visually inspite of good vision (**visual agnosia**), but will pick up almost all objects and **explore them orally**.
- They also show **hypersexuality and hyperphagia** (ominiphagic).
  - The striking abnormality is to **examine everything orally**.
- Animal fails to ignore peripheral stimuli (**hypermetamorphosis**), and therefore, **respond to every stimulus and explore everything**.

Similar picture is observed in human beings following bilateral surgical **removal of temporal lobes, cerebral atrophies and meningoencephalitis** following toxoplasmosis, herpes simplex or AIDS.

Exam Questions

1. Describe the connections and functions of limbic system.
2. Draw a diagram to depict Papez circuit. Describe the functions of aminergic and cholinergic systems of the brain.
3. Describe the physiology of motivation and emotion. Add a note on Klüver-Bucy syndrome.

Multiple Choice Questions

1. The nucleus involved in formation of Papez circuit is:
A. Pulvinar B. Intralaminar
C. VPL nucleus D. Anterior nucleus of Thalamus

2. Window of limbic system:
A. Hypothalamus B. Amygdale
C. Hippocampus D. Thalamus

3. Functions of limbic system are all EXCEPT:
A. Emotion B. Memory
C. Higher functions D. Planned motor activity

4. Which of the following statements about 'Sham Rage' is not true?
A. Caused by hypothalamic stimulation
B. Abolished by decortications
C. Pathological rage reaction
D. Association with sympathetic stimulation

5. Which of the following is not a feature of Kluver-Bucy syndrome?
A. Hypersexuality
B. Hypophagia
C. Visual agnosia
D. Respond to every stimulus and explore everything

6. Which of the following neurotransmitter is mainly involved in motivation?
A. Serotonin
B. Histamine
C. Dopamine
D. Epinephrine

7. Which of the following is main center of motivation?
A. Nucleus accumbens
B. Amygdala
C. Hippocampus
D. Septum

Answers

1. D **2.** B **3.** D **4.** B **5.** B **6.** C **7.** A

Chapter 114

PY10.9

Physiology of Learning and Memory

Learning Objectives

On completion of study of this chapter:

The student will be able to (must know):

1. Define and classify learning and memory and give examples for each category.
2. Briefly explain the mechanism and significance of conditioned reflexes.
3. Describe the mechanism of learning and memory.
4. Name the brain areas involved in different types of learning and memory.
5. Outline the physiological basis of abnormalities of learning and memory.

The student may also be able to (desirable to know):

1. Describe physiological basis abnormalities of learning and memory.

DEFINITIONS

Learning

Learning is defined as **acquirement of information or knowledge by experience** that results in the alteration of behavior.

- Learning is the sincere *attitude and readiness to perform an assigned task.*
- It depends mostly on **motivation** that creates adequate interest and attention to promote learning.

Memory

Memory is defined as **retention of learned information and experiences**. The stored information should be retrieved and utilized at any time in life whenever needed. Thus, memory has **four stages**:

1. **Registration of memory that includes proper perception and attention:** Failure of learning and memory occurs due to impaired perception and attention because the material to be learned is never registered and assimilated (Application Box 113. 1).
2. **Integration and retention:** Learned experiences are processed and integrated by various structures in CNS and then retained at appropriate place in the brain in the form of short-term or long-term memory.
3. **Recognition and recall:** At the appropriate time and place, memory is recalled for proper use.
4. **Reutilization:** Memory (the learned experience) is utilized for improvement of further learning.

Application Box 113.1

Anterograde and retrograde amnesias: When information can't be correctly registered and can't be retained for more than few minutes, anterograde amnesia (failure of learning) occurs, and when there is defect in recall and reproduction of memories that have been formed several days, weeks or years before, retrograde *amnesia* occurs (for details, see below).

TYPES OF MEMORY

Memory is broadly divided into explicit or **declarative memory** and implicit or **nondeclarative memory**.

I. **Explicit or declarative memory** (memory of facts i. e. semantic memory, and memory of events (episodic memory)
   1. Short-term memory
   2. Long-term memory

II. **Implicit or nondeclarative memory**
   1. Priming
   2. Procedural memory
      - Skills and habits
   3. Associative learning
      a. Classical conditioning
      b. Operant conditioning
   4. Nonassociative learning
      a. Habituation
      b. Sensitization

Explicit memory and many forms of implicit memory involve short-term and long-term memory.

Explicit Memory

The explicit memory, also known as **declarative memory** is connected with awareness.

- It has **two forms**: the memories of events (*episodic memory*), and the memories of facts (*semantic memory*).
- The **declarative memory** is dependent on the **hippocampus** and other parts of the medial temporal lobes of the brain for its retention.

Short-Term Memory

- Short-term memory is the memory that *lasts for seconds to hours*, during which processing in the hippocampus and elsewhere lays down long-term changes in synaptic strength.
- **Working memory** is a form of short-term memory that makes information available for a brief period.
  - As a result of repeated training, short-term memory can be transferred into long-term memory, which depends on a process called **consolidation**.
- During short-term memory, the memory traces are subject to disruption by trauma and various drugs.

Long-Term Memory

- Long-term memory is the one that *stores information for years together*, and sometimes for life.
- Long-term memory traces are remarkably resistant to disruption.
- This is broadly divided into explicit and implicit memory. Some forms of implicit memories also involve short-term and long-term memories.

Implicit Memory

The implicit memory is not associated with awareness and is therefore also called as **reflexive or nondeclarative memory**.

1. It includes **skills, habits, priming and conditioned reflexes** etc.
2. Explicit memory is initially required to develop implicit memory. For example, a learner of motorcycle riding initially remembers the steps of changing the gear (he changes gears with conscious knowledge) till it becomes a reflexive habit to do so (he changes gear without awareness). Once skill is acquired, the acts become unconscious and automatic.

Priming

Priming is the facilitation of recognition of words or objects **by prior exposure** to them. An example is improved recall of a word when presented with first few letters of it.

Procedural Memory

Includes **skills and habits**, which once acquired become unconscious and automatic.

Nonassociative Learning

The organism learns about a single stimulus. Examples are habituation and sensitization.

Habituation:

- Habituation is a simple form of learning in which ***repeated application of a neutral stimulus elicits less and less response.***
- Habituation implies learning and therefore can be studied for its cellular mechanisms.
  - It can be **short-term**, or it can be **prolonged** if exposure to the benign stimulus is repeated many times.
- Habituation is a classic example of **nonassociative learning**.

Sensitization:

- Sensitization is the opposite reaction in which ***repeated application of stimulus evokes greater and greater response.***
  - Sensitization occurs especially when the stimulus to which habituation has developed is **coupled with a pleasant or unpleasant stimulus.**
  - For example, application of noxious stimulus to gill results in greater withdrawal of gill (an increased responsiveness).
- Sensitization may occur as a **transient response**, or if it is reinforced by additional pairings of the noxious stimulus and the initial stimulus, it can exhibit **features of short-term or long-term memory**.

Associative Learning

The organism learns about the **relation of one stimulus with other**. The classical example is *conditioned response*.

Conditioned Reflexes

Definition

Reflex response to a stimulus that hardly elicited any response in the past, but presently the **response to the stimulus is acquired by pairing the stimulus with another stimulus** that normally produces the response, is called a conditioned response.

Types of Conditioned Reflexes

There are **two types** of conditioned responses: **classical conditioning and operant conditioning**.

- Conditioned reflexes have two components that *are associated with* **emotional responses** and **motor responses**.
- The emotional responses are regulated by **amygdala** and the motor responses are controlled by **cerebellum**.

Classical Conditioning

1. In classic conditioning, in the beginning, there is a stimulus that **normally elicits a specific innate response** (the response which is already present

without training).
- The stimulus is called **unconditioned stimulus** (UCS).

2. Later, an arbitrary stimulus that normally does not produce any response, on application does produce a **significant response** when ***paired with*** the UCS.
    - The stimulus is called **conditioned stimulus** (CS).
3. The typical example of classic conditioning is the **Ian Pavlov's experiment** on salivation in dog. First, Pavlov produced salivation in dog by placing a piece of meat in its mouth. Then, he rang a bell just before placing meat in dog's mouth, and repeated the procedure a number of times till the animal was made to salivate with bell-ringing, and finally without even placing meat in the mouth.
    - In this experiment, salivation in dog by **placing meat in the mouth is the UCS** and **bell ringing is the CS**.
    - **Salivation in response to CS** (sound of the bell) occurred by pairing it sufficient number of times with UCS (placing meat in the mouth).
4. Finally, CS produces the response even in the absence of UCS, which is initially evoked only by UCS.

Significant contribution of Scientist

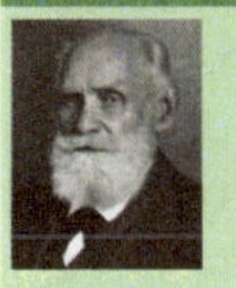

Ivan Petrovich Pavlov (1849 – 1936), a skillful experimental physiologist, Pavlov described the concepts of **conditioned reflex action**. He is popularly known for the conditioned experiments of salivation he carried on dogs. He received the **Nobel Prize in Physiology or Medicine** in 1904.

Inhibition of Conditioned Reflex: Conditioned reflexes can be inhibited in **two ways**: internal and external inhibitions.
- If the CS is presented indefinitely without UCS, the response decreases and eventually stops. This is called **internal inhibition** or extinction.
- Conditioned reflex response can also be abolished if animal is disturbed externally just after the application of CS. This is called **external inhibition**.

Reinforcement of Conditioned Reflex: It is difficult to maintain conditioned reflex indefinitely.
- However, if CS is paired repeatedly with UCS from time to time, **conditioned reflex becomes permanent** (***reinforcement*** *of conditioned reflex*).
- **Conditioned reflex can also be strongly formed** by associating UCS with a **pleasant or unpleasant affect**. Accordingly, there are two types of reinforcements: Positive and negative reinforcement.
    - If the UCS is associated with a pleasant affect, **positive reinforcement** occurs and if associated with an unpleasant affect, **negative reinforcement** occurs (Application Box 114.2).

Application Box 114.2

Physiological utility of conditioned reflexes: A number of autonomic changes (somatic and visceral) can be achieved by conditioning. For example, heart and blood pressure can be decreased by appropriate conditioning. This method has been successfully tried for the treatment of hypertension. The conditioning of visceral responses is known as **biofeedback**.

Operant Conditioning

1. In this type of conditioning, animal is trained to carry out a task for either **to receive a reward or to avoid a punishment**.
2. The UCS may be a **pleasant or unpleasant event**. The CS is applied as a signal in the form of light or sound that alerts the animal to perform.
3. **B. F. Skinner** had extensively studied this type of conditioning. The animal, usually a rat is kept in the **Skinner box**, in which provision is made in such a way that pressing a bar results in delivery of food pallet, or prevention of an electric shock.
    - Initially, the response occurs by chance. However, later response occurs with greater probability as reward follows the response (animal learns that food is obtained by pressing the bar or the shock is prevented).
    - Thus, the reinforcement may be a **positive reinforcement** (by pressing bar animal gets food), or a **negative reinforcement** (by pressing bar animal prevents electric shock).
4. Conditioned motor response results in **avoidance of electric shock**.
    - Therefore, this is also called **conditioned avoidance reflex** or **aversion conditioning** (Application Box 114.3).
5. Another example of negative reinforcement (conditioned avoidance reflex) if **food aversion conditioning**, in which animal severely develops aversion to a particular food, if the taste of food (UCS) is coupled with injection of a chemical that develops physical illness (CS).

Application Box 114.3

Physiological utility of operant conditioning: Aversion conditioning occurs in human beings. Food aversion is very strong in humans if the food is associated with illness developed by application of a CS. It develops strongly even in single pairing of UCS with CS, and even persists after separation of CS from UCS. This helps in avoiding ingestion of poisonous foods.

MECHANISMS OF LEARNING AND MEMORY

Mechanisms underlying learning and memory may be divided into **cellular (molecular), neural and biochemical mechanisms**.

Molecular Mechanisms

Learning and memory are initiated and established by several neurochemical changes like increased synaptic connection, neurotransmitter secretion, formation of intracellular second messenger, protein synthesis and gene activation.

Sensitization and Habituation

Habituation: Habituation occurs due to **decreased neurotransmitter release** from the presynaptic sensory ending in response to repeated application of a particular stimulus.

- ***Serotonin secretion decreases*** from the modulator neuron.
- The stimuli gradually **inactivate calcium channel** resulting in **decreased calcium content** at the presynaptic terminal that in turn inhibit neurotransmitter release.

Sensitization: Sensitization occurs due to **prolongation of action potential** in the sensory endings that results in **increase in intracellular calcium**, which in turn **increases neurotransmitter release**.

- **Serotonin released from modulator neurons** has been identified to be the mediator.
- **In sensitization**, serotonin secretion is increased at the target sensory neurons.
  - In the sea snail Aplysia, the noxious stimulus causes **discharge of serotonergic neurons** that end on presynaptic endings of sensory neurons.
- Thus, sensitization is due to **presynaptic facilitation**.
  - Serotonin *activates cyclic AMP* in the sensory neuron terminal. Cyclic AMP phosphorylates one set of K^+ channels that **closes the K^+ channels**.
  - This results in slowing of repolarization and prolongation of action potential.
  - This facilitates **voltage dependent calcium influx** into the sensory terminal that increases release of transmitter by exocytosis.
- The **short-term prolongation** of sensitization is due to a ***calcium-mediated change*** in adenylyl cyclase that leads to a greater production of cAMP.
- The **long-term potentiation** also involves ***protein synthesis*** and ***growth*** of the presynaptic and postsynaptic neurons and their connections.

Conditioned Reflexes

In classical conditioning, pairing of UCS with CS causes biochemical changes in target neurons. The basic mechanism involved is the **prolongation of action potential** that causes **presynaptic facilitation**.

- For the classic conditioned reflex to develop, it is important that the **UCS should come soon after the CS** to cause a temporal association.
- The UCS acts on neurons that are activated by CS.
  - UCS **increases calcium in the presynaptic terminal**.
  - The long-term increase in presynaptic calcium alters **adenylyl cyclase activity**.
- Thus, when CS **activates the presynaptic neuron**, adenylyl cyclase is activated to a greater extent that forms **more and more cAMP**.
  - Increased cAMP causes ***phosphorylation of a set of K^+ channels*** *and closes the channel.*
  - This slows the repolarization and **prolongs the action potential**.

Post-tetanic Potentiation

This is the production of **enhanced postsynaptic potentials** in response to stimulations. This enhancement lasts upto 60 seconds and occurs after a brief (tetanizing) train of stimuli in the presynaptic neuron.

- The tetanizing stimulation causes **Ca^{++} to accumulate** in the presynaptic neuron to such a degree that the intracellular binding sites that keep cytoplasmic Ca^{++} low, are overwhelmed.

Learning and Long-Term Potentiation

The physiological process of learning is inadequately explained due to the complex mechanisms involved in it.

1. Repeated stimulation of presynaptic neurons results in change in excitability of postsynaptic neurons by altering the rate of discharge, **new protein synthesis and neurotransmitter release**. These changes are found to be associated with learning.
2. Long-term potentiation (LTP) is an important process for establishment of learning and memory.
   - Unlike post-tetanic potentiation, it is initiated by an **increase in intracellular Ca^{++}** in the postsynaptic rather than the presynaptic neuron.
   - Increased excitability and ***change in intracellular protein*** formation by repeated synaptic stimulation are known mechanisms of LTP.
3. In LTP, the initial step is the **phosphorylation of a number of proteins** that are stimulated by formation of receptor-mediated second messengers.
   - Phosphorylation of proteins activates various **intracellular enzymes** and alters **neuronal excitability**.
4. In the later stage of LTP, the **synaptic connections** between neurons increase.

LTP occurs in the **hippocampus** in mammals. This is a process of potentiation of impulse transmission in neuronal pathways in hippocampus that lasts for **days to weeks** when they are stimulated at a high frequency. The potentiation is **mediated by calcium influx**.

Hippocampal LTP: Hippocampal LTP is of **two types**: the mossy fiber LTP and Schaffer collateral LTP.

1. **The mossy fiber LTP** is NMDA independent.

- It is mediated by presynaptic mechanisms that involve cAMP and I_h, a hyperpolarization-activated cation channel.

2. **The Schaffer collateral LTP** is initiated by increased ***intracellular calcium*** in the postsynaptic neuron and depends on NMDA receptors.
   - Increased calcium level makes glutamate receptors accessible to glutamate molecules.

In the amygdala, NMDA-independent LTP is produced in GABAergic neurons.

Long-Term Depression

Though long-Term Depression (LTD) was first described in the hippocampus, it was subsequently demonstrated in all the fibers as for LTP.

- LTD is just the opposite of LTP. It is mainly characterized by a **decrease in synaptic strength**.
  - It is demonstrated by slower stimulation of presynaptic neurons and there is smaller rise in intracellular Ca^{++} compare to that as occurs in LTP.
- **In cerebellum**, LTD requires ***phosphorylation of the GluR2 subunit*** of AMPA (α–Amino-3-hydroxy-5-Methylisooxazole-4-Propionic acid) receptors, which may be involved in motor learning.

Neural Mechanisms

Brain Regions Involved

Three brain regions that have been thoroughly studied in experimental animals (especially in monkey and rat) to understand learning and memory are: prefrontal cortex, inferotemporal cortex and hippocampus.

Prefrontal Cortex

- Removal of the frontal lobes in monkeys resulted in delayed response to different memory tasks. It was suggested that spatial short-term memory resides in the frontal lobes.
- It was further investigated by ablation studies that spatial short-term memory (see below) is the function of **dorsolateral frontal cortex**.
- Thalamic fibers concerned with memory project to prefrontal cortex and from there *to the basal forebrain*. From basal forebrain, fibers project to *amygdala, hippocampus and neocortex*. These fibers are **mainly cholinergic fibers**.

Inferotemporal Cortex

- Lesion of this part of the cortex interferes with visual discrimination, whereas tactile, auditory or olfactory cues remain unaffected.
- The integrity of pre-frontal and inferotemporal cortices is required for performance of tasks that are relatively difficult. Thus it appears that neural substrates for learning are task specific.

Hippocampus

- Hippocampus is an important component of the Papez circuit, which is extensively connected with, hypothalamus, thalamus, amygdala and septum.
- The *combined lesions of the hippocampus and the amygdala produce significant amnesia* than the individual lesions.
  - The neural basis of learning involves the substrates of reward.
  - The hippocampus and medial forebrain bundle are important structures of the reward system.
- Prefrontal cortex, the seat of working memory is connected with hippocampus and parahippocampal portion of medial temporal lobe.
- Bilateral destruction of ventral hippocampus in humans causes **striking deficit in short-term memory**. They have intact working memory and remote memory.
  - They are capable of learning new tasks and retaining pre-lesion remote memories.
  - However, they can not form new long-term memory.
- Hippocampal connections with mammillary body (hypothalamus), amygdala and thalamus are also involved in memory.
- *Lesion of mammillary body or thalamus causes impairment of recent memory*. Hippocampal connection with amygdala is *concerned with emotions related to memory*.

By MRI and evoked potential studies, recently it has been observed in humans that **activity in left parahippocampal cortex and left frontal lobe** increases when they recall words and activity in right parahippocampal cortex and right frontal lobe increases when they recall pictures.

- New neurons are formed in hippocampus in response to learning and memory (Application Box 114.4)

> **Application Box 114.4**
>
> **New brain cells are formed in hippocampus:** Now it has been documented that the new neurons are formed from stem cells throughout life in two brain structures: the olfactory bulb and the hippocampus. The process of formation of new neurons is called neurogenesis. In hippocampus, neurogenesis has been observed with learning and memory and decrease in the number of new neurons formed in hippocampus is proposed to decrease the hippocampal memory production.

Neural Mechanisms of Declarative and Procedural Memory

Declarative Memory

Declarative memory refers to the **memory of events and facts and the ability to knowingly access them**.

- Declarative memory is integrated in ***medial portion of the temporal lobe***.
- Patients, who have undergone bilateral medial temporal lobectomy, for example for the treatment of intractable temporal lobe epilepsy) lose their declarative

memories or become incapable in forming new declarative memory, but retain procedural memory.

Procedural Memory

Procedural memory refers to the **ability to learn and remember new skills and procedures.**

- Procedural memory is integrated in **different parts** of the brain, depending on type of tasks learned and remembered.
  - Learning and remembering **new motor skills and habits** require the ***striatum, motor cortex, and cerebellum.***
- Remembering **emotional components** associated with tasks and skills require the ***amygdala.***
- Learning the **conditioned reflexes** requires the ***cerebellum and cortex.*** The medial temporal lobe is not involved in procedural memory.

Neural Mechanisms of Short-Term and Long-Term Memory

Short-Term Memory

Learned experiences that are newly and recently acquired **can be easily recalled** using short-term memory. For example, before an individual dials a telephone number, first he sees the number and repeats that mentally till the number is dialed, and then he forgets the number quickly once he starts talking on phone. This is a form of **working memory.**

- However, if the number is repeatedly used or is an important number, the number is stored in the memory for a longer duration.
  - Thus, the permanent storage of information is based **on its importance or its repeated use** or on whether it is associated with an **important or emotional event.**
- For memory to become more permanent, processing occurs in subcortical areas that mainly **involve hippocampus.**

Working Memory: Working memory makes the information available for a brief period.

1. The center for working memory is the **prefrontal cortex.**
2. Working memory has **two components**: *verbal component* that retains the verbal memory and *visuospatial component* that retains the visual and spatial aspects of the objects (**spatial short-term memory**).

Long-Term Memory

The short-term memory is converted to long-term memory mainly by ***three ways***:

i) By **repeating the process** of learning frequently.
ii) By **adding more than one sensory modality** to the process of learning, for example writing and at the same time also hearing a newly acquired acknowledge.
iii) By **associating the process** of a particular learning with a ***meaningful emotional event.***

Consolidation: The process of permanent storage of memory is called **consolidation.**

1. **Hippocampus** plays an important role in consolidating memory, which is ***reinforced by an emotional state*** that is associated with the learning or the experience.
2. The **medial temporal lobe** is important for long-term declarative memory formation, especially the ***hippocampal and parahippocampal cortices.*** However, the hippocampus is *not required for* subsequent retrieval of long-term memory.
3. Long-term memories are **stored in various parts of the neocortex.**
   - Various components of long-term memory reside **in concerned cortical regions.** For example, visual and auditory parts of memories are located in visual and auditory cortex respectively.
   - Therefore, once long-term memories are established, they can ***readily be recalled by association with similar events*** (visual, auditory, olfactory or somatosensory) later in life.

Intercortical Transfer of Memory: Memory is transferred from one cortical hemisphere to the other **through corpus** callosum and the **commissural fibers** (anterior and posterior).

- If these fibers are sectioned, then the no memory transfer occurs.
- If an animal (cat or monkey) is shown and taught some task with one eye (other eye blindfolded), and then the blindfold is transferred to the other eye, the animal remembers the task and can perform it.
- But, if the optic chiasm and corpus callosum is cut, it can't perform the task as it can't remember what has been learned with the other eye. This is called **split brain animal.**

Neural Mechanisms of Learning

Prefrontal cortex is critical for coordinating the process of learning and memory.

1. The cerebral cortex processes information related to learning and communicates them to the limbic structures.
   - The prefrontal cortex gathers sensory information from the somatosensory, visual and auditory cortices.
   - **Prefrontal cortex** integrates inputs related to ***language and mathematical ability*** in the light of previously acquired learning.
2. The prefrontal cortex is considered as the ***site of working memory.***
   - New experiences are processed in the prefrontal cortex.

- The processed information is then transmitted **to the hippocampus**.

3. **Consolidation of information** *occurs in hippocampus* over several hours into a lasting from.
4. Then, the learned experience is ***stored in the association cortices***, from where it can be retrieved whenever needed.

Role of Cholinergic Neurons in Memory

Acetylcholine is the major transmitter in learning and memory, and other cognitive function.

1. **Cholinergic neurons** that are present plentily in **basal forebrain region** project heavily to the hippocampus and different parts of cerebral cortex.
   - The cell bodies of these cholinergic neurons are **highly concentrated in basal forebrain nuclei** especially in the **nucleus basalis of Meynert** and the **nucleus accumbens.**
   - Cholinergic fibers are also **main projecting neurons** from brainstem reticular formation (mainly from pedunculopontine nucleus) to the thalamus and spinal cord.
   - More than 90% of projections from brainstem to thalamic nuclei are cholinergic.
2. **Loss of cortical and subcortical cholinergic neurons**, especially in the basal forebrain region is associated with **dementia**, an impairment of memory, abstract thinking, and judgment.

Brain areas for Integration of Various forms of Memory

1. **Explicit or declarative memory** (facts and events): Medial temporal lobe

Short-term memory : Hippocampus
Working memory : Prefrontal cortex
Long-term memory : Various parts of neocortex

2. **Implicit or nondeclarative memory**

Priming : Neocortex
Procedural memory : Striatum
(Skills and habits)
Associative learning (Classical and operant conditioning)
Emotional responses : Amygdala
Skeletal musculature : Cerebellum
Nonassociative learning : Reflex pathways
(Habituation & sensitization)

Biochemical Basis

Changes underlying learning is the **repeated transmission of impulses** along neural circuits that results in permanent changes in the concerned neurons.

- One important consequence is the **new protein formation** in the nerve cells.
- **Increased RNA synthesis** in response to learning has been well documented.
- Recently it has been suggested that ***activation of specific gene*** is responsible for learning.

Strangeness and Familiarity

Stimulation of some parts of the temporal lobes causes change in interpretation of one's surroundings such as the subject **feels strange** in a familiar place or **familiarity** with the new events.

- Such of strangeness or familiarity helps the normal individual to adjust to different environments. But, inappropriate feeling of familiarity with new events or surroundings is clinically known as the **déjà vu phenomenon**, (a French word, which means 'already seen'.
- This phenomenon may occur in normal individuals. However, this usually occurs as **an aura** that precedes the ***onset of temporal lobe epilepsy***.

APPLIED PHYSIOLOGY

Amnesia

Amnesia means **impairment of memory**. There are *two forms* of amnesia: retrograde amnesia and anterograde amnesia.

Retrograde Amnesia: Loss of memory for ***events that just precede the head injury*** *or the disease* is called retrograde amnesia.

1. Usually, the loss occurs only for short-term memory.
2. Retrograde amnesia occurs commonly in head injury in which patient **develops concussion**.

Anterograde Amnesia: Inability to recall the memory or to form new memories ***after the event*** (head injury, mental shock or disease) is called anterograde amnesia. Anterograde amnesia also follows head injury but the duration covered by the amnesia usually shortens with time.

Dementia

Dementia is a syndrome consisting of several intellectual inabilities.

- The **deficits occur for many cognitive functions including learning and memory**.
- It occurs in many conditions that affect cortical functions. The commonest is the **senile dementia**.
- Pathological dementia is commonly seen in neurodegenerative diseases like *Alzheimer's disease*.
- However, **drug induced dementia** and **alcoholic dementias** are not uncommon.

Alzheimer's Disease

Alzheimer's disease is the common degenerative disease of the brain characterized mainly by **premature and progressive dementia**.

Etiology

There is **severe loss of cholinergic neurons** projecting from basal forebrain to neocortex, amygdala and hippocampus.

- Especially, fibers **projecting from nucleus basalis of Meynert** (substantia innominata) are severely affected.
- Cerebral atrophy mainly involves **frontal, temporal and parietal lobes**.
- **Pronounced neuronal loss** occurs in hippocampus, entorhinal cortex, parahippocampal gyri and subiculum.

Pathology

Three pathologic features are characteristic of the disease.

1. Presence of ***neurofibrillary "tangles"*** in the nerve cell cytoplasm is the cytopathologic ***hallmark of the disease***.
   - These tangles are fiber-like strands composed of hyperphosphorylated form of ***microtubular protein*** "tau".
   - They appear like pairs of helical filaments.
2. Other characteristic feature is the appearance of ***neuritic plaques*** scattered throughout the cerebral cortex.
   - The plaques contain amyloid protein (amyloid β protein or *Aβ protein*) as the central core surrounded by degenerating nerve terminals.
3. ***Granulovacular degeneration*** of neurons, especially in pyramidal layer of hippocampus.

Role of APP: Normally, **amyloid precursor protein** (APP) is secreted from nerve cells. APP is hydrolyzed by the enzyme γ-secretase to **form Aβ protein**. This protein is hydrolyzed at ***three different sites*** by α-secretase, β-secretase, and γ-secretase, respectively.

- If APP is hydrolyzed by α-secretase, nontoxic peptide products are produced.
- But, if APP is hydrolyzed by β-secretase and γ-secretase, polypeptides with 40 to 42 amino acids are produced, that are toxic in nature.
- The most toxic among them is **A**$\beta\sigma_{1\text{-}42}$.

These **toxic polypeptides** form extracellular aggregates that can bind to AMPA receptors. They also bind to Ca^{2+} ion channels and increase Ca^{2+} influx.

1. They also **induce inflammatory responses and produce intracellular tangles.**
   - Eventually, the affected cells die.
1. Excessive and abnormal **hydrolysis of APP** results in more production of ***Aβ proteins*** that form **neuritic plaques**.
3. Neuritic plaques induce inflammatory reactions, tangle formation, oxidative damage and neuronal degeneration (especially cholinergic neurons).

Features

1. Usually the patient is above 50 years.
2. **Progressive development of forgetfulness** is the major symptom.
3. The disease starts with **loss of short-term memory** and later followed **by loss of other cognitive functions**.
4. **Dysnomia** (forgetting words especially names), visuospatial disorientation, and **paranoia** and other personality changes usually occur.

Treatment

1. Cerebral vasodilators, stimulants, and high dose of vitamin B, C, E have beneficial effects.
2. Trials of oral physostigmine, choline, lecithin and cholinergic precursor and agonists have yielded some results.

Exam Questions

1. Describe the mechanisms of learning and memory.
2. Describe neural mechanisms of learning and memory. Add a note on conditioned reflexes.
3. Describe molecular mechanisms of learning and memory. Add a note on Alzheimer's disease.

Multiple Choice Questions

1. The mechanism of learning and memory, include all EXCEPT:
A. Changes in level of neurotransmitter at synapse
B. Increasing protein synthesis
C. Recruitment by multiplication of neurons
D. Spatial reorganization of synapse

2. The processing of short-term memory to long-term memory is done (consolidation of long term memory occurs) in:
A. Prefrontal cortex B. Hippocampus
C. Neocortex D. Amygdala

3. Associative learning is:
A. Associated with consciousness
B. Includes skill and habits
C. Relation of one stimulus to another
D. Facilitation of recognition of words

4. Striatum damage affects primarily:
A. Procedural memory B. Short term memory
C. Long term memory D. Explicit memory

Answers 1. C 2. B 3. C 4. A

Chapter 115

PY10.9

Physiology of Language and Speech

Learning Objectives

On completion of study of this chapter:

The student will be able to (must know):

1. Name the speech areas in the brain and give their functions.
2. Trace the pathway for speech.
3. Understand the theory of speech production.
4. Name speech and language disorders and understand the physiological basis.

The student may also be able to (desirable to know):

1. Describe the neurophysiology of language and speech

LANGUAGE AND SPEECH AREAS IN THE BRAIN

There are **four main areas** in the brain that play important role in the processing of language and speech. These **four areas** are collectively known **language zone** that are present around the Sylvain fissure (therefore, also called **perisylvian areas**).

Two are called *receptive areas* and two are called *executive areas* (Fig. 115.1).

All these areas are located in association cortex, adjacent to cortical areas that are essential in language formation.

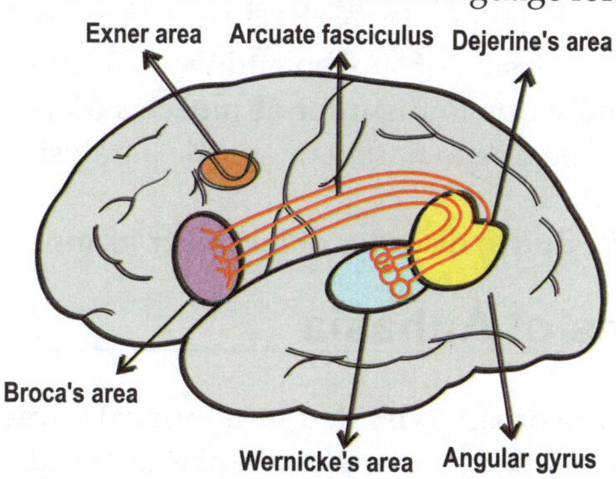

Fig. 115.1: Areas in the brain concerned with language functions.

Receptive Areas

The receptive areas are also called sensory speech areas as they receive and process the sensory information for speech.

- They are **Wernicke's area** (area 22) that subserves the ***perception of spoken language*** and the **angular gyrus** (area 39) that subserve the ***perception of written language***.
- **Area 41 and 42** also are included in receptive areas that take part in ***processing spoken language.***

Wernicke's Area

The area is so named as it was described by **Carl Wernicke** in 1874.

1. Wernicke's area is located in the upper part of the temporal lobe, the area that is in the **parietal-temporal-occipital association cortex**.
2. This is the **major association area for processing sensory information** from the somatic sensory, visual and auditory cortices.
3. Wernicke's area is essential for the **comprehension, recognition, and construction** of words and language.
4. Patients with **lesion in Wernicke's area** may speak, but the words they frame and put together will **have no meaning**.

Angular Gyrus (Area 39)

This is the **second receptive area** that occupies the angular gyrus in the inferior parietal lobule anterior to the visual receptive area. This is also called **Dejerine's area**. This subserves the **perception of written language**.

Executive or Expressive Areas

The executive areas are also called **motor speech areas** as they execute the expression of speech. They are **Broca's area** (area 44 and 45) and **Exner writing area**.

Broca's Area

Broca's area is concerned with **motor aspects of speech**, hence called **motor speech area** (area 44 and 45). This area was described by Paul Broca in 1865.

- It is present in the frontal lobe, which is located in the **prefrontal association cortex**, adjacent to the motor cortex.
- Broca's area regulates functions of the **muscles of the lips, tongue, pharynx and larynx**.
- Patients with **lesion of Broca's area** are capable of comprehending a spoken or written word but they are **not able to say the word**.

Exner Writing Area

Exner writing area is located in the ***posterior part of the frontal lobe*** (though some disagreement exists for this concept). The **visually perceived words are given expression** in writing through this area.

Thus, there are **two parallel systems** for speech. One is for understanding the spoken words and producing speech, and the other for understanding written word and producing writing.

Arcuate Fasciculus

The sensory and motor areas are intricately connected with each other. Especially, a rich network of nerve fiber, the arcuate fasciculus, which passes through the isthmus of temporal lobe and posterior end of the sylvian fissure, **connects Wernicke's area with Broca's area**.

- This fasciculus ***coordinates the understanding and execution of speech and the language skills***.
- Broca's area is further connected with lower rolandic cortex by short association fibers that in turn ***innervate speech apparatus*** (muscles of mouth, tongue and throat).

THEORY OF SPEECH PRODUCTION

Angular gyrus receives visual and auditory inputs and makes **preliminary processing** of these information.

1. Angular gyrus **projects to Wernicke's area**, which is concerned with the **comprehension of visual and auditory information**.
2. Wernicke's area **projects to Broca's area** through arcuate fasciculus, which further processes information received from Wernicke's area into **elaborate process of vocalization** (programming of articulation).
3. Broca's area ***projects to motor cortex*** that brings about the **motor activities of speech apparatus**, which finally produces speech (Fig. 115.2).

Language function is closely associated with the **concept of cerebral dominance**. It is a highly lateralized function of the brain **residing in the left hemisphere** in right handed persons. This dominance is observed also in left-handed individuals (for details see next chapter).

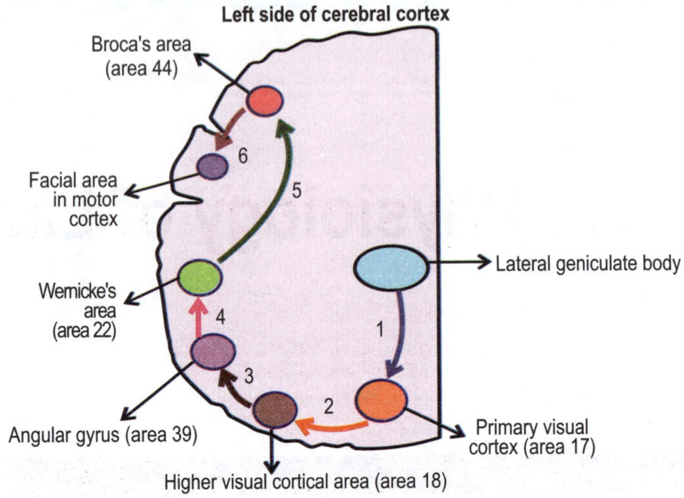

Fig. 115.2: Pathway for speech for naming a visual object.

DISORDERS OF SPEECH & LANGUAGE

Speech and language disorders may be divided into **four categories**.

1. Aphasia or dysphasia

Loss or impairment of production and/or comprehension of spoken or written language due to an acquired lesion of the brain is called aphasia.

2. Disturbances of speech secondary to other global disease

Disturbances of speech or language with diseases that globally affect higher mental function like dementia, in which speech and language functions are impaired as part of the general loss. For example, in Alzheimer's disease gradual loss of all aspects of language function occurs without any specific aphasia. In this category, commonly, **palilalia** (extreme perseveration) and **echolalia** (patient repeats the words he hears like a parrot) are observed.

3. Dysarthria

Defect in articulation of speech with intact mental function and comprehension of spoken and written language. This occurs purely due to **disorder of muscles of articulation**, which may be due to flaccid or spastic paralysis.

4. Aphonia

Loss of voice due to disorder of larynx or its innervation.

Types of Aphasia

Aphasias are broadly divided into **four categories**: Motor aphasia, sensory aphasia, global aphasia and dissociative language syndromes.

Motor Aphasia (Broca's Aphasia)

This is also called **nonfluent aphasia** or **expressive aphasia**.

- This occurs in disease processes that **affect Broca's area**.
- The **primary deficit is in the language output** or speech production, with relative preservation of comprehension.
  - In its **mildest form**, motor speech deficit manifests as ***poverty of speech*** (cortical dysarthria) with preservation of comprehension and ability to write.
  - In **advanced form**, there is ***complete loss*** of power of speaking.
- There is *no paralysis of speech apparatus* as patient can chew, swallow, clear the throat, cry or even vocalize without word.
- Usually, lower part of face, and arm of the right side are weak.

Sensory Aphasia (Wernicke's Aphasia)

This is also called **fluent aphasia** or **receptive aphasia**. This occurs in disease processes that **affect Wernicke's area**. The syndrome comprises of **two main features**:

1. **Impairment of comprehension** of speech, and
2. Relatively fluent, but ***paraphasic speech*** (use of malformed and inappropriate words).

The impairment of comprehension is basically an **inability to differentiate word elements** or phonemes both spoken and written, which indicates the **involvement of auditory and visual association areas**.

- Defect in language manifests by **inability to repeat** written or spoken word.
- Despite fluency in speech, the language is remarkably **devoid of speech**.
- They also **can't understand** of what is said to them.
- The motor apparatus required for expression of language remains intact. **Written letters** are often combined into ***meaningless words***.

Global Aphasia

This occurs due to destruction of large part of language zones involving **both Broca's and Wernicke's areas**.

- The lesion usually occurs due to occlusion of the left internal carotid artery or middle cerebral artery.
- **All aspects of speech and language are affected**.
- At best they may say few simple words, but characteristically they fail to carry out a series of simple commands or name objects.
- They **can't read, write or repeat** what is said to them.
- Usually this syndrome is associated with varying degrees of right hemiplegia, hemianesthesia, and homonymous hemianopia.

Dissociative Language Syndromes

Dissociative language syndromes refer to language deficit that do not result from lesion of cortical language areas, but **from disruption of pathways joining them**. Included in this category are: conduction aphasia, pure word deafness, pure word blindness, pure word mutism, anomic aphasia and transcortical aphasia.

Conduction Aphasia: Occurs due to **separation of auditory and motor language areas** without damaging these areas.

1. Characteristically, **repetition is severely affected** for both single words and nonwords in the face of preserved comprehension.
2. There is fluency and paraphasia in self-initiated speech as seen Wernicke's aphasia.
3. Writing is invariably impaired.

Pure Word Deafness: This is also called **auditory verbal agnosia**, is characterized by impairment of auditory comprehension and repetition and an **inability to write following dictation.**

1. Spontaneous writing and ability to comprehend written language are preserved, that differentiated it from Wernicke's aphasia.
2. They may declare that they may not hear, ***audiometry discloses no hearing defect***.
3. Usually the **lesion is bilateral in superior temporal gyrus.**

Pure Word Blindness: This is also called **visual verbal agnosia**, is characterized by inability to read aloud, to understand written script and to name colors. Therefore, this is also called ***visual verbal color anomia.***

1. Understanding the spoken language, repetition of what is heard, writing spontaneously and to dictation, and conversation are all intact.
2. The striking feature is that capacity to write fluently is retained, but he **can't read what has been written**.
   - This called **alexia without agraphia.**
3. Lesion usually affects **left visual cortex**, geniculocalcarine tract and the connection of the visual cortex of the dominant hemisphere with the language areas.

Pure Word Mutism: The loss of capacity to speak while perfectly retaining the ability to write, to understand spoken words, to read silently with comprehension, and to repeat spoken words is called pure word mutism or **aphemia**. This is also called **pure motor aphasia of Déjerine**. This occurs due vascular lesion or localized injury to the dominant frontal lobe.

Anomic Aphasia: In anomic aphasia, there is no difficulty with speech or understanding the auditory information, but there is **difficulty in understanding written language or picture**.

1. This occurs due to **lesion of angular gyrus in categorical hemisphere** without affecting language areas.

2. The visual information is not transmitted to Wernicke's area.

Transcortical Aphasia: Isolation of language areas due to hypoxic injury as occurs in carbon monoxide poisoning or prolonged hypotension results in this syndrome.

1. Either the motor speech area or the sensory speech area is isolated from rest of the cortex in the same hemisphere.
2. Accordingly it results in **transcortical motor aphasia** (inability to initiate conversational speech with preservation of comprehension and repetition) or **transcortical sensory aphasia** (deficit auditory and visual word, but speech remain fluent and repetition is remarkably preserved).

Other Language Disorders

Agraphias

Agraphia is the **loss of previously possessed ability to communicate through writing**.

1. Though writing is an integral component of language function, many people speak without learning to read or write. Therefore, if someone has already learned writing, and then he loses this ability, agraphia is said to be present.
2. Pure agraphia is very rare.
3. There are **different types of agraphias**: aphasic agraphia, constructional agraphia, apraxic agraphia and linguistic agraphia (beyond the scope to discuss here).

Disorder of Articulation

Impairment of articulation is called **dysarthria**. Articulation consists of contraction of pharynx, palate, tongue and lips that alter the vocal sounds.

1. In pure dysarthria, there is no abnormality of cortical language mechanisms.
2. They *understand perfectly* whatever is heard, and have no difficulty in reading and writing.
3. It is commonly due to **neuromuscular problems**.

Disorder of Phonation

Aphonia is impairment of phonation. It occurs due to **paralysis of vocal cords**. Paralysis of respiratory movements can also produce aphonia because insufficient air is provided for phonation.

Exam Questions

1. Describe the brain areas for speech and language. Give a note on language disorders.
2. Describe the mechanism of speech production. Give a note on ahpasias.

Multiple Choice Questions

1. **Wernicke's area is:**
   A. Area 22
   B. Area 39
   C. Area 42
   D. Area 44
2. **Broca's area is:**
   A. Area 22
   B. Area 39
   C. Area 42
   D. Area 44
3. **Broca's area is present in:**
   A. Superior temporal gyrus
   B. Precentral gyrus
   C. Post central gyrus
   D. Inferior frontal gyrus
4. **Broca's area is concerned with:**
   A. Word formation
   B. Comprehension
   C. Repetition
   D. Reading
5. **Motor aphasia refers to defect in:**
   A. Peripheral speech apparatus
   B. Verbal expression
   C. Auditory comprehension
   D. Verbal comprehension
6. **Of words and language, Wernicke's area is concerned with:**
   A. Comprehension
   B. Recognition
   C. Construction
   D. All of the above
7. **In pure word deafness, the lesion is likely in:**
   A. Superior temporal gyrus
   B. Angular gyrus
   C. Calcarine gyrus
   D. Frontal cortex
8. **In pure word blindness, the lesion is likely in:**
   A. Superior temporal gyrus
   B. Angular gyrus
   C. Geniculocalcarine tract and visual cortex
   D. Frontal cortex

Answers 1. A 2. D 3. D 4. A 5. B 6. D 7. A 8. C

Chapter 116

Neocortex (Association Cortex), Cerebral Asymmetry, Lobes of the Brain and Cortical Plasticity

Learning Objectives

On completion of study of this chapter:

The student will be able to (must know):

1. Name the association cortical areas and list the functions of neocortex.
2. Understand the concept of cerebral asymmetry.
3. Name the lobes of the brain, major areas present in each lobe and give their functions.
4. List the deficit produced by lesion of each lobe of the brain.
5. Appreciate the concept of cortical plasticity.

The student may also be able to (desirable to know):

1. Describe the functional organization and function of neocortex.

NEOCORTEX (ASSOCIATION CORTEX)

Functional Organization

There are **four neocortical or association cortical areas** (Fig. 116.1): Prefrontal association cortex, parietal-occipital-temporal association cortex, temporal association cortex and limbic association cortex.

Frontal or Prefrontal Association Cortex: This consists of rostral part of cerebral hemisphere in front of the premotor area.

Parietal-Temporal-Occipital Association Cortex: This extends between the somatosensory and visual cortices above, and posterior portion of temporal cortex below.

Temporal Association Cortex: This extends from the lower portion of the temporal lobe to the limbic system.

Limbic Association Cortex: The cortical areas associated with limbic system are included in limbic association cortex.

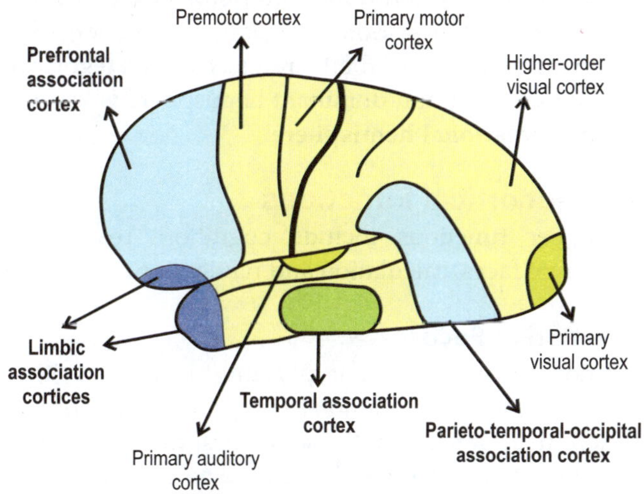

Fig. 116.1: Cortical association areas.

Feedback Control System of Neocortex

The association cortices are part of the **six-layered cortical areas** of gray matter that spreads in the cerebral hemispheres. The connections within the neocortex are a complex network of neurons. Like other cortical areas such as motor cortex, there are **pyramidal and nonpyramidal cells** in association cortices.

A **complex feedback control system** exists within the neocortex.

1. The **descending axons** of pyramidal cell send collaterals that project via association neurons **back to the dendrites** of the cells from which they originate.
   - This forms the anatomical basis for **feedback control**.
   - The other collaterals connect the adjoining cells.
2. The dendrites of cells in the deeper layers receive **inputs from thalamus, reticular formation, and other cortical areas**.

3. Afferents **from thalamus** terminate mainly in *layer IV of the cortex*.
4. The neurons and their connections in the cortex have enormous ability to adapt, called **cortical plasticity**.

Neocortical Functions

Language Functions

The functions of language and speech in humans i.e. to understand the spoken and written words and to express ideas in speech and writing are mainly the function of association cortex located in the perisylvian region or language areas (for details, refer previous chapter).

- However, the language function is **dependent more on one cerebral hemisphere** than on the other.
  - The hemisphere, which is concerned with language, is called as **dominant hemisphere**, and the other hemisphere as **non-dominant hemisphere**.
- Due to its categorization in language function, the dominant hemisphere is better referred to as **categorical hemisphere,** and non-dominant hemisphere is known as **representational hemisphere**.

Other Neocortical Functions

Other higher functions include cognition, reasoning, recognition of faces, calculation and navigation.

Recognition of Faces

Recognition of faces is an important function as it is essential for social and emotional interaction. This is the **function of representational hemisphere**, which is usually the right hemisphere (described below).

- Integration and storage of information regarding recognition of faces occur in the right inferior temporal lobe, that receives visual inputs from objects, particularly the visual impression of faces.
- Lesion in this area results in **prosopagnosia**, the inability to recognize faces.
- They can recognize known people by their voices, but not by seeing their faces.

Calculation

Two brain regions are involved in arithmetic calculations:
1. **inferior part of the left frontal lobe**, the area concerned with actual calculations, and
2. **areas around the intraparietal sulci** of the parietal lobes of both sides, areas concerned with memorizing numbers and finger counting.

Lesion of frontal lobe results in **acalculia** (impairment of mathematical ability).

Navigation

Navigation means **sense of direction-findings**.

- This is a special spatial skill. It is **more developed in man** than in woman. Men usually try to find out the directions themselves when they are lost, whereas women do seek others help for the same.
- **Right side hippocampus**, which is concerned with learning, and the **right caudate nucleus**, which is concerned with movement are the areas involved in navigation.

The actual sites and mechanisms for cognition and reasoning are not known.

CEREBRAL ASYMMETRY (CEREBRAL DOMINANCE)

Concept of Cerebral Asymmetry

Two hemispheres serving discrete functions have been referred to as cerebral asymmetry. Especially, the **functions of language and speech** in humans are more localized in one cerebral hemisphere than in the other.

The hemisphere, which is concerned with language functions, has traditionally been called as **dominant hemisphere**, and the opposite hemisphere as **non-dominant hemisphere**.

1. **One hemisphere is categorized** for language functions.
   - However, this does not mean that the non-dominant hemisphere is less developed.
   - Due to this categorization in language function, the dominant hemisphere is better referred to as **categorical hemisphere**.
2. The other (non-dominant) hemisphere is rather focused in functions **concerned more with visuospatial relations**, i. e., recognizing faces, drawing pictures, identifying objects by their form, recognizing musical themes etc.
   - Therefore, non-dominant hemisphere is better referred to as non-categorical or **representational hemisphere**.
3. Thus, the **categorical hemisphere**, which is usually the *left hemisphere*, is specialized for the ***verbal and sequential processing*** of higher functions and the **representational hemisphere**, which is usually the *right hemisphere*, is specialized in ***nonverbal, nonmathematical and non-sequential processing*** of higher functions, mainly in **visuospatial tasks** such as observing faces.
4. Also, categorical hemisphere ***mediates mathematical learning*** and representational hemisphere ***mediates musical perception***.

Cerebral Lateralization: It is not only the language and visuospatial functions that exhibit preference for their location in one hemisphere, but also the other functions.

- For example, ***volitional control of movement*** *is integrated more in left pre-central motor cortex.*

- **Asymmetry exists also for cognitive and other higher functions** in the cerebral cortex. This was observed by surgical section of corpus callosum (**the split-brain preparation**), which was first undertaken to prevent spread of activation of opposite cortex during an epileptic fit. Studies in subjects with congenital absence of corpus callosum have also revealed the same.
- **Roger Sperry,** the founder of the split-brain preparation had noted in 1950s that "intellectual **left hemisphere is highly evolved** and a relatively retarded right hemisphere generally lack higher cognitive function".
- Hemispheres serving such discrete functions is also called **cerebral lateralization**.

Relation with Handedness

Specialization of hemisphere is **linked to handedness.**

1. About 90% of human populations are right-handed. In **96% of right-handed individuals, left hemisphere is the categorical or dominant hemisphere** (only in 4%, the right hemisphere is dominant).
2. In left-handed individuals also the **left hemisphere is the categorical hemisphere in 70%** and right hemisphere is dominant only in 15% with no clear lateralization in rest 15%.
    - Therefore, the **left hemisphere is often regarded as the dominant hemisphere** (specialized in language functions) and the *right hemisphere as nondominant hemisphere* (specialized in visuospatial functions).
3. Broadly it is stated that the **left hemisphere is meant for vocalization** (speech) and **right hemisphere for recognition of faces.**
4. It has also been observed that **language disorders are more common in left-handers**, though they are more **talented in spatial functions** like music and art.

Anatomical and Biochemical Basis

The functional differences between the two hemispheres may be correlated with their **anatomical variations.**

- The **planum temporale**, an area in the superior temporal gyrus involved in language-related auditory processing, is significantly **larger in the left hemisphere.**
- It has also been confirmed by imaging studies that the **upper surface of the left temporal lobe**, the area primarily concerned with speech and language functions is ***larger in right-handed individuals.***
    - In patients, it has been observed that the **reduction in size of left superior temporal gyrus** is correlated with the ***degree of disorders of thoughts and language.***
- There is also **biochemical differences between the two hemispheres**, though the neurochemical basis of language and other cognitive functions is not clearly known.
    - The **dopamine concentration is high** in the nigrostriatal pathway on the left side of basal ganglia in right-handed individuals.

Effects of Lesions

A small **lesion of the language areas** (as described in previous chapter) ***in the categorical hemisphere produces significant language deficits,*** whereas widespread lesion of the same areas in the representational hemisphere does not.

1. **Lesion in the parietal lobe** of the ***representational hemisphere produces visuospatial deficits*** like *astereognosis* (inability to identify objects by palpating them with eyes closed) and agnosias (***Agnosia*** is loss of ability to interpret sensory stimuli with intact sensory modality).
2. Especially, **lesion of the inferior parietal lobule** in representational hemisphere produces unilateral inattention, called **hemineglect.**
    - These individuals ignore stimuli originating from *the contralateral half of their bodies* though they do not have any primary visual, auditory, or somatosensory deficits.
    - In severe cases, they *do not dress half their bodies,* shave half their faces, eat from half of the plate or even read half of each page.
3. **Mental depression** is more common in patients with diseases affecting ***categorical hemisphere,*** whereas patients may be **euphoric** when diseases involve ***representational hemisphere.***

Physiological Significance

The functional asymmetry perhaps is the **ingenious way of economizing the brain tissue.** By distributing important functions separately to two hemispheres, possibly nature has effectively doubled the capabilities of the brain for its given size.

PY10.7

FUNCTIONS OF DIFFERENT LOBES OF THE BRAIN

Each hemisphere of the brain consists of **four lobes:** Parietal lobe, temporal lobe, occipital lobe and frontal lobe (Fig. 116.2).

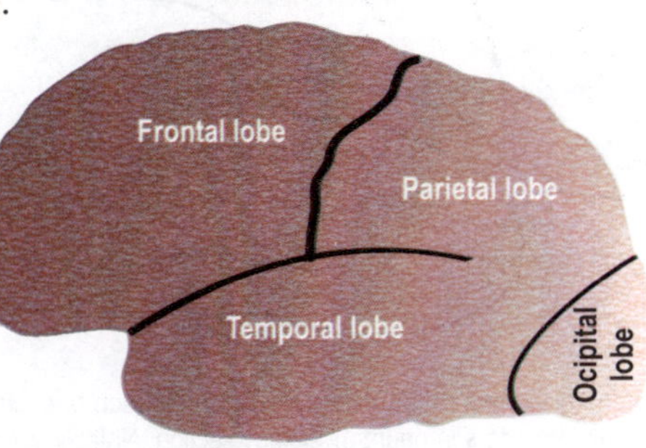

Fig. 116.2: Four lobes (frontal, parietal, temporal, and occipital) of the brain.

Parietal Lobe

Location and Divisions

Parietal lobe lies posterior to the central sulcus and rostrodorsal to lateral sulcus (sylvian fissure). It is divided into **two regions**:

1. **The anterior region** that mainly contains **primary somatosensory cortex** (S I), i. e., the **Brodmann's area 3, 1, and 2.**
2. **The posterior region** that contains other sensory areas, which is considered to be the **association sensory cortex.**
   - This includes the **area 5 and 7** in the upper part, and **area 39 and 40** in the lower part (Fig. 116.3).

Functions

1. **Area 3, 1 and 2** are meant for ***perception of sensations***, especially the cortical sensations (stereognosis, tactile localization and two-point discrimination), fine touch, proprioception and vibration.
2. **Area 5** is more involved in ***processing of somatosensory information*** to produce movement.
3. **Area 7** primarily ***processes visual information*** in order to produce not only ***movement***, but also ***arousal, attention and emotion.***

Effects of Lesions

Lesion of parietal lobe results in following syndromes:

Hemineglect: Patient **neglects contralateral parts of the body** and contralateral portion of the external world.

- In extreme cases, they do not dress half their body, eat only from half of the plate or even read half of each page.

Language Defects: Patients with a left parietal lesion have difficulty with the second half but not the first half of words, both in writing and speaking.

- Some patients with parieto-occipital lesions write only with consonants and omit vowels.

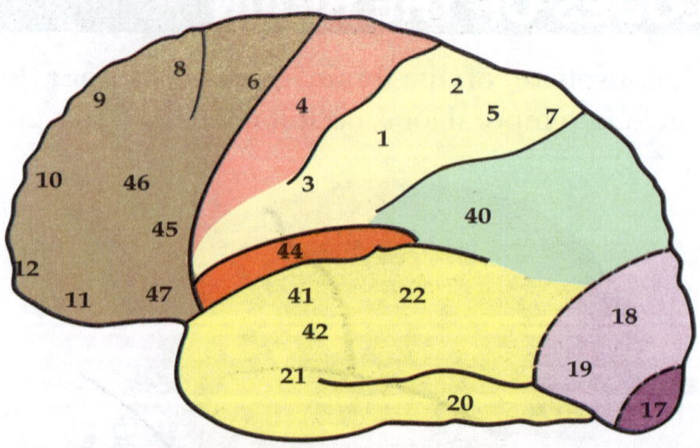

Fig. 116.3: Brodmann's areas in the cerebral cortex. Function of each area has been described in different chapters in neurophysiology section. Notably important are motor areas (areas 4 and 6), sensory areas (areas 1–3, 5, and 7), visual areas (areas 17 and 18), motor speech area (area 44), sensory speech area (area 22), and auditory areas (41 and 42).

Motor Defects: The most striking defect is inability to reach accurately for objects.

- **Lesion of area 5** causes deficit **in tactile reaching**, and **lesion of area 7** causes deficit **in visual reaching.**

Sensory Deficits: Loss of all cortical sensations resulting in **astereognosis, and loss of tactile localization and two-point discrimination,** and severe impairment of fine touch, vibration and proprioception, if S-I is damaged.

- Pain, temperature and crude touch are least affected.
- If area 5 and 7 are also involved, impairment occurs in learning and retention of tasks.

Deficit in Spatial Perception: Motor and sensory deficits in posterior parietal lobe lesion (mainly area 5 and 7) are produced secondary to a defect in spatial perception.

- Brain receives sensory information but unable to integrate for spatial orientation that results in both inaccurate reaching and wrong interpretation of tactile cues.
- There will be *difficulty in dealing with three-dimensional space*.
- Bilateral parietal lesion causes **spatial disorientation** (patient can't find his way even in familiar surrounding).

Attentional Deficit: Motor and sensory deficits in posterior parietal lobe lesion may also be due to a defect in attention.

- Like hemineglect, there will be **hemi-inattention.**
- They ignore stimuli from contralateral side.

Constructional Apraxia: Bilateral parietal lesion, there is **inability to copy an object or even a simple design.**

- This is called constructional apraxia (apraxia means inability to perform organized movements in the absence of paralysis).
- In bilateral lesion, also there will be **abolition of visual placing**, though tactile placing will be retained.

Temporal Lobe

Divisions and Functions

Temporal lobe is divided into **three regions**: Superior temporal gyrus, inferior temporal gyrus and mediobasal portion of temporal lobe.

Superior Temporal Gyrus:

This consists of **Brodmann's area 22, 41, and 42** (Fig. 116.3). This is primarily **concerened with audition** (Fig. 116.4). Area 41 and 42 constitute primary auditory cortex that receives inputs from medial geniculate body (MGB) and projects to area 22, which is **crucial for understanding speech.**

- Area 22 receives input from prestriate visual areas and project to frontal lobe, parietal lobe and cingulate gyrus.
- Thus area 22 processes visually perceived words and symbols.

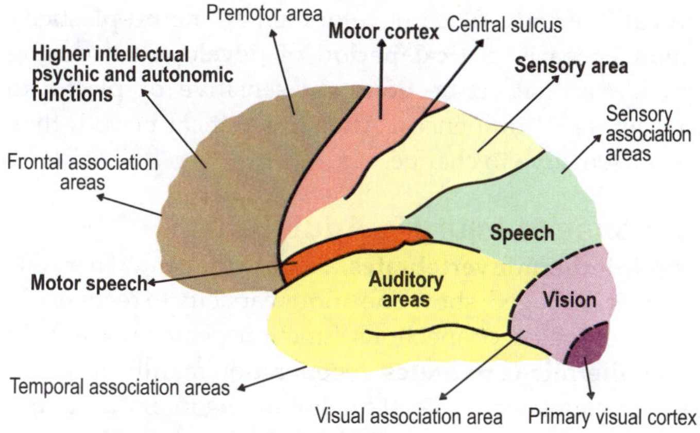

Fig. 116.4: Major functions of different lobes of brain.

Inferior Temporal Gyrus

This consists of **Brodmann's area 20, 21, and 37**. This is primarily ***concerened with vision***.

- It receives input from prestriate visual areas, pulvinar area of thalamus and parietal lobe.
- It projects to prestriate visual areas, amygdala, entorhinal cortex and basal ganglia.

Mediobasal Portion of Temporal Lobe

It is mainly the anterior part of temporal lobe that consists of **amygdala, hippocampus**, other limbic structures, prepyriform cortex and other cortical areas concerned with olfaction.

- This part of temporal lobe is concerned with **limbic functions and olfaction**.

Effects of Lesions

The important deficits observed following lesion of temporal lobe are:

Prosopagnosia: This is the **inability to recognize known** faces, though the patient can identify people by hearing their voices.

- Even he may not identify his own face (seeing a mirror). This is not a perceptual deficit.
- The lesion involves inferior temporal lobe. Patient usually also have **achromatopsia** (cerebral color blindness).

Auditory Deficits: The deficit occurs mainly in **auditory discrimination learning.**

- Though, temporal lobe receives heavy inputs from MGB, the lesion in superior temporal gyrus produces *deficits only in distinguishing between complex sounds* (auditory tasks).

Visual Deficits: Lesion affecting inferior temporal lobe results in deficit in **visual discrimination learning.**

- Difficulty not only occurs for learning new visual discrimination tasks, but also the previously learned tasks are not remembered.
- Though visual perception is less affected, visual memory is significantly disturbed.

Memory Deficit: Lesion of left temporal lobe affects **verbal memory** and lesion of right temporal lobe affects **nonverbal memory**.

- Short-term memory depends on lateral temporal cortex.
- If hippocampus and amygdala are affected in temporal lobe lesion, *deficit occurs in long-term memory.*

Klüver-Bucy Syndrome: Removal of temporal lobe of both the sides results in Klüver-Bucy syndrome as first described by Klüver and Bucy in experimental animals.

Frontal and Prefrontal Lobes

Divisions and Functions

The part of the cortex rostral to central sulcus (**precentral sulcus**) and medial to sylvian fissure is the frontal lobe. It is divided into **three parts**: precentral region, transitional region and prefrontal association cortex.

Precentral Region

Precentral region contains primary **motor cortex** (area 4) and **premotor cortex** (area 6). These areas **control movements, both skilled and postural**.

Transitional Region

Transitional region is the area between precentral gyrus and prefrontal cortex. This includes area 44 and area 8. **Area 44** is the motor speech area that **controls motor activities of speech apparatus**, and **area 8** is the frontal eye field that **controls eye movement**.

Prefrontal Association Cortex (Prefrontal Lobe)

Prefrontal association cortex includes **area 9–14**.

- This is subdivided into **orbital region** (area 11-14 and 47), and **dorsolateral region** (area 9, 10, 45, and 46).
- **Area 24** of prefrontal lobe (in cingulated gyrus) is a part of Papez circuit, which plays an important role in **genesis and control of emotion**.

Effects of Lesion

Effects of lesions of frontal lobe are as follows:

Motor Deficit: Lesion of motor cortex results in **hypertonia at rest** and inability to react in term of past experience.

- Postural reflexes are preserved except hopping and placing reactions.
- Central feature of frontal lobe lesion is *inability to perform a delayed response task and perseveration.*

Limbic Dysfunctions: Limbic dysfunctions, especially **emotional shallowness** occurs in prefrontal lesion. There is also impairment of memory and learning capacity.

Personality Changes: **Lack of initiative and inability to assess personal performance** are striking changes in personality in frontal lobe lesion.

- Other features are tactlessness, change in social habits, impaired concentration, disturbance in judgment, and tendency towards irresponsible behavior.

Prefrontal Lobotomy & Frontal Lobe Syndrome: When the connection of thalamus with prefrontal lobe is cut (This is called prefrontal lobotomy), the major areas of prefrontal lobe (area 8, 9, 10, 11, 12, 44-47) are disconnected.

This is associated with frontal lobe syndrome, which is characterized by:

1. Difficulty in planning due to flight of ideas.
2. Sense of well-being (euphoria), and failure to understand the seriousness of others feeling.
3. Loss of recent memory with impairment of moral and social sense.
4. Loss of attention and ability to concentrate.
5. Decreased mental drive and lack of initiation.
6. Emotional instability.
7. May be associated with hyperphagia, and urinary and fecal incontinence.

Occipital Lobe

This is the area of the brain **posterior to the parieto-occipital sulcus**. It is mainly ***concerned with vision***.

- It contains **area 17** (the primary visual cortex), and **18 and 19** (the association visual cortex or higher order of visual cortex).

CORTICAL PLASTICITY

The basic element of the nervous system is the neuron. The neural connections are determined genetically, and once established, remain almost throughout life. However, in some special circumstances, synaptic connections can be modified in CNS, especially in the brain. This ability to modify is referred to as **cortical plasticity**, or more broadly the **neural plasticity**. But, in what situations and by what mechanism do the neurons modify?

There are **three known major circumstances** of neural plasticity: 1. postnatal modifications, 2. changes as a consequence to injury to the brain, and 3. the plasticity during learning or experience.

Postnatal Development

Postnatal modifications of neuronal connectivity occur as a result of interactions with the environment.

- **Environmental effects** affect development and alteration of many neural connections.
- During this early phase of development, many neural changes occur, changes in **cellular, axonal and synaptic parts** of the neuron.
- **Number of synapses increases** during development until maximum levels are gradually reached in early adulthood.

Critical Period: The developmental neuro-plasticity exhibit an **early critical period** of development during which neuronal connections are sensitive or plastic to environmental influences. After this critical period, they are not sensitive to change.

Response to Injury in Adult Brain

In poikilothermic vertebrates, axons in the central nervous system if damaged, show enormous capacity to regenerate. The regenerated connections function nearly normal. **In homeothermic vertebrates**, regeneration mainly occurs in the peripheral nervous system. Following injury to central nervous system, the regeneration is incomplete. However, **significant modifications** do occur.

1. For example, the phenomenon of **axonal sprouting** that occurs following spinal transection.
   - *Axonal sprouting also occurs in other structures* in central nervous system, including hippocampus, septum, cerebellum and red nucleus.
2. In some cases, the new connections have indeed formed **functional connections**.
   - For example, the **cerebellar projection** to red nucleus is preferentially to the soma and proximal dendrites of the neurons, whereas the **cortical projection** to red nucleus primarily ends on distal dendrites.
3. If the cerebellar efferent fibers to red nucleus are damaged, then the **cortical projection fibers sprout** to establish more proximal connections at the synaptic sites that have been vacated by degeneration of the cerebellorubral fibers.
   - These new connections increase the influence of the motor cortex on the red nucleus and **contribute to the recovery of motor function**. This is the best example of cortical plasticity.

However, not all pathways are equally capable of sprouting.

Learning and Memory

The capacity of certain neurons **to change their behaviour as a function of environmental inputs** is a very important property of the nervous system. This serves the basis of learning and adaptive behaviors.

1. **Learning** refers to a process of *change in behavior as a result of experience.*
2. **Memory** is the *storage of information* of the experience-induced modification.

The storage of information involves actual physical changes in neurons. **Change in synaptic connections and cellular changes** are the bases of learning and memory. This is another example of cortical plasticity.

Exam Questions

1. Describe the functional organization and function of neocortex. Write a note on cerebral asymmetry.
2. Describe the connections and functions of different lobes of the brain. Add a note on cortical plasticity.

Multiple Choice Questions

1. Which of the following is not a function of neocortex?
A. Language and speech
B. Intellect and personality
C. Learning and memory
D. Motor control

2. Area for arithmetic calculation resides in:
A. Inferior part of left frontal lobe
B. Parietal lobe
C. Temporal lobe
D. Cingulate gyrus

3. Lesion of inferior parietal lobule in representational hemisphere produces:
A. Agnosia
B. Prosopagnosia
C. Hemineglect
D. Visual defects

4. Left lobe is responsible for
A. Appreciation of Music
B. Spatial orientation
C. Visual stimuli processing
D. Written and spoken languages

5. Neurophysiological defects present in right lobe involvement are all, EXCEPT:
A. Visuospatial defect
B. Anosognosia
C. Dyscalculia
D. Dysgraphia

6. Attention and concentration are mediated by:
A. Hypothalamus
B. Frontal lobe
C. Parietal lobe
D. Basal ganglia

7. If the patient is able to recognize person by name but not by face, the lesion is in:
A. Post parietal region
B. Occipital
C. Frontal lobe
D. Temporal lobe

8. Hemineglect occurs in lesion of:
A. Temporal lobe
B. Prefrontal lobe
C. Parietal lobe
D. Frontal lobe

9. Inability to recognize know face is called:
A. Prosopagnosia
B. Visual agnosia
C. Facial agnosia
D. Sensory agnosia

10. Superior temporal gyrus is concerned with:
A. Motor learning
B. Audition
C. Personality
D. Visual emotion

Answers 1. D 2. A 3. C 4. D 5. C 6. B 7. D 8. C 9. A 10. B

Chapter 117

Cerebrospinal Fluid and Blood-Brain Barrier

Learning Objectives

On completion of study of this chapter:

The student will be able to (must know):

1. Remember the functional anatomy of ventricular system and subarachnoid space.
2. Outline the mechanism of formation, circulation and absorption of cerebrospinal fluid (CSF).
3. Give the composition and functions of CSF and list the differences between plasma and CSF.
4. Draw a schematic diagram and identify the components of blood brain barrier (BBB)
5. Outline the structure and functions of BBB and list the structures present outside BBB.
6. Appreciate the clinical importance of BBB.
7. Learn importance of CSF examination effects of increased CSF pressure.

The student may also be able to (desirable to know):

1. Describe the regulation of CSF formation, circulation and absorption.

CEREBROSPINAL FLUID

Functional Anatomy

Ventricular System & Subarachnoid Space

Ventricular System

There are **four ventricles** in the brain. two lateral ventricles, a third ventricle and a fourth ventricle (Fig. 117.1).

1. **Lateral ventricles** are the largest ones that are located symmetrically in the cerebral hemispheres.
2. The **third ventricle** is located in the diencephalons, and the **fourth ventricle** is enclosed in the pons and medulla.
   - The two lateral ventricles communicate with the third ventricle through two independent openings called the **foramina of Monro**.
   - The third ventricle communicates with fourth ventricle through a narrow passage called the **aqueduct of Sylvius**.
2. The **fourth ventricle** narrows down caudally as it enters the spinal cord that continues as the central canal in the cord.

Each ventricle contains a bunch of epithelial-vascular tissue known as the **choroid plexus**.

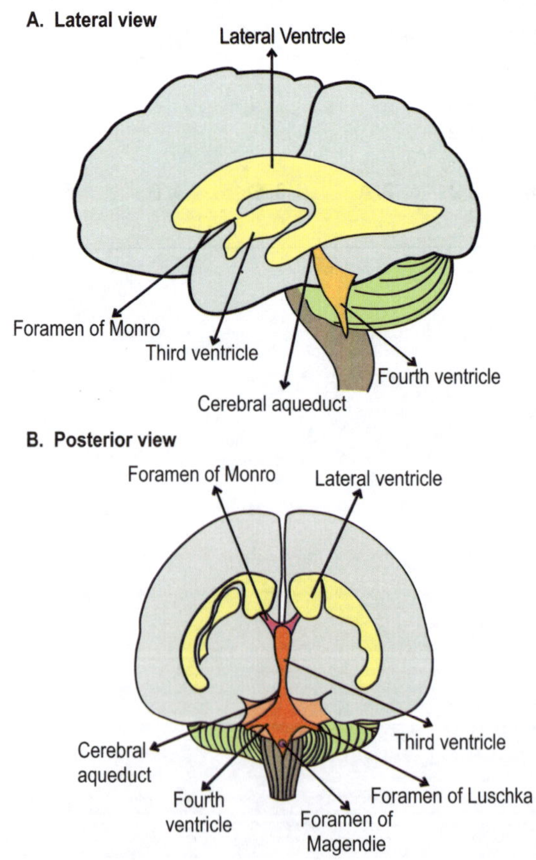

Fig. 117.1: Ventricles in the brain.

Subarachnoid Space

The brain and spinal cord are covered by three layers of the connective tissues, called **meninges**.

- The innermost layer, which is in close contact with the brain tissue, is called the **pia mater**. Next to pia mater is the **arachnoid mater** and outermost layer is the **dura mater**, which is in close contact with the inner wall of the skull.
- There are *two potential spaces* between these layers. The space between the pia mater and arachnoid mater is called the **subarachnoid space**, and the space between the arachnoid mater and the dura mater is the **subdural space**.

Features of subarachnoid space:

1. The subarachnoid space is enlarged at few places to form **cisterns**.
2. There are *four major cisterns* and many minor cisterns.
3. **The major cisterns** are:
   i) **Superior cistern**, located dorsal to midbrain
   ii) **Cerebellomedullary cistern**, located between cerebellum and medulla (this is a large one, therefore also called **cisterna magna**)
   iii) **Pontine cistern**, located near pons
   iv) **Interpeduncular cistern**, located at the cerebral peduncles.
4. **The minor cisterns** are cistern of the optic disc, cistern of lamina terminalis, cistern of corpus callosum, perimesencephalic cisterns, cistern of lateral sulcus and the lumbar cistern.
   - The **lumbar cistern** is the large spinal subarachnoid space extending between L_2 and S_2 vertebra (Clinical Note 117.1).

Clinical Note 117.1

Site for lumbar puncture: In the spinal cord, the lumbar cistern is a potentially large spinal subarachnoid space that extends from L_2 to S_2 vertebra. Therefore, the preferred site for lumbar puncture to collect CSF is intervertebral space between L_1 and L_2 as it is easy to introduce the needle here than lower down in the vertebral column.

Arachnoid Granulations

Arachnoid granulations are a collection of villi that project from the arachnoid into the subdural venous sinuses.

- Thus, the subarachnoid space communicates with the venous blood through arachnoid granulations.

Communication between Ventricles and Subarachnoid Space

The cerebral ventricles communicate with the subarachnoid space through openings (foramens) in the fourth ventricle.

- One opening is in the midline, called the **foramen of Magendie** and two openings are placed laterally, called the **foramen of Luschka**.
- Through these openings CSF formed in the ventricles enter subarachnoid space.

Formation, Circulation & Absorption of CSF

Formation of CSF

Choroid plexuses located in the floor of lateral, third and fourth ventricles are the **major source** of CSF. However, CSF continues to be formed even after choroid plexuses are removed.

- The other sources of CSF are the blood vessels of subependymal regions and pia.

Rate of Formation

In an adult, the intracranial volume is about 1700 ml, of which brain measures 1200-1400 ml, **CSF accounts for 70-160 ml**, and blood in cerebral vessels is about 150 ml.

- Thus, CSF occupies **less than 10%** of the volume of total intracranial space.
- The **rate of formation of CSF is about 0.35 ml/min** or, 20 ml/hour or, **500ml/day**.
- As a whole, CSF is totally replaced four to five times daily.

Mechanism of Formation

CSF is formed by a combination of passive diffusion, active transport and facilitated diffusion.

1. **Passive diffusion:** The thin walled vessels of choroid plexuses allow passive diffusion of substances from blood plasma into extracellular space surrounding choroidal cells.
2. **Active transport:** The choroid epithelium secretes sodium ions by active transport. This is achieved by **Na^+-K^+ pump** operating in the apical surface of the plexus that **pumps Na^+ into the ventricular cavity** (Fig. 117. 2).
   - **Chloride ions** move into the CSF passively in response to electrical gradient generated by Na^+ movement.
   - **Cl^-–K^+ exchanger** also exchanges chloride for K^+ in the apical membrane.
   - The sodium and chloride ions **create the osmotic gradient** for flow of water into the ventricles.
   - In the basal surface, chloride is exchanged for bicarbonate, and H^+ is exchanged for Na^+.
   - **Secretion of bicarbonate** is essential to maintain pH of brain ECF by neutralizing the acidity created by secretion of H^+.
3. **Facilitated diffusion:** Penetration of substances into brain is *directly proportional to their lipid solubility*. Ionized compounds like hexoses and amino acids are relatively insoluble in lipid. They enter by **facilitated diffusion**, which is stereospecific

(carrier binds only with a solute having specific configuration).

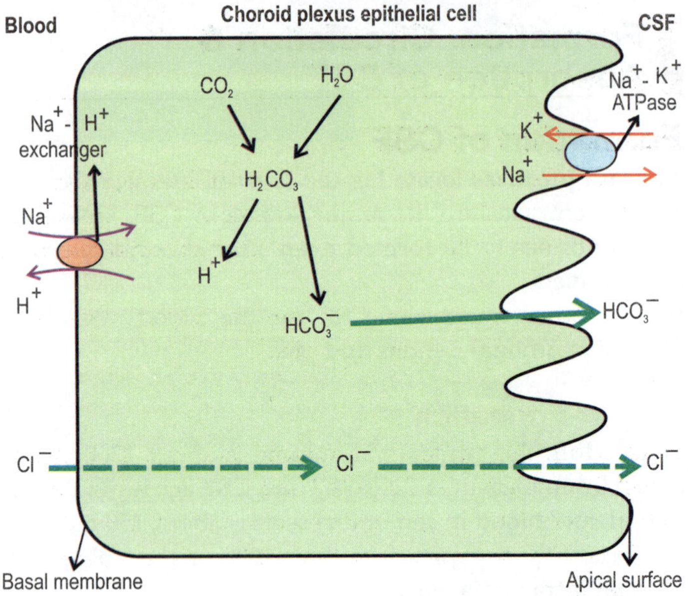

Fig. 117.2: Mechanism of cerebrospinal fluid (CSF) formation in the choroidal epithelial cells in the brain.

Steps of Formation

CSF formation occurs **in two steps**: ultrafiltration and active secretion.

1. **Ultrafiltration** of plasma occurs across the fenestrated capillary wall into the ECF that baths the basal surface of epithelial cells of choroid plexus.
2. Choroidal epithelial cells transport ions and solutes into CSF, mainly by **active secretion**.

Composition of CSF

The osmolality and concentration of sodium ion in CSF are equal with that of plasma, whereas chloride ion concentration is higher, and potassium and bicarbonate ion concentration is lower (Table 117.1). The concentration of glucose and protein in CSF is lower than that of plasma.

Table 117.1 | Composition of CSF compared to that of plasma.

	CSF	Plasma
Protein (g/dL)	0.03	7
Sodium mEq/L)	145	145
Chloride (mEq/L)	115	100
Potassium (mEq/L)	2.8	4.5
Bicarbonate (mEq/L)	25	24.5
Glucose (mg/dL)	60	100
Amino acids (mM)	0.7	2.7
pH	7.3	7.4
Osmolarity (mOsm/L)	290	290

Circulation and Absorption of CSF

Circulation of CSF

Harvey Cushing described circulation of CSF as the third circulation in the body (first is blood and second is lymphatic).

1. The CSF is mainly **formed in the lateral ventricle**, from where it flows downward **into the third ventricle** through foramen of Monro, and from the third ventricle **into the fourth ventricle** though aqueduct of Sylvius.
2. Finally, CSF comes out of fourth ventricle through the foramen of Magendie and Luschka to **enter the subarachnoid space.**
3. In the subarachnoid space, CSF moves **upwards towards the cerebral hemispheres** and **downwards towards the spinal cord** (Fig. 117.3).

Thus, obstruction of foramen of Monro results in distension of lateral ventricles, occlusion of aqueduct of Sylvius causes distension of third ventricle, and blockage of foramina of Magendie and Luschka initially distends fourth ventricle and later the entire **ventricular system is distended**.

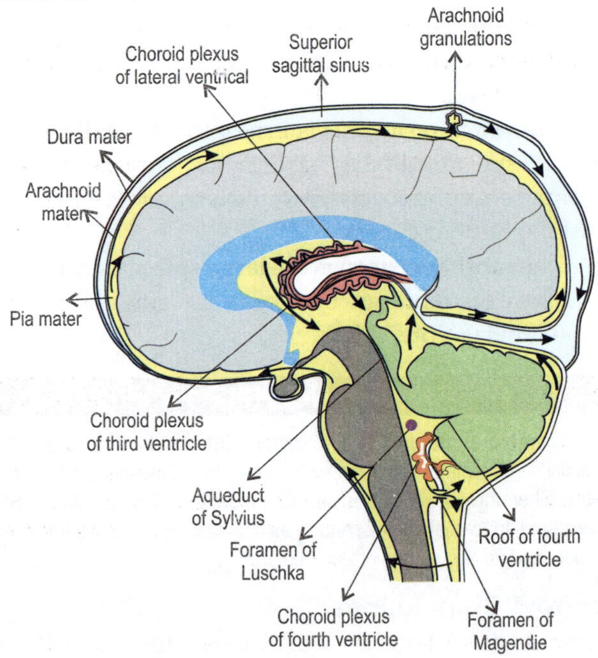

Fig. 117.3: Route of circulation of CSF in the ventricles and cisterns in the brain.

Absorption of CSF

Absorption of CSF occurs through **the arachnoid villi**. Arachnoid villi project into the subdural venous sinuses (Flowchart 117.1).

- The **main factor** that facilitates the movement of the fluid is the **oncotic pressure** (colloid osmotic pressure of plasma, which is 25 mm Hg) that is higher than that of CSF because CSF has very less proteins.
- The **other factor** promoting this mechanism is the **hydrostatic pressures** of CSF, which is about **0.5-5 mm Hg higher** than that in the subdural venous sinuses.

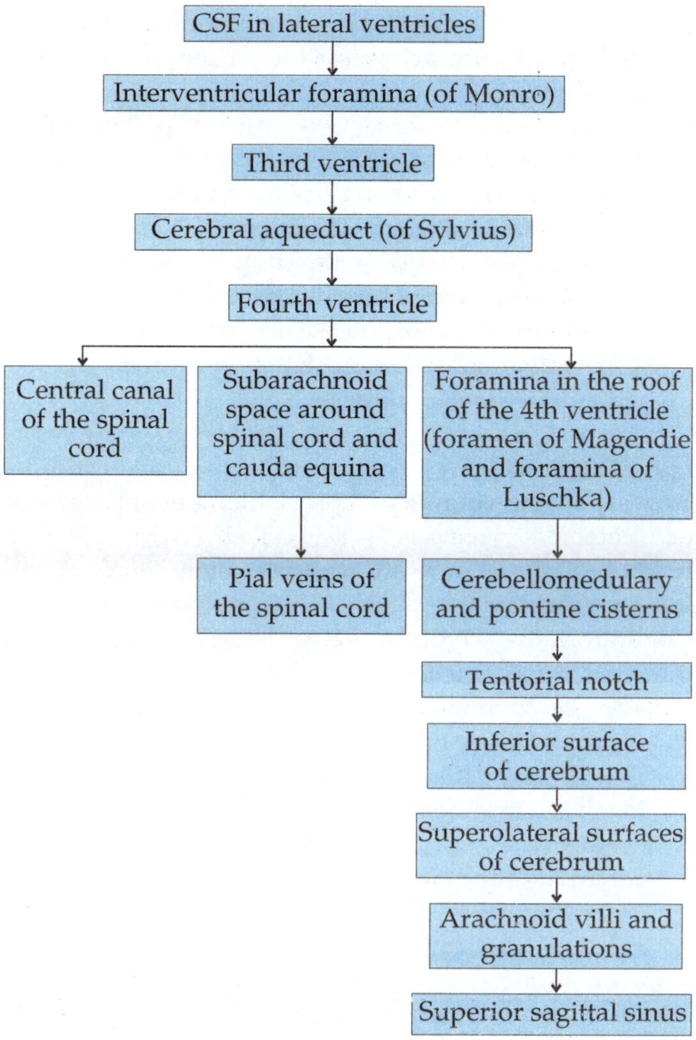

Flowchart 117.1: Circulation and absorption of CSF.

CSF Pressure

In recumbent position, the normal intracranial pressure (ICP), which reflects the CSF pressure as measured by lumbar puncture is normally about **8 mm Hg** or 110 mm H_2O.

1. However, **in the standing posture**, ICP is less (may be close to zero) and CSF pressure is more as the column of CSF added incrementally to the pressure in the lumbar subarachnoid space.
   - Therefore, CSF pressure is **recorded in recumbent posture**.
2. It is important to note that in normal conditions, the **major determinant of CSF pressure is the cerebral venous pressure**, not the resistance to CSF outflow.
   - CSF pressure is in equilibrium with capillary or pre-venous pressure.
3. Increase in **arterial pressure has little effect** on capillary pressure due to autoregulation and therefore, does not significantly increase CSF pressure.
4. In contrast, **increase in venous pressure exerts immediate effect** on CSF pressure by increasing pressure in intracerebral veins, venules and dural sinuses.
   - This forms the **physiological basis for Queckenstedt test** (see below).
5. CSF pressure increases in any space occupying lesion of skull cavity.

Functions of CSF

1. **Protection from mechanical injury:** A major function of CSF is to **protect brain from mechanical injury**.
   - Brain floats in CSF, and therefore the weight of the brain is decreased to about 50 g from its actual weight of 1400 g due to the effect of buoyancy. The buoyancy is due to the difference in specific gravity of brain (1.040) and CSF (1.007).
   - Due to higher specific gravity, brain **floats freely in CSF** rather than resting heavily on the skull box.
   - Thus, the risk of routine acceleration-deceleration injuries is eliminated and also the impact of major injuries is greatly diminished (Clinical Note 117.2).

Clinical Note 117.2

Contrecoup phenomenon: When the buoyancy effect of CSF is not adequate to protect, the brain gets injured following a hit. Surprisingly, the brain injury occurs on the opposite side of hit. This is called as the *contrecoup injury*. This happens because skull moves with the head along the direction of hit but the brain lags behind slightly due to its inertia. A vacuum is created between the brain and the skull. When skull comes to rest, the side of the brain opposite the blow hits the skull due to the combined effect of inertia and vacuum.

2. **Provides microenvironment for brain cells:** Brain is metabolically fragile. Neurons in the brain are highly sensitive to changes in oxygen, glucose, pH, temperature etc. in their external environment.
   - However, the CSF ***ensures constancy in the external environment of neurons***.
   - CSF accomplishes this by buffering the changes in blood on one side with the brain interstitial fluid on the other.
3. **Role in homeostasis:** CSF is indirectly involved in regulation of respiration, blood pressure, water intake and visceral function by bringing about the chemical changes like hydrogen ion concentration (pH), osmolality etc. in cerebral interstitial fluid.
   - The changes in blood PO_2, PCO_2 and pH are transmitted to ***chemo-sensitive respiratory neurons and central chemoreceptors*** via CSF for appropriate homeostatic responses.
4. **Removal of proteins and waste products:** There are no lymphatic channels in brain and spinal cord.
   - CSF removes ***proteins and waste products of metabolism***, especially H^+, lactate and CO_2 through its sink action.
   - In the brain, small amount of protein that leaks into the interstitial fluid is drained by the CSF and returned to the blood stream.

- Thus, the CSF serves the function of lymphatics in brain.

Applied Physiology

Lumbar Puncture

Sampling of CSF by lumbar puncture (LP) is an important diagnostic tool in neurology. Composition (cells, protein, glucose etc), color and pressure of CSF provide important information about the **nature of brain pathology**.

- In adults, LP is performed by inserting a needle preferably through the interspace between L_3 and L_4 into the spinal subarachnoid space, below the end of the spinal cord.

Examination of CSF

Normal CSF is transparent and colorless. Presence of turbidity indicates excess of proteins and cells. Determination of types of cells, and estimations of protein and glucose concentration are very useful.

In Meningitis: Meningeal inflammation (meningitis) due to infection is characterized by ***presence of more proteins and cells*** in CSF. The glucose concentration is low as microorganisms utilize glucose, but protein concentration is high due to increased capillary permeability that increases ultrafiltration of protein.

- ***In bacterial meningitis*** polymorphs are more, in ***tubercular meningitis*** lymphocytes are more (***cob-web appearance*** due to increased fibrin clot) and in ***viral meningitis*** moderate increase occurs in lymphocytes (but no decrease in glucose).
- The **culture of CSF** confirms the nature of the infection.

Cerebral Hemorrhage: CSF is bloody or yellow in appearance (with red cells) and protein is raised.

Encephalitis: CSF is usually clear. ***Lymphocyte and protein are high.***

Brain tumor: CSF is clear. It, may be associated with mild increase in lymphocyte and protein.

Poliomyelitis: Clear and colorless CSF. Significant ***increase in lymphocytes*** occurs with moderate increase in protein.

Brain Abscess: Clear or slightly turbid CSF. Normal lymphocyte count (0 to 5 cells). Mild increase in protein may occur.

Spinal cord tumor: Clear or yellow CSF. Significant increase in protein may be a feature.

Queckenstedt Test

During lumbar puncture, if the needle is connected to a manometer it records CSF pressure. If the patient is lying on his side, the pressure ranges from 100 to 180 cm H_2O or 7 to 13 mm Hg.

- Queckenstedt test is performed to demonstrate ***spinal subarachnoid block***, if present.
- For this test, the patient in lying posture (on his side), the **jugular veins are pressed** to see the ***pattern of rise in CSF pressure***.
- Compression of jugular vein causes an **immediate rise in intracranial CSF pressure**, which is rapidly transmitted to the lumbar subarachnoid space, unless there is spinal subarachnoid block.
  - Normally, the rise is **rapid up to 100 to 200 mm H_2O**, and the pressure returns to normal within 10 seconds following release of compression.
- If the spinal subarachnoid **block is present**, the rise and fall ***are slow or absent***.

Hydrocephalus

Increase in the volume of CSF resulting in enlargement of cerebral ventricles is called hydrocephalus. Hydrocephalus is of **two categories**: communicating and noncommunicating.

Communicating Hydrocephalus: Hydrocephalus due to impaired absorption of CSF is called communicating type, because the communication between the ventricles and subarachnoid space is intact.

- This is also called ***normal pressure hydrocephalus***, which is a misnomer as the ICP is often intermittently elevated.
- Communicating hydrocephalus occurs due to ***damage to arachnoid villi***, which commonly happens following infection or inflammation of meninges.

Non-communicating Hydrocephalus: Hydrocephalus occurs ***due to obstruction of the foramens*** that drain CSF.

- The ICP is usually very high in this type of hydrocephalus. Therefore, this is also called ***obstructive hydrocephalus*** or **high-pressure hydrocephalus**.
- The manifestation depends on the site of obstruction.
  - **Obstruction of foramen of Monro** results in distension of lateral ventricles, **obstruction of aqueduct of Sylvius** causes distension of third and lateral ventricles, and **obstruction of foramina of Magendie and Luschka** initially distends fourth ventricle but later enlarges entire ventricular system.
- The **usual site of obstruction is aqueduct of Sylvius**.

Effects of Increased CSF Pressure

The chronic rise in CSF pressure compresses and damages the brain.

- Any **space-occupying lesion** of cranial cavity like brain tumor increases ICP. The usual finding is the ***papilledema***, and engorgement and edema around the optic disc (Clinical Note 117.3).

IMPORTANT NOTE

lumbar puncture should be avoided if the ICP/CSF pressure is high: In raised ICP, lumbar puncture **should be avoided** as it may be life threatening.

- CSF comes out rapidly when it is under high pressure through lumbar puncture needle, which suddenly releases pressure in cranial cavity.
- This may **suck cerebellum and medulla** into the foramen magnum, causing their herniation.
- The herniation of cerebellum and medulla, the phenomenon also called as coning, damages the vital centers (cardiovascular and respiratory centers) in the medulla leading to **sudden cardio-respiratory arrest.**

Clinical Note 117.3

Fundus examination is a must in increased ICP: Whenever increased ICP is suspected, *fundus examination* must be performed to ensure that no papilledema is present before the lumbar puncture is performed. Otherwise, coning may cause sudden cardiorespiratory depression.

Clinical features in children (Fig. 117.4):

1. Large size of head and bossing of forehead.
2. Wide separation of cranial sutures
3. Enlarged and tense anterior fontanelle
4. Dilated veins on scalp.
5. Eyes look downward with setting sign appearance.
6. Progressive motor loss and cranial nerve palsy.

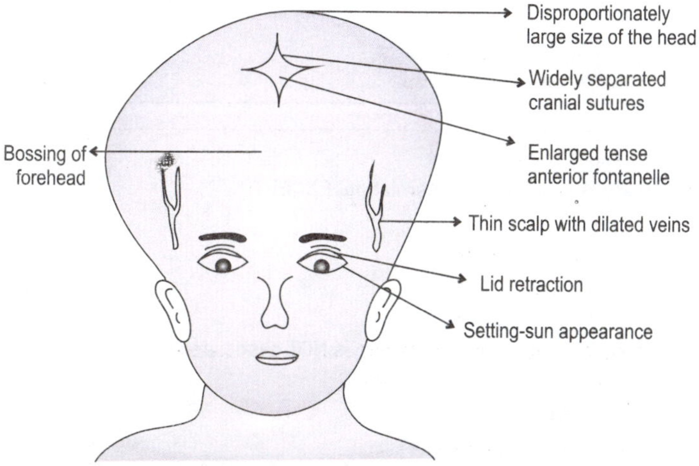

Fig. 117.4: Features of hydrocephalus.

BLOOD-BRAIN BARRIER

A special barrier that exists between the blood and the brain tissue is the blood brain barrier (BBB). A similar barrier exists between the blood and CSF, the **blood CSF barrier**.

Anatomical Basis of BBB

BBB is formed by **tight junctions between** endothelial cells of capillaries of the brain and **foot processes of astroglia** (refer Fig. 39.1, Chapter39 'Cerebral Circulation').

Circumventricular Organs

Normally, BBB is deficient in some regions of the brain that are collectively called as circumventricular organs (Fig. 117.5). Thus, they **remain outside BBB.**

The important circumventricular organs are:

1. Organum vasculosum of lamina terminalis (OVLT)
2. Subfornical organ (SFO)
3. Area postrema in medulla oblongata
4. Posterior pituitary and median eminence (ventral part) of hypothalamus
5. The pineal gland.

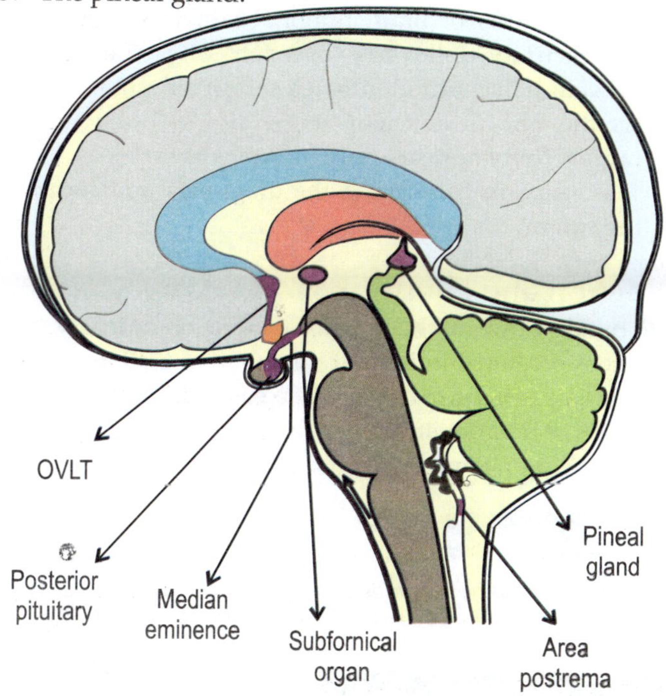

Fig. 117.5: Location of circumventricular organs. OVLT: organum vasculosum of lamina terminalis.

Functions of BBB

1. Neurons depend on a normal concentration of various ions in the fluid bathing them, especially Na^+, K^+, Ca^{++}, H^+ and Mg^{++}. Alteration in these ion concentrations in ECF of brain tissue results in severe consequences. BBB **maintains constancy of these ions** in brain fluids.
2. Many toxins either produced endogenously or administered exogenously circulate in blood. These ***toxins are harmful*** to the neurons that are highly sensitive. BBB **protects neurons** from these harmful substances.
3. BBB **prevents escape of neurotransmitters** from brain into circulation.
4. Disruption of BBB helps in **identifying the location and extent of lesions** in the brain.
5. BBB influences **drug permeability** into the brain.

Clinical Importance

Kernicterus

BBB is **not fully developed during infancy and early childhood. Bilirubin** has special affinity for basal ganglia.

- Therefore, if there is **hyperbilirubinemia during infancy**, as occurs in *hemolytic diseases of newborn* like **erythroblastosis fetalis**, free bilirubin enters the brain and **deposited in basal ganglia** and damage the structure.

- The condition is known as kernicterus.

Brain Tumor

BBB is **absent at the site of a brain tumor**.

- For diagnosis of brain tumor, **brain is scanned for radioactivity** following injection of a radioactive substance like radio-iodinated serum albumin.
- As the BBB is deficient at the site of brain tumor, **radioactivity appears only in tumor area**.
- This helps in confirming the **diagnosis and locating the tumor**.

Infection and Injury

BBB breaks down in the regions of infection or injury.

Therefore, **antibiotics** that do not cross BBB in normal individuals ***penetrate brain tissue*** easily in patients with infection or inflammation.

This helps in **appropriate use of medicines** in treatment of the disease.

Use of Hypertonic Solution

BBB is temporarily weakened by exposing the cerebral capillaries to hypertonic solutions. The hypertonic fluid causes **shrinking of the endothelial cells**, which in turn makes the tight junctions leaky (less tight). This property of BBB is exploited in treatment of brain diseases.

- Before administration of drugs that are aimed to penetrate brain tissue, a **hypertonic solution is injected** into the carotid artery.
- This **weakens BBB** and helps in **achieving proper concentration** of the drug in brain.

CSF-Brain Barrier

Strictly, there is **no CSF-brain barrier** because the **ependymal cells** that line the ventricles and the **pia mater are highly permeable**.

- Therefore, when a drug or an anesthetic agent is injected into the CSF by lumbar puncture can easily reach the brain and spinal cord.

Exam Questions

1. Describe the mechanism of formation, route of circulation, and functions of CSF. Add a note on hydrocephalus.
2. Describe the structure and functions of blood-brain barrier (BBB). Give a note on clinical importance of BBB.

Multiple Choice Questions

1. **CSF does not pass through:**
   A. Ventricles B. Venous sinuses
   C. Epidural spaces D. Subarachnoid space
2. **CSF is principally secreted by:**
   A. Choroid plexus
   B. Arachnoid granulation
   C. Floor of fourth ventricle
   D. Periaqueductal grey
3. **The normal adult CSF pressure is:**
   A. 1-2 mm Hg B. 6-12 mmHg
   C. 15-30 mm Hg D. 730 mmHg
4. **Low CSF protein may be seen in all of the following conditions, EXCEPT:**
   A. Recurrent lumbar puncture
   B. Hypothyroidism
   C. Pseudotumor cerebri
   D. infants
5. **Regarding CSF all the following statements are true, EXCEPT:**
   A. its pH is less than blood
   B. No neutrophils present normally
   C. Formed by arachnoid villi
   D. Persistent leakage can cause headache
6. **CSF pressure is mainly regulated by:**
   A. Rate of CSF formation
   B. Rate of CSF absorption
   C. Cerebral blood flow
   D. Venous pressure
7. **All are seen in cerebral herniation, EXCEPT:**
   A. Neck stiffness
   B. Loss of consciousness
   C. Pupil dilation
   D. Autonomic disturbances
8. **Increase in intracranial pressure is NOT associated with:**
   A. Deterioration of consciousness
   B. Tachycardia
   C. Respiratory depression
   D. Increase in BP
9. **"Blood brain barrier' is present at all of the following sites, EXCEPT:**
   A. Hebenular nucleus
   B. Subfornical organ
   C. Cerebellum
   D. Pontine nucleus
10. **Circumventricular organ is:**
    A. Anterior pituitary
    B. Posterior pituitary
    C. Pineal gland
    D. Hypothalamus

Answers

1. C	2. A	3. B	4. B	5. C
6. B	7. A	8. B	9. B	10. B

Section XII

Special Senses

In the silence of your heart, there is always peace and joy..

The Mother
(of Sri Aurobindo Ashram, Pondicherry, INDIA)

Chapter 118

PY10.17

Functional Anatomy of Eye

Learning Objectives

On completion of study of this chapter:

The student will be able to (must know):

1. Appreciate the functional anatomy of the eye to understand physiology of the eye.
2. Name the layers of sclera, cornea and retina and give their functions.
3. Understand the role of choroid, ciliary body and iris in visual functions.
4. Learns the importance of fovea centralis, fundus and optic disc.
5. Give the normal value of intraocular pressure and its physiological significance.

The student may also be able to (desirable to know):

1. Describe the structure and functions of choroid, ciliary body and iris.
2. Describe the formation and drainage of aqueous and vitreous humor.

LAYERS OF THE EYE

The eyeball is a fluid filled spherical organ with a diameter of 24 mm. A cross section through the human eye (Fig. 118.1) shows that the eyeball consists of **three concentric layers** housing the optical system.

1. **The outermost layer** is transparent in its anterior part called **cornea** and the rest opaque area is known as **sclera**.
2. **The middle** vascular and pigmented uveal tract forms **choroid** and **ciliary body** in its posterior part and **iris** in its anterior part.
3. **The innermost layer** is called **retina,** which contains the photoreceptors in association with a neuronal network that is absent in the anterior segment.

The interior of the eyeball is divided into **three spaces**, ***anterior chamber***, ***posterior chamber*** and the ***posterior cavity***.

- The fluid present in the anterior cavity (in the anterior and posterior chambers) is called **aqueous humor** and the posterior cavity contains **vitreous humor**.

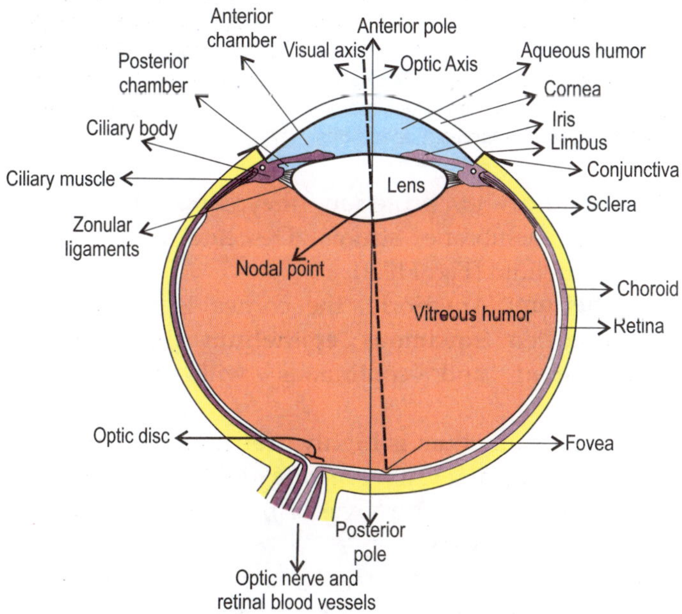

Fig. 118.1: The horizontal section of the right human eye, showing the major parts and their relative positions.

Sclera and Cornea

Sclera

As we look at the eye, part of the sclera is seen as white area surrounding central dark region.

1. The sclera is a white tough **avascular fibrous coat** composed of collagen fibers with little elastic tissue in adult.
   - It provides protection for the contents of the eyeball.
2. The **extraocular muscles** regulating the eyeball movements in different directions are **inserted on the sclera**.
   - It is covered by a thin layer of mucous membrane called **bulbar conjunctiva**.
3. The mucous membrane extends to the inner surface of the eyelids and is known as **palpebral conjunctiva**.

Inflammation of the conjunctiva is called **conjunctivitis** that occurs due to infection or allergy with symptoms of redness of the eyes and discharge.

Cornea

The anterior one-sixth of the sclera, which is **transparent and more convex** is called cornea.

- It is supplied by the sensory nerve endings of the trigeminal nerve. Light rays enter the eyeball through the cornea.
- The *curvature of the cornea contributes to* **most of the refractive power of the eye**.
- The sclero-corneal junction is known as **limbus**. The **cornea is an avascular tissue** (Application Box 118.1) composed of five layers.

> **Application Box 118.1**
>
> **Corneal transplant is usually successful:** Inflammation of the cornea is known as keratitis that may result in corneal ulcer. Corneal opacities may occur due to infection or injury. In these cases if the vision is grossly impaired, *corneal transplantation* shows encouraging result. As the cornea is avascular, blood-borne antibodies cannot reach the grafted tissue to cause transplant rejection. Therefore, it is one of the most common and **most successful transplant operations.**

From anterior to posterior, they are: epithelium, Bowman's membrane, stroma, Descemet's membrane and endothelium (Fig. 118.2).

i. **Epithelium:** Anteriorly, the cornea is covered by a **stratified squamous epithelium** that is thin, transparent and continuous with the bulbar conjunctiva.
   - The epithelium is **highly proliferative** in nature. If damaged, it can ***regenerate and heal rapidly***.
   - The complete turnover of the epithelium occurs in about a week.

ii. **Bowman's membrane:** This is the basement membrane of the epithelium.
   - If damaged, the Bowman's membrane *heals with a scar* resulting in blurred vision.

iii. **Stroma or substantia propria:** It consists of *highly structured thin collagen fibrils* in a mucopolysaccharide matrix.
   - The fibrils are of equal diameter, spaced at regular intervals and form a hexagonal lattice that confers transparency to the cornea.
   - The stroma constitutes **90 percent of the corneal thickness**.

iv. **Descemet's membrane:** It is a thin elastic membrane lining the posterior part of stroma.
   - The Descemet's membrane is **resistant to infection and can regenerate if damaged**.

v. **Endothelium:** It consists of a single layer of leaky endothelial cells and covers the posterior surface of Descemet's membrane.
   - The endothelium **prevents the excess hydration of the cornea**.
   - It removes the electrolytes and water flows passively out of the stroma.

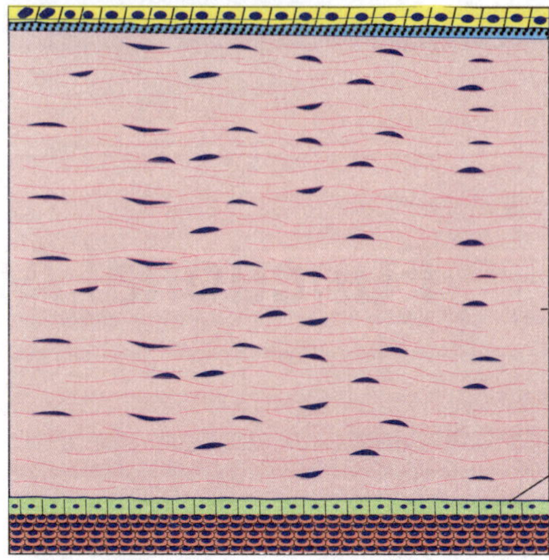

Fig. 118.2: Layers of cornea

Lacrimal Gland

- The lacrimal gland present at the lateral corner of the eye secretes a complex liquid known as **tear that keeps the cornea moistened**. When the eyes are open, this allows *oxygen to diffuse* from the atmosphere to the corneal cells, as they do not have blood supply.
- The tears *flush away the foreign particles* and their **lysozymes and antibodies prevent infection.**
- It is drained through the naso-lacrimal duct located at the medial corner of the eye.
  - In the absence of emotional or external stimuli, blinking helps in spreading of the film of tear over cornea and keep it moistened.
  - Some amount of water from the tear gets evaporated through the corneal epithelium to air.
- **Partial dehydration of the cornea is necessary for its transparency** but a totally dry cornea soon loses its transparency and a hydrated cornea becomes chalky white.
- Thus, *precise regulation of the stromal water content is essential for the clarity of vision.*

Choroid, Ciliary Body and Iris

Choroid

1. The **chorioid lines the inner aspect of sclera**. It contains many blood vessels that provide *nourishment to the structures of the eye.*
   - The choroidal blood vessels increase in size from within outwards.
2. The **membrane of Bruch** lines the inner side of the choroid and separates it from the retina.

- Beneath this membrane, the choroidal blood vessels divide to form capillaries that *supply nutrition to the outer portion of the retina by diffusion*.
- The space between the choroid and sclera is called **suprachoroidal or epichoroidal space**.

3. The blood vessels of choroid are bound together by connective tissue containing pigmented cells called **chromatophores**.
   - In albinism, pigments may be congenitally absent in the choroid.
4. The sensory supply to the choroid is from the trigeminal nerve fibers and autonomic neurons have vasomotor function.
5. Inflammation of the choroid is known as **choroiditis** that invariably involves the retina causing *chorioretinitis*.

Ciliary Body

The ciliary body is present between the iris and the choroid. It is a triangular structure with its base directed forwards and medially and its apex is continuous with the choroid posteriorly. The iris arises from the middle of the base and projects medially.

Parts of Ciliary Body: The ciliary body consists of ***two parts***: the **ciliary muscle** on the outer side and the **ciliary processes** at the inner side.

1. The **ciliary muscle** is made up of circular and radial multiunit smooth muscle fibers that are supplied by the ciliary ganglion, which in turn gets activated by the Edinger Westphal nucleus of the oculomotor nerve.
   - The ciliary body attaches to the peripheral ends of the zonule (**suspensory ligaments**) that ***hold the lens in position*** (Fig. 118.1). The *contraction of the ciliary muscles* pulls the zonule medially causing relaxation of the ligaments and the *lens becomes more convex*.
2. From the inner aspect of the ciliary body several fine projections arise, called **ciliary processes** that are lined by ciliary epithelium and contain many capillaries interspersed with connective tissues.
   - The ciliary processes ***secrete aqueous humor***. The ciliary body extends backwards upto **ora serrata**, the point where the retina begins.

The Inflammation of the ciliary body is known as **cyclitis** that invariably involves the iris causing **iridocyclitis**.

Iris

Projecting from the ciliary body, iris is a **thin, pigmented, circular, contractile diaphragm** that hangs over the anterior surface of the lens.

- The iris has a central aperture, the **pupil,** *through which light rays enter into the eye*.
- The iris along with the anterior margin of the lens **separates the anterior from the posterior chamber** of the eyeball.
- Inflammation of iris is called **iritis**.

From anterior to posterior, the iris shows **three layers**. They are: i) endothelium, ii) stroma and muscles and iii) epithelium.

Endothelium: It covers the anterior surface of the iris and is peripherally continuous with the endothelium on the posterior surface of cornea.

1. The iris consists of **circular and radial multiunit smooth muscles** embedded in a loose pigmented, highly vascular connective tissue stroma.
2. The ***abundant pigment*** makes the iris impervious to light and confers a ***characteristic colour to the eye***.

Stroma: The stroma contains a rich meshwork of blood vessels that run in radial direction.

1. The circular muscles (**sphincter pupillae**) are present close to the pupillary margin and are supplied by the ***parasympathetic fibers*** *of the occulomotor nerve*.
   - They contract in response to **parasympathetic stimulation** resulting in pupillary constriction (**miosis**) that decreases the amount of light entering into the eye (Fig. 118.3).
   - **Pupillary constriction cuts off more diffracted rays and decreases spherical and chromatic aberrations**; thereby, the focus becomes better and the sharpness of the retinal image increases.

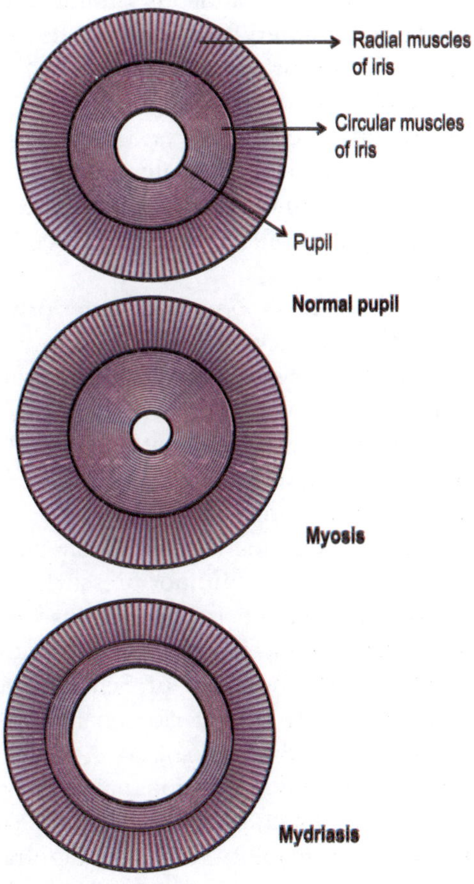

Fig. 118.3: Change in pupillary diameter in response to varying intensities of light. During miosis, the circular muscles of iris contract causing pupillary constriction. During mydriasis, causing pupillary dilation.

2. The **sympathetic fibers** from the cervical sympathetic chain supply the radial muscles (**dilator pupillae**) that are arranged radially near the root of the iris.
    - **Sympathetic stimulation** produces *contraction of radial muscles that causes pupillary dilation* (**mydriasis**) letting more amount of light in.

Epithelium: The posterior surface of the iris is covered by a double layer of pigmented epithelium.

Intrinsic Muscles of Eye

The ciliary and iris muscles are known as the intrinsic muscles of the eye.

Aqueous Humor, Lens and Vitreous Humors

Aqueous Humor

The aqueous humor is a **protein-free clear fluid** from which the lens and cornea derive their metabolic requirements.

- In the ciliary processes, it is continuously formed from plasma by the mechanism of ***ultrafiltration, diffusion and active transport*** and a complete turnover occurs in about an hour.
- Its **composition is similar to that of plasma**, but *lacks in proteins* and has *higher concentrations of ascorbic acid*.

The ciliary processes form aqueous humor and pour it into the **posterior chamber**, from where it flows through the pupil into the **anterior chamber** (Fig. 118.4).

Posterior Chamber: It is a triangular space enclosed anteriorly by the back of the iris and posteriorly by the anterior surface of the lens. Laterally, its base is formed by the ciliary body. Medially the apex is situated at the point where the pupillary margin comes in contact with the lens.

Anterior Chamber: It is bounded anteriorly by the posterior surface of the cornea; and posteriorly by the anterior surface of the iris and the anterior surface of the lens that is not covered by the iris.

1. Both these chambers are filled with aqueous humor.
2. The **aqueous pressure** is about 15-18 mm Hg higher than the intracranial pressure.
    - This pressure helps to maintain the shape of the eye and keeps the vitreous humor pressurized.
3. From the anterior chamber, the aqueous humor gets absorbed by the spongy meshwork of trabercular tissue and is drained into the **canal of Schlemn,** a venous channel at the angle of anterior chamber (junction between the iris and the cornea).

Rise in IOP: Decreased absorption of aqueous humor leading to rise in intraocular pressure (IOP) can occur due to reduced permeability through the trabercular tissue (**open-angle glaucoma)** or due to obstruction of the passage by anterior displacement of iris (**closed- angle glaucoma**).

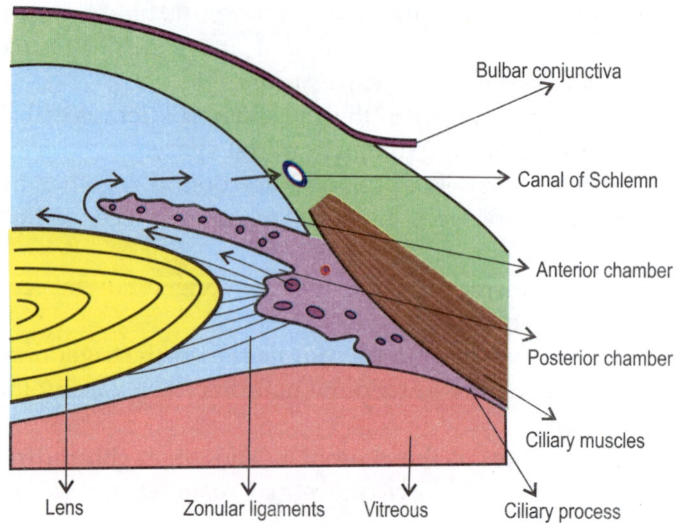

Fig. 118.4: Direction of flow of aqueous humor.

Lens

The lens is a biconvex transparent **avascular highly elastic structure** held in place behind the iris and in front of vitreous body by the suspensory ligaments.

1. The main function of the lens is to **converge the light rays and focus them on the retina.**
2. The crystalline lens **develops from the ectoderm**. It is enclosed in a thin *tough transparent elastic capsule,* formed from the secretion of epithelial cells.
3. It is composed of **transparent collagen fibrils**, which are arranged in layers like that of an onion.
    - The cells of the lens are rich in the protein ***α-crystalline*** that increase the density and enhance the focusing power of the lens.
    - The glucose present in the aqueous humor (60 mg %) is the principal source of energy for the lens.
4. The **capsule of the lens is semipermeable** that allows the nutrients to diffuse through it.
    - The lens gets its *oxygen supply from the aqueous humor* that contains dissolved oxygen.
5. **At rest**, the lens ligaments are stretched and the *anterior surface is les convex* than the posterior one.
6. **When the eye tries to focus**, the radial fibers of the ciliary muscles contract and pull the ciliary body forward.
    - This decreases the tension in the suspensory ligaments and relaxes the lens capsule causing the **anterior surface to bulge forward** *and become more convex, thereby* ***increasing the refractive power of the lens***.
    - This helps to **focus objects over a wide range**, from 10 cm to as far as 6m.
6. **In young people,** ***the lens contributes about 17 diopters to the total refractive power of the eye.***
7. **In children**, the lens can have a greater curvature and a greater refractive power.
8. **With advancing age,** the lens starts to lose its high-water content, becomes tougher and less elastic.

- This results in **decreased convexity** of the lens following relaxation of the suspensory ligaments.
- The lens also becomes gradually **less transparent** with age.

Cataract: Development of any degree of opacity in the lens or its capsule is known as **cataract**.

- It usually occurs with **aging** (degenerative or ***senile cataract***) or secondary **to diseases** like diabetes mellitus.
- Complete opacity of the lens is known as **mature cataract** and before that it is called immature cataract.
- Absence of the lens in the eye (from its normal position) is known as **aphakia**, as occurs due to operative removal of the lens following cataract or due to dislocation of the lens.

Vitreous Humor

The vitreous humor or **vitreous body** is a transparent avascular tissue of gelatinous consistency that occupies the **posterior cavity** of the eye. The portion of the vitreous present behind the posterior surface of the lens, acts as a cushion for the lens.

1. This **jelly-like mass** contains loose collagenous fibers and **vitrein**, a highly hygroscopic protein that is formed during early embryonic life and is not replaced thereafter.
2. **In fetal life**, the **hyaloid artery** runs antero-posteriorly in the middle of the vitreous and nourishes the vitreous as well as the fibro-vascular sheath of the lens.
3. In the later months of intra-uterine life, the artery gets obliterated and **shortly after birth it disappears** leaving an empty narrow channel known as ***hyaloid canal.***
   - **Persistent hyaloid artery** is a *congenital anomaly* that causes defective vision.
4. The avascular vitreous may show **degenerative changes in old age and high myopia**, in which cases, it loses its gel like consistency and **gets liquefied.**

Light traverses several media in the eye to reach the retina: The incident light rays travel from air to pass through ***several transparent media*** before it reaches the retina; they are:

i. A thin film of tear
ii. Cornea
iii. Aqueous humor
iv. Lens
v. Vitreous humor.

Retina

The retina is a thin transparent membrane containing the **photoreceptors cells** (rods and cones) and many-layered **neuronal network** that takes part in initial stages of image processing.

1. When light rays are focused on the retina, **it stimulates the photoreceptors**, which send the signal to the next order of neurons.
   - The chain of neurons at various levels in the optic pathway process the signal, which when arrives at the visual cortex generates the visual sensation.
2. The retina surrounds the vitreous in its inner surface and is covered by the choroid externally.
3. It extends forwards to the anterior end of the choroid where its termination is known as **ora serrata**.

The retina consists of i) **outer pigmented epithelial layer** that lies in close proximity to the choroid and ii) **inner neural layer** that is confined to the posterior three quarters of the retina.

Pigment Epithelium

The pigment epithelium is **rich in melanocytes** and is continuous with the epithelium of the iris. It has the following functions.

i. **Prevents scattering of light:** The photoreceptor layer of retina is present next to the pigment epithelium. Some of the light rays do not strike the photoreceptors as they travel in the gap between two receptors. They strike the underlying pigment epithelium.
   - The opaque melanin pigments ***adsorb light rays*** (photons) that are not first captured by photoreceptors, preventing their reflection back to the retina.
   - Thus, the pigment epithelium ***averts the blurring of visual images*** and preserves their sharpness and clarity.
   - Absence of melanin in albinism causes visual problems (Application Box 118.2)

ii. **Phagocytosis:** The pigment epithelial cells *phagocytose fragments of membrane* that are continuously shed from the outer segments of the photoreceptors.
   - So, the pigment epithelium helps in the ***renewal process of photoreceptors*** by removing the degenerated membrane.
   - The sloughed and degraded photoreceptor discs engulfed by the pigment epithelium are known as phagosomes.

iii. **Storage of vitamin A:** The pigment epithelium ***stores large quantities of vitamin A***, which is required for the synthesis of visual pigment rhodopsin, a protein present abundantly in rods.

Application Box 118.2

Visual problems in albinism: In albinism, melanin pigment is congenitally absent in all parts of the body, including the eye. In albinos, lack of melanin in the pigment epithelium as well as in the choroid causes nystagmus, photophobia and defective vision. They perceive a higher light intensity compared to a normal person, and are advised to wear sunglasses to reduce the intensity.

Visual problems in albinism: In albinism, melanin pigment is congenitally absent in all parts of the body, including the eye. In albinos, lack of melanin in the pigment epithelium as well as in the choroid causes nystagmus, photophobia and defective vision. They perceive a higher light intensity compared to a normal person, and are advised to wear sunglasses to reduce the intensity.

Neural Layers

The retina is very thin (about **200 μm thick** in humans) sheet of tissue that shows **ten different layers** (Fig.118.5). From outer to inner, they are:

1. Layer of pigment epithelium
2. Layer of rods and cones
3. External limiting membrane
4. Outer nuclear layer
5. Outer plexiform layer
6. Inner nuclear layer
7. Inner plexiform layer
8. Layer of ganglion cells
9. Layer of nerve fibers
10. Internal limiting membrane

Physiological Aspects

i) The visual receptors (**rods and cones**) synapse with **bipolar cells**, which in turn synapse with ganglion cells. In each eye, there are about ***120 million rods, 6 million cones and only 1 million ganglion cells***.

ii) The photoreceptors converge on **bipolar cells** and bipolar cells converge on **ganglion cells**; the *functional convergence is more than 100: 1.*

iii) **Horizontal cells** are interneurons present in the outer plexiform layer, where they send out processes and interconnect adjacent receptor cells as well as give input to the bipolar cells.

iv) **Amacrine cells** are interneurons present in the inner plexiform layer, where they send out processes and interconnect adjacent ganglion cells.
- The horizontal and amacrine cells form both presynaptic and postsynaptic connections.
- The interneurons have only dendrites but no axons. The retinal neurons also form gap junctions with the adjacent neurons.

v) Interspersed between the neural elements are present the supporting glial cells, called the **Müller cells** that have a nutritive function.
- The processes of these cells form the internal limiting membrane that separates the retina from the vitreous and an external limiting membrane in the receptor layer.

vi) The nerve fibers of the ganglion cells congregate to form the **optic nerve** that come out of the eye ball through the **optic disc**.

vii) When the neural layer gets separated from the pigment layer, the condition is called **retinal detachment**.
- The patient suffers from blindness and is treated by rejoining the layers by laser surgery or cryosurgery (Application Box 118.3)

viii) **In premature babies**, if oxygen is administered at high concentration (more than 40 percent) as a life saving measure, there occurs vascular proliferation from the peripheral retina causing ***retrolental opacity***, a condition known as **retro-lental fibroplasia**.

Application Box 118.3

Retinal detachment cause blindness: The central retinal artery and veins enter the eyeball with the optic nerve and supply the bipolar and ganglion cells present in the inner layers of retina. The rods and cones present in the outer layers of retina derive their nourishment from the choroidal capillaries by diffusion. Therefore, rods and cones suffer from hypoxic injury and vision is affected in retinal detachment.

Light traverses retinal layers to reach the photoreceptors: The incident light rays pass through the layer of blood vessels, ganglion cell axons and neurons of retina before it strikes the photoreceptors (rods and cones); the only exception is the fovea centralis, where light rays reach directly.

- Passage of light across different layers of retina does not affect the visual image quality much as the retina is quite thin and the layers are very transparent.

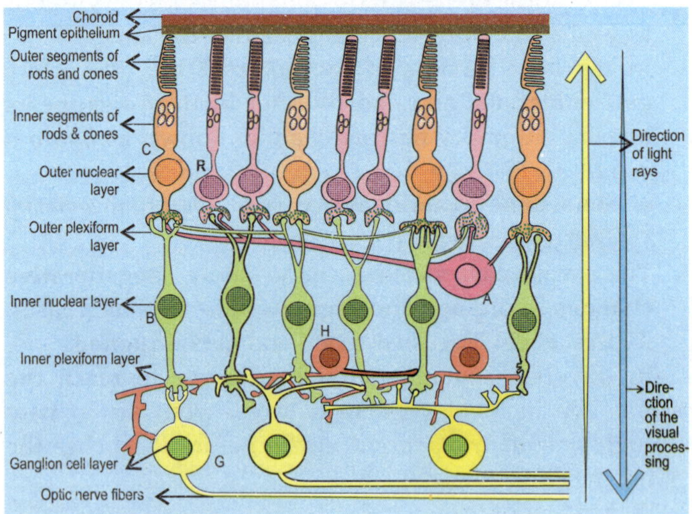

Fig. 118.5: Layers of retina.

Fovea Centralis

If a line is drawn straight along the visual axis, at the posterior pole of the eye, a small yellowish spot of about 1-2 mm in diameter is present, called the **macula lutea** (*in Latin* macula = spot; lutea = yellow). This area is specialized for sharp colour vision. Its central part has a small depression of about 0.4 mm in diameter, called the *fovea centralis* (fovea = shallow pit). **The fovea is the most sensitive part of the retina having maximum visual acuity** because of the following reasons:

- Its layer of photoreceptors contains *large number of tightly packed small sized cones* only.
- The *other neural layers of retina are displaced laterally* to the side of the fovea, so that light rays directly reach the exposed photoreceptors
- In the fovea region, *the ratio of cone cell to ganglion cell is 1:1*, i.e. a cone cell synapses with a single bipolar cell, which in turn synapses with only one ganglion cell.
  - Thus, the receptive field of a ganglion cell is smallest in the fovea region and it increases toward periphery of the retina.
- Unlike at other regions of the retina, the ganglion cell axons, the *central artery of retina and central retinal vein pass at the sides of macula*, not over it.
  - The macula gets its nutrition from the choroidal blood vessels by diffusion, as retinal blood vessels are absent in the macular region.

Optic Disc

The optic disc is located about 3 mm medial to and slightly above the posterior pole of the eye.

1. It is an **area in the retina devoid of the photoreceptors.**
   - Therefore, while mapping the peripheral field of vision, a **blind spot** is observed at the temporal visual field.
2. The **ganglion cell fibers and the central retinal veins** come out of the eye and the **central artery of retina** enter into the eye through the optic disc.
3. In ophthalmoscopy it **looks white** in colour, as it contains bundles of myelinated nerve fibers.

Fundus

This is the posterior portion of the interior of the eye as seen through an ophthalmoscope. The normal fundus gives a **red background** owing to the presence of choroidal blood vessels.

1. The microcirculation of the eye, i.e. the branches of the central artery and vein that ramify and spread over the superficial layers of retina can be **directly viewed** through the lens with the help of an ophthalmoscope.
   - **The fundus is the only region in the body where arterioles are readily visible.**
   - Therefore, this window is useful for the diagnosis of ocular diseases as well as conditions not directly related to ocular functions.
2. The **progress of several systemic diseases** like diabetes mellitus, hypertension and other diseases that affect the vessel wall can be assessed by examining the changes in retinal blood vessels.
   - In diabetes mellitus and hypertension, ***degeneration and exudation*** occur that appear as opacities against the transparent background.
   - In atherosclerosis, the ***narrowing of the vessel lumen*** is observed.

Intraocular Pressure

The intraocular pressure (IOP) is **10-20 mmHg.**

- The volume of lens, aqueous, vitreous, blood inside the vessels and the elasticity of the three layers contribute to the development of this pressure.
- **It maintains the shape of the eyeball.**
- The IOP keeps the retina pressed against the choroid so that **retinal surface is even** for the formation of a clear image.
- IOP is measured by **tonometry**.
- The variation in IOP mainly depends on the **amount of aqueous humor present at any given moment.**
- Increased IOP causes **glaucoma** and in long-term leads to degeneration of the retina.

Exam Questions

1. Name the layers of retina. Describe the importance of fovea centralis and optic disc.
2. Describe the formation and circulation of aqueous humor. Add notes on: a) vitreous humor and b) intraocular pressure.

Multiple Choice Questions

1. All of the following are true for the lens of the eye, EXCEPT:

A. It has no blood supply
B. Possesses higher refractive index at the center than the periphery
C. It develops from the endoderm
D. It composed of transparent collagen fibrils

2. Compared to plasma, Aqueous humor has higher concentration of

A. Protein B. Lactic acid
C. Glucose D. Potassium

3. Normal intraocular pressure is:

A. 5-10 mmHg B. 10-20 mmHg
C. 20-30 mmHg D. 30-40 mmHg

4. Amacrine cells secrete

A. Acetylcholine B. Noradrenaline
C. Adrenaline D. Glutamate

5. All of the following are true for intraocular pressure (IOP), EXCEPT:

A. Volume of lens contributes to IOP
B. IOP keeps the retina pressed against the choroid
C. IOP depends on the amount of aqueous humor present
D. Decrease in IOP in long term leads to degeneration of the retina

Answers

1. C 2. B 3. B 4. A 5. D

Chapter 119

PY10.17

Image Forming Mechanisms

Learning Objectives

On completion of study of this chapter:

The student will be able to (must know):

1. Learn the physical principles of optics.
2. Define refractive power of the eye and the concept of reduced eye.
3. Explain the mechanism of accommodation.
4. Say what is near point, near response, and the mechanism of alteration in pupil size.
5. Define myopia, Hypermetropia, astigmatism and presbyopia and understand the physiological basis of causation and prevention of these defects of image forming mechanism.

The student may also be able to (desirable to know):

1. Describe the physiology of optics and the defects in image forming mechanism.

When light rays from an object fall on the eye, the image of the object is focused on the retina by the following **three mechanisms**:

1. **Refraction** of light rays by cornea and lens.
2. Ciliary muscle activity-causing **accommodation** of lens.
3. **Change in pupil size** by iris muscles.

REFRACTION OF LIGHT RAYS

When light rays traveling through a transparent medium pass into a second transparent medium with a different density (e.g. air to water), they **bend at the interface.** This *change of direction of light rays* at the junction between the two interfaces is called refraction.

The **degree and direction of bending** depend on the following factors.

i. The **angle at which the ray strikes the surface** of the second medium (curvature of the interface).
    - If the ray strikes at an angle of 90°, there is no bending and the ray passes straight.
    - Oblique rays bend more sharply.
    - If the surface of the next medium **is curved**, based on the type (concave or convex) and degree of curvature (greater the radius of curvature, more is the bending), parallel rays of light bend in different angles and travel in the new medium in different directions.

ii. **Difference in density** between the two mediums. When the rays pass from a less dense to a dense medium (e.g. air to water), bending is towards the midline.

iii. **Wavelength** of light.
    - Light rays of longer wavelength get refracted more than lights of shorter wavelength.
    - The visible light has wavelengths ranging from **400 nm to 750 nm**.

Refractive Index (RI)

The **ratio of speed of light in a given medium to that in air is called the refractive index** of that medium. Light travels rapidly in a less dense medium (e.g. air) and slowly in a denser medium (e.g. lens). The refractive index (RI) of air being taken as 1, the RI of other media is as follows: cornea (1.38), aqueous humor (1.33), lens (1.38) and vitreous humor (1.33).

Principles of Optics

The light rays coming from a distant source of light (more than 6 m) are assumed to be parallel and the rays coming from a distance of less than 6 m are diverging rays.

1. A **convex/positive lens** has increasingly more bending power (from center to periphery) and brings parallel light rays to a common point, called **focal point** (Fig. 119.1A).

- A converging lens can form a real image.
- The lens present in the eye is a biconvex lens.

2. The line joining the centers of the two spheres parts of which form the lens surfaces is called the **principal axis** of the lens.
   - The **optical center** of the lens is a point on the principal axis through which light rays pass without being deviated.
   - When parallel rays of light strike the surface of the lens, they converge to meet at a point behind the lens called the **principal focus.**
   - The distance between the optical center of a lens and the principal focus is called the **focal distance.**
3. In case of a **biconcave lens,** the light rays striking the surface of the lens diverge and they appear to diverge from the principal focus situated in front of the lens (Fig. 119.1B).

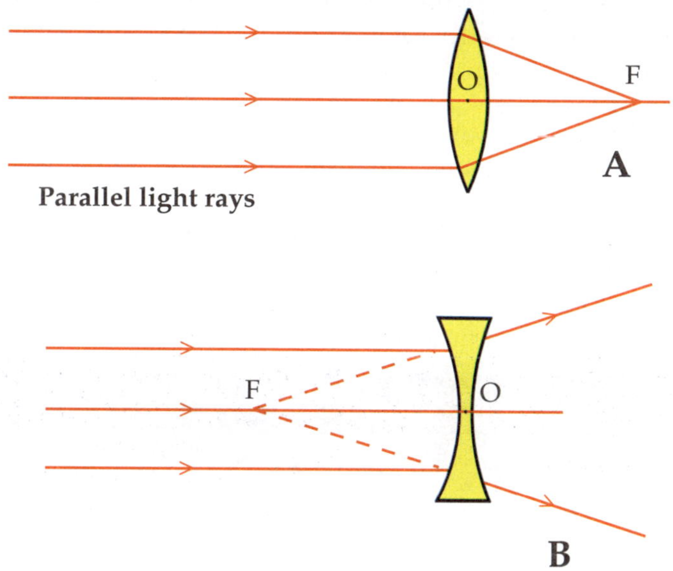

Figs. 119.1: Refraction of light rays by (A) convex and (B) concave lenses.

Refractive Power

The refractive power of a lens is expressed in **diopters** (D), which is the reciprocal of the focal distance of a lens in meters. A lens with a focal length of one meter has a refractive power of 1/1= 1D. Similarly, lenses with focal lengths of 2m, 0.5m and 0.25 m have refractive powers of 0.5 D (1/2), 2 D (1/0.5), and 4D (1/0.25) respectively. In other words, the **greater the lens curvature, the greater is its refractive power**; here, the principal focus is nearer and the focal distance is smaller.

1. As light rays enter the eye, they get **refracted by the cornea.**
2. The light rays are further **refracted at both surfaces of the lens** so that they come into exact focus on the retina.
3. The eye has a **total refractive power of 60 D**; out of which **43 D is contributed by the cornea** and only **17 D by lens.**
   - The ***cornea has the greatest refractive power*** because the ***change in density between the two media is maximum*** *in it i.e. 1 to 1.33.*
   - When the head is immersed **in water**, the refractive power contributed by the cornea *becomes zero* because water has the same refractive index as cornea.

Reduced Eye

The process of refraction is explained with the help of a **schematic eye or reduced eye** (Fig. 119.2). The path of light rays and the image formed on the retina is diagrammatically represented by assuming that all refractions occur at the anterior surface of the cornea, between a medium with RI 1.0 (air) and a medium with RI 1.33 (water).

1. The **nodal point (optical center of the eye)** is situated *7 mm behind the anterior surface of the cornea* and coincides with the *junction of the middle and posterior third of the lens.*
   - The light rays from an object that pass through the nodal point *do not get refracted,* whereas other rays get refracted at the anterior surface of the cornea and are brought to focus on the retina.
   - As the eye is about 24 mm in length, the distance of the nodal point from the retina (focal length) is about 24 – 7 = 17 mm (0.017m).
   - The refractive power of the schematic eye will be **1 divided by its focal length** in meters i.e. 1/0.017 = 59 D. This value is same with the refractive power of the normal human eye, when measured with X-ray.
2. As shown in the diagram, the light rays coming from the object AB, get refracted and form an image A′B′ on the retina. The rays arising from B pass through the nodal point (N) without any refraction; ANB and A′NB′ are similar triangles. The angle subtended by the object AB at the nodal point (<ANB) is known as the **visual angle.**

The **size of the retinal image** can be calculated if, the height of the object and its distance from the eye (observer) is known.

$$\frac{\text{Size of object}}{\text{Size of image}} = \frac{\text{distance of object from nodal point}}{\text{distance of image from nodal point}}$$

If the object is 1 meter high and 10 meters away from the eye, the size of the image will be

$$\frac{1\times 1000\text{ mm}}{\text{Size of image}} = \frac{10\times 1000\text{ mm}}{17\text{ mm}}$$

Size of image = 17/ 10 = 1.7 mm

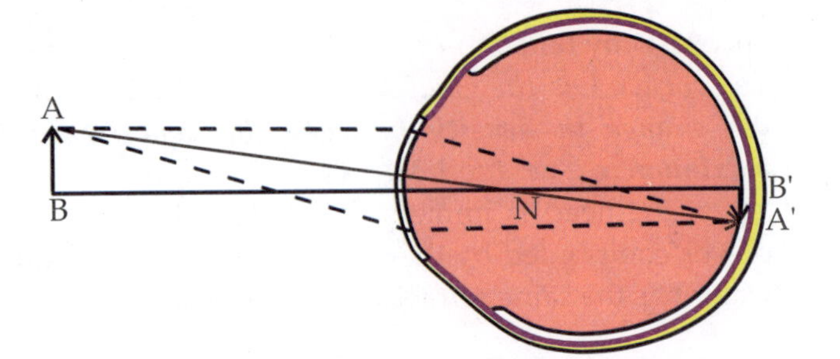

Fig. 119.2: Reduced eye. AB: the object; N: nodal point; A'B': the image formed on the retina. All refractions are assumed to occur on the surface of cornea (refraction by lens is not taken into account).

Retinal Image

The emergent rays from the posterior surface of the lens form a **real, inverted and much smaller image** on the retina.

1. The image is **upside down** (Fig. 119.2).
2. Also, there is **left to right reversal of the image** i.e. light rays from the left side of an object strikes the right side of the retina, and from right side of an object strikes the left side of the retina.
   - That means a tree will be focused as branches down and base up; a man lying down with head on left side will be focused as man with head on right side.
3. But actually, ***we do not see an inverted world*** because **neural processing helps the brain to perceive visual images with upright appearance**. This phenomenon is inherent to us since birth.

ACCOMMODATION

Basically, to be able to see an object clearly, the object should be present at the focal point of the focusing apparatus. Like a camera, the eye can focus on objects at varying distances by changing its point of focus.

1. As the *cornea is a fixed structure whose curvature does not change*, its **refractive power is constant** in air medium.
2. The ability of the eye to alter its focal distance is due to the **malleable lens** that can *change its curvature of the anterior surface* by **contraction of the ciliary muscles** (the radius of curvature changes from 12 mm to 6 mm).
3. The curvature of the posterior surface of lens does not change much (6 mm at rest to 5 mm in full accommodation).
4. In a normal resting eye, the ciliary muscles are relaxed, the lens is stretched and the eye is focused on distant objects at more than 6 m. To focus an object present within 6 m, the eye has to increase its refractive power, a process called **accommodation**, in which the *curvature of the lens is increased* (Fig. 119.3).
5. During accommodation, the **ciliary muscle contracts**, pulls the ciliary body forward and medially towards the lens. The *suspensory ligaments relax, the tension exerted on the lens capsule decreases* and the *elastic lens becomes more convex*.

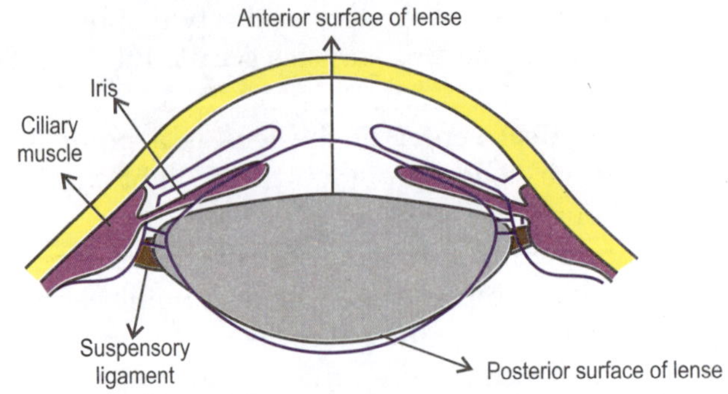

Fig. 119.3: Changes during accommodation. The ciliary muscle contracts, so that the ciliary body moves forward and medially. As a result, the suspensory ligaments relax, decreasing the tension exerted on the lens capsule. The elastic lens becomes more convex; the curvature of anterior surface increases more than the posterior surface.

Near Point

It is defined as the **nearest point to the eye, at which an object can be clearly seen**. At this point, accommodation is exerted to its maximum. The ciliary muscle has contracted to its maximum and the suspensory ligaments have maximally relaxed. If an object is kept at a distance less than this, it appears blurred and can be visible clearly with the help of a convex lens.

- The **maximum accommodation ability of the eye decreases throughout life,** and so the near point recedes, slowly during the initial 35- 40 years of life and then rapidly afterwards (Table 119.1).

Table 119.1 | Effect of age on state of near point and accommodation ability.

Age (in years)	Near point (in cm)	Accommodation ability (in diopters)
10	9	11
20	10	10
30	13	8
40	18	6
50	50	2
60	85	1.5
70	100	1

This *gradual loss of accommodation* is due to **progressive loss of elasticity of the lens**. With advancing age, the lens becomes harder that results in decreased ability of the lens to increase its curvature in response to the contraction of the ciliary muscles.

Near Response

When an individual changes his gaze from a distant object to a near object, **three changes** occur in his eye. They are:

i. **Increase in curvature of the anterior surface of the lens** (accommodation)
ii. **Convergence of the visual axes** (as the eyeballs rotate medially); more near the object, greater the inward rotation.

iii. **Constriction of the pupil**.

SIZE OF THE PUPIL

1. In bright light, the **pupil constricts to a minimum diameter of 2 mm** and in dark, it **dilates to about 8 mm**. As the area of a circle depends upon the square of its radius, the pupil can change its area to 16 fold in conditions of extreme illumination.
2. The small size of pupil **decreases spherical and chromatic aberration** by eliminating the peripheral rays and increases the depth of focus.
3. The **optimum vision is achieved with a pupillary diameter of 2 to 3 mm**.

Chromatic Aberration: As light travels in a medium, its velocity depends on its wavelength. Lights with longer wavelength (e.g. red color light) get refracted more and lights with shorter wavelength (e.g. violet color light) get refracted less. Thus, **lights of different colors get focused at different points on the retina**. This is known as chromatic aberration.

Spherical Aberration: Spherical aberration occurs due to **non-uniform refractive index of the lens** at its center and the periphery. Light rays that pass through the lens near its periphery get refracted more than the rays that enter through its central portion. Thus, lights of a single wavelength **get focused at different points on the retina**. This is known as spherical aberration.

DEFECTS OF THE IMAGE FORMING MECHANISM

The refractive condition of a normal eye is known as **emmetropia** and the eye is known as an emmetropic eye, in which the parallel rays of light from a distant object are focused on the retina without accommodation (Fig.119.4A).

- If the refractive state differs from the normal, it is known as **ammetropia**, in which parallel rays are focused in front or behind the retina resulting in a blurred image.
- If this occurs in children, one of the images is suppressed, causing loss of vision in one eye. This is called **amblyopia ex anopsia.**
- Ammetropia is of three types: myopia, hypermetropia and astigmatism.

The **refractive errors of the eye** *may be due to abnormality in the following.*

i) Axial length of the eye
ii) Refractive power
  - Curvature of the surface of the cornea or the lens,
  - Refractive indices of the media,
  - Position of the lens.

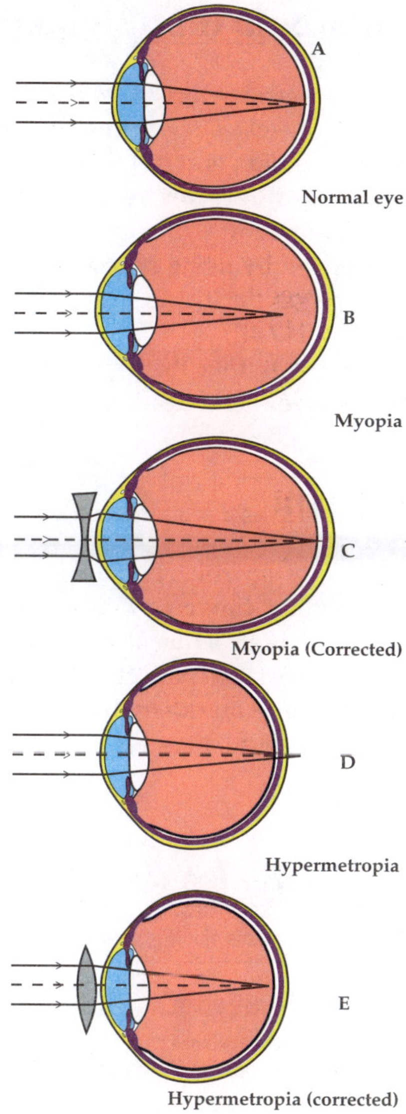

Figs. 119.4: Common defects of the image forming mechanism. (A) Normal eye; (B) Myopia, where the light rays are focused in front of the retina; (C) Correction of myopia by using a biconcave lens; (D) Hypermetropia, where the light rays are focused behind the retina; (E) Use of a biconvex lens helps to focus light rays on the retina and corrects hypermetropia.

Myopia (Short-Sightedness)

It is a refractive error in which *parallel rays of light from a distant object are brought into a* **focus in front of the retina** when the accommodation is at rest (Fig. 119.4B).

The **causes** of myopia can be **genetic or acquired**.

1. Congenitally, the eyeball may be elongated, i.e. the **antero-posterior diameter of the eye is increased**.
2. Myopia is acquired, when increased duration of close works over years like reading, working on computer or sewing etc. continuously activates the accommodation process, especially the *lens becomes more convex.*

Myopia can be **corrected by using spectacle with biconcave lens** that diverges the incident rays before they strike the cornea (Fig. 119.4C).

Hypermetropia (Far-Sightedness)

It is a refractive error in which *parallel rays of light from a distant object are brought into a* **focus behind the retina** when the accommodation is at rest (Fig. 119.4D).

1. It occurs mainly due to **decreased antero-posterior diameter of the eye**.
2. It can be **corrected by using spectacles with biconvex lens** that converges the incident rays before they strike the cornea (Fig. 119.4E).
3. The near point is farther than normal, so the patient needs the biconvex lens (reading glass) at an earlier age.

Astigmatism

It is a refractive error in which parallel rays of light from a distant object **cannot converge to a point focus** on the retina due to **unequal refraction at different meridians**.

1. The corneal surface is not perfectly spherical; therefore, the **curvature of one meridian differs from the other**. Accordingly, the light rays are focused at different points on the retina causing blurring of image.
2. It can also occur **if the lens curvature is not uniform** or if the **lens is pushed out of alignment**.
3. It is **corrected by using a cylindrical lens**.

Presbyopia

This is a physiological phenomenon seen in all persons at about the **age of 40 years** in which the **near point of vision recedes** beyond the normal reading or working distance due to **progressive loss of plasticity of the lens**.

1. As the **near point recedes** beyond the point at which one is used to do close work or read ordinary prints, which is about 28 cm from the eye, the person has difficulty in reading, writing and performing close work (e.g. threading a needle).
2. It is **corrected by using a convex lens** for near vision, and concave lens for distant vision, usually prescribed in the form of **bifocal lenses**, so that when the person wants to change his focus from a near to distant object, each time he need not take off the glasses.

Exam Questions

1. Describe the physical principles of optics with reference to refractive index and refractive power. Add a note on reduced eye.
2. Describe the mechanism of accommodation. Add a note on near point.
3. Describe the mechanisms of image formation and the defects in image formation. Add a note on retinal image.

Multiple Choice Questions

1. The distance between the optical of the eye and anterior surface of the cornea is about:
A. 17 mm B. 15 mm
C. 7 mm D. 2 mm

2. If the eye has a total refractive power of 60 D, the lens contributes about:
A. 17 D B. 23 D
C. 33 D D. 43 D

3. When the head is immersed in water, the refractive power contributed by cornea becomes:
A. 43 D B. 33 D
C. 17 D D. 0 D

4. When water enters the eye, the vision becomes blurred because:
A. Water medium poorly transmits light
B. Corneal surface becomes irregular
C. No refraction occurs at water at water layer in front of cornea
D. No refraction occurs at cornea

5. Refraction mainly occurs at the:
A. Anterior surface of cornea
B. Anterior surface of lens
C. Posterior surface of cornea
D. Posterior surface of lens

6. The closest that a normal eye can focus in a child aged 10 years is:
A. 3 cm B. 9 cm
C. 13 cm D. 25 cm

7. All of the following occur during near response, *except*:
A. Contraction of the suspensory ligaments
B. Contraction of the cilliary muscles
C. Constriction of the pupil
D. Convergence of the visual axes

8. Which of the following statement is TRUE?
A. Anteroposterior diameter of the eye is decreased in myopia
B. Hypermetropia is corrected by a biconcave lens
C. Astigmatism occurs if the lens is pushed out of alignment
D. In presbyopia, lens plasticity is not altered

9. The optimum vision is achieved by a pupillary diameter of:
A. 1–2 mm
B. 2–3mm
C. 4–5 mm
D. 5–6 mm

10. The pupillary area can change to a maximum:
A. 2 fold
B. 4 fold
C. 8 fold
D. 16 fold

Answers

1. C 2. A 3. D 4. D 5. A 6. B 7. A 8. C 9. B 10. D

Chapter 120

PY10.17

Photoreceptor Mechanisms

Learning Objectives

On completion of study of this chapter:

The student will be able to (must know):

1. Illustrate the structure and functions of rods and cones.
2. Name the photopigments and give their functions.
3. Describe the mechanism of genesis of photoreceptor potentials in rods and cones.
4. Outline the major steps of phototransduction.
5. Say how are the photoreceptor activities restored to the resting state.

The student may also be able to (desirable to know):

1. Describe biochemical and physiological mechanisms of phototransduction.

STRUCTURE OF PHOTORECEPTORS

Rods

The rod cell is so named because of its long, slender, and cylindrical appearance (Fig. 120.1).

1. Its **outer segment** contains numerous disks composed of cell membrane in which the molecules of the photopigment **rhodopsin** are embedded. The disks are separated from the cell membrane.
   - The **double membrane disks** are flattened and piled up on each other in a regular manner like a stack of coins.
2. From the upper part of the outer segment, old disks are regularly shed and removed by phagocytosis by the pigment epithelium, and replaced with new disks synthesized at the inner edge of the outer segment.
   - This **renewal is a continuous and rapid process**, at a rate of about ***30 disks per day.***
3. The rod cell synapses with several rod bipolar cells.

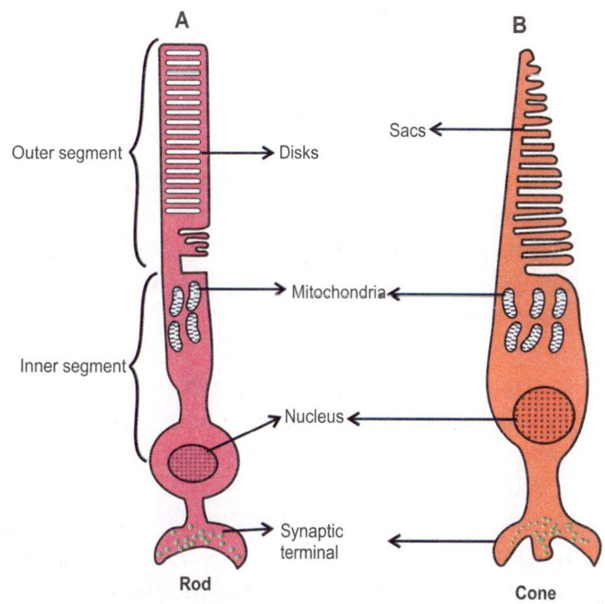

Fig. 120.1: Structure of A: rod, and B: cone.

Cones

Cones have a broad inner segment and a tapered outer segment that gives them a conical appearance (Fig. 120.1). The ***foveal cones are smaller*** *and thinner than the extrafoveal cones.*

1. The **outer segment** is formed by infoldings of the cell membrane.
   - The membrane invaginations look similar to the **rod disks**, but they are not separated from the cell membrane, and their size increases from tip to the inner edge of the outer segment.
   - The **photopigments are present on these membrane infoldings**.
2. The ***renewal process*** *in cones is more diffuse* and occurs at ***multiple sites*** in its outer segment.

Photopigments

There are **four different photosensitive compounds** present in the retina, **one in the rods** and **three in the cones**.

- The photopigment is made up of **retinene$_1$**, the actual light-sensitive component of the photopigments and **opsin**, an integral membrane protein.
- The **retinine (chromophore molecule)** is the same in each of the photopigments but the **opsin differs** in each of the four pigments. The retinines are also called **retinals**, as they are the aldehyde of vitamin A.

Rod Pigment (Rhodopsin)

The photosensitive pigment in the rods that absorbs light is called **rhodopsin or visual purple**.

1. It is a **G protein** coupled serpentine receptor for light.
   - It is a globular protein with a molecular weight 41,000. Rhodopsin molecules are very tightly packed with a density of 30,000 molecules per square micrometer of the membrane; consequently, they make up ***90% of the total protein in disk membranes***.
2. It is made up of **retinene and an opsin**, called **scotopsin**.
   - **Opsin** is a single polypeptide that spans the membrane seven times.
   - **Retinene** remains parallel to the surface of the membrane being encircled by the opsin chain.
3. The **peak spectral sensitivity** for rhodopsin is **500 nm**.

Cone Pigments

Three types of cone pigments are present in the retina. The pigments differ in the wavelength of light that optimally excites them.

1. The peak spectral sensitivity for the **red-sensitive pigment** is 560 nm; for the **green-sensitive pigment** is 530 nm; and for the **blue-sensitive pigment**, it is about 420 nm.
2. Each cone cell contains **one of the three cone pigments**; accordingly, there are **red, green and blue cones**.
   - Each pigment contains retinene$_{-1}$ and an opsin that has seven membrane spanning domain like scotopsin; but structures of opsins and the way they bind to retinene differs.

Melanopsin

This pigment is **present in some photoreceptors that do not contain rhodopsin or the cone pigments**. The receptors *converge on to specific ganglion cells*, whose fibers travel in the optic nerve and project to the **suprachiasmatic nuclei and pretectal nuclei**.

- These nuclei are concerned with the **regulation of circadian rhythms and pupillary light reflexes**.
- In the absence of the gene for melanopsin, or in damage to the receptors or to the pathways, the above responses are abolished.

MECHANISM OF PHOTOTRANSDUCTION

When light strikes the eye, a hyperpolarizing potential is generated in the rods and cones, known as **photoreceptor potential**. The conversion of the light energy to neural signal by the visual pigments in the photoreceptors is known as **phototransduction**.

- Light induces a **conformational change** in the photopigment and the associated G protein that alters membrane potential by **lowering the cGMP level**.
- The change in membrane potential at the synaptic terminal modulates the discharge of the neurotransmitter **glutamate** and thus, initiates a response in the next order of neuron.
- The mechanism of phototransduction can be better appreciated by understanding the processes taking place in the absence of light.

Processes Occurring in the Dark

The **Na^+ channels** on the membrane of the outer segment of the photoreceptors are **cGMP-dependent**.

1. In the absence of light, a constitutively active **guanylyl cyclase** hydrolyses **GTP to cGMP**, which maintains the Na^+ channels in the open state, allowing **Na^+ influx**.
2. Inside the rod cell, **Na^+ flows from the outer segment toward the inner segment** along its concentration gradient, as the cytoplasmic Na^+ concentration of the inner segment is maintained at a lower level by the action of **Na^+-K^+ ATPase.**
3. Outside the cell ***sodium flows from the ECF close to inner segment*** *and from ECF close to the outer segment along a favorable gradient* (Fig. 120.2).
   - Thus, in the outer segment, continuous inflow of sodium is maintained producing a decrease in membrane potential that in turn keeps the ***voltage-gated calcium channels open*** in the synaptic terminal.
4. The **calcium-mediated exocytosis** of synaptic vesicles results in a steady release of the neurotransmitter **glutamate**.
   - Thus, the photoreceptor cell is **depolarized at rest**.

Genesis of Photoreceptor Potential

In Rods

In the dark, the retinene$_1$ in the rhodopsin remains in a less stable form, known as 11-**cis-retinal.**

1. When light strikes the eye, it **absorbs a photon** and gets isomerized to **all-trans-retinal**, which is a more

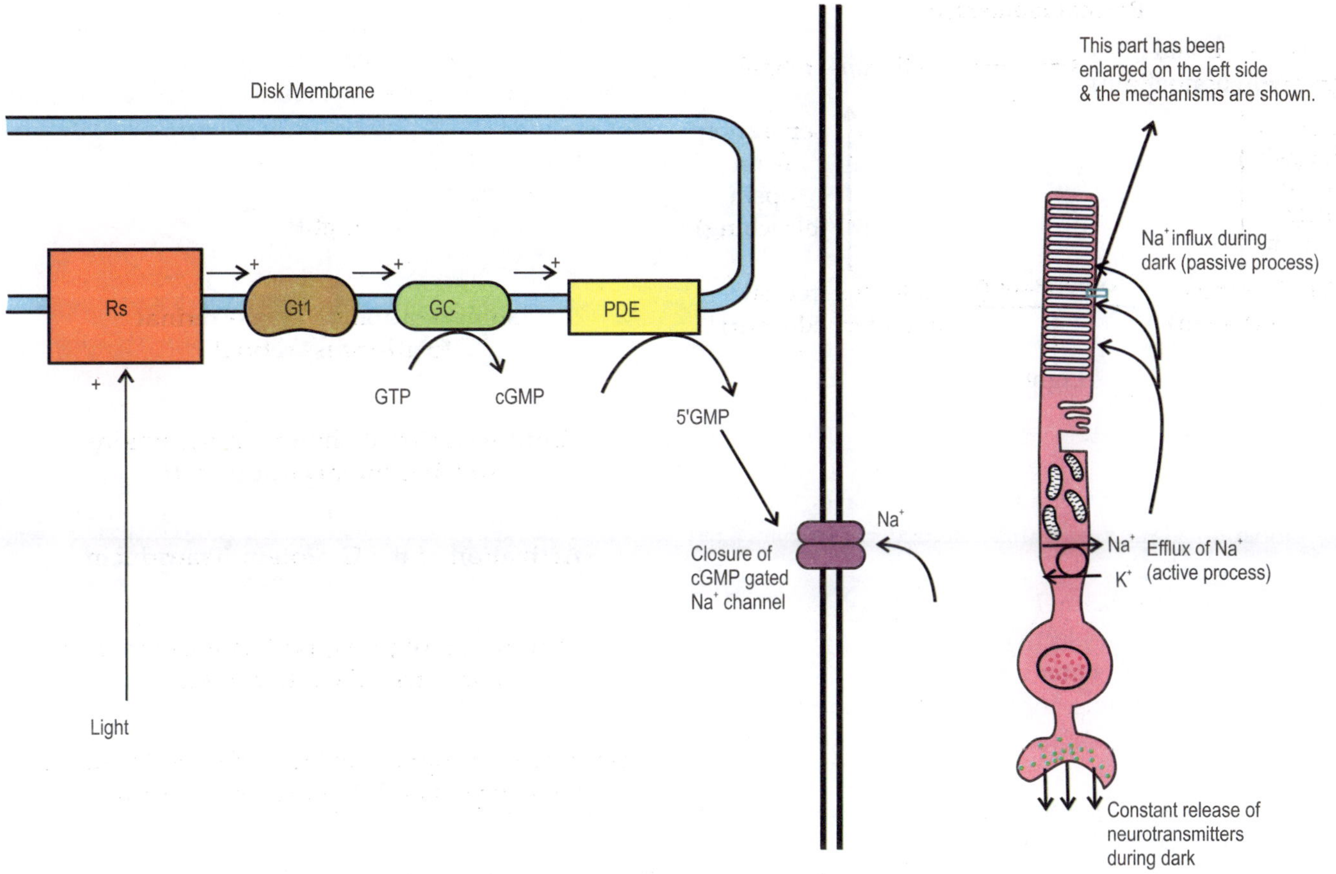

Fig. 120.2: Mechanism of phototransduction. Light activates rhodopsin that stimulates the G protein. Gt1 activates PDE, which converts cGMP into 5'GMP and brings in closure of cGMP-gated Na^+ channels. Guanylyl cyclase hydrolyzes GTP to cGMP. Na^+-K^+ ATPase decreases cytoplasmic Na^+ level by pumping out Na^+ from the outer segment of the photoreceptors. Na^+ enters the inner segments along concentration gradient through the cGMP-gated Na^+ channels. Rs: rhodopsin; GC: guanylyl cyclase; PDE: phosphodiesterase.

stable form.

- This isomerization induces conformational change and converts rhodopsin to **metarhodopsin II**, which in turn activates an associated G protein, called **Gt1** or **transducin.**
- During the activation process, GDP is exchanged for GTP, causing separation of α subunit from β, γ subunit.

2. **Transducin** stimulates **cGMP phosphodiesterase** that converts cGMP to 5'GMP (Fig. 120.2).
   - The *decreased cGMP level* in the cytoplasm leads to **closure of cGMP-gated Na^+ channels**.
   - This produces a hyperpolarizing membrane potential as compared to the potential in the dark, resulting in decreased neurotransmitter release at the terminal synapse.
   - Thus, **the photoreceptor becomes hyperpolarized on stimulation**.
3. The phototransduction pathway **gets amplified** during the cascade of reactions increasing the response several fold.
   - The absorption of 1 photon stimulates 1 metarhodopsin molecule that activates 700 transducins causing hydrolysis 1400 cGMP molecules.

In Cones

The mechanism of phototransduction in cones is similar to that in the rods except that the **G protein is Gt2**, which stimulates the enzyme cGMP phosphodiesterase.

Restoration of the Resting State

Soon after isomerization, **all-trans-retinal is separated** from opsin. As a result, the reddish color imparted to opsin by the photopigment disappears and opsin becomes pale yellow. Hence, the process is called **bleaching**.

1. The all-trans-retinal moves to the pigment epithelium, where the enzyme **retinal isomerase** converts it into **11-cis-retinal**.
   - The **photopigment then gets translocated** to the outer segment of the rods to **recombine with opsin**, replenishing the rhodopsin store (Fig. 120.3).
   - It takes a **few minutes** for one regeneration cycle to get completed.
2. Following activation of phosphodiesterase by the G protein, the intrinsic GTPase activity of the α subunit hydrolyzes GTP to GDP, terminating the action of G protein.

- The stimulating activity of transducin *comes to an end* by its binding to **β-arrestin**, a cytosolic protein.

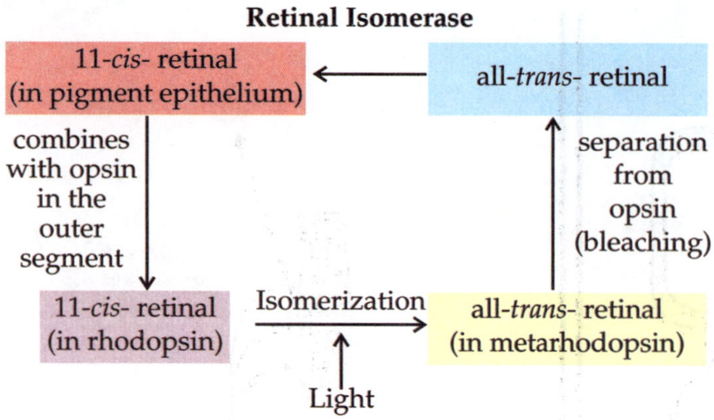

Fig. 120.3: Changes occurring in retinene-1 during light and dark.

- The enzyme **rhodopsin kinase** causes phosphorylation of light-activated rhodopsin and thus, ***deactivates it.***

3. The **cGMP-gated channel** present in the photoreceptor membrane is a nonselective cation channel, through which **Na^+ and Ca^{2+} enter** into the cell.
   - **When light strikes** the eye, **these channels close** and the concentration of **Na^+ and Ca^{2+} decreases in the cell.**
   - The *reduced Ca^{2+} concentration* ***stimulates guanylyl cyclase*** and inhibits phosphodiesterase, resulting in **raised cGMP level.**
   - Thus, cytoplasmic cGMP concentration is maintained by the activity of guanylyl cyclase and phosphodiesterase, both of which are finely regulated by cytoplasmic Ca^{2+} concentration.
4. **In the dark,** Ca^{2+} influx *exerts an inhibitory effect* on guanylyl cyclase, so that cGMP concentration does not become very high.
   - Ca^{2+} is removed from the outer segment by a Na^+-Ca^{2+} exchanger.
5. Thus, *in the resting state, the* ***photoreceptors are partially depolarized*** and increased amount of neurotransmitters are released at the synaptic endings.

The mechanism of phototransduction is summarized in Fig. 120.4.

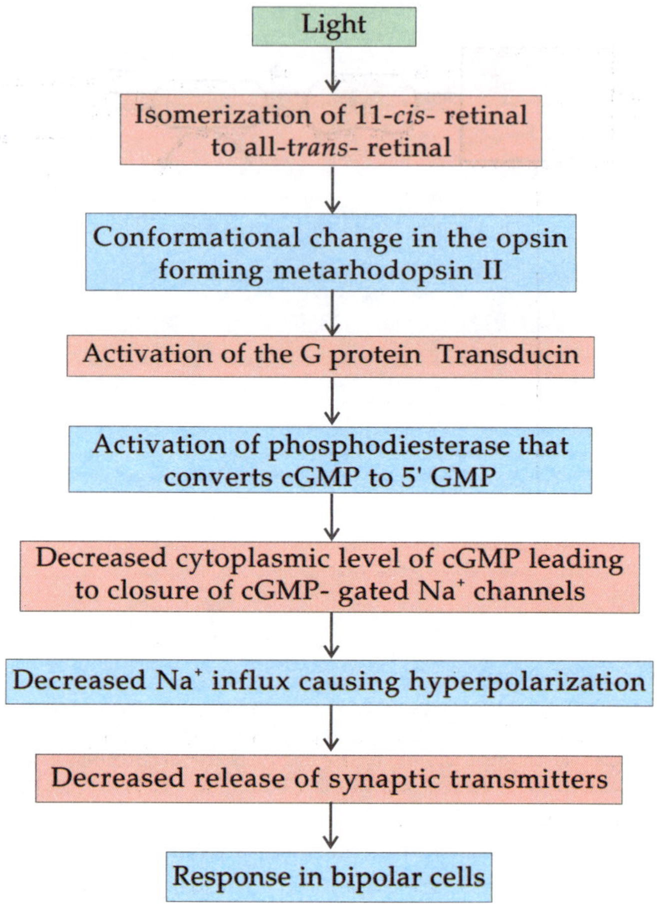

Fig. 120.4: Steps of phototransduction.

Exam Questions

1. Draw labelled diagrams of rods and cones, and describe the mechanism of phototransduction.
2. Describe the mechanisms of genesis of photoreceptor potentials. Give a note on how are the photoreceptors restored to resting state?

Multiple Choice Questions

1. **The receptor potential of rod cells differs from other sensory receptors that it shows**
   A. Depolarization
   B. Hyperpolarization
   C. Increased conductance of sodium
   D. Decreased negativity
2. **Transducin is required for**
   A. Smell B. Somatic sensation
   C. Audition D. Vision
3. **On exposure to dark, photoreceptors release**
   A. Glutamate B. Adrenaline
   C. Acetylcholine D. Histamine
4. **Which of the following combines with opsin to form Rhodopsin in the absence of light**
   A. 11-cis –retinol B. 11-cis-retinaldehyde
   C. All-trans-retinaldehyde D. All –trans – retinol
5. **All of the following are differences between rods and cones EXCEPT**
   A. Acuity
   B. B. Wavelength
   C. Signal transduction
   D. Light sensitivity

Answers

1. B 2. D 3. A 4. B 5. C

Chapter 121

Visual Pathway and Visual Cortex

Learning Objectives

On completion of study of this chapter:

The student will be able to (must know):

1. Draw a labeled diagram of visual pathway and name the visual defects produced by lesions at different levels.
2. Briefly describe the responses of retinal neurons to photic stimulation.
3. Name the ganglion cells and give their functions.
4. Illustrate the topographical organization in lateral geniculate body.
5. Name the visual cortical areas and give their functions.
6. Say what is ocular dominance column and what is its importance.

The student may also be able to (desirable to know):

1. Describe the connections and functions of different components of visual pathway.
2. Describe the structural organization and functions of visual cortex.

VISUAL PATHWAY

The visual sensations arise in **rods and cones** (end organs), from which they are transmitted to the bipolar cells that convey the sensation to the ganglion cells.

1. From the retina, the fibers of the ganglion cells congregate to form the **optic nerve** as they come out through the optic disc.
   - Each optic nerve carries about *1 million fibers* from each retina.
   - The optic nerve travel to the optic chiasm, where about half the fibers of each eye cross over to the opposite side. After the chiasm, fibers travel as **optic tract** to the **lateral geniculate body** (LGB).
2. Fibers from the **temporal half of retina do not cross the midline** and travel in the optic tract of the same side.
   - Fibers from the **nasal half of retina decussate at the chiasm** and travel in the *optic tract of the opposite side* (Fig. 121.1A to D).
   - Thus, each optic tract contains fibers arising from temporal half of retina of the same side and nasal half of the retina of the opposite side. In other words, **left optic tract contains fibers from the left half of the retina** (right visual field) and **right optic tract contains fibers from the right half of the retina** (left visual field).
   - The **macular fibers decussate** *in a similar manner* at the chiasm, i.e. nasal half of the fibers decussate at the chiasm and temporal half of macular fibers travel uncrossed in the optic tract.
3. The direct and crossed fibers in the optic tract pass to the alternating lamina **of the LGB** and end there.
4. From the neurons of the LGB, the axons project to the ipsilateral primary visual cortex or V1 (**Brodmann's area 17**), located on the sides of the calcarine fissure on the medial aspect of the occipital lobe of the brain.
   - The fibers carrying visual impulses from the LGB to the calcarine cortex are called **geniculocalcarine tract**.
   - As these fibers spread out from LGB, they are known as **optic radiation**.
   - Since V1 is also known as striate cortex, these fibers are named as **geniculostriate tract**.
5. From the LGB, **macular fibers** project to the posterior pole of the occipital lobe.
6. The optic nerve fibers project to several **other areas of the brain** like association visual cortex, superior colliculus, pretectal nucleus, and suprachiasmatic nucleus of hypothalamus.
   - These fiber systems participate in regulation of other functions like **circadian rhythm associated with vision**.

IMPORTANT NOTE

Divergence in Visual Pathway: There are about one million fibers in optic nerve, **two million fibers** in geniculocalcarine tract and **1000 million fibers in the visual cortex; a good example of divergence.**

PY10.18

Effects of Lesion: The effects of lesion at various levels of the visual pathway are shown in the Fig. 121.1A to D and the visual deficits due to lesion are described as 'Visual Field Defects' in Chapter 122.

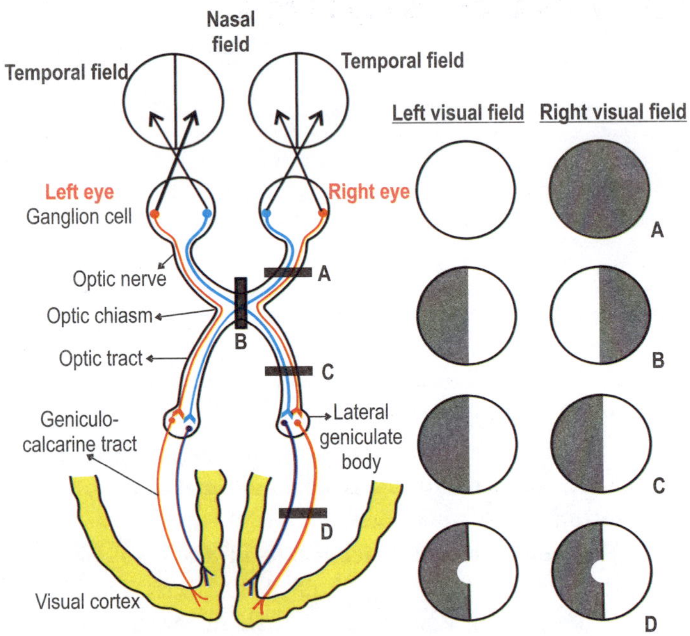

Figs. 121.1: Effects of lesions at various levels of visual pathway. (A) Lesion of right optic nerve produces blindness in right eye; (B) Lesion of optic chiasm produces bitemporal hemianopia; (C) Lesion of right optic tract produces left homonymous hemianopia; (D) Lesion of right geniculocalcarine tract produces left homonymous hemianopia with macular sparing.

Processing of the Visual Signal

Responses of the Retinal Neurons

Photoreceptors

The threshold for rods is lower than that for cones. Therefore, **rods are more sensitive** (*can respond to a single photon of light*).

1. **In rods**, the response is proportionate to the stimulus intensity, but after reaching a maximum, the response does not increase.
   - Thus, **rods are receptors for dim light** and *detect absolute illumination at lower range of stimulus intensity.*
2. **The cones** require high level of illumination for activation and then, their response become proportionate to the stimulus intensity.
   - So, the **cones are receptors for bright light** and they *detect changes in stimulus intensity*.
3. Thus, the human eye can operate over a wide range of light intensities.
   - However, the **response of rods is slower** (*sharp onset, slow offset*) than that of cones (*sharp onset, sharp offset*).
4. When a light stimulus is placed in the receptive field of a **photoreceptor, it produces a hyperpolarizing response** that is transmitted to the bipolar cell.

Bipolar Cell

Bipolar cells link the photoreceptors to ganglion cells.

1. Some of the bipolar cells show a **depolarizing potential** that is excitatory to the ganglion cells, whereas other cells show a **hyperpolarizing potential** that is inhibitory.
2. Based on their morphology and function, the bipolar cells have been **classified into 12 types**.
3. The cells show **on-center and off-center response** like the ganglion cells, as described below.

Horizontal Cell

The photoreceptors also give input to the horizontal cells, which respond with a **hyperpolarizing membrane potential.**

1. With their branching dendrites, they **link rods and cones to other photoreceptors**.
2. Also, the dendrites of the horizontal cells spread laterally and produce inhibition of the bipolar cells on which they synapse.

Amacrine Cell

Amacrine cells exhibit a **depolarizing response**.

1. The amacrine cells spread laterally and synapse on the ganglion cells to which they provide excitatory input.
2. They are classified into **29 types** based on their connections with the ganglion cells in the inner plexiform layer.

Neural Network: Thus, in the retina, the bipolar cells, horizontal cells and amacrine cells comprise the ***neural network layer***, in which considerable processing of visual information takes place. The cells form **gap junctions** with the adjacent cells, so that signals spread in the form of electrotonic potentials rather than propagated action potentials.

Ganglion Cells

They integrate the information received from bipolar and the amacrine cells and respond with a **depolarizing potential** that propagates along the axon (optic nerve).

1. In the resting state, the ganglion cell has a discharge rate of 20-50 spikes/s.
2. The **response** shown by the ganglion cells is of **two types** and accordingly, there are **two types of cells**:
   i) On-center ganglion cells, and
   ii) Off-center ganglion cells.

3. **Receptive field** of a ganglion cell is the area of the visual field in which presence of a light stimulus modulates the discharge pattern of a ganglion cell.
   - The **central retinal neurons** have ***smaller receptive fields***, whereas **peripheral retinal neurons** have ***larger receptive fields***.
4. The **on-center** ganglion cell increases its spike rate in response to a central small circular light stimulus in its receptive field **(on-response)** and when an annulus of light around the center is turned on, its spike rate decreases **(off-response)** (Fig.121.2).
5. In the **off-center** ganglion cell, spike rate decreases when the central stimulus is turned-on and its spike rate increases in response to the surround illumination.
   - Thus, the **on-center ganglion cell** is stimulated ***in response to an excitatory center with an inhibitory surround***, whereas an **off-center ganglion cell** is stimulated ***in response to an inhibitory center with an excitatory surround***.
   - Due to this **center-surround antagonism**, the ganglion cells have been called as **contrast detectors**.
6. **During the off-response** of the on-center ganglion cell, the annulus of light activates a ring of photoreceptors that **stimulates the horizontal cells** (present on both sides of the receptor circle) on which they synapse. The horizontal cells in turn **inhibit the nearby photoreceptors** by ***lateral inhibitory inputs***.
   - In this manner, the **centrally present photoreceptors get inhibited** by the surrounding horizontal cells.
   - Thus, decrease in activity of the neighboring cells by stimulation of a specific cell is known as **afferent** or **lateral inhibition**.
   - This is an important component of information processing during which, **signal transmission** through a ***particular pathway is allowed***, whereas, propagation of action potential through the ***adjacent pathways is inhibited***.
   - Examples of afferent inhibitions are common in spinal cord. In the retina, ***this improves the sharpness*** at the periphery of an image and ***increases contrast***.
7. **Based on size**, there are **two types of ganglion cells** present in the retina: large ganglion cells (**Magno, or M cells**), and small ganglion cells (**Parvo, or P cells**).
   - **The M cells** are concentrated in the peripheral retina and they ***mediate functions of the rod system***. Their axons have a large diameter with a large receptive field.
   - **The P cells** are concentrated in the central retina and exhibit lateral inhibition. They ***mediate the function of cone system*** (colour vision). They have small diameter axons and small receptive fields.
8. Axons of the M ganglion cells **project to the magnocellular layer** of the LGB; and the P ganglion cells **project to the parvocellular layer** and interlaminar region of the LGB.
   - The **function of M cells** is to add potentials from different kinds of cones and transmit the integrated response in the form of action potential. The M cells convey ***information regarding movement and stereopsis*** to the LGB.
   - The **P cells analyze and subtract** response from one type of cone from response from another. They send the ***information regarding color, texture and shape*** of an object to the LGB.

Important features of retinal neurons:

1. The photoreceptors get **hyperpolarized on activation**.
2. **Input to the retina is received** by the photoreceptors and the ganglion cells are the output cells.
3. **Processing of visual signals** mainly occurs in the neuronal network layer.
4. The responses of the cells of the neuronal network layer **are integrated** in the ganglion cell layer.
   - Ganglion cells **generate the action potentials**.
5. The photoreceptors and the ganglion cells are **spontaneously active in the resting state**, so that, any change in visual stimulus brings in a response in them.
6. The visual information (largely from the rods) **converges on the ganglion cells**. This decreases the contrast of an image, but **improves the sensitivity**.

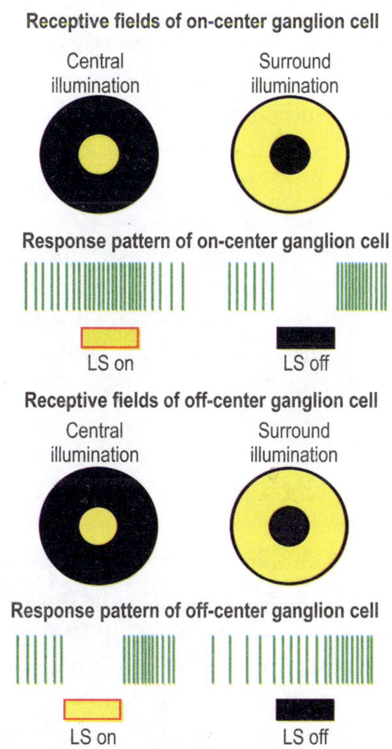

Fig. 121.2: Response patterns of an on-center and an off-center ganglion cell. The firing rate of on-center ganglion cell increases in response to a central small circular light stimulus in its receptive field (on-response) and when an annulus of light around the center is turned on, its firing rate decreases (off-response). In the off-center ganglion cell, spike rate decreases by central illumination and increases in response to surround illumination. LS: Light stimulus.

In Lateral Geniculate Body

Organization and Topography

Most of the fibers of the optic tract terminate in lateral geniculate body (LGB) of thalamus.

1. The LGB is divided into **six well-defined layers numbered 1 to 6** from ventral to dorsal direction.
    - The ventrally placed **layers 1 and 2** have large cells and accordingly are called **magnocellular** that receive input **from M ganglion cells** (Fig. 121.3).
    - **Layers 3,4,5,6** are called **parvocellular** as they contain small cells and receive input from the P ganglion cells. The interlaminar region of the LGB receives inputs from the P ganglion cells.
2. Each LGB receives half of the inputs from both retina through the optic tract and the inputs from each eye project distinctly to specific layer of LGB.
    - Inputs from **nasal retina of contralateral eye projects to layers 1,4 and 6.**
    - Inputs from **temporal retina of ipsilateral eye project to layers 2, 3 and 5.**
3. There is a precise **topographic map** of the retina in each layer of the LGB, i.e. for each point of retina that is excited; there is a specific part of the LGB that receives the potential and responds to it.
    - Thus, the right half (temporal half) of right retina is **represented thrice** in the right LGB; once in layer 2, again in layer 3, and once more in layer 5.
    - Similarly, the right half (nasal half) of left retina is **represented thrice** in the right LGB; once in layer 1, once in layer 4, once in layer 6.
    - Along a perpendicular line through the layers of LGB, **all the cells have the same visual field** (Fig. 121.3).
    - Moreover, this ***point-for-point representation*** follows an orderly pattern.
    - When a visual stimulus activates a group of photoreceptors that are adjacent to each other, the **photoreceptors excite the adjacent cells** in the LGB.
    - The fibers from the **upper part of the retina** project to the ***medial half of LGB***, and fibers from the **lower part of the retina** project to the ***lateral half of LGB.***
4. The **macular area** (central retina) projects to the ***posterior LGB***, whereas the peripheral retina projects more anteriorly.
    - The macular area has the **highest representation** in the LGB compared to the peripheral retina.
5. The neurons of LGB **respond to a point stimulus.**
    - When the stimulus is a bar of light, they respond to each point of the bar.
6. Apart from the inputs from retina, LGB receives maximum inputs **from the visual cortex and other brain areas.**
    - The **visual cortex inputs** provide necessary feedback regarding ***perception of orientation and movement of an object.***

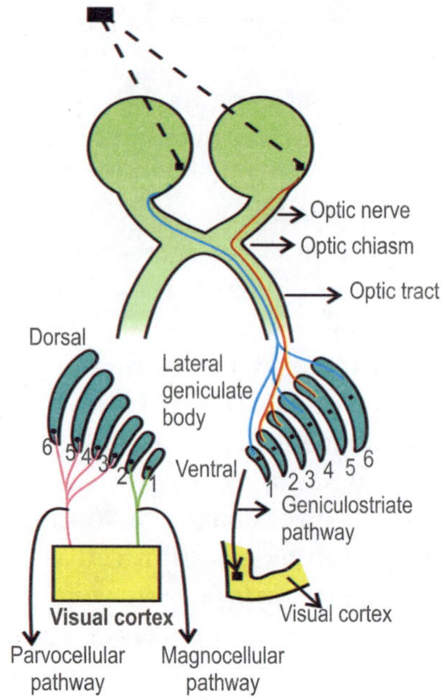

Fig. 121.3: Anatomy of geniculostriate pathway. A rectangular stimulus in the left visual field projects to all six layers of the right lateral geniculate body (LGB). The neurons (represented as black boxes in the figure) receiving this visual impulse are present along a perpendicular line through the layers of LGB. From there, the visual signal is transmitted to a single point in the right visual cortex. On the left side, the origin of parvocellular and magnocellular pathways from the LGB is shown.

- The output from LGB goes to visual cortex as ***geniculostriate fibers.***
- From the cell bodies in **layers 1 and 2**, the fibers form the magnocellular pathway that is concerned with ***detection of movement, depth and flicker.***
- The fibers form the cell bodies ***in layers 3-6,*** carries the impulses regarding ***color, texture, shape and finer detail.***

7. Axons that originate from the **interlaminar region of the LGB** carry the impulses ***for color vision.***

VISUAL CORTEX

Primary Visual Cortex

Organization and Topography

The primary visual cortex (V1) is the **Brodmann's area 17,** located on the sides of the calcarine fissure. It is also known as the **visuo-sensory area** as it receives the sensory information regarding vision.

1. The fibers from the LGB project to the visual cortex in a **topographic manner.**
    - The **geniculocalcarine tract fibers** mainly terminate on the medial part of occipital cortex, above and below the calcarine fissure.
    - The fibers **from the medial part of the LGB** representing upper quadrants of both retinas travel in the dorsal part of the optic radiation and project to the upper lip of the calcarine fissure.

- The fibers from the **lateral part of the LGB** representing the lower quadrants of both retinas form the ventral part of the optic radiation and project to the lower lip of the calcarine fissure.

2. The cortical area devoted to receive **afferents from macula** is much greater than other areas.
   - Thus, **macula has a much larger cortical representation** than peripheral retina.
   - In the visual cortex, the fibers from LGB carrying ***macular afferents terminate more posteriorly*** in the calcarine fissure and the fibers from LGB carrying impulses from ***peripheral retina terminate anteriorly*** in the calcarine fissure (Fig. 121.4).
3. Like other cortical areas, the visual cortex is divided into **six parallel layers**, numbered 1-6.
   - The magnocellular and parvocellular fibers from the LGB project to the **deeper layer 4C** of the visual cortex. *This layer receives information regarding movement, location, orientation, texture, shape and color of an object.*
   - The fibers from the interlaminar region of the LGB project to the **superficial layers 2,3** of the visual cortex. The cells of layers 2,3 are ***rich in enzyme cytochrome oxidase*** and form clusters, known as ***blobs*** that receive information regarding color of an object.
   - The **cells from layer 4** also project to the neurons in layers 2 and 3. The neurons that have their cell bodies in layers 2 and 3, project to the other cortical regions and to the neurons in layer 5.
   - The neurons that have their cell bodies in **deeper layer 5**, project to the superior colliculus, pulvinar and other brainstem nuclei.
   - The neurons in **layer 6** projects to the LGB.

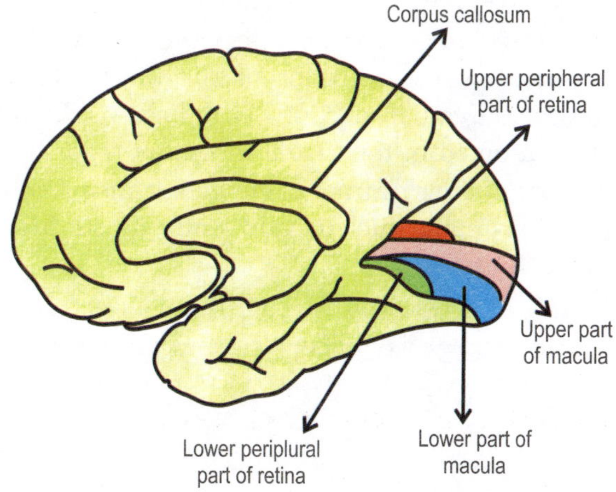

Fig. 121.4: Medial view of the right cerebral cortex. The painted area shows the projection of retinal fibers into the calcarine cortex.

Responses

Like the bipolar cells, ganglion cells and cells of LGB, the cells of visual cortex exhibit **on-center and off-center responses**. But unlike these cells that respond to a point stimulus, the neurons of visual cortex **respond to a linear stimulus like lines, edges or bars of light**. Thus, the stimulus can be a **bar of light against dark background** or a **dark bar against a light background**.

1. The **neurons of layer 4** of the visual cortex respond to a stimulus that is positioned at any angle i.e. they have **no preferred orientation**. But, the cells in other layers are responsive to the orientation of the bar stimulus. Based on this, the cells are classified into **simple, complex and hypercomplex cells.**

Simple Cell: A simple cell responds best to a **particular orientation of the bar stimulus**.

- When the stimulus is rotated as little as 10° from the precise position, the response decreases.

Complex Cells: The complex cells show a low resting discharge rate, whereas the simple cells discharge only on stimulation.

- The complex cells respond best when a bar stimulus moves laterally without change in its orientation.
- Thus, the complex cells are **concerned with movement and velocity of the stimulus** and less with its central location.

Hypercomplex Cells: There are also hypercomplex cells that respond best to a **moving bar with a precise orientation but also with a defined length**.

- Some respond better to a stimulus having a **specific angle** (for example, a L- shaped or tongue-shaped stimulus) or having **two borders**.

2. Thus, the visual cortex receives information regarding **orientation, movement, depth, velocity as well as color** of an object and help in **depth perception and stereopsis** *(**binocular depth perception**)*.
3. Usually, the simple cells project to the complex cells and the hypercomplex cells receive inputs from the complex cells.
   - So, the **receptive fields of the simple cells are smaller** than those of the complex cells and receptive fields **of the hypercomplex cells are larger** than those of the complex cells.
4. When a microelectrode is inserted perpendicularly into the visual cortex, the cells that come across have the same orientation (**orientation column**).
   - The adjacent columns of cells differ 5° to 10° in their orientation in an organized manner.
   - Thus, the simple and complex cells are called ***feature detectors***.
5. All cortical neurons have their **receptive fields in the contralateral visual field.**
   - Each neuron of the layer 4 receives input from only one eye.
   - Also, the cells receiving input from one eye alternate with the cells receiving input from the other eye.
   - When radioactive dye is injected into one eye, the dye reaches visual cortex by axoplasmic transport.

The cortical picture presents a **typical banded pattern**. These alternate columns of cells are known as **ocular dominance columns.**

6. Many of the simple and complex cells of the visual cortex receive input from both the eyes.
   - Thus, the **visual cortex integrates inputs from both the eyes.**
7. The primary visual cortex (V1) **projects to various cortical areas.**
   - Area V8 receives the information about color vision; area V3A and MTV5 are concerned with movement of an object.
   - The LO area is for recognition of larger objects, whereas the functions of area V4v and V7 are not known.
   - The V2, V3 and VP area receive inputs from larger visual fields and are involved in continuous processing of the information.

The effects of lesions of visual cortex are described under visual field defects.

Other Visual Areas

Visual Association Areas

1. **Area 18 and 19** are the **visual association areas.**
2. They are located on the lateral part of the occipital cortex.
3. They receive visual **information from primary visual cortex** and are concerned with **interpretation of the visual stimulus.**
4. They help in appreciating the **finer attributes of the objects** like perception of **form, texture, shape, depth, location** and orientation of the object.
5. **Lesions** of the association areas produce **impairment of these higher visual functions.**

Frontal Eye Field

- The frontal eye field (**Area 8**) is present in the frontal gyrus.
- It controls **saccadic eye movements.**
- Convergence, divergence and near response is influenced by activity in an area anterior to the frontal eye fields.

Superior Colliculi

The superior colliculus is divided into **superficial and deep layers.**

1. The **superficial layers** receive inputs from the optic tract fibers and visual cortex and in turn project to various thalamic nuclei like anterior thalamic nucleus, pulvinar and lateral geniculate body.
   - The neurons of the superficial layer receive inputs from both the eyes and they *discharge in response to a stimulus moving quickly in a particular direction.*
   - Thus, the superior colliculi **coordinate simultaneous bilateral eye movements,** like *saccades and convergence* and keep the **eyeball in focus.**
2. The **deep layers** of superior colliculi receive visual inputs from its superficial layers, inputs from the ***auditory fibers and somatosensory inputs from different body parts.***
   - Also, the neurons of the deep layers regulate the ***head and eye position.***
   - The sensory stimuli are integrated in the deep layers for various reflex activities that involve **appropriate head movement and change in eye opposition.**

Pretectal Nucleus

1. Fibers from the optic tract project to the pretectal nucleus and cause **activation of the Edinger-Westphal nucleus.**
2. These fibers mediate pupillary reflexes and are involved in the **regulation of visual fixation.**

Suprachiasmatic Nucleus

1. It is a small nucleus in the medial hypothalamus, located just above the optic chiasm.
2. It receives fibers from the optic nerve and synchronizes **sleep-wake cycle,** secretion of hormones like cortisol, and other circadian rhythms with light-dark cycle.
3. Information from the visual receptors regarding light intensity during diurnal cycle gets transmitted to the suprachiasmatic nucleus and entrains its **biological clock** activity.

Exam Questions

1. Draw a diagram of visual pathway and depict the effect of lesions at various levels of pathway. Briefly describe the processing of visual signals in ganglion cells.
2. Describe the organization and topography in lateral geniculate body. Add a note on geniculocalcarine projections.
3. Describe the cortical visual areas. Add a note on orientation column and ocular dominance column.

Multiple Choice Questions

1. Which order neuron is the Bipolar cell in the visual pathway?

A. First B. Second
C. Third D. Fourth

2. The only neurons in the retina showing action potentials are

A. Bipolar cell B. Rods and cones
C. Ganglion cell D. Amacrine cell

Answers: 1. B 2. C **MCQs Continued in page number 967.**

Chapter 122

Visual Acuity, Visual Field, Light and Dark Adaptations, and Visual Reflexes

Learning Objectives

On completion of study of this chapter:

The student will be able to (must know):

1. Define and list the factors affecting visual acuity.
2. Understand the physiological basis of tests for visual acuity.
3. Define visual field & learn its mapping.
4. Name the visual field defects produced by lesion at different levels of visual pathway.
5. Describe mechanisms of light adaptation & dark adaptation.
6. Name the visual reflexes and trace the pathways of each visual reflex.

The student may also be able to (desirable to know):

1. Describe the physiological basis of visual filed defects produces by lesions at different levels of visual pathway.
2. Describe the details of mechanisms and significance of light and dark adaptations.

VISUAL ACUITY

Visual acuity is defined as the **ability of the eye to identify two closely placed points as two distinct points**.

- The shortest distance, by which two objects can be separated and still be visualized as two different objects, is known as the **minimum separable distance**.
- Visual acuity expresses the **resolving power of the eye**, that is, the extent to which the eye can perceive the details and contours of an object.
- **Visual acuity is the function of the cones.** There are different tests for testing visual acuity for distant vision and near vision.

Factors Affecting Visual Acuity

Optical Factors

These factors mainly determine the degree of visual acuity. They include the **structures that take part in the image forming mechanisms** of the eye and help in focusing an object, such as:

1. Curvature of the cornea
2. Curvature of the lens
3. Plasticity of the lens
4. Condition of the ciliary muscle and lens ligaments.

Retinal Factors

Visual acuity depends on the **functional status of the cones.** As the cones are concentrated more at the fovea, **visual acuity is highest at the fovea** and decreases toward the periphery.

Stimulus Factors

Various features of an object affect the visual acuity, such as:

1. Size of the object
2. Distance of the object from eye
3. Color of the object
4. Contrast between the object and the background
5. Shape of its borders
6. Brightness of the object
7. Duration for which the object remains in view.

Visual acuity increases as the **size of the object increases** and distance of the object from eye decreases. Thus, visual acuity is **directly proportional to the visual angle**.

Tests for Visual Acuity **PY10.20**

Test for Distant Vision and Near Vision

Visual acuity is tested with the help of **Snellen's chart** and near point of vision is tested by **Jaeger's chart**. The details of these tests are described in Textbook of Practical Physiology, by GK Pal and Pravati Pal, 5th Edition, 2020.

VISUAL FIELD

The area of the external world that can be seen when the gaze is fixed is known as the visual field of that eye.

1. The visual field is limited on the medial side by the bridge of the nose and superiorly by the roof of the orbit, so that the field is not circular.
   - The visual field plotted with one eye is known as **monocular visual field**.
   - The visual field of both eyes overlap in the center and is called **binocular visual field** (Fig. 122.1).
   - An object present in the binocular visual field can be seen by both eyes simultaneously.
2. Each visual field is divided into a **nasal** (medial) and a **temporal** (lateral) portion. For each eye, light rays from an object situated in the nasal field stimulate the temporal retina and light rays from an object situated in the temporal field stimulate the nasal retina.
3. Also, light rays from objects located at the upper part of the visual field stimulate the lower part of retina and those from the lower part of the visual field stimulate the upper part of retina.

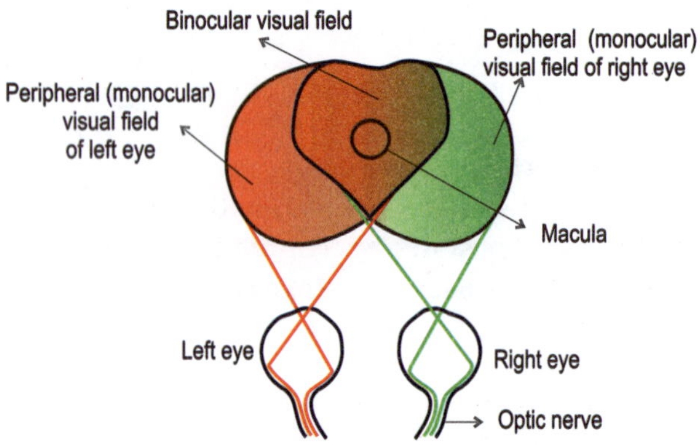

Fig. 122.1: The monocular and binocular visual fi elds.

Binocular Vision

When a person looks at an object with both eyes, the light rays coming from the object stimulate both the retinas.

- The action potentials transmitted by the neural pathways from both retinas **get fused at the visual cortex,** so that the brain perceives them as single image.
- Thus, viewing an object as a single one with both eyes is called *binocular vision.*

Corresponding Points

1. The two points on the retinas on which the light rays from an object fall simultaneously to make binocular vision possible, are known as **corresponding points**.
   - The foveas and all points lying at the same distance and in the same direction from the foveas are corresponding points.
   - For a distant object, the eyeballs move symmetrically and for a near object, the eyeballs converge to allow the light rays to fall on corresponding points.
2. When light rays fall on noncorresponding points, double vision (**diplopia**) results. For example, while looking at an object if you slightly push one eyeball out of the line, diplopia occurs.
3. When the light rays from any object do not fall on the corresponding points for a prolonged period, especially in **children below the age of 6** years, diplopia is not seen as one of the images get suppressed (**suppression scotoma**). This is a cortical phenomenon.
   - This suppression **does not develop in adults**.
   - It should be detected and treated early; otherwise there occurs permanent loss of visual acuity in the eye, in which the image is suppressed.
   - Diplopia also occurs when the **medial rectus or lateral rectus muscles are damaged** or over-activated.

Mapping of Visual Field PY10.20

This is done to diagnose visual field defects.

For Peripheral Field:

1. The **peripheral visual field** is mapped by an instrument called **perimeter** and the process is known as **perimetry,** in which each eye is mapped separately.
2. The perimeter chart paper has circles called **isopters** around the central point, drawn at 10° intervals across the radius from 0° to 90°.
   - There are radial lines called **meridians** that join the periphery at 10° intervals.
3. During the procedure one eye is covered, while the test eye is fixed on a central fixation point.
   - A small contrast target is moved slowly from the periphery to the center in selected meridians along the arc of the instrument, completing the full circle.
   - The spot, where the target becomes first visible is marked in the chart paper.

For Central Field:

1. The **central visual field** comprises of the area within 30° from the central fixation point. It is mapped with **Bjerrum's screen**.
2. The area where the target is not seen is designated as **blind spot or scotoma.**
3. The **scotoma area** is mapped by noting the spot where the object disappeared to the point, where again it reappeared.
4. The **physiological blind spot** due to optic disc is observed on the temporal visual field.

Visual Field Defects PY10.18

Blindness of visual field is known as **anopia. Hemianopia** means half-blindness, which can be **homonymous** (same side of both visual fields) or **heteronymous.**

1. **Lesion of optic nerve** cuts off impulse transmission from that eye and produces **blindness** in that visual field (Refer Fig. 121.1A, Chapter 121).

2. **Lesion of optic chiasm** damages the nasal fibers from both eyes and produces **bitemporal (heteronymous) hemianopia** (Refer Fig. 121.1B).
   - This usually occurs in tumors of anterior pituitary, especially of the growth hormone secreting somatotrophs, in which the enlarged pituitary presses upon the optic chiasm and produces bitemporal hemianopia, a feature of acromegaly.
3. **Lesion of one side temporal fibers** produces blindness of that side nasal field.
   - For example, lesion of **right-side temporal fibers** produces ***right nasal hemianopia***.
   - Lesions of **both side temporal fibers** produce ***binasal hemianopia***.
4. **Lesion of optic tract** damages ipsilateral temporal fibers and contralateral nasal fibers resulting in ***homonymous hemianopia***.
   - Lesion of **left optic tract** produces right homonymous hemianopia; and lesion of **right optic tract** produces left homonymous hemianopia (Fig.121.1C).
5. **Lesion of geniculocalcarine tract** damages ipsilateral temporal fibers and contralateral nasal fibers resulting in **homonymous hemianopia with macular sparing** as macular fibers travel dorsal to the optic radiation and escape the damage (Fig.121.1D).
   - The visual field defects are similar to that of optic tract.
6. **Lesion of occipital cortex** damages ipsilateral temporal fibers and contralateral nasal fibers **with macular sparing.**
   - It produces **scotoma** (blind patches) in the homonymous visual fields, which are usually quadrantic in nature (upper or lower quadrant of either half of visual field).
   - **The macular fibers are spared** unless the damage is widespread because i) the macular fibers project separately in the visual cortex, and ii) they have a much larger representation compared to rest of the retina.

VISUAL ADAPTATIONS

Visual adaptation is of two types: light adaptation, and dark adaptation.

Light Adaptation

When a person suddenly moves from a dimly lighted area to broad daylight, initially the light seems very bright and uncomfortable, and the image appears blurred.

- The visual system activates several mechanisms to adjust to the bright light so that vision improves after some time. This is known as light adaptation.
- **Light adaptation takes about 5 minutes.**
- As an immediate reaction to sudden bright light, the **pupil constricts** and the amount of light entering the retina is reduced.

Mechanisms of Light Adaptation

There are **two mechanisms** of light adaptation: neural and chemical.

Neural Adaptation

1. Following a light stimulus, the **sensitivity of retinal photoreceptors decreases** that manifests in the form of **decreased burst of activity to a constant stimulus.**
2. The **horizontal cells** may have a ***feedback inhibitory effect*** upon the photoreceptors.
   - Besides, with the increase in light intensity, the **amplitude of receptor response does not rise** proportionately.
   - This mechanism plays a greater role in **quickly bringing down** the sensitivity of the photoreceptors, so that light adaptation is mainly a neural phenomenon.

Chemical Adaptation

1. In bright light, **rhodopsin is rapidly converted to all-trans-retinal and opsin.**
   - Due to this bleaching, **rod responsiveness decreases** considerably as rhodopsin becomes less available. As the rods fail to respond further to bright light, **cones come into play.**
   - Thus, with increased light intensity, **rods become deactivated and cones get stimulated.**
2. When **rhodopsin level falls by 7 percent**, vision is taken over by the cones. The image ***appears less bright*** as cones are less sensitive to light than the rods.
3. Further, in the hyperpolarized rods, there is **reduced Ca^{2+} influx** that removes the inhibitory effect on guanylyl cyclase.
   - As a result, the **cGMP level is restored** that increases the sensitivity of photoreceptors after some time.

Chemical mechanisms have a lesser role in light adaptation.

Dark Adaptation

1. If a person stays for some time in bright sunlight and then moves into a dimly lighted room, he experiences a temporary blindness that improves after a few minutes. During this time his eye adjusts to the low levels of illumination, a phenomenon known as dark adaptation.
2. Maximum dark adaptation occurs **in about 20 minutes.**
3. In dim light, the pupil dilates to allow the maximum possible light through the eye to have optimal vision.

Mechanisms of Dark Adaptation

There are two mechanisms of light adaptation: neural and chemical.

Neural Adaptation

1. The **first phase of adaptation** occurs due to ***decrease in threshold of the cones*** *that occurs within 5- 10 minutes.* This **increases retinal sensitivity** to 100 times.
2. In the **second phase of adaptation**, *the* ***rod threshold falls*** *reaching its maximum in about 20 minutes* (Fig. 122.2) and the retinal sensitivity increases by 1000-10,000 times.

As the rods are more sensitive than the cones, in the low levels of illumination of the darkened room, **visual capacity depends mainly on the rods.**

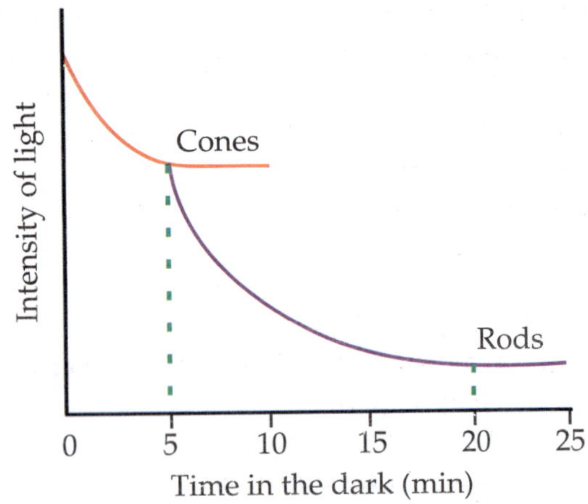

Fig. 122.2: Dark adaptation. Maximum fall in cone sensitivity occurs in 5 minutes; maximum fall in rod sensitivity occurs in 20 minutes.

Chemical Adaptation

1. In the dark, there occurs **regeneration of the photopigment rhodopsin.**
   - During the exposure to bright light, due to conversion of rhodopsin to all-trans-retinal and opsin, no rhodopsin is available that can be activated by light.
   - Hence, rods become insensitive to light.
2. **Rods cannot respond completely again** *until rhodopsin is restored to its resting state.* This process requires several minutes, during which the level of rhodopsin rises increasing the sensitivity of the rods proportionately.
3. In the retina, the rod concentration is more in an area that is about 15-20 degrees from the fovea.
   - The dark-adapted retina is most sensitive to light in this region.
   - As a whole, **the dark-adapted retina is 10,000 times more sensitive than the light adapted one.**
4. **Vitamin A** is required for the synthesis of retinine. So, ***vitamin A deficiency*** *adversely affects the dark adaptation ability*, the condition known as ***night blindness***, in which the person has impaired vision in the evening and dim light.

Factors Affecting: The time taken to accomplish full dark adaptation depends on the **intensity, duration and wavelength** of light to which the eyes were exposed when the person was in bright light. If the **light was very bright** or if the eyes were **exposed for longer period**, the dark adaptation requires longer time. Longer wavelength of light like red colour stimulates the cones to a fair extent, but rods are relatively insensitive to it. So a person **previously exposed to red light becomes rapidly dark-adapted** (Application Box 122.1).

> **Application Box 122.1**
>
> **Pilots are advised to wear red goggles:** The aircraft pilots and radiologists who work in dim light are advised to wear red goggles when they are in bright light, so that the rods are less bleached and their sensitivity is maintained. When they enter the dimly lit room, they do not have to wait for 20 minutes as rods are soon dark-adapted.

VISUAL REFLEXES

PY10.17

Light Reflex

When light is focused on one eye, the pupils of both eyes constrict; this is called light reflex.

1. The pupillary constriction occurring in the stimulated eye is called **direct light reflex** and in the other eye is called **consensual light reflex** (Flowchart 122.1).
2. The **latent period** of the response is about 0.2 –0.5 sec.
3. **Afferent pathway:** The first order neurons from the retinal ganglion cells project to the pre-tectal nucleus; from here the second order neurons start and proceed to the mid-brain Edinger-Westphal nucleus.
4. **Efferent pathway:** The parasympathetic fibers of the oculomotor nerve form the first order neurons that originate from mid-brain Edinger-Westphal nucleus and project to the ciliary ganglion. The second order neurons start from here and innervate the sphincter pupillae.

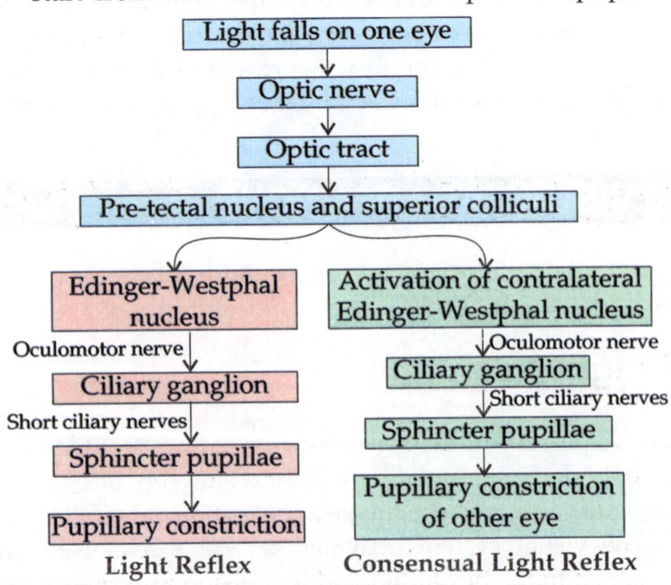

Flowchart 122.1: Pathway of direct light reflex and consensual light reflex.

Accommodation Reflex

The pupils of both eyes constrict on looking at a near object; this is called accommodation reflex (Flowchart 122.2).

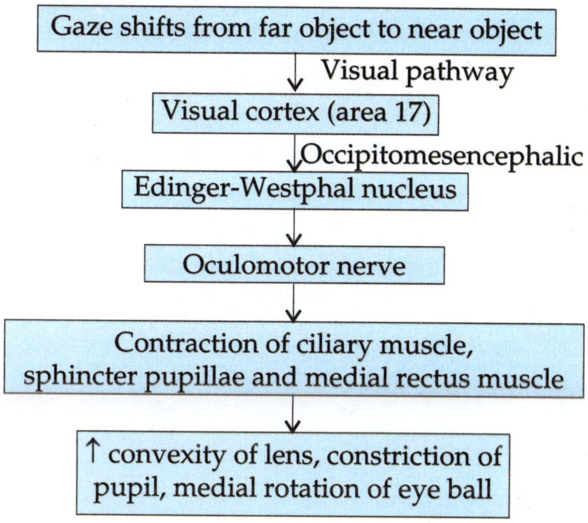

Flowchart 122.2: Pathway of accommodation reflex.

1. **Afferent pathway:** The first order neurons from the retinal ganglion cells project to the LGB; from here, the second order neurons start and project to the area 17, from where the third order neurons start and proceed to the mid-brain Edinger-Westphal nucleus.
2. **Efferent pathway:** From the striate cortex via the occipito-mesencephalic pathway, impulse travels to the oculomotor nerve nucleus and then to the sphincter pupillae, ciliary muscle and medial rectus.

Argyll Robertson Pupil

1. In neurological lesions in the pretectal-superior colliculi region of the mesencephalon, the fibers mediating light reflex are damaged.
2. This is the classical pupillary abnormality in neurosyphilis; but it is not seen now days, because syphilis can be effectively treated at its early stage.
3. Here the **light reflexes (both direct and consensual) are lost**, but **accommodation reflex is present** (ARP: accommodation reflex present, *to remember*) because the fibers for accommodation reflex take a different course.

Exam Questions

1. List the factors that affect visual acuity and visual field. Briefly describe how central field of vision can be mapped.
2. Describe the mechanism of light adaptation and dark adaptation. Add a note on light reflex and accommodation reflex.

Multiple Choice Questions (for both Chapter 121 and 122)

3. Lateral inhibition is exerted by
A. Horizontal cells B. Amacrine cells
C. Bipolar cells D. Ganglion cells

4. The parvocellular pathway, from the lateral geniculate body to the visual cortex, carries signals for the detection of
A. Movement, depth and flicker
B. Color vision, shape and fine details
C. Temporal frequency
D. Luminance contrast

5. True stereopsis is perceived due to the following:
A. Overlay of contours B. Motion parallax
C. Bi-nasal disparity D. Linear perspective

6. Visual acuity decreases with:
A. Decrease in distance of object from the eye
B. Increased activation of retinal neurons at fovea centralis
C. Increased duration of the object that remains in view
D. Decrease in size of the object

7. Which of the following tests near vision?
A. Ishihara chart B. Snellen's chart
C. Jaeger chart D. Edridge chart

8. Binocular vision results when:
A. Light rays fall on noncorresponding points
B. A binocular is used to visualize an object
C. Light rays from an object do not fall on the corresponding points for a long time
D. An object is viewed as a single object with both eyes

9. The central visual field is mapped with:
A. Lister's Perimeter B. Tonometer
C. Snellen's chart D. Bjerrum screen

10. Bitemporal hemianopia occurs when the lesion is present in:
A. Right optic nerve B. Temporal retina
C. Optic chiasm D. Left geniculocalcarine tract

11. Macular sparing occurs because:
A. Macula is protected by neural layers of retina
B. Macula is a very small structure
C. Macular fibers have a larger representation in the visual cortex
D. Macula has the highest blood supply

12. All of the following are mechanisms of dark adaptation, *except*:
A. Increase in threshold of cones within 5–10 minutes
B. Rod threshold falls to a maximum in 20 minutes
C. Retinal sensitivity increases 1000 times
D. Rhodopsin is regenerated

Answers

3. A 4. B 5. C 6. D 7. C 8. D 9. D 10. C 11. C 12. A

Chapter 123

Color Vision

Learning Objectives

On completion of study of this chapter:

The student will be able to (must know):

1. Give the characteristics of colors.
2. Understand the physiological basis of color vision.
3. Describe Young-Helmholtz theory of color vision.
4. Classify color blindness and understand the physiological basis of color blindness.
7. Mention the tests for color blindness.

The student may also be able to (desirable to know):

1. Describe single-opponent theory and double-opponent theory of color vision.
2. Describe the theories of color vision.

The human eye is sensitive to the light rays in the visible spectrum. There are **seven colors** in the visible spectrum, called spectral colors. They are **violet, indigo, blue, green, yellow, orange and red** (VIBGYOR), with wavelengths ranging from 400-750 nm. Human eye does not respond to electromagnetic radiations beyond the visible spectrum, for e.g. ultraviolet (< 400 nm) and infrared (> 750 nm) rays.

Characteristics of Color

There are **three characteristics of color**: intensity, hue and saturation. In abnormalities of color vision, one or more of these characteristics are decreased.

Primary Colors

There are **three primary colors**: red, green and blue.

- Any color can be produced by mixing various proportions of these three colors.
- The primary colors when mixed in equal proportions produce white color.

Complementary Color

Each color has a complementary color.

- When any color is mixed with its complementary color, the **mixture appears white**.
- For example, purple and green, orange and blue, yellow and dark blue are complementary colors.

Effect of Illumination

The color perceived depends not only on the wavelength but also other factors like **illumination**. When the spectral colors are seen in dim light, the brightest part of the spectrum is green, as the rods are most sensitive to the green light.

- When viewed in high illumination, for e.g. in daylight, the brightest part of the spectrum is yellow, as the cones have maximum sensitivity in the yellow region.
- Thus, the brightest part of the spectrum **shifts to left during scotopic vision** and **shifts to right during photopic vision**.
- This shift of the maximum sensitivity to the visible spectrum with change in illumination is known as **Purkinje shift phenomenon.**

Effect of Background Color

The color perceived by the eye depends on the background color. For example, green letters against a green background is hardly visible, whereas they are seen as green against yellow or red background.

Effect of Intensity

For the same wavelength of light, when the intensity of the color is increased or decreased, different shades of the color are perceived.

Receptors: Cones are receptors for color vision. The information about color sensation is processed at different levels of the visual pathway. The color perceived by a person is determined by the **type, number and degree of cone stimulation** as well as the **number and pattern of action potentials** in the neural pathways.

PY10.17

THEORIES OF COLOR VISION

There are **two theories** of color vision: pigment theory and opponent theory.

Pigment Theory

This theory is also known as **Young-Helmholtz theory** as it was proposed in 1801 by Thomas Young and later modified by Hermann von Helmholtz. It is also known as **Retinal or Trichromatic theory**.

1. There are the **three types of cones** and each has a pigment with a different absorbance spectrum.
- The **red-sensitive pigment** absorbs light maximally in the yellow portion of the spectrum, the **green-sensitive pigment** absorbs maximally in the green portion and the **blue-sensitive pigment** absorbs maximally in the blue-violet portion.
2. Traditionally, the cones and cone pigments are called **red, green and blue** respectively. Now, they are called **L** (long-wavelength), **M** (middle-wavelength) and **S** (short-wavelength) as they show optimal sensitivity to lights of wavelengths of **560 nm**, **530 nm**, and **420 nm** respectively.
3. As evident from the graph, each type of **cone pigment can absorb a wide range of wavelengths** (Fig. 123.1).
   - Also, a particular color (light of a fixed wavelength) produces different levels of stimulation in various cones.
4. The visual cortex **compares the relative frequency** of action potentials in the activated cone pathways and deciphers the wavelength and thereby, makes out the color.
   - For example, a green monochromatic light with a wavelength of 530 nm produces excitation of the red, green and blue cones at a ratio of 31:67:36, and interpreted as green.
5. The change in intensity is perceived by appreciating the change in wavelength. Stimulation of only one type of cones does not encode any color perception. **At least two types of cones are required for color vision.**
6. According to the Young-Helmholtz theory, the color vision is due to **presence of three types of cones** each maximally sensitive to one of the three primary colors.
   - Therefore, normal color vision depends on the integrity of the cones.
   - Absence or malfunction of one or more than one type of cone cells lead to different forms of color blindness.

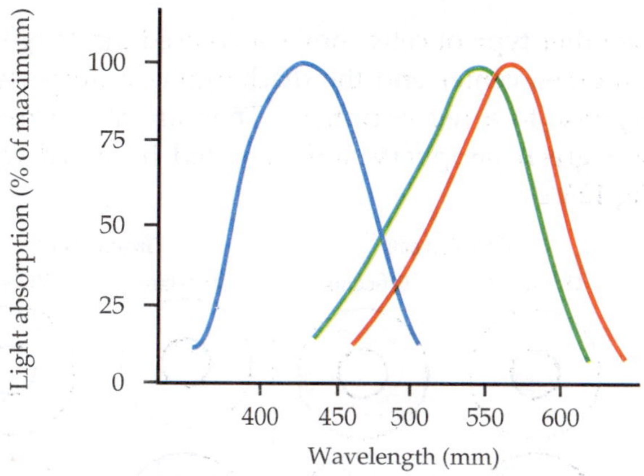

Fig. 123.1: Mean absorption spectra of the three-cone pigments in the human retina.

7. The **fovea mediates color vision** as it contains densely packed cones.
   - However, fovea contains only **M and L types of cones.**
   - Thus, it can distinguish fine spatial details of a colored object, but its capacity to discriminate different colors is less compared to the extra-foveal regions.
   - As already described above, the color perception is altered by the illumination, background color and intensity of the light.

Genes: The **gene for human rhodopsin** is located on **chromosome 3**. The **gene for the blue-sensitive cone** pigment is located on **chromosome 7**. The **genes for the red-sensitive and the green-sensitive cone** pigments are arranged in tandem on the **q arm of the X-chromosome**.

- Humans, apes and old-world monkeys are **trichromats**; i.e., they have **all the three cone systems.**
- **Many mammals are dichromats**; i.e., they have only two cone pigments, a blue-sensitive and a red-sensitive pigment.

Opponent Theory

This theory is also known as **Hering's theory of color vision** as it was proposed by Hering. It is based on his observation that there is **no greenish-red or bluish-yellow color**.

- The red and green colors oppose each other, and the blue and yellow colors are opposed.
- The ganglion cells, the cells of the LGB and the neurons of the visual cortex show color-opponent property.

Single-Opponent Property

1. The ganglion cells and the cells of LGB are **single-opponent type**. There are two subtypes.
2. Some cells are excited when a red stimulus is present in the center of the receptive field, and inhibited when a green stimulus is present in the periphery of the receptive field. Also, these cells are inhibited by a green center and excited by a red periphery.

3. The other type of cells shows increased discharge rate to a green center and the discharge rate decreases in response to a red periphery. They are also activated by a green periphery and inhibited by a red center (Fig.123.2).

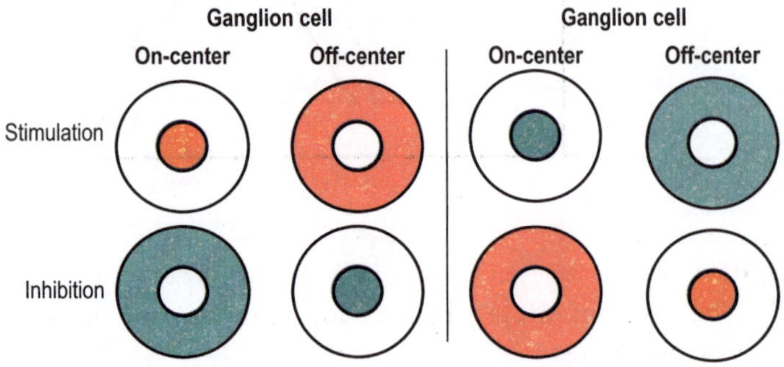

Fig. 123.2: Discharge pattern of single-opponent cells. Red-sensitive on-center cells are excited by red center and inhibited by green periphery. Red-sensitive off-center cells are excited by red periphery and inhibited by green center. Green-sensitive on-center cells are excited by green center and inhibited by red periphery, whereas the off-center cells are excited by green periphery and inhibited by red center.

Double-Opponent Property

1. The cells of the visual cortex are **double-opponent type**. They are of **two types**.
2. One type of cells is excited by a **red center with green periphery**; and inhibited by a **green center with red periphery**.
3. The other type of cells is **excited by a green center** with red periphery; and **inhibited by a red center** with green periphery (Fig.123.3).

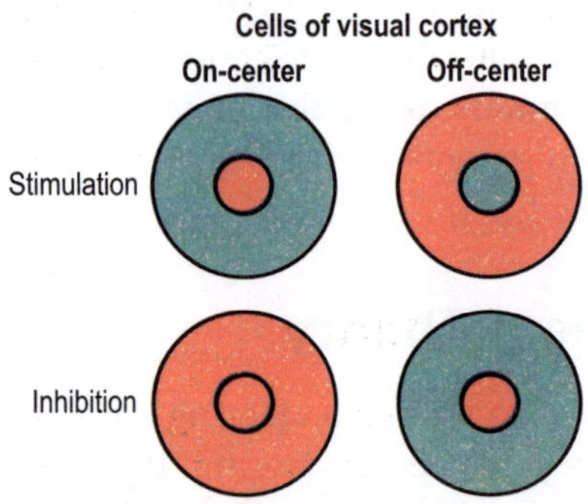

Fig. 123.3: Discharge pattern of double-opponent cells. One type of cells is excited by a red center with green periphery, and inhibited by a green center with red periphery. The other type of cells is excited by a green center with red periphery, and inhibited by a red center with green periphery.

Transmission and Encoding of Color Signals

1. The **P ganglion cells** receive information regarding color from the cone cells and transmit to the parvocellular layer of the LGB.
   - Processing of impulses start at the ganglion cell level where inputs from different types of cones are added or input from one type of cone is subtracted from the input from another cone.
2. Impulses **from the LGB** are transmitted to the deep layer **4 C of V1 and blob region** of the visual cortex through specific neural pathways.
   - The blob region of visual cortex contains clusters of cells that have high concentration of the enzyme cytochrome oxidase.
3. A **red-green pathway** transmits the subtracted inputs of the L- and M-cone responses; a **blue-yellow pathway** signals the differences between the S-cone and the sum of L- and M-cone responses, and a **luminance pathway** that transmits the added inputs of the L- and M-cone responses.
4. Information from the deep layer 4 C of V1 and the blobs is transmitted to the V8 region of the visual cortex.

COLOR BLINDNESS

Total loss of color vision is known as achromatopsia. In partial loss of color vision, the inability to distinguish certain colors is termed as color blindness. It affects 8% males and 0.4% females. The most common type is red-green color blindness. Color blindness is described with the help of the following terms.

Use of prefix: Prefixes like *prot-*, *deuter-* and *trit-* are used to describe the red-, blue- and green- cone system defects respectively.

Use of suffix: The suffix **anomaly** means color weakness and the suffix **anopia** means color blindness.

Classification

Color blindness is classified in the following manner.

I. Trichromats: This is the most common type. About 6% of affected males are trichromats. These are **individuals with all three-cone systems**, but **one of the cone systems is defective**. Thus, the ability of the individual to recognize one of the primary colors is decreased. Accordingly, trichromats can have one of the following defects:

- Deuteranomaly (most common)
- Protanomaly
- Tritanomaly

II. Dichromats: About 2% of affected males are dichromats. These are individuals with **two-cone systems and the third cone system is absent**. Thus, a dichromats can have any of the following:

- Deuteranopia (most common)
- Protanopia
- Tritanopia

III. Monochromats: These are individuals with **only one cone system** present. Thus, they cannot appreciate any color, because minimum two cone systems are required to appreciate a color. They see only black and white and shades of gray.

Etiology

The cause can be **inherited** (genetic) or **acquired**, due to lesion or drugs.

Genetic: Color blindness is inherited as an **X-linked recessive** disorder.

1. As **males contain XY chromosomes** in their germ cells, they **develop color blindness** if the X chromosome contains the defective gene.
   - On the other hand, the **females** develop color blindness only when both the X-chromosomes are defective, which is **rare**.
2. The female having one defective X chromosome remains **symptom free**, but **transmits the disease to half of her sons**.
   - Thus, **females are the carriers** and **males are the sufferers**.
   - All the daughters of a color-blind person become carriers and half of their sons suffer from the disease.
   - Thus, color blindness manifests in **every second-generation males.**

Deuteranomaly and **protanomaly** are the ***most common defects***. Tritanomaly and tritanopia are rare and occur equally in both males and females.

Lesion: Following lesion of the striate cortex (area V8), the individual suffers from complete loss of color vision (achromatopsia).

Drugs: Drugs like **sildenafil** (Viagra) inhibits the enzyme phosphodiesterase. Thus, individuals develop ***transient blue-green color weakness*** till the effect of the drug lasts.

Tests for Color Blindness **PY10.20**

Color vision is tested by the following ways.

Ishihara Chart: It is the most routinely used test for color blindness in clinics.

1. It consists of **lithographic plates** in which numerals or pathways are drawn in colored spots against a background of spots of different colors and sizes (Fig.123.4).
2. The subject reads the number and traces the pathway. The colors of the numerals or tracings and the background colors are arranged in such a way that a colour-blind person reads them differently or traces a different pathway from a normal person.

Edridge-Green Lantern Test: In this test, the light from a lantern is shown through different colored glass pieces fixed on a rotation disc and the subject is asked to name the colors.

Holmgren's Wool-Matching Test: The subject is asked to perform a **series of color matching** from a collection of **wools of different colors**.

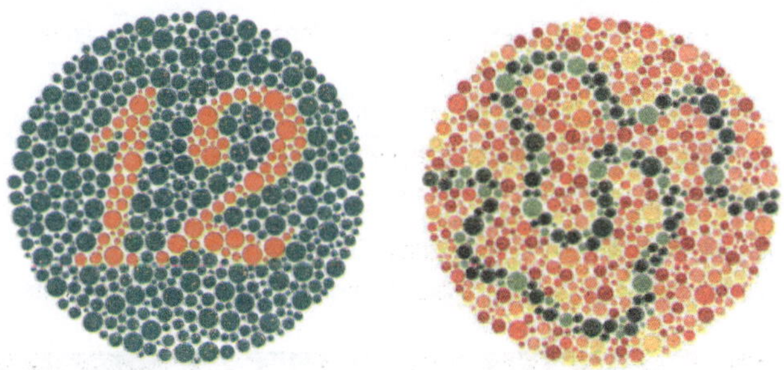

Fig. 123.4: Ishihara chart.

Exam Questions

1. Describe the theories of color vision. Add a note on color blindness.

Multiple Choice Questions

1. Protanopes have difficulty in recognizing the following color
A. Red
B. Green
C. Blue
D. Black

2. The wavelength range visible to human eye is
A. 440 - 840 nm
B. 440 - 740 nm
C. 380 – 840 nm
D. 380 - 740 nm

3. Blurring of vision is commonly seen in albinos because of:
A. Degeneration of choroid
B. Defective pigment epithelium layer of retina
C. Defective phototransduction mechanism in rods and cones
D. Degeneration of fovea

4. Trichromats are individuals with:
A. Three cone system
B. Normal color vision
C. Two normal and one weak cone system
D. Deuteranomaly

5. The blobs of visual cortex are associated with:
A. Saccadic eye movements
B. Orientation
C. Ocular dominance
D. Color vision

6. Which of the following is TRUE for color vision?
A. Depends on intensity discrimination
B. Independent of wavelength of light
C. Minimum at fixation point
D. Involves opponent color neurons

Answers: 1. A 2. D 3. B 4. A 5. D 6. D

Chapter 124

Movements of the Eye

Learning Objectives

On completion of study of this chapter:

The student will be able to (must know):

1. Name extraocular muscles, and give their innervation and functions.
2. List the types of ocular movements.
3. Outline the effects of paralysis of extraocular muscles.
4. Define nystagmus and appreciate the types of nystagmus.
5. Leans the basic of EOG, ERG and VEP.

The student may also be able to (desirable to know):

1. Describes the physiological basis of abnormalities of eye movements..

EXTRAOCULAR MUSCLES

The extra ocular muscles (EOM) originate on the bone of the orbit and insert on the sclera. They are lateral rectus, medial rectus, superior oblique, inferior oblique, superior rectus and inferior rectus (Fig.124.1).

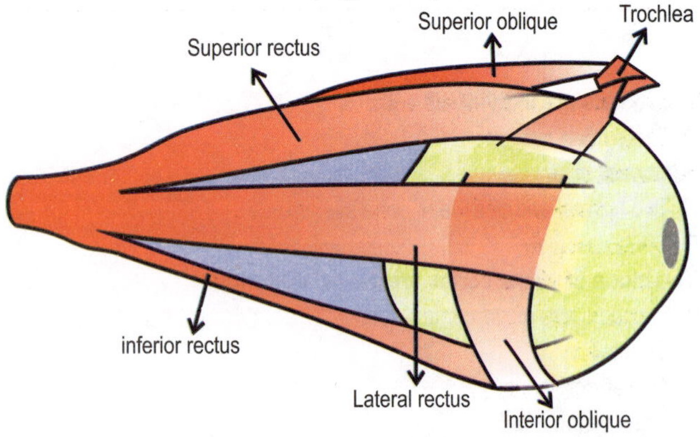

Fig. 124.1: Extraocular muscles.

Nerve Supply of EOM

The lateral rectus muscle is supplied by the abducent nerve and the superior oblique by the trochlear nerve (LR_6, SO_4). The **oculomotor nerve innervates rest of the extra ocular muscles.**

Action of EOM

Normally, the eye can move 50° medially, 30° upwards and 50° downwards.

- When the **eyeball is placed temporally** (abducted position), the superior rectus causes elevation and the inferior rectus causes depression of the eyeball.
- When the **eyeball moves nasally** (adducted position), the superior oblique depresses it and inferior oblique elevates it.
- In the **mid position** of the eyeball, the lateral and medial recti cause lateral and medial movement of the eyeball respectively (Fig.124.2).

The actions of the various extraocular muscles are shown in the table 124.1.

Cardinal Movements: The vertical and horizontal movements of the eyeball made from the mid position of the gaze are called cardinal movements.

Conjugate movement: When a person looks at an object, the eyeballs move symmetrically and the visual axes of both eyes meet at one point. This is known as conjugate movement of the eyes. It is possible due to **integration of the afferent inputs of the III, IV and VI cranial nerves** at the level of the brainstem.

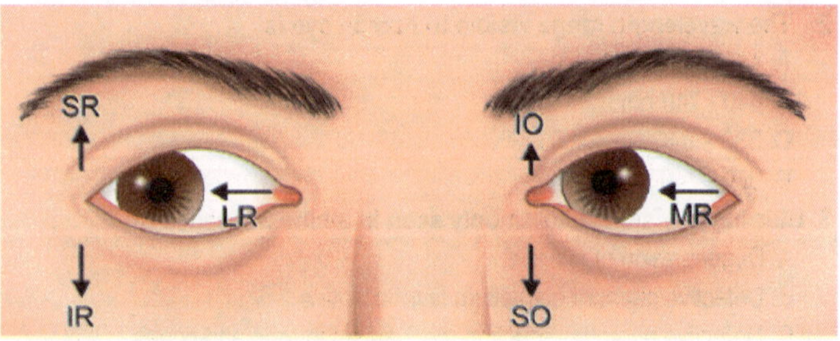

Fig. 124.2: Action of the various extraocular muscles.

TYPES OF OCULAR MOVEMENTS

There are four types of eye movements: saccades, smooth pursuit movements, vergence and vestibular movements. The first three movements are described in relation to a stationary head.

Saccades: These are **rapid, jerky movements that occur when the gaze shifts** from one object to the other.

- Their function is to keep the **new object in focus** by changing the orientation of the eyeball.
  - Thus, they prevent the adaptation of neurons in the visual pathway and reduce the strain on the extra ocular muscles by bringing out the change.
- When the gaze is fixed on an object for longer period, the extra ocular muscles remain contracted to maintain the position of the eyeball and this may lead to muscle fatigue.
- These movements are regulated in the **frontal cortex and superior colliculi**.

Smooth Pursuit Movements: These are **tracking movements** of the eyes as they follow moving objects. These movements are integrated in the cerebellum.

- Saccades and pursuit movements are commonly experienced while looking out of the window of a moving train.
  - As one looks at an object, initially, pursuit movement follows the object and the eyeball rotates sideways till its maximum.
- When the object cannot be viewed anymore, the eyeball rapidly moves to the earlier position to fix the gaze on a new object.

Vergence: These movements occur when an object comes near or moves far from the eye.

- For example, if an object comes near in the midline, both eyeballs turn medially (**convergence**), and if it goes away, both eyeballs rotate laterally (**divergence**).
- So, for a single eyeball, when an object moves closer in the nasal field of vision, convergence occurs; and when it moves closer in the temporal field of vision, divergence occurs.

Vestibular Movements: When the head moves, to keep the object in focus, the eyeball moves in response to stimuli arriving from the semicircular canals. Vestibular movements occur while standing/sitting on an unsteady platform (e.g. a ship) and looking at an object.

Nystagmus

The involuntary, rhythmical, oscillatory movement of the eyeball is known as nystagmus.

Physiological Nystagmus

1. When the **gaze is fixed on a stationary object**, there occur continuous contractions of a few muscle fibers producing minute oscillations at a rate of ***30-80 cycles per second***. This is called *physiological nystagmus*.

1. Due to this small tremor like movements, the **image constantly moves** over a small area of the retina. As the same neuron does not get stimulated continuously, the adaptation of neurons in the visual pathway is prevented.
2. Though the stimulus first activates the photoreceptors, it is the **neurons that get adapted earlier** than the photoreceptors. *If the image falls on the same spot of the retina, the neural discharge gradually decreases and the object disappears from view.*
3. Thus, the physiological nystagmus helps the eyes **to see the object clearly for a longer duration**.
   - As the oscillations help to fix the gaze on an object, they are also called **fixation movements**.

When the eyes follow a rapidly moving object, **optokinetic nystagmus** is seen. The eyes slowly follow the object and then quickly come back to the initial position of gaze by a rapid saccade.

Pathological Nystagmus

In some pathological conditions, these oscillatory movements become noticeable. Nystagmus can be due to disorders of vestibular system or lesion of the neural pathways controlling the ocular movements.

ABNORMALITIES OF EYE MOVEMENTS

Abnormalities of eye movements are summarized in Table 124.1. In case of paralysis of eye muscles, abnormalities like diplopia, strabismus and loss of accommodation occur.

Depth Perception

- The two eyes are positioned slightly away from each other. So, each eye receives a little different image of the same object compared to the other.
- Fusion of both images at the level of visual cortex helps to view the object as a single one, but the difference helps in depth perception (stereoscopic vision).
- The depth perception ability is greatly reduced in case of blindness of one eye.

INVESTIGATIONS

Electrooculography

Electrooculography (EOG) records the **effect of light and dark adaptation on the retinal resting potential** generated at the pigment epithelium.

1. The eyeballs move laterally for placing electrodes at

the inner and outer canthi.

Table 124.1 | The Innervation, function and effect of paralysis of external ocular muscles.

Muscle	Innervation	Function	Effect of paralysis
Lateral rectus	Abducent (VI cranial nerve)	Outward movement of the eyeball (Abduction)	Due to the unopposed action of the healthy medial rectus muscle, the following features are seen i) inability to move the eye outwards ii) Diplopia (on trying to look in outward direction) iii) Convergent squint
Superior oblique	Trochlear (IV cranial nerve)	Downward movement of the adducted eyeball	i) inability to move the adducted eye downwards ii) Diplopia (while looking down from mid position of gaze)
Medial rectus	Oculomotor (III cranial nerve)	Inward movement of the eyeball (Adduction)	In lesion of oculomotor nerve, - due to unopposed action of VI and IV cranial nerves, there is outward and downward deviation of the eyeball • Paralysis of individual muscle is rare. However, if occurs, the action of the affected muscle is lost The other features of oculomotor nerve palsy are: • Ptosis (drooping of eye lid) • Dilated & fixed pupil • Loss of accommodation (as the oculomotor nerve supplies eyelid, constrictor pupil and ciliary muscles)
Superior rectus	Oculomotor (III cranial nerve)	Upward movement of the abducted eyeball	
Inferior rectus	Oculomotor (III cranial nerve)	Downward movement of the abducted eyeball	
Inferior oblique	Oculomotor (III cranial nerve)	Upward movement of the abducted eyeball	

2. The retinal resting potential is 6 mV across the pigment epithelium with the receptors side being electrically positive and the choroidal side electrically negative.
3. EOG is useful in the diagnosis of **retinal dystrophies and degenerative diseases** like retinitis pigmentosa.

Electroretinography

Recording of **electrical activities of the retina** by stimulating it with a ***flash of light*** is called electroretinography (ERG).

1. With fully dilated pupil and following application of local anesthetic, it is performed by placing contact lens electrode (recording electrode) on the cornea, reference electrode on the skin of the forehead, and reference electrode over the earlobe.
2. Electroretinogram (ERG) has an initial rapid downward negative deflection **a-wave** that appears after a latent period, followed by a bigger upward positive deflection **b-wave** of short duration, and following this, a prolonged small amplitude positive **c-wave** (Fig. 124.3).
3. The **a-wave** originates from the **retinal photoreceptors**; the **b-wave** originates from the ***bipolar cells*** and the **c-wave** originates from the ***pigment epithelium.***
4. ERG assesses the **functional integrity of the retina**.
   - It gives information about the rods located at the periphery of the retina and their connections.
   - It is helpful in the diagnosis of retinal detachment, retinal dystrophy, vitamin A deficiency etc.

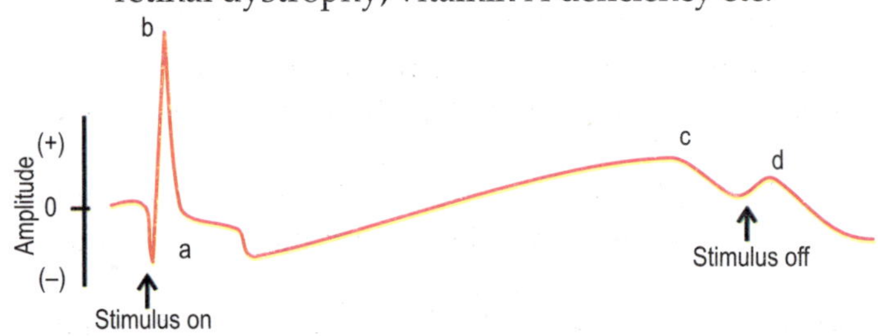

Fig. 124.3: The waves of electroretinogram

Visual Evoked Potentials PY10.19

Visual evoked potentials (VEPs) are the electrical potential differences recorded from the scalp in response to visual stimuli.

- VEPs are generated in the **visual pathway from retina to the visual cortex** in response to light or **pattern stimulation** of the eye.
  - They indicate the intactness of the entire visual system; however, can only detect the abnormality, but cannot exactly localise the site of the lesion in the visual pathway.
- A chain of waves is produced at various latencies, out of which **P100 is a large positive potential** that occurs after 100 milliseconds after application of the stimulus.
- Abnormalities in the **latency and amplitude** of various waveforms are helpful in the diagnosis of various diseases like optic neuritis, optic atrophy, refractive errors, color blindness etc.

(Details of VEP are given in GK Pal's Practical Physiology Book)

Exam Questions

1. Describe the innervation, and functions of extraocular muscle. Add a note on nystagmus.

Chapter 125

PY10.15

Functional Anatomy and Functions of the Ear

Learning Objectives

On completion of study of this chapter:

The student will be able to (must know):

1. List the functions of middle ear.
2. Name the auditory ossicles and ossicular muscles, and give their functions.
3. Appreciate the functions of tympanic membrane and tympanic reflex.
4. Understand the physiology of cochlea and organ of Corti.
5. Illustrate the structure of cochlear hair cell and the mechanism of activation of hair cells.

The student may also be able to (desirable to know):

1. Describe the functions of middle ear.
2. Describe the functional organization and functions of organ of Corti.

EXTERNAL EAR

It consists of the auricle (**pinna)** and external auditory canal. The small portion of cartilage in front of the opening of the auditory canal is known as **tragus**. The external ear collects sound waves and channels them inward.

Pinna

The pinna is a **flap of elastic cartilage** covered by skin. In humans, the pinna is fixed, but in many animals, it is movable, and can be oriented in the direction of sound. The rim of the auricle is called the **helix** and the lower soft tissue portion is called the **lobule**.

The pinna has the following functions:

i) It **funnels the sound waves** into the auditory canal to reach the tympanic membrane.
ii) It helps to establish the **direction of sound waves**; i.e. to know whether they are from the front or the back or from the above or below.

External Auditory Canal

Auditory canal (meatus) is a **2.5 cm long tube** in the temporal bone extending from the auricle to the eardrum (Fig. 125.1).

1. It **conducts the sound waves to the middle ear**. The external one-third of the canal is cartilaginous and the internal two third is bony.
2. The canal contains sebaceous glands that secrete **cerumen** (earwax) and **fine hairs** that line its wall.
   - The oily cerumen and the hairs prevent entry of dust and foreign particles into the ear.
   - Excessive production of sebum along with lack of proper cleaning of the external meatus leads to hardening and **impaction of the wax** that block the passage and produces conduction deafness.
3. The *pinna and the external auditory canal together* produce a **15 dB increase in the sound intensity** due to their characteristic shape.

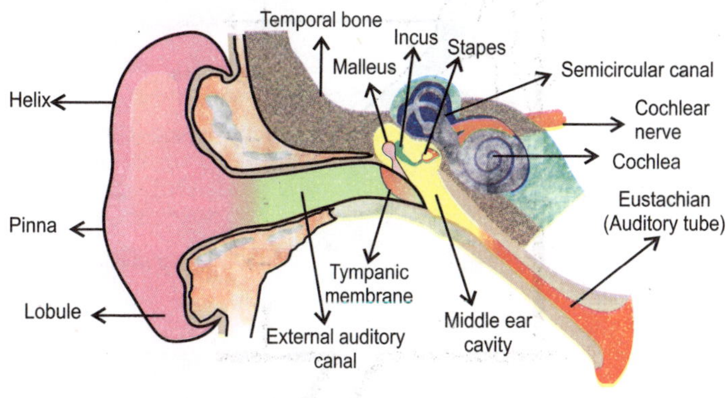

Fig. 125.1: Structure of the human ear.

MIDDLE EAR

1. The middle ear (tympanic cavity) is a rectangular air-filled compartment in the temporal bone (Fig. 125.2).
2. It is lined by epithelial cells and has **four walls, a floor and a roof**.
   - The **anterior wall** opens to the exterior via the eustachian tube at the level of the nasopharynx.
   - The **posterior wall** communicates with the mastoid air cells (air cavities in the mastoid process of the temporal bone) through a space called the tympanic antrum. When infections of the middle ear spread to the mastoid air cells, they cause **mastoiditis**.
   - The **medial wall** contains two small membrane-covered openings (the oval window and the round window) and separates the middle ear from the internal ear.
   - The **lateral wall** is formed by the tympanic membrane that separates the external ear from the middle ear.
3. The ***bony floor*** separates the middle ear from the jugular fossa.
4. The ***roof*** of the middle ear is formed by **tegmen tympani** that separates it from the middle cranial fossa.
5. The middle ear contains **three bony ossicles** and **two ossicular muscles**.

Tympanic Membrane

Tympanic membrane (**eardrum**) is a thin elastic semitransparent conical membrane about **50-90 mm^2 in surface area**, with its apex (called **umbo**) toward the middle ear.

1. It is made up of collagen and elastic fibers.
2. Its inner surface is lined by mucous membrane and its outer surface is covered by skin.
3. Inflammation of the tympanic membrane is known as *tympanitis*.

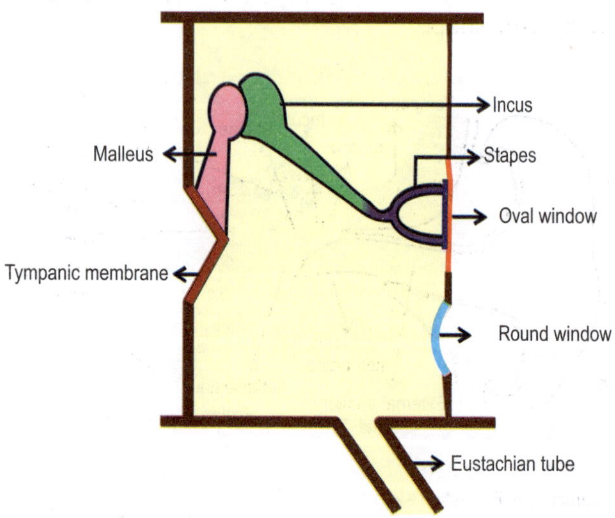

Fig. 125.2: Middle ear cavity

Functions

1. The eardrum receives the sound waves arriving from the external ear. When sound waves strike the tympanic membrane, it vibrates almost at the same frequency as that of the sound waves.
   - Thus, *it is extremely sensitive to the pressure changes and* **acts as a resonator**.
2. The vibrations of the membrane get transmitted to the tiny bone (malleus) attached to it.
   - It stops vibrating soon after the cessation of the sound waves; therefore, **it critically dampens the sound waves**.
3. Though thin, it stands as a mechanical barrier and prevents the entry of foreign particles, dust and secretions from the outer ear to the middle ear.

Auditory Ossicles

These are three small bones, the **malleus (hammer), the incus (anvil), and the stapes (stirrup)**. They extend across the middle ear cavity one joined to the other (Fig. 125 .2).

1. The **handle of the malleus** (manubrium) is attached to the internal surface of the tympanic membrane. The malleus articulates with the body of the incus that in turn articulates with the head of the stapes.
2. The footplate of the stapes is attached to the oval window (fenestra vestibuli).
   - The **pressure waves travel through the ossicular chain** and produce **vibrations of the footplate of stapes**, which then transmits the vibrations **to the perilymph of the inner** ear through oval window.
3. In a disease called **otosclerosis**, there is bony **fixation of the stapes** to the walls of the fenestra vestibuli, resulting in *severe deafness due to loss of the vibrating capacity of the stapes*.
4. The round window is present below the oval window and is enclosed by a flexible membrane called the **secondary tympanic membrane**.

Ossicular Muscles

Stapedius and tensor tympani are ***two tiny skeletal muscles*** attached to the **stapes and the malleus** respectively.

Functions

1. The **tensor tympani** muscle pulls the handle of the malleus inwards, thereby *increases tension of the tympanic membrane*. This makes the membrane **more responsive to the sound waves**.
2. The stapedius is the smallest skeletal muscle in the body. *In response to loud noise*, it contracts and pulls the footplate of stapes out from the oval window, therefore, **dampens the vibrations transmitted to the inner ear** (Application Box 125.1).

3. In paralysis of the stapedius muscle, the patient is abnormally sensitive to loud noises, known as **hyperacusis**.

Application Box 125.1

Tympanic reflex: Also called **acoustic reflex**, this is a protective reflex that decreases the damage to the inner ear from loud sound. In response to a prolonged loud noise, the tensor tympani and the stapedius contract reflexively (simultaneously in both the ears), causing the outward movement of the malleus and the inward movement of the stapes. This makes the ossicular chain much closer to each other and articulation sites very tight.
- As a result, the vibration transmitted through the ossicles to the inner ear is reduced, decreasing the degree of stimulation of the receptors (hair cells) present in the inner ear.
- Thus, the reflex checks over-stimulation of hair cells and prevents the damage to the cochlea.
- The reflex does not protect the ear from abrupt and brief loud sound like gunshot or bomb blast, as the activation time for the reflex is 40-160 ms.

The middle ear muscles also **contract in response to low frequency sound waves**. This helps to filter the low frequency waves and augments the transmission of waves of 1000-2000 Hz (the range of voice communication).
- The *masking of most of the low frequency environmental noise* allows the human voices to be audible inspite of noise in the environment. The muscles are active prior to and during vocalization. This **minimizes hearing of one's own voice.**
- They contract before and during any movement that may stimulate the ossicles like chewing, swallowing, yawning, walking and gross bodily activities and thereby, **suppresses the sounds produced by these movements.**
- Contraction of tensor tympani and stapedius related to speech and movements are not reflex responses as they contract prior to these events.

To summarize, the **middle ear muscles have the following functions**. They:

I. **Prevent the damage** to the cochlea.
  - **Improve sound transmission** to the cochlea in the range of voice communication while decreasing responses to frequencies above and below this range.

iii. **Suppress the self- generated sounds**.

Eustachian Tube

This connects the middle ear with the pharynx and **equalizes the air pressures on both sides of the tympanic membrane.**
- This helps the membrane to vibrate at the same frequency as the sound waves.
- The pharyngeal end of the tube is normally closed by a valve-like mechanism, but muscle movements open it during swallowing, yawning or sneezing, and the pressure in the middle ear equilibrates with the atmospheric (pharyngeal cavity) pressure (Application Box 125.2).

Application Box 125.2

Eustachian Tube Dysfunctions: Altered pressure on either side of the tympanic membrane can stretch it and cause pain. For e.g. **during rapid** ascent in an airplane, the fall in atmospheric pressure causes the tympanic membrane to be pushed out by the higher pressure in the middle ear. The middle ear pressure does not fall due to the closed eustachian tube.
- During diving in water or rapid descent in a plane, the tympanic membrane is pushed in due to increased outside pressure.
- If the tube is blocked due to common cold, the air in the middle ear is gradually absorbed and the tympanic membrane is sucked in, causing pain and loss of hearing.
- The discomfort and pain in the ear due to pressure difference are relieved by swallowing saliva or air.

Functions of the Middle Ear

1. **Receives sound waves** from the external ear by the tympanic membrane
2. **Transmission of sound waves** to the inner ear through the tympanic membrane and the ossicular chain.
3. **Amplification of sound waves:** The force of sound waves that strike the tympanic membrane increases several times as it reaches the footplate of stapes and oval window. This occurs due to two factors.
   i. The surface area of the tympanic membrane (50 mm^2) is much larger than that of the oval window (3 mm^2), the **ratio being 17:1.** The total force of a sound wave exerted on the tympanic membrane is transmitted to the oval window. But due to the decrease in the surface area, the **pressure (force per unit area) increases 17 times.**
   ii. The ossicular chain acts as lever while transmitting the vibration of sound waves. As the handle of malleus is 1.3 times longer than the long process of incus, there is a lever ratio of 1.3:1 that **enhances the force 1.3 times.**

Thus, the **total amplification of sound** waves occurs about 17× 1.3 = 22 times. In this manner the middle ear performs the job of **impedance matching** (Application Box 125.3).

4. **Equalization of air pressure** through the eustachian tube.
5. **Protects against prolonged, loud sound** by activation of *tympanic reflex*.

Application Box 125.3

Impedance matching: When sound waves travel from air to water, about 99.9% of the sound energy gets reflected away from the surface of water. So, the conduction of sound from air to fluid meets with considerable **acoustic impedance** (resistance).
- If the sound waves were to strike the oval window directly (without traversing through the tympanic membrane and the ossicular chain), only 0.5% of the sound energy would have reached the endolymph in the inner ear.
- The *amplification process helps to compensate for the loss.* This is known as impedance matching and the middle ear is therefore often called an impedance-matching device.

INNER EAR

The internal (inner) ear is situated in the petrous part of the temporal bone. It is called **labyrinth** due to presence of complicated series of canals. Structurally, it is divided into an outer bony labyrinth that houses an inner membranous labyrinth.

1. The **bony labyrinth** contains a fluid called **perilymph** that surrounds the membranous labyrinth.
   - The composition of perilymph is similar to that of cerebrospinal fluid.
2. The **membranous labyrinth** is a series of fluid-filled membranous tubes and sacs, which mimic the shape of bony labyrinth. The fluid present in the membranous labyrinth is called **endolymph** that is rich in K^+ and resembles intracellular fluid.
   - The membranous labyrinth consists of the **auditory apparatus** (cochlea) and the **vestibular apparatus** (the saccule, utricle and the semicircular canals).
3. The function of cochlea is transduction of the sound energy into action potentials in the cochlear nerve fiber. The vestibular apparatus is described under motor physiology.

Tympanic Membrane

The cochlea (meaning **snail's shell**) is a snail shaped fluid-filled coiled tube. It has an outer bony spiral canal that houses an inner membranous cochlear duct.

Bony Cochlea

1. The bony cochlea is part of the bony labyrinth. In humans, the cochlea is 35 mm in length and makes two and three fourth (2¾) turns around a central bony core called the **modiolus**.
2. Cochlear vessels and nerves traverse through the base of modiolus. Around the modiolus, a thin plate of bone called spiral lamina give attachment to the basilar membrane.

Membranous Cochlea

1. The membranous cochlea (**cochlear duct**) is like a tube that follows the spiral shape of bony cochlea. It is **filled with endolymph** and is part of the membranous labyrinth (Fig.125.3).
2. In the cross sectional view of the cochlea, the **Reissner's membrane** and the **basilar membrane** divide the cochlea into three fluid-filled compartments known as **scala vestibuli, scala media and scala tympani** (Fig.125.4).

Scala Vestibuli: Scala vestibuli is the gap above the Reissner's membrane, **filled with perilymph**. At the base of the cochlea, it is separated from the middle ear by the oval window. At the apex of the cochlea, it is continuous

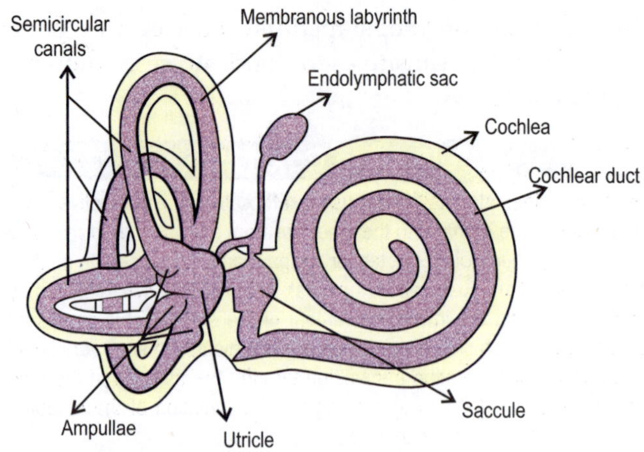

Fig. 125.3: The membranous labyrinth.

with scala tympani through a small opening called **helicotrema**.

Scala Media: Scala media is the compartment between Reissner's and basilar membranes. The space is **filled with endolymph** that is secreted by a layer of fibrous vascular tissue known as **stria vascularis** present along the lateral wall of scala media.

- The stria vascularis pumps K^+ into and Na^+ out of the scala media as its cells have a high concentration of Na^+-K^+ ATPase. So, the endolymph is **rich in potassium**.
- The cochlear duct is triangular in cross section.
- The Reissner's membrane, basilar membrane and the stria vascularis form the three walls of the cochlear duct.
- The basilar membrane houses the organ of Corti that locates the receptor cells for hearing.
- The two membranes join at the apex of the cochlear duct, leaving a narrow gap between the membranous and bony cochlea, known as **helicotrema.**

Scala Tympani: Scala tympani is the space below the basilar membrane, **filled with perilymph**. At the base of the cochlea, it is separated from the middle ear by the round window, which is enclosed by a flexible membrane called the **secondary tympanic membrane**.

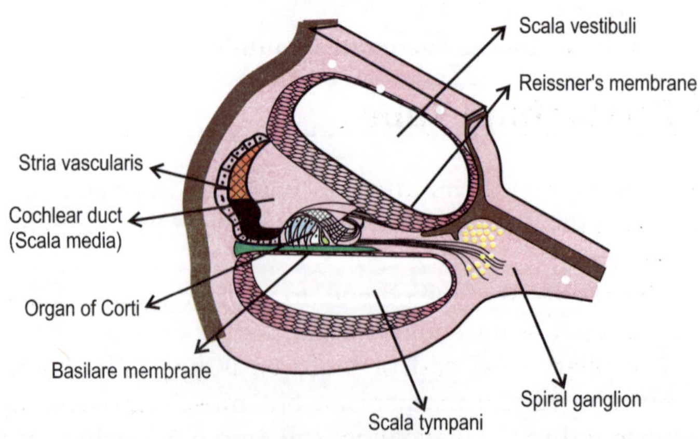

Fig. 125.4: The cross-sectional view of the cochlea, showing the three compartments.

Organ of Corti

The Organ of Corti or the spiral organ is the specialized structure **located on the basilar membrane** containing the receptors for hearing, the **hair cells** (Fig.125.5). It consists of hair cells, the associated nerve terminals, supporting cells, tunnel of Corti, basilar membrane, tectorial membrane and reticular lamina.

1. When sound waves reach the organ of Corti, It acts as a **transducer to convert the mechanical form of energy into action potentials in the cochlear nerve**.
2. There are **two (inner and outer) groups of hair cells** situated on the basilar membrane, separated by the *rods of Corti*.
3. The triangular gap between the rods of Corti is known as the **tunnel of Corti**.
4. The **inner hair cells** (closer to the modiolus) are about 3500 in human cochlea. They form a single row and extend the entire length of cochlea.
5. Lateral to the tunnel of Corti, there are present three rows of **outer hair cells**, about 20,000 in number.
6. The hair cells are surrounded by the supporting or ***sustentacular cells***. The apical ends of the hair cells contain cilia (hair) that pass through the reticular lamina supported by the rods of Corti.
7. The cilia of the outer hair cells project into a thin flexible gelatinous **tectorial membrane** that covers the rows of hair cells, whereas the cilia of the inner hair cells do not touch the membrane. The viscous membrane contains collagen and glycoprotein and is firmly attached only along its medial edge.

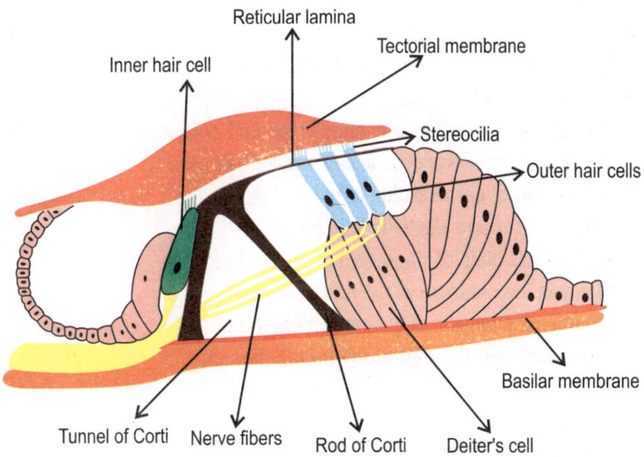

Fig. 125.5: The Organ of Corti

Hair Cells

Structure

The structures of inner and outer hair cells are anatomically similar, but the **outer hair cell is longer than the inner hair cell.**

1. The hair cell is a cup shaped structure with **fine cilia** (hairs) at its apical end (Fig.125.6), and its basal end makes synaptic connections with the afferent fibers.
   - Unlike the hair cells in vestibular apparatus, **there is no kinocilum in the cochlear hair cells** and the cilia are known as **stereocilia.**
2. The height of stereocilia is about 4 to 10 μm and they are 0.2 to 0.8 μm in diameter with a narrow base. The bases of the stereocilia are inserted into the apical part of the hair cell.
3. Each stereocilium has a core of cross-linked and closely packed **actin filaments** that are surrounded by myosin molecules. There are about **50-100 stereocilia** present at the apical surface of the hair cell.
   - The tips of cilia are linked to each other by minute strands called **tip-links.** Mechanically *sensitive cation channels* **(transduction channels)** are present at the junction of cilia with the **tip-links.** The tip-links help the bundle of stereocilia to **move as a unit**.
4. Along the basilar membrane, the size of inner hair cells does not change, but the *size of outer hair cells gradually increases from the base to the apex* of the cochlea.
5. The stereocilia of inner hair cells (about 50 in number) are present in three parallel rows, whereas that of outer hair cells (about 100 in number) are present in **three rows in a W-shaped formation.**
6. The height of the stereocilia gradually increases toward the lateral edge of the hair cell; therefore, the ***row of stereocilia toward the stria vascularis is tallest.***
   - The tips **form a slope**, the lower end being towards the modiolus.
   - The tips of stereocilia of outer hair cells are embedded in the tectorial membrane whereas those of inner hair cells are just short of contact with the tectorial membrane.
   - Along the basilar membrane, the *height of stereocilia progressively increases* from the base toward apex of cochlea.

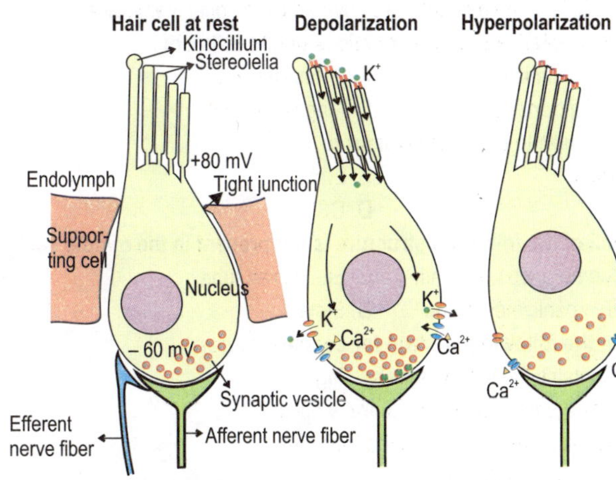

Fig. 125.6 A: Structure of cochlear hair cell; B. Depolarization of hair cell occurs as stereocilia bend towards longest stereocilium. C. Repolarization of hair cell occurs as stereocilia bend away from longest stereocilium.

Innervations of Hair Cells

Each nerve fiber forms synapse with only one hair cell, but **a single hair cell** gets synaptic connection **from 8–30 nerve fibers.**

1. The **inner hair cells** are the actual receptor for hearing. Though they constitute only 15–20% of the hair cell population, they **receive about 90–95% of the afferent nerve endings.**
2. On the other hand, only 5-10% of the afferent neurons innervate the bases of the outer hair cells.
3. The axons of the afferent nerves form the **auditory (cochlear) division** of the VIII cranial and project to the brain stem.
4. The efferent neurons (olivocochlear axons) arise from the superior olivary complex in the brain stem. They mainly give projections to the bases of the outer hair cells and form few synapses with the afferent axons of the inner hair cells.

Exam Questions

1. Describe the functions of the middle ear. Add a note on auditory ossicles.
2. Draw a labelled diagram of organ of Corti. Describe the mechanisms of activation of Cochlear hair cells.

Multiple Choice Questions

1. The increase in sound intensity due to the pinna and the external auditory canal is:

A. 1 dB B. 2 dB
C. 5 dB D. 15 dB

2. All of the following are true for the tympanic membrane, EXCEPT:

A. Acts as a resonator
B. Surface area is 5-9 mm^2
C. Its outer surface is covered by skin
D. Critically dampens the sound waves

3. All of the following are functions of middle ear, EXCEPT:

A. Equalization of air pressure
B. Transmission of sound wave
C. Transduction of sound wave
D. Amplification of sound wave

4. The resting membrane potential of cochlear hair cell is:

A. -15 mV B. -60 Mv
C. -90 mV D. +80 mV

5. All of the following are true for hair cells, EXCEPT:

A. A single hair cell synapses with one afferent neuron
B. Inner hair cells receive 90% of the afferent innervations
C. Inner hair cells are about 3500 in human cochlea
D. Cillia of the hair cells are covered by tectorial membrane

6. The depolarization of hair cells is due to influx of

A. Sodium ion B. Potassium ion
C. Calcium ion D. Magnesium ion

7. Endolymph in ear is equivalent to

A. Blood B. Lymph
C. ICF D. CSF

8. Which of the following structure is not present in the middle ear?

A. Membranous labyrinth B. Eustachian tube
C. Tympanic membrane D. Stapes

9. All of the following are true for cochlea, *except*:

A. Contains the receptor for hearing
B. Has a broad base and a narrow apex
C. Takes 3 1/4 turn around the modiolus
D. Contains perilymph

10. All of the following are true for tympanic reflex, EXCEPT:

A. There occurs inward movement of malleus and outward movement of stapes
B. Is due to contraction of tensor tympani and stapedius
C. Develops in 40 msec and completes in 160 msec
D. Decreases damage to the inner ear from loud sound

11. Secondary tympanic membrane:

A. Has no role in hearing
B. Mediates vibration of basilar membrane
C. Restricts the vibration of the Reissner's membrane
D. Covers the oval window

12. During transmission of sound waves, the pressure within the middle ear increases by:

A. 2 fold
B. 4 fold
C. 12 fold
D. 22 fold

13. Cochlear hair cells are activated by:

A. Bending of stereocilia towards the longest stereocillia
B. Compression of hair cells
C. Voltage difference between endolymph and perilymph
D. Bending of inner hair cells towards outer hair cells

14. The function of ear ossicles is to:

A. Amplify the sound waves to 1.3 times
B. Pull the foot plate of stapes out of the oval window
C. Maintain the pressure within middle ear
D. Increase the tension of tympanic membrane

15. In otosclerosois, the pathology mainly lies in:

A. Malleus
B. Incus
C. Stapes
D. Tympanic membrane

16. The abnormal sensitivity to loud noise (hyperacusis) occurs due to:

A. Paralysis of tensor tympany
B. Paralysis of stapedius
C. Damage to malleus
D. Damage to tympanic membrane

Answers: **1.** D **2.** B **3.** C **4.** B **5.** A **6.** B **7.** C **8.** A **9.** C **10.** A **11.** B **12.** D **13.** A **14.** A **15.** C **16.** B

Chapter 126

PY10.15

Auditory Pathways

Learning Objectives

On completion of study of this chapter:

The student will be able to (must know):

1. Draw a labelled diagram of auditory pathway.
2. List the functions of inferior colliculus and medial geniculate body
4. Name auditory cortical areas and give their functions.

The student may also be able to (desirable to know):

1. Describe the connections and functions of auditory pathways

FUNCTIONAL ORGANIZATION

The **auditory pathways** in general have **five order of neurons.** However, the neuronal arrangement is a complex one

1. **First orders of neurons** (cochlear division of 8th cranial nerve) start from the hair cells and project to the ipsilateral dorsal and ventral *cochlear nuclei* of the medulla oblongata.
   - The cochlear nerves are bipolar neurons whose cell bodies are present in the **spiral ganglion** located in the modiolus.
2. **Second orders of neurons** start from the cochlear nuclei and project to the *superior olivary nuclei* (bilaterally) and to the *nuclei of trapezoid body* (contra-laterally) (Fig. 126.1).
   - Some of the fibers from the dorsal cochlear nuclei (second order neurons) ascend contra-laterally in the lateral lemniscus to the inferior colliculi.
3. **Third-order neurons** from the superior olivary nuclei ascend bilaterally in the lateral lemniscus to the *inferior colliculi* of the midbrain.
   - Fibers from trapezoid body ascend ipsilaterally in the lateral lemniscus to the inferior colliculi.
   - Some of the fibers from the superior olivary nuclei (third order neurons) project to the medial geniculate body.
   - Fibers in the lateral lemniscus give collaterals to the **reticular nuclei and cerebellum.**
4. **Fourth-order neurons** project bilaterally from the inferior colliculi to the **medial geniculate body** (MGB) of the thalamus.
5. **Fifth-order neurons** start from the MGB and terminate in the **primary auditory cortex** (areas 41 and 42) situated in the superior temporal gyrus (Flowchart 126.1).

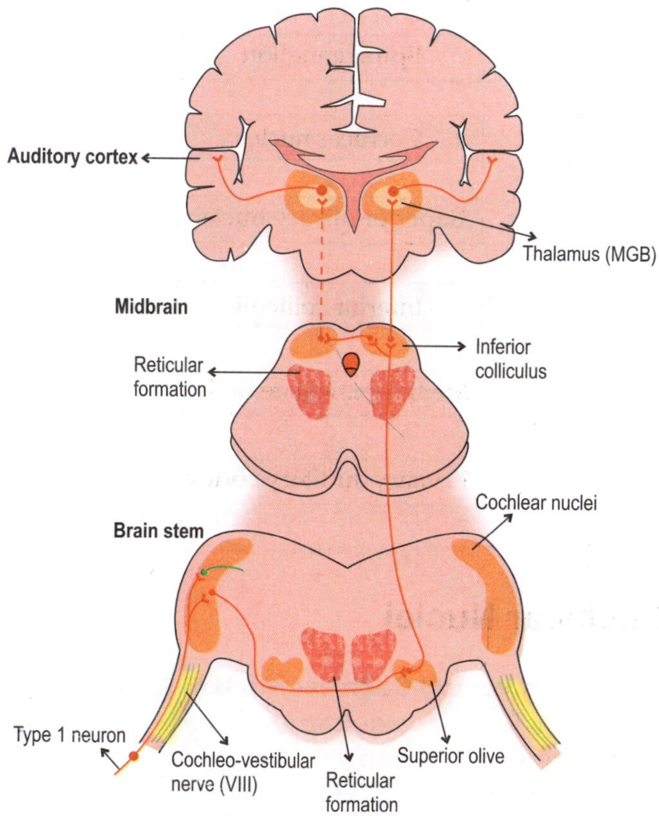

Fig. 126.1: Auditory pathway. Note the five orders of neurons in the pathway.

Specialities of Auditory Pathway:

1. Characteristically, the middle order neurons in the auditory pathway give **extensive bilateral projection**.
   - This helps to preserve the auditory capacity even if one of the centers is affected.
2. Moreover, the fibers do not project to single nucleus, rather to **multiple higher centers**.
   - For example, all the second order neurons do not project only to the superior olivary nuclei. This is in contrast to the specific nature of projection of the fibers of the visual pathway.
3. In the auditory pathway, the neurons while ascending up give *collaterals to the reticular nuclei and cerebellum*.
   - Thus, the body becomes alert and adjusts its posture to protect itself from the source of sound stimulus that may be harmful.
4. There is an orderly **tonotopic organization** of the fibers in the auditory pathway.
   - That means each fiber responds to a given tone and arrangement of fibers is based on the tone of sound.
   - The systematic pattern of fibers is evident from the first order neurons and right up to the primary auditory cortex.
5. Fibers descend down heavily from auditory cortex to **medial geniculate body, inferior colliculus and cerebellum**

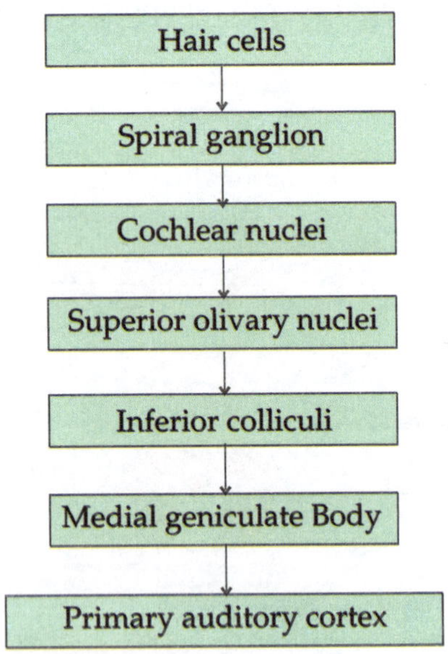

Flowchart 126.1: Schematic diagram of auditory pathway.

Cochlear Nuclei

Dorsal and Ventral Cochlear Nuclei

The *innermost part of the cochlear nuclei* receives inputs from neurons **responding to high tone** that originates from the basal part of cochlea. The *peripheral part of the cochlear nuclei* receives inputs from neurons **responding to low tone** that originates from the apical part of cochlea.

Superior Olivary Complex

The superior olivary complex is the **first nucleus** in the auditory pathway that **integrates binaural stimuli**, which means auditory signals from both ears converge on single neurons.

- It receives information **from the trapezoid body** for comparing timing of auditory stimuli arriving at both ears.
- All these contribute to the **localization of the source of sound**.
- Superior olivary complex receives the ascending sensory fibers and acts as the auditory relay center.
- It **projects bilaterally to the inferior colliculi**.
- It also gives rise to the efferent fibers called **olivocochlear bundle**.

Inferior Colliculus and MGB

The inferior colliculus is divided into a **central nucleus** (situated in its core) and a **peripheral region** that has pericentral and external nuclei. The core neurons are **tonotopically organized** from superficial to deep layers for low to high frequency sounds.

Peripheral Part: The peripheral part receives somatosensory information from the medial lemniscus and spinothalamic tract and visual input from the superior colliculus.

- Inferior colliculus *projects to midbrain reticular formation and periaqueductal gray*, thus **mediates the arousal and attention to auditory stimuli**.
- It projects to the *vermal part of the cerebellum* that contributes to **maintenance of posture in response to sound**. For example, startling reaction to noise or dancing to music.

Central Nucleus: The central nucleus projects to laminated part of MGB, which projects to **deep layers of auditory cortex**.

- The peripheral nuclei project to nonlaminated part of MGB, which projects to superficial layers of auditory cortex.
- MGB and auditory cortex **mediate conscious perception of sound**.

AUDITORY CORTICAL AREAS

Primary Auditory Cortex

The primary auditory cortex (**Brodmann's area 41**) is located in the sylvian fissure, in the superior portion of the temporal lobe.

1. The **auditory map of cochlea has a point for point representation** in the cortex of the animals. In the primary auditory cortex of humans, *high tones are represented posteromedially* and *low tones are represented in its anterolateral part*.
2. Similar to the visual cortex, the auditory cortex has **isofrequency columns**. When an electrode enters

vertically, it comes across neurons all of which code for the same frequency.

Other Auditory Cortical Areas

There are other auditory cortices as well as auditory association areas that integrate auditory inputs with motor speech area (words to be spoken after listening), with visual areas (words to be written after listening), with motor areas (playing an instrument after listening to the music) and so on. These cortical areas show **distinct hemispheric specialization**.

1. Usually the *left hemisphere is concerned with the analytical aspect* whereas the *right hemisphere processes the subjective or abstract features* of the auditory signals. Thus, they exhibit marked **cortical asymmetry** while processing the auditory inputs.
2. Besides, the auditory areas show great **cortical plasticity**.
   - Based on the modified inputs arriving in the auditory cortices, the size and extent of the different areas change by the learning and experience of the individual.
   - It is a known phenomenon that people who become **blind at an early age have a greater acuity of hearing**; they can better localize the source of a sound stimulus than people with normal vision.
   - Also, **trained musicians** who can better perceive and differentiate various tones have *larger auditory areas* responding to tone.

Brodmann's Area 22

Brodmann's area 22 processes auditory signals related to speech. In the right hemisphere, it **processes the intensity, pitch and melody** of speech. In the left side, it helps in **understanding the words** that is being spoken.

Planum Temporale: Planum temporale, a part of the posterior superior temporal gyrus **processes auditory signals related to language**. This area is larger in the left hemisphere than in the right cerebral hemisphere. However, the left side planum temporale in musicians is bigger than that in a normal person.

Efferent Pathways

(Descending Fibers from Auditory Cortex)

Pathways

The efferent fibers originating from auditory cortex **project to the medial geniculate body, inferior colliculus and cerebellum** via pons.

- The fibers from inferior colliculus project to the **superior olive and cochlear nuclei**.
- The efferent fibers arising from the superior olivary complex are known as the **olivo-cochlear bundle**.
- These fibers descend down and innervate the outer group of hair cells of the ipsilateral as well as contralateral organ of Corti.
- The ***olivo-cochlear fibers are cholinergic*** that secrete acetylcholine at their nerve endings that hyperpolarizes them.

Functions

1. **Stimulation** of these efferent fibers *hyperpolarizes the outer hair cells* and elongates them, whereas **inhibition** of the efferent fibers *depolarizes the outer hair cells* and shortens them.
2. The flexibility is due to presence of a membrane protein called **prestin,** a motor protein in the outer hair cell membrane.
3. The olivo-cochlear fibers modulate the transmission of nerve impulses in the afferent fibers.
   - This **enhances the pitch discrimination ability and increases amplitude & clarity of sound waves**.
4. The efferent modulation also augments the capacity to distinguish sounds in the presence of noise and protect the inner hair cell by dampening their responses to loud music.
5. The olivocochlear fibers also give projection to the **cochlear nucleus**, where they influence the transmission of impulses from first order to second order neurons.
6. The descending fibers from the higher nuclei also **influence the ascending fibers**.

Exam Questions

1. With the help of a suitable diagram, trace the auditory pathways. Add a note on auditory cortex.

Multiple Choice Questions

1. All of the following are included under auditory cortical areas, EXCEPT:

A. Brodmann area 22
B. Brodmann area 41
C. Brodmann area 42
D. Planum Temporale

2. Which of the following is NOT a speciality of auditory pathway?

A. Middle order neurons project ipsilaterally
B. Fibers project to multiple higher centres
C. Fibers show an orderly tonotopic organization
D. Ascending fibers give projection to cerebellum

3. The primary auditory cortex is situated in:

A. Parietal lobe B. Temporal lobe
C. Occipital lobe D. Limbic lobe

Answers: 1. C 2. A 3. B

Chapter 127

PY10.15

Mechanisms of Hearing

Learning Objectives

On completion of study of this chapter:

The student will be able to (must know):

1. Mention the properties of sound waves.
2. Understand the meaning and importance of masking.
3. Give a brief description of transmission of sound waves in the middle ear and inner ear.
4. Explain the transduction mechanism of sound waves.
5. Learn the mechanism of genesis of receptor potential in hair cells.
6. List the special features and properties of basilar membrane.
7. Comprehend the concept of travelling wave hypothesis.
8. Describe the mechanism of hearing.
9. List the differences between the cochlear microphonics and action potentials.

The student may also be able to (desirable to know):

1. Describe the role of cochlea in hearing
2. Explain the cochlear microphonics.

SOUND WAVES

Sound waves are alternate compression and rarefaction of molecules that strike the tympanic membrane to produce the sensation of sound. The waves originate from a vibrating source (like vocal cord, tuning fork etc.) and travel through an elastic medium like air or water.

Speed

- Sound waves travel in the air at a speed of 340 m/s at 20 °C at sea level.
- The speed is **more in hot environment and high altitude**.
- The speed decreases with decrease in temperature.
- Sound waves travel with a **much greater speed in water** and the speed is *more in seawater than fresh water* (In fresh water, the sound waves travel with a speed of 1400m/s).

Frequency

- The frequency of sound waves is expressed as the **number of waves per second**. Its unit is **Hertz** (1 **Hz** = 1 cycle per second). The audible range of frequency for human ear is 20 to 20,000 Hz, but the ear is more sensitive to sounds with frequencies of 1000-4000 Hz.
- The frequency is also expressed as tone or pitch. A sinusoidal sound wave having one frequency is called a **pure tone**; for example, 50 Hz or 100 Hz.
- A **complex sound** wave contains more than one frequency; they are perceived as musical sounds if regularly repeated and as noise when there is no regular pattern. Speech is a complex sound.

Pitch: The **subjective sensation produced by the frequency of sound** is known as pitch. The *greater the frequency, the higher is the pitch*.

- During conversation, the male and female pitch is about 120 Hz and 250 Hz respectively. Therefore, *female voice is shriller* and is audible from a greater distance.
- A person can differentiate about 2000 pitches and this capacity can improve with training. **Pitch discrimination is best between 1000 -3000 Hz**. The human ear can sense a difference in frequency of **as little as 3 Hz** in this range.

Wavelength: The **distance between the two adjacent peaks** is known as the wavelength of sound. It is inversely related to frequency.

Loudness

- The **amplitude of sound waves** determines the loudness or intensity of the sound. The *greater the amplitude, the louder is the sound*.
- Frequency also affects loudness. So, the hearing threshold varies with frequency. Sound intensity is measured in units called **decibels (dB)**.

- The sound intensity in bel is the logarithm of the ratio of the intensity of the sound heard and the standard sound (1 dB = 0.1 bel). So,

$$\text{Number of decibel} = 10 \log \frac{\text{Intensity of the sound heard}}{\text{Intensity of standard sound}}$$

As this is in logarithmic scale, a sound of 0 decibel means the intensity is equal to that of the standard. Each 10 dB interval corresponds to a 10-fold increase in sound intensity.

- The human audibility curve ranges from 0-100 dB and the human ear is more sensitive to intensity of about 60 dB at a frequency of 1000 - 4000 Hz.

Hearing Threshold

The threshold of hearing is 0 dB at 1000 Hz for a normal young adult in a noise free environment. The sound is felt as well as heard at a level of 140 dB. The decibel scales for common sounds are given below. As the intensity of sound is proportionate to the square of sound pressure, 0 dB is equal to 2×10^4 dynes/cm^2 (hearing threshold).

140 dB Pain and damage to the ear
120 dB uncomfortable to the ear
80 dB Shouting
60 dB Normal conversation
20 dB Whispering
0 dB Hearing threshold

Masking

The hearing threshold for a given sound increases in the presence of background sounds or noise. This phenomenon is known as masking.

Mechanism of Masking

1. As the background sounds stimulate the auditory receptors and nerve fibers, they are in a *relative or absolute refractory state when the given sound arrives*. So, the **sensitivity of the auditory apparatus to a given tone decreases in the presence of other sounds**.
2. The degree to which a given sound can be masked *depends on the frequency of the masking sound*. Low-frequency sounds masks high- frequency sounds more effectively. A fairly broad-spectrum noise (**white noise**) serves as a useful mask for a wide range of test frequencies.

This is a **common experience in the factory areas** where sound due to machineries makes it difficult for two people to talk in a normal voice. Even in so called calm environment, some amount of auditory stimuli is present which exert a masking effect on the ears. Therefore, in **conduction deafness sound is better heard in the defective ear.** The hearing threshold increases in a soundproof room.

Transmission of Sound Waves

Transmission through Outer & Middle Ear

Sound waves travel in the external ear canal to the tympanic membrane. In the middle ear, the vibrations of the tympanic membrane get transmitted through the chain of ossicular bones, become amplified and reach the footplate of stapes.

Ossicular Conduction: *Sound waves are transmitted* from the external ear to the internal ear primarily ***through tympanic membrane and the ossicular chain*** causing vibration of the footplate of stapes. This is known as **ossicular conduction.**

Air Conduction: From the tympanic membrane, sound waves are also transmitted ***through the air of the middle ear cavity*** and vibrate the secondary tympanic membrane to reach the perilymph of the scala tympani. This is known as **air conduction**. The force of vibration is much reduced as it arrives at the surface of perilymph. Moreover, the *stronger vibration reaching through oval window is a greater stimulus* for the hair cells. So, **air conduction has a very negligible role in normal hearing**.

Bone Conduction: From the environment, sound waves get **mechanically transmitted through the bones** and reach the inner ear. Bone conduction is better appreciated when a vibrating tuning fork is placed on the bone of the skull, especially the mastoid process. It is used to diagnose hearing loss due to defective transmission of sound waves through the external and middle ear.

Transmission through Inner Ear

- Sound waves are transmitted from the footplate of stapes to the fluid of the inner ear. The stapes moves inward and outward causing similar movement of the membrane of the oval window.

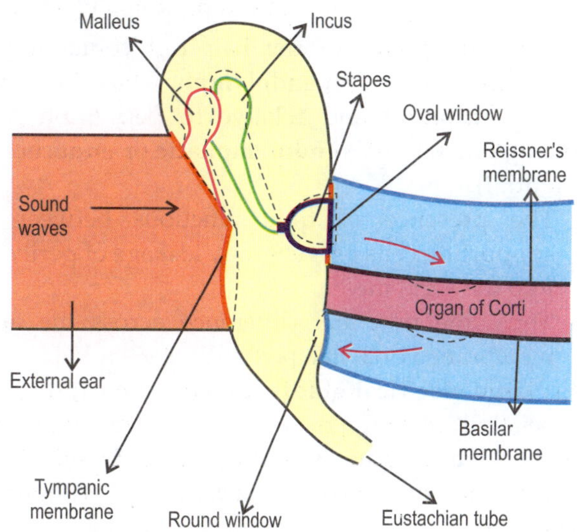

Fig. 127.1: Transmission of pressure wave through the outer, middle, and inner ear. The resultant displacements of the tympanic membrane, auditory ossicles, and the membranes of inner ear are shown by dashed lines. Arrows indicate the direction of pathway of sound wave.

- The perilymph is incompressible as the cochlea is encased in a rigid bone. When the stapes moves inward, the **pressure in the perilymph of scala vestibuli increases.**
- This *depresses the Reissner's membrane* that in turn produces *depression of the basilar membrane*. The pressure wave is then transmitted to the perilymph of the scala tympani and finally produces **outward movement of the round window into the middle ear** (Fig.127.1).
- When the stapes moves outward, there occurs upward bulging of basilar membrane and the round window is pulled inward. The up and down movement of the basilar membrane produce *upward and downward movement of the organ of Corti.*

TRANSDUCTION OF SOUND WAVES

The mechanical energy (pressure waves) of sound is **converted into receptor potentials** in the hair cell and finally gets conducted as action potentials in the auditory pathways.

Resting State of Hair Cell

In the resting state, **two potentials** are recorded from the ear.

i) **Resting membrane potential** of the hair cell
ii) **Endocochlear potential**

The basolateral **resting membrane potential** of the hair cell is – 60 mV. It is due to the continuous efflux of K^+ across its basolateral membrane.

1. The ***basolateral surface*** of the hair cell is bathed in perilymph, which has a low K^+ concentration and zero potential (an electrically neutral fluid like ECF).
2. The ***apical surface*** of the hair cell containing the stereocilia is bathed in **endolymph**, which has a **high K^+ concentration** and relative to perilymph has a potential of +80 mV (**endolymphatic** or **endocochlear potential**).
    - The presence of tight junctions between the supporting cells prevents any leakage of perilymph into the scala media.
    - Thus, the potential difference across the apical membrane is 140 mV [+80 mV – (–60 mV)].
3. This **large electrical gradient favors the cation influx** especially K^+ through the transduction channels. In the absence of any auditory stimulus the hair cell remains at rest, with the stereocilia straight up, without any deflection.
4. In the resting state however, about **15% of the cation channels are open** allowing a steady leak of K^+ into the cell.

Genesis of Receptor Potential in Hair Cells

Process of Depolarization

The hair cell is a mechanoreceptor, which is **very sensitive to the direction and degree of movement of cilia**. The appropriate stimulus for hair cell is the lateral bending of cilia. A deflection of stereocilia of as little as 0.5 nm generates a response in the hair cell.

1. When the **shorter stereocilia bend toward the taller stereocilia** (toward the stria vascularis) the **cation channels open**, allowing entry of K^+ (mostly) and Ca^{+2} into the hair cell (refer, Fig. 125.6, Chapter 125).
2. The resulting depolarization causes **opening of voltage-gated Ca^{+2} channels** at the base of the hair cell.
    - Increased cytoplasmic calcium concentration causes **movement and fusion of vesicles** with the synaptic specialization at the base of the hair cell.
3. This results in **release of glutamate** into the synaptic cleft producing action potentials in the afferent nerve fibers.
    - The number of action potentials increases with the increased release of neurotransmitter.
4. Following depolarization, a molecular motor made up of myosin drags the channel to the resting state and relaxes the stretched tip-links.
5. The resting membrane potential is **restored by diffusion of K^+** along the electrochemical gradient through the leaky K^+ channels at the basolateral membrane.

Process of Repolarization

1. When the **stereocilia are pushed away from the taller stereocilia** (toward the modiolus), the apical transduction **channels close**, leading to hyperpolarization (refer, Fig. 125.6, Chapter 125).

There occurs no change in membrane potential when the stereocilia bend at right angles, and the maximum change takes place when they are positioned at 45°angle (midway). Thus, the hair cell acts as a fine transducer in which, depolarization or hyperpolarization depends on the direction of movement of hairs; and the magnitude of change in membrane potential depends on the distance they travel toward or away from the mid position.

Role of Cochlea

When the sound waves arrive at the inner ear, the basilar membrane, the hair cells and the tectorial membrane act in an integrated fashion to convert the mechanical form of energy into appropriate action potentials for the precise perception of sound.

- The cochlea *also encodes the frequency and amplitude of sound waves* that is further processed in the auditory pathway higher up in the cortex.
- Thus, the cochlea acts as a fine transducer as well as a frequency analyzer.

Special Features of Basilar Membrane

The structure and property of basilar membrane is not same throughout its length.

1. Although the cochlea as a whole becomes narrower toward the apex, the **basilar membrane is narrow at the base and wider towards the apex** (Fig. 127.2).
   - Also, it is **stiff at the base** and becomes gradually **elastic towards the apex**.
   - Its stiffness decreases 100-fold from base to apex.
2. These mechanical characteristics enable the membrane to **respond differently to the wide range of sound frequencies** along its length.
   - When sound wave of a given pitch arrives, only *hair cells situated at a particular location* along the membrane are maximally stimulated as maximum bowing of basilar membrane occurs at that area and a ***fixed set of afferent fibers discharge***.
   - Thus, **each successive spot** along the basilar membrane **is most sensitive to a slightly different frequency**.
   - As there occurs encoding of specific tones at specific places, this is known as **place coding** or **place theory** in the auditory system.
   -

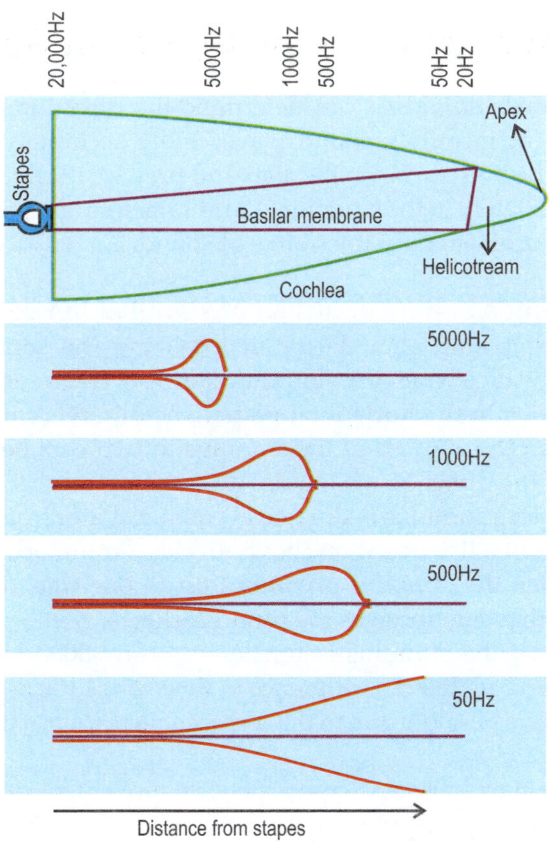

Fig. 127.2: High-frequency sound waves cause maximal displacement of the basilar membrane near its base, and low-frequency sound waves cause maximal displacement at the apical end, near the helicotrema.

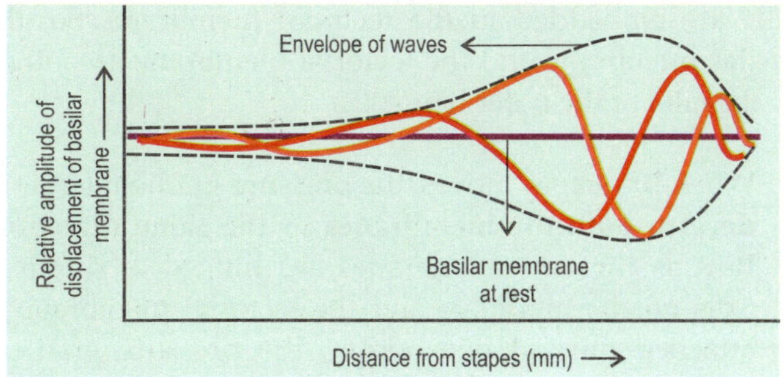

Fig. 127.3: Traveling wave. The orange and red lines represent the waves at two instants of time, respectively.

3. The basilar membrane is the first site for **pitch discrimination**.
   - The hair cells toward the apical region maximally respond to low frequency sound waves and those toward the basal region maximally respond to high frequency sound waves.
   - Thus, different frequencies can be mapped in a serial manner along the length of the basilar membrane.
   - This orderly representation of tone is maintained in the cochlear neurons as well as in the neurons of the auditory pathway. This is called the **tonotopic organization**.
2. The basilar membrane also **responds to different intensities of sound waves**.
   - Loud sound causes greater displacement of the basilar membrane that generates increased number of action potentials in the cochlear nerve.

Traveling Wave

As the stapes moves in and out, it generates a **series of traveling waves** in the perilymph of scala vestibuli. The organ of Corti including the basilar membrane **vibrates in accordance with the undulation** created in the perilymph, i.e. **it distorts in the form of a traveling wave**. As the wave travels along the basilar membrane from its base to apex, it ***attains maximum amplitude*** at a point depending on its frequency and then falls rapidly (Fig. 127.3).

1. **High-frequency sounds cause maximal displacement** of the membrane near its base, near the oval window and ***low-frequency sounds generate waves that attain maximum amplitude*** at its apical end, near the helicotrema (Fig. 127.2).
2. Thus, the perception of different tones by the brain depends upon the **type of wave generated** in the cochlear fluid and the basilar membrane. This phenomenon is also known as **traveling wave hypothesis**.

Shearing Force Bends Cilia

The upper parts of the hair cells are tightly held by the reticular lamina and the tips of the hairs of the outer hair cells are embedded in the tectorial membrane. So, the basilar membrane and the tectorial membrane are joined by the cilia of the outer hair cells.

- When the stapes moves, the pressure gradient tends to **deform both the membranes in the same direction**. But, as the two membranes are hinged at different axes on the modiolus and the tectorial membrane is attached only at one border, the pressure gradient **creates a lateral shearing force** that causes **bending of the cilia**.
  - The hairs of the inner hair cells do not touch the tectorial membrane, but they bend by the movement of endolymph between the inner hair cells and the tectorial membrane.
- ***When the basilar membrane moves up***, the stereocilia bend away from the modiolus, and the **hair cells depolarize**.
- ***When the basilar membrane moves down***, the stereocilia bend towards the modiolus, and the **hair cells repolarize**.

COCHLEAR POTENTIALS

In addition to the **resting potentials** recorded from the ear (endolymphatic potential and resting membrane potential of the hair cell), three **dynamic potentials** are seen when an auditory stimulus arrives at the cochlea. These are **cochlear microphonic** (CM), **summation potentials** (SP) and **nerve action potentials** (AP). These potential can be detected by placing electrodes on the round window or in areas near the cochlea and the procedure is known as electrocochleography.

Cochlear Microphonics

- Cochlear microphonic CM is the **electrical response that represents the summated intracellular potentials of many hair cells**.
- It is generated instantaneously due to the **large current flow** across the apical surface of the hair cells along a favorable electrical gradient.
  - Each and every auditory stimulus produces CM and it follows the pattern of vibration of the basilar membrane precisely. So, CM is an ***oscillatory event*** that has the same frequency as the auditory stimulus.
  - It is proposed to originate **primarily from the outer hair cells** since it almost disappears after lesions that destroy the outer hair cells but spare the inner hair cells.

The differences between CM and action potentials are listed in Table 127.1.

Summation of Potentials

This dynamic cochlear potential can be a positive summation potential (+SP) or negative summation potential (– SP). The **bending of cilia** may cause +SP and –SP may have a neural origin. **Positive SP can be masked**, whereas negative SP cannot be masked.

Table 127.1 | **Difference between cochlear microphonics and action potentials.**

Cochlear Microphonics (CM)	Action Potentials (AP)
- Have no latency	- Have latency
- Have no refractory period	- Have refractory periods
- Occur before the commencement of action potential	- AP occurs after CM
- When the stimulus rate is high, the rate of CM formation is more than that of the action potential	- Rate of AP generated is less compared to that of CM
- CMs do not fatigue	- AP of Neurons also don't fatigue
- The recording of CM can be a positive or a negative deflection with the reversal of polarity of the stimulus (from condensation-rarefaction to rarefaction-condensation)	- the AP is always a positive deflection
CM cannot be masked	- AP is completely masked by a broad-spectrum noise

Localization of the Source of Sound

A normal individual can determine the direction of the source of incoming sound waves quite accurately. This helps the body to be on the alert and prepare itself to react appropriately to the situation. Various factors are involved in the localization of the source of sound.

Difference in time of arrival of stimulus in two ears

This is an important factor in localizing the source of sound waves when the stimulus **is of low frequency** and originates **in the horizontal plane**. The difference in time between the arrivals of the stimulus in two ears helps to decide the direction of sound.

1. When a stimulus is situated at equal distance from both ears of a listener, it reaches both ears simultaneously.
2. When the ***stimulus originates off to one side***, the ear on that side receives the sound earlier.
3. When the stimulus frequency is below 3000 Hz, the brain can detect a difference in time of as little as 20 µs. This is possible due to the remarkable response time of hair cells.
4. The hair cells can sense repetitive movement of up to 100,000 times per second.

Difference in intensity that reaches the two ears

In the horizontal plane, the stimulus intensity is ***perceived more in the ear that is nearer to the stimulus***. When the stimulus frequency is above 3000 Hz, this factor plays a **greater role in sound localization.**

Role of Pinna

Many animals like cat and deer can turn their pinna to **focus hearing in a particular direction without changing head position.** In humans, this capacity is absent. Sound wave enters the auditory canal both directly and after being reflected by the pinna and the sound that we hear is a combination of the two.

- The shape of the pinna/tragus tends to *accentuate or attenuate certain sound frequencies depending on the angle at which sound waves approach the ear.*
- Thus, the pinna is essential in humans for **sound localization in the vertical plane.** In the horizontal plane, as the pinna is curved little forward the sound coming from the back differs in quality from the sound that comes from the front.

The time of arrival of stimulus and its intensity decides the pattern of action potentials from each ear. This causes maximal or minimal activation of neurons in the auditory centers that receive inputs from both ears.

- As the superior olivary nucleus is the first station to receive bilateral input, it is the first center for localization of the source of sound.
- The auditory cortex finally compares the input from both ears and determines the direction of sound.
- In lesions of auditory cortex, sound localization is very much affected.

Exam Questions

1. Describe the mechanism of hearing.
2. Describe the process of transduction of sound waves in the cochlea.
3. Describe the genesis of receptor potential in the hair cells. Add a note on travelling wave hypothesis. List the differences between cochlear microphonics and action potential.

Multiple Choice Questions

1. The neurotransmitter released from the hair cell at the synaptic cleft is:
A. Acetylcholine B. Glutamate
C. Glycine D. Dopamine

2. Which of the following is the first site of pitch discrimination?
A. Basilar membrane B. Tympanic membrane
C. Oval window D. Reissner's membrane

3. Endocochlear potential is:
A. +45 mV B. −45 mV
C. −60 mV D. +85 mV

4. The human ear is most sensitive to a frequency of:
A. 100-300 Hz B. 300-500 Hz
C. 1000-4000 Hz D. 10000-20000 Hz

5. Pain and damage to the ear occurs at a sound wave crosses:
A. 60 dB B. 80 dB
C. 100 dB D. 140 dB

6. The number of pitches that a normal person can differentiate is about:
A. 100 B. 1000
C. 2000 D. 5000

7. The speed of sound in air at 0°C is:
A. 33 meters/sec B. 340 meters/sec
C. 500 meters/sec D. 1000 meters/sec

8. The minimum intensity of sound at 1000 Hz that the human ear can perceive in a noise free environment is:
A. 0 dB B. 20 dB
C. 60 dB D. 100 dB

9. Scala media is filled with:
A. Perilymph B. Endolymph
C. Lymph D. CSF

10. When the stimulus frequency is below 3000Hz, the brain can detect a difference in time of
A. 2μs B. 20μs
C. 200 μs D. 2 ms

11. Compared to action potentials, the cochlear microphonics
A. Have no latency
B. Have no refractory period
C. Can be completely masked
D. Have higher rate when the stimulus rate is high

12. In the basilar membrane, high frequency sound waves cause
A. Maximal displacement near its apex
B. Maximal displacement in the middle
C. Maximal displacement near its base
D. No displacement at any place

Answers

1. B 2. A 3. D 4. C 5. D 6. C 7. B 8. A 9. B 10. B
11. C 12. C

Chapter 128

PY10.16

Hearing Defects and Hearing Tests

Learning Objectives

On completion of study of this chapter:

The student will be able to (must know):

1. Classify hearing defects and name the causes for each defect.
2. Give the physiological basis of each test to assess hearing defects.
3. Name the hearing tests, understand their procedure and interpretation.
4. Understand the principle of audiometry and BAEP.

The student may also be able to (desirable to know):

1. Describe the physiological basis of hearing defects and the tests to assess them.

HEARING DEFECTS

Deafness

Deafness is divided into the following types: **conductive deafness** and **sensorineural deafness**. When both conductive and sensorineural deafness are present, it is known as **mixed deafness.**

Conductive Deafness

Conduction deafness occurs due to impaired transmission or amplification of sound to the cochlea due to disease of the external or middle ear. The sound waves are conducted to the cochlea by the skull bones (bone conduction) and produce vibration of the basilar membrane. So, the hearing loss is usually partial. The common causes are:

1. **Blockade of external auditory canal:** This occurs as a result of impaction of wax, or foreign bodies. Less common causes are atresia or tumor of the auditory canal.
2. **Thickening of the tympanic membrane** following repeated middle ear infections. Sometimes perforation may occur due to infection or trauma.
3. **Acute and chronic otitis media**
4. **Immobility of the ossicles.** This may occur as a result of adhesions due to repeated middle ear infections or bony ankylosis. When the stapes is fixed to the oval window in an abnormally rigid manner, it is known as **otosclerosis**.
5. **Destruction of the auditory ossicles.**
6. **Eustachian tube obstruction** leads to absorption of the air from the middle ear cavity by the lining mucosa. This results in negative intratympanic pressure producing a retracted tympanic membrane.

Sensorineural Deafness

This occurs as a result of diseases of the cochlea or of the 8th cranial nerve. The degree of hearing impairment depends on the extent to which the structures are affected. When deafness occurs due to lesion of the cochlear nuclei or their central connections, it is known as central deafness. It occurs rarely and is associated with marked neurological deficits.

The common causes of sensorineural deafness are:

1. **Toxic degeneration of the hair cells** caused by chronic treatment with **drugs** such as aminoglycoside antibiotics (streptomycin, kanamycin, gentamycin). These drugs **block the mechanosensitive channels** in the stereocilia of hair cells, subsequently ***leading to their degeneration***. They also *affect the hair cells of the vestibular apparatus*, so **nerve deafness** along with abnormal vestibular functions occurs. Some **other drugs** like salicylates, quinine, cytotoxic drugs and certain diuretics also produce deafness.
2. **Senile degeneration of the hair cells:** There occurs gradual cumulative loss of hair cells and neurons due to effect of aging. This is known as **presbycusis.** It is seen in about one-third of population over 75.

3. **Damage to the outer hair cells** *by prolonged exposure to loud noise* e.g. loud music, revved-up motorcycles and engine roar of jet planes. Usually, deafness begins with loss of sensitivity for high intensity sounds.
4. **Tumors** of the vestibulocochlear nerve (acoustic neuroma) or tumors in the cerebellopontine angle pressing on the cochlear nerve.
5. **Trauma or** *fracture of the base of the skull*
6. **Labyrinthitis**
7. **Meniere's disease** is characterized by episodic vertigo, deafness and tinnitus.

Mixed Deafness

Mixed deafness can be due to trauma, infection or tumor that affect both middle ear and inner ear. Deafness due to **genetic mutations** is classified into *syndromic* (when it is associated with abnormalities in other systems) and *nonsyndromic* (when deafness is the only abnormality).

The mutations can occur in the following proteins and cause nonsyndromic deafness.

- **Connexon 26**, which helps in normal recycling of K^+ through supporting cells,
- **Myosin-VIIa**, which is associated with actin in the hair cell processes,
- **Myosin-Ib,** which causes movement of the cation channels at the tip links,
- **Myosin-VI**, which plays a role in the formation of the cilia,
- **α-tectin**, which is the major protein in tectorial membrane.

Mutations in the following proteins cause syndromic deafness.

- **Sulfate transport protein**: Its mutation results in Pendred's syndrome (deafness and goiter).
- **KVLQT1**, a K^+ channel protein that is present in the stria vascularis and maintains the high K^+ concentration of the endolymph and a normal QT interval in the heart. Its mutation produces long QT syndrome (deafness and a longer QT interval that predisposes to ventricular arrhythmias)
- *Barttin*, the mutation of which causes deafness and renal manifestation of Bartter's syndrome.

Tinnitus: It is the perception of sound in the absence of any sound in the environment. It may be buzzing, roaring or ringing type and can be pulsatile. It is usually associated with conductive or sensorineural deafness.

Treatment of Deafness

Complete restoration of hearing is possible in cases where the cause can be treated successfully; for example, removal of wax or tumor and treating otitis media with antibiotics.

Hearing Aids: Hearing aids are useful to restore the hearing capacity to some extent in cases of deafness due to partial decrease in functions of middle ear or cochlea.

- These are electronic devices **attached to the ear** that amplify the sound waves.

Cochlear Implants: These are tiny electronic devices **implanted under the skin over the mastoid bone**. They translate the sound waves into electrical signals that are directly transmitted to the auditory pathways bypassing the damaged structures. As they take up the role of hair cells in sound transduction, they are also called **artificial ears**.

- The implants are used for people with deafness due to disease or injury that has **destroyed hair cells of organ of Corti**.
- These days cochlear implants are quite successful to restore almost normal hearing.

PY10.20

TESTS FOR HEARING

Tuning Fork Tests

Rinne's Test

Normally, sound conducted through **air and the ossicular system is louder than that conducted through skull bones** to the inner ear.

1. First, the bone conduction (BC) is tested by placing the base of the vibrating tuning fork on the mastoid process. The subject hears the sound and indicates by raising his finger, when he no longer hears the sound.
2. The vibrating tuning fork is then held near the ear and a normal person continues to hear the sound for some time. This tests the air conduction (AC).
3. So, **AC is more than BC in a normal person** or *in partial nerve deafness*.
4. In case of **conduction deafness**, *bone conduction is normal* but he does not hear any sound when the fork is placed near the ear. So, BC is more than AC.
5. In case of total nerve deafness, AC and BC both are absent and no sound is heard.

Weber's Test

Normally, environmental *noise is transmitted to the inner ear by ossicular conduction* along with the sound the person listens to, and tends to mask it; but it has no effect on sound conducted through the bone of the skull.

1. If the base of a vibrating tuning fork is placed at the center of the forehead, or the vortex of the skull, a **normal person will hear it equally in both ears**, but a person with **conduction deafness** will *hear it louder in the diseased ear*, because the environmental noise does not reach the inner ear of that side.
2. On the other hand, the subject with **nerve deafness** *hears the sound louder in the normal ear*.

Schwabach's Test

This test employs the same principle as the Weber's test.

The bone conduction of the patient is compared with that of a normal person. If the *bone conduction of the patient is better than normal*, he has **conduction deafness**, but if his *bone conduction is less than normal*, he has **nerve deafness**.

Audiometry

The assessment of hearing using electronic equipments is known as audiometric test. The tests can be subjective (results are based on patient's answer) and objective.

Pure Tone Audiometry: This is one of the most generally used subjective tests for assessing hearing. The machine is called audiometer and the recording is called audiogram. This test is useful to detect or rule out conduction deafness.

1. The audiometer **emits pure tones of various frequencies**, which the subject listens to through the earphones (for air conduction) or by an electronic vibrator fixed to the mastoid process (for bone conduction).
2. The test is performed in a soundproof room and each ear is tested separately beginning with the better ear. A total of 6-10 different tones with frequencies ranging from 250 to 8000 are tested and the threshold decibels against each tone are plotted for each ear.
3. When hearing loss is present, the ***non-test ear is masked*** *by sounds of broad-spectrum* to have proper evaluation.
4. During the bone conduction test, the non-test ear is masked with some narrow band of noise centered on the test frequency as vibrations on any part of the skull easily get heard at the untested ear.

Speech Audiometry: **Other** subjective hearing tests are **speech audiometry** (measures the patient's ability to recognize and repeat correctly lists of words that are presented to him), **alternate binaural loudness balance test, loudness discomfort level test** and **tone decay test**.

Brainstem Auditory Evoked Responses (BAER) PY10.19

The potentials recorded from the auditory pathway in response to a brief auditory stimulation are known as BAERs. As the stimulus travels from the cochlea to higher up, it generates action potentials in all the nerve fibers. BAERs assesses functional status of the auditory pathway up to the mid brain.

1. The waveforms of BAEP are named I, II, III, IV and V (Fig. 128.1).
2. **Wave I** originates from peripheral portion of eighth cranial nerve adjacent to the cochlea.
3. **Wave II** arises from cochlear nucleus. Action potentials in the superior olivary nucleus generate **wave III**.
4. **Wave IV** arises from lateral lemniscus.
5. **Wave V** originates from inferior colliculi. Absence or reduced amplitude of a waveform indicates lesion of the area that gives rise to that wave.

BAEP is useful in **assessing hearing loss in infants and small children**. It is also useful in **localizing brainstem lesions**, diagnosing tumors at various levels of the auditory pathway, coma, brain death and strokes affecting the brain stem.

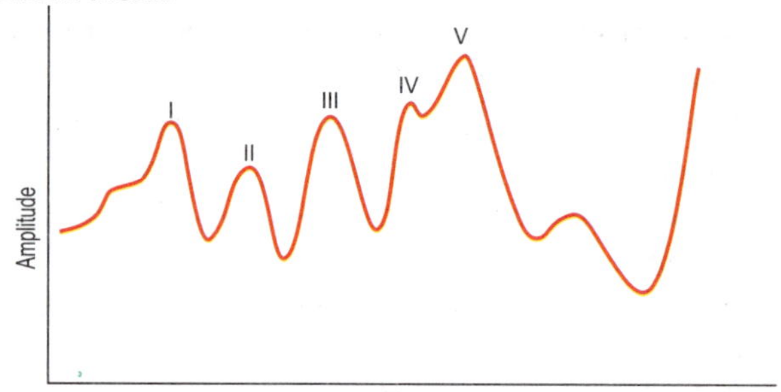

Fig. 128.1: Brainstem auditory evoked potential recorded in a normal individual.

Exam Questions

1. Describe various tests for hearing. Describe how to differentiate the sensorineural deafness and conductive deafness.
2. Briefly describe brainstem auditory evoked potential. Add a note on audiometry.

Multiple Choice Questions

1. All of the following conditions result in conductive deafness, EXCEPT:
A. Thickening of tympanic membrane
B. Immobility of the ossicles
C. Labyrinthitis
D. Chronic otitis media

2. All of the following conditions result in sensorineural deafness, EXCEPT:
A. Damage to the outer hair cells by prolonged loud noise
B. Chronic treatment with aminoglycosides
C. Senile degeneration of the hair cells
D. Destruction of the auditory ossicles

3. Which of the following conditions result in conductive deafness?
A. Chronic treatment with streptomycin
B. Presbycusis
C. Tumor of vestibulocochlear nerve
D. Eustachian tube obstruction

4. Which of the following conditions result in sensorineural deafness?
A. Meniere's disease
B. Acute otitis media
C. Impaction of wax in external auditory canal
D. Otosclerosis

Answers

1. C 2. D 3. D 4. A

Chapter 129

Physiology of Smell

Learning Objectives

On completion of study of this chapter:

The student will be able to (must know):

1. Give the structure and functions of olfactory epithelium and olfactory receptor cells.
2. Name the neurons in the olfactory bulb, and organization of olfactory glomeruli.
3. Trace the olfactory pathways.
4. Briefly describe the physiology of olfaction.
5. List factors affecting olfaction.

The student may also be able to (desirable to know):

1. Connections and functions of cortical olfactory areas.
2. Describe the mechanisms and factors affecting olfaction.

The sense of smell is known as olfaction. The receptors for smell are **chemoreceptors** located in the **olfactory mucosa of the nasal epithelium**. The olfactory system is the only sensory system that **does not relay in the thalamus** on its way to the cortex, and it has asymmetric cortical representation.

SITE OF OLFACTION

Olfactory Epithelium

The **olfactory receptor cells** are located in a specialized area of the nasal mucosa lining the roof of the nasal cavity called the **olfactory epithelium** or the olfactory mucus membrane.

1. It is a patch of yellowish-pigmented mucus membrane extending laterally to the superior concha and medially to the upper third of the median septum (Fig. 129.1).
2. It occupies an area of about 2.5 sq.cm in each nostril in humans and is covered by mucus produced by the **Bowman's glands**.
   - The area is **large in animals** like dogs in which the sense of smell is pretty well developed (**macrosmatic** animals).
   - Human beings are **microsmatic**.
3. The olfactory epithelium contains **10-20 million receptor cells** interspersed between **supporting cells** and **progenitor cells**.
   - The progenitor cells are stem cells that form new receptor cells by mitosis.

Vomeronasal Organ: In rodents and other mammals, another patch of *olfactory mucus membrane present along the nasal septum,* called vomeronasal organ, senses pheromones secreted from the mating partner.

- Axons from the vomeronasal organ **project to the accessory olfactory bulb** and from there primarily to areas in the amygdala and hypothalamus.
- These areas are concerned with reproduction and feeding behavior.

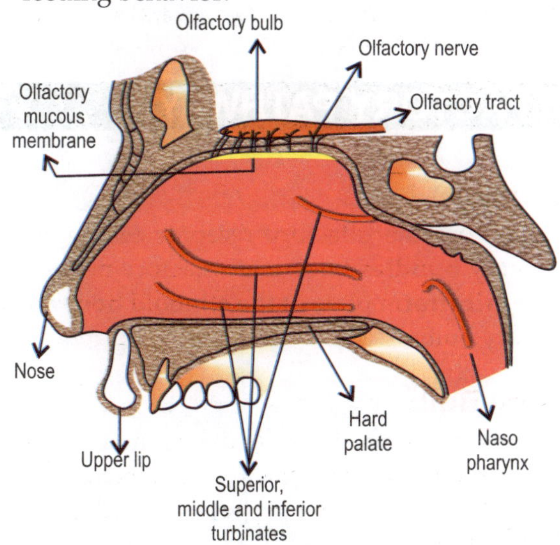

Fig. 129.1: Location of the olfactory mucus membrane.

Olfactory Receptor Cell

The olfactory receptor cell is a **bipolar neuron**.

1. It has a short thick dendrite with an expanded end called an **olfactory rod** that gives off **10-20 cilia** (Fig. 129.2).
2. Each cilium is about 2 μm long and 0.1 μm in diameter. The cilia are unmyelinated and **project into the mucus** where they interact with odorants dissolved in the mucus.

Olfactory Neurons: Unlike other neurons in the body, the olfactory neurons (also the taste receptor cells) are unique as they **regenerate**.

- The olfactory neurons are **replaced in about 60 days** as basal cells proliferate to form new receptor cells.
- A growth factor called **bone morphogenic protein** (BMP) exerts an inhibitory effect on this renewal process.
- Another unique feature of olfactory mucosa is that it is one place in the body where the ***nervous system is exposed to the external environment***.

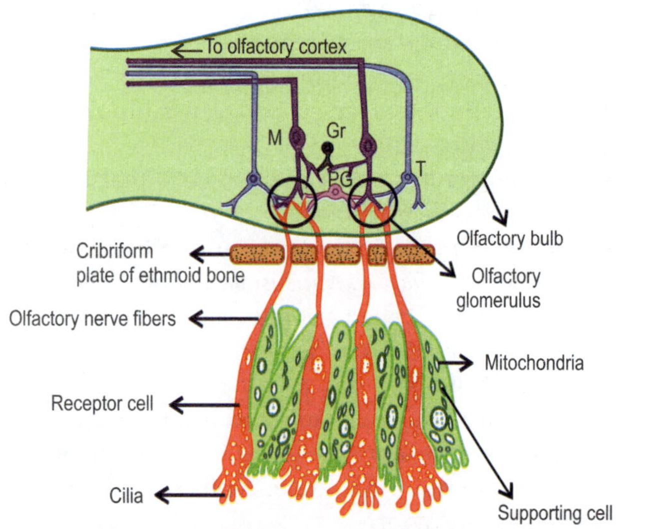

Fig. 129.2: Olfactory receptor cells and the olfactory pathway. M: Mitral cell; Gr: Granule cell; T: Tufted cell; PG: Periglomerular cell.

OLFACTORY PATHWAYS

Olfactory Nerves

The axons from the olfactory receptor cells gather into about **twenty bundles** known as olfactory nerves, which **pierce the cribriform plate of the ethmoid bone** and enter the olfactory bulbs.

Olfactory Bulb

Above the cribriform plate of the ethmoid bone, and below the orbital surface of the frontal lobe on each side, the portion of the brain that projects forward is known as the olfactory bulb.

Four types of neurons are present in the olfactory bulb:

1. Small tufted cells
2. Large mitral cells,
3. Periglomerular cells
4. Granule cells.

The first two are second-order neurons, and the last two are *interneurons*

Olfactory Glomeruli

These are globular formations present in the olfactory bulb, where terminals of **olfactory nerve synapse with the dendrites of tufted cells and mitral cells.**

1. As many first order neurons converge on the few second order neurons, the **high convergence ratio** increases the ***olfactory sensitivity***.
2. The periglomerular cells ***inhibit adjacent glomeruli*** and the granule cells ***inhibit mitral and tufted cells***.
   - The latter is an example of **feedback inhibition** i.e. the mitral and tufted cells stimulate granule cells (the neurotransmitter released is glutamate) and the granule cells in turn cause inhibition of mitral and tufted cells.
   - The inhibition is by ***releasing GABA***.

Olfactory Tract

The axons of mitral and tufted cells extend to the olfactory cortical areas as olfactory tract.

Cortical Olfactory Areas

While entering to the brain the fibers of the olfactory tract **divide into lateral and medial olfactory stria**. The fibers terminate in the apical dendrites of the pyramidal cells of the **olfactory cortex**.

Lateral Olfactory Stria: The lateral olfactory stria projects to the ***piriform cortex, amygdala, entorhinal cortex, anterior olfactory nucleus*** *and olfactory tubercle.*

1. Fibers from these areas project to the **orbitofrontal cortex** via thalamus, **frontal cortex, hippocampus, hypothalamus** and contralateral olfactory bulb (Fig. 129.3).
   - Sniffing activates the piriform cortex.
   - The **amygdala evokes emotional responses** associated with **smell.**
   - The **entorhinal cortex** is concerned with olfactory **memories.**
   - The **lateral and anterior orbitofrontal cortex** of the frontal lobe is concerned with ***conscious perception and differentiation of odors***.
2. Olfaction is asymmetrically represented in the orbitofrontal cortex as **right-side olfactory cortex is bigger** than the left.
   - **In lesion of orbitofrontal cortex**, the capacity to discriminate odors is lost.

Medial Olfactory Stria: The **medial olfactory stria** projects to **amygdala, septum and hypothalamus** that mediates various ***autonomic responses*** associated with smell.

1. Olfactory fibers also project to the **dorsal motor nucleus of vagus** that mediates ***parasympathetic responses*** to smell (e.g. secretion of saliva, gastric juice and pancreatic juice during the cephalic phase).

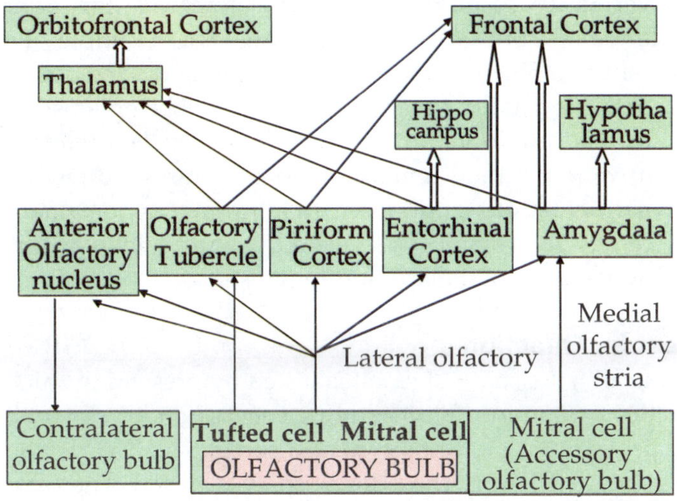

Fig. 129.3: Olfactory pathway. From olfactory bulb, axons of the tufted cells and mitral cells travel in the lateral olfactory stria, which project to the anterior olfactory nucleus, olfactory tubercle, piriform cortex, entorhinal cortex, and amygdala. The axons of the mitral cells from the accessory olfactory bulb form the medial olfactory stria and project to the amygdala. Information from these areas except the anterior olfactory nucleus travel to the orbitofrontal cortex via thalamus, frontal cortex, hippocampus, and hypothalamus. The anterior olfactory nucleus projects to the contralateral olfactory bulb.

PHYSIOLOGY OF OLFACTION

PY10.13

Mechanism of Olfaction

Role of Mucus and Odorant-Binding Protein

Olfactory receptors are activated only when the odoriferous substances are **dissolved in the thin layer of mucus** covering the olfactory epithelium and come in contact with the cilia of the olfactory receptors. Generally, odoriferous substances are **small molecules** with a few carbon atoms.

1. The **water-soluble odorants** dissolve in the mucus overlying the olfactory epithelium to reach the cilia of the olfactory receptors.
2. The **lipid-soluble odorants** bind to an **Odorant-Binding Protein (OBP)** to get transported in the hydrophilic mucus and reach the receptors.

- The OBP is secreted into the mucus by the lateral nasal gland.

Olfactory Transduction

There are about **1000 different odorant receptors** and all of them are coupled to heterotrimeric **G proteins**.

1. When the odorant binds to the receptor, the G protein is activated that leads to **opening of cation channels** causing influx of calcium (major mechanism), activation of **adenylyl cyclase-cAMP system**, where the G protein is called G_{olf}, and stimulation of **phospholipase C-IP$_3$, DAG system** occurs.
2. Activation of one of these systems produces **depolarization of the olfactory receptor cells** leading to generation of ***action potentials*** along the olfactory nerve fiber.

Sharpening of Impulses: Electrophysiological studies show that there is a **continuous background firing** of impulses through the olfactory tract, and the introduction of **odors increases the frequency** of these impulses. The dendrites of the periglomerular cells and granule cells spread laterally and produce **inhibition of the olfactory glomeruli** on which they synapse. This **sharpens and focuses** the action potentials in the mitral and tufted cells. The remarkable capacity to discriminate over 10,000 different odors depends upon the **following factors.**

i) There are **many types of odorant receptors**.
ii) The olfactory neuron arising **from one type of odorant receptors project to one glomerulus** and the neuron arising from ***another type of odorant receptors project to a different glomerulus***.

Factors Affecting Olfaction

1. **Type of odorant stimulus:** If the odorant chemicals are volatile, they are easily transported by air into the nose and are quickly recognized. A strong odor has a ***high lipid or water solubility***.
2. **Threshold of olfactory receptors:** The olfactory receptors are extremely ***sensitive to minute concentrations of some of the odoriferous substances***. For example, methyl mercaptan, which gives garlic its odor, can be smelt at concentrations as low as 0.000,000,4 mg per liter of air.
   - Usually, *women are more sensitive to smell* than men and their sensitivity to odors *increases further at the time of ovulation*.
   - The threshold for olfaction increases with advancing age, both for male and female.
3. **Intensity of stimuli:** Humans can discriminate over 10,000 different odors. But their *ability to distinguish changes in intensity of odors is* ***less significant***.
   - The change in concentration of odors must be over 30 percent to be perceived, compared with a 1 percent change in the visual system.
4. **Olfactory adaptation:** When the olfactory receptors are *exposed to a continuous stimulus*, they **adapt rapidly**. It is well known that when somebody enters a scented room, he becomes aware of the odor, but after some time, the *perception of the odor declines and ceases over time*.
   - Adaptation occurs due to activation of **cyclic nucleotide-gated (CNG) ion channels** by calcium-calmodulin complex.
   - When CNG A4 is knocked out, adaptation is slowed.

Reflexes Associated with Olfaction

1. **Sniffing** at the arrival of a new odor.
2. **Salivation**, or **gastric secretion, and pancreatic secretion** at the smell of food.
3. **Sneezing, lacrimation** and in extreme case, **respiratory inhibition** in response to irritant odors. Chemicals like chlorine, ammonia, menthol and peppermint stimulate the naked nerve endings of trigeminal pain fibers that are present in the olfactory mucus membrane. Thus, these odors produce unpleasant and burning sensation.
4. **Vomiting** in response to a foul smell.

PY10.14

APPLIED PHYSIOLOGY

Hyposmia and Anosmia

Depending on the extent of structural and/or functional loss, the sense of smell may be **diminished** (hyposmia) or **absent** (ansomia).

- Hyposmia or anosmia may result from common cold (commonest cause), old age, fracture of the cribriform plate damaging the olfactory epithelium, injury to the olfactory nerve or olfactory bulb, atrophic rhinitis and in receptor abnormalities.
- In **Kallmann's syndrome**, anosmia is associated with hypogonadism.

Dysosmia or Parosmia

When the sense of smell is **distorted** (dysosmia) or **perverted** (parosmia), the patient perceives the odor differently from a normal person. For example, he perceives offensive odors as pleasing and vice versa. Parosmia is usually a feature of temporal lobe epilepsy.

- In this condition, an irritating ***lesion in the olfactory areas*** of the temporal lobe causes **olfactory hallucinations** commonly manifesting as imaginary repulsive smell associated with involuntary movements of the lips and tongue.

Test for Olfaction

PY10.20

Clinically, the sense of smell is tested by presenting small bottles containing familiar odor e.g. asafetida, clove oil or peppermint oil, to each nostril separately. The person is asked to identify the odor with eyes closed. The odor should not be an irritating substance like ammonia; else it will stimulate the 5th **cranial nerve**. This is a qualitative test to assess olfactory function. Quantitatively, olfaction is tested by the **olfactometer**.

Exam Questions

1. With the help of a schematic diagram, trace the olfactory pathways. Briefly describe the mechanism of olfaction.
2. Describe the structure and functions of olfactory receptor cells. Briefly describe the factors affecting olfaction.

Multiple Choice Questions

1. The number of receptor cells in the olfactory epithelium is:
A. 1-2 million B. 3-5 million
C. 10-20 million D. 30-40 million

2. During quiet breathing, the inspired air:
A. Does not reach the olfactory epithelium
B. Reaches directly the olfactory epithelium
C. Cannot provide oxygen to the olfactory epithelium
D. Move up by convection current to reach the olfactory epithelium

3. Which of the following is NOT true about vomeronasal organ?
A. Is present in all mammals
B. Is necessary for successful mating behaviour
C. Has axons projecting to the accessory olfactory bulb
D. Gives information finally to the amygdala

4. Which of the following is NOT true about olfactory receptor cells?
A. Has a short thick dendrite called olfactory rod
B. The olfactory rod gives rise to 10-20 cilia
C. The cilia are myelinated
D. The cilia interact with the odorants

5. Which of the following statemmnet is NOT true about olfaction?
A. Adaptation occurs due to knocking out of CNG ion channel
B. Humans can discriminate over 10,000 different odours
C. Odorant receptors are coupled to G-protein called Golf
D. The lipid soluble odorants bind to odorant-binding protein

6. Olfactory receptor cells are:
A. Pseudounipolar neurons B. Modified epithelial cells
C. Bipolar neurons D. Multipolar neurons

7. Which is incorrectly matched?
A. Eyes - Rods and cones B. Olfaction - Hair cells
C. Tongue - Na+ channels D. Carotid body - Chemoreceptor

8. Which of the following sensation has the smallest range of intensity discrimination?
A. Somatosensory B. Hearing
C. Smell D. Taste

9. All of the following are brain areas receive olfactory sensation, EXCEPT:
A. Piriform cortex B. Amygdala
C. Anterior nucleus of thalamus D. Anterior olfactory nucleus

10. All of the following are reflexes associated with olfaction, EXCEPT:
A. Vomiting B. Sneezing
C. Salivation D. Defecation

Answers

1. C	2. D	3. A	4. C	5. A	6. C
7. B	8. C	9. C	10. D		

Chapter 130

Physiology of Taste

Learning Objectives

On completion of study of this chapter:

The student will be able to (must know):

1. Give the structure and functions of taste buds, and gustatory receptor cells.
2. Draw a schematic diagram of taste pathways.
3. Understand the mechanism of gustatory transduction for various testants.
4. List the factors influencing taste sensations.

The student may also be able to (desirable to know):

1. Describe the physiology of gustation.
2. Describe the physiological basis of abnormalities of taste sensation.

The sense of taste is known as **gustation**. Like smell, it is classified under **visceral senses** and the gustatory receptors are **chemoreceptors.**

RECEPTOR ORGANS (TASTE BUDS)

The receptor organs for taste are called **taste buds** that house the chemoreceptors responsible for taste. They respond to gustatory stimuli (**tastants**) and mediate the taste sensation.

- There are a total of about **10,000 taste buds**.
- The number decreases with advancing age.

Location

The **taste buds** are located mainly on the tops of the numerous **fungiform papillae** and along the sides of the less numerous **circumvallate** and **foliate papillae** of the tongue. A few taste buds are present in the mucosa of the palate, epiglottis, pharynx, larynx and esophagus. A **papilla** is a small, elevated projection on the dorsum of tongue.

1. The small **fungiform papillae** are located at the **tip** and along the **edges** of the anterior two thirds of the tongue.
   - Each papilla contains up to five taste buds at its top.
2. The **circumvallate and foliate papillae** are large and each contains up to 100 taste buds along its sides.
   - In the **posterior third** of the tongue, the circumvallate papillae are located in the walls of a V-shaped trough and the foliate papillae are located at the edge of the V.
3. The dorsum of the tongue is covered by small conical threadlike **filiform papillae** that do not contain taste buds.

Also, there are **no taste buds in the under surface of the tongue.**

Structure

The taste buds are oval shaped multicellular structures about 70 μm high and 50μm in diameter. The following types of cells are present in a taste bud: **basal** cells, **supporting** (sustentacular) cells and the **gustatory receptor** cells (Fig.130.1).

Types of Cells: The gustatory receptor cells or taste cells are of **three types**: **dark cells, light cells and intermediate cells**, also known as **type I, type II and type III** cells respectively.

1. The cells lie mostly buried in the surface of the tongue; the chemicals reach the receptor cells through an opening in the apical surface of the taste bud called the **taste pore** (gustatory pore).
2. The **supporting cells** do not have any afferent synaptic connections.
3. The **basal cells** are formed from the epithelial cells surrounding the taste bud.
   - They are the **undifferentiated stem cells** from which new receptor cells are constantly formed by differentiation and proliferation replacing the old receptor cells.

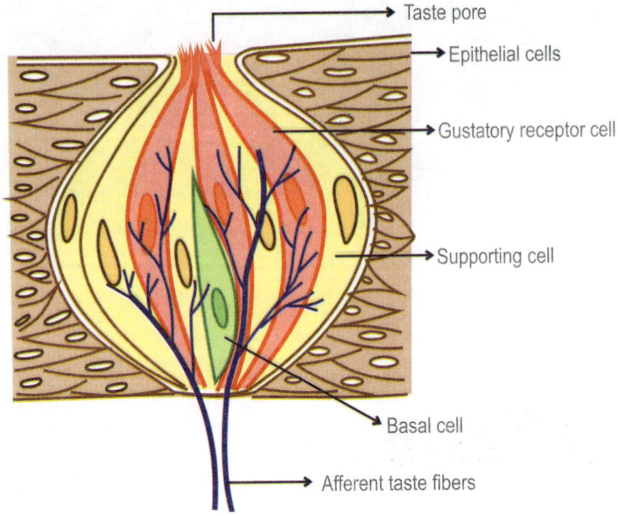

Fig. 130.1: Structure of a taste bud.

Gustatory Receptor Cell

The taste receptor cell is a **modified epithelial cell**. The receptor cell is elongated and extends full length of the taste bud.

1. At its apical end, a single, hair like **microvillus** (gustatory hair) projects to the external surface through the taste pore, where it comes in contact with the ***gustatory stimuli*** or **tastant**.
    - The **microvilli increase the surface area** of the receptor cells. The receptor cells are the **most numerous taste bud cells** (50-75%).
2. A taste bud contains **about 50-150 taste receptor cells** that are surrounded by the supporting cells.
3. The apical regions of the receptor cells and the supporting cells are joined by tight junctions so that only the microvilli come in contact with the fluids in the oral cavity.
4. Unlike the olfactory system, the gustatory receptor cells are ***not primary afferent neurons***. At their basal end, the receptor cells form synapse with the nerve endings of primary sensory axons (first order neuron).
    - Each taste bud is innervated by **50 afferent fibers** and each afferent fiber receives input from about five taste buds.

Regeneration of Cells: The receptor cells have a **life span of about 10 days**. Like the olfactory receptors they degenerate and are continuously **replenished by new receptor cells** from the basal cells.

- In this process, the synaptic connections of the old cell also degenerate and the new ones are formed.
- It has been observed that sectioning the afferent nerve fiber leads to degeneration of the taste buds supplied by it; and when the nerve regenerates, **new taste buds are formed** near the nerve endings.
- It is reported that the nerve terminals release **growth factors** and exert a **trophic effect on the taste buds**, as well as confer on them chemical specificity.

Innervation

1. The fungiform papillae receive sensory innervation from **chorda tympani**, a branch of the facial nerve.
2. The circumvallate and foliate papillae are innervated by **sensory fibers from the glossopharyngeal nerve**.
3. The taste buds in the palate are supplied by the greater superficial petrosal branch of the facial nerve, whereas the taste buds in other parts are innervated by the vagus nerve.

PY10.13

PHYSIOLOGY OF GAUSTATION

Taste Pathways

The chorda tympani branch of the facial nerve and the glossopharyngeal nerve carry sensations from the taste buds in the anterior two thirds and posterior one third of the tongue respectively. The taste sensations from other areas travel in the vagus nerve.

1. The afferent fibers (first order neurons) enter the medulla oblongata and terminate in the nucleus tractus solitarius (Fig. 130.2).
2. From there, the second-order neurons arise and ascend in the ipsilateral medial lemniscus to terminate in the ventral posteromedial (VPM) nucleus of thalamus.
3. From the thalamus, the third-order neurons arise and travel in the thalamic radiation to project to the face and tongue areas of the ipsilateral primary sensory cortex (foot plate of the post-central gyrus) (Flowchart 130.1).
4. The third-order neurons also project to the anterior insular cortex and frontal operculum; these areas in turn project to lateral orbitofrontal cortex.
5. While ascending up in the medial lemniscus, the second-order axons give branches to the ***reticular formation, the limbic system, hypothalamus and the locus ceruleus.***

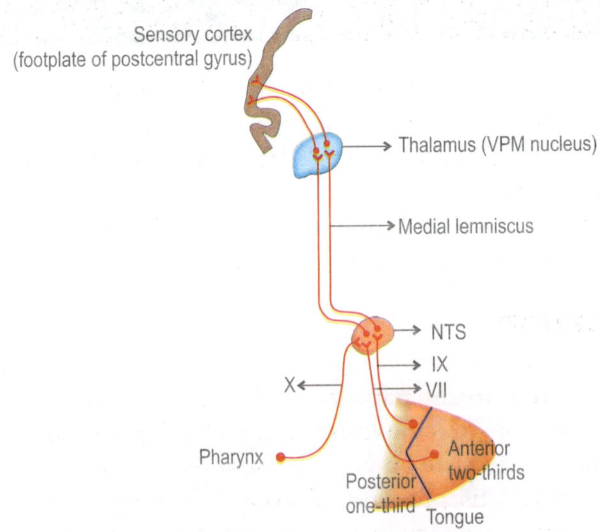

Fig. 130.2: Taste pathway. Note that fibers project to the thalamus and cortex of same side. (NTS: Nucleus tractus solitarius; VPM: Ventral posteromedial).

Tongue Ant. 2/3rd by (chorda tympani) VII, and Post. 1/3 by X cranial nerves

↓

NTS (via medial lemniscus)

↓

VPM nucleus of thalamus (ipsilateral)

↓

Sensory cortex
(Ipsilateral foot plate of post central gyrus)

Flowchart 130.1: Taste pathway. NTS: nucleus tractus solitarius; VPM: Ventral postero-medial thalamic nucleus.

Type of Tastes

Traditionally, **four basic taste sensations** have been described: **sweet, salty, sour and bitter**.

- Recently, a fifth type called **umami** (delicious in Japanese) has also been included in the list of basic tastes. The umami taste is pleasant and sweet but differs from standard sweet taste.
- The different **sub-modalities** of taste sensations are believed to arise from various combinations of these primary taste sensations blended with simultaneous stimulation of touch, temperature and pain receptors in the oral and lingual mucosa, as well as olfactory sensations.

Though the tip of the tongue is sensitive to sweet; anterior edges to salt, the sides to sour and the back of tongue is sensitive to bitter taste, the ***regional specificity for taste on the tongue is less***, and **all tastes are sensed from all parts of the tongue.**

Mechanisms of Gustatory Transduction

The receptors for taste are **chemoreceptors** that respond to chemicals arriving on the lingual epithelium. A gustatory stimulus produces depolarization of the receptor cell.

- In the oral cavity, when the chemicals released from dissolved food particles **come in contact with the microvilli**, they bind to specific receptors and activate them.
- There is a graded depolarization of the receptor cell, defined as its **receptor potential.**
  - The depolarization when adequate opens voltage-gated calcium channels causing **Ca^{+2} influx.**
  - The raised intracellular Ca^{+2} level results in **exocytosis of the neurotransmitter glutamate** from the basal end of the receptor cell into the synaptic cleft.
- **Glutamate** promotes generation of action potentials in the sensory axons.

Thus, the process of generation of action potentials by the gustatory stimuli acting on the taste buds is known as gustatory transduction.

Receptor Mechanism: Most of the receptors respond to **more than one of the primary tastes**; only they have differences in sensitivity to the various tastants. The chemicals are of diverse structure, and the receptors have multiple mechanisms and second messenger systems to signal the different taste modalities.

- Many of the chemicals act by stimulating the gustatory G protein, **gustducin.**
- Usually, depolarization of a receptor occurs either due to increase in membrane **permeability to Na^+, or closure of K^+ channels, or increase in Ca^{+2} concentration.**

Recently, **a protein** that binds the tastants molecules has been cloned. It is secreted by **Ebner's glands.** The protein concentrates the tastants molecules and transports them to the membranes of the microvilli.

Salty Taste

The salty taste is elicited by Na^+, present most commonly in NaCl, the table salt.

1. The **salt-sensitive receptors** have epithelial Na^+ channels (**ENaC**) in their membrane, which allows Na^+ entry when extracellular Na^+ concentration increases.
2. The increased intracellular Na^+ level results in **depolarization of the receptor cell**. It has been found that following application of the Na^+ channel-blocking diuretic **amiloride** on the tongue, the ability to taste salt ***is not completely abolished.***
   - This indicates that apart from the ENaC-mediated mechanism, there is **some other mechanism** for depolarization.
3. All inorganic **anions taste salty**, but the cation may have varied effect.
   - **Potassium salts are bitter and salty**; lead and beryllium salts taste sweet and mercuric salts taste metallic.
4. **Lysyltaurine** is a more potent salty agent than NaCl.

Sour Taste

The sour taste is triggered by hydrogen ions, the adequate stimulus being a pH of less than 4 of the solution.

1. **Hydrogen ions block the K^+ channels** in the apical cell membrane.
2. The decreased K^+ permeability produces depolarization of the receptor cell.
3. The **ENaCs** also allow entry of H^+ and the inward positive current leads to depolarization.
4. The sour taste may also be due to stimulation of **HCN**, a hyperpolarization-activated **cyclic nucleotide-gated cation channel** receptor and other receptors.
   - All acids are sour and the intensity of perception depends on the degree of dissociation of the acid

(i.e. the number of free hydrogen ions). However, some organic acids give mixed sensations.

5. Citric acid is sweet and sour, and picric acid is bitter and sour.

Umami Taste

The umami taste is **produced by glutamate**, which is present in purine 5-ribonucleotides such as inositol monophosphate (IMP) and guanosine monophosphate (GMP) in the diet.

1. **Glutamate is present as a flavor-enhancer** in monosodium glutamate (MSG), a food additive used extensively in Asian cooking.
2. Glutamate binds to and activates a cation channel that **permits Na^+ and Ca^{++} entry** causing depolarization of the receptor cell.
   - Glutamate also activates a ***metabotropic glutamate receptor***, **mGluR4** resulting in a **decrease in cAMP level**. However, further mechanism of depolarization following receptor stimulation is not clear.

Bitter Taste

The bitter taste is elicited by a variety of unrelated substances, many of which are poisons and the bitter taste serves as a **protective warning** to avoid them. As per the large variety of chemicals, the receptors and the mechanisms of their activation are also many.

1 Many of the bitter compounds act by binding to receptors coupled to G protein and produce depolarization by activating the G protein-mediated second messenger cascades. The **number of receptors** linked to G protein is as many as **24 in humans**.

2. **Strychnine** binds to a receptor of T2R family linked to the G protein gustducin and stimulate phosphodiesterase.
   - The resultant decrease in the level of cAMP produces depolarization.
   - Some compounds activate G protein linked to another class of receptor and activate phospholipase C to increase the formation of **IP_3 and DAG** that trigger the release of Ca^{+2} from the endoplasmic reticulum.
   - The raised intracellular **Ca^{+2} concentration** leads to depolarization and release of neurotransmitter.
   - The mechanism of action of the bitter tasting amino acid **leucine** is G protein-mediated.
3. **Quinine** is the yardstick for bitterness
   - It acts by direct stimulation of the G protein bypassing the receptor.
   - Some compounds produce inhibition of the phospholipase that metabolizes cGMP.
4. Substances like **morphine, nicotine and caffeine** taste bitter.
5. Many **non-alkaloids** taste bitter e.g. urea, magnesium, potassium, calcium and ammonium salts.
   - Calcium binds directly to K^+ channels and block them leading to depolarization.

Sweet Taste

Sweet substances act by the **G protein gustducin.** About 20% of taste cells express G protein-coupled receptors of **$T1R_3$ family**. Some of them also express the G protein, named **gustducin**.

1. The stimulation of G protein-coupled receptor activates membrane adenylyl cyclase and **increases cAMP level**.
2. The raised intracellular cAMP activates protein kinase A that promotes **phosphorylation of K^+ channels** on the basolateral membranes.
3. This results in **closure of K^+ channels** and depolarization of the cell.
4. Some sweet substances increase **intracellular IP_3 level and promote Ca^{++} release** from the endoplasmic reticulum, thereby cause depolarization.

Most sweet substances are **organic**; specially **all sugars** tend to elicit a sweet taste (e.g. glucose, sucrose, fructose). **Sucrose** is taken as a standard for sweet substances. Several **non-sugar substances** also taste sweet, e.g. salts of lead and beryllium, chloroform, aspartame and saccharin. As **salts of lead** are sweet, ingestion of toxic amount of these salts can happen. The **α-amino acids are sweet**, but polypeptides are often bitter. The proteins **thaumatin and monellin** are much sweeter.

Encoding of Gustatory Stimuli

An adequate gustatory stimulus depolarizes the receptor cell and generates action potentials in the afferent nerve fibers. **Most of the receptor cells respond to more than one of the primary taste stimuli**. Each afferent fiber forms ***synapse with a number of receptor cells***. Thus, the afferent neuron receives information regarding a variety of taste stimuli.

- Each afferent neuron *fires optimally in response to one of the five primary taste stimuli*.
- The neurons in gustatory cortex are stimulated in response to the pattern of action potentials in the afferent neuron.
- Thus, the encoding of the gustatory sensation is not a simple labeled-line, chemical sensory system.

Taste Thresholds and Intensity Discrimination

Taste Thresholds

The **lowest concentration of a gustatory stimulus** to which the taste buds respond by depolarization is known as the threshold concentration of that substance. The threshold concentrations for different types of tastants vary (Table 130.1). The **thresholds of bitter compounds are usually low**.

1. As most of these are poisons, taste buds detect them even at a very low concentration and warn us from further ingestion.
2. Generally, ***women are less sensitive*** *to sour taste and* ***more sensitive*** *to sweet and salt taste* as their threshold for these sensations vary with men.
3. The threshold concentrations of substances eliciting a particular taste exhibit a wide range of variation. **Sucrose is 8 times sweeter** than glucose.
4. The **artificial sweetener saccharin** (threshold concentration - 23 μ mol/L) is **67 times** sweeter than sucrose. The proteins **thaumatin and monellin** (threshold concentration 0.01 μ mol/L) are **100,000 times** sweeter than sucrose.

Intensity Discrimination

As in olfaction, the ability of humans to discriminate differences in the intensity of tastes is poor. A 30% change in the concentration of the substance being tasted is required before an intensity difference is perceived. Humans can discriminate 4000- 10,000 tastants.

Table 130.1 | Taste thresholds of some tastants

Tastants	Taste	Threshold concentration (μ mol/L)
Strychnine Hydrochloride	bitter	1.6
Quinine	bitter	8
Hydrochloric acid	sour	100
Sodium chloride	salt	2000
Sucrose	sweet	10,000
Glucose	sweet	80,000

Factors Influencing Taste Sensation

1. **Age:** The taste sensation decreases after the age of 50. The **number of taste buds starts decreasing** due to the enhanced degeneration process.
2. **Gender:** Generally, **women** are less sensitive to sour taste and *more sensitive to sweet and salt taste*.
3. **Concentration of the tastants:** The intensity of the taste sensation depends on the concentration of the tastants solution. A concentrated solution elicits a stronger taste sensation than a diluted one.
4. **Area of stimulation:** The intensity of the taste sensation depends on the **number of taste buds** stimulated.
   - When a tastant solution is applied to a small area of the tongue, it produces a weaker sensation.
   - On application of the same solution *to larger area of tongue* produces a more intense sensation. This is due to activation of a ***greater number of afferent fibers.***
5. **Temperature of the tastants:** Increased temperature over some ranges tends to enhance the perceived taste sensitivity, especially for cooked food and spicy food.
   - For example, *perception of sweet taste is increased when the food is not warm.*
6. **Duration of stimulation:** The taste receptors show a slow but definite **adaptation.**
   - If a tastant solution is applied to one area of the tongue for a longer duration, the intensity of taste sensation gradually decreases.
   - This occurs due to **decrease in discharge of afferent nerve fibers over time.**
7. **Effect of other tastants:** When two or more stimuli are applied simultaneously, or one after the other, one may affect the perception of the other.
   - This is due to **facilitation or blockade at receptor level.**
   - For example, sweet taste enhances with little bit of salt, salty taste can be reduced by mixing with sour and sour taste decreases when taken with sugar.
   - Also, when a bitter stimulus is applied before any other tastants, the bitter taste lingers and dominates over other tastes.
8. **Effects of taste modifying substances:** A plant protein known as **miraculin** changes the taste of acids from sour to sweet.
   - **Gymnemic acid** when applied to the tongue abolishes the sensation of sweet, but does not affect other taste sensations.
9. **Effects of drugs:** Some drugs **containing sulfhydryl groups**, such as *captopril and penicillamine* tend to cause temporary loss of taste.
10. **Nutrient Deficiencies:** The preference for salty food arises in salt deficiency and calorie deficiency produces preference for sweet food.
11. **Culture and habit:** As the food habit is different in various cultures, the brought up and habit of a person also affects his taste.
12. **After-affects:** If *illness occurs following ingestion of a new food,* aversion develops toward that food. This may be due to structural and functional alterations in higher order and cortical neurons, a central phenomenon.

PY10.14

APPLIED PHYSIOLOGY

Abnormalities of Taste Sensations

Ageusia and Hypogeusia

Absence of the sense of taste is known as **ageusia**, and diminished taste sensitivity is known as **hypogeusia**. These conditions can occur due to the following causes:

- **Xerostomia** (dryness of mouth): Due to lack of salivary secretion, the chemicals in food are not dissolved in saliva and cannot reach the receptor cell. In Sjögren's syndrome, an autoimmune inflammatory disease, there is progressive loss of salivary glands.
- **Drugs** like captopril, cisplantin and penicillamine
- Tobacco use for a prolonged period
- Deficiency of vitamin B_3 or zinc
- **Damage to receptor cells** as occurs in old age or due to radiation therapy and herpes virus
- **Injury to gustatory pathway neurons**: Due to trauma or neoplasm, stroke, or systemic diseases like diabetes mellitus and hypothyroidism.

Selective Taste Blindness: Some persons show insensitivity to the taste of certain substance, whereas perception of other tastants remains unaltered. This is known as **selective taste blindness**. For example, some individuals do not perceive the taste of the bitter tasting chemical phenyl thiocarbamide, but the taste sensations of sweet, sour, salt and other bitter stimuli are normal. The condition is *inherited as an autosomal recessive* trait and may be due to lack of formation of a particular receptor protein.

Dysgeusia

Distorted sense of taste is known as **dysgeusia or parageusia**, in which the perception of taste is different from what is being presented (for e.g. a salty food may taste bitter), or there is perception of a taste without any tastants in the oral cavity (**hallucination of taste**). Dysgeusia is a feature of **temporal lobe epilepsy**.

Following adrenalectomy in man, there is an increased sensitivity to taste sensation.

Tests for Taste Sensation PY10.20

The tests are done by serial **application of different types of tastant solution** over the surface of a protruded tongue. The person is asked to indicate the type of taste perceived by showing a card and the tongue is thoroughly rinsed after application of each tastant solution.

Reflexes Associated with Taste

On arrival of the tastant molecules at the vicinity of the taste buds, there occurs *reflex stimulation of salivary secretion* sometimes called **taste-salivary reflex.** The afferent goes via the 7th, 9th, and 10th cranial nerves to the nucleus tractus solitarius, which project to the superior and inferior salivary nuclei of the facial and glossopharyngeal nerves. The efferent fibers from there innervate the salivary glands.

Presence of food in the mouth also stimulates gastric and pancreatic secretion by activating vagal efferent fibers, thereby prepares the alimentary tract for the digestion of the food if swallowed. These reflexes are the basis of the **conditioning reflexes** described by Pavlov and others.

Exam Questions

1. List the factors affecting taste sensation. With the help of a suitable diagram, trace the pathway for taste.
2. Draw a diagram of taste bud. Describe the mechanism of gustatory transduction.

Multiple Choice Questions

1. The taste buds are present in all of the following papillae, EXCEPT:
A. Foliate B. Cuneate
C. Circumvallate D. Fungiform

2. Which of the following is NOT true about gustatory receptor cell?
A. Is a modified epithelial cell
B. A taste bud contains 50-150 receptor cells
C. It is the primary afferent neuron
D. Has a life span of about 10 days

3. Umami taste sensation is produced by
A. Noradrenaline B. Glutamate
C. Glycine D. Acetylcholine

4. Which of the following mechanisms mediates bitter taste?
A. G protein B. Epithelial Na^+ channel
C. Guanylyl cyclase D. Tyrosine kinase

5. The taste buds carrying bitter taste sensation are situated in the following area of the tongue:
A. Sides B. At the tip
C. Behind the tip D. Posterior part

6. Salty taste is due to:
A. H+ channels B. G protein
C. Na+ channel D. Ca+2 channels

7. Which of the following are chemoreceptors?
A. Rods B. Cones
C. Taste buds D. Muscle spindle

8. Which of the following produces maximum sweet tase taste?
A. Monellin B. Glucose
C. Sucrose D. Saccharin

Answers:

1. B 2. C 3. B 4. A 5. D
6. C 7. C 8. A

Section XIII

Integrative Physiology

(Environmental Physiology, Exercise and Sports Physiology, Space Physiology, General Topics, Nutrition, Aging and Yoga)

"*What cannot be acquired or conquered during life*
can certainly not be done after death.
The physical life is the true field for progress and realization.

The Mother"
(of Sri Aurobindo Ashram, Pondicherry, INDIA)

Chapter 131

Structure and Functions of the Skin

Learning Objectives

On completion of study of this chapter:

The student will be able to (must know):

1. Name the layers of skin and cell types in each layer.
2. Name the glands of skin and give their distribution and functions.
3. Name the appendages of skin and give their functions.
4. List the functions of skin.

The student may also be able to (desirable to know):

1. Describe the structural organization and functions of skin.

FUNCTIONAL ANATOMY

As skin has many *secretory and synthetic functions*, it is also called as **an organ** of the body.

- As it covers the whole-body part, it is considered as the **largest organ** of the body.
- The total weight of the skin is about **3.5 kg**.

Layers of the Skin

The skin is divided into **two main layers**: epidermis and dermis.

Epidermis

The epidermis is formed by **stratified squamous epithelium**. It consists of **five layers** (Fig. 131.1). From superficial to deep, they are: stratum corneum, stratum lucidum, stratum granulosum, stratum spinosum, stratum germinativum (basale). There are ***no blood vessels in the epidermis***.

Stratum Corneum: Stratum corneum is *composed of dead cells containing keratin*.

1. Nuclei are almost absent in many cells.
2. They are continuously shed off from the skin.
3. It is particularly thick in palm and sole, where the skin is thicker than other parts of the body.

Stratum Lucidum: Stratum lucidum appears homogenous throughout.

1. It is composed of flattened cells that contain **eleidin**, a protein, which is the precursor of **keratin**.
2. These cells degenerate and migrate superficially to form the stratum corneum.

Stratum Granulosum: Stratum granulosum layer contains cells that are *rich in granules*.

1. The granules are formed by **keratohyaline**.
2. This layer consists of multiple layers of rhomboidal cells.

Stratum Spinosum: Stratum spinosum is formed by multiple layers of polyherdral cells, called prickle cells due to presence of spine-like processes on their surface.

1. These cells migrate towards the surface forming the three superficial layers to it, one after another.
2. **Langerhans cells** that participate in defence mechanism are present in this layer.

Stratum Germinativum: Stratum germinativum is the ***deepest layer of epidermis***.

1. This is also called **stratum basale**.
   - Cells are arranged in a single layer on a basement membrane. Active mitosis occurs in the cells of this layer and the cells gradually shift through the above four layers towards the surface.
2. **Melanocytes**, the cells that synthesize and secrete melanin are present in this layer of the skin. Melanocytes have **melanosomes and melanin granules** that are located mainly in the cytoplasmic or dendritic processes.
   - In melanocytes, tyrosinase converts tyrosine into 3,4-dihyroxyphynylalanine (**DOPA**), which is converted into melanin.
   - **Melanin** is stored in the vesicles in melanocytes.

Dermis

Dermis is the inner layer of the skin. Many glands, hair follicles and few smooth muscles along with fibroblasts and histiocytes are present in the dermis. Dermis is composed of **two layers**: a superficial papillary layer and a deep reticular layer.

Papillary Layer: The papillary layer is a compact layer that forms papillae. Papillae from this layer project into the epidermis. The papillae contain blood vessels, nerve endings and lymphatics.

Reticular Layer: The reticular layer consists of fat and loose areolar tissue impregnated with reticular and elastic fibers. This layer merges with the subcutaneous layer of fat and binds the skin with deeper structures.

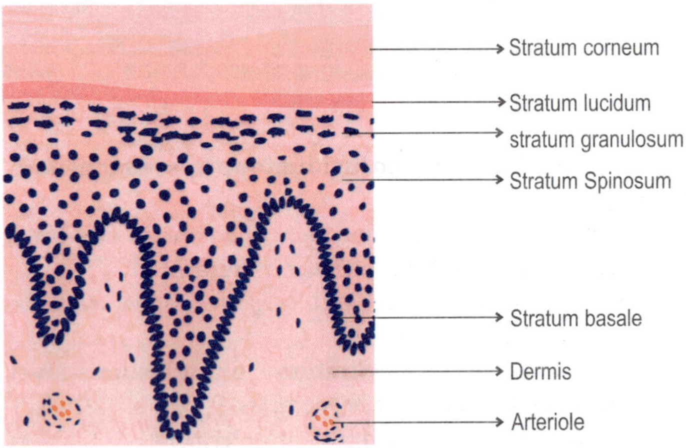

Fig. 131.1: Layers of the skin. Note, epidermis is formed by five layers. From superficial to deep, these are stratum corneum, stratum lucidum, stratum granulosum, stratum spinosum and stratum germinativum (basale).

Glands in the Skin

The glands in the skin are mainly the **sweat glands** and **sebaceous glands**.

Sweat Glands

Sweat glands are present all over the skin *except in ear drum*, lips and glans penis. They are of **two types**: merocrine and apocrine.

Merocrine Glands: The merocrine glands are known as eccrine glands. They are present in the skin all over the body.

- They are **simple tubular glands**. The tubules of the gland are very long and coiled.
- These are the sweat glands in the skin, and present in large number.
- Thus, sweat is formed mainly from the eccrine glands.

Apocrine Glands: The apocrine glands are present on mons pubis, axilla, circum-anal area and areola of breasts.

- The **ceruminous and mammary glands** belong to this category of cutaneous glands.
- The secretion from these glands starts after puberty and impart characteristic odor to the body.

Sebaceous Glands

Sebaceous glands are small pear-shaped alveolar glands (Fig. 131.2).

1. They open at the hair follicles or directly to the skin.
2. Obstruction of secretion from these glands is responsible for **acne formation**, which is seen at puberty due to increased activity of dehydroepiandrosterone.

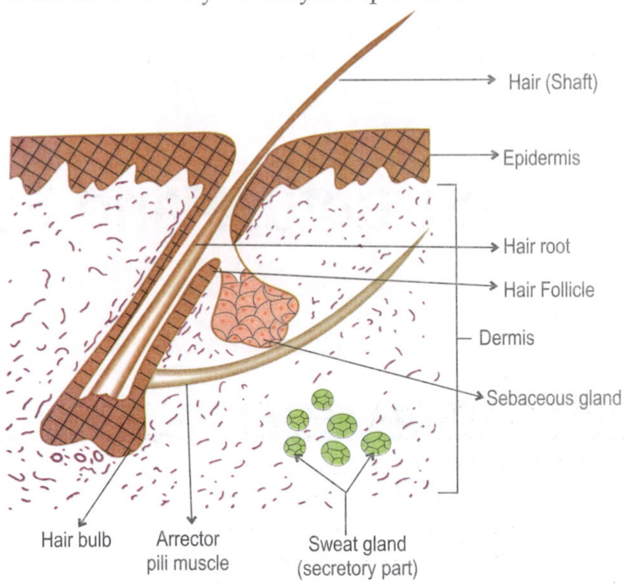

Fig. 131.2: Glands in the skin and structure of hair.

Skin Appendages

Skin appendages include **hairs and nails.**

Hairs

Different types of hairs are seen in fetus and in postnatal life. On the body of the fetus, the hairs are soft that are called **lanugo hairs**. After birth, **two types of hairs** are seen: vellous and terminal hairs.

Vellous Hairs: The vellous hairs are soft hairs found on the body of infants and children.

Terminal Hairs: The terminal hairs grow during puberty and replace the vellous hairs of childhood. However, vellous hairs persist on the face of adult females.

Hairs have root, shaft and follicle

Hair Follicle: The hair follicle consists of an epithelial root sheath, which is continuous with the stratum germinativum.

- The **arrector pilorum muscle** is attached to the follicle.
- Contraction of this muscle causes erection of hair during sympathetic stimulation. Sebaceous glands also open to the hair follicle.

Nails

Nails are modified skin at the tip of digits. Nail consists of a root, a body and the free margin. The root is continuous with the stratum germinativum layer of the epidermis.

- In fact, constant proliferation of cells from stratum

germinativum, continuous growth of nail occurs.

- These cells in the nail become flat and keratinized.

N.B: The innervation of skin and cutaneous circulation have been discussed in Chapter 39.

FUNCTIONS OF THE SKIN

1. **Body protection:** Skin is the outer covering that forms protective layer on the body. It provides ***mechanical protection against infection***. Therefore, *loss of skin in burns leads to severe sepsis*. Skin is also impervious to many substances in the air and water. Thus, the body is protected from toxic materials in the environment.
2. **Temperature regulation:** Secretion of sweat contributes significantly to temperature regulation. It causes *evaporation of water* from the skin. Skin also allows *insensible perspiration*, which helps in temperature regulation. **Sebum**, the secretion of sebaceous glands makes the skin greasy that prevent the skin from drying.
3. **Sensory organs:** There are many sensory receptors in the skin (**exteroceptors**) that help to collect information from the environment.
   - Hair follicles are rich in such receptors. Therefore, hairs are more sensitive sensory structures.
   - All types of receptors such as pain, touch, temperature, etc. are present in skin.
4. **Vitamin synthesis:** In exposure to sunlight, skin synthesizes 7-dehydrocholesterol, the precursor of vitamin D_3.
5. **Contributes to central blood volume:** Cutaneous vascular bed accommodates a good quantity of blood volume. Hence, ***constriction of blood vessels in the skin contributes to central blood reservoir***, from where blood can be diverted to vital organs at the time of need.
   - In circulatory shock, blood is diverted from cutaneous and splanchnic bed to cerebral and coronary circulations to perfusion of brain and heart respectively. This is achieved by **sympathetic vasoconstriction**, an immediate compensatory mechanism activated by shock.
   - Also, cutaneous vasoconstriction or dilation plays an important role in **temperature regulation** (for details, refer the next chapter).
6. **Water and electrolyte balance:** Sweat secreted from the skin contains water and salt. Hence, excessive sweating leads to dehydration and sodium deficiency.
   - Hormones like aldosterone affect water and electrolyte excretion from skin.
   - Sweat also acts as a medium for excretion of waste materials from the body.
7. **Protection from UV rays:** Skin protects the body against the damaging effects of ultraviolet (UV) rays of sunlight. Melanin pigment in the skin helps in this process.
8. **Immunity:** Skin plays a crucial role in nonspecific defence of the body. Sebum secreted from sebaceous glands is acidic and contains microbicidal agents.
   - Clasmatocytes in the skin are cells of mononuclear phagocyte system that trap and kill organism.
   - Skin is the **natural dressing of the body**. Therefore, loss of skin as occurs in burns or injury allows pathogenic bacteria to enter the body, which produces septicemia if uncontrolled.
9. **Route for drug administration:** Many lipid soluble drugs like steroids and fat-soluble vitamins are applied over the skin.
   - **Topical ointments** are applied on the skin as their absorption is poor from the skin, hence they **act locally**.
   - However, drugs are used as **subcutaneous implants** when their release into circulation is required at a lower rate over a period of months or years. Estrogen-progesterone contraceptive implants are examples.
10. **Diagnosis of diseases:** Apart from skin diseases, many diagnostic signs of systemic diseases are recorded from the skin surface.
    - For example, typical skin changes that occur in systemic lupus erythematosus.
    - **Degree of anemia, jaundice and cyanosis** are detected from skin and mucus membrane.
11. **Beauty of the Body:** The beauty of the body primarily depends on the health of the skin. Prettiness of an individual not only lies in his or her complexion and construction of the body, but also on the physical condition of the skin that makes the body surface shining and attractive. An unhealthy skin imparts poor appearance to the body, irrespective of its color. Therefore, health of the skin is the real wealth of the being.

Exam Questions

1. Describe the structure and functions of skin.
2. Describe the types of gland and hairs in the skin.

Chapter 132

Regulation of Body Temperature and Acclimatization to Hot and Cold Environments

Learning Objectives

<u>On completion of study of this chapter:</u>

The student will be able to (must know):

1. List the factors affecting body temperature.
2. List the mechanisms of heat generation and transfer, & preservation and heat loss from the body
3. Describe the mechanisms of regulation of body temperature.
4. Elucidate the role of hypothalamus in temperature regulation.
5. Enumerate the responses activated by exposure to heat and exposure to cold.
6. Outline the processes of acclimatization in hot and cold environment.
7. Understand the pathophysiology of fever and the effects of fever on the body.
8. Know the mechanisms of heat syncope, heat exhaustion and heat stroke.
9. List the major causes and effects of hypothermia.

The student may also be able to (desirable to know):

1. Describe the mechanisms of adaptation to hot and cold environments.
2. Explain the physiological basis of hyperthermia and hypothermia

PY11.1

TEMPERATURE REGULATION

In homeotherms, temperature regulating mechanisms **create an optimal internal environment** for smooth functioning of the body.

- In them, an effective **thermoregulatory system** prevents body from damaging consequences of pathological alterations in body temperature. Such a system works on the **principle of visceral reflex mechanisms.**
- Therefore, the **components of a temperature controlling system** consist of a general reflex mechanism, that includes: sensor (thermal sensor), afferent pathway, integrating center(s), efferent pathway and effector organs.
- The **effector organs** are skeletal muscle, skin and sweat glands that control heat mainly by generating and transferring heat from the body.

Factors Influencing Body Temperature

Normal Body Temperature & its Recording: The normal body temperature of an adult is approximately 37°C, which corresponds to 98.6°F. However, the temperature varies from 36.6°C to 37.2°C or 98°F to 99°F (Table 132.1).

1. Though, **axillary temperature** is recorded in clinics by using a clinical thermometer, it is ideal to record sublingually (**oral temperature**).
   - The temperature recorded ***from body surface*** is called **shell temperature**, which varies between 31°C to 34°C on different parts of the body and at different times.
   - Normally, axillary temperature is 0.5°C less than sublingual temperature.
   - In infants and children, rectal temperature is recorded.
2. The temperature recorded from ***inner body structures*** is called **core temperature**, which is about 37°C.
   - The core temperature is not easily affected by environmental conditions.
   - **Rectal, vaginal and esophageal recordings** of temperature represent *core temperature.*

Therefore, **oral temperature** recording is preferred clinically, which is more or less close to inner body temperature.

Table 132.1 | Normal and abnormal body temperatures.

	Centigrade	Fahrenheit
Normal	36.6 – 37.2°C	98 – 99°F
Subnormal	< 36.6 °C	< 98°F
Febrile (pyrexia)	> 37.2°C	99°F or more
Hyperpyrexia	> 41.6°C	> 107°F
Hypothermia	< 35°C	< 95°F

Body temperature is affected by **following factors**:

Time of the Day: In human beings, body temperature is maintained by a circadian 24-h cycle, known as body-temperature rhythm that varies approximately by 0.8°C.

1. The body temperature is usually **lowest in the early morning** between 3 to 6 a.m. and **maximum in the evening between 4 to 6 p.m.** (Fig. 131.1).
2. This circadian rhythmicity is an intrinsic mechanism and is independent of the sleep-wakefulness cycle.

State of Physical Activity: Increased physical activity generates excess heat by **increasing rate of metabolism.**

- Temperature is elevated during physical activity and remains elevated during recovery period. This increased body heat triggers appropriate heat-loss mechanisms.

Age: Newborns, infants and elderly people are less capable of maintaining body temperature especially in an altered state of environmental condition.

1. **Sweating and shivering are poorly developed in newborns.** Therefore, they fail to regulate body temperature and behave like a poikilotherm.
2. The *surface-to-mass ratio is also high in infant and children*, which render them susceptible to wide fluctuations in core temperature on exposure to extreme weathers.
3. **Elderly people** have decreased metabolic rate, reduced muscle mass, atrophied sweat gland, decreased cardiovascular reserve to dissipate heat and impaired ability to sense heat and cold.
   - Therefore, they are also subjected to greater fluctuations in core temperature on exposure to external challenges for their reduced ability to generate and dissipate heat.

Gender: In women during their reproductive life, under the influence of progesterone, body temperature **increases by about 0.5°C** following ovulation (in the **post-ovulatory phase** of the menstrual cycle). This is called rise in basal body temperature, which is an **indicator of ovulation.**

- Females are less influenced than males by external temperature due to the presence of more subcutaneous fat in them.

State of Sympathetic Activity: People with **higher basal sympathetic tone**, irrespective of other factors *have higher body temperature* due to increased catecholamines that increase body metabolism.

- Therefore, individuals with **sympathetic personality** have higher body temperature than parasympathetic personality.

Body Size: Heat generation and dissipation depend **on the ratio of body mass to body surface area.**

- Therefore, in smaller animals, body heat is more than in larger animals, and so also in human beings.

Type of Meal: Food rich in protein generates more heat due to **higher SDA (specific dynamic action) of proteins.**

- Animal **proteins produce more heat** than plant proteins.

Environmental Conditions: Environmental temperature and humidity and state of atmospheric circulation of air influence body temperature by altering evaporation of heat from the body.

Types of Clothing: Nature of clothing influences body temperature.

- Usually, **silken and linen clothing** increase body temperature by **preventing heat loss from the body.** *Cotton clothing has opposite effect*.
  - Therefore, generally it is advised to wear cotton dresses in summer and silk and linen dresses in winter.

Sleep: During sleep, body temperature is less due to central as well as peripheral mechanisms.

In sleep, **heat production is less** due to *decreased sympathetic and physical activities*, and also due to *decreased sensitivity of the thermostat*.

Emotion and Excitement: Emotional reactions and excitements increase body temperature.

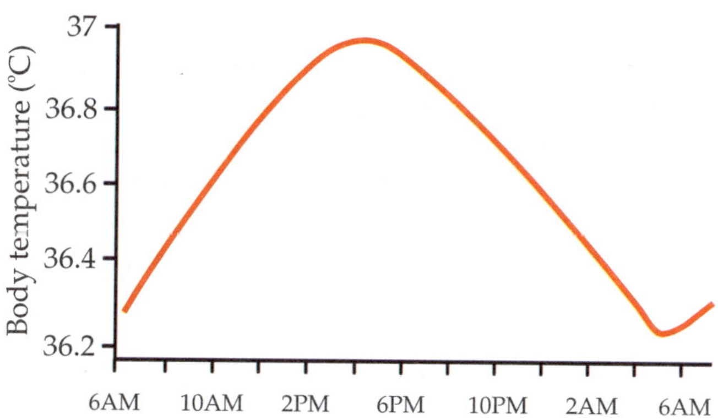

Fig. 132.1: Diurnal variation in body temperature.

Principles of Heat Generation & Transfer

Heat Generation

Rate of Heat Production: In normal individuals, rate of heat production varies between 80 kcal/h at rest to 600 kcal/h during exercise. This is intimately associated with the **rate of metabolism** that generates heat.

1. The **resting metabolic rate** (RMR) provides basal energy.
2. Any extra muscular activity such as walking adds to the overall metabolic heat production.
   - Increased process of digestion and absorption following a meal is the example of **state of increased metabolism.**
3. ***Many hormones*** such as thyroxine, norepinephrine, epinephrine and glucagon increase the rate of cellular metabolism.

Rate of Heat Generation: **In resting conditions,** body's energy requirement is low. Therefore, the rate of heat production is less, which is **about 80 kcal/h**.

1. Conversely, **during exercise,** the rate of heat generation is more, which is proportionate to the intensity of exercise.
   - This may be as high as ***600 kcal/h*** as occurs in severe exercise such as fast walking for about one hour.
2. The thermal load in physical exercise increases the core temperature of the body by about **1°C for every 10 minutes of exercise** if heat loss is not activated adequately.
3. Usually, the body increases the rate of heat dissipation to match its heat generation.

Heat Transfer

Heat transfer from the tissue to the circulating blood depends on **four factors**: the rate of energy production, the temperature of the tissue, temperature of the incoming blood to the tissue and the amount of blood flowing through the tissue.

1. The **rate of O_2 consumption** by the tissue is a *measure of metabolic rate of the tissue*. On average, 1.5 to 2 ml of O_2 per minute is consumed by one kg of muscle tissue.
   - The principal source of heat in the body is the **skeletal muscle**, which can increase its rate of heat production to more than 100-fold.
2. However, the remarkable increase in tissue temperature in exercise is **relatively short-lived** for following **two reasons**:
   - The increase in muscle temperature **reverses the temperature gradient** between muscle and the blood perfusing it. Therefore, after few minutes of exercise, **heat flows from muscle to blood**.
   - Dilation of blood vessel of skeletal muscle decreases vascular resistance in muscle. This, plus increased cardiac output **rapidly increase blood flow through the exercising muscle**, which is proportionate to the intensity of exercise. Blood flow increases upto 30-fold, which accounts for the major **transfer of heat from active muscle to blood**.

However, as exercise continues, muscle temperature increases to a ***new steady-state level***. This causes continuous transfer of more heat from exercising muscle to blood. Thus, it keeps increasing the core temperature of the body as warm venous blood leaves active muscles and enters the body core.

Transfer of Heat from Body Core to the Skin

The excess of heat carried away from active tissue to the blood, temporarily increases core temperature. Body prevents the core from overheating by transferring heat to the surface.

1. Heat is **transferred from core to the skin**, which is relatively cool. Skin is the largest organ in the body. Most of the heat generated in the body flows to the skin **by convection in the blood**. The blood flow to the skin can increase markedly due to **thermogenic vasodilation**.
2. Therefore, under physiological conditions, alteration in cutaneous blood flow is the primary determinant of heat flow from body core to body surface (skin). Hence, the *capacity to restrict blood flow to the body surface* is an **essential defense mechanism against cooling** of the body in hypothermia.
3. Similarly, the *ability to promote skin blood flow* is an **essential defense against hyperthermia**.
4. Some heat is also transferred from the body core by the evaporation of water from the respiratory tract, which is proportional to the **rate of pulmonary ventilation**.

Heat Loss from Skin to the Environment

Transfer of heat from skin to environment occurs by radiation, conduction, convection, and evaporation (see below).

Clothing Limits Heat Transfer: Clothing **insulates the body from environment** and impairs heat transfer between body core and the environment. However, *with light clothing, heat is also transferred* from a warmer body to a cooler environment by means of radiation, conduction, convection and evaporation that take place from the clothing surface rather than directly from the skin. Hence, *more clothing to cover larger area of skin and use of thicker clothing* are major ways of protecting body temperature in cold atmosphere.

Heat Balance

This is the balance between **heat preservation and heat dissipation**.

Heat Preservation

Preservation of heat in the body depends on **heat production** in the body and **heat gain** from the environment.

Mechanisms of Heat Production

At rest, heat production depends on **basal metabolic activity, muscular activity, specific dynamic action of food and nonshivering thermogenesis**.

Basal Metabolic Activity: The rate of **basal metabolism** is the major cause of heat production in the body. **In this process, food substrates are oxidized to produce energy.**

1. One gram of carbohydrate, protein and fat yield about 4, 4, and 9 calories respectively. Most of the metabolic energy is *converted into heat in the body*. This is called **metabolic heat**.

2. Though muscle and skin contribute to about 56% of body mass, their contribution to heat production is only 18% (Table 132.2).
3. However, **during physical exercise,** *90% of heat is produced by muscular activity*.

Table 132.2 | Body structures contributing to body mass and heat production at rest.

Structures	Contribution to % of body mass	Contribution to % of heat production
Trunk viscera	34	56
Brain	2	16
Muscle and skin	56	18*
Other structures	8	10

* Note that during physical exercise, 90% of heat production is contributed by muscle.

Muscular Activity: As noted above, enormous quantity of heat is produced by skeletal muscle during exercise.

1. However, also at rest, the basal muscular activity to some extent contributes to heat production. This is mainly by the *activity of respiratory muscle, cardiac muscle and basal tone of skeletal muscle*.
2. **On exposure to cold**, skeletal muscle activity increases that increases heat production by several fold. This is called **shivering thermogenesis**.

SDA of Food and Digestion of Food: During digestion and assimilation of food, the energy produced is converted into heat.

1. The metabolic rate and thus, the heat production increases by about 15% after a meal. This is called **specific dynamic action** (SDA) of food or **thermic effect of food**, which lasts for several hours after food intake.
2. SDA is **maximum for protein**. Therefore, ingestion of **protein-rich food has more thermic effect**.
3. The act of eating increases heat production due to increased muscular activity of chewing and swallowing.

Nonshivering Thermogenesis: Hormones such as **catecholamines and thyroxine** increase body metabolism.

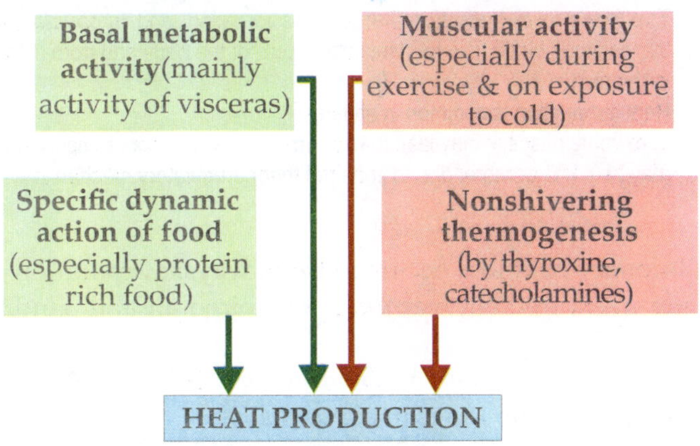

Fig. 132.2: Mechanisms of heat production in the body.

- Therefore, these hormones ***contribute to basal heat production***. This is called nonshivering thermogenesis. Excess secretion of these hormones increases body temperature (Fig. 132.2).

Mechanisms of Heat Gain from the Environment

Heat gain from environment occurs by **three mechanisms**: radiation, conduction and convection. Heat gain also occurs by means of ingestion and ventilation.

Radiation: Heat transfer by radiation occurs between the skin and solid bodies in the environment.

1. The body gains or loses heat by radiation at a rate that is *proportional to the temperature difference between the skin and the radiating body*.
2. **Solar radiation** (radiation directly from the sun) is the major source of human or animal body imbibing heat from the environment.

Conduction: Heat transfer by conduction occurs when the body touches a **solid material of different temperature.**

- For example, body lying on hot sand conducts heat from the sand.

Convection: Transfer of heat into the body ***from a hot fluid or air*** is called convection.

- For example, when body is immersed in warm or hot water, heat is conducted into the body.

Ingestion and Ventilation: Ingestion of hot food and drinks (tea, coffee) allows heat to enter the body. Breathing hot air from external environment as in hot climate, increases body temperature.

Heat Dissipation

Heat is lost from body through skin (**cutaneous heat loss**), lungs (**pulmonary heat loss**) and excretory organs (**excretory heat loss**). From skin, heat is dissipated into the atmosphere by means of radiation, conduction, convection and evaporation.

Cutaneous Heat Loss

From skin, heat is dissipated into the atmosphere by means of radiation, conduction, convection and evaporation.

Radiation: Heat transfer by radiation occurs between two objects having difference in their temperature. In winter, the radiant heat loss from the body to low radiant temperature of the environment accounts for substantial loss of heat from the body.

1. Radiation of heat from the body accounts for **about 50% of heat loss** from the body (Table 132.3) when the body is at rest in a neutral thermal indoor environment (the environment in which air temperature, air flow and humidity to the naked body does not lead to shivering or sweating).
2. The loss of heat by radiation increases with decreased environmental temperature.

Table 132.3 | Mechanisms of heat loss from the body.

Mechanism	Heat loss in calories	% loss
Radiation	1500	50
Conduction & convection	600	20
Evaporation - From Skin - Pulmonary Loss	690 210	20 7
Loss in inspired air	60	2
In feces and urine	30	1
Total	**3000**	**100**

Conduction: Conduction transfers heat from the body when the *body touches a solid material of different temperature.*

- For example, placing an ice pack on the body surface causes heat loss by conduction. However, clothing causes minimal heat loss.

Convection: Heat transfer by convection occurs *when body is exposed to a uid or air with temperature different from the body.*

- The convective heat loss is proportional to the difference between skin and ambient temperature. **Exposure to cold air or water** causes convective heat loss from the body (Application Box 132.1).

Application Box 132.1

Hypothermia killed people of Titanic disaster: When the body is immersed in water, heat exchange essentially occurs by convection. Immersion of body in chilled water leads to speedy loss of heat from the body leading to ***rapid hypothermia***. Therefore, it was believed that most of the deaths in the historic *Titanic shipwreck* disaster were due to hypothermia rather than drowning.

Evaporation: Dissipation of all of the extra heat during exercise can occur by evaporating sweat from the skin surface.

- The rate of evaporation does not depend on the temperature gradient, rather proportionate to the **water vapor–pressure gradient** between skin and environment.
- Evaporation from skin accounts for loss of about 600 cal (20% of heat) from the body. Evaporation occurs in two forms: **sweating and perspiration** (Fig. 132.3).

Sweating: Evaporation of 1 g of water from the skin removes about 0.6 kcal from the body.

- As the sweat glands of the body release about 30 g (approximately 30 ml) of fluid per minute or 2 liters/h to the skin surface, **evaporation can remove 18 kcal/min,** from the body.
  - Thus, almost all of the heat produced during severe exercise could be removed by evaporation under normal conditions by sweating.
  - However, the efficiency of heat transfer from the skin to the environment depends on many physiological and environmental factors such as humidity and skin temperature.
- **When humidity is high**, the water vapor-pressure gradient between skin and environment becomes low. This decreases evaporation and therefore, facilitates accumulation of excess heat produced during exercise. Hence, humidity impairs exercise performance.
- **When humidity is low**, as in desert conditions, heat loss by evaporation occurs easily, even in the presence of high ambient temperature.

Perspiration: Perspiration is **insensible water loss.** Diffusion of fluid from the body to epidermis occurs continuously, which is evaporated from the body surface, even in the absence of external sweating.

- This is called perspiration. It is not sensed by the body as sweating does not occur.
- It usually does not depend on external conditions (Application Box 132.2).
- It accounts for loss of about **400 kcal heat per day**.

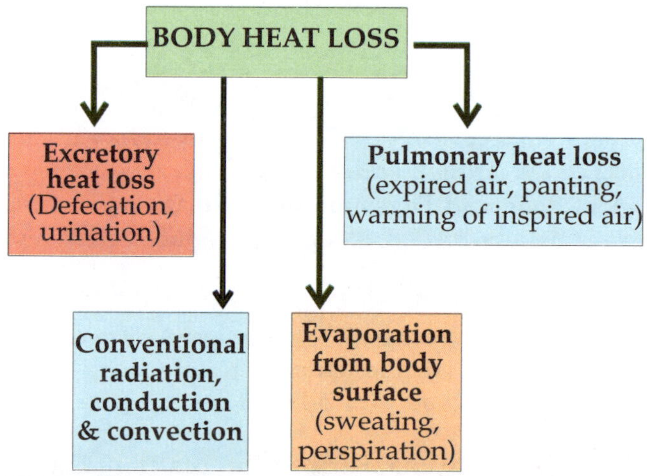

Fig. 132.3: Mechanisms of heat loss from the body.

Application Box 132.2

Heat exhaustion is common in athlete: In athlete, dissipating the thermal load is essential for prolonging exercise. A physiotherapist and a sports physician must understand these basic principles to treat thermal illnesses.

- In **heat exhaustion** as occurs in excessive heat exposure, core temperature may be as high as 39°C as body cannot dissipate the heat load.
- This leads to ***dehydration*** that reduces sweating, and ***hypovolemia*** that reduces blood flow from muscle to core of the body and from there to the skin.
- Heat exhaustion is common in athletes.
- In extreme cases, it may lead to **heat stroke**, in which core temperature may be 41°C or more, due to impaired thermoregulatory mechanisms.

Pulmonary Heat Loss

Pulmonary heat loss occurs in **three ways**: evaporation of water in expired air, warming of inspired air and panting (Fig. 132.3).

Evaporation of Water in Expired Air: About **300 ml of water** is lost from lungs in expired air.

- This is because **water is evaporated in expired air.** Also the expired air is warm and the **heat is lost in**

expired air.

- All these account for about loss of 200 kcal of heat. In animals, especially in dogs, it is the primary mechanism of heat loss.

Warming of Inspired Air: Air breathed in from atmosphere is cooler than the body temperature.

- Therefore, in the air passage warming of inspired air occurs. In this process, 2% of heat is lost from the body.

Panting: Panting is the **rapid and shallow breathing through the mouth cavity.**

- It is typically seen in **dog and few other mammals.** As mouth cavity is kept open in such breathing, evaporation of water increases from the mouth.
- Thus, heat is lost in this process. However, normally panting does not occur in humans.

Excretory Heat Loss

Any substance (fluid, semisolid or solid) lost from the body is warm.

- Stool coming out of large intestine and urine coming out of urinary tract are warm as they come out of the inner core of the body. In this process of removal of excretory products, heat is lost from the body.

Balance Between Production and Loss of Heat

Balance between heat loss and heat production, *keeps the core temperature constant*. Heat is mainly *produced by metabolism*.

1. Metabolic heat moves from the tissue to the core, then from core to the skin, and finally from skin to the environment.
2. **Increase in metabolism or interference of transfer of heat** at any part of this heat dissipation system leads to *increase in core temperature*.
3. When metabolic production of heat equals heat loss, the **heat storage is nil** and the core temperature is constant.
4. **Core temperature rises** when the *heat storage is positive*, as occurs in exercise, *prolonged immersion in warm water*, and *excessive heat exposure*.

REGULATION OF BODY TEMPERATURE

In human beings, body temperature is ***regulated by two systems***: behavioral thermoregulation and physiological thermoregulation. **PY11.8**

1. **The behavioral thermoregulation** requires conscious effort to regulate body temperature by changing the conditions of physical environment that includes modification of shelter, heating or cooling of the space by air-conditioning or other means, and by use of appropriate clothing etc.
2. **The physiological thermoregulation** uses various bodily mechanisms that precisely control body temperature though it fails to regulate over a wide range of environmental temperature.

Physiological Thermoregulation System: Physiologically, body temperature regulation occurs by a **feedback reflex system** that includes **temperature sensors** (thermoreceptors), **afferent pathway** that carry sensory information from thermoreceptors to the brain, a **hypothalamic control center**, **efferent pathway** that principally forms a part of the autonomic nervous system, and **thermal effector organs** that either control heat transfer of heat between the body and environment or regulate the heat production in the body.

Thermal Sensors

Thermal sensors are **thermoreceptors** that are located in ***two crucial structures*** in the body: the **skin and the hypothalamus.**

Cutaneous Thermoreceptors

The cutaneous thermoreceptors are present in the skin and mucus membrane. Few thermoreceptors are also located in visceral organs. They sense change in ambient temperature.

There are **two distinct thermoreceptors**: warmth and cold receptors.

Warmth Receptors: Warmth receptors constitute only about **10% of thermoreceptors.**

- They are stimulated at higher temperature.
- When local temperature increases to 44–46°C, warmth receptors increase their firing rate steadily.

Cold Receptors: About **90% of thermoreceptors** in skin are cold receptors.

- They typically increase their firing rate when local temperature decreases from approximately 40°C to 24°C.

Receptor Responses

Two **types of receptor responses** are observed in thermoreceptors: **static and dynamic**.

- When temperature change is sustained, a stable change occurs in the sensor's firing rate. This is called **tonic or static response**.
- When change in temperature is a temporary one, the response of thermoreceptors becomes **phasic or dynamic**.

Cutaneous sensors provide information about immediate change in ambient temperature to hypothalamic thermoregulatory center.

Hypothalamic Thermoreceptors

Hypothalamus plays an important role in temperature regulation. About **10% of hypothalamic neurons** exhibit an increased activity in response to change in local temperature.

- Hypothalamic thermoreceptors play a crucial role in conditions in which **rate of heat production and dissipation changes dramatically** as happens during exercise.
- Failure on the part of hypothalamus to detect such changes and mediate such responses **leads to rapid alteration in core temperature** resulting in grievous consequences.
- In hypothalamus, unlike that in the skin, **warmth receptors greatly outnumber cold receptors**.

Hypothalamic Temperature Regulating Neurons

Hypothalamic neurons that are involved in regulation of body temperature are broadly divided into **three categories**: sensor neurons, heat-loss neurons and heat production neurons.

Sensor Neurons: These are hypothalamic thermoreceptors that are located in **anterior hypothalamus**.

- As described above, warmth sensitive cells are more than the cold sensitive cells.
- They collect information about temperature from both peripheral and central thermoreceptors.

Heat-loss Neurons: Neurons that on activation induce loss of heat are located in **anterior hypothalamus.**

- Therefore, **anterior hypothalamus** is called heat loss center.
  - On stimulation, this center produces **vasodilation and sweating** that promote heat loss.
  - **Lesion of this center produces hyperthermia**, especially on exposure to hot environment.
- **Preoptic area** is also classified under heat loss center.

Heat-production Neurons: The neurons that on activation activate mechanisms that prevent loss of heat and produce internal heat are located in **posterior hypothalamus.**

- Therefore, posterior hypothalamus is called **heat production center**.
  - On activation, it produces **cutaneous vasoconstriction and shivering** that increase body temperature.
- **Lesion of this center leads to hypothermia**, especially on exposure to cold environment.

Role of Hypothalamic Centers

Change in the temperature of the environment close to the skin alters both the **tonic and the phasic components** of thermoreceptor activity.

1. The impulses generated in cutaneous thermoreceptors **ascend up in the sensory pathway** in the spinal cord.
   - **Through collaterals** from the ascending pathways information reach hypothalamus.
2. **Hypothalamus integrates thermal information** received from skin and from other parts of the body including the hypothalamus.
3. Hypothalamus, compares the prevailing thermal situation with the standardized set of thermal condition of the body, and accordingly **directs appropriate command signal** in the efferent pathway to alter the rate of the heat transfer from the body by either generating and preserving the heat, or by dissipating the heat.
   - For its major role in regulation of body temperature, hypothalamus is designated as **THERMOSTAT** of the body.
4. The **thermosensitivity of hypothalamus** is 8 – 10 times greater the thermosensitivity of skin.

Nature of Responses

The responses are both **reflexive and feedback** in nature. Reflex responses occur mostly to cutaneous receptor stimulation and feedback responses occur mostly to change in core temperature.

Reflex Responses: The cutaneous sensors provide information about ambient temperature that affects rate of body's heat transfer.

- These are the reflex responses to change in skin temperature, which may be **anticipatory in nature.**

Feedback Responses: Thermoregulatory responses to changes in internal body temperature, as occur during exercise, are mainly **negative feedback** in nature.

- These effects modify the rate of heat transfer that restores the core temperature to normal level.
- They **minimize change in core temperature** and consequent changes in metabolic activity.

Mechanism of Hypothalamic Integration

The major effector mechanisms for temperature regulation are located in hypothalamus. This hypothalamic thermostat has a **set point for body temperature**.

1. The set point is set with a narrow range of temperature with average set temperature of 98.6°F or 37°C.
2. Any deviation from this set temperature is received by the thermostat as an **error signal**.
3. Thermal error signal influences hypothalamic integration centers to generate appropriate **thermal effector signals** (Fig. 132.4).

Role of Hypothalamic Centers

Responses activated by thermal effector signals are mediated by various **autonomic, somatic and endocrine mechanisms.** The target effector organs mainly include

cutaneous blood vessels, sweat glands and skeletal muscles.

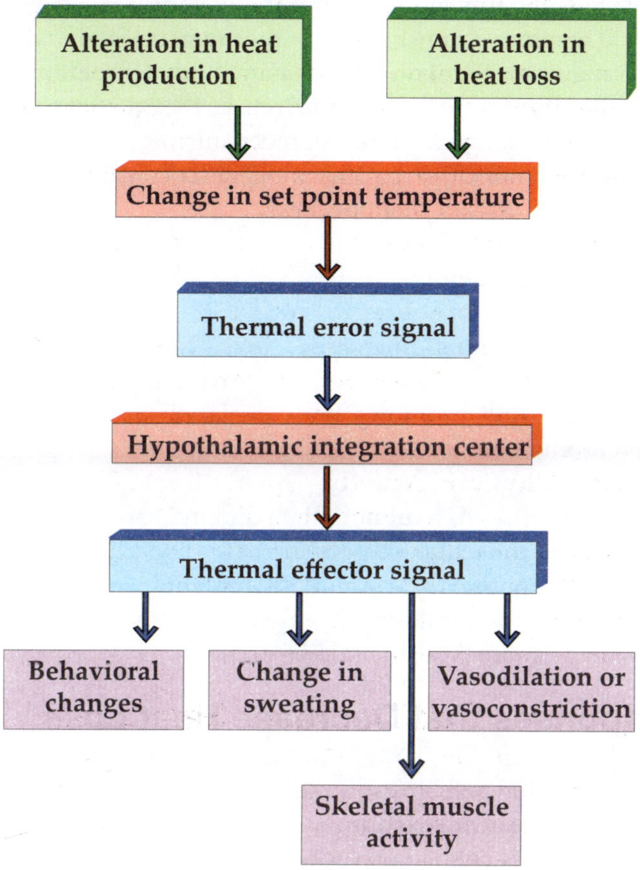

Fig. 132.4: Mechanism of hypothalamic integration following change in set point temperature.

These responses may be broadly grouped into **two categories**: responses activated by heat and responses activated by cold (Table 132.4).

Table 132.4 | Responses activated by change in temperature.

A. Responses activated on exposure to heat
1. Responses that promote heat loss
- Cutaneous vasodilation
- Sweating
- Increased respiration or panting
2. Responses that reduce heat production
- Decreased appetite
- Decreased physical activity
B. Responses activated on exposure to cold
1. Responses that promote heat gain
- Shivering (shivering thermogenesis)
- Increased physical activity
- Increased secretion of catecholamines (nonshivering thermogenesis)
- Increased appetite
2. Responses that decrease heat loss
- Cutaneous vasoconstriction
- Change in body's attitude
- Piloerection

Responses Activated by Heat

On exposure to hot environment, body temperature increases. Body tries to reduce its temperature by activating the **mechanisms that promote heat loss** and the **mechanisms that reduce heat production**.

Responses that Promote Heat Loss

Three major responses promote heat loss from the body: cutaneous vasodilation, sweating and increased breathing.

Cutaneous Vasodilation

On exposure to heat, the major mechanism activated for heat dissipation is cutaneous vasodilation.

- Skin blood flow ***increases upto ten-fold*** above the resting level. By increasing flow of blood from deeper parts of the body to the skin (the body surface), core heat is transferred to the surface.
    - This is called **heat flow**.
- Heat flow to the skin is the ***primary mechanism of heat dissipation*** to the environment.

Thus, by adjusting the caliber of cutaneous arterioles, body facilitates blood flow, and therefore heat flow, from the core to the skin surface, the principal site of heat dissipation.

Mechanisms: Cutaneous blood flow is controlled by sympathetic nervous system.

- Active vasodilation in cutaneous vascular bed is achieved by sympathetic inhibition (**neural vasodilation**).
- Impulses from heat-loss center of hypothalamus inhibit sympathetic discharge to the cutaneous blood vessels.
- Vasodilation also occurs due to locally released kinins from sweat glands (**chemical vasodilation**) and direct effect of heat on blood vessel (**thermogenic vasodilation**).

Sweating

In moderate heat load, the primary mechanism of heat transfer is by increasing cutaneous blood flow.

- **When heat load is adequately large**, the autonomic response activates the eccrine sweat glands to secrete sweat onto the skin surface.
    - This promotes evaporation from skin surface that facilitates heat loss.
- The secretory segment of the sweat gland is innervated by cholinergic sympathetic fibers.
    - The **activity of sympathetic fibers** to sweat gland is increased by hypothalamic drive.
- Sweating is almost nil in cold weather, which may **reach 700 ml/h or more** in a very hot weather.
    - Associated loss of salt from the body causes **sodium depletion** (Application Box 132.3).

Increased Respiration

In hot weather, respiration is stimulated. Normally, in the process of breathing, hot air comes out of the lung that removes body heat to the environment.

- Respiratory stimulation occurs due to both **sympathetic and thermogenic activation**.
    - Therefore, expired air is felt warmer than the atmospheric air.
- **Panting** as occurs in animals like dogs also facilitates heat loss from the oral cavity.

Application Box 132.3

Sweating causes salt and water loss: Though concentration of salt is variable in sweat, sweat is always hypotonic to plasma. Therefore, **sweating always increases osmolality of plasma**. The NaCl concentration remains high following sweating until the lost water is replaced. The **hepernatremic dehydration** predisposes to heatstroke (see below).

Responses that Reduce Heat Production

Heat production is reduced by **loss of appetite** and **reduced physical activity**.

Decreased Appetite: In a hot environment, **anorexia** develops.

- Decreased food intake decreases the amount of heat produced by metabolism and SDA of food.

Decreased Physical Activity: In extreme hot weather, physical activities are reduced. The individual loses interest to work and develops **lethargy**.

- Decreased muscular activity decreases heat production.

Responses Activated by Cold

On exposure to cold environment, body temperature decreases. Body tries to elevate its temperature by activating the mechanisms **that promote heat gain**. Heat is gained by processes that *promote heat production* and the processes *that reduce heat loss*.

Responses that Promote Heat Production

Heat generation is increased by shivering and nonshivering thermogenesis, increased physical activity and increased intakes.

Shivering Thermogenesis: On immediate exposure to cold, shivering is initiated in responses to impulses from posterior hypothalamus.

- Shivering is an immediate thermogenic mechanism in severe cold. Shivering is involuntary **rhythmic contractions of skeletal muscle**.
- It increases metabolic rate by three to four times of that of basal level.

Nonshivering Thermogenesis: Increased *cellular metabolism associated with uncoupling of oxidative phosphorylation* increases body temperature. This is called nonshivering thermogenesis or **chemical thermogenesis**.

1. This occurs mainly due to **secretion of catecholamines** in response to sympathetic stimulation.
2. The quantity of **brown fat** in the body determines the level of chemical thermogenesis. This is because the cells of brown fat are ***rich in mitochondria*** that carry out uncoupled oxidation.
    - Also, brown fat has ***rich sympathetic innervation***.
    - In infants and children, brown fat is present in considerably large amount than in adults.
    - Therefore, nonshivering thermogenesis **is the major mechanism of increasing body temperature in infants and young children**, as they do not have well developed shivering mechanism.
3. **In adults,** nonshivering thermogenesis contributes to about only ***10% of thermogenesis***.
4. Chemical thermogenesis also occurs due to **increased thyroxine secretion**.
    - In chronic exposure to cold, TSH secretion from hypothalamus increases that causes thyroid hyperplasia and increased thyroxine secretion.
    - **Thyroxine** promotes body metabolism and heat production.

Increased Physical Activity: Apart from shivering, physical activities like rubbing the palm increase in cold.

- **Increased muscular activity** increases body heat.

Increased Appetite: Cold stimulates appetite.

- **Increased food intake** increases heat production by increasing metabolism and SDA of food.

Responses that Decrease Heat Loss

Heat loss from the body is decreased by cutaneous vasoconstriction, piloerection and change in body posture.

Cutaneous Vasoconstriction: The immediate response to cold exposure is cutaneous vasoconstriction.

1. Cutaneous vasoconstriction is mediated by **sympathetic nerves in response to discharge from posterior hypothalamus**.
2. Vasoconstriction in skin elicits reduction in cutaneous blood flow to about half the resting rate of cutaneous blood flow.

Change in Body's Attitude: In severe cold, body flexes maximally (**curling up of the body**), especially in sleep and in lying posture. This reduces the surface area of the body for heat loss.

Piloerection: Cold induces contraction of piloerector muscle at the hair root that causes piloerection.

1. The skin becomes like **goose skin** and *entraps a layer of air* in the hairs.
2. This acts as an insulator and reduces the transfer of heat from the body.

Role of Training

Temperature regulation occurs by **two drives**: cutaneous drive and hypothalamic drive.

1. **Cutaneous drive** is the skin blood flow and other factors like sweating modulate effector response in response to change in core temperature.
2. Core temperature changes the sensitivity of hypothalamus, the **hypothalamic drive**.

Interaction between two drives: Cutaneous drive is controlled by the hypothalamic drive. Under normal conditions, peripheral responses increase linearly with an increase in hypothalamic drive.

- **Increase in skin temperature** has **two effects**: shifts the temperature threshold downward, and increases the sensitivity of the peripheral response to particular level of hypothalamic drive. Training produces similar effects in an athlete, i.e., **increases heat loss for a given hypothalamic drive**.
- **When skin temperature is lowered**, the temperature threshold is shifted upward and ***sensitivity of peripheral responses to hypothalamic drive is also decreased***. Dehydration that limits the ability to sweat has similar effects.

ACCLIMATIZATION TO TEMPERATURE CHANGES IN ENVIRONMENT

PY11.2

Heat Acclimatization

Physiological changes that occur due to *prolonged or repeated exposure to a particular stressful environment* are called acclimatization.

Systemic Changes

Acclimatization responses include cardiovascular changes, and changes in sweating, body temperature and fluid and electrolyte balance.

Cardiovascular Adaptations

Cardiovascular change is mainly the **reduction in heart rate**. The reduction in heart rate occurs to the extent that maintains minimum level of activity. Usually, this occurs within a week's time.

Changes in Sweating

Changes in sweating occur more slowly. The *core temperature threshold for sweating is reduced*. Therefore, sweating occurs earlier and at a lower core temperature.

1. **Sweating rate becomes high** for a given level of core temperature as sensitivity of sweat glands increases to cholinergic stimulation.
2. Thus, sweat rate becomes high and the higher sweat rate remains for sustained period.

Changes in Core and Skin Temperatures

The changes in sweating reduce the level of core and skin temperature during exercise.

1. This enables the individual to **perform exercise for a longer duration**.
2. The *core temperature threshold for cutaneous vasodilation and sweating is reduced*, which maintains adequate transfer of heat from the body core to the skin.

Changes in Fluid and Electrolyte Balance

After the initial acute water and sodium loss due to profuse sweating, the plasma volume is restored, which then slowly increases. However, after one or two week's time, the volume change disappears.

1. Sweat **glands conserve sodium** by secreting sweat with less sodium. All these effects are mediated through **increased aldosterone secretion**, which occurs due to initial hyponatremia.
2. Sweat gland response to aldosterone is slower than the response of kidney, and *aldosterone escape phenomenon as seen in kidney tubule does not occur in sweat glands*.
3. Thus, sweat glands **keep on preserving body sodium** substantially till acclimatization continues. In unacclimatized person, continuation of excess sweating results in water and electrolyte loss.

Consequence of Heat Acclimatization

The major consequence of heat acclimatization is due to the **persistence of sodium-retaining property of sweat glands**.

1. Therefore, **sweat contains less salt** irrespective of its amount secreted. Hence, loss of a given volume of sweat *does not result in proportionate loss in salt from the body*.
2. This leads to **smaller decreases in ECF volume** for a particular volume of sweat loss.
3. However, effects of heat acclimatization *vanish rapidly* when the individual is lastingly shifted from the hot environment or when he is not exposed to such environments repeatedly.

Cold Acclimatization

The cold acclimatization depends on the nature, degree and duration of the cold exposure. The changes mainly occur in blood vessels, metabolism and tissue temperature.

Cardiovascular Changes

Two important changes that occur on exposure to severe cold for a longer duration are **cold induced vasodilation and the Lewis-Hunting response.**

Cold-induced Vasodilation

When skin temperature is below 15°C for a longer duration, cold-induced vasodilation occurs, which increases cutaneous blood flow.

- This is observed **mainly in areas rich in arteriovenous anastomoses** as in hands and feet.
- The mechanism of this vasodilation is not exactly known, but it may be due to the *inhibitory effect of cold on the vascular smooth muscle*.

- The degree of vasodilation response is not adequate in individuals who have less experience of previous exposures to cold.

Lewis-Hunting Response

On repeated exposure to cold, cold-induced vasodilation begins early and the degree of response becomes more. This produces greater cutaneous blood flow.

- In addition, **vasoconstriction alternating with vasodilation** occurs in succession.
- This **rhythmic pattern of vasoconstriction-vasodilation** resulting in ***decreased and increased blood flow*** is called the Lewis-Hunting response.
  - It is typically seen in individuals those who **regularly dip their body parts in cold water** like fishermen working in rivers in winter season.
- This response that intermittently increases blood flow to the part **protects the part from cold injury**.

Metabolic Changes

Though, generally it is believed that human beings acclimatize to cold environment by *increasing their metabolic rate*, reports of experimental studies in humans and animals do not reveal such findings.

1. Instead, reports indicate that on chronic cold exposure, additional decrease occurs in core temperature and also a fall is seen in temperature threshold for shivering, and a **decline in metabolic response**.
2. These changes are **aimed at preserving metabolic energy**, which may be helpful during prolonged stay in a cold environment.

Decreased Heat Conductance

The conductance of heat from inner core of the body to skin surface is lowered in repeated exposure to cold.

- This causes **tissue insulation** in cold acclimatization.
  - This is another factor that *contributes to decresed metabolic response* in cold acclimatization.
- The increased tissue insulation is *not related to the degree of subcutaneous fat* as it is also seen in very lean subjects.
- The exact mechanism of tissue insulation is not known, but, it may be due to **enhanced countercurrent heat exchange** in the acclimatized subjects.

APPLIED PHYSIOLOGY

PY11.3

Fever

Fever or **pyrexia** is the increase in body temperature above normal range. It is the common feature of most of the diseases that occur due to infection and inflammation. .

Pathogenesis of Fever: Toxins released from infecting organism or traumatized tissue stimulate the inflammatory cells like monocytes and macrophages to release cytokines, **the endogenous pyrogens.**

1. Cytokines act on organum vasculosum of lamina terminalis (OVLT) which in turn stimulate preoptic area to **increase the local production of prostaglandins especially prostaglandin E_2 (PGE_2).**
2. There are **four types of prostaglandin receptors** in hypothalamus: **EP_1, EP_2, EP_3 and EP_4. EP_3** mainly mediates the effects of PGE_2.
   - PGE_2 alters the firing rate of the central thermoregulatory controller, raising the thermostat set point (Flowchart 132.1).

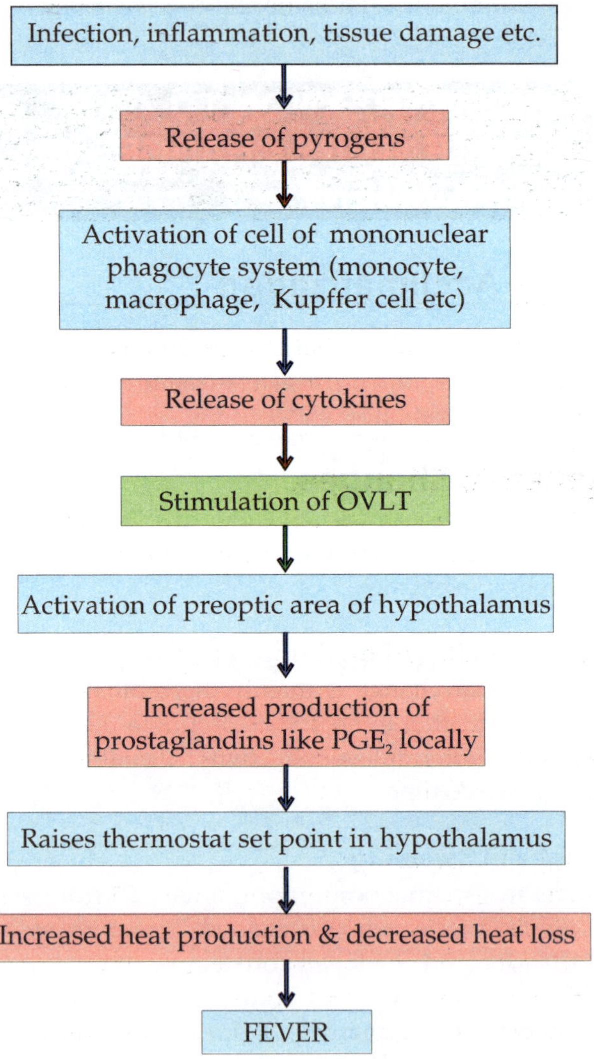

Flowchart 132.1: Mechanism of genesis of fever.

3. Raised hypothalamic set point **activates the mechanisms that stimulate heat production and inhibit heat loss** (Clinical Note 132.1).

Effects of Fever: Fever is considered as **the defence mechanism of the body against the disease.** It eliminates the disease process by following mechanisms:

1. Fever **kills the organism** by its thermogenic effects. For

example, high fever in malaria kills malarial parasites. Also, fever is bacteriostatic.

2. Fever *induces enzymatic activity* that in turn kills the invading organism.
3. Fever *enhances production of antibodies* that kill the microorganisms.

IMPORTANT NOTE

Fever causes negative nitrogen balance: Fever for a longer duration is harmful to the body as it produces **negative nitrogen balance and alkalosis**. Very high pyrexia causes unconsciousness by suppressing brain centers.

Clinical Note 132.1

PG E_2 inhibitors reduce fever: Endogenous pyrogens produce fever by increasing the local synthesis and release of prostaglandin E_2 in hypothalamus. Therefore, aspirin and many other nonsteroidal anti-inflammatory drugs decrease body temperature by inhibiting hypothalamic production of prostaglandins.

Conditions of Heat Stress

Heat stress is the condition of **excessive hyperthermia** in which impact of heat on the body becomes acute and severe. It commonly occurs in **extremely hot and humid weather**. Loose clothing helps in preventing heat stress.

IMPORTANT NOTE

Loose clothing protects from radiative hyperthermia: The most effective protection against radiative hyperthermia is **to cover the skin with loose white clothing**, which *screens the radiation of heat* from the environment and at the same time *allows movement of air underneath the clothing* that maintains loss of heat by evaporation and convection.

The **common forms** of heat stress are: heat syncope, heat exhaustion and heat stroke.

Heat Syncope

Heat syncope is a **state of circulatory failure that occurs due to excessive heat**.

- The **major pathophysiologic dysfunction** is due to ***venous pooling of blood*** that decreases venous return.
  - **Venodilation** occurs as a compensatory increase in skin blood flow in prolonged exposure to heat.
  - The consequent *decrease in end-diastolic volume* **lowers cardiac output and blood pressure**.
- **In severe form**, it may cause loss of consciousness.
- As thermoregulatory mechanisms are intact, usually **core temperature is not raised**.
  - Skin mostly remains wet and cool.
- In addition to transferring patient from hot environment immediately, **treatment aims at improving the diastolic filling** of the heart.

Heat Exhaustion

Heat exhaustion is a common condition of heat stress. It occurs due to **imbalance in cardiovascular homeostasis in a hot environment**. This is also called **heat collapse**.

1. Collapse is usually *precipitated during exercise*.
2. **Decreased diastolic filling** of ventricle is the primary pathophysiologic mechanism of heat exhaustion.
3. However, exact mechanism of decreased venous return is not known, though **hypovolemia** is proposed to be the major contributing factor.
4. Hypotension activates baroreceptors reflex and therefore prevents fainting.

Features: Features of heat exhaustion include nausea, vomiting, tachycardia, weakness, confusion, headache, ataxia and vertigo. The patient *sweats profusely*. In severe cases, dilation of pupil may develop and patient may faint.

Treatment: The **fluid replacement and rest** usually improve the condition. ***Salt intake*** helps.

Though, usually body temperature is normal or slightly elevated in heat exhaustion, hyperthermia and dehydration frequently lead to heatstroke. Hence, it is better to **keep the patient in a cool environment**.

Heat Stroke

Heat stroke is the *most perilous disorder* of heat stress. It is characterized by **high core temperature, neurological deficits** and loss of consciousness. **Convulsion** is the frequent association.

There are **two forms of heatstroke**: classical and exertional.

1. For **classical heatstroke**, the major cause is a ***very high environmental heat*** that supersedes thermoregulatory mechanisms of the body.
2. For **exertional heatstroke**, the major cause is ***accelerated production of metabolic heat***. Usually, exertion in a high ambient temperature predisposes to heatstroke.

The exact **pathophysiologic mechanism** of heatstroke is not known. Though **hyperthermia** is the major culprit, ***state of physical exercise*** is an important contributor. A *triggering factor* could be **release of endotoxin from bacterial flora** which may occur due to intestinal ischemia that allows the toxins to enter circulation and activate inflammatory responses.

Treatment Should be Prompt: Damage to kidney, liver and skeletal muscle are usual **complications**. In heatstroke, patient rapidly becomes comatose. The skin is dry and body temperature is usually above 106°F. In fact, it is a **medical emergency** and requires prompt treatment.

1. **Immediate therapy** includes **rapid reduction in body temperature**, which is effectively accomplished by immersion of the body in cold water.
2. Prompt hydration and maintenance of a patent airway prevents complications to develop.

Malignant Hyperthermia

Malignant hyperthermia is a rare condition of **very high increase in body temperature** that usually occurs on **exposure to anesthetics or depolarizing neuromuscular blockers**.

- Halothane anesthesia is known to cause in susceptible individuals.
- There is a genetic predisposition.
- The **plasma calcium concentration rises abnormally** that severely *activates myosin ATPase activity*.
- The consequent hyperactivity and hypermetabolic processes rapidly increase core temperature.

Treatment is by immediate use of **dantrolene sodium** that decreases the release of calcium from the sarcoplasmic reticulum.

Hypothermia

The common cause of hypothermia is **prolonged exposure to severely cold environment** or prolonged **immersion in cold water**.

- Hypothermia occurs **earlier and in more severe form in cold water** than in cold air.
  - Hypothermia in infants and elderly people is severe than in adults.
- **A thick layer of insulating fat decreases loss of heat** to the water.
  - Therefore, **swimmers in cold water apply a thick layer of grease** on the skin surface before swimming.

When body temperature is **less than 25°C**, ill effects of hypothermia develop. Decreased body metabolism, enzymatic activity, slowing of heart and respiration, and slowing reflex activities are features of hypothermia. If very severe, loss of consciousness occurs, which may further lead to death.

Exam Questions

1. Describe the mechanism of regulation of body temperature.
2. List factors that affect body temperature. Describe the mechanisms of heat generation and transfer and mechanisms of heat dissipation.
3. Describe the role of hypothalamus in temperature regulation. Add a note on malignant hyperthermia.
4. Describe the mechanisms of heat acclimatization and cold acclimatization. Add a note on heat stroke.

Multiple Choice Questions

1. Hyperthermia is a state in which:
A. Temperature >41.5°C
B. > 40°C with autonomic dysfunction
C. No change in hypothalamic thermostat
D. One which normalizes with antipyretic

2. Lesion of preoptic nucleus of hypothalamus causes:
A. Hyperphagia B. Hyperdipsia
C. Hyperthermia D. Hyperglycemia

3. Sweating, a result of exertion, is mediated through:
A. Adrenal hormone
B. Sympathetic cholinergic
C. Sympathetic adrenergic
D. Parasympathetic cholinergic

4. Heat loss from the body depends mostly on:
A. Thermoregulatory center
B. Warming of air during inspiration
C. On the environmental temperature
D. Radiation and evaporation

5. The first physiological response to high environmental temperature is:
A. Sweating
B. Vasodilatation
C. Decreased heat production
D. Decreased nonshivering thermogenesis

6. Under physiological conditions, heat acclimatization is accomplished by all, EXCEPT:
A. Decreased renal blood flow
B. Increased urine sodium
C. Increased aldosterone secretion
D. Excessive sweating

7. Nonshivering thermogenesis in adults is due to:
A. Thyroid hormone
B. Brown fat between the shoulders
C. Noradrenaline secretion
D. Muscle metabolism

8. Nonshivering thermogenesis is mediated by:
A. α1 receptor B. β2 receptor
C. β3 adrenergic receptor and UCP-1 D. UCP-2

9. All the following can occur in a neonate for heat production, EXCEPT:
A. Shivering
B. Breakdown of brown fat with adrenaline secretion
C. Universal flexion like a fetus
D. Cutaneous vasoconstriction

10. The hormone associated with cold adaption is:
A. Growth hormone B. Thyroxine
C. Insulin D. Melanocyte-stimulating hormone

11. Which of the following sites does not contain brown adipose tissues?
A. Scapula B. Subcutaneous tissue
C. Around blood vessel D. Around adrenal cortex

Answers

1. C 2. C 3. B 4. C 5. B 6. B 7. C 8. C 9. A 10. B 11. B

Chapter 133

Physiology of Exercise and Sports Science

Learning Objectives

On completion of study of this chapter:

The student will be able to (must know):

1. List the differences between isotonic and isometric exercises, and their benefits.
2. Classify the degrees of exercise based on heart rate, oxygen consumption and work done.
3. List the factors affecting exercise and explain the mechanisms of fatigue in exercise.
4. List the energy sources in exercise.
5. Define VO2max and name the factors that affect VO2max.
6. Define anerobic threshold and briefly explain its importance.
7. Describe the respiratory changes in exercise.
8. Draw a schematic diagram depicting CV changes in mild, moderate and severe exercise.
9. Describe the cardiovascular changes in exercise.
10. Appreciate the importance of aerobic training, and list the advantages of training.

The student may also be able to (desirable to know):

1. Describe the physiological mechanisms and changes in exercise.

Types of Exercises

Physiological changes during exercise depend on the type of exercise. Exercises have traditionally been classified into **two categories**: isotonic and isometric.

Isotonic Exercise: Exercise that involves isotonic muscle contraction is categorized as isotonic exercise.

- In isotonic muscle contraction, muscle length changes; therefore, the ***external work is done***. Hence, this is also called **dynamic exercise**.
- Walking, jumping and jogging are the examples of isotonic exercises.

Isometric Exercise: This type of exercise involves isometric muscle contractions.

- As in isometric contraction, muscle length remains same, ***no external work is done***. Hence, this is also called **static exercise**.
- Trying to lift a heavy weight and pushing against a wall are examples of isometric exercise.

Degrees of Exercise PY3.15

Exercise has been graded into mild, moderate, severe and very severe depending on level of **heart rate increase, rate of oxygen consumption and the amount of work done.**

Mild Exercise: In mild exercise, the **rise in heart rate is about 25%.**

- That means, if the pre-exercise basal heart rate is 80/min, it increases to about 100/min.
- The oxygen consumption is 0.5 L/min to 1 L/min and the work done is 150–350 watts.

Moderate Exercise: In moderate exercise, the **rise in heart rate is about 50%.**

- Heart rate increases from its pre-exercise value of 80/min to about 120/min.
- The oxygen consumption is 1 L/min to 2 L per min and the work done is 350–550 watts.

Severe Exercise: Heart rate rises to about **80%.**

- That means, if the pre-exercise basal heart is 80, it increases to 144.
- The oxygen consumption is 1.8 L/min to 2.5 L/min. and the work done is 550–700 watts.

Very Severe Exercise: In very severe exercise, the rise in heart rate is **close to 100%,** which reaches to about 160/min.

- The oxygen consumption is more than 2.5 L per min. and the work done is usually more than 700 watts.

FACTORS AFFECTING MUSCLE WORK

In physical exercise, it is the skeletal muscle that works. The degree and duration of exercise (muscle work) depends on the following factors:

1. Type of muscle contraction
2. Size of the muscle
3. Type of muscle fibers
4. Strength of muscle
5. Motor units
6. Ability to sustain fatigue
7. Level of training
8. Environmental conditions

Types of Muscle Contraction

1. In isometric contraction, the muscle does not shorten, whereas in isotonic contraction, muscle shortening occurs. **Isotonic contractions** are of *two types*: concentric and eccentric. **In concentric type of isotonic contraction**, muscle shortens while exerting a force, for example, during climbing up stairs.
2. **In eccentric contraction**, lengthening of muscle occurs while resisting an external load, for example, during walking down stairs.

Size of the Muscle

As the exercise is performed by skeletal muscles, it is the muscle mass that contributes significantly to the quantity and quality of exercise. The type of exercise also contributes to muscle mass. Thus, muscle mass and exercise are reciprocally related.

Type of Muscle Fibers

There are two types of skeletal muscle fibers: type I and type II. Type I fiber is **slow-twitch** or **oxidative type**, and type II fibers are **fast-twitch** or **glycolytic type**.

1. Generally, **type II fibers** *shorten rapidly* than type I fibers and the velocity of shortening depends on myosin ATPase activity.
2. ***In concentric type of muscle contractions***, the velocity of shortening declines rapidly with increasing load. That means, when the load is more, muscle shortens slowly.
3. **Type I muscle fibers** *have lower velocity of shortening at a given load*.
4. Practice of **aerobic** (isotonic or free-hand type) exercises slowly increases number of type I or oxidative type muscles and isometric exercises increase type II muscles in the body.

Strength of Muscle

Strength of the muscle is a single most important factor for rate and duration of exercise. Vice versa, muscle strength increases by exercise.

Role of Motor Units

A **motor unit** consists of a ***single motor nerve and all the muscle fibers*** innervated by it (refer to Fig. 22.6; Chapter 22). A motor unit is a *functional unit of muscle contraction* as all muscle fibers in a motor unit contract at the same time in response to discharge of the motor neuron of the unit.

1. Intensity of muscle contraction can be increased by increasing the number of motor units that fire simultaneously. This is achieved by **recruitment of motor units**.
   - Thus, recruitment of additional motor units **increases the velocity of muscle contraction**.
2. This pattern of recruitment of motor units in which smaller motor units are recruited first (at lower intensity of discharge) and larger motor units later is known as the **size principle** (Application Box 133.1).

> **Application Box 133.1**
>
> **Applications of size principle:** Size principle has two important applications: 1). With increased effort for work, force of contraction increases in a graded fashion with gradual recruitment of more motor units. 2). Sustaining mild to moderate tension for a longer duration is easier than to sustain maximal tension.

Ability to Sustain Fatigue

Fatigue is the ***inability to maintain force generated by muscle***. Fatigue occurs due to central and peripheral causes.

1. **Central causes** include failure of transmission of information from motor cortex or other cortical areas to muscle. However, central defects for fatigue are rare.
2. **Peripheral causes** are impaired neuromuscular transmission, defect in generation of action potential in the muscle fiber, decreased excitation-contraction coupling, and decreased availability of O_2 or glycogen to meet the energy requirement that impair the ability to generate force.

Fatigue in Isometric Exercise: Fatigue in isometric contraction is of **high-frequency type.** In maximal effort of isometric exercise, all muscle fibers including fast-twitch fibers are **recruited rapidly**.

In **fast-twitch or glycolytic muscle fibers**, fatigue occurs within seconds to minutes, which is due to:

- Immediate decrease in glycogen, decline in pH locally in muscle, and impaired conduction of action potentials along the muscle fiber due to accumulation of K^+ in the T-tubular system that comes from ECF.
- But this high-frequency fatigue **lasts for a short duration**.
  - Therefore, the muscle can generate another isometric contraction following the previous one.
- However, if contraction occurs in quick succession,

the maximum isometric tension developed decreases gradually.

Training has little effect on high frequency fatigue: For example, weightlifting can enhance muscle strength but cannot provide resistance to fatigue.

Fatigue in Isotonic Exercise: Fatigue in isotonic contraction is of **low-frequency type.**

- This occurs during repeated isotonic muscle contractions that mainly recruit slow-twitch or oxidative fibers.
- The frequency of motor-neuron discharge to cause fatigue is much less than the frequency required for maximal isometric contraction.
- Fatigue develops slowly over a period of many minutes to hours, which occurs due to impaired excitation-contraction coupling following *depletion of the intracellular* Ca^{2+}.

Training for aerobic exercises **imparts resistance to low-frequency fatigue** and therefore, *promotes exercise endurance* especially when moderate effort is repeatedly applied to perform the exercise. Thus, ***training enhances performance and decreases fatigability***.

Level of Training

Appropriate training promotes exercise performance and impairs fatigability. Aerobic training enhances isotonic exercise endurance.

Environmental Conditions

Environmental temperature and humidity are two important conditions that influence exercise. *Hot and humid environment decreases physical performance.*

1. Body temperature increases during exercise that **activates heat dissipation mechanisms** by mainly promoting cutaneous vasodilation and sweating.
   - The rate of heat production in the body increases in proportion to the intensity of exercise.
   - To transfer heat from the body to the environment, skin blood flow and sweating increase proportionately. The ***evaporative heat loss*** is thus increased.
2. **In increased ambient humidity**, *evaporative loss is impaired*, which further increases body heat (for details, see the previous chapter) and impairs exercise performance.
3. **Physical training decreases the degree of hyperthermia** induced by exercise by first reducing the threshold for sweating so that sweating begins earlier and later by increasing sweating sensitivity so that more sweating is produced at a given temperature level.

Thus, **training enhances evaporative heat loss**. The resulting dehydration caused by evaporative heat loss should be managed by ***fluid replacement*** during prolonged exercise.

Energy Source in Exercise

During physical activity, **chemical energy is converted to mechanical work**. The energy is derived from muscle metabolism. The rate of metabolism in skeletal muscle is low at rest. The energy sources in exercise are: ATP, phosphocreatine, fatty acids, glycogen and lactic acid.

N.B.: Details of energy source provided by ATP and phosphocreatine have been described in Chapter 22, under subheading "Energy sources in skeletal muscle"

Triglycerides and Fatty Acids: Though storage of O_2 in the body is negligible, sufficient reserve of fuel is available to sustain exercise for a longer duration.

- The **stored energy is derived from triglycerides** in the adipose tissue and **intramuscular stores of fatty acids**.
- In prolonged exercise, free fatty acids (FFA) *account for approximately 60% of total supply* of fuel to the muscle.

Muscle and Liver Glycogens: Muscle glycogen is another source of energy.

- Normally, 300 to 400 g of glycogen can be stored in muscles, which at the time of need can **provide about 1500 kcal of energy**.
- However, *hepatic glycogen is of little use* for acute muscular contractions as it is not made available immediately for the muscle cells.
- Nevertheless, as exercise continues, glycogen is released from liver for utilization by the exercising muscle.

In prolonged exercise, liver glycogen that releases glucose into blood by glycogenolysis becomes the fuel source for the exercising muscle (Application Box 133.2). **When exercise reaches its steady state**, the oxidation of glucose released from muscle and liver glycogen accounts for about 50% of the energy supply, and rest of energy source is the oxidation of fatty acid.

Application Box 133.2

Carbohydrate diet prior to exercise postpones fatigue in runners: In a normal well-built individual, muscle glycogen storage averages about 15 to 18 g/kg of muscle, which is reduced to about 3 g/kg of muscle after a marathon running. To avoid early onset of fatigue due to muscle glycogen depletion, the runner ***should have more muscle glycogen at the beginning of running.*** Consumption of carbohydrate-rich diet few days or at least a day prior to the competition will increase resting muscle glycogen and delays the onset of fatigue.

FACTORS AFFECTING MUSCLE WORK

The major changes in exercises are change in oxygen uptake, cardiovascular changes, respiratory changes, and changes in tissue. All these changes are **primarily meant to increase oxygen supply** to the tissue and **to promote oxygen utilization** by the tissue. Oxidation of fuel is required for supply of energy during exercise.

O_2 Uptake During Exercise

VO_2 max

The O_2 consumption by the whole body during rest is about 250 ml/min. It increases to 15–20 times during maximal exercise (Table 133.1).

1. The *maximum amount of O_2 that can be consumed* by an individual is called as **maximal O_2 consumption or VO_2 max.**
   - The average VO_2 max in an adult is ***about 3 L/min*** and in ***athlete about 5 L/min***.
   - This is an important physiological indicator of an individual's capacity to carry out aerobic exercise as it represents ***highest attainable rate of aerobic metabolism*** during performance.
2. In a normal individual, usually it is ***limited by the rate of increase in cardiac output*** rather than increase in ventilatory capacity or diffusion capacity.
3. However, the ***ability of the tissue to extract and utilize O_2*** and the ***size of total muscle mass*** contribute to it.
4. It reaches its peak during young adulthood and then declines slowly with advancement of age.

Table 133.1 |Oxygen consumption by whole body at different level of activities.

Degree of activity	O2 consumption (L/min)
Rest	0.25
Slow walking	0.8
Fast walking	1.5
Prolonged jogging	2
Fast running	3

Phases of Muscular Exercise

Based on O_2 uptake, the entire period of a physical exercise is divided into ***three phases***: adaptation phase, steady phase and recovery phase.

Adaptation Phase

This is the early part (first 2 to 5 minutes) of muscular exercise during which ***oxygen consumption increases linearly to reach its VO_2 max level***.

1. However, the O_2 consumption in this stage *is much less than its demand* for the body.
2. Therefore, **oxygen deficit** occurs at the beginning of exercise and *continues throughout exercise*. Hence, energy supply above VO_2 max is fulfilled by the anaerobic pathway.

Steady Phase

This phase of exercise is characterized by ***plateau state of VO_2 max***, which indicates that *O_2 consumption is at its maximum and steady state*. However, excess energy requirement in the presence of oxygen deficit is met with by anaerobic pathway like breakdown of creatine phosphate and muscle glycogen.

1. Due to anaerobic metabolism, ***lactic acid level rises sharply*** in blood *decreasing the blood pH*. Acid in blood is buffered by the bicarbonate buffer and in the process more CO_2 is produced that causes hyperventilation.
2. Therefore, the energy supply by anaerobic metabolism ***is limited by his capacity to withstand metabolic acidosis*** produced by the accumulation of lactic acid.
3. *Trained athletes produce less quantity of lactic acid* for any given level of work and have also the greater ability to tolerate for lactic acidosis.

Recovery Phase

This refers to the *period following completion or termination of exercise* during which ***extra amount of O_2 is consumed***. The extra amount of O_2 consumed during recovery phase is called **oxygen debt**.

1. The degree of O_2 debt is proportionate to the extent to which energy demand during exercise exceeds the capacity of aerobic synthesis of energy store.
2. The O_2 debt is meant ***to remove the excess lactate*** produced by anaerobic metabolism, ***to replenish the ATP*** and phosphorylcreatine store, ***to replace the O_2*** that comes from myoglobin.

Respiratory Changes PY11.4

The **primary objective** of respiratory changes is *to facilitate O_2 consumption of the body to meet the metabolic need during exercise*. Also, hyperventilation *removes excess of CO_2* produced during exercise. Therefore, arterial pO_2 and pCO_2 are maintained almost at the normal level even during the strenuous exercise. The ***major respiratory changes*** are increased ventilation and increased O_2 uptake by the lungs.

Increase in Ventilation

The major respiratory change in exercise is increase in ventilation. The increased ventilation matches the metabolic demand of exercise and ventilation may increase to about twenty-fold.

1. The ventilation **increases almost linearly** with the increase in intensity of exercise (Fig. 133.1) until the **anaerobic threshold is reached.**
2. **Anaerobic threshold** is the degree of exercise that produces an elevation of blood lactate levels that results from a shift from aerobic to anaerobic metabolism.
   - The anaerobic threshold is also called **lactate threshold,** as lactate concentration rises gradually with exercise intensity.
   - Lactic acidosis stimulates the ventilation further and therefore *the rise in ventilation becomes supralinear*.

3. **In athletes,** lactate threshold occurs ***at higher level*** than in non-athletes.
   - The anaerobic threshold occurs at approximately 60% of the maximal exercise level, irrespective of the physical fitness of the individual.
4. **Above the anaerobic threshold,** the increase in ventilation is ***proportionate to the increase in O_2 consumption*** as lactic acid produced imparts additional respiratory drive.
5. As removal of CO_2 exceeds its production that occurs due to additional hyperventilation, ***arterial pCO_2 falls*** significantly below the resting level during strenuous exercise.

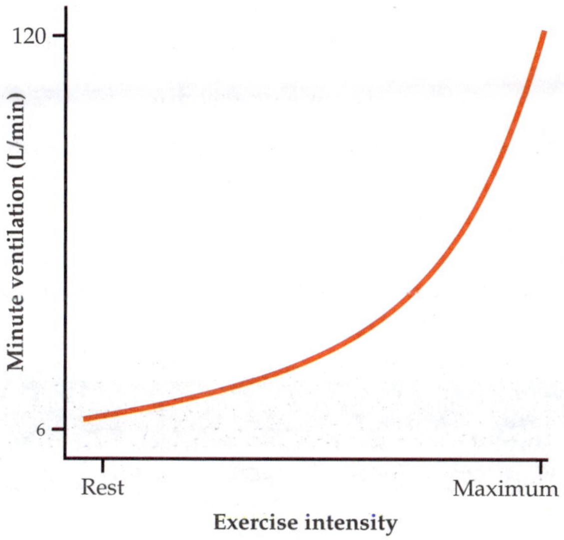

Fig. 133.1: Rate of increased ventilation in different grades muscular exercise.

Increase in Rate and Depth of Respiration

Increase in ventilation occurs due to **increase in both rate and depth of respiration**.

1. **At rest** in adults, the rate of respiration is 12–18 /min and the tidal volume is about 500 ml. Therefore, the minute ventilation (rate × tidal volume) is 6 to 7 L/min. During exercise, both rate and depth of respiration increase.
2. **In mild to moderate exercise**, with increase in intensity of exercise, the tidal volume (depth of respiration) increases rapidly with the increase in rate of respiration. However, *tidal volume increases to its limited maximum value* beyond which ventilation is largely increased by *increase in the rate of respiration* when vigorous exercise is continued for a longer period.
3. **In severe exercise** like running fast for an hour, minute ventilation increases **to 80–100 L/min** as rate of respiration may increase to about 40/min and the tidal volume to 2.5 L (Table 133.2).
4. However, even during **most strenuous exercise**, the **minute ventilation remains below the maximum breathing capacity** of the individual, which is normally 100–120 L/min.

Table 133.2 | Minute ventilation in different types of exercise

Types of exercise	Minute ventilation (L/min)
Rest	6
Slow walking	20
Fast walking	40
Prolonged jogging	50
Fast running	80

Mechanisms and Effects of Increased Ventilation

Exact mechanism for increased ventilation is still not clearly known. However, the effects are possibly mediated through neural, chemical and thermal mechanisms.

1. Ventilation increases abruptly at the beginning of the exercise, and then followed by a brief pause, again increases gradually to reach a steady state as the exercise is continued.
2. **The initial rise is mediated via neural mechanism** and gradual increase in the **later phase is mediated by chemical mechanism**.

Neural Mechanisms

Neural mechanism plays an important role at the beginning of exercise.

1. Ventilation increases abruptly at the beginning of the exercise due to **psychic stimuli** originating in the limbic system.
2. Also, **impulses originating from proprioceptors** (especially from receptors in the muscle, joints and ligaments) contribute.
3. Neural factors also contribute to **anticipatory hyperpnoea** before the onset of exercise.

Chemical Mechanisms

Humoral mechanism contributes to the **gradual increase in ventilation** in the later phase of exercise. The **arterial pO_2, pCO_2, pH and K^+** play role in this process.

1. Though the alveolar and arterial pO_2 are maintained at normal levels throughout exercise and in different degrees of exercise, and arterial pCO_2 and pH are maintained in mild to moderate exercise (Table 133.3), it is believed that these chemical factors play role in exercise hyperventilation.
2. However, the exact mechanism by which they stimulate ventilation is not exactly known. It is suggested that **accentuations of the normal oscillations in pO_2 and pCO_2,** synchronous with respiration stimulate the carotid body chemoreceptors that in turn stimulate ventilation.

Arterial pO_2: Alveolar and arterial pO_2 **remain almost normal** throughout the period of exercise. Inspite of rapid utilization of O_2 by exercising muscle, arterial pO_2 is maintained due to proportionate increase in ventilation.

1. In the later stage in strenuous exercise, **lactic acidosis** due to anerobic metabolism stimulates ventilation and maintains arterial pO_2.
2. Though pO_2 remains constant in exercise (Fig. 133.2), oxygen is believed to play some role in inducing ventilation as experimentally it is observed that increase in ventilation is less in magnitude while breathing air than while breathing 100% oxygen.
3. Also, *increase in ventilation is proportionate to increase in oxygen consumption*.

Arterial pCO_2: Despite increase in production of CO_2 from metabolically active tissue in exercise, the **arterial pCO_2 remains normal in mild to moderate exercise**. This is because hyperventilation removes extra CO_2 produced by muscle metabolism.

1. However, ventilation is stimulated due to *increase in chemoreceptor sensitivity to CO_2 or to fluctuation in CO_2*.
2. When exercise continues beyond lactate threshold, further stimulation of ventilation removes more CO_2 than the amount of CO_2 produced.
3. Therefore, **in strenuous exercise pCO_2 falls** (Fig. 133.2). Inspite of decline in pCO_2, ventilation is stimulated by fall in pH (Application Box 133.3).

Arterial pH: Lactic acidosis is produced due to **excess anerobic metabolism** in severe exercise. With continuation of strenuous exercise, excess of lactic acid produced is buffered and in the process of buffering, CO_2 is formed. This extra CO_2 further stimulates ventilation.

1. Thus, with increased production of lactic acid, the **generation of CO_2 is more** and therefore, there is proportionate increase in ventilation. Due to increased ventilation, accumulation of CO_2 in the blood is prevented.
2. Consequently, the buffering of the acid is called **isocapnic buffering**, as CO_2 change relatively little. However, further continuation of exercise **beyond lactate threshold** (exhaustion of lactate buffering) decreases blood pH due to accumulation of more lactic acid. This heralds the onset of metabolic acidosis.
3. **Overload of lactic acid** causes *supralinear stimulation of ventilation* (see above).
4. Stimulation of ventilation occurs via **activation of peripheral chemoreceptors** in carotid and aortic bodies. During this period of exercise, arterial pCO_2 falls significantly secondary to extra-hyperventilation (Fig. 133.2).
5. However, the decline in arterial pCO_2 induced by excessive ventilation becomes the **physiological mechanism for respiratory compensation** of metabolic acidosis (for details, refer the chapter "Acid-Base Balance".

Plasma K^+ level: During moderate to severe exercise, K^+ is released from exercising skeletal muscles. Increased plasma K^+ **stimulates peripheral chemoreceptors** that aids to hyperventilation induced by other chemical factors.

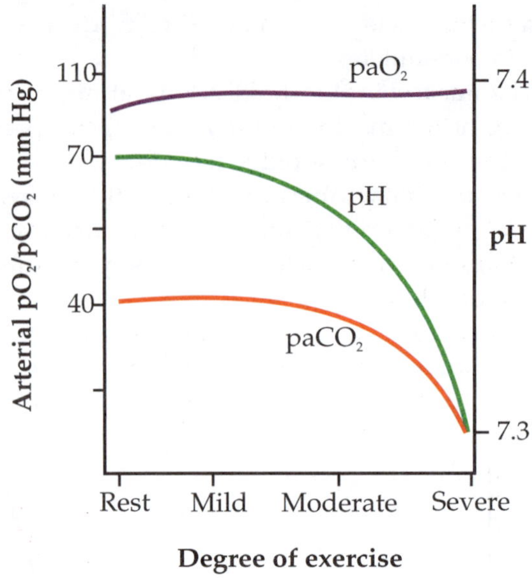

Fig. 133.2: Change in arterial pO_2, pCO_2, and pH in different degrees of exercise.

Thermogenic Mechanism

Exercising muscles generate heat and increase body temperature. Increased temperature in sustained exercise contributes to stimulation of ventilation.

Table 133.3 | Alveolar and arterial pO2 and arterial pCO2 and pH in different types of exercise.

Types of Exercise	pAO_2	paO_2	$paCO_2$	pH
Rest	103	100	40	7.4
Slow walking	103	100	40	7.4
Fast walking	105	100	38	7.4
Prolonged jogging	106	100	36	7.4
Fast running	110	100	25	7.32

Note: For pO_2, A = alveolar; a = arterial

Application Box 133.3

Ventilation-perfusion ratio: As oxygen is utilized rapidly by actively exercising muscles, the pO_2 of venous blood is grossly reduced. Hence, blood returning to lungs is severely depleted of oxygen. The decreased pulmonary arterial pO_2 is another stimulus for stimulation of ventilation. Though pulmonary arterial blood flow increases during exercise, the increase in ventilation is more than the increase in blood flow. Therefore, ventilation-perfusion ratio rises from 0.8 at rest to about 4 in severe exercise.

Increase in O_2 Uptake

Hyperventilation in exercise increases oxygen uptake in the lungs. This helps maintain arterial oxygenation. Maximal O_2 uptake may be about **20 times the resting O_2 uptake**. In severe exercise, oxygen uptake is raised from 250 ml/min at rest to about 4 L/min.

Mechanisms of Increased Oxygen Uptake

1. **Increased alveolar-to-arterial gradient of pO_2:** In exercise, skeletal muscles extract more O_2 from the

arterial blood and therefore O_2 *content of the venous blood reaching the lungs is decresed* by about five times (to about 3 ml/100 ml of blood from its resting value of about 15 ml/100 ml). This further **increases the pO_2 gradient** from the alveolar air to pulmonary capillary blood. Hence, O_2 uptake in the lungs increases radically.

2. **Increased perfusion of lungs:** Increased cardiac output in exercise *increases pulmonary blood flow to approximately six times*. As more blood passes through the lungs per unit time, more quantity of O_2 is automatically picked up by the lungs.
3. Increased diffusion capacity of alveolocapillary membrane: Increased pulmonary blood flow causes **opening of several capillaries** in the lungs that are normally closed at rest. This promotes better alveolar perfusion. Opening up of more capillaries *increases the surface area available for diffusion* in the presence of more oxygen that has already been made available due to increased ventilation. Thus, diffusion capacity of the lungs increases to about three times. This raises the rate of oxygen diffusion from 21 ml/min/mm Hg at rest to about 65 ml/min/mm Hg during exercise.

Importance of Maximal O_2 Uptake

The VO_{2max} (maximal oxygen uptake by the lungs) is an **index of the functional capacity of the individual to sustain exercise.**

1. The VO_{2max} in a moderately active adult male is 35 to 40 ml O_2/min/kg body weight.
2. In a strong athlete, VO_{2max} may be as high as 80 to 90 ml O_2/min/kg body weight, which is about 20-fold increase of their resting VO_2. T
3. Therefore, while assessing athletic potential of an individual, it is imperative to measure the VO_{2max} along with measurement of other work efficiencies.
4. In chronic lung and heart diseases, VO_{2max} may be as low as 10 ml O_2/min/kg body weight. At high-altitude VO_{2max} is decreased.

O_2 Store of the Body

The O_2 store of the body is **only about one liter**. This mainly represents the O_2 bound to hemoglobin.

- This much of O_2 can maximally support a mild exercise for one minute, a moderate exercise for 30 seconds and a heavy exercise for 15 seconds, and maximal exercise for less than 5 seconds.
- Therefore, for the exercise to continue for more than 15 to 30 seconds, the body must transport O_2 from the atmosphere to the mitochondria in the muscle at a rate proportionate to the O_2 utilization by the exercising muscle.
- In exercise, increased *alveolar ventilation promotes oxygenation of blood* and *increased cardiac output ensures adequate supply of oxygenated blood* to the muscles.

Factors That Limit O_2 Uptake by Muscles

Five major processes are involved in the transport of O_2 from the atmosphere to the mitochondria in exercising muscle. Therefore, alteration in any of these mechanisms by physiological or pathological processes could retard final O_2 uptake by the exercising tissue.

These steps are:

1. **Pulmonary ventilation** that facilitates O_2 delivery to the alveoli in lungs.
2. **Pulmonary perfusion** that promotes pick-up of O_2 from the alveoli.
3. **Ventilation-perfusion ratio** contributing to oxygenation (O_2 content) of arterial blood.
4. **Dynamism of circulation** that delivers O_2 from lungs to the muscle.
5. **Extraction of O_2** from blood by the exercising muscle.

The final muscle oxidative metabolism depends on the adequacy of muscle blood flow, O_2 delivery to muscle, the pO_2 gradient between blood and muscle mitochondria, and aerobic metabolic capacity of the muscle cells.

Cardiovascular Changes

The primary aim of cardiovascular changes in exercise is to **supply adequate oxygenated blood** to exercising muscle at a rate that meets their metabolic demand. This is achieved by following cardiovascular responses:

1. Increase in the cardiac output
2. Increase in the skeletal muscle blood flow
3. Redistribution of blood flow in the body
4. Changes in blood pressure
5. Changes in blood volume.

Increase in Cardiac Output

Ability of the cardiovascular system to transport O_2 to the exercising muscle determines VO_{2max}.

1. The **increase in cardiac output** that determines the rate of O_2 delivery to the tissue **is the limiting step in oxygen extraction.**
2. During exercise, the cardiac output increases from its resting level of 5 L/min **to about 25 L/min.**
   - In athletes, the maximal increase in cardiac output is greater than in nonathletes.
   - During a strenuous exercise, **in strong athletes,** cardiac output can increase upto **35–50 L/min.**
3. The increase in cardiac output **is proportionate to increase in oxygen consumption.**

Increase in cardiac output occurs due to increase in **both heart rate and stroke volume** (Table 133.4).

Table 133.4 | Increase in heart rate (HR), stroke volume (SV) and cardiac output (CO) in different physical activities, in a middle-aged.

	HR/min	SV (ml)	CO (L/min)
Rest	75	70	5.2
Slow walking	100	85	8.5
Fast walking	130	100	13
Prolonged jogging	150	110	16.5
Fast running	190	120	23

Increase in Heart Rate

The heart at rest is called **basal heart rate** (BHR). BHR is a good index of parasympathetic activity (vagal tone). However, BHR is a poor index of endurance fitness, as BHR is influence by genetic and others factors too.

1. Heart rate increases linearly with the severity and duration of exercise.
2. The **maximal heart rate** (maximum increase in heart rate) achieved is **determined by the age of the subject**.
3. This is also called **target heart rate** (THR) that forms the ***basis of treadmill test*** while assessing cardiac status of an individual.
    - The approximate THR in an adult aged 40 years is 190.
    - **THR decreases with age**.
    - THR also depends on the basal heart rate, physical fitness and gender of the individual.
4. Increase in heart rate after exercise takes time to return to normal (Clinical Note 133.1)

Mechanisms:

Tachycardia in exercise occurs due to following mechanisms:

1. ***Increased sympathetic discharge:*** The increase in heart rate occurs even before exercise begins, which is called **anticipatory tachycardia**. This occurs due to psychic stimuli that originate from limbic system and activates sympathetic discharge via hypothalamus. During exercise, increase in motor activity produces tachycardia by stimulating sympathetic system.
2. ***Muscle-heart reflex:*** Peripheral reflexes that originate from the exercising muscles and joints increase the heart rate, which is known as **muscle-heart reflex**. This causes tachycardia as soon as the exercise begins.
3. ***Hormonal mechanisms:*** Release of **catecholamines** from adrenal medulla in response to sympathetic stimulation and plasma chemical changes contribute to increase in heart rate.

Clinical Note 133.1

Heart rate normalizes slowly: After the cessation of exercise, tachycardia continues for a longer period than the persistence in increased blood pressure. The heart rate takes considerable time to return to resting levels as the hormonal effects and body temperature take time to normalize.

4. ***Thermogenic stimulation:*** When exercise is continued, heat is produced from exercising muscles. The increased body temperature stimulates pacemaker activity and increases heart rate.

Increase in Stroke Volume

The stroke volume increases simultaneously along with heart rate. **In isometric exercise** both heart rate and stroke volume increase, but **increase in stroke volume is much less**. In isotonic exercise, the increase in stroke volume is more than the increase in heart rate. In athletes, increase in stroke volume is the major mechanism to increase cardiac output (Application Box 133.4).

Mechanisms: Stroke volume increases by following mechanisms:

1. ***Increased sympathetic discharge:*** Increased sympathetic activity **increases myocardial contractility** that increases stroke volume.
2. ***Increased EDV:*** End-diastolic volume (EDV) increases due to increased venous return. Venous return increases due to increased activities of **skeletal muscle pump, thoracic pump, and abdominal pump**. Also, sympathetic venoconstriction *increases venous return*. Increased venous return increases stroke volume by Frank-Starling mechanism.

Application Box 133.3

Athletes increase CO by increasing SV: The vagal tone is high in strong athletes. They increase a target cardiac output (CO) by mainly increasing the stroke volume, whereas nontrained individuals increases cardiac output mainly by increasing heart rate. Thus, **at any level of cardiac output athletes have lower heart rate** than nonathletes.

Increased Skeletal Muscle Blood Flow

At rest, skeletal muscle blood flow is 2–4 ml/100 gm of tissue/min, which accounts for about **16% of total cardiac output** as the total muscle blood flow is approximately 850 ml/min.

1. During strenuous exercise, the skeletal muscle blood flow can increase to about 50–80 ml/100 gm/min, about **20 times** the resting level.
2. This primarily occurs due to **arteriolar dilation and opening up of capillaries**.
    - In skeletal muscle at rest, many capillaries are closed and blood flow occurs mainly via thoroughfare vessels.
    - During exercise, opening of capillaries not only increases blood flow but also increases **surface area for gas exchange**.

Mechanisms that Increase Muscle Blood Flow

Skeletal muscle blood flow increases by **three mechanisms**: autonomic, metabolic and hormonal factors.

Autonomic Control: Sympathetic innervation of skeletal

muscle is cholinergic, which is called ***sympathetic vasodilator system***.

- These fibers heavily terminate on arterioles and cause arteriolar dilation on activation.
- This increases muscle blood flow during exercise.

Metabolic Control: In prolonged exercise, accumulation of metabolites in the exercising muscles causes dilation of their blood vessel.

- The **metabolites** are carbon dioxide, lactic acids, potassium ions, decreased local oxygen content, accumulation of hydrogen ions in the tissue, and local rise in temperature.
- Metabolites cause **dilation of arterioles and precapillary sphincters**.
- The **metabolic vasodilation** maintains blood flow during recovery from exercise.

Humoral Control: The skeletal blood vessels contain both **α adrenergic and β receptors**, respectively. These two receptors counter each other in their action and therefore, may not contribute significantly to the increase in skeletal blood flow during exercise. However, some authors do believe that adrenaline through the β-receptor mediated vasodilation contribute to increase in muscle blood flow before, during and after the exercise.

Blood flow through non-exercising muscles also increases during exercise though the flow is less than in exercising muscles.

Redistribution of Blood Flow

Increased skeletal muscle blood flow is not only due to increased cardiac output but also to redistribution of blood flow. Sympathetic **vasoconstriction in visceral and cutaneous vascular bed** diverts enough blood to the exercising skeletal muscles. However, vasodilation in coronary and cerebral circulation maintains blood flow to these two crucial vital organs.

Visceral Blood Flow: Sympathetic discharge to visceral structures causes **constriction of blood vessels in visceral organs**. This significantly contributes to ***divert blood flow to skeletal muscles***.

- Renal blood vessels also constrict that decreases renal blood flow to about 80% in severe exercise. Therefore, *prolonged and severe exercise may impair kidney functions*.
- Hence proteinuria may occur in strenuous exercise.

Cutaneous Blood Flow: Cutaneous blood flow is also decreased due to ***sympathetic cutaneous vasoconstriction***.

- This also contributes to divert blood flow to exercising muscles.
- However, **in prolonged exercise**, increased body temperature causes ***thermogenic vasodilation*** to promote dissipation of heat generated during exercise.

Cerebral Blood Flow: Though sympathetic vasoconstriction occurs in cerebral vessels, the degree of vasoconstriction is less, and metabolic vasodilation immediately following the increased sympathetic activity maintains cerebral blood flow.

Coronary Blood Flow: During exercise, sympathetic vasodilation occurs in coronary blood vessels due to presence of a greater number of β receptors in coronary arteries.

- Also, **metabolic factors** contribute.
- Increased coronary blood flow is nature's autoregulatory process to supply adequate nutrient and oxygen to the cardiac muscle to maintain increased cardiac output throughout the period of exercise.

Adipose Tissue Blood Flow: Blood flow to adipose tissue increases during exercise.

This **helps in lipolysis to mobilize fatty acids** from triglyceride stores in fat depots to the exercising muscles.

Blood Pressure Changes

Systolic Blood Pressure

Systolic pressure **always increases in exercise** proportionate to increase in cardiac output (Fig. 133.3). This occurs due to *sympathetic induced cardio acceleration*.

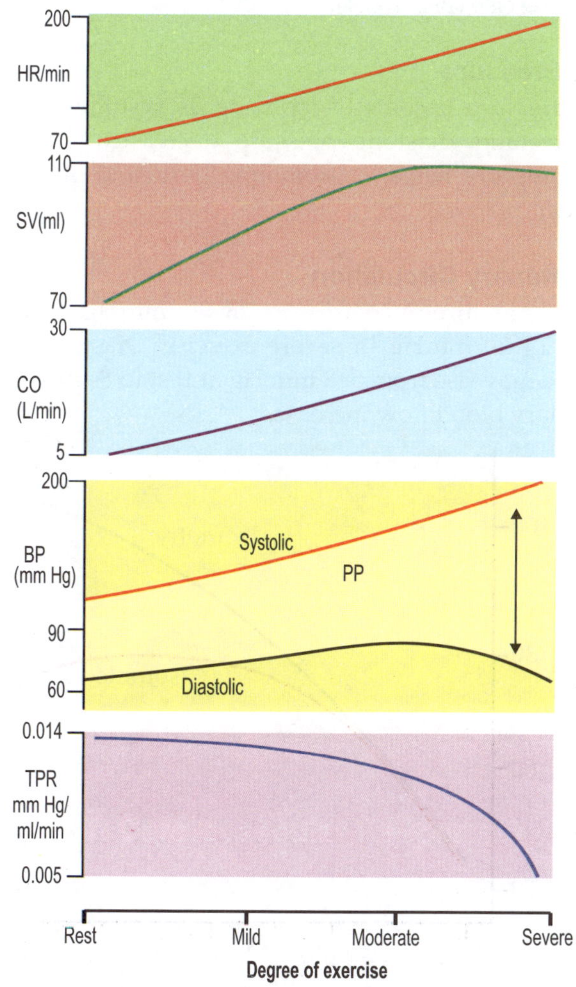

Fig. 133.3: Cardiovascular changes in isotonic exercise. (HR: heart rate; SV: stroke volume; CO: cardiac output; BP: blood pressure; TPR: total peripheral resistance; PP: pulse pressure).

Diastolic Blood Pressure

Change in diastolic pressure ***depends on the degree of exercise***. Diastolic pressure depends on peripheral resistance, which primarily depends on the diameter of blood vessel.

1. **In mild to moderate exercise,** vasoconstriction induced by sympathetic activation *increases diastolic pressure*.
2. **In moderate to severe exercise**, vasodilation *decreases peripheral resistance*, which in turns *decreases diastolic pressure*.
3. Vasodilation occurs in exercise by **three mechanisms**: sympathetic cholinergic vasodilation of skeletal blood vessels, metabolic vasodilation and thermogenic vasodilation (see above).

Mean Blood Pressure

Mean pressure increases in mild to moderate exercise that helps in promoting blood flow to skeletal muscle through dilated vessels.

- In severe and continued exercise, *mean pressure gradually falls as diastolic pressure falls*.
- However, in isometric exercise mean pressure continued to increase throughout the period of exercise (Fig. 133.4).

Pulse Pressure

Pulse pressure becomes very wide as systolic pressure increases and diastolic pressure decreases. **Increased pulse pressure** helps in promoting perfusion of skeletal muscles.

In Pulmonary Circulation

Systolic pressure increases to 25–30 mmHg from its resting 15–20 mmHg in severe exercise. Diastolic blood pressure may rise from 5–8 mm Hg at rest to 8–10 mmHg. Pulmonary blood flow increases.

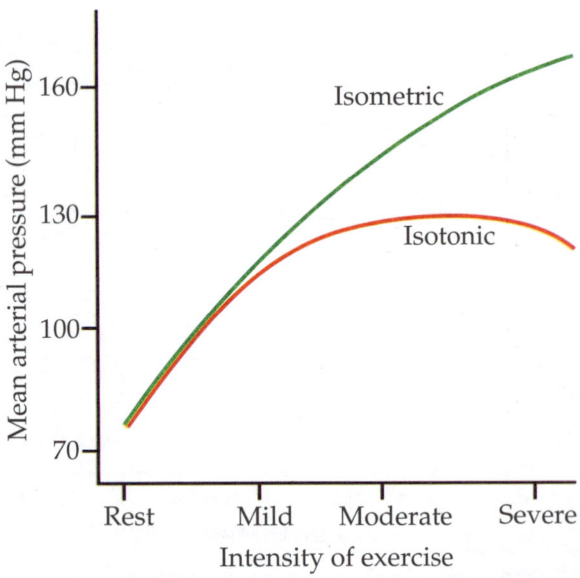

Fig. 133.4: Change in mean arterial pressure in isometric and isotonic exercises.

Cardiovascular Changes in Isometric Exercise

1. **Heart rate increases** as soon as exercise begins and continues to increase throughout exercise. Tachycardia at the beginning of exercise is mainly due to **vagal withdrawal** though sympathetic stimulation contributes to tachycardia in the later part of exercise.
2. However, **increase in stroke volume is relatively less** as vagal inhibition is the major means of cardiac changes.
3. **Systolic and diastolic pressure increase sharply**.
4. Mean pressure **remains elevated throughout** the entire period of exercise (Fig. 133.4). As exercising muscle remains tonically contracted during isometric exercise, **skeletal muscle blood flow is grossly reduced** due to mechanical vasocompression (Application Box 133.4).

Application Box 133.4

Isometric exercise is harmful for hypertensive patients: As blood pressure remains elevated throughout the entire period of isometric exercise, people suffering from hypertension and vascular anomalies should not perform these exercises. Also, people with heart diseases should not practice isometric exercises as they put maximum stress on the heart. However, isotonic exercise is advised for management of hypertension.

Change in Blood Volume

Efficiency of maintaining arterial blood pressure during exercise depends on effective blood volume, which depends on total blood volume and venomotor tone that determine venous return to the heart. Effective **circulating volume falls** during prolonged exercise, especially when exercise is performed in hot environment. In strenuous exercise, blood volume decreases 15–20% that causes hemoconcentration. Blood volume decreases due to **four factors**:

1. Increased hydrostatic pressure **increases capillary filtration** that facilitates escape of fluid from vascular compartment into extravascular space.
2. Accumulation of **osmotically active metabolites** in the tissue reverses the normal filtration gradient. Thus, water moves into the interstitial tissue space.
3. Increased **sweating and evaporation** from skin during exercise contributes to fall in effective blood volume. The rate of water loss from the skin may be upto 30 ml/min in severe exercise.
4. In prolonged exercise, **redistribution of blood volume** to the skin to increase cutaneous blood flow for heat transfer from the body decreases effective blood volume. Cutaneous vasodilation is an effective means of dissipation of heat from the body generated during exercise.

Hemoconcentration due to decreased blood volume **increases blood viscosity** (Clinical Note 133.2). However, oxygen carrying capacity increases as relative red cell concentration becomes more.

Clinical Note 133.2

Ingesting salt with water facilitates recovery: Dehydration due to exercise should be treated by water containing salt. The more effective means of restoring body fluid volume following severe exercise is to ingest NaCl with water volume. **Successful rehydration** occurs effectively and early, when water is ingested with salt. Rapid recovery of fluid volume provides a better ability to regulate body temperature in exercise-collapse.

Other Changes

Changes in Tissues

The changes at the tissue level are aimed at extracting large amount of O_2 from blood, utilizing O_2 in the exercising tissue and facilitating removal of CO_2 from the tissues to the blood. These objectives are achieved by following mechanisms:

1. **Increased blood flow:** Increased blood flow to skeletal muscles **supplies more O_2** to the tissue. **Opening up of muscle capillaries** increase perfusion and surface for exchange of gasses between blood and the muscle.
2. **Increased pO_2 gradient:** As exercising muscle rapidly utilize O_2, **the gradient of O_2** between capillary blood and muscle tissue **is increased**. This facilitates O_2 extraction from capillary blood into the tissue fluid.
3. **Increased oxidative metabolism:** The muscle metabolism is increased by *activation of oxidative enzymes*.
4. **Right shift of O_2-Hb dissociation curve:** Due to increased tissue metabolism, **CO_2** accumulate in the tissue, **temperature** increases locally and red blood cell **2,3-DPG** increases. All these factors shift O_2-Hb dissociation curve to the right, which causes **three-fold increase in O_2 extraction** from blood.

Endocrinal Responses

During exercise, many hormones are secreted in large quantity. Not only these hormones mediate acute physiological effects of exercise, but also participate in long term adaptation to exercise.

Catecholamines: Secretion of catecholamines from adrenal medulla increases in severe exercise.

- These hormones promote **availability of fuels to the exercising muscles by mobilizing fatty acids** from adipose tissue and glucose from liver.

Glucagon: Secretion of glucagon is increased in prolonged exercise.

- By **facilitating glycogenolysis** it mobilizes glucose from glycogen and by **promoting lipolysis** it mobilizes fatty acids from the adipose tissue.

Antidiuretic Hormone: Secretion of ADH is increased during exercise.

- ADH helps in **water retention by increasing water reabsorption from kidney**.
- This compensates for water loss from the body that occurs in the form of sweating during exercise for dissipation of heat.

ACTH and Cortisol: ACTH secretion is increased during strenuous exercise.

- This increases glucocorticoid secretion and helps in mobilizing fat.
- Cortisol reduces the impact of exercise stress.

Endorphin: Secretion of endorphin increases greatly during exercise.

- Endorphin is known to increase mood and bring happiness.
- This **reduces the exercise stress**, and **alleviates post-exercise pain**.

AEROBIC TRAINING

The primary aim of training is to increase the resistance to fatigue. Therefore, this is also called **endurance training**.

1. Aerobic training **increases VO_{2max}** and **promotes elimination of excess** heat produced during exercise. By increasing VO_{2max}, the rate of ATP production increases more aerobically.
2. When VO_2 is less than 50% of the maximum, essentially all of the net energy release in active muscle is aerobic.
    - Thus, O_2 demand and the metabolic load of muscle are met without disturbing acid-base balance.
    - Increase in VO_{2max} raises the threshold of exercise intensity for lactic acid production.
3. Thus, training alters both the **O_2 transport and O_2-acceptance systems**.
4. Training has minimal effects on respiratory responses and more effects on cardiovascular responses.

Systemic Effects

Respiratory Effects

Effects on O_2 Delivery and Extraction

Aerobic training **improves both O_2 delivery and extraction**. There is large increase in VO_{2max} with training. Though there is no evidence to suggest *increase in Hb concentration* in physical training, **O_2 carrying capacity of blood increases** with training. Also, tissue extraction of O_2 is marginally high in training.

Effects on Cardiovascular Responses

On Cardiac Output and Plasma Volume

Training **increases stroke volume and decreases maximal heart rate**.

1. The net effect is greater increase in maximal cardiac output. Therefore, athletes achieve a target increase in cardiac output by increasing stroke volume.

2. Increase in stroke volume is mainly due to **increased myocardial contractility**, which occurs due to elevation in key oxidative enzymes in the mitochondria of type I muscle fibers.
   - Also, expansion of the plasma compartment occurs in training that increases the preload and therefore, increases ventricular filling.
3. As heart is more efficient in increasing stroke volume than heart rate, **higher stroke volume reduces the myocardial metabolic load** for any level of physical activity.
4. **Red blood cell volume** increases with aerobic training.
   - However, greater expansion of plasma-volume reduces the hemoglobin content resulting in **physiological sports anemia**.
5. The increased blood volume promotes the ability to achieve greater cutaneous blood flow in unfavorable conditions like hot environment.

Other Effects

On O_2 Diffusion into Muscle

With training, **O_2 extraction from blood to tissue increases**. This is because, trained muscles accommodate more blood flow as they have *more new capillaries*.

1. **Increased capillary density** increases greater surface area for O_2 diffusion and reduces the diffusion distance for O_2 between the capillary blood and membrane of muscle cells.
2. This also, **increases the transit time** of blood to pass through the muscle capillaries that allows more time for O_2 extraction.
3. Training also increases total skeletal-muscle blood flow.

Effects on Mitochondrial Enzymes

Oxidative enzyme activity in the muscle mitochondria is enhanced in training.

1. The **mRNA number and activity increase** in muscle cell that increases transcription of muscle proteins.
2. The **enzymes activated** by training are succinate dehydrogenase, NADH dehydrogenase and cytochrome oxidase.
3. This provides an **increased ability to oxidize** free fatty acids and other fuels.

Effect on Insulin Sensitivity

Aerobic training **increases tissue sensitivity to insulin**. This promotes glucose transport into the muscle. This helps in **sparing muscle glycogen**.

Advantages of Training

Aerobic training improves performance of athletes and sports persons.

Table 133.5 | Energy expenditure of various exercises.

Exercise	Energy spent (kcal/min)
Active standing	3
Cooking	4
Making bed	4
Slow walking (3 km/h)	4
Fast walking (6 km/h)	6
Dancing	7
Active gardening	8
Climbing stairs	11
Prolonged jogging	12
Swimming (50 m/min)	15
Running (12 km/h)	16

1. This is because the endurance activity **facilitates muscle oxidative capacity**. Regular training is essential not only for maintaining physical fitness of sports persons but also of army-men and police personnel.
2. Also in general population, health of individuals practicing regular physical training remains always better than untrained individuals.
3. It also **slows the process of aging**. Regular physical exercise **promotes psychological health.**
4. This is attributed to increased *secretion of endorphins* in response to exercise that is known to alleviate mental stress and produce a sense of well-being.
5. Thus, regular physical training is the key to a **healthier and happier life**.

PY11.5

Therapeutic Benefits of Regular Exercise

Physiological Consequences of Sedentary Life: Lack of exercise (sedentary life) leads to obesity and obesity related diseases. Also, sedentary life is the root cause of metabolic syndrome and many other psychosomatic diseases. Practice of regular exercise is an important component of management of many diseases.

1. Practice of regular exercise is known to **reduce insulin resistance**. Tissue sensitivity to insulin and glucose tolerance improves with exercise. Exercise increases the ***number of insulin receptors and promotes activity of glucose transporters***. Hence, exercise therapy is very useful in the treatment of diabetes mellitus.
2. Regular exercise is known to **decrease sympathetic tone**. Therefore, exercise like morning walk is the best mode of treatment of hypertension.
3. Exercise **improves coronary perfusion** and causes **neovascularization** of myocardium. Therefore, regular practice of slow and mild exercise (without exerting much pressure on heart) helps patients suffering from chronic myocardial infarction.
4. Exercise, if practiced regularly, **decreases body fat**

mass. Especially, **brisk walking in the early morning** is very effective in this regard. Physical activities like walking, running, swimming, dancing and jogging are known to induce energy expenditure that in the long run is very effective in reducing obesity (Table 133.5). Therefore, this is the best way to check obesity and obesity-induced disorders.

5. Exercise **prevents osteoporosis**. Regulated exercise programme **stimulates osteoblastic activity**, facilitates bone mineral metabolism and preserves the geometry. *Immobilization and inactivity stimulate osteoclastic activity* and produce bone loss.
6. Specific exercises are prescribed for **treatment of osteoarthritis** as they improve muscle strength and joint stability.
7. Regular exercise is used **for stress and psychological problems**, as endorphins released during exercise are known to improve mood.

Exam Questions

1. Describe the respiratory and cardiovascular changes in a moderate isotonic exercise.
2. List the factors affecting muscle work and briefly describe the energy sources in exercise. Add a note on VO_2max.
3. Describe the CV changes in exercise. Adda note on physiologic effects of training.

Multiple Choice Questions

1. All of the following are true about VO2 max, EXCEPT:
A. It is about 3L/min in an adult
B. Limited by rate of increase in cardiac output
C. Limited by rate of increase in diffusion capacity
D. Represents highest attainable rate of aerobic metabolism

2. Which of the following is NOT true? Oxygen debt is meant to:
A. To remove the excess lactate produced by anerobic metabolism
B. To remove the excess CO_2 produced by anerobic metabolism
C. To replenish the phosphorylcreatine store
D. To replace the O_2 that comes from myoglobin

3. In moderate exercise, the respiratory rate is increased due to response of:
A. Proprioception receptor in the joints
B. Increased PCO2 in arterial blood
C. Increased PO2 in arterial blood
D. J-receptor stimulation

4. Aerobic capacity is increased by:
A. Prolonged exercise to be done routinely
B. Strenuous exercise
C. Regular 30 minutes exercise
D. Spurt of exercise

5. Exercise causes which of the following?
A. Increased blood flow to the muscles after half minute
B. Increase in cerebral blood flow due to increase in systolic blood pressure
C. Increased in body temperature
D. Decreased O2 consumption

6. Which of the following is true regarding physiological changes in the brain during moderate exercise?
A. Blood flow decreased
B. Blood flow increased
C. Blood flow remains unaltered
D. Blood flow initially increases and then decreases

7. Autoregulation means the process that:
A. Maintains the blood flow   B. Varies with change in pressure
C. Is regulated by local metabolites   D. Is well developed in the skin

8. In isometric exercise, all are increased, except:
A. Heart rate   B. Cardiac rate
C. Mean arterial pressure   D. Systemic vascular resistance

9. Exercise that strengthen the muscle, is:
A. Isotonic   B. Isometric   C. Aerobic   D. None

10. The main cause of increased blood flow to exercising muscle is:
A. Raised blood pressure
B. Vasodilation due to local metabolites
C. Increased sympathetic discharge to all peripheral blood vessels
D. Increased heart rate

11. All are true regarding blood supply increase in muscle during exercise, except:
A. Decreased beta-adrenergic stimulation
B. Local metabolites
C. Increased arterial pressure
D. Cholinergic stimulation

12. All are the features of exercise, except:
A. Left shift of Hb-O2 dissociation curve
B. Increase blood supply to muscle
C. Increase stroke volume
D. Increase O2 extraction

13. Physiological changes during severe exercise are all, except:
A. Hyperventilation in the beginning
B. Hyperkalemia
C. Decreased PaO2
D. Decreased PaCO2

14. In exercising muscle; true about metabolism is:
A. Same in aerobic and anaerobic
B. Fatty acids are used mainly
C. Glycogen and phosphocreatine kinase are used anaerobically
D. All of the above

15. Exercise is also prescribed as an adjuvant treatment of depression. Most probably it acts by:
A. Increasing pulse pressure   B. Improving hemodynamics
C. Inducing good sleep   D. Raising endorphin levels

16. All of the following are therapeutic benefits of regular exercise, EXCEPT:
A. Improved coronary pperfusion   B. Increased sympathetic tone
C. Reduced insulin resistance   D. Increased osteoblastic activity

Answers

1. C 2. B 3. A 4. C 5. C 6. C 7. A 8. D 9. B 10. B 11. A 12. A
13. C 14. C 15. D 16. B

Chapter 134

Aviation and Space Physiology

Learning Objectives

On completion of study of this chapter:

The student will be able to (must know):

1. Define positive G and negative G and understand the concept of these gravitational forces.
2. Calculate centrifugal acceleratory force.
3. Say what is black-out of vision and red-out of vision.
4. List the effects of positive and negative G on body.

The student may also be able to (desirable to know):

1. Describe the effects and their mechanisms of chronic stay in SF.

Aviation physiology and space-flight physiology are examples of such extremes of conditions. Many of the basic problems of space medicine such as hypoxia, dysbarism, thermal support, acceleration and response to great altitudes have been studied long before. As man has ascended to higher and higher altitudes in aviation, mountain climbing and space vehicles, it imperative to understand the effects of altitude and low gas pressures on the human body.

- Flight, diving, and space traveling all involve **pressure changes, forced changes in body position, controlled breathing sources**, and dependence on life support equipment.
- However, **space flight** poses unique medical problems due to prolonged exposure to a combination of **stressful stimuli, such as acceleration forces, radiation, and weightlessness**.

AVIATION PHYSIOLOGY DURING FLIGHT

In flight, there are **rapid changes in velocity and direction of motion** and therefore several types of acceleratory and decceleratory forces act on the body. However, as the person is sitting in a pressurized cabin in the flight, the impacts on the body are minimal.

At the **beginning of flight**, there is *linear acceleration*, at the **end of flight** there is *deceleration*, and during the flight every time the vehicle turns, **centrifugal acceleration** is experienced. As ascent and descent occur quite rapidly, the impacts experienced are transient. But the centrifugal acceleration is experienced throughout the flight journey.

Centrifugal Acceleratory Forces: When an airplane makes a turn, the force of centrifugal acceleration is determined by the following relation:

$f = mv^2/r$

where, '*f*' is centrifugal acceleratory force,

'*m*' is the mass of the object,

'*v*' is velocity of travel, and

'*r*' is radius of curvature of the turn.

As the velocity increases, the **force of centrifugal acceleration increases** in proportion to the square of the velocity. Also, the force of acceleration is **directly proportional to the sharpness of the turn**.

+G and –G

When an aviator is sitting in his seat, the force with which he is pressing against the seat results from the **pull of gravity** and is equal to his weight. The **intensity of this force is said to be +1G** because it is equal to the pull of gravity. If the force with which he presses against the seat becomes **five times** his normal weight during pull-out from a dive, the force acting on the seat **is +5 G.**

1. **Positive G** forces are **anything that exceeds 1 G**. This is well experienced during acceleration in flight.
2. The negative force is any **G force exerted in opposite direction**, i.e., when the body is *accelerating towards the earth faster than the force of gravity*.

- If the airplane goes through an outside loop so that the person is held down by his seat belt, **negative G** is applied to his body.
- If the force with which he is held down by his belt is equal to the weight of his body, the negative force is –1G. If he decelerates much faster than this, it becomes –2G, –3G according the speed of deceleration.

Effects of Positive G

As blood is highly mobile in the blood vessels and blood being fluid can easily be translocated by centrifugal forces, the most important effect of **centrifugal acceleration** is seen **on the cardiovascular system**. When an aviator is subjected to *positive G*, blood is centrifuged toward the lowermost part of the body.

1. **If the person is in standing position** and centrifugal acceleratory force is +5 G, the pressure of blood in the veins of the feet is greatly increased to about 450 mm Hg.
2. **If the person in the sitting position**, the pressure becomes nearly 300 mm Hg.
   - As pressure in the **vessels of the lower limb** increases, these vessels **passively dilate** so that a major portion of the blood from the upper body is translocated into the lower vessels.
   - Heart cannot pump unless blood returns back to it. Hence, during +G as the greater the quantity of blood is "**pooled" in in the lower part** of the body, the less blood is available for the cardiac output. **Cardiac output decreases** that in turn **decreases blood pressure**.
   - Thus, when about +3.3 G is suddenly applied to a sitting person, blood pressure falls below 22 mm Hg for the first few seconds after the acceleration begins, but systolic pressure of about 55 mm Hg and a diastolic pressure of 20 mm Hg **returns back within 10 to 15 seconds**.
   - The prompt recovery is mainly due to **activation of the baroreceptor reflexes**.
3. Acceleration greater than 4 to 6 G causes **"blackout" of vision** within a few seconds and unconsciousness shortly thereafter.
   - If this great degree of acceleration is continued, the person will die.

Effects on Vertebrae. Extremely high acceleratory forces can cause **fracture of vertebrae**, when exerted for even for a fraction of a second. The degree of positive acceleration that the average **person can withstand** in the sitting position before vertebral fracture occurs is **about 20 G.**

Effects of Negative G

The effects of negative G on the body is experienced, when body is accelerated towards earth faster. An aviator can usually go through outside loops up to negative acceleratory forces of **–4 to –5 G** without causing much permanent harm, although intense **temporary hyperaemia** of the head usually occurs. Occasionally, **psychotic disturbances** lasting for 15 to 20 minutes occur as a result of **brain edema**.

However, if negative G forces is so great (–20 G, for instance) and centrifugation of the blood into the head is more, the cerebral blood pressure reaches 300 to 400 mm Hg, sometimes causing **small vessels on the surface of the head and in the brain to rupture**.

But, usually, the intracranial vessels **withstand rupture** due to following reason:

- When blood is centrifuged toward the cranial vessels, simultaneously the cerebrospinal fluid is also centrifuged toward the head. This greatly increases the pressure of the cerebrospinal fluid. **Increased CSF pressure** acts as a cushioning buffer on the outside of the brain vessels and prevents the intracerebral vascular rupture.
- As the eyes are not protected by the cranium, **intense hyperaemia occurs** in eyes during strong negative G.
- As a result, temporarily the person is ***blinded with eyes often becoming red***, the condition called **the "red-out" of vision.**
- This problem, is usually faced during a parachute jump and if there is a faster decent to the earth.

However, during air flight as the person sits in the pressurized cabins, the effects of positive and negative G are not much experienced.

SPACE PHYSIOLOGY

Foundation of space physiology was laid in the 1970s, with three sequential **Skylab missions** of increasing duration (28, 56, and 84 days) happened, each mission with three astronauts, and enough data were collected to understand the problems of spacecraft. There were reports of negative calcium balance with bone density loss, muscle atrophy, cardiovascular and hemodynamic changes, metabolic, endocrine, and sleep disturbances, and space physicians concluded that astronauts undergo **rapid senescence** in space. However, there were rapid recoveries from these changes after coming back to earth.

As there is no atmosphere in outer space, an **artificial atmosphere is produced** in a spacecraft for the astronauts. The oxygen concentration inside the cabin must be kept high enough and the carbon dioxide concentration low enough to prevent suffocation. In modern space shuttle, gases equal to those in normal air are used, with four times as much nitrogen as oxygen and a total pressure of 760 mm Hg. The presence of nitrogen in the mixture greatly diminishes the likelihood of fire and explosion.

The problems in the space are due to weightlessness or microgravity and exposure to high external radiation.

Weightlessness and Microgravity

A person in an orbiting satellite or a nonpropelled spacecraft experiences **weightlessness,** or a state of **near-zero G force**, which is sometimes called **microgravity.** That is, the person is not drawn toward the bottom, sides, or top of the spacecraft but simply **floats inside its chamber**.

- The cause of this is not failure of gravity to pull on the body because gravity from any nearby heavenly body is still active.
- Rather, the gravity acts on both the spacecraft and the person at the same time so that **both are pulled with exactly the same acceleratory forces and in the same direction.** For this reason, the person simply is not attracted toward any specific wall of the spacecraft.

Problems are Related to Duration of Weightlessness

If the period of weightlessness is not too long, the physiologic problems of weightlessness will not be of much significance. However, if is chronic for more than months, problems are likely to occur. Problems are mainly due to **three effects of weightlessness**:

1. **Motion sickness** during the first few days of travel
2. **Translocation of fluids** within the body because of **failure of gravity** to maintain normal hydrostatic pressure.
3. **Diminished physical activity**, as there is no strength of muscle contraction needed to oppose the force of gravity.

In first days of space travel, more than 50 percent of astronauts experience motion sickness, with nausea and s vomiting, which is probably due to an **unfamiliar pattern of motion signals** arriving in the equilibrium centers of the brain, and simultaneously there are lack of gravitational signals.

The **major effects** of prolonged stay in space could be:

1. Decrease in blood volume
2. Decrease in red blood cell mass.
3. Decrease in muscle strength and work capacity
4. Decrease in maximum cardiac output
5. Loss of calcium and phosphate from the bones and loss of bone mass.

Such problems are often observed in people who are bed ridden for an extended period of time. In astronauts, in addition to **lack of exercise**, the is **lack of effect of gravity on the body**, especially on musculoskeletal system. Hence, specialized exercise programs are carried out by astronauts during prolonged stationing in the shuttle during space missions.

N.B.: The details of effects of microgravity on body systems are described in 'Comprehensive Textbook of Medical Physiology' 2nd Edition (2019), by GK Pal, Jaypee Publication.

Exam Questions

1. Define +G and −G. Describe the effects of microgravity on body systems.

Multiple Choice Questions

1. **Microgravity can produce all of the following cardiovascular effects, EXCEPT:**
   A. Decreased heart rate
   B. Decreased mean arterial pressure
   C. Decreased systemic vascular resistance
   D. Decreased vascular permeability
2. **Microgravity can produce all of the following effects on eye and vision, EXCEPT:**
   A. Decreased near sight when exposed for few days
   B. Decreased intraocular pressure
   C. Swollen and bent optic nerve sheath
   D. Decreased visual acuity
3. **Which of the following statements is TRUE?**
   A. Positive G is exerted when a person sitting in an aircraft accelerates towards earth faster than gravity
   B. Positive G is when +1G is applied to the body
   C. When –3G applied to the body becomes –2G, it is called positive G
   D. Positive G forces are anything that exceeds 1G
4. **All of the following can be features of positive G, except:**
   A. Black out of vision B. Brain edema
   C. Fracture of vertebrae D. Decreased diastolic blood pressure
5. **All of the following can be features of negative G, except:**
   A. Red out of vision
   B. Increased CSF pressure
   C. Rupture of small vessels in the brain
   D. Fracture of vertebrae
6. **Staying at space station for prolonged period can result in:**
   A. Decreased nitric oxide release
   B. Decreased activation of renin-angiotensin system:
   C. Decrease in type H cells
   D. Increase in osteoprogenitor cells
7. **Staying at space station for prolonged period can result in all of** the following, except:
   A. Decreased osteocalcin level
   B. Increased ADH release
   C. Decreased osteoclastic activity
   D. Decrease in oxygen consumption
8. **All of the following are effects of radiation injury, EXCEPT:**
   A. Disseminated intravascular coagulation
   B. Decreased white blood cell count
   C. Decreased blood vessel density
   D. Decreased reactive oxygen species generation

Answers

1. D 2. B 3. D 4. B 5. D 6. C
7. C 8. D

Chapter 135

PY7.5

Principles of Acid-Base Homeostasis

Learning Objectives

On completion of study of this chapter:

The student will be able to (must know):

1. Define pH, pK, acid, alkali and buffer, and have a basic concept of acid-base balance.
2. Name the buffer systems of the body and give their mechanism of buffering.
3. Briefly describe the regulation of acid-base balance.
4. Learn the basics of metabolic acidosis & alkalosis and respiratory acidosis & alkalosis.

The student may also be able to (desirable to know):

1. Describe the details of acid-base balance of the body.
2. Describe the physiological abnormalities in acid-base disorders.

GENERAL CONCEPT

The pH of body fluids is maintained within a **narrow range** as blood pH is maintained between **7.35 to 7.45.**

- This is due to **fine adjustment between production of acids and bases and their disposal** from the body.
- The balance is due to integrated functions of **buffer systems** that are mainly executed by **lungs and kidneys**.
- Therefore, *pulmonary and renal dysfunctions invariably lead to acid-base abnormalities.*

In the present chapter, we shall give a brief outline of acid-base physiology, core concepts of acid-base homeostasis and basic pathophysiology of acid-base disorders. However, for details of acid-base balance, a textbook of biochemistry may be referred.

Definitions

The pH: The pH of a solution is defined **as negative logarithm of the hydrogen ion concentration** in the solution.

The pK and K_a: The pK is defined as **negative logarithm of the ionization constant of an acid** (K_a) in a solution. The pK is the pH at which the concentration of acid and its conjugate bases are in equal proportion for a buffer. The lower the pK, the stronger is the acid.

The Acid and Alkali: Acid is defined as a substance that adds H^+ to the body fluids and alkali or base is defined as a substance that removes H^+ from the body fluids.

The Buffer: A pH buffer of a solution is defined as a **system of weak acid and its salt conjugate base or a weak base and its conjugate acid that minimizes the change in the pH of the solution within a narrow range** when a strong acid or base is added to it.

Concept of Acid-Base Balance

Acids and bases are generated continuously in the body. There are also mechanisms that buffer (trap and neutralize) the acids and bases. Hence, the balance between acid and base is accomplished by maintaining the equilibrium between their production in the body and removal from the body.

- Acid base balance is achieved through the **coordinated functions of kidneys and lungs**.
- ***Various metabolisms*** in the body add acids to the body fluids.
- Also, ***skeletal muscles*** add acid to the body during exercise in anaerobic conditions.
- The various **types of acids produced in our body are** carbonic acid, sulfuric acid, phosphoric acid, lactic acid etc.

Volatile vs. Nonvolatile Acids: In adults, acid or base added to the body fluids is **determined primarily by the diet**.

1. In a normal diet, approximately 15 to 20 mole of acid is added daily, which is converted into carbon dioxide. Therefore, this acid is called **volatile acid**.
   - The CO_2 produced by metabolism is removed through expired air.
   - Therefore, the effect of CO_2 on body and especially on acid base balance is well coordinated.
2. **The normal processes of metabolism such as oxidation of sulfur containing amino acids, incomplete oxidation of energy substrates (lactic acid by glycolysis, ketoacid by fatty acid beta oxidation etc) and oxidation of these intermediates (gluconeogenesis of lactate, ketone body oxidation etc) all together produce large amount of acids that cannot be removed** by lungs.
   - Therefore, these acids are called as **nonvolatile acid**.
   - The nonvolatile acid is handled by kidney.
3. Typically, **diets rich in proteins** such as meat, fish and milk produce acid more than base.

The pH-Buffer Systems PY1.7

The pH of a fluid system is protected and stabilized by action of buffers. A pH buffer in a solution is the one that minimizes the alteration in pH produced when an acid or a base is added to the solution. A buffer is mixture of weak acid and a salt of its conjugate base or a weak base and the salt of its conjugate acid. The efficiency of buffer system is explained by the **Henderson-Hasselbalch equation** (described in 1908), which is:

$HA \leftrightarrow H^+ + A^-$

According to Henderson-Hasselbalch equation, in a buffer system, the undissociated acid (HA) is in equilibrium when its concentration of anion equals the concentration of cations. At equilibrium, the rate of dissociation of an acid to form $H^+ + A^-$ and the rate of association to from H^+ and A^- to from HA are equal. The **dissociation constant** (K_a) or equilibrium constant is the product of cations and anions divided by undissociated acid, i. e.,

$$K_a = \frac{H^+ \times A^-}{HA}$$

The strength of an acid is **determined by of the level of K_a**. The ***higher the dissociation constant, stronger is the acid*** as it is more ionized. This is because the magnitude of acidity depends on concentration of free H^+ in the solution. The examples of strong acids are hydrochloric acid, phosphoric acid, nitric acid and sulfuric acid. Weak acids have low K_a and ionize slowly. Examples of weak acids are lactic acid, carbonic acid, ammonium and dihydrogen phosphate. Whenever, an acid of higher strength than HA is added to the system, the H^+ concentration is raised.

The value of a buffer is expressed in terms of β units. **One β unit** is the amount of base or acid required to bring the change of pH by about one unit.

- If the concentration of acid and base are equal for a buffer then its pH is equal to its pK.
- A good buffer resists the changes in pH in the interval of ± 1 pH unit of its pK. That is why the pK value of a good buffer **should be near to body pH** value.
- For effective buffering, the **ratio of acid to base should be 1:10** or **base to acid be 10:1**. Buffers are more effective at higher concentrations. For example, a 10 mmol/L buffer solution is far more effective compared to 1 mmol/L of the same buffer solution.

There are **four buffer systems** in our body:

1. Bicarbonate-carbonic acid buffer system
2. Plasma protein buffer system
3. Phosphate buffer system
4. Hemoglobin buffer system

The **first three act mainly in the extra-cellular fluid** and the **last two and first one act in the intracellular fluid**, especially in red cells.

Bicarbonate-Carbonic Acid Buffer System

This is the most important buffer system **of the plasma**. It is also a buffer **in red cells**. This buffer is the main buffer system in plasma. Though **its pK is 6.1** and **ratio of base to acid in plasma is 20:1**, it is an effective plasma buffer due to its high concentration (>20 mmol/L). Also this system works effectively in conjunction with lungs to retain or eliminate acid in terms of CO_2 whenever required.

Buffering by bicarbonate system depends on:

1. Removal or retention of acid via lungs in the form of carbon dioxide, and
2. Titration of nonvolatile acids by the bicarbonates in the renal tubules.

In plasma, the partial pressure of carbon dioxide is relatively constant so that it can be expelled or retained in body via lungs. The HCO_3^--H_2CO_3 buffer system easily generates or assimilates it and therefore resists the change in the pH.

Plasma Protein Buffer System

This accounts for **95% of non-bicarbonate buffers in plasma**. The albumin component of plasma protein acts as the buffer.

- The **histidine residue** of albumin is responsible for its buffering action.
- As the pK value of histidine is 7.3, albumin (each albumin molecule contains 16 histidine residues) acts as an **excellent buffer at physiological pH** of blood.
- For each molecule of bicarbonate ion generated, one molecule of non-bicarbonate buffer disappears.
- Therefore, **non-bicarbonate buffer is essential to maintain the bicarbonate concentration**.

Phosphate Buffer System

Phosphate buffer system has both organic and inorganic components.

Organic Component: The organic phosphate is the **major buffer system in the intracellular fluid.**

It consists of AMP, ADP, ATP, and 2,3-DPG.

- As 2,3-DPG is more in red cells, it accounts for about 15% of the non-bicarbonate buffer system in RBC.

Inorganic Component: Inorganic component of the phosphate buffer consists of **disodium hydrogen phosphate** (Na_2HPO_4) and **sodium dihydrogen phosphate** (NaH_2PO_4) with a ratio of 4:1.

- The pK value is 6.8. Though, it represents only 5% of the non-bicarbonate buffer system in plasma, *in the intracellular fluid its buffering contribution is appreciable.* Phosphate buffer plays important role especially in the renal tubule in **acidification of urine**.

Hemoglobin Buffer System

This is the non-bicarbonate buffer that plays a **major buffering role in red cells.**

- Out of total **buffering load in red cells**, it accounts for **approximately 85%,** and rest 15% is by 2,3-DPG, which is a phosphate buffer.
- The **histidine residue in Hb** is responsible for its buffering action.
- In lungs, with oxygenation of Hb, the H^+ ion is liberated and buffering capacity of Hb is decreased due to the decrease in pK value. However, when O_2 is released from oxyhemoglobin complex in the tissue, Hb binds to H^+ and forms HHb, a weaker acid.

REGULATION OF ACID BASE BALANCE

Two major mechanisms in the body regulate acid base balance: respiratory mechanism and renal mechanism.

Respiratory Mechanism

The respiratory mechanism is mainly operated by change in the rate and depth of respiration in response to the inputs from **central and peripheral chemoreceptors**. Chemoreceptors respond to acid base imbalance immediately.

1. **During acidosis**, bicarbonate ions are sequestered. The carbonate salt formed from it gets converted into carbon dioxide.
    - Thus, pCO_2 increases in plasma.
    - The decrease in plasma pH or the increase in pCO_2 is sensed by peripheral chemoreceptors.
2. The central receptors sense change in pH of CSF.
    - Chemoreceptor stimulation in turn **stimulates respiratory center that produces hyperventilation** and subsequent *expulsion of excess CO_2*.
    - This decreases pCO_2, and fall in pCO_2 is rapidly equilibrated across blood brain barrier.
3. The CSF pH increases. Till CSF pH returns to normal it takes time for the respiration to become normal.

Renal Mechanism

Kidneys maintain acid base balance by reabsorbing the filtered HCO_3^- and by excreting the non-volatile acid produced by metabolism. The details of handling of acid and base by kidney tubules and and acidification of urine are describes in Chapter 91.

ABNORMALITIES OF ACID BASE BALANCE

Failure of acid-base balance could either lead to acidosis or alkalosis.

Acidosis occurs as a result of increased addition of acid or decreased removal of acid or an increased loss in base.

Alkalosis occurs as a result of increased addition of base or decreased removal of base or an increased loss of acid. Alkalosis represents elevated arterial pH, and an increased pCO_2 that occurs due to the subsequent compensatory alveolar hypoventilation to reduce the pH. Usually, alkalosis is due to failure of kidneys to excrete bicarbonate at their normal capacity.

Abnormalities of acid-base balance are typically classified into **four groups**.

1. Metabolic acidosis
2. Respiratory acidosis
3. Metabolic alkalosis
4. Respiratory alkalosis

The summary of primary changes and compensatory responses in these four acid-base disorders are summarized in Table 135.1. Their details are given in respective chapters of kidney and respiratory physiology.

Table 135.1 | Differences in primary and compensatory changes in various types of acid base disorders.

Acid-base disorder	Primary changes	Final compensatory changes
Metabolic acidosis	Decrease in the concentration of bicarbonate ion	Decrease in the partial pressure of CO_2
Metabolic alkalosis	Increase in the concentration of of bicarbonate ion	Increase in the partial pressure of CO_2
Respiratory acidosis (Acute form)	Increase in the partial pressure of CO_2	Increase in the concentration of bicarbonate ion by 1 mmol/L for each 10mm Hg rise in pCO_2

Table 135.1 contd...		
Respiratory acidosis (Chronic form)	Increase in the partial pressure of CO_2	Increase in the concentration of bicarbonate ion by 3.5 mmol/L for each 10mm Hg rise in pCO_2
Respiratory alkalosis (Acute form)	Decrease in the partial pressure of CO_2	Decrease in the concentration of bicarbonate ion by 2 mmol/L for each 10mm Hg fall in pCO_2
Respiratory alkalosis (Chronic form)	Decrease in the partial pressure of CO2	Decrease in the concentration of bicarbonate ion by 5 mmol/L for each 10mm Hg fall in CO2

Exam Questions

1. Describe the mechanisms of acid-base homeostasis. Add a note on metabolic acidosis.

Multiple Choice Questions

1. In metabolic acidosis, which of the following changes are seen

Increased K^+ excretion
Decreased K^+ excretion
Increased Na^+ excretion
Increased Na^+ reabsorption

2. Which of the following is the most effective buffer system of the body?

A. Plasma protein
B. Phosphate
C. Hemoglobin
D. Bicarbonate-carbonic acid

3. Presence of which of the following is responsible for the buffering action of Hb?

A. Histidine B. Valine
C. Serine D. Leucine

4. Causes of metabolic alkalosis include the following, EXCEPT:

A. Prolonged vomiting
B. Continuous gastric aspiration
C. Hyperventilation
D. Ingestion of antacids

5. Which of the following conditions will produce high anion gap acidosis?

A. Diarrhea B. Renal tubular acidosis
C. Renal failure D. Ureterosigmoidostomy

6. Metabolic alkalosis is characterized by:

A. High hydrogen ion concentration in plasma
B. Increased pCO2
C. Elevated chloride level in serum
D. Low potassium level

7. Which of the following parameters indicate compensated state in a case of respiratory alkalosis?

A. High pCO2
B. Low anion gap
C. Low bicarbonate
D. Low potassium level

8. Causes of respiratory alkalosis include the following, EXCEPT:

A. Chronic obstructive pulmonary disease
B. Hyperthyroidism
C. High altitude
D. Hyperpyrexia

Answers

1. B 2. D 3. A 4. C 5. C 6. D 7. B 8. A

Chapter 136

Body Fluid Volume Homeostasis

Learning Objectives

On completion of study of this chapter:

The student will be able to (must know):

1. Understand the mechanisms of water balance of the body.
2. Understand the control of volume is important for homeostasis.

WATER BALANCE

Control of volume of body fluids is directly linked with water balance of the body. Therefore, before discussing regulation of body fluid volumes, first let us understand the mechanism of *water balance*. Normally, water balance is achieved by matching the water gain with water loss.

Water Gain

Body gains water from **two sources**: exogenous and endogenous.

Exogenous Water Gain

Exogenous water gain occurs mainly by two processes: drinking of water and water ingested with food. The exogenous water intake normally ranges from 2 to 10 liters per day.

Water Drinking

Drinking of water is the major form of water gain.

- It ranges from **0.5 to 8 liters /day** depending mainly upon the environmental conditions. Fluid drinking is more in hot and humid weathers, and less in cold climate.
- However, social and personal habits considerably influence this.
- Water intake is mainly controlled by the **thirst centers in the brain**. Change in plasma volume and osmolality influences thirst center and control water ingestion.

Ingestion of Water in Food

Water is a major constituent of foodstuffs. Water is present in all food preparations and fruits. Though water content of food is highly variable, it is present in high quantity in liquid preparations such as soup, dal, rasam, sambar, mohr, fish curry, vegetable curries etc.

- However, social habits and personal preferences contribute to it.
- On average, water ingested in food (in break fast, lunch, snacks and dinner) varies from **1 to 5 liters per day**.

Endogenous Water Gain

Water is one of the ***products of metabolism*** (other products are ATP, CO_2 and temperature). During the process of tissue oxidation, *water is continuously produced* in the body and this endogenous production of water accounts for 300–500 ml of water added per day to the body fluids.

Water Loss

Water loss from the body occurs mainly in four forms: urine, feces, sweat and as insensible loss.

Loss in Urine

Urinary loss of water is a major form of water output from the body. About **one liter of water is excreted** from the body in urine per day. However, this varies with liquid intake, environmental conditions and salt intake.

- Kidney plays important role in water balance by altering water excretion in urine, which primarily depends on the **concentration of ADH in plasma**.
- ADH contributes to urine volume that may vary from 0.5 to 18 L/day.
- This **indirectly determines urine osmolality**, which varies from **50 to 1200 mOsm/kg H_2O** with the corresponding change in urine volume.
- Osmolality of tubular fluid also decides water output in urine. Increased tubular fluid osmolality as occurs in diabetes mellitus increases urinary water loss.

Fecal Loss

Normally, about **200 ml of water per day** is excreted in feces. The ingested water is mainly absorbed in the intestine.

- Increased absorption of water leads to constipation and decreased absorption causes diarrhea.
- In diarrhea, water is also lost in vomiting.

Loss in Sweat

Water is routinely lost from the body in the form of sweat. Sweating is greatly influenced by **environmental temperature and the level of physical activity**.

- The rate of sweat production per day is about 0.1 L at ambient temperature of 23°C, 1.5 L at 38°C and 5 L at 45°C.
- Exercise in hot weather increases water loss in sweating.

Insensible Water Loss

In addition to loss in sweating, water is continuously **evaporated from the skin surface**.

- Water is also continuously evaporated from respiratory passage in breathing.
- These losses constitute the insensible water loss.

Positive and Negative Water Balance

The net water gain or loss leads to alteration in many physiological functions as it produces increase or decrease in volume of fluid compartments and accordingly produces dilution or concentration of body fluids.

1. **Positive water balance** occurs when *water gain is more than its loss*. This causes hemodilution, therefore, decreases in osmolality of plasma, decreases red cell count and produces hyponatremia.
2. **Negative water balance** occurs when *water loss is more than its gain*. This leads to dehydration and causes hemoconcentration. It increases plasma osmolality. Due to hemoconcentration, there is relative increase in red cell count.

Factors Influencing Water Balance

Water intake and output are controlled mainly by **two factors**: plasma osmolality and blood volume.

Plasma Osmolality

Plasma osmolality is an important factor for water balance. Alteration in osmolality is detected **by osmoreceptors in hypothalamus** that stimulates thirst. Increased plasma osmolality is also a primary stimulus for ADH secretion.

Factors that Affect Plasma Osmolality: Plasma osmolality depends on the presence of osmotically active molecules in plasma, especially ***NaCl, proteins and glucose***. Among them, most effective in influencing osmolality is NaCl. However, abnormal increase in protein and glucose in plasma also exerts considerable osmotic effect.

Blood Volume

Alteration in blood volume is detected by **volume receptors** in atria that send impulses to hypothalamus and pituitary **to secrete ADH**. However, *increased osmolality is a better stimulus than hypovolemia* for stimulation of thirst and ADH secretion.

Factors that Affect Blood Volume: Blood volume depends on the **plasma volume and the hematocrit**. Increase in water content of plasma causes plasma expansion and increase in cell count, especially red cell count increases blood volume. Conversely, in opposite conditions, blood volume decreases.

EFFECTIVE CIRCULATING VOLUME

Effective circulatory volume (ECV) is the blood volume in the arterial system that causes effective perfusion of the tissues. This is also called **effective blood volume**. This excludes the stagnated blood present in some visceral organs and inactive muscles, which does not participate in perfusion. The pressure in the circulation that helps in this perfusion is called *effective perfusion pressure*. Approximately 20% of blood volume forms the ECV. The ECV is monitored by the volume sensors located entirely within the vascular tree.

1. **In physiological conditions**, ECV reflects the ECF volume and arterial volume, and ECV contributes to cardiac output and arterial pressure. Change in volume of ECF, changes vascular volume and therefore, **changes ECV, cardiac output and arterial pressure**.
2. **In pathological conditions,** in which expansion of ECF is the major pathophysiological change of the disease as occur in congestive heart failure, nephrotic syndrome and hepatic cirrhosis, the ECV does not completely depend on ECF volume. In such conditions, inspite of expansion of ECF volume, *ECV may remain normal or*

even reduced. Kidneys sense change in ECV not ECF, therefore, decrease in ECV causes renal retention of Na^+ and H_2O that further aggravates fluid accumulation and **edema formation.** ECV and Na^+ balance are closely linked. Therefore, retention of Na^+ causes expansion of ECV and depletion of Na^+ contraction of ECV.

Volume Sensors

Volume sensors or ***ECV sensors*** are volume receptors located in the vascular tree that respond to stretch of the vessel wall. These are basically the vascular baroreceptors that are generally classified into two categories: low pressure baroreceptors and high-pressure baroreceptors.

Low-Pressure Volume Receptors: are located in low pressure side of circulation, especially in atria, and pulmonary vasculature.

High-Pressure Volume Receptors: are present in high-pressure compartment of circulation. These receptors include the baroreceptors present in carotid sinus, aortic arch and left ventricle.

Volume sensors are also present in liver (hepatic volume receptors), brain (central nervous system Na^+ sensors) and in JG apparatus.

Effects of Stimulation of Volume Receptors

Low-pressure volume receptors respond ***mainly to fullness of vascular tree***, i. e. vascular volume. Afferents from these receptors travel in vagus nerve and terminate in nucleus tractus solitarius (NTS) in the medulla. Fibers also contact ADH secreting neurons in posterior pituitary. Therefore, stimulation of these receptors leads to:

1. Sympathetic activation and
2. ADH release.

High-pressure volume receptors respond ***primarily to the arterial pressure***. Afferents from these receptors from carotid sinus and aortic arch travel in 9th and 10th cranial nerves to terminate in NTS in medulla. They inhibit sympathetic discharge and activate vagal output.

Stimulation of receptors of JG apparatus ***activates the renin-angiotensin mechanism***. Activation of hepatic sensors, regulate gastrointestinal Na^+ absorption and stimulation of CNS Na^+ receptors, may be located in the hypothalamus regulate renal sympathetic nerve activity.

Exam Questions

1. Describe the mechanism of water balance of the body. Add a note on volume sensors.

Multiple Choice Questions

1. **Which of the following are true about body water?**
   A. Water constitutes 60% of the body weight
   B. Plasma volume constitutes 10% of the total body water
   C. ECF volume can be determined by dilution methods
   D. 10% is intracellular water
2. **Which of the following is true statement about ion composition in body?**
   A. Intracellular & Extra cellular ions compositions are same
   B. Phosphorus & Mg^{++} are major ions intracellularly
   C. Na^+, Cl^- principal ions in E.C.F
   D. Kidney tightly regulates Na^+, K^+, Cl^- compositions
3. **True statement regarding extracellular fluid to intracellular fluid is:**
   A. ECF is rich K^+
   B. ECF is more than ICF
   C. ECF is rich in organic anion
   D. High Na^+:K^+ ratio is seen
4. **Normal plasma osmolality is:**
   A. 250 – 270 mOsm/Kg H_2O
   B. 260 – 280 mOsm/Kg H_2O
   C. 280 – 295mOsm/Kg H_2O
   D. 290 – 310 mOsm/Kg H_2O
5. **Daily loss of water from skin in absence of sweating (insensible water loss) per day is:**
   A. 1 litre B. 1.5 litres
   C. 200-300 ml D. 500-700 ml
6. **Hyponatremia refers to plasma sodium less than (mEq/l):**
   A. 154 B. 145 C. 140 D. 135
7. **True about free water clearance is:**
   A. Regulated by ADH B. Regulated by aldosterone
   C. Increased by furosemide D. None of the above
8. **All of the following statements are correct about potassium balance, EXCEPT:**
   A. Most of potassium is intracellular
   B. Three quarter of the total body potassium is found in skeletal muscle
   C. Intracellular potassium is released into extracellular space in response to severe injury
   D. Acidosis leads to movements of potassium from extracellular to intracellular fluid compartment
9. **Which of the following is not a cause of hyperkalemia?**
   A. Hemolysis
   B. Metabolic acidosis
   C. Renal failure
   D. Primary hyperaldosteronism
10. **All of the following are causes of hypokalemia, EXEPT:**
    A. Metabolic alkalosis
    B. Starvation
    C. Adrenal insufficiency
    D. Insulin therapy

Answers

1. A	2. B	3. D	4. C	5. C	6. D
7. A	8. D	9. D	10. C		

Chapter 137

Growth and Development, Physiology of Stress and Aging

Learning Objectives

<u>On completion of study of this chapter:</u>

The student will be able to (must know):

1. Draw a schematic diagram of growth curve.
2. List the factors that regulate growth and behavioral aspects of development.
3. Learn the assessment of psychological development.
4. Understand the physiology of stress and how stress causes disease.
5. Understand the physiological basis of different types of dwarfisms.
6. Describe the theories of aging.

The student may also be able to (desirable to know):

1. Describe the physiology of growth and development.
2. Describe the physiology of stress.

The terms growth and development are closely and mutually dependent. generally, **growth** refers to increase in the physical size, as the infant grows into childhood and then into adulthood, whereas **development** refers to the maturation, which is the improvement in the capacity of the organ systems and body parts.

GROWTH AND DEVELOPMEMNT **PY11.6**

Though there is a usual **pattern of growth** for the whole body in general, different parts of the body do not follow a uniform pattern of growth. Especially, **growth pattern is different for gonadal, neural and lymphoid tissues**. Accordingly, the growth curves are different for these different body tissues.

General Growth Curve **PY11.9**

General growth is the growth of the body as a whole, which include increase in height and weight, and growth of the musculoskeletal, cardiovascular, respiratory, gastrointestinal, endocrine and excretory systems.

- Though the growth rate is different at different stages of life, there are **two periods of rapid growth**.
- The period of rapid growth is called **growth spurt**.

The two general growth spurts are **infantile** (during infancy) and **pubertal** (during late puberty) spurts.

Infantile Growth Spurt **PY11.10**

Height and weight are good indices of growth in infants and children. After few days of **initial weight-loss** following birth, the neonate gradually starts gaining weight.

- During infancy, **birth weight is almost doubled at sixth month** and increased to approximately **three times at one year of age**.
- In post-natal life, the height gain is maximal during first two years of life, which is about 25 cm per year.
- Then, height gain almost decreases speedily to 5–10 cm per year for next 8–10 years (Fig. 137.1).

Physiology During Neonatal Period and Infancy

Immediately after birth many cardiovascular and respiratory changes occur to adopt to the environment outside the uterus. The details are described in Chapter 40. Behavioral development is described below.

- The neuronal development occurs maximally during first year of life. Therefore, nutritional deficiency in infancy leads to mental retardation.
- Visceral development is also faster in infancy.

Pubertal Growth Spurt

Full pubertal development ranges between **12–18 years of life.**

- Weight gain is rapid during this period, which occurs at about **3 to 4 kg gain per year between 12 and 18 years of age.**

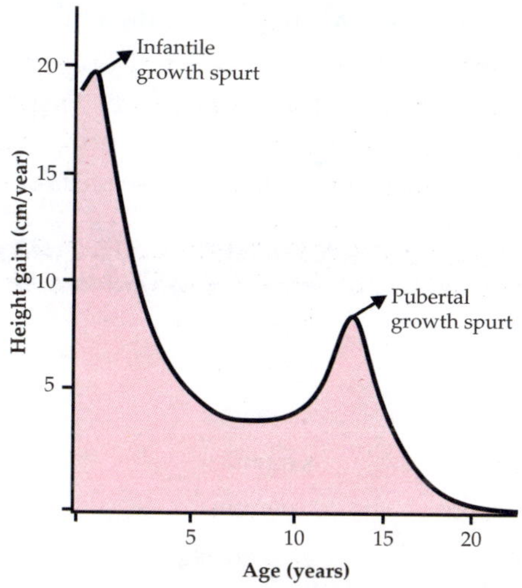

Fig. 137.1: Percentage increase in height till young adulthood.

- During puberty, **rapid growth occurs in the musculoskeletal system**. Therefore, both height and weight increase during the period.
- Height gain increases from its **prepubertal 5 cm/year** to about **10 cm per year during puberty**.
- Growth spurt appears 2 to 3 years earlier in girls. Cessation of height-gain occurs immediately after puberty due to **closure of epiphysis induced by sex hormones**.

Neural Growth Curve

Neural growth includes the growth of brain, spinal cord, and eye.

1. These organs grow rapidly during infancy.
2. In first year of postnatal life, the brain attains about 70% of the adult size (Fig. 137.2). Rest 30% growth occurs in next 3 to 5 years to attain fully developed size by 5th to 6th year of life.
3. The head circumference increases proportionately in first year and then in next 5 years of age.

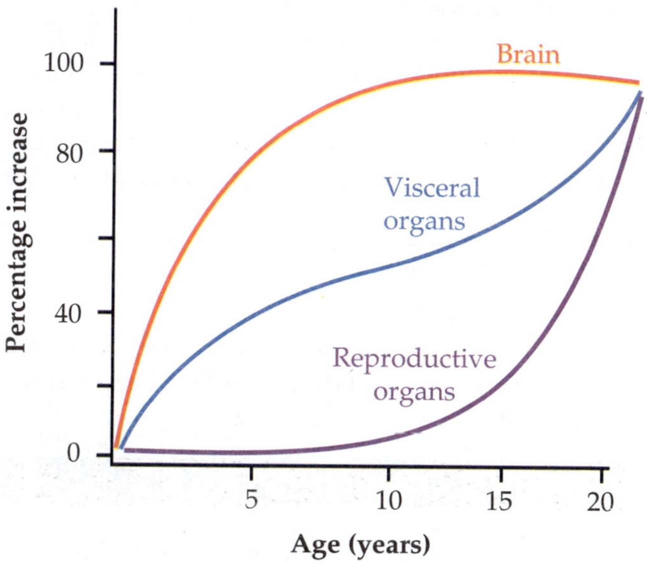

Fig. 137.2: Percentage increase in height till young adulthood.

Gonadal Growth Curve

The reproductive organs, especially gonads and accessory sex organs remain rudimentary throughout childhood. They start growing at puberty and rapidly **between 14 to 18 years of age**.

Lymphoid Growth Curve

Lymphoid tissues grow very rapidly during infancy and childhood. Lymphoid organs include lymph nodes, spleen, tonsils, adenoids, thymus and lymphatic tissues of the intestine.

1. At puberty, these organs undergo partial involution.
2. The tonsils and adenoids attain maximum size **at the age of 6–10 years**.
3. Though tonsillitis is common in children, a surgeon should not be tempted to remove these structures surgically just based on their big size.

Regulation of Growth

Patterns of growth and development vary between races and communities. However, the important factors affecting growth are: hormonal, nutritional, social, environmental and genetic factors.

Hormonal Factors

The important hormones which affect the growth and development are: **Growth hormone, insulin-like growth factor, thyroxine, gonadal hormones and insulin.**

Details of these hormones on growth have been described in the respective chapters in Section VIII (Endocrine physiology).

Nutritional Factors

Growth of tissues depends on the supply and utilization of all ingredients of nutrition. Proteins, fats, carbohydrates, vitamins, minerals and trace elements are essential components of **balanced diet** and contribute to growth and development in various ways.

1. Though proteins are the building blocks for tissues, others are cementing substance. Therefore, for optimal growth, all are equally important.
2. **Nutritional requirement is therefore more during active periods of growth**. Nutritional deficiency during childhood is the commonest cause of growth retardation in developing countries.
3. In children, growth becomes faster after a period of food deprivation (Application Box 137.1)

Application Box 137.1

Catch-up growth: In children, following a period of illnesses or starvation, the rate of growth becomes faster than normal. This accelerated growth aims at catching up the level of growth prior to illness. Therefore, it is called catch-up growth. However, the exact mechanism of catch-up growth is not known.

Environmental Factors

Environmental **temperature and humidity, light-dark cycle and altitude** have considerable effects on growth development. The people living in temperate zone have small height and less built than people living at normal temperature and sunlight.

Social Factors

Social factors play important role in growth and development during childhood. Not only physical growth, but also psychological growth takes place during the formative years of development. **Proper love and care** from parents and relatives are very essential for mental development of a child. **Harmony in the family** is very crucial in this development. Quarrels between parents, divorce, family disturbances and economic deficiency are causes of psychological abnormalities in children.

Genetic Factors

Irrespective of other factors, genetic inheritance is the major determinant of height and body constitution.

Behavioral Development

Behavioral development of a child depends on **environmental, social and genetic factors. Both physical and environmental factors** are essential behavioral attainment.

Aspects of Behavioral Development

Behavioral development can be divided into four aspects: motor, language, psychosocial and adaptive behaviors.

Motor Behavior: Motor behavior is the behavioral response that involves motor activities like change in posture, standing, walking etc.

- In infants, it starts with grasp reflex, and gets improved slowly with ability to walk and run (Table 137.1).

Language Behavior: Language is the best form of communication.

- It manifests with facial expression, phonation, vocalization of words, and formation of phrases or sentences.
- This needs coordinated functioning of speech apparatus with neural signals originating in speech areas.
- Speech is a **mixture of sensory and motor behavior**. It is greatly modified by social influences.

Psychosocial Behavior: Psychosocial development depends mainly on social and cultural environments and neurological maturation of the child.

- Emotional responses to environmental stimuli, control of bowel and bladder habits, proper sleeping, taking bath, ability to feed oneself and develop self-dependence are important milestones of psychosocial development.

Adaptive Behavior: Ability to adjust with different environmental situations includes not only psychosocial development, but also smoother sensory-motor coordination like hand-eye co-ordination that help to perform and protect in various adverse situations.

Table 137.1 | Chronology of development at childhood.

Milestones	Age
Raises head	3 months
Head stabilizes	4 months
Sits with support	5 months
Sits without support	7 months
Crawls on belly	7½ months
Crawls on knees and elbow	8 months
Stands with help	8½ months
Stands without help	1 year
Walks with support	1 year two months
Walks without support	1½ years

Measurement of Psychological Development

Mental and psychological developments are measured by developmental and intelligence quotients.

Developmental Quotient

Developmental quotient (DQ) is the **measure of developmental parameters with respect to age**. Development of adaptive and psychological behaviors compared with age of the child.

$$DQ = \frac{\text{Maturity age}}{\text{Chronological age}} \times 100$$

Intelligence Quotient

Intelligence quotient (IQ) measures the **intellectual abilities of a child**, which requires some degree of maturity of the mind. Usually, such mental maturity starts growing after the age of five. Therefore, IQ can be tested only after this age, whereas DQ can be tested at any age.

$$IQ = \frac{\text{Mental age}}{\text{Chronological age}} \times 100$$

Developmental Deficiencies

Developmental deficiencies at childhood lead to **dwarfism**. Details of different types of dwarfism have been described in the Chapter 71 'Growth Hormone'

PY8.5

PHYSIOLOGY OF STRESS

Stress is defined as any condition or type of a change that causes physical, emotional or psychological strain on the individual. It is a threat, real or implied, to the psychological or physiological integrity of an individual.

Stressor is a stimulus, condition or event that causes stress.

IMPORTANT NOTE

Allostasis: It is the processes of adaptation to acute stress, involving the output of stress hormones that act to restore homeostasis.

Allostatic load: It is the price that the body pays for being forced to respond to adverse psychological or physical situations.

Stress Triad: Hans Selye, the pioneer researcher on stress had demonstrated the **stress triad** consisting of, i) hyperemia and enlargement of the adrenals, ii) atrophy of the thymus and lymph nodes, and iii) hemorrhagic gastric erosions and ulcers.

General Adaptation Syndrome

Hans Selye's proposal of a general adaptation syndrome focused mainly on adrenal glands and the role of steroid. He demonstrated three distinct stages in the general adaptation syndrome.

1. **Alarm:** The period during which the stressor disrupts homeostasis.
2. **Resistance:** During this period, the body activates the responses to adjust to the stress.
3. **Exhaustion:** Failure of adaptation due to continued stress, especially if severe leads to tissue damage, disease, and even death.

It was proposed that many diseases are the product of a lack of an adaptive response or maladaptation.

Stress System

Types of Stress

Stress may be **acute** (short lived for minutes to hours), **subacute** (exists for a little more period, which could be for days) or **chronic** (sustained for a long period of time, may be for months and years).

Stressors

Stressors could be different kinds of events, situations, or stimuli. Broadly, stressors are of **three types**:

1. **Physical stressors:** Example are restraint, audiogenic stress, pain, hemorrhage, infection, etc.
2. **Psychological stressors:** This could be the failure to satisfy internal drives, failure to achieve or perform upto satisfaction, predator-related cues, aversive environmental stimuli, etc.
3. **Social stressors:** Such as death of a partner or a close relation, divorce, unemployment, etc.

Effects of Stress

The individuals respond differently to the same stress. This depends on the body's perception of stress and the response to stress.

Perception of Stress

The perception of physical stressors occurs in the **brainstem and hypothalamus**, and perception of psychological stressors occurs in the **prefrontal cortex and limbic system**. In addition, there are many **neuronal circuits** associated with each of the structures.

- The central nucleus of the amygdala is involved in autonomic response integration.
- The paraventricular nucleus of the hypothalamus is involved in the activation of hypothalamic-pituitary-adrenal (HPA) axis.
- The locus coeruleus is involved in sympathoadrenal medullary (SAM) activation.

Response to Stress

Two major systems involved in the response of the body to stress: sympathetic-adrenomedullary axis and hypothalamic-pituitary axis.

Sympathetic-Adrenomedullary Axis Activation: The brain structures involved in this system include among others, the locus coeruleus, the rostral ventrolateral medulla, and the paraventricular nucleus of the hypothalamus.

- Projections from these structures project to the preganglionic sympathetic neurons on intermediolateral grey matter in the thoracolumbar regions of the spinal cord.
  - Some of the presynaptic neurons **innervate the adrenal medulla** that secrets catecholamines, especially **adrenaline**.
- This effector system provides rapid but relatively **short-lived responses**.

Hypothalamic-Pituitary Axis Activation: The paraventricular nucleus of the hypothalamus secretes corticotropin-releasing hormone (CRH), oxytocin and vasopressin.

- CRH stimulates synthesis and release of adrenocorticotropic hormone (ACTH) from anterior pituitary.
- ACTH acts on the adrenal cortex and stimulates secretion of glucocorticoids.
- This hormonal response is relatively slow but more sustained .

General Effects

The activation of the sympathetic nervous system and the release of adrenaline from the adrenal medulla generally evokes the **fight-or-flight response**.

- This includes a mobilization of fuels, an increase in the rate and contractility of the heart, and an increased blood flow to skeletal muscle, among others.
- The immune system is activated.
- Cortisol increases the availability of substrates (glucose, free fatty acids, and amino acids) from their endogenous stores.

- Cortisol also stimulates appetite and increases food intake.

IMPORTANT NOTE

Chronic stress causes obesity, insulin resistance and suppression of immunity: Individuals subjected to high levels of cortisol for prolonged periods eat more, gain weight and increase their fat stores. They also develop insulin resistance that initiates metabolic and cardio-vascular disease. As cortisol has immunosuppressive effects, in chronic stress due to exposure to high levels of cortisol, immunity is inhibited.

Acute Stress and Eustress: Acute stress and eustress are **beneficial** as they activate the body and protect the body

Chronic and Severe Stress: Chronic and severe stress are **harmful** as they inhibit immunity and increase secretion of proinflammatory cytokines that damage the body (Clinical Note 137.1)

Clinical Note 137.1

Stress as cause of disease and promotes aging: Stress has been implicated in a large number of diseases. Individuals exposed to chronic stressful conditions may adopt unhealthy behavior and predispose themselves to cardiovascular diseases (hypertension, ischemic heart disease), exacerbation of asthma, obesity, and depression and anxiety, and even malignancy.

PY11.7

PHYSIOLOGY OF AGING

Theories of Aging

The biological **changes of aging** are clearer than the mechanisms that mediate it. The common changes include:

1. Chromosomal abnormalities
2. Increased DNA cross-linking
3. Increased frequency of single-strand breaks in DNA
4. Decrease in DNA methylation
5. Loss of DNA telomeric sequences.
6. Increased posttranslational changes in proteins.
7. Deamidation, oxidation, and nonenzymatic glycation of proteins.
8. Deformation in mitochondrial structure

Aging is **multifactorial**. There are many theories of aging that are not completely compatible in their explanation. However, they can be broadly divided into two categories: genetic theories and random damage theories.

Genetic Theories of Aging

Genetic theories of aging are based on **programmed senescence**, which means that at the time of birth the time of aging and death has been predetermined. That means the aging is preprogrammed by a biological timetable. Three genetic theories have been developed recently:

Mutation Theory

The first one is the mutation theory. Usually, animals die much before completion of their expected life span due to adverse effects of natural forces. Therefore, this theory suggests the importance of mutations that retards long survival. The mutations pile up in the genes that are transferred from generations to generations.

Theory of Pleiotropic Antagonism

The second one is the theory of pleiotropic antagonism, which proposes that aging is caused by the **harmful effects of genes**. These unfavorable genetic effects are preserved for the purpose of survival and these properties are imparted prior to reproduction.

Ecological Theory

The ecological theory applies to the ecological conditions **where external hazards** are less. In such favourable environments, the mutation is such that the aging process is retarded to allow the animal to reproduce and protect the offsprings.

Random Damage Theories

The random damage theories explain that the aging is due to the **loss of balance between ongoing damage and repair**. The continuous tissue damage in the body occurs due to constant production of free radicals, and by the processes of oxidation and glycation.

- However, the damage is immediately repaired by regenerating an anti-stress mechanisms. With advancement of age, especially after the age of 40 years, capacity to repair cells, tissues and organs decline.
- Regenerative senescence was also suggested to be due to the arrest of the cell cycles at the G_1/S phase.
- This is the phase in cell cycle at which synthesis of DNA starts. Thus DNA synthesis is impaired.

Role of Cell Replication

In recent times, the **length of telomeric DNA** has also been associated to cell replication. Telomeric DNA is present at the ends of chromosomes. Telomeric DNA has following important functions:

1. Prevents chromosomal instability.
2. Slows chromosomal fragmentation and rearrangement.
3. Anchors chromosomes to nuclear matrix.
4. Acts as a buffer between coding regions of DNA and the ends of the chromosomes.
5. It is also necessary for cell divisions.

There are about a total of 2000 base pairs of the telomere. During each cell division, approximately 50 base pairs are lost. Thus, cell division decreases length of telomeric DNA.

- **Telomeric shortening** causes loss of gene accessibility. Gene accessibility is necessary to repair the cell damage that occurs continuously by metabolic processes. Thus, **telomeric shortening slows the repair process.**

- Along with cytoplasmic factors that mediate arrest of DNA synthesis, telomeric shortening limits the ability of the cell to divide, which prevent replacement of cells that are lost by apoptosis.

In the past, **many mechanisms** have been postulated for aging. These are: **somatic mutation theory** which postulates that aging occurs due to cumulative spontaneous mutations, **the error catastrophe theory** which proposes that aging results from errors in the synthesis of proteins critical to the synthesis of genetic material, and **the intrinsic mutagenesis theory** which hypothesizes that aging is due to the intrinsic DNA rearrangements. However, *none of these theories have satisfied* the physiological bases of aging. However, calorie intake and free radicals are known to play important role in aging.

Role of Calorie Intake

Strongly implicated in aging is calorie consumption. Increased calorie intake after the age of 40 has been proved to facilitate aging. It has been observed that **calorie restriction delays the onset of aging**. The calorie restriction by about 30% of the total calorie intake has been documented to have following effects:

1. Increase in average life expectancy and maximum life span.
2. Delay in onset of age-associated diseases.
3. Decrease in deterioration of physiologic processes like immune responsiveness, glucose metabolism, muscle atrophy etc.
4. Influence on gene expression, protein turnover and cross-linking.

The impact of general calorie restriction is different from specific dietary restriction like restriction for fat etc. However, calorie restriction must be supplemented with vitamins and antioxidants to prevent aging.

Role of Free Radicals and Oxidative Stress

Due to metabolism, **free radicals** like peroxide and hydroxyl radicals are continuously produced in the body. These radicals damage the cells and tissues by the process of oxidation.

- The free radicals **damage DNA and proteins and cause peroxidation of lipids in the membranes**. This is called oxidative stress. However, simultaneously a scavenging system of antioxidants also exists in the body that neutralizes the toxic effects of free radicals.
- **Antioxidants** include glutathione, vitamin E, vitamin A and vitamin C. Oxidative stress becomes more when production of oxidants is more than the generation of antioxidants (for details of free radicals, see below). Oxidative stress promotes aging.

Atherosclerosis

Atherosclerosis is the process of narrowing of lumen of blood vessels due to **deposition of lipid materials on the inner endothelial lining of blood vessels**.

- Atherosclerosis is the physiological process that **starts almost at infancy**. In childhood, atherosclerosis starts in aorta and larger arteries. As age advances, atherosclerosis starts in smaller arteries and arterioles.
- Due to atherosclerosis, blood supply to organs and tissues of the body decreases that causes structural and functional degenerations. This is the **natural process of degeneration** (aging) and death.
- However, the process of degeneration is facilitated by **accelerated atherosclerosis** in which **fibrofatty plaques** are deposited in greater amount in the blood vessel lumen and hyperplasia of smooth muscle of blood vessels occur. This causes **premature aging** and death.

The **predisposing factors** for accelerated atherosclerosis are:

1. Hyperlipidemia (hypercholesterolemia, hypertriglyceridemia)
2. Obesity
3. Diabetes mellitus
4. Hypertension
5. Smoking
6. Excess eating (increased calorie intake) after 40 years of age
7. Chronic stress
8. Lack of exercise

Geriatric Changes

Though there is no clear-cut demarcation of age to say that the individual has entered into geriatric age group, usually age more than 60 years is considered for the purpose. The body physiology changes in geriatric age group. The increase in blood pressure, osteoporotic changes in bones, decreased digestive functions, decreased immunity, decreased audiovisual acuity, loss of memory and decreased sensory and motor responses are common physiological changes in old age (Table 137.1). Increased incidence of diabetes, hypertension, malignancies and GI dysfunctions are common in elderly.

Table 137.1 | Physiological changes in geriatric age groups.

Organ system	Physiological changes	Effects
General	Increased fat mass of the body Decreased body water content	Proneness for atherosclerotic diseases Susceptibility to rapid dehydration

Table 137.1: Conted...

Respiratory	Decreased compliance of chest wall and lung parenchyma	Decreased ventilation and decreased pO_2
pO2	Decreased activity of cough reflex	Easy aspiration
Cardiovascular	Decreased arterial compliance Decreased β receptor sensitivity Decreased SA nodal activity Decreased baroreceptor sensitivity	Increased systolic pressure Decreased cardiac output Decreased heart rate Impaired blood pressure regulation, especially in response to standing
GI system	Decreased hepatic function Decreased gastric acidity Decreased colonic motility	Impaired intermediary metabolisms Impaired digestion Constipation
Hematologic	Decreased bone marrow activity	Anemia
Immune system	Decreased T cell function Increased autoantibodies, antinuclear	Decreased defenses False-positive rheumatoid factor, antinuclear autoimmune disease
Renal	Decreased GFR Impaired capacity for urine concentration and dilution	Impaired excretion of waste products, increased serum creatinine Decreased ability to excrete salt or fluid
Endocrine	Impaired insulin secretion Decreased thyroxine secretion and thyroxine clearance Increased ADH release and decreased aldosterone secretion Decreased testosterone secretion and Vitamin D activation	Increased glucose level in response to illness Decreased body metabolism Impaired Na^+ and water excretion Impotence Osteopenia, easy fractures
Nervous system	General brain atrophy Decreased catecholamine secretion Decreased brain dopaminergic synthesis Decreased righting reflexes Decreased stage 4 sleep Impaired thermal regulation	Forgetfulness, confusion Psychological gloominess Stiff gait and postures On walking body sways, may even fall Get up very early morning, insomnia, sleep apnea Decreased body temperature
Musculoskeletal	Decreased muscle mass Decreased bone density	Weakness Osteopenia, easy fracture
Genitourinary	Atrophy of vaginal mucosa In males, prostrate enlargement	Dyspareunia, bacterial infections Urinary incontinence
Eyes and ears	Presbyopia Opacification of lens Decreased sound conduction	Decreased accommodation Decreased vision Decreased audition

Exam Questions

1. Describe the process of growth and development during infancy and childhood. Describe the regulation of growth.
2. Describe the Physiology of Stress
3. Describe the theories of aging.

Multiple Choice Questions

1. **All of the following are aspects of behavioral development, EXCEPT:**
   A. Adaptive B. Language
   C. Physical D. Motor
2. **For calculation of IQ, along with chronological age, which of the following is included?**
   A. Dental age B. Bone age
   C. Maturity age D. Mental age
3. **Which of the following organ has the maximum % of growth in first two years of life:**
   A. Brain B. Gonads
   C. Kidney D. Liver
4. **Which of the following hormones does not much affect physical growth?**
   A. Insulin B. Somatomedins
   C. Thyroxine D. Glucagon
5. **All of the following are the stages of general adaptation syndrome, EXCEPT:**
   A. Exhaustion B. Resistance C. Activation D. Alarm
6. **Which of the following is not an effect of chronic stress?**
   A. Insulin resistance B. Suppression of immunity
   C. Eosinophilia D. Obesity
7. **All of the following are genetic theories of aging, EXCEPT:**
   A. Ecological theory B. Elimination theory
   C. Mutation theory D. Theory of pleotropic antagonism
8. **All of the following contribute to aging, EXCEPT:**
   A. Excess calorie intake B. Increased oxidative stress
   C. Decreased telomere length D. Decreased atherosclerosis
9. **All of the following are decreased in geriatric age group, EXCEPT:**
   A. Fat mass of the body B. Water content
   C. Arterial compliance D. GFR

Answers

1. C 2. D 3. A 4. D 5. C 6. C
7. B 8. D 9. A

Chapter 138

Physiology of Nutrition and Obesity

Learning Objectives

On completion of study of this chapter:

The student will be able to (must know):

1. Understand the basic principles of nutrition for preserving good health.
2. Remember the sources and daily requirements of all nutrients including vitamins.
3. List the composition of balanced diet.
4. Understand the physiological basis of disorders of nutrition. .

The student may also be able to (desirable to know):

1. Describe the role of various vitamins in human health and disease.

Basic Concept

PY5.8

The **objectives of good nutrition** are to:

1. Restore and provide energy
2. Maintain and control physiological processes of the body
3. Promote growth and development
4. Repair the tissue damages
5. Prevent degeneration of the tissues
6. Minimize the impact of diseases on the body.
7. Maintain immunity and fight infection

Dietary Requirements: In general, **a standard diet for an adult** should contain 50% carbohydrate, 20% fat, 20% protein and 10% fibers. With advancement of age, the fat and carbohydrate intake should be reduced and the fiber intake should be increased.

1. The total caloric intake mainly depends on the individual's ability to use and store energy and on the level of physical activity. In general, men require more calories per kg of body weight than women. **Calorie is supplied by carbohydrate and fat.**
2. In addition, lipids are **primary component of the cell membrane and intracellular signal transduction pathways** (such as diacylglycerol and inositol triphospate). Fats also enhance satiety, help in the absorption of vitamins from intestine, prevent tissue degeneration and protect against some malignancies.
   - Therefore, the present trend of low-fat intake to prevent arteriosclerosis-induced diseases and diabetes should not be vigorous to the extent of causing cell degeneration.
3. Though, the **daily protein requirement** in adult humans is **approximately 0.8 g/kg body weight**, it is more in growing children, in adults following major surgeries, athletes, during pregnancy and lactation, and during recovery from diseases.
   - Therefore, the diet should contain all **essential amino acids and minimum proteins** that are required for tissue maintenance and repair. Proteins also play key role in host defense mechanisms.
4. **Vitamins and minerals** are not energy sources, but are necessary for enzymatic reactions, growth and metabolisms.

ESSENTIAL NUTRIENTS

The essential nutrients in balanced diet are **carbohydrates, proteins, fats, vitamins and minerals**. Carbohydrates provide energy, proteins build the body and give strength, lipids provide energy and control growth, vitamins regulate growth and metabolism and minerals promote tissue repair and growth.

Carbohydrates: The carbohydrates are the **major source of energy**. Complete breakdown of **1 gm of carbohydrate yields 4 kcal**. When carbohydrate is consumed in excess, obesity develops due to conversion of carbohydrate into fat in the body.

Lipids: Breakdown of **1 gm of fat yields 9 calories**. The **main lipids in the diet are triglycerides**. Some amount

Table 138.1 | Recommended dietary allowance (RDA) for Indians as per ICMR, 1990

Categories	Particulars or Age	Body Weight (kg)	Energy (Kcal/d)	Protein (g/d)	Calcium (mg/d)	Iron (mg/d)	Vitamin A (mg/d)	Vitamin C (mg/d)	Folic Acid (mg/d)	Vitamin B12 (mg/d)
Adult man	Moderate work	60	2875	60	400	28	600	40	100	1
Woman	Moderate work	50	2225	50	400	30	600	40	100	1
	Pregnant		2525	65	1000	38	600	40	400	1
	Lactation	2775	75	1000	30	950	80	150	1.5	
Infant	0-6 months	5.4	108 kcal/kg	2.05g/kg	500		350	25	25	0.2
	6-12 months	8.6	98 kcal/kg	1.65 g/kg	500		350	25	25	0.2
Children	1-3 yr	12.2	1240	22	400	12	400	40	30	1
	4-6 yr	19.0	1690	30	400	18	400	40	40	1
	7-9 yr	26.9	1950	41	400	26	600	40	60	1
Boys	10-12 yr	35.4	2190	54	600	19	600	40	70	1
Girls	10-12 yr	31.5	1970	57	600	34	600	40	70	1
Boys	13-15 yr	47.8	2450	70	600	28	600	40	100	1
Girls	13-15 yr	46.7	2060	65	600	41	600	40	100	1
Boys	16-18 yr	57.1	2640	78	500	30	600	40	100	1
Girls	16-18 yr	49.9	2060	63	500	50	600	40	100	

of cholesterol is also present. Triglyceride is the glycerol attached to three molecules of fatty acids. The different triglycerides differ in structure depending on the **degree of saturation**, the **length of the carbon chain** and the **presence or absence of essential fatty acids**.

Protein: The minimum daily intake of protein should be **1 g/kg body weight**. The requirement is more in infants, children and adolescents and during pregnancy, lactation and recovery from diseases

Vitamins: Vitamins act as cofactors in many enzymatic reactions such as decarboxylation, carboxylation etc. They act as oxidizing and reducing agents in oxido-reductive processes. Vitamins decrease the risk of various cancers by their antioxidant property. Antioxidant vitamins are β-carotene, vitamins C and E. Adequate vitamin E intake lowers the risk for coronary artery disease.

Minerals and Electrolytes: The minerals that are important in body functions are **calcium, phosphorus, iron, iodine, zinc, copper and selenium**. Deficiency of minerals occurs due to the same general reasons as vitamin deficiency.

Details of all these nutrients have been given in Biochemistry books, Due to 'Integrated Curriculum in Teaching" , they are repeated here in physiology book.

RECOMMENDED DIETARY ALLOWANCES

The recommended dietary allowance (RDA) of a nutrient is the quantity, which meets the known nutritional needs of a normal healthy population. RDAs depend on age, gender, body weight, climate, physiological states especially in women (pregnancy, lactation etc), and physical activity of the individual (Table 183.1). Therefore, RDA varies from regions to regions and countries to countries. Various illnesses affect the RDA. RDA helps in framing balanced diet for a population.

Balanced Diet PY4.3

A balanced diet is a satisfactory diet that provides **adequate quantities of all essential nutrients**. It depends mainly on the age, sex, body weight and level of physical activity of the individual.

- It should provide energy intake, and desirable minimum protein intake on the basis of RDA.
- For example, for a 50 kg moderately active woman, the diet should provide 2225 kcal and at least 50 g protein everyday.
- As 50g protein provides 200 kcal; the remaining 2025 kcal should be obtained from carbohydrates and fats.
- The diet should also provide at least the RDA of vitamins and minerals.

Daily Dietary Allowances: As **recommended by ICMR**, the daily allowances for various age groups in both males and females are summarized in Table 138.1.

This can generally be achieved by:

1. A mixture of cereals and pulses as the major source of energy. This ensures adequate calorie and protein. If the grains are not highly refined, it also ensures adequate fiber intake.
2. **Role of dietary fibers:** The fibers in the diet facilitate intestinal motility, reduce fat intake and prevent constipation. Vegetables and fruits should be about 400g per day per person. This ensures adequate vitamin

and mineral intake. Dietary fibers have recently been reported to prevent intestinal malignancy.

3. Some milk and milk products should be included in the diet.
4. For children and pregnant women, some nonvegetarian food like fish, egg or meat should be included.

DISORDERS OF NUTRITION

Malnutrition

Malnutrition is common in children, and occurs in two forms: **marasmus and kwashiorkor**.

- The total starvation causing **depletion of calorie** leads to **marasmus in children**.
- Sometimes calorie is adequate but **food may be grossly deficient** in proteins and vitamins; the condition known as **kwashiorkor in children**.
  - Accordingly the condition is called **protein-energy malnutrition**.
- Usually, when **edema is present, is called kwashiorkor**, and **when edema is absent, is called marasmus**.

Obesity

PY8.5

Obesity is a complex **disorder of appetite regulation** (details given in Chapter 111) **and energy metabolism**. Genes that predispose to obesity in humans and animals have already been identified indicating the importance of genetic factor in the development of this disorder. **Secondary obesity** occurs in various diseases like hypothyroidism, Cushing syndrome etc, as part of **metabolic syndrome**. Understanding the neural mechanism of feeding behavior focuses light on the management of **primary obesity**.

Exam Questions

1. Describe the basic requirements of various nutrients for an average active adult male. Add a note on balanced diet

Multiple Choice Questions

1. All of the vitamins are fat soluble, EXCEPT:
A. Vitamin K
B. Vitamin D
C. Vitamin C
D. Vitamin E

2. All of the following are essential fatty acids, EXCEPT:
A. Lauric acid
B. Lenoleic acid
C. Linolenic acid
D. Arachidonic acid

3. The calories produced by 1g of fat is:
A. 4
B. 6
C. 9
D. 15

4. All of the following are essential amino acids, EXCEPT:
A. Valine
B. Proline
C. Leucine
D. Phenylalanine

5. The most important role of vitamin E is:
A. To produce clotting factors
B. Antidote of selenium poisoning
C. Anticoagulant
D. Antioxidant

6. Biochemical function of vitamin K is:
A. Converting proline to hydroxyproline
B. Conversion of prothrombin to thrombin
C. Gamma carboxylation of clotting factors
D. Inhibition of lipid peroxidation in biomembranes

7. The water-soluble vitamin synthesized in human body is:
A. Ascorbic acid
B. Pyridoxine
C. Niacin
D. Pantothenic acid

8. All are features of pellagra, except:
A. Skin lesions
B. Break down of scars
C. Diarrhea
D. Decreased mental agility

9. Methylmalonic aciduria is sensitive index of deficiency of:
A. Vitamin B2
B. Vitamin B12
C. Vitamin B6
D. Niacin

10. All of the following are functions of vitamin C, EXCEPT:
A. Conversion of tyrosine to noradrenaline
B. Conversion of tryptophan to serotonin
C. Facilitation of formation of ferritin in tissues
D. Inhibition of oxidation-reduction reactions

11. All of the following are features of Vitamin A deficiency, EXCEPT:
A. Ageusia
B. Xerophthalmia
C. Keratomalacia
D. Nyctalopia

12. All of the following are features of wet beriberi, EXCEPT:
A. Wenicke's encephalopathy
B. Wide pulse pressure
C. Cardiomegaly
D. Tachycardia

Answers

1. C 2. A 3. C 4. B 5. D 6. C 7. C 8. B 9. B 10. D 11. A 12. A

Chapter 139

Physiology of Yoga and Meditation

Learning Objectives

On completion of study of this chapter:

The student will be able to (must know):

1. List the benefits of practice of yoga.
2. Name the common asanas and list the advantages of practicing asanas.
3. Classify pranayamas and learn basic principle of pranayama practice.
4. Realize the improvement of sympathovagal balance by slow pranayamas.
5. Remember the benefits of practice of surya namaskar.
6. Illustrate the application of yoga in improving quality of life.
7. Name the types of meditations and their benefits.

The student may also be able to (desirable to know):

1. Describe the physiology of yoga and meditation.

Yoga is the complete union with the Divine and manifestation of Divine qualities in human life. In other words, it is a conscious effort to attain and lead the Divine life. Thus, yoga is the evolution of human consciousness into divine consciousness.

- **Sri Aurobindo** has said '**Yoga is a rapid and concentrated evolution of being, which can take effect in one-life time, while unassisted natural evolution would take many centuries or many births to attain the full divinity**'.
- **Swami Vivekananda** has said "**Yoga is a means of compressing one's evolution into a single life, or even a shorter time than that**".

Thus, yoga is to hasten the evolution of the human being into a divine being in less period.

Schools of Yoga: There are several systems of yoga, the four have been widely accepted.

1. Hatha yoga
2. Raja yoga
3. Tantra yoga
4. Integral yoga

HATHA YOGA

Hatha yoga includes practice of asanas, pranayamas, surya namaskar and kriyas. It mostly aims at perfection of the body. A true practitioner (hatha-yogi) not only achieves a healthy body and a greater longevity but also gains mastery over functions of the body. However, in general, it neglects perfection of the mind. Therefore, hatha yoga by and large attains improvement of physical health without much refinement of the mind.

- Though recent **medical research on yoga therapy** has revealed the usefulness of asanas, pranayamas and surya namaskar in the treatment of many life-style disorders, research in larger cohorts, follow-up studies in with lager sample size, and clinical trials are needed to establish therapeutic benefits of these yoga practices.

Asanas

Asanas are different **body postures**. Anatomically, keeping the body in a particular posture, allows the physical structures to adapt to that particular position of the body to assist and maintain the posture. Standing, sitting and lying are the three common postures of human activities. However, postures are changed in seconds to minutes during routine activities.

1. Postures are changed by **movements of body parts** that occur due to **contraction of agonist muscles and relaxation of antagonist muscles** that change the **angle at various joints**.
2. Postures are maintained by the effect of gravity that acts as a stimulus to cause **contraction of appropriate extensor group of muscles** of joint that keep the **joint in extension**. The details of regulation of posture are discussed in physiology of motor system.

3. The ability to immediately make flexion or extension at a joint is the primary requirement of posture and movement.
   - Therefore, **flexibility of the joint**, which depends on integrity of joint ligaments, tendons, joint capsule and adequacy of the fluid in the joint space, should be preserved to maintain the mobility of the body as a whole.
   - Further, **force generated in the muscle** should be adequate to support a posture and **bones should be strong enough** to maintain a posture, especially in erect position.
   - Therefore, musculo-skeletal framework should be healthy enough to provide strong support to joints to conduct and maintain a posture.
4. Asanas provide flexibility to joints and muscles.

General Benefits of Asanas

Practice of yogasana keeps the person physically fit by improving following functions of the body.

1. **Improves flexibility of joints**, maintains power and suppleness of muscles, provides strength to bones.
2. Different yogasana postures modulate **blood flow to visceral organs** and improve their functions.
3. Controls **secretion from endocrine glands** and therefore profoundly influences body metabolisms.
4. Asanas such as ardhachandrasana, padahastasana, tribhujasana, matsyasana, nauasana, paschimottanasana, dhanurasana, chakrasana, yoga mudra and abdominal breathing that greatly affect abdominal pressure and movement, **improve insulin secretion and sensitivity**. Thus. these asanas are proposed to be beneficial in diabetes.
5. Asanas such as matsyasana, sarvangasana, halasana, dhanurasana, that affect neck movement and stretchability **improve thyroid secretion** and therefore greatly affect metabolisms.
6. Many asanas by controlling thoraco-abdominal movements and blood to visceral organs, improve **exocrine secretions, liver functions, GI motility and secretions.** Thus, yogasana improves appetite and balances digestion and metabolism.
7. Asanas that affect movement of trunk and rotation of body along the main axis improve the **flexibility of vertebral joints** and reduce stiffness of the back muscles.
8. Asanas that cause forward and backward bending of the body torso, **reduce fat in the abdomen** and pelvic regions.
9. Asanas that influence thoracoabdominal movement, control **ventilation and respiratory functions**. These asanas balance sensitivity of airways and are useful in the treatment of asthma.
10. Asanas such as sarvangasana and sirshasana that **increase blood flow to brain improves memory, learning, general intelligence and cognition**. Also, these asanas improve functions of the nervous system.
11. Yogasana has profound influence on **hemodynamics, circulation and cardiovascular functions**. Regular practice of asanas maintains heart functions and blood pressure.
12. Asanas like sarvangasana, paschimottanasana, abdominal breathing and shavasana **ensures relaxation of body and mind and promote sleep**. They decrease stress and anxiety, improve autonomic balance and reduce heart rate and blood pressure.

List of Asanas and Practice Schedule

Basic principles and Precautions

1. Should be practiced in a well-lit and well-ventilated room or in the open space like in the ground, terrace or roof top etc.
2. Should ideally be done in the morning between 4 am to 8 am or in the evening between 4pm to 8 pm. Nice to have a daily or routine schedule for asanas.
3. Bowel and bladder should be evacuated before yogasana practice.
4. Should not be done in full stomach (stomach should be empty).
5. Should not mix asanas with other form of exercises in a single session
6. Do not strain body to attain a full position for the asanas. If there is a resistance for full-bending of the body for a particular asana, it can be achieved slowly by bending little by little more every day.
7. Do not be in a hurry to complete the session.
8. Breathe comfortably during asanas.
9. Usually, in a complete asana schedule, forward and backward bending asanas are done alternately to allow the body to balance between the acute change of postures.

List of Asanas

There are **more than 100 asanas**. However, ideally, the **list of 29 asanas** as described below can be practiced daily. Before practice of asanas, **warm-up (free hand) exercise for** about 5 min should be done.

Vrikshasana (Vrikhsa or Tree pose)

Steps: Stand erect with feet together

- Straighten out arms fully and raise the arms sideways to the overhead.
- Stretch and raise your feet and stand on toes (Fig. 139.1).
- Stretch the body fully in upward direction with knees straight and abdomen pulled in.

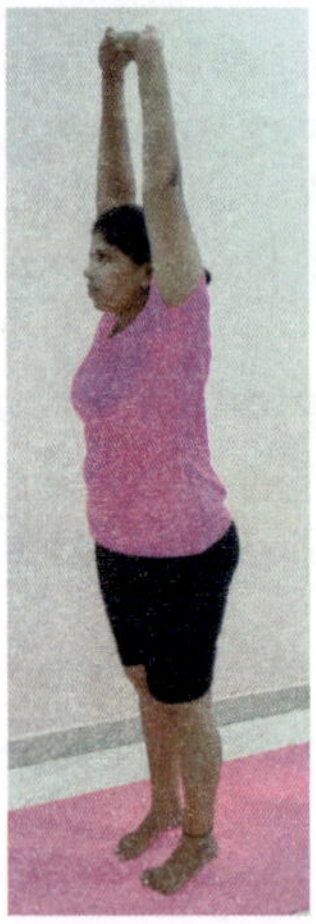

Fig. 139.1: Vrikshasana

Benefits: Stretches the muscles and joints and prepares the body for the various asanas.

- Also improves the general balance of the body.

Ardhachandrasana

Steps: Stand erect with feet together

Raise arms from front with hands together.

- Bend the body backward slowly and comfortably as far as possible (Fig. 139.2).
- Keep knees straight, and arms close to ears and arms kept straight.

Benefits: Perfects the control and balance of the body and gives the feeling of lightness.

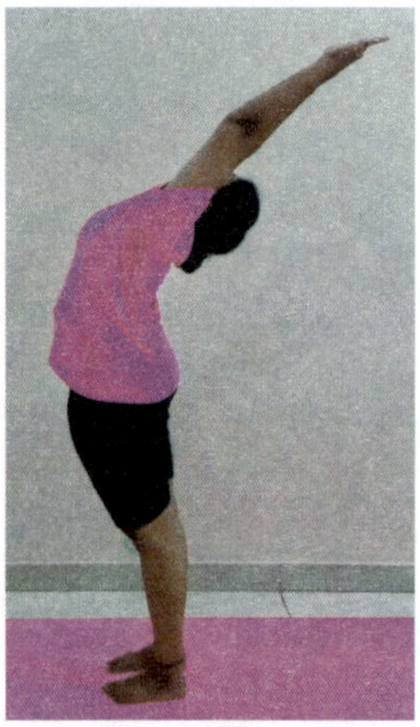

Fig. 139.2: Ardhachandrasana (Half-moon pose)

- Improves mobility and flexibility of vertebral joints and promotes spinal flexibility
- Strengthens the hip joint.
- Enables muscular athletes to tense and strengthen their abdominal muscles in the stretched condition, thus preventing what is known as 'Athlete's abdominal cramps'.
- Increases appetite, enhances body energy and raises vitality.

Padahastasana

Steps: Stand erect with feet together.

- Raise arms overhead.
- Bend down slowly with head between arms
- Keep knees straight and try to hold the ankles, bringing head close to the knees as much as possible (Fig. 139.3).

Benefits: Lightens the body

- Removes fat, especially from abdomen.

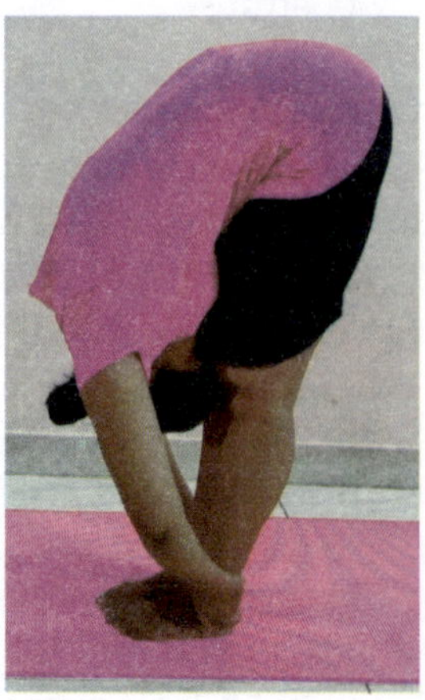

Fig. 139.3: Padahastasana (Hand-to-feet pose)

- Increases GI functions, increases digestive power.
- It is a very energizing posture.
- Ensures greater blood supply to the head, removes fatigue due to excessive brain (mental) work.

Trikonasana

Steps: Stand with feet well apart, body weight equally on both feet, with knees straight.

- Raise right arm sideways up touching right ear, palm facing left.
- Bend trunk laterally to the left – don't push abdomen forward or hips backward, right arm straight and as close to head as possible.

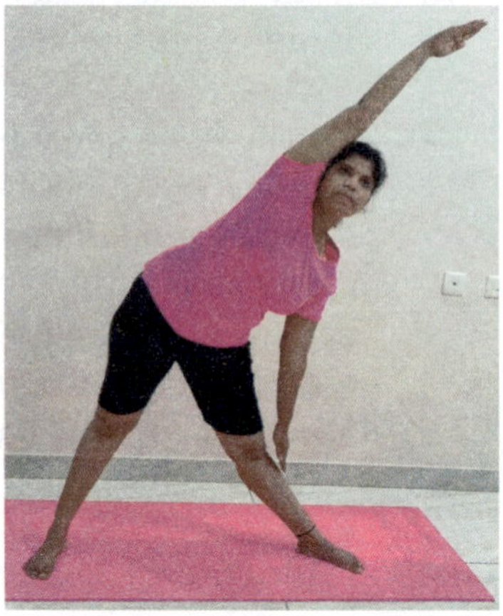

Fig. 139.4: Trikonasana

- Don't take support with left hand, left hand should hang down straight.
  - This forms a triangle of the body, remain in this posture for 30 seconds (Fig. 139.4).
- Repeat same movements with left arm and bend to the right.

Benefits: Gives a good lateral bending to the spine and helps to keep vertebral joints flexible and healthy.

Tribhujasana

Steps: Stand with feet well apart, body weight equally on both feet, arms sideways, palms down.

- Bend forward with back and arms horizontal, palms down, head up.
- Twist trunk to right, left hand touching or close to right foot, right arm in line with right leg, look at fingers of right hand (Fig. 139.5).

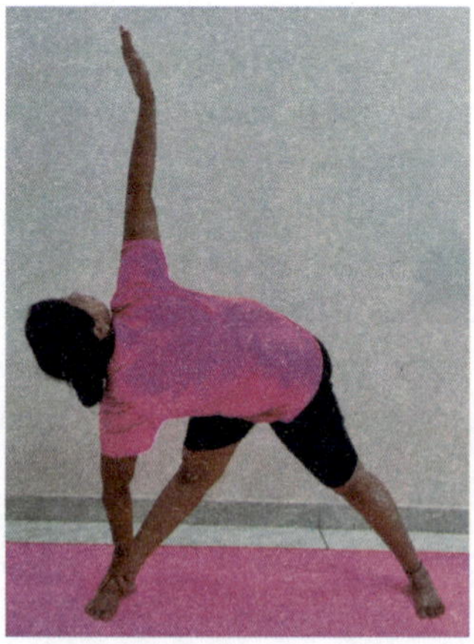

Fig. 139.5: Tribhujasana (body assumes three-limb pose)

- Hold for 1 minute. Then come back to previous position. Repeat asana turning trunk on the other (left) side.

Benefits: Gives a good rotational movement to the vertebrae and spine.

- Vitalizes (activates) the kidney and other abdomino-pelvic organs.

Utkatasana

Steps: Stand erect, feet slightly apart, toes slightly turned out.

- Bend from the knees (as in sitting on a chair), knees slightly out and vertically over toes.
- Keep back straight, arms stretched forward (horizontal and parallel) palms down, head up (Fig. 139.6).

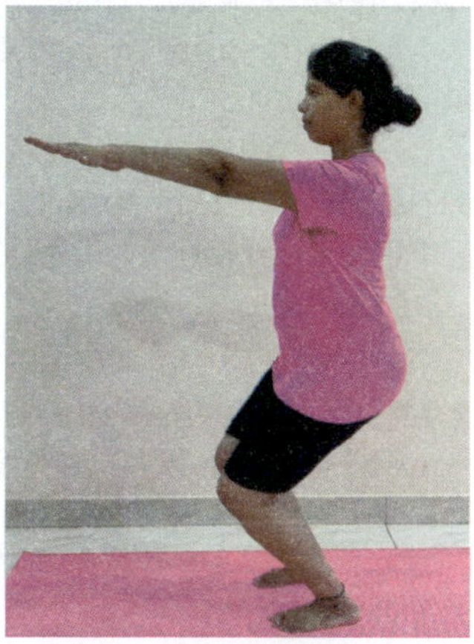

Fig. 139.6: Utkatasana

Benefits: Strengthens leg muscles.

- Lightens the body and brings it under control.
- A special benefit is that its practice strengthens the knee joints and ensures joint circulation that keeps cartilages healthy.

Sarvangasana

Steps: Lie on your back, arms kept alongside.

- Raise both legs together, taking support of hands on the hips and elbows on the ground.
- Straighten the body – feet, knees, hips and back form one vertical column from the base of the neck to the tip of the toes.
- Keep the leg and feet stretched, toes pointed, chin pressed against the chest (Fig. 139.7).
- Take normal breathing.

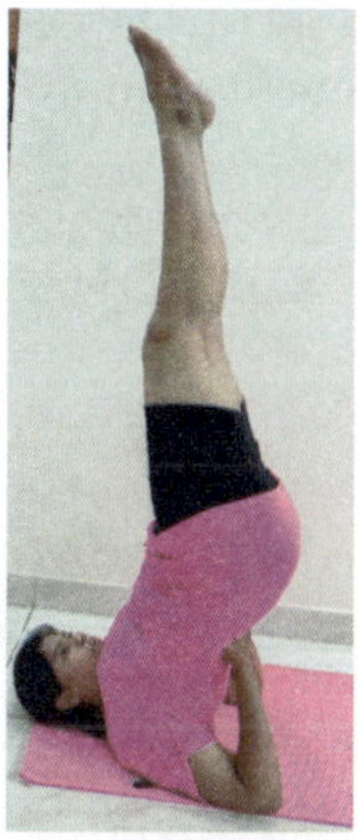

Fig. 139.7: Sarvangasana

Benefits: Promotes secretion of the thyroid gland leading to healthy functioning of body metabolism, circulatory, respiratory, alimentary and genito-urinary systems.

- Keeps the vertebrae and spine flexible.
- Prevents the bones from early ossification.
- Supplies large quantities of blood to the spinal roots of the nerves, thereby giving them sufficient nourishment.

Matsyasana (Fish pose)

Steps: Sit with legs as in Padmasana, i.e., with knees bent, feet on opposite thighs heels towards the abdomen.

- Lie on your back.
- Placing hands near the head for support lift your back above the ground.
- Keep the top of your head on the ground over a padded surface, e.g. a towel (Fig. 139.8, i and ii).
- Keep your hands on your feet. Take normal breathing.

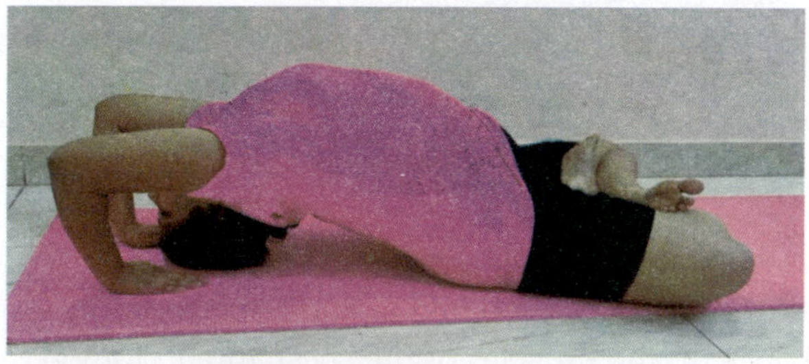

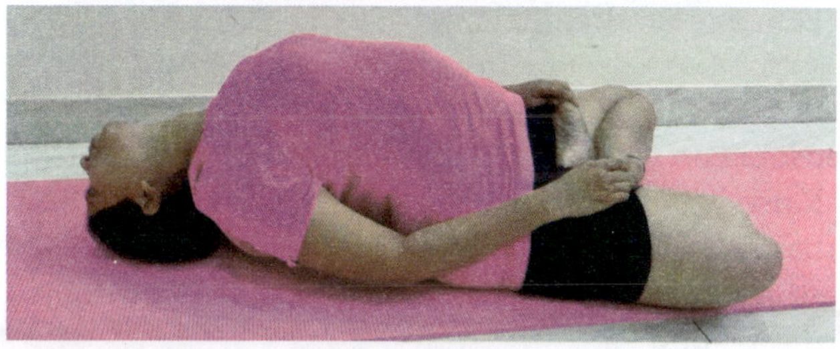

Fig. 139.8: Matsyasana (Step i) Matsyasana (Step ii)

Benefits: Makes the neck flexible and strong

- Increases the size of the rib cage, widens the windpipe and thus helps in breathing capacity.
- Relieves and relaxes the neck after sarvangasana.

Paschimottanasana

Steps: Lie on your back, legs straight, arms overhead, hands together, palms facing up.

- Sit up, take hands overhead and keep back straight
- Then bend forward, try to hold the big toes, head between arms and touching the knees (Fig. 139.9).

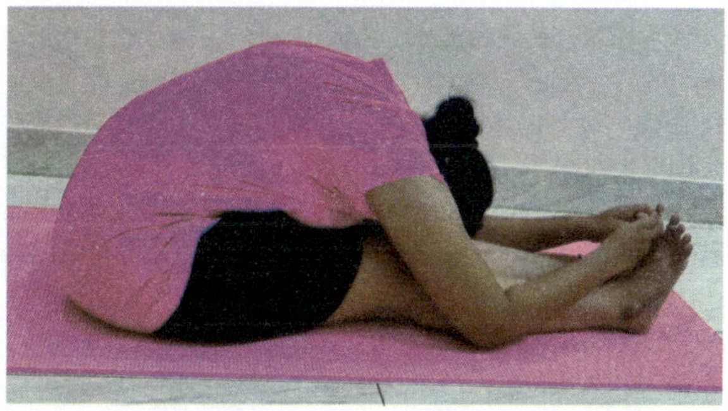

Fig. 139.9: Paschimottanasana

Benefits: Reduces abdominal fat.

- Removes wind from the intestines.
- Facilitates GI functions and increases appetite.

Nauasana

Steps: Lie on your stomach, legs straight, toes pointed, arms stretched overhead, hands together, palms on the ground.

- Raise legs (knees straight) arms (hands together), chest and head to form a boat-like arch (Fig. 139.10).
- Do not hold your breath.

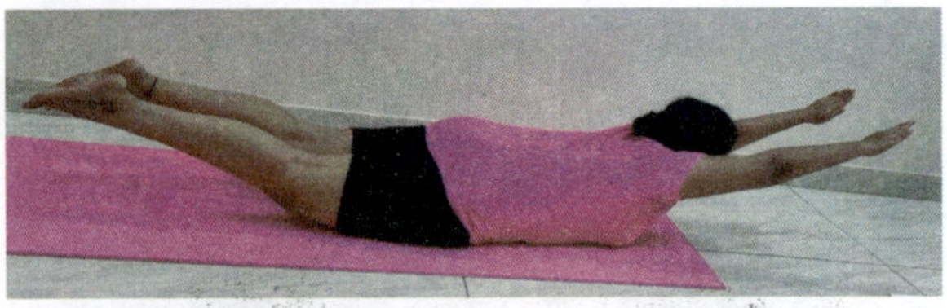

Fig. 139.10: Nauasana (Boat pose)

Benefits: Improves GI function and appetite.

- Tones up the muscles of the chest and abdomen.
- Dissolves abdominal fat.

Halasana (plough pose)

Steps: Lie on your back, arms alongside.

- Raise legs as in Sarvangasana (you may take help of hands on the hips), then lower them overhead, knees straight, ankles stretched, toes pointed and touching the ground.
- Arms stay on grounds as in beginning, palms on the ground.
- The posture resembles the shape of a plough (Fig. 139.11).

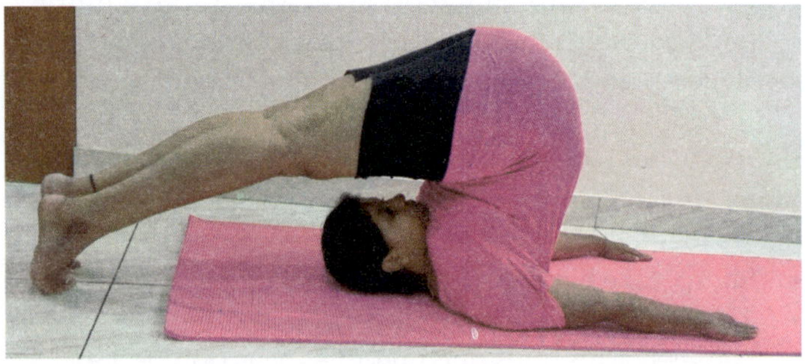

Fig. 139.11: Halasana

Benefits: Makes the vertebral joints and spine flexible.

- Creates energy and increases the supply of blood to the muscles of the back.
- Facilitates thyroid secretion, thus improves metabolism and systemic functions of CVS, CNS, reproduction.
- Aids the functioning of thymus gland, thus improves immunity.
- Helping retain the individual's youthful physical characteristics for a longer period.

Salabhasana

Steps: Lie on your stomach, hands under thighs, palms up, forehead on the ground, feet together, toes pointed.

- Raise legs gradually as high as you can (Fig. 139.12).
- Keep the knees straight. Do not take support of your hands.

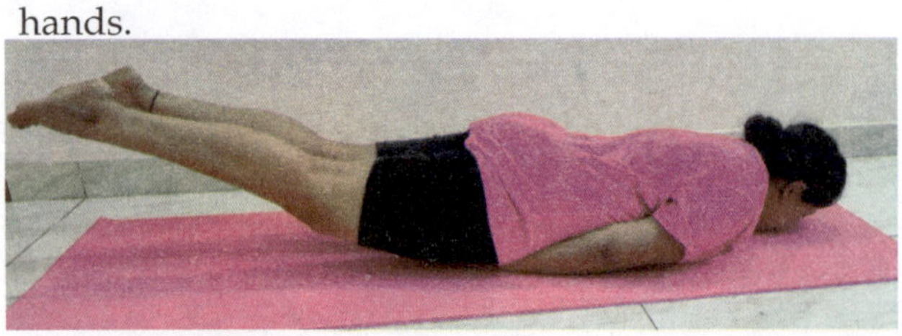

Fig. 139.12: Salabhasana

Benefits: Helps remove all sorts of muscular pains in the lower region of the back.

- Makes the lumbar vertebrae flexible.

Janushirasana

Steps: Sit with legs stretched out in front, back straight.

- Place right foot against left thigh, heels as close to groin as possible.
- Raise arms overhead, hands together, thumbs locked.
- Bend down to hold left foot or toes from both sides, head as close to left knee as possible.
- Left knee should be straight, right knee on the ground (Fig. 139.13). Repeat this asana with opposite leg positions.

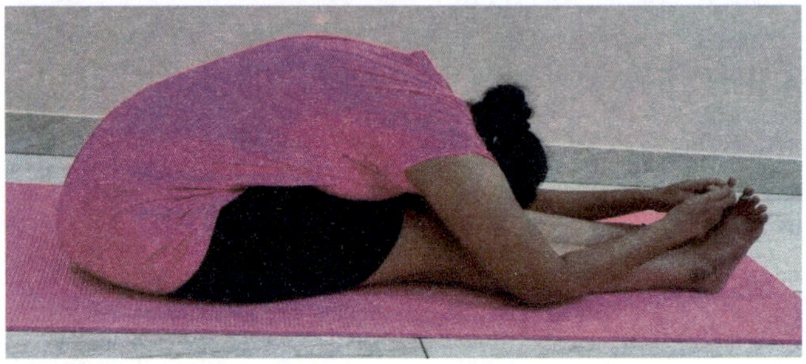

Fig. 139.13: Janushirasana

Benefits: Improves GI functions and increases digestive power.

- Improves genito-urinary functions.
- Cures urinary bladder and urethral problems.

Dhanurasana

Steps: Lie on your stomach.

- Bend knees, hold the ankles.
- Pull with your hands and push with your legs, knees together, till the trunk forms an arch with only the stomach on the ground (Fig. 139.14).
- Look up.
- After releasing the posture, lie for a while in Shavasana.

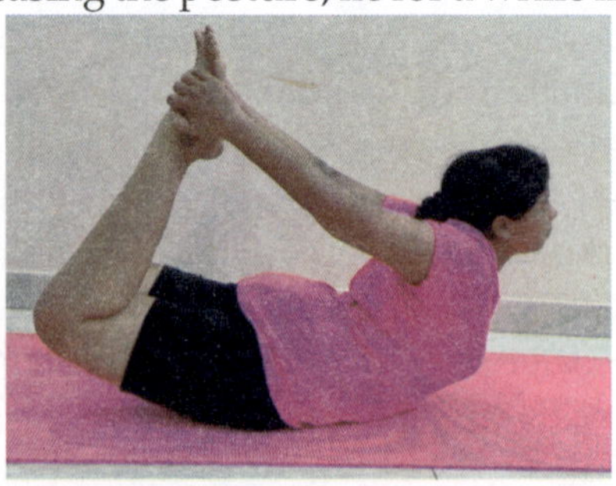

Fig. 139.14: Dhanurasana (Bow pose)

Benefits: Reduces abdominal fat.

- The compressing of abdomen against the spinal column, pressing the nerves with the scapulae (the winged bones at the back attached to the arms) minimizes blood circulation while in the asana.
  - But when the pose is released, a greater supply of blood is ensured to those very regions, improving abdominal and pelvic organ functions.

- Increases vital-spinal flexibility and definitely raising the vitality.

Yogamudra

Steps: Sit with legs as in padmasana i.e., knees bent, feet on opposite thighs, heels towards the abdomen, back straight.

- Hold your hands behind the back and on the ground, shoulders squared head up.
- Slowly bend forward to touch the ground with the forehead in front of the shins (Fig. 139.15).
- Don't raise hips.

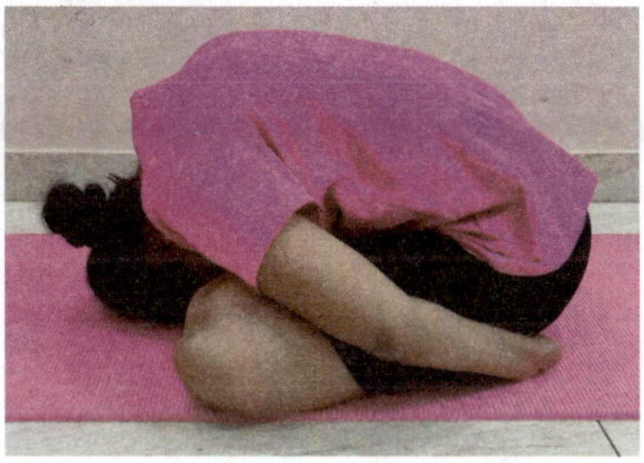

Fig. 139.15: Yogamudra

Benefits: Improves circulation to head and neck.

- In general, the oxygenation of the blood is greatly enhanced by this mudra.

Chakrasana

Steps: Lie on your back.

- Bend knees, place feet apart and close to hips, place hands overhead, palms beside ears and shoulders.
- Push with hands and, without moving feet, raise trunk as high as possible to curve the back into an arch, look on the ground between the hands (Fig. 139.16).

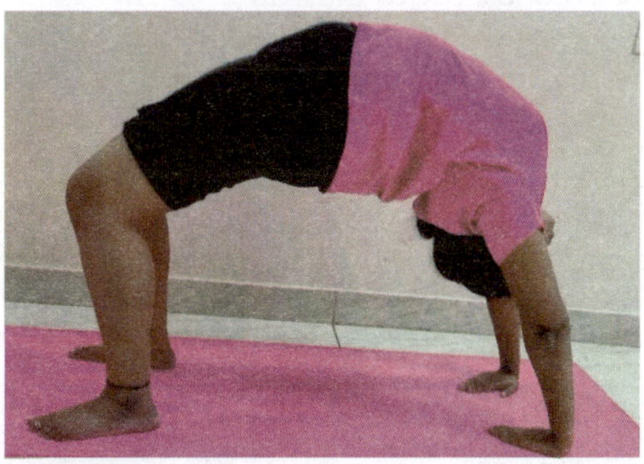

Fig. 139.16: Chakrasana

Benefits: Builds a flexible back by strengthening vertebral column.

- Stimulates the nerves roots of vertebral column.
- Improves visceral functions by massaging abdominal organs.
- One of the powerful back-bending postures.

Utthitapadasana

Steps: Lie on your back, arms alongside.

- Raise legs to 45 degrees, knees together, toes pointed.
- Keep lower back pressed to the ground (Fig. 139.17). Normal breathing as far as possible.

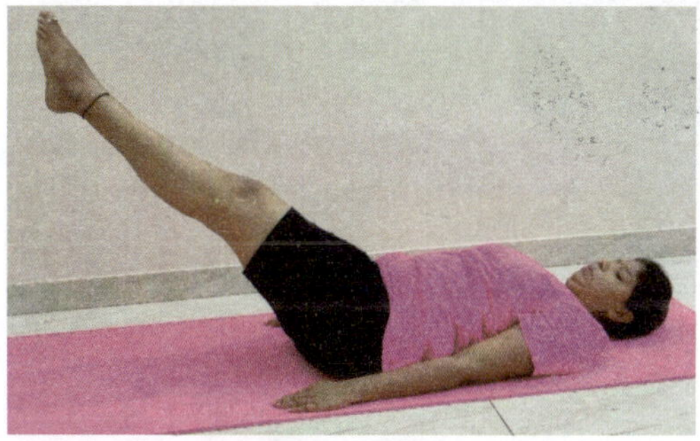

Fig. 139.17: Utthitapadasana (Feet raising pose)

Benefits: Strengthens the abdominal muscles.

- Strengthens muscle of legs.
- Improves GI function and helps cure indigestion.

Bhujangasana

Steps: Lie on your abdomen, forehead on the ground, hands under shoulders.

- Raise your upper body by the strength of the back muscles, head up (Fig. 139.18).
- Don't take help of the hands, they may remain on the ground or held on the back over the hips.

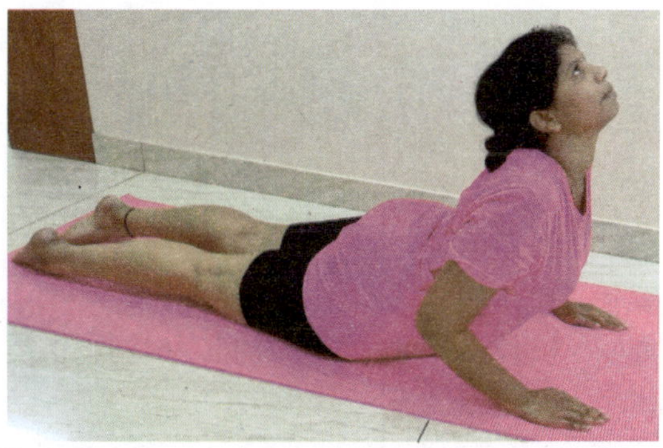

Fig. 139.18: Bhujangasana

Benefits: Helps in keeping the dorsal vertebra and spine flexible and strong.

- Backache due to overstrain can be relieved.
- Helps considerable reduction in abdominal fat.

Pavanamuktasana Series

(½ minute each: right, left, and both legs – lying and sitting)

Steps: Lie on your back.

- Bend one knee, hold it close to the chest, other leg straight, head on the ground.
- Repeat with the other knee.
- Repeat with both knees. Sit with legs stretched in front,

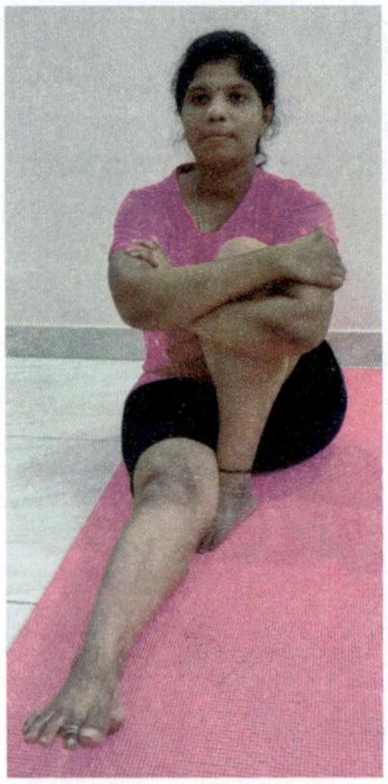

Fig. 139.19: Pavanamuktasana (Step 3)

bring one foot close to hips. Hug the knee to chest, other leg stretched on the ground, back straight, head normal (Fig. 139.19).

- Repeat with the other knee.
- Repeat with both knees.

Benefits: Removes gas from the large intestine.

- Reduces abdominal fat.
- Increases the flexibility of the knees and hips.

Bhadrasana

Steps: Sit holding feet together, heels as close to groin as possible, knees as close to ground as possible.

- Back as erect as possible, head up chin down, normal breathing.

Benefits: Specially recommended for those suffering from genito-urinary disorders.

- Cures bladder and prostate dysfunctions.
- The pelvis, the abdomen and the back get stimulated through a plentiful supply of blood.
- Keeps the kidneys, the prostate and the bladder healthy.

Ardhamatsyendrasana (1 minute each side)

Steps: Sit with legs stretched out in front.

- Bend right knee, place right foot on left side of left knee, left leg straight.
- Hold left leg with left hand – keep right knee on the left of left arm.
- Turn trunk to right, look back over right shoulder, right hand on ground for support or behind the back as close to left thigh as possible.
- The right hand can be lifted from the ground and kept on the waist as close to left thigh as possible (Fig. 139.20)
- Repeat with left knee bent and trunk turning to left.

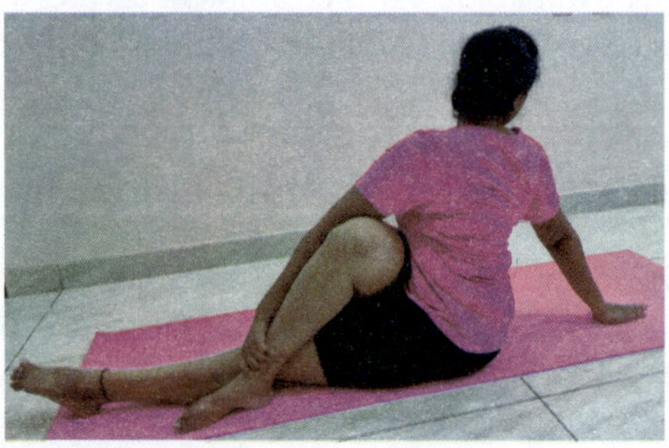

Fig. 139.20: Ardhamatsyendrasana

Benefits: Increases the flexibility of the vertebrae and spine.

- Massages the abdomen and internal organs and improves visceral functions.

Gomukhasana

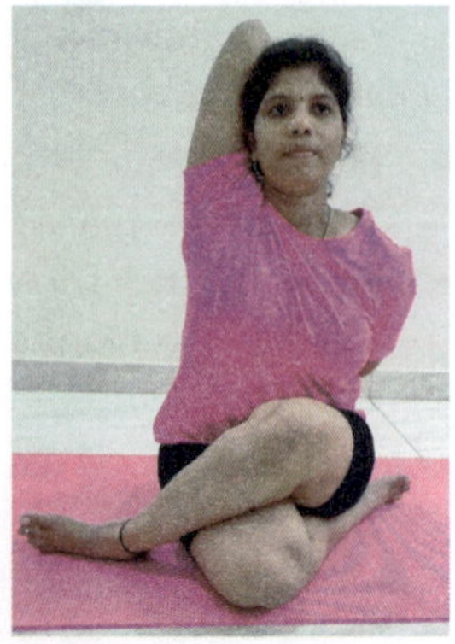

Fig. 139.21: Gomukhasana

Steps: Sit with right knee on left, back and head erect, feet on either side of the hips.

- Hold hands behind the back, right elbow pointing upward and left elbow pointing downward (Fig. 139.21).
- Repeat with left knee on right, left elbow pointing upward.

Benefits: Helps proper functioning of the gonad glands.

- It can be practiced to a great advantage just before retiring by those suffering from sleeplessness in which case the timing may be increased to half an hour on each side.

Ushtrasana

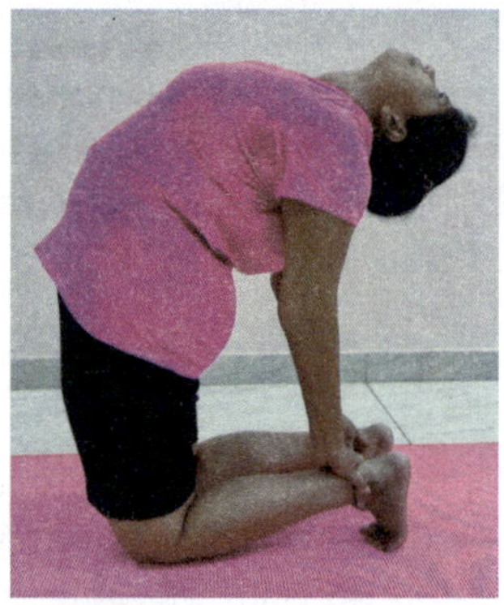

Fig. 139.22: Ushtrasana (Camel pose)

Steps: Kneel.

- Hold your ankles, push with your hands, arms straight, to raise your chest and form an arch, look up, head relaxed behind (Fig. 139.22).

Note: Start Ardhakurmasana immediately after this asana.

Benefits: Makes the spine supple.

2. Increases blood flow to the brain.
3. Good for back problems.

Ardhakurmasana

Steps: From Japanese sit (hips on or between the heels, knees together) bend down, arms stretched forward, forehead and palms on ground (Fig. 139.23).

- Body completely relaxed.
- Normal breathing.

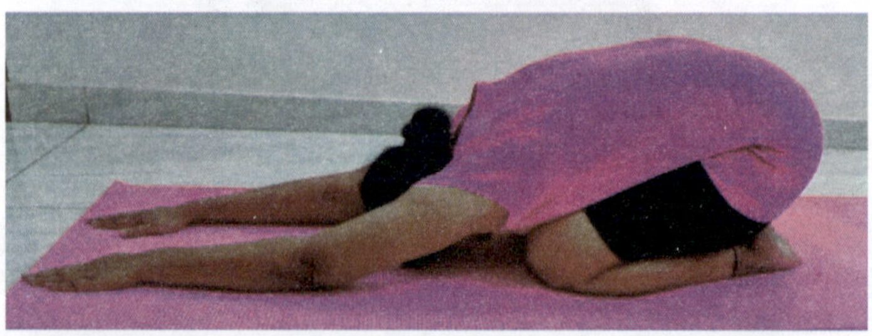

Fig. 139.23: Ardhakurmasana

Benefits: Removes fat in the abdomen and buttocks.

- Helps to improves digestion.

Shashakasana

Steps: Japanese sit.

- Place top of the head on the ground as close to knees as possible, hold your heels and raise the hips until the arms are straight (Fig. 139.24).
- Normal breathing.

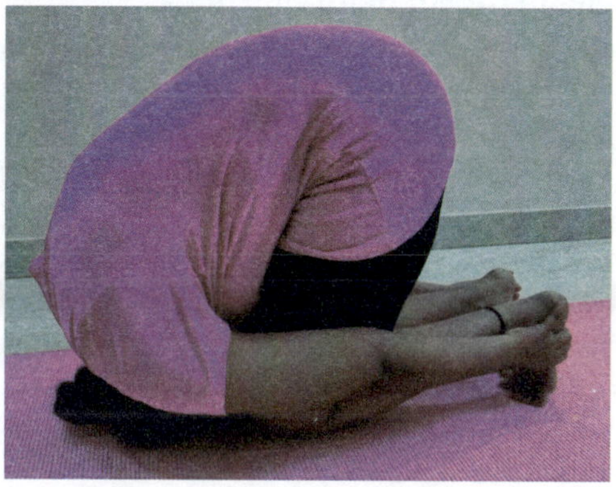

Fig. 139.24: Shashakasana

Benefits: Increases digestive power.

- Helps the functioning of the liver and spleen.
- Makes the vertebrae and spine flexible.

Sirshasana

Steps: Place top of the head and elbows on the ground, palms at the back of the head, fingers locked – head and elbows form a triangle.

Legs taken up to vertical in line with the rest of the body, feet stretched, toes pointed – entire weight on the top of the head.

- Normal breathing. After coming down rest in Shavasana for one full minute.

Benefits: Gives a rich supply of blood to the brain and good nourishment.

- A powerful neuro-tonic, it invigorates and energizes the nervous system.
- Aids the digestive power and also helps to purify the blood.

Veerasana

Steps: Japanese sit.

- Hands on knees, abdomen drawn in, chest up, back straight, shoulder squared, head erect.
- Normal breathing.

Benefits: Aids in digestion

- Helps cure sciatica.

Shavasana

Steps: Lie on your back, feet slightly apart, toes slightly turned out, hands a little away from the body, palms up (Fig. 139.25).

- Breathe normally, through the nose.
- Deliberately loosen up each and every muscle.
- Imagine you are a floating cloud or a piece of cloth on the floor.
- You can concentrate in your heart and feel relaxed. You must feel relaxed.
- Continue as long as one is comfortable

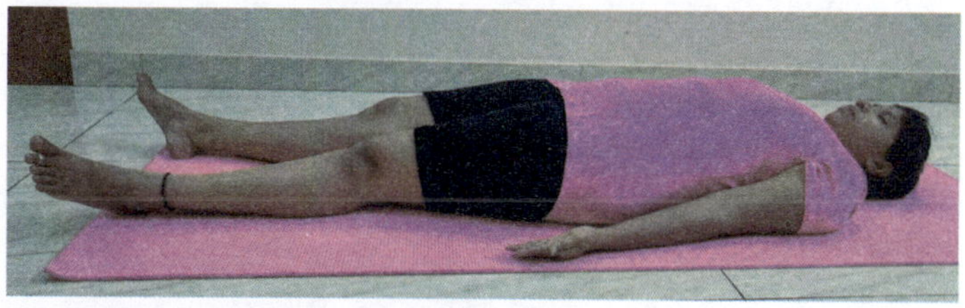

Fig. 139.25: Shavasana (corpse or dead-body pose)

Benefits: Makes the muscles soft and pliable and enables the blood flow to return to its normal pace.

- Relaxes the body and mind.
- Relieves stress and anxiety.
- Stabilizes autonomic activity.

A Brief Schedule of Asana Practice

The day there is less time for yoga practice, **15 min** of asanas may be practiced: Sarvangasana, Matsyasana, Paschimottanasana, Nauasana, Halasana, Salabhasana, Pavanamuktasana, Ardhamatsyendrasana and Shavasana.

Pranayama

Pranayama (prana + ayama) is the controlled breathing in which the practitioner regulates his breathing (ayama) for imbibing cosmic energy (prana) from the atmosphere through structured and meticulous inspirations. In normal breathing, the duration of inspiration is longer than expiration.

- Normally, the **duration of expiration is less than half** of the duration of inspiration.
- During inspiration, **heart rate is more due to less vagal tone** and during expiration heart rate is less due to more vagal tone. This phenomenon is known as **sinus arrhythmia**.
- In pranayama, duration of expiration is more than that of inspiration, which strengthens the vagal tone.

Types of Pranayama

Pranayama is classified into two categories: Fast pranayamas and slow pranayamas.

Fast Pranayamas: In fast pranayamas such as **kapalabhati, bastrika, and bellows breathing**, the respirations are faster but deep.

- Usually by practicing fast pranayamas, **sympathetic discharge increases**.
- Sympathetic tone also increases by **suryanadi pranayama** (right nostril breathing).

Slow Pranayamas: The slow type of pranayamas are

anuloma-viloma (alternate nostril breathing), **chandranadi** (left nostril breathing), **sitkari** (cooling breaths), and **bhramari** (breathing with vibrations through ear).

- In slow pranayama, respirations are slower, deeper, and prolonged with more duration of expiration.
- By reducing inspiration and lengthening expiration, the vagal tone is increased.

Benefits of Pranayama

1. Increases vagal tone and improves sympathovagal balance

Mechanisms of increased vagal tone by slow pranayamas:

1. In slow pranayamas, the duration of expiration is gradually increased by the practitioner in the proportion of (inspiration-expiration ratio) 1;1, 1:2, 1:3, 1:4 and so on. With gradual increase in expiration, the **duration of vagal activation becomes gradually more** as per the process of sinus arrythmia. This improves vagal discharge and **increases vagal tone**. Thus, heart rate is reduced and heart rate variability (HRV) is improved.
2. In slow pranayamas, gradual and graded **increase in lung volume and rib cage** increases nerve traffic from thoracic cage proprioceptors that strengthen vagal tone through the **central limbic-hypothalamic influence of the sensory projections** to thalamus and cortex.
3. Slow pranayamas **augment cerebral blood flow and oxygenation** that improves neuronal activities of the brain centers including those present in the limbic areas, hypothalamus, and medulla, the centers autonomic discharge. This improve sympathovagal outflow by facilitating vagal discharge.

Thus, slow pranayamic breathings **improve sympathovagal balance**.

- Especially, practice of **chandranadi pranayama** (left-nostril breathing) and **anuloma-viloma pranayama** (alternate nostril breathing) is very effective in increasing vagal tone and decreasing sympathetic tone.
- The practice of **fast pranayama and suryanadi pranayama** (right nostril breathing) increases sympathetic activity.

2. Improvement of visceral, endocrine, metabolic and reproductive functions

By improving sympathovagal balance they improve **visceral functions**, increase **insulin secretion and sensitivity**, improve thyroid secretion and **control metabolism**, improve **genito-urinary functions and reproductive functions**.

3. Alleviation of CV Risks

Pranayama is directly linked to autonomic activity, regulation of heart rate, and heart rate variability (HRV). **Decrease in heart rate** by practice of yoga **improves HRV**.

- Although resting heart rate varies widely in general population between 60 to 100 beats/min, persistent tachycardia has been reported to decrease HRV, which is an established CV risk.
  - It has been recently reported that heart **rate more than 75/min increases CV risk**.
  - As slow pranayamas are **very effective in reducing heart rate and blood pressure**, they profoundly decrease CV risks.

4. Improvement higher brain functions

Pranayama incenses neuronal functions, in the brain and peripheral nervous system. It increases **learning, memory, cognition and higher intellectual functions**.

5. **Improves lifespan:** Slow breathing increase longevity.

IMPORTANT NOTE

> **Breathing rate decides your longevity:** It has been noted in *Hathayoga Pradipika* that at the time of birth, the **number breaths for the entire lifetime is allotted** for everyone. If he breathes fast, he lives less years, and if he breathes slow, he lives longer, as the total number of breathings are fixed for one's life. Hence, it is upto the person to pace his breathing and decide his longevity.

Pranayama Schedule

Though there are many types of pranayamas, the following pranayama schedule of **four pranayamas** (kapalabhati, anuloma-viloma, chandranadi and brhamari) with each about 5 min duration may be practiced.

Kapalabhati Pranayama

Steps:

- Sit in any meditative posture preferably in Sukhasana/ Padmasana/ Vajrasana.
- Close the eyes and relax the whole body.
- Inhale deeply through both nostrils, expand the chest.
- Expel the breath with **forceful contractions of the abdominal muscles** and relax (Fig. 139.26).
- Do not strain. Continue active/forceful exhalation and passive inhalation.
- Complete 30 rapid breaths, then take a deep breath and exhale slowly.
- This is one round of Kapalabhati.
- Each round shall be followed by deep breathing.
- Repeat 2 to 5 rounds.

Breathing: Forceful exhalation by contracting the abdominal muscles, without any undue movements in the chest and shoulder region. Inhalation should be passive throughout the practice.

Number of rounds: Beginners can practice up to 3 rounds of 20 breaths each. The count and rounds can be increased gradually over a period of time.

Benefits: Kapalabhati purifies the frontal air sinuses; helps to overcome cough disorders.

- It is useful in treating cold, rhinitis, sinusitis, asthma and bronchial infections.

- It rejuvenates whole body, and keeps the face young and vibrant.
- It balances and strengthens the nervous system and tones up the digestive system.

Caution: It should not be practiced if there is bleeding in the nose, during attacks of migraine, stroke, acute hernia and acute gastritis.

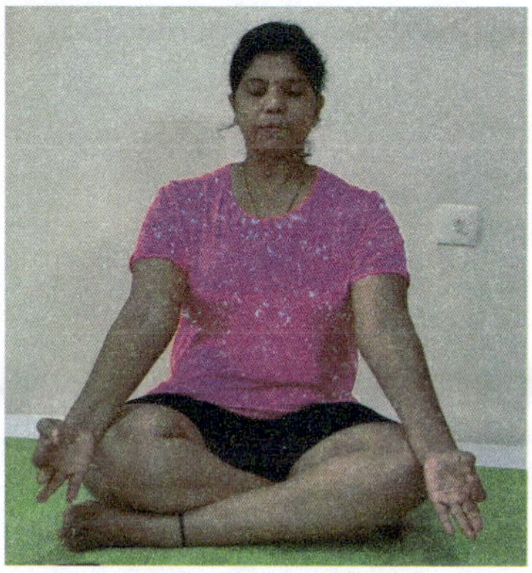

Fig. 139.26: Kapalabhati pranayama. Note forceful contraction of abdominal muscles during fast breathing.

Nadisodhana or Anuloma-Viloma Pranayama

The main characteristic feature of this pranayama is alternate breathing through the left and right nostrils without or with retention of breath (*kumbhaka*).

Steps: Sit in any meditative posture.

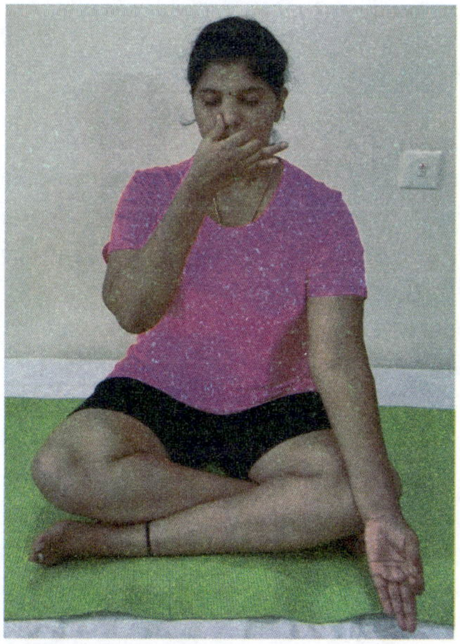

Fig. 139.27: Nadisodhana pranayama.

- Keep the spine and head straight, relax the body with few deep breaths.
- Sit in Nasagra mudra (as shown in the picture below).
- Place the ring and small fingers on the left nostril; keep the middle and index finger on forehead. Place the right thumb on the right nostril (Fig. 139.27).
- Breathe in from the left nostril; then close the left nostril with the small and ring fingers and release the thumb from the right nostril; exhale through the right nostril.
- Next, inhale through the right nostril.
- At the end of inhalation, close the right nostril, open the left nostril and exhale through it.
- This complete process is one round of the Nadisodhana or Anuloma-Viloma Pranayama
- Repeat 5 rounds.

Nasagra mudra (Please note the position of thumb and ring finger on both nostrils)

Ratio and timing: For beginners, the duration of inhalation and exhalation should be equal.

- Gradually make 1:2; inhalation: exhalation

Breathing: Breath should be slow, steady and controlled. It should not be forced or restricted in any way.

Benefits: The main purpose of this pranayama is to purify the principle channels of carrying energy called *nadis*; hence nourishes the whole body.

- Induces tranquility and helps to improve concentration.
- Increases vitality and **lowers the level of stress and anxiety**.
- It alleviates cough disorders.
- Balances sympathetic and vagal activity and **promotes sympathovagal homeostasis**.
- **Improves memory.**

Chandranadi Pranayama (Left-nostril breathing)

The main characteristic feature of this pranayama is breathing through the left without breathing in right and without retention of breath.

Steps: Sit in any meditative posture.

- Keep the spine and head straight, relax the body with few deep breaths.
- Sit in Nasagra mudra (as shown in the picture above).
- Place the ring and small fingers on the left nostril; keep the middle and index finger on forehead. Place the right thumb on the right nostril and close the right nostril (Fig. 139.27).
- Breathe through left nostril with the right nostril closed.
- Take deep inhalation through left nostril and then exhale slowly with exhalation time more than inhalation. Exhalation time can be slowly prolonged.
- This completes one round of Chandranadi Pranayama
- Repeat 10 rounds of left nostril breathing.

Benefits: The main purpose of this pranayama is to purify chandranadi, the channel of purification and coolness of the body.

- Induces tranquility and improves concentration.
- Increases vitality and lowers the level of stress and anxiety.
- Decreases sympathetic and **improves vagal activity**.
- **Improves memory**.
- **Decreases heart rate and blood pressure**, effective in treatment of hypertension.

- By increasing vagal discharge, it **increases insulin secretion** and sensitivity. Effective in management of diabetes.

Bhramari Pranayama

The word 'Bhramari' is derived from *bhramara* which means a black bee.

During the practice of this pranayama, the sound produced resembles the buzzing of a black bee.

Steps: Sit in any meditative posture with eyes closed.

- Inhale deeply through the nose.
- Close the ears both sides with respective index fingers as demonstrated in the figure below (Fig. 139.28).
- This is also called Sanmukhi Mudra.
- Exhale slowly in a controlled manner while making a deep, steady humming sound such as that of black bee. This is one round of Bhramari. Repeat 5 rounds.

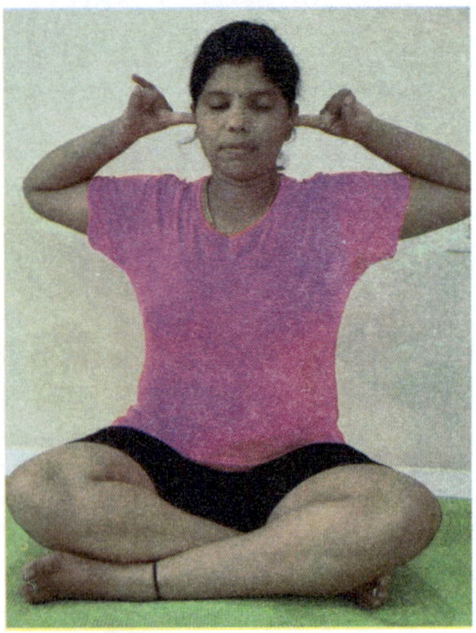

Fig. 139.28: Bhramari Pranayama

Benefits: The practice of Bhramari relives stress and helps in alleviating anxiety, anger and hyperactivity.

- The resonance effect of humming sound creates a soothing effect on the mind and nervous system.
- It is a great tranquilizer; found good in the management of stress related disorders.
- It is a useful preparatory *pranayama* for concentration and meditation.
- Balances autonomic activity with increased vagal activity.
- Known to **increase nitric oxide** level and decrease BP.

Precaution: Don't practice it in acute nose and ear infections.

Surya Namaskar

Surya namaskar or the **sun salutation** is done in the morning, when sun is rising. This can also be done at the sun set. It consists of 12 steps and each step is an asana. With each step, breathing (inspiration and expiration) alternates, and each step is performed slowly with deeper breathing. Thus, surya namaskar is a combination of asana and pranayama.

Benefits: Surya namaskar has both the benefits of asana and pranayama.

1. Improves **flexibility of joints**, suppleness of musculoskeletal system, especially **of the vertebral joints and reduce neck and back stiffness.**
2. Different yogasana postures in 12 steps modulate **blood flow to visceral organs** and improve their functions.
3. Controls **secretion from endocrine glands** (including insulin and thyroxine) and therefore profoundly influences body metabolisms.
4. Improves exocrine secretions, **liver functions, GI motility and secretions.**
5. Reduces fat in the abdomen and reduces obesity.
6. Increases blood flow to brain and improves **memory, learning, general intelligence**.
7. Improves **cardiovascular and respiratory** functions.
8. **Improves autonomic balance** and functions of internal organs.

N.B.: Authors are thankful to **Mrs. Prabhavathi P.,** Yoga Instructor, Puducherry, for agreeing to publish all her poses of Asanas and Pranayamas, in this Textbook of Medical Physiology.

OTHER FORMS OF YOGA

Raja Yoga

Raja yoga basically aims at **perfection of the mind**. Patanjali, the master of raja yoga, has advocated yoga into **eight limbs**, hence called **Ashtanga Yoga**. The eight limbs are: yama, niyama, asana, pranayama, pratyahara, dharana, dhyana and samadhi.

Yama: Yama consists of **five principles:** ahimsa (non-violence), satya (stick to truth only), asteya (non-stealing), brahmacharya (celibacy), aparigraha (non-receiving, or not being greedy)

Niyama: Niyama also consists of ***five principles***: shaucha (cleanliness, purification of body and mind), santosh (be satisfied with what you get), tapas (austerities, or disciplining our movements), swadhyaya (study of spiritual scriptures) and ishwar-pranidhan (surrender to the Divine).

Asana & Pranayama: Described above.

Pratyahara: Pratyahara is withdrawal of senses to free the mind. It is mainly the material withdrawal, the withdrawal from physical enjoyments.

Dharana: Dharana is the concentration of the mind on a particular point, which may be an object, a sound or an idea.

Dhyana: Dhyana is the meditation, in which mind is

allowed to flow towards the point of concentrations.

Samadhi: This is the state of super-consciousness. The individual enters into a transcendent consciousness, and withdraws from external objects.

Tantra Yoga

The tantra yoga is based on the principles that **all creation is Divine** manifestation and all worldly activities are **Divine play**. It does not reject the world as an illusion but considers it as a manifestation of the Divine. Therefore, one should wholeheartedly participate in the cosmic play and enjoy them without attachment.

Integral Yoga

Yoga of the Gita

The Gita taught us the triple path of work, knowledge and devotion as a synthesis of yoga. The yoga through knowledge, or ***jnana yoga***, the yoga through devotion, or ***bhakti yoga***, and the yoga through works, or ***karma yoga*** are the triple paths of yoga.

Integral Yoga

Integral yoga is the **yoga of Sri Aurobindo**. It accepts the central principle of triple path of yoga of the Gita, but does not stop at salvation. It proposes the **transformation of the being** as a whole; the mental transformation, the vital transformation and finally the physical transformation. Therefore, this is also called **yoga of transformation**.

Integral yoga of Sri Aurobindo is based on the concept of evolution, according to which if life has evolved from matter and mind has evolved from life, then mind is bound to be evolved into a state of **supermind**. The man has to ***evolve into a higher consciousness***, what Sri Aurobindo says ***Supramental Consciousness***. Therefore, his yoga is also called the **Supramental Yoga**.

1. There are three fundamental practices: ***aspiration*** for higher spiritual life, ***rejection*** of lower qualities of nature and ***surrender*** to the Divine.
   - Sri Aurobindo descended the **Supramental Force** from the supracosmic level to the earth subtle atmosphere to transform human nature and the body.
2. The **Supramental Force** is the force of the Divine Mother. Hence, this yoga is also called the **Yoga of the Divine Mother**.
3. **Surrender to the Divine Mother** is the central condition in this yoga. With the surrender, the Divine Mother pours in the being the supernatural powers and the spiritual experiences needed for progress.
4. Surrender gives the confidence that the Divine takes care of everything of the being, and therefore there is no need to worry for anything. Hence, what is required from man is to **surrender to the Supreme** and to become a sincere worker of the Divine. This knowledge **Lord Krishna** had taught to Arjuna in the midst of Mahabharata (Kurukshetra) War. He instructed Arjuna.... *"Sarba Dharma Parihstajya Mamekam Sharanam Braja"*, which means 'Oh Arjuna, abandon everything, and just surrender to me', ... ***rest all I shall deliver***.
5. A truly surrendered life makes the life stressless and progressive and brings the true happiness. To lead this stress-free and happy life is the **best way to prevent aging**.

PY11.12

MEDITATION

Definition

Meditation is a practice where an individual uses a technique such as mindfulness, or focusing the mind on a particular object, thought or activity to train attention and awareness, and achieve a mentally clear and emotionally calm and stable state. Meditation is practiced in all religions in different names, using different techniques.

Types of Meditation

There are different kinds of meditation, practiced in different sects of yoga. However, generally they are grouped into **six categories**:

1. **Mindfulness Meditation:** The practitioner pays attention to his thought as they pass through his mind.
   - He does not judge the thought, they just become aware (mindful) of the thoughts.
   - This is an adaptation from traditional Buddhist meditation.
2. **Focused Meditation:** Focusing the attention on a single object during the whole meditation session.
   - The focus may be breathing, physical sensation, or a visual image.
   - This form of meditation enhances mental acuity and focus.
   - This form of meditation is practiced in Himalayan yoga and Mantra Yoga.
3. **Relaxing or Body-Scan Meditation:** Body scan meditations focus on consciously relaxing different parts of the body.
4. **Walking Meditation:** Instead of using the breath as the object of awareness, walking meditation encourages you to focus on each footstep in order to be fully present.
   - This involves becoming aware of the movement of each foot; noticing the action of lifting, lowering, and having each foot touch the ground, one step after another.
   - Like body-scan meditation, walking meditation allows you to cultivate a sense of mind-body awareness by

focusing on your body›s physical sensations as it moves.

5. **Transcendental Meditation:** Transcendental meditation involves focusing on a specific mantra or phrase by repeating it during meditation.

- The mantra acts as the object of awareness for the practitioner, just like breathing is the object of awareness for mindfulness meditation.
- A mantra can be something as simple as saying "Om" or a phrase like "I am worthy."
- This is quite popular in USA and other western world.

6. **Loving-kindness Meditation:** Loving kindness is a form of meditation geared towards cultivating compassion for yourself and others.

- Negative attitudes are replaces by positive and empathetic feelings.
- During this meditation, one can direct phrases of goodwill and a positive intention to yourself, loved ones, and even for difficult people in your life.

Effects of Meditation on the Body

Effects on EEG

In the **short-term meditation**, following changes are observed in the EEG.

A decrease in the delta waves (between 1 and 3Hz): Delta waves originate in the thalamus and cortex. As delta waves are increased in deep sleep, this finding suggests that delta waves may play a role in meditations that increase attentiveness.

An increase in theta waves: This is seen across a range of meditative practices and appears to be associated with the extent of training and experience with the meditation practice.

- Frontal midline theta waves may be associated with increased internal attentiveness.
- Anterior cingulate gyrus could be the source of the increase in frontal midline theta waves.
- Increase in theta waves is correlated with diminished sympathetic nervous activity.

An increase in alpha waves: This may be seen in frontal, parietal and occipital areas during focused and Om-chanting types of meditation.

Long-term Effects of Meditation

Effects on Brain Functions: Meditation increases cortical thickness and subcortical grey and white matter. Changes in the prefrontal cortex, anterior cingulate cortex and insula have been more expressed.

- Refines the functions of amygdala and ventral striatum that are involved in **emotional processing**.
- Enhances **sleep quality**, and reduces perceived stress.
- Meditation **improves cognition** and is the targets for therapeutic neuromodulation.

Cardiovascular and Other Functions:

1. ***Reduction in blood pressure:*** There are reports of reduction in blood pressure with meditation. It is now recommended as non-therapeutic method of blood pressure reduction.
2. ***Reduction in stress:*** Meditation reduces markers of stress and inflammation.
3. ***Reduction in cerebral aging:*** Reduction of grey matter with age is less in individuals who are long term meditation practitioners.
    - This raises the possibility that sustained meditation may help maintain brain tissue, preserve cognitive, and emotional reserves, and reduce the risk of dementia and possibly other age-related neurodegenerative diseases.

Improvement in respiratory functions: This may be due to improvements in breathing patterns, muscle relaxation, and reduction in stress. Improves lung functions

The following message of **The Mother of Sri Aurobindo Ashram** on "**How to Remain Young**" is ever eternal in its force and action.

HOW TO REMAIN YOUNG?

(The Message of 'The Mother' of Sri Aurobindo Ashram, Pondicherry, India)

It is not the number of years you have lived that makes you grow old. You become old when you stop progressing.

As soon as you feel you have done what you had to do, as soon as you think you know what you ought to know, as soon as you want to sit and enjoy the results of your effort, with the feeling you have worked enough in life, then at once you become old and begin to decline.

When, on the contrary, you are convinced that what you know is nothing compared to all which remains to be known, when you feel that what you have done is just the starting-point of what remains to be done, when you see the future like an attractive sun shining with the innumerable possibilities yet to be achieved, then you are young, however many are the years you have passed upon earth, young and rich with all the realizations of tomorrow.

And if you do not want your body to fail you, avoid wasting your energies in useless agitation. Whatever you do, do it in a quiet and composed poise. In peace and silence is the greatest strength.

Multiple Choice Questions

1. Air is breathed through nostril in all pranayamas EXCEPT?
   A. Surya Bhedana B. Sitali
   C. Bhastrika D. Ujjai
2. All of the following Asana bends the spinal column backward, EXCEPT:
   A. Matsyasana B. Bhujangasana
   C. Dhanurasana D. Paschimottanasana
3. Which of the following Asana bends the spinal column forward?
   A. Pada-hastasana B. Ardhachndrasana
   C. Sarvangasana D. Ushtrasana
4. Which of the following is under Patanjali's eight limbs of yoga?
   A. Nirodha B. Chitta
   C. Dhauti D. Dharana
5. All of the following pranayamas increase vagal tone, EXCEPT:
   A. Kapalabhati B. Sitkari
   C. Bhramari D. Chandranadi
6. Cleansing of the nasal passage is done by
   A. Kapalabhati B. Dhauti
   C. Neti D. Nauli
7. As per yogic text, human beings are enmeshed in how many Sheaths (Koshas)?
   A. 4 B. 5
   C. 6 D. 7
8. Which of the following Chakra is connected to the pineal gland?
   A. Swadhisthana B. Vishuddha
   C. Ajna D. Anahata
9. Which of the following Chakra is connected to the Thyroid gland?
   A. Swadhisthana B. Vishuddha
   C. Manipura D. Ajna
10. Which of the following Chakra is connected to the pancreas and liver?
    A. Swadhisthana B. Vishuddha
    C. Muladhara D. Manipura
11. The exhalation phase in pranayama is known as
    A. Rechaka
    B. Kumbhaka
    C. Trataka
    D. Puraka
12. Which of the following is NOT classified under the four Vedas?
    A. Atharvaveda
    B. Yajurveda
    C. Guruveda
    D. Samaveda
13. Which of the following is TRUE?
    A. Inhaling by right nostril increases vagal tone
    B. Inhaling by left nostril increases sympathetic tone
    C. Slow pranayamas improve sympathovagal balance
    D. Slow pranayamas decrease heart rate variability (HRV)
14. All of the following are under Patanjali's eight limbs of yoga, EXCEPT:
    A. Pratyahara
    B. Pranayama
    C. Niyama
    D. Nauli
15. All of the following are fast pranayamas, EXCEPT:
    A. Anuloma-viloma
    B. Bellows breathing
    C. Suryanadi
    D. Bhastrika
16. All of the following are basic principles of integral yoga, EXCEPT:
    A. Aspiration
    B. Rejection
    C. Surrender
    D. Samadhi

Answers

1. B 2. D 3. A 4. D 5. A 6. C 7. B 8. C 9. B 10. D 11. A 12. C
13. D 14. D 15. A 16. D

"All good physicians are physiologists and all good physiologists are physicians".
G. K. Pal

Index of Normal Values

A. Blood

1. Hemogram

Total RBC count

Men : 4.5–6 million/mm^3

Women : 4–5.5 million/mm^3

Hemoglobin

Men : 14–18 g/dl

Women : 12–16 g/dl

Packed cell volume (Hematocrit)

Men : 40–50%

Women : 37–47%

Mean corpuscular volume (MCV) : 78–96 fl

Mean corpuscular hemoglobin (MCH) : 27–33 pg

Mean corpuscular Hb conc (MCHC) : 30–37%

Colour index :0.85 0 1.10

Total leucocyte count : 4000–11,000/mm3

Differential count

Neutrophils : 50–70%

Eosinophils : 1–4%

Lymphocyte : 20–40%

Monocyte : 2–8%

Basophils : 0–1%

Total platelet count : 150,000–400,000/mm3

Reticulocyte count : 0.5–1% of red cells

ESR

a) Westergren method

Men 3–5 mm at the end of 1 h

Women 5–12 mm at the end of 1 h

b) Wintrobe method)

Men 0–9 mm at the end of 1 h

Women 0–20 mm at the end of 1 h

Osmotic fragility of red cells : Hemolysis begins at 0.45% of NaCl and completes at 0.35% of NaCl.

2. Coagulation studies

Bleeding time (Duke method) : 1–5 min.

Clotting time (capillary tube method) : 2–8 min.

Fibrinogen : 200–400 mg%

Fibrin degradation product : 10 mg/dl

Activated partial thromboplastin time (APTT) : 25–40 sec.

Thrombin time : 15–20 sec.

Clot retraction time : 50% by 1 h
Whole blood clot lysis time : > 24 h

3. Gases

PO2

Arterial blood (PaO_2) : 80–100 mmHg
Venous blood : 25–40 mmHg

PCO2

Arterial blood ($PaCO_2$) :35–45 mmHg
Venous blood : 40–50 mmHg

4. pH : 7.35–7.45

B. Serum

Bilirubin

Adult : 0.2–0.8 mg %
Newborn : 0.5–5 mg %
At 3 days after birth : 1–10 mg %

Creatinine : 0.6-1.8 mg %
Calcium : 9–11 mg/dl
Iron : 50–150 mg/dl
Plasma glucose (fasting) : 70–110 mg/dl (111–125 mg% is prediabetes)
Plasma glucose (postprandial, 2 hours) : < 140 mg%
Plasma glucose (random) : < 200 mg%

Electrolytes

Sodium : 136–145 meq/L
Potassium : 3.5–5 meq/L
Chlorides : 96–106 meq/L
Phosphorus (inorganic) : 2.5–4.5 mg/dl

Cholesterol : 120–200 mg/dl
Osmolality : 280–295 mosm/kg of water

C. Urine

Glucose

Qualitative : Absent
Quantitative : 16–300 mg/24 h

Protein

Qualitative : Absent
Quantitative : 10–150 mg/24 h

Bilirubin Absent
Hemoglobin Absent
Creatine : 0–200 mg in 24 h
Creatinine : 15–25 mg/kg body weight/day
Uric acid : 250–750 mg/24 h
Urobilinogen : 0.05–3.5 mg/24 h
Sodium : 40–220 meq/24 h
Potassium : 25–125 meq/24 h
Chloride : 10–200 mmol/l
Calcium (normal diet) :100 – 300 mg/24 h
Osmolality : 100–900 mosm/l
pH : 4.6–8.0 (average 6)

D. Cerebrospinal fluid

Glucose : 50–70 mg/dl
Protein : 10–30 mg/dl
Bilirubin : Absent
Cells : 0–5/mm3 (usually lymphocytes)
Chloride : 110–125 mmol/l
Pressure : 7–20 cm of water
pH : 7.34–7.43

E. Semen

Liquefaction : Completes at 15 min.
Morphology : Minimum 60% normal
Motility : Minimum 75% motile
pH : 7.2–8.0
Count : 50 million/ml
Volume : 2–5 ml

F. Synovial fluid

Cells : 200 cells/mm3
Glucose : Same as serum
Hyaluronic acid : 2.5–4 g/dl
Proteins : 2.5 g/dl
pH : 7.32–7.64
Crystals : Absent

G. Stool

Fat :3–5 g/day
Nitrogen :2.2 g/24 h
Stercobilinogen : 40–280 mg/24 h
Corpoporphyrin :15–500 mg/24 h

H. Cardiovascular parameters

Heart rate : 60 to 100 per min.
Cardiac output : 5 litres per min (each ventricle)
Systolic BP : 100–119 mmHg (120–139 mmHg is prehypertension)
Diastolic BP : 60–79 mmHg (80–89 mmHg is prehypertension)
Pulse pressure : 20–50 mmHg
Mean arterial pressure: 20–50 mmHg

Bibliography

1. Kaushansky K, Litchman MA, Prchal JT, Levi MM, Press OW, Burns LJ, Caliguri MA. 2020. *William's Hematology*; 9th edition. London: McGraw-Hill.
2. Pal GK and Pal P. 2020. *Textbook of Practical Physiology*; 5th edition. Hyderabad: Universities Press.
3. Renu S, Pati HP, Mahapatra M (eds.). 2018. *de Gruchy's Clinical Hematology in Medical Practice*; 6th edition. London: Science.
4. Bannister R and Mathews CJ (eds.). 2013. *Autonomic Failure: A Textbook of Clinical Disorders of the Autonomic Nervous System*; 5th edition. London: Oxford University Press.
5. Barett KE, Barman SM, Brooks HL and Yuan J (eds.). 2020. *Ganong's Review of Medical Physiology*; 26th edition. New York: McGraw-Hill.
6. Glynn M and Drake W (eds.), 2019. *Hutchison's Clinical Methods*; 23rd edition. London: WB Saunders.
7. Jameson JL, Fauci AS, Kasper DL, Hauser SL, Longo DL, and Loscalzo J (eds.). 2018. *Harrison's Principles of Internal Medicine*; 20th edition. New York: McGraw-Hill.
8. Koeppen BM, Stanton BA. 2018. *Berne and Levy Physiology*; 7th edition. New York: Elsevier.
9. Mishra UK and Kalita J. 2019. *Clinical Neurophysiology*; 4th edition, New Delhi: Elsevier.
10. Pal GK, Pal P and Nanda N. 2019. *Comprehensive Textbook of Medical Physiology*; 2nd edition, New Delhi: Jaypee Publications.
11. Singh V. 2020. *Textbook of Anatomy (Vol. 1 to 3)*; 3rd edition. New Delhi: Elsevier.
12. Papadakis MA and Me Phee SJ (eds.). 2020. *Current Medical Diagnosis and Treatment*; 45th edition. New York: McGraw-Hill-Lange.
13. Singh V. 2016. *Textbook of Clinical Neuroanatomy*; 4th edition. New Delhi: Elsevier.
14. Gunasegaran JP. *Textbook of Histology*; 4th edition. New Delhi: Elsevier.
15. Bhattacharya GK. *Concise Pathology*; 4th edition. New Delhi: Elsevier.

Index

A

B

C

D

E

F

G

H

L

M

N

O

P

Q

R

S

T

U

V

W

X

Y

Z